T0231121

Acute Care of the Cancer Patient

Acute Care of the Cancer Patient

Andrew D. Shaw
Bernhard J. Riedel
Allen W. Burton
Alan I. Fields
Thomas W. Feeley

The University of Texas M.D. Anderson Cancer Center
Houston, Texas, U.S.A.

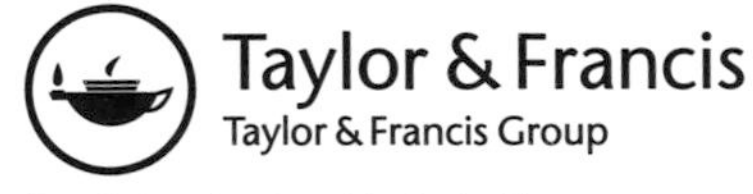

Boca Raton London New York Singapore

Published in 2005 by
Taylor & Francis Group
6000 Broken Sound Parkway NW, Suite 300
Boca Raton, FL 33487-2742

Printed in the United States of America on acid-free paper
10 9 8 7 6 5 4 3 2 1

International Standard Book Number-10: 0-8247-2689-8 (Hardcover)
International Standard Book Number-13: 978-0-8247-2689-8 (Hardcover)

Library of Congress Cataloging-in-Publication Data

Catalog record is available from the Library of Congress

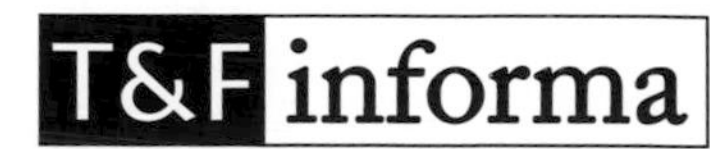

Taylor & Francis Group is the Academic Division of T&F Informa plc.

Visit the Taylor & Francis Web site at
http://www.taylorandfrancis.com

This book is dedicated to the memory of Douglas Carter (1918–1999), a man whose integrity, flexibility and courage typified the qualities of those who would do battle with this dreadful disease. Let no operation be left untried, no drug remain untested and no compassion be spared for those who have no choice but to fight.

Introduction

The M.D. Anderson Cancer Center is a branch of The University of Texas with 1,000 faculty who focus their entire activities on our mission to eliminate cancer. Our integrated programs in patient care, research, education and prevention provide a wealth of knowledge on clinical care, gained partially from the outcome of extensive research and partly from experiences that have been incorporated into our practices.

This knowledge becomes especially important when skilled medical specialists who are not primarily cancer physicians are called upon to participate, and often temporarily lead, in care delivery for a cancer patient. The continuum of care provided by multidisciplinary teams of surgeons, medical oncologists, and radiation oncologists is frequently punctuated by acute episodes requiring these medical specialists to intervene, with both expertise and speed.

Unstable patients, who ordinarily would not be subjected to extensive surgery, must be stabilized and supported as best as possible when surgery is the only alternative for extending life. We deliberately expose patients to aggressive noninvasive treatments that compromise their ability to fight infection, maintain homeostasis, and prevent bleeding. When these types of complications occur, they become life threatening and require expert intervention. Here the cancer specialist is dependent upon his or her colleague's knowledge of the special problems that often complicate the cancer patient's care.

This book addresses the needs of physician specialists who inevitably become "team members" in the multidisciplinary care of the cancer patient. Most of the chapters focus upon the specialties of internal medicine, anesthesiology, and critical care. The special aspects of caring for pediatric patients and for end-stage cancer patients requiring palliative care are also addressed.

In addition, cancer specialists will find a wealth of information and experience, enabling better anticipation and fulfillment of their patients' needs.

The recommendations presented in this volume are documented from the research literature when available. Equally important, they draw upon the vast experience of internists, anesthesiologists, critical care specialists and oncologists at a major cancer center. In 2004, M.D. Anderson physicians saw over 60,000 cancer patients, including over 24,000 new patients, from all over the USA and worldwide. Over 12,000 patients participated in therapeutic clinical trials. We performed 12,463 surgeries, 250,035 courses of radiation therapy, and had over 750,000 patient visits in our clinics. All 13,000 employees, including faculty and staff, are striving to improve cancer care and our understanding of this disease.

As our population ages, the incidence of cancer will double, even though the chances for curing individual patients are improving substantially. In my own lifetime, the 5-year disease-free survival rate has nearly doubled to 60 percent. New targeted therapies that hold great promise are under investigation. More and older patients who are symptomatic, even critically ill, will have treatment options that offer the possibility of prolonged life or even cure. The team effort required to sustain these patients will become more difficult, but also more promising. It is this hope for increased curability that motivates oncologists to push forward with new, aggressive treatments that often require intensive and rapidly responsive supportive care. Thus, acute cancer care is a timely and relevant topic.

I am pleased that the outstanding faculty at M.D. Anderson, together with collaborators from other institutions, have made this excellent book available to all who undertake the care of patients with cancer.

John Mendelsohn, M.D.
President
The University of Texas
M.D. Anderson Cancer Center
Houston, Texas, U.S.A.

Preface

This book has been written in an effort to collect in one place the knowledge and expertise of the many individuals who provide acute medical care for cancer patients while they receive chemotherapy, radiation treatment and/or undergo surgical resection. Over the past five years we have received many "curbside consults" from colleagues and friends in other institutions about how we do certain things or approach difficult oncological problems, all with the theme "there's no book, so I called to ask." We have thus attempted to organize the "para-oncological" problems of cancer patients into logical groups, and then provide a contemporaneous account of what the issues are and how they are solved in each author's unit. We have divided the book into five sections, according to how we deal with these issues on a daily basis. Thus the first section describes the general principles of oncological practice — a primer for the non-specialist. The second section describes the perioperative care of patients undergoing cancer resection surgery, with surgical, anesthesiological and critical care perspectives in most cases. In the third section of the book we address the acute medical problems encountered by cancer patients, with an emphasis on critical care medicine and physiology. Section four deals with pediatric issues, while the final section covers the problems of pain management and palliative care. Each chapter has been written by one or more individuals whom we would trust to care for ourselves or our families, and thus whose opinions we trust. We feel that this is the ultimate test of faith in any one physician's skill, and was thus a natural benchmark when deciding whom we would invite to write each chapter. All of our authors have surpassed our expectations, and we think the result is a truly global collection of experience, skill and knowledge that was previously available only on individual cerebral hard drives. Inevitably there are differences in style when a book is written by more than 100 authors; however, we have tried to maintain consistency of philosophy wherever possible.

We hope that this book provides guidance to those who seek it, reassurance to those who are doubtful, and a challenge to those who may choose to do things a different way. It is our view that there are many ways to practice medicine, and not all are suitable in all places, for all patients, and for all physicians. Thus we have tried to emphasize themes, principles and approaches rather than to provide a recipe for every different situation. Please write and let us know what we did badly, so we may improve it next time around.

Andrew D. Shaw
Bernhard Riedel
Allen W. Burton
Alan I. Fields
Thomas W. Feeley

Contents

Contributors

Karen O. Anderson Department of Symptom Research, The University of Texas M.D. Anderson Cancer Center, Houston, Texas, U.S.A.

Tayab R. Andrabi Department of Anesthesiology, The University of Texas M.D. Anderson Cancer Center, Houston, Texas, U.S.A.

Richard J. Andrassy The University of Texas M.D. Anderson Cancer Center, Houston, Texas, U.S.A.

James F. Arens Department of Anesthesiology, The University of Texas, M.D. Anderson Cancer Center, Houston, Texas, U.S.A.

Ashok Balasubramaian Division of Endocrinology, Metabolism and Diabetes, Baylor College of Medicine, Houston, Texas, U.S.A.

Jacqueline Bickham Department of Neuro-Oncology (Psychiatry Section), The University of Texas M.D. Anderson Cancer Center, Houston, Texas, U.S.A.

Martin L. Blakely Division of Pediatric Surgery, The University of Tennessee Health Science Center, Memphis, Tennessee, U.S.A.

Robert J. Bohinski Department of Neurosurgery, The University of Cincinnati College of Medicine and The Mayfield Clinic and Spine Institute, Cincinnati, Ohio, U.S.A.

W. Botnick Perioperative Services, The University of Texas M.D. Anderson Cancer Center, Houston, Texas, U.S.A.

Gregory H. Botz Department of Critical Care, The University of Texas M.D. Anderson Cancer Center, Houston, Texas, U.S.A.

Jay B. Brodsky Departments of Anesthesia and Cardiothoracic Surgery, Stanford University School of Medicine, Stanford, California, U.S.A.

Lyle D. Broemeling Department of Biostatistics, The University of Texas M.D. Anderson Cancer Center, Houston, Texas, U.S.A.

Troy S. Browne Intensive Care and High Dependency Unit, Tauranga, New Zealand

Carleen A. Brunelli Department of Research Administration, Children's Hospital Boston, Boston, Massachusetts, U.S.A.

Thao P. Bui Department of Anesthesiology and Pain Management, The University of Texas M.D. Anderson Cancer Center, Houston, Texas, U.S.A.

Allen W. Burton Section of Cancer Pain Management, Department of Anesthesiology and Pain Medicine, The University of Texas M.D. Anderson Cancer Center, Houston, Texas, U.S.A.

Humberto Caldera Department of Medicine, Veterans Affairs Medical Center, West Palm Beach, Florida, U.S.A.

Todd Canada Division of Pharmacy, The University of Texas M.D. Anderson Cancer Center, Houston, Texas, U.S.A.

A. C. Carr Department of Anaesthesia and Intensive Care Medicine, St. George's Hospital Medical School, London, U.K.

Anees Chagpar Department of Surgical Oncology, The University of Texas M.D. Anderson Cancer Center, Houston, Texas, U.S.A.

Arturo Chavez-Reyes Department of Bioimmunotherapy, The University of Texas M.D. Anderson Cancer Center, Houston, Texas, and Departamento de Microbiologia e Inmunologia, Universidad Autonoma de Nuevo Leon, Monterrey, Mexico, U.S.A.

Silwan Chedid The University of Texas M.D. Anderson Cancer Center, Houston, Texas, U.S.A.

Karen Chen Department of Critical Care, The University of Texas M.D. Anderson Cancer Center, Houston, Texas, U.S.A.

Davy C. H. Cheng Department of Anesthesia and Perioperative Medicine, London Health Sciences Centre, St. Joseph's Health Care, University of Western Ontario, London, Ontario, Canada

John L. Chow Departments of Anesthesia and Cardiothoracic Surgery, Stanford University School of Medicine, Stanford, California, U.S.A.

Charles S. Cleeland Department of Symptom Research, The University of Texas M.D. Anderson Cancer Center, Houston, Texas, U.S.A.

Lisa E. Connery Department of Anesthesiology, University of Wisconsin Medical School, University of Wisconsin Hospital and Clinics, Madison, Wisconsin, U.S.A.

Janice N. Cormier Department of Surgical Oncology, The University of Texas M.D. Anderson Cancer Center, Houston, Texas, U.S.A.

Daniel R. Couriel Department of Blood and Marrow Transplantation, The University of Texas M.D. Anderson Cancer Center, Houston, Texas, U.S.A.

Douglas B. Coursin Department of Anesthesiology, University of Wisconsin Medical School, University of Wisconsin Hospital and Clinics, Madison, Wisconsin, U.S.A.

Denise Daley Department of Anesthesiology and Pain Management, The University of Texas M.D. Anderson Cancer Center, Houston, Texas, U.S.A.

D. M. Dent Departments of Anaesthesia and Surgery, University of Cape Town, Cape Town, South Africa

George Despotis Departments of Pathology and Immunology and Anesthesiology, Washington University School of Medicine, St. Louis, Missouri, U.S.A.

Ed Diaz Department of Head and Neck Surgery, The University of Texas, M.D. Anderson Cancer Center, Houston, Texas, U.S.A.

Burton F. Dickey Department of Pulmonary Medicine, The University of Texas M.D. Anderson Cancer Center, Houston, Texas, U.S.A.

Jessica S. Donington Departments of Anesthesia and Cardiothoracic Surgery, Stanford University School of Medicine, Stanford, California, U.S.A.

P. M. Dougherty Department of Anesthesiology and Pain Medicine, The University of Texas M.D. Anderson Cancer Center, Houston, Texas, U.S.A.

Ahmed Elsayem Department of Palliative Care and Rehabilitation for Medicine, The University of Texas M.D. Anderson Cancer Center, Houston, Texas, U.S.A.

M. Fanshawe Departments of Anaesthesia and Perioperative Medicine and Anaesthesiology and Critical Care, Royal Brisbane Hospital, University of Queensland, Brisbane, Australia

David Ferson Department of Anesthesiology, The University of Texas M.D. Anderson Cancer Center, Houston, Texas, U.S.A.

Isaiah J. Fidler Department of Cancer Biology, The University of Texas M.D. Anderson Cancer Center, Houston, Texas, U.S.A.

Alan I. Fields Division of Pediatrics, The Children's Cancer Hospital at The University of Texas M.D. Anderson Cancer Center and Division of Anesthesiology and Critical Care, The University of Texas M.D. Anderson Cancer Center, Houston, Texas, U.S.A.

Kevin W. Finkel Division of Renal Diseases and Hypertension, Houston Medical School and Section of Nephrology, The University of Texas M.D. Anderson Cancer Center, Houston, Texas, U.S.A.

Anne L. Flamm The Clinical Ethics Service, The University of Texas M.D. Anderson Cancer Center, Houston, Texas, U.S.A.

John R. Foringer Division of Renal Diseases and Hypertension, Houston Medical School and Section of Nephrology, The University of Texas M.D. Anderson Cancer Center, Houston, Texas, U.S.A.

John C. Frenzel Department of Anesthesiology and Pain Medicine, The University of Texas M.D. Anderson Cancer Center, Houston, Texas, U.S.A.

Robert F. Gagel Department of Endocrine Neoplasia and Hormonal Disorders, The University of Texas M.D. Anderson Cancer Center, Houston, Texas, U.S.A.

James Gajewski Department of Blood and Marrow Transplantation, The University of Texas M.D. Anderson Cancer Center, Houston, Texas, U.S.A.

Kerri J. George Baylor College of Medicine and Texas Children's Hospital, Houston, Texas, U.S.A.

Dhaval R. Ghelani Department of Intensive Care Medicine, The Queen Elizabeth Hospital, Woodville, Adelaide, South Australia, Australia

Shubhra Ghosh Department of Blood and Marrow Transplantation, The University of Texas M.D. Anderson Cancer Center, Houston, Texas, U.S.A.

Nancy L. Glass Baylor College of Medicine and Texas Children's Hospital, Houston, Texas, U.S.A.

Ziya Gokaslan Department of Neurosurgery, Johns Hopkins University, Baltimore, Maryland, U.S.A.

Lawrence T. Goodnough Departments of Pathology and Medicine, Stanford University School of Medicine, Stanford, California, U.S.A.

Bruce M. Greenwald Division of Pediatric Critical Care Medicine, Weill Medical College of Cornell University, New York, New York, U.S.A.

Yolanda Gutierrez-Puente Department of Bioimmunotherapy, The University of Texas M.D. Anderson Cancer Center, Houston, Texas, and Departamento de Microbiologia e Inmunologia, Universidad Autonoma de Nuevo Leon, Monterrey, Mexico, U.S.A.

George M. Hall Department of Anaesthesia and Intensive Care Medicine, St. George's Hospital Medical School, London, U.K.

Peter Hsu Department of Anesthesiology, The University of Texas M.D. Anderson Cancer Center, Houston, Texas, U.S.A.

Kelly K. Hunt Department of Surgical Oncology, The University of Texas M.D. Anderson Cancer Center, Houston, Texas, U.S.A.

M. F. M. James Departments of Anaesthesia and Surgery, University of Cape Town, Cape Town, South Africa

Nora A. Janjan Division of Radiation Oncology, The University of Texas M.D. Anderson Cancer Center, Houston, Texas, U.S.A.

Tami Johnson Division of Pharmacy, The University of Texas M.D. Anderson Cancer Center, Houston, Texas, U.S.A.

Spencer S. Kee Department of Anesthesiology and Pain Medicine, The University of Texas M.D. Anderson Cancer Center, Houston, Texas, U.S.A.

Todd Kelly Department of Critical Care, The University of Texas M.D. Anderson Cancer Center, Houston, Texas, U.S.A.

Debra L. Kennamer Department of Anesthesiology, The University of Texas M.D. Anderson Cancer Center, Houston, Texas, U.S.A.

Jerald J. Killion Department of Cancer Biology, The University of Texas M.D. Anderson Cancer Center, Houston, Texas, U.S.A.

Alicia Kowalski Department of Anesthesiology and Pain Management, The University of Texas M.D. Anderson Cancer Center, Houston, Texas, U.S.A.

Oscar de Leon-Casasola Department of Anesthesiology, University at Buffalo and Department of Anesthesiology and Pain Medicine, Roswell Park Cancer Institute, Buffalo, New York, U.S.A.

Xinsheng Liao Department of Bioimmunotherapy, The University of Texas M.D. Anderson Cancer Center, Houston, Texas, U.S.A.

Jeff Lipman Departments of Intensive Care Medicine and Anaesthesiology and Critical Care, Royal Brisbane Hospital, University of Queensland, Brisbane, Australia

Andrew MacLachlan Department of Anesthesiology, The University of Texas M.D. Anderson Cancer Center, Houston, Texas, U.S.A.

David C. Madoff Department of Interventional Radiology, The University of Texas M.D. Anderson Cancer Center, Houston, Texas, U.S.A.

Mario Maldonado Division of Endocrinology, Metabolism and Diabetes, Baylor College of Medicine, Houston, Texas, U.S.A.

Paul F. Mansfield Division of Surgical Oncology, The University of Texas M.D. Anderson Cancer Center, Houston, Texas, U.S.A.

Ian McLellan University Hospitals of Leicester NHS Trust, University of Leicester, Leicester, U.K.

Rodrigo Mejia Division of Pediatrics, The Children's Cancer Hospital at the University of Texas M.D. Anderson Cancer Center and Division of Anesthesiology and Critical Care, The University of Texas M.D. Anderson Cancer Center, Houston, Texas, U.S.A.

Tito R. Mendoza Department of Symptom Research, The University of Texas M.D. Anderson Cancer Center, Houston, Texas, U.S.A.

Michael J. Miller Department of Plastic Surgery, The University of Texas M.D. Anderson Cancer Center, Houston, Texas, U.S.A.

Rashmi N. Muller Department of Anesthesiology, University of Texas Medical Branch, Galveston, Texas, U.S.A.

James L. Murray Department of Bioimmunotherapy, The University of Texas M.D. Anderson Cancer Center, Houston, Texas, U.S.A.

Chaan S. Ng Department of Radiology, The University of Texas M.D. Anderson Cancer Center, Houston, Texas, U.S.A.

N. Nguyen Shriners Orthopedic Hospital, Houston, Texas, U.S.A.

Peter Norman Department of Anesthesiology and Pain Management, The University of Texas M.D. Anderson Cancer Center, Houston, Texas, U.S.A.

C. Lee Parmley The University of Texas M.D. Anderson Cancer Center, Houston, Texas, U.S.A.

Timothy M. Pawlik Department of Surgical Oncology, The University of Texas M.D. Anderson Cancer Center, Houston, Texas, U.S.A.

Sandra L. Peake Department of Intensive Care Medicine, The Queen Elizabeth Hospital, Woodville, Adelaide, South Australia, Australia

Raphael E. Pollock Department of Surgical Oncology, The University of Texas M.D. Anderson Cancer Center, Houston, Texas, U.S.A.

Kristen Pytynia Department of Head and Neck Surgery, The University of Texas M.D. Anderson Cancer Center, Houston, Texas, U.S.A.

Issam I. Raad Department of Infectious Diseases, Infection Control, and Employee Health, The University of Texas M.D. Anderson Cancer Center, Houston, Texas, U.S.A.

Arun Rajagopal Section of Cancer Pain Management, Department of Anesthesiology, The University of Texas M.D. Anderson Cancer Center, Houston, Texas, U.S.A.

Pedro Ramirez The University of Texas M.D. Anderson Cancer Center, Houston, Texas, U.S.A.

Suresh K. Reddy Department of Palliative Care and Rehabilitation for Medicine, The University of Texas M.D. Anderson Cancer Center, Houston, Texas, U.S.A.

Cielito C. Reyes-Gibby Department of Symptom Research, The University of Texas M.D. Anderson Cancer Center, Houston, Texas, U.S.A.

Laurence D. Rhines Department of Neurosurgery, The University of Texas M.D. Anderson Cancer Center, Houston, Texas, U.S.A.

Anthony H. Risser Department of Symptom Research, The University of Texas M.D. Anderson Cancer Center, Houston, Texas, U.S.A.

Kenneth V. I. Rolston Department of Infectious Diseases, Infection Control and Employee Health, Section of Infectious Diseases, The University of Texas M.D. Anderson Cancer Center, Houston, Texas, U.S.A.

Richard E. Royal Division of Surgical Oncology, The University of Texas M.D. Anderson Cancer Center, Houston, Texas, U.S.A.

Marc A. Rozner Departments of Anesthesiology and Cardiology, The University of Texas M.D. Anderson Cancer Center, Houston, Texas, U.S.A.

Edward B. Rubenstein Medical Supportive Care, The University of Texas M.D. Anderson Cancer Center, Houston, Texas, U.S.A.

Amar Safdar Department of Infectious Diseases, Infection Control, and Employee Health, The University of Texas M.D. Anderson Cancer Center, Houston, Texas, U.S.A.

Rajagopal V. Sekhar Division of Endocrinology, Metabolism and Diabetes, Baylor College of Medicine, Houston, Texas, U.S.A.

Hemant N. Shah Section of Cancer Pain Management, Department of Anesthesiology and Pain Medicine, The University of Texas M.D. Anderson Cancer Center, Houston, Texas, U.S.A.

Vickie R. Shannon Department of Pulmonary Medicine, The University of Texas M.D. Anderson Cancer Center, Houston, Texas, U.S.A.

Andrew D. Shaw Department of Critical Care Medicine, The University of Texas M.D. Anderson Cancer Center, Houston, Texas, U.S.A.

Sanjay Singh Department of Radiology, The University of Texas M.D. Anderson Cancer Center, Houston, Texas, U.S.A.

S. Eva Singletary Department of Surgical Oncology, The University of Texas M.D. Anderson Cancer Center, Houston, Texas, U.S.A.

Ashish Sinha Department of Anesthesiology, Louisiana State University Health Science Center, New Orleans, Louisiana, U.S.A.

Martin L. Smith Department of Critical Care, The University of Texas M.D. Anderson Cancer Center, Houston, Texas, U.S.A.

Nicole D. Switzer Department of General Internal Medicine, The University of Texas M.D. Anderson Cancer Center, Houston, Texas, U.S.A.

Rudranath Talukdar Department of Palliative Care and Rehabilitation for Medicine, The University of Texas M.D. Anderson Cancer Center, Houston, Texas, U.S.A.

S. G. Tan Changi General Hospital, Singapore

Ravi Taneja Department of Anesthesia and Perioperative Medicine, London Health Sciences Centre, University of Western Ontario, London, Ontaria, Canada

Dilip Thakar Division of Anesthesia and Critical Care, The University of Texas M.D. Anderson Cancer Center, Houston, Texas, U.S.A.

Paula Trahan-Rieger American Society of Clinical Oncology Headquarters, Alexandria, Virginia, U.S.A.

Jonathan Trent The University of Texas M.D. Anderson Cancer Center, Houston, Texas, U.S.A.

J. Tring University Hospitals of Leicester NHS Trust, University of Leicester, Leicester, U.K.

Mylene T. Truong Department of Radiology, The University of Texas M.D. Anderson Cancer Center, Houston, Texas, U.S.A.

Anne Tucker Division of Pharmacy, The University of Texas M.D. Anderson Cancer Center, Houston, Texas, U.S.A.

H. Michael Ushay Division of Pediatric Critical Care Medicine, Weill Medical College of Cornell University and Laura Rosenberg Pediatric Observation Unit, Memorial Sloan-Kettering Cancer Center, New York, New York, U.S.A.

Saroj Vadhan-Raj Department of Bioimmunotherapy, The University of Texas M.D. Anderson Cancer Center, Houston, Texas, U.S.A.

Alan D. Valentine Department of Neuro-Oncology (Psychiatry Section), The University of Texas M.D. Anderson Cancer Center, Houston, Texas, U.S.A.

Steven Waguespack Department of Endocrine Neoplasia and Hormonal Disorders, The University of Texas M.D. Anderson Cancer Center, Houston, Texas, U.S.A.

Michael J. Wallace Department of Interventional Radiology, The University of Texas M.D. Anderson Cancer Center, Houston, Texas, U.S.A.

James D. Wilkinson Department of Epidemiology and Public Health, University of Miami School of Medicine, Miami, Florida, U.S.A.

Alan W. Yasko Department of Anesthesiology and Pain Management, The University of Texas M.D. Anderson Cancer Center, Houston, Texas, U.S.A.

Edward T. H. Yeh Department of Cardiology, The University of Texas M.D. Anderson Cancer Center, Houston, Texas, U.S.A.

S. Wamique Yusuf Department of Cardiology, The University of Texas M.D. Anderson Cancer Center, Houston, Texas, U.S.A.

Zdravka Zafirova Department of Anesthesia and Critical Care, University of Chicago, Chicago, Illinois, U.S.A.

Leonard A. Zwelling Office of Research Administration, The University of Texas M.D. Anderson Cancer Center, Houston, Texas, U.S.A.

1

Cancer Growth, Progression, and Metastasis

JERALD J. KILLION and ISAIAH J. FIDLER

Department of Cancer Biology, The University of Texas M.D. Anderson Cancer Center, Houston, Texas, U.S.A.

I. EVOLUTION OF THE PRIMARY TUMOR

The major clinical challenge for cancer therapy remains the eradication (or prevention) of metastatic disease. A principal barrier to destruction of disseminated cancer is the heterogeneous nature of cancer; tumors contain subpopulations of cells that are able to subvert host defenses and recruit infiltrating cells that supply needed growth factors and blood supply. Moreover, metastatic lesions can become autonomous with respect to homeostatic mechanisms of normal tissue architecture (1–3). Neoplastic transformation involves genetic alterations such as the activation or disregulation of oncogenes (4). There are probably continuous selection pressures for cells that are able to circumvent normal growth control mechanisms. The continual evolution of genetically unstable neoplasms eventually favors the emergence of cell subpopulations with metastatic potential. By the time of diagnosis of the primary tumor, malignant neoplasms contain multiple cell populations that are heterogeneous with respect to a variety of biological properties such as cell-surface characteristics, antigenicity, immunogenicity, growth rate, karyotype, sensitivity to chemotherapeutic drugs, and the ability to invade and metastasize (2,5–8). The existence of these subpopulations of cells presents a dilemma for the clinician. The emergence of drug-resistant variants during or subsequent to chemotherapy has been documented as having differences in the response of primary and metastatic tumors to therapeutic agents (2). The obstacle to chemotherapy that heterogeneity imposes may also affect the success of immunotherapy or the use of biological response modifiers (2,9–11).

Actually, the concept that tumors are heterogeneous is not new. Paget (12) analyzed the postmortem data of women who died of cancer and noticed the high frequency of metastasis to the ovaries and different incidence of skeletal metastases associated with different primary tumors. Paget concluded that the organ distribution of metastases is not a matter of chance and suggest that metastases develop only when the "seed" (certain tumor cells with metastatic ability) and the "soil" (colonized organs providing a microenvironment for growth advantage) are compatible. In recent years, Paget's hypothesis has received considerable experimental and clinical support (13–16). A current definition of the "seed and soil" hypothesis encompasses three principles. First, neoplasms are biologically heterogeneous (1,13). Second, the process of metastasis is highly selective, favoring the survival and growth of a small subpopulation of cells that pre-exist in the parent neoplasm (17). Third, the outcome of metastasis depends on multiple interactions of metastatic cells with homeostatic mechanisms. The majority of malignant tumors actually usurp homeostatic mechanism to gain growth advantage. Neoplastic angiogenesis is an excellent example.

II. TUMOR ANGIOGENESIS

Because a tumor mass >0.25 mm in diameter exceeds the oxygen and nutrient diffusion limits of its vascular supply, to survive and grow, it must generate additional vasculature, i.e., angiogenesis (18–20). The process of angiogenesis consists of a series of sequential steps that result in the establishment of a new vascular bed. To generate capillary sprouts, endothelial cells proliferate, migrate, degrade the basement membrane, and form a structure, i.e., a new lumen organization (21). To stimulate angiogenesis, both tumor cells and host infiltrate cells (such as macrophages) secrete a variety of factors. More than a dozen of proangiogenic molecules have been reported, including basic fibroblast growth factor (bFGF), vascular endothelial growth factor (VEGF, also known as vascular permeability factor) (22–25), interleukin-8 (IL-8), angiogenin, angiotropin, platelet-derived growth factor (PDGF), transforming growth factor-α (TGF-α), transforming growth factor-β (TGF-β), epidermal growth factor (EGF), and tumor necrosis factor-α (TNF-α) (18–23). However, many tissues and tumors also generate factors that inhibit angiogenesis, such as angiostatin, endostatin, thrombospondins, interferon-α (IFN), and interferon-β (IFN-β) [O′R (26), O′ (27), Thrombosp (28–31)]. The angiogenic phenotype of an organ or a tumor is therefore determined by the net balance between positive and negative regulators of neovascularization (32). In normal tissues, factors that inhibit angiogenesis predominate (e.g., IFN-β), whereas in rapidly dividing tissues, factors that stimulate angiogenesis predominate. The type 1 interferons (α and β) are potent inhibitors of transcription of proangiogenic molecules, such as bFGF, matrix metalloproteinases 2 and 9 (MMP-2, MMP-9) and have antiangiogenic activity in treatment of vascular hemangiomas in humans and orthotopic murine tumor models (reviewed in Ref. 33).

Moreover, the structure and architecture of tumor vasculature can dramatically differ from those found in normal organs (34–36). Indeed, blood vessels in tumors are different than those found in wound healing and inflamed tissues. The blood flow through tumors can be tortuous and constantly modeled by regions of necrosis, rapid cell division, and presence of infiltrate cells. Receptors for VEGF (KDR in humans, Flt-1 in mice) are expressed specifically by tumor endothelium, as well as by the angiopoietin tyrosine kinase receptor, Tie-2 (37). In addition, receptors for PDGF and EGF are found on tumor endothelial cells (38–40).

The endothelium is fragile and upregulation of survival factors (such as Bcl-2 and survivin) by molecules found in abundance within the tumor microenvironment, such as VEGF and bFGF, help prevent apoptosis of new endothelium (41–44). There is increased leakiness to macromolecules (perhaps due to the presence of VEGF) (45,46), and vessels often lose distinct features of arteriole, capillary, and venule formation. Modern techniques, such as phage-display targeting, have defined "vascular addresses" that may be distinct for different organs, as well as tumors in those organs, and perhaps offer attractive targets for antivasculature therapy (47).

Angiogenic heterogeneity exists within a single tumor (zonal or intralesional) between different metastases even in a single organ and different neoplasms of the same histologic type is also documented (48,49). For example, the expression of proangiogenic molecules (and, therefore, blood vessel density) in murine or human tumors growing at orthotopic sites in athymic mice is zonal, i.e., demonstrates intralesional heterogeneity. Small tumors (3–4 mm in diameter) expressed more bFGF and IL-8 than large tumors (>10 mm in diameter), whereas more VEGF is expressed in large tumors. Immunostaining showed a heterogeneous distribution of these angiogenic factors within the tumor; expression of bFGF and IL-8 was highest on the periphery of a large tumor, where cell division was maximal. VEGF expression was higher in the center of the tumor (48). Similarly, heterogeneous dependence on angiogenesis was reported for cell subpopulations isolated from human melanoma xenografts having differential expression of hypoxia-inducing factor-1 (49).

Heterogeneity of blood vessel distribution in surgical specimens of human cancers is well documented (50,51). Benign neoplasms are sparely vascularized and tend to grow slowly in contrast to highly vascularized and rapidly growing malignant tumors (51). However, the distribution of vessels in a tumor is not uniform, and Weidner et al. (50,51) cautioned that, to predict the aggressive nature of human cancers, one must determine the mean vessel density (MVD) in the "areas of most intense neovascularization," i.e., tumors exhibit intralesional and zonal heterogeneity for MVD. Similarly, the expression of proangiogenic molecules in surgical specimens of human colon carcinoma was determined by in situ hybridization technique. Matrix metalloproteinase-9 and bFGF were overexpressed at the periphery of the tumor where cells were rapidly dividing, whereas VEGF expression was higher in the center of the lesions (52).

The extent of angiogenic heterogeneity in malignant neoplasms is also regulated by the organ microenvironment. For example, human renal carcinoma cells implanted into the kidney of athymic mice produced a high incidence of lung metastasis, whereas those implanted subcutaneously did not (53). Histopathologic examination of the tissues revealed that the tumors grown in the subcutis of nude mice had few blood vessels when compared with the tumors in the kidney. The subcutaneous tumors also had a significantly lower level of mRNA transcripts for bFGF than the tumor in the kidney, and the expression of the naturally occurring angiogenic inhibitor, IFN-β (which downregulates bFGF), was high in epithelial cells and fibroblasts surrounding the subcutaneous tumors. This was not detected in or around the tumors grown in the kidney (54). The production of IL-8 by melanoma cells is regulated by complex interactions with skin keratinocytes (55). Interleukin-8 expression can be increased by coculture of melanoma cells with skin keratinocytes, and this expression is inhibited by coincubation of melanoma cells with hepatocytes from the liver (56). The organ microenvironment also influences the expression of VEGF. Human gastric cancer cells implanted into the stomach were highly vascularized and expressed high levels of VEGF when compared with implantation in to an ectopic (subcutaneous) site, such as the skin. In addition, metastasis only occurred from the tumor implanted in the stomach (57).

The molecular cross-talk that occurs with tumor cells and endothelium within the tumor microenvironment results in sufficient recruitment of a vascular supply that has physiological properties that allow migration and eventual escape of subpopulations of tumor cells able to complete a cascade of events necessary for metastasis.

III. DETERMINANTS OF METASTASIS

The process of metastasis consists of a series of sequential steps, which can only be completed by an extremely small proportion of cells within the primary tumor (5). Metastasis begins by invasion into host stroma surrounding the primary neoplasm. This is facilitated by the production of enzymes such as the metalloproteinases, cathepsin B, and plasminogen activators (58–60). The invasive process is completed by dissolution of the basement membrane, enhanced motility of some tumor cells, and eventual penetration of blood vessels or lymphatics (61). Reduced expression of the E-cadherin–catenin complex is critical for intercellular adhesion and maintenance of both normal and malignant tissue architecture. Reduced expression of this cohesive complex is associated with tumor invasion, metastasis, and unfavorable prognosis (62). During blood-borne metastasis, tumor cells must survive transport in the circulation, interact with immune cells, and eventually express favorable adhesion molecules that allow arrest in a distant capillary bed. Using radiolabeled melanoma cells, it was found that, at 24 hr after entry of tumor cells into the circulation, $<1\%$ of the cells were viable and $<0.1\%$ eventually formed an experimental metastasis (63). This strengthens the concept that the mere presence of circulating tumor cells does not in itself constitute a prognosis for metastases. The subsequent interactions of metastatic cells with cells of the vascular endothelium include not only nonspecific lodgment of cell emboli, but also the formation of stable adhesions between tumor cells and small-vessel endothelial cells. Extravasation from the luminal side of the blood vessel and subsequent continued growth of the metastatic cell population require response to motility factors, enhanced enzyme expression, upregulation of growth factor receptors, and induction of an angiogenesis within the local environment (reviewed in Ref. 13). Organ-specific properties of the tumor cells result in interactions that enhance tumor growth and survival. For example, subsequent to a partial hepatectomy, the liver undergoes raid cell division termed "regeneration" without simultaneous cell division occurring in other organs, like the kidneys. In contrast, subsequent to nephrectomy, the contralateral kidney compensates by hypertrophy and hyperplasia, but the liver does not (64). When human colon carcinoma cells were implanted in nude mice that were subjected to nephrectomy, partial hepatectomy, or sham-surgery (as a control), it was observed that liver regeneration in nude mice actually stimulated the growth of the colon carcinoma, whereas nephrectomy specifically stimulated the growth of human renal cell carcinoma (64). Human colon carcinoma cells capable of growing in the liver parenchyma (Dukes' stage D) express a higher number of functional receptors for TGF-α (a ligand for the EGF-receptor) and hepatocyte growth factor (c-met) than do cells with low metastatic potential (Dukes' stage B) (65,66).

This concept was expanded to include an examination of the expression of metastasis-related genes such as E-cadherin, MMP-2, MMP-9, bFGF, VEGF, and IL-8. Analysis of the results indicated that these genes could be the predictors of patient survival and metastatic potential of a patient's colorectal carcinoma (67–69), gastric carcinoma (70), prostate carcinoma (71), pancreatic carcinoma (72), lung cancer (73), renal cell carcinoma (74), and ovarian cancer (75). Furthermore, the ratio between expression of collagenase type IV (mean of the expression of MMP-2 and MMP-9) and E-cadherin (the MMP–E-cadherin ratio, measured at the periphery of each tumor analyzed) correlated with malignant phenotype; a lower MMP–E-cadherin ratio was associated with significantly longer survival and reduced disease recurrence. Studies using DNA microarray analysis on primary breast tumor specimens found that gene expression profiles are strong predictors of prognosis (76).

IV. IMPLICATIONS FOR THERAPY OF CANCER

A. Molecular Targeting in Clinical Studies

The hallmark of the malignant diagnosis is invasion of cytologically abberant cells into the surrounding normal tissue architecture. The primary tumor contains subpopulations of cells that are heterogeneous with respect to a variety of biological, immunological, biochemical, and metastatic properties. This heterogeneity results in the need for multilevel treatment strategies, as conventional therapies are selected for resistant cells. The identification of molecular interactions between tumor cells and tumor endothelium that promote tumor growth also identifies potential avenues for targeted therapy. Moreover, therapeutic strategies may identify unique targets on both tumor cells and their associated blood vessels. New drug development has focused upon targeting growth factor receptors and proangiogenic molecules found in the tumor microenvironment.

Inhibition of growth factor receptors has been accomplished with two main approaches: antibody inhibition of receptor signaling and highly specific inhibitors of intracellular activation (autophosphorylation) of the receptors. These receptors and mutant derivatives of the family of these receptors are often constitutively activated or overexpressed in cancer cells and confer chronic signaling for cell proliferation. The HER2/Neu family of receptors is often found in breast cancer and serves as a target for trastuzumab, the anti-HER2 antibody. This therapy has been used as a single agent, and best results in HER2+ patients were observed when this form of anti-EGF therapy was combined with conventional chemotherapy (77,78). Encouraging clinical results have been obtained using the anti-EGF-R antibody, IM-C225 (cetuixmab), in combination with chemotherapy or radiation in treatment of patients with recurrent or refractory squamous cell carcinoma of the head and neck (79).

Rapid clinical approval was obtained for a small molecule inhibitor of the BCR-ABL kinase (related to c-kit and the PDGF-receptor) for imatinib mesylate (Gleevec, STI-571) in therapy of chronic myeloid leukemia (80) with subsequent approval for use in gastrointestinal stromal tumors (81). These initial and dramatic results motivated clinical evaluation of a myriad of tyrosine kinase inhibitors (TKIs) that are highly specific for different families of growth factor receptors (reviewed in Ref. 82). ZD1839 (Iressa), a TKI of EGF-R, has been approved for advanced non-small cell lung cancer. Phase I and II trials indicated promising activity of this compound, even though patients were not selected for EGF-R expression (83). Therapies that rely upon specific expression of target molecules will eventually show much more efficacy in the patient population when molecular profiles of responders and nonresponders are defined (83).

Interestingly, animal experiments have defined mechanisms regarding the use of inhibitors of proangiogenic factors (and their receptors) that result in a concept of two-compartment targeting, i.e., therapy directed against dividing tumor cells and tumor-associated endothelium. This "dual" targeting occurred using both antibody and small molecule-mediated inhibition of growth factor receptor signaling.

B. Blockade of Epidermal Growth Factor Receptor Signaling

Bruns et al. (84) demonstrated regression of human pancreatic carcinoma growing orthotopically in nude mice by therapy with IM-C225 antibody plus gemcitabine. Although both gemcitabine and IM-C225 had activity in this model and are used as single agents, superior results, as measured by tumor burden and incidence of liver metastasis, were achieved by combination therapy. Of particular interest was the finding that apoptosis of tumor-associated endothelial cells was induced by treatment with IM-C225 (due to a coordinate downregulation of VEGF and IL-8 production of the pancreatic carcinoma cells by binding of the IM-C225 antibody). This striking observation, namely, inhibition of growth factor production or receptor signaling could lead to endothelial cell apoptosis, was confirmed using IM-C225 in an orthotopic bladder tumor model using combination therapy with paclitaxel (85).

The use of small molecule inhibitors of growth factor receptor signaling (TKI) has been extensively studied in animal tumor models. Using the orthotopic pancreatic model of human cancer in nude mice, Bruns et al. (86) reported that the modest activity of single agent use of either PKI-166 (EGF-R TKI) or gemcitabine was markedly improved by the combination of these agents (reduction in tumor burden of 85%). This combination therapy also inhibited lymph node and liver metastasis. This form of therapy resulted in apoptosis of both tumor cells and tumor-associated endothelium.

The selective nature of EGF-R expression within tumors was demonstrated when human prostate tumor cells were injected into the tibia of nude mice (87). Immunohistochemical analysis revealed that the PC-3MM2 cells growing adjacent to the bone expressed high levels of EGF-R and activated EGF-R, whereas tumor cells in the adjacent musculature did not. Moreover, endothelial cells within the bone tumor lesions, but not within uninvolved bone or tumors in the muscle, expressed high levels of activated EGF-R. Oral administration of PKI-166 or PKI-166 plus paclitaxel reduced the incidence and size of bone tumors and the destruction of bone. The combination therapy resulted in a significant inhibition of phosphorylation of EGF-R on tumor and endothelial cells and induced significant apoptosis of endothelial cells within the tumor lesions.

Baker et al. (88) used four different orthotopic animal models, namely, bladder carcinoma, (253J-BV, EGF/TGF-α+), pancreatic carcinoma (L3.6pl, EGF/TGF-α+), EGF/TGF-α-negative renal cell carcinoma (SN12-PM6), and EGF/TGF-α+ renal cell carcinoma (RBM1-IT). Treatment with orally administered PKI-166 alone, intraperitoneal paclitaxel alone (253J-BV), gemcitabine alone (SN12-PM6), or combination of PKI-166 and chemotherapy produced 60%, 32%, or 81% reduction in the tumor volume of 253J-BV bladder tumors, respectively, and 26%, 23%, or 51% reduction in the tumor volume of SN12-PM6 kidney tumors, respectively. Immunohistochemical analyses demonstrated downregulation of phosphorylated EGF-R in the EGF/TGF-α+ and the EGF/TGF-α– tumors taken from mice treated with PKI-166, although apoptosis of tumor-associated endothelial cells was observed in mice whose tumors secreted EGF/TGF-α. These data strongly suggested that optimal combination therapy occurred in tumors that were positive for the respective growth factor receptors and secreted the ligand (which upregulated the receptor on tumor-associated endothelium, thus being vulnerable to TKI-mediated apoptosis). This dual targeting is not limited to EGF-R inhibition.

C. Blockade of Vascular Endothelial Growth Factor Receptor Signaling

Using a mouse-specific antibody (DC101) against the VEGF receptor, Bruns et al. (89) demonstrated inhibition of tumor growth, decrease in metastasis, and induction of apoptosis in both tumor cells and the tumor-associated endothelium in the human pancreatic tumor model in nude mice. Together, these data suggest that either deprivation of growth factors (caused by a decrease in their production) or blockade of receptor signaling leads to dual targeting within the tumor microenvironment. Solorzano et al. (90) demonstrated the inhibition of growth and liver metastasis of human pancreatic cancer implanted into the pancreas of nude mice by combination therapy with gemcitabine and PTK787/ZK222584, an inhibitor of the VEGF receptor. While both agents were active and used alone, superior results in reduction of tumor volume and incidence of lymph node and liver metastasis were achieved with combination therapy of gemcitabine plus PTK787. In addition, apoptosis of tumor cells and tumor-associated endothelial cells was observed. The use of TKI was taken a step further when Baker et al. (91) showed that combining PTK787 (VEGF-R TKI) plus PKI-166 (EGF-R TKI) in combination with gemcitabine resulted in a 97% reduction of pancreatic tumor volume in the orthotopic animal model, and the efficacy correlated with a decrease in circulating proangiogenic molecules (VEGF, IL-8) decreases in staining for dividing cells as measured by proliferating cell nuclear antigen and increases in apoptosis of tumor cells and endothelial cells.

D. Blockade of Platelet-Derived Growth Factor Receptor Signaling

Recent studies have shown that the use of TKI of PDGF-R signaling, STI-571, in combination with paclitaxel reduced the tumor incidence and bone lysis of human prostate cancer cells injected into the tibia of nude mice (92). This was associated with decreased phosphorylation of PDGF-R on tumor cells and tumor-associated endothelial cells and induction of apoptosis in both cell types. The benefits of targeting both pericytes (stromal supporting cells for endothelium, see Ref. 37) and endothelial cells within the tumor with kinase inhibitors have also been discussed (93).

E. Antiangiogenic Properties of Interferon-α

The antiangiogenic properties of IFN-α have been defined by studies using syngeneic murine tumor models and human tumors implanted into nude mice. As found with the chronic administration of IFN-α in hemangiomas (33), frequent, low doses of free-form IFN-α administered to mice implanted with syngeneic bladder carcinoma cells result in downregulation of angiogenesis-related genes (bFGF, MMP-9) and reduction of tumor burden (94). This was not observed with high-dose IFN-α, demonstrating that the optimal therapeutic dose was not the maximally tolerated dose. These studies were expanded to include therapy of pancreatic cancer in nude mice (low dose IFN-α plus gemcitabine), and the 87% reduction in tumor volume observed using combination therapy was demonstrated to be due to inhibition of the expression of bFGF, MMP-9 and induction of apoptosis in both tumor cells and tumor-associated endothelium (95). Similar findings were reported using low-dose schedules of pegylated IFN-α in combination with paclitaxel in human ovarian cancer implanted into the peritoneal cavity of nude mice (96) and combination therapy with pegylated IFN-α and docetaxel in an orthotopic tumor model of human prostate cancer (97).

Molecular-based targeting of both tumor-associated endothelium and tumor cells will eventually depend upon the identification of unique profiles of human cancers that can be defined prior to therapy. In addition to targeting dividing endothelial cells, additional targets may be identified for existing tumor vasculature (as opposed to strict targeting of angiogenic endothelium) (98).

REFERENCES

1. Fidler IJ, Hart IR. Biological diversity in metastatic neoplasms: origins and implication. Science 1982; 217: 998–1003.
2. Fidler IJ, Balch CM. The biology of cancer metastasis and implications for therapy. Curr Prob Surg 1987; 24: 131–233.
3. Killion JJ, Fidler IJ. The biology of tumor metastasis. Semin Oncol 1989; 16:106–115.
4. Bishop MJ. The molecular genetics of cancer. Science 1987; 235:305–311.
5. Poste G, Fidler IJ. The pathogenesis of cancer metastasis. Nature 1980; 283:139–146.
6. Heppner G. Tumor heterogeneity. Cancer Res 1984; 44: 2259–2265.
7. Nicolson GL. Generation of phenotypic diversity and progression in metastatic tumors. Cancer Metastasis Rev 1984; 3:25–42.
8. Killion JJ, Kollmorgen GM. Isolation of immunogenic tumor cells by cell-affinity chromatography. Nature 1976; 259:674–676.
9. Kerbel RS. Implications of immunological heterogeneity in tumors. Nature 1979; 280:358–360.
10. Killion JJ. Immunotherapy with tumor subpopulations. II. Therapy of drug-resistant L1210 leukemia and E14 lymphoma. Cancer Immunol Immunother 1979; 5: 21–26.
11. Malkovska V, Sondel PM, Malkovsky. Tumor immunotherapy. Curr Opin Immunol 1989; 1:883–890.
12. Paget S. The distribution of secondary growths in cancer of the breast. Lancet 1889; 1:571–573.
13. Fidler IJ. Critical factors in the biology of human cancer metastasis: twenty-eighth G.H.A. Clowes memorial award lecture. Cancer Res 1990; 50:6130–6138.
14. Fidler IJ. Experimental orthotopic models of organ-specific metastasis by human neoplasms. Adv Mol Cell Biol 1994; 9:191–215.
15. Price JE. Host–tumor interaction in progression of breast cancer metastasis. In Vivo 1994; 8:145–154.
16. Hart IR. "Seed and soil" revisited: mechanisms of site-specific metastasis. Cancer Metastasis Rev 1982; 1: 5–16.
17. Fidler IJ, Kripke ML. Metastasis results from preexisting variant cells within a malignant tumor. Science 1977; 197:893–895.
18. Fidler IJ, Ellis LM. The implication of angiogenesis to the biology and therapy of cancer metastasis. Cell 1994; 47:185–188.
19. Folkman J. Angiogenesis in cancer, vascular, rheumatoid, and other disease. Nat Med 1995; 1:27–31.
20. Liotta LA, Steeg PS, Stetler-Stevenson WG. Cancer metastasis and angiogenesis: an imbalance of positive and negative regulation. Cell 1991; 64:327–336.
21. Auerbach W, Auerbach R. Angiogenesis inhibition: a review. Pharmacol Ther 1994; 63:265–311.
22. Folkman J, Klagsbrun M. Angiogenic factors. Science 1987; 235:444–447.
23. Bouck N, Stellmach V, Hsu SC. How tumors become angiogenic. Adv Cancer Res 1996; 69:135–174.
24. Folkman J. Seminars in medicine of the Beth Israel Hospital, Boston, MA. Clinical applications of research on angiogenesis. N Engl J Med 1995; 333:1757–1763.
25. Cockerill GW, Gamble JR, Vadas MA. Angiogenesis: models and modulators. Int Rev Cytol 1995; 159: 113–160.
26. O'Reilly MS, Holmgren L, Shing Y, Chen C, Rosenthal RA, Moses M, Lane WS, Cao Y, Sage EH, Folkman J. Angiostatin: a novel angiogenesis inhibitor that mediates the suppression of metastases by a Lewis lung carcinoma. Cell 1994; 79:185–188.
27. O'Reilly MS, Boehm, T, Shing Y, Fukai N, Vasios G, Lane WS, Flynn E, Birkhead JR, Olsen BR, Folkman J. Endostatin: an endogenous inhibitor of angiogenesis and tumor growth. Cell 1997; 88:277–285.
28. Miyata Y, Koga S, Takehara K, Kanetake H, Kanda S. Expression of thromobspondin-derived 4N1K peptide-containing proteins in renal cell carcinoma tissues is associated with a decrease in tumor growth and angiogenesis. Clin Cancer Res 2003; 9:1734–1740.
29. Folkman J. How is blood vessel growth regulated in normal and neoplastic tissue? G.H.A. Clowes memorial award lecture. Cancer Res 1986; 46:467–473.
30. Fidler IJ, Ellis LM. The implications of angiogenesis for the biology and therapy of cancer metastasis. Cell 1994; 79:185–188.
31. Singh RK, Llansa N, Bucana CD, Sanchez R, Koura A, Fidler IJ. Cell density-dependent regulation of basic fibroblast growth factor expression in human renal cell carcinoma cells. Cell Growth Differ 1996; 7:397–404.

32. Hanahan D, Folkman J. Patterns and emerging mechanisms of the angiogenic switch during tumorigenesis. Cell 1996; 86:353–364.
33. Fidler IJ. Regulation of neoplastic angiogenesis. J Natl Cancer Inst Monogr 2000; 28:10–14.
34. Ebhard A, Kahlert S, Goede V, Hemmerlein B, Plate KH, Augustin HG. Heterogeneity of angiogenesis and blood vessel maturation in human tumors: implications for antiangiogenic tumor therapies. Cancer Res 2000; 60:1388–1393.
35. Nels V, Denzer K, Drenchahn D. Pericyte involvement in capillary sprouting during angiogenesis in situ. Cell Tissue Res 1992; 270:469–474.
36. Nor JE, Polverni PJ. Role of endothelial cell survival and death signals in angiogenesis. Angiogenesis 1999; 3: 101–116.
37. Liu, W, Ahmad SA, Reinmuth N, Shaheen RM, Jung YD, Fan F, Ellis LM. Endothelial cell survival and apoptosis in the tumor vasculature. Apoptosis 2000; 5: 323–328.
38. Uehara H, Kim SJ, Karashima T, Shepherd DL, Fan D, Tsan R, Killion JJ, Logothetis C, Mathew P, Fidler IJ. Effects of blocking platelet-derived growth factor-receptor signaling in a mouse model of experimental prostate cancer bone metastases. J Natl Cancer Inst 2003; 19:458–470.
39. Veenendall LM, Jin H, Ran S, Cheung L, Navone N, Marks JW, Waltenberger J, Thorpe P, Rosenblum MG. In vitro and in vivo studies of a VEGF121/r Gelonin chimeric fusion toxin targeting the neovasculature of solid tumors. Proc Natl Acad Sci USA 2002; 99: 7866–7871.
40. Suhardja A, Hoffman H. Role of growth factors and their receptors in proliferation of microvascular endothelial cells. Microsc Res Tech 2003; 60:70–75.
41. Wang JH, Wu QD, Bouchier-Hayes D, Redmond HP. Hypoxia upregulates Bcl-2 expression and suppresses interferon-gamma induced antiangiogenic activity in human tumor derived endothelial cells. Cancer 2002; 15: 2745–2755.
42. Mesri M, Morales-Ruiz M, Ackermann EJ, Bennett CF, Pober JS, Sessa WC, Altieri DC. Suppression of vascular endothelial growth factor-mediated endothelial cell protection by surviving targeting. Am J Pathol 2001; 158:1757–1765.
43. Gerber HP, Dixit V, Ferrara N. Vascular endothelial growth factor induces expression of the antiapoptotic proteins Bcl-2 and A1 in vascular endothelial cells. J Biol Chem 1998; 273:13313–13316.
44. Karsan A, Yee E, Poirier GG, Zhou P, Craig R, Harlan JM. Fibroblast growth factor-2 inhibits endothelial cell apoptosis by Bcl-2-dependent and independent mechanisms. Am J Pathol 1997; 151:1775–1784.
45. Jain RK. Transport of molecules across tumor vasculature. Cancer Metastasis Rev 1987; 6:559–563.
46. Dvorak HF. Leaky tumor vessels: consequences for tumor stroma generation and for solid tumor therapy. Prog Clin Biol Res 1990; 354A:317–330.
47. Pasqualini R, Arap W, McDonald DM. Probing the structural and molecular diversity of tumor vasculature. Trends Mol Med 2002; 8:563–571.
48. Kumar R, Kuniyase H, Bucana CD, Wilson MR, Fidler IJ. Spatial and temporal expression of angiogenic molecules during tumor growth and progression. Oncol Res 1998; 10:301–311.
49. Yu JL, Rak JW, Carmeliet P, Nagy A, Kerbel RS, Coomber BL. Heterogeneous vascular dependence of tumor cell populations. Am J Pathol 2001; 158: 1225–1234.
50. Weidner N, Semple JP, Welch JR, Folkman J. Tumor angiogenesis and metastasis-correlation in invasive breast cancer. N Engl J Med 1991; 324:1–8.
51. Weidner N, Folkmna J, Pozza F, Bevilacqua P, Allred EN, Moore DH, Meli S, Gasparini G. Tumor angiogenesis: a new significant and independent prognostic indicator in early-stage breast carcinoma. J Natl Cancer Inst 1992; 84:1875–1887.
52. Kitadai Y, Bucana CD, Ellis LM, Anzai H, Tahara E, Fidler IJ. In situ hybridization technique for analysis of metastasis-related genes in human colon carcinoma cells. Am J Pathol 1995; 147:1238–1247.
53. Singh RK, Bucana CD, Gutman M, Fan D, Wilson MR, Fidler IJ. Organ site-dependent expression of basic fibroblast growth factor in human renal cell carcinoma cells. Am J Pathol 1994; 145:365–374.
54. Singh RK, Gurman M, Bucana CD, Sanchez R, Llansa N, Fidler IJ. Interferons alpha and beta down-regulate the expression of basic fibroblast growth factor in human carcinomas. Proc Natl Acad Sci USA 1995; 92: 4562–4566.
55. Herlyn M. Human melanoma: development and progression. Cancer Metastasis Rev 1990; 9:101–112.
56. Gurman M, Singh RK, Xie K, Bucana CD, Fidler IJ. Regulation of interleukin-8 expression in human melanoma cells by the organ environment. Cancer Res 1995; 55:2470–2475.
57. Takahasi Y, Mai M, Wilson MR, Ellis LM. Site-dependent expression of vascular endothelial growth factor, angiogenesis and proliferation in human gastric carcinoma. Int J Oncol 1996; 8:701–705.
58. Sloane BF, Honn KV. Cysteine proteinase and metastasis. Cancer Metastasis Rev 1984; 3:249–265.
59. Jones PA, DeClerck YA. Extracellular matrix destruction by invasive tumor cells. Cancer Metastasis Rev 1982; 1:289–319.
60. Liotta LA, Rao CN, Barksy SH. Tumor invasion and the extracellular matrix. Lab Invest 1983; 49:636–649.
61. Liotta LA, Stetler-Stevenson WG. Metalloproteinases and cancer invasion. Semin Cancer Biol 1990; 1: 99–106.
62. Bremnes RM, Veve R, Hirsch FR, Franklin WA. The E-cadherin cell–cell adhesion complex and lung cancer invasion, metastasis, and prognosis. Lung Cancer 2002; 36:115–124.
63. Fidler IJ. Metastasis: quantitative analysis of distribution and fate of tumor emboli labeled with

125I-5-iodo-2′-deoxyuridine. J Natl Cancer Inst 1970; 45:773–782.
64. Gutman M, Singh RK, Price JE, Fan D, Fidler IJ. Accelerated growth of human colon cancer cells in nude mice undergoing liver regeneration. Invasion Metastasis 1994; 14:362–371.
65. Radinsky R, Bucana CD, Ellis LM, Sanchez R, Clearly KR, Brigati DJ, Fidler IJ. A rapid colorimetric in situ messenger RNA hybridization technique for analysis of epidermal growth factor receptor in paraffin-embedded surgical specimens of human colon carcinomas. Cancer Res 1993; 53:937–943.
66. Radinsky R, Risin S, Fan D, Dong Z, Bielenberg, D, Bucana CD, Fidler IJ. Level and function of epidermal growth factor receptor predict the metastatic potential of human colon carcinoma cells. Clin Cancer Res 1995; 1:19–31.
67. Kitadai Y, Ellis LM, Tucker SL, Greene GF, Bucana CD, Cleary KR, Takahashi Y, Tahara E, Fidler IJ. Multiparametric in situ mRNA hybridization analysis to predict disease recurrence in patients with colon carcinoma. Am J Pathol 1996; 149:1541–1551.
68. Kitadai Y, Ellis LM, Takahashi Y, Bucana CD, Anzai H, Tahara E, Fidler IJ. Multiparametric in situ messenger RNA hybridization analysis to detect metastasis-related genes in surgical specimens of human colon carcinomas. Clin Cancer Res 1995; 1:1095–1102.
69. Kitadai Y, Bucana CD, Illis LM, Anzai H, Tahara E, Fidler IJ. In situ mRNA hybridization technique for analysis of metastasis-related genes in human colon carcinoma cells. Am J Pathol 1995; 147:1238–1247.
70. Anzai H, Kitadai Y, Bucana CD, Sanchez R, Omoto R, Fidler IJ. Expression of metastasis-related genes in surgical specimens of human gastric cancer can predict disease recurrence. Eur J Cancer 1998; 34:558–565.
71. Greene GF, Kitadai Y, Pettaway CA, von Eschenback AC, Bucana CD, Fidler IJ. Correlation of metastasis-related gene expression with metastatic potential in human prostate carcinoma cells implanted in nude mice using an in situ messenger RNA hybridization technique. Am J Pathol 1997; 150:1572–1582.
72. Kuniyasu H, Ellis LM, Evand DB, Abbruzzese JL, Fenoglio CJ, Bucana CD, Cleary KR, Tahara E, Fidler IJ. Relative expression of E-cadherin and type IVC collagenase genes predicts disease outcome in patients with resectable pancreatic carcinoma. Clin Cancer Res 1999; 5:25–33.
73. Herbst RS, Yano S, Kuniyasu H, Khuri FR, Bucana CD, Guo F, Liu D, Kemp B, Lee JJ, Hong WK, Fidler IJ. Differential expression of E-cadherin and type IV collagenase genes predicts outcome in patients with stage I non-small cell lung carcinoma. Clin Cancer Res 2000; 6:790–797.
74. Slaton JW, Inoue K, Perrotte P, El-Naggar AK, Swanson DA, Fidler IJ, Dinney CP. Expression levels of genes that regulate metastasis and angiogenesis correlate with advanced pathological stage of renal cell carcinoma. Am J Pathol 2001; 158:735–743.
75. Herrera CA, Xu L, Bucana CD, Silva VG, Hess KR, Gershenson DM, Fidler IJ. Expression of metastasis-related genes in human epitheilial ovarian tumors. Int J Oncol 2002; 20:5–13.
76. Van't Veer LJ, Dai H, van de Vijver MJ, He YD, Hart AA, Mao M, Peterse HL, van der Kooy K, Marton MJ, Witteveen AT, Schreiberr GJ, Kerkhoven RM, Roberts C, Linsley PS, Bernards R, Friend SH. Gene expression profiling predicts clinical outcome of breast cancer. Nature 2002; 415:530–536.
77. Arteaga CL. Trastuzumab, an appropriate first-line single-agent therapy for HER2-overexpressing metastatic breast cancer. Breast Cancer Res 2003; 5:96–100.
78. Christodoulou C, Klouvas G, Pateli A, Mellou S, Sgouros J, Skarlos DV. Prolonged administration of weekly paclitaxel and trastuzumab in patients with advanced breast cancer. Anticancer Res 2003; 23: 737–744.
79. Herbst RS, Hong WK. IMC-C225, an anti-epidermal growth factor receptor monoclonal antibody for treatment of head and neck cancer. Semin Oncol 2002; 29: 18–30.
80. Peggs K, Mackinnon S. Imatinib mesylate—the new gold standard for treatment of chronic myeloid leukemia. New Engl J Med 2003; 348:1048–1050.
81. Patel SR. Recent advances in systemic therapy of soft tissue sarcomas. Expert Rev Anticancer Ther 2003; 3: 179–184.
82. Fabbro D, Ruetz S, Buchdunger E, Cowan-Jacob SW, Fendrich G, Liebetanz J, Mestan J, O'Reilly T, Traxler P, Chaudhuri B, Fretz H, Zimmermann J, Meyer T, Caravatti G, Furet P, Manley PW. Protein kinases as targets for anticancer agents: from inhibitors to useful drugs. Pharmacol Ther 2002; 93:79–98.
83. Ranson M, Thatcher N. Commentary on ZD1839 (Iressa) in non-small cell lung cancer. Lung Cancer 2003; 40:77–78.
84. Bruns CJ, Harbison MT, Davis DW, Portera CA, Tsan R, McConkey DJ, Evans DB, Abbruzzese JL, Hicklin DJ, Radinsky R. Epidermal growth factor receptor blockade with C225 plus gemcitabine results in regression of human pancreatic carcinoma growing orthotopically in nude mice by antiangiogenic mechanisms. Clin Cancer Res 2000; 6:1936–1948.
85. Inoue K, Slaton JW, Perrotte P, Davis DW, Bruns CJ, Hicklin DJ, McConkey DJ, Sweeney P, Radinsky R, Dinney CP. Paclitaxel enhances the effects of the anti-epidermal growth factor receptor monoclonal antibody ImClone C225 in mice with metastatic human bladder transitional cell carcinoma. Clin Cancer Res 2000; 6: 4874–4884.
86. Bruns CJ, Solorzano CC, Harbison MT, Ozawa S, Tsan R, Fan D, Abbruzzese J, Traxler P, Buchdunger E, Randinsky R, Fidler IJ. Blockade of the epidermal growth factor receptor signaling by a novel tyrosine kinase inhibitor leads to apoptosis of endothelial cells and therapy of human pancreatic carcinoma. Cancer Res 2000; 60:2926–2935.

87. Kim SJ, Uehara, H, Karashima T, Shepherd DL, Killion JJ, Fidler IJ. Blockade of epidermal growth factor receptor signaling in tumor cells and tumor-associated endothelial cells for therapy of androgen-independent human prostate cancer growing in the bone of nude mice. Clin Cancer Res 2003; 9:1200–1210.
88. Baker CH, Kedar D, McCarty MF, Tsan R, Weber KL, Bucana CD, Fidler IJ. Blockade of epidermal growth factor receptor signaling on tumor cells and tumor-associated endothelial cells for therapy of human carcinomas. Am J Pathol 2002; 161:929–938.
89. Bruns CJ, Shrader M, Harbison MT, Portera C, Solorzano CC, Jauch KW, Hicklin DJ, Radinsky R, Ellis LM. Effect of the vascular endothelial growth factor receptor-2 antibody DC101 plus gemcitabine on growth, metastasis and angiogenesis of human pancreatic cancer growing orthotopically in nude mice. 2002; 102:101–108.
90. Solorzano CC, Baker CH, Bruns CJ, Killion JJ, Ellis LM, Wood J, Fidler IJ. Inhibition of growth and metastasis of human pancreatic cancer growing in nude mice by PTK787/ZK222584, an inhibitor of the vascular endothelial growth factor receptor tyrosine kinases. Cancer Biother Radiopharm 2002; 16:359–370.
91. Baker CH, Solorzano CC, Fidler IJ. Blockade of vascular endothelial growth factor receptor and epidermal growth factor receptor signaling for therapy of metastatic human pancreatic cancer. Cancer Res 2002; 62:1996–2003.
92. Uehara H, Kim SJ, Karashima T, Shepherd DL, Fan D, Tsan R, Killion JJ, Logothetis C, Mathew P, Fidler IJ. Effects of blocking platelet-derived growth factor-receptor signaling in a mouse model of experimental prostate cancer bone metastases. J Natl Cancer Inst 2003; 95:458–470.
93. Bergers G, Song S, Meryer-Morse N, Bergsland E, Hanahan D. Benefits of targeting both pericytes and endothelial cells in the tumor vasculature with kinase inhibitors. J Clin Invest 2003; 111:1287–1295.
94. Slaton JW, Perrotte P, Inoue K, Dinney CPN, Fidler IJ. Interferon-α-mediated down-regulation of angiogenesis-related genes and therapy of bladder cancer are dependent on optimization of biological dose and schedule. Clin Cancer Res 1999; 5:2726–2734.
95. Solorzano CC, Hwang R, Baker CH, Bucana CD, Pisters PW, Evans DB, Killion JJ, Fidler IJ. Administration of optimal biological dose and schedule of interferon alpha combined with gemcitabine induces apoptosis in tumor-associated endothelial cells and reduces growth of human pancreatic carcinoma implanted orthotopically in nude mice. Clin Cancer Res 2003; 9: 1858–1867.
96. Tedjarati S, Baker CH, Apte S, Huang S, Wolf JK, Killion JJ, Fidler IJ. Synergistic therapy of human ovarian carcinoma implanted orthotopically in nude mice by optimal biological dose of pegylated interferon alpha combined with paclitaxel. Clin Cancer Res 2002; 8: 2413–2422.
97. Huang SF, Kim SJ, Lee AT, Karashima T, Bucana C, Kedar D, Sweeney P, Mian B, Fan D, Shepherd D, Fidler IJ, Dinney CP, Killion JJ. Inhibition of growth and metastasis of orthotopic human prostate cancer in athymic mice by combination therapy with pegylated interferon-alpha-2b and docetaxel. Cancer Res 2002; 62: 5720–5726.
98. Thorpe PE, Chaplin DJ, Blakey DC. The first international conference on vascular targeting: meeting overview. Cancer Res 2003; 63:1144–1147.

2

Principles of Clinical Cancer Staging

S. EVA SINGLETARY

Department of Surgical Oncology, The University of Texas M.D. Anderson Cancer Center, Houston, Texas, U.S.A.

I. INTRODUCTION

The first half of the 20th century was marked by a growing recognition that not all tumors at a given anatomic site share the same prognosis or require the same type of treatment. In the breast, for example, the radical mastectomy recommended by Halsted in the 19th century was needlessly disfiguring for some women with small tumors, while doing little to affect survival for those with advanced disease. This growing recognition of the heterogeneity of cancer resulted in attempts to define characteristics that would be useful in assessing prognosis and determining appropriate treatment for individual tumors.

By the 1940s, there was a widespread consensus that the major anatomical attributes of a tumor that determine its behavior are: size of the primary tumor (T), presence and extent of regional lymph node involvement (N), and presence of distant metastases (M). Starting in 1942, Pierre Denoix began the development of a cancer-staging system based on these attributes (1). Clinical stage classifications for cancers of the breast and larynx were first presented in 1958 (2). Recommendations for 23 other body sites were published in brochures by the International Union against Cancer (UICC), and consolidated into the "TNM Classification of Malignant Tumors" published by the UICC in 1968 (3). Second and third editions were published in 1974 and 1978, and the third edition was enlarged and revised in 1982.

The American Joint Committee on Cancer (AJCC) was first organized in 1959 as the American Joint Committee for Cancer Staging and End-Point Results Reporting, with the goal of developing a clinical-staging system that was acceptable to the American medical profession. The first formal edition of the cancer-staging manual from the AJCC appeared in 1977. The second edition, published in 1983, revised and expanded the earlier edition, and also moved to ensure conformity between the AJCC system and the UICC system. By ensuring this conformity, a uniform "language" is maintained for the exchange of clinical information among national and international treatment centers. Subsequent revisions of the TNM-staging system have been driven by significant advances in diagnosis and treatment, with the underlying goals of improving the assessment of prognosis and the ability to make appropriate treatment decisions. The latest revision of the TNM-staging system was published in 2002 (4,5) and officially adopted for use in tumor registries in January 2003.

The TNM-staging system includes four classifications: clinical, pathologic, retreatment, and autopsy. Clinical classification (TNM or cTNM) is based on evidence that is gathered before initial treatment of the primary tumor, and is used to make treatment recommendations. Pathologic classification (pTNM) includes the results of clinical staging, as modified by evidence obtained from surgery and from pathologic examination of the primary tumor, lymph nodes, and distant metastases (if present). It is used to assess prognosis and to make recommendations for adjuvant treatment. Retreatment classification (rTNM) includes all information available at the time when further treatment is needed for a tumor that has recurred after a disease-free interval. Autopsy classification (aTNM) is used for cancers discovered after the death of a patient, when the cancer was not detected prior to death.

The T, N, and M classifications are separately defined for tumors at each anatomic site. Although TNM staging offers a valuable platform for assessing tumors at most sites, certain cancers require a different approach to staging. Both Hodgkin's and non-Hodgkin's lymphoma, for example, are staged by distribution and symptomatology, rather than local extent of the disease. Primary tumors of the central nervous system have not been amenable to TNM staging. In the brain, the size of the tumor is not as important for outcome as the histology and location. There are no lymph nodes in the brain, so an "N" classification is not possible. Finally, most patients with brain cancer tend to have a short survival time, so distant metastases do not have time to develop or cannot pass through the blood–brain barrier.

This review will cover the general principles used in clinical staging with the TNM system (4,5). Besides its current importance for primary treatment selection, clinical staging will have growing importance in cancer treatment as clinicians explore noninvasive modalities for tumor ablation. Noninvasive approaches currently under study include percutaneous radiofrequency ablation, cryosurgery, laser ablation, and MRI-guided focused sonography. Accurate clinical staging will be critical to ensure proper patient selection for such procedures, and will also be increasingly important in determining appropriate adjuvant treatment, since the primary tumor will be destroyed during the initial procedure.

II. PRINCIPLES OF CLINICAL CANCER STAGING USING THE TNM SYSTEM

A. General Rules

The natural history of a specific tumor is determined by a variety of factors. Cancers that develop in the same site (e.g., breast or prostate) and have similar histology can be expected to have roughly similar patterns of growth. Beyond that, increasing size of the tumor is one of the key indicators of outcome. As the primary tumor becomes larger, it is more likely to be associated with lymph node involvement and, ultimately, distant metastases. For some tumors, other factors have been found to significantly influence prognosis, and are also considered. For example, histologic grade is considered in the staging of soft-tissue sarcoma and prostate adenocarcinoma, and histologic type and patient age are considered in the staging of thyroid carcinoma.

Evidence for T, N, and M categories is acquired before any treatment of the primary tumor (including neoadjuvant systemic therapy), using the results from clinical examination. (If classification is performed during or following neoadjuvant therapy or other initial multimodality therapy, which might alter the original pathology, the TNM or pTNM categories are identified by a "y" prefix, e.g., ypTNM.) A variety of imaging studies and additional tests (endoscopy, surgical exploration, curettage, etc.) are used as appropriate for specific sites (see Table 1, for examples). All

Table 1 Evidence Used for Clinical Cancer Staging

Cancer site	Staging evidence
Salivary gland	Neurologic evaluation of cranial nerves; radiologic studies (MRI or CT) to examine deep tissue extent, bone invasion
Thyroid	Indirect laryngoscopy, radioisotope thyroid scan, MRI, or CT
Colon and rectum	Sigmoidoscopy, colonoscopy with biopsy, special examinations to demonstrate extracolonic metastases (chest films, liver function tests, liver scans)
Gall bladder	Ultrasound, CT, surgical exploration.
Melanoma	"T" classification based on thickness and ulceration, as determined by excisional biopsy (punch biopsy, fusiform ellipse, or saucerization)
Cervix	Colposcopy, endocervical curettage, hysteroscopy, cystoscopy, proctoscopy, intravenous urography, x-ray of lungs and skeleton
Prostate	Digital rectal exam, transrectal ultrasound, sextant needle biopsy
Kidney	CT, laparoscopy, biopsy of distant sites

cases must be confirmed microscopically for TNM staging. A biopsy (excisional, fine needle aspiration, core) is used to determine histologic type and grade, and to establish a diagnosis of cancer. The clinical stage of the primary tumor is not changed on the basis of additional information gathered during treatment. If there is any doubt about the appropriate T, N, or M category, the less advanced category is chosen.

B. The "T" Classification

The size of the primary tumor is clinically assessed through direct visualization, palpation, or imaging studies, and is represented as the linear measurement of the greatest dimension. Biopsy results are not used for clinical assessment of tumor size. The clinical estimation of tumor size by palpation may differ from that obtained on imaging studies. For example, it is relatively common to obtain different size estimates by physical examination and mammography in patients with breast cancer (6,7). In such cases, an average of the two values may be used (8). Clinical tumor size is classified as:

TX Primary tumor cannot be assessed
T0 No evidence of primary tumor
Tis Carcinoma in situ
T1, T2, T3, T4 Increasing size and/or local extent of the primary tumor

In cases where there are multiple simultaneous tumors in one organ, the T category is assigned according to the size of the largest tumor, rather than a combination of tumor sizes. The clinical record should indicate either the presence of multiple tumors [e.g., T2 (m)] or the number of tumors [e.g., T2 (5)].

C. The "N" Classification

The N classification reflects metastases of the primary tumor to regional lymph nodes. Lymph nodes are clinically assessed through palpation or imaging studies or through biopsy (e.g., FNA) of suspicious nodes. They are classified as:

NX Regional lymph nodes cannot be assessed
N0 No regional lymph node metastases
N1, N2, N3 Increasing involvement of regional lymph nodes

Direct extension of a tumor into a lymph node is classified as a lymph node metastasis. Metastasis in any lymph node other than a regional node is considered to be a distant metastasis. Although biopsy of suspicious nodes is used for some tumors (e.g., thyroid carcinoma), sentinel lymph node assessment is *not* considered a part of clinical staging. The sentinel lymph node is the first node (or nodes) to receive drainage from the primary tumor, and its status (positive or negative for metastases) is predictive of the status of the other lymph nodes in that basin. Sentinel lymph node dissection is considered as part of the pathologic classification.

D. The "M" Classification

Distant metastases are typically detected through the use of imaging or through surgical exploration, often initiated as a result of patient symptomatology. They are classified as:

MX Distant metastasis cannot be assessed
M0 No distant metastasis
M1 Distant metastasis

The M1 category can be further categorized to reflect the site of the distant metastasis: pulmonary (PUL), osseous (OSS), hepatic (HEP), etc.

E. Assigning a Stage

After assigning a T, N, and M category, the categories are combined into stages. The clinical stage assigned to a specific tumor is used to select the appropriate initial treatment for that tumor. The TNM stages range from Stage 0 to IV. Carcinoma in situ is categorized as Stage 0 and, for most sites, the presence of distant metastases is categorized as Stage IV. Stages I, II, and III represent increasing anatomic extent of the tumor, characterized by increasingly poor outcomes. The TNM stages are defined such that the tumors represented in each stage are relatively homogeneous with regard to survival. Survival rates associated with different stages are defined separately for different cancer sites.

III. CHANGES IN THE TNM-STAGING SYSTEM

A. The Importance of Stability

The TNM-staging system is not a static set of rules. Since its inception, it has evolved because of advances in detection, diagnosis, and treatment for every tumor site. Significant advances in clinical imaging have enabled physicians to use these noninvasive technologies to more accurately determine tumor size and nodal involvement. Improved survival as the result of developments in systemic treatment has resulted in alterations to both clinical and pathologic staging in some cases. For example, metastases to the supraclavicular lymph nodes (SCLN) in patients with breast cancer are associated with a poor prognosis, and the 1997 revision of the TNM-staging system classified

SCLN metastases as distant metastases (M1), resulting in a designation of Stage IV (9). Such patients were generally considered to be end-stage and were given only palliative care. However, Brito et al. (10) found that when SCLN-positive breast cancer patients received aggressive multimodal treatment, their survival time was equivalent to that seen in Stage IIIB patients without distant metastases. Thus, in the new edition of the TNM-staging system, metastases to the SCLN are classified as N3c rather than M1.

However, changes in the TNM system are not undertaken lightly. The TNM-staging system represents a shorthand whereby clinical experience can be accurately conveyed to other practitioners, and the results of clinical studies in different institutes and different countries can be compared directly. The use of TNM staging in the United States is a mandatory requirement for admission to cancer-approved hospitals, and TNM staging is used in the accrual and sorting of cancer outcome data in national data bases. Thus, it is important for the TNM system to remain relatively consistent over extended time periods, and to incorporate only those changes that are supported by strong clinical data and represent a current consensus among medical practitioners.

To assess the difficulties that can arise even when necessary changes are made to the TNM-staging system, Woodward et al. (11) examined records from 1350 breast cancer patients who had received mastectomy and doxorubicin-based chemotherapy at M.D. Anderson Cancer Center. They assigned pathologic stage according to both the 1988 and the 2003 AJCC-staging criteria. Only about 60% of the patients who were Stage II in the 1988 classification system were still Stage II with the 2003 system. A significant percentage of patients with Stage IIb disease were upstaged to Stage IIIa in the new system, resulting in improved survival for both Stage II and Stage III.

B. The Future of the TNM System

1. Morphological Markers

In addition to amendments to the existing TNM system, researchers have investigated the potential usefulness of adding additional morphological and nonmorphological variables to the staging system. For some sites, this has already been done. Histology, patient age, and tumor grade are currently used in staging for some sites. The incorporation of grade has also been considered for breast cancer staging, and this will likely occur in the near future (4). Additional tumor characteristics, such as vascular invasion of tumor emboli into the lymphatic spaces or blood vessels, or patient characteristics, including ethnicity, may also prove to be useful.

2. Nonmorphological Markers

The use of nonmorphological markers in the staging of cancer has been actively pursued over the last 10 years. This research has been fueled by developing technologies in immunogenetics and molecular biology, with the ultimate goal of being able to define cancer prognosis on an individual basis for each patient.

The major drawback in the use of molecular markers for cancer staging has been the sheer complexity involved. The process of tumorigenesis involves the synergistic interplay of dozens of genes and gene products that regulate cell proliferation, apoptosis, tumor suppression, etc. Table 2 shows a list of 24 molecular markers that have been investigated to determine prognostic significance in breast cancer. A comprehensive review of the literature indicated that only two of these markers (cathepsin-D and Ki-67 labeling index) appeared to be independently correlated with survival in patients with early stage breast cancer (12). Even for these two markers, there is considerable controversy,

Table 2 Potential Molecular Markers for Prognosis in Breast Cancer

Marker type	Potential molecular markers
Proliferation	Ki-67 labeling index
	Proliferation cell nuclear antigen
Apoptosis	bcl gene family
Tumor suppressor genes	P53
	Nm23
Oncogenes	c-myc
	h-ras
Proteases	Cathepsin-D
	Urokinase-type plasminogen activator
	Matrix metalloproteinases
Breast cancer specific genes	BRCA1
	BRCA2
Growth factors	Epidermal growth factor receptor
	HER2/*neu*
	Transforming growth factor-alpha
	Insulin-like growth factor
	IGF-binding protein
Regulation of the cell cycle	Cyclin D1
	Cyclin D2
	Cyclin E
	Telomerase
Other	Estrogen/progesterone receptor
	ps2
	Heat shock proteins

in part due to technical difficulties in obtaining measurements that are consistent between laboratories and, sometimes, within the same laboratory. For example, Tandon et al. (13) published a report in which cathepsin-D was reported to be a good prognostic factor for early stage breast cancer, but were unable to duplicate this finding in a later study that used a different immunologic reagent to detect cathepsin-D (14).

A potential approach to dealing with the complexity of genetic interactions involved in tumorigenesis lies with the new technique of microarray analysis to create a genetic fingerprint of the tumor. In this technique, RNA from tumor cells is isolated and used to prepare complementary RNA (cRNA), which is then labeled and hybridized to microarray panels containing up to 25,000 oligonucleotides. Positive labeling, indicating binding of an oligonucleotide to a cRNA molecule, indicates that the genetic material was being actively expressed in the tumor cells. Van't Veer et al. (15) have used RNA-based microarrays to investigate the relationship between gene expression profiles and breast cancer prognosis. Using RNA isolated from 98 primary breast tumors, they hybridized onto microarrays containing probes from 25,000 genes. They established a profile of 70 genes associated with prognosis. Not surprisingly, a poor prognosis was associated with upregulation of genes related to the cell cycle, invasion, metastasis, angiogenesis, and signal transduction. In a follow-up study from the same researchers (16), the 70-gene expression profile was a more powerful predictor of 10-yr overall survival rates for young patients with breast cancer than standard prognostic indicators based on clinical and histologic criteria. While these studies were carried out using tumor samples obtained from surgical excision, it seems likely that these techniques can be readily adapted to use samples obtained through biopsy, and thus be useful for clinical staging. Microarray analysis may become an important tool in determining optimal treatment strategies for patients based on an individualized assessment of tumor aggressiveness.

Another approach that may refine our ability to establish accurate clinical staging involves the use of immunohistochemical or molecular biologic techniques to identify isolated tumor cells/clusters of cells. These isolated tumor cells are frequently identified during histologic examination of lymph nodes, where their significance has been the subject of much debate (4). Isolated tumor cells have also been identified in peripheral blood, where it is hypothesized that they may be significantly correlated with degree of malignancy. A recent study by Huang et al. (17) used nested reverse transcriptase–polymerase chain reaction to analyze mRNA expression of cancer-specific antigens [carcinoembryonic antigen, cytokeratin-19 (CK19)], cytokeratin-20) in peripheral blood from patients with gastrointestinal carcinoma, patients with inflammatory gastrointestinal disease, and healthy volunteers. Among patients with gastrointestinal carcinoma, 74.2% were positive for at least one marker, while only one blood sample from a healthy control was positive for a marker. A similar approach has been used in several studies examining the correlation between CK19-positive peripheral blood cells and outcome in patients with breast cancer. In a report from Stathapoulou et al. (18), CK19 mRNA was detected in the peripheral blood of 3.7% of healthy controls, 30% of patients with early breast cancer, and 52% of patients with metastatic breast cancer. By multivariate analysis, detection of peripheral blood CK19-positive cells was an independent prognostic factor for disease relapse and death. Kahn et al. (19) reported CK19-positive peripheral blood samples from 30% of patients with node-negative breast cancer, 36% of patients with node-positive breast cancer, and 71% of patients with metastatic disease.

IV. CONCLUSIONS

For almost 50 years, the TNM-staging system has been the best available tool for assessing prognosis and determining treatment options for a variety of human cancers. Its usefulness has been the result of a careful balance between the need to preserve a stable system and the requirement for change to represent current clinical consensus. For much of the 50 years, revisions to TNM have been largely concerned with fine-tuning the assessment of tumor size and regional and distant metastases. Gradually, however, the system has been diversifying, as different markers (e.g., tumor grade, serum factors) have shown themselves to be of prognostic significance for specific types of cancer. In the current environment of explosive change in our technical abilities to find and analyze tumor cells, it is to be expected that the diversification of the TNM system will increase in the future. With the incorporation of new tools of molecular biology, the staging system of the future is likely to approach the goal of becoming patient-specific.

REFERENCES

1. Denoix PF. Tumor, node and metastasis (TNM). Bull Inst Nat Hyg (Paris) 1944; 1:1–69.
2. UICC Committee on Clinical Stage Classification and Applied Statistics. Clinical stage classification and presentation of results, malignant tumors of the breast and larynx. Paris: International Union Against Cancer, 1958.

3. UICC Committee on Clinical Stage Classification and Applied Statistics. TNM Classification of Malignant Tumors. Geneva: International Union Against Cancer, 1968.
4. Greene FL, Page DL, Fleming ID, Fritz AG, Balch CM, Haller DG, Morrow M, eds. AJCC Cancer Staging Manual. 6th ed. New York: Springer, 2002.
5. Sobin LH, Wittekind C, eds. International Union Against Cancer (UICC): TNM Classification of Malignant Tumors. 6th ed. New York: Wiley, 2002.
6. Fornage BD, Tonbas O, Morel M. Clinical, mammographic, and sonographic determination of preoperative breast cancer size. Cancer 1987; 60:765–771.
7. Pain JA, Ebbs SR, Hern RP, Lowe S, Bradbeer JW. Assessment of breast cancer size: a comparison of methods. Eur J Surg Oncol 1992; 18:44–48.
8. Wittekind C, Henson DE, Hutter RVP, Sobin LH, eds. TNM Supplement. 2nd ed. New York: Wiley, 2001.
9. Fleming ID, Cooper JS, Henson DE, Hutter RVP, Kennedy BJ, Murphy GP, O'Sullivan B, Sobin LH, Yarbro JW, eds. AJCC Cancer Staging Manual. 5th ed. New York: Lippincott-Raven, 1997.
10. Brito RA, Valero VV, Buzdar AU, Booser DJ, Ames F, Strom E, Ross M, Theriault RL, Frey D, Kau SW, Asmer L, McNeese M, Singletary SE, Hortobagyi GN. Long-term results of combined-modality therapy for locally advanced breast cancer with ipsilateral supraclavicular metastases: The University of Texas M.D. Anderson Cancer Center experience. J Clin Oncol 2001; 19:628–633.
11. Woodward WA, Strom EA, McNeese MD, Perkins GH, Schechter NR, Singletary SE, Theriault RL, Hortobagyi GH, Hunt KK, Buchholz TA. Changes in the 2003 AJCC staging for breast cancer dramatically affect stage-specific survival. J Clin Oncol 2003; 21:3244–3248.
12. Mirza AN, Mirza NO, Vlastos G, Singletary SE. Prognostic factors in node-negative breast cancer: a review of studies with sample size more than 200 and follow-up more than 5 years. Ann Surg 2002; 235:10–26.
13. Tandon AK, Clark GM, Chamness GC, Chirgwin JM, McGuire WL. Cathepsin-D and prognosis in breast cancer. N Engl J Med 1990; 322:297–302.
14. Ravdin PM, Tandon AK, Allred DG, Clark GM, Fuqua SA, Hilsenbeck SH, Chamness GC, Osborne CK. Cathepsin-D by western blotting and immunohistochemitry: failure to confirm correlations with prognosis in node-negative breast cancer. J Clin Oncol 1994; 12:467–474.
15. Van't Veer LJ, Dai H, van de Vijver MJ, He YD, Hart AA, Mao M, Peterse JL, van der Kooy K, Marton MJ, Witteveen AT, Schreiber GJ, Kerkhoven RM, Roberts C, Linsley PS, Bernards R, Friend SH. Gene expression profiling predicts clinical outcome of breast cancer. Nature 2002; 415:530–536.
16. Van de Vijver MJ, He YD, Van't Veer LJ, Dai H, Hart AA, Voskuil DW, Schreiber GJ, Peterse JL, Roberts C, Marton MJ, Parrish M, Atsma D, Witteveen A, Glas A, Delahaye L, van der Velde T, Bartelink H, Roden S, Rutgers ET, Friend SH, Bernards R. A gene-expression signature as a predictor of survival in breast cancer. New Eng J Med 2002; 347:1999–2009.
17. Huang P, Wang J, Guo Y, Xie W. Molecular detection of disseminated tumor cells in the peripheral blood in patients with gastrointestinal cancer. J Cancer Res Clin Oncol 2003; 129:192–198.
18. Stathapoulou A, Vlachonikolis I, Mavroudis D, Perraki M, Kouroussis C, Apostolaki S, Malamos N, Kakolyris S, Kotsakis A, Xenidis N, Reppa D, Georgoulias V. Molecular detection of cytokeratin-9-positive cells in the peripheral blood of patients with operable breast cancer: evaluation of their prognostic significance. J Clin Oncol 2002; 20:3404–3412.
19. Kahn HJ, Yang LY, Blondal J, Lickley L, Holloway C, Hanna W, Narod S, McCready DR, Seth A, Marks A. RT-PCR amplification of CK19 mRNA in the blood of breast cancer patients: correlation with established prognostic parameters. Breast Cancer Res Treat 2000; 60:143–151.

3

Principles of Surgical Cancer Care

JANICE N. CORMIER and RAPHAEL E. POLLOCK

Department of Surgical Oncology, The University of Texas M.D. Anderson Cancer Center, Houston, Texas, U.S.A.

I. INTRODUCTION

Surgery is the oldest and continues to be the primary modality of cancer therapy. Over the last few decades, cancer treatment has improved dramatically due to an improved understanding of the natural history of malignancy, contemporary diagnostic imaging, novel adjuvant and multimodality therapies, advanced surgical, anesthetic and critical care techniques, and the creation of an unique surgical discipline, surgical oncology, to embrace this ever-expanding body of knowledge (1).

The curative role of surgery in cancer therapy is a development of the last century (2). Original attempts at conservative tumor resection resulted in extremely high rates of local recurrence and subsequent patient mortality. In the late 19th century, complete en bloc resections and amputations were used to treat patients with malignant lesions. Although these techniques yielded improved results, the procedures were ablative and mutilating. The early foundations of radical surgery included the Halsted radical mastectomy and the Moynihan abdominoperineal resection for rectal cancer (3). These operations emphasized the need to remove regional lymph nodes. With the advent of effective complementary treatment modalities, notably radiation therapy in the 1920s, and chemotherapy in the 1950s, the trend of surgical tumor resection once again became conservative. Even in the contemporary era of multimodality cancer therapy, surgery continues to be the mainstay of treatment for patients with solid tumors. In general, the addition of adjuvant chemotherapy alone or in combination with radiation therapy, for patients with a high likelihood of recurrence due to microscopic residual disease has improved disease-free survival and prolonged quality of life for patients who have been rendered free of gross disease by prior surgical resection.

Surgical techniques and expertise are applicable to many facets of oncology care including prevention, diagnosis, definitive treatment, and palliation. Advances in oncology have expanded the field such that a relatively new specialty in surgical oncology has emerged. The surgical oncologist is a surgeon who not only treats cancer but is familiar with the natural history of particular tumors, as well as all aspects of treatment principles including radiation therapy, chemotherapy, and newer modalities including available clinical trials.

II. HISTORICAL PERSPECTIVE

In the second century A.D., Galen published his classification of tumors and cautioned that cancer was a systemic disease not amenable to cure by surgery. It was not until the 18th century that advances in anatomic pathology by Morgagni, Le Dran, and Da Salva established that there was an initial period of local tumor growth prior to distant dissemination. However, in the era prior to the advent of safe general anesthetics, cancer surgery consisted primarily of amputation or cauterization of surface tumors of the trunk or extremities because patients were unwilling to submit to the pain of tumor surgery when there was little likelihood of positive survival impact.

The first recorded elective tumor resection was performed in 1809 by an American surgeon, Ephraim McDowell. He successfully removed a 22-lb ovarian tumor from a patient who subsequently survived 30 years. McDowell's work, which included 12 more ovarian resections, stimulated greater interest in elective surgery for cancer patients. In 1842, ether was first used for general anesthesia and the first published account of ether anesthesia (1846) was for the elective removal of a tongue carcinoma.

Even with the advent of antisepsis and general anesthesia, surgical tumor resection in the second half of the 19th and early 20th centuries was associated with high patient mortality rates. Cancer was rarely diagnosed in the early stages; consequently, few patients were considered candidates for curative surgery. Surgeons who attempted excision of malignant lesions were hindered by crude instruments, rudimentary anesthesia, and lack of antibiotics. Additionally, there was no appreciation for the importance of margin negative resection and surgeons relied on gross visual assessment of the tumor perimeter. Gradual recognition of principles of meticulous surgical technique, gentle tissue handling, and applications of Listerian principles led to rapid advancements in the field of surgical oncology. Pioneers such as Albert Theodore Bilroth (first gastrectomy, laryngectomy, and esophagectomy) and William Stewart Halsted (en bloc resection, radical mastectomy) led to the advent of contemporary surgical oncology (2).

III. PATIENT ASSESSMENT

A. Staging

Accurate cancer staging is essential (see Chapter 2). The goal of clinical staging is to define the extent of disease in order to recommend therapy, advise about prognosis, avoid unnecessary interventions, and perform comparisons of new treatment regimens. Tumor staging is a system used to describe the anatomic extent of a specific malignant process in an individual patient. Staging systems cluster relevant prognostic factors about the primary tumor, such as size, grade, location, as well as information about dissemination to regional sites (e.g., lymph nodes) or distant metastatic loci. The American Joint Committee on Cancer (AJCC) (4) and the Union Internationale Contre Cancer (International Union Against Cancer, UICC) have adopted a shared TNM system that defines a cancer in terms of the primary tumor (T), the presence or absence of nodal metastases (N), and the presence or absence of distant metastases (M). For some tumor types, such as soft tissue sarcoma, a G for grade of malignancy is added to the system in recognition of its prognostic importance in particular diseases. High-grade tumors are less differentiated and tend to metastasize more readily.

The TNM system has four classifications; clinical, pathologic, retreatment, and autopsy. The *clinical* classification (cTNM) represents the extent of the disease *prior* to first definitive treatment as determined from physical examination, imaging studies, endoscopy, biopsy, surgical exploration, and any other relevant findings. Surgical staging may be required prior to undertaking major surgical procedures, such as laparoscopic staging prior to pancreaticoduodenectomy or gastrectomy, or para-aortic lymph node biopsy prior to esophagectomy. The *pathologic* classification (pTNM) incorporates the additional information derived from pathologic examination of a completely resected specimen which is useful in planning adjuvant therapy. The *retreatment* classification (rTNM) is used to stage a cancer that has recurred following a disease-free interval and the *autopsy* classification (aTNM) is based on postmortem examination.

B. Preoperative Considerations

Determining the risks associated with a given operation is a complicated and inexact process based on a number of factors (5,6). The physical status of the patient, including nutritional assessment and comorbid conditions, morbidity inherent to a specific operation, and the intent of surgical procedure (curative vs. palliative) are all pertinent to this assessment. The technical complexity of an operation and the relative experience of the involved health-care personnel can all impact on the complications of a procedure. The risk assessment for cancer patients should balance the risks associated with disease progression and those associated with the treatment (6).

The preoperative cancer patient is frequently in relatively poor physical condition. Patients often present with poor nutritional status, considerable pain, physiologic abnormalities (e.g., electrolyte disorders), and significant comorbid conditions. The etiology of anorexia in a cancer patient may be multifactorial: interference with normal alimentary function, as is often encountered with cancers of the mouth, pharynx, esophagus, intestinal tract; pain that may contribute to anorexia; systemic tumor effects. Nutritional deficiencies should be corrected prior to surgery if possible, with hyperalimentation or total parenteral nutrition (TPN). Reconstitution of nutritional stores is a slow process, and the risks and benefits of delaying therapy vs. restoring positive nitrogen balance must be considered. Consideration should also be given to re-establishing depleted blood volume and correcting electrolyte abnormalities prior to major surgical resections. Physiologic status related to cardiopulmonary reserve and hepatic and renal function should also be assessed and optimized. Surgical morbidity and mortality following extensive cancer operations will predictably be problematic if critical physiologic and biochemical deficiencies are not corrected in advance.

Operative morbidity and mortality are defined as events that occur within 30 days of an operative procedure. For patients with cancer, the underlying disease as well as the procedure itself must be considered in the preoperative risk assessment. Various scales for risk assessment, such as the five-level physical status classification of the American Society of Anesthesiologists and the five-step performance status scale of the Eastern Cooperative Oncology Group, may be useful in assessing the appropriateness of a given operation for a specific patient. Advanced age alone should not disqualify a patient from a potentially curative surgical procedure.

The risk assessment for palliative surgical procedures is particularly difficult. The high incidence of postoperative complications must be weighed against the potential for symptom control. For example, palliative surgery in the context of intestinal obstruction secondary to carcinomatosis has a 20–30% perioperative mortality. In such circumstances, the risk-to-benefit ratio and ultimate surgical objectives must be defined as clearly as possible and accepted by patient, family, and surgeon.

A patient's psychologic make-up and life situation must also be considered in treatment planning. The potential risks and benefits of all available treatment options must be examined, and a patient who is unable to accept the morbidity associated with a given treatment should be offered other options. In particularly difficult situations, consultation with a psychiatrist experienced in cancer (a psycho-oncologist) may help a patient and family deal with the reality of the disease and its treatment. This is particularly true for surgical procedures that significantly alter a patient's appearance, such as mastectomy or colostomy.

The experience of the surgeon and the clinical team has been defined as critical factors in surgical outcomes for cancer patients and should be included in risk assessment (6,7). There have been a number of studies that have demonstrated significant variations in operative survival based on hospital case volume (7). Particularly for high-risk surgical interventions such as pancreaticoduodenectomy, esophagectomy, gastrectomy, pelvic exenterations and hepatic resections, these studies indicate that the more cases performed at an institution the better the results (7,8). There have also been a few studies performed in patients with cancer that have suggested that patient long-term survival is impacted by the training and expertise of the operating surgeon regardless of whether interventions are high risk or low risk (e.g., procedures for breast cancer) (9–12).

IV. ROLES FOR SURGERY

A. Prevention

There has been much effort on the part of the medical community and various organizations and advocacy groups to educate the public on the early signs and symptoms that may indicate the presence of early malignancies that are more likely to be cured (1). This awareness along with the adoption of screening programs has resulted in an increased proportion of early stage, curable malignancies (13).

The identification of genetic mutations that predispose to subsequent cancer development has emerged as a means of risk assessment. The utility of prophylactic surgical treatments must be examined carefully on an individual basis. There is a growing list of indications for the role of prophylactic surgery in conditions such as cryptorchidism associated with subsequent testicular carcinoma, ulcerative colitis or familial polyposis associated with colon carcinoma, multiple endocrine neoplasia syndromes associated with the development of medullary carcinoma of the thyroid, oral leukoplakia associated with subsequent development of squamous cell carcinoma, and familial breast and ovarian cancer. In familial conditions with a high incidence of cancer, it is often the responsibility of the surgeon to educate the family of the risks to other family members.

B. Diagnosis

The diagnosis of solid tumors requires localization and biopsy for histologic confirmation. Historically, significant errors have been made when biopsy confirmation of malignancy was not obtained prior to treatment, as in the radical mastectomies that were performed for benign conditions. Contemporary practice requires that actual slides be obtained and reviewed at an institution prior to the commencement of therapy. This is particularly important for rare neoplasms in which an erroneous interpretation may have been made in the initial pathologic assessment.

There are a variety of biopsy techniques available which can be used to obtain tissue for histologic diagnosis including fine-needle aspiration, core biopsy, incisional biopsy, and excisional biopsy. Several general principles should be followed in the acquisition of tissues suspected of malignancy (14). First, the biopsy site, whether needle tracks or surgical scars should be carefully selected so that it can easily be excised as part of the subsequent definitive surgical resection. Second, adjacent tissue planes should not be contaminated during biopsy as a result of poor technique such as inadequate hemostasis. Third, the choice of biopsy technique should be selected based on the sample of tissue required for adequate evaluation by the pathologist. Lastly, biopsy material should be handled with care from the time of resection, in which precise orientation must be defined by the surgeon, and subsequent handling and processing.

Fine-needle aspiration (FNA) is a cytologic technique in which cells are aspirated from a tumor using a needle and syringe with the application of negative pressure. It is an acceptable method of diagnosing most solid tumors, particularly when the results correlate closely with clinical and imaging findings. However, the resulting aspirated tissue consists of disaggregated cells rather than intact tissue and should be performed for primary diagnosis of tumors only at centers with experienced cytopathologists. Because of the lack of intact tumor architecture, the diagnosis of malignancy depends entirely on the detection of abnormal intracellular features, such as nuclear pleomorphism, increasing the margin of error over other biopsy techniques. Fine-needle aspiration biopsy is the procedure of choice to confirm or rule out the presence of a metastatic focus or local recurrence.

Superficial lesions are often subjected to fine-needle aspiration biopsy in the clinic setting. Deeper tumors may require an interventional radiologist to perform the technique under sonographic or computed tomography guidance. The technique generally involves use of a 21- to 23-gauge needle that is introduced into the mass after appropriate cleansing of the skin and injection of local anesthetic. Negative pressure is applied, and the needle is pulled back and forth several times in various directions. After the negative pressure is released, the needle is withdrawn and the contents of the needle are used to prepare a smear. A cytopathologist then examines the slides to determine whether sufficient diagnostic material is present. If insufficient diagnostic material is obtained, a core needle biopsy should be performed.

Core needle biopsy is a safe, accurate, and economical diagnostic procedure. Core biopsies are performed with a large-bore needle, such as the Vim Silverman or Tru Cut type. This technique retrieves a small piece of intact tumor tissue, which allows the pathologist to study the invasive relationship between cancer cells and the surrounding microenvironment. The tissue sample obtained from a core needle biopsy is usually sufficient for several diagnostic tests, such as electron microscopy, cytogenetic analysis, and flow cytometry. Computed tomography guidance can enhance the positive yield rate of a core needle biopsy by accurately pinpointing the location of the tumor. Precise localization in the tumor mass is particularly important to avoid sampling nondiagnostic necrotic or cystic areas of the tumor. Computed tomography guidance also permits access to tumors in otherwise inaccessible anatomic locations or near vital structures.

Open or incisional biopsy involves removal of a small portion of the tumor mass. It is a reliable diagnostic method that allows adequate tissue to be sampled for definitive and specific histologic identification. It is best performed under circumstances where the incisional wound can be totally excised in continuity with the definitive surgical resection, in the event that any tumor cells are spilled at the time of biopsy. When adequate tissue for diagnosis cannot be obtained by fine-needle aspiration biopsy or core biopsy, incisional biopsy is indicated for deep or superficial tumors larger than 3 cm. Because open biopsy may have complications, incisional biopsies are usually performed as a last resort. Open biopsy should ideally be performed by the surgeon who will perform the definitive surgical resection. For extremity tumors, the biopsy incision should be oriented longitudinally to allow subsequent wide local excision to encompass the biopsy site, scar, and tumor en bloc. A poorly oriented biopsy incision often mandates an excessively large surgical defect for subsequent wide local excision. Another mandate of surgical technique is that adequate hemostasis must be achieved at the time of biopsy to prevent dissemination of tumor cells into adjacent tissue planes by hematoma.

Excisional biopsy completely removes the local tumor mass. It is used for small, discrete masses that are 2–3 cm in diameter, where complete removal will not interfere with a subsequent wider excision that may be required for definitive local control. Surgeons should always orient biopsy specimens with sutures or metal clips so that if removal is incomplete and further excision is needed, positive margins can be accurately identified in situ. Excisional biopsies are commonly used for polypoid lesions of the colon, thyroid and breast nodules, small skin lesions, and when the pathologist cannot make a definitive diagnosis from tissue removed by incisional biopsy. Excisional biopsies rarely provide any benefit over other biopsy techniques and may cause postoperative complications that could ultimately delay definitive therapy. Ill-conceived incisions can unnecessarily contaminate tissue planes, necessitating wider radiotherapy fields or more extensive subsequent resection. The classic example involves tumors of the extremities, which are best biopsied using longitudinal incisions that can be encompassed at the time of definitive en bloc resection. The final caveat is that surgical biopsy incisions should be performed with meticulous hemostasis as postoperative hematomas can create widespread dissemination of tumor cells with contamination of adjacent tissue planes.

Special consideration with regard to anatomic location and specimen processing should be given to surgical lymph node biopsies. Selection of axillary nodes may be preferable to groin nodes if both are enlarged due to a decreased likelihood of postoperative infection. Cervical lymph nodes should not be biopsied until a careful search for a primary tumor has been made using nasopharyngoscopy, esophagoscopy, and bronchoscopy since the etiology of cervical adenopathy is usually metastasis from laryngeal, oropharyngeal, and nasopharyngeal tumors. In contrast, supraclavicular nodes more frequently represent metastases from primary tumors of the thoracic, abdominal cavities, or breast. For patients with unknown primary tumors and/or suspected lymphoma, cytogenetic analysis requires sterile tissue processing.

C. Treatment of Primary Tumors

Surgery remains the most effective treatment of localized solid tumors. In general, en bloc resection encompassing all gross and microscopic tumor is the goal and often requires resection of adjacent anatomic structures or organs. Over the last two decades, there have been major improvements in operative technique as well as the optimization of multimodality therapy enhancing the ability to achieve surgical resection. These techniques have significantly reduced the overall morbidity and mortality associated with the surgical treatment of solid neoplasms. Specific examples include breast-conserving surgery for patients with breast carcinoma (15), limb salvage procedures for patients with bone and soft tissue sarcomas (16), improved techniques such as total mesorectal excision for clearance of rectal tumors (17), and procedures with preserve sexual potency and urinary continence for patients with prostate cancer (18).

Once a decision has been made to proceed with surgical therapy, the operative procedure must be carefully planned recognizing that the opportunity for cure is often limited to the first surgical resection. When a previous biopsy has been performed, the entire biopsy scar and any drain exit sites should be encompassed within the operative field when possible. Intraoperative considerations include the potential risk of implanting cancer if the tumor is inadvertently violated during an operative procedure. Local recurrence can occur despite all efforts to isolate the tumor or avoid spilling cancer cells into the operative field. Reasons for local recurrence include malignant cells present in local lymphatics or blood-borne cells, which implant into a wound. Manipulation of the tumor at any time during the surgical procedure can greatly increase the number of cancer cells recovered from the bloodstream. Likewise, it is also important to use appropriately large incisions to minimize excessive manipulation of the tumor.

1. Types of Cancer Operations

Local resection with removal of an adequate margin of normal peritumoral tissue may be adequate treatment for some neoplasms including wide excision of primary melanoma, early stage colon cancers as well as low-grade neoplasms such as basal cell carcinomas and mixed tumors of the parotid gland. In contrast, neoplasms that infiltrate adjacent tissues, such as soft tissue sarcomas, esophageal and gastric carcinomas, must be excised with a wide margin of normal tissue. Even tumors, which appear encapsulated at the time of resection, often demonstrate pseudocapsules composed of a compression zone of normal tissue interspersed with neoplastic cells when examined microscopically. Simple enucleation of these tumors results in local recurrence in virtually all cases.

Wide local resection of some tumors requires sacrificing major vessels, nerves, joints, or bones. Occasionally, even amputation may be necessary as an initial surgical procedure if a curative result is to be obtained. The extent of operation must be based solely on the extent of resection needed to achieve negative tumor margins. During the operation, pathologic evaluation of resected margins may indicate the need to alter the initial operative plan. These decisions are often difficult and require experienced judgment. It is usually better to proceed with a potentially curative tumor extirpation unless there is unequivocal histologic confirmation that the lesion has extended beyond the boundaries of curative surgical resection. Issues of reconstruction should be approached separately and often require the participation of plastic and reconstructive surgeons and other surgical specialists who have been consulted prior to the resection.

Many neoplasms metastasize via the lymphatics, and operations have been designed to remove the primary neoplasm along with draining regional lymph nodes. Circumstances that favor this type of operative approach are when the lymph nodes draining the neoplasm are adjacent to the tumor bed or when there is a single avenue of lymphatic drainage that can be removed without sacrificing vital structures. When there is demonstrable metastatic spread to adjacent nodal basins, it is generally agreed that en bloc regional lymph node dissection is appropriate. However, in many such cases, the tumor has already spread beyond regional nodes and cure rates may be quite low. Regional lymph node involvement should not be viewed as a contraindication to surgical resection because en bloc removal of the involved lymph nodes may offer the only chance for cure and/or significant palliative local control. Nodal involvement should be viewed as a possible indication for adjuvant therapies, such as radiation or chemotherapy.

The value of elective or prophylactic lymph node dissection has been challenged, particularly with respect to radical nodal resections in gastric, pancreatic, esophageal, rectal, and lung cancer (3). It is not clear whether cure rates are enhanced when subclinically positive lymph nodes are removed. Actively accruing randomized clinical trials in a number of disciplines are currently addressing this question. Regardless of whether or not there is a direct therapeutic benefit, knowledge of regional node tumor status can have an impact on tumor staging and subsequent treatment recommendations. The ability to identify and assess sentinel lymph nodes has revolutionized cancer staging for patients with melanoma and breast cancer. As many as 30% of previously negative regional lymph nodes are identified to harbor occult metastases by contemporary histologic analysis of sentinel lymph nodes (19). Therapeutic lymph node dissection and adjuvant therapy can now be directed to patients with confirmed microscopic nodal disease. Current controversy pertains to the utility of subsequent complete nodal dissection in subsets of patients with minimal micrometastatic disease detected in sentinel lymph nodes.

Improvements in surgical technique, anesthesia, and supportive care allow radical operative resections to be performed for locally advanced tumors. Such heroic procedures, if safely executed, can be justified in select situations with curative intent. For example, pelvic exenteration that entails the removal of all pelvic organs (bladder, uterus, and rectum) is a potentially curative procedure for patients with recurrent cancers of the cervix and well-differentiated locally extensive adenocarcinomas of the rectum. Reconstruction following exenteration involves creation of a colostomy, urinary tract drainage, and possible tissue coverage in the perineum. Experienced multidisciplinary surgical teams are often required for the best functional outcome. In addition to technical expertise, postoperative emotional support and rehabilitation services are often required.

In select patients, surgical resection of locally recurrent neoplasms may produce long periods of remission. For example, surgical procedures are frequently successful in controlling recurrent soft tissue sarcomas, anastomotic recurrences of colon cancer, certain basal and squamous carcinomas of skin and local breast cancer recurrence following segmental mastectomy. Clinical judgment must be exercised when considering surgical resection of a locally recurrent tumor in a patient with synchronous metastatic disease. Under normal circumstances surgical resection should not be contemplated unless the entire local recurrence can be completely excised and there is some form of effective therapy available to treat the metastases.

2. *Emerging Surgical Techniques*

Several new procedures have become part of the armamentarium of the surgical oncologist. Sentinel lymph node mapping and biopsy have become the standard of care for staging patients with breast cancer and melanoma. Laparoscopic surgery, which has been in existence for years, is being defined in relation to oncology by way of clinical trials. Isolated regional perfusion with chemotherapy continues to be evaluated. Newer technologies, such as radiofrequency ablation (RFA) and breast ductal lavage, are currently being evaluated.

a. *Sentinel Lymph Node Biopsy*

Sentinel lymph node (SLN) biopsy techniques have become established techniques for the staging assessment of patients with breast carcinoma (20) and melanoma (21). Expanded indications for this technique are being evaluated in a number of other tumor histologies including gastrointestinal (22–25), genitourinary (26,27), gynecologic (28,29), and head and neck (30) malignancies.

In melanoma, remarkable progress has been made such that sentinel lymph node positivity in patients with clinically negative axillae is the most important single known prognostic factor for subsequent melanoma recurrence (31).

The role of sentinel lymph node biopsy also continues to mature in carcinoma of the breast. Recent refinements in technique have rendered application of this technology less cumbersome with the administration of radiolabeled sulfur colloid that is used to identify the sentinel node 24 hr prior to surgical biopsy, relieving time constrictions inherent in immediate preoperative injection. Intraoperative assessment of sentinel node status using touch preparation techniques (32) has also been investigated as a means of obtaining immediate information allowing definitive surgical nodal dissections while preserving nodal tissue as compared to frozen section analysis for other clinical and research applications. Neoadjuvant chemotherapy has recently been shown not to affect sentinel node biopsy accuracy, rendering surgical consolidation less morbid in patients so treated (33). Other new applications such as in ductal carcinoma in situ (DCIS) are apparent in results from recent studies suggesting a 12% positive rate in the higher risk patients with DCIS, such as those with microinvasion (34). It can be anticipated that sentinel node biopsy technology will continue to develop as new uptake markers are applied and as analytic schema such as microarray technology are coupled with this minimal surgical approach.

b. Laparoscopic Surgery

Laparoscopic surgery has been used for the diagnosis, staging, and treatment of patients with malignancy. Despite contemporary radiologic imaging, laparoscopy has been demonstrated to have utility in tumor staging, particularly with upper gastrointestinal malignancies (35). A laparoscopic evaluation can provide additional information about the primary tumor nodal disease, as well as detect small hepatic and peritoneal diseases that cannot be appreciated on radiologic imaging. The addition of ultrasound techniques have been shown to increase the sensitivity of tumor staging beyond laparoscopy alone and radiologic imaging (36,37). Clinical trials are ongoing to determine the utility of laparoscopic oncologic resections.

c. Isolated Regional Perfusion

Isolated perfusion is a technique that was devised to administer concentrated dose of chemotherapy to tumors. The majority of the experience has been in isolated limb perfusion for in-transit melanoma and as a means of providing a limb sparing alternative for patients with locally advanced soft tissue sarcomas.

Isolated limb perfusion involves isolating the main artery and vein of the perfused limb from the systemic circulation. The choice of anatomic approach is determined by tumor site; external iliac vessels are used for thigh tumors, femoral or popliteal vessels for calf tumors, and axillary vessels for upper-extremity tumors. The vessels are dissected, and all collateral vessels are ligated. The vessels are then cannulated and connected to a pump oxygenator similar to that used in cardiopulmonary bypass. A tourniquet or Esmarch band is applied to the limb to achieve complete vascular isolation. For the lower limb, the Esmarch band is anchored at the anterior–superior iliac spine with the aid of a pin inserted into the pelvic bones. For the upper limb, the pin is anchored at the scapular and pectoral levels. Chemotherapeutic agents are then added to the perfusion circuit and circulated for 90 min. Systemic leakage from the perfused limb is monitored continuously by monitoring ^{99}Tc-radiolabeled human serum albumin injected into the perfusate. Radioactivity above the precordial area is recorded with a Geiger counter. The temperature of the perfused limb is maintained during the entire procedure by external heating and warming of the perfusate to 40°C. At the end of the procedure, the limb is washed out, the cannulas are extracted, and the blood vessels are repaired.

Despite a 40-year history of isolated limb perfusion being used, many questions remain to be answered. The choice of chemotherapeutic agent in the perfusion circuit, the benefits of hyperthermia, and the effectiveness of hyperthermic perfusion in the neoadjuvant or adjuvant setting remain to be elucidated. Studies published to date have involved heterogeneous patient groups and diverse chemotherapeutic agents.

With a similar intent, optimal cytoreduction and intraperitoneal hyperthermic peritoneal perfusion has been used for the treatment of patients with peritoneal implants from a variety of tumor histologies including pseudomyxoma peritonei (38), gastrointestinal carcinomatosis (39), intra-abdominal mesothelioma (40), ovarian cancer (41), and sarcomatosis (42).

d. Radiofrequency Ablation

Radiofrequency ablation is a technique by which tumor tissue is selectively destroyed by the transfer of heat energy from an electrode placed within the tumor and delivered as an alternating current. This approach has been used extensively in the context of unresectable primary and secondary hepatic malignancy (43). The technique has also been successfully utilized as an initial treatment in bilobar liver disease in conjunction with synchronous or sequential hepatic resection and in the treatment of hepatocellular carcinoma in patients with cirrhosis (44).

Based on the success of RFA in treating malignancy of the liver, attempts are being made to broaden its indications with investigations in the treatment of unresectable pancreatic carcinoma, retroperitoneal sarcoma, and other malignant diseases. A recent report has demonstrated the utility of RFA in early stage breast carcinoma where the need to preserve tissue may be a concern to many patients (45). This is currently being evaluated in clinical trials in which patients undergo core needle biopsy to assess for residual viable tumor 4 weeks after RFA, and then undergo sequential or modified mastectomy only if the core needle biopsy is positive (46). Patients with negative core biopsies will receive radiation therapy without mastectomy. Approaches such as these indicate potential approaches for eliminating tumors without the necessity of ablative surgical resections in the future.

e. *Breast Ductal Lavage*

Breast ductal lavage is emerging as another minimally invasive surgical procedure to identify cellular abnormalities in the epithelial lining of the breast ductal system. The procedure consists of identifying fluid-yielding breast ducts by initial aspiration, followed by placement of small catheters into the fluid-yielding duct with infusion and then aspiration of normal saline effluent. The effluent is collected and examined using standard cytopathology techniques (47). The technique has been demonstrated to be sensitive in populations of patients at high risk for breast cancer. The ability to perform minimally invasive procedures that increase the sensitivity of detecting cellular atypia may ultimately become incorporated into surveillance strategies for asymptomatic patients at risk for developing breast cancer.

3. *Surgery as a Component of Multimodality Therapy*

Tumors that are at high risk for local and/or distant recurrence are often treated with multimodality therapies. The use of combined modality therapy (surgery in combination with radiation and chemotherapy) was pioneered by pediatric oncologists in the management of childhood neoplasms. Tumors such as retinoblastoma, Wilms' tumor, and embryonal rhabdomyosarcoma can often be cured using combinations of radiation, chemotherapy, and surgery. For example, the cure rate for patients with Wilms' tumor is 75% if surgical therapy is followed by radiation and chemotherapy, an increase of 40% over operation alone.

Until recently, the effectiveness of multimodality therapy was only occasionally demonstrable for adult neoplasms. Clinical trials have confirmed the benefit of combination surgical resection and radiation therapy for the local control of localized breast cancers (15) and skeletal and soft tissue sarcomas. In the past, surgical resection of these tumors as a single treatment resulted in frequent local recurrences. The addition of radiation to more conservative surgical resections (segmental mastectomy and limb-sparing tumor resection) can achieve rates of local control similar to mastectomy and amputation. With both types of neoplasms, survival and local recurrences were the same for patients treated with multimodality therapy; however, patients were spared the physical deformity and psychological stress associated with radical surgical procedures (3,48).

Surgical resection and radiation are the most successful means of treating cancer localized to the primary site and/or regional lymph nodes. Since these forms of therapy exert their effects loco-regionally, it is not usually considered curative once a tumor has metastasized beyond these sites. Chemotherapy, immunotherapy, and hormonal therapy are treatments that can potentially kill tumor cells that have metastasized to distant sites. These systemic modalities have a greater chance of cure in patients with minimal (or even subclinical) tumor burden as compared with those with clinically evident disease. Consequently, surgery and radiation therapy may be useful in decreasing a given patient's tumor burden, thereby maximizing the impact of subsequent systemic approaches. Evidence of such treatment benefit is the survival benefit seen in patients with stage III colon cancer who receive 5-FU and leukovorin following surgical resection.

An emerging element of the multimodality approach for some tumors is immunotherapy, treatment aimed at activation of the immune system. The concept of immunostimulation with biologic response modifiers or nonspecific immunomodulators is not new in cancer therapy. Nearly a century ago, William B. Coley developed the basis for nonspecific cancer immunotherapy using mixed bacterial vaccines (Coley's toxin). Since then, whole cell or cell fragment tumor vaccines have been introduced for active specific immunotherapy of neoplastic disease, and some of these have reached clinical applications. In melanoma, immunotherapy alone or in combination with chemotherapy is often used as an adjuvant to surgery for the treatment of regional disease or in attempts to prolong the survival of patients with distant metastases. Cytokines, such as interferon-α and interleukin-2, are also being used to modulate the immune response and have proven effective in some diseases, such as myeloid leukemia and hairy cell leukemia, melanoma, and renal cell carcinoma.

Historically, surgery was performed first in the sequence of therapies for solid neoplasms with the addition of radiation and/or chemotherapy following adequate healing of the surgical wound. There is increasing evidence that suggests that definitive surgical resection should follow chemotherapy and/or radiation. Postoperative surgical sites may be relatively hypoxic and resistant to radiation therapy, whereas the chemotherapeutic regimen may be tailored for efficacy with tumors in situ. Surgical resection may then be employed to remove residual tumor. Frequently, sequencing chemotherapy and radiotherapy prior to surgical resection can cause shrinkage of tumor mass due to destruction of chemo- and radiosensitive tumors resulting in less ablative surgical resections with improved function. These concepts have been applied to patients with breast cancer, bone and soft tissue sarcomas and other neoplasms.

Treatment sequencing requires the input of a multidisciplinary team, which includes radiation, medical, and surgical oncologists. The surgical oncologist must be able to co-ordinate and integrate the efforts of the entire oncologic team if he or she is to retain a primary role in the management of the cancer patient.

D. Patterns of Tumor Spread

In general, tumors disseminate via direct infiltration of surrounding tissues, lymphatic invasion, vascular dissemination, or implantation in serous cavities. A combination of dissemination routes is also possible and the sequence may not be predictable. For example, patients with breast cancer or melanoma may manifest distant metastatic disease in the lungs, liver, or skeleton without ever developing evidence of lymph node metastases.

Direct extension through tissue planes is characteristic of adenocarcinomas of the stomach or esophagus, which can extend for a considerable distance (10–15 cm) along tissue planes beyond the palpable tumor mass. Soft tissue sarcomas are often described to have "finger-like" projections into the surrounding tissues resulting in high local recurrence rates for tumors that are not excised with wide margins. Also, central nervous system tumors may result in death by infiltrating surrounding brain tissue and affecting vital functions.

Tumor cells can readily enter the lymphatics and traverse these channels by permeation or embolization to lymph nodes. Lymphatic involvement is extremely common in epithelial neoplasms of all types, except basal cell carcinoma of the skin, which metastasizes to regional lymphatics in less than 0.1% of cases. Growth of tumor cells along the course of a lymphatic channel (permeation) is commonly seen in patients with breast cancer with involvement of the skin lymphatics and in patients with carcinoma of the prostate who demonstrate perineural lymphatics invasion. Lymphatic embolization is of great clinical importance in a number of neoplasms. Tumor cells traverse the lymphatic channels to regional lymph nodes and deposit initially in the subcapsular space. Eventually, the tumor cells are able to permeate the sinusoids and replace the nodal parenchyma. It is thought to spread directly from node to node. When tumor involved lymph nodes become enlarged, tumor can extend beyond the capsule into the perinodal fat, often indicating an ominous prognosis.

Lymphatic drainage from the lower extremities and intra-abdominal organs ultimately empties into the thoracic duct by way of the cisterna chyli. Ultimately, lymph flows into the left jugular vein creating a direct route for tumor cells to pass from the lymphatic system into the bloodstream. Alternatively, tumor cells may reach the bloodstream by direct invasion of blood vessels, most commonly through capillaries or veins. Vascular invasion is common in both carcinomas and sarcomas and is associated with a poor prognosis. Some types of neoplasms have a particular tendency to grow as a solid column along the course of veins. For example, renal cell carcinoma can grow into the renal vein and inferior vena cava extending to the right atrium. In such situations, en bloc removal requiring resection with cardiopulmonary bypass may still result in long-term survival or even cure.

Tumor cells occasionally gain entrance to serous cavities by growing through the wall of an organ. Many tumor cells can grow in suspension without a supporting matrix and may spread freely within the peritoneal cavity by attaching to serous surfaces. Widespread peritoneal seeding is common with gastrointestinal neoplasms including pseudomyxoma peritonei and ovarian tumors. Similarly, malignant gliomas may spread widely within the CNS via the cerebrospinal fluid.

Although much is known about the routes of tumor spread, the mechanisms underlying this process remain unclear. Some cancers are metastatic at the time of primary diagnosis, whereas other tumors of the same histologic type may remain localized for years. In some instances, metastases may dominate the presenting clinical picture, whereas the primary tumor remains latent and asymptomatic or even undetectable. For example, cerebral metastases from silent cancers in the bronchus or the breast are often mistaken for primary benign central nervous system neoplasms.

An en bloc tumor resection is intended to remove the primary neoplasm along with contiguous lymphatic and vascular channels that may contain tumor. Potential cure is achieved by the mechanical removal of all cancer cells. However, in many instances cancer cells can be found in operative washings, blood or lymphatics without subsequent distant recurrence indicating that the metastatic process is inefficient. Host immune mechanisms may also have a role in the salvage of patients undergoing resection of metastases in distant organs, such as the lung or liver. Particularly, in patients who undergo resection of metastatic disease, it is likely that they harbor subclinical metastases in other sites, which are presumably destroyed by host immune mechanisms such that at least a subset of postresection patients subsequently become disease-free long-term survivors.

E. Surgical Emergencies

A number of surgical emergencies can emerge as a result of enlarging tumors including exsanguinating hemorrhage, perforated viscus, abscess formation, or impending obstruction of a hollow viscus, such as gastrointestinal organs, critical blood vessels, or respiratory structures. Additionally, surgical intervention may also be indicated to decompress tumors invading the central nervous system or destroying critical neurologic components by exerting pressure in closed spaces.

Specific issues pertaining to the evaluation of cancer patients for emergency surgical interventions include the effects of recent myelosuppressive chemotherapy. Potential catastrophes can sometimes be avoided by performing elective procedures on patients expectantly, just after they have gone through the nadir of their most recent myelosuppressive chemotherapy. In truly emergent situations, patient and families must be made aware of the increased surgical risks and the potential benefits of the proposed surgery, which is frequently only palliative.

F. Surgical Palliation

1. Metastatic Disease

It is recognized in general that if patients require heroic resections to obtain loco-regional control of their primary disease, it is likely that the disease has already disseminated to distant sites. Metastatic disease disseminated to vital organs is the cause of death in the majority of patients with cancer. Despite this, the removal of metastatic lesions in the lung, liver, or brain has occasionally produced prolonged survival and/or cure. Occasionally, even multiple metastases may be successfully resected. Extensive radiologic assessment should be performed prior to embarking on surgical resection of metastatic disease to ensure that metastatic spread is limited to region of the proposed surgery.

Examples of particular scenarios in which surgical resection has been demonstrated to be successful in patients with metastatic cancer include liver metastases in patients with colorectal carcinoma and pulmonary metastases in patients with sarcoma. Metastatectomy is considered in patients with colorectal cancer in whom the primary tumor has been controlled, there is no evidence of extrahepatic metastases, with resectable liver metastases (isolated primarily to hepatic lobe). Although only a minority of patients with colon cancer metastatic to the liver will meet these requirements of operability, approximately 25% of operable patients will survive more than 5 years following resection. The results for resection of pulmonary metastases for sarcoma have also been very satisfactory. For example, resection of a solitary or limited pulmonary metastasis for some tumor types, such as osteogenic sarcoma, results in a higher survival rate than does resection of primary bronchogenic carcinoma of the lung. Resection of pulmonary metastases may be indicated even when more than one metastatic lesion is present, particularly for tumors that have responded to systemic therapy or have a long doubling time.

2. Palliative Procedures

A surgical oncologist is often faced with a dilemma when a cancer has spread beyond the possibility of cure. Patients are generally deemed incurable if they have widespread distant metastases or evidence of extensive local tumor infiltration of critical anatomic structures. The goal of therapy in such situations is to treat symptomatic disease progression and maintain maximum activity and quality of life as long as possible (6,49). Histologic proof of distant metastases should be obtained before a patient is considered incurable. Occasionally, an exploratory celiotomy or thoracotomy may be necessary to determine the histology of ambiguous lesions in the lungs or liver. Within each anatomic region of the body, there are specific criteria defining whether a patient is unequivocally incurable. Although tumor invasion of some organs and contiguous structures may imply a poor prognosis, such scenarios may not indicate absolute incurability. In equivocal situations, patients should be explored with the intention and preparation for surgical cure.

A palliative operation may be justified to relieve pain, hemorrhage, obstruction, or infection. Particularly, invasive interventions must be balanced by "realistic expectations of achieving low morbidity and achieving durable palliation"(49). Palliative surgery may also be considered in circumstances when there are no better nonsurgical means of palliation with the potential for improving quality of life, even if it does not result in prolonged survival. In a review by Wagman (49), the primary considerations for patients and physicians considering a palliative procedure include: the complexity of the procedure, the duration of the hospitalization as well as overall recovery period, the likelihood of achieving the palliative goal, the interim evaluations that will be required to sustain palliation, the likely durability of palliation, and the anticipated malignant disease progression. Examples of palliative surgical procedures include: (1) colostomy, enterostomy, or gastrojejunostomy to relieve gastrointestinal obstruction; (2) cystectomy to control hemorrhagic tumors of the bladder; (3) amputation for control of intractable pain; (4) soft tissue resections (e.g., mastectomy) for infection control of primary tumors for patients with metastatic disease; and (5) colon resection to prevent obstruction in the presence of hepatic metastases.

Cytoreduction, treatment that incompletely eradicates tumor, is a special application of palliative surgery. The basis for cytoreductive surgery is that in some patients extensive yet isolated local spread of malignancy precludes gross total resection of all disease. In such circumstances, removal of bulky symptomatic tumor often improves function and quality of life and theoretically may improve response to systemic therapies by reducing overall tumor burden (50). The benefits of cytoreductive surgery have been demonstrated in a number of tumor histologies including ovarian neoplasms (51), germ cell tumors (52), some gastrointestinal tumors (53), and metastatic neuroendocrine tumors (54). The risks associated with cytoreductive surgery can be significant and the particular tumor biology must be examined prior to embarking on an extensive cytoreductive resection (50). McCarter and Fong (50) outline several principles for identifying patients likely to benefit from cytoreductive surgery including patients with symptomatic, slow-growing tumors (favorable biologic behavior), likely to respond to additional therapies, and in whom cytoreductive resection can be performed safely.

In addition to surgical resection, a number of less invasive cytoreductive techniques have emerged including cryoablation, RFA, ethanol injection, and embolization, as a means of treating patients that are not candidates for surgical resection (54). Methods for applying these techniques safely and effectively using percutaneous applications are under investigation.

G. Special Situations

1. *Vascular Access*

Vascular access is commonly required in cancer patients requiring long-term nutritional and hematologic support, as well as for the administration of systemic therapies. Catheter technology has progressed over the past 35 years and there are a large variety of vascular access devices that can be inserted percutaneously depending on the intended use. Multi-lumen catheters are available which allow the simultaneous administration of otherwise incompatible agents, such as some blood products, antibiotics, and chemotherapies.

Catheter placement can be accomplished at the bedside, in the radiology procedure suite, or in the operating room and must be performed as a sterile surgical procedure. Postcatheter placement chest radiographs are required to confirm catheter tip location and rule out the presence of iatrogenic complications. Catheterization is associated with venous thrombosis so that for patients that require serial catheters, nuclear flow studies performed prior to subsequent catheterizations may detect chronic subclinical occlusion in a potential candidate recipient vessel.

There have been little data available upon which to base a decision of whether to use percutaneous venous access or a subcutaneously implantable venous access system. Results of a recently published Canadian randomized trial suggests that the majority of participants can receive satisfactory venous access percutaneously, with the added expense of an implantable system reserved for those patients who fail percutaneous access strategies (55). This latter approach has been the standard of practice at the University of Texas M.D. Anderson Cancer Center for more than a decade with comparably satisfactory results.

V. RECONSTRUCTION AND REHABILITATION

Developments in reconstructive surgery have remarkably improved the quality of life for many cancer patients following surgical resection of tumors (56). The routine application of microvascular anastomotic techniques has enabled the free transfer of composite grafts containing skin, muscle, and/or bone to surgical defects. Examples of these dramatic improvements in the combined surgical management of complex cancer problems include breast reconstruction after mastectomy (57,58), tissue transfers as part of radical resection of extremity tumors (59–61), aerodigestive reconstruction (62,63), and perineal reconstruction following radical pelvic surgery (64,65). Research is ongoing to define the applications of tissue engineering to extend the reconstructive armamentarium (66). It may be possible in the future to custom grow nerve, fat, muscle, bone cartilage, or other body components as replacement tissues for reconstruction of oncologic surgical defects.

VI. THE SURGICAL ONCOLOGIST

Surgical oncologists are surgeons who devote most of their time to the study and treatment of malignant neoplastic disease. They must possess the necessary knowledge, skills, and clinical experience to perform both the standard as well as extraordinary surgical procedures often required for patients with cancer. However, surgical oncology is more of a cognitive than a technical surgical specialty. With the exception of a small cluster of index operations, such as regional pancreatectomy, limb salvage and retroperitoneal sarcoma surgery, isolated limb perfusion, and multisegment liver resection, most of the surgical procedures that are performed by surgical oncologists are similar to those performed by a surgeon not oncologically trained. What frequently differentiates these two types of surgeons is the knowledge of contemporary multimodality cancer care. Surgical oncologists must be able to diagnose tumors accurately and to differentiate aggressive neoplastic lesions from benign reactive processes. In addition, surgical oncologists should have a firm understanding of radiation oncology, medical oncology, pathology, and hematology.

Surgical oncologists have a shared role with medical oncologists as the "primary-care physicians" of cancer treatment. Almost all cancer patients will initially be managed by one of these two specialists who will bear the ultimate responsibility for co-ordinating appropriate multimodality care for the individual patient. As a member of a multidisciplinary team, the role of the surgical oncologist is to co-ordinate and assist with all aspects of a patient care including tumor diagnosis, surgical resection, follow-up and often palliative interventions. The cancer surgeon is commonly charged with the responsibility of establishing a tissue diagnosis by selection of biopsy technique, communicating biopsy findings to the patient, completing staging procedures and initiating the interaction with other members of the multimodality oncology team. During these initial interactions with patients and family, it is most often the cancer surgeon who educates and explains the sequence and rationale of the various treatment components that can be used to manage their specific malignancy. In this role, a cancer surgeon must be aware of the different therapeutic options, the natural history of a given malignancy, and how these factors will be integrated into a well-conceived and appropriate multimodality treatment algorithm.

Beyond the initiation of diagnosis and treatment, a surgical oncologist is also involved in decisions about follow-up care and surveillance to detect tumor recurrence. In this regard, the cancer surgeon, unlike almost any other surgical specialist, makes a patient commitment for the acute as well as the long-term components of their disease process (10).

Given the complexity of contemporary multidisciplinary approaches to the cancer patient, free-standing cancer centers have developed facilities to provide the needed planning expertise, clinical care, patient support services, and access points to clinical trials. These comprehensive cancer centers are frequently affiliated with academic medical institutions and offer the complete spectrum of oncologic therapies, clinical trials, rehabilitation and social services, as well as basic and translational research programs.

As part of a larger surgical community, the surgical oncologist is a critical conduit of cancer information to colleagues in general surgery and other surgical specialties. This function is often performed at academic surgical meetings, such as those of the American College of Surgeons or the Society of Surgical Oncology, as well as by service in directing hospital-based tumor boards and direct consultation on behalf of individual cancer patients. Because of their leading role in the initial diagnosis of cancer, it is not surprising that surgical oncologists are also frequently in leadership roles in cancer prevention and screening programs. Nation-based multimodality clinical trial groups also depend on surgical oncology expertise to help in trial design, establishing the criteria of surgical quality control, educating trial participants regarding standards of surgical care, as well as assistance in accurate data collection, analysis, and presentation of trial results.

VII. CONCLUSIONS

Within the next decade, cancer is predicted to replace cardiovascular disease as the most prevalent killer of Americans on an annual basis. At present, surgery remains the most promising treatment modality with the greatest chance of cure for solid tumors. As multimodality treatments increase in number and grow in complexity, surgical oncologists will have to become increasingly involved in basic science, technology development, and clinical trial design. Understanding the natural history of specific malignancies will require an expanded knowledge base about genetics and the molecular biology that drives solid tumor proliferation and metastasis. The contemporary surgical approach encompasses appropriate margins of resection including regional nodal basins with morbidity in proportion to the benefits of reducing recurrence (3). Cancer prevention and early diagnosis are the mainstays of increasing survival, whereas advances in adjuvant systemic therapies including molecularly targeted therapies may provide hope for those with advanced disease. Surgical oncologists must be flexible and examine new techniques scientifically as they become available. Risk assessments must be performed for all procedures, keeping in mind that doing nothing may at times be beneficial.

REFERENCES

1. Bremers AJ, Rutgers EJ, van de Velde CJ. Cancer surgery: the last 25 years. Cancer Treat Rev 1999; 25: 333–353.

2. Hill GJ. II. Historic milestones in cancer surgery. Semin Oncol 1979; 6:409–427.
3. Cady B. Fundamentals of contemporary surgical oncology: biologic principles and the threshold concept govern treatment and outcomes. J Am Coll Surg 2001; 192:777–792.
4. American Joint Committee on Cancer. Cancer Staging Manual. 6th ed. New York: Springer, 2002:221–226.
5. Rahlfs TF, Jones RL. Risks and outcomes in oncology patients undergoing anesthesia and surgery. Int Anesthesiol Clin 1998; 36:141–149.
6. Rew DA. Risk analysis in surgical oncology—part II: risk and the practicing surgeon. Eur J Surg Oncol 2000; 26:705–710.
7. Hillner BE, Smith TJ, Desch CE. Hospital and physician volume or specialization and outcomes in cancer treatment: importance in quality of cancer care. J Clin Oncol 2000; 18:2327–2340.
8. Begg CB, Cramer LD, Hoskins WJ, et al. Impact of hospital volume on operative mortality for major cancer surgery. JAMA 1998; 280:1747–1751.
9. Hodgson DC, Fuchs CS, Ayanian JZ. Impact of patient and provider characteristics on the treatment and outcomes of colorectal cancer. J Natl Cancer Inst 2001; 93:501–515.
10. Helsper JT. Impact of the surgeon on cancer management outcomes. J Surg Oncol 2003; 82:1–2.
11. McArdle CS, Hole D. Impact of variability among surgeons on postoperative morbidity and mortality and ultimate survival. BMJ 1991; 302:1501–1505.
12. Gillis CR, Hole DJ. Survival outcome of care by specialist surgeons in breast cancer: a study of 3786 patients in the west of Scotland. BMJ 1996; 312:145–148.
13. Cady B. Basic principles in surgical oncology. Arch Surg 1997; 132:338–346.
14. Rosenberg SA. Principles of cancer management: surgical oncology. In: Vincent T, DeVita J, Hellman S, Rosenberg SA, eds. Cancer: Principles and Practice of Oncology. Philadelphia: Lippincott Williams & Wilkins, 2001:253–264.
15. Fisher B, Anderson S, Bryant J, et al. Twenty-year follow-up of a randomized trial comparing total mastectomy, lumpectomy, and lumpectomy plus irradiation for the treatment of invasive breast cancer. N Engl J Med 2002; 347:1233–1241.
16. Rosenberg SA, Tepper J, Glatstein E, et al. The treatment of soft-tissue sarcomas of the extremities: prospective randomized evaluations of (1) limb-sparing surgery plus radiation therapy compared with amputation and (2) the role of adjuvant chemotherapy. Ann Surg 1982; 196:305–315.
17. Heald RJ, Ryall RD. Recurrence and survival after total mesorectal excision for rectal cancer. Lancet 1986; 1: 1479–1482.
18. Sokoloff MH, Brendler CB. Indications and contraindications for nerve-sparing radical prostatectomy. Urol Clin North Am 2001; 28:535–543.
19. Cote RJ, Peterson HF, Chaiwun B, et al. Role of immunohistochemical detection of lymph-node metastases in management of breast cancer. International Breast Cancer Study Group. Lancet 1999; 354:896–900.
20. Giuliano AE, Jones RC, Brennan M, et al. Sentinel lymphadenectomy in breast cancer. J Clin Oncol 1997; 15:2345–2350.
21. Morton DL. Lymphatic mapping and sentinel lymphadenectomy for melanoma: past, present, and future. Ann Surg Oncol 2001; 8:22S–28S.
22. Tanaka K, Kobayashi M, Konishi N, et al. Laparoscopic intraoperative detection of micrometastatic sentinel nodes by immunohistochemical staining in patients with early gastric cancer. Surg Endosc 2003; 28:28.
23. Tien HY, McMasters KM, Edwards MJ, et al. Sentinel lymph node metastasis in anal melanoma: a case report. Int J Gastrointest Cancer 2002; 32:53–56.
24. Yasuda S, Shimada H, Chino O, et al. Sentinel lymph node detection with Tc-99m tin colloids in patients with esophagogastric cancer. Jpn J Clin Oncol 2003; 33: 68–72.
25. Bilchik AJ, Nora DT, Sobin LH, et al. Effect of lymphatic mapping on the new tumor-node-metastasis classification for colorectal cancer. J Clin Oncol 2003; 21:668–672.
26. Tanis PJ, Lont AP, Meinhardt W, et al. Dynamic sentinel node biopsy for penile cancer: reliability of a staging technique. J Urol 2002; 168:76–80.
27. Wawroschek F, Wagner T, Hamm M, et al. The influence of serial sections, immunohistochemistry, and extension of pelvic lymph node dissection on the lymph node status in clinically localized prostate cancer. Eur Urol 2003; 43:132–137.
28. DuBeshter B, Deuel C, Gillis S, et al. Endometrial cancer: the potential role of cervical cytology in current surgical staging. Obstet Gynecol 2003; 101:445–450.
29. De Hullu JA, Van Der Zee AG. Sentinel node techniques in cancer of the vulva. Curr Womens Health Rep 2003; 3:19–26.
30. Pitman KT, Ferlito A, Devaney KO, et al. Sentinel lymph node biopsy in head and neck cancer. Oral Oncol 2003; 39:343–349.
31. Solorzano CC, Ross MI, Delpassand E, et al. Utility of breast sentinel lymph node biopsy using day-before-surgery injection of high-dose 99mTc-labeled sulfur colloid. Ann Surg Oncol 2001; 8:821–827.
32. Henry-Tillman RS, Korourian S, Rubio IT, et al. Intraoperative touch preparation for sentinel lymph node biopsy: a 4-year experience. Ann Surg Oncol 2002; 9:333–339.
33. Breslin TM, Cohen L, Sahin A, et al. Sentinel lymph node biopsy is accurate after neoadjuvant chemotherapy for breast cancer. J Clin Oncol 2000; 18:3480–3486.
34. Klauber-DeMore N, Tan LK, Liberman L, et al. Sentinel lymph node biopsy: is it indicated in patients with high-risk ductal carcinoma-in-situ and ductal

carcinoma-in-situ with microinvasion? Ann Surg Oncol 2000; 7:636–642.
35. Conlon KC, Minnard EA. The value of laparoscopic staging in upper gastrointestinal malignancy. Oncologist 1997; 2:10–17.
36. Finch MD, John TG, Garden OJ, et al. Laparoscopic ultrasonography for staging gastroesophageal cancer. Surgery 1997; 121:10–17.
37. John TG, Greig JD, Carter DC, et al. Carcinoma of the pancreatic head and periampullary region. Tumor staging with laparoscopy and laparoscopic ultrasonography. Ann Surg 1995; 221:156–164.
38. Sugarbaker PH. Cytoreductive surgery and perioperative intraperitoneal chemotherapy as a curative approach to pseudomyxoma peritonei syndrome. Tumori 2001; 87:S3–S5.
39. Glehen O, Mithieux F, Osinsky D, et al. Surgery combined with peritonectomy procedures and intraperitoneal chemohyperthermia in abdominal cancers with peritoneal carcinomatosis: a phase II study. J Clin Oncol 2003; 21:799–806.
40. Ma GY, Bartlett DL, Reed E, et al. Continuous hyperthermic peritoneal perfusion with cisplatin for the treatment of peritoneal mesothelioma. Cancer J Sci Am 1997; 3:174–179.
41. Atkins CD. Intraperitoneal chemotherapy for stage III ovarian cancer. J Clin Oncol 2003; 21:957; author reply 957–958.
42. Rossi CR, Foletto M, Mocellin S, et al. Hyperthermic intraoperative intraperitoneal chemotherapy with cisplatin and doxorubicin in patients who undergo cytoreductive surgery for peritoneal carcinomatosis and sarcomatosis: phase I study. Cancer 2002; 94:492–499.
43. Curley SA, Izzo F, Delrio P, et al. Radiofrequency ablation of unresectable primary and metastatic hepatic malignancies: results in 123 patients. Ann Surg 1999; 230:1–8.
44. Curley SA, Izzo F, Ellis LM, et al. Radiofrequency ablation of hepatocellular cancer in 110 patients with cirrhosis. Ann Surg 2000; 232:381–391.
45. Izzo F, Thomas R, Delrio P, et al. Radiofrequency ablation in patients with primary breast carcinoma: a pilot study in 26 patients. Cancer 2001; 92:2036–2044.
46. Singletary SE, Fornage BD, Sneige N, et al. Radiofrequency ablation of early-stage invasive breast tumors: an overview. Cancer J 2002; 8:177–180.
47. Dooley WC, Ljung BM, Veronesi U, et al. Ductal lavage for detection of cellular atypia in women at high risk for breast cancer. J Natl Cancer Inst 2001; 93: 1624–1632.
48. Karakousis CP. Radical versus conservative cancer surgery: an anachronism? J Surg Oncol 2001; 77:221–224.
49. Wagman LD. Palliative surgery: a modern perspective. J Surg Oncol 2002; 80:1–3.
50. McCarter MD, Fong Y. Role for surgical cytoreduction in multimodality treatments for cancer. Ann Surg Oncol 2001; 8:38–43.
51. Eisenkop SM, Friedman RL, Wang HJ. Complete cytoreductive surgery is feasible and maximizes survival in patients with advanced epithelial ovarian cancer: a prospective study. Gynecol Oncol 1998; 69:103–108.
52. Richie JP. Surgical aspects in the treatment of patients with testicular cancer. Hematol Oncol Clin North Am 1991; 5:1127–1142.
53. Gomez Portilla A, Deraco M, Sugarbaker PH. Clinical pathway for peritoneal carcinomatosis from colon and rectal cancer: guidelines for current practice. Tumori 1997; 83:725–728.
54. Miller CA, Ellison EC. Therapeutic alternatives in metastatic neuroendocrine tumors. Surg Oncol Clin N Am 1998; 7:863–879.
55. Bow EJ, Kilpatrick MG, Clinch JJ. Totally implantable venous access ports systems for patients receiving chemotherapy for solid tissue malignancies: a randomized controlled clinical trial examining the safety, efficacy, costs, and impact on quality of life. J Clin Oncol 1999; 17:1267.
56. Bland KI. Oncologic and plastic surgeons: colleagues, collaborators, teammates. Plast Reconstr Surg 1998; 102:1733–1747.
57. Petit J, Rietjens M, Garusi C. Breast reconstructive techniques in cancer patients: which ones, when to apply, which immediate and long term risks? Crit Rev Oncol Hematol 2001; 38:231–239.
58. Newman LA, Kuerer HM, Hunt KK, et al. Feasibility of immediate breast reconstruction for locally advanced breast cancer. Ann Surg Oncol 1999; 6:671–675.
59. Bickels J, Wittig JC, Kollender Y, et al. Distal femur resection with endoprosthetic reconstruction: a long-term followup study. Clin Orthop 2002; 1(400):225–235.
60. Zenn MR, Levin LS. Microvascular reconstruction of the lower extremity. Semin Surg Oncol 2000; 19: 272–281.
61. Hornicek FJ, Gebhardt MC, Sorger JI, et al. Tumor reconstruction. Orthop Clin North Am 1999; 30:673–684.
62. Haughey BH, Taylor SM, Fuller D. Fasciocutaneous flap reconstruction of the tongue and floor of mouth: outcomes and techniques. Arch Otolaryngol Head Neck Surg 2002; 128:1388–1395.
63. Losken A, Carlson GW, Culbertson JH, et al. Omental free flap reconstruction in complex head and neck deformities. Head Neck 2002; 24:326–331.
64. Arkoulakis NS, Angel CL, DuBeshter B, et al. Reconstruction of an extensive vulvectomy defect using the gluteus maximus fasciocutaneous V-Y advancement flap. Ann Plast Surg 2002; 49:50–54.
65. Rietjens M, Maggioni A, Bocciolone L, et al. Vaginal reconstruction after extended radical pelvic surgery for cancer: comparison of two techniques. Plast Reconstr Surg 2002; 109:1592–1597; discussion 1598–1599.
66. Miller MJ. Osseous tissue engineering in oncologic surgery. Semin Surg Oncol 2000; 19:294–301.

4

Principles of Chemotherapy

SILWAN CHEDID and JONATHAN TRENT
The University of Texas M.D. Anderson Cancer Center, Houston, Texas, U.S.A.

I. INTRODUCTION

Chemotherapy may be used as the sole therapy for malignancy, but is more commonly used in combination with surgery, radiotherapy, or both. This strategy enhances local control and eradicates occult metastases. The dosage and schedule of chemotherapeutic agents are a balance between efficacy and toxic effects on vital organ systems. Many patients receiving chemotherapy may require elective or even emergent surgery, and the perioperative team members must have a clear understanding of the actions, interactions, and potential toxic effects of each agent in the chemotherapeutic regimen. The preoperative evaluation of the patient should include a detailed history of the exact type and dosing information for each antineoplastic agent used. Organ systems most likely to have been and to be affected should be thoroughly evaluated.

This chapter includes a brief discussion of the basic principles of chemotherapy, synopses of chemotherapeutic mechanisms of action and drug resistance, and a review of select classes of chemotherapeutic agents, namely: alkylating agents, platinum agents, antimetabolites, anthracyclines, topoisomerase inhibitors, microtubule inhibitors, and miscellaneous agents.

II. TUMOR GROWTH

Most antineoplastic drugs are designed to interfere with cell division by interfering with DNA synthesis, replication, transcription, and translation. Cells that are replicating more quickly are also usually more sensitive to chemotherapeutic agents. This balance between cell death and cell replication dictates the degree of response to treatment with a given agent.

Tumor cell kinetics and doubling time are not constant in all cancer cells within an affected individual. Moreover, the proliferating proportion of tumor cells varies among cancers, from 90% in some hematalogic malignancies (for example, lymphoma) to less than 20% in some solid tumors. However, within the tumor's proliferating subpopulation, the doubling time remains constant. As the tumor mass increases, the percentages of nondividing and dying cells will increase.

The smallest mass detectable on chest radiography (approximately 1 cm in diameter) represents approximately 1 g of tissue (1×10^9 cells). In such cases, the neoplastic cells have been present for some time, but vital organs are often not damaged until the tumor mass increases to 1×10^{12} to 10^{13} cells (approximately 1 to 10 kg of tissue). For cell division to be sustained within the body, the growing tumor must induce neoangiogenesis to supply the tumor cells with adequate nutrients and oxygen; otherwise, necrosis will ensue. The resulting new blood vessels differ from the body's normal vasculature in that they are often densely packed, tortuous, and chaotically distributed.

Many solid tumors contain large quantities of nonproliferating cells that are resistant to the cytotoxic effects of chemotherapy. Proliferating cells are preferentially susceptible to chemotherapeutic agents; quiescent cells may also be killed, albeit less efficiently. This selectivity partially explains why many solid tumors are refractory to chemotherapeutic intervention. In addition, pre-existing genetically distinct tumor cell subclones may display accelerated growth and an ability to metastasize, a property often associated with larger primary tumors (1).

III. CHEMOTHERAPY AND THE CELL CYCLE

Different chemotherapeutic agents affect cells at different points in the cell's replicative cycle. Combining chemotherapeutic agents that target cells at different points in the cell cycle can be very effective, with additive or even synergistic effects in some cases. Certain normal cells such as those found in the bone marrow, hair follicle, and gastrointestinal mucosa are continually replenishing their numbers by traversing through the cell cycle. Chemotherapy may damage these normal cells resulting in side effects such as myelosuppression, alopecia, and mucositis.

A patient's tumor is composed of cells formed as a result of mitosis and consists of three subpopulations: cells that are nondividing and terminally differentiated, cells that are progressing through the cell cycle toward cell division, and resting cells that may return to the cell cycle (i.e., stem cells). All malignant solid tumors are composed of all three-cell populations.

Tumor cells that are proliferating traverse the mitotic cell cycle, which is composed of the G1, S, G2 and M phases. Cells that are resting (G0 phase) are able to divide again by re-entering the cell cycle at the G1 phase. Preliminary synthetic cellular processes occur, preparing cells to enter the DNA synthetic (S) phase. Specific protein signals regulate the cell cycle and allow replication of the genome, where the DNA content becomes tetraploid. After completion of the S phase, the cell enters a second resting phase, G2, before undergoing mitosis. The cell progresses to mitotic (M) phase, where the chromosomes separate and the cell divides (2,3).

Chemotherapeutic agents can be classified according to the phase of the cell cycle in which they are active (Table 1). This is not an arbitrary classification scheme. Agents whose action is consistent throughout all phases of the cell cycle (e.g., alkylating agents) have a linear dosage–response curve: the greater the dosage of the agent, the larger the percentage of cell kill. In contrast, drugs whose action is specific to a particular cell cycle phase plateau in their ability to kill cells since some cells will not be in that phase of the cell cycle. The percentage of cell kill will not increase with increasing drug dosage.

Table 1 Agents That Kill Tumor Cells in Specific Phases of the Cell Cycle

G1 phase	S phase	G2 phase	M phase
Asparaginase	Capecitabine	Bleomycin	Docetaxel
Corticosteroids	Cytarabine	Irinotecan	Etoposide
	Doxorubicin	Mitoxantrone	Paclitaxel
	Fludarabine	Topotecan	Teniposide
	Fluorouracil		Vinblastine
	Gemcitabine		Vincristine
	Hydroxyurea		Vinorelbine
	Mercaptopurine		
	Methotrexate		
	Prednisone		
	Procarbazine		
	Thioguanine		

IV. COMBINATION CHEMOTHERAPY

Chemotherapy combinations have been devised in order to maximize cell killing by using agents that target different points in the cell cycle, rather than combining agents that target the cells in the same phase. Combining different chemotherapeutic agents accomplishes at least three objectives: It provides overlapping and sometimes synergistic cell kill within the range of toxicity tolerated by the patient for each drug, it provides coverage for resistant tumor cell subclones in a heterogeneous tumor population, and it slows the development of new drug-resistant tumor cell subclones (4). Several general principles guide selection of agents used in combination regimens: (a) Drugs known to be active as single agents should be chosen, with preference for agents that induce complete remission. (b) Drugs with different mechanisms of action should be chosen, to allow for additive or synergistic effects on tumor cells. (c) Drugs with differing dose-limiting toxicities should be chosen, to allow for each drug to be given at the full therapeutic dosage. (d) The treatment-free interval between cycles should be the shortest time that allows for recovery of the most sensitive normal tissue. (e) Drugs with different patterns of resistance should be combined to maximize killing of cells that may be resistant to a single agent.

V. DOSAGE INTENSITY

Dosage intensity is a phenomenon that has been observed to be a beneficial strategy in retrospective studies of colon cancer, ovarian cancer, breast cancer, and lymphoma (5). For chemotherapy-sensitive cancers, the factor limiting the capacity to cure is insufficient dosing. Suboptimal doses of chemotherapy most often result from the development of chemotherapy-related side effects. As the dosage of an agent is reduced, the cure rate significantly decreases, and there is an appreciable decline in the complete remission rate. Therefore, chemotherapy-sensitive cancer patients are commonly given, doses approaching the maximal tolerated dosage.

VI. DRUG RESISTANCE

Cancer is a genetic disease. Cancer cells are inherently more prone to genetic mutations than are normal cells, and spontaneous mutations occur in subpopulations of cells before exposure to chemotherapy. Some of these subpopulations are drug resistant and continue to proliferate after chemotherapy has eliminated the sensitive cell lines. The Goldie–Coldman hypothesis asserts that the probability of a tumor population containing resistant cells is a function of the total number of cells present (6,7). Several mechanisms for chemotherapeutic failure have been identified and are described below.

A. Single-Drug Resistance

Cell lines may become resistant to a single-drug class or to multiple drugs, depending on the type of resistance. Mechanisms by which tumors become more resistant to a single agent are increased production of catabolic enzymes to degrade drugs, direct drug inactivation by glutathione, reduced ability to repair DNA strand breaks, and alterations in transport proteins.

Exposure to a drug can result in gene amplification of DNA for specific catabolic enzymes. Upregulation of catabolic enzymes and the resulting decrease in effective drug levels causes drug resistance. Examples include increases in dihydrofolic reductase, which metabolizes methotrexate (8); deaminase, which deactivates cytarabine (9); and glutathione, which inactivates alkylating agents (10). Glutathione is not only essential for DNA synthesis but is a scavenger of free radicals and appears to play a role in drug resistance. The hypothesized mechanisms of glutathione-mediated drug resistance are inactivation of alkylating agents through direct binding, increased metabolism, detoxification, and repair of DNA damage.

Increased topoisomerase inhibition results in both inhibition of DNA replication and failure to repair strand breaks. DNA strands are wound together and attached to the nuclear matrix at regularly spaced domains. Topoisomerases bind to these domains, forming a "cleavable complex" that allows DNA to unwind in preparation for cell division. Topoisomerases later participate in the resealing of DNA molecules during cell division. Inhibition of topoisomerase causes both inhibition of DNA replication and failure to repair strand breaks (11). Camptothecin derivatives, such as irinotecan and topotecan, exert their effect by inhibiting topoisomerase I. Epipodophyllotoxin derivatives, such as etoposide, inhibit topoisomerase II. Both of these agents cause stable, and therefore lethal, DNA strand breaks. Alternatively, resistance to topoisomerase inhibitors may develop with decreased drug access to the enzyme, alteration of the enzyme structure or activity, increased rate of DNA repair or as the result of the action of a multidrug-resistance protein (12,13).

Drug exposure can also induce production of transport proteins that effectively lower intracellular concentrations of a drug and thus lead to drug resistance, possibly owing to smaller amounts of a drug entering a cell or larger amounts being carried out because of adaptive changes in cell membrane transport. Examples include methotrexate transport and multidrug-resistance gene-1 (MDR-1) (14).

B. Multidrug Resistance

Resistance can also arise to multiple drugs simultaneously. Induction or amplification of MDR-1 can result in multidrug resistance through increased production of a pump that rapidly transport hydrophobic chemicals out of the cell (14). Another product of normal cells that confers resistance to chemotherapy is P-170, found in healthy renal, colonic, and adrenal cells (15). P-170 can be induced by and mediates the transport of actinomycin D, anthracyclines, colchicines, epipodophyllotoxin, and vinca alkaloids.

Overexpression of certain gene products, such as BCL-2, suppress apoptosis. This suppression of apoptosis not only removes a major mechanism by which antineoplastic agents kill cells, but also allows cancer cells to accumulate genetic defects, resulting in preferential selection of more aggressive cancer cells (16).

VII. CHEMOTHERAPEUTIC AGENTS

Many patients with cancer who undergo elective or emergent surgery also will undergo or have undergone chemotherapy at some point in their treatment. The clinical benefits of chemotherapy are often limited by the toxic effects of these agents on vital organ systems (Tables 2 and 3). Members of the perioperative team must have a clear understanding of the actions, interactions, and toxic effects of the various chemotherapeutic agents that have been or will be used. During the perioperative evaluation, the exact type and dosages of chemotherapeutic agents used should be reviewed and the organ systems most likely to be affected should be carefully evaluated.

Chemotherapeutic agents can be grouped into several major classes on the basis of their underlying antineoplastic mechanism of action or the source from which they are derived. Table 2 lists several commonly used antineoplastic agents by class, along with the toxic effects associated with each drug. Rational use of systemic anticancer therapies is based on an understanding of tumor cell biology and clinical pharmacology. The choice of an appropriate chemotherapeutic agents depends, in part on the inherent sensitivity of a specific disease to the various classes of drugs that are currently available and on the ability to administer the agents

Table 2 Toxic Effects of Chemotherapeutic Agents Grouped by Class

Class	Agent(s)	Toxic effect(s)
Alkylating agents	Busulfan, chlorambucil, cyclophosphamide, ifosfamide, mechlorethamine, melphalan, thiotepa	Myelosuppression, pulmonary infiltrates, pulmonary fibrosis, hemorrhagic cystitis, alopecia, nausea, emesis
	Lomustine, carmustine	Myelosuppression, emesis
	Procarbazine, dacarbazine, temozolomide, hexamethylmelamine	Anorexia, myelosuppression, peripheral neuropathy
Platinum agents	Cisplatin	Nausea and emesis, nephrotoxicity, hypomagnesemia, neurotoxicity
	Carboplatin	Myelosuppression, emesis
Antimetabolites	Cytarabine, fludarabine, floxuridine, fluorouracil, 6-mercaptopurine, methotrexate, 6-thioguanine	GI mucositis, myelosuppression, alopecia, neurotoxicity
Anthracyclines	Doxorubicin, daunorubicin, epirubicin, idarubicin, mitoxantrone	GI mucositis, alopecia, myelosuppression, cardiotoxicity
Topoisomerase inhibitors	Etoposide, teniposide	Myelosuppression, alopecia, GI mucositis, blisters, neuropathy, anaphylaxis
	Irinotecan, topotecan	Myelosuppression, diarrhea, electrolyte disorders
Microtubule inhibitors	Paclitaxel, docetaxel	Myelosuppression, stomatitis, neuropathy, anaphylaxis, edema
	Vinblastine	Myelosuppression, GI toxicity, neuropathy, blisters, alopecia, hypertension, pulmonary toxicity
	Vincristine	Peripheral neuropathy, paralytic ileus, syndrome of inappropriate secretion of antidiuretic hormone, rash, alopecia, bladder atony
	Vinorelbine	Myelosuppression, alopecia
Other agents	Plicamycin	Myelosuppression, hypocalcemia, hepatotoxicity
	Mitomycin C	Myelosuppression, GI mucositis, hypercalcemia
	Dactinomycin	GI mucositis, myelosuppression, alopecia
	Bleomycin	Nausea, emesis, alopecia, pulmonary fibrosis
	Asparaginase	GI toxicity, somnolence, confusion, fatty liver
	Hydroxyurea	Myelosuppression
	Mitotane	Adrenal insufficiency, emesis, diarrhea, tremors
	Streptozocin	Hypoglycemia
	Levamisole	Rash, arthralgia, myalgia, fever, neutropenia
	Leucovorin	Allergy

Table 3 Types and Degrees of Toxic Effects of Chemotherapeutic Agents

Drug	Toxicity			
	Hematologic	Hepatic	Nephrotoxic	Cardiac
Actinomycin	3[a]	0	0	1
Amsacrine (AMSA)	2	1	0	3
Ara-C (cytarabine)	3	3	0	0
L-Asparaginase	0	3	0	0
Azathioprine	–	3	0	2
Bleomycin	0	0	0	1
Busulfan	–	1	0	0
Carboplatin	3	0	0	0
Carmustine (BCNU)	3	3	2	0
Chlorambucil	2	1	0	0
Cyclophosphamide	3	1	0	0
Dacarbazine (DTIC)	1	2	0	0
Deoxycoformycin	1	2	1	0
Daunomycin/doxorubicin	3	0	0	3
Etoposide/teniposide	2	2	0	0
Fludarabine	2	1	1	0
Fluorouracil	1–2	2	0	1
Hexamethylmelamine	1	0	0	0
Hydroxyurea	3	0	0	0
Ifosfamide	2	0	2	0
Lomustine (CCNU)	3	3	2	0
Melphalan	3	1	0	0
Mercaptopurine	2	3	0	0
Methotrexate	1–2	3	2	0
Mithramycin	1	3	3	0
Mitomycin C	1	0	2	1
Mitotane	–	0	0	0
Mitoxantrone	2	1	0	0
Nitrogen mustard	3	0	0	0
Procarbazine	2	0	0	0
Streptozocin	1	3	3	0
Taxol (paclitaxel)	3	2	0	3
Thioguanine (6-TG)	2	2	0	0
Thiotepa	–	0	0	0
Vincristine	1	2	0	1
Vinblastine	3	0	0	0
Vindesine	2	0	0	0

[a] Toxicity ratings: 0, rare or very mild; 1, occasional, usually not severe; 2, moderately severe; 3, frequent or severe. –, Type of toxicity not reported to date in the general medical literature.

either as single agents or in combination, based on their combined toxic effects on critical organ systems.

A. Alkylating Agents

Alkylating agents were the first nonhormonal chemotherapeutic agents. Introduced in the 1940s, these agents have been increasingly used both as a primary treatment for cancer and, more important, as an adjuvant therapy to be administered in association with surgery or radiotherapy or both. The alkylating agents are a large group of agents that can impair cell function by transferring alkyl groups to amino, carboxyl, sulfhydryl, and phosphate groups. The common feature of these compounds is that they are composed of monofunctional or bifunctional alkyl groups linked to a core structure that confers pharmacologic and toxicologic differences on the alkylating moieties. The four drugs which have replaced nitrogen mustard in common clinical practices are L-phenylalanine mustard (LPAM; melphalan), ifosfamide, chlorambucil, and cyclophosphamide.

The common mechanistic feature of alkylating agents is that, upon entering cells, the alkyl groups bind to DNA, RNA, and proteins. This alkylation results in abnormal nucleotide sequences, miscoding of messenger RNA, cross-linked DNA strands that cannot replicate, breakage of DNA strands, and other damage to the transcription and translation of genetic material. These agents depend on cell pro liferation for activity but are not cell cycle-phase-specific.

1. *Cyclophosphamide, Ifosfamide, Chlorambucil, Mechlorethamine, and Melphalan*

Both cyclophosphamide and chlorambucil are orally bioavailable and are administered either intravenously or orally; ifosfamide is utilized by the intravenous route. Except for the requirement for hepatic metabolism of cyclophosphamide and ifosfamide, which prolongs its primary elimination as well as the disappearance of its metabolites (approximately 8 hr), elimination of the alkylating agents in the blood is rapid (less than 2 hr) owing to chemical decomposition.

The toxicity of alkylating agents is primarily hematopoietic. Some alkylating agents, such as mechlorethamine, have a more prominent effect on granulocytes; other agents, such as melphalan, induce relatively greater thrombocytopenia, although granulocytopenia often also occurs. The nadir of hematologic counts usually occurs 8–14 days after drug administration. The cyclophosphamide and ifosfamide metabolite acrolein can irritate the bladder mucosa, requiring strict attention to hydration and urine flow; ifosfamide metabolites, may also produce renal tubular injury. All alkylating agents can cause alopecia, nausea, emesis, and infertility. These agents are also associated with the rare development of treatment-related second malignancies. Clear evidence shows that alkylating agents are associated with the development of secondary leukemias, the frequency of which is related to the amount of alkylating agent received. The presumed mechanism of this effect is damage to the normal bone marrow stem cells resulting in mutagenic changes (17).

Alkylating agents are among the most widely used antineoplastic agents and form an important part of curative therapeutic regimens for lymphomas and important surgical adjuvant regimens for breast cancer and soft-tissue sarcomas. Alkylating agents are also the class of drugs with the steepest dose–response curves in vitro and, therefore, are also the antineoplastic drugs that are most readily dose escalated. Thus, these drugs are frequently employed in high dose chemotherapeutic regimens administered with autologous or allogeneic bone marrow support.

2. *Nitrosoureas*

Nitrosoureas are lipid soluble and appear to be the most effective agents for use in malignancies of the central nervous system (CNS). Their lipid solubility is believed to enhance penetration of these agents through the blood–brain barrier and hence delivery into the CNS. These agents have a unique pattern of toxicity for normal tissues, although their mechanism of tumor cell killing seems to be DNA cross-linking similar to that of the classic alkylating agents. Nitrosoureas tend to exert their most pronounced toxic effects on the hematopoietic system at a later time than do classic alkylating agents. After nitrosourea therapy with carmustine (bischloroethylnitrosourea, BCNU), for example, the nadir of myelosuppression occurs at days 30–36, although drug disappearance from the circulation is rapid; further, nitrosoureas appear to have the ability to damage bone marrow stem cells more effectively than do other classic alkylating agents. Nitrosoureas are also more commonly associated with pulmonary interstitial fibrosis than are other alkylating agents and can produce cumulative renal injury.

Other alkylating agents in clinical practice include busulfan, an alkane sulfonate used for treatment of chronic myelogenous leukemia, and dacarbazine, which methylates as well as binds to DNA and is used to treat soft-tissue sarcomas and malignant melanoma.

B. Platinum Agents

1. *Cis-platinum*

The finding that platinum salts are toxic to bacteria led to the discovery that such salts are also quite effective antineoplastic agents. The classic platinum coordination complex is the drug cisplatin (*cis*-diamminedichloroplatinum II), whose action is similar to those of alkylating agents. The platinum compound covalently links to biologically important macromolecules, for example the primary target for cisplatin damage in proliferating cells is DNA. "Platinated" DNA contains intra- and interstrand crosslinks that disrupt DNA function and replication. The clearance of cisplatin is primarily through endogenous inactivation via binding to biologic macromolecules, and the half-life of the unchanged parent molecule in plasma is short; hepatic metabolism and renal excretion play little role in the elimination of the drugs. The toxicity of cisplatin can be significant, with toxic effects that may include severe nausea and emesis; renal tubular impairment; damage to cochlear hair cells, with high-frequency hearing loss; and peripheral nerve damage resulting in a sensorimotor neuropathy. However, careful attention to enhanced intravenous hydration and urine output can largely ameliorate the neurotoxicity of cisplatin, and the recent development of improved antiemetic regimens has dramatically reduced the emetogenic side effects of cisplatin administration. Myelosuppression induced by cisplatin, although modest, must also be carefully monitored.

The introduction of cisplatin into oncologic therapeutics has led to a remarkable change in the therapy for disseminated testicular germ cell cancer, significantly increasing the curability of this disease, as well as the management of advanced ovarian, small and nonsmall cell lung cancers, osteosarcomas, and squamous cancers of the head and neck.

2. *Carboplatin*

Carboplatin (diamine 1,1-cyclobutanedicarboxylato-platinum II) is structurally similar to cisplatin, but differs markedly in its pharmacokinetics and spectrum of toxicity. The half-life of carboplatin is longer than that of cisplatin, and the clearance of carboplatin is determined primarily by renal excretion. Carboplatin is substantially less toxic to the kidneys and has a lesser propensity for causing nausea and emesis. Similarly, no neurotoxicity occurs with carboplatin except at high doses. Unlike cisplatin, carboplatin is associated with greater bone–marrow suppression. Platelets are affected more than are granulocytes. Generally, the antitumor activity of carboplatin appears to be equivalent to that of cisplatin, except in the treatment of germ cell malignancies. However, the precise dosage equivalents of these two drugs are uncertain. In combination chemotherapy, carboplatin's myelosuppressive effects can necessitate dosage reduction of both carboplatin and other myelosuppressive agents used at the same time. Tumor resistance to these agents appears to be related to the capacity of cells to repair nucleic acid damage and to inactivate the drugs by conjugation with glutathione (18,19).

C. Antimetabolites

Members of a substantial group of highly effective chemotherapeutic drugs known as antimetabolites disrupt the intermediary metabolism of malignant cells. These compounds can inhibit important enzymes or serve as inhibitory substances, resulting in incorporation of a "fraudulent" molecule into biologically active molecules. Several antimetabolites are widely used as part of curative chemotherapeutic regimens for treatment of childhood malignancies, acute leukemias, lymphomas, osteosarcomas, and for palliation in patients with common solid tumors.

1. *Methotrexate*

Methotrexate, the most widely used folate antagonist, is the prototype of the antimetabolite class. First developed for treatment of childhood leukemias in the late 1940s, methotrexate, a folate analogue, binds to and inhibits dihydrofolate reductase (DHFR), thereby inhibiting DNA replication. Methotrexate is water-soluble and is cleared by glomerular filtration, with a terminal half-life of 8 hr. Impaired renal function and pleural effusions can considerably alter the pharmacokinetics and toxicity of methotrexate. Because methotrexate impairs the genesis of reduced folates, the toxicity and efficacy of the agent can, in part, be inhibited by concomitant administration of exogenous reduced folates, such as leucovorin (citrovorum factor). However, when the toxic effects of methotrexate, such as renal dysfunction, myelosuppression, or mucositis, become clinically evident, reduced folates play little role in their resolution. Methotrexate has broad activity in the treatment of acute lymphocytic leukemia, osteosarcoma, and head and neck cancer (20).

2. *Fluoropyrimidines*

The fluoropyrimidines 5-fluorouracil (5-FU) and 5-fluorodeoxyuridine (FUdR) alter metabolic conversion and, in the presence of reduced folates, bind to the DNA synthetic enzyme thymidylate synthase in place of the normal substrate, uracil, forming a covalent complex and inactivating the enzyme. Fluoropyrimidines can also be directly incorporated into RNA in place of uracil, leading to impaired RNA processing. They are cleared rapidly by hepatic metabolism, with a half-life in plasma of 10–15 min; the large capacity of the liver to detoxify these drugs provides a pharmacologic advantage when they are infused directly into the liver, causing a high local drug concentration with modest or no systemic drug exposure or toxicity. Hepatic artery infusion of fluoropyrimidines is modestly successful in the treatment of hepatic metastases from colorectal cancer. Recently, patients with partial or complete deficiencies of dihydropyrimidine dehydrogenase, the key enzyme in fluoropyrimidine catabolism, have been described; these individuals are at markedly increased risk of developing severe side effects after treatment with fluoropyrimidine. The toxicity of fluoropyrimidines is manifested as reversible, usually mild myelosuppression and potentially severe diarrhea and stomatitis, with very occasional cerebellar dysfunction and minimal alopecia, principally occurring 8–14 days after completion of therapy. Fluoropyrimidines are important components of combination regimens utilized for breast cancer and are the most active compounds in a wide variety of gastrointestinal malignancies. Because the binding of fluoropyrimidines to thymidylate synthase can be enhanced by increasing the intracellular concentration of reduced folates, 5-FU and leucovorin have been combined. This combination has proved to be one of the most active regimens for the treatment of colorectal cancer in both the advanced disease and the adjuvant settings. However, treatment with this combination is associated with an increased risk of severe mucositis or diarrhea (21).

3. *Cytosine Arabinoside*

Cytosine arabinoside (Ara-C) is a "fraudulent" nucleoside consisting of a purine cytosine linked to arabinose, a sugar that is not naturally produced by humans. The Ara-C is metabolized by the same enzymes necessary for synthesis of cytosine triphosphate (CTP), which is incorporated into DNA. Incorporation of the fraudulent base Ara-C inhibits DNA replication and repair, and leads to impaired cellular proliferation, in part through induction of apoptosis. The efficacy of Ara-C is directly related to the rate of formation of Ara-CTP, a process that can be enhanced by administering the drug at high dosages. Ara-C is rapidly catabolized in the liver, peripheral tissues, and serum by the enzyme cytidine deaminase, with a terminal half-life of 2 hr. The major toxic effects of Ara-C are bone–marrow suppression, stomatitis, and intrahepatic cholestasis. Higher doses of Ara-C may have toxic effects on the CNS consisting of disorientation, cerebellar dysfunction, and coma. The primary use of Ara-C is in the treatment of acute myelogenous leukemia (22,23).

4. *Gemcitabine*

Like Ara-C, the cytidine analogue gemcitabine (2′2′-difluorodeoxycytidine; dFdC), is activated by deoxycytidine kinase and detoxified by cytidine deaminase. Gemcitabine exerts antineoplastic effects by incorporation of its major intracellular metabolite into DNA. The dose-limiting toxicity of gemcitabine is myelosuppression, with neutropenia occurring more frequently than thrombocytopenia. Fever, skin rash, and flu-like symptoms may occur. Gemcitabine has been shown to improve the quality of life of patients with advanced pancreatic cancer and has a palliative benefit in the treatment of nonsmall cell lung cancer, soft-tissue sarcomas, ovarian cancer, and breast cancer (24).

D. Anthracyclines

The anthracyclines doxorubicin and daunorubicin were isolated from *Streptomyces* species and thus have been termed antitumor antibiotics. However, these drugs interact significantly with a wide range of biochemical systems in tumor cells; many of these interactions contribute to their broad antineoplastic activity. Anthracyclines appear to exert their antitumor activity, at least in part, by the following mechanisms: binding to the nuclear enzyme topoisomerase II to form a "cleavable complex" that interferes with the ability of the enzyme to reduce torsional strain in DNA; generation of reactive oxygen species that interfere with mitochondria functions and critical macromolecules; and activation of signal transduction pathways that ultimately lead to stimulation of apoptosis. The pharmacokinetics of doxorubicin and daunorubicin, as well as epirubicin, the anthracycline analogue most frequently used in Europe, demonstrate triexponential decay, with a long terminal half-life in plasma (approximately 10 hr). All anthracyclines are metabolized primarily by the liver and excreted, in part, into the bile; individuals with liver dysfunction may exhibit considerably enhanced anthracycline toxicity because of delayed drug clearance. The toxicity profile of anthracyclines includes myelosuppression and damage to oral and gastrointestinal mucosa, resulting in stomatitis and diarrhea. Alopecia is a universal effect of anthracycline administration. Anthracycline antibiotics are also potent vesicants; extravasation of these agents into soft-tissue results in extensive necrosis and soft-tissue damage. Consequently, great care must be exercised when anthracyclines are administered intravenously. Continuous infusion must be done through indwelling central venous catheters.

A unique toxicity of anthracyclines is cumulative, dose-dependent myocardial damage. This toxicity is enhanced by the high iron content of myocardial tissue. Recent studies that have employed either gated cardiac blood pool scanning or endomyocardial biopsy as end points for functional or histopathologic confirmation of cardiac toxicity of doxorubicin have demonstrated that the incidence of measurable heart damage begins to climb when the cumulative dose exceeds 350–400 mg/m^2 if the drug has been administered by short intravenous infusion (a "bolus" injection is often given over 30 min). Thus, in patients who begin therapy with normal cardiac function, anthracyclines can be administered with low risk of myocardial dysfunction. However, in individuals with a history of hypertensive heart disease or prior left chest wall irradiation, the maximum safe dose of doxorubicin may be lower. Data indicate that infusional therapy with anthracyclines (e.g., 72- to 96-hr continuous infusion) allows for a much higher cumulative dose to be administered with diminished risk of cardiac toxicity. Dexrazoxane is a novel agent that chelates iron, minimizing the myocardial toxicity of doxorubicin administered as a bolus.

Anthracyclines have a broad range of antineoplastic activities and form an important component of combination therapies for non-Hodgkin's lymphoma, Hodgkin's disease, breast cancer, osteosarcoma, soft-tissue sarcomas, and a variety of pediatric solid tumors. Daunorubicin, idarubicin, and doxorubicin are also the most active drugs for the treatment of lymphoid and myeloid leukemias (25,26).

E. Topoisomerase Inhibitors

1. Podophyllotoxins

Etoposide (VP-16) and teniposide (VM-26) are the two podophyllotoxin derivatives now commonly used. The antiproliferative effects of podophyllotoxin derivatives have been known for many years. These agents exert their anticancer activity through interaction with the enzyme topoisomerase II, which facilitates the uncoiling of DNA before DNA replication. VP-16 and VM-26 are metabolized by the liver; about 40% of a dose of etoposide is excreted by the kidney. The terminal half-lives of both drugs are 8–10 hr in plasma after intravenous administration.

VP-16 is the most frequently used podophyllotoxin and can be administered either intravenously or orally. Recent data suggest that continuous low-dose oral VP-16 is active when intermittent schedules have failed. The primary toxic effects of these agents are leukopenia, thrombocytopenia, and mild to moderate alopecia; at high dosages, stomatitis occurs. An unfortunate late effect of VP-16 is the development of secondary leukemia. VP-16 is active in germ cell tumors, small cell carcinomas of the lung, Hodgkin's and non-Hodgkin's lymphomas, and myeloid and lymphoid leukemias (27,28).

2. Campothecins

Camptothecin and its derivatives inhibit the nuclear enzyme topoisomerase I, a protein that plays a critical role in relieving torsional strain in DNA during replication, and thus resulting in cell death. The camptothecin derivatives topotecan and irinotecan (CPT-11) are useful for the treatment of advanced ovarian and colorectal carcinoma, respectively. The major toxic effect of topotecan is myelosuppression, especially neutropenia, which occurs approximately 10 days after administration. Irinotecan is excreted into the urine and bile; SN-38, the active metabolite of irinotecan, is also excreted into the bile. In addition to neutropenia, treatment with irinotecan can produce two forms of diarrhea that may be dose-limiting: the early type of diarrhea, which occurs within hours of drug administration, is probably cholinergic and is associated with cramping and diaphoresis; it can be prevented by pretreatment with atropine. More difficult to control is the late-onset diarrhea that is frequently seen after the second or third weekly dose of irinotecan; this effect can produce dehydration if not aggressively managed with loperamide and fluid replacement. Topotecan has demonstrated moderate activity in patients with platinum-refractory ovarian cancer. Irinotecan clearly can produce objective remission in patients with fluoropyrimidine-refractory colorectal cancer (29,30).

F. Microtubule Inhibitors

1. Vinca Alkaloids

The two most commonly utilized vinca alkaloids, vincristine, and vinblastine are complex molecules whose mechanism of action is based on disruption of microtubular function through microtubular aggregation. This action results in disruption of the formation of the mitotic spindle and inhibition of cells progressing through the cell cycle at the stage of mitosis. Vinca alkaloids are metabolized primarily by the liver, and their toxicity is considerably enhanced in individuals with severe hepatic dysfunction. The primary toxicity of vincristine is neurologic. Vincristine administration may result in a peripheral neuropathy or ileus. The peripheral neuropathy is related to nerve damage associated with axonal microtubular disruption, while the ileus is thought to be due to damage to autonomic nerves supplying the gastrointestinal tract.

Vinca alkaloids are components of effective combination therapies for a wide variety of tumors. They are most active in hematologic malignancies and germ cell tumors. Activity in small, non-small cell lung cancer, and breast cancer is limited but does occur. The primary toxic effect of vinblastine is myelosuppression affecting both granulocytes and platelets; neuropathy is an uncommon side effect of vinblastine administration (31,32).

2. Taxanes

Paclitaxel was the first clinically useful compound in the taxane class of antimicrotubule agents. The drug was originally isolated from the bark of the pacific yew, *Taxus brevifolia*, but is now semisynthetically derived. This agent has a wide spectrum of antineoplastic activity and a unique mechanism of cytotoxicity. Paclitaxel interacts with microtubules but, rather than inhibiting their formation as the vinca alkaloids do, stabilizes microtubules and inhibits their dissolution, upsetting the dynamic balance between microtubule formation and dissolution upon which many intracellular processes depend. The most obviously affected process is mitosis, which requires microtubules for chromosome separation and cell division. Although both paclitaxel and vinca alkaloids inhibit microtubular function, cells resistant to one class of drugs are not always resistant to the other. Paclitaxel is cleared primarily by the liver; dosage adjustment is required for patients with moderate elevations of hepatic enzymes. The primary toxic effects of paclitaxel are myelosuppression and peripheral neuropathy. Toxic effects of paclitaxel that complicate its development are hypotension and anaphylactoid reactions, which appear to be related to the vehicle in which paclitaxel is prepared (Cremophor-EL). The hypersensitivity reactions have been averted by administration of antihistamines and corticosteroids. Paclitaxel is active in refractory ovarian cancer, small and nonsmall cell lung cancers, and breast cancer.

The taxane analogue docetaxel is a product of semisynthetic approaches. Docetaxel, like paclitaxel, is metabolized by the liver. Because of its enhanced solubility, docetaxel is prepared in a vehicle different from that of paclitaxel and thus does not produce as many immediate hypersensitivity reactions. However, unlike paclitaxel, docetaxel can produce a capillary leak syndrome characterized by peripheral edema, ascites, or pleural effusion. Prior premedication with dexamethasone can decrease and delay the onset of this syndrome (33,34). There is incomplete cross-resistance between docetaxel and paclitaxel. Docetaxel is very active in the treatment of breast, lung, and ovarian cancers.

G. Other Agents

1. *Actinomycin D*

A byproduct of *Streptomyces*, Actinomycin D is used for the treatment of childhood malignancies, particularly soft-tissue sarcomas and neuroblastoma. The drug's mechanism of action is inhibition of RNA and protein synthesis that occurs after DNA intercalation, with RNA chain elongation being principally affected. The drug is excreted in part by the kidney and into the bile as the unchanged parent molecule with a long terminal half-life (over 30 hr). The major toxic effects of actinomycin D are myelosuppression, which may be severe; alopecia; nausea and emesis; diarrhea and mucositis; and the potential for extravasation injury if the drug leaks from a vein into the surrounding soft tissues (35).

2. *Mitomycin C*

Like actinomycin D, mitomycin C was isolated from a species of *Streptomyces* yeast. This unique molecule combines quinine and aziridine moieties, both of which play important roles in the agent's reductive intracellular activation to a potent alkylating species and in the generation of reactive oxygen molecules. Under hypoxic conditions, reductive alkylation appears to be responsible for tumor cell killing. Mitomycin C is metabolized by the liver and excreted in part by the kidney, with a terminal half-life of 30–60 min. Its major toxic effects include myelosuppression (which may be delayed up to 4–5 weeks after treatment), alopecia and stomatitis, hemolytic–uremic syndrome, extravasation injury, and exacerbation of anthracycline-induced cardiac toxic effects. The major therapeutic roles of mitomycin C are in the treatment of superficial bladder cancer, for which the drug is administered by direct instillation, and in palliative therapy for gastrointestinal, breast, and nonsmall cell lung cancers (36,37).

3. *Bleomycin*

Bleomycin is a complex mixture of peptides isolated from the *Streptomyces verticillus* fungus plays an important role in the treatment of testicular germ cell neoplasms and non-Hodgkin's lymphoma. The agent's unique mechanism of tumor cell killing involves the formation of metal–bleomycin complex, which rapidly binds oxygen; the activated metal (usually ferrous iron)–oxygen–bleomycin complex is stabilized by and actively cleaves DNA, producing both single and double strand breaks. Bleomycin is metabolized by a hydrolase that is found in both normal and malignant cells but at low concentrations in skin and lung, two organs that are particularly sensitive to the drug. Bleomycin is excreted in the urine, with an elimination half-life in plasma of approximately 3 hr; the pharmacokinetics of the drug is markedly altered in patients with abnormal renal function. Bleomycin produces little myelosuppression, but its administration is frequently associated with fever and occasionally with acute allergic reaction. The major side effect of bleomycin is a cumulative pulmonary toxicity, the etiology of which remains unclear; however, the clinical picture of bleomycin-induced lung damage is well known and is characterized by nonproductive cough and shortness of breath, with minimal findings on physical examination, and occasionally patchy interstitial infiltrate on chest radiography. Pulmonary function studies demonstrate a reduced diffusion capacity, especially in patients who have received a total dose greater than 240 mg. Pulmonary function testing is recommended prior each cycle of therapy (every 3–4 weeks). Discontinuation of the drug may lead to complete resolution of signs and symptoms of respiratory impairment over a period of months to years; however, all patients exposed to bleomycin remain at risk of developing acute respiratory failure postoperatively if exposed to high oxygen tensions during the perioperative period (38,39).

VIII. DEFINITION OF RESPONSE

The word "response" is used by oncologists to determine whether a therapy is shrinking a given solid tumor. This is commonly used as a surrogate marker to determine the efficacy of a given chemotherapy in solid tumors. Radiographic imaging or physical examination is used to determine the baseline size of a tumor prior to chemotherapy. After a certain number of treatments (usually 2 cycles of chemotherapy, or 6–8 weeks), the size of the solid tumor is once again measured. Treatment continues until the patient does not tolerate further chemotherapy, or there is evidence that the tumor has grown. In 1994, the task force reviewed and updated the criteria used to evaluate response to treatment of solid tumors. The task force concluded that for a baseline lesion to be termed measurable the longest diameter must be $\geq$20 mm using conventional imaging or $\geq$10 mm with spiral CT scanning, all lesions with smaller diameters are considered nonmeasurable. All the following lesions are also considered nonmeasurable: ascites, bone lesions, cystic lesions, inflammatory breast disease, leptomeningeal disease, lymphangitis, pericardial effusion, pleural/pericardial effusion, and cutis/pulmonis, as well as any abdominal masses that are not confirmed and followed up using imaging techniques. Tumors located in a previously irradiated area might be considered measurable.

To assess overall tumor burden, the sum of the longest diameters of all measurable lesions up to a maximum of five lesions per organ and 10 lesions total should be calculated and recorded (these tumors are considered the target lesions). All other lesions or sites of disease should be recorded as baseline "nontarget" lesions.

The definition of "tumor response" has changed somewhat from the original definition in the *WHO Handbook*. Using only the longest diameter for all lesions, a *complete response* is currently defined as the disappearance of all target lesions; a *partial response* is at least a 30% decrease in the sum of the longest diameters of all target lesions, taking as a reference the sum of the longest diameters of the target lesions since the treatment started. *Stable disease* is shrinkage insufficient to meet the definition of, partial response or increase in tumor diameters insufficient to qualify for progressive disease, taking as a reference the smallest sum of the longest diameter since the treatment started. *Progressive disease* is at least a 20% increase in the sum of the longest diameters of all target lesions, taking as a reference the smallest sum of the longest diameters recorded since the treatment started, or as the appearance of one or more new lesions.

IX. CONCLUSION

Cancer chemotherapy has had a profound influence on the treatment and survival of patients with both primary and metastatic cancers. Since these agents have potentially lethal side effects, yet must be used at an adequate therapeutic dose, the clinicians caring for these patients are engaged in a delicate balance of risks and benefits. Knowledge of the type of cancer, the stage of disease in the individual patient, and the side effects of the chemotherapeutic agents must be used to achieve maximal therapeutic benefit with minimal adverse events. This information will enhance the likelihood of success in the care of patients with cancer.

REFERENCES

1. Shackney SE, McCormack GW, Cuchural GJ Jr. Growth rate patterns of solid tumors and their relation to responsiveness to therapy: an analytical review. Ann Intern Med 1978; 89:107–121.
2. Hartwell LH, Weinert TA. Checkpoints: controls that ensure the order of cell cycle events. Science 1989; 246:629–634.
3. Hartwell LH, Kastan MB. Cell cycle control and cancer [rev] [101 refs]. Science 1994; 266:1821–1828.
4. DeVita VT Jr, Young RC, Canellos GP. Combination versus single agent chemotherapy: a review of the basis for selection of drug treatment of cancer. Cancer 1975; 35:98–110.
5. Levin L, Hryniuk WM. Dose intensity analysis of chemotherapy regimens in ovarian carcinoma. J Clin oncol Off J Amer Soc Clin Oncol 1987; 5(5):756–767.
6. Goldie JH, Coldman AJ. Quantitative model for multiple levels of drug resistance in clinical tumors. Cancer Treatment Rep 1983; 67(10):923–931.
7. Goldie JH, Coldman AJ. A mathematic model for relating the drug sensitivity of tumors to their spontaneous mutation rate. Cancer Treatment Rep 1979; 63(11–12):1727–1733.
8. Schrecker AW, Mead JA, Greenberg NH, Goldin A. Dihydrofolate reductase activity of leukemia L1210 during development of methotrexate resistance. Biochem Pharmacol 1971; 20(3):716–718.
9. Steuart CD, Burke PJ. Cytidine deaminase and the development of resistance to arabinosyl cytosine. Nat New Biol 1971; 233(38):109–110.

10. Puchalski RB, Fahl WE. Cancer Research, U.O. Expression of recombinant glutathione s-transferase pi, Ya, or Yb1 confers resistance to alkylating agents. Proc Natl Acad Sci USA 1990; 87(7):2443–2447.
11. Hsiang YH, Hertzberg R, Hecht S, Liu LF. Camptothecin induces protein-linked DNA breaks via mammalian DNA topoisomerase I. J Biol Chem 1985; 260(27): 14873–14878.
12. Benedetti P, Fiorani P, Capuani L, Wang JC. Camptothecin resistance from a single mutation changing glycine 363 of human DNA topoisomerase I to cysteine. Cancer Res 1993; 53(18):4343–4348.
13. Knab AM, Fertala J, Bjornsti MA. Mechanisms of camptothecin resistance in yeast DNA topo isomerase I mutants. J Biol Chem 1993; 268(30): 22322–22330.
14. Gros P, Fallows DA, Croop JM, Housman DE. Chromosome-mediated gene transfer of multidrug resistance. Mol Cell Biol 1986; 6(11):3785–3790.
15. Weide R, Dowding C, Paulsen W, Goldman J. The role of the MDR-1/P-170 mechanism in the development of multidrug resistance in chronic myeloid leukemia. Leukemia 1990; 4(10):695–699.
16. Strasser A, Huang DC, Vaux DL. The role of the bcl-2/ced-9 gene family in cancer and general implications of defects in cell death control for tumourigenesis and resistance to chemotherapy. Biochimica et biophysica acta 1997; 1333(2):F151–F178.
17. Sandoval C, Pui CH, Bowman LC, Heaton D, Hurwitz CA, Raimondi SC, Behm FG, Head DR. Secondary acute myeloid leukemia in children previously treated with alkylating agents, intercalating topoisomerase II inhibitors, and irradiation. J Clin Oncol Off J Amer Soc Clin Oncol 1993; 11(6):1039–1045.
18. Lind MJ, Thatcher N. Alkylating agents. Curr Opinion Oncol 1989; 1:192–197.
19. Meyn RE, Murray D. Cell cycle effects of alkylating agents. Pharmacol Therapeutics 1984; 24:147–163.
20. Chabner BA, Myers CE, Coleman CN, Johns DG. The clinical pharmacology of antineoplastic agents (first of two parts). New England J Med 1975; 292: 1107–1113.
21. Myers CE. The pharmacology of the fluoropyrimidines. Pharmacol Rev 1981; 33:1–15.
22. Stentoft J. The toxicity of cytarabine. Drug Safett 1990; 5:7–27.
23. Hamada A, Kawaguchi T, Nakano M. Clinical pharmacokinetics of cytarabine formulations. Clin Pharmacokinetics 2002; 41:705–718.
24. Hui YF, Reitz J. Gemcitabine: a cytidine analogue active against solid tumors. Amer J Health Syst Pharmacy 1997; 54:162–170; quiz 197–168.
25. Danesi R, Fogli S, Gennari A, Conte P, Del Tacca M. Pharmacokinetic-pharmacodynamic relationships of the anthracycline anticancer drugs. Clin Pharmacokinetics 2002; 41:431–444.
26. Hortobagyi GN. Anthracyclines in the treatment of cancer. An overview. Drugs 1997; 54(suppl 4):1–7.
27. Gray R, Slevin ML. The clinical pharmacology of etoposide. BMJ 1991; 302:1100–1101.
28. Carney DN. The pharmacology of intravenous and oral etoposide. Cancer 1991; 67:299–302.
29. Mathijssen RH, Sparreboom, A, Verweij J, Karlsson MO. Pharmacology of topoisomerase I inhibitors irintoecan (CPT-11) amd topotecan. J Clin Oncol 2002; 20:3293–3301.
30. Verweij J, Loos WJ, de Bruijn P, Nooter K, Sparreboom A, Abang AM. The clinical pharmacology of topoisomerase I inhibitors. Br J Cancer 2002; 87:144–150.
31. Budman DR. New vinca alkaloids and related compounds. Seminars Oncol 1992; 19:639–645.
32. Rahmani R, Zhou XJ. Pharmacokinetics and metabolism of vinca alkaloids. Cancer Surveys 1993; 17: 269–281.
33. Crown J. The taxanes: an update [comment]. Lancet 2000;355:1176–1178.
34. Rowinsky EK, Donehower RC. Paclitaxel (taxol) [erratum appears in N Eng J Med 1995 Jul 6; 333(1)75]. New England J Med 1995; 332:1004–1014.
35. Sekine I, Fukuda H, Kunitoh H, Saijo N. Cancer chemotherapy in the elderly. Jap J Clin Oncol 1998; 28:463–473.
36. Bradner WT, Mitomycin C. A clinical update. Cancer Treatment Rev 2001; 27:35–50.
37. Sugai M, Komatsuzawa H, Hong YM, Suginaka H, Tomasz A, Verweij J, Mitomycin C. Mechanism of action, usefulness and limitations. Proc Natl Acad Sci USA 1995; 92:285–289.
38. Johnson RK, Mattern MR, Wang X, Hecht SM, Beck HT, Ortiz A, Kingston DG. Bleomycin: new perspectives on the mechanism of action. J Nat Products 2000; 63:217–221.
39. Dorr RT. Bleomycin pharmacology: mechanism of action and resistance, and clinical pharmacokinetics. Seminars Oncol 1992; 19:3–8.

5

Endocrine Evaluation and Management of the Perioperative Cancer Patient

STEVEN WAGUESPACK and ROBERT F. GAGEL

Department of Endocrine Neoplasia and Hormonal Disorders, The University of Texas M.D. Anderson Cancer Center, Houston, Texas, U.S.A.

MARIO MALDONADO, RAJAGOPAL V. SEKHAR, and ASHOK BALASUBRAMAIAN

Division of Endocrinology, Metabolism and Diabetes, Baylor College of Medicine, Houston, Texas, U.S.A.

I. INTRODUCTION

There are a variety of endocrine and metabolic disorders that impact the management of the perioperative or critically ill patient in the cancer environment. Most are similar to clinical disorders seen in the general population; a subset is unique to patients with cancer and may be caused by the malignancy or by its treatment. This chapter will describe succinctly the major endocrine disorders in patients with cancer and focus on those areas of endocrinology and metabolism most likely to impact upon the perioperative patient.

A. Preoperative Evaluation

Several endocrine system disorders can have a major impact on perioperative morbidity and mortality. These include diabetes mellitus, diabetes insipidus (DI), hypopituitarism, thyroid disorders, abnormalities of adrenal medullary and cortical function, and calcium and electrolyte disorders. Failure to identify these disorders in the preoperative period can lead to acute medical problems in the intra- or postoperative periods. Most of these disorders can be easily identified and treated if recognized in advance. Initial evaluation should include simple questions focused on personal or family history for these disorders (Table 1).

II. MANAGEMENT OF THE CANCER PATIENT WITH DIABETES MELLITUS

With over 151 million patients diagnosed worldwide, diabetes mellitus has become a leading cause of morbidity and mortality (1). Not surprisingly, it coexists frequently with another highly prevalent disorder, i.e. cancer.

A. Glucose Metabolism During Acute Illness

Acute illness, as well as surgical procedures, in healthy persons causes several physiological alterations that may lead to hyperglycemia and its complications. Stress responses associated with illness or surgery result in elevations of hormones such as glucagon, epinephrine, cortisol, and growth hormone (GH) that

Table 1 Preoperative Evaluation for Endocrine and Metabolic Disorders

History
Personal or family history of:
Diabetes mellitus or hypoglycemia, polyuria or polydipsia
Hyper- or hypothyroidism or thyroid hormone replacement
Hypertension or hypotension, tachycardia, adrenergic symptoms
Adrenal cortical surgery, excessive cortisol production
Pituitary surgery or symptoms of hypopituitarism, polyuria, DI
Kidney stones, tetany, hypercalcemia, or other symptoms of hyper- or hypocalcemia
Physical examination
Physical findings suggestive of endocrine disorders
Hypertension or hypotension may indicate pituitary or adrenal disorder; bradycardia or tachycardia may indicate thyroid or adrenal disorder
Skin—examination for scars of prior pituitary, thyroid, or adrenal surgery; signs of corticoid excess (bruising, centripetal obesity, loss of muscle mass, rounded facies) or deficiency (increased pigmentation in Addison disease or pallor in hypopituitarism)
Eyes—visual field abnormalities
Thyroid—enlargement or nodularity
Cardiovascular system—bradycardia or tachycardia may indicate thyroid disorder
Genitalia—small testicular size may indicate pituitary insufficiency
Laboratory
Routine—glucose, electrolytes, blood urea nitrogen, creatinine
Tests suggested by historical or physical findings—free thyroxine, TSH, gonadotropins, prolactin, GH, insulin-like growth factor I, serum testosterone, 8 AM serum cortisol, plasma catecholamines and metanephrines

counter the effects of insulin. Increased circulating levels of these hormones result in a hypercatabolic state, with lipolysis, ketogenesis, glycogenolysis, and gluconeogenesis, resulting in increased circulating levels of free fatty acids, glucose, and ketone bodies. Medications used to treat acute illnesses may alter glucose metabolism by decreasing insulin secretion, increasing insulin resistance, or increasing the clearance of antidiabetic medications (Table 2) (2). The end result is hyperglycemia.

Hyperglycemia inhibits host defenses against infections by diminishing chemotaxis, phagocytosis, granulocyte adhesion, and bactericidal function (3,4). It also leads to osmotic diuresis, leading to whole body and cellular dehydration, which is associated with increased morbidity and mortality. Hyperglycemia can also cause endothelial dysfunction, which may contribute to adverse cardiovascular outcomes (5). Thus, in a hospitalized patient who already has a variably compromised immune system or cardiovascular status, hyperglycemia and insulin resistance increase the risks for infection and vascular disease.

At the other end of the glycemic spectrum, hospitalized patients face many situations that may increase their propensity to develop hypoglycemia . The patient may be kept fasting for prolonged periods in preparation for surgical or diagnostic procedures, or the disease itself or its treatment may cause anorexia, nausea, and/or vomiting, limiting caloric intake. If renal insufficiency, liver failure, or sepsis develops, the capacity for glycogenolytic or gluconeogenic responses to hypoglycemia is impaired and the plasma clearance of hypoglycemic medications, including insulin, may be prolonged. The patient then becomes very prone to developing hypoglycemia. Several medications commonly administered to hospitalized patients may also cause hypoglycemia by increasing the circulating levels of insulin, transiently improving insulin sensitivity, depleting glycogen stores, or impeding gluconeogenesis (Table 2) (2).

1. *Special Considerations in the Patient with Cancer*

Many neoplastic disorders are associated with changes in carbohydrate metabolism. Impaired glucose tolerance has been described as an early and prominent metabolic complication of cancer (6). The plasma levels of GH, a counter regulatory hormone, may be elevated, aggravating whole body insulin resistance (7). Glucocorticoids are frequently used to treat cancer patients, and these agents can cause significant hyperglycemia in a diabetic or glucose intolerant patient (7). Cancer patients are frequently immunosuppressed, making them susceptible to infections. Infections can aggravate hyperglycemia, which in turn complicates effective treatment of the infections. Hospitalized cancer patients are also prone to developing hypoglycemia, especially if they have pre-existing diabetes and are taking oral antidiabetic agents or insulin. Such

Table 2 Medications That Alter Glucose Metabolism

Hyperglycemia	Hypoglycemia
α-Interferon	α-Agonists
β-Adrenergic agonists	β-Blockers
β-Blockers	ACE inhibitors
Alcohol and illicit drugs	Acetaminophen
Amiodarone	Aluminum hydroxide
Amoxapine	Anabolic steroids
Atypical antipsychotic agents	Diphenhydramine
Aripiprazole	Disopyramide
Clozapine	Doxepin
Olanzapine	Encainide
Quetiapine	Ethanol
Risperidone	Fibric acid derivatives
Ziprasidone	Fluoxetine
Calcium channel blockers	Ganciclovir
Central α-blockers	Haloperidol
Cyclosporine	Indomethacin
Dilantin	Isoproterenol
Dopamine	Lidocaine
Droperidol	Lithium
Ephedrine	Monoamine oxidase inhibitors
Epinephrine	Octreotide
Glucocorticoids	Orphenadrine
Growth hormone	Ouabain
L-Dopa	Para-aminosalicylic acid
Lithium	Pentamidine
Loop diuretics	Quinidine
Morphine	Quinolones
Nucleoside reverse transcriptase inhibitors	Salicylates
Octreotide	Tricyclic antidepressants
Oral contraceptives	Trimethoprim-sulphamethoxazole
Phenothiazines	Warfarin
Protease inhibitors	
Quinolones	
Thiazides	
Thyroid hormone	

common complications of cancer or its treatment as anorexia, nausea, vomiting, and ileus can result in decreased caloric intake and nutrient absorption, setting the stage for hypoglycemia (7).

2. *Goals of Glycemic Control*

A growing body of data from carefully conducted clinical trials suggests that the attainment and maintenance of normoglycemia or near-normoglycemia is associated with significantly improved outcomes when compared with a more relaxed approach (8–11). It is reasonable to extrapolate from these data that normalizing plasma glucose levels should also be the goal in a hospitalized patient with complications associated with cancer. Some experts advocate a less aggressive glycemic target of 140–200 mg/dL (12) or 150–250 mg/dL (7). However, there are no well-controlled studies on optimal levels of glycemic control in hospitalized cancer patients, although there are excellent outcome studies that support the use of tight glycemic control in hospitalized patient with other illnesses (8–11). Hence, we advocate a glycemic target of 100–140 mg/dL, with due care to avoid hypoglycemia. This can be achieved effectively and safely by careful bedside glucose monitoring coupled with rational insulin therapy.

3. *Terminally Ill Patients*

In these patients, intensive glucose control may not be warranted due to the increased discomforts of multiple insulin injections and the risk of hypoglycemia. On the other hand, uncontrolled hyperglycemia may result in unnecessary and preventable complications such as ketoacidosis or hyperosmolality. A reasonable approach therefore would be to maintain blood glucose in a range of 140–200 mg/dL.

B. Preoperative Assessment of the Cancer Patient for Diabetes Mellitus

The preoperative assessment of the patient with diabetes must take several important issues into account as listed below.

1. *Type of Diabetes*

a. *Type 1 Diabetes Mellitus*

It should go without saying that a patient known to have type 1 diabetes has no endogenous insulin production and therefore needs continuous insulin replacement. A cardinal principle is that such a patient needs insulin even in the fasted state in order to prevent severe hyperglycemia and ketoacidosis. Hence, meal-based "sliding scale" regimens of short-acting insulins without a constant supply of basal insulin are completely inadequate. Table 3 provides some recommendations for specific circumstances in hospitalized patients with type 1 diabetes.

b. *Type 2 Diabetes Mellitus*

These patients may still have endogenous insulin production, so they may not require exogenous insulin. Still, it is important to monitor the blood glucose levels during the hospitalization, as they may develop significant hyperglycemia. Many apparently "type 2" diabetic patients lose β-cell function several years after

Table 3 Recommendations for the Management of Diabetes Mellitus in Specific Circumstances

	Diabetes mellitus	
Circumstances	Type 1	Type 2
Intraoperative and prolonged procedures	Major operation or procedure: continuous IV insulin and glucose infusions	Major operation or procedure: continuous IV insulin and glucose infusions
	Minor operation or procedure: 50–75% of long acting insulin, monitor glucose levels. If glucose >140 mg/dL, consider continuous IV insulin and glucose infusions	Insulin requiring, minor operation or procedure: 1/2 to 2/3 of long acting insulin, monitor glucose levels. If glucose >140 mg/dL, consider continuous IV insulin and glucose infusions.
		Noninsulin requiring: hold oral medications, monitor glucose levels. If glucose >140 mg/dL, consider continuous IV insulin and glucose infusions
Intensive care unit	Continuous IV insulin and glucose infusions	Continuous IV insulin and glucose infusions
Parenteral nutrition and continuous tube feeding	Continuous IV insulin	Continuous IV insulin
Glucocorticoid therapy	Small dose: increase basal insulin and monitor glucose levels. If glucose >140 mg/dL, consider continuous IV insulin and glucose infusions	Small dose, insulin requiring: increase basal insulin and monitor glucose levels. If glucose >140 mg/dL, consider continuous IV insulin and glucose infusions
	Intermediate dose: increase basal and preprandial insulin and monitor glucose levels. If glucose >140 mg/dL, consider continuous IV insulin and glucose infusions	Small dose, noninsulin requiring: monitor glucose levels. If glucose >140 mg/dL, consider long acting insulin
	High dose: continuous IV insulin and glucose infusions	Intermediate dose, insulin requiring: increase basal and preprandial insulin and monitor glucose levels. If glucose > 140 mg/dL, consider continuous IV insulin and glucose infusions
		Intermediate dose, noninsulin requiring: start basal insulin and monitor glucose levels. If glucose >140 mg/dL, consider continuous IV insulin and glucose infusions
		High dose insulin and noninsulin requiring: continuous IV insulin and glucose infusions

diagnosis, and these patients will require continuous exogenous insulin. If the patient is not insulin-dependent, and no significant change in the diet is anticipated, oral antidiabetic medications should be continued. If the patient is to be kept fasting for any reason, the oral agents should be withheld. The patient on metformin therapy is at high risk of developing lactic acidosis, so this medication should be withheld if the patient has or is expected to experience any situation that might lead to a lowering of the glomerular filtration rate (e.g., renal insufficiency, cardiac or hepatic failure, volume depletion, hemorrhage). Sulfonylureas also should be withheld if the patient has renal insufficiency or liver failure. Thiazolindinedione drugs should be withheld if the patient has cardiac failure or hepatitis. The alpha-glucosidase inhibitors should be withheld if the patient has diarrhea. Table 3 provides recommendations for some specific conditions.

2. *Management of Exogenous Insulin*

a. *Insulin Administration in a Stable Patient*

In a patient who is already taking insulin, the same dosage and frequency of insulin injections should be maintained as long as there are no major changes in daily caloric intake. If the patient is to be kept fasting for any length of time beyond the usual sleeping hours, or if caloric intake is expected to decrease significantly, short-acting insulin should be withheld, but subcutaneously administered long-acting or "basal" insulin should be continued or initiated at 50–60% of the total usual daily dose of insulin. This dose should be "titrated" appropriately on the basis of close monitoring of blood glucose at the bedside. A continuous source of calories is essential to prevent hypoglycemia, if the patient is to be treated with daily intermediate- or long-acting insulin preparations.

b. *Continuous Insulin Infusions*

Many patients who require intensive care, or who are undergoing surgery or a prolonged procedure, are better managed with a continuous, intravenous infusion of insulin together with potassium and glucose. There is considerable experience with the use of this combination infusion, which permits flexibility of treatment with ease of attaining normoglycemia. Table 4 displays a typical algorithm we use to guide the adjustments needed to achieve and maintain normoglycemia.

C. Perioperative Management of Diabetes Mellitus

The length and type of diabetes should guide perioperative management. Table 3 summarizes different approaches for specific circumstances.

Patients with type 1 diabetes require a continuous supply of exogenous insulin to preserve life. For minor procedures, short acting insulin should be withheld and 50–75% of the basal insulin requirement should be administered in the form of NPH or Lente insulin, with frequent monitoring of blood glucose during the procedure. Continuous insulin and glucose infusions should be considered, if the blood glucose levels remain >140 mg/dL. For longer procedures, infusions of insulin and glucose are ideal. Type 2 diabetic patients who are completely insulin dependent should be managed as if they have type 1 diabetes. For the noninsulin requiring type 2 diabetic patient undergoing a minor procedure, oral hypoglycemic medications should be

Table 4 Intravenous Insulin and Glucose Infusion Rates in the ICU

Capillary blood glucose (mg/dL)	Insulin infusion[a] rate (U/hr)	Glucose infusion[b] rate (cc/hr)	Additional glucose (IV push)/action
<80	0	50	25 cc of 50% dextrose
80–100	1.0	40	–
101–140	2.0	30	–
141–200	3.0	20	–
201–250	6.0	10	–
251–300	8.0	5	–
301–350	10.0	2.5	Call physician
351–400	13.0	2.5	Call physician
401–450	15.0	2.5	Call physician
>450	18.0	2.5	Call physician

[a] In 100 cc of normal saline, add 100 U of regular insulin and 60 mEq of KCl.
[b] 10% Dextrose.

Table 5 Scale for Premeal Insulin, Lispro or Aspart

Capillary blood glucose (mg/dL)	Insulin dose (U)	Addition glucose or action	Size of meal (calories)	Additional insulin dose (U)
<60	0	25 cc of 50% dextrose (intravenous push) page physician		
60–80	0	30 cc of orange juice	<300	−2
81–100	2	–	300–500	0
101–140	3	–	501–700	+1
141–200	4	–	701–800	+2
201–250	5	–	801–1000	+3
251–300	6	–		
>300	7	Call physician		

held, with frequent glucose monitoring; if blood glucose levels remain consistently >140 mg/dL, continuous insulin and glucose infusions should be considered. For longer procedures, the noninsulin requiring type 2 diabetic patient is also better managed with the continuous insulin and glucose infusions.

D. Postoperative Management

1. Bedside Glucose Monitoring

Capillary blood glucose testing at the bedside is essential in the management of any hospitalized patient with diabetes. The frequency of bedside glucose testing with a glucometer should be determined by the patient's condition and specific clinical situation. At a minimum, in a nonintensive-care setting such as for a stable patient admitted for elective surgery or an uncomplicated illness, bedside glucose testing should be performed before each meal and at bedtime. Tables 5 and 6 present specific recommendations for the use of short acting pre-meal insulin and adjustment of night-time insulin doses based on blood glucose values. For patients who are not likely to be consuming regular meals or who are receiving continuous intravenous insulin, monitoring should be more frequent.

Table 6 Sliding Scale for the Adjustment of the Bedtime Insulin Dose

Prebreakfast capillary blood glucose (mg/dL)	Change in insulin dose (U)
<60	−3
60–80	−2
81–100	−1
101–140	0
141–200	+1
201–250	+2
251–300	+3
301–350	+4
351–400	+5
>400	+6

2. Special Considerations in Patients Receiving Glucocorticoids

Patients with various malignancies are frequently treated with high doses of glucocorticoids, which can lead to severe hyperglycemia and ketoacidosis. It is of paramount importance to anticipate this effect, intensify blood glucose monitoring, and prepare to increase insulin doses when therapy with glucocorticoids is planned. It is usually necessary to increase the dosage of twice-daily NPH insulin rapidly to keep up with increasing hyperglycemia during the active treatment phase. For nondiabetic patients, the risk for developing diabetes should be assessed before initiating glucocorticoid therapy (Table 3).

III. MANAGEMENT OF THE CANCER PATIENT WITH THYROID DISEASE

The production and secretion of thyroid hormones are regulated by the hypothalamus, pituitary, and the thyroid gland. The hypothalamus secretes thyrotropin-releasing hormone (TRH), which stimulates the thyrotroph cells in the anterior pituitary to secrete thyroid-stimulating hormone (TSH). Thyroid-stimulating hormone, in the presence of an optimal supply of dietary iodine, stimulates the synthesis and release of thyroxine (T4) and triiodothyronine (T3) from the thyroid. T3, the active hormone, is also generated at the target organs by selective 5′-deiodination of T4. T3 feeds back on the hypothalamus and anterior pituitary to downregulate TRH and TSH secretion. This exquisitely regulated system maintains circulating T4 and T3 levels within narrow physiologic limits. The plasma concentrations of T4 and T3 (and of their "free" or unbound components) are also affected by binding proteins, predominantly thyroxine binding globulin produced by the liver.

Maintenance of a normal "euthyroid" state depends on the proper functioning of all of these regulatory steps. Therefore, pathologic conditions that specifically disrupt each of these steps can result in hyper- or hypothyroidism. Unfortunately, the TRH–TSH–T4–T3 axis can also be affected by a variety of drugs, as well as by both acute and chronic stress or illness, resulting in the so-called "euthyroid sick" state. It is important to differentiate "true" disorders of thyroid function from those in which thyroid function test values are altered due to nonthyroidal illness.

Severe thyrotoxicosis can lead to a life-threatening condition associated with high mortality sometimes termed "thyroid storm", whereas severe hypothyroidism can evolve into the serious condition of myxedema coma. However, it is important to recognize that milder degrees of thyroid dysfunction can also complicate the clinical course of patients undergoing surgical operations.

Mild hyperthyroidism and hypothyroidism are extremely common, affecting 6% and 12% of the elderly, respectively. They often go undiagnosed before the patient presents for surgery. The symptoms of hyperthyroidism may be muted, especially in the elderly or chronically ill. Even "subclinical" hyperthyroidism is associated with a doubling of the risk of cardiac arrhythmias in the elderly and a small increase in the risk of systemic embolism. Furthermore, acute illness, surgical procedures, administration of iodine in radiocontrast materials, and induction of anesthesia can precipitate severe, life-threatening thyrotoxicosis in a patient with subclinical hyperthyroidism. Therefore, it is important to detect and diagnose hyperthyroidism and hypothyroidism, be alert to situations in the intra- and perioperative periods that might precipitate a thyrotoxic or myxedematous crisis, and treat these conditions promptly and appropriately.

A. Preoperative Assessment for Thyroid Disease

1. Patients with known hyperthyroidism should be rendered euthyroid before elective surgery, to avoid precipitating thyroid storm. Standard measures to control hyperthyroidism include the use of thionamides such as propylthiouracil (PTU) or methimazole and beta-blockers, or, if time permits, they include ablation of the gland with radioactive iodine. This management is best undertaken by an experienced endocrinologist with the knowledge that it may take as long as 6–8 weeks to achieve euthyroidism. In the more acute setting of an urgently required surgical procedure, high doses of PTU or methimazone and beta-blockers should be administered, with additional measures to block the release of preformed thyroid hormones from the gland and/or the peripheral conversion of T4 to T3, such as administration of iodine in the form of saturated solution of potassium iodide (SSKI), sodium ipodate or Lugol's iodine, glucocorticoids, and in rare circumstances, lithium. Treatment becomes more complicated in the patient with a dysfunctional bowel or severe upper small intestinal obstruction, since the first-line antithyroid drugs, PTU and methimazole, are not available in parenteral form. However, both the antithyroid agents and sodium iodide are very well absorbed via the rectal route, even in patients with severely compromised small intestinal function. These measures are effective and may achieve sufficient control to permit emergent surgery without serious metabolic decompensation. In rare situations, where it is necessary to proceed with a particular oncologic treatment on an emergent basis that cannot be safely performed in the presence of hyperthyroidism, an emergent thyroidectomy may be appropriate following extensive beta-adrenergic blockade.
2. Hypothyroidism is extremely common (13,14) and causes widespread dysfunction of physiologic functions and metabolism. It is associated with impaired myocardial contractility, diminished cardiac output, depressed baroreceptor function, decreased oxygen consumption, increased peripheral vascular resistance (15), hypoglycemia, hyperlipidemia (16), and hyponatremia. Patients with untreated hypothyroidism also have expanded plasma volumes and reduced GFR (17), with distinctly abnormal rates of hepatic drug metabolism (18,19). Hypothyroidism also induces a hypercoagulable state (20). Importantly, many of these metabolic and physiologic disturbances—e.g., the impaired ventilatory responses (21)—can be reversed by thyroid hormone replacement therapy for as short a period as 1 week.
3. Hypothyroid patients should be treated to achieve euthyroidism before planning elective surgery. The treatment options include levothyroxine (LT4, half-life 7 days) and LT4 plus liothyronine (T3, half-life 36 hr) (Goodman). Levothyroxine is the preferred treatment in stable patients not requiring urgent surgery

and, at the proper dose, will render a patient euthyroid in several weeks. In an emergent situation, such as in the patient with myxedema coma, it may be necessary to use a combination of LT4 and T3 to reverse organ dysfunction more rapidly. However, caution must be exercised in administering these hormones, especially in combination, in very ill patients. Treatment in such circumstances requires the experience of an endocrinologist to avoid potentially severe adverse cardiac effects such as myocardial ischemia or infarction (22). Varying doses and routes of administration of thyroid hormones have been used to treat myxedema coma. Arlot et al. (23) compared the oral and parenteral routes of thyroxine administration and found that although absorption is variable with oral T4 administration, clinical response occurs quickly even in patients with ileus; the intravenous route involves high peaks of plasma T4 and T3 with the peripheral conversion of T4 to T3 allowing gradual T3 delivery to organ systems, and the levels diminished slowly over 5–9 days.

4. Primary hypothyroidism may be associated with primary adrenal insufficiency. Hypothyroid patients also exhibit a blunted response to glucocorticoids, even to "stress doses" of steroid. Hence, it is advisable to test patients with recently diagnosed hypothyroidism for adrenal insufficiency and to consider administering glucocorticoids in addition to thyroxine replacement during the intraoperative and postoperative periods.

B. Intraoperative and Postoperative Assessment

1. *Hyperthyroidism*

a. Patients with known hyperthyroidism, who have achieved a biochemically euthyroid status as a result of appropriate management, are not at increased risk for anesthetic complications. Patients with undetected or untreated thyrotoxicosis are at risk for severe complications including the precipitation of thyroid storm (15,24–30). Other thyroid-related complications of specific concern to the anesthesiologist include difficulties in endotracheal intubation and maintaining a patent airway in patients with large goiters and retrosternal extensions of the thyroid, cardiac dysfunction including tachyarrhythmias, ventilatory and respiratory compromise. Further, liver dysfunction, hypermetabolism, altered protein binding, and other effects of uncontrolled hyperthyroidism may interfere with the clearance of anesthetic drugs and must be monitored carefully with appropriate changes in dosing. Conventional doses of propofol may achieve only subtherapeutic serum levels of the drug in hyperthyroid patients due to increased volumes of distribution and clearance, and the effects of propofol may be attenuated by the use of beta-blockers. Hence, increased dosing of propofol may be required during surgery in such patients (31–33)

b. Thyroid storm is easily precipitated in the suboptimally treated or undiagnosed hyperthyroid patient due to the stress of surgery or infection (25,26,32a,34,35–37). Burch and Wartofsky have proposed a clinical score to help diagnose thyroid storm, but there is really no definitive set of signs or laboratory tests to define the condition. Thyroid storm should be suspected whenever a patient has signs, symptoms, and thyroid function test results consistent with thyrotoxicosis, together with any marked decompensation of an organ system—e.g., severe heart failure, intractable tachyarrhythmia, extreme volume loss, marked hepatic dysfunction, or acute, global central nervous system dysfunction. It has been noted to occur upon induction of anesthesia and in association with malignant hyperthermia in a patient with well-controlled Grave's disease undergoing subtotal thyroidectomy. These patients responded well to a high dose of dantrolene during the perioperative period (26,36). In another instance, thyroid storm presented as unconsciousness in a patient after emergent Caesarian section (25). Hyperthyroidism and possible thyroid storm should be suspected in any patient developing unexplained tachycardia during surgery. The principles of managing thyroid storm are as described earlier for hyperthyroidism in the setting of urgent surgery; however, the chronology of treatment is very important. When there is a reasonable possibility of thyroid storm, the first step is to administer a large dose of PTU (1–2 g) or methimazone (60–80 mg) by any enteral route, in order to inhibit thyroid hormone synthesis. After ~1 hr, this should be followed by administration of a large enteral dose of iodine, such as SSKI (3–4 drops), Lugol's iodide (8–12 drops), or sodium ipodate (1–3 g), to block the release of preformed thyroid hormone. An intravenous bolus of radiocontrast dye is also an effective way to supply a large dose of iodine. Administering iodine before the initial dose of the antithyroid drug may actually exacerbate thyrotoxicosis, and hence the order of treatment is crucial. Both the antithyroid drug and the iodine preparation should be continued at the same or slightly lower doses for every 6–8 hr, until the patient has stabilized. Additional measures include intravenously administered beta-blocker (esmolol) for tachyarrhythmia or acute heart failure, cooling blankets for hyperthermia, normal saline to maintain blood volume, stress-dose glucocorticoids, and, in general, close monitoring and intensive support.

c. The risks, complications, and management of hyperthyroid patients undergoing nonthyroidal surgery have already been considered. Surgical removal of all or part of the thyroid gland itself, for treatment of hyperthyroidism, requires special consideration. Although in the U.S.A. surgical treatment for Graves' disease, the most common cause of hyperthyroidism, has been largely replaced by radioiodine ablation, surgery is still offered to patients unable or unwilling to undergo medical therapy. The surgical approaches to treat hyperthyroidism include subtotal thyroidectomy and total thyroidectomy. In either case, it is imperative that the patient be rendered euthyroid prior to surgery, using the methods described earlier, in order to avoid the risk of precipitating thyroid storm. With these precautions, hyperthyroidism due to Graves' disease and toxic nodular goiter may be treated successfully by surgical thyroidectomy. Amiodarone-induced thyrotoxicosis has also been treated surgically using local anesthesia because of the higher risk of complications associated with general anesthesia. A meta-analysis by Palit et al. (38). found an appreciable rate of persistent hypothyroidism among patients undergoing total thyroidectomy and a 7.9% failure rate in patients undergoing subtotal thyroidectomy. The surgical complications included permanent paralysis of the recurrent laryngeal nerve (in 0.9%) and permanent hypoparathyroidism in up to 1.6% of patients.

2. *Hypothyroidism*

a. Hypothyroidism has generally been considered a contraindication to surgery, but the anesthetic and surgical risks for a mildly hypothyroid patient are probably less than for a patient with hyperthyroidism. An early study by Ladenson et al. (39) examined perioperative complications in hypothyroid patients and found that intraoperative hypotension occurred frequently during noncardiac surgery, and that cardiac surgery was complicated by heart failure more often than in euthyroid patients. Postoperative complications were also found to be higher in hypothyroid patients and included gastrointestinal and neuropsychiatric complications, difficulty in weaning from ventilatory support, and hyponatremia. However, other studies have found that patients with mild hypothyroidism undergoing surgery do not appear to be at increased risk for perioperative complications (40). More recent retrospective studies on the risks of percutaneous transluminal coronary angioplasty also did not detect increased morbidity or mortality in patients with either overt or subclinical hypothyroidism who underwent this procedure (41,42). However, patients with more severe hypothyroidism (defined by TSH >90 mU/L) may have an increased risk of ventilatory complications that appear to reverse with replacement therapy (21).

b. In conclusion, patients undergoing surgery must be carefully screened and evaluated for thyroid disease. The presence of hyperthyroidism is associated with increased risk in the peri- and postoperative period and must be fully treated before proceeding with surgery. Mild hypothyroidism is not a contraindication to surgery; however, severe hypothyroidism (TSH >90 mU/L) must be treated before surgery.

IV. DISORDERS OF THE ADRENAL GLAND

A. Adrenal Insufficiency

1. *Clinical Features*

Overt features of adrenal cortical insufficiency include nausea and vomiting, hypotension, electrolyte abnormalities (hyponatremia, hyperkalemia, metabolic acidosis), dehydration (elevated blood urea nitrogen and creatinine), hypoglycemia, and hyperpigmentation; the latter is caused by chronic elevation of adrenocorticotrophic hormone (ACTH)-related peptides with melanocyte stimulating activity. Unfortunately, the only features that are strongly suggestive of adrenal insufficiency are the combination of hyponatremia, hyperkaemia, and metabolic acidosis in a hypotensive patient. More commonly, in the cancer patient, there are few overt features of adrenal insufficiency and the clinician must infer the possibility of corticosteroid deficiency from certain historical and clinical features. The diagnosis should be considered in patients who have been treated with suppressive doses of corticosteroids (>7.5 mg prednisone equivalents/day or recurrent depot injections of potent corticosteroids) for a month or lower doses for a longer period of time. Metastasis of cancer to the adrenal gland is common in certain malignancies (renal cell, lung, breast, and melanoma, among others). In addition, the diagnosis should be considered in those with systemic fungal infections or tuberculosis, anticoagulated patients, and patients with hypothalamic or pituitary metastasis.

2. Diagnosis

a. Primary Adrenal Insufficiency

A high-dose cosyntropin test should be performed, as outlined in Table 7. A serum cortisol of >18 μg/dL basally or after synthetic ACTH indicates a normal response. In the context of a preoperative assessment, a lesser response should prompt intraoperative and postoperative corticosteroid replacement. Although not all patients with a lesser response will have adrenal insufficiency, a more detailed assessment may not be possible in the compressed context of a preoperative

Table 7 Testing for Adrenal Insufficiency and Stress Dose Steroids

Tests for adrenal insufficiency
If there is no time to perform diagnostic testing and the patient is critically ill, draw a baseline cortisol and ACTH before giving steroids; alternatively, give 4 mg of dexamethasone IV and perform testing within a few hours
Primary adrenal insufficiency
High-dose cosyntropin (Cortrosyn®) stimulation test
Measure a baseline serum cortisol (±ACTH), inject 250 μg of cosyntropin IV/IM, and measure serum cortisol 30 and 60 min later
Normal response is cortisol > 18–20 μg/dL (500–550 nmol/L)
Central adrenal insufficiency
Low-dose cosyntropin (Cortrosyn®) stimulation test
Measure a baseline serum cortisol (±ACTH), inject 1.0 μg of cosyntropin IV, and measure serum cortisol 20 and 30 min later
Normal response is cortisol >18–20 μg/dL (500–550 nmol/L)
Overnight metyrapone (Metopirone®) test
Give metyrapone 3000 mg with food at 11–12 PM; at 8 AM the next morning, draw a serum cortisol (±ACTH) and 11-desoxycortisol (compound S)
Normal response is cortisol <5 μg/dL and 11-desoxycortisol > 7 μg/dL
Insulin tolerance test
Obtain baseline cortisol (±ACTH); give 0.05–0.1 U/ kg of regular insulin IV; draw serum cortisol levels every 15 min for 1 hr; sugar should be < 40 mg/dL to provide an adequate stimulus
Normal response is cortisol > 18–20 μg/dL (500–550 nmol/L)
Stress steroid dosing (should be individualized on the basis of patient's clinical history and current status)
During minor physiologic or surgical stress
Take the usual daily steroid dose (if already on steroids)
Or
Administer 25 mg of hydrocortisone IV/IM on-call to the operating room
During moderate physiologic or surgical stress
Take triple the usual steroid dose (if already on steroids at physiologic doses)
Or
Administer 50 mg of hydrocortisone IV/IM on-call to the operating room and
Administer 25–50 mg of hydrocortisone IV q8 hr (or as continuous drip)
During major physiologic or surgical stress
Administer 50–100 mg of hydrocortisone IV/IM on-call to the operating room and
Administer 50–100 mg of hydrocortisone IV q8 hr (or as continuous drip)

evaluation. If the diagnosis of adrenal insufficiency is considered during a surgical procedure, obtaining a serum cortisol prior to the administration of corticosteroids will allow the clinician to separate adrenal insufficiency from other causes of hypotension during the postoperative period.

b. Secondary or Central Adrenal Insufficiency

Table 7 provides several testing procedures for assessing the intactness of the hypothalamic–pituitary–adrenal (HPA) axis. It will be discussed in greater detail in the following section that addresses hypopituitarism.

3. Management

a. Primary adrenal insufficiency should be managed with a combination of corticosteroid and mineralocorticoid. Hydrocortisone or cortisone acetate in doses of 20–25 mg in the morning and 10–15 mg in the evening will provide satisfactory long-term corticosteroid replacement. These steroids are generally considered more physiologic than corticosteroids with a longer half-life (prednisone 5 mg in the morning and 2.5 mg in the evening, or dexamethasone) that have been used extensively in the past. Aldosterone is replaced with fludrocortisone (Florinef®) 0.05–0.1 mg/day.
b. Corticosteroid coverage is addressed in Table 7. The duration of corticosteroid coverage should be based on the extent and length of the surgical procedure. For example, a patient with a minor surgical procedure may require supplemental corticosteroid coverage only for the procedure, returning to baseline corticosteroid coverage the following day. More complicated surgical procedures (neurosurgical, thoracic, or abdominal procedures) may require stress doses of corticosteroids for several days or longer. Stress doses of corticosteroids should be used in critically ill or infected patients until their physiologic status has returned to normal; corticosteroids should be tapered, once the patient appears to be stable, by halving the doses of corticosteroids each day until baseline replacement doses have been achieved.
c. Management of the patient with suspected adrenal insufficiency. Adrenal insufficiency may be suspected in patients with unexplained hypotension during the intraoperative or postoperative period, particularly when there is an inadequate response to pressors. It is appropriate to treat such patients with stress doses of corticosteroids (mentioned earlier); obtaining a serum cortisol immediately prior to infusion of corticosteroid is useful for determining post hoc whether a state of adrenal insufficiency existed.
d. Management of the patient who has received chronic corticosteroid therapy: There is a spectrum of risk for adrenal insufficiency associated with the usage of chronic corticosteroid. A spectrum of recommendations for adequate replacement is shown in Table 8. In general, if there is uncertainty about the dosage or duration of corticosteroid treatment (for

Table 8 Assessing the Risk of Adrenal Insufficiency in Patients on Chronic Steroids

Risk for adrenal insufficiency	Patient characteristics	Recommended action
Low	Any dose of GC for < 3 weeks Daily doses of < 20 mg/day of hydrocortisone or its equivalent[a] Alternate-day dosing	Continue usual steroid dose
High	Supraphysiologic dosing for >3 weeks Daily doses of >80 mg/day of hydrocortisone or its equivalent[a] Clinical Cushing's syndrome	Treat with perioperative stress steroid coverage until usual home dose can be resumed (see Table 7)
Undetermined	Daily doses between 20 and 80 mg/day of hydrocortisone or its equivalent[a] Patients on high daily doses of inhaled or topical steroids	Observe closely while continuing home dose, empirically cover with stress steroids, or test using a 1 µg ACTH stimulation test (see Table 7)

Note:[a] 20 mg Hydrocortisone = 5 mg prednisone = 4 mg methylprednisolone = 0.5 mg dexamethasone.
Abbreviations: AI, adrenal insufficiency; GC, glucocorticoid
Source: Adapted from Ref. 50.

patients on corticosteroid coverage at the time of preoperative evaluation), patients should be tested preoperatively to assess the adequacy of the HPA axis (Table 7) or placed on the appropriate stress doses of corticosteroids during the operative and postoperative periods (Table 7).

B. Glucocorticoid Excess: Cushing Syndrome

1. Clinical Features and Perioperative Management

a. Features of Cushing syndrome that are of importance during the perioperative period include the presence of hypertension, hypokalemic metabolic alkalosis, diabetes mellitus, and propensity for infection. Several different mechanisms of glucocorticoid excess can be envisioned: ACTH dependent (pituitary Cushing disease caused by an ACTH producing pituitary tumor or ectopic ACTH by benign or malignant nonpituitary tumors) or production of cortisol by a benign or malignant adrenal cortical tumor. Optimally, patients with excessive production of cortisol should be pretreated with inhibitors of corticosteroid synthesis for a period of days to weeks to normalize the serum cortisol concentration and other metabolic abnormalities. Treatment with metyrapone, 2–4 g/day orally in divided doses, combined, if necessary, with ketoconazole 300–600 mg/day will normalize cortisol production and reverse most of the metabolic abnormalities over a period of days to a few weeks. It is important to treat the patient with 1–2 mg dexamethasone/day during therapy with corticosteroid synthesis inhibitors to prevent adrenal insufficiency. In patients on inhibitors of adrenal corticosteroid synthesis, stress doses of corticosteroids should be given during and after the operative period (see the section on Adrenal Insufficiency). In Cushingoid patients, where emergent or semiemergent surgery is necessary, hypertension, hyperglycemia, and hypokalemic metabolic alkalosis should be corrected by use of antihypertensive agents, insulin therapy, and replacement of potassium prior to the surgical procedure. Postoperative management of a patient with Cushing syndrome can be complicated by poor wound healing, muscle weakness, poor intestinal motility, difficult-to-manage diabetes mellitus, wound or other infections and fluid retention, resulting in prolongation of the postoperative recovery period.
b. Once the patient has stabilized following the operative period, the goal should be to maintain the serum cortisol in the normal physiologic range of 10–20 μg/dL by titrating doses of metyrapone or ketoconazole.

C. Pheochromocytoma

1. Clinical Features

a. Pheochromocytoma is a neoplastic process of the adrenal gland, rarely malignant, characterized by excessive production of catecholamines. Approximately 75% of pheochromocytomas are sporadic and therefore unilateral. In 15–25% of cases, patients may have hereditary pheochromocytoma [multiple endocrine neoplasia types 1 and 2, von Hippel Lindau syndrome, neurofibromatosis, and hereditary paraganglioma syndromes types 2 and 4], an important distinction because they may be bilateral and multicentric. Most pheochromocytomas, both nonhereditary and hereditary, produce norepinephrine, creating a clinical phenotype characterized by attacks of hypertension, headaches, palpitations, and jitteriness. These symptoms and signs may be intermittent or sustained.
b. Measurement of plasma or urine catecholamines or metanephrines remains the mainstay for diagnosis of pheochromocytoma (43). Plasma catecholamines or metanephrine values are almost always abnormal; in rare patients with small tumors, catecholamine or metanephrine abnormalities may be intermittent, requiring measurements during an attack to make a diagnosis. Localization of a pheochromocytoma is accomplished by either CT or MRI scanning of chest and abdomen with rare pheochromocytomas in the pelvis; in most symptomatic pheochromocytomas or catecholamine-producing paragangliomas, the tumor will be localized by these imaging studies (44). Occasionally, additional radionuclide scans (utilizing radiolabeled octreotide or meta-iodo-benzyl guanidine) are helpful to identify a small tumor not visualized by CT or MRI scanning (45).
c. Preoperative management of pheochromocytoma is straightforward: either inhibit synthesis of catecholamines or interfere with their

interaction with adrenergic receptors. Treatment with alpha-methyl tyrosine (Demser®), a tyrosine hydroxylase inhibitor, inhibits synthesis of catecholamines. It should be started at a dose of 250 mg once or twice a day and titrated upward to control hypertension and other symptoms of pheochromocytoma. It is important to initiate therapy several weeks prior to a planned surgical procedure to allow time to titrate the dose of alpha-methyl tyrosine to an effective dose (usually 1–2 g/day). In addition, most patients should also be treated with a combination of alpha- and beta-adrenergic antagonists. The authors prefer to use a short acting alpha-adrenergic antagonist such as prazosin (Minipress®), starting at 1 mg once or twice a day and titrating upward; others prefer a longer-acting agent such as phenoxybenzamine (Dibenzyline®; starting dose of 10 mg/day with titration). In addition, beta-adrenergic antagonists may reduce tachycardia or ventricular arrhythmias. Therapy with an alpha-adrenergic antagonist should be initiated concomitantly or before beta-adrenergic therapy. Occasionally, initiation of adrenergic therapy is associated with hypotension, sometimes severe enough to require intravenous fluids. It is important to start pharmacologic therapy several weeks prior to a planned surgical procedure, particularly in hypertensive patients. Controlling the hypertension diminishes vasoconstriction and re-establishes normal intravascular volume, thereby eliminating the hypotension associated with rapid vasodilation following removal of a pheochromocytoma.

d. There are several challenges associated with intraoperative management of a patient with a pheochromocytoma. The first is the unsuspected pheochromocytoma, an event that occurs infrequently but must be dealt with in the context of another surgical procedure, labor and delivery, or removal of an adrenal tumor not thought to be a pheochromocytoma. In situations where the situation is unstable, it may be advisable to stop the surgical procedure and stabilize the patient prior to a reoperation. In most cases, treatment with short-acting intravenous alpha- or beta-adrenergic antagonists or nitroprusside will control blood pressure and other cardiovascular manifestations and permit continuation of the surgical procedure. In such cases, hypotension may follow removal of the pheochromocytoma, necessitating volume replacement and short-term pressor therapy. The second is the inevitable intermittent release of catecholamines associated with induction of anesthesia and manipulation of the tumor. The anesthesiologist must be prepared to manage transient episodes of hypertension or arrhythmia by a combination of intravenous nitroprusside or alpha- and beta-adrenergic antagonists.

e. Hypotension in the postoperative period is uncommon in pretreated patients. If it occurs, it should be treated with fluids and pressors.

V. HYPERCALCEMIA AND HYPOCALCEMIA

A. Hypercalcemia

1. Malignancy-related hypercalcemia is the most common cause of hypercalcemia in the context of a cancer hospital. The differential diagnosis includes humoral hypercalcemia of malignancy, most commonly caused by overproduction of parathyroid hormone-related protein (PTHrp) by a malignant tumor, bone metastasis, increased production of 1,25-dihydroxyvitamin D3 in lymphoma or associated with fungal infection or tuberculosis. Multiple myeloma may cause hypercalcemia through increased bone resorption. Hyperparathyroidism occurs with an incidence of 1 in 1000 in the general population and should be considered in hypercalcemic patients with or without cancer. Finally, hyperthyroidism and Addison disease can rarely cause hypercalcemia.
2. Measurement of the immunoreactive serum intact parathyroid hormone concentration is central to the evaluation process. Patients with hyperparathyroidism will have elevated serum ionized or total calcium and intact PTH measurements and a normal or elevated serum 1,25-dihydroxyvitamin D_3. Patients with all other types of hypercalcemia will have a suppressed intact PTH value. It is possible to separate hyperparathyroidism from other causes in most cases using this approach. There are rare patients, particularly in the context of oncology, who may have more than one cause for their hypercalcemia (lymphoma and 1° hyperparathyroidism or breast cancer and 1° hyperparathyroidism). The routine evaluation of a patient with hypercalcemia in the context of cancer should include a serum ionized or total

calcium, intact PTH and PTHrp measurements, serum and urine protein electrophoresis and immunoelectrophoresis, thyroid hormone levels, and serum 1,25-dihydroxyvitamin D_3 and 25-hydroxyvitamin D_3 measurements. If there are clinical signs suggestive of adrenal insufficiency, a cosyntropin test should be performed (Table 7).

3. Hypercalcemia associated with an elevated intact PTH should be further evaluated by obtaining a sestamibi scan and an ultrasound of the neck to identify a parathyroid adenoma. If the diagnosis is confirmed the parathyroid adenoma should be surgically removed. In patients who have hypercalcemia caused by cancer, an attempt should be made to differentiate between humoral hypercalcemia of malignancy (PTHrp-mediated or myeloma) and 1,25-dihydroxyvitamin D_3-mediated hypercalcemia (lymphoma and fungal or tuberculous infections). Humoral hypercalcemia of malignancy will respond to intravenous pamidronate [60–90 mg intravenously over 2 hr or zoledronic acid 4 mg intravenously over 30 min], whereas 1,25-dihydroxyvitamin D_3-mediated hypercalcemia will respond to corticosteroids (10–20 mg prednisone/day). Hydration (half-normal saline at 100–200 cc/hr) will reverse dehydration and hasten the clearance of calcium. Lowering of the serum calcium concentration may require 48–72 hr following initiation of therapy. Complete removal of a tumor producing PTHrp will lead to normalization of the serum calcium concentration.
4. It is inadvisable to perform surgery on a hypercalcemic patient; the surgical procedure should be delayed until the serum calcium is normalized or lowered <11 mg/dL. The one exception to this may be a patient with a parathyroid adenoma, in whom normalization of the serum calcium can be expected to occur rapidly following removal of a parathyroid adenoma.

B. Hypocalcemia

1. Hypocalcemia is uncommon in the oncologic setting, although a low total serum calcium may occur as a result of hypoalbuminemia, a common occurrence in cancer patients. The total serum calcium concentration can be corrected for a low albumin concentration by adding the value obtained by multiplying 0.8 mg/dL times the difference between a normal albumin value (4 gm/dL) and the observed value. For example, the corrected serum calcium concentration in a patient with an observed serum calcium concentration of 7.5 mg/dL and a serum albumin concentration of 2 gm/dL is given by 7.5 mg/dL + 0.8 (4 − 2 gm/dL) which is equal to a corrected calcium concentration of 9.1 mg/dL, a normal value. Alternatively, one could obtain an ionized calcisum measurement.
2. The differential diagnosis includes vitamin D deficiency caused by malabsorption or defects in synthesis of vitamin D, hypoparathyroidism [autoimmune, genetic (pseudohypoparathyroidism) or acquired during head and neck surgery for squamous cell or thyroid carcinoma] or severe magnesium (Mg^{++}) deficiency. Preoperative identification of hypocalcemia should lead to a detailed evaluation of calcium metabolism to exclude parathyroid hormone deficiency or resistance (pseudohypoparathyroidism) or vitamin D deficiency. The serum calcium concentration should be normalized prior to anesthesia and surgery. This is best accomplished emergently by a calcium infusion or by a combined replacement with oral calcium supplementation and vitamin D therapy over a 3–5 day period.
3. Hypocalcemia following head and neck surgery is always caused by a transient or permanent hypoparathyroidism. The serum calcium should be checked in the night after surgery. Symptomatic hypocalcemia (perioral numbness or tetany) can be treated with a continuous infusion of calcium gluconate (3 g/L) with an infusion rate of 100 cc/hr. This can be tapered as an oral calcium or calcitriol effect is manifested. If the serum calcium is between 7.5 and 8.5 mg/dL, the oral calcium should be initiated at 1–2 g of elemental calcium twice daily; a serum calcium <7.5 mg/dL should be treated with 2–3 g of elemental calcium orally twice daily and calcitriol of 0.5–1 μg/day. It is preferable to initiate calcitriol therapy early in the course of hypocalcemia; 2–3 days may be required before the serum calcium is normalized. If parathyroid function returns to normal (usually occurs within the first 24–48 hr, if it is to occur), the calcitriol can be stopped.
4. After initiating calcium and vitamin D analog therapy, it is important to continue to monitor the serum calcium concentration weekly for several weeks, monthly for 6 months, and

then every 3–6 months, once a stable dose of calcium and vitamin D has been established.

VI. PERIOPERATIVE MANAGEMENT OF THE PATIENT WITH PITUITARY DISEASE

A. General Concepts

1. Patients with disorders of the anterior and/or posterior pituitary pose a unique challenge to the clinician. Because there are multiple hormones to consider, the perioperative and intensive care management of the pituitary patient require a systematic approach, so that each patient can be optimally managed based on his/her unique underlying hormonal status.
2. The most important pituitary hormones to assess in the surgical patient are TSH, ACTH, and arginine vasopressin (AVP). Although clinically relevant to the outpatient management of pituitary patients, disorders of GH, gonadotropins (LH or FSH), prolactin (PRL), and oxytocin secretion do not generally need to be addressed in the perioperative period, unless the surgical procedure directly addresses a disorder of one of these hormones. Next, in a patient with pituitary dysfunction, the most common deficiencies are GH and the gonadotropins (LH and FSH) (46), followed by TSH and ACTH when there is more extensive pituitary involvement. This hierarchy of pituitary hormone loss is helpful to the clinician; for example, a patient is unlikely to have ACTH (and subsequent cortisol) deficiency, if all other anterior pituitary function is normal. Likewise, a patient with GH, gonadotropin, and TSH deficiencies is at very high risk for having concomitant ACTH deficiency.
3. Other clinical "pearls" to consider in the evaluation of pituitary function include: (i) levothyroxine replacement in the patient with ACTH deficiency can unmask adrenal insufficiency and precipitate an adrenal crisis; therefore, every effort should be made to clarify the patient's adrenal status, if one is going to treat central hypothyroidism (defined as hypothyroidism with a low TSH concentration) and (ii) the treatment of cortisol deficiency can unmask AVP deficiency; therefore patients with central adrenal insufficiency should be alerted to look for signs of DI when starting glucocorticoid replacement.

B. Patient with Previously Diagnosed Hypopituitarism

1. Prior to elective surgery, the patient with pre-existing hypopituitarism should be evaluated for the adequacy of thyroid, corticosteroid, and vasopressin replacement. Measurements of thyroid hormone and electrolytes should be made. Although the clinical signs and symptoms of pituitary hormone deficiencies are more subtle and less severe than those that accompany diseases affecting the end organ, adequate hormone replacement is important for a smooth operative course.
2. Hypothyroid patients are at increased operative risk, and an attempt should always be made to render the patient euthyroid, documented by a normal free T4 concentration preoperatively, to ensure an uneventful operation and recovery. A low TSH value is expected in central hypothyroidism; measurement is unnecessary and a low value may confuse the clinician unaware of the pituitary disorder, leading to cessation of thyroid replacement. An individual discovered to have a mildly low free T4 (20% below normal) secondary to TSH deficiency can be cleared for surgery. However, more profound thyroid hormone deficiency should be corrected (with an ultimate levothyroxine dose of 1.6 μg/kg per day) prior to any elective surgery. This can typically be accomplished in a few weeks, but it may take longer in those individuals with coronary artery disease or congestive heart failure where rapid thyroid replacement could lead to myocardial ischemia or arrhythmias.
3. In the hypothyroid patient who requires emergency surgery, lower anesthetic doses should be administered, necessitating inclusion of the anesthesiologist in the preoperative discussions. Recovery from anesthesia, which may be prolonged, must be carefully monitored, and the indiscriminate use of narcotics and sedatives should be avoided (47). Finally, hypothyroid patients have a decreased ability to excrete free water, and their fluid and electrolyte management should be closely managed, particularly if the patient has a coexistent disorder of vasopressin secretion.
4. Levothyroxine, the most commonly used preparation to treat hypothyroidism, has a half-life of 6–7 days. Therefore, in the patient on chronic therapy, it can be held for a few days without any clinical consequence. However, if a postoperative patient is able to take oral medications, the

preoperative dose of thyroid replacement should be administered. For the ICU patient or patient on prolonged bowel rest after surgery, levothyroxine can be administered intravenously once daily, typically at 50% of the oral dose.

5. Surgery is a significant physiologic stress that activates the HPA axis. Plasma ACTH and cortisol levels normally increase at the time of incision and are secreted continuously during surgery, with the greatest production of these hormones during reversal of anesthesia and the immediate postoperative recovery period (48). Serum ACTH and cortisol concentrations typically return to baseline values within 1–2 days (49). The adrenal glands produce about 50 mg/day of cortisol during minor surgery and 75–150 mg/day with major surgery (49); although cortisol secretion rates can reach 200–500 mg/day in severe stress, it would be unusual to see similar secretion rates after surgery (50,51). Therefore, if the patient has preexisting ACTH/cortisol deficiency, it is imperative to cover the patient with stress dose steroids during the surgery and recovery period (Table 7). If a patient has multiple anterior pituitary hormone deficiencies (e.g., GH, gonadotropin, and TSH deficiencies) and is not on corticoid replacement, the patient should be assessed for adrenal insufficiency prior to surgery (Table 7). If this is not feasible, the patient should be empirically covered during the perioperative period so as to ensure that symptomatic adrenal insufficiency does not occur. Any patient with known pituitary disease, who develops hypotension after surgery and who is not on steroids, should also be treated with stress steroids after appropriate testing is obtained (Table 7). Of note, unlike primary adrenal insufficiency, those persons with ACTH deficiency do not gene rally require treatment with a mineralocorticoid (i.e., fludrocortisone), because the renin–angiotensin–aldosterone axis is intact in these individuals.
6. In the patient already on corticosteroid replacement, hydrocortisone can be administered immediately prior to surgery and then every 8 hr. Alternatively, a continuous hydrocortisone infusion can be utilized. The exact dosing of perioperative steroid coverage should be tailored to the patient's medical history, preoperative steroid dose, and the amount of stress anticipated by the given surgical procedure (Table 7). Once the patient is taking adequate liquids and medications by mouth, oral steroids should be substituted. For the first 1–2 postoperative days (in cases of moderate to major stress), an increased dose of corticosteroid is administered. If the patient continues to do well and is without fever or other complications, normal maintenance doses can be resumed.
7. The replacement of GH and sex steroids is not necessary in the acute inpatient management of the patient with pituitary disease. In the critically ill patient, anabolic agents such as GH and androgens have previously been used to counteract the catabolic response (52). These studies have had limited success and in one report, the use of high dose GH actually increased morbidity and mortality (53). Of note, these studies were not conducted in patients with hypopituitarism. There is currently no compelling evidence to support the continuation of sex steroids and GH in patients during the perioperative period. In addition, the risk of venous thrombosis is sufficiently great in the postoperative patient to warrant withholding estrogen therapy in the hypogonadal female patient. Finally, in the patient taking a dopamine agonist to treat hyperprolactinemia, therapy can typically be withheld briefly and restarted once the patient is discharged from the hospital.

C. Patient with a Sellar or Suprasellar Mass Whose Pituitary Status Is Unknown

1. The neurosurgical patient who has a mass within or in the region of the sella turcica requires special consideration during the preoperative and postoperative periods. These patients should be evaluated by an endocrinologist prior to elective surgery. In cases where there is rapid visual loss, cranial nerve palsy, hydrocephalus, or pituitary apoplexy, urgent surgery usually precludes a detailed evaluation. A complete endocrinologic evaluation assures the identification of hypopituitarism and syndromes of endocrine hormone excess. A history and physical exam and the following screening labs should be performed: an 8 AM fasting IGF-1, prolactin, electrolytes, LH, FSH, testosterone or estradiol, TSH, free T4, ACTH, and cortisol. For pituitary tumors, the risk of preoperative hypopituitarism correlates directly with the size of the tumor; the patient with a pituitary microadenoma ($\leq$1 cm) is unlikely to have compromised pituitary functioning, whereas approximately 70–90% of patients with

macroadenomas (>1 cm) will have deficiencies of one or more hormones (54). A caveat: DI is rarely seen in pituitary adenomas, regardless of size, but is more likely to be present in the patient with other tumors (craniopharyngioma, germinomas) or infiltrative diseases (Langerhans' cell histiocytosis, sarcoidosis) (55).

2. Postoperative care should address both endocrine and nonendocrine issues. CSF leakage, meningitis, worsening of vision, and CNS hemorrhage are uncommon events and will generally be addressed by the neurosurgeon (54). The postoperative endocrine issues include the management of fluid balance and the assessment of long-term hormone requirements.
3. In patients undergoing neurosurgery for a sellar/suprasellar mass, there are two main perioperative issues to consider: the management of postoperative fluid/sodium balance and the determination of postoperative hormone therapy. The most immediate endocrine sequela of neurological surgery is the development of either central DI or the syndrome of inappropriate antidiuretic hormone (SIADH). Hyponatremia (caused by excessive or unregulated secretion of AVP) may occur in up to 25% of patients 7 days postsurgery and DI (deficiency of AVP) occurs in ~20% of patients (54,56). The detailed management of these disorders is described in subsequent sections. Typically, if a patient exhibits hypopituitarism before surgery, postoperative hypopituitarism is likely, although ~6% of patients with preoperative pituitary deficiencies will experience some recovery of pituitary function after surgery (55). Hormone replacement in this setting is generally the same as those for patients with previously diagnosed hypopituitarism. In all patients who have undergone pituitary surgery, hypopituitarism should be considered a possibility and specific testing should be performed. Clinical features that can assist the clinician in identifying the patients at highest risk for long-term pituitary dysfunction include the size and type of tumor, the extent of surgery, the presence or absence of post-op DI, and the amount of normal pituitary tissue removed (as identified by histopathological evaluation of the surgical specimen).
4. A thorough evaluation and treatment plan is often not relevant during the immediate post-op period because of edema and healing. Typically, the need for long-term hormone therapy is determined 6–8 weeks after surgery. However, the clinician must decide whether or not to discharge these patients on corticosteroid replacement. Two approaches are used. First, one can empirically discharge every patient on maintenance doses of hydrocortisone and reassess adequacy of cortisol production, as described in Table 1, following cessation of corticosteroids at least 24 hr earlier. An alternative is to give stress steroids perioperatively and then discontinue hydrocortisone in the hospital, once the patient is stable, assessing an AM cortisol level 24 hr later; patients with cortisol levels >15 μg/dL can be discharged without corticoid replacement, although they should be educated about the signs and symptoms of adrenal insufficiency. Those patients with values <15 μg/dL can be sent home on hydrocortisone with plans for reassessing 6–8 weeks after surgery.
5. Each patient with permanent hypopituitarism should be provided specific instructions on the use of "stress" doses of corticosteroids and should also be offered a "MedicAlert" or similar bracelet, available from http://www.medicalert.org.

D. Unique Situations

1. Pituitary Apoplexy

a. Pituitary apoplexy refers to the potentially life-threatening clinical syndrome that results from an acute hemorrhage into or infarction of a pituitary adenoma or rarely from these same events in an otherwise normal pituitary gland. The classical presentation is one of an abrupt onset of severe headache, visual defects, typically with ophthalmoplegia, and/or alteration of mental status. A high clinical suspicion is warranted in these cases, as prompt treatment with glucocorticoids and neurosurgical intervention is often necessary to preserve vision and life (57,58). It appears that the risk for pituitary apoplexy may be higher in those patients who are anticoagulated (59) or who undergo combined pituitary stimulation tests prior to surgery (60). Therefore, the benefit of such interventions should be weighed against the theoretical risks in patients known to have pituitary adenomas.
b. It is important for the anesthesiologist and neurosurgeon to recognize the possibility of hypopituitarism and initiate "stress" doses of corticosteroid replacement (Table 7).

2. *Cushing Syndrome*

a. The preoperative assessment of the Cushing patient is geared towards optimizing treatment of the multiple medical morbidities that coexist with hypercortisolism, including diabetes mellitus, cardiac failure, infection, hypertension, and electrolyte abnormalities (hypokalemic metabolic alkalosis). Severe cortisol excess can transiently suppress normal anterior pituitary hormone production (61); therefore, these patients may need hormone replacement initially but may spontaneously recover after successful treatment of the underlying disorder causing Cushing syndrome. In severely affected patients, medical therapy to decrease cortisol production may be of value to reduce postoperative complications (see section on Glucorticoid Excess: Cushing syndrome).

b. Patients with Cushing disease have excessive corticosteroid production and do not need perioperative steroid administration. Furthermore, adequate treatment, i.e. successful removal of the pituitary adenoma, will result in secondary adrenal insufficiency because of long-term suppression of the HPA axis. Some centers treat Cushing patients with glucocorticoids perioperatively (54), whereas other centers do not (55). It is reasonable to withhold steroids after surgery to assess whether or not the hypercortisolism is cured. Some centers even recommend performance of a low dose dexamethasone test at this time (62). In those patients who are successfully treated, the cortisol level (obtained at least 24 hr after surgery and 24 hr after the last dose of hydrocortisone) will be $< 3\,\mu g/dL$ and the patient will have symptoms of adrenal insufficiency, such as anorexia, weakness, nausea, etc. If the patient does not develop symptoms or signs of adrenal insufficiency postoperatively, pituitary tumor treatment failure is suggested. Those with low postoperative cortisol values have a higher probability of long-term remission (62a). These general comments are also relevant for Cushing syndrome caused by ectopic ACTH production (bronchial carcinoids) or cortisol production by adrenal tumors (benign or malignant adrenal cortical tumors).

c. Patients with chronic glucocorticoid excess may have poor tissue healing, prolonged ileus following abdominal surgery, a higher risk for infection, hypercoagulability, and venous thromboembolism (63), and appropriate steps should be taken to address each of these problems.

3. *Acromegaly*

a. Patients with acromegaly are at increased risk for cardiovascular/cerebrovascular disease and should have the appropriate medical clearance prior to surgery. Whether acromegalics should receive specific therapy to lower GH and IGF-1 levels prior to surgery is not clear (64).

b. Long-term effects of GH excess on soft tissues may cause macroglossia; obstructive sleep apnea is common, and intubation in these patients may be more difficult (65). Furthermore, acromegalic patients may have more difficulty breathing with the nasal packs after trans-sphenoidal surgery (55).

c. The anesthesiologist should also be aware that anesthetic requirements may be altered in acromegalic patients (65).

d. Diabetes mellitus is identified in about a quarter of acromegalic patients, and the blood glucose concentration should be normalized in the preoperative period. This can be either accomplished with oral diabetes agents or with insulin (see the section on Perioperative Management of Diabetes Mellitus). Successful removal of a pituitary adenoma will often result in reversal of diabetes mellitus in the postoperative period.

e. After successful tumor resection, GH levels drop within a few hours; therefore, measurement of GH in the postoperative period may be useful in determining the likelihood of cure. The success rate of surgery is highest in those patients with the smallest tumors. IGF-1 levels should not be measured immediately after surgery because of the longer half-life of this molecule. Surgical cure may result in a significant mobilization of tissue fluid and diuresis, easily confused with acquired DI (54).

4. *Prolactinomas*

Most prolactinomas are treated medically with a dopamine agonist. In the rare patient who has surgery for a prolactin-secreting tumor (serum prolactin usually $> 200\,ng/mL$), the management issues are similar to those for other pituitary tumors.

5. *Patient on Chronic Corticosteroid Therapy: 2° Adrenal Insufficiency*

a. The chronic use of exogenous glucocorticoids may suppress the HPA axis. Even patients who are no longer taking these agents, but who were on prolonged treatment with supraphysiologic doses within the preceding year, may be at risk for secondary adrenal insufficiency. Although clinically relevant adrenal insufficiency is unlikely to occur in this setting and there is good evidence that stress steroid coverage may not always be needed (66,67), each of these patients should be considered individually.

b. Surgeons and anesthesiologists should be aware that there are well-documented examples of HPA axis suppression caused by oral, inhaled, or topical steroids. If it is not possible to perform an adequate preoperative evaluation, consideration should be given to "stress" dose coverage or initiation of corticosteroid replacement intraoperatively at the first sign of adrenal insufficiency (usually hypotension during the intraoperative period). In the preoperative assessment of these patients, the main issue to address is whether or not the patient's dose and duration of steroid therapy have predisposed them to clinically relevant adrenal insufficiency (Table 8). Other important aspects to consider in patients on chronic corticosteroids are the impaired wound healing and other postoperative complications that may be secondary to that treatment (50).

c. The exact dose at which suppression of the HPA axis occurs in a given individual is unknown, and previous studies have demonstrated the difficulty in predicting suppression on the basis of the dose or extent of therapy (49,50,68). Nevertheless, if one approaches this question physiologically, it may be possible to predict for a given individual. The typical physiologic replacement dose of hydrocortisone in an average adult (1.73 m^2) would be 20 mg of hydrocortisone per day. Doses >20 mg taken for more than 3 weeks may place the patient at risk for adrenal insufficiency (see Refs. 49,69,70 for a discussion). Table 7 offers some general guidelines.

E. Patient with a Disorder of Sodium and Water Balance

1. *General*

It is not uncommon for the clinician to encounter disorders of fluid and sodium balance, particularly in hospitalized patients and those with cancer (47,71). There are a multitude of etiologies that contribute to such processes, and a complete review of hyponatremia and hypernatremia is beyond the scope of this chapter. Therefore, the following discussion will center on the management of disorders of AVP excess (SIADH) and deficiency (DI), common problems in the perioperative period.

2. *Syndrome of Inappropriate Antidiuretic Hormone Secretion*

a. SIADH refers to the abnormal production or action of AVP, resulting in an excess of total body free water relative to sodium. Excess secretion of antidiuretic hormone is manifested by hyponatremia (serum Na <135 mEq/L) and by definition, the urine is inappropriately concentrated (urine osmolality >100 mOsm/kg, usually >300 mOsm/kg)in the presence of low serum osmolality (<289 mOsm/kg), euvolemia, and normal liver, kidney, and adrenal function. In SIADH, there is decreased aldosterone production and possibly increased secretion of natriuretic peptides (72). This results in increased renal sodium excretion (>20 mEq/L, usually >40 mEq/L). This helps to distinguish SIADH from hypovolemic and hypervolemic hyponatremia, where the urine sodium is typically <20 mEq/L unless there is an underlying process contributing to renal salt wasting (e.g., those patients on diuretics). Inappropriate secretion of antidiuretic hormone is a diagnosis of exclusion; other processes that can cause euvolemic hyponatremia, including adrenal insufficiency and profound hypothyroidism, should be excluded. The hemodilution associated with SIADH commonly lowers hematocrit and serum concentrations of uric acid and BUN (73). Measurement of AVP and water loading tests to differentiate SIADH from other conditions are rarely helpful (47).

b. The causes of SIADH are outlined in Table 9. The perioperative management of hyponatremia should focus on understanding cause and implementing therapy. Critically ill or

Table 9 Causes of SIADH

Tumor related
Extrapulmonary small cell carcinoma
Lymphoma
Meningeal carcinomatosis
Metastatic brain tumors
Olfactory neuroblastoma (esthesioneuroblastoma)
Pancreatic carcinoma
Primary brain tumors
Prostate carcinoma
Small cell lung carcinoma and other pulmonary tumors
Thymic tumors
Nonmalignant conditions
Acute psychosis
Acute respiratory failure/positive pressure ventilation
AIDS
Encephalitis
Hydrocephalus
Idiopathic, particular in the elderly
Meningitis
Nausea and pain
Pneumonia
Postoperative state (major abdominal or thoracic surgery; pituitary surgery)
Stroke
Subarachnoid hemorrhage and other intracranial hemorrhages
Traumatic brain injury
Drugs
First generation sulfonylureas (Chlorpropamide)
Carbamazepine
Cisplatin
Cyclophosphamide
Desmopressin/Vasopressin
Melphalan
Methylenedioxymethamphetamine ("ecstasy")
Nonsteroidal anti-inflammatory agents
Opiates
Oxytocin
Phenothiazines
Prostaglandin-synthesis inhibitors
Selective serotonin reuptake inhibitors (SSRIs)
Tricyclic antidepressants
Vinblastine
Vincristine

postoperative patients may have several processes contributing to hyponatremia, necessitating a thorough evaluation. Early clinical findings of hyponatremia include malaise, anorexia, muscle cramps, nausea, vomiting, confusion, lethargy, and headache; this can progress to cerebral edema and severe neurologic manifestations such as seizures, respiratory arrest, coma, and death. In the patient with a gradual onset of hyponatremia, the brain can adapt to the hypotonic state, and these symptoms do not typically occur unless the serum sodium is < 120 mEq/L. However, these same neurologic findings may occur at higher sodium levels, particularly if there is a rapid descent of the serum sodium concentration. Although SIADH may spontaneously improve after treatment of the underlying disease or withdrawal of the offending medication, medical therapy is frequently instituted to prevent a further fall in serum tonicity and attendant neurologic sequelae.

c. In the patient with significant neurologic manifestations or profound hyponatremia, the sodium should be increased 1–2 mEq/hr (see the following for discussion of complications of increasing the serum sodium too quickly) using hypertonic saline (3% NaCl) (Table 10), preferably in an ICU setting. Initial therapy is aimed at improving neurologic symptoms, and frequently, even a minimal rise in the sodium levels will improve the clinical situation. Once the patient's

Table 10 Management of SIADH and Hyponatremia

Demeclocycline (Declomycin®)
Produces reversible nephrogenic DI
300–600 mg BID
Lithium carbonate
Produces reversible nephrogenic DI
600–1800 mg/day in divided doses
Narrow therapeutic window
Fludrocortisone (Florinef®)
Increased renal sodium retention
0.1–0.3 mg/day
High salt diet and/or oral NaCl
Increased solute intake helps to augment water loss
Start 1–3 gm/day
Urea
Increased solute intake helps to augment water loss
30 gm/day
Vasopressin 2 receptor antagonists
Inhibit ADH action at the V2 receptor
In clinical trials
Hypertonic saline (formula derived from Ref. 74)
Can use with a loop diuretic (enhances free water clearance)
Total amount of 3% NaCl to infuse (mL) = Desired change in serum Na × 1000 / ΔNa
[a]ΔNa (change in serum sodium per liter infused) = 513[a]-Serum sodium / Total body water (L)[b] + 1

[a] Amount of sodium (mmol) in 1 L of 3% NaCl.
[b] TBW (L)= Weight (kg)× 0.6 (children, nonelderly men); 0.5 (nonelderly women, elderly men); or 0.45 (elderly women).

symptoms have improved, the rate of infusion should be slowed with a gradual rise toward the range of 125–130 mEq/L, combining hypertonic saline with a loop diuretic such as furosemide to limit treatment-induced expansion of extracellular fluid volume and to promote electrolyte-free water excretion (74). Normal saline should not be used in the acute management of hyponatremia (74).

d. In the asymptomatic patient, SIADH is initially treated with fluid restriction (500–1000 mL daily in adults; 1 L/m^2 per day or two-thirds maintenance in children). Intake and output should be monitored closely to ensure compliance with fluid restriction and to maintain an oral intake of at least 500 mL/day below the average urine volume (in adults). If unsuccessful, other strategies can be employed (Table 10). The most commonly used agent is the tetracycline antibiotic, demeclocycline, which interferes with the effect of AVP at the level of the renal tubule. A period of $\geq$5 days may be required for a maximal effect (47).

e. The rapid correction of hyponatremia by any means can cause central pontine myelinolysis or osmotic demyelination syndrome. It is characterized by severe and often irreversible neurologic sequelae such as dysarthria, dysphagia, psychiatric disturbances, spastic paraplegia or quadriplegia, seizures, pseudobulbar palsy, and altered mental status (75). Therefore, in the patient with chronic hyponatremia, the goal of treatment should be not to increase the serum sodium levels by $>$0.5 mEq/L per hour (or 12 mEq/L per day) (76). However, some experts recommended an even more conservative therapeutic goal of an increase of no more than 8 mEq/L per day (74).

3. *Cerebral Salt Wasting*

Although it remains controversial and incompletely understood, the cerebral salt wasting (CSW) syndrome is a clinical entity characterized by hyponatremia and volume depletion in patients with intracranial disorders, particularly neurosurgical patients. Cerebral salt wasting is defined as significant renal salt wasting as a consequence of intracranial disease. This combination causes hyponatremia and decreased extracellular fluid volume (77). It is differentiated from SIADH by the presence of volume depletion (clinical signs of dehydration or low central venous or pulmonary wedge pressure). In SIADH, there will be evidence of hemodilution and lower than normal uric acid and blood urea nitrogen measurements, whereas these are likely to be increased in CSW. This differentiation is important, because CSW requires volume replacement. It is believed that CSW results from the primary overproduction of natriuretic peptides (78).

4. *Diabetes Insipidus*

a. Diabetes insipidus is characterized by the excessive production of a dilute urine (polyuria) with a compensatory increase in thirst (polydipsia). The diagnosis of DI should be considered only in those individuals with daily urinary volumes $>$3 L/day (in children $>$1.5 L/m^2 per day) who also complain of extreme thirst. Thirst and polyuria that persist throughout normal sleeping hours are particularly compelling evidence for DI. It is generally caused by inadequate production of AVP (central DI) or a defect of AVP action on the renal tubular cell (nephrogenic DI) (Table 11). Patients with DI who have an intact thirst mechanism and free access to water should not develop derangements in serum sodium or osmolality. On the other hand, when an individual with DI is fasted, has an altered thirst mechanism, or develops an altered mental status that precludes adequate fluid intake, there is a risk for development of hypernatremia and hyperosmolality.

b. The diagnosis of DI should be considered in any patient with polyuria accompanied by significant polydipsia, particularly those with a sellar/suprasellar mass or who have had recent surgery affecting the hypothalamic–pituitary region. However, DI is but one cause of frequent urination or excessive thirst. For example, DI may be difficult to distinguish from primary polydipsia, in which AVP secretion is appropriately decreased by excessive free water intake. In the patient who has had a trans-sphenoidal pituitary adenoma resection and who is an obligate mouth breather due to the nasal packings, polyuria result from the excessive fluid intake used to alleviate symptoms of a dry mouth. Furthermore, postoperative patients will often have postoperative diuresis secondary to intraoperative fluid expansion.

c. In the outpatient setting, the diagnosis of DI can be established by the measurement of paired urine and serum electrolytes and

Table 11 Causes of DI

- *Central DI*
  - Autoimmune
  - Congenital
    - DIDMOAD/Wolfram syndrome
    - Familial autosomal dominant
    - Septo-optic dysplasia
    - Cytomegalovirus infection
  - Granulomatous diseases
    - Sarcoidosis
    - Mycobacterial infection
  - Idiopathic
  - Neoplastic
    - Germinoma
    - Langerhans cell histiocytosis
    - Metastatic tumors
      - Lung and breast
    - Craniopharyngioma
    - Leukemia/myelodysplastic syndrome
    - Other suprasellar tumors
  - Pituitary ischemia
    - Shock
    - Brain death
  - Postsurgical
  - Trauma
- *Nephrogenic DI*
  - Congenital
    - X-linked
      - V_2 receptor mutations
    - Autosomal recessive
      - Aquaporin-2 mutations
  - Drugs
    - Amphotericin B
    - Demeclocycline
    - Lithium
    - Methoxyflurane
    - Vincristine
  - Electrolyte disorders
    - Hypercalcemia
    - Hypokalemia
  - Renal disease
    - Amyloidosis
    - Medullary sponge kidney
    - Obstructive uropathy
    - Polycystic kidney disease
    - Sickle cell disease
- *Other*
  - Pregnancy-increased vasopressinase

osmolality in the morning following an overnight fast. A normal serum sodium concentration and osmolality in the presence of a urine osmolality >300 mOsm/kg excludes significant DI. The higher the urine osmolality after an overnight fast, the lower the likelihood of DI is. Individuals with significant symptoms of polydipsia and polyuria, particularly during the night, may be at risk for development of volume depletion from a prolonged fast. In these situations, it may be necessary to hospitalize the patient or to conduct the fast under controlled conditions in the outpatient setting. The water deprivation test, performed with frequent monitoring of laboratory parameters, urine output, vital signs, and weight, remains the gold standard for the diagnosis of DI. Once the urine osmolality has reached a plateau (a rise in urine osmolality <50 mOsm/kg over two successive hourly collections), the patient is given aqueous vasopressin to separate central from nephrogenic DI. A rise in the urine osmolality of >50% following vasopressin administration indicates a central deficiency of AVP. Measurement of an AVP level just prior to the administration of vasopressin may also be helpful; a low AVP concentration in this context is indicative of central DI.

d. In outpatients, the treatment should focus on alleviation of symptoms of polyuria and polydipsia. In most cases, serum tonicity will be maintained in those with access to fluids. In

Table 12 Management of DI and Hypernatremia

- *Aqueous vasopressin (Pitressin®)*
  - 20 U/mL
  - 5–10 U SQ/IM q4–6 hr
  - Shorter duration of action (4–6 hr)
  - Can be used as a continuous drip to a maximum of 0.01 U/kg per hour (significant pressor activity when used intravenously)
- *Desmopressin acetate (DDAVP®)*
  - Duration of action 8–12 hr
  - Synthetic analog of AVP
  - Intranasal rhinal tube (10 μg/0.1 mL)
  - 0.05–0.4 mL (5–40 μg) divided one to two times per day
  - Nasal spray (one spray = 10 μg = 0.1 mL)
  - One to four sprays (10–40 μg) divided one to two times per day
  - For injection: 4 μg/mL
  - 2–4 μg SQ/IM divided one to two times per day
  - Tablets (0.1 and 0.2 mg)
  - 0.2–1.2 mg divided two to three times per day
- *Hypotonic fluids (formula derived from Ref. 74)*:
  - Total amount of D5W to infuse (mL) $= \text{Desired change in serum Na} \times 1000 / {}^{a}\Delta\text{Na}$
  - ${}^{a}\Delta\text{Na}$ (change in serum sodium per liter infused) $= 0^{a} - \text{Serum sodium} / \text{Total body water (L)}^{b} + 1$

[a] Amount of sodium (mmol) in 1 L of D5W (may substitute 77 for 0.45% NS, etc.).
[b] TBW (L)= Weight (kg) × 0.6 (children, nonelderly men); 0.5 (nonelderly women, elderly men); or 0.45 (elderly women).

the hospitalized patient with DI, fluid intake and output must be closely monitored. Central DI is treated by the administration of desmopressin, a synthetic analog of AVP (79) (Table 12). Oral and intranasal routes of administration are available, and the dose and frequency of administration are adjusted so that symptoms are alleviated and breakthrough urination occurs prior to the next scheduled dose, the latter eliminating the risk of excessive water retention that can result in hyponatremia. In hospitalized patients, additional parenteral compounds are available for routine use (Table 12). In the intensive care unit, a vasopressin drip may also be used to maintain antidiuresis.

e. Patients who develop DI after a neurosurgical procedure may show a typical triphasic response: DI followed by SIADH followed by recurrence of DI (79). Severe hyponatremia may occur during the second phase (highest risk about 1 week after surgery), and caution should be used when treating central DI immediately after surgery. Patients with DI in this setting should be advised to drink fluids only to quench their thirst lest they develop hyponatremia. This is a particular concern in the neurosurgical patient with a nasal pack. In the rare individual with hypodipsia, scheduled free water intake may be required to maintain serum sodium levels and osmolality.

f. Nephrogenic DI can be a difficult problem in the hospitalized patient. Treatment includes adequate fluid intake, diuretics, salt restriction, and nonsteroidal anti-inflammatory drugs (79). Severe or symptomatic hypernatremia should be treated with the replacement of the free water deficit using hypotonic fluid administration (Table 12). Rapid correction of prolonged hypernatremia and hyperosmolality in this context can result in cerebral edema and, therefore, hypotonic fluids should be infused at a rate designed to reduce the serum sodium concentration to a maximum of 0.5 mEq/L per hour (74).

REFERENCES

1. Zimmet P, Alberti KG, Shaw J. Global and societal implications of the diabetes epidemic. Nature 2001; 414:782–787.
2. Pandit MK, Burke J, Gustafson AB, Minocha A, Peiris AN. Drug-induced disorders of glucose tolerance. Ann Intern Med 1993; 118:529–539.
3. Rosenberg CS. Wound healing in the patient with diabetes mellitus. Nurs Clin North Am 1990; 25:247–261.
4. McMahon MM, Bistrian BR. Host defenses and susceptibility to infection in patients with diabetes mellitus. Infect Dis Clin North Am 1995; 9:1–9.
5. Tomas E, Lin YS, Dagher Z, Saha A, Luo Z, Ido Y, Ruderman NB. Hyperglycemia and insulin resistance: possible mechanisms. Ann N Y Acad Sci 2002; 967:43–51.
6. Tayek J. A review of cancer cachexia and abnormal glucose metabolism in humans with cancer. J Am Coll Nutr 1992; 11:445–456.
7. Poulson J. The management of diabetes in patients with advanced cancer. J Pain Symptom Manage 1997; 13:339–346.
8. Malmberg K. Prospective randomised study of intensive insulin treatment on long term survival after acute myocardial infarction in patients with diabetes mellitus. DIGAMI (Diabetes Mellitus, Insulin Glucose Infusion in Acute Myocardial Infarction) Study Group. Br Med J 1997; 314:1512–1515.
9. Malmberg K, Norhammar A, Ryden L. Insulin treatment post myocardial infarction: the DIGAMI study. Adv Exp Med Biol 2001; 498:279–284.
10. Diaz R, Paolasso EA, Piegas LS, Tajer CD, Moreno MG, Corvalan R, Isea JE, Romero G. Metabolic modulation of acute myocardial infarction. The ECLA (Estudios Cardiologicos Latinoamerica) Collaborative Group. Circulation 1998; 98:2227–2234.
11. van den Berghe G, Wouters P, Weekers F, Verwaest C, Bruyninckx F, Schetz M, Vlasselaers D, Ferdinande P, Lauwers P, Bouillon R. Intensive insulin therapy in the surgical intensive care unit. N Engl J Med 2001; 345:1359–1367.
12. Levetan CS, Magee MF. Hospital management of diabetes. Endocrinol Metab Clin North Am 2000; 29:745–770.
13. Kanaya AM, Harris F, Volpato S, Perez-Stable EJ, Harris T, Bauer DC. Association between thyroid dysfunction and total cholesterol level in an older biracial population: the health, aging and body composition study. Arch Intern Med 2002; 162:773–779.
14. Mya MM, Aronow WS. Subclinical hypothyroidism is associated with coronary artery disease in older persons. J Gerontol A Biol Sci Med Sci 2002; 57: M658–M659.
15. Murkin JM. Anesthesia and hypothyroidism: a review of thyroxine physiology, pharmacology, and anesthetic implications. Anesth Analg 1982; 61:371–383.
16. Duntas LH. Thyroid disease and lipids. Thyroid 2002; 12:287–293.
17. Villabona C, Sahun M, Roca M, Mora J, Gomez N, Gomez JM, Puchal R, Soler J. Blood volumes and renal function in overt and subclinical primary hypothyroidism. Am J Med Sci 1999; 318:277–280.
18. Sarich TC, Wright JM. Hypothyroxinemia and phenytoin toxicity: a vicious circle. Drug Metabol Drug Interact 1996; 13:155–160.

19. O'Connor P, Feely J. Clinical pharmacokinetics and endocrine disorders. Therapeutic implications. Clin Pharmacokinet 1987; 13:345–364.
20. Muller B, Tsakiris DA, Roth CB, Guglielmetti M, Staub JJ, Marbet GA. Haemostatic profile in hypothyroidism as potential risk factor for vascular or thrombotic disease. Eur J Clin Invest 2001; 31: 131–137.
21. Ladenson PW, Goldenheim PD, Ridgway EC. Prediction and reversal of blunted ventilatory responsiveness in patients with hypothyroidism. Am J Med 1988; 84: 877–883.
22. Hiasa Y, Ishida T, Aihara T, Bando M, Nakai Y, Kataoka Y, Mori H. Acute myocardial infarction due to coronary spasm associated with L-thyroxine therapy. Clin Cardiol 1989; 12:161–163.
23. Arlot S, Debussche X, Lalau JD, Mesmacque A, Tolani M, Quichaud J, Fournier A. Myxoedema coma: response of thyroid hormones with oral and intravenous high-dose L-thyroxine treatment. Intensive Care Med 1991; 17:16–18.
24. Wolfson B, Smith K. Cardiac arrest following minor surgery in unrecognized thyrotoxicosis: a case report. Anesth Analg 1968; 47:672–676.
25. Pugh S, Lalwani K, Awal A. Thyroid storm as a cause of loss of consciousness following anaesthesia for emergency caesarean section. Anaesthesia 1994; 49:35–37.
26. Bennett MH, Wainwright AP. Acute thyroid crisis on induction of anaesthesia. Anaesthesia 1989; 44:28–30.
27. Robson NJ. Emergency surgery complicated by thyrotoxicosis and thyrotoxic periodic paralysis. Anaesthesia 1985; 40:27–31.
28. Ragaller M, Quintel M, Bender HJ, Albrecht DM. [Myxedema coma as a rare postoperative complication]. Anaesthesist 1993; 42:179–183.
29. Sherry KM, Hutchinson IL. Postoperative myxoedema. A report of coma and upper airway obstruction. Anaesthesia 1984; 39:1112–1114.
30. Mizuno J, Nakayama Y, Dohi T, Tokioka H. [A case of hypothyroidism found by delayed awakening after the operation]. Masui 2000; 49:305–308.
31. Tsubokawa T, Yamamoto K, Kobayashi T. Propofol clearance and distribution volume increase in patients with hyperthyroidism. Anesth Analg 1998; 87:195–199.
32. Matsumoto S, Unoshima M, Takeshima N, Yamamoto H, Yoshitake S, Noguchi T. [Hemodynamic effects of propofol as an anesthesia induction agent in hyperthyroidism patients on chronic beta-blocker]. Masui 2000; 49:976–980.
32a. Burch HB, Wartofsky L. Life-threatening thyrotoxicosis. Thyroid strom. Endocrinol Metab Clin North Am 1993; 22:263–277.
33. Nishio W, Takahata O, Yamamoto Y, Mamiya K, Iwasaki H. [Perioperative management using propofol in a patient with uncontrolled preoperative hyperthyroidism]. Masui 2001; 50:655–657.
34. Yoshida D. Thyroid storm precipitated by trauma. J Emerg Med 1996; 14:697–701.
35. Burger AG, Philippe J. Thyroid emergencies. Baillieres Clin Endocrinol Metab 1992; 6:77–93.
36. Nishiyama K, Kitahara A, Natsume H, Matsushita A, Nakano K, Sasaki S, Genma R, Yamamoto Y, Nakamura H. Malignant hyperthermia in a patient with Graves' disease during subtotal thyroidectomy. Endocr J 2001; 48:227–232.
37. So PC. Unmasking of thyrotoxicosis during anaesthesia. Hong Kong Med J 2001; 7:311–314.
38. Palit TK, Miller CC III, Miltenburg DM. The efficacy of thyroidectomy for Graves' disease: a meta-analysis. J Surg Res 2000; 90:161–165.
39. Ladenson PW, Levin AA, Ridgway EC, Daniels GH. Complications of surgery in hypothyroid patients. Am J Med 1984; 77:261–266.
40. Weinberg AD, Brennan MD, Gorman CA, Marsh HM, O'Fallon WM. Outcome of anesthesia and surgery in hypothyroid patients. Arch Intern Med 1983; 143:893–897.
41. Sherman SI, Ladenson PW. Percutaneous transluminal coronary angioplasty in hypothyroidism. Am J Med 1991; 90:367–370.
42. Mantzoros CS, Evagelopoulou K, Moses AC. Outcome of percutaneous transluminal coronary angioplasty in patients with subclinical hypothyroidism. Thyroid 1995; 5:383–387.
43. Lenders JW, Keiser HR, Goldstein DS, Willemsen JJ, Friberg P, Jacobs MC, Kloppenborg PW, Thien T, Eisenhofer G. Plasma metanephrines in the diagnosis of pheochromocytoma. Ann Intern Med 1995; 123: 101–109.
44. Laursen K, Damgaard-Pedersen K. CT for pheochromocytoma diagnosis. Am J Roentgenol 1979; 134: 277–280.
45. Fujita A, Hyodoh H, Kawamura Y, Kanegae K, Furuse M, Kanazawa K. Use of fusion images of I-131 metaiodobenzylguanidine, SPECT, and magnetic resonance studies to identify a malignant pheochromocytoma. Clin Nucl Med 2000; 25:440–442.
46. Kelly DF, Gonzalo IT, Cohan P, Berman N, Swerdloff R, Wang C. Hypopituitarism following traumatic brain injury and aneurysmal subarachnoid hemorrhage: a preliminary report. J Neurosurg 2000; 93: 743–752.
47. McGlynn T, Simons R. Endocrine disorders. Kammerer W, Gross RMedical Consultation; The Internist on Surgical, Obstetric, and Psychiatric Services. 2nd ed. Philadelphia: Lippincott, Williams & Wilkins, 1990: 275–309.
48. Udelsman R, Norton JA, Jelenich SE, Goldstein DS, Linehan WM, Loriaux DL, Chrousos GP. Responses of the hypothalamic–pituitary–adrenal and renin–angiotensin axes and the sympathetic system during controlled surgical and anesthetic stress. J Clin Endocrinol Metab 1987; 64:986–994.

49. Lamberts SW, Bruining HA, de Jong FH. Corticosteroid therapy in severe illness. N Engl J Med 1997; 337:1285–1292.
50. Welsh GA, Manzullo E, Orth DN. The surgical patient taking corticosteroids. In: Rose BD, ed. UpToDate. Online 11.2 ed. Wellesley, MA: UpToDate, 2003.
51. Salem M, Tainsh RE, Jr, Bromberg J, Loriaux DL, Chernow B. Perioperative glucocorticoid coverage. A reassessment 42 years after emergence of a problem. Ann Surg 1994; 219:416–425.
52. Hadley JS, Hinds CJ. Anabolic strategies in critical illness. Curr Opin Pharmacol 2002; 2:700–707.
53. Takala J, Ruokonen E, Webster NR, Nielsen MS, Zandstra DF, Vundelinckx G, Hinds CJ. Increased mortality associated with growth hormone treatment in critically ill adults. N Engl J Med 1999; 341:785–792.
54. Singer PA, Sevilla LJ. Postoperative endocrine management of pituitary tumors. Neurosurg Clin N Am 2003; 14:123–138.
55. Vance ML. Perioperative management of patients undergoing pituitary surgery. Endocrinol Metab Clin North Am 2003; 32:355–365.
56. Olson BR, Gumowski J, Rubino D, Oldfield EH. Pathophysiology of hyponatremia after transsphenoidal pituitary surgery. J Neurosurg 1997; 87:499–507.
57. Rolih CA, Ober KP. Pituitary apoplexy. Endocrinol Metab Clin North Am 1993; 22:291–302.
58. da Motta LA, de Mello PA, de Lacerda CM, Neto AP, da Motta LD, Filho MF. Pituitary apoplexy. Clinical course, endocrine evaluations and treatment analysis. J Neurosurg Sci 1999; 43:25–36.
59. Fuchs S, Beeri R, Hasin Y, Weiss AT, Gotsman MS, Zahger D. Pituitary apoplexy as a first manifestation of pituitary adenomas following intensive thrombolytic and antithrombotic therapy. Am J Cardiol 1998; 81:110–111.
60. Otsuka F, Kageyama J, Ogura T, Makino H. Pituitary apoplexy induced by a combined anterior pituitary test: case report and literature review. Endocr J 1998; 45:393–398.
61. Watanabe K, Adachi A, Nakamura R. Reversible panhypopituitarism due to Cushing's syndrome. Arch Intern Med 1988; 148:1358–1360.
62. Chen JC, Amar AP, Choi S, Singer P, Couldwell WT, Weiss MH. Transsphenoidal microsurgical treatment of Cushing disease: postoperative assessment of surgical efficacy by application of an overnight low-dose dexamethasone suppression test. J Neurosurg 2003; 98: 967–973.
62a. Bochicchio D, Losa M, Buchfelder M, Institute of Endocrine Sciences OMIMI. Factors influencing the immediate and late outcome of Cushing's disease treated by transsphenoidal surgery: a retrospective study by the European Cushing's Disease Survey Group. J Clin Endocrinol Metab 1995; 80(11):3114–3120.
63. Jackson JA, Trowbridge A, Smigiel M. Fatal pulmonary thromboembolism after successful transsphenoidal hypophysectomy for Cushing's disease. South Med J 1990; 83:960–962.
64. Ben-Shlomo A, Melmed S. Clinical review 154: the role of pharmacotherapy in perioperative management of patients with acromegaly. J Clin Endocrinol Metab 2003; 88:963–968.
65. Seidman PA, Kofke WA, Policare R, Young M. Anaesthetic complications of acromegaly. Br J Anaesth 2000; 84:179–182.
66. Glowniak JV, Loriaux DL. A double-blind study of perioperative steroid requirements in secondary adrenal insufficiency. Surgery 1997; 121:123–129.
67. Bromberg JS, Alfrey EJ, Barker CF, Chavin KD, Dafoe DC, Holland T, Naji A, Perloff LJ, Zellers LA, Grossman RA. Adrenal suppression and steroid supplementation in renal transplant recipients. Transplantation 1991; 51:385–390.
68. Schlaghecke R, Kornely E, Santen RT, Ridderskamp P. The effect of long-term glucocorticoid therapy on pituitary–adrenal responses to exogenous corticotropin–releasing hormone. N Engl J Med 1992; 326: 226–230.
69. Esteban NV, Loughlin T, Yergey AL, Zawadzki JK, Booth JD, Winterer JC, Loriaux DL. Daily cortisol production rate in man determined by stable isotope dilution/mass spectrometry. J Clin Endocrinol Metab 1991; 72:39–45.
70. Kerrigan JR, Veldhuis JD, Leyo SA, Iranmanesh A, Rogol AD. Estimation of daily cortisol production and clearance rates in normal pubertal males by deconvolution analysis. J Clin Endocrinol Metab 1993; 76:1505–1510.
71. Yeung SJ, Lazo-Diaz G, Gagel RF. Metabolic and endocrine emergencies. In: Yeung SJ, Escalante CP eds. Oncologic Emergencies. 1st ed. Hamilton, Ontario: BC Decker Inc, 2002:103–144.
72. Kamoi K, Ebe T, Kobayashi O, Ishida M, Sato F, Arai O, Tamura T, Takagi A, Yamada A, Ishibashi M, et al. Atrial natriuretic peptide in patients with the syndrome of inappropriate antidiuretic hormone secretion and with diabetes insipidus. J Clin Endocrinol Metab 1990; 70:1385–1390.
73. Miller M. Syndromes of excess antidiuretic hormone release. Crit Care Clin 2001; 17:11–23.
74. Adrogue HJ, Madias NE. Hyponatremia. N Engl J Med 2000; 342:1581–1589.
75. Lampl C, Yazdi K. Central pontine myelinolysis. Eur Neurol 2002; 47:3–10.
76. Sterns RH. The management of symptomatic hyponatremia. Semin Nephrol 1990; 10:503–514.
77. Harrigan MR. Cerebral salt wasting syndrome. Crit Care Clin 2001; 17:125–138.
78. Betjes MG. Hyponatremia in acute brain disease: the cerebral salt wasting syndrome. Eur J Int Med 2002; 13:9–14.
79. Singer I, Oster JR, Fishman LM. The management of diabetes insipidus in adults. Arch Intern Med 1997; 157:1293–1301.

6

Principles of Bioimmunotherapy: Interferon, Interleukins, Growth Factors, Monoclonal Antibodies, Antisense

YOLANDA GUTIERREZ-PUENTE and ARTURO CHAVEZ-REYES

Department of Bioimmunotherapy, The University of Texas M.D. Anderson Cancer Center, Houston, Texas, and Departamento de Microbiologia e Inmunologia, Universidad Autonoma de Nuevo Leon, Monterrey, Mexico, U.S.A.

SAROJ VADHAN-RAJ, XINSHENG LIAO, and JAMES L. MURRAY

Department of Bioimmunotherapy, The University of Texas M.D. Anderson Cancer Center, Houston, Texas, U.S.A.

PAULA TRAHAN-RIEGER

American Society of Clinical Oncology Headquarters, Alexandria, Virginia, U.S.A.

I. INTRODUCTION

The evolving field of biotherapy represents the fourth modality of cancer care. Biotherapy has represented one of the first attempts to target cancer therapies more specifically toward the cancerous cell (1). The understanding of cancer as a multifactorial disease that results from mutations in specific classes of genes controlling the cell's life cycle will ultimately lead to ever newer and more specific forms of cancer therapy in the future. Categories of agents included under the umbrella of biotherapy are the interferons (IFNs), interleukins (ILs), hematopoietic growth factors, monoclonal antibodies, vaccines, and antisense technology.

The roots of biotherapy used therapies based on stimulation of the immune system. The use of immunotherapy as treatment for malignant disease can be traced back to the 19th century and even earlier. Immunotherapy, defined broadly, is a form of therapy that uses the immune system, its cells, and molecules, which serve as messengers among cells involved in immune responses to battle disease. The mission to understand and control the relationship between the immune system and cancer is linked to three observations that have withstood the test of time: spontaneous remissions in patients with cancer, the increased incidence of cancer in immunosuppressed patients, and the presence of lymphoid infiltrates in solid tumors (2).

In the 1980s, scientific advancement in the way biological agents were identified, isolated, produced, and used improved tumor responses to biotherapy and positioned it as a viable cancer-treatment modality. Advances in four areas were critical in establishing biotherapy as a promising treatment entity: (1) an increased understanding of the intricate complexities of the immune system, (2) refinement of recombinant deoxyribonucleic acid (DNA) and hybridoma technology, (3) laboratory methods to produce large quantities of immune effector cells in culture, and (4) isolation and purification of new biologic products aided by advances in computer hardware and software.

II. DEFINITION AND CLASSIFICATION OF BIOTHERAPY

Biotherapy encompasses the use of agents derived from biological sources or of agents that affect biological responses (3). Primarily, these are products derived from the mammalian genome. In 1983, the National Cancer Institute, Division of Cancer Treatment Subcommittee on Biologic Response Modifiers, defined biological response modifiers (BRMs) as "agents or approaches that modify the relationship between tumor and host by modifying the host's biologic response to tumor cells with a resultant therapeutic effect" (4). This term distinguishes a class of agents composed of native and altered endogenous proteins that result in a specific desired cellular response. Most BRMs are either lymphokines or cytokines (5). The terms used to describe these agents and approaches have changed as scientific advances have increased our understanding of them. Historically, the term "immunotherapy" was used because the major focus of this therapeutic approach was modulation of the immune response. Although modulation of the immune response remains a major focus, the terms "biotherapy" or "biological therapy" have replaced "immunotherapy" because the scope of the field has widened to include "gene therapy." In actuality, most BRMs are a form of "gene therapy" since they are produced using recombinant DNA technology. Biological response modifiers, or more commonly biological agents—the agents used in this therapeutic modality—have pleiotropic effects, that is, they possess multiple actions. They are capable of producing immunologic actions, other biological effects, or a combination of these activities. Biotherapy is generally used as a global term to refer to all of these activities.

The specific categories of BRMs are described below in the order of their discovery and clinical uses. In addition, a summary of the most common side effects of each BRM is presented. This latter information should be of use to both anesthesiologists and critical care physicians.

A. Interferons

In the early 1930s, it was a known fact that cells infected with viruses were capable of protecting other cells from viral infection. In 1957, Isaacs and Lindemann (6) discovered the protein that partly explained this phenomenon and named it IFN because of its ability to "interfere" with viral replication. Within a few years, researchers began to identify the unique biological properties of this molecule (e.g., its antiproliferative and immunomodulatory cellular effects). As of 2003, five major species of IFN are known: alpha (α), beta (β), gamma (γ), omega (ω), and tau (τ) (7). Interferon-ω and interferon-τ remain in the early stages of study and not yet approved for therapeutic use in humans (7,8).

Cantell et al. (9) in Finland developed techniques for purifying IFN-α from donated human blood. This method proved to be costly as well as time and resource intensive and resulted in an impure product. However, it did provide the opportunity to begin to test this molecule as an antitumor agent in the late 1970s and early 1980s. The development of recombinant DNA technology in 1980 and the birth of the biotechnology industry led to the production of highly purified IFN molecules through recombinant technology. In 1981, the first human trials with recombinant IFN-α began in the United States (U.S.). Since then, research has led to the U.S. Food and Drug Administration (FDA) approval of IFN-α as treatment for multiple diseases and approval of IFN-β and IFN-γ as treatment for one disease each (see Table 1) (10,11).

The IFN family comprises a very complex set of proteins and glycoproteins. To date, two types and five species of IFNs have been described: Type I, which includes IFN-α, -β, -ω, and -τ and Type II, which includes IFN-γ. Interferons are termed pleiotropic cytokines, meaning they have multiple biological effects. Type I IFNs differ from Type II IFNs in their structure and their interaction with cell-surface receptors. Type I IFNs are more effective in inducing an antiviral state in cells, whereas type II IFNs are linked to the proper functioning of the immune system. Additionally, Type I IFNs share a common ligand-binding site, induce common biological effects, and are generally defined by the cell that produces them. Both IFN-α and IFN-ω are derived primarily from leukocytes, and IFN-β is derived from fibroblasts. Interferon-τ is derived from trophoblasts. Interferon-γ is secreted by CD8+ T cells and some CD4+ T cells. These cells secrete IFN-γ only when activated by IL-2 and IL-12 (7,8).

For IFN-α, the type principally used in treating patients with cancer, these effects can be summarized as antiviral, antitumor effects, immuomodulatory, and antiangiogenic activity. Virally infected cells synthesize and release IFN into the extracellular space. Interferon then binds to receptors on other cells and is internalized. The IFN-induced cells then produce several enzymes that can regulate the process of viral

Table 1 Type I and II Interferons in Clinical Use

Species	Subtype	Trade name	Manufacturer	FDA-approved indications
Alpha (α)	Recombinant alpha-A (IFN-α2a)	Roferon-A®	Hoffmann-LaRoche	Hairy-cell leukemia AIDS-related Kaposi's sarcoma Chronic myelogenous leukemia Chronic hepatitis C
	Recombinant alpha-2 (IFN-α2b)	INTRON-A®	Schering-Plough	High-risk melanoma Non-Hodgkins Lymphoma Hairy-cell leukemia AIDS-related Kaposi's sarcoma Condylomata acuminata Chronic hepatitis C Chronic hepatitis B (adult and pedi)
	Lymphoblastoid (IFN-αN1)	Wellferon®	Wellcome Foundation	Not commercially available in the United States – Approved for hepatitis C in patients 18 year
	Human leukocyte derived (IFN-αN3)	Alferon®	Interferon Sciences	Condylomata acuminata
	Recombinant consensus (IFN-Con_1)	Infergen®	Amgen	Chronic hepatitis C
Beta (β)	Recombinant beta-1a (IFN-β1a)	Avonex®	Biogen	Multiple sclerosis
	Recombinant beta-1a	Rebif®	Serono	Multiple sclerosis
	Recombinant beta-1b (IFN-β1b)	Betaseron®	Chiron/Berlex	Multiple sclerosis
Gamma (γ)	Interferon gamma-1b (IFN-γ1b)	Actimmune®	Intermune	Chronic granulomatous disease

[a] Denotes common side effects.

protein synthesis. Among the IFN-induced proteins important in the antiviral actions of IFNs are the RNA-dependent protein kinase (PKR), the 2′, 5′-oligoadenylate synthetase (OAS) and RNase L, and the Mx protein GTPases. Indirectly, the IFNs may mediate antiviral effects by stimulating cytotoxic T lymphocytes (CTLs) to lyse virally infected cells (12).

The alpha IFNs also exhibit antitumor or direct effects though cytostatic (i.e., prolongation of the cell cycle) effects on tumor cells which is thought to be achieved by modulation of OAS or cellular oncogenes. Interferon-α may also act synergistically with IFN-γ to promote cell lysis (8). Recently, research has demonstrated that IFN-α has proapoptotic effects in human tumor cells lines (13). Lastly, IFN-α exherts indirect antitumor effects through upregulation of Class I histocompatibility antigens (i.e., making cells more recognizable by the immune system) and through the stimulation of other immune cells such as natural killer cells, cytotoxic T cells and activation of macrophages (7,8).

Angiogenesis or neovascularization is now known to play a significant role in tumor metastasis. In addition to enabling the metastatic spread of tumor cells, the process of angiogenesis is also believed to reduce the tumor's accessibility to chemotherapeutic drugs (14). Endogenous IFN is one of the many negative regulators of angiogenesis. Of clinical note, IFN-α has demonstrated efficacy in the treatment of hemangiomas (15).

The IFNs have been referred to as the "prototype" biological agent and have undergone extensive molecular, preclinical, and investigational scrutiny. Interferon-α therapy now has an established role in the treatment of several advanced malignancies. For reviews of the use of IFN as cancer therapy, see Refs. 7, 8, 16, 17. Numerous phase II and phase III trials have demonstrated its efficacy as a single agent. Additional studies have shown its ability to induce responses in refractory neoplasms and to modify chromosomal disorders in disease such as chronic myelogenous leukemia (CML).

In 1986, just a few years after its introduction as an anticancer agent, the first IFN-α was approved by the FDA for its significant role in the treatment of hairy cell leukemia (HCL). Although there are now more effective treatments for HCL (e.g., cladrabine), it represents an important milestone as the first disease for which a biological agent received regulatory approval (11).

Shortly thereafter, in 1989, IFN-α received its second FDA approval for the treatment of acquired immunodeficiency syndrome (AIDS)-related Kaposi's sarcoma (KS). It has been useful in patients with predominantly mucocutaneous disease. It is most effective in patients with limited lymphadenopathy, no history of opportunistic infections, absence of B symptoms (fever, night sweats, cachexia, and diarrhea), and an intact immune system (CD4 count greater than $200/mm^3$). Although initially approved as high-dose therapy [36 million international units (MIU) daily as induction therapy], current research is focusing on the use of lower doses and IFN in combination with antiviral agents (18,19).

Additional oncology indications in the United States for IFN-α include treatment of CML, as adjuvant therapy for melanoma, and for non-Hodgkin's lymphoma (NHL) (10,11). During the last four decades, the optimal first-line treatment for CML in chronic (stable) phase has progressed from alkylating agents, to hydroxyurea (HU), and then to IFN-α which was first approved for this indication in the late 1980s. Allogeneic stem-cell transplantation, which offers the chance of prolonged leukemia-free survival to about 20% of all CML patients, is the only certain approach to cure. Recently, the FDA approved imitimab, a new inhibitor specific for tyrosine kinase of the Bcr–Abl oncoprotein as frontline therapy for CML. Research will continue to investigate the role of IFN, both alone and in combination, in context with new and emerging therapies (20).

Melanoma, diagnosed and treated at its earliest stages, can be cured by surgery alone. However, when metastatic beyond the regional nodes, it is almost uniformly fatal. Adjuvant therapy targeted toward the treatment of microscopic residual disease after surgical resection has been the focus of numerous clinical investigations because this is the stage at which it is possible to have the greatest impact on disease-free and overall survival. Based on response rates in the range of 15% for patients with metastatic melanoma, many studies have centered on the use of IFN in the adjuvant setting. The reader is referred to Refs. 7, 8, 21, 22 for a review of these studies. In 1995, based on the results of an Eastern Cooperative Group (ECOG) trial, IFN-α2b was approved at high doses for the adjuvant treatment of melanoma. Since then, numerous studies worldwide have continued to evaluate the role of IFN in different doses, schedules, and as combination therapy. Overall, it appears that high-dose IFN increases disease-free survival, but does not prolong overall survival. Data continue to indicate that high-dose IFN-α2b should be offered to appropriately select intermediate- and high-risk patients with melanoma not involved in an experimental protocol (21).

In the past 15–20 years, IFN-α has been shown to be effective in the treatment of non-Hodgkin's lymphoma, with response rates of 40–50%. These encouraging single-agent results have led to the incorporation of these agents into combination programs. Interferon-α2b was approved by the FDA in 1997 for use with CHOP-like regimens in patients with advanced low-grade follicular NHL. The approval was based on research by the French co-operative group, Groupe d'Etude des Lymphomes Folliculaires (GELF) (23). Interferon has been incorporated into combination chemotherapy programs either as a maintenance strategy or as concurrent therapy. Most studies have shown a favorable impact of IFN on failure-free survival but not on overall survival. Some studies have shown no impact at all. A major barrier has been management of IFN-associated side effects. Many practitioners feel that the modest favorable impact of IFN is offset by the fatigue and other side effects of the drug, even though a quality-of-life analysis has concluded that the incorporation of IFN is worthwhile (24). In a variety of malignancies (e.g., multiple myeloma, T-cell malignancies, renal cell cancer, bladder cancer, and squamous carcinomas of the skin and cervix in combination with the retinoids), the use of IFN remains experimental (7).

Interferon has efficacy in a variety of other diseases as well. In viral diseases, IFN-α has clinical applications for the treatment of hepatitis B, hepatitis C (7,25), and condylomata acuminata. Chronic granulomatous disease (CGD) is an inherited abnormality of certain cells of the immune system that "ingest" bacteria and kill them (phagocytic cells). The abnormality results in chronic infection by certain types of bacteria that result in severe, recurrent infections of the skin, lymph nodes, liver, lungs, and bone. Because treatment with IFN-γ led to a 70% reduction of serious infections in patients with this disease, this agent was approved in 1990 (7,26). In 1993, IFN-β was approved for the treatment of relapsing-remitting (RR)-multiple sclerosis (MS). Interferon therapy provides hope for an effective treatment for MS since the disease was first described in 1868 (10,11,27,28).

The toxicity profile of IFN-α is dependent on the dose, the route of administration, and the treatment schedule (7,29). The majority of side effects associated with IFN are constitutional. They include fatigue, fever, chills, myalgias, headache, and anorexia. This constellation of side effects is often referred to as flu-like symptoms. They are reported almost universally following initial administration of treatment. The appearance of subsequent tachyphylaxis or tolerance depends on the dose, the route, and the schedule of administration. The chronic side effect of fatigue can be the most clinically challenging and patients often report a negative impact on quality of life (30).

In summary, IFN-α was the first pure human protein found to be effective in the treatment of cancer. The most important future direction for research on IFNs and possibly their greatest value will be in prolonging the disease-free interval and, ultimately, survival. Numerous studies have demonstrated improvement in these areas. The hope remains that as biotherapy with IFN becomes applied to earlier-stage disease, greater gains in survival and disease-free interval may be sustained. The challenge remains to maximize the use of this drug while reducing the patient's experience of side effects.

B. Interleukins

The ILs are a family of cytokines that represent a major communication network in living organisms. Interleukins are proteins that exist as natural components of the human immune system and they are produced by monocytes, endothelial cells, astrocytes/glial cells, fibroblasts, bone marrow stromal cells, and thymocytes as well as lymphocytes. The primary function of ILs is the immunomodulation and immunoregulation of leukocytes; however, most ILs are capable of inducing multiple biological activities in a variety of target cells (31).

The term "interleukin" was originally used to define substances produced by leukocytes that had activity on other leukocytes. However, this early definition fails to adequately describe the production and range of activities now attributed to the family of ILs. As a result, of the many ILs described in early research, each had several names, each of which describes a different function. In 1986, the Sixth International Congress of Immunology decided that new cytokines would be named according to their biological properties but that, on identification of the amino-acid sequence, a sequential IL number would be assigned (32). To qualify as an IL, the cytokine must be documented to have a unique amino-acid sequence and functional activity involving leukocytes. The evidence is evaluated by the Nomenclature and Standardization Committee of the International Cytokine Society and the Union of Immunological Societies, which then make a recommendation to the World Health Organization (33). There is no ranking in terms of importance or specific activity.

Over 25 ILs have so far been identified and isolated as of June 2003 and are undergoing either preclinical or clinical evaluation (34,35). Only IL-2 and IL-11 have been approved by the FDA for use in patients with cancer. Interleukin-2 is indicated for treatment of metastatic renal cell cancer (metastatic RCC) and metastatic melanoma. Interleukin-11 has been approved for use in preventing severe thrombocytopenia and in decreasing the need for platelet transfusions following myelosuppressive therapy (10,11).

Various ILs may produce autocrine, paracrine, or endocrine actions within the body. Autocrine action refers to the binding and activation of the same cell that produced the IL. Paracrine action describes the binding and activation of nearby cells. Endocrine action occurs when ILs are secreted and bind to distant cells in the body (31). Primarily, the ILs affect local or regional cells rather than distant cells as seen in endocrine actions.

The complex balance between cellular activation and immunoregulation is orchestrated by the secretion of ILs and the resultant effects of the immune system on cells. Actions produced by the ILs may by redundant, synergistic, or antagonistic. Redundant actions are similar actions that may be produced by different ILs. Synergistic activity occurs when more than one IL is essential to produce activity in a particular target cell. Antagonistic effects occur when an IL inhibits the target-cell activity induced by another cytokine (36).

Interleukin-2 is a lymphokine first described in 1976 as a T-cell growth factor (37). Produced primarily by activated T-helper (T_h) cells, IL-2 is a messenger-regulatory molecule that has profound immunomodulatory effects in the body. The regulation of IL-2 production is dependent on the activation of T cells by antigens. Its biologic effects are numerous and include stimulation of the growth and maturation of subpopulations of T cells, including cytotoxic T cells (killer T cells), and the proliferation of natural killer cells. It is capable of enhancing humoral immune responses and stimulates the production of other immune messenger molecules as well. Its potent stimulation of immune responses led to clinical investigation in a variety of diseases; however, the majority of clinical successes thus far have been seen in patients with renal cell cancer and melanoma. It is the first agent available for the treatment of metastatic cancer that functions solely through stimulation of the immune system.

Initial clinical trials with IL-2 were high-dose bolus regimens, and often included the administration of immune effector cells. Although some complete responses were achieved, the side effects were substantial and the regimen was not easily replicated in the community setting. Interleukin-2 first received regulatory approval for the treatment of adults with metastatic RCC in 1992 based on combined data from randomized clinical trials. Two hundred and fifty-five patients with metastatic RCC were treated with single-agent IL-2 in seven clinical studies conducted at 21 institutions. In 1998, IL-2 was approved for the treatment of metastatic melanoma based on studies involving 270 patients with metastatic melanoma treated with single-agent IL-2 in eight clinical studies conducted at 22 institutions. In these clinical trials, IL-2 was given by 15 min intravenous (IV) infusion every 8 hr for up to 5 days (maximum of 14 doses). No treatment was given on days 6–14 and then dosing was repeated for up to 5 days on days 15–19 (maximum of 14 doses). These two cycles constituted one course of therapy. Patients could receive a maximum of 28 doses during a course of therapy. In practice >90% of patients had doses withheld. Metastatic RCC patients received a median of 20 of 28 scheduled doses of IL-2. Metastatic melanoma patients received a median of 18 of 28 scheduled doses of IL-2 during the first course of therapy (38).

Because of the significant toxicity associated with high-dose regimens, current research has focused on regimens using subcutaneous administration of IL-2 in the ambulatory setting or infusion by an ambulatory pump both in renal cancer and melanoma, the goal being to decrease toxicity and maintain clinical responses. With these regimens, IL-2 doses are lower, generally in the range of 3–10 MIU/m^2, given 3–5 days/week over several weeks. Patients may also receive concomitant therapy with IFN-α and/or chemotherapy. Low-dose IL-2 therapy has produced disappointing clinical response rates in melanoma. Although the response rates to low-dose IL-2 have been better in renal cell carcinoma, the quality of these responses relative to those seen with high-dose IL-2 therapy remains a concern. The addition of IL-2 to chemotherapeutic regimens (biochemotherapy) has been associated with overall response rates (ORRs) of up to 60% in patients with metastatic melanoma, but this has yet to be translated into a confirmed improvement in survival. Clinical trials have not demonstrated superiority for combinations of IL-2 and IFN-α than high-dose IL-2 alone. It remains to be determined whether further modifications of IL-2-based regimens or the addition of newer agents to IL-2 will produce better tumor response and survival (39,40).

The side effects profile for patients who receive IL-2 therapy differs depending on the dose, route, and schedule of IL-2 given. In general, high-dose IL-2 therapy produces more severe toxic effects which have the potential to involve nearly every major organ system. Patients who are to be treated with IL-2 should have normal cardiac, pulmonary, hepatic, and CNS function at the start of therapy. For a summary of toxicities, see Table 2 at the end of this chapter.

In summary, IL-2 has demonstrated efficacy in two very difficult-to-treat diseases, RCC and metastatic melanoma. Future investigations of IL-2 will involve combination regimens that include other cytokines, activated lymphocytes, vaccines, and chemotherapeutic agents for these two malignancies and a variety of malignancies and other diseases. Doses, routes of administration, and schedules will be altered to attempt to achieve greater efficacy with less toxic effects. In some patients who have received therapy with IL-2 or RCC or metastatic melanoma, startling and durable complete remissions have been seen. However, the percentage of patients achieving this response is low. In the future, new technologies, such as microarray technology, may help clinicians determine, which subset of patients will best respond to therapy with IL-2.

C. Hematopoietic Growth Factors

Myelosuppression is a common dose-limiting factor for many cancer patients receiving cytotoxic treatment, and contributes to the need for hospitalization, IV antibiotic administration, transfusion of blood products, dose reduction, and treatment delays. In addition, it may have significant negative effects on patient's quality of life or even response to treatment. Over the past several years, a great deal of progress has been made in understanding the process of hematopoiesis by which mature cellular elements of blood are formed (41). Hematopoietic growth factors are a family of regulatory molecules that play important roles in the growth, survival, and differentiation of blood progenitor cells, as well as in the functional activation of mature cells. In the last decade, several hematopoietic growth factors have become available for attenuating hematologic toxicity of chemotherapy. Table 3 lists the recombinant human hematopoietic growth factors that have been approved by the FDA for clinical use: granulocyte colony-stimulating factor [G-CSF, filgrastim (Neupogen)], yeast-derived granulocyte–macrophage colony-stimulating factor [GM-CSF, sargramostim (Leukine)], erythropoietin [EPO (Epogen, Procrit)], and interleukin-11 [IL-11, oprelvekin (Neumega)]. More recently, two new growth factors of second generation, pegfilgrastim and darbepoetin alfa with a long serum half-life, have received FDA approval in oncology setting. In addition, several other hematopoietic cytokines are under clinical development (34,42).

Granulocyte colony-stimulating factor is lineage specific for the production of functionally active neutrophils. It has been extensively evaluated in several clinical scenarios. It was first approved in 1991 for clinical use to reduce the incidence of febrile neutropenia in cancer patients receiving myelosuppressive chemotherapy. This broad initial indication has since been expanded even further to include many other areas of oncologic practice, such as mobilization of progenitor

Table 2 Side Effects of Biologic Agents

System	Interferons	Interleukin-2	Hematopoietic growth factors	Monoclonal antibodies	Vaccines	Antisense-oligos
Central nervous system	Impaired concentration, headache, lethargy, confusion, depression	Impaired concentration, headache, lethargy, confusion, anxiety, psychoses, depression	Rare	Rare	Rare	Rare
General	Constitutional symptoms,[a] fatigue[a]	Constitutional symptoms,[a] fatigue,[a] weight gain during therapy, followed by weight loss[a]	Mild constitutional symptoms, fatigue (mostly with GM-CSF)	Constitutional symptoms, allergic reactions, rare anaphylaxis	Constitutional symptoms,[a] chills, fatigue[a]	Fever,[a] malaise
Cardiovascular	Hypotension, tachycardia, arrhythmias, rare myocardial ischemia	Hypotension,[a] edema,[a] ascites arrhythmias, decreased systemic vasculoresistance[a]	Rare hypertension with epoetin alfa	Hypotension, chest pain	Rare	Rare
Pulmonary	Rare	Dyspnea, pulmonary edema	Rare occurrence of dyspnea with first dose of GM-CSF	Dyspnea, wheezing	Rare	Rare
Renal/hepatic	Proteinuria, elevated liver enzymes[a]	Oliguria,[a] increased BUN, creatinine,[a] proteinuria, azotemia, increased bilirubin, SGOT, SGPT, LDH	Rare elevation of LDH, alkaline phosphatase with G-CSF	Rare	Rare	Elevation of liver enzymes
Gastro-intestinal	Nausea/vomiting, diarrhea, anorexia[a]	Nausea/vomiting,[a] diarrhea,[a] anorexia,[a] mucositis	Rare	Nausea/vomiting	Rare	Nausea and vomiting,[a] mucositis,[a] diarrhea
Genitourinary	Impotence, decreased libido	Decreased libido	Rare	Rare	Rare	Rare
Integumentary	Alopecia, rash	Rash,[a] dry desquamation,[a] erythema,[a] pruritus,[a] inflammatory reaction at injection sites[a]	GM-CSF/G-CSF: inflammation at injection site, rare occurrence of rash	Urticaria, rash, pruritus	Pruritus, inflammatory reaction at injection sites	Rare
Hematologic	Leukopenia,[a] anemia, thrombocytopenia	Anemia,[a] thrombocytopenia, lymphopenia,[a] eosinophilia[a]	Leukocytosis,[a] eosinophilia (GM-CSF).[a] Note—expected biologic effect of HGF used	In hematologic malignancies, leukopenia	Rare	Platelet aggregation,[a] thrombocytopenia bleeding[a]
Musculo-skeletal	Myalgias,[a] arthralgias[a]	Myalgias, arthralgias	Bone pain[a] with GM- and G-CSF	Rare arthralgias	Myalgias	Bone pain,[a] myalgias,[a] arthralgias[a]

[a] Denotes common side effects.
Source: From Ref. 41a.

Table 3 FDA-Approved Hematopoietic Growth Factors/Cytokines

Cell lineage	Growth factor/cytokine	Trade name	Approval date	Manufacturer/distributor
Myeloid lineage	G-CSF (filgrastim)	Neupogen	1991	Amgen
	GM-CSF (sargramostim)	Leukine	1991	Immunex/Berlex
	Pegfilgrastim	Neulasta	2002	Amgen
Erythroid lineage	Epoetin alfa	Epogen	1989 (Nephrology)	Amgen
		Procrit	1993 (Oncology)	OrthoBiotech
	Darbepoetin alfa	Aranesp	2001 (Nephrology)	Amgen
			2002 (Oncology)	
Megakaryocytic lineage	Interleukin-11 (oprelvekin)	Neumega	1997	Genetics Institute/Wyeth

cells, stimulation of neutrophil recovery following high-dose chemotherapy with stem-cell support. In addition, G-CSF is indicated to increase neutrophil production in endogenous myeloid disorders, such as congenital neutropenic states. The recommended dose of recombinant human G-CSF (Neupogen) is 5 μg/kg/day. Granulocyte colony-stimulating factor is used at a higher dose (10 μg/kg/day) for mobilization of progenitor cells and following bone marrow transplantation (BMT). Outside of the context of stem-cell mobilization and transplantation, however, there is no data indicating that doses in excess of 5 μg/kg/day are ever required.

Myeloid growth factors have been remarkably well tolerated based on extensive clinical experience with these cytokines over the past decade. The predominant side effect observed with the use of G-CSF is mild-to-moderate bone pain, which is usually seen at the initiation of G-CSF therapy or at the very beginning of neutrophil recovery. Occasionally, the pain can be severe with vigorous marrow response to CSF stimulation, and may require analgesics for control (41,42).

Granulocyte–macrophage colony-stimulating factor, primarily a myeloid-lineage-specific growth factor, stimulates the production of neutrophils, monocytes, and eosinophils. It received a more narrow FDA approval in 1991 for clinical use in patients with nonmyeloid malignancies undergoing autologous BMT. Since that initial indication, GM-CSF has also been approved for an expanded range of conditions, such as mitigation of myelotoxicity in patients with leukemia who are undergoing induction chemotherapy. To date, no large-scale randomized trials have compared the efficacy of the two CSFs in the same clinical setting. Future comparative trials may help determine the optimal clinical utility of these CSFs in different clinical situations.

The recommended dose of yeast-derived GM-CSF following autologous BMT is 250 μg/m^2/day given by a 2-hr IV infusion. In phase I and II studies in the chemotherapy setting, activity has been observed at doses ranging from 250 to 750 μg/m^2/day. In patients with MDS, neutrophil responses have been seen at much lower doses. Yeast-derived GM-CSF (sargramostim) is generally well tolerated at recommended doses. In the transplant setting, no excessive toxicity is seen in patients treated with this form of GM-CSF, as compared with controls. In other settings, the most commonly reported side effects of GM-CSF have included constitutional symptoms, such as fever, bone pain, myalgia, headaches, and chills. These side effects are seen more frequently when GM-CSF is administered at higher doses and by continuous IV infusion than when given at recommended doses by the SC route. In patients with MDS, the dose can be titrated to the smallest effective level to avoid untoward side effects (41,42).

Erythropoietin was the first hematopoietic growth factor to become commercially available for clinical use in the United States. Recombinant human EPO has been approved for the treatment of anemia of chronic renal failure in predialysis or dialysis patients, anemia associated with zidovudine (Retrovir) therapy in patients infected with human immunodeficiency virus (HIV), anemia in cancer patients receiving chemotherapy, and anemia in patients scheduled for elective, noncardiac, and nonvascular surgery.

The anemia caused by chemotherapy is due mainly to drug effects on bone marrow precursor cells and is proportional to chemotherapy dose intensity. In addition, with platinum agents, anemia may be related to renal effects on these drugs on EPO production. Several trials, both randomized and nonrandomized, support the finding that EPO can significantly reduce transfusion requirements and improve patient's reported quality of life (41,43). Overall, about 60% of cancer patients receiving chemotherapy respond to EPO treatment. Therefore, patient selection is important to ensure the cost effectiveness of EPO therapy. Available data suggest that patients with baseline anemia or a fall in hemoglobin value >2 g/dL after the first cycle of chemotherapy are more likely to need blood transfusions. The best predictors of a clinical response to EPO therapy are an early rise in hemoglobin values and an increase in reticulocyte counts. The current FDA approved initial dose of EPO in cancer patients is 150 U/kg SC three times a week, which can be increased to 300 U/kg three times weekly if an adequate response does not occur after 4 weeks of therapy. However, a more common practice, based on data from several clinical trials, is to administer EPO at a dose of 40,000 units SC once weekly to be increased to 60,000 units weekly in nonresponders. Patients who do not respond after 8 weeks of EPO therapy (despite a dose increase) are unlikely to respond to higher doses. Erythropoietin has been well tolerated in cancer patients receiving chemotherapy. Hypertension associated with a significant rise in hemoglobin has been observed rarely in cancer patients receiving EPO therapy. Occasionally, seizures have been observed in patients with underlying CNS disease and in the context of a significant rise in blood pressure (41,43).

Severe thrombocytopenia requiring platelet transfusions is an uncommon acute problem with standard dose chemotherapy; however, it can represent a cumulative problem with the many chemotherapeutic regimens especially in heavily pretreated patients. Several hematopoietic cytokines with thrombopoietic activity have been evaluated in clinical trials. These include IL-l, IL-3, IL-6, IL-11, thrombopoietin (TPO), megakaryocyte growth and development factor (MGDF), and PIXY 321. Most of these cytokines have shown modest thrombopoietic activity and mediate a multitude of biological effects, including some undesirable effects. To date, IL-11 is the only thrombopoietic cytokine that has received FDA approval for clinical use (41,44).

Interleukin-11 is a pleiotropic cytokine which acts synergistically with other hematopoietic growth factors, such as TPO, IL-3, and stem cell factor (c-kit ligand), to promote the proliferation of hematopoietic progenitor cells and to induce maturation of megakaryocytes. It was approved by the FDA to prevent severe thrombocytopenia and to reduce the need for platelet transfusions following myelosuppressive chemotherapy in patients with nonmyeloid malignancies who are at risk of severe thrombocytopenia (45). The recommended dose of IL-11 in adults is 50 μg/kg SC once daily and is continued until the postnadir platelet count is $\geq$50,000/mm^3. Dosing beyond 21 days per treatment cycle is not recommended. Patients treated with IL-11 commonly experience mild-to-moderate fluid retention, as manifested by peripheral edema and/or dyspnea. In some patients, pre-existing pleural effusions have increased during IL-11 administration. In addition, moderate decreases in hemoglobin values (thought to be related to dilutional anemia) have also been observed. Interleukin-11 should be used with caution in patients with a history of cardiac arrhythmias, since palpitations, tachycardia, and atrial arrhythmias have been reported in some patients receiving this agent (44,45).

Thrombopoietin is a lineage-dominant hematopoietic cytokine that regulates proliferation and maturation of cells of the megakaryocyte/platelet lineage. Results of initial clinical trials using truncated or full-length forms of the TPO molecule indicate that TPO is a powerful stimulus for the production of megakaryocytes and normal platelets in humans and that it enhances platelet recovery following chemotherapy (46–48). However, clinical development of MGDF, a truncated version of TPO, was halted due to the occurrence of neutralizing antibodies directed against TPO. However, similar antibodies have not been detected with the full-length version of recombinant human TPO. Recombinant human thrombopoietin (rhTPO) is a full-length molecule that is glycosylated. This carbohydrate moiety, although, not required for thrombopoietic activity, it contributes to a long circulating half-life to the molecule (18–32 hr). Thus, a single dose of rhTPO results in a platelet increase that is sustained for long time, with a peak response around day 12 and return of the counts close to a baseline at 3 weeks. This delayed peak response has contributed in part to a complexity in development of this molecule (49,50). With the regimens that cause late nadir (e.g., carboplatin), rhTPO-administered postchemotherapy has been shown to be effective in attenuating the severity of thrombocytopenia and the need for platelet transfusions (48). However, with the regimens that cause early nadir, rhTPO-administered postchemotherapy has not shown consistent effect. Recently, it has been shown that administration of rhTPO both before and after chemotherapy reduced the severity of thrombocytopenia (51). Thus, future trials will need to optimize the dose/schedule of this agent in chemotherapy and other settings where severe thrombocytopenia is problematic. Recent studies have also shown utility of this growth factor in increasing plateletpheresis yield in normal donors and in cancer patients for cryopreservation and autologous platelet transfusions to support during chemotherapy-induced severe thrombocytopenia (52,53). This strategy may be quite useful in the management and, in certain high-risk patients, in the prevention of alloimmunization and platelet refractoriness.

Recently, longer-acting hematopoietic growth factors, pegfilgrastim (Neulasta) and darbepoetin alfa (Aranesp) have been developed. Both these molecules were created to provide therapeutic agents with a long half-life to reduce the frequency of administration (54–60).

Pegfilgrastim is manufactured by the conjugation of a 20-kDa polyethylene glycol (PEG) moiety to the amino terminal residue of filgrastim. Pegfilgrastim's mechanism of action is similar to filgrastim (54). Filgrastim is cleared from the circulation by a combination of renal and neutrophil-mediated clearance. Pegylation of filgrastim makes its molecular size greater and thus reduces its renal clearance, which then results in a greater dependence on neutrophil-mediated clearance. Elimination half-life of filgrastim is approximately 3.5 hr, whereas, plasma half-life of pegfilgrastim is approximately 46–62 hr in healthy volunteers. However, in cancer patients receiving chemotherapy, clearance is directly related to neutrophil recovery which supports the rationale for administering pegfilgrastim once per cycle of chemotherapy (55–57). In the phase III trials, pegfilgrastim administered once per cycle at a dose of 6 mg fixed dose or 100 mcg/kg provided neutrophil support similar to that with filgrastim administered daily. Pegfilgrastim is FDA approved for the indication of prevention of infections, as manifested by febrile neutropenia, in patients with nonmyeloid malignancy receiving myelosuppressive chemotherapy.

Darbepoetin alfa has a half-life approximately three times longer than that of epoetin alfa (58). Early observations indicated that increasing the sialic acid content of epoetin alfa would increase its biological activity. Darbepoetin alfa was created by using site-directed mutagenesis to allow for the attachment of two additional sialic-acid-containing carbohydrate chains. Despite the structural differences, darbepoetin alfa binds to the same receptor as endogenous erythropoietin and exerts the same receptor-mediated erythropoietic action. Darbepoetin alfa has been approved for the treatment of anemia in patients with renal failure and in patients with nonmyeloid malignancies with chemotherapy-related anemia. Clinical trials in cancer patients receiving chemotherapy have shown that darbepoetin is safe and effective when administered at every 1-, 2-, or 3-week intervals (59,60). The results of these trials have shown that darbepoetin alfa administered at every 2 weeks has similar efficacy to epoetin alfa administered every week. The randomized comparative trials are ongoing.

In conclusion, the availability of hematopoietic regulatory molecules have reduced hematologic toxicity and related complications in cancer patients receiving cytotoxic treatment. Although this first generation of growth factors has been widely used, the necessity of frequent administration has posed an inconvenience and compliance issues for some patients. The recent introduction of the new molecules with a longer serum half-life would simplify patient management. The future directions with the growth factors would likely involve use of the new agents designed with the need for infrequent dosing, less potential for immunogenicity and toxicity, and expanding role in improving overall treatment outcome.

D. Monoclonal Antibodies and Immunoconjugates

In the early 1900s, Paul Ehrlich envisioned that antibodies could be used as "magic bullets" to deliver drugs and toxins to tumor cells. This dream was not realized until 1975 when Köhler and Milstein (61) published a seminal article describing a method to produce large quantities of antibodies recognizing a single antigen (Ag). The technique involved fusing B-lymphocytes from mice immunized with tumor cells or cell lysates to an "immortal" murine plasma cell resulting in a "hybridoma" capable of secreting unlimited quantities of pure "monoclonal" antibodies (Mab). Following selection in "HAT-free" medium hybridomas could be grown continuously in cell culture or as mouse ascites; supernatants were then screened for the Mab(s) of choice.

Monoclonal antibodies can mediate antitumor effect either directly or indirectly (Table 4). They may lyse tumors through interaction of the Fc end with human complement or immune effector cells resulting in antibody-dependent cell-mediated cytotoxicity (ADCC). Several Mab have been capable of regulating cell growth through receptor–ligand interactions, or as anti-idiotype vaccines. Indirect mechanisms include the use of immunoconjugates consisting of Mab coupled to radionuclides, drugs, toxins, or cytokines to target tumors (62).

The advent of hybridoma technology resulted in large quantities of pure Mab specific for tumor-

Table 4 Strategies for In Vivo Use of Monoclonal Antibodies as Anticancer Therapy

Antibody alone
Complement mediated cytotoxicity (CMC)
Antibody-dependent cell-mediated cytotoxicity *ADCC*
Regulatory (ligand/receptor) interactions
Anti-idiotype vaccine
Immunoconjugates
Radiolabeled antibodies
Immunotoxins
Chemotherapy-antibody conjugates
Cytokine immunoconjugates
Cellular immunoconjugates

Source: From Ref. 62.

associated Ag. In the early 1980s and 1990s, a number of clinical trials were performed in cancer patients (reviewed in Refs. 63, 64). Although toxicity was minimal, unmodified murine Mab were largely unsuccessful in mediating antitumor effects. This was due to several problems which could be categorized under the following headings (Table 5): (1) properties of the tumor Ag, (2) properties of the target cell, (3) properties of the Mab themselves, and (4) immunologic mechanisms. With respect to (1), Ag shedding and/or low levels of expression on tumors resulted in inadequate Mab binding to tumor, formation of immune complexes, and rapid clearance from the circulation. Binding of Mab to tumors often resulted in internalization of the Mab/Ag complex with failure of re-expression of Ag (termed "modulation"). The majority of Mab upon binding to tumors were unable by themselves to initiate downstream intracellular events which resulted in tumor lysis or apoptosis. With respect to problems (3) and (4), murine Mab were extremely immunogenic in humans resulting in the formation of human antimouse antibodies (HAMA) (65), or were unable to mediate immune effector functions such as ADCC or complement-mediated lysis.

Several major innovations occurred which addressed each of the above issues (66): (1) recombinant DNA techniques such as phage libraries resulting in the ability to produce mouse–human "chimeric" or "humanized" Mab were developed (Fig. 1). By insertion of the mouse variable region genes along with the human constant region genes into an expression vector, "chimeric" Mab could be produced containing the mouse variable region and human constant region of light and heavy chains, respectively. Similarly, the insertion of complementarity-determining (CD) regions [i.e., the sections of variable light (V_L) chain which interact with Ag] into the human variable/constant region framework resulted in the production of "humanized" Mab. Recently, completely human Mab have been made using transgenic mice containing human immunoglobulin genes (67). Chimeric and humanized Mab are much less immunogenic and are more capable of mediating effector functions, (2) humanized Mab were produced against growth factor receptors such as the epidermal growth factor receptor (EGFr) family, which upon binding to receptor could inhibit ligand binding and subsequent intracellular signaling events, eventually leading to apoptosis or cell death (Fig. 2), and () stable, more potent immunoconjugates—Mab bound to radioisotopes, drugs, or toxins—were developed. These innovations resulted in a number of newer Mab/immunoconjugates which mediated more potent antitumor effects and were less able to induce antihuman antibodies.

The first Mab to be approved and licensed by the FDA for treatment of cancer was rituximab

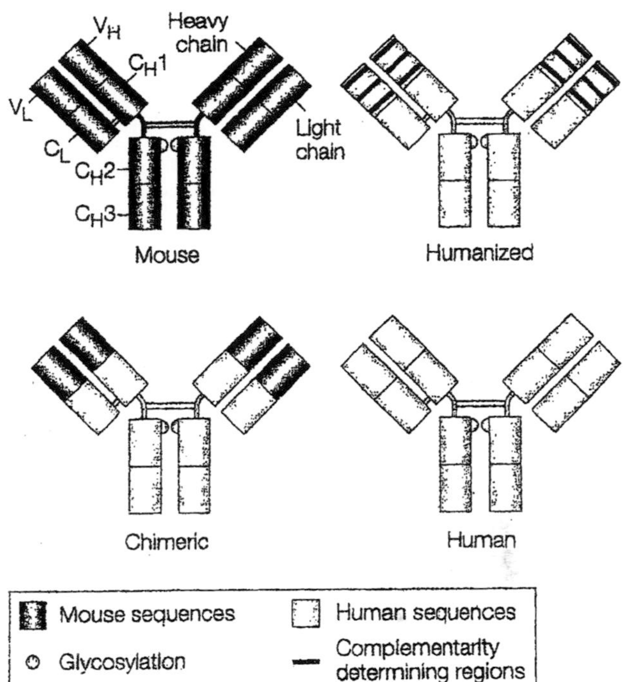

Figure 1 Types of Mab: *Murine Mab*: Derived by hybridoma technology. *Chimeric Mab*: Obtained by joining the antigen-binding variable domains (V_L, V_H) of a mouse Mab to human constant domains (C_L, C_H). *Humanized Mab*: Grafting antigen-binding loops, or complementary determining (CD) regions from a moise Mab into a human IgG. *Human Man*: Obtained from very large, single-chain variable fragments (scFvs), Fab phage display libraries, or transgenic mice that contain human Ig genes. *Source*: Adapted from Ref. 66.

Table 5 Barriers to Effective Therapy with Unmodified Monoclonal Antibodies

Properties of antigen	*Properties of monoclonal antibodies*
Secretion/shedding of antigen	Immunogenicity
Low-level expression	Correct isotype
Modulation	Ability to trigger apoptosis
Permissive for lysis/apoptosis	Accessibility to tumor masses
	Effector mechanisms
Properties of target cell	Quantity
Cellular defense mechanisms	Activation
	Recruitment to tumor sites

Source: Adapted from Ref. 69a.

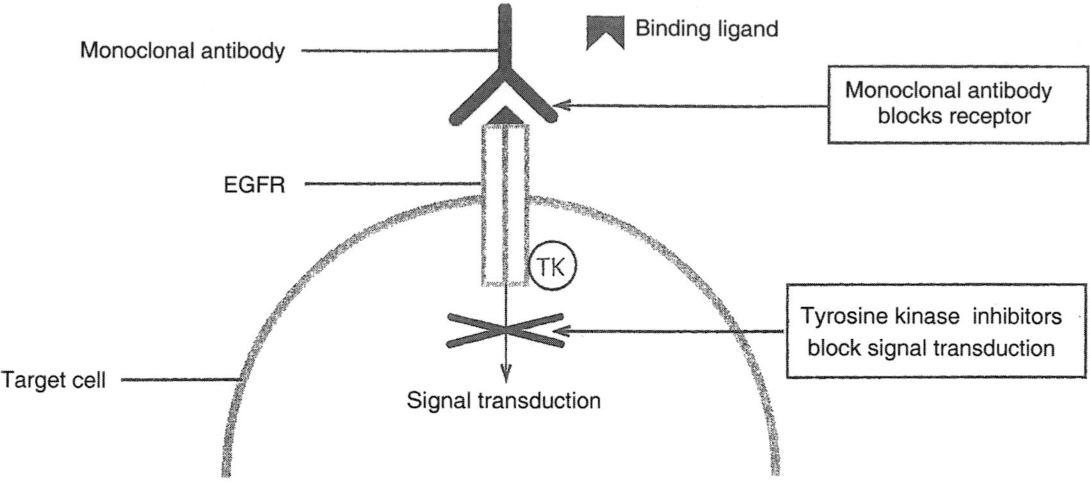

Figure 2 Mechanisms of anti-EGFr Mab inhibition: Mab binding to receptor blocks ligand interactions which results in inhibition of tyrosine kinase activation along with several proliferative signaling pathways that are associated with antiapoptotic, pro-proliferative signaling processes. *Source*: Adapted from Bristol-Myers Squibb Oncology.

(Rituxan™). Rituximab is a chimeric Mab which binds to the CD20 Ag, a differentiation Ag found on developing and mature B cells. Over 90% of non-Hodgkin's lymphomas express CD20 (68).

In a pivotal phase II trial, McLaughlin et al. (69) treated low-grade NHL patients refractory to chemotherapy with weekly infusions of rituximab for a duration of 4 weeks. The ORR was 48%. More importantly, durable responses occurred as late as 6 months after treatment and lasted for a median of 11 months. Side effects were mild and included minor allergic-type reactions. Ten percent of patients had grade 3–4 toxicity including neutropenia, thrombocytopenia, hypotension, bronchospasm, angioedema, and recurrence of pre-existing cardiac conditions. Ninety-seven percent completed all four infusions.

Since FDA approved rituximab has had potential in combination with chemotherapy (70), resulting in higher initial response rates and more prolonged time to progression (TTP). Rituximab has also shown promise in other hematologic malignancies and autoimmune diseases such as chronic lymphocytic leukemia (71), immune thrombocytopenic purpura (72), and autoimmune hemolytic anemia (73). A presumptive mechanism for its efficacy in the latter two diseases is prolonged B-cell lymphopenia with decrease in auto-antibody formation.

Trastuzumab (Herceptin™) is a humanized Mab which has been recently approved for the treatment of metastatic breast cancer. Trastuzumab binds to the HER2/neu oncoprotein receptor, a member of the EGFr family (74). The receptor is expressed in 30% of breast cancers and is associated with a poor prognosis (75). By binding to the EGFr receptor, the Mab inhibits ligand binding and subsequent downstream signaling pathways involved in tumor mitogenesis, motility, and invasion (Fig. 2).

Cobleigh et al. (76) performed a phase II trial of trastuzumab in which patients received a loading dose of 4 mg/kg i.v. followed by 2 mg/kg weekly. Toxicity was minimal and the ORR was 15%. Based on preclinical data that demonstrated that trastuzumab had additive or synergistic effects on tumors when combined with chemotherapy (77), a randomized, multicenter phase III trial was performed in which response rate, TTP, and overall survival (OS) were compared for patients who received adriamycin/cytoxan (AC) or taxol (T) alone at the time of first relapse for metastatic disease to a combination of either AC + Herceptin (H) or T + H. The ORR, TTP, and OS were significantly better for both AC + H and T + H compared to either drug alone (78). A downside to treatment with the combination of AC + H, however, was an increased incidence of cardiac toxicity. Additional trials of other chemotherapy drugs including platinum compounds and Herceptin appear promising and Mab/drug combinations are being compared to chemotherapy alone in the adjuvant situation. Another Mab from the EGFr receptor family which has been shown to synergize with chemotherapy and/or radiation is cetuximab, an IgG1 chimeric Mab which binds to the EGFr. Cetuximab has recently shown promise when combined with chemotherapy for the treatment of head and neck cancer and pancreatic cancer (79,80).

Several other Mab have been approved for cancer treatment especially for hematological malignancies. For a review, see Ref. 81.

Mab have also shown promise when conjugated to radionuclides, drugs, or toxins. Ibritumomab tiuxetan (Zevalin™), an anti-CD20 murine Mab chelated to the radioactive isotope yttrium-90 (^{90}Y), was shown to induce significant tumor responses in low-grade NHL patients in phase I/II trials (82). A randomized phase III trial comparing Zevalin to rituximab demonstrated a superior ORR (80% vs. 56%) and CR rate (30% vs. 16%) for Zevalin. The TTP for each agent was similar at 11 months (83). In combined studies of Zevalin (84), toxicity was primarily hematologic and consisted of grade 4 reversible neutropenia, thrombocytopenia, and anemia in 30%, 10%, and 3% of patients, respectively. Based on these encouraging results, Zevalin has been recently approved for the treatment of recurrent/refractory low-grade follicular NHL. Similar results have been observed with anti-CD20 murine Mab coupled to iodine-131 (Bexxar™) (85). Clinical trials of high-dose radioimmunotherapy with ^{131}I-labeled anti-CD20 Mab followed by peripheral blood stem-cell reconstitution have been impressive, with complete response rates close to 80% and the majority of NHL patients surviving beyond 5 years free of recurrent disease (86). Additional trials combining Zevalin or Bexxar with standard or high-dose chemotherapy are in progress.

A number of preclinical and clinical studies have evaluated the effect of plant [i.e., ricin (R) and gelonin (G)] or bacterial [i.e., diphtheria (DT) and pseudomonas exotoxin (PE)] toxins coupled to Mab for their effects on inhibition of tumor growth (reviewed in Ref. 87). The majority of toxin molecules consist of an alpha (α) chain, which upon internalization into the cell inhibits protein synthesis, and a beta (β) chain, which binds to galactose residues on the cell and assists entry of the α chain. Immunotoxins have been constructed by coupling the Mab to the α chain or the whole molecule along with a "blocking" sugar residue to inhibit nonspecific binding of the β chain to cells. Fewer toxin conjugates have been approved to date due to their modest antitumor effects along with significant toxicities, including a "vascular leak" phenomenon and liver abnormalities. Despite these problems, one toxin, DAB-IL-2 (Ontak™), has been approved for the treatment of hairy-cell leukemia. Ontak is not actually a whole Mab but consists of recombinant DNA resulting from a fusion of genes for IL-2 and PE.

Several Mab conjugated to drugs such as adriamycin or oligomycin (88,89) have been tested in the clinic. Mylotarg™, consisting of an anti-CD33 Mab (gemtuzumab) which binds to an acute leukemia Ag conjugated to oligomycin has been approved for the treatment of acute myelogenous leukemia (90).

Mab have also been evaluated as anti-idiotype vaccines (reviewed in Ref. 90) or for other nonmalignant conditions, including prevention and treatment of transplant rejection (91), respiratory syncytial virus (RSV) infections (92), rheumatoid arthritis (93), and septic shock (94).

In summary, the use of Mab for cancer treatment and other conditions appears extremely promising. Future directions include the development of "bifunctional" Mab (Fig. 3). Identification of novel targets such as vascular endothelial growth factor (VEGF) (95), along with novel routes of Mab administration [i.e., intraperitoneal (96,97) and intracranial (98)], should solidify Mab/immunoconjugates along with IFN, IL-2, and growth factors as the fourth major modality of cancer treatment.

E. Vaccines

Tumor vaccines refer to a means of active immunization against tumors in contrast to adoptive immunotherapy where immune cells or products are given, either for secondary prevention of tumor recurrence, or induction of tumor regression. Therapeutic anticancer vaccines differ from traditional vaccines against viruses and bacteria for primary prevention of infection. Furthermore, traditional vaccines are mostly designed to induce antibody stimulation by B cells while tumor vaccines are designed to stimulate T-cell responses.

Antitumor immunity is mostly mediated by T lymphocytes. CD8+ CTLs, and to lesser degree CD4+ T cells ("helper" cells), have been found to mediate most of the antitumor effects in animal models (99). In humans, the most convincing evidence of endogenous immune responses against cancer has been observed in melanoma and CML. In CML patients, antiproteinase 3 CD8 cells are found only in patients with sustained remission after IFN treatment and bone marrow transplantation, modalities to stimulate T-cell responses, but not in patients who are not in remission and who were treated with chemotherapy (100). For melanoma, CD4 and CD8 lymphocytes have been detected infiltrating tumor sites, circulating in the peripheral blood and residing in lymph nodes of melanoma patients (101,102). In recent years, many antigens recognized by these T cells (tumor-associated antigens, TAAs) have been molecularly cloned from cDNA expression libraries of the tumor cells. They can be divided into three categories: differentiation antigens that are expressed in malignant cells as well as in normal counterparts (such as Mart-1/Melan A, tyrosinase,

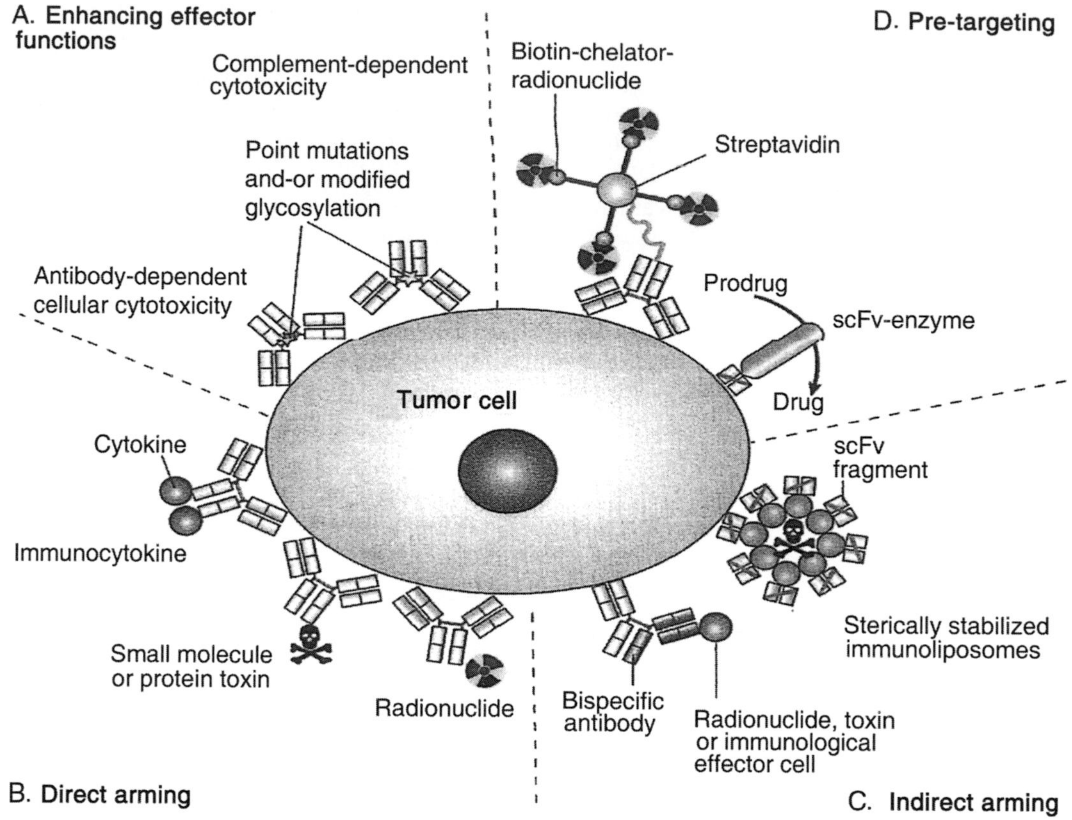

Figure 3 Strategies for enhancing the potency of antitumor antibodies: (A) Enhancing effector function by point mutations in the Fc region. (B) Direct arming with drugs, radionuclides, toxins, and cytokins. (C) Indirect arming by bifunctional Mab or attaching Ab fragment to drug-loaded liposomes. (D) Pretargeting enzyme-linked Mab to tumor followed by enzyme activation (prodrug approach). *Source*: Adapted from Ref. 66.

gp100, and proteinase 3), cancer testis antigens that are expressed in testis and cancer cells, but not in any normal somatic cells (such as Mage antigens), and cancer-specific antigens that are the consequence of mutations of a particular protein in the tumor (103).

Most of the TAAs are intracellular proteins. In order for the T cells to recognize the antigens, the antigen proteins are processed by the cells into short peptides (epitopes) and presented on tumor cells and antigen-presenting cells in association with the major histocompatibility complex (MHC). T cells then recognize the peptide–MHC complexes in an HLA restricted fashion. The most potent cells that can stimulate CTLs are dendritic cells (DCs) that are capable of capturing large amounts of antigen and expressing high level of peptide–MHC and costimulatory molecules to stimulate CTLs. Identification of TAAs, their HLA restricted epitopes, techniques to procure and manipulate CTLs and DCs have provided unprecedented opportunities to treat some cancers immunologically.

The clinical success of immunotherapy has long been evidenced in the setting of bone marrow transplantation pioneered by Dr. E. Donnal Thomas of the Fred Hutchinson Cancer Research Center, who found allogeneic immune response to be crucial in curing leukemia (104). Infusion of antigen-specific CTLs led to regression of tumor nodules bearing the target antigens (105). Although these treatments served to prove the principle of immunotherapy, they carry high degree of toxicity or complexity in preparing the cells. The study of tumor immunology revealed an interesting relationship among the tumor cells and immune cells, in that patients can mount CTL response against tumor antigens through cross-presentation of TAAs by DCs to CD8 T cells (Fig. 4). However, the natural CTL response is not sufficient to eradicate tumors and many such CTLs are incapable of tumor killing (102). Vaccination through DCs is believed to be an attractive intervention point to change the relationship between T cells and tumor cells without much toxicity and complexity of CTL preparation.

There are two different vaccination approaches: direct delivery of antigens to the subjects, where the antigens are picked up by DCs in vivo and presented

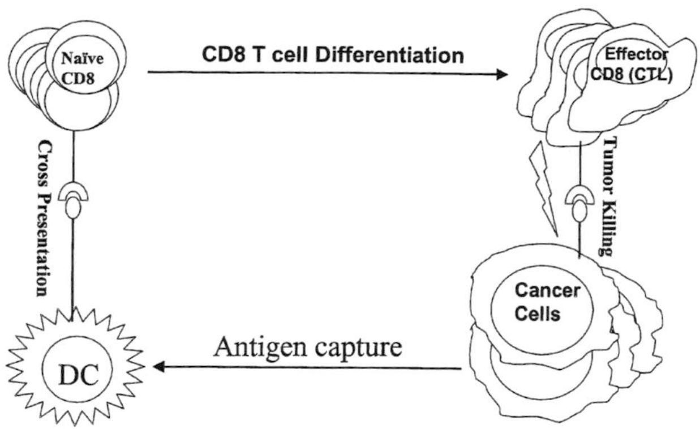

Figure 4 Relationship among tumor cells, dendritic cells and CD8+ T cells. DCs pagocytose apoptosing or necrotic tumor cells, crosspresent the TAAs to naïve CD8 T cells and stimulate them to become CTLs. In patients, such stimulated CTLs may not function well, so tumor cells continue to grow. Vaccination with DCs loaded with TAAs is aimed to CD8 response and tumor regression.

to T cells, and a cell therapy approach, where antigen loaded-DCs are prepared ex vivo and injected into the subject. Peptides and plasmid DNA can be delivered in the former approach, whereas the latter approach can deliver antigens in the forms of peptide, DNA, RNA, apoptotic tumor cells, necrotic tumor cells, cell lysate, and tumor–DC hybrid cells.

The direct delivery approach has the advantage of ease of administration. Peptides can be injected alone or with adjuvants such as incomplete Freud adjuvant, QS-21, or GM-CSF, to subcutaneous tissue. The injected peptides are picked up by DCs and presented to T cells. T-cell stimulations have been observed with this approach and even tumor nodule regressions have been observed on patients (106). Since peptides are HLA restricted, delivery of whole antigen would bypass this limitation. A novel approach employs delivery of attenuated intracellular bacteria such as *Salmonella*, *Shigella*, and *Listeria* species that are transformed with the tumor antigen. After the bacteria are given orally, they transmigrate across mucosa and are phagocytosed by DCs. The DCs can then crosspresent the antigens to T cells (Fig. 4) (107). Such an approach has been shown to stimulate T-cell responses in animals. Clinical trials are planned and it would be very interesting to observe whether this technique is efficacious in cancer patients.

Most clinical trials have taken the form of cell therapy although there is no clear evidence for its superiority to the direct delivery approach. There are two functional states of DCs, immature and mature. Dendritic cells residing in the subcutaneous tissues or submucosa are immature DCs capable of antigen capture. They become capable of T-cell stimulation only when they become mature DCs after stimulation with inflammatory signals (108). How to mature the DCs seems critical in T-cell stimulation and in the breaking of "immune tolerance," particularly for antigens expressed on normal tissues. The cell therapy approach may render a better ex vivo manipulation on this process than the direct delivery approach. An example of such an advantage is illustrated in the case of HLA-A1 restricted MAGE-A3 peptide vaccination, where the cell therapy approach generated polyclonal T-cell stimulation while the direct injection approach only gave rise to monoclonal stimulation (109). Table 6 lists clinical trial results using both approaches.

In the cell therapy approach, it seems that the effectiveness of the vaccine is mostly governed by maturation status of DCs and how antigens are loaded onto the DCs. For an antigen whose gene has been isolated and immunogenic epitopes have been identified, the choice of antigen forms may include peptide, protein, DNA, or RNA encoding the antigen. Peptides are suitable for mass production and easy to load onto DC. Clinical trials of peptide vaccines have resulted in the stimulation of cytotoxic T cells with regression of some tumor nodules (Table 6). However, peptides tend to stimulate CTLs with low TCR avidity, and it is difficult to pulse DCs with multiple peptides covering most of Class I and Class II alleles. This problem can be bypassed by loading the DC with protein, DNA, or RNA encoding the whole antigen protein. Although proteins are difficult to prepare, DNA and RNA can be easily obtained in large quantity, and be molecularly engineered to stimulate both $CD4^+$ and $CD8^+$ T cells. Most of techniques to introduce DNA rely on viral vectors that may be complicated with issues such as safety and immunogenicity against the vector. Recently, adenovirus vector- and alpha virus-based vaccines have been tested in animals and they seem promising. In addition, nonviral DNA transfection techniques are being developed utilizing electroporation, lipid, or polymer. It would be interesting to see how efficient any of these techniques will be in eliciting T-cell responses against tumor. RNA-transfected DCs have many advantages because expression of antigens from mRNAs is transient and is not dependent on promoters or vectors, as compared with DNA-vector-based vaccines, therefore eliminating vector immunogenicity and potential insertional mutagenesis and oncogenesis due to persistent expression of pro-oncogenic tumor antigens, such as E7 of HPV. In addition, RNA-transfected DCs have been shown to be more potent in stimulating CTL activity than DNA transfected DC (119) and peptide pulsed DCs (X. Liao,

Table 6 Examples of Tumor Vaccine Clinical Trials

Antigen used	Adjuvant	No. of points	T cell response	Clinical response	Ref.
MAGE-A3.A1 peptide	None	25	Monoclonal	4 PR, 3 CR	106,109
Tyrosinase A2 peptide	QS-21	9	2	0	110
NY-ESO-1 A2 peptide	No	9	7	1 Nodule PR 4 Nodules CR	111
Gp100 A2 peptide	No	7	7	0	112
Melanoma peptides	DC	16	11	2 CR, 3 PR	113
MAGE-3 A1 peptide	DC	11	8	8 PR	114
MART-1 A2 peptide	DC	7	1	1 PR	115
Melanoma peptides	DC	14	5	2 PR	116
PSA RNA	DC	13	13	6 SD	117
Renal Ca cells	DC hybrid	17		4 CR, 2 PR	118

Abbreviations: CR, complete response; PR, partial response; SD, stable disease; DC, dentritic cell.

submitted for publication). Clinical trials using RNA-transfected DCs in prostate cancer and colon cancer showed little toxicity and some efficacy in clearing the circulating cancer cells (117). For suspected antigens that are not identified, one can load the DCs with whole cellular content, either DCs pulsed with tumor cell lysate (120) or whole cellular RNA (121,122), or in the form of tumor cell–DC fusion (118).

In summary, there is no doubt that T cells play a critical role in regression of some cancers, and DCs are the most effective way to stimulate them. Although the principle of tumor vaccine has been proven, it is very important to note that tumor vaccine development is still in its infancy. Successful development of tumor vaccines as a part of cancer treatment regimen has to await the resolution of some important issues, such as tumor heterogeneity, and efficient T-cell expansion after immunization. Other important areas for research include testing of sufficient adjuvants, the use of costimulatory molecules to boost CD4 T-cell responses, and methods to overcome host tolerance and enhance CD8 T-cell proliferation and function at the tumor site. Attention to these details should hopefully make vaccines an important part of the biotherapy armamentarium.

F. Gene Therapy: Antisense Oligodeoxynucleotides

The notion of synthesizing short single-stranded DNA segments to inhibit the expression of specific genes was suggested for more than two decades ago. The earliest attempt to inhibit gene expression using antisense oligodeoxynucleotides (oligos) was reported in 1978 (123).

Antisense oligos are short sequences of DNA that selectively bind target mRNA molecules by Watson–Crick base pairing, which results in the inhibition of mRNA processing or translation. This inhibition occurs through various mechanisms including prevention of mRNA transport, splicing, and translational arrest (Fig. 5) (124). If that protein is essential for the survival of the cell, then blocking its production should bring about the death of the cell (125). Several genes known to be important for the regulation of apoptosis, cell growth, metastasis, and angiogenesis have been identified as potential targets for cancer therapy.

Antisense technology is attractive for several reasons. First, antisense drugs have the potential to offer affinity and specificity many orders of magnitude higher than the traditional chemotherapy drugs. Second, these drugs have the potential to target any mRNA molecule. This is because natural phosphodiester oligos are rapidly hydrolyzed in vivo by nucleases (126,127). The majority of experimental work and all the clinical trials have been performed using phosphorothioate oligos (128). In contrast, the phosphorothioate oligo analogs (in which sulfur substitutes one of the nonbridging oxygen atoms in the phosphate backbone) are more stable because they are more resistant to endo- and exonucleases (129,130).

By inhibiting the target gene expression, antisense oligos can induce sequence-dependent toxicity. However, antisense oligos have also been found to induce sequence independent toxicity. Antisense oligos may inadvertently inhibit the expression of a gene that is not the initial target because of its sequence homology to the original target. Furthermore, the first generation of phosphorothioate oligos can produce anticoagulant effects (131,132) and complement activation. Neither of these toxicities has contributed to major clinical problems, and can be managed by maintaining peak plasma concentrations below threshold concentrations

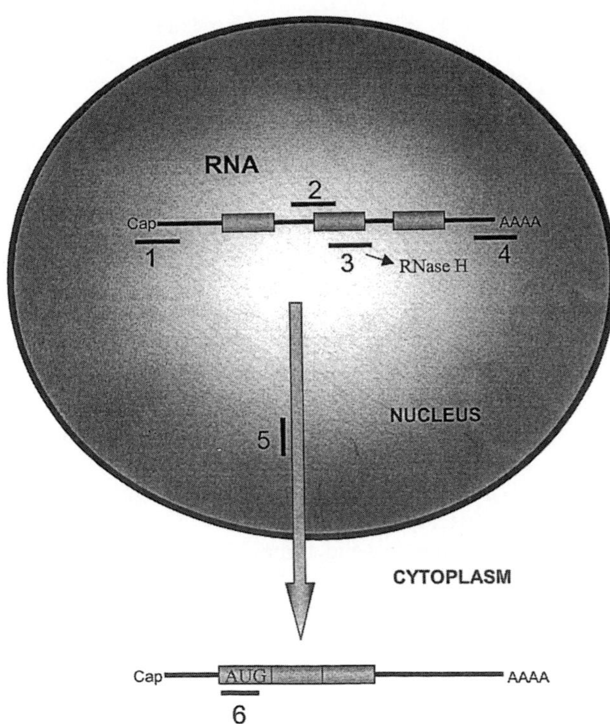

Figure 5 Mechanisms by which antisense oligonucleotides inhibit protein expression: **1**, inhibiting 5′-Cap formation; **2**, inhibiting RNA splicing; **3**, activating RNase H; **4**, inhibiting mRNA polyadenilation; **5**, inhibiting mRNA transport, **6**, inhibiting protein translation.

(133). But this may prevent administration of sufficient doses for the antisense oligos to induce significant tumor inhibition.

It is possible that a new antisense will produce a surprising toxicity not previously seen with other antisense oligos (134). With proper planning, the toxicity studies can be initiated before completion of the preclinical pharmacology studies so that the toxicology studies do not cause delays in getting the new antisense drug into clinical trials.

The application of antisense oligos as therapeutic agents in oncology has been proposed for more than two decades. Several oncogene products, most notably *bcl-2*, *c-raf-1*, protein kinase C-[alpha], and *H-ras*, have been evaluated as targets for therapeutic inhibition, and oligos designed to inhibit the expression of these gene have been studied extensively in phase I and II clinical trials. Inhibition of target expression in tumor (non-Hodgkin's lymphoma) and surrogate tissues has been demonstrated in several of these trials (135,136). Continuous infusion over 2–3 weeks appears preferable to weekly administration for toxicity and downregulation of target gene expression.

The first antisense oligo to be evaluated in clinical trials was targeted to the tumor suppressor gene *p53* and was administered to patients with acute myelogenous leukemia and myelodysplastic syndrome (137). Antisense oligos against the *bcl-2* oncogene (G3139; Genta Inc., San Diego, CA) were next evaluated in a phase I study with 11 patients who had prostate cancer. The serine/threonine kinase *c-raf* has been the subject of three phase I trials using distinct treatment schedules; five cases of grade 3 anemia were found in a thrice-weekly regimen of *c-raf* antisense (ISIS 5132; Isis Pharmaceuticals, Inc., Carlsbad, CA) (138). Antisense oligos targeted to protein kinase C-[alpha] # ISIS 3521, have been studied extensively in phase I and II clinical trials, as a continuous intravenous infusion in 21 patients with different cancers (139). Also, an antisense inhibitor of *H-ras* translation (ISIS 2503; Isis Pharmaceuticals, Inc.) has been evaluated alone and in combination with conventional chemotherapy in three phase I trials.

The efficacy data available suggest that antisense therapy alone could limit disease progression in some patients, but rarely induces major tumor responses. The specificity and tolerability of these oligos prompted the investigation of combining antisense oligos with chemotherapy, and early combination studies have yielded results of interest. Antisense oligos against *bcl-2*, *c-raf-1*, and protein kinase C-[alpha] continue to be the major focus of ongoing clinical trials.

In summary, there is increasing evidence that antisense can work in a sequence-specific manner in patients and finally live up to their promise. Antisense strategies which aim at restoration of apoptosis signaling, alteration of signaling pathways involved in cell proliferation, or targeting to the tumor's microvasculature may prove particularly useful in combination with conventional cancer therapeutic agents. By lowering the apoptotic threshold of cancer cells, antisense oligos could prove to be a very attractive strategy to overcome chemotherapy and radiation resistance. Currently much effort is devoted to making second generation of antisense oligo analogues that have higher antisense activity but reduced nonspecific toxicity.

III. BIOTHERAPY-RELATED SIDE EFFECTS

Select characteristics of biotherapy-related side effects differ from those associated with chemotherapy. As with chemotherapy, most biotherapy-related toxic effects are dose related; that is, the intensity of the toxic effects increases as the dose is elevated. However, different from some chemotherapeutic agents such as doxorubicin, biotherapy-related toxic effects are typically noncumulative, in that there is not a ceiling dose beyond which a patient can receive no further therapy. Furthermore, most biotherapy-related side effects, myelosuppression included, are readily reversed on cessation of therapy. The timing of side effects also may differ from that of chemotherapy. For example, certain side effects may occur early in therapy and are often termed "acute." Others are manifested late in therapy and are classified as "chronic." Although most side effects are not life threatening, they often have a tremendous impact on the patient's quality of life. The chief side effects associated with each biological agent are shown below (Table 2).

IV. CONCLUSIONS

Advances in molecular biology have essentially made the human genome available as a source of potentially therapeutic biological agents (3,140). Constant discovery of new agents and the refinement of molecules through genetic-engineering techniques will continue to provide new therapeutic avenues. The "molecularization of medicine" has led to a more thorough understanding of the molecular basis of disease and disease pathogenesis. This has led in turn to the development of recombinant proteins for the treatment of disease. Within this context, a more complete understanding of the biology of cancer will lead to increasingly selective therapy and ultimately to repair of underlying cellular defects. Gene therapy is one aspect of this potential that continues to grow, with the number of new strategies and protocols increasing at an exponential rate.

The next 20 years will represent one of the most exciting eras in the management of cancer. The ability to determine the cellular defect for a given cancer and then to design effective therapy may one day become reality. Biotherapy has the potential to be a part of this revolution. Doctors caring for patients receiving biotherapy will be continually challenged to remain abreast of changes in a rapidly expanding field and to chart new territory in developing strategies of care for these patients through clinical practice and research.

REFERENCES

1. Rieger PT. Biotherapy: an overview. In: Rieger PT, ed. Biotherapy: A Comprehensive Overview. 2nd ed. Sudbury: Jones & Bartlett Publishers, 2001:3–37.
2. Oettgen H, Old L. The history of cancer immunotherapy. In: DeVita V, Hellman S, Rosenberg S, eds. Biologic Therapy of Cancer. Philadelphia: W.B. Saunders, 1991:87–119.
3. Oldhan R. Cancer biotherapy: general principles. In: Oldham R, ed. Principles of Cancer Biotherapy. 3rd ed. Dordrecht, The Netherlands: Kluwer Academic Press, 1998:1–15.
4. Mihich E, Fefer A. ed. Biological Response Modifiers: Subcommittee Report National Cancer Institute Monograph. Washington: National Cancer Institute, 1983:63.
5. Mazanet R, Morstyn G, Foote M. Development of biological agents. In: Schilsky R, Milano G, Ratain M, eds. Principles of Antineoplastic Drug Development and Pharmacology. New York: Marcel Dekker Inc, 1996:55–73.
6. Isaacs A, Lindemann J. Virus interference I. The interferon. Proc R Soc Serv 1957; B147:258–267.
7. Cuaron L, Thompson J. The interferons. In: Rieger PT, ed. Biotherapy: A Comprehensive Overview. 2nd ed. Sudbury: Jones & Bartlett, 2001:125–191.
8. Decatris M, Santhanam S, O'Byrne K. Potential of interferon-α in solid tumours part 1. Biodrugs 2002; 16(4):261–281.
9. Cantell KS, Hirvonen S, Kauppinen HL. Production and partial purification of human immune interferon. Methods Enzymol 1986; 119:54–63.
10. Food and Drug Information—Center for Biologics Evaluation and Research. Product Information. Accessed Dec 5, 2003 http://www.fda.gov/cber/index.html.
11. Medical Economics Staff, ed. Physicians' Desk Reference 2003. Medical Economics Company Inc.: Montvale, NJ.
12. Samuel CE. Antiviral actions of interferons. Clin Microbiol Rev 2001; 4:778–809.
13. Barber GN. The interferons and cell death; guardians of the cell or accomplices of apoptosis. Semin Cancer Biol 2000; 10(20):103–111.
14. Folkman J. Role of angiogenesis in tumor growth and metastasis. Semin Oncol 2002; 29(6 suppl 16):15–18.
15. Ezekowitz RAB, Mulliken JB, Folkman J. Interferon alpha-2a therapy for life-threatening hemangiomas of infancy. N Engl J Med 1992; 326(22):1455–1463.
16. Kirkwood J. Cancer immunotherapy: the interferon-alpha experience. Semin Oncol 2002; 29(3 suppl 7):18–26.
17. Jonasch E, Haluska FG. Interferon in oncological practice: review of interferon biology, clinical applications, and toxicities. Oncologist 2001; 6(1):34–55.
18. Morris AK, Valley AW. Overview of the management of AIDS-related Kaposi's sarcoma. Ann Pharmacother 1996; 30(10):1150–1163.
19. Krown SE, Li P, Von Roenn JH, Paredes J, Huang J, Testa MA. Efficacy of low-dose interferon with antiretroviral therapy in Kaposi's sarcoma: a randomized phase II AIDS clinical trials group study. J Interferon Cytokine Res 2002; 22(3):295–303.
20. Goldman JM. Therapeutic strategies for chronic myeloid leukemia in the chronic (stable) phase. Semin Hematol 2003; 40(1 suppl 2):10–17.
21. Terando A, Sabel MS, Sondak VK. Melanoma: adjuvant therapy and other treatment options. Curr Treat Options Oncol 2003; 4(3):187–199.

22. Kirkwood J. Adjuvant IFNα2 therapy of melanoma. Lancet 1998; 351:1901–1903.
23. Solal-Celigny, Lepage PE, Brousse N, Tendler CL, Brice P, Haioun C, Gabarre J, Pignon B, Tertian G, Bouabdallah R, Rossi JF, Doyen C, Coiffier B. Doxorubicin-containing regimen with or without interferon alpha-2b for advanced follicular lymphomas: final analysis of survival of toxicity in the Groupe d'Etude des Lymphomes Folliculaires 86 trial. J Clin Oncol 1998; 16(7):2332–2338.
24. McLaughlin P. Progress and promise in the treatment of indolent lymphomas. Oncologist 2002; 7(3): 217–225.
25. McHutchison JG, Fried MW. Current therapy for hepatitis C: pegylated interferon and ribavirin. Clin Liver Dis 2003; 7(1):149–161.
26. Interimmune. Actimmune–Gamma Interferon 1b (Package Insert). Brisbane: InterMune, Inc., 2001.
27. Rudick RA. Contemporary immunomodulatory therapy for multiple sclerosis. J Neuroophthalmol 2001; 21(4):284–291.
28. Filippini G, Munari L, Incorvaia B, Ebers GC, Polman C, D'Amico R, Rice GP. Interferons in relapsing remitting multiple sclerosis: a systematic review. Lancet 2003; 361(9357):545–552.
29. Kirkwood JM, Bender C, Agarwala S, Tarhini A, Shipe-Spotloe J, Smelko B, Donnelly S, Stover L. Mechanisms and management of toxicities associate with high-dose interferon alpha-2g therapy. J Clin Oncol 2002; 20(17):3703–3718.
30. Dean G. Fatigue. In: Rieger PT ed. Biotherapy: A Comprehensive Overview. 2nd ed. Sudbury: Jones & Bartlett, 2001:547–575.
31. Abbas AK, Pober JS, Lichtman AH. Cellular and Molecular Immunology. 5th ed. Philadelphia: W.B. Saunders, 2003.
32. Dinarello C, Mier J. Current concepts: lymphokines. N Engl J Med 1987; 317(15):940–945.
33. Oppenheim J. Forward. In: Thomson A, ed. The Cytokine Handbook. 3rd ed. San Diego, CA: Academic Press, 1998:xviii–xxii.
34. Hurst SD, Muchamuel T, Gorman DM, Gilbert JM, Clifford T, Kwan S, Menon S, Seymour B, Jackson C, Kung TT, Brieland JK, Zurawski SM, Chapman RW, Zurawski G, Coffman RL. New IL-17 family members promote Th1 or Th2 responses in the lung: in vivo function of the novel cytokine IL-25. J Immunol 2002; 169(1):443–453.
35. Fickenscher H, Hor S, Kupers H, Knappe A, Wittmann S, Sticht H. The interleukin-10 family of cytokines. Trends Immunol 2002; 23(2):89–96.
36. Goldsby RA, Kindt TJ, Osborne BA. Kuby immunology. Cytokines [Chap. 12]. 4th ed. New York: W.H. Freeman, 2000.
37. Morgan D, Ruscetti F, Gallo R. Selective in vitro growth of T lymphocytes from normal human bone marrows. Science 1976; 193(4257):1007–1008.
38. Chiron. Package insert. PROLEUKIN® (aldesleukin), recombinant human interleukin-2 (rhIL-2). Emeryville, CA.
39. Atkins MB. Interleukin-2: clinical applications. Semin Oncol 2002; 29(suppl 7):12–17.
40. Mier JW, Atkins MB. Interleukin-2. In: DeVita VT Jr, Hellamn S, Rosenberg SA, ed. Cancer Principles and Practice of Oncology: 6th ed. Philadelphia: Lippincott–Williams & Wilkins, 2001:471–478.
41. Demetri GD, Vadhan-Raj S. Hematopoietic Growth Factors. Cancer Management: A Multidisciplinary Approach. 4th ed. 2000; 38:747–761.
41a. Rieger PT. Biotherapy: The fourth modality of therapy. In: Barton-Burke, M, ed. Cancer Chemotherapy: A Nursing Process Approach. Boston: Jones & Bartlett Publishers, 1996.
42. Anderson JR, Anderson PN, Armitage JO, Beckhardt S, Bennett CL, Bodey GP, Crawford J, Davidson NE, Demetri GD, Hamm JT, Hillner B, Kardinal CG, Levine MN, Miller JA, Ochs JJ, Santana VM, Schiffer CA, Shea TC, Smith TJ, Vadhan-Raj S, Wade JL III, Weeks JC, Winn RJ. Recommendation for the use of hematopoietic colony-stimulating factors: evidence-based, clinical practice guidelines. J Clin Oncol 1994; 14(6):2471–2508.
43. Rizzo JD, Lichtin AE, Woolf SH, Seidenfeld J, Bennett CL, Cella D, Djulbegovic B, Goode MJ, Jakubowski AA, Lee SJ, Miller CB, Rarick MU, Regan DH, Browman GP, Gordon MS. Use of epoetin in patients with cancer: evidence-based clinical practice guidelines of the American Society of Clinical Oncology and the American Society of Hematology. J Clin Oncol 2002; 20(19):4083–4107.
44. Vadhan-Raj S. IL-11: is there evidence to evaluate risks, benefits, and impact on patient outcomes? Oncology 1999; 13(11A).
45. Tepler I, Elias S, Smith JW II, Hussein M, Rosen G, Chang AY, Moore JO, Gordon MS, Kuca B, Beach KJ, Loewy JW, Garnick MB, Kaye JA. A randomized placebo-controlled trial of recombinant human IL-11 in cancer patients with severe thrombocytopenia due to chemotherapy. Blood 1996; 87(9):3607–3614.
46. Vadhan-Raj S, Murray LJ, Bueso-Ramos C, Patel SR, Reddy SP, Hoots WK, Johnston T, Papadopolous NE, Hittelman WN, Johnston DA, Yang TA, Paton VE, Cohen RL, Hellman SD, Benjamin RS, Broxmeyer HE. Stimulation of megakaryocyte and platelet production by a single dose of recombinant human thrombopoietin in patients with cancer. Ann Intern Med 1997; 126(9):673–681.
47. Basser RL, Rasko JE, Clarke K, Cebon J, Green MD, Grigg AP, Zalcberg J, Cohen B, O'Bryne J, Menchaca DM, Fox RM, Begley CG. Randomized, blinded, placebo-controlled phase I trial of pegylated recombinant human megakaryocyte growth and development factor with filgrastim after dose-intensive chemotherapy in patients with advanced cancer. Blood 1997; 89: 3118–3128.

48. Vadhan-Raj S, Verschraegen CF, Bueso-Ramos C, Broxmeyer HE, Kudelka AP, Freedman RS, Edwards CL, Gershenson D, Jones D, Ashby M, Kavanagh JJ. Recombinant human thrombopoietin attenuates carboplatin-induced severe thrombocytopenia and the need for platelet transfusions in patients with gynecologic cancer. Ann Intern Med 2000; 132(5):364–368.
49. Vadhan-Raj S. Clinical experience with recombinant human thrombopoietin in chemotherapy-induced thrombocytopenia. Semin Hematol 2000; 37(2 suppl 4): 28–34.
50. Schiffer CA, Anderson KC, Bennett CL, et al. Platelet transfusion for patients with cancer: clinical practice guidelines of the American Society of Clinical Oncology. J Clin Oncol 2001; 19(5):1519–1538.
51. Vadhan-Raj S, Patel S, Bueso-Ramos CE, Papdopolous N, Burgess A, Broemling LD, Broxmeyer HE, Benjamin RS. Importance of pre-dosing of recombinant human thrombopoietin to reduce chemotherapy induced thrombocytopenia. J Clin Oncol, In press.
52. Vadhan-Raj S, Kavanagh JJ, Freedman RS, Folloder J, Currie LM, Bueso-Ramos C, Verschraegen CF, Narvios AB, Conner J, Hoots WK, Broemeling LD, Lichtiger B. Safety and efficacy of transfusions of autologous cryopreserved platelets derived from recombinant human thrombopoietin to support chemotherapy-associated severe thrombocytopenia: a randomised cross-over study. Lancet 2002; 359(9324): 2145–2152.
53. Kuter DJ, Goodnough LT, Romo J, DiPersio J, Peterson R, Tomita D, Sheridan W, McCullough J. Thrombopoietin therapy increases platelet yields in healthy platelet donors. Blood 2001; 98:1339–1345.
54. McKenna PJ, Korach E, Andresen J. Filgrastim-SD, a sustained duration form of filgrastim. (rhuG-CSF) has similar effects on neutrophil function compared to filgrastim [abstr]. Blood 1998; 92(10) (suppl 1):379a.
55. Johnston E, Crawford J, Blackwell S, Bjurstrom T, Lockbaum P, Roskos L, Yang BB, Gardner S, Miller-Messana MA, Shoemaker D, Garst J, Schwab G. Randomized, dose-escalation study of SD/01 compared with daily filgrastim in patients receiving chemotherapy. J Clin Oncol 2000; 18(13):2522–2528.
56. Holmes FA, O'Shaughnessy JA, Vukelja S, Jones SE, Shogan J, Savin M, Glaspy J, Moore M, Meza L, Wiznitzer I, Neuman TA, Hill LR, Liang BC. Blinded, randomized, multicenter study to evaluate single administration pegfilgrastim once per cycle versus daily filgrastim as an adjunct to chemotherapy in patients with high-risk Stage II or Stage III/IV breast cancer. J Clin Oncol 2002; 20(3):727–731.
57. Green M, Koelbl H, Baselga J, Kubista E, Guillem V, Gascon P, Siena S, Lalisang R, Krippl P, Clemens M, Zani V, Bashir S, Renwick J, Liang B, Piccart M. A randomized, double-blind, phase 3 study evaluating fixed-dose, once-per-cycle pegylated filgrastim (SD/01) vs daily filgrastim to support chemotherapy for breast cancer [abstr]. Proc Am Soc Clin Oncol 2001; 20:23a.
58. Glaspy JA, Jadeja JS, Justice G, Kessler J, Richards D, Schwartzberg L, Tchekmedyian NS, Armstrong S, O'Bryne J, Rossi G, Colowick AB. Darbepoetin alfa given every 1 or 2 weeks alleviates anaemia associated with cancer chemotherapy. Br J Cancer 2002; 87: 268–276.
59. Kotasek D, Berg R, Poulsen E, Colowick A. Randomized, double-blind, placebo controlled, phase I/II dose finding study of ARANESP administered once every three weeks in solid tumor patients [abstr]. Blood 2000; 96:294a.
60. Vansteenkiste J, Pirker R, Massuti B, Barata F, Font A, Fiegl M, Siena S, Gateley J, Tomita D, Colowick AB, Musil J. Double-blind, placebo-controlled, randomized Phase III trial of darbepoetin alfa in lung cancer patients receiving chemotherapy. J Natl Cancer Inst 2002; 94(16):1211–1220.
61. Köhler G, Milstein C. Continuous culture of fused cells secreting antibody of predefined specificity. Nature 1975; 256:495–497.
62. Dillman RO. Monoclonal antibodies in the treatment of malignancy: basic concepts and recent developments. Cancer Invest 2001; 19(8):833–841.
63. Murray JL. Current clinical applications of monoclonal antibodies. Cancer Bull 1991; 43:152–162.
64. Dillman RO. Monoclonal antibodies in treating cancer. Ann Intern Med 1989; 111:592–603.
65. Khazaeli MB, Conry RM, LoBuglio AF. Human immune response to monoclonal antibodies. J Immunol 1994; 15:42–54.
66. Carter P. Improving the efficacy of antibody-based cancer therapies. Nature Rev 2001; 1:118–129.
67. Fishwild DM, O'Donnell SL, Bengoechea T, Hudson DV, Harding F, Bernhard SL, Jones K, Kay RM, Higgins KM, Schramm SR, Lonberg N. High avidity human IgGκ monoclonal antibodies from a novel strain of minilocus transgenic mice. Nat Biotechnol 1996; 14:845–851.
68. Press O, Appelbaum F, Ledbetter J, Martin P, Zarling J, Kidd P, Thomas E. Monoclonal antibody 1F5 (anti-CD20) serotherapy of human B-cell lymphomas. Blood 1987; 69:548–591.
69. McLaughlin P, Grillo-Lopez A, Link B, Leby R, Czuczman M, Williams M, Heyman M, Bence-Bruckler I, White, Cabanillas F, Jain V, Ho A, Lister J, Wey K, Shen D, Dallaire B. Rituximab chimeric anti-CD20 monoclonal antibody therapy for relapsed indolent lymphomas: half of patients respond to a 4-dose treatment program. J Clin Oncol 1998; 16:2825–2833.
69a. Dyer and Osterborg. In: Chesen B, ed. Chronic Lymphocytic Leukemias. NY: Marcel Dekker 2001.
70. Czuczman M, Grillo-Lopez A, White C, Saleh M, Gordon L, LoBuglio F, Jonas C, Klipperstein D, Dallaire B, Varns C. Treatment of patients with low-grade B-cell lymphoma with the combination of chimeric anti-CD20 monoclonal antibody and CHOP chemotherapy. J Clin Oncol 1999; 17:268–276.
71. O'Brien SM, Kantarjian H, Thomas DA, Giles FJ, Freireich EJ, Cortez J, Lener S, Keating MJ. Rituxi-

mab dose-escalation trial in chronic lymphocytic leukemia. J Clin Oncol 2001; 19:2165–2170.

72. Hegde UP, Wilson WH, White T, Cheson B. Rituximab treatment of refractory fludarabine-associated immune thrombocytopenia in chronic lymphocytic leukemia. Blood 2002; 100(6):2260–2262.
73. Zecca M, Nobili B, Ramenghi U, Amendola G, Rosito P, Jankovic M, Perrotta S, Pierani P, De Stefano P, Bonora MR, Locatelli F. Rituximab for the treatment of refractory autoimmune hemolytic anemia in children. Blood 2003; 101(10):3857–3861.
74. Baselga J, Mendelsohn J. Receptor blockade with monoclonal antibodies as anti-cancer therapy. Pharmacol Ther 1994; 64(1):127–154.
75. Slamon DJ, Clark GM, Wong SG, Levin WJ, Ullrich A, McGuire WL. Human breast cancer: correlation of relapse and survival with amplification of the HER-2/neu oncogene. Science 1987; 235(4785):177–182.
76. Cobleigh MA, Vogel CL, Tripathy D, Robert NJ, Scholl S, Fehrenbacher L, Wolter JM, Paton V, Shak S, Lieberman G, Slamon DG. Multinational study of the efficacy and safety of humanized anti-HER2 monoclonal antibody in women who have HER2-overexpressing metastatic breast cancer that has progressed after chemotherapy for metastatic disease. J Clin Oncol 1999; 17(9):2639–2648.
77. Baselga J, Norton L, Albanell J, Kim YM, Mendelsohn J. Recombinant humanized anti-HER2 antibody (Herceptin) enhances the antitumor activity of paclitaxel and doxorubicin against HER2/neu overexpressing human breast cancer xenografts. Cancer Res 1998; 58(13): 2825–2831.
78. Slamon DJ, Leyland-Jones B, Shak S, Fuchs H, Paton V, Bajamonde A, Fleming T, Eiermann W, Wolter J, Pegram M, Baselga J, Norton L. Use of chemotherapy plus a monoclonal antibody against HER2 for metastatic breast cancer that overexpresses HER2. N Engl J Med 2002; 344(11):783–792.
79. Burtness BA, Li Y, Flood W, Mattar BI, Forastiere AA. Phase III trial comparing cisplatin (C)+ placebo (P) to C + anti-epidermal growth factor antibody (EG-R) C225 in patients (pts) with metastatic/recurrent head and neck cancer (HNC) [abstr]. Proc Am Soc Clin Oncol 2002; 21(suppl 1):226a.
80. Burris HA III, Moore MJ, Anderson J, Green MR, Rothenberg ML, Modiano MR, Cripps MC, Portenoy RK, Storniolo AM, Tarassoff P, Nelson R, Dorr FA, Stephens CD, Von Hoff DD. Improvements in survival and clinical benefit with gemcitabine as first-line therapy for patients with advanced pancreas cancer: a randomized trial. J Clin Oncol 1997; 15(6):2403–2413.
81. Alpaugh K, von Mehren M. Monoclonal antibodies in cancer treatment: a review of recent progress. Biodrugs 1999; 12(3):209–236.
82. Wiseman GA, White CA, Stabin M, Dunn WL, Erwin W, Dahlbom M, Raubitschek A, Karvelis K, Schultheiss T, Witzig TE, Belanger R, Spies S, Silberman DHS, Berlfein JR, Ding E, Grillo-Lopez A. Phase I/II ^{90}Y-Zevalin (yttrium-90 ibritumomab tiuxetan, IDEC-Y2B8) radioimmunotherapy dosimetry results in relapsed or refractory non-Hodgkin's lymphoma. Eur J Nucl Med 2000; 27(7):766–777.
83. Witzig TE, Gordon LI, Cabanillas F, Czuczman MS, Emmanouilides C, Joyce R, Pohlman BL, Bartlett NL, Wiseman GA, Padre N, Grillo-Lopez AJ, Multani P, White CA. Randomized controlled trial of yttrium-90-labeled ibritumomab tiuxetan radioimmunotherapy versus rituximab immunotherapy for patients with relapsed or refractory low-grade, follicular, or transformed B-cell non-Hodgkin's lymphoma. J Clin Oncol 2002; 20(10):2453–2463.
84. Witzig TE, White CA, Gordon LI, Wiseman GA, Emmanouilides C, Murray JL, Lister, Multani PS. Safety of yttrium-90 ibritumomab tiuxetan radioimmunotherapy for relapsed low-grade, follicular, or transformed non-Hodgkin's lymphoma. J Clin Oncol 2003; 21(7):1263–1270.
85. Wahl RL, Zasadny KR, MacFarlane D, Francis IR, Ross CW, Estes J, Fisher S, Regan D, Kroll S, Kaminski MS. Iodine-131 anti-b1 antibody for B-cell lymphoma: an update on the Michigan phase I experience. J Nucl Med 1998; 39(suppl):21S–23S.
86. Lui SY, Eary JF, Petersdorf SH, Martin PJ, Maloney DG, Appelbaum FR, Matthews DC, Bush SA, Durack LD, Fisher DR, Gooley TA, Bernstein ID, Press OW. Follow-up of relapsed B-cell lymphoma patients treated with iodine-131-labeled anti-CD20 antibody and autologous stem-cell rescue. J Clin Oncol 1998; 16(10):3270–3278.
87. Frankel AE, Kreitman RJ, Sausville EA. Targeted toxins. Clin Cancer Res 2000; 6(2):326–334.
88. Tolcher AW, Sugerman S, Gelman KA, Cohen R, Saleh M, Isaacs C, Young L, Healey D, Onetto N, Slichenmyer W. Randomized phase II study of BR96-doxorubicin conjugate in patients with metastatic breast cancer. J Clin Oncol 1999; 17(2):247–484.
89. Berger MS, Leopold LH, Dowell JA, Korth-Bradley JM, Sherman ML. Licensure of gemtuzumab ozogamicin for the treatment of selected patients 60 years of age or older with acute myeloid leukemia in first relapse. Invest New Drugs 2002; 20(4):395–406.
90. Bhattacharya-Chatterjee M, Chatterjee SK, Foon KA. The anti-idiotype vaccines for immunotherapy. Curr Opin Mol Ther 2001; 3(1):63–69.
91. Waldmann T, O'Shea J. The use of antibodies against the IL-2 receptor in transplantation. Curr Opin Immunol 1998; 10(5):507–512.
92. Scott L, Lamb H. Palivizumab. Drugs 1999; 58(2): 305–311.
93. Maini RN, Breedveld FC, Kalden JR, Smolen JS Davis D, Macfarlane JD, Antoni C, Leeb B, Elliott MJ Woody JN, Schaible TF, Feldmann M. Therapeutic efficacy of multiple intravenous infusions of anti-tumor necrosis factor alpha monoclonal antibody combined with low-dose weekly methotrexate in rheumatoid arthritis. Arthritis Rheum 1998; 41(9):1552–1563.

94. Quezedo Z, Banks S, Natanso C. New strategies for combating sepsis: the magic bullets missed the mark... but the search continues. Trends Biotechnol 1995; 13(2):56–63.
95. Fox WD, Higgins B, Maiese KM, Drobnjak M, Cordon-Cardo C, Scher HI, Agus DB. Antibody to vascular endothelial growth factor slows growth of an androgen-independent xenograft model of prostate cancer. Clin Cancer Res 2002; 8(10):3226–3231.
96. Rosenblum MG, Verschraegen CF, Murray JL, Kudelka AP, Gano J, Cheung L, Kavanagh JJ. Phase I study of ^{90}Y-labeled B72.3 intraperitoneal administration in patient with ovarian cancer: effects of dose and EDTA coadministration on pharmacokinetics and toxicity. Clin Cancer Res 1999; 5:953–961.
97. Meredith RF, Partridge EE, Alvarez RD, Khazaeli MB, Plott G, Russell CD, Wheeler RH, Lui T, Grizzle WE, Schlom J, LoBuliio AF. Intraperitoneal radioimmunotherapy of ovarian cancer with lutetium-f177-CC49. J Nucl Med 1996; 37(9):1491–1496.
98. Laske DW, Muraszko KM, Oldfield EH, DeVroom HL, Sung C, Dedrick RL, Simon TR, Colandrea J, Copeland C, Katz D, Greenfield L, Groves ES, Houston LL, Youle RJ. Intraventricular immunotoxin therapy for leptomeningeal neoplasia. Neurosurgery 1997; 41:1039–1049.
99. Greenberg PD. Adoptive T cell therapy of tumors: mechanisms operative in the recognition and elimination of tumor cells. Adv Immunol 1991; 49:281–355.
100. Molldrem JJ, Lee PP, Wang C, Felio K, Kantarjian HM, Champlin RE, Davis MM. Evidence that specific T lymphocytes may participate in the elimination of chronic myelogenous leukemia. Nat Med 2000; 6:1018–1023.
101. Yannelli JR, Hyatt C, McConnell S, Hines K, Jacknin L, Parker L, Sanders M, Rosenberg SA. Growth of tumor-infiltrating lymphocytes from human solid cancers: summary of a 5-year experience. Int J Cancer 1996; 65: 413–421.
102. Lee PP, Yee C, Savage PA, Fong L, Brockstedt D, Weber JS, Johnson D, Swetter S, Thompson J, Greenberg PD, Roederer M, Davis MM. Characterization of circulating T cells specific for tumor-associated antigens in melanoma patients. Nat Med 1999; 5:677–685.
103. Rosenberg SA. Progress in human tumour immunology and immunotherapy. Nature 2001; 411:380–384.
104. Appelbaum FR. Haematopoietic cell transplantation as immunotherapy. Nature 2001; 411:385–389.
105. Yee C, Thompson JA, Byrd D, Riddell SR, Roche P, Celis E, Greenberg PD. Adoptive T cell therapy using antigen-specific CD8+ T cell clones for the treatment of patients with metastatic melanoma: in vivo persistence, migration, and antitumor effect of transferred T cells. Proc Natl Acad Sci USA 2002; 99:16168–16173.
106. Marchand M, van Baren N, Weynants P, Brichard V, Dreno B, Tessier MH, Rankin E, Parmiani G, Arienti F, Humblet Y, Bourlond A, Vanwijck R, Lienard D, Beauduin M, Dietrich PY, Russo V, Kerger J, Masucci G, Jager E, De Greve J, Atzpodien J, Brasseur F, Coulie PG, van der Bruggen P, Boon T. Tumor regressions observed in patients with metastatic melanoma treated with an antigenic peptide encoded by gene MAGE-3 and presented by HLA-A1. Int J Cancer 1999; 80:219–230.
107. Dietrich G, Spreng S, Favre D, Viret JF, Guzman CA. Live attenuated bacteria as vectors to deliver plasmid DNA vaccines. Curr Opin Mol Ther 2003; 5:10–19.
108. Banchereau J, Briere F, Caux C, Davoust J, Lebecque S, Liu YJ, Pulendran B, Palucka K. Immunobiology of dendritic cells. Annu Rev Immunol 2000; 18:767–811.
109. Coulie PG, Karanikas V, Lurquin C, Colau D, Connerotte T, Hanagiri T, Van Pel A, Lucas S, Godelaine D, Lonchay C, Marchand M, Van Baren N, Boon T. Cytolytic T-cell responses of cancer patients vaccinated with a MAGE antigen. Immunol Rev 2002; 188:33–42.
110. Lewis JJ, Janetzki S, Schaed S, Panageas KS, Wang S, Williams L, Meyers M, Butterworth L, Livingston PO, Chapman PB, Houghton AN. Evaluation of CD8(+) T-cell frequencies by the Elispot assay in healthy individuals and in patients with metastatic melanoma immunized with tyrosinase peptide. Int J Cancer 2000; 87:391–398.
111. Jager E, Gnjatic S, Nagata Y, Stockert E, Jager D, Karbach J, Neumann A, Rieckenberg J, Chen YT, Ritter G, Hoffman E, Arand M, Old LJ, Knut A. Induction of primary NY-ESO-1 immunity: CD8+ T lymphocyte and antibody responses in peptide-vaccinated patients with NY-ESO-1+ cancers. Proc Natl Acad Sci USA 2000; 97:12198–12203.
112. Lee KH, Wang E, Nielsen MB, Wunderlich J, Migueles S, Connors M, Steinberg SM, Rosenberg SA, Marincola FM. Increased vaccine-specific T cell frequency after peptide-based vaccination correlates with increased susceptibility to in vitro stimulation but does not lead to tumor regression. J Immunol 1999; 163:6292–6300.
113. Nestle FO, Alijagic S, Gilliet M, Sun Y, Grabbe S, Dummer R, Burg G, Schadendorf D. Vaccination of melanoma patients with peptide- or tumor lysate-pulsed dendritic cells. Nat Med 1998; 4:328–332.
114. Thurner B, Haendle I, Roder C, Dieckmann D, Keikavoussi P, Jonuleit H, Bender A, Maczek C, Schreiner D, von den Driesch P, Brocker EB, Steinman RM, Enk A, Kampgen E, Schuler G. Vaccination with mage-3A1 peptide-pulsed mature, monocyte-derived dendritic cells expands specific cytotoxic T cells and induces regression of some metastases in advanced stage IV melanoma. J Exp Med 1999; 190: 1669–1678.
115. Panelli MC, Wunderlich J, Jeffries J, Wang E, Mixon A, Rosenberg SA, Marincola FM. Phase 1 study in patients with metastatic melanoma of immunization with dendritic cells presenting epitopes derived from

the melanoma-associated antigens MART-1 and gp100. J Immunother 2000; 23:487–498.

116. Mackensen A, Herbst B, Chen JL, Kohler G, Noppen C, Herr W, Spagnoli GC, Cerundolo V, Lindemann A. Phase I study in melanoma patients of a vaccine with peptide-pulsed dendritic cells generated in vitro from CD34(+) hematopoietic progenitor cells. Int J Cancer 2000; 86:385–392.

117. Heiser A, Coleman D, Dannull J, Yancey D, Maurice MA, Lallas CD, Dahm P, Niedzwiecki D, Gilboa E, Vieweg J. Autologous dendritic cells transfected with prostate-specific antigen RNA stimulate CTL responses against metastatic prostate tumors. J Clin Invest 2002; 109:409–417.

118. Kugler A, Stuhler G, Walden P, Zoller G, Zobywalski A, Brossart P, Trefzer U, Ullrich S, Muller CA, Becker V, Gross AJ, Hemmerlein B, Kanz L, Muller GA, Ringert RH. Regression of human metastatic renal cell carcinoma after vaccination with tumor cell-dendritic cell hybrids. Nat Med 2000; 6:332–336.

119. Strobel I, Berchtold S, Gotze A, Schulze U, Schuler G, Steinkasserer A. Human dendritic cells transfected with either RNA or DNA encoding influenza matrix protein M1 differ in their ability to stimulate cytotoxic T lymphocytes. Gene Ther 2000; 7:2028–2035.

120. Geiger JD, Hutchinson RJ, Hohenkirk LF, McKenna EA, Yanik GA, Levine JE, Chang AE, Braun TM, Mule JJ. Vaccination of pediatric solid tumor patients with tumor lysate-pulsed dendritic cells can expand specific T cells and mediate tumor regression. Cancer Res 2001; 61:8513–8519.

121. Nair SK, Morse M, Boczkowski D, Cumming RI, Vasovic L, Gilboa E, Lyerly HK. Induction of tumor-specific cytotoxic T lymphocytes in cancer patients by autologous tumor RNA-transfected dendritic cells. Ann Surg 2002; 235:540–549.

122. Su Z, Dannull J, Heiser A, Yancey D, Pruitt S, Madden J, Coleman D, Niedzwiecki D, Gilboa E, Vieweg J. Immunological and clinical responses in metastatic renal cancer patients vaccinated with tumor RNA-transfected dendritic cells. Cancer Res 2003; 63: 2127–2133.

123. Zamecnik PC, Stephenson ML. Inhibition of Rous sarcoma virus replication and cell transformation by a specific oligodeoxynucleotide. Proc Natl Acad Sci USA 1978; 75:280–284.

124. Hoke GD, Draper K, Freier SM, Gonzalez C, Driver VB, Zounes MC, Ecker DJ. Effects of phosphorothioate capping on antisense oligonucleotide stability, hybridization and antiviral efficacy versus herpes simplex virus infection. Nucleic Acids Res 1991; 19(20): 5743–5748.

125. Stein CA, Narayanan R. Antisense oligodeoxynucleotides. Curr Opin Oncol 1994; 6:587–594.

126. Cotter FE, Johnson P, Hall P, Pocock C, al Mahdi N, Cowell JK, Morgan G. Antisense oligonucleotides suppress B-cell lymphoma growth in a SCID-hu mouse model. Oncogene 1994; 9(10):3049–3055.

127. Crooke ST. Therapeutic applications of oligonucleotides. Ann Rev Pharmacol Toxicol 1992; 32:329–376.

128. Akhtar S, Kole R, Juliano RL. Stability of antisense DNA oligodeoxynucleotide analogs in cellular extracts and sera. Life Sci 1991; 49:1793–1801.

129. Crooke RM, Graham MJ, Cooke ME, Crooke ST. In vitro pharmacokinetics of phosphorothioate antisense oligonucleotides. J Pharmacol Exp Ther 1995; 275: 462–473.

130. Milligan JF, Matteucci MD, Martin JC. Current concepts in antisense drug design. J Med Chem 1993; 36:1923–1937.

131. Henry SP, Novotny W, Leeds J, Auletta C, Kornbrust DJ. Inhibition of coagulation by a phosphorothioate oligonucleotide. Antisense Nucleic Acids Drug Dev 1997; 7:503–510.

132. Sheehan JP, Phan TM. Phosphorothioate oligonucleotides inhibit the intrinsic tenase complex by an allosteric mechanism. Biochemistry 2001; 40:4980–4989.

133. Henry SP, Giclas PC, Leeds J, Pangburn M, Auletta C, Levin AA, Kornbrust DJ. Activation of the alternative pathway of complement by a phosphorothioate oligonucleotide: potential mechanism of action. J Pharmacol Exp Ther 1997; 281(2):810–816.

134. Black LE, Farrelly JG, Cavagnaro JA, Ahn CH, DeGeorge JJ, Taylor AS, DeFelice AF, Jordan A. Regulatory considerations for oligonucleotide drugs: updated recommendations for pharmacology and toxicology studies. Antisense Res Dev 1994; 4(4): 299–301.

135. Kitada S, Miyashita T, Tanaka S, Reed JC. Investigations of antisense oligonucleotides targeted against *bcl-2* RNAs. Antisense Res Dev 1993; 3:157–169.

136. Kitada S, Takayama S, De Riel K, Tanaka S, Reed JC. Reversal of chemoresistance of lymphoma cells by antisense-mediated reduction of *bcl-2* gene expression. Antisense Res Dev 1994; 4:71–79.

137. Bayever E, Iversen PL, Bishop MR, Sharp JG, Tewary KH, Arneson MA, Pirruccello SJ, Ruddon RW, Kessinger A, Zon G. Systemic administration of a phosphorothioate oligonucleotide with a sequence complementary to p53 for acute myelogenous leukemia and myelodysplastic syndrome: initial results of a phase I trial. Antisense Res Dev 1993; 3(4):383–390.

138. Stevenson JP, Yao KS, Gallagher M, Friedland D, Mitchell EP, Cassella A, Monia B, Jesse Kwoh T, Yu R, Holmlund J, Andrew Dorr F, O'Dwyer PJ. Phase I clinical/pharmacokinetic and pharmacodynamic trial of the *c-raf-1* antisense oligonucleotide ISIS 5132 (CGP 69846A). J Clin Oncol 1999; 17:2227–2236.

139. Yuen AR, Halsey J, Fisher GA, Holmlund JT, Geary RS, Kwoh TJ, Dorr A, Sikic BI. Phase I study of an antisense oligonucleotide to protein kinase C-alpha (ISIS 3521/CGP 64128A) in patients with cancer. Clin Cancer Res 1999; 5(11):3357–3363.

140. Russell C, Clarke L. Recombinant proteins for genetic disease. Clin Genet 1999; 55:389–3394.

7

Bone Marrow Transplantation Complications Requiring Therapy in the Intensive Care Unit

HUMBERTO CALDERA

Department of Medicine, Veterans Affairs Medical Center, West Palm Beach, Florida, U.S.A.

JAMES GAJEWSKI

Department of Blood and Marrow Transplantation, The University of Texas M.D. Anderson Cancer Center, Houston, Texas, U.S.A.

I. INTRODUCTION

Bone and marrow transplantation is a therapeutic modality of hematopoietic support enabling the administration of dose-intensive chemotherapy and/or radiation therapy for the treatment of hematologic malignancies and some solid tumors (1–3). Once the transplant has engrafted, donor-derived immunopoiesis gives therapeutic benefits by reducing the risk of relapse in some malignancies (4–7).

According to the source of the stem cells, transplants are divided in: (1) *autologous* transplant, in which the patient receives his/her own cells; (2) *syngeneic* transplants, from identical twins; and (3) *allogeneic* transplant, in which the cells come from individuals genetically different from the patient, including family members, unrelated donors, or cord blood.

The most frequent types of allogeneic bone marrow transplantations performed are those involving human leukocyte antigen (HLA) type-identical siblings. Alternative stem cell sources for those patients without available HLA-identical siblings include: partially HLA-matched family members, matched unrelated donors, and related or unrelated umbilical cord blood (8–12).

Autologous and syngeneic transplants are associated with less risk because the cells will not be immunologically rejected or mediate an immunologic reaction, whereas allogeneic transplants have a greater risk of morbidity and mortality due to the complications related to graft-versus-host disease (GVHD), immunosuppressive drugs, and infection. The incidence and severity of these complications are higher in recipients of unrelated grafts, compared to HLA-matched siblings.

Intensive chemotherapy and/or radiation therapy followed by bone marrow transplantation are associated with many potential complications, including regimen-related toxicities, infections due to neutropenia or post-transplant immunodeficiency, bleeding due to thrombocytopenia, and in the allogeneic setting transplant rejection and GVHD. The transplant-related mortality rate in autologous and allogeneic transplants is about 5–10% and 10–15%, respectively.

The medical management of these patients is very complex and requires a multidisciplinary approach. A bone marrow transplant team includes specialized nursing care, nutritional, pharmacist, and physical therapy support; and close collaboration with virtually all of the medical subspecialties. Despite improvement in transplantation procedures and supportive care, a large number of bone marrow transplant recipients will require at some time intensive care management due to transplant-related complications.

In this chapter, we will summarize some unique clinical situations that can often complicate recipients of blood or marrow transplantation and that require prompt recognition and management by the intensive care team. A more detailed description of GVHD-related complications will be described separately (see Chapter 39).

II. OUTCOME OF BONE MARROW TRANSPLANTATION RECIPIENTS REQUIRING INTENSIVE CARE

Despite adequate selection of transplantation candidates and improvements in supportive care and prophylactic strategies to prevent infections and bleeding complications, a significant proportion of patients undergoing autologous and allogeneic blood and marrow transplantation will develop respiratory failure and other complications requiring intensive care unit (ICU) management and/or mechanical ventilation. It is estimated that 10–40% of patients receiving a transplant will require ICU care, primarily due to respiratory failure (13–19).

Survival rate in transplanted patients with respiratory failure, especially in those requiring mechanical ventilation, is very poor. Single institution studies report a six-month survival ranging from 3% to 5% (14,16–18) to 15% at best (13). Data from MD Anderson Cancer Center showed that although 18% of patients on mechanical ventilation survived the admission to ICU, only 5% were alive at 6 months (5/26 with diffuse alveolar hemorrhage (DAH), 4/33 with pneumonia). Prolonged mechanical ventilation and development of respiratory failure more than 30 days post-transplantation were associated with poorer outcome (18).

Several attempts have been made to identify predictive factors that may allow for better patient risk-stratification and patient/family counseling when intensive care services and/or mechanical ventilation are needed. The Acute Physiologic And Chronic Health Evaluation an (APACHE) II score has been studied in this regard. In a retrospective analysis involving 116 patients, an APACHE score of 45 or more predicted 100% mortality, whereas a less than 35 score underestimated survival in 46% of the cases (13); at least another trial had similar observations (20). At the MD Anderson (18) and other centers (14,15) experience, however, the APACHE II score underestimated mortality and had no correlation with survival.

Respiratory failure requiring mechanical ventilation is the biggest risk factor predicting poor outcome in patients admitted to ICU. Sepsis causing multiorgan failure (14,15), prolonged ICU stay (20), prolonged intubation, and development of pneumonia later than 30 days post-transplantation (18) are also associated with poor survival.

Noninvasive mechanical ventilation has not been yet extensively studied in the transplant setting. A recent promising report (21) showed improved 30-day ICU survival (56%) in oncologic patients—including autologous stem cell transplantation recipients—treated with noninvasive mechanical ventilation as opposed to invasive mechanical ventilation.

Pneumonias caused by bacterial, fungal (especially aspergillosis and *Pneumocystis carinii*), or viral pathogens are responsible for most cases of respiratory failure in post-transplanted patients, followed by DAH. In this chapter, we will elaborate on the clinical aspects and management of DAH and pneumonias caused by cytomegalovirus and community respiratory viruses (influenza, parainfluenza, respiratory syncytial virus (RSV), rhinovirus, adenovirus). Bacterial and fungal pneumonias are (see Chapter 37) described elsewhere in this book.

III. DIFFUSE ALVEOLAR HEMORRHAGE

Pulmonary complications frequently occur after high-dose chemotherapy and autologous or allogeneic stem cell support (22,23). DAH is a noninfectious pulmonary complication that usually manifests as cough, progressive dyspnea, hypoxia, and diffuse consolidation on the chest radiograph in the early post-transplantation period.

Based on results from bronchoscopies and bronchoalveolar lavage (BAL) studies in post-stem cell transplantation patients with pulmonary complications, it has been demonstrated that DAH is the leading noninfectious cause of respiratory failure and admission to the ICU in the transplantation setting (18,23–25).

The diagnostic criteria for DAH are: (a) widespread alveolar injury (multilobar pulmonary infiltrate), symptoms and signs of pneumonia, increased alveolar to arterial oxygen gradient in the arterial blood examination; (b) absence of an infectious cause to explain the clinical picture; and (c) BAL showing progressively bloodier return from three separate subsegmental bronchi or the presence of 20% or more hemosiderin-laden macrophages in the lung tissue (22,23,26,27).

Radiographic manifestations of DAH are nonspecific and usually precede clinical symptoms. In a study reported by Witte et al. (28) evaluating 39 cases of DAH; initial radiologic manifestations were evident 11 days post-transplantation. All patients had abnormalities in the central portions of the lung, primarily middle and lower portions. The initial pattern was interstitial in two-thirds of the patients and alveolar in the rest. More than 80% of the patients had progressive disease with diffuse bilateral radiographic abnormalities involving all lung fields within a week after the diagnosis (28).

The incidence of DAH has been reported to be between 1% and 21% in autologous transplantation, and 2–17% in allogeneic recipients (19,22,23,27,29–41).

Treatment of DAH includes intensive care and ventilatory support. Due to the suspected inflammatory nature of this condition, steroids have been used as primary medical therapy. The University of Nebraska Group (33) reported a retrospective analysis suggesting that high-dose corticosteroid therapy (more than 30 mg of methylprednisolone or its equivalent) compared to low-dose steroids or best supportive care was associated with decreased incidence of respiratory failure and improved survival.

More recently, Lewis et al. (32) reported that 10 of 15 patients treated with methylprednisolone 250 mg to 2 g/day had at least a transient improvement in the respiratory symptoms, however mortality was very high (74%) and no different that prior reports (23).

Smaller reports (36,40,42) have also demonstrated at least transient respiratory improvements with high-dose steroids, although the mortality rate remained higher than 50%.

Recombinant Factor VII (rFVIIa), an activated form of plasma coagulation factor VII that has been approved for the treatment of bleeding in hemophiliac patients, has recently gained attention as a potential treatment for steroid-refractory DAH. Treatment with rFVIIa on boluses of 90 μg/kg has been documented to effectively stop alveolar bleeding in several cases reported by several investigators (29,43,44), even when patients were rechallenged after a second bleeding episode (29).

The outcome of 12 patients with DAH treated at the MD Anderson Cancer Center has been recently reported (45). Fifty-eight percent of the patients were intubated due to respiratory failure. At a median of 1 day after the diagnosis was made, all patients were treated with rFVIIa (median dose and duration were 84 mg/kg/dose for 3.5 days), concurrent high-dose steroids (at least 2 mg/kg/day), aminocaproic acid, platelet transfusion, and antibiotics. Six out of eight patients (75%) that developed DAH "early" after transplantation (less than 30 days) and one out four patients (25%) with "late" DAH (more than 30 days after BMT) survived the event and were discharged from the hospital.

This data suggest that treatment with rFVIIa may be more effective in treating patients with DAH in the early post-transplantation period. Patients who develop DAH late post-transplantation may not have same outcome, probably due to concurrent infectious complications (45). Optimal dosage and duration of treatment with rFVIIa have not yet been established. Elevated costs (up to $200,000 for a 16-day course) remain the most significant limitation for this therapy.

In summary, DAH remains a deadly complication after high-dose chemotherapy and autologous or allogeneic stem cell transplantation. Clinical suspicious and suggestive radiological signs mandate immediate bronchoscopic evaluation. Once the diagnosis is established, aggressive support and medical management must start. At our center, we immediately start high-dose methylprednisolone (1 g IV every day for 3 days, followed by slow taper). Desmopressin (DDAVP), antibiotics, platelet transfusions, and aminocaproic acid are used as adjunct therapy. Randomized clinical trials are needed to assess the role and timing for treatment of DAH with rFVIIa, especially in patients that do not respond to steroid therapy.

IV. VIRAL PNEUMONIAS

The RSV is a very important cause of serious respiratory illness in recipients of autologous and allogeneic stem cell transplantation; it is the commonest and deadliest pathogen among community-acquired viral respiratory infections in the transplant population (46,47).

These infections usually occur during community outbreaks in the fall-winter months (48). Typically patients will have upper respiratory symptoms that can quickly progress to severe pneumonia (in about 50% of the cases) that may be fatal in up to 60–80% of the cases (46–54). Progression from upper respiratory infection to pneumonia is more likely to occur in the early post-transplantation and pre-engraftment periods (48–50,53).

Early recognition is probably the most important factor affecting the outcome of these patients. At our center, all post-transplant patients with acute upper respiratory infections (URI), defined by rhinorrhea, nasal or sinus congestion, otitis media, pharyngitis or cough with a clear chest radiograph, are screened with nasopharyngeal to rule/out the presence of the infection by rapid RSV antigen assay (either by ELISA or indirect immunofluorescence).

Treatment with ribavirin, a synthetic nucleoside analogue with in vivo activity against RNA and DNA viruses (55), has been shown to be effective in the treatment of RSV URI/pneumonia when given parenterally (46,54) or aerosolized, either alone (46,51,52,56,57) or in combination with intravenous immunoglobulin (48,50,53,54).

At the MD Anderson Cancer Center, RSV-URIs are treated with aerosolized ribavirin (2 g) administered via face-mask (patients isolated inside scavenging tents) for 2 hr, every 8 hr. If the patient develops pneumonia, ribavirin is given at 6 g/day over 18 hr every day. Intravenous immunoglobulin (500 mg/kg) is given every other day for the duration of the therapy. The length of treatment will depend on the immunologic status of the patient, clinical response, and duration of viral shedding; typically, a high-risk patient will be treated for 10–14 days. This strategy has resulted in improved responses and survival (48,53).

Early recognition is probably the most important factor affecting the outcome of RSV infections. All post-transplant patients with acute URI, defined by rhinorrhea, nasal or sinus congestion, otitis media, pharyngitis or cough with a clear chest radiograph, must be screened with nasopharyngeal lavage to rule-out the presence of the infection by rapid RSV antigen assay (either by ELISA or direct immunofluorescence). Once the presence of the virus is established, treatment must be promptly started.

Other agents have been proven to be effective in treating RSV infections. The RSV immune globulin (RespiGam) infused as a single dose (1500 mg/kg) to pediatric post-transplant patients resulted in 91% survival (58). Palivizumab, an RSV-specific monoclonal antibody derived from a murine monoclonal antibody (59), has been approved by the FDA for the prophylaxis against hospitalization for RSV infection in high-risk children (premature infants and infants with chronic lung disease) (60,61). At the Fred Hutchinson Cancer Center, 15 patients with RSV infections (URI $n = 3$, pneumonia $n = 12$) were treated with aerosolized ribavirin plus a single intramuscular injection of palivizumab (15 mg/kg). Eighty-three percent of the patients with pneumonia and all with URI survived for 28 days (59). Due to the prohibitively high costs of these drugs, efficacy needs to be demonstrated in larger controlled trials before their routine use in adult patients can be considered.

Although less frequently detected, other respiratory viruses (Rhinovirus, adenovirus, influenza, and parainfluenza) have been associated with fatal pneumonias in recipients of stem cell transplantation.

Parainfluenza virus (PIV) infections have been documented in 2–7% of recipients of bone marrow transplantation by major transplant centers (62–65). In the largest of those studies (62), PIV-3 was the most frequently isolated pathogen. Most patients present with URI symptoms, however, 30–40% will have either concurrent pneumonia at the time of diagnosis or will progress to pneumonia early in the course of the disease. Diagnosis is usually made from direct antibody fluorescence from nasopharyngeal or bronchoalveolar secretions. Steroid therapy (62) and allogeneic vs. autologous transplantation (63) have been described as risk factors for the development of pneumonia. Thirty to thirty-five percent mortality rate have been reported in the early post-transplantation period (62–65), and the Seattle group reported 75% mortality at day 180 (62). Mortality rate seems to be higher in patients with concurrent infections, especially with aspergillosis (62,63).

Treatment of PIV pneumonia with ribavirin (aerosolized or intravenously) with or without intravenous immune globulin has been ineffective (62). Prevention of exposure and surveillance are the most useful strategy at the moment.

Influenza A or B infections can occur during community outbreaks in transplant recipients. Whimbey et al. (66) reported a 29% incidence of infection among transplant recipients during the 1991–92 influenza epidemic in Houston, Texas. Six of eight affected patients developed pneumonia with a 17% mortality rate. Influenza infections (particularly type A) accounted for about 10–18% of all viral respiratory infections in bone marrow transplant recipients during seasonal outbreaks in Seattle (1990–96) (46) and Houston (1992–94) (67). Due to small number of cases reported, little is known about therapeutic strategies. Oral treatment with amantadine and rimantadine has not been effective in these patients (66,68). Anecdotal responses to ribavirin have been reported.

Recent publications by the MD Anderson Cancer Center Group reported the incidence and outcome of adenovirus (69) and rhinovirus (70) infections in bone marrow transplantation recipients. Three percent of patients undergoing transplantation between 1990 and 1998 were diagnosed with adenovirus infection; 20 out of 76 patients developed either pneumonia ($n = 15$) or disseminated infection with pneumonia ($n = 5$). Mortality rate in this group was 75% (15/20) and strongly influenced by type of transplant (allogeneic vs. autologous), presence of GVHD, and treatment with two or more immunosuppressive agents (69). In our hands, ribavirin therapy did not show to be effective in these patients. Twenty-two blood and marrow transplant recipients were diagnosed with rhinovirus infection at the MD Anderson Cancer Center between 1992 and 1997 (70). Seven patients developed pneumonia that was fatal in all cases. All developed profound fulminant respiratory failure at a median of 12 days after onset of URI symptoms.

Prevention of infection from community respiratory viruses in blood and marrow transplantation recipients is paramount. The Center for Disease Control and Prevention has developed guidelines in this regard (71,72).

a. Health care workers and visitors with URI symptoms should be restricted from contact with transplant recipients or candidates.
b. Transplant recipients with upper or lower respiratory infection symptoms should be placed under contact isolation to avoid transmission to health care workers, visitors, or other patients, until the cause of infection has been identified. Optimal isolation precautions must be applied once the precise diagnosis is made.
c. Transplant candidates with URI symptoms should postpone the starting of the conditioning regimen until the symptoms are resolved.

Specific measures regarding prevention of RSV infection include (71,72):

a. Respiratory secretions of any hospitalized transplant candidate or recipient with URI symptoms should be tested by rapid diagnostic tests and viral cultures for RSV.
b. In hospitalized transplant candidates or recipients with respiratory symptoms, if two diagnostic samples, taken 2 days apart fail to diagnosed the pathogen, a BAL should be obtained.
c. Patients must be aggressively treated early after identification of the virus to prevent progression to pneumonia.

The following measures should be taken for the prevention of influenza infections in blood and marrow transplant recipients (71,72):

a. Influenza vaccination of close contacts starting the season before the planned transplant and for the next 2 years. Vaccination should continue beyond 24 months if patient remains immunocompromised (i.e., receiving immunosuppressant drugs).
b. Seasonal influenza vaccination strongly recommended for health care workers in contact with blood and marrow transplant recipients.
c. Lifelong seasonal influenza vaccination is recommended for all transplant candidates/recipients (start 6 months after transplantation).
d. All transplant recipients (<6 months post-transplantation) should receive chemoprophylaxis with amantadine or rimantadine during community or nosocomial influenza A outbreaks.
e. During nosocomial outbreaks caused by an influenza A strain not included in the current vaccine, health care workers, healthy family members, and close contacts should take amantadine or rimantadine prophylaxis until the end of the outbreak. A neuraminidase inhibitor (zanamavir, oseltamavir) may be offered if amantadine or rimantadine not tolerated, if the strain is resistant to amantadine, or if the outbreak is caused by influenza B.

V. CYTOMEGALOVIRUS PNEUMONIA

Interstitial pneumonia caused by cytomegalovirus (CMV) is a major cause of morbidity and mortality in recipients of allogeneic and autologous blood and marrow transplantation (73–77). The clinical presentation resembles that of *P. carinii* pneumonia, with fever, cough, hypoxemia, and diffuse interstitial radiologic changes (78).

The most significant risk factor for the development of CMV pneumonia is seropositivity prior to transplant. The frequency of CMV infection is probably similar in recipients of both autologous and allogeneic transplantation (approximately 40–50%) (73,74), however, CMV pneumonia occurs more frequently in the allogeneic setting, especially in high-risk patients, like those with extensive chronic GVHD and recipients of T-cell depleted transplants (73,76). Other risk factors, including older age, conditioning with total body irradiation, treatment with antithymocyte globulin, and viruria, have been mentioned (76).

Without effective antiviral prophylaxis and therapy, CMV pneumonia can occur in up to 20% of recipients of allogeneic stem cell transplantation, with a greater than 85% mortality (73,79–81). If patients are treated before respiratory insufficiency develops, the mortality rate ranges from 30% to almost 70%. If therapy starts once mechanical ventilation is required, then the mortality rate is almost universally 100%, with only anecdotal cases surviving the infection (73–77). It has been postulated that the mortality rate is higher among patients receiving total body irradiation in the conditioning regimen (75,77).

There are two strategies for preventing CMV pneumonia in seropositive patients undergoing blood or marrow transplantation (73). A commonly used strategy is prophylactic therapy with ganciclovir or foscarnet (especially in neutropenic patients) for the first 3 months after the transplant; a second approach involves pre-emptive therapy for subclinical CMV infections, as determined by the detection of CMV virus in the blood or BAL. Patients that are treated with the prophylactic strategy are at risk of developing "late" CMV pneumonia (73,82), which is usually complicated by concurrent infections and carries a very high mortality. We suggest that prolonged or even life-long surveillance should be followed in high-risk patients (chronic extensive GVHD and recipients of T-cell depleted transplants).

The standard prophylaxis therapy at the MD Anderson Cancer Center consists of ganciclovir 5 mg/kg every 12 hr from day –8 to –2 prior to the transplantation and 5 mg/kg/day 5 days a week from engraftment until day plus 100. Intravenous acyclovir [5 mg/kg every 8 hr] is given from day –1 until engraftment. Intravenous immune globulin (500 mg/kg) is given weekly from day –7 until day plus 100, then monthly for 1 year. Foscarnet (60 mg/kg/day) is substituted for ganciclovir if patients develop neutropenia (ANC<1000/mm^3).

Treatment for CMV pneumonia includes ganciclovir (5 mg/kg every 12 hr) and intravenous immune globulin (500 mg/kg) every other day for 21 days or longer. If patient has neutropenia unresponsive to growth factors, foscarnet (60 mg/kg every 8 hr) is substituted for ganciclovir. A new antiviral agent, valganciclovir, which is an oral prodrug of ganciclovir with a 10-fold greater oral bioavailability (83), has become available and is now being used as part of our pre-emptive therapy.

VI. POSTERIOR REVERSIBLE LEUKOENCEPHALOPATHY SYNDROME (PRES)

In 1996, Hinchey et al. (84) described this syndrome, characterized by headache, decreased alertness, altered mental functioning, seizures, and visual loss. Patients presenting with these symptoms had abnormal imaging studies of the brain, showing edema that was predominantly seen in the posterior portions of the white matter. These changes were reversible in all patients.

The original report included 15 patients: four with hypertensive encephalopathy, three with glomerulonephritis, one with hepatorenal syndrome, three with pre-eclampsia, and eight were receiving immunosuppressant agents (cyclosporine, interferon, or tacrolimus) for aplastic anemia, malignant melanoma, or bone marrow or solid organ transplants. Fourteen out of 15 patients had white matter abnormalities in the occipital and/or posterior parietal lobes. The neurological changes resolved within 2 weeks in all patients after antihypertensive therapy (when indicated) and withdrawal of immunosuppressant drugs (84).

Most patients will present with subacute onset of headache, altered mental status, ranging from drowsiness to stupor, seizures, vomiting, confusion, decreased speech, and abnormal visual perception. Sometimes, the initial presentation could be seizures, usually generalized. Multiple seizures are more common than single events. Even though patients may develop deep coma, most patients will remain responsive to stimuli. Visual changes commonly include blurred vision, although hemianopia, visual neglect, and frank cortical blindness may occur (84,85).

The typical radiological changes can be detected by computed tomography or magnetic resonance imaging of the brain (preferred). Fluid attenuated inversion recovery (FLAIR) is a magnetic resonance sequence used to suppress signals from the CSF. This technique is better than T2-weighted imaging in detecting small periventricular lesions. A nonvascular distribution of the lesions detected by FLAIR technique is highly suggestive of PRES. This modality should be the imaging of choice when suspecting this syndrome in post-transplant patients taking immunosuppressive therapy (85–87).

The mechanism for which immunosuppressant drugs may cause this syndrome is unknown, and is usually not related to elevated drug levels. Cyclosporine may frequently cause hypertension, but only 3–5% of patients receiving this drug for GVHD prophylaxis develop neurological complications (88,89). It is possible that cyclosporine may cause endothelial injury directly or indirectly (through its products) disrupting the blood brain barrier (90), with a tendency to do so in the vertebrobasilar system and its branches, which could, in turn, result in posterior cerebral vascular damage (88).

Most cases of PRES in the post-transplantation period have been attributed to cyclosporin and tacrolimus therapy (84,85,91,92). The syndrome has also been described early in the transplantation process, after the infusion of the stem cells, and may be caused by dimethylsulfoxide (DMSO) used for the cryopreservation of the stem cells (93).

Posterior reversible leukoencephalopathy syndrome should be suspected in patients receiving immunosuppressant drugs after stem cell or organ transplantation and must be promptly recognized to avoid permanent brain damage. Aggressive management of hypertension, treatment of seizures, supportive care usually in the ICU, and discontinuation of the immunosuppressive therapy will usually result in complete resolution of the syndrome in the majority of the cases. Patients will not require chronic antiepileptic therapy following resolution of the symptoms and imaging abnormalities (85).

VII. TRANSFUSION ISSUES IN BONE MARROW TRANSPLANT RECIPIENTS

Blood group barriers are often mismatched in bone marrow transplantation. Major ABO incompatibility occurs when the recipient possesses antibodies capable of react with red cell antigens on the surface of the donor's red cells (e.g., group A donor, group O recipient). In minor ABO incompatibility, the donor has hemagglutinins capable of react with antigens on the recipient's red cells (group O donor, group A recipient). In some situations (group B donor, group A recipient) both major and minor ABO incompatibilities coexist.

In cases of major ABO incompatibilities, red cells are removed from the donor graft, leaving the product with a 3–4% hematocrit that can be usually handled by a normal adult with only minor complications. Major transfusion reactions can occasionally be seen when the recipient has been sensitized to the donor's red cells, such as mother/child transplant.

With minor ABO incompatibility, there is risk of both immediate and delayed hemolysis with infusion of the marrow graft. Immediate reactions are an issue when large volumes are to be infused (adult to child transplant). A delayed hemolytic reaction can occur at approximately days 5–8 post-transplant, when the lymphocytes start producing antibodies directed against recipient antigens (94,95).

In the case of major or minor ABO incompatible graft, only group O red cells should be transfused. Platelets products should have plasma that is compatible with both the recipient and the donor. If there is risk for incompatibility, the platelet products should be reduced to minimize antibody exposure. Only after the donor graft is firmly established, these transfusion policies can be changed.

More recently, with the use of nonmyeloablative transplantation (so-called minitransplant), post-transplant-mixed chimeric states are occurring more frequently. Transfusion implications of this phenomenon have not yet been studied, but there is at least a theoretical risk for increased post-transplant hemolysis (96).

VIII. THROMBOTIC THROMBOCYTOPENIC PURPURA (TTP)

Microangiopathic hemolytic anemia (TTP or hemolytic–uremic syndrome (HUS)) can often complicate bone marrow transplantation recipients. Although the exact mechanism for the development of TTP/HUS in transplanted patients remains unknown, several factors have been implied, including endothelial cell injury by the conditioning regimen, CMV infection, immunosuppressive drugs (especially cyclosporine) used for the prevention and treatment of GVHD, and possibly a direct graft-versus-host effect in the endothelium (97–100).

Establishing the clinical diagnosis of TTP/HUS after BMT becomes a real challenge to the clinician, since anemia, thrombocytopenia, renal impairment, and neurological changes are very common and may be seen in many different situations in transplanted patients.

The true incidence of TTP in bone marrow transplant patients is unknown and may be over or underestimated, reflecting flexibility in applying diagnostic criteria among different centers and published series. The largest retrospective analysis published by the Italian Group of Bone Marrow Transplantation (101) included 4334 patients and showed an incidence of 0.1% and 0.5% in the autologous and allogeneic transplants groups, respectively. Other series report incidences ranging from 0% to 7% in autologous patients and from 2% to 14% in recipient of allogeneic transplantations (97,98,102–104).

There are not clear risk factors for the development of TTP/HUS in bone marrow transplant patients; however, there is an increased incidence in recipients of transplants from unrelated or not fully matched donors (97,101,102,104). Microangiopathic hemolytic anemia is more likely to occur in patients having transplant-related complications like acute GVHD and sepsis, and in those taking intensive immunosuppression for the prevention of GVHD (101,103).

Disseminated aggregates of microthrombi consisting of platelets and von Willebrand factor (vWF) are found in idiopathic TTP (105). Highly adhesive, unusually large vWF multimers are demonstrated in the plasma of patients with idiopathic TTP (106). An inhibiting autoantibody against vWF-cleaving protease plays a causative role in a large number of patients with congenital and idiopathic TTP (107–109). The presence of these antibodies could not be demonstrated in 10 patients with post-transplant TTP (97), furthermore, vWF-cleaving protease activity was normal in all patients, and unusually large vWF multimers were found in only 3 of 10 patients. The available data suggest that the primary mechanism for post-transplant TTP may be endothelial injury rather than vWF protease deficiency (97,110).

Plasma exchange is the most used strategy for the treatment of transplant-related TTP/HUS. Deciding who needs treatment and when to start is a very difficult challenge, since some of the clinical features of the disease may not be present at the beginning or may be attributed to other causes (102). Cyclosporin itself can cause red cell fragmentation, platelet count may be already low in the early post-transplantation course, neurological assessment may be very difficult in the setting of sepsis or acute GVHD, renal function may be affected by several drugs, and the level of lactic dehydrogenase can be elevated due to multiple causes in the post-transplant population (111).

Treatment of microangiopathic hemolytic anemia in post-transplant patients consists of stopping cyclosporin immediately, aggressively treats any underlying disorder (CMV infection, sepsis, GVHD, etc.), and initiates plasma exchange (101–104). Long-term survival after plasma exchange varies between the different series, and has been reported to be as low as 0% (103) and as high as 50% in the Italian series (101). Number of plasma exchange sessions, duration of therapy, and parameters to assess response (platelet count vs. lactic dehydrogenase level) remains to be defined in clinical trials. It seems that patients that develop a clinical picture closer to HUS than to TTP may be far better, and that TTP occurring early in the post-transplant period carries a worse prognosis (101).

Defibrotide has been recently reported to be effective in the treatment of post-transplant TTP/HUS in a small phase II trial, with a reported benefit in 6 out of 12 patients (112). The drug is a polydeoxyribonucleotide salt with an antithrombotic and thrombolyitic effect that has been successfully used for the treatment of veno-occlusive disease, deep vein thrombosis, and vasculitis.

In conclusion, the pathogenesis of post-transplant TTP is unclear. The small number of patients studied and reported in the literature suggests that endothelial damage may be the most important pathologic event, however, a contributing role of a vWF-related protease has not yet been completely ruled out, and further data are awaited to clarify this issue. Until then, patients with suspected TTP/HUS should be promptly treated with plasma exchange and any suspected offending agent must be immediately stopped. Aggressive supportive care, including treatment of infections and GVHD, must be provided. Duration and number of plasma exchange sessions will be guided by patient's response to therapy. The combination of plasma exchange with other strategies, like defibrotide, must be addressed in clinical trials. The role for other antiplatelet drugs like glycoprotein IIB-IIIA inhibitors and factor X remains to be determined in clinical trials.

IX. CENTRAL VENOUS CATHETER-RELATED COMPLICATIONS

Central venous catheters are placed in all patients receiving autologous and allogeneic stem cell transplantation; they allow for the delivery of multiple drugs and blood products required by these patient population, however they can be the source for complications, mainly thrombosis and local site and systemic infections, including bacteremia, endocarditis, septic thrombophlebitis, and other metastatic infections (113). Due to the use of prophylactic antibiotics over the last decade, there has been and increase in the number of infections caused by gram-positive organisms in cancer patients, now accounting for about 60% of the cases; many of these infections come from indwelling central venous catheters (114–116).

The incidence of infectious complications caused by central venous catheters is higher in ICUs, with the consequent increase in duration of hospitalization, mortality rate, and expense. The Infectious Disease Society of America has recommended guidelines for the prevention of these infections (113). Adequate training of health care providers regarding insertion and maintenance of the catheter, skin antisepsis with 2% chlorhexidine, and the use of antiseptic/antibiotic-impregnated catheters is addressed by the guidelines.

Catheters impregnated with chlorhexidine and silver sulfadiazine and catheters impregnated with minocyclin and rifampin are the most frequently types of used antimicrobial-impregnated catheters (117). The use of these catheters has been shown to reduce the incidence of catheter-related infections in several trials, especially in centers where the rate of infections is 2% or higher (118,119). Some have suggested that the rifampin-impregnated catheter may be more effective than the chlorhexidine ones (120), however, the Infectious Disease Society's guidelines recommend that either one should be used for catheters that are going to be inserted for more than 6 days, which is the case in all transplant patients.

Catheter-related infections may originate from: (a) the exit site, leading to contamination of the external surface of the catheter, (b) the catheter hub, leading to internal colonization, or (c) the blood stream (hematogenous seeding). Subclavian catheters are less likely to get infected, compared to internal jugular and femoral vein sites (117).

The management of catheter-associated infections has been also addressed in guidelines published by the Infectious Disease Society of America (121). Once the infection is suspected, blood cultures must be taken from the catheter and peripheral sites. A positive culture from the catheter may indicate contamination from the hub, catheter colonization, or bloodstream infection. Empirical antibiotic therapy should start promptly to cover for *Staphilococcus epidermidis* or *Staphilococcus aureus* infections. In transplant patients, broad-spectrum antibiotics against gram-negative organisms should be added.

If there is any purulence or erythema around the catheter, an exit infection is likely and the catheter must be removed; other indications for removal include septic emboli, hypotension associated with catheter use, nonpatent catheter, and if no response to antibiotics is apparent after 2–3 days. Debridement of infected tissue is advisable for atypical mycobacterium infection. Infections caused by fungal organisms, and due to *Bacillus* species, *Pseudomonas aeruginosa*, *Stenotrophomonas maltophilia*, or vancomycin-resistant enterococci are better treated with removal of the catheter (121).

If the patient is not in septic shock and antibiotics have been initiated, the catheter should be changed over the wire to avoid insertion-related complications (122,123). If the patient is in septic shock, and no other source of infection is evident, the catheter should be removed and replaced on a new site. A positive culture from a catheter tip means that the patient has either catheter colonization or catheter-related bloodstream infection; in that case, a catheter changed over the wire should be placed at another location.

X. MUCOSITIS

Blood and marrow transplant patients are often afflicted with mucositis as a consequence of the preparative regimen and from such drugs as methotrexate in the GVHD prophylaxis. Post-transplant mucositis poses increased risk for intubation and airway compromise. For those patients receiving methotrexate, a risk is possible for those with gene rearrangement or polymorphism, for subtypes of the gene methylene tetrahydrofolate reductase (MTHFR) C677T (124–133). Additional risk factors include use of dental appliances, history of oral lesions, history of smoking, differences in oral care, and elevated weight. Patients who are scheduled to receive methotrexate should have an assessment for sleep apnea risk. A combination of oral methotrexate and obstructive sleep apnea may place patients at a high risk for sudden pulmonary events. In recent data studying mucositis prevention, cytokine shields such as keratinocyte growth factor have been used and have had some preliminary positive results. Mucositis post-transplant has left clinicians hesitant to place nasogastric tubes for feeding and to perform diagnostic endoscopic studies to assess for infection. The newer nonmyeloablative transplants may have a lower risk of mucositis. However, this remains to be seen, as many feel that post-transplant methotrexate is a major risk and perhaps the use of lower doses of post-transplant methotrexate has actually improved outcomes.

REFERENCES

1. Thomas E, Storb R, Clift RA, et al. Bone marrow transplantation. N Engl J Med 1975; 292:832–843.
2. Elias A, Armitage JO. Bone marrow transplantation. N Engl J Med 1994; 331:617.
3. O'Reilly RJ. Allogeneic bone marrow transplantation: current status and future directions. Blood 1983; 62:942–946.
4. Lum LG. The kinetics of immune reconstitution after human marrow transplantation. Blood 1987; 69: 369–380.
5. Fefer A, Cheever MA, Thomas ED, et al. Bone marrow transplantation for refractory acute leukemia in 34 patients with identical twins. Blood 1981; 57: 421–430.
6. Sullivan KM, Weiden PL, Storb R, et al. Influence of acute and chronic graft-versus-host disease on relapse and survival after bone marrow transplantation from HLA-identical siblings as treatment of acute and chronic leukemia. Blood 1989; 73:1720–1728.
7. Horowitz MM, Gale RP, Sondel PM, et al. Graft-versus-leukemia reaction after bone marrow transplantation. Blood 1990; 75:555–562.
8. Beatty PG, Clift RA, Mickelson EM, et al. Marrow transplantation for related donors other than HLA-identical siblings. N Engl J Med 1985; 313:765–771.
9. Gajewski J, Cecka M, Champlin R. Bone marrow transplantation using HLA-matched unrelated donors. Blood Rev 1990; 4:132–138.
10. Kernan NA, Bartsch G, Ash RC, et al. Retrospective analysis of 462 unrelated marrow transplants facilitated by the National Marrow Donor Program (NMDP) for treatment of acquired and congenital disorders of the lymphohematopoietic system and congenital metabolic disorders. N Engl J Med 1993; 328: 593–602.
11. Gluckman E, Rocha V, Boyer-Chammard A, et al. Outcome of cord blood transplantation from related and unrelated donors. Eurocord transplant group and the European blood and marrow transplantation group. N Engl J Med 1997; 337:373–381.
12. Kurtzberg J, Laughlin M, Graham MC, et al. Placental blood as a source of hematopoietic stem cells for transplantation into unrelated recipients. N Engl J Med 1996; 335:157–166.
13. Jackson SR, Tweeddale MG, Barnett MJ, et al. Admission of bone marrow transplant recipients to the intensive care unit: outcome, survival and prognostic factors. Bone Marrow Transplant 1998; 21:697–704.
14. Afessa B, Tefferi A, Hoagland HC, et al. Outcome of recipients of bone marrow transplants who require intensive-care unit support. Mayo Clinic Proc 1992; 67(2):117–122.
15. Torrecilla C, Cortes JL, Chamorro C, et al. Prognostic assessment of the acute complications of bone marrow transplantation requiring intensive therapy. Intensive Care Med 1988; 14(4):393–398.

16. Denardo SJ, Oye RK, Bellamy PE. Efficacy of intensive care for bone marrow transplant patients with respiratory failure. Crit Care Med 1989; 17(1):4–6.
17. Crawford SW, Petersen FB. Long-term survival from respiratory failure after marrow transplantation for malignancy. Am Rev of Respir Dis 1992; 145(3):510–514.
18. Huaringa AJ, Leyva FJ, Giralt SA, et al. Outcome of bone marrow transplantation patients requiring mechanical ventilation. Crit Care Med 2000; 28(4):1014–1017.
19. Ho VT, Weller E, Lee SF, et al. Prognostic factors for early severe pulmonary complications after hematopoietic stem cell transplantation. Biol Blood Marrow Transplant 2001; 7:223–229.
20. Paz HL, Crilley P, Weinar M, et al. Outcome of patients requiring medical ICU admission following bone marrow transplantation. Chest 1993; 104(2):527–531.
21. Azoulay E, Alberti C, Bornstain C, et al. Improved survival in cancer patients requiring mechanical ventilatory support: impact of noninvasive mechanical ventilatory support. Crit Care Med 2001; 29(3):519–525.
22. Afessa B, Tefferi A, Litzow MR, et al. Diffuse alveolar hemorrhage in hematopoietic stem cell transplant recipients. Am J Respir Crit Care Med 2002; 166:641–645.
23. Robbins RA, Linder J, Stahl MG, et al. Diffuse alveolar hemorrhage in autologous bone marrow transplant recipients. Am J Med 1989; 87:511–518.
24. Feinstein MB, Mokhtari M, Ferreiro R, et al. Fiberoptic bronchoscopy in allogeneic bone marrow transplantation: findings in the era of serum cytomegalovirus antigen surveillance. Chest 2001; 120(4):1094–1100.
25. Huaringa AJ, Leyva FJ, Signes-Costa J, et al. Bronchoalveolar lavage in the diagnosis of pulmonary complications of bone marrow transplant patients. Bone Marrow Transplant 2000; 25(9):975–979.
26. De Lassence A, Fleury-Feith J, Escudier E et al. Alveolar hemorrhage: diagnostic criteria and result in 194 immunocompromised host. Am J Respir Crit Care Med 1995; 151:157–163.
27. Agusti C, Ramirez J, Picado C, et al. Diffuse alveolar hemorrhage in allogeneic bone marrow transplantation: a postmortem study. Am J Respir Crit Care Med 1995; 151:1006–1010.
28. Witte RJ, Gurney JW, Robbins RA, et al. Diffuse pulmonary alveolar hemorrhage after bone marrow transplantation: radiographic findings in 39 patients. Am J Roent 1991; 157(3):461–464.
29. Hicks K, Peng D, Galewski J. Treatment of diffuse alveolar hemorrhage after allogeneic bone marrow transplant with recombinant factor VIIa. Bone Marrow Transplant 2002; 30:975–978.
30. Cordonnier C, Bernaurdin JF, Bierling P, et al. Pulmonary complications occurring after allogeneic bone marrow transplantation: a study of 130 consecutive transplanted patients. Cancer 1986; 58:1047–1054.
31. Jules-Elysee K, Stover DE, Yahalom J, et al. Pulmonary complications in lymphoma patients treated with high-dose therapy autologous bone marrow transplantation. Am Rev Respir Dis 1992; 146:485–491.
32. Lewis ID, DeFor T, Weisdorf DJ. Increasing incidence of diffuse alveolar hemorrhage following allogeneic bone marrow transplantation: cryptic etiology and uncertain therapy. Bone Marrow Transplant 2000; 26:539–543.
33. Metcalf JP, Rennard SI, Reed EC, et al. Corticosteroids as adjunctive therapy for diffuse alveolar hemorrhage associated with bone marrow transplantation: University of Nebraska Medical Center Bone Marrow Transplant Group. Am J Med 1994; 96:327–334.
34. Nevo S, Swan V, Enger C, et al. Acute bleeding after bone marrow transplantation: incidence and effect on survival: a quantitative analysis of 1402 patients. Blood 1998; 91:1469–1477.
35. Baker WJ, Vukelja SJ, Burrell LM, et al. High-dose cyclophosphamide, etoposide and carboplatin with autologous bone marrow support for metastatic breast cancer: long-term results. Bone Marrow Transplant 1998; 21:775–778.
36. Chao NJ, Duncan SR, Long GD, et al. Corticosteroid therapy for diffuse alveolar hemorrhage in autologous bone marrow transplant recipients. Ann Intern Med 1991; 114:145–146.
37. Frankovich J, Donaldson SS, Lee Y, et al. High-dose therapy and autologous hematopoietic cell transplantation in children with primary refractory and relapsed Hodgkin's disease: atopy predicts idiopathic diffuse lung injury syndromes. Biol Blood Marrow Transplant 2001; 7:49–57.
38. Jabro G, Koc Y, Boyle T, et al. Role of splenic irradiation in patients with chronic myeloid leukemia undergoing allogeneic bone marrow transplantation. Biol Blood Marrow Transplant 1999; 5:173–179.
39. Mulder PO, Meinesz AF, de Vries EG, et al. Diffuse alveolar hemorrhage in autologous bone marrow transplant recipients. Am J Med 1991; 90:278–281.
40. Raptis A, Mavroudis D, Suffredini A, et al. High-dose corticosteroid therapy for diffuse alveolar hemorrhage in allogeneic bone marrow stem cell transplant recipients. Bone Marrow Transplant 1999; 24: 879–883.
41. Seiden MV, Elias A, Ayash L, et al. Pulmonary toxicity associated with high dose chemotherapy in the treatment of solid tumors with autologous marrow transplant: an analysis of four chemotherapy regimens. Bone Marrow Transplant 1992; 10:57–63.
42. Haselton DJ, Klekamp JG, Christman BW, et al. Use of high-dose corticosteroids and high-frequency oscillatory ventilation for treatment of a child with diffuse alveolar hemorrhage after bone marrow transplantation: case report and review of the literature. Crit Care Med 2000; 28:245–248.
43. Blatt J, Gold SH, Wiley JM, et al. Off-label use of recombinant factor VIIa in patients following bone marrow transplantation. Bone Marrow Transplant 2001; 28:405–407.
44. White B, Martin M, Kelleher S, et al. Successful use of recombinant FVIIa (Novoseven) in the management of pulmonary hemorrhage secondary to aspergillus

infection in a patient with leukemia and acquired FVII deficiency. Br J Haematol 1999; 106:254–255.
45. Ippoliti C, Hey D, Donato ML, et al. Use of activated recombinant factor VII (rFVIIa) for treatment of pulmonary hemorrhage in stem cell transplantation recipients. Proc ASCO 2003; 22:841 (3378a).
46. Bowden RA. Respiratory virus infections after marrow transplant: the Fred Hutchinson Cancer Research Center experience. Am J Med 1996; 102(3A):27–30.
47. Khushalani NI, Bakri FJ, Wentling D, et al. Respiratory syncytial virus infection in the late bone marrow transplant period: report of three cases and review. Bone Marrow Transplant 2001; 27:1071–1073.
48. Ghosh S, Champlin RE, Englund J, et al. Respiratory syncytial virus upper respiratory tract illnesses in adult blood and marrow transplant recipients: combination therapy with aerosolized ribavirin and intravenous immunoglobulin. Bone Marrow Transplant 2000; 25: 751–755.
49. Harrington RD, Hooton TM, Hackman RC, et al. An outbreak of respiratory syncytial virus in a bone marrow transplant center. J Infect Dis 1992; 165(6): 987–993.
50. Whimbey E, Champlin RE, Englund JA, et al. Combination therapy with aerosolized ribavirin and intravenous immunoglobulin for respiratory syncytial virus disease in adult bone marrow transplant recipients. Bone Marrow Transplant 1995; 16(3):393–399.
51. Fouilliard L, Mouthon L, Laporte JP, et al. Severe respiratory syncytial virus pneumonia after autologous bone marrow transplantation: a report of three cases and review. Bone Marrow Transplant 1992; 9(2):97–100.
52. Ljungman P. Respiratory virus infections in bone marrow transplant recipients: the European perspective. Am J Med 1997; 102(3A):44–47.
53. Ghosh S, Champlin RE, Ueno NT, et al. Respiratory syncytial virus infections in autologous blood and marrow transplant recipients with breast cancer: combination therapy with aerosolized ribavirin and parenteral immunoglobulins. Bone Marrow Transplant 2001; 28:271–275.
54. Machado CM, Vilas Boas LS, Mendes AVA, et al. Low mortality rates related to respiratory virus infecions after bone marrow transplantation. Bone Marrow Transplant 2003; 31:695–700.
55. Sparrelid E, Ljungman P, Ekelof-Andstrom E, et al. Ribavirin therapy in bone marrow transplant recipients with viral respiratory tract infections. Bone Marrow Trasnsplant 1997; 19:905–908.
56. Markovic S, Adlakha A, Smith T, et al. Respiratory syncytial virus pneumonitis-induced diffuse alveolar damage in an autologous bone marrow transplant recipient. Mayo Clinic Proc 1998; 73(2):153–156.
57. van Dissel JT, Zijlmans JM, Kroes AC, et al. Respiratory syncytial virus, a rare cause of severe pneumonia following bone marrow transplantation. Ann Hematol 1995; 71(5):253–255.
58. DeVincenzo JP, Hirsch RL, Fuentes RJ, Top FH Jr. Respiratory syncytial virus immune globulin treatment of lower respiratory tract infection in pediatric patients undergoing bone marrow transplantation – a compassionate use experience. [Clinical Trial. Journal Article. Multicenter Study] Bone Marrow Transplantation 2000; 25(2):161–165.
59. Boeckh M, Berrey MM, Bowden RA, et al. Phase 1 evaluation of the respiratory syncytial virus-specific monoclonal antibody palivizumab in recipients of hematopoietic stem cell transplants. J Infect Dis 2001; 184:350–354.
60. Impact-RSV Study Group. Palivizumab, a humanized respiratory syncytial virus monoclonal antibody, reduces hospitalization from respiratory syncytial virus infection in high-risk infects. Pediatrics 1998; 102: 531–537.
61. Malley R, DeVicenzo J, Ramilo O, et al. Reduction of respiratory syncytial virus (RSV) in tracheal aspirates in intubated infants by use of humanized monoclonal antibody to RSV F protein. J Infect Dis 1998; 178: 1555–1561.
62. Nichols WG, Corey L, Gooley T, et al. Parainfluenza virus infections after hematopoietic stem cell transplantation: risks factors, response to antiviral therapy, and effect on transplant outcome. Blood 2001; 98:573–578.
63. Lewis VA, Champlin R, Englund J, et al. Respiratory disease due to parainfluenza virus in adult bone marrow transplant recipients. Clin Infect Dis 1996; 23: 1033–1037.
64. Wendt CH, Weisdorf DJ, Jordan MC, et al. Parainfluenza virus respiratory infection after bone marrow transplantation. N Engl J Med 1992; 326(14):921–926.
65. Whimbey E, Vartivarian SE, Champlin RE, et al. Parainfluenza virus infection in adult bone marrow transplant recipients. Eur J Clin Microbiol and Infect Dis 1993; 12(9):699–701.
66. Whimbey E, Elting LS, Couch RB, et al. Influenza A virus infection among hospitalized adult bone marrow transplant recipients. Bone Marrow Transplant 1994; 13(4):437–440.
67. Whimbey E, Champlin RE, Couch RB, et al. Community respiratory virus infections among hospitalized adult bone marrow transplant recipients. Clin Infect Dis 1996; 22(5):778–782.
68. Hayden FG. Prevention and treatment of influenza in immunocompromised patients. Am J Med 1997; 102(3A): 55–60.
69. La Rosa AM, Champlin RE, Mirza N, et al. Adenovirus infections in adult recipients of blood and marrow transplants. Clin Infect Dis 2001; 32:871–876.
70. Ghosh S, Champlin R, Couch R, et al. Rhinovirus infections in myelosuppressed adult blood and marrow transplant recipients. Clin Infect Dis 1999; 29(3): 528–532.
71. Dykewicz CA. Guidelines for preventing opportunistic infections among hematopoietic stem cell transplant recipients: focus on community repiratory virus

infections. Biol Blood Bone Marrow Transplant 2001; 7:19S–22S.
72. Center for Disease Control and Prevention. Guidelines for preventing opportunistic infections among hematopoietic stem cell transplant recipients: recommendations of CDC, the Infectious Disease Society of America, and the American Society of Blood and Marrow Transplantation. Biol Blood Marrow Transplant 2000; 6:659–734.
73. Nguyen Q, Champlin R, Giralt S, et al. Late cytomegalovirus pneumonia in adult allogeneic blood and marrow transplant recipients. Clin Infect Dis 1999; 28:618–623.
74. Konoplev S, Champlin RE, Giralt S, et al. Cytomegalovirus pneumonia in adult autologous blood and marrow transplant recipients. Bone Marrow Transplant 2001; 27:877–881.
75. Ljungman P, Engelhard D, Link H, et al. Treatment of interstitial pneumonitis due to cytomegalovirus with ganciclovir and intravenous immune globulin: experience of European bone marrow transplant group. Clin Infect Dis 1992; 14(4):831–835.
76. Enright H, Haake R, Weisdorf D, et al. Cytomegalovirus pneumonia after bone marrow transplantation. Risk factors and response to therapy. Transplantation 1993; 55(6):1339–1346.
77. Ljungman P, Biron P, Bosi A, et al. Cytomegalovirus interstitial pneumonia in autologous bone marrow transplant recipients. Infectious disease working party of the European group for bone marrow transplantation. Bone Marrow Transplant 1994; 13(2):209–212.
78. Salomon N, Perlman DC. Cytomegalovirus pneumonia. Sem Resp Infect 1999; 14(4):353–358.
79. Meyers JD, Flournoy N, Thomas ED. Risk factors for cytomegalovirus infection after human bone marrow transplantation. J Infect Dis 1986; 153:478–488.
80. Winston DJ, Ho WG, Champlin RE. Cytomegalovirus infections after allogeneic bone marrow transplantation. Rev Infect Dis 1990; 12(suppl 7):S776–792.
81. Meyers JD, Ljungman P, Fisher LD. Cytomegalovirus excretion as a predictor of cytomegalovirus disease after marrow transplantation: importance of cytomegalovirus viremia. J Infect Dis 1990; 162:373–380.
82. Boeck M, Leisenring W, Riddell SR, et al. Late cytomegalovirus disease and mortality in recipients of allogeneic hematopoietic stem cell transplants: importance of viral load and T-cell immunity. Blood 2003; 101:407–414.
83. Reusser P. Oral valganciclovir: a new option for treatment of cytomegalovirus infection and disease in immunocompromised hosts. Expert Opinion Investigational Drugs 2001; 10(9):1745–1753.
84. Hinchey J, Chaves C, Appignani B, et al. A reversible posterior leukoencephalopathy syndrome. N Engl J Med 1996; 334(8):494–500.
85. Garg RK. Posterior leukoencephalopathy syndrome. Postgrad Med J 2001; 77:24–28.
86. Port JD, Beauchamp NJ. Reversible intracerebral pathological entities mediated by vascular autoregulatory dysfunction. Radiographics 1998; 18:353–367.
87. Inoha S, Inamura T, Nakamizo A, et al. Magnetic resonance imaging in cases with encephalopathy secondary to immunosuppressive agents. J Clin Neurosci 2002; 9(3):305–307.
88. Schwartz RB, Bravo SM, Klufas RA, et al. Cyclosporine neurotoxicity and its relationship to hypertensive encephalopathy. Am J Radiol 1995; 165:627–631.
89. Fiorani L, Bandini G, D'Alessandro R, et al. Cyclosporin A neurotoxicity after allogeneic bone marrow transplantation. Bone Marrow Transplant 1994; 14:175–176.
90. Kochi S, Takanaga H, Matsuo H, et al. Effect of cyclosporin A or tacrolimus on the function of blood–brain barrier cells. Eur J Pharmacol 1999; 372:287–295.
91. Furukawa M, Terae S, Chu BC, et al. MRI in seven cases of tacrolimus (FK-506) encephalopathy: utility of FLAIR and diffusion-weighted imaging. Neuroradiology 2001; 43:615–621.
92. Takahata M, Hashino S, Izumiyama K, et al. Cyclosporin A-induced encephalopathy after allogeneic bone marrow transplantation with prevention of graft-versus-host disease by tacrolimus. Bone Marrow Transplant 2001; 28:713–715.
93. Higman MA, Port JD, Beauchamp NJ Jr, et al. Reversible leukoencephalopathy associated with re-infusion of DMSO preserved stem cells. Bone Marrow Transplant 2000; 26:797–800.
94. Hows J, Beddow K, Gordon-Smith E, et al. Donor-derived red blood cell antibodies and immune hemolysis after allogeneic bone marrow transplantation. Blood 1986; 67:177–181.
95. Gajewski JL, Petz LD, Calhoun L, et al. Hemolysis of transfused group O red blood cells in minor ABO-incompatible unrelated-donor bone marrow transplants in patients receiving cyclosporin without post-transplant methotrexate. Blood 1992; 79: 3076–3085.
96. Lapierre V, Oubouzar N, Auperin A, et al. Influence of the hematopoietic stem cell source on early immunohematologic reconstitution after allogeneic transplantation. Blood 2001; 97:2580–2586.
97. Elliot MA, Nichols WL Jr, Plumhoff EA, et al. Post-transplantation thrombotic thrombocytopenic purpura: a single center experience and a contemporary review. Mayo Clin Proc 2003; 78:421–430.
98. Pettit AR, Clark RE. Thrombotic microangiopathy following bone marrow transplantation. Bone Marrow Transplant 1994; 14:495–504.
99. Maslo C, Peraldi MN, Desenclos JC, et al. Thrombotic microangiopathy and cytomegalovirus disease in patients infected with human immunodeficiency virus. Clin Infect Dis 1997; 24:350–355.
100. Holler E, Kolb HJ, Hiller E, et al. Microangiopathy in patients on cyclosporin prophylaxis who developed acute graft-versus-host disease after HLA-identical bone marrow transplantation. Blood 1989; 73:2018–2024.

101. Iacopino P, Pucci G, Arcese W, et al. Severe thrombotic microangiopathy: an infrequent complication of bone marrow transplantation. Bone Marrow Transplant 1999; 24:47–51.
102. Fuge R, Bird JM, Fraser A, et al. The clinical features, risk factors and outcome of thrombotic thrombocytopenic purpura occurring after bone marrow transplantation. Br J Haematol 2001; 113:58–64.
103. Paquette RL, Tran L, Landaw EM. Thrombotic microangiopathy following allogeneic bone marrow transplantation is associated with intensive graft-versus-host disease prophylaxis. Bone Marrow Transplant 1998; 22:351–357.
104. Roy V, Rizvi MA, Vesely SK, George JN. Thrombotic thrombocytopenic purpura-like syndromes following bone marrow transplantation: an analysis of associated conditions and clinical outcomes. Bone Marrow Transplant 2001; 27:641–646.
105. Asada Y, Sumiyoshi A, Hayashi T, et al. Immunohistochemistry of vascular lesion in thrombotic thrombocytopenic purpura, with special reference to factor VIII related antigen. Thromb Res 1985; 38:469–479.
106. Moake JL, McPherson PD. Abnormalities of von Willebrand factor multimers in thrombotic thrombocytopenic purpura and the hemolytic–uremic syndrome. Am J Med 1989; 87:9N–15N.
107. Furlan M, Robles R, Galbusera M, et al. von Willebrand factor-cleaving protease in thrombotic thrombocytopenic purpura and the hemolytic–uremic syndrome. N Engl J Med 1998; 339:1578–1584.
108. Tsai HM, Lian EC. Antibodies to von Willebrand factor-cleaving protease in acute thrombotic thrombocytopenic purpura. N Engl J Med 1998; 339:1585–1594.
109. Levy GG, Nichols WC, Lian EC, et al. Mutations in a member of the ADAMTS gene family cause thrombotic thrombocytopenic purpura. Nature 2001; 413:488–494.
110. van der Plas RM, Schiphorst ME, Huizinga EG, et al. von Willebrand factor proteolysis is deficient in classic, but not in bone marrow transplantation-associated, thrombotic thrombocytopenic purpura. Blood 1999; 93:3798–3802.
111. Anderlini P, Przepiorka D, Seong D, et al. Clinical toxicity and laboratory effects of granulocyte-colony-stimulating-factor (filgrastim) mobilization and blood stem cell apheresis from normal donors, and analysis of charges for the procedures. Transfusion 1996; 36: 590–595.
112. Corti P, Uderzo C, Tagliabue A, et al. Defibrotide is a promising treatment fro thrombotic thrombocytopenic purpura in patients undergoing bone marrow transplantation. Bone Marrow Transplant 2002; 29:542–543.
113. O'Grady NP, Alexander M, Dellinger EP, et al. Guidelines for the prevention of intravascular catheter-related infections. Clin Infect Dis 2002; 35: 1281–1307.
114. Chandrasekar PH, Arnow P. Cefepime versus ceftazidime as empiric therapy for fever in neutropenic patients with cancer. Ann Pharmacother 2000; 34:98–95.
115. Johanson PJ, Sternby E, Ursing B. Septicemia in granulocytopenic patients: a shift in bacterial etiology. Scand J Infect Dis 1992; 24:357–360.
116. Rolston KVI, Berkey P, Bodey GP, et al. A comparison of imipenem to ceftazidime with or without amikacin as empiric therapy in febrile neutropenic patients. Arch Intern Med 1992; 152:283–291.
117. McGee DC, Gould MK. Preventing complications of central venous catheterization. N Engl J Med 2003; 348: 1123–1133.
118. Raad I, Darouiche R, Dupuis J, et al. Central venous catheters coated with minocycline and rifampin for the prevention of catheter-related colonization and bloodstream infections: a randomized, double-blind trial. Ann Intern Med 1997; 127:267–274.
119. Maki DG, Stolz SM, Wheeler S, Mermel LA. Prevention of central venous catheter-related bloodstream infection by use of an antiseptic-impregnated catheter: a randomized, controlled trial. Ann Intern Med 1997; 127:257–266.
120. Darouiche RO, Raad II, Heard SO, et al. A comparison of two antimicrobial-impregnated central venous catheters. N Engl J Med 1999; 340:1–8.
121. Hughes WT, Armstrong D, Bodey GP, et al. 2002 guidelines for the use of antimicrobial agents in neutropenic patients with cancer. Clin Infect Dis 2002; 34:730–751.
122. Martinez E, Mensa J, Rovira M, et al. Central venous catheter exchange by guidewire for treatment of catheter-related bacteremia in patients undergoing BMT or intensive chemotherapy. Bone Marrow Transplant 1999; 23: 41–44.
123. Michel LA, Bradpiece HA, Randour P, Pouthier E. Safety of central venous catheter change over guidewire for suspected catheter-related sepsis: a prospective randomized trial. Int Surg 1988; 73:180–186.
124. Bellm LA, Epstein JB, Rose-Ped A, et al. Patient reports of complications of bone marrow transplantation. Support Care Cancer 2000; 8:33–39.
125. Stiff P. Mucositis associated with stem cell transplantation: current status and innovative approaches to management. Bone Marrow Transplant 2001; 27(suppl 2):S3–S11.
126. Sonis ST, Oster G, Fuchs H, et al. Oral mucositis and the clinical and economic outcomes of hematopoietic stem-cell transplantation. J Clin Oncol 2001; 19:2201–2205.
127. Woo SB, Sonis ST, Monopoli MM, et al. A longitudinal study of oral ulcerative mucositis in bone marrow transplant recipients. Cancer 1993; 72:1612–1617.
128. Ulrich CM, Yasui Y, Storb R, et al. Pharmacogenetics of methotrexate: toxicity among marrow transplantation patients varies with the methylenetetrahydrofolate reductase C677T polymorphism. Blood 2001; 98: 231–234.
129. Seto BG, Kim M, Wolinsky L, et al. Oral mucositis in patients undergoing bone marrow transplantation. Oral Surg Oral Med Oral Pathol 1985; 60:493–497.

130. Weisdorf DJ, Bostrom B, Raether D, et al: Oropharyngeal mucositis complicating bone marrow transplantation: prognostic factors and the effect of chlorhexidine mouth rinse. Bone Marrow Transplant 1989; 4:89–95.
131. Zerbe MB, Parkerson SG, Ortlieb ML, et al. Relationships between oral mucositis and treatment variables in bone marrow transplant patients. Cancer Nurs 1992; 15:196–205.
132. McGuire DB, Altomonte V, Peterson DE, et al. Patterns of mucositis and pain in patients receiving preparative chemotherapy and bone marrow transplantation. Oncol Nurs Forum 1993; 20:1493–1502.
133. Dodd MJ, Miaskowski C, Shiba GH, et al. Risk factors for chemotherapy-induced oral mucositis: dental appliances, oral hygiene, previous oral lesions, and history of smoking. Cancer Invest 1999; 17:278–284.

8

Palliative Radiotherapy: Clinical and Radiobiologic Considerations

NORA A. JANJAN

Division of Radiation Oncology, The University of Texas M.D. Anderson Cancer Center, Houston, Texas, U.S.A.

I. INTRODUCTION

Over 70% of all cancer patients develop symptoms from either their primary or metastatic disease. Approximately half the patients diagnosed with cancer will develop metastatic disease (1–4). There is a profound need for expertise in palliative care in oncology. Quality of life is now recognized as an endpoint of secondary importance only to survival (5–8).

The physical symptoms among 350 hospice inpatients with cancer were found to correlate with patient characteristics, general condition, tumor location, and medications. The mean number of symptoms correlated directly with the performance status; the performance status was 10–20 with seven symptoms, 30–50 with six symptoms, and ≥ 60 with four symptoms (9). Quality of life measurements have also been shown to predict for survival and add to the prognostic information derived from the Karnofsky Performance Status (KPS) and extent of disease. Among 208 patients with terminal cancer, the overall median survival was 15 weeks. Physical symptoms that include pain, dry mouth, constipation, change in taste, lack of appetite and energy, feeling bloated, nausea, vomiting, weight loss, feeling drowsy, or dizzy portend a poorer prognosis (10). Shorter survival times were independently associated with the following factors: primary site (lung cancer versus breast and gastrointestinal cancers), liver metastases, comorbidities, weight loss of greater than 8 kg in the previous 6 months, and clinical estimation of a less than 2-month survival by the treating physician. Laboratory assessments including serum albumin levels of less than 3.5 dg/L, lymphocyte counts of less than 1×10^9/L, LDH levels of more than 618 U/L also were associated with a poor prognosis. After these independent factors were accounted for in the analysis, other factors, like the performance status, did not independently impact on prognosis.

Many studies have shown that physicians are often reluctant to prescribe adequate levels of analgesics unless it is anticipated that the patient has 6 months or less to live (1,11–13). However most physicians are often unable to correctly predict prognosis. A review of five studies involving a total of 468 patients who were considered to have less than 6 months to live demonstrated that physicians correctly predicted prognosis about half of the time with a range of 22–70% (14,15). In these studies, the actual median survival was 3.5 weeks (range 2–5 weeks) as compared to the estimated median survival of 6 weeks (4.5–8 weeks) by the physician.

Some of the uncertainties in predicting prognosis were overcome in a project, the Study to Understand Prognoses and Preferences for Outcomes and Risks of Treatments (SUPPORT). This study first retrospectively evaluated and developed a model to predict prognosis based on the outcomes of 4301 patients. The model was then prospectively tested using 4028 patients (14,15). Once developed, the model to predict prognosis was applied by physicians among 1757 cases to estimate the likelihood that a patient would survive 2 to 6 months. Using this model, physicians were able to predict survival within 9% of the actual survival. But, patients with metastatic cancer generally overestimated their survival in this study. Once patients acknowledged that they had a 10% chance of dying within 6 months, they were much more likely to prefer comfort care instead of antineoplastic treatments that caused toxicity in an attempt to extend life. Despite over more than a decade of efforts to educate physicians and patients about palliative care options and about end-of-life issues, many patients in this recent study continued to receive ineffective cancer treatments, defined having response rate of 20% and they died in the hospital.

Barriers to effective pain treatment include lack of assessment, patient reluctance to report pain and to use analgesics, and physician reluctance to prescribe opioids (1,11–13,16–18). The mean pain score, using a Visual Analogue Scale where 10 is the worst pain imaginable, was 5.2 among 45 inpatients referred for consultation to the pain service; 56% of patients had pain scores ≥ 5 and 20% had pain scores ≥ 8 on presentation. All patients had used opioids previously and 41 were receiving opioids at the time of consultation. Within 24 hr using medical management, the mean pain intensity was 2.7 ($p < 0.05$).

The debility that results from cancer and its treatment is a significant issue on a socioeconomic level. Among more than 9700 community-based Medicare beneficiaries, poorer health, more limitations of the activities of daily living, and greater levels of health utilization were documented among the 1647 individuals who had cancer (19). Limitations in activities included difficulty in walking (38%), getting out of a chair (21%), completing heavy housework (34%), and shopping (17%). Poorer health was observed more frequently in lung, breast, prostate, and colon cancer patients. Lung, bladder, and prostate cancers predicted for increased health care utilization, and lung cancer most frequently limited the activities of daily living. The mean annual Medicare reimbursement for lung cancer was more than twice that for colon, breast, and prostate cancers. Even though the decrease in functional capacity for cancer patients is generally not as prolonged as with other chronic diseases like arthritis, stoke, and emphysema, the annual health care costs for cancer patients were greater than the health care costs for other chronic diseases (20). Assuming that not all of the individuals identified with the diagnosis of cancer in this Medicare review had active disease at the time of the analysis, then an even greater percentage of cancer patients with active disease are functionally impaired and use more health care resources.

Among 108 patients referred to an outpatient multidisciplinary bone metastases clinic. The median age of the population was 55 years and 69% of the patients were less than 65 years of age. The time since diagnosis of the primary tumor ranged from 2 weeks to 23 years; the median time since diagnosis was 22 months and 30% of patients had been diagnosed within the past 6 months (18). Pain was the presenting symptom in 74% of patients at diagnosis. On average, pain was rated as moderate to severe in 79% and severe in 23% of patients; at its worst, pain was rated as severe by 78% and intolerable by 22% of the patients. Only 45% of patients experienced good relief from the prescribed analgesics and 23% indicated that the prescribed analgesics were ineffective. Despite this, 21% of patients worked full-time and 6% were employed part-time; 13% were homemakers, and only 16% of patients considered themselves to be disabled.

It is important to recognize that terminal illness imposes also substantial economic and other burdens on our patients and those who care for them. Among six randomly selected cities across the United States, 988 terminally ill patients and 893 caregivers were interviewed. Needs for transportation, nursing care, personal care, and economic costs were evaluated (21). The leading causes of terminal illness were cancer (51.8%), heart disease (18%), and chronic obstructive pulmonary disease 10.9%. The mean age was 66.5 years (range 22–109 years), and 59.4% were at least 65 years of age. Among all patients, 50.2% experienced substantial pain, 17.5% were bedridden for more than 50% of the day, 70.9% had shortness of breath while walking one block or less, 35.5% had urinary or fecal incontinence, and 16.8% had depressive symptoms. In the previous 6 months, only 33.5% had not been hospitalized, and 22.3% required a hospital stay that involved the intensive care unit, 36.8% had undergone a surgical procedure. Overall, 35% of patients had substantial care needs that resulted in an expenditure of more than 10% of their household income on health care; 16% of families had to take out a loan, spend their savings, or obtain an additional job to cover medical costs. Patients with substantial needs were more likely to consider euthanasia and administering care significantly impacted the life of over 35% of caregivers. Importantly, physicians who listened to the needs of patients and their caregivers had significantly fewer burdens of care. Only 28% of families felt burdened by the illness if the physician was involved in the needs of terminal care as compared to 42% whose physicians did not listened to the needs of the family ($p = 0.005$). However, few medical textbooks prepare physicians in end-of-life care. On average, textbooks cited 2% of their total pages to end-of-life care (22). A review of the 50 top-selling textbooks from multiple medical specialties found that only 24% of textbooks, and specifically only 38% of oncology textbooks, had helpful information in end-of-life care.

Approximately 300,000 patients nationwide receive palliative radiation costing $900 million per year. About 100,000 patients receive curative radiation therapy costing a total of $1.1 billion per year (23,24). The National Institutes of Health estimate that the overall cost for cancer in the year 2000 was $180.2 billion. This included $60 billion for direct medical costs, $15 billion resulting from lost productivity due to illness, and $105.2 billion caused by lost productivity due to death (25). These analyses become increasingly important because health care costs represent a key economic and political issue. The charge is to find palliative care strategies that relieve suffering, increase personal independence and prevent complications of the disease, and its treatment in the most cost-effective way.

Issues regarding the estimation of prognosis are important to the development of a palliative care plan, and they impact on pain control. Physicians need to develop a palliative care plan so that the patients do not spend a disproportionate percentage of their survival getting palliative treatment. But, palliative treatment needs to provide durable relief of symptoms for the duration of the patient's life. To address the importance of pain control, the Joint Commission on Accreditation of Healthcare Organizations (JCAHO) has incorporated a set of standards for the assessment and management of pain that went into effect January 1, 2001. These standards include that all patients have the right to appropriate assessment and management of pain, and that patients be taught that pain management is an integral part of their cancer treatment.

Unlike other aspects of cancer therapy, tumor control and survival are not the endpoints of therapeutic success in palliative care. Palliative cancer treatment is given to maintain comfort (2–8,26,27). With palliative care, cancer is treated like a chronic disease in which medical efforts try to prevent or manage the symptoms of the disease. The goal of palliative care is to relieve symptoms effectively and efficiently with the fewest treatment-related symptoms, and to maintain the maximum quality of life for the duration of the patient's life. Keeping the goals of palliative care in mind, palliative therapy targets symptomatic areas or areas at risk for incurring morbidity with progressive disease. Therapeutic approaches should be used to provide durable control of symptoms and maintain functional integrity. Treatment of the cancer can be localized, like surgery or radiation, or systemic like radiopharmaceuticals, and chemo-hormonal therapy.

Control of cancer-related pain with the use of analgesics is imperative to allow comfort during and while awaiting response to therapeutic interventions. Pain represents a sensitive measure of disease activity (28–33). Symptoms that recur after palliative radiation most commonly result from localized regrowth of tumor. Close follow-up should be performed after any palliative therapeutic intervention to initiate diagnostic studies to identify progressive or recurrent disease.

Ineffective therapies that incur morbidity and cost, and provide little to no palliative benefit should not be administered. The factors that determine the effectiveness of palliative therapy include the percentage of patients who experience persistent/recurrent symptoms, and if these symptoms can be relieved with other therapeutic modalities that are easier to administer, that have fewer side effects, and that include less cost.

II. PALLIATIVE RADIATION TECHNIQUES

The symptoms most commonly relieved with palliative radiation are pain, bleeding, and obstruction. A number of clinical, prognostic, and therapeutic factors must be considered to determine the optimal treatment approach. Depending on prognostic factors and known treatment-related side effects, palliative treatment can range from the use of all three treatment modalities (surgery, radiation, and chemotherapy) to single therapeutic modality like radiation alone.

Radiotherapy techniques vary considerably based upon the involved and adjacent normal structures. Basic to an understanding of applied techniques and potential morbidity during a course of radiation are the following principles (34). Radiation therapy is delivered in units designated as the Gray. Relating this to the previously used term rad, equivalent doses can be expressed as 1 Gray (Gy), 100 centigray (cGy), and 100 rad; 1 rad equals 1 cGy.

Radiation may be delivered by either *external beam therapy* (linear accelerators, Cobalt 60 units) or *brachytherapy* using radioactive isotopes applied directly to the region involved by the tumor. External beam therapy is administered with a prescribed number of daily fractions over several weeks, while brachytherapy is a continuous application of radiation to the tumor bed over a number of minutes to days. A variety of radiation energies and biological characteristics are now available to help localize treatment to the areas at risk and exclude uninvolved normal tissues.

A. External Beam Irradiation

Included within the classification of external beam radiation are *photons* that are penetrating forms of radiation, and *electrons*, delivering treatment to superficial areas. Other specialized types of external radiation beams available at only a few centers and they include *proton beam* therapy (administering radiation with high precision to well-defined small areas of tumor involvement like pituitary or midbrain lesions) and *neutrons* (used by a few centers to treat bulky unresectable or recurrent tumors).

The concept of integral dose relates the amount of radiation deposited to uninvolved normal tissues located between the skin surface and tumor; the goal in any radiation plan is to minimize integral dose by selecting the appropriate beam energy (Table 1). The D_{max} radiation dose is the depth at which 100% of the prescribed radiation is deposited. Higher energy photon radiation, like 18 mV photons, reduces integral dose because it deposits more radiation to deeper structures while delivering relatively little radiation to superficial tissues.

Multiple radiation portals, each of which is treated daily, are also routinely used in radiotherapy to reduce integral dose. Table 2 demonstrates an example of the impact on integral radiation dose when 200 cGy are prescribed at 10 cm depth from a 6 mV linear accelerator. When only the anterior radiation portal is used to deliver radiation in the example, the integral dose is high because more superficial tissues receive nearly 50% more than the prescribed radiation dose at the site of the tumor located 10 cm below the skin surface; at 1.5 cm from the skin surface, the daily radiation dose is 294 cGy per fraction and the total dose is 5880 cGy as compared to the 200 cGy per fraction and total radiation dose of 4000 cGy at the tumor. Radiation tolerance is primarily based on the daily radiation dose; as the daily radiation dose increases, the total radiation dose that can be given to normal tissues decreases. Because of this, treatment with an anterior field alone would result in significant side effects due to the high integral dose. It is important to realize that giving the first half of the radiation course from the anterior (AP) field alone, and the second half of the radiation course from the posterior (PA) field alone would not reduce radiation side effects. Although the total radiation dose would be more even using an AP field during the first half and a PA field during the last half of a radiation dose, side effects still may be severe because of the high daily (integral) dose of radiation.

Table 1 Concept of Integral Dose Demonstrated by Radiation Dose Distributions for Three Different Energies: Cobalt 60, 6, and 18 MV Photons[a]

Skin surface (cm)	Cobalt 60 (%)	6 MV (%)	18 MV (%)
0.5	100	30	25
1.0	98	90	50
1.5	95	100	90
2.0	93	98	96
2.5	90	97	98
3.0	88	95	98
3.5	85	92	100
5.0	80	88	96
10	55	68	80

[a] D_{max}, the maximum dose, refers to the depth at which 100% of the prescribed dose is located below the skin surface. The greater the D_{max}, the greater the skin sparing associated with less of an integral dose.

When the radiation is delivered each day from both an AP and PA radiation portal, the radiation dose given in the portal is the sum of the radiation dose from each field (Fig. 1). The integral dose in the case presented decreases significantly with AP and PA treatment fields because the daily radiation dose throughout the treatment field is within 6% (with a daily dose of 211 cGy per fraction at 16.5 cm below the anterior skin surface) of the prescribed dose of 200 cGy per fraction (Fig. 2). Likewise, the maximum total radiation dose in the field is 4220 cGy, just 220 cGy more than the prescribed radiation dose at the tumor (Fig. 3). Newer treatment approaches, like conformal radiation therapy, exploit this relationship by treating up to eight different radiation fields each day. Reducing integral dose is a principal concept of radiation treatment planning because it allows higher radiation doses to the tumor and less radiation to the surrounding normal tissues.

External beam irradiation is administered from specialized machines which emit gamma rays from a housed isotope (cobalt 60) or x-rays (linear accelerators), which are more than 1000 times as powerful as those used in diagnostic radiology, that are generated by electricity. The availability of higher energy radiation beams, and the development of a variety of different radiation energies was critical to the advancement of radiation therapy. These advancements allowed more precise deposition of the radiation in the area of the tumor while sparing surrounding uninvolved normal tissues.

Placing this in perspective, the first machines used in radiation therapy emitted *orthovoltage* radiation. In contrast to the 18 meV linear accelerators currently available, the low radiation energy of orthovoltage radiation ranges between 125 and 250 keV (Fig. 4). Orthovoltage is delivered generally in one or two fractions through a cone that is directly applied to the

Table 2 Impact on Integral Radiation Dose when 200 cGy Prescribed at Midline (10 cm Depth; Patient Diameter is 20 cm) from a 6 mV Linear Accelerator Single Anterior Radiation Field delivering 200 cGy at Midline (10 cm)

Distance from skin surface (cm)	6 MV photons (%) (of prescribed radiation)
0.5	30
1.0	90
1.5	**100**
2.0	98
2.5	97
3.0	95
3.5	92
5.0	88
10	**68**
15.0	51
16.5	48
17.5	44
18.5	42
19.5	40

Radiation dose = 200 cGy at 10 cm depth; percentage depth dose = 68%; radiation dose at 1.5 cm (D_{max} or 100%) is the radiation dose Rx'ed/0.68 or 294 cGy j; radiation dose at other depths is the D_{max} dose (294 cGy) × % isodose. (See Table 1.)

Single anterior radiation field delivering 200 cGy at midline (10 cm)

Depth from anterior skin surface (cm)	Dose from AP	Total dose × 20 fractions
0.5	88 cGy (294 × 0.30)	1760 cGy (88 × 20)
1.5	**294 cGy (200/0.68)**	**5880 cGy (294 × 20)**
2.5	285 cGy (294 × 0.97)	5700 cGy (285 × 20)
3.5	279 cGy (294 × 0.92)	5580 cGy (279 × 20)
5.0	259 cGy (294 × 0.88)	5180 cGy (259 × 20)
10	**200 cGy (294 × 0.68)**	**4000 cGy (200 × 20)**
15	150 cGy (294 × 0.51)	3000 cGy (165 × 20)
16.5	141 cGy (294 × 0.48)	2820 cGy (144 × 20)
17.5	129 cGy (294 × 0.44)	2580 cGy (129 × 20)
18.5	123 cGy (294 × 0.42)	2460 cGy (126 × 20)
19.5	118 cGy (294 × 0.40)	2360 cGy (118 × 20)

Parallel opposed (P and PA) radiation fields treated each day delivering 200 cGy at midline (10 cm)

Depth from anterior skin surface (cm)	Dose from AP	Dose from PA	Total dose per fraction (AP + PA) (cGy)	Total dose × 20 fractions (AP + PA) (cGy)
0.5	44 cGy (147 × 0.30)	59 cGy (147 × 0.40)	103	2060
1.5	**147 cGy (100/0.68)**	**62 cGy (147 × 0.42)**	**209**	**4180**
2.5	143 cGy (147 × 0.97)	65 cGy (147 × 0.44)	208	4160
3.5	140 cGy (147 × 0.92)	71 cGy (147 × 0.48)	211	4220
5.0	129 cGy (147 × 0.88)	75 cGy (147 × 0.51)	204	4080
10.0	**100 cGy (147 × 0.68)**	**100 cGy (147 × 0.68)**	**200**	**4000**
15.0	75 cGy (147 × 0.51)	129 cGy (147 × 0.88)	204	4080
16.5	71 cGy (147 × 0.48)	140 cGy (147 × 0.92)	211	4220
17.5	65 cGy (147 × 0.44)	143 cGy (147 × 0.97)	208	4160
18.5	62 cGy (147 × 0.42)	147 cGy (100/0.68)	209	4180
19.5	59 cGy (147 × 0.40)	44 cGy (147 × 0.30)	103	2060

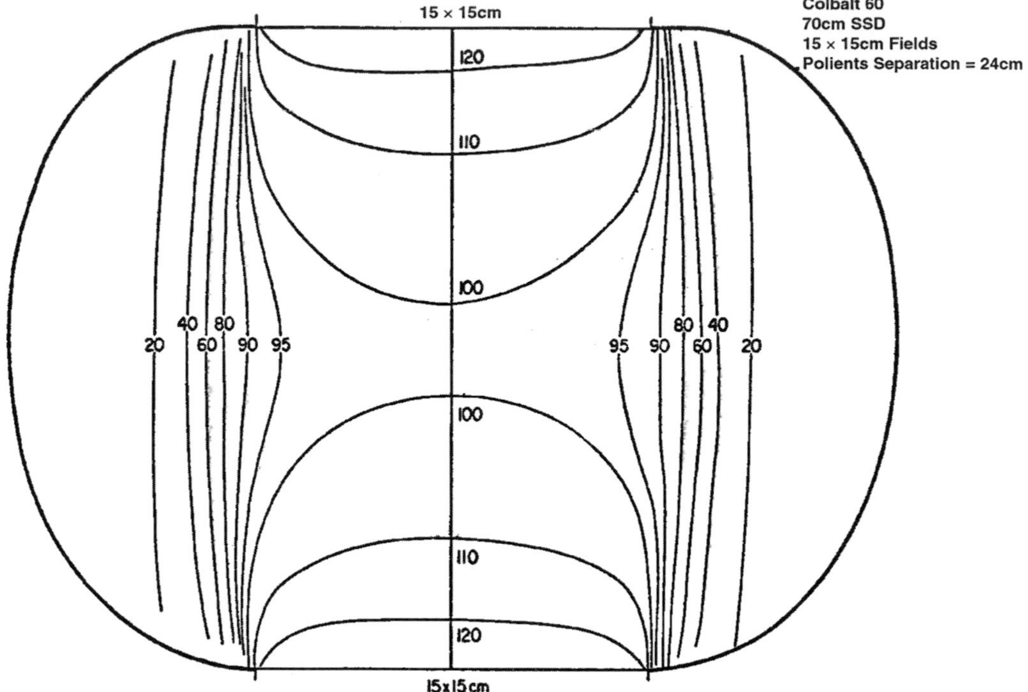

Figure 1 The radiation isodose distribution for a 15 cm × 15 cm radiation field using anterior and posterior (AP and PA) parallel opposed portals with cobalt 60. In this case, the patient has a 24 cm diameter. Each number represents a percentage of the prescribed radiation dose. If 200 cGy was prescribed to the 100% isodose line, then 240 cGy would be delivered to the 120% isodose line near the skin surface and only 180 cGy would be given at the edge of the radiation field at the 90% isodose line. The edges of the field receive less radiation dose because there is opportunity for the radiation dose to interact with adjacent radiated tissue at the blocked edge than in the middle of the field.

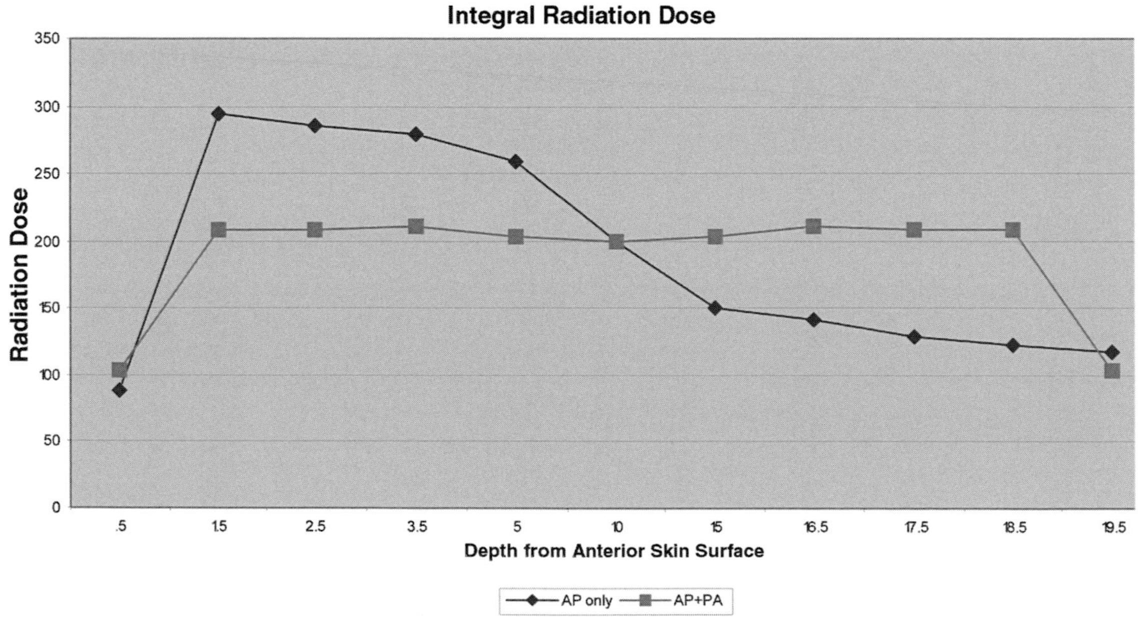

Figure 2 Graphic comparison of the integral dose, defined as the radiation dose deposited between the skin surface and the tumor. In this case, the tumor is 10 cm below the skin surface. If radiation were only given from the anterior treatment portal, the daily radiation dose to the skin would result in complications because of the high radiation dose per fraction as well as the high total dose of radiation.

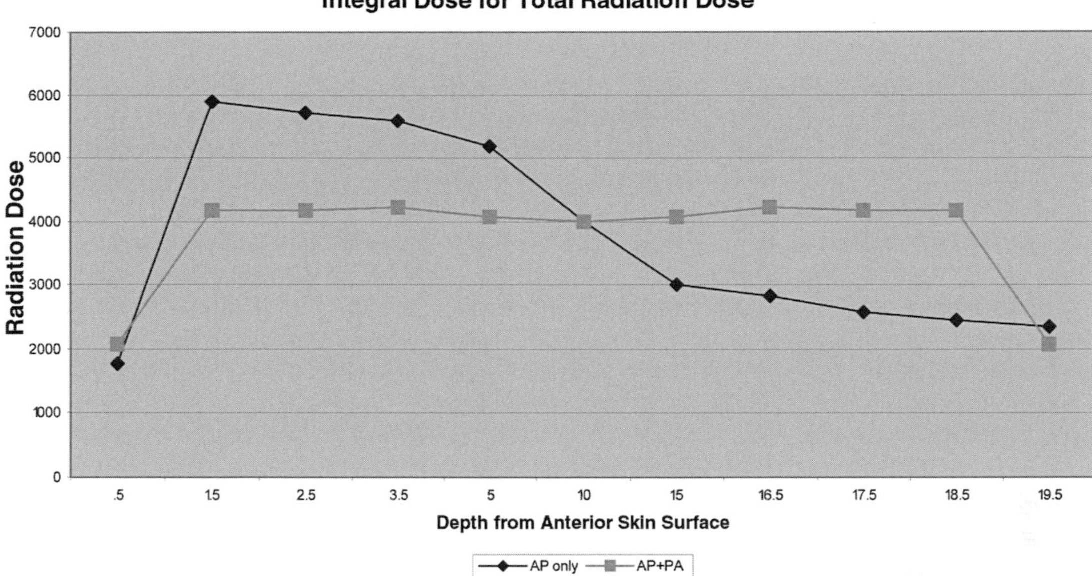

Figure 3 Graphic comparison of the total radiation dose given when a single anterior radiation field is used instead of parallel opposed radiation fields (AP and PA fields) treated every day. With the AP field alone, the skin would receive 30% more radiation than the parallel opposed treatment approach to achieve the same radiation dose at the tumor.

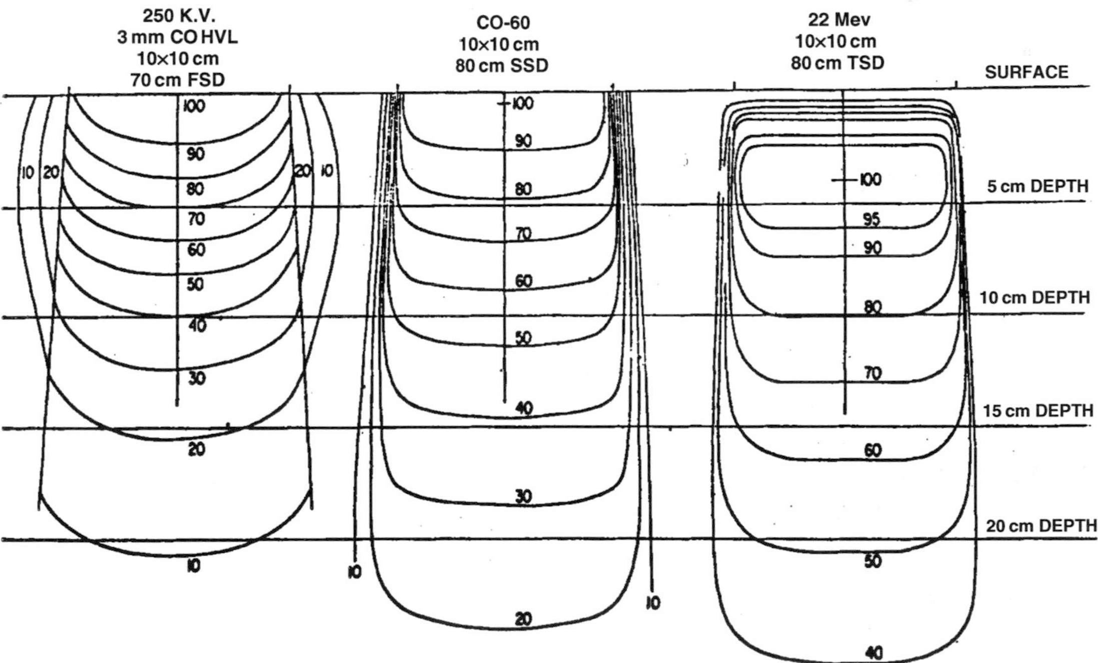

Figure 4 The different radiation isodose distributions for 10 cm × 10 cm radiation fields. The three beams compared include orthovoltage radiation with a 250 keV radiation beam (*left*), a cobalt 60 unit (*middle*), and a 22 MeV linear accelerator (*right*). The 250 keV unit has no skin sparing and little depth of penetration of the radiation beam. The cobalt 60 unit is ideal to treat head and neck cancers so that adequate radiation is given to superficial lymph nodes and scars in the postoperative setting. Because the diameter of the head and neck region is limited, a highly penetrating photon beam is not advisable. Twenty-two mega-electron-volt photons are ideal for deep-seated tumor like in the pelvis and abdomen because of skin sparring and deep penetration of the photon beams.

tumor. Orthovoltage has limited applications, but it continues to be highly effective in reducing bleeding from rectal and cervical cancers. Protracted courses with orthovoltage radiation, however, resulted in late radiation complications that included osteonecrosis. Osteonecrosis developed because of the increased absorption of low-energy radiation by tissues that have a high atomic number, like the bone. This characteristic allows the differentiation between bones and soft tissues in diagnostic radiology, but the radiation doses used in the treatment of cancer are several magnitudes greater than those used for diagnostic purposes. This increased absorption of radiation in bone or other tissues of high atomic number does not, however, occur in current megavoltage radiation beams because of the higher energies used (Fig. 5).

A wide variety of *photon* energies are available. This allows selective administration of treatment to the tumor and minimizes radiation to uninvolved tissues. As a standard, available photon beam energies range from Cobalt 60 to 22 MeV photons. Cobalt 60 delivers 100% of the prescribed radiation dose, indicated as the maximum radiation dose (D_{max}), 0.5 cm below the skin surface. Six megavolt x-rays from a linear accelerator have a D_{max} of 1.5 cm, and 18 MeV photons have a D_{max} of 3.5 cm below the skin. Tissues 0.5 cm below the skin surface treated with 18 MeV photons receive only 30% of the prescribed radiation dose. This demonstrates the relationship in radiation physics that there is more sparing of superficial structures (skin and subcutaneous tissues) from radiation with higher photon energies even though the beam deeply penetrates into the tissue.

Electron beam radiation is an important therapeutic option in the treatment of superficial tumors. The penetration of the beam can roughly be estimated by dividing the energy by different numerical factors. For example, 80% of the radiation dose from a 9 MeV electron beam is deposited within 3 cm of the surface (9 divided by 3) while essentially all of the radiation is given within 4.5 cm of the skin (9 divided by 2) with no radiation penetrating beyond that depth. A variety of electron beam energies are available to allow precise localization of the radiation to superficial lesions while sparing underlying critical structures. Electron beam radiation is routinely used in head and neck cancer to treat the posterior cervical lymph nodes while avoiding treatment of the underlying spinal cord.

Proton beam therapy and "radiosurgery" are more limited in application and availability; however, the concept is to precisely deposit a large amount of radiation to a well-defined volume of tumor while sparing

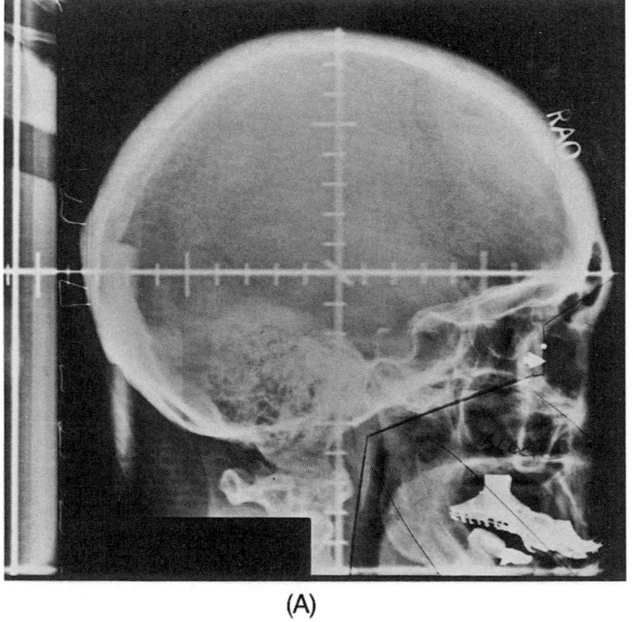

(A)

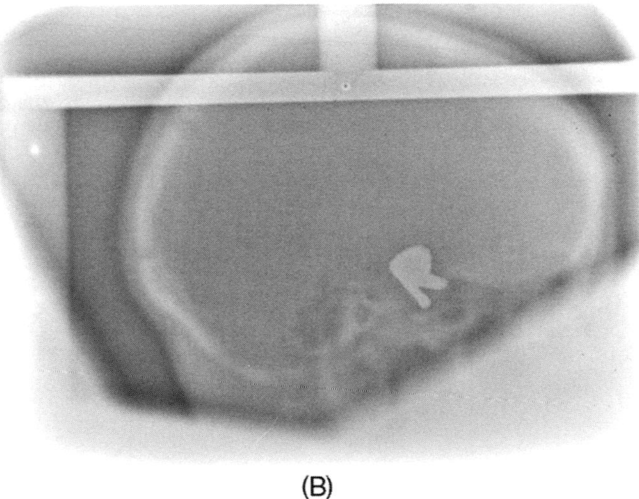

(B)

Figure 5 (A) A diagnostic x-ray taken during simulation of the radiation fields. There is a significant difference in the contrast between the bones and the soft tissues due to the low energy of the photons used in diagnostic x-rays. Because calcium has a high atomic number, this results in the bones absorbing a dose of radiation that is about three times more than the radiation dose absorbed by the soft tissues (photoelectric effect). (B) An image taken during a radiation treatment. Because of the high energy of the radiation photons used during radiation therapy, the contrast between the bones and soft tissues is less apparent. Because the energy of the radiation is so high, the bones and soft tissues absorb about the same dose of radiation (Compton effect).

intervening tissues. Precision of proton beam therapy is to the level of the millimeter, requiring exact mapping of the tumor volume and potential microscopic areas of involvement. An additional advantage of proton irradiation is the improvement of relative biologic effectiveness of this type of radiation because of the characteristic Bragg–Peak distribution of radiation within a narrow volume of tissue (Fig. 6). Chordomas and localized intracranial tumors, especially around the optic chiasm, have been treated with proton irradiation. Because of its precision, research is ongoing to define further applications of proton therapy, especially in pediatric tumors and previously irradiated recurrent tumors.

Neutron radiation is primarily used among patients who have undergone previous aggressive cancer therapy resulting in the presence of resistant clonogens, or with large tumor burdens. Neutron radiation is more efficient than photons in killing tumor cells because neutron radiation is less dependent on oxygen radicals to cause irreversible radiation damage. The radiobiological effectiveness (RBE), describes the relative efficiency of different radiation beams in terms of a ratio of doses, to produce the same level of cellular damage. Based on this ratio, a single fraction of neutron radiation has an RBE of 1.5, as compared to an RBE of 3.0 for photons (35). This characteristic reflects a reduced initial shoulder of radiation resistance on the cell survival curve and the decreased influence of oxygen on radiosensitivity with neutron irradiation (Fig. 7). All solid tumors greater than 180 μm in size contain hypoxic cells. Although promising in preclinical evaluation and in treatment of unresectable tumors, only a few centers continue to have neutrons.

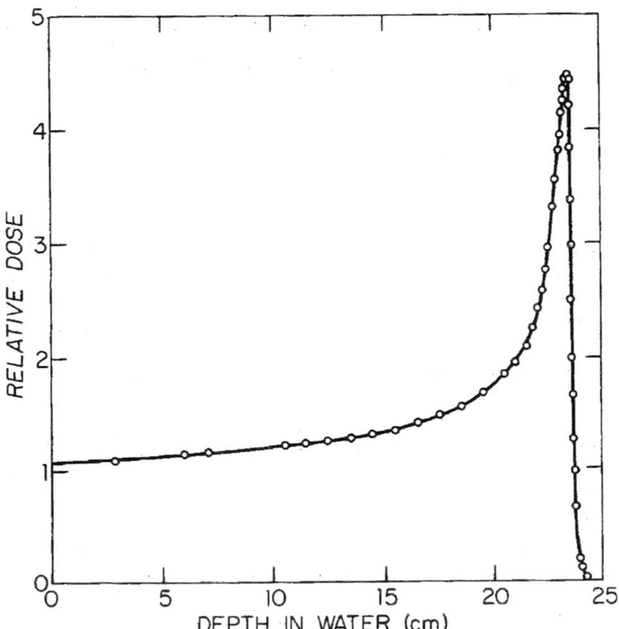

Figure 6 The Bragg–Peak effect in radiation associated with proton radiation. Only the designated tumor area received the prescribed dose of radiation, and the surrounding normal tissues are spared radiation. Although currently used to treat intracranial tumors and pediatric cases, proton radiation may have application in palliative care for the retreatment of tumors.

Because radiation therapy is frequently used to palliate localized sites of disease, many radiotherapeutic options are needed for tumors that cause localized symptoms. The clinical status of the patient is accounted for in the treatment setup and in the number of radiation treatments that are prescribed. The radiation dose-fractionation schedule and technique also considers the site and volume irradiated, and the integration of other therapies. Conformal and intensity modulated radiation therapy, intraoperative radiation, brachytherapy, and endocavitary therapy are all techniques that can better localize radiation dose and reduce side effects, especially in a previously irradiated area.

B. Reirradiation

Issues regarding reirradiation are especially important in palliative therapy. Experimental data suggest that acute responding tissues, like mucosa and small bowel, recover radiation injury in a few months and can tolerate additional radiation therapy. However, there is considerable variability in recovery from radiation among late reacting tissues like the spinal cord and brain (36). This recovery depends on the technique used, the organ irradiated, the volume irradiated, the initial total dose of radiation, the radiation dose given with each fraction, and the time interval between the initial and second courses of radiation (37).

Correlating with existing clinical experience, limited toxicities occur with reirradiation when there is careful attention to treatment techniques and radiobiological factors. Radiotherapeutic techniques that localize the radiation dose to the recurrent tumor and limit the dose to the surrounding normal tissues allow the reirradiation of recurrent tumors. Other techniques include conformal external beam radiation and intensity modulated radiation therapy (IMRT), intraoperative radiation therapy (IORT) brachytherapy, and endocavitary radiation (38–44).

1. Conformal Radiation Therapy/IMRT

Conformal radiation techniques precisely localize the radiation dose using external beam radiation from a linear accelerator. Because very low doses of radiation are given through a number of beams, no one area of

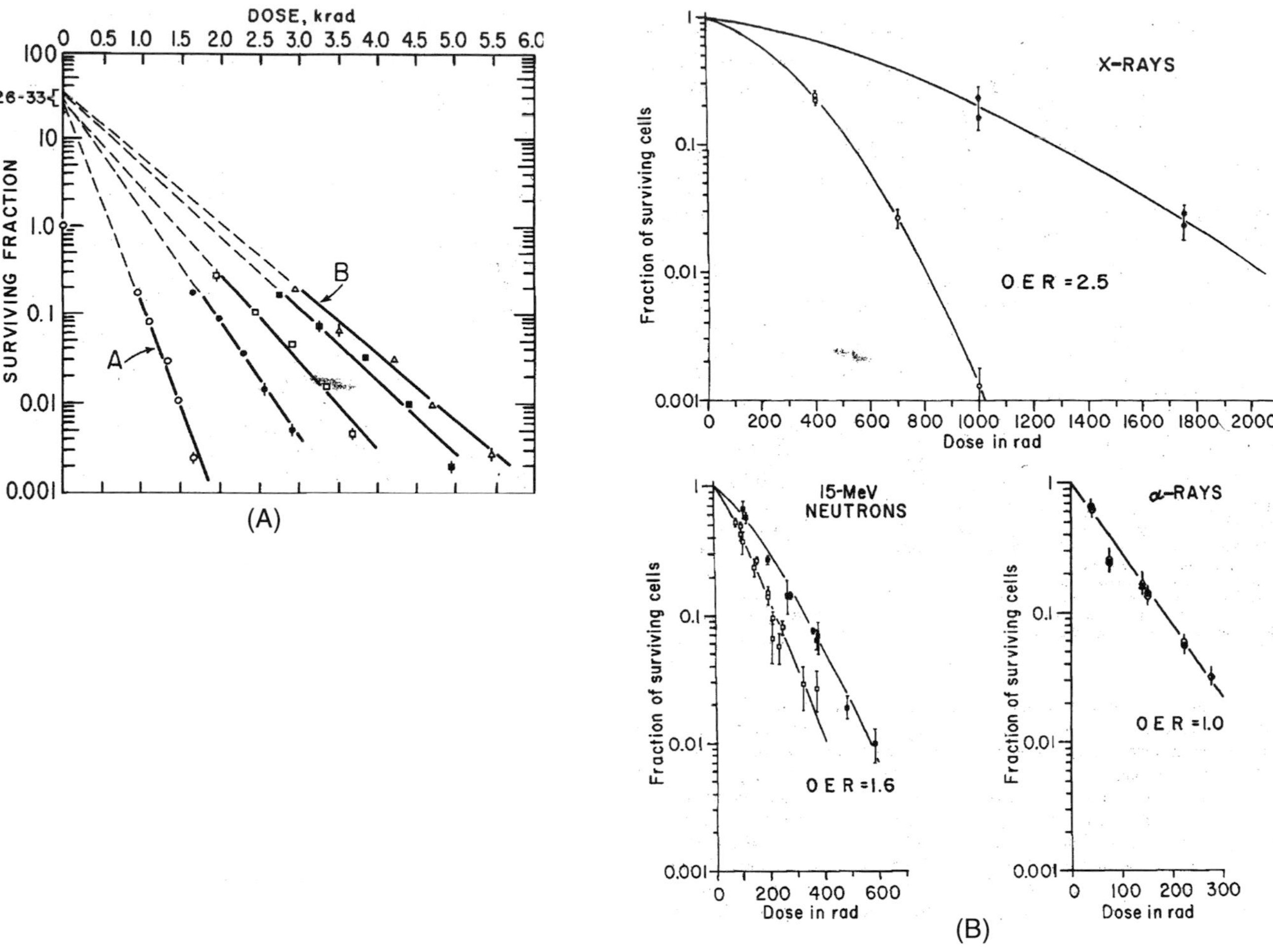

Figure 7 (A) The dependence of radiation sensitivity on oxygen tension known as the oxygen enhancement ratio (OER). (B) The radiobiologic effect (RBE) of photon and neutron radiation. Because neutron radiation is less dependent on oxygen, tumors are more sensitive to neutron radiation. Neutron radiation has been used in palliative care to treat recurrent or unresectable tumors.

normal tissue receives a significant dose of radiation. The tumor, though, is given the sum of the radiation from the beams and receives a high dose of radiation. This technique has allowed high doses of radiation to be given, and has allowed for reirradiation of normal tissues without significant side effects.

Intensity modulated radiation therapy is a form of conformal external beam radiation that even more precisely administers radiation. It is possible to deliver different doses of radiation to specific areas in a single radiation fraction. For example, with IMRT the center of the tumor may receive 2.20 Gy with each radiation treatment to a total dose of 66 Gy over 30 fractions in 6 weeks, while the periphery of the tumor may receive 2.0 Gy with each radiation treatment to a total dose of 60 Gy. At the same time, the normal tissues within 2 cm of the tumor (clinical tumor volume to account for possible microscopic tumor extension) may receive 1.8 Gy with each radiation treatment to a total dose of 54 Gy. Intensity modulated radiation therapy provides the radiobiologic advantage of giving a high daily dose of radiation localized within the center of a tumor while giving a well-tolerated lower daily dose of radiation to the surrounding tissues at the same time. Localizing high daily and total doses of radiation in the tumor, IMRT is able to kill more cancer cells with higher radiation doses without harming the surrounding tissues. Any shape or configuration of radiation dose, like an hourglass, can be designed with IMRT. Because of these factors, this radiotherapeutic tool is extremely helpful in delivering high radiation doses to inoperable tumors over a shorter period of time, and in treating tumors that recur in a previously irradiated field.

2. *Intraoperative Radiation Therapy (IORT)*

Intraoperative radiation has also been used as a supplement to external beam radiation or as the only therapy when further external beam radiation is not possible. Intraoperative radiation therapy administers radiation totaling 10–20 Gy in a single fraction to a localized region during the surgical procedure.Adjacent tissues, like the bowel, receive no radiation because they are displaced from the radiation field (41–44). Electron beam radiation is generally used with intraoperative radiation because it penetrates only the first few centimeters of tissue. Studies have demonstrated that IORT results in significant improvements in control of symptoms and the tumor, but the level of success is dependent on the volume of residual tumor treated.

3. *Brachytherapy and Endocavitary Radiation*

Brachytherapy involves placement of radioactive sources within a tumor bed and it represents another means of administering well-localized radiotherapy to limit dose to adjacent uninvolved structures. Uninterrupted radiation is delivered precisely to the tumor bed over a determined number of minutes to hours. Brachytherapy has been used as definitive treatment of localized disease, as a boost in conjunction with external beam irradiation, and for the treatment of disease recurring in an area previously irradiated.

Practical advantages of brachytherapy include reduced overall treatment time, and sparing of uninvolved surrounding structures that also allows reirradiation. Theoretical advantages of brachytherapy include the direct placement of radiation in the operative bed that is at risk for microscopic residual disease, and better oxygenation of surgical bed before the development of postoperative fibrosis. Because brachytherapy localizes the radiation dose within a 3 cm radius of the catheters, considerably less normal tissue is irradiated with brachytherapy when compared to external beam radiotherapy (Fig. 8). Reirradiation is then possible because the radiation from brachytherapy is well localized and does not injure surrounding previously irradiated tissues (38–40). The localization of radiation dose with brachytherapy is based on the inverse-square law. In this, the radiation dose rapidly decreases as the distance increases from the radiation source (Fig. 9). For example, only one-fourth the radiation dose is given to tissues that are located 2 cm away from the radiation source. Tissue hypoxia significantly reduces radiosensitivity; with brachytherapy, radiation is administered before hypoxic scar tissue develops in the wound. The inverse-square law and tissue hypoxia are critical to limiting the radiation dose needed for reirradiation of recurrent tumors. Like IMRT, the inverse-square law allows for higher doses of radiation to be given directly to the tumor, while limiting the radiation dose to the surrounding tissues.

Brachytherapy sources can be placed either temporarily or permanently within the tumor. There are a wide variety of brachytherapy sources and strengths that can be used (Table 3). Low-dose rate brachyther-

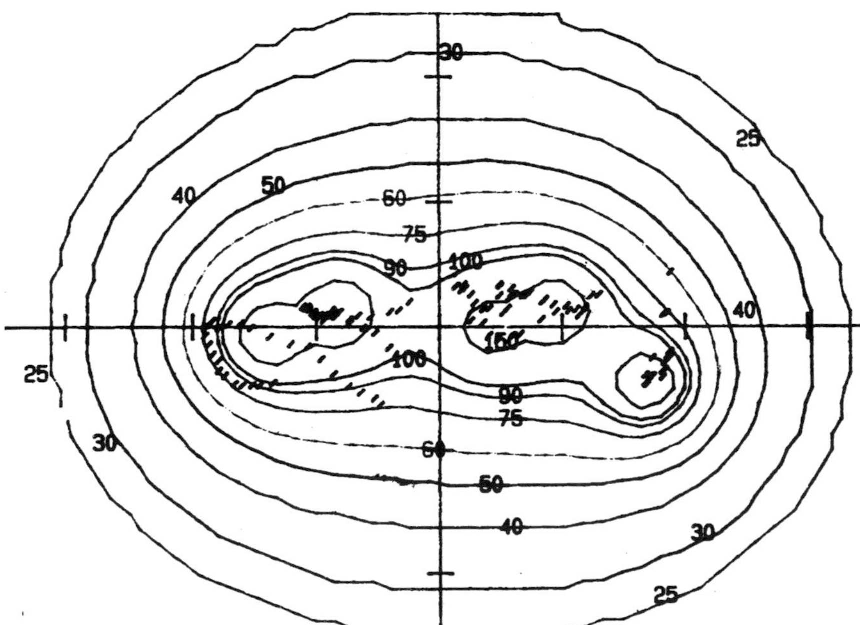

Figure 8 An isodose plan for brachytherapy in a tumor bed. The small dashes represent radiation seeds. Notice that within 2 cm on the x-axis only 70% of the prescribed radiation dose is given and on the y-axis, the tissues receive only 30% of the prescribed radiation dose.

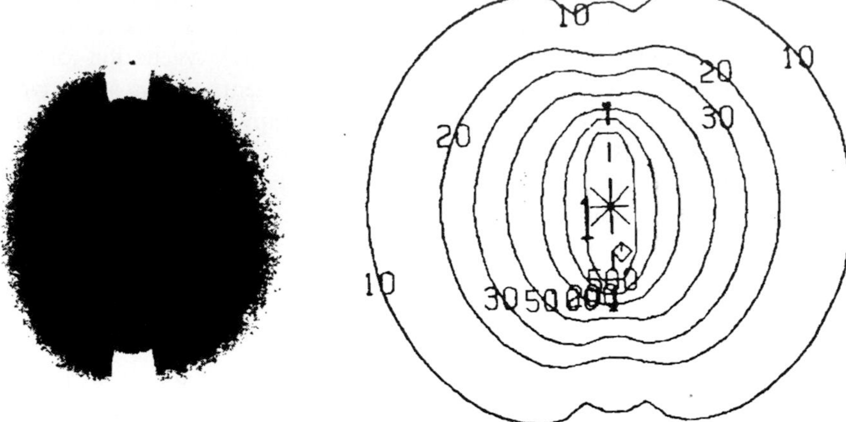

Figure 9 The emitted radioactivity and the radiation dose distribution from a radioactive source. Because the radiation is so localized and placed adjacent to or within tumors, high radiation doses can be administered even in cases of reirradiation.

apy places a lower energy radiation source either adjacent to (temporary implant) or inside tumors (permanent implant). Temporary implants place radioactive sources in catheters that remain in the surgical wound for generally 2–5 days and can deliver 20–50 Gy over that time frame. The sources are then removed, much like a surgical drain. Sources commonly used for low-dose rate brachytherapy include iridium-192 for temporary implants, and iodine-125 and gold-198 for permanent implants.

Table 3 Characteristics of Isotopes Used in Brachytherapy

Isotope	Energy	Half-life
Radium	2.29 MeV	1620 years
Cesium 137	0.662 MeV	30 years
Cobalt 60	1.17 MeV	5 years
Iridium 192	0.34 MeV	75 days
Iodine 125	30 keV	60 days
Gold 198	0.412 MeV	2.7 days
Strontium 90	2.2 MeV (beta)	28 years

Note: All of these are gamma emitting isotopes except strontium 90 which emits beta particles. Beta radiation penetrates tissue poorly, as evidenced by a half value layer of 1 mm in tissue and the fact that only 3% of the dose is measured at a distance of 5 mm from the surface of the source. Strontium 90 is generally used in the eye to treat ptyergia. Iodine 125 is characterized as a weak gamma-emitting isotope (average energy of 30 keV or 0.03 MeV) used in permanent implants. Cesium 137 is generally used in intracavitary implants in gynecologic malignancies and iridium 192 is used for interstitial implants. The term milligram radium equivalent relates to the amount (millicuries) of the isotope that would be necessary to deliver the same amount of radiation as 1 mg of radium, which continues to represent the standard in brachytherapy.

High-dose rate brachytherapy places an intense radioactive radiation source adjacent to a tumor for a few minutes. High-dose rate brachytherapy is often used to treat tumors involving the biliary tract, esophagus, cervix, and bronchus. Relief of dysphagia and bronchial obstruction ranges between 70% and 85% in a number of published reports when brachytherapy has been used in the treatment of esophageal cancer. A combination of a short course of external beam radiation (30Gy in 10 fractions) plus high-dose rate brachytherapy used as a localized radiation boost relieves dysphagia or bronchial obstruction for several months (38–40). Relative contraindications to performing brachytherapy for esophageal cancer include a tumor length of 10 cm or more, extension to the gastroesophageal junction or cardia, skip lesions, extensive extraesophageal spread of disease, macroscopic regional adenopathy, tracheoesophageal fistula, cervical esophageal involvement, or stenosis that cannot be bypassed.

Brachytherapy and endocavitary radiation can be used alone, or more commonly, in conjunction with external beam radiation for pelvic tumors. Administering highly localized doses of radiation, brachytherapy can provide high doses of radiation directly to well-defined volumes to palliate bleeding and obstructive symptoms. Most often, these approaches are used among patients who are unable or unwilling to undergo surgical resection.

C. Palliative Radiation Treatment Schedules

Despite the wide variety of available treatment approaches, external beam radiation remains the most common application of radiotherapy. The administration of external beam irradiation is analogous to the prescription of medications based upon pharmacologic principles of dosing. A balance is required between the dose required to kill the tumor and the radiation dose tolerated by the normal tissues; this is similar to the limitations imposed by renal tolerance to certain classes of antibiotics or by bone marrow and gastrointestinal tolerance to chemotherapy.

The concept of fractionated radiation allows treatment of the cancer while not exceeding the tolerance of the surrounding normal tissues. The four "R's" of radiation biology are repair of sublethal damage, reoxygenation, repopulation, and reassortment of cells within the cell cycle (35). These four factors are key to deciding the radiation schedule to optimize tumor regression while minimizing effects to normal tissues.

With fractionated radiation normal tissues are able to *repair* sublethal radiation effects between treatments. With large daily doses of radiation, a large number of tumor cells are killed, but repair of normal tissues is lower (Fig. 10). Because the normal tissues are unable to repair the radiation damage of large daily doses of radiation, the total radiation dose that can be given is also much lower (35).

Equivalent normal tissue effects can be achieved with a variety of radiation treatment schedules. The

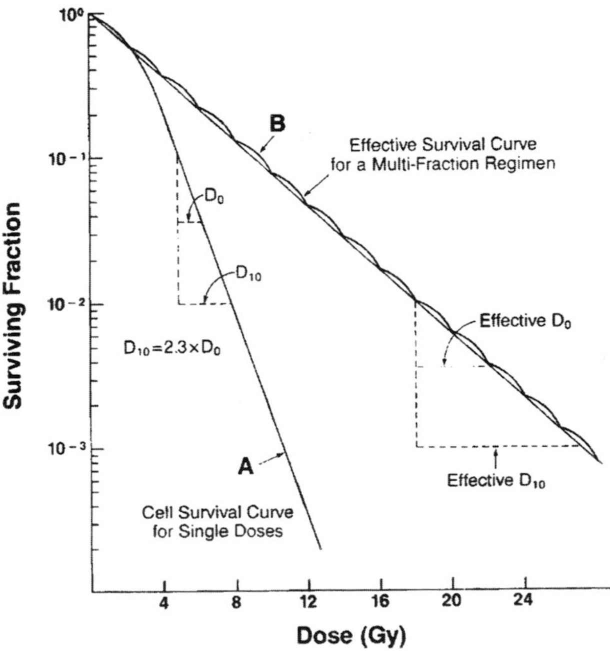

Figure 10 Cell survival after a single large fraction of radiation and multiple small doses of radiation. Because of sublethal damage and repair, a significantly greater total dose of radiation is needed to achieve tumor control when multiple radiation fractions are used.

following clinical radiation schedules are used to treat spine metastases: 2000 cGy is delivered in five fractions, 3000 cGy is administered in 10 fractions, 3500 cGy in 14 fractions or 4000 cGy in 20 fractions. The late radiation effects on the spinal cord uninvolved by tumor would be equal to giving 2800, 3600, and 3900 cGy, respectively at 200 cGy per fraction. This shows that as the radiation dose per fraction increases, the late radiation toxicities biologically exceed the total radiation dose administered to the tumor. This effect is more exaggerated as the radiation dose per fraction increases from the standard 200 cGy per fraction (45). Relating back to the example on integral dose in Table 2, administration of 5880 cGy at 294 cGy per fraction would result in severe long-term radiation effects because this would be biologically equal to a total radiation dose of 7200 cGy at 200 cGy per fraction to a large area of small bowel (46). In summary, as the radiation dose per fraction increase the normal tissues are damaged more than the tumor cells.

The total dose of radiation necessary to eradicate a tumor is a function of the volume of disease and the number of tumor cells killed with each radiation fraction. The tumor volume is the sum of viable and nonviable cells. In most tumors, the potential number of tumor cells is directly proportional to the tumor volume. In some tumors, like soft tissue sarcomas, there is a large necrotic fraction and the rate of cell loss and removal of dead tumor cells from the tumor volume is low. The viable cells may be less responsive to radiation because of the low oxygen tension in the nearby necrotic region. The radiosensitivity of cells also varies during the cell cycle. Cells are most resistant to radiation when they are in the late S-phase, and in the late G1/G0 phase. Radiation resistance results from either rapidly proliferating tumors that spend most of their time in S-phase or a slowly proliferating tumor where many cells are in G1/G0.

Less total radiation dose is required to control microscopic residual disease than bulk disease. For example, the 2-year rate of local control following radiation alone in the treatment of cervical node metastases in head and neck cancer is directly related to the node diameter and total dose. Using 200 cGy per daily fraction of radiation, over 95% of patients with only microscopic residual cancer achieve tumor control, and over 85% of patients with lymph node diameters of less than 2 cm in size are controlled with a median dose of 6600 cGy. But, only 69% of nodes measuring between 2.5 and 3.0 cm are controlled after 6900 cGy and 59% of nodes larger than 3.5 cm are controlled after 7000 cGy. Large tumors have a large hypoxic fraction of cells (35). Hypoxic cells are relatively resistant to radiation effects; it takes three times the dose of radiation to control hypoxic tumors as it does well-oxygenated tumors (Fig. 7). With fractionated radiation, hypoxic areas are able to *reoxygenate* to some degree during the course of treatment.

Additionally, tumor cells and normal tissues vary widely in their tolerance to radiation because of cellular *repopulation*. Radiation doses need to be high enough to kill tumor cells but low enough to allow normal tissues to repair and repopulate. Very low doses of radiation have limited acute effects on normal tissues. No inflammation of the skin or mucosa occurs when the radiation dose is less than 2000 cGy when given in 200 cGy fractions over 2 weeks. But this total dose of radiation is not sufficient to permanently kill tumor cells due to repopulation of the tumor cells. In the past, a course of radiation was interrupted after 2 weeks of treatment in order to minimize the side effects of treatment that predictably occur in the list 3 also of radiation therapy. These so-called "split-courses of radiation" that allowed repair and repopulation of normal tissues and improved tolerance to radiation have been abandoned because tumor control rates were compromised by tumor repopulation during the interruption in the treatment (47,48). In fact, tumor repopulation was found during radiobiologic evaluations to be accelerated after 2 weeks of radiation because of tumor reoxygenation.

Tolerance to radiation also depends on the type of tissue treated. There are two types of normal tissues. *Acute reacting tissues*, which are rapidly proliferating tissues like mucosal surfaces, usually develop an inflammatory radiation reaction during the course of treatment. *Late reacting tissues*, which do not proliferate like brain, liver, and muscle, generally do not develop a significant inflammatory reaction during the radiation course. Acute radiation reactions do not predict the extent of late radiation effects. Scar tissue is the most common form of late radiation effect. These effects are similar to those seen in wound healing. The alpha–beta ratio is a calculation that relates to the ability of normal tissues to repair the damage caused by radiation (35). With low daily doses of radiation over several weeks, more acute radiation effects are seen during the course of radiation. When high daily doses of radiation are given over a short period of time, the most significant radiation side effects occur months to years later after the radiation is completed.

Relating normal tissue tolerance to a 5% risk of a treatment-related complication at 5 years, the tolerance doses (TD 5/5) of each organ have been reported by a National Cancer Institute task force (51). The TD 5/5 ranges from 1000 cGy for the eye, 1750 cGy for the lung, 4500 cGy for the brain, and 7000 cGy for the larynx when the entire organ is treated. Radiation tolerance is a function both of the type and the volume of tissue irradiated. When only one-third of the organ is irradiated, these values equal 4500 cGy for the lung, 6000 cGy for the brain, and 7900 cGy for the larynx.

With palliative radiation, shorter external beam radiation schedules are generally used that administer a higher radiation dose with each radiation fraction. This is known as hypofractionation (Table 3). Tumor cell kill is proportional to the radiation dose that is administered. Therefore, symptomatic relief is more quickly achieved because of the large number of tumor cells that are killed in a short period of time with large daily doses of radiation.

A shorter course of therapy also has a significant impact on quality of life. This short course of treatment not only provides more prompt relief of tumor-related symptoms, but it limits the amount of time needed for the patient to come back and forth for radiation treatments. This is particularly important because the median survival is less than 6 months among patients with poor prognostic factors. However, higher radiation doses, that provide more durable pain relief, are considered warranted for patients with good prognostic factors who require treatment over the spine and other critical sites.

In contrast to the low daily radiation doses (1.8–2 Gy) given with each treatment during conventional radiation schedules to total radiation doses of 50–60 Gy over 5–6 weeks, large daily radiation fractions are given with *hypo*fractionated radiation schedules used for palliative radiation. Because of normal tissue tolerance to radiation, the total radiation dose that can be administered is low when high doses of radiation are given with each daily fraction. Hypofractionated radiation schedules can range from 2.5 Gy per fraction administered over 3 weeks for a total radiation dose of 35 Gy to a single 8 Gy dose of radiation (49,50). Most frequently, 30 Gy is administered in 10 fractions over 2 weeks. The decision for the radiation schedule depends on the radiation tolerance of the tissues in the field and the prognosis.

A variety of other radiation schedules have been developed that administer very high total doses of radiation, but use small daily doses of radiation, given twice a day, in an attempt to improve local regional control of the tumor. This approach is now also being used in palliative radiation, especially in cases of reirradiation, because the radiation effects to normal tissues are reduced. As shown in Table 4, *hyper*fractionated radiation administers two small radiation doses, usually 120 cGy per fraction, each day with a 6-hr separation between doses to allow for normal tissues to repair the effects of radiation between the doses of radiation (35,49,50). Studies have shown that the

Table 4 (A) Different Radiation Schedules. (B) Relative Relationships of Radiation Dose Per Fraction, and Total Dose in a Variety of Radiation Schedules.

(A) Comparison of radiation dose and fraction schedules	*Conventional*	*Hyperfractionation*	*Accelerated*	*Hypofractionation*
Intent	Curative	Curative	Curative	Palliative
Number of fractions per day	1	2 [↑]	1/day for the first 3–4 weeks of XRT [↔] Then 2/day (large field + boost field around the tumor) for the last 1–2 weeks of XRT [↑]	1 [↔]
Number of fractions	25–30	60–70 [↑]	30–35 [↑]	1–15 [↓]
Dose per fraction	1.8–2 Gy	1.2 Gy BID [↓]	1.8–2 Gy to a large field [↔] 1.5 Gy to a boost field [↓]	8 [1 fraction] to 2.5 Gy [15 fraction] [↑]
Number of weeks	5–6	7–9 [↑]	5–6 [↔]	1–3 [↓]
Total radiation dose	45–60 Gy	70–84 Gy [↑]	52–65 Gy [↑]	8–35 Gy [↓]

(B) Total dose: number of fractions *Low*		*High*	
Hypofractionation	Conventional fractionation	Hyperfractionation	Accelerated fractionation
8–35 Gy	50–60 Gy	70–80 Gy	55–65 Gy
1–15 fractions	25–30 fractions	60–70 fractions	28–35 fractions
1 day–3 weeks	5–6 weeks	7–8 weeks	5–6 weeks

[a]Arrows represent a comparison to conventional fractionation. [b]When a high dose of radiation is given per fraction, the total dose must be low and given in a small number of fractions.

6-hr separation is critical because it takes 6-hr for repair of radiation effects in the normal tissues to be complete. If the radiation doses were given less than 6-hr apart, then the late radiation effects would be more significant. The total radiation doses with hyperfractionation for curative radiation range from 70 Gy to more than 80 Gy. These radiation doses of 70 Gy to more than 80 Gy with hyperfractionation result in late normal tissue effects that are equivalent to a total radiation dose of 58–68 Gy with a conventional radiation schedule that uses one daily fraction of 180–200 cGy. Although the total radiation doses with hyperfractionation in the palliative setting are generally lower, the most significant advantage is in the reduction in the development of late side effects to normal tissues like small bowel injury.

Loosely defined, any course of radiation that relieves symptoms is palliative treatment. More commonly, palliative radiation is designated for patients with incurable disease due to extensive local tumor infiltration and/or metastatic disease. Short courses of radiation are used in these cases. However, symptomatic patients with an extensive primary tumor but who do not have distant metastases or have limited metastatic disease may have a prolonged survival. Therefore, the radiation schedule that is used to relieve symptoms must be indexed to the types of tissues treated, the potential for tumor resection and/or overall prognosis.

D. Demographics

Within this decade, 11 million cases of cancer were diagnosed and 5 million people have died from cancer. Approximately half the patients diagnosed with cancer will develop metastatic disease. Over 70% of all cancer patients develop symptoms from either their primary or metastatic disease (1–4,24). Prognosis is influenced by the overall metastatic burden, and the number and location of the sites involved by disease. When metastases are found also in the lung, liver, and/or central nervous system, the prognosis is especially poor (10,51–59).

The demographics for cancer are changing because of effective screening procedures and are exemplified in prostate and breast cancers. Currently prostate cancer is the second leading cause of death from cancer among men represents that more than one million men >50 years of age in the United States (60–62). Because of an aging population and availability of screening procedures, the incidence of prostate cancer is increasing significantly. However, the clinical presentation of prostate cancer has changed in the past 20 years with routine use of digital rectal examination (DRE) and PSA screening. In the 1970s, only 50% of cancers were confined to the prostate gland and metastases were present in 30% of cases at diagnosis. When patients were referred to an urologist for symptoms before, only 70% of cases had disease confined to the prostate gland. However, with routine screening, using DRE and PSA, more than 90% of cases have disease confined to the gland.

The risk for the subsequent development of distant metastases is significantly lower when the primary tumor is controlled. Survival rates after an isolated recurrence of disease in prostate cancer are influenced by the initial stage of the disease and the disease-free interval from initial treatment (61–64). In over 70% of cases of locally recurrent prostate cancer, radiation can control symptoms that include hematuria, urinary outflow obstruction, ureteral obstruction, and lower extremity edema (61). With or without local recurrence, the survival rate is most compromised by the presence of distant metastases. The survival rates at 5 and 10 years after pelvic recurrence alone equals 50%, and 22%, respectively. With distant metastases, the survival rate at 5 years is 20% and less than 5% at 10 years (62). Pain is the presenting symptom in only 11% of newly diagnosed prostate cancer patients (55,56,63). However, pain will develop in 75% of prostate cancer patients during the course of their disease (63). Radiographically identified bone metastases develop in 20% of patients with stage A_2 [T_{1b}] and B [T_2] disease, 40% of patients with stage C [T_3], and 62% of patients with stage D_1 [T_4] disease presentations (55,62,64).

Palliation represents a large component of cancer treatment and includes the use of therapeutic and supportive care measures. Treatment with palliative intent is intended to control the symptoms of disease when the disease cannot be eradicated. Unlike other aspects of cancer therapy, tumor control and survival are not the endpoints of therapeutic success in palliative care. The goal of palliative care is to effectively and efficiently relieve symptoms, and to maintain the maximum quality of life for the duration of the patient's life (2–9). Factors that determine the effectiveness of palliative radiation include the percentage of patients who experience persistent/recurrent symptoms in the radiated area, whether additional treatment is possible and provides relief of persistent/recurrent symptoms, and treatment-related morbidity. The palliative interventions recommended depend on the patient's clinical status, burden of disease and the location of the symptomatic site.

At M.D. Anderson Cancer Center, about 40% of all radiation therapy consultations were for palliative care. This pattern of practice has been consistent for over 35 years and it has specifically been the same over the past 10 years (65). In the 20 years between 1978 and 1998, 60,156 patients received radiation therapy at M.D. Anderson Cancer Center, and 23,082 (38%) were referred for palliative care. Of these, 8632 patients received palliative radiation for bone metastases constituting 14% of all patients treated with radiation, and 37% of all patients referred for palliative radiation. Since 1993, about 425 patients are referred for palliative radiation for bone metastases each year. The primary sites of disease are breast cancer (23%), lung cancer (25%), prostate cancer (12%), and other sites (40%).

The symptoms most commonly relieved by radiation are pain, bleeding, and obstruction. The symptomatic site is more important to the radiation treatment plan than whether it results from locally advanced or metastatic tumor. Similar radiation portals are used to palliate bronchial obstruction due to a primary lung cancer, recurrent breast cancer, or metastatic melanoma. The number of radiation fractions prescribed for treatment with palliative intent will depend on prognosis and not on primary histology. Common sites palliated by radiation, either alone or in combination with other treatments, include tumor involvement of the lung, pelvis, skin and subcutaneous tissues, brain and bone.

Bone metastases are the most common cause of cancer-related pain, and over 70% of patients with bone metastases are symptomatic. Among hospitalized patients, over 50% of patients experience severe pain due to bone metastases (4). One of the most important goals in the treatment of bone metastases is to relieve suffering and return the patient to independent function (66,67). The location of the metastasis influences the types of palliative intervention necessary, especially in weight-bearing bones and bones responsible for ambulation and activities of daily living. Complete pain relief (CR) after radiation is achieved in 88% of limb lesions, 73% of spine metastases, and 67% of pelvic metastases (68).

The three most common cancers, lung, breast, and prostate cancers, have high rates of metastatic spread to bone and visceral structures (51,52,54,64,69). Occasionally, musculoskeletal pain is an indicator of an undiagnosed malignancy. Among 491 patients with new or recurrent complaints of bone pain and no known underlying malignancy, 4% of the entire group and 9% of patients more than 50 years in age subsequently had metastatic cancer diagnosed (53). Of the group that had any abnormality noted on bone scan, 20% had evidence of metastatic cancer, and all of these occurred in patients more than 50 years of age. Among all the patients evaluated, pain was localized 52% in the back, 16% in the hips or pelvis, and 15% in the extremities. Among cancer patients, diffuse pain was identified in 57%, 18% had neck or upper T-spine pain, and 18% had pain in the hips, pelvis, or the extremities. Subsequently diagnosed malignancies were in the lung (32%) and prostate (16%).

Bone scans are the most sensitive and specific method of detecting bone metastases, but magnetic resonance imaging (MRI) is the best available technique for evaluating the bone marrow, neoplastic invasion of the vertebrae, the central nervous system, and peripheral nerves (70–72). Bone or other metastases rarely fail to be detected when radiographic diagnosis is pursued. When radiographic confirmation of malignancy is equivocal, bone biopsy should be considered (73).

Bone metastases in prostate and breast cancers involve the axial skeleton more than 80% of the time because of the predilection of these tumors to involve the red marrow. Metastatic invasion of the bone cortex rarely happens without red marrow involvement (70–74). For this reason, the spine, pelvis, and ribs are generally involved before metastases become evident in the skull, femora, humeri, scapula, and sternum. The mechanisms involved in the metastatic spread of cancer to the bone are complex. The predilection of specific types of tumors, like prostate cancer, that metastasize to bone is not well understood.

After bone metastases are diagnosed, the median survivals are 12 months for breast cancer, 6 months with prostate cancer, and 3 months with lung cancer. In breast cancer, the median survival rate is 48 months when metastases are confined to the skeletal system, but it decreases to only 9 months if visceral metastases are also present (10,75). In prostate cancer, the distribution of bone metastases on scintigraphy also has prognostic significance. The rate of survival is significantly longer when the metastases are restricted to the pelvis and lumbar spine, and among patients who respond to salvage hormone therapy (62,64,69). Any metastatic involvement outside the pelvis and lumbar spine results in lower rates of survival irrespective of response to salvage hormone therapy. Although the length of survival can vary significantly after the development of bone metastases, two factors are constant. First, the presence of bone metastases predicts for progression of disease to other sites and second, bone metastases are the most common cause of cancer-related pain (51,52,55,56,61,62,64,69,75).

Multidisciplinary evaluation of patients with metastatic disease of bone allows comprehensive management of the symptoms and helps coordinate administration of a wide range of available antineoplastic therapies (18). Pain, risk for pathological fracture, and spinal cord compression are the most common indications to treat bone metastases with localized therapy including radiation and surgery. Because external beam radiation provides treatment only to a localized symptomatic site of disease, it is frequently used in coordination with systemic therapies like chemotherapy, hormonal therapy, and bisphosphonates.

Radiopharmaceuticals are another systemic option that treats diffuse symptomatic bone metastases. Because the radiation is deposited directly at the involved area in the bone, radiopharmaceuticals, like strontium-89 or samarium-153, can also be used to treat bone metastases when symptoms recur in a previously irradiated site (76–89). Radiopharmaceuticals can also act as an adjuvant to localized external beam irradiation and reduce the development of other symptomatic sites of disease.

Control of cancer-related pain with the use of analgesics is imperative to allow comfort during and while awaiting response to antineoplastic interventions. Pain represents a sensitive measure of disease activity. Close follow-up should be performed to insure control of cancer and treatment-related pain, and to initiate diagnostic studies to determine the cause of persistent, progressive, or recurrent symptoms. The limited radiation tolerance of the normal tissues, like the spinal cord, that are adjacent to a bone metastasis make it impossible to administer a large enough dose of radiation to eradicate a measurable volume of tumor. Palliative radiation should result in sufficient tumor regression off critical structures to relieve symptoms. Symptoms that recur after palliative radiation most commonly result from localized regrowth of tumor in the radiation field.

E. Site Specific Palliative Radiation

The site and volume of tumor involvement are the most important considerations in the development of a palliative radiation treatment plan because of the radiation tolerance of adjacent normal tissues to treatment. Unlike the comprehensive radiation treatment portals used in curative therapy that include adjacentlymph node regions, palliative radiation generally only encompasses the radiographically evident tumor volume. Radiation treatment planning must minimize possible toxicities, and account for prior courses of radiation. Toxicities are reduced by limiting the volume irradiated, and through the application of dosimetric principles that reduce integral dose.

1. Localized Bone Metastases

Radiation of localized bone metastases relieves symptoms and helps prevent pathological fracture. There has been much controversy about palliative radiation schedules for localized symptomatic bone metastases. The Radiation Therapy Oncology Group (RTOG) conducted a prospective trial that included a variety of treatment schedules. In order to account for prognosis, patients were stratified on the basis of whether they had a solitary or multiple sites of bony metastases. The initial analysis of the study concluded that low-dose, short-course treatment schedules were as effective as high-dose protracted treatment programs (90). For solitary bone metastases, there was no difference in the relief of pain when 20 Gy using 4 Gy fractions were compared to 40.5 Gy delivered as 2.7 Gy per fraction. In patients with multiple bone metastases, the following dose schedules were compared 30 Gy at 3 Gy per fraction, 15 Gy given as 3 Gy per fraction, 20 Gy using 4 Gy per fraction, and 25 Gy using 5 Gy per fraction. No difference was identified in the rates of pain relief between these treatment schedules. Partial relief of pain was achieved in 83%, and complete relief occurred in 53% of the patients studied. Over 50% of these patients developed recurrent pain, and 8% of patients developed a pathologic fracture rate.

In a reanalysis of the data, a different definition for complete pain relief was used and accounted for the continued administration of analgesics. Using this definition, the relief of pain was significantly related to the number of fractions and the total dose of radiation that was administered (91). Complete relief of pain was achieved in 55% of patients with solitary bone metastases who received 40.5 Gy at 2.7 Gy per fraction as compared to 37% of patients who received a total dose of 20 Gy given as 4 Gy per fraction (Table 5). A similar relationship was observed in the reanalysis of patients who had multiple bone metastases. Complete relief of pain was achieved in 46% of patients who received 30 Gy at 3 Gy per fraction vs. 28% of patients treated to 25 Gy using 5 Gy fractions.

Three important issues are identified from this RTOG experience. First, the results of the reanalysis demonstrate the importance of defining what represents a response to therapy. Second, this revised definition of response showed that the total radiation dose did influence the degree that pain was relieved (90,91). Third, the RTOG experience identified the amount of time that was needed to experience relief of pain after radiation for bone metastases (Table 6). It is important to note that only half of the patients who were going to respond had relief of symptoms at 2–4 weeks after radiation (90,91). This underscores the need for continued analgesic support after completing radiation. Consistently, it took 12–20 weeks after radiation to accomplish the maximal level of relief. That period of time may reflect the time needed for reossification.

Radiographic evidence of recalcification is observed in about one-fourth of cases, and in 70% of the time recalcification is seen within 6 months of completing radiation and other palliative therapies (92–94). Therefore, it is critical to determine the time and parameters of response. Pretreatment characteristics also can influence the level of response. Neuropathic pain is a significant clinical variable that reduces the response to palliative radiation (95–97).

The parameters of response to palliative treatment also are multifactorial. An evalution was done every 2 weeks for 2 months among 49 patients, with an ECOG score of 1, who received palliative radiation therapy (20, GY/5 fractions). Treatment was most commonly administered to the pelvis (43%) and lumbar spine (17%), and 16% of the group had more than one site irradiated. The majority of patients had improvements in their pain scores (98). Four weeks after completing radiation, 37% of patients were taking more analgesic than at baseline (flare reaction), but analgesic requirements subsequently declined in most patients. By week 4, 63% were more active 4, and 83% had functional improvement by week 8. Quality of life improved in 42% by week 4 and was stable or improved in all patients by week 8. Overall response to palliative radiation for bone

Table 5 Dose Response Evaluation from the Reanalysis of the RTOG Bone Metastases Protocol

	Dose/fx(Gy)	Total dose (Gy)	Tumor dose at 2 Gy/fx	CR (%)	*p* Value
Solitary bone metastases					$p < 0.0003$
	2.7	40.5	42.9	55	
	4.0	20.0	23.3	37	
Multiple bone metastases					$p < 0.0003$
	3.0	30	32.5	46	
	3.0	15.0	16.2	36	
	4.0	20.0	23.3	40	
	5.0	25.0	31.25	28	

[a]Listed are the dose per fraction (dose/fx), total radiation dose, the radiobiological equivalent dose if administered at 2 Gy/fx, the complete response rate (CR) using the definition that accounts for the use of analgesics and that accounts for retreatment. *Source*: From Ref. 90.

Table 6 Percentage of Patients Who Responded to Radiation Relative to Time, Designated in Weeks after Completion of Radiation Therapy

			Weeks post-XRT			
Total dose (Gy)	Dose per fraction (Gy)	Tumor dose at 2 Gy/fx	< 2 (%)	2–4 (%)	4–12 (%)	12–20 (%)
Solitary metastases						
40.5	2.7	42.9	7	29	53	77
20.0	4	23.3	16	50	66	82
Multiple metastases						
30.0	3	32.5	19	48	73	84
15.0	3	16.2	34	70	84	93
20.0	4	23.3	28	53	75	88
25.0	5	31.25	22	41	72	80

[a]This prospective trial, conducted by the RTOG, randomized radiation dose and number of fractions and stratified the randomization on the basis of solitary or multiple bone metastases. Also listed is the radiobiological equivalent dose if administered at 2 Gy per fraction. *Source*: From Refs. 79, 80.

metastases equaled 67%, with 37% having a partial response and 30% having a complete response at 12 weeks (99). But integrating the pain scores with the analgesic requirements, the overall response rate declined to 45%. Because most patients have multiple sites of metastatic disease, a decline in analgesic requirements does not represent a good index of response to localized radiation.

At consultation, the pain levels among 518 patients were classified as moderate in 31% and severe in 45%, but 34% of these patients had no analgesics or only codeine was prescribed for their pain (100). However, 87% of 2132 bone metastases patients, and 71% of patients without bone metastases received opioids at some point during their final year of life. Corresponding figures for the use of long-acting opioids were 53% and 24%. Long-acting opioids were used over 25% of the days survived in the outpatient setting with bone metastases during last year of life (101). By comparison, patients without bone metastases only used long-acting opioids 14% of the days they lived in the outpatient setting. However, during the last month of life, 61% of bone metastases patients and 29% of patients with metastatic cancer to sites other than bone needed long-acting analgesics.

Therefore, functional parameters may prove more reliable than analgesic dose in evaluating response to palliative therapy. An international consensus on palliative radiotherapy endpoints for future clinical trials has been developed. Issues addressed involved the definition of pain relief relative to continued analgesic use, time to and duration of response, the need for reirradiation, and the validity and reliability of instruments used to assess symptoms (102). Research was needed to determine the accuracy of pain reports from caregivers, what constitutes a partial response, better methods of predicting survival, and cost-effectiveness of treatment.

2. *Single Fraction Radiation*

A single large radiation fraction is as effective in relieving pain as other radiation schedules that have more treatments. In more than 10 prospective randomized trials conducted in Europe, no difference was reported in either how quickly symptoms resolved or in the duration of pain relief when a single dose of radiation was compared a radiation schedule with multiple radiation fractions (103–120). In each case, symptom relief lasted 3 months in 70% of patients, 6 months in 37%, and 12 months in 20% of cases. Like the RTOG study, about 69% responded at 4 weeks, and response rates plateau, totaling 80%, at 8 weeks. Complete response rates after a single 8 Gy fraction total 15% at 2 weeks, 23% at 4 weeks, 28% at 8 weeks, and 39% at 12 weeks postradiation. Because survival is determined by the location and number of sites of metastatic disease rather than the number of radiation fractions used for a localized area of disease, overall survival rates for a single fraction of radiation are equivalent to a course of palliative radiation with multiple fractions.

A meta-analysis of 18 prospective randomized trials evaluated three approaches to palliative radiation dose schedules. These three approaches to palliative radiation dose schedules included different doses of single-fraction radiation therapy, comparisons of single-fraction vs. multiple-fraction radiotherapy, and comparisons of different doses of multiple-fraction radiotherapy. This comparison showed no difference in response rates based on radiotherapy dose (107). The median period of pain relief ranged between 11 and 24 weeks, and no difference was, found in the 1–4-week median time to pain relief. A significant difference, however, was seen between remineralization of lytic lesions at 6 months follow-up and was 173% after 30 Gy in 10 fractions; compared to 120% after a single 8 Gy fraction; but the pretreatment and post-treatment risk of pathological fracture was not determined (120). Factors found retrospectively to influence the use of a single vs. multiple radiation fractions for bone metastases included patient age, performance status, anatomical site, and year of radiation therapy (119).

The RTOG also conducted a prospective randomized trial consisting of 949 breast and prostate cancer patients comparing 30 Gy in 10 fractions to a single 8 Gy fraction for bone metastases. The pretreatment characteristics of the 847 analyzable patients were equally balanced between treatment arms including 56% having a weight-bearing painful site, 72% having severe pain, 27% who were receiving bisphosphonates, and 57% with a solitary painful site. Acute toxicity was mild with a total of only two patients experiencing a grade-4 toxicity and 24 with a grade-3 toxicity (118). But, there was significantly more grade-2 to grade-4 toxicity, 17% vs. 10%, in the 30 Gy arm. Median survival was 9 months with 41% of patients alive at 1 year. No difference was observed in pain relief at 3 months. The rates of complete pain relief (CR) and partial pain relief (PR) were 15% and 50% for the 8 Gy arm, and 18% and 48% for the 30 Gy arm. At 3 months, one-third of patients no longer required analgesics.

A shorter radiation schedule, like a single fraction, is advantageous for patients with poor prognostic factors. *First*, it is easier for patients with a poor KPS to complete therapy. *Second*, response and survival rates are equal for single and multifraction therapy at 3 months, and median survival is less than 6 months among patients with poor prognostic factors and average around 24 months among patients with metastatic disease (107,108,111,112,115,116,119). This is an important consideration when the number of weeks of survival is evaluated relative to the number of weeks receiving palliative treatment. *Third*, the option of retreatment after a single fraction of radiation may also provide an advantage among patients with good prognostic factors as a means to periodically reduce tumor burden and control symptoms in noncritical anatomic sites. *Fourth*, a single fraction of radiation is more cost effective. The cost of radiation therapy is reduced by 41% when a single fraction of radiation therapy is compared to a 10-fraction course of palliative radiation. Finally, the cost of radiation therapy is less expensive than the continued cost of analgesics (121). An analysis of the Dutch prospective study also showed cost benefit for a single fraction of radiation when compared to multiple radiation fractions, even when retreatment is included in the costs of the single-fraction arm, or when compared to the continued use of analgesics (115,116).

Metastatic cancer is now being treated as a chronic disease. Treatment is given to prevent or relieve symptoms of the disease. None of the radiation schedules used for palliation eradicates the disease and symptoms will recur with regrowth of the tumor. Reirradiation for persistent or recurrent pain is often precluded when higher radiation doses are administered, but reirradiation is possible after a single fraction of radiation (103–106,122). Reirradiation was necessary in 25% of patients who received a single 8 Gy radiation fraction, but all of these patients were reported to respond to the second dose of radiation. When a single fraction of 4 Gy was compared to a single 8 Gy fraction, the rate of response was slightly lower and fewer acute radiation reactions were noted, but a greater proportion of patients required reirradiation (105). With reirradiation, the overall rate of response was equivalent for 8 and 4 Gy fractions. A single fraction of radiation can then be repeatedly used to suppress symptoms when they recur.

The projected length of survival is the critical issue for radiation dose and schedule for palliative radiation. In one study, only 12 of 245 patients were alive at the time of analysis with approximately 50% alive at 6 months, 25% at 1 year, 8% at 2 years, and 3% at 3 years after palliative radiation. For breast cancer patients, the survival rates at these time points after palliative radiation were 60%, 44%, 20%, and 7%, respectively. For prostate cancer, the survival rates were 60% at 6 months, 24% at 1 year and there were no patients who survived 2 years (123). In the RTOG trial, the median survival for solitary bone metastases was 36 weeks and was 24 weeks for multiple bone metastases (90,91). The RTOG study also demonstrated that the level of pain correlated with prognosis among patients with multiple bone metastases. This survival difference may be an important observation because unrelieved pain and the resultant sequelae of immobility may contribute to mortality as well as morbidity.

The influence of improved control of pain on overall survival was demonstrated in a prospective randomized trial among 202 patients with intractable pain. Improved pain control was achieved in 85% of patients with intrathecal analgesics as compared to 71% with optimized medical management (124). Significantly less toxicity due to analgesic therapy occurred with intrathecal analgesics; compared to baseline, the toxicity rate decreased by 50% with intrathecal analgesics versus 17% for medical management. Intrathecal analgesics also were associated with decreases in fatigue and depression. With comparable stages of disease in the two groups, the overall survival at 6 months was 54% with intrathecal analgesics compared to 37% with optimized medical management. While the performance status has long been associated with prognosis, this is one of the first studies to demonstrate how medical intervention to improve the performance status by relieving pain impacts survival.

For patients with metastatic disease, time is critical. The time under radiation needs to be considered as the opportunity cost of palliative treatment (125). If the median survival of a patient with bone metastases is 6 months (180 days), the patient will spend 0.6% of the remaining survival time under radiation treatment when a single fraction of radiation is given. If 10 radiation fractions are given, 8% of the remaining survival and if 20 fractions are prescribed 16% of the remaining survival will be consumed by radiation therapy. Even if retreatment with a second single fraction is required, the patient will continue to spend about 1% of the survival time under radiation therapy. For lung cancer patients with a 3-month survival rate, 1% of the remaining time is spent with a single fraction of radiation as compared to 16% if 10 fractions are given, or 30% if 20 fractions are prescribed.

Acute radiation toxicities are a function of the dose per fraction, total dose, and the area and volume of tissue irradiated. If mucosal surfaces like the upper aerodigestive tract, bowel, and bladder can be excluded from the radiation portals, acute radiation side effects can be significantly reduced whether a single or multiple fractions are prescribed. A more protracted course of radiation is still used for patients with good prognostic factors who require treatment over the spine and other critical sites (111,119,126–132). But, for most patients who receive palliative radiation, a single fraction of radiation provides an efficient and effective therapeutic option.

3. *Pathologic Fracture*

The most significant morbidity of bone metastases relates to pathological fracture and spinal cord compression. Pain that persists or that recurs after palliative radiation should be evaluated to exclude progression of disease, possible extension of disease outside the radiation portal that results in referred pain, and bone fracture. Reduced cortical strength can result in compression, stress, or microfractures. Plain radiographs have a 91% concordance rate in detecting post-treatment disease progression and fractures in comparison to the 57% specificity rate of bone scans performed after radiotherapy (93).

Pathologic fractures occur in about 20% of patients with bone metastases (67,133–139). Proximal long bones are more commonly involved than distal bones. Consequently, pathologic fractures occur 50% of the time in the femur and 15% in the humerus (Fig. 11). The femoral neck and head are the most frequent locations for pathologic fracture because of the propensity for metastases to involve proximal bones and the stress of weight placed on this part of the femur. Patients with bone scan evidence of metastases in the femur or humerus at the time of diagnosis of bone metastases are significantly more likely to fracture these bones when compared to other patients with bone metastases located in other bones sites when metastatic is diagnose (138). Pathological fracture occurred in one of eight patients with bone scan evidence of humeral disease as compared to one in 35 patients without humeral involvement at diagnosis of bone metastases. More than 80% of pathologic fractures occur in breast (138), kidney, lung, and thyroid cancers.

Approximately 20% of metastatic lesions in long bones will result in pathologic fracture that requires surgical intervention. Patients with pathologic fracture due to bone metastases generally have clinical outcomes following surgical repair that are comparable to patients sustaining a traumatic fracture (67,134,135). Prognosis is poor, however, if hypercalcemia is present and if parenteral narcotics are required to control pain from other sites of bone metastases; in these cases, the decision for surgical intervention should be based on the severity of and the symptoms associated with the fracture (67). As shown in Fig. 12, postoperative radiation is often given after surgical fixation of a pathologic fracture to reduce risk of progressive disease in the bone that could result in instability of the internal fixation (134).

A retrospective analysis of 859 patients was performed that divided patients into four groups based on extent of disease at the diagnosis of bone metastases. These groups included bone metastases only, bone and soft tissue disease, bone and pleuro-pulmonary disease, bone and liver disease. Survival from diagnosis of bone only metastases was the longest of any group; the shortest survival was 5.5 months for patients with liver and bone metastases (138). The time to vertebral fracture was the shortest for the bone only metastases group, but there was no difference in the time to pathological long bone fractures. Because of an extended survival, most fractures occurred in the bone only metastases group (17%) as compared to a 5% risk for pathological long bone fracture in the bone and liver metastases group.

Treatment of pathologic fracture or impending fracture depends on the bone involved and the clinical

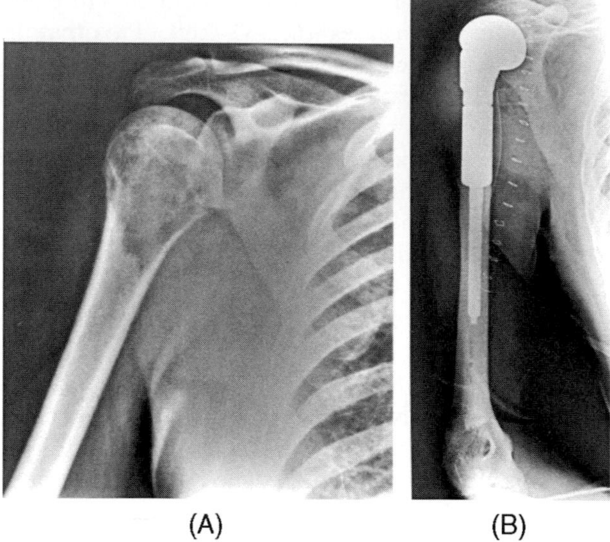

Figure 11 (A) An extensive lytic lesion in the proximal humerus. Prophylactic internal fixation was performed to prevent pathological fracture (B). This patient, who complained primarily of pain in the hip, would have been placed on crutches to reduce stress on the involved femur. A bone scan and x-rays, obtained to exclude other sites of metastatic involvement, identified this lesion in the humerus. The humerus would have certainly fractured if all the patient's weight had been displaced to the upper extremities with crutches.

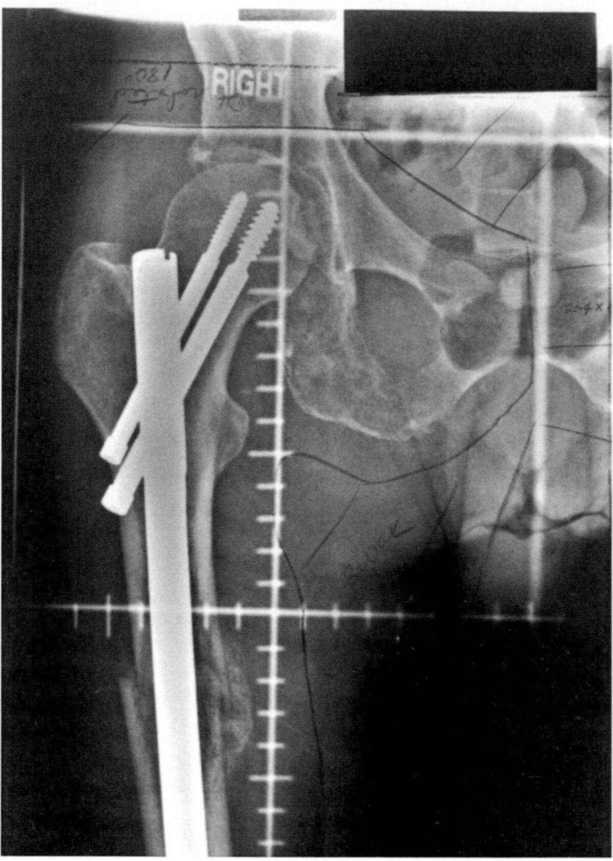

Figure 12 Typical radiation portal following fixation of a pathologic fracture of the femur. Radiation is administered to treat residual disease around the internal fixation device, pubis, and acetabulum.

status of the patient. Indications for surgical intervention of pathologic fracture or impending fracture include these factors: (1) an expected survival of more than 6 weeks; (2) an ability to accomplish internal stability of the fracture site; (3) no coexistent medical conditions that preclude early mobilization; (4) metastases involving weight-bearing bones; and (5) lytic lesions more than 2–3 cm in size or metastases that destroy more than 50% of the cortex (67,136,137). It is unclear whether osteolytic metastases are more likely to fracture than osteoblastic lesions because osteoblastic lesions, by definition, have an osteolytic component so that new bone can be formed.

The cost of treatment was evaluated for 2 years among 28 prostate cancer patients with bone metastases in The Netherlands who were receiving hormonal therapy. Approximately one skeletal-related event occurred per patient per year totaling 54 events (139). External beam radiation was administered 33 times, and 21 patients were treated with radiopharmaceuticals. Eight patients were hospitalized; four for spinal cord compression and four for pathological fracture. The average cost of care for patients with prostate cancer metastatic to bone was €13,051 per patient and about half of this cost was due to the treatment of skeletal related events.

4. *Spinal Cord Compression*

Pain is the initial symptom in approximately 90% of patients with spinal cord compression, and the development of spinal cord compression is associated with a poor overall prognosis. Paraparesis or paraplegia occurs in over 60%, sensory loss is noted in 70–80%, and 14–77% have bladder and/or bowel disturbances (140–169). The extent of the epidural mass influences prognosis because a complete spinal block results in greater residual neurologic impairment than a partial block. The time from the original diagnosis to the development of metastatic spinal disease averages 32 months, and the average time is reported to be 27 months from diagnosis of skeletal metastases to spinal cord compression. Median survival among patients with spinal cord compression ranges between 3 and 7 months with a 36% probability for a 1-year survival. For specific types of cancer, the mean survival time is 14 months for breast cancer, 12 months in prostate cancer, 6 months in malignant melanoma, and 3 months in lung cancer once epidural spinal cord compression is diagnosed (126,133). The vertebral column is involved by metastatic tumor in 40% of patients who die of cancer. Approximately 70% of vertebral metastases involve the thoracic spine, 20% the lumbosacral region, and 10% the cervical spine. From a tumor registry of 121,435 patients, the cumulative probability of at least one episode of spinal cord compression occurring in the last 5 years of life was 2.5% (158). The diagnosis of spinal cord compression was associated with a doubling of the time spent in hospital in the last year of life.

Weakness can signal the rapid progression of symptoms and 30% of patients with weakness become paraplegic within 1 week. Rapid development of weakness, defined as occurring in less than 2 months, most commonly occurs in lung cancer while breast and prostate cancers can progress more slowly. Neurological deficits can develop within a few hours in up to 20% of patients with spinal cord compression (99–126,143,159,161). The rate of development of motor symptoms correlates with therapeutic improvement (159,161). Motor function improved among 86% of patients who had >14-day time to development of symptoms. Only 29% improved when motor deficits developed over 8–14 days before the diagnosis of spinal cord compression. Improvements occurred in only 10% if motor deficits developed over 1–7 days. The severity of weakness at presentation is the most significant factor for recovery of function (159,161). Ninety percent of patients who are ambulatory at presentation will be ambulatory after treatment. Only 13% of paraplegic patients will regain function, particularly if paraplegia is present for more than 24 hr before the initiation of therapy. Over 30% of patients who develop spinal cord compression are alive 1 year later and 50% of these patients will remain ambulatory with appropriate therapy.

Among 153 consecutive cases of spinal cord compression in one study, 37% of patients had breast cancer, 28% had prostate cancer, 18% had lung cancer, and 17% had other solid tumors. The time between primary tumor diagnosis and development of spinal cord compression was dependent on tumor type with the shortest time associated with lung cancer and the longest time for breast cancer. Lung cancer patients had the most severe functional deficit with more than 50% totally paralyzed. Breast cancer patients were ambulatory 59% of the time. More severe disturbances in gait occurred when the time between the interval from the diagnosis of the primary tumor and spinal cord compression was short. Total blockage of the spinal cord occurred in 54%, and 46% had partial blockage (162). Total paralysis was present in 43 patients, 31 could move their legs but could not walk, 19 were able to walk with assistance, and 60 could walk unassisted. Sensory examination of the legs was normal in 34, slight disturbances were present in 84, and total lack of pain perception occurred in 35 patients. After radiation, 40 were totally paralyzed, 20 could move their legs without being able to walk, 17 were able to walk with assistance, and 76 had unassisted gait. The median survival time was 3.4 months. Survival was dependent on time from primary tumor diagnosis, and ambulatory function at diagnosis and after treatment.

Pain can be present for months to days before neurological dysfunction evolves. Unlike degenerative joint disease which primarily occurs in the low cervical and low lumbar regions, pain due to epidural spinal cord compression can occur anywhere in the spinal axis, and is aggravated by recumbency. Any cancer patient with back pain, especially with known metastatic involvement of the vertebral bodies, should be suspected as having spinal cord compression. The risk of spinal cord compression exceeds 60% among patients with back pain and plain film evidence of vertebral collapse due to metastatic cancer (141,126–132,142–146). Epidural spinal cord disease is documented in 17% of asymptomatic patients who have an abnormal bone scan but normal plain films. When vertebral metastases are present both on bone scan and plain film, 47% of asymptomatic patients will have epidural disease (143). An MRI to rule out spinal cord compression should be performed in symptomatic patients with osteoblastic changes on plain film even if the vertebral contour and bone scan are normal (Fig. 13).

Radiographic determination of the involved spinal levels is critical to radiation treatment planning. Clinical determination of the location of epidural spinal cord compression is incorrect in 33% of cases (126–128). Plain film radiographs will show involvement of more than one spinal level in about one-third of patients. If the results of MRI, tomographic studies, and surgical findings are included, over 85% of patients will have multiple sites of vertebral involvement (126–132,142,143,145,156,165). Bone scans fail to detect bone metastases 13% of the time (156). When there was evidence of spinal metastases on bone scan, 49% had more extensive disease on MRI (156). While spinal cord compression is caused by soft tissue epidural metastases in 75% of cases, the remaining 25% of cases are caused by bone collapse (155). Computed tomography (CT) finds metastases most commonly in the posterior portion of the vertebral body, and the destruction of the pedicles occurs only in combination

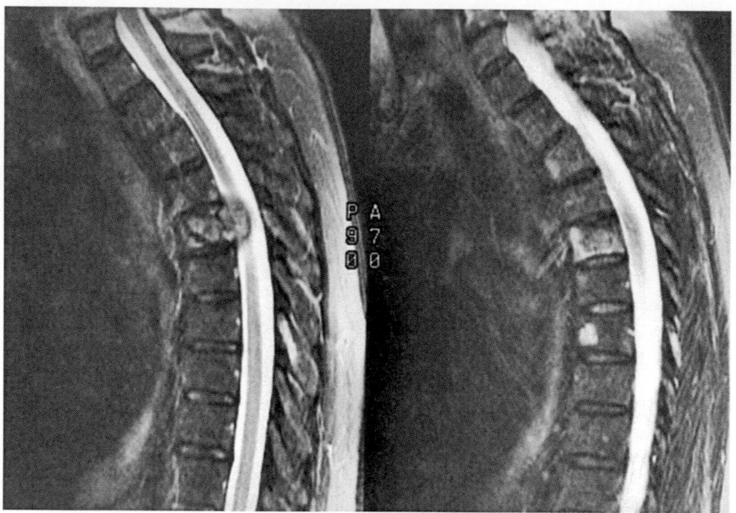

Figure 13 Magnetic resonance imaging of the spine demonstrating epidural spinal cord compression.

with involvement of the vertebral body (145). With plain x-rays, however, the destruction of the pedicles is most common finding that identifies spine metastases. Osteoblastic bony expansion, commonly seen in both prostate and breast cancers, can result in spinal cord compromise as well as osteolytic vertebral compression fractures (Fig. 14) (144,155). MRI findings have also correlated well with stage of multiple myeloma, the β_2 microglobulin level, the type of chain, and the response to therapy (165).

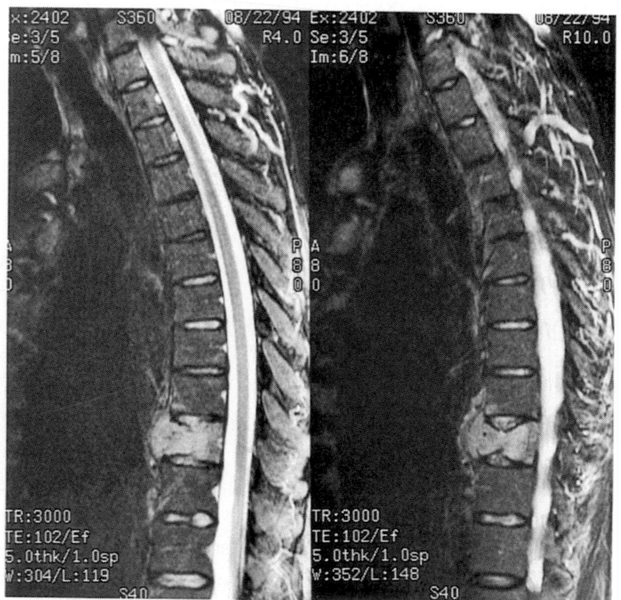

Figure 14 Osteoblastic involvement, demonstrated on magnetic resonance imaging of the spine, associated with vertebral collapse with breast cancer.

Treatment of spinal cord compression includes emergent corticosteroids, radiotherapy and/or neurosurgical intervention. Radiotherapy is the treatment of choice for most cases of spinal cord compression and is a radiotherapeutic emergency (Fig. 15). Functional outcome is dependent on the level of symptoms at the time radiation is administered (126–132,142,143,157,163). In these cases, 73% of patients have pain relief following treatment. Among 108 breast cancer patients, the mean time to pain relief was 35 days. Recurrent symptoms at a different spinal level occurred in more than three-fourths of patients and within 6 months of the initial treatment (163).

A statistically significant improvement in functional outcome occurs with laminectomy and radiotherapy in treatment of epidural spinal cord compression over either modality alone for selected clinical presentations. Laminectomy has been recommended to promptly reduce tumor volume in an attempt to relieve compression and injury of the spinal cord and provide stabilization to the spinal axis. The rate of tumor regression following radiotherapy is too slow in these cases to effect recovery of lost neurologic function, and radiation therapy cannot relieve compression of the spinal column due to vertebral collapse. After radiation alone to treat a partial spinal cord block, 64% of patients regain ambulation, 33% have normalization of sphincter tone, 72% are pain free, and median survival is 9 months (129,131,132,142,143,160). With a complete spinal cord block, only 27% will have improvement in motor function and 42% will continue to have pain after radiation alone. In paraparetic patients who undergo laminectomy and radiation, 82% regain the ability to walk, 68% have improved sphincter function, and 88% have relief of pain.

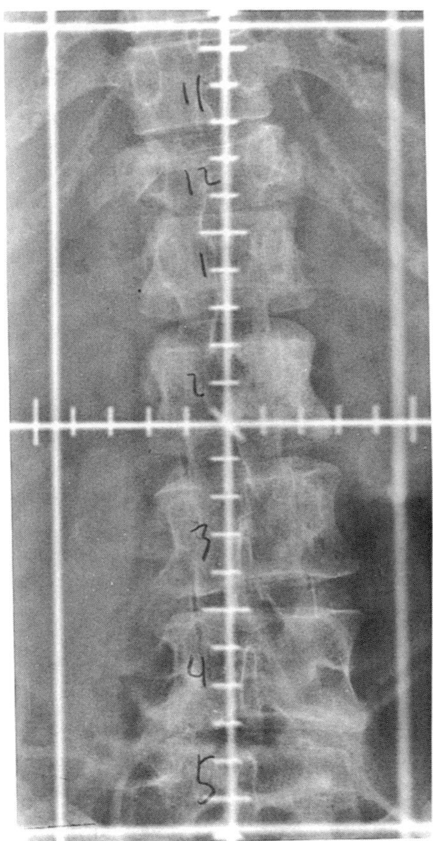

Figure 15 Typical radiation portal to treat disease involvement in the vertebral bodies and epidural region.

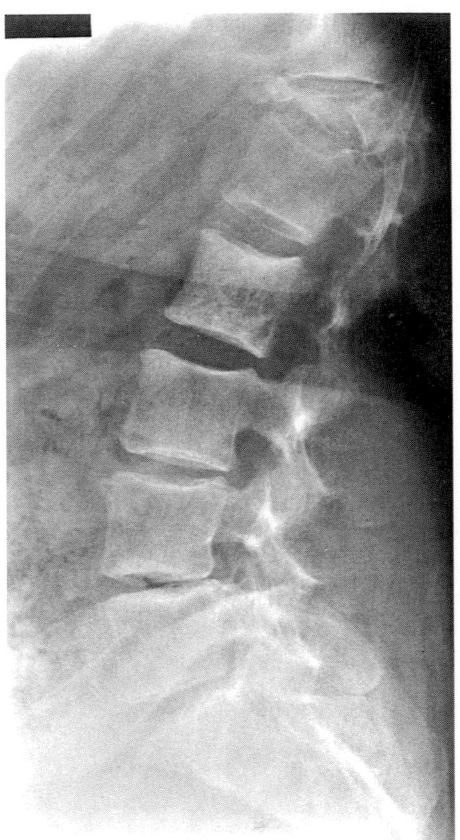

Figure 16 Compression fracture of the 12th thoracic vertebral body following an initial pain-free interval after palliative radiation. Vertebral weakness with rapid tumor regression resulting in the compression fracture which caused recurrent back pain due to spinal instability.

Laminectomy is indicated with rapid neurologic deterioration, tumor progression in a previously irradiated area, stabilization of the spine, paraplegic patients with limited disease and good probability of survival, and to establish a diagnosis (126–128) (130–132,146). Adjuvant radiotherapy is often given to treat microscopic residual disease after neurosurgical intervention (126,127,130,143). Surgical restoration of the vertebral alignment may be required due neurologic compromise and pain caused by progressive vertebral collapse. Vertebral collapse may occur due to cancer or vertebral instability after cancer therapy (Fig. 16). Appropriate diagnostic studies and intervention should be pursued with persistent pain because the neurologic compromise and pain from vertebral instability can be as devastating as that with epidural spinal cord metastases (131,146).

5. *Radiation Tolerance of the Spinal Cord*

The potential for the development of radiation myelitis with total radiation doses which exceed 40 Gy at 2 Gy per fraction represents the limiting factor in the treatment of large tumor burdens near or involving the spinal canal. Furthermore, the length of spinal cord that needs to be irradiated significantly affects the radiation tolerance of the spinal cord (149–151,164,166). Persistent pain after radiotherapy for vertebral metastases should be investigated to exclude the possibility of progressive disease in or outside the radiation portal, or mechanical spinal instability because of a vertebral compression fracture. Changes seen in the bone marrow on MRI after palliative radiotherapy initially includes decreased cellularity, edema and hemorrhage followed by fatty replacement and fibrosis. These well-defined changes on MRI after radiotherapy can be distinguished from those seen with progressive disease (145,152,153).

Histopathologic changes experimentally observed after fractionated irradiation of the spinal cord include white matter necrosis, hemorrhage, and segmental parenchymal atrophy that are consistently associated with abnormal neurologic signs (151). Other pathologic responses involve focal fiber loss and white matter vacuolation. Two separate mechanisms of radiation injury can occur and result from white matter damage and vasculopathies. White matter damage is associated with diffuse demyelination and swollen axons that can be focally necrotic and have associated glial reaction. Vascular damage experimentally has been shown to be age dependent, and can result in hemorrhage, telangiectasia, and vascular necrosis (149–151). Low doses of radiation experimentally has been shown to interfere with the formation of syringomyelia and glial scar that facilitate the recovery of paraplegic animals (166).

Six major types of injury have been experimentally shown to result from radiation to the spinal column. Five of these occur in the spinal cord and one in the dorsal root ganglia. The most severe spinal lesions, all of which are due to vascular damage and result in neurological dysfunction, include white matter necrosis, hemorrhage, and segmental parenchymal atrophy. The two less severe spinal lesions included focal fiber loss and scattered white matter vacuolation due to damage to glial cells, axons, and/or the vasculature; these less severe sequelae are seen with lower total doses of radiation and are less likely to result in neurological dysfunction. In dorsal root ganglia, radiation damage included intracytoplasmic vacuoles and loss of neurons and satellite cells that could affect sensory function. These findings are distinct from the demyelination of the posterior columns associated with the self-limiting Lhermitte's syndrome (150). Meningeal thickening and fibrosis can also be observed after radiation, but the clinical significance of this is unknown. Ependymal and nerve root damage from radiation is rare.

Clinical and experimental experience has failed to demonstrate any difference in radiosensitivity in different segments of the spinal cord (149). The risk of radiation myelitis in the cervico-thoracic spine is less than 5% when 6000 cGy is administered at 172 cGy per fraction, or 5000 cGy is given with daily fractions of 200 cGy per fraction. Especially among patients who have received chemotherapy or need to have a significant length of spinal cord irradiated, the total dose to the spinal cord is generally limited to 4000 cGy administered at 200 cGy per fraction to minimize any risk of irreversible radiation injury to the spinal cord. A steep curve based on total radiation dose predicts the risk of developing radiation myelopathy; a small increase in total radiation dose can result in a large increased risk for radiation myelopathy (149,151). Retreatment of a previously irradiated segment of spinal cord results in high risk for radiation-induced myelopathy because other neurological pathways cannot compensate for an injury to a specific level of the spinal cord. Experimental data also have shown that the time course and the extent of long-term recovery from radiation are incomplete and are dependent on the specific type and age of tissue.

The radiation tolerance of the spinal cord can be compromised by prior injury. Difficulty arises in separating the pathologic and radiotherapeutic injuryto spinal cord compression. Vasogenic edema of the spinal cord and nerve roots can be caused by compression injury. Metastatic epidural compression results in vasogenic spinal cord edema, venous hemorrhage, loss of myelin, and ischemia. Vasogenic edema results in an increased synthesis of prostaglandin E_2 that can be inhibited by steroids or nonsteroidal anti-inflammatory agents (149–151).

Surgery often is the only available option for therapy because previously administered radiation may preclude further radiotherapy in the region of the malignant spinal cord compression. This is often the case in lung cancer because metastases are located in the thoracic spine in over 70% cases, and many of these patients have received mediastinal irradiation (148). Early involvement by the radiotherapist in the management of the patients with suspected spinal cord involvement is important to allow time to obtain prior radiotherapy records to determine if further radiation is possible and expedite the clinical decision making process. Reirradiation has been performed among selected patients with cumulative radiation doses of 68 Gy (167,168). Using stereotactic conformal radiotherapy and intensity-modulated radiation therapy to total doses of 39 Gy, reirradiation results in 95% local control at 12 months follow-up (167). Half of patients had neurologic improvement, and 13 of 16 patients had relief of pain. No significant late toxicity was reported.

Based on clinical and radiographic grounds, leptomeningeal carcinomatosis must also be considered in the diagnostic evaluation. Leptomeningeal carcinomatosis occurs more commonly than expected. For example, only half of breast cancer patients with leptomeningeal carcinomatosis will be diagnosed before death (126,132,143,154,169). Performing a lumbar puncture is a relative barrier to the diagnosis. At least three cerebral spinal fluid (CSF) samples are necessary to cytologically exclude the diagnosis of leptomeningeal disease because in 10–40% of patients, the initial CSF sample fails to document tumor cells (169). MRI can identify leptomeningeal disease among patients with normal CSF cytology, and is sensitive and specific in locating regions of nodular leptomeningeal involvement. Except in the case of nodular leptomeningeal involvement where localized radiotherapy may be of benefit as an adjuvant, intrathecal chemotherapy is generally the treatment of choice (154).

F. Treatment of Diffuse Bone Metastases

Systemic radionuclides and bisphosphonates have been used among patients with disseminated bone metastases. Both approaches are useful in augmenting the therapeutic effect of localized radiation, and in preventing asymptomatic bony lesions from progressing. Although usually not a significant consideration in localized radiation, adequate bone marrow reserve is required for systemic radionuclides. Bone marrow scans can be performed to determine the volume of functioning marrow and assess the feasibility of delivering radionuclides (76–89,170–175).

1. Radiopharmaceuticals

The most commonly used radiopharmaceutical in the treatment of bone metastases is strontium-89. Many reports indicate effective palliation of pain lasting more than 6 months in 60–80% of patients with breast and prostate cancers (76–80,82,83,170,171). Improvements in functional status and quality of life have been observed, and about 20% of patients have complete resolution of pain. Pain control has been reported to be superior among patients with disseminated prostate cancer treated both with strontium-89 and local radiotherapy as compared to localized irradiation alone. Experience from a number of clinical trials has demonstrated strontium-89 to be an effective therapy that is easily administered in an outpatient setting. An important contraindication to the use of radiopharmaceuticals is when epidural disease is associated with vertebral metastases because the activity of radiopharmaceuticals is limited to bone and disease outside the bone is untreated.

Strontium-89 combines with the calcium component of hydroxyapatite in osteoblastic lesions. Because the activity of strontium-89 is limited to bone, there are no systemic toxicities. Myelotoxicity, resulting in a 25% decline of initial platelet and white blood cell counts, is usually transient and represents the only significant toxicity associated with strontium-89 (84,171). Marrow suppression caused by radioisotopes is either caused by penetrating gamma radiation or by a radioisotope with a long half-life. Even though strontium-89 emits a beta particle of low penetrance and low energy (1.46 MeV), myelosuppression can occur. Radiation doses to metastatic bony lesions with strontium-89 can range from 3 to over 300 Gy. The radiation dose absorbed by the normal bone marrow is 2–50 times less than the dose administered by strontium-89 to the osteoblastic lesion. The half-life of strontium-89 in normal bone is about 14 days and its half-life in the diseased bone is 51 days. Hematotoxicity is more pronounced in patients with pretreatment platelet counts of $\leq 60 \times 10^3$, white blood counts of $\leq 2.5 \times 10^3$, or with $\geq 30\%$ involvement of the red marrow bearing bone (84,173). Compromise of the red marrow bearing bone can be a consequence of tumor or prior radiation and chemotherapy.

Response to strontium-89 therapy has been documented both subjectively and objectively. Subjective response, manifested as symptomatic improvement, was reported by over 80% of prostate cancer patients using a validated survey. Objective evidence of response was documented by reductions in alkaline and acid phosphatase levels that were also associated with a decrease in the uptake of metastatic lesions on sequential bone scans (76–80,82,83,170,171).

Prior therapies for prostate cancer, including local radiation therapy and systemic chemotherapy, or hormone therapy, do not influence toxicity or affect clinical response to strontium-89. Administered as an adjuvant to localized external beam radiotherapy in metastatic prostate cancer, strontium-89 has been shown to improve pain relief and delay progression of disease in prospective randomized clinical trials. Almost twice as many patients treated with strontium-89 a systemic radiopharmaceutical were reported to be pain free at 3 months in follow-up when compared to patients treated with localized external beam radiation. Analgesics were no longer required by 17% of patients treated with strontium-89, while only 2% of the patients treated with localized radiotherapy alone were able to discontinue analgesic use. Quality-of-life assessments demonstrated increased physical activity along with improved pain relief after strontium-89 was administered in conjunction with localized external beam radiation therapy. Cost–benefit analysis has also suggested an advantage to the administration of strontium-89 with reductions in costs of hospitalization for tertiary care (76,77,85,171).

Several other radiopharmaceuticals are available for clinical application including samarium-153, gallium nitrate, phosphorus-32, and rhenium-186 (79,81,84) (86–88,170,173). The therapeutic mechanism of action relates to the physical and biologic half-life in the bony lesion, the mean energy, and the delivered dose of the radiopharmaceutical. Table 5 summarizes some of the physical characteristics and clinical data for various radionuclides. Phosphorus-32 and strontium-89 emit pure beta rays (little penetration in tissue) while rhenium-186 and samarium-153 emit both beta rays and relatively high energy gamma-ray photons that penetrate tissue for some distance (103–159 keV).

Because samarium-153 has a gamma-ray component, it is possible to directly image the distribution of the radiation dose. The scans after injection of samarium-153 are comparable to diagnostic scans obtained with technetium-99m. The mean skeletal uptake is over 50% of the dose (79,81,84,86–88). Non-skeletal sites receive negligible radiation doses and complete clearance of radiation, not absorbed by the disease, occurs within 6–8 hr of administration. In a double-blind placebo controlled clinical trial, samarium-153 has been shown to be an effective agent in palliating painful bone metastases in breast cancer patients. Pain relief occurred within 1 week and lasted at least 16 weeks after administration. Approximately 65% of patients responded within the first 4 weeks and 43% had relief of pain of at least 16 weeks duration. No significant bone marrow toxicities have been observed. Recommended doses range between 1.0 and 1.5 mCi/kg. In over one-third of patients, multiple administrations are possible.

Sequential x-rays and bone scans after hormonal and radiopharmaceutical therapy for breast and prostate cancers demonstrate a response (93,94). Approximately one-third of patients will have evidence of increased pain 1 to 4 weeks after demonstration and increased tracer uptake on bone scans (flare) obtained 8–16 weeks after treatment. Of these patients with a flare response on bone scan, 72% will experience a response to the treatment. By comparison, only 36% will have a relief of pain when a limited to no flare response is observed.

Despite this experience, recent trials using strontium-89 have failed to demonstrate significant benefit. One study, evaluating 95 patients and using physician-assessed responses to therapy indicated no improvement. However, half of the patients, when surveyed directly, had significant relief of pain at 3 months, and 34% had improved social function (174). This is consistent with the well established differences between physician and patient reports of pain level. Furthermore, strontium-89 administration resulted in highly significant reductions in serum alkaline phosphatase, reaching a nadir at 3 months. No reductions, in PSA levels occurred, and strontium-89 did not improve survival. Improved progression-free survival occurred in a subgroup, having the characteristics of prostate cancer, with few bone scan detected metastases, and low alkaline phosphatase levels. Strontium-89 did not incur benefit among 203 prostate cancer patients based on pain relief, biochemical reduction, or treatment toxicity in a recent EORTC study based on study population characteristics (175).

G. Visceral Metastases

The symptoms caused by visceral metastases result in bleeding, obstruction, edema as well as pain. Palliative radiation can relieve these symptoms in about 70% of cases. Radiation therapy treatment planning is especially important to exclude mucosal surfaces and reduce treatment-related toxicity. Minimizing treatment-related toxicities in symptomatic and often frail patients referred for palliative radiation is critical.

This is especially important when mucosal surfaces of the head and neck region, and the esophagus are included in the radiation portal. Among the most radiosensitive visceral structures are the small bowel, stomach, lung, and skin. Radiation toxicities resulting from the small bowel include diarrhea. Nausea and vomiting can result when the stomach is in the radiation portal. Radiation pneumonitis, manifested by cough and scarring of the lung can occur especially when large volumes of lung are in the treatment field. Dry and moist desquamation can be painful and allow secondary infection.

1. Lung

Locally advanced primary or metastatic involvement of the lung often requires palliative intervention because cure is possible in only a few of these cases. A variety of symptoms, some of them emergent, can manifest due to tumor involvement of the lung (176). Pain can result from tumor invasion of the ribs and nerve roots of the chest wall. Vertebral involvement can be associated with spinal cord compression. Obstructive pneumonitis and hemoptysis can result from bronchial obstruction. Mediastinal infiltration can cause superior vena cava syndrome. All of these clinical presentations can be palliated with external beam radiation that encompasses the disease that is evident on diagnostic images and that treats pain referred along involved nerve roots.

Radiation schedules that administer 20 Gy in 5 fractions or 30 Gy in 10 fractions over 2 weeks are typically prescribed to previously unirradiated sites. If the area has been previously irradiated, techniques that exclude critical anatomic structures, like the spinal cord, are applied. Other approaches can be used when the symptomatic site is well localized and accessible. Brachytherapy, which applies radioactive sources next to tumors, can be used to treat bronchial obstruction and bleeding by placing a radioactive source directly against the tumor under bronchoscopic guidance. In these cases, large doses of radiation can be delivered over a few minutes by a high-dose rate brachytherapy unit.

2. Abdomen

There are many types of clinical presentations that require palliative management for tumors that involve the gastrointestinal region. Recurrent rectal cancer is the most common, but pain associated with the infiltration and biliary obstruction caused by pancreatic cancer often requires palliative therapy. Nausea and vomiting due to obstruction at many locations along the gastrointestinal tract may require surgical decompression if other less invasive approaches are not successful. Metastases from gastrointestinal malignancies can occur in any location, become symptomatic, and require palliative care.

The most common presenting symptoms of gastric and esophageal cancers are upper abdominal discomfort, weight loss, hematemesis and weakness from anemia. Exophytic tumors can cause significant bleeding. Infiltrative tumors can invade the celiac plexus and cause severe back pain like that observed with pancreatic cancer. Tumor infiltration resulting in linitis plastica is associated with an extremely poor prognosis. Epigastric pain from gastric cancer can also result from acid secretion. Early satiety, hematemesis, and melena occur less commonly. Obstructing lesions in either the antrum or cardia can cause vomiting or dysphagia, respectively. Several series indicate that 50–75% of patients experience improvement of bleeding, gastric outlet obstruction, and pain.

Treatment-related side effects are known, and medications should be prophylactically administered. The importance of aggressive supportive care in the setting of a multidisciplinary care team cannot be over emphasized. This is illustrated by the GITSG experience. Even though the chemoradiation group eventually had a better outcome, six of 45 patients in that group died because of sepsis or nutritional inadequacy. Prior to initiation of chemoradiation of gastric cancer, laparoscopic placement of a jejunostomy-feeding tube may be necessary to support the extended need for nutrition and hydration. Prophylactic antiemetic therapy, like that given with administration of systemic therapy, should be given prior to and during the course of radiation and chemotherapy as needed. A proton pump inhibitor and/or H-2 blocker, or other antiemetics are also recommended during the course of chemoradiation.

The most common presenting symptoms of pancreatic cancer are jaundice, weight loss due to anorexia and exocrine insufficiency, and abdominal pain. Jaundice is usually a presenting symptom with pancreatic head lesions. Pain occurs more commonly among lesions arising in the body or tail of the pancreas. Direct extension of tumor to the first and second celiac ganglia posteriorly leads to characteristic sharp pain, which is perceived as back pain. Pain is a symptom of locally advanced disease. It is typically described as sharp and knifelike located in the mid epigastric region with radiation to the back and is often a clinical indicator of unresectable disease.

The dose limiting structures surrounding the pancreas include the stomach, duodenum, small bowel, kidneys, spinal cord, and liver. Despite the generally poor overall prognosis with pancreatic cancer, most treatment programs for pancreatic cancer will administer radiation over 4–6 weeks to deliver 45–60 Gy. However, at M.D. Anderson Cancer Center, we found no survival advantage to the use of higher doses of radiation in the definitive treatment of pancreatic cancer. Routinely, 30 Gy, administered in 10 radiation fractions, is given and well tolerated for both definitive and palliative therapy. Furthermore, this fractionation schedule limits the time under treatment that is of particular importance in the palliative setting. In our experience with 5FU and either preoperative chemoradiation and pancreaticoduodenectomy using 50.4 Gy and rapid-fractionation chemoradiation totaling 30 Gy, and pancreaticoduodenectomy plus postoperative adjuvant chemoradiation totaling 50.4 Gy, it was found that no patient who received preoperative chemoradiation experienced a delay in surgery because of chemoradiation toxicity (177). In contrast to the rapid fractionation group treated with 30 Gy over 2 weeks, hospitalization, due to acute gastrointestinal toxicity, was required by one-third of the preoperative patients who received 50.4 Gy over 5.5 weeks. Also 24% of patients did not receive intended postoperative chemoradiation because of delayed recovery following pancreaticoduodenectomy.

3. *Pelvis*

Hemorrhage, and visceral, lymphovascular and nerve root obstruction present most commonly with locally advanced or metastatic disease in the pelvis. Treatment may require emergent radiotherapeutic and/or surgical interventions. Hemorrhage is commonly associated with tumors involving the rectum and genitourinary tracts, like the cervix or bladder. As with tumors in the lung, radiation is an effective means of stopping active bleeding. Colorectal cancers are often diagnosed among patients with unexplained bleeding. Obstruction by colorectal tumors may require stent placement to maintain the integrity of the visceral lumen while administering radiation (176). Occasionally, a diverting colostomy will be required to bypass intestinal obstruction or fistula formation.

Because rectal tumors are generally locally advanced, preoperative radiation is given in 25 treatments over 5–6 weeks if no or limited metastatic disease is evident; this is intended to stop bleeding, render the patient operable, and provide a chance for cure. Radiation schedules at M.D. Anderson Cancer Center have included 35 Gy/14 fractions, 30 Gy/10 fractions, and 30 Gy/6 fractions given twice weekly for 3 weeks (178). In our experience, a diverting colostomy was required by 16% of patients prior to radiation. No significant treatment-related toxicities were observed. Whether administered as conventional or hypofractionated radiation with 5-fluorouracil, symptoms from the primary tumor resolved in 94% of cases. The endoscopic complete response rate was 36%. Twenty-five patients underwent primary tumor resection. Although the two-year survival was greater in the group that underwent resection (46% vs. 11%), the colostomy-free survival was greater in the unresected group (79% vs. 51%). Durable control of pelvic symptoms was not significantly different and was 81% for palliative chemoradiation and 91% for preopera tive chemoradiation. Predictors for a worse prognosis included pelvic pain at presentation, biologic equivalent dose at 2 Gy/fraction of <35 Gy, and poor tumor differentiation (179). Among patients with locally advanced rectal cancer who also had liver metastases at presentation, the median survival was 17 months when treated with palliative radiation and chemotherapy.

The influence of tumor factors on response to therapy and survival was also demonstrated at the Princess Margaret Hospital (180). The most frequent palliative radiation schedule for locally advanced rectal cancer administered 50 Gy in 20 fractions in 4 weeks using a four-field technique. The 5-year survival was directly dependent on the extent of the tumor; 48% with mobile, 27% with partially fixed, and only 4% of patients with fixed tumors were alive at 5 years. Tumor extent also predicted for response to radiation; 50% of mobile, 30% of partially fixed, and only 9% of fixed tumors achieved a complete clinical response to radiation. The rate of tumor regression was slow; only 60% achieved a complete response by 4 months and 9 months was required by 90% of those who had a complete response. Of the complete responders, approximately half of the mobile and partially fixed, and over 70% of the fixed tumors developed progressive disease. Salvage surgery to relieve symptoms was accomplished without significant complication in over 90% of patients who developed progressive or recurrent disease.

Tumors involving the cervix can hemorrhage and require emergent radiotherapeutic intervention. Superficial x-rays are applied directly to the bleeding cervix through a cone that treat the bleeding site and do not compromise later radiation of other pelvic structures (176). Usually radiation doses between 5 and 10 Gy are administered in 1–3 applications of cone therapy. Brachytherapy also can be used to treat gynecologic tumors especially in the vagina, cervix, and endometrium.

Bladder cancers or tumors that secondarily invade the bladder can also result in significant bleeding that can be palliated by external beam radiation. Urinary obstruction commonly occurs with locally advanced pelvic cancers, especially with prostate and cervical cancers. Occasionally, placement of a urinary stent or urostomy/nephrostomy will be required until sufficient tumor regression can be accomplished by radiation to re-establish integrity of the urinary tract (176). As with the bowel and gynecologic tracts, a vesical fistula, resulting from either the tumor itself or from tumor regression, remains a concern.

The pelvic lymph nodes and major blood vessels may become obstructed by tumor. This most frequently is seen when tumor arise in pelvic structures but can also occur with pelvic metastases from breast and other cancers. Lymphovascular obstruction results in painful edema that is refractory to diuretic and other therapies. When severe, fluid and electrolyte imbalances can occur. Pelvic radiation can relieve lymphovascular obstruction through tumor regression.

Pelvic tumors can also invade the sacral plexus and result in intractable pain. Tumor can tract along nerve roots and can be associated with bony invasion of the sacrum. Pain due to visceral and/or lymphovascular obstruction often responds more rapidly to palliative radiation than the neuropathic pain seen with sacral plexus involvement. Other radiotherapeutic approaches, like brachytherapy, are extremely limited when the cancer persists or recurs after external beam radiation. Interventional pain management techniques are frequently required to control pain associated with sacral plexus involvement.

4. *Skin and Subcutaneous Tissues*

Tumors can cause ulceration of the skin and subcutaneous tissues that are often painful and distressing due to constant drainage. Representing a source for the development of sepsis in immunocompromised patients, localized radiation can be applied to destroy tumor and allow re-epithelialization of the skin. Radiation that treats only the skin and subcutaneous tissues (electron beam therapy) is generally used to avoid radiation side effects to underlying uninvolved normal structures. Although usually 10 radiation treatments are given, the course of radiation can be abbreviated further ranging from 1 to 5 days. Occasionally these lesions are treated with brachytherapy. The radioactive sources can be placed in a mold that sits on top of the tumor and delivers treatment over a few minutes (high-dose rate) or a few days (low-dose rate).

5. Brain Metastases

Radiation is used to relieve the symptoms of headache, seizure, nausea/vomiting, and neurologic dysfunction associated with brain metastases. Surgery, either alone or in combination with radiation, is often performed when a solitary brain metastasis is present, if the performance status is good and if the cancer burden is otherwise limited (181). Radiation is generally given over 2–3 weeks with daily fractions of 2.5–3 Gy per day; total radiation doses range from 25 Gy after resection to 30 Gy with unresectable disease and a poor prognosis.

H. Therapeutic Recommendations

Radiation remains an important modality in palliative care. A number of clinical, prognostic, and therapeutic factors must be considered to determine the most optimal treatment regimen in palliative radiotherapy. Adequate management of cancer-related pain is important both during and after completing palliative irradiation. Efficient and effective palliative treatment is imperative for locally advanced and metastatic cancer in order to relieve symptoms, improve function, and minimize disease-related morbidity.

Symptoms that persist after palliative radiation should be evaluated to exclude progression of disease in the treated area, possible extension of disease outside the radiation portal, or treatment-related side effects. For example, reduced cortical strength after treatment of bone metastases can result in compression, stress, or microfractures.

More specific criteria need to be delineated for prognosis to determine the appropriate treatment regimen for metastases. A staging system within the category of metastatic disease should incorporate the performance status, type and extent of bone and visceral involvement, time to disease progression, the primary tumor site, and account for prior failed therapies. Therefore, the response to and outcomes after radiation therapy must specifically defined relative to the radiated and unirradiated sites of disease, and the other antineoplastic and supportive care therapies administered.

Radiation therapy is an important means of treating localized symptoms related to tumor involvement by providing a wide range of therapeutic options. Radiobiological principles, the radiation tolerance of adjacent normal tissues, and the clinical condition influence the selection of radiation technique, dose, and fraction size. Validated symptom assessment tools, management of symptoms, prognostic factors, and radiobiological principles are priorities to deliver the most efficient and efficacious treatment schedule according to the clinical presentation.

Palliative irradiation should be integrated in a multidisciplinary therapeutic approach because of the need to treat associated symptoms and other underlying medical problems. Antineoplastic therapy can provide tumor regression, relief of cancer-related symptoms, and maintain functional integrity. Control of cancer-related pain with the use of analgesics is imperative to allow comfort during and while awaiting response to radiation and other therapies. Pain represents a sensitive measure of disease activity. Close follow-up should be performed to insure control of cancer and treatment-related pain, and assess for progressive disease or recurrent disease.

REFERENCES

1. Cleeland CS, Gonin R, Hatfield AK, Edmonson JH, Blum RH, Stewart JA, Pandya KJ. Pain and its treatment in outpatients with metastatic cancer. N Engl J Med 1994; 330:592–596.
2. Jacox AK, Carr DB, Payne R, eds. Management of Cancer Pain. Clinical Practice Guideline No. 9. Rockville, MD: Agency for Health Care Policy and Research (AHCPR publication no. 94-0592), 1994.
3. Jacox A, Carr DB, Payne R. New clinical practice guidelines for the management of pain in patients with cancer. N Engl J Med 1994; 330:651–655.
4. Brescia FJ, Portenoy RK, Ryan M, Krasnoff L, Gray G. Pain, opioid use, and survival in hospitalized patients with advanced cancer. J Clin Oncol 1992; 10:149–155.
5. Porzsolt F. Goals of palliative cancer therapy: scope of the problem. Cancer Treat Rev 1993; 19(suppl A):3–14.
6. Rubens RD. Approaches to palliation and its evaluation. Cancer Treat Rev 1993; 19(suppl A):67–71.
7. Porzsolt F, Tannock I. Goals of palliative cancer therapy. J Clin Oncol 1993; 11(2):378–381.
8. Cella DF, Tulsky DS. Quality of life in cancer: definition, purpose, and method of measurement. Cancer Invest 1993; 11:327–336.
9. Morita T, Tsunoda J, Inoue S, Chihara S. Contributing factors to physical symptoms in terminally ill cancer patients. J Pain Symptom Manage 1999; 18: 338–346.
10. Chang VT, Thaler HT, Polyak TA, Kornblith AB, Lepore JM, Portenoy RK. Quality of life and survival—the role of multidimensional symptom assessment. Cancer 1998; 83:173–179.
11. Von Roenn JH, Cleeland CS, Gonin R, et al. Physicians attitudes and practice in cancer pain management: a survey from the Eastern Cooperative Oncology Group. Ann Intern Med 1993; 119:121–126.

12. Paice JA, Toy C, Shott S. Barriers to cancer pain relief: fear of tolerance and addiction. J Pain Symptom Manage 1998; 16:1–9.
13. Cleeland CS, Janjan NA, Scott CB, Seiferheld WF, Curran WJ. Cancer pain management by radiotherapists: a survey of Radiation Oncology Group physicians. Int J Radiat Oncol Biol Phys 2000; 47: 203–208.
14. Lamont EB, Christakis NA. Some elements of prognosis in terminal cancer. Oncology 1999; 13: 1165–1170.
15. Zhong Z, Lynn J. Review of the Lamont/Christakis article. Oncology 1999; 13:1172–1173.
16. Manfredi PL, Chandler S, Pigazzi A, Payne R. Outcomes of cancer pain consultations. Cancer 2000; 89:920–924.
17. Pargeon KL, Hailey BJ. Barriers to effective cancer pain management: a review of the literature. J Pain Symptom Manage 1999; 18:358–368.
18. Janjan NA, Payne R, Gillis T, Podoloff D, Libshitz HI, Lenzi R, Theriault R, Martin C, Yasko A. Presenting symptoms in patients referred to a multidisciplinary clinic for bone metastases. J Pain Symptom Manage 1998; 16:171–178.
19. Stafford RS, Cyr PL. The impact of cancer on the physical function of the elderly and their utilization of health care. Cancer 1997; 80:1973–1980.
20. Cohen HJ. Cancer and the functional status of the elderly. Cancer 1997; 80:1883–1886.
21. Emanuel EJ, Fairclough DL, Slutsman J, Emanuel LL. Understanding economic and other burdens of terminal illness: the experience of patients and their caregivers. Ann Intern Med 2000; 132:451–459.
22. Rabow MW, Hardie GE, Fair JM, McPhee SJ. End of life care content in 50 textbooks from multiple specialties. JAMA 2000; 283:771–778.
23. Hanks GE. The crisis in health care costs in the United States: some implications for radiation oncology. Int J Radiat Oncol Biol Phys 1992; 23:203–206.
24. Dale RG, Jones B. Radiobiologically based assessments of the net costs of fractionated radiotherapy. Int J Radiat Oncol Biol Phys 1996; 36:739–746.
25. Greenlee RT, Hill-Harmon MB, Murray T, Thun M. Cancer statistics, 2001. CA Cancer J Clin 2001; 51: 15–36.
26. Cassel EJ. The nature of suffering and the goals of medicine. N Engl J Med 1982; 306:639–645.
27. World Health Organization. Cancer Pain Relief. Geneva, Switzerland: World Health Organization, 1986.
28. Janjan NA. Radiation for bone metastases—conventional techniques and the role of systemic radiopharmaceuticals. Cancer 1997; 80:1628–1645.
29. Fielding LP, Henson DE. Multiple prognostic factors and outcome analysis in patients with cancer–communication from the American Joint Committee on cancer. Cancer 1993; 71:2426–2429.
30. Liu L, Meers K, Capurso A, Engebretson TO, Glicksman AS. The impact of radiation therapy on quality of life in patients with cancer. Cancer Practice 1998; 6:237–242.
31. Joranson DE, Ryan KM, Gilson AM, Dahl JL. Trends in medical use and abuse of opioid analgesics. JAMA 2000; 283:1710–1714.
32. Ward SE, Berry PE, Misiewicz H. Concerns about analgesics among patients and family caregivers in a hospice setting. Res Nurs Health 1996; 19:205–211.
33. Weissman DE. Doctors, opioids, and the law: the effect of controlled substances regulations on cancer pain management. Semin Oncol 1993; 20(2 suppl 1): 53–58.
34. Khan FM. Dose distribution and scatter analysis. In: The Physics of Radiation Therapy. Baltimore: Williams and Wilkins, 1984:157–178.
35. Hall E. Dose response relationships for normal tissues. In: Radiobiology for the Radiologist. 4th ed. Philadelphia: JB Lippincott, 1994:45–75.
36. Nieder C, Milas L, Ang KK. Tissue tolerance to reirradiation. Semin Radiat Oncol 2000; 10:200–209.
37. Morris DE. Clinical experience with retreatment for palliation. Semin Radiat Oncol 2000; 10:210–221.
38. Shasha D, Harrison LB. The role of brachytherapy for palliation. Semin Radiat Oncol 2000; 10:221–239.
39. Erickson B, Janjan N, Wilson JF. Brachytherapy: more versatile, more important for local control. Intern Med 1993; 14:33–46.
40. Janjan NA, Waugh KA, Skibber JM, Curley SA, Carrasco CH, Lawrence D, Richli WR, Thomas J, Berner P, Lawyer A, Horton JL. Control of unresectable recurrent anorectal cancer with Au198 seed implantation. J Brachytherapy Int 1999; 15:115–129.
41. Bussieres E, Gilly FN, Rouanet P, Mahe MA, Roussel A, Delannes M, Gerard JP, Dubois JB, Richaud P. Recurrences of rectal cancers: results of a mutlimodal approach with intraoperative radiation therapy. Int J Radiat Oncol Biol Phys 1996; 34:49–56.
42. Martinez-Monge R, Nag S, Martin EW. Three different intraoperative radiation modalities (electron beam, high-dose-rate brachytherapy, and iodine-125 brachytherapy) in the adjuvant treatment of patients with recurrent colorectal adenocarcinoma. Cancer 1999; 86:236–247.
43. Mohiuddin M, Marks GM, Lingareddy V, Marks J. Curative surgical resection following reirradiation for recurrent rectal cancer. Int J Radiat Oncol Biol Phys 1997; 39:643–649.
44. Mohiuddin M, Regine WF, Stevens J, Rosato F, Barbot D, Biermann W, Cantor R. Combined intraoperative radiation and perioperative chemotherapy for unresectable cancers of the pancreas. J Clin Oncol 1995; 13:2764–2768.
45. Barton M. Tables of equivalent dose in 2 Gy fractions: a simple application of the linear quadratic formula. Int J Radiat Oncol Biol Phys 1995; 31:371–378.

46. Minsky BD, Conti JA, Huang Y, Knopf K. Relationship of acute gastrointestinal toxicity and the volume of irradiated small bowel in patients receiving combined modality therapy for rectal cancer. J Clin Oncol 1995; 13:1409–1416.
47. Cox JD, Pajack TF, Asbell S, Russell AH, Pederson J, Byhardt RW, Emami B, Roach M. Interruptions of high-dose radiation therapy decrease long-term survival of favorable patients with unresectable non-small cell carcinoma of the lung: analysis of 1244 cases from 3 Radiation Therapy Oncology Group (RTOG) trials. Int J Radiat Oncol Biol Phys 1993; 27:493–498.
48. Cox JD, Pajak TF, Marcial VA, Coia L, Mohiuddin M, Fu KK, Selim HM, Byhardt RW, Rubin P, Ortiz HG, et al. Interruptions adversely affect local control and survival with hyperfractionated radiation therapy of carcinomas of the upper respiratory and digestive tracts. New evidence for accelerated proliferation from Radiation Therapy Oncology Group Protocol 8313. Cancer 1992; 69:2744–2748.
49. Cox JD. Fractionation: a paradigm for clinical research in radiation oncology. Int J Radiat Oncol Biol Phys 1987; 13:1271–1281.
50. Cox JD. Large-dose fractionation (hypofractionation). Cancer 1985; 55(9 suppl):2105–2111.
51. Greenwald HP, Bonica JJ, Bergner M. The prevalence of pain in four cancers. Cancer 1987; 60:2563–2569.
52. Sherry MM, Greco FA, Johnson DH, Hainsworth JD. Breast cancer with skeletal metastases at initial diagnosis—distinctive clinical characteristics and favorable prognosis. Cancer 1986; 58:178–182.
53. Jacobson AF. Musculoskeletal pain as an indicator of occult malignancy. Arch Intern Med 1997; 157: 105–109.
54. Abbas F, Scardino PT. The natural history of clinical prostate carcinoma. Cancer 1997; 80:827–833.
55. Borre M, Nerstrom B, Overgaard J. The natural history of prostate carcinoma based on a Danish population treated with no intent to cure. Cancer 1997; 80:917–928.
56. Vuorinen E. Pain as an early symptom in cancer. Clin J Pain 1993; 9:272–278.
57. Reuben DB, Mor V, Hiris J. Clinical symptoms and length of survival in patients with terminal cancer. Arch Int Med 1988; 148:1586–1591.
58. Fielding LP, Henson DE. Multiple prognostic factors and outcome analysis in patients with cancer—communication from the American Joint Committee on Cancer. Cancer 1993; 71:2426–2429.
59. Portenoy RK, Miransky J, Thaler HT, Hornung J, Bianchi C, Cibas-Kong I, Feldhamer E, Lewis F, Matamoros I, Sugar MZ, Olivieri AP, Kemeny NE, Foley KM. Pain in ambulatory patients with lung or colon cancer. Cancer 1992; 70:1616–1624.
60. Pienta KJ, Esper PS. Risk factors for prostate cancer. Ann Int Med 1993; 118:793–803.
61. Perez CA, Cosmatos D, Garcia DM, Eisbruch A, Poulter CA. Irradiation in relapsing carcinoma of the prostate. Cancer 1993; 71:1110–1122.
62. Lai PP, Perez CA, Lockett MA. Prognostic significance of pelvic recurrence and distant metastases in prostate carcinoma following definitive radiotherapy. Int J Radiat Oncol Biol Phys 1992; 24:423–430.
63. Chisholm GD, Rana A, Howard GCW. Management options for painful carcinoma of the prostate. Semin Oncol 1993; 20(suppl 2):34–37.
64. Yamashita K, Denno K, Ueda T, Komatsubara K, Kotake T, Usami M, Maeda O, Nakano S, Hasegawa Y. Prognostic significance of bone metastases in patients with metastatic prostate cancer. Cancer 1993; 71:1297–1302.
65. Janjan NA. An emerging respect for palliative care in radiation oncology. J Palliative Med 1998; 1:83–88.
66. Powers WE, Ratanatharathorn V. Palliation of bone metastases [Chapter 82]. In: Perez CA, Brady LW eds. Principles and Practice of Radiation Oncology. 3rd ed. Lippincott Raven Publishers, 1998:2199–2219.
67. Bunting RW, Boublik M, Blevins FT, Dame CC, Ford LA, Lavine LS. Functional outcome of pathologic fracture secondary to malignant disease in a rehabilitation hospital. Cancer 1992; 69:98–102.
68. Arcangeli G, Micheli A, Arcangeli F, Giannarelli D, Pasta O, Tollis A, Vitullo A, Ghera S, Benassi M. The responsiveness of bone metastases to radiotherapy: the effect of site, histology and radiation dose on pain relief. Radiother Oncol 1989; 14:95–101.
69. Knudson G, Grinis G, Lopez-Majano V, Sansi P, Targonski P, Rubenstein M, Sharifi R, Gruinan P. Bone scan as a stratification variable in advanced prostate cancer. Cancer 1991; 68:316–320.
70. Steiner RM, Mitchell DG, Rao VM, Schweitzer ME. Magnetic resonance imaging of diffuse bone marrow disease. Radiol Clin North Am 1993; 31:383–409.
71. Algra PR, Bloem JL, Tissing H, Falke THM, Arndt JW, Verboom LJ. Detection of vertebral metastases: comparison between MR imaging and bone scintigraphy. Radiographics 1991; 11:219–232.
72. Le Bihan DJ. Differentiation of benign versus pathologic compression fractures with diffusion-weighted MR imaging: a closer step toward the "holy grail" of tissue characterization? Radiology 1998; 207:305–307
73. Nielsen OS, Munro AJ, Tannock IF. Bone metastases: pathophysiology and management policy. J Clin Oncol 1991; 9:509–524.
74. Mercadante S. Malignant bone pain: pathophysiology and treatment. Pain 1997; 69:1–18.
75. Sherry MM, Greco FA, Johnson DH, Hainsworth JD. Metastatic breast cancer confined to the skeletal system. Am J Med 1986; 81:381–386.
76. Porter AT, McEwan AJB, Powe JE, Reid R, McGowan DG, Lukka H, Sathyanarayana JR,

Yakemchuk VN, Thomas GM, Erlich LE, Crook J, Gulenchyn KY, Hong KE, Wesolowski C, Yardley J. Results of a randomized phase III trial to evaluate the efficacy of strontium 89 adjuvant to local field external beam irradiation in the management of endocrine resistant metastatic prostate cancer. Int J Radiat Oncol Biol Phys 1993; 25:805–813.
77. Porter AT, McEwan AJB. Strontium 89 as an adjuvant to external beam radiation improves pain relief and delays in disease progression in advanced prostate cancer: results of a randomized controlled trial. Semin Oncol 1993; 20:38–43.
78. Robinson RG, Preston DF, Schiefelbein M, Baxter KG. Strontium 89 therapy for the palliation of pain due to osseous metastases. JAMA 1995; 1995; 274: 420–424.
79. Serafini AN, Houston SJ, Resche I, Quick DP, Grund FM, Ell PJ, Bertrand A, Ahmann FR, Orihuela E, Reid RH, Lerski RA, Collier BD, McKillop JH, Purnell GL, Pecking AP, Thomas FD, Harrison KA. Palliation of pain associated with metastatic bone cancer using samarium-153 lexidronam: a double-blind placebo-controlled clinical trial. J Clin Oncol 1998; 16:1574–1581.
80. Rogers CL, Speiser BL, Ram PC, Shaw JA, Thomas TA. Efficacy and toxicity of intravenous strontium-89 for symptomatic osseous metastases. J Brachytherapy Int 1998; 14:133–142.
81. De Klerk JMH, Zonnenberg BA, van het Schip AD, van Dijk A, Han SH, Quirijnen JMSP, Blijham GH, van Rijk PP. Dose escalation study of rhenium-186 hydroxyethylidene disphosphonate in patients with metastatic prostate cancer. Eur J Nucl Med 1994; 21:1114–1120.
82. Sciuto RMaini CL, Tofani A, Fiumara K, Scelsa MG, Broccatelli R. Radiosensitization with low-dose carboplatin enhances pain palliation in radioisotope therapy with strontium-89. Nucl Med Commun 1996; 17: 799–804.
83. Bolger JJ, Dearnaley DP, Kirk D, Lewington VJ, Mason MD, Quilty PM, Reed NSE, Russell JM, Yardley J. Strontium-89 (metastron) versus external beam radiotherapy in patients with painful bone metastases secondary to prostatic cancer: preliminary report of a multicenter trial. Semin Oncol 1993; 20(suppl 2):32–33.
84. Bayouth JE, Macey DJ, Kasi LP, Fossella FV. Dosimetry and toxicity of samarium-153-EDTMP administered for bone pain due to skeletal metastases. J Nucl Med 1994; 35:63–69.
85. McEwan AJB, Amyotte GA, McGowan DG, MacGillivray JA, Porter AT. A retrospective analysis of the cost-effectiveness of treatment with metastron in patients with prostate cancer metastatic to bone. Eur Urol 1994; 26(suppl 1):26–31.
86. Alberts AS, Smit BJ, Louw WKA, van Rensburg AJ, van Beek A, Kritzinger V, Nel JS. Dose response relationship and multiple dose efficacy and toxicity of samarium-153-EDTMP in metastatic cancer to bone. Radiother Oncol 1997; 43:175–179.
87. Franzius C, Schuck A, Bielack SS. High-dose samarium-153 ethylene diamine tetramethylene phosphonate: low toxicity of skeletal irradiation in patients with osteosarcoma and bone metastases. J Clin Oncol 2002; 20:1953–1954.
88. Anderson PM, Wiseman GA, Dispenzieri A, Arndt CA, Hartmann LC, Smithson WA, Mullan BP, Bruland OS. High-dose samarium-153 ethylene diamine tetramethylene phosphonate: low toxicity of skeletal irradiation in patients with osteosarcoma and bone metastases. J Clin Oncol 2002; 20:189–196.
89. Windsor PM. Predictors of response to strontium-89 (metastron) in skeletal metastases from prostate cancer: report of a single centre's 10-yr experience. Clin Oncol 2001; 13:219–227.
90. Tong D, Gillick L, Hendrickson FR. The palliation of symptomatic ossesous metastases—final results of the study by the Radiation Therapy Oncology Group. Cancer 1982; 50:893–899.
91. Blitzer PH. Reanalysis of the RTOG study of the palliation of symptomatic osseous metastasis. Cancer 1985; 55:1468–1472.
92. Ford HT, Yarnold JR. Radiation therapy—pain relief and recalcification. In: Stoll BA, Parbhoo S, eds. Bone Metastases: Monitoring and Treatment. New York, NY: Raven Press, 1983:343–354.
93. Hortobagyi GN, Libshitz HI, Seabold JE. Osseous metastases of breast cancer—clinical, biochemical, radiographic, and scintigraphic evaluation of response to therapy. Cancer 1984; 53:577–582.
94. Vogel CL, Schoenfelder J, Shemano I, Hayes DF, Gams RA. Worsening bone scan in the evaluation of antitumor response during hormonal therapy of breast cancer. J Clin Oncol 1995; 13:1123–1128.
95. Rutten EHJM, Crul BJP, van der Toorn PPG, Otten AWI, Dirksen R. Pain characteristics help to predict the analgesic efficacy of radiotherapy for the treatment of cancer pain. Pain 1997; 69:131–135.
96. Kelly JB, Payne R. Pain syndromes in the cancer patient. Neurol Clin 1991; 9:937–953.
97. Portenoy RK. Cancer pain management. Semin Oncol 1993; 20:19–35.
98. Wilson PC, Levin W, Bezjak A, Heath C, Williams D, Sharma N, Cops F, McLean M, Soban F, Wong R. Palliative radiation for bone metastases-does pain response reflect full clinical benefit? Int J Radiat Oncol Biol Phys 2002; 54:309
99. Chow E, Wong R, Hruby G, Connolly R, Franssen E, Fung KW, Andersson L, Schueller T, Stefaniuk K, Szumacher E, Hayter C, Pope J, Holden L, Loblaw A, Finkelstein J, Danjoux C. Prospective patient-based assessment of effectiveness of palliative radiotherapy for bone metastases. Radiother Oncol 2001; 61:77–82.
100. Yau, V, Chow E, Davis L, Holden L, Schueller T, Danjoux C. Pain management in cancer patients with

bone metastases remains a challenge. J Pain Symptom Manage 2004; 27:1–3.
101. Berger A, Dukes E, Smith M, Hagiwara M, Seifeldin R, Oster, G. Use of oral and transdermal opioids among patients with metastatic cancer during the last year of life. J Pain Symptom Manage 2003; 26:723–730.
102. Chow E, Wu JSY, Hoskin P, Coia L, Bentzen SM, Blitzer P. International consensus on palliative radiotherapy endpoints for future clinical trials in bone metastases. Radiother Oncol 2002; 64:275–280.
103. Barak F, Werner A, Walach N, Horn Y. The palliative efficacy of a single high dose of radiation in treatment of symptomatic osseous metastases. Int J Radiat Oncol Biol Phys 1987; 13:1233–1235.
104. Cole DJ. A randomized trial of a single treatment versus conventional fractionation in the palliative radiotherapy of painful bone metastases. Clin Oncol 1989; 1:59–62.
105. Hoskin PJ, Price P, Easton D, Regan J, Austin D, Palmer S, Yarnold JR. A prospective randomised trial of 4 Gy or 8 Gy single doses in the treatment of metastatic bone pain. Radiother Oncol 1992; 23:74–78.
106. Price P, Hoskin PJ, Easton D, Austin A, Palmer SG, Yarnold JR. Prospective randomised trial of single and multifraction radiotherapy schedules in the treatment of painful bone metastases. Radiother Oncol 1986; 6:247–255.
107. Wu JSY, Wong R, Johnston M Bezjak A, Whelan T, on behalf of the Cancer Care Ontario Practice Guidelines Initiative–Supportive Care Group. Meta-analysis of dose-fractionation radiotherapy trials for the palliation of painful bone metastases. Int J Radiat Oncol Biol Phys 2003; 55:594–605.
108. Kal HB. Single reactions radiotherapy is as effective as multiple fractions for palliating painful bone metastases. Cancer Treat Rev 2003; 29:345–347.
109. Jeremic B. Single fraction external beam radiation therapy in the treatment of localized metastatic bone pain. A review. J Pain Symptom Manage 2001; 22:1048–1058.
110. Fiorca F, De Marco G, Camma C, Venturi A, Candela M, Fiorica G, Falchi A, Cartei F. Short fractionation radiotherapy versus multiple fractionated radiotherapy in patients with bone metastases: a meta-analysis of randomized clinical trials. Int J Radiat Oncol Biol Phys 2003; 57(suppl):S446–S445.
111. Chow E, Lutz S, Beyene J. A single fraction for all, or an argument for fractionation tailored to fit the needs of each individual patient with bone metastases? Int J Radiat Oncol Biol Phys 2003; 55:565–567.
112. Sze WM, Shelley MD, Held I, Wilt TJ, Mason MD. Palliation of metastatic bone pain: single fraction versus multifraction radiotherapy—a systematic review of randomized trials. Clin Oncol 2003; 15: 345–352.
113. Yarnold JR, on behalf of the Bone Pain Trial Working Party. 8 Gy single fraction radiotherapy for the treatment of metastatic skeletal pain: randomized comparison with a multifraction schedule over 12 months of patient followup. Radiother Oncol 1999; 52:111–121.
114. Steenland E, Leer J, van Houwelingen H, Post WJ, van den Hout WB, Kievit J, de Haes H, Martijn H, Oei B, Vonk E, van der Steen-Banasik E, Wiggenraad RGJ, Hoogenhout J, Warlam-Rodenhuis C, van Tienhoven G, Wanders R, Pomp van Reign J, van Mierlo T, Rutten E. Radiother Oncol 1999; 52: 101–109.
115. Van den Hout WB, van der Linden YM, Steenland E, Wiggenraad RG, et al. Sinvle versus multiple-fraction radiotherapy in patients with painful bone metastases: cost-utility analysis based on a randomized trial. J Natl Cancer Inst 2003; 95:222–229.
116. Steenland E, Leer JW, van Houselingen, et al. The effect of a single fraction compared to multiple fractions on painful bone metastases: a global analysis of the Dutch bone metastasis study. Radiother Oncol 1999; 52:101–109.
117. McQuay HJ, Collins SL, Carroll D, Moore RA. Radiotherapy for the palliation of painful bone metastases. Cochrane Database Syst Rev 2000; 2:pCD002067.
118. Hartsell WF, Scott C, Bruner DW, Scarantino CW, Ivker R, Roach M, Suh J, Demas W, Movasa B, Petersen I, Konski A. Phase III randomized trial of 8 Gy in 1 fraction vs. 30 Gy in 10 fractions for palliation of painful bone metastases: preliminary results of RTOG 97-14. Int J Radiat Oncol Biol Phys 2003; 57(suppl):S124.
119. Haddad P, Wong R, Wilson P, McLean M, Levin W, Bezjak A. Factors influencing the use of single versus multiple fractions of palliative radiotherapy for bone metastases: a 5-yr review and comparison to a survey. Int J Radiat Oncol Biol Phys 2003; 57(suppl):S278.
120. Koswig S, Budach V. Remineralization and pain relief in bone metastases after different radiotherapy fractions (10 times 3 Gy vs. 1 time 8 Gy). A prospective study. Strahlenther Onkol 1999; 175:500–508.
121. Macklis RM, Cornelli H, Lasher J. Brief courses of palliative radiotherapy for metastatic bone pain. Am J Clin Oncol 1998; 21:617–622.
122. van der Linden Y, Lok J, Steeland E, Martijn H, Martijn C, Leer J. Re-irradiation of painful bone metastases. A further analysis of the Dutch bone metastasis study. Int J Radiat Oncol Biol Phys 2003; 57(suppl):S222.
123. Gaze MN, Kelly CG, Kerr GR, Cull A, Cowie VJ, Gregor A, Howard GCW, Rodger A. Pain relief and quality of life following radiotherapy for bone metastases: a randomised trial of two fractionation schedules. Radiother Oncol 1997; 45:109–116.
124. Smith TJ, Staats PS, Deer T, Stearns LJ, Rauck RL, Boortz-Marx RL, Buchser E, Catala E, Bryce DA, Coyne PJ, Pool GE, for the Implantable Drug Delivery Systems Study Group. J Clin Oncol 2002; 20: 4040–4049.

125. Chow E, Coia L, Wu J, Janjan N, Kirkbride P, Hoskin P, Blitzer P. This house believes that multiple-fraction radiotherapy is a barrier to referral for palliative radiotherapy for bone metastases. Curr Oncol 2002; 9:60–66.
126. Boogerd W, van der Sande JJ. Diagnosis and treatment of spinal cord compression in malignant disease. Cancer Treat Rev 1993; 19:129–150.
127. Byrne TN. Spinal cord compression from epidural metastases. N Engl J Med 1992; 327:614–619.
128. Grant R, Papadopoulos SM, Greenberg HS. Metastatic epidural spinal cord compression. Neurol Clin 1991; 9:825–841.
129. Maranzano E, Latini P, Checcaglini F, Ricci S, Panizza BM, Aristei C, Perrucci E, Beneventi S, Corgna E, Tonato M. Radiation therapy in metastatic spinal cord compression—a prospective analysis of 105 consecutive patients. Cancer 1991; 67:1311–1317.
130. Janjan NA. Radiotherapeutic management of spinal metastases. J Pain Symptom Manage 1996; 1:47–56.
131. Loblaw DA, Laperriere NJ. Emergency treatment of malignant extradural spinal cord compression: an evidence-based guideline. J Clin Oncol 1998; 16: 1613–1624.
132. Boogerd W. Central nervous system metastasis in breast cancer. Radiother Oncol 1996; 40:5–22.
133. Paterson AHG. Bone metastases in breast cancer, prostate cancer and myeloma. Bone 1987; 8(supp 1): 17–22.
134. Townsend PW, Smalley SR, Cozad SC, Rosenthal HG, Hassanein RES. Role of postoperative radiation therapy after stabilization of fractures caused by metastatic disease. Int J Radiat Oncol Biol Phys 1995; 31:43–49.
135. Heisterberg L, Johansen TS. Treatment of pathologic fractures. Acta Orthop Scand 1979; 50:787–790.
136. Fidler M. Incidence of fracture through metastases in long bones. Acta Orthop Scand 1981; 52:623–627.
137. Oda MAS, Schurman DJ. Monitoring of pathological fracture. In: Stoll BA, Parbhoo S, eds. Bone Metastases: Monitoring and Treatment. New York, NY: Raven, 1983:271–288.
138. Plunkett TA, Smith P, Rubens RD. Risk of complications from bone metastases in breast cancer. Eur J Cancer 2000; 36:476–482.
139. Groot MT, Boeken Kruger CGG, Pelger RCM, Uyl-de Groot CA. Costs of prostate cancer, metastatic to the bone, in The Netherlands. Eur Urol 2003; 43: 226–232.
140. Bates T, Yarnold JR, Blitzer P, Nelson OS, Rubin P, Maher J. Bone metastases consensus statement. Int J Radiat Oncol Biol Phys 1992; 23:215–216.
141. Bates T. A review of local radiotherapy in the treatment of bone metastases and cord compression. Int J Radiat Oncol Biol Phys 1992; 23:217–221.
142. Turner S, Marosszeky B, Timms I, Boyages J. Malignant spinal cord compression: a prospective evaluation. Int J Radiat Oncol Biol Phys 1993; 26:141–146.
143. Boogerd W, van der Sande JJ, Kroger R. Early diagnosis and treatment of spinal metastases in breast cancer: a prospective study. J Neurol Neurosurg Psychiatry 1992; 55:1188–1193.
144. Wada E, Yamamoto T, Furuno M, et al. Spinal cord compression secondary to osteoblastic metastasis. Spine 1993; 18:1380–1381.
145. Algra PR, Heimans JJ, Valk J, Nauta JJ, Lachniet M, Van Kooten B. Do metastases in vertebrae begin in the body or the pedicles?—imaging study in 45 patients. Am J Roentgenol 1992; 158:1275–1279.
146. Landmann C, Hunig R, Gratzi O. The role of laminectomy in the combined treatment of metastatic spinal cord compression. Int J Radiat Oncol Biol Phys 1992; 24:627–631.
147. Kim RY, Smith JW, Spencer SA, Meredith RF, Salter MM. Malignant epidural spinal cord compression associated with a paravertebral mass: its radiotherapeutic outcome on radiosensitivity. Int J Radiat Oncol Biol Phys 1993; 27:1079–1083.
148. Bach F, Agerlin N, Sorensen JB, et al. Metastatic spinal cord compression secondary to lung cancer. J Clin Oncol 1992; 10:1781–1787.
149. Jeremic B, Djuric L, Mijatovic L. Incidence of radiation myelitis of the cervical spinal cord at doses of 5500 cGy or greater. Cancer 1991; 68:2138–2141.
150. Wen PY, Blanchard KL, Block CC, et al. Development of Lhermitte's sign after bone marrow transplantation. Cancer 1992; 69:2262–2266.
151. Powers BE, Thames HD, Gillette SM, Smith C, Beck ER, Gillette EL. Volume effects in the irradiated canine spinal cord: do they exist when the probability of injury is low? Radiother Oncol 1998; 46:297–306.
152. Sugimura H, Kisanuki A, Tamura S, et al. Magnetic resonance imaging of bone marrow changes after irradiation. Invest Radiol 1994; 29:35–41.
153. Yankelevitz DF, Henschke C, Knapp PH, Nisce L, Yi Y, Cahill P. Effect of radiation therapy on thoracic and lumbar bone marrow: evaluation with MR imaging. Am J Roentgenol 1991; 157:87–92.
154. Russi EG, Pergolizzi S, Gaeta M, Mesiti M, D'Aquino A, Delia P. Palliative radiotherapy in lumbosacral carcinomatous neuropathy. Radiother Oncol 1993; 26: 172–173.
155. Saarto T, Janes R, Tenhunen M, Kouri M. Palliative radiotherapy in the treatment of skeletal metastases. Eur J Pain 2002; 6:323–330.
156. Altehoefer C, Ghanem N, Hogerle S, Moser E, Langer M. Comparative detectability of bone metastases and impact on therapy of magnetic resonance imaging and bone scintigraphy in patients with breast cancer. Eur J Radiol 2001; 40:16–23.
157. Hoskin PJ, Grover A, Bhana R. Metastatic spinal cord compression: radiotherapy outcome and dose fractionation. Radiother Oncol 2003; 68:175–180.
158. Loblaw DA, Laperriere NJ, Mackillop WJ. A population-based study of malignant spinal cord compression in Ontario. Clin Oncol 2003; 15:211–217.

159. Rades D, Heidenreich F, Karstens JH. Final results of a prospective study of the prognostic value of the time to develop motor deficits before irradiation in metastatic spinal cord compression. Int J Radiat Oncol Biol Phys 2002; 53:975–979.
160. Hatrick NC, Lucas JD, Timothy AR, Smith MA. The surgical treatment of metastatic disease of the spine. Radiother Oncol 2000; 56:335–339.
161. Rades D, Blach M, Bremer M, Wildfang I, Karstens JH, Heidenreich F. Prognostic significance of the time of developing motor deficits before radiation therapy in metastatic spinal cord compression: one-year results of a prospective trial. Int J Radiat Oncol Biol Phys 2000; 48:1403–1408.
162. Helweg-Larsen S, Sorensen PS, Kreiner S. Prognostic factors in metastatic spinal cord compression: a prospective study using multivariate analysis of variables influencing survival and gait function in 153 patients. Int J Radiat Oncol Biol Phys 2000; 46:1163–1169.
163. Prie L, Lagarde P, Palussiere J, El Ayoubi S, Dilhuydy JM, Durand M, Vital JM, Kantor G. Radiation therapy of spinal metastases in breast cancer: retrospective analysis of 108 patients. Cancer/Radiotherapie 1997; 1:234–239.
164. Maranzano E, Bellavita R, Floridi P, Celani G, Righetti E, Lupattelli M, Panizza BM, Frattegiani A, Pellicciolі GP, Latini P. Radiation induced myelopathy in long-term surviving metastatic spinal cord compression patients after hypofractionated radiotherapy: a clinical and magnetic resonance imaging analysis. Radiother Oncol 2001; 60:281–288.
165. Moineuse C, Kany M, Fourcade D, Aziza R, Attal M, Mazieres B, Laroche M. Magnetic resonance imaging findings in multiple myeloma: descriptive and predictive value. Joint Bone Spine 2001; 68:334–344.
166. Ridet JL, Pencalet P, Belcram M, Giraudeau B, Chastang C, Philippon J, Mallet J, Privat A, Schwartz L. Effects of spinal cord x-irradiation on the recovery of paraplegic rats. Exp Neurol 2000; 161:1–14.
167. Milker-Zabel S, Zabel A, Thilmann C, Schlegel W, Wannenmacher M, Debus J. Clinical results of retreatment of vertebral bone metastases by stereotactic conformal radiotherapy and intensity-modulated radiotherapy. Int J Radiat Oncol Biol Phys 2003; 55:162–167.
168. Grosu AL, Andratschke N, Nieder C, Molls M. Retreatment of the spinal cord with palliative radiotherapy. Int J Radiat Oncol Biol Phys 2002; 52:1288–1292.
169. Bach F, Bjerregaard B, Soletormos G, et al. Diagnostic value of cerebrospinal fluid cytology in comparison with tumor marker activity in central nervous system metastases secondary to breast cancer. Cancer 1993; 72:2376–2382.
170. Holmes RA. Radiopharmaceuticals in clinical trials. Semin Oncol 1993; 20:22–26.
171. Porter AT, Ben-Josef E. Strontium 89 in the treatment of bony metastases. In: DeVita VT, Hellman S, Rosenberg SA, eds. Important Advances in Oncology Philadelphia, PA: JB Lippincott Co, 1995:87–94 [Chapter 7].
172. Preston DF, Baxter KG, Dusing RW, Spicer JA. Clinical experience with strontium 89 in prostatic and breast cancer patients. Semin Oncol 1993; 20:44–48.
173. Eary JF, Collins C, Stabin M, Vernon C, Petersdorf S, Baker M, Hartnett S, Ferency S, Addison SJ, Appelbaum F, Gordon EE. Samarium 153-EDTMP biodistribution and dosimetry estimation. J Nucl Med 1993; 34:1031–1036.
174. Smeland S, Erikstein B, Aas M, Skovlund E, Hess SL, Fossa SD. Role of strontium-89 as adjuvant to palliative external beam radiotherapy is questionable: results of a double-blind randomized study. Int J Radiat Oncol Biol Phys 2003; 56:1397–1404.
175. Oosterhof GON, Roberts JT, de Reijke TM, Engelholm SA, Horenblas S, von der Maase H, Neymark N, Debois M, Collette L. Strontium 89 chloride versus palliative local field radiotherapy in patients with hormonal escaped prostate cancer: a phase III study of the European Organization for Research and Treatment of Cancer Genitourinary Group. Eur Urol 2003; 44:519–526.
176. Kagan AR. Palliation of visceral recurrences and metastases [Chapter 83]. In: Perez CA, Brady LW, eds. Principles and Practice of Radiation Oncology. 3rd ed. Lippincott Raven Publishers, 1998: 2219–2226.
177. Spitz FR, Abbruzzese JL, Lee JE, Pisters PWT, Lowy AM, Fenoglio CJ, Cleary KR, Janjan NA, Goswitz MS, Rich TA, Evans DB. Preoperative and postoperative chemoradiation strategies in patients treated with pancreaticoduodenectomy for adenocarcinoma of the pancreas. J Clin Oncol 1997; 15:928–937.
178. Janjan NA, Breslin T, Lenzi R, Rich TA, Skibber JM. Avoidance of colostomy placement in advanced colorectal cancer with twice weekly hypofractionated radiation plus continuous infusion 5-fluorouracil. J Pain Symptom Manage 2000; 20:266–272.
179. Crane CH, Janjan NA, Abbruzzese JL, Curley S, Vauthey JN, Sawaf HB, Dubrow R, Allen P, Ellis LM, Hoff P, Wolff RA, Lenzi R, Brown TD, Lynch P, Cleary K, Rich TA, Skibber J. Effective pelvic symptom control using initial chemoradiation without colostomy in metastatic rectal cancer. Int J Radiat Oncol Biol Phys 2001; 49:107–116.
180. Brierly JD, Cummings BJ, Wong CS, Keane TJ, O'Sullivan B, Catton CN, Goodman P. Adenocarcinoma of the rectum treated by radical external radiation therapy. Int J Radiat Oncol Biol Phys 1995; 31:255–259.
181. Kagan AR. Palliation of brain and spinal cord metastases [Chapter 81]. In: Perez CA, Brady LW, eds. Principles and Practice of Radiation Oncology. 3rd ed. Lippincott Raven Publishers, 1998:2187–2198.

9

Clinical Trials in Oncology: Organization and Oversight

CARLEEN A. BRUNELLI

Department of Research Administration, Children's Hospital Boston, Boston, Massachusetts, U.S.A.

LEONARD A. ZWELLING

Office of Research Administration, The University of Texas M.D. Anderson Cancer Center, Houston, Texas, U.S.A.

I. PHILOSOPHY AND PRINCIPLES OF CLINICAL RESEARCH

Debate over distinguishing research from standard therapy has been ongoing for decades. In fact, the Belmont Report discusses the importance of separating the two to make sure that the ethical principles of respect, beneficence and justice are applied to all individuals participating in research (1). The two types of interventions, research and standard clinical care, must also be differentiated to determine which interventions need to be overseen by an Institutional Review Board (IRB).

There are two schools of thought about whether clinical research is part of the continuum of clinical care. The first school ascribes to the belief that clinical research is part of a continuum of care that considers clinical research as therapy. As was recently pointed out in a paper by Miller and Rosenstein in the *New England Journal of Medicine*, this is exemplified by the University of Texas M.D. Anderson web site, which they are quoted as saying "a clinical trial is just one of many treatment options at M.D. Anderson" (2).

The second school of thought places a firm barrier between what is clinical care and what is research. There are a number of reasons to support this position.

- Clinical research is subject to special oversight by federal agencies (e.g., the Office of Human Research Protections, the Food and Drug Administration) that clinical care is not.
- Unlike clinical care, clinical research must be reviewed and overseen by an IRB.
- All clinical investigators have a dual allegiance. In legal terms, they have two, competing fiduciary roles. In the most obvious role as a patient advocate, the patient's well being is the doctor's primary concern. However, when a physician, particularly one who has been caring for a patient for some time and has built up a trusting doctor–patient relationship, dons the role of a clinical investigator, he assumes a fiduciary relationship where his interests may clash with that of his primary role as patient advocate. As a clinical investigator, he must adhere to the terms of the IRB-approved protocol. His fiduciary role here is to the trial plan, the trial's sponsor and the IRB. He may not be able to enroll one of his

long-standing patients on his own trial, even if he believes that the trial drug might benefit the patient, if the patient is not fully eligible for the trial. Furthermore, it is difficult for a physician who has been caring for a patient for many years to offer that patient an opportunity to participate in a trial, particularly a randomized, placebo-controlled trial, and not have that patient interpret this offer as a therapeutic recommendation. Yet, it cannot be a therapeutic recommendation because the physician cannot know to which arm of the trial the patient will be assigned and a proper informed consent process dictates presenting all aspects, including unresolved or unknown aspects of the trial, to perspective participants. These dynamics are unlikely in the routine course of clinical care.

- The data keeping and reporting necessary for clinical research exceeds that needed for routine patient care. Thus, a significant personnel and administrative infrastructure is needed for clin ical research that is not needed for routine care. This can be expensive, yet its absence can lead to serious noncompliance with federal code and potentially increased risk to trial subjects. Each of these outcomes can lead to a loss of research funds, suspensions of research programs, and damaged reputations of both institutions and physicians.

We firmly ascribe to the second of these schools of thought. Although we fully understand that in oncology, more than in most subspecialties, care resembles the performance of protocol-based clinical research, there are just too many good reasons to view clinical care and clinical research as distinct activities.

It is with this in mind that we describe an infrastructure to support clinical research that disrupts the administration of good clinical care as little as possible, but insists on an environment that makes compliance with federal code as easy as possible. This chapter will describe our answers to the challenges of performing clinical research in a center where research is considered "one of many treatment options," in fact, the one many people come to find.

II. INSTITUTIONAL REVIEW BOARDS AND THE DEPARTMENT OF HEALTH AND HUMAN SERVICES

A. History

The Belmont Report outlines what the National Commission for the Protection of Human Subjects of Biomedical and Behavioral Research determined to be the basic ethical principles that should serve as the foundation for all biomedical research involving human subjects. This report is the result of a meeting that occurred at the Smithsonian Institution's Belmont Conference Center in 1976 and discussions spanning several years thereafter.

The Belmont Report discusses the basic ethical principles of respect for persons, beneficence and justice, and how they should be applied to the informed consent process, the assessment of risk vs. benefit, and the equitable selection of subjects for participation in research projects. Since its publication, the Belmont Report has played a role in the design and implementation of policies and procedures related to the protection of human subjects in research.

The Department of Health and Human Services (DHHS) enforces Title 45 Code of Federal Regulations Part 46, Protection of Human Subjects. These regulations, codified in 1974, are "... a rigorous and formalized system of regulation and guidelines... included in the former Department of Health, Education and Welfare's regulation" (3). 45 CFR 46 implements certain sections of the Public Health Service Act including: Sec. 491(a) which requires entities applying for funds for human subject research to assure that they will protect the rights of the subjects; Sec. 491(b) (1) which required DHHS to establish a section to respond to the inquiries for guidance from researchers; and Sec. 491(2) which required DHHS to also set up policies and procedures to receive and respond to information about violations of the rights of research subjects (4). In addition to the guidance and oversight function, DHHS was charged with implementing Sec. 492A(a) describing the requirements for IRB review and approval of research (5).

Oversight of clinical research is the shared responsibility of a select number of federal departments and agencies, the institutions where research is conducted, the IRBs that review the research, and the investigators and their research teams, which perform the research. In 1991, 16 federal departments and agencies, including the DHHS that conduct, support, and regulate human subject research adopted the regulations embodied in the Federal Policy found in 45 CFR 46. These regulations have since been referred to as the Common Rule (6). The Common Rule provides guidance to IRBs, investigators, and institutions on appropriate methods to review and conduct research. The joint effort of these groups was undertaken to provide uniformity to the guidelines and oversight for federally funded research. It eased the burden on investigators performing research under the oversight of more than one agency by standardizing the regulations to which investigators adhere.

It is of interest to note that the Food and Drug Administration (FDA), one of the most visible agencies that oversees human subject research, has not adopted the Common Rule. However, the agency has modified its IRB and informed consent regulations (21 CFR 50) to concur with the Common Rule without adopting the rule as a whole.

B. Regulations

The Common Rule is the most well known and often cited of the regulations governing the conduct of clinical research. This is primarily because it applies to all federally funded research. The Common Rule provides a clear outline of (a) how IRBs should be structured, (b) how they should conduct their initial and continuing review, (c) what the role of the institution is and (d) what steps need to be taken when instances of serious or continuing noncompliance are found. It is imperative to remember that all federal regulations, including the Common Rule, provide the floor, not the ceiling, for institutional policy. It is not uncommon to find institutions with policies that are more stringent than what is required by the federal guidelines or by their Assurance Document.

In addition to the Common Rule, there can be other applicable sections of the Code of Federal Regulations that may govern the conduct of clinical research depending on which agency is providing the funding or if the study is being conducted to support any type of application to the FDA. When more than one agency and set of regulations are involved, the research must meet the requirements of each agency or department. And, as with all regulations, there are gray areas open to interpretation in the Common Rule and different agencies can offer different interpretations.

The FDA has the most extensive set of regulations relating to human subject research in addition to those covering the functions of the IRB and the informed consent process. Due to the nature of the FDA's role in ensuring the safety and efficacy of new therapies prior to allowing commercialization, Title 21 of the CFR covers the preparation, submission, and review process of Investigational New Drug Applications (IND). Furthermore, 21 CFR provides complete guidance on the responsibilities of the IND sponsor, the trial monitors and the principal investigators. Failure to comply with these regulations can lead to punishment beginning with withdrawal of an IND up to and including the debarment of an investigator.

Although some investigators believe the CFR changes on a regular basis, the fact is such changes are rare. It is the environment in which research is conducted that changes constantly. The most extensive change to the human subject research regulations occurred with the implementation of the privacy section of the Health Insurance Portability and Accountability Act (HIPAA) in April 2003 (7). By increasing the control individuals (e.g., patients, research subjects) have over their protected health information, HIPAA expanded some components of the Common Rule to research that is neither funded nor conducted by a federal agency and therefore not previously subject to the Common Rule. Although HIPAA impacted all health providers conducting research, the new regulation had a far greater impact on research previously exempt from 45 CFR 46 (Common Rule).

For example, any hospital, clinic, medical practice or other entity conducting human subject research that was privately funded did not have to establish an IRB or ethics board that ensured research participants were informed that their private health information would be used for research. The weighing of risk vs. benefit to the participant may not have been in accordance with the accepted standards outlines in 45 CFR 46. Furthermore, the discussions between a health care provider and a patient may not have provided the potential participant with adequate information to make a decision regarding their participation in the research.

In addition to adding another layer of regulations to institutions and researchers, it brought the DHHS Office of Civil Rights (OCR) into the regulatory arena for human subject research. Along with the HIPAA regulations, the OCR listed civil as well as criminal penalties including fines and incarceration for failure to comply with the privacy regulations. Only time will tell how the OCR interprets HIPAA. To date, no precedents have been set with regard to complying with these new regulations or punishment for not complying.

C. Operations

The Office for Human Research Protections (OHRP) oversees the Common Rule (45 CFR 46), which applies to all research that is conducted or supported by the DHHS. Due to the large number of research facilities in this country, it is obvious that OHRP cannot provide on-site monitoring for research compliance at all of these locations. Instead, OHRP has implemented a system of Assurance Documents by which an institution makes certain promises to OHRP regarding their human subject research program.

This formal document, which serves as a "contract" between the institution and OHRP, is now in template form and begins with the research entity's promise to abide by the Common Rule and the Belmont Report. The document continues by listing the institution's or signatory's IRBs registered with OHRP that are responsible for overseeing the research and identifies all the sites or facilities conducting research overseen by the listed IRBs. The Assurance is signed by the IRB chairperson and the institution's signatory official for human subject research.

In addition, the Assurance Document provides OHRP with information regarding compliance monitoring, education of IRB members, support staff and investigators, and the institutional resources available to support these functions. The Office for Human Research Protections now requires education for the IRB chairperson, the institutional official responsible for human subject research and for the IRB administrator of record prior to approving the Assurance Document.

Institutions are responsible for providing the resources required to support one or more IRBs as described in 45 CFR 46. Failure on the part of the institution to provide adequate support of the IRB to appropriately discharge its duties can result in a failure of the clinical research oversight system leading to a revocation of the Assurance Document by OHRP and a cessation of the research. The public relations damage done in such situations can be far more costly than the loss of research dollars.

There is a fine line between institutional support of the IRB and intrusion on the committee's autonomy. The IRB must conduct its business in an environment that is independent of all undue influence from institutional administrators and departments (45 CFR 46.112). Therefore, it is most appropriate for the individuals that staff the IRB and its functions to be part of an independent department as opposed to having an affiliation with any academic department. This allows them to work in an environment of institutional support free from conflicts or attachments with any individual research team. This organizational structure decreases the chances of preferential treatment to any group, whether intended or not.

Institutional policies and procedures should be established, implemented, and published to guide the IRB and the research teams. As we discussed in the opening paragraphs, the design of the research infrastructure must be able to identify and accommodate the difference between research and standard clinical care in a way that allows both to continue in an uninterrupted fashion. To achieve the appropriate level of compliance, the intricacies of the Common Rule and other pertinent federal regulations must be clearly understood by researchers and administrators alike. This knowledge, together with an understanding of the research being conducted by a particular institution, provides the basis for designing the framework of the infrastructure to support the research enterprise.

Although the Code of Federal Regulations changes infrequently, federal agencies commonly publish guidance on how institutions should interpret or implement policies to ensure compliance and publish them on their websites (www.fda.gov, www.hhs.gov/ohrp, www.opa.osophs.dhsi.gov, www.dhhs.gov). The infrastructure, policies, and procedures that work today are not guaranteed to work tomorrow. Flexibility and openness to change are critical factors required to guarantee the future of any research enterprise and the infrastructure supporting it.

III. SCIENTIFIC REVIEW

The purpose of a scientific review process is to evaluate the scientific content of research requiring a clinical protocol. This is usually done prior to the human subjects protection review at an IRB. However, most IRBs consider the validity of the science of any protocol part of their purview as it does impact the area of human subjects protection.

A clinical protocol is the instrument for conducting and evaluating the research. This includes all protocols originated by physician–investigators; all protocols sponsored by the National Cancer Institute (NCI), pharmaceutical and biotechnology companies, and co-operative groups; all large multi-institutional trials; and any other clinical investigation requiring IRB oversight including those studying human tissue or using surveys.

Comprehensive cancer centers supported by a cancer center support grant (CCSG) from the NCI should have a protocol review and monitoring system (PRMS) to perform the scientific review function. The PRMS, as described by the CCSG Guidelines, should be designed and operated to ensure that the clinical research performed is of the highest quality possible. The primary elements of the PRMS at our institution are: the scientific review process by either the Clinical Research Committee (CRC) for treatment protocols or the Psychosocial, Behavioral or Health Services Research Committee (PBHSRC) for quality of life and prevention studies; a Protocol Data Management System (PDMS) which is the centralized clinical trial database used for protocol activation and termination, patient registration with eligibility checklists; and twice yearly electronic accrual audits.

The CRC reviews and approves all aspects of the scientific research that is incorporated into a protocol plan. This includes specific aims, background, and rationale; methods used to validate the scientific questions being asked; appropriateness of the biostatistical analysis to establish the success or failure of an experiment; appropriateness of radiologic and pathologic procedures; the amount of nursing care required by the protocol; and evaluation of pharmaceutical information provided in the protocol.

The purpose of the PBHSRC is to evaluate the scientific content of all research that addresses areas of investigation related to psychosocial, behavioral and health services research including methodological and outcome studies in psychosocial and behavioral research, health services research, pain assessment and management, descriptive studies of psychosocial functioning and studies of patient and clinician decision-making. Examples of methodological studies include pain assessment approaches in acute postoperative and chronic cancer pain and the development of quality of life instruments. Endpoints of outcomes research, for example, include: quality of life; cost-effectiveness, utility, and benefit; smoking cessation; dietary change and other behavioral modification interventions.

In this regard, the PBHSRC and the CRC are scientific reviewing agents for the Surveillance Committee (the MDACC IRB) for protocols defined by the scope of committee functions mentioned above and are a critical component of the PRMS.

IV. QUALITY ASSURANCE

When the regulatory burden on institutions and researchers is combined with the increased scrutiny of the conduct of clinical trials by patients, advocates, and the media, constant vigilance is essential to ensure compliance. Inherent in the policies and procedures implemented to oversee human subject research should be methods for monitoring the conduct of clinical research. Monitoring should include ensuring the research is conducted according to the IRB-approved protocol, federal and institutional guidelines, and a mechanism to report to any institutional officials and federal department or agency heads when serious breaches of compliance are found.

A. Auditing

Our Office of Protocol Research Quality Assurance (OPRQA) was established in 1996 to develop a system of protocol auditing, an ombudsman reporting system, and an institutional mechanism for follow-up on issues of clinical research data quality. Clinical research training of faculty and research personnel is also done by this office. These systems were developed to ensure that clinical research performed at The University of Texas M.D. Anderson Cancer Center (UTMDACC) meets standards of the highest quality and is thereby consistent with the mission of the institution.

This office is a part of the Office of Research Administration and reports to the Vice President for Research Administration (VPRA) through the Chief Research and Regulatory Affairs Officer (CRRAO). The function of this office is further augmented by the OPRQA Oversight Committee, consisting of UTMDACC faculty members. This official body operates within a medical review-advisory capacity, and reports to the President of the University of Texas M.D. Anderson Cancer Center.

The OPRQA Audit Program assures that the data used to analyze study results (e.g., database spread sheets, Protocol Data Management System data, and case report forms) are an accurate reflection of the primary data source (e.g., medical record). The audit program assesses protocol compliance in the following categories: informed consent, eligibility, treatment, response, toxicity, general data quality, and compliance with institutional guidelines and federal regulations for the protection of human subjects.

A focused audit may occur to address protocol compliance in any of the specified area(s) of clinical trial performance usually in response to a perceived problem or external concern. In a random audit, all areas will be reviewed for a certain percentage of study cases. Random audits are part of the overall institutional QA program.

Although the scope of OPRQA spans the entire spectrum of UTMDACC clinical trials, emphasis for internal auditing is placed on those trials that do not undergo monitoring or auditing by an external agency (e.g., the NCI or pharmaceutical sponsor).

The role of an institution's audit program is:

- To verify the accuracy and integrity of the research data collected;
- To determine protocol compliance using source documentation;
- To verify adherence to the IRB-approved protocol and to federal and institutional requirements;
- To enhance the delivery of accurate and reliable clinical trials data and results according to good clinical practice (GCP);
- To provide educational support to the clinical research staff regarding issues related to data management and quality assurance;
- To gauge quality indicators regarding protocol performance

B. Monitoring

The quality assurance unit of any institution should also provide monitoring services if it is deemed necessary in the IRB-approved data and safety monitoring plan for any protocol that is not monitored by an outside entity. Unlike a protocol audit, which is conducted "after the fact," monitoring is an ongoing process that enables the detection and correction of any problems or issues of noncompliance to be detected and corrected at the earliest stages of a protocol's life. Monitoring procedures are to assure the adequate protection of the rights of human subjects, the safety of all subjects involved in clinical investigations, and the integrity of the resulting data submitted to the FDA.

Accountability is especially important in instances where UTMDACC is the sponsor of the IND or Investigational Device Exemption (IDE). The MDACC OPRQA conducts the monitoring function for all NCI sponsored protocols that are not monitored by an industry sponsor, Contract Research Organization (CRO) or other entity outside UTMDACC. In addition, OPRQA monitors all IND studies and provides reports to the VPRA and CRARAO who represent the UTMDACC as the institutional sponsor.

Guidelines for the monitoring roles and responsibilities are based on the FDA's *Guideline for the Monitoring of Clinical Investigations*, which "reflects principles recognized by the scientific community as desirable approaches to monitoring clinical research involving human subjects" and represents a "standard of practice that is acceptable to the FDA" (8).

The monitoring process begins with a dialogue between the monitoring team and the research team prior to opening a protocol for enrollment (protocol "activation"). During this preactivation meeting, the discussion should focus on the requirement described in the FDA Form 1572; the posting of the protocol on the clinicaltrials.gov website; the regulatory binder; review of eligibility and the protocol in general; review of protocol-specific source documents and adverse event reporting requirements. The protocol-specific monitoring plan and timeline for monitoring visits should be scheduled at this time.

Monitoring timelines should be developed on a protocol-by-protocol basis depending on the risk inherent in the protocol and the expected accrual rate. Guidance on the timeline to be followed can also be obtained from the IRB-approved data and safety monitoring plan that is in each protocol. Monitoring reviews should occur frequently enough to assure that:

- The investigational plan is being followed
- Changes to the protocol have been approved by the IRB and FDA before being implemented
- Accurate, complete and current records are being maintained
- Accurate, complete and timely reports are being made to the IRB and to the sponsor
- The investigator is carrying out the agreed upon activities and has not delegated them to inappropriate or unspecified staff.

To do this, source documentation should be reviewed and used to independently verify study data. Data quality should be assessed by measuring it against the standards for optimal data as delineated in the research protocol. Investigator compliance with regulatory requirements and guidelines for Good Clinical Practice (GCP) should also be assessed. The documentation of informed consent, eligibility, pretherapy requirements, treatment administration, study evaluation and follow-up, severe adverse event reporting, efficacy, and the general quality of the data should be examined for each case reviewed.

The Clinical Trials Monitor should submit a written report of each monitoring visit to the PI and the sponsor or other agent responsible for the conduct of the study. Reports should include a summary of what the monitor reviewed, any significant findings, actions taken or to be taken, and/or actions recommended to secure compliance. If the monitoring report documents any finding of unexpected toxicities or instances of noncompliance with GCP, IRB policies and procedures, or failure to follow the study protocol, a copy of the report should also be presented to the IRB for review.

C. Accrual Audits

Monitoring the scientific progress of clinical trials is another major function of the PRMS core of the UTMDACC CCSG. This is accomplished using the Protocol Data Management System (PDMS). All patients who sign a consent form to participate in a clinical trial must be registered to the protocol in the (PDMS). All eligibility questions must be answered and if the participant is not 100% eligible, the system will reject the registration and send the registrant to the Quality Assurance Office for assistance in getting IRB approval to over-ride the eligibility criteria or to use a single use (compassionate) treatment mechanism.

Prior to protocol activation, the target accrual number and the estimated accrual rate are also entered into the system. A program has been developed that compares the actual accrual with the estimated accrual on protocols that have been activated. This program also reports on protocols that have been IRB-approved but not yet activated in the system. Every six months, an accrual audit is done to review those protocols that have no accrual, slow accrual, and those that are IRB-approved but have not yet been activated. The PI of every protocol that is not accruing participants at the expected rate is queried as to whether or not the protocol is of sufficient priority to remain open.

While special exemptions are given to protocols involving rare diseases or pediatric patients, and those awaiting funding, the entire list of slow accruing protocols and the principal investigator's response to the QA inquiry is reviewed by the CRC or PBHSRC to determine whether they should remain open for another six months or be closed to new patient entry.

In addition to the accrual audits, patient evaluability is audited on a monthly basis as an indicator of the quality of the research being conducted. When a patient is taken off study, it is required that information as to whether the patient was inevaluable, evaluable for toxicity only, response only, or both, be entered.

D. When Something Goes Wrong...

When something goes wrong, and it is inevitable that it will, the first step is to review what happened and, if indicated, take immediate steps to ensure the safety of the trial participants. If an unexpected toxicity occurs or other event that is related to the experimental agent or therapy, then it may be necessary to hold study drug until further discussion with the sponsors, the IRB or the FDA occur.

If the event is not related to toxicity, but found to be an error related to the conduct of the trial, there are several avenues that must be investigated.

- Is there a problem with the institution's administrative processes and procedures that allowed the event to occur? If so, how can the system be strengthened to ensure the same type of event is prevented in the future?
- Was there a lack of communication between members of the research team or others involved in delivering the protocol treatment?
- Did the event result from a lack of understanding or knowledge of the protocol, institutional policies or federal regulations or did the researcher disregard the rules and regulations?

What happens next depends on the severity of the incident and the type of information collected during the review of the incident. Dealing with infrastructure problems are the easiest. As the cutting edge of research moves forward, new situations and therapies will put stresses on the infrastructure, as will increases in volumes when a research enterprise grows. At some point, the stress will cause a failure in the system. Monitoring metrics related to volumes on a regular basis is a convenient way to track areas that may need additional resources to keep up. However, a seasoned administrator knows that at some point, all systems will fail for one reason or another.

In the area of human subjects protection, the failure of infrastructure must be addressed expeditiously by the institution's leadership. Without action, not only patient welfare, but also the institution's privilege to perform clinical research are at risk.

Problems developing from lack of communications or miscommunications are more difficult to resolve due to the personalities that might be involved. However, issues can often be handled quite diplomatically at the department level after being reported to the IRB. Again, depending on the severity of the issue, the IRB may require an update or report on the process that brought the issue to resolution.

The most difficult problems to deal with are those that are investigator related. Due to the highly charged political nature of the academic environment, it is appropriate, indeed absolutely essential, to have written policies and procedures describing how to deal with issues of investigator noncompliance. These events generally stem from either a lack of education or a blatant disregard for the regulations. Educational issues can be resolved through the educational programs within the institution or at national seminars. Ignoring the regulations or repeated acts of serious noncompliance must be dealt with firmly since the entire research enterprise can be put at risk based on a single individual's carelessness.

After developing a plan to implement the necessary changes to ensure that the same event is not repeated, the severity of the incident, its effect on patient safety, and the degree to which it did not comply with the federal code must be estimated to determine if the event falls into the category that would require notifying OHRP or any other regulatory or funding agency. Each institution's Assurance Document discusses the need to notify federal agencies of certain events. Self-monitoring and self-reporting are the basis for OHRP's oversight process of institutions and their IRBs. It has been our experience that the process of acknowledging problems, implementing solutions, and notifying OHRP builds a trusting relationship between institutions and federal agencies. It also tends to minimize punitive actions by federal agencies.

V. INSTITUTIONAL CULTURE

The design of the research infrastructure and its associated policies and procedures are tangible components of the research enterprise that impact the extent and ease with which compliance is achieved in a research facility. However, there are also intangible factors that impact research compliance that are far more difficult to discern without extended interactions in the institution. These factors vary from facility to facility and must be clearly understood prior to developing and implementing systems and policies related to research compliance.

The most important of these intangible factors is the culture of the institution. All institutions, including public, private, and academic research facilities, have a culture. It cannot be seen, heard, or read about, but its impact can be felt by *all* employees. In today's research environment, it is a prerequisite that each research institution adopt a culture in which compliance with federal and institutional regulations is the expected standard. To do otherwise will jeopardize the future of the research enterprise.

A. The Role of Senior Management

Since the culture of an institution emanates from the very top of the organization, it is imperative that senior management set the tone and let others know the level of research compliance that is expected. This must be a continuous process and the most senior levels of the institution should demonstrate their support and backing for decisions made by the IRBs and the administrators overseeing the research compliance infrastructure.

This support must be broadcast to the institution in a clear and unwavering manner. There can be no exceptions to the rules. It is only through such participation of the senior management of an institution that any true impact on the culture can be attained.

B. The Role of Research Administration

It is the responsibility of research administration to:

- design and implement systems that enable clinical research to be conducted according to federal, state, and institutional guidelines;
- to make these systems as user friendly as possible;
- to provide education programs on federal regulations, the protection of human subjects and GCP for principal investigators, research nurses, and data managers;
- to convey to all researchers important information related to human subject research in a clear and transparent manner.

The process by which research policies and procedures are designed and implemented has a tremendous impact on their acceptance and their compliance rate. This is one area in which academia and industry differ more significantly than in other areas. In a traditional academic environment, the faculty expect to have far greater input into the design and implementation of the infrastructure and rules that govern them than researchers in pharmaceutical or biotechnology companies. In an industrial enterprise or other nonacademic setting, policies and procedures are far more likely to be made by individuals at the vice presidential level in conjunction with the legal department and forwarded by memo to the managerial staff for implementation. Input from the affected individuals is often far less than that expected by faculty in academia.

For acceptance in the academic environment to occur, plans must be vetted by several faculty governance and oversight committees. This can be time consuming and difficult as the committee members are often not experts in the federal regulations which serve as the foundation for the new policy or change. Furthermore, research compliance is often viewed by the faculty as a barrier to the progress of their research programs. Administrators must take care to educate and not alienate these groups because without their support, adherence to the new policy is unlikely. To make the collaboration between research administration and faculty successful, administrators must be understanding of the needs of the researchers and the researchers must understand and appreciate the need for change.

Here, we digress for a moment and revisit the culture of the institution and how it impacts the implementation of the research infrastructure. In an environment in which investigators are aware that they will be held accountable for research compliance, the process of designing and implementing new policies and procedures is less strenuous since the only issue that arises is "how" to implement since the "if we implement" has been taken out of the equation.

VI. EDUCATION PROGRAMS

A. Faculty

In addition to educating academic committee members, education of the researchers themselves is critical to a successful research program. Frequently, the first introduction an individual has to clinical research is during a fellowship program. Although medical schools and their associated training programs provide intensive education in disease processes and patient care, clinical research is not a topic covered with any regular frequency. This issue perpetuates the problems of clarifying the differences between patient care and research, especially in instances where part of the research includes standard care.

For these reasons, it is essential in today's environment that institutions provide a formal education program for all faculty members involved in research that covers the basic concepts of clinical research, and the Belmont Report and the Nurenberg Code on which these concepts are based. Since 2002, the National Institute of Health has also required that all essential personnel on research grants and contract provide evidence of training in the protection of human research subjects (5).

For clinicians, understanding the Belmont Report, Nurenberg Code, and the federal regulations is not sufficient. It is essential that they understand the concepts of GCP. Often the only difference between treating an individual with standard therapy or on a clinical trial, after obtaining informed consent, is the documentation required and the necessity of adhering to the IRB-approved protocol.

During investigations of noncompliance, research administrators often encounter the justification that the agents being used were commercially available. The federal regulations governing clinical research and GCP have one set of standards that apply to all clinical research, whether the test agent is commercially available or not. This again highlights the absolute necessity that physicians understand when they are conducting research and when they are treating a single patient.

For these reasons, the educational programs that should be developed for clinicians and their research teams should include detailed discussions of the correct way to document the research process including informed consent, patient eligibility, interim patient evaluation, tumor measurements, dose adjustments, adverse events, and drug accountability. The required documentation for two different individuals receiving the same treatment, with one person on study and one not on study can be completely different. And it is this reality that must be made clear. Furthermore, this documentation should be in the medical record as well as the case report form.

B. Research Nurses and Data Managers

Often, the research nurses and data managers are on the front lines of clinical research programs. They are frequently responsible for collecting information from the patient and the patient's local physicians, entering the study results in databases or case report forms, collecting and submitting adverse event to the sponsors and IRB, and documenting other aspects of the trial in the medical record reports and PI's clinical study files. It is therefore imperative that they also receive formal education so that they understand and appreciate the intricacies of clinical research and how it differs from standard medical care.

These members of the research team, like principal investigators, need to be well versed in the federal regulations and GCP, especially as it applies to the collection of data and the documentation of the conduct of the trial. In addition, it is essential that all aspects of adverse event collection, documentation and reporting be an integral part of the training for research nurses and data managers. They are frequently the interface between the research administration office and the patients.

As part of the education programs for all members of the research teams, separate instructions should be provided for any electronic information systems (IS) used for protocol authoring, monitoring, and reporting. These IS generally vary from institution to institution which requires that the training be ongoing throughout the year to train new staff members as they are hired.

VII. CONCLUSIONS

Performing human subject research is not a right, it is a privilege. As with all other privileges, certain requirements and standards must be met to retain the ability to continue to conduct human subject research. It is up to research institutions to set the standards and up to researchers to meet or exceed these standards. Since we believe that clinical research and standard care are not a continuum, but separate activities, those well versed in the latter, may not be well versed in the former. Creating an infrastructure that supports compliance, educates faculty and staff, and fosters a culture of quality will lead to better research, and ultimately, to effective and safe new treatments.

REFERENCES

1. The Belmont Report. Ethical Principles and Guidelines for Protection of Human Subject's Research. U.S. Government Printing Office, DHEW Publication (0S78–0012) reprinted in the Federal Register April 18, 1979; 44:23192.
2. Miller FG, Rosenstein DL. The therapeutic orientation to clinical trials. N Engl J Med 2003; 348:1383–1386.
3. Clinton WJ. Memorandum for the Vice President and the Heads of Executive Departments and Agencies February 17, 1994.
4. The Health Research Extension Act of 1985, Public Law 99–158, November 20, 1985.
5. The National Institutes of Health Revitalization Act of 1993, Public Law 103–43, June 10, 1993.

6. Federal Policy for the Protection of Human Subjects (Basic DHHS Policy for Protection of Human Research Subjects). 45 CFR 46 Subpart A, 1991.
7. Health Insurance Portability and Accountability Act. Standards for Privacy of Individually Indentifiable Health Information. 45 CFR Parts 160 and 164, August 14, 2002.
8. Guideline for the Monitoring of Clinical Investigations. U.S. Department of Health and Human Services, Food and Drug Administration. Docket number 82D-0322, 1998.
9. Required education in the protection human research participants. National Institute of Health. Notice OD-00–039, June 5, 2000.

10

Clinical Trials in Oncology: Study Design

LYLE D. BROEMELING
Department of Biostatistics, The University of Texas M.D. Anderson Cancer Center, Houston, Texas, U.S.A.

I. INTRODUCTION

A clinical trial is a medical experiment where patients are studied in order to improve medical interventions. Modern medicine and statistics meet in the design, implementation, and analysis of clinical trials, and patients involved in such trials have the opportunity to receive the latest and most promising care. Since 1950s, the properly designed clinical trial has resulted in the development of medical interventions that have had a dramatic and significant effect on the care of the cancer patient. Trials span treatment, prevention, screening, and quality of life studies, and involve all the various disease groups in cancer.

Briefly, there are four basic types of clinical trials, designated as Phase I, Phase II, Phase III, or Phase IV. Phase I trials test a new treatment (e.g., drug or surgical intervention) that has been explored earlier in animals. The Phase I trial usually studies a small number of patients and has the primary objective of testing a new treatment for safety. Often the main objective of Phase I trials is to determine a safe dose to administer the treatment. Phase II studies are of two varieties. A Phase IIa trial includes one group of patients and focuses on determining if the treatment has any benefit to the patient, while in Phase IIb trials, the intervention has shown some effect in earlier studies, and the goal is to determine the extent of that benefit. Phase IIb trials can be one-arm (single treatment group) or multiarm (two or more treatment groups), some may have a dose-finding component, and they may or may not be randomized. Randomization is the random assignment of study participants to different groups. Phase IIb trials are inherently comparative, either to an historical control or to a concurrent intervention.

Interventions that have shown promise in Phase I and II trials are subsequently studied in Phase III trials. These trials usually involve a large number of patients and compare the new treatment and a standard medical treatment. Patients are usually randomized between two or more treatment groups. Phase IV studies are also large trials that evaluate the long-term safety and effectiveness of a new treatment. Table 1 presents a summary of the basic characteristics of the various study designs.

Clinical trials in anesthesiology and critical care play an important role in support of the patient in a cancer center. For example, determining the optimal dose of an anesthetic in a Phase I trial is important in the surgical management of the patient. We will review such a trial involving the postoperative emergence of patients from anesthesia. In addition, we will describe examples of Phase II and Phase III study

Table 1 Summary of Basic Types of Clinical Trials

Phase	Primary objective	Typical number of patients
I	Safety Dose finding How treatment affects the human body	≤30
IIa	Efficacy	30–60
IIb	Extent of efficacy	30–60
III	Compare new treatment to standard treatment	100–1000's
IV	Long-term safety and effectiveness	100–1000's

designs in the approval of human activated protein C for care of patients with severe sepsis. For brevity, we will not discuss Phase IV trials further.

This chapter provides an overview of the different types of clinical trials and introduces the reader to various designs for implementing the trials. These include the $3+3$ and the continual reassessment methods (CRM) in Phase I studies; designs such as Simon's two-stage and Bayesian designs which allow for early stopping in Phase II studies; and finally designs for large Phase III studies that compare the efficacy of two interventions based on survival.

II. CLINICAL TRIAL DESIGN

The planning of clinical trials is critical to the ultimate ability of the trial to provide information that can be of use in medical treatment. The study protocol carefully describes the details of how a clinical trial is to be implemented. Almost all parts of the protocol are relevant to the statistical design of the trial, and clinicians and statisticians work together to ensure that studies are designed in a proper scientific manner utilizing the latest in statistical methodology. See Ref. 1 for a discussion of statistical contributions to clinical trials.

The protocol should include the following components: (1) an explanation of the scientific basis for the study; (2) a summary of the results of all previous trials and experiments of the study intervention; (3) the patient eligibility and ineligibility criteria; (4) a list of the major and minor endpoints, including their definitions and how and when they will be measured; (5) the definitions of evaluable and intent-to-treat populations; (6) the estimated patient accrual rates by site; (7) a statistical section that outlines a detailed power analysis, a description of early stopping rules, methods for randomizing patients, and proposed statistical analysis; and (8) nonstatistical stopping rules for safety considerations.

Described below are how one might design Phase I, Phase II, and Phase III trials for studies in anesthesiology and in critical care.

A. Phase I Designs

Phase I trials evaluate how a treatment is to be administered and how that treatment affects the human body. First, consider a Phase I study which evaluates safety among a set of doses of a new treatment. The study will be designed to determine the maximum tolerable dose (MTD), which is the dose, whereby at higher doses the safety of the patient would be compromised. We are assuming in this example that as the dose level increases, the probability of toxicity increases and the probability of efficacy also increases. The main endpoint in a Phase I study is some measure of toxicity experienced by the patient as a result of the treatment, while the secondary endpoint is some measure of efficacy. To define the toxicity endpoint, the investigator characterizes the dose-limiting toxicity (DLT), which is a set of toxicities that are severe enough to prevent giving more of the treatment at higher doses. The investigator bases the DLT on knowledge of the disease, treatment, and the patients who are eligible for the trial. Investigators are guided by the NCI list of common toxicities or in some other manner that is appropriate for the particular study. Phase I trial objectives may include the study of the pharmacokinetics and pharmacodynamics of the drug; however, we will not emphasize this here. Primarily, the goal of Phase I studies is to profile the toxicity of the drug or intervention using a set of doses and a well-defined DLT.

Prior to implementing a Phase I trial, the investigator must have decided upon the treatment route of administration and schedule. Also required for estimating the MTD are the patient population defined via the eligibility and ineligibility criteria, a starting dose and a set of dose levels to test, the DLT, and the dose escalation. The dose escalation includes decisions on how to select the MTD among a set of doses. The chosen starting dose is based on other similar Phase I studies and/or information from animal experiments. Once the investigator has chosen the dose levels to be tested, the dose escalation can be described. Dose spacing can be based on the idea of a Fibonacci sequence, a modified Fibonacci sequence, or and adaptive or fixed increment approach (2).

There are many dose escalations, including the commonly used $3+3$ design and the CRM. Since the early days of the NCI, investigators have used traditional

Table 2 Example of a 3 + 3 Dose Escalation Scheme

Patients with DLT at a given dose level	Escalation decision rules		
0 out of 3	Enter 3 patients at next higher dose If dose is highest to be tested, then MTD is undeclared		
1 out of 3	Enter 3 more patients at same dose	If 0 of 3 experience DLT, then enter 3 patients at the next highest dose	If only 3 patients have been treated at next lower dose, enter 3 additional patients at the next lower dose
		If ≥1 of 3 experience DLT, then dose exceeds MTD and is declared the maximally administered dose	If next lower dose is lowest dose to be tested, then MTD is undeclared
≥2 of 3	Dose exceeds MTD and is declared the maximally administered dose	If only 3 patients have been treated at next lower dose, enter 3 additional patients at the next lower dose. If next lower dose is lowest dose to be tested, then MTD is undeclared	
≤1 out of 6 at highest dose level below the maximally administered dose	Dose is the MTD		
≥2 out of 6	Dose exceeds MTD and is declared the maximally administered dose	If only 3 patients have been treated at next lower dose, enter 3 additional patients at the next lower dose. If next lower dose is lowest dose to be tested, then MTD is undeclared	

escalating rules such as the 3 + 3 design for determining the MTD in oncology trials, while the CRM is a newer development (2) that is becoming more popular. The 3 + 3 design is based on cohorts of size 3 or 6, and there are several versions; however, all are based on a plan similar to that given below.

Table 3 illustrates the dose escalation of a 3 + 3 design (3). The first cohort of three patients are administered the starting dose. None of the patients experienced a DLT; therefore, the second cohort of three patients are administered the treatment at dose level 2. Once again, none of the patients experienced a DLT; therefore, a third cohort of patients is administered the treatment at dose level 3. At this dose, one of the patients had a DLT, so the dose is not escalated to dose level 4. Instead, the next cohort of three patients is administered the treatment at dose level 3. This means that six patients were observed at the third dose level. Because no new DLTs were observed, three patients were entered at dose level 4. Two of the three patients had a DLT; thus, investigators declare the previous dose (level 3) as the MTD.

Note that the 3 + 3 design does not depend on statistical considerations for escalating the dose. For example, the probability of a DLT is not considered and neither is the idea of the target toxicity level (TTL), the probability of a DLT that one is willing to accept. For example, in the graph below of the dose–toxicity profile with six dose levels, the TTL is 0.33. This means that we would only want to accept a dose level where the maximum chance of a DLT is 33%. The dose nearest to the TTL of 0.33 is dose level 4, which is the MTD. Any dose level above four would produce a probability of DLT in excess of 0.33.

Because the 3 + 3 design does not incorporate the TTL, statisticians have proposed other dose escalations, and among these, the CRM is becoming the most widely used. O'Quigley (4) developed the CRM, which employs a dose–toxicity model and Bayesian estimation for choosing the MTD. This design estimates the dose–toxicity profile of the treatment, and thus the MTD corresponding to a prespecified TTL among a set of doses. Note the 'true' dose–toxicity profile is unknown, and the investigator's goal is to estimate it. The CRM allows the investigator to compute the probability of a DLT at any of the dose levels as expressed by a logistic regression model:

$$\begin{aligned}&\Pr[\mathrm{DLT}|\mathrm{dose}\ d, \theta]\\&\quad = \exp(3 + \theta d)/[1 + \exp(3 + \theta d)]\end{aligned} \tag{1}$$

where d is the dose level and θ an unknown parameter that measures the effect of the dose on the probability of a DLT. In this model, the dependent variable is binary and is zero if patient does not have a DLT; otherwise, it equals to one. The independent variable is the dose level, and in this example (Fig. 1), as the dose level increases the probability (the proportion of patients with a DLT) also increases.

The dotted horizontal line corresponds to the known TTL; thus, if we knew the true dose–toxicity profile, we would know the MTD. Of course, the MTD will never be known with certainty because of the limitations of information obtained from a small number of patients.

Dose escalation with the CRM is as follows:

1. Specify prior information for the parameter of the model. That is, using the information from the investigator, propose an initial dose–toxicity profile. This will, in turn, induce a prior distribution for the parameter of the model.
2. Given the current information about the parameter, treat one patient at the dose level closest to the current estimate of the TTL.
3. Observe the toxicity outcome of patient.
4. Update the dose–toxicity profile.
5. Repeat the steps above until the maximum number of patients is reached.

Notice that once the toxicity of a patient is observed, the dose–toxicity model above (1) is updated and hence the estimate of the MTD is updated. In this dose escalation plan, information from all the patients is used and the trial is not stopped early. There are some variations to this design (2). For example, the trial must begin with the first dose level and the trial can be stopped early at dose d when the probability of a DLT at dose d is sufficiently close to the TTL.

Table 3 Example of 3 + 3 for Determining the Maximum Tolerated Dose (MTD)

Cohort of 3 patients	Dose level				
	1	2	3	4	5
1	0/3				
2		0/3			
3			1/3		
4			0/3		
5				2/3	
			MTD		

B. Phase II Designs

Once a particular treatment or intervention has been studied with a Phase I trial and the MTD has been

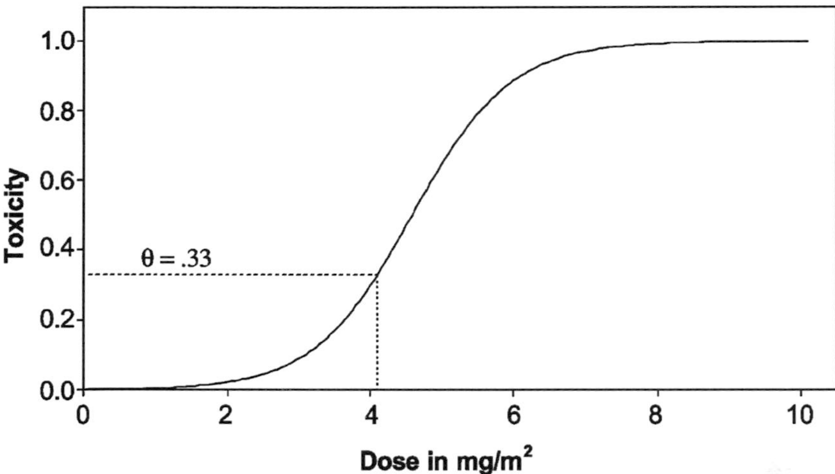

Figure 1 Dose–toxicity relationship.

selected and we are quite satisfied that the treatment will be safe, studies of the treatment may progress to Phase II trials to determine if the treatment holds sufficient promise. Typically, the target population is patients with a specific disease, disease site, histology, or stage, or patients undergoing some surgical or anesthetic procedure. Often the treatment dose is the MTD determined from previous Phase I trials. Although limited dose finding is sometimes allowed to accommodate different patient populations, the primary endpoints are measures of efficacy, while safety would be a secondary endpoint.

The efficacy information from a Phase I trial is also quite important and largely determines the type of Phase II trial to be designed. If little is known about the efficacy, a Phase IIa trial can be performed with the goal of determining a certain minimum efficacy. On the other hand, if the efficacy information from Phase I trials indicates that the intervention does indeed have some treatment benefit, a Phase IIb trial may be implemented to determine if the treatment has sufficient benefit compared to some standard treatment, either historical (from past patient data) or from ongoing therapy.

Designs for Phase IIa trials include the Gehan's two-stage (2), Simon's two-stage (2), some Bayesian alternatives (5), and various multistage designs such as the Ensign and Chen designs. See Ref. 2. Simon's two-stage and some Bayesian alternatives will be discussed here, because by far, the Simon's two-stage design is the most popular for a Phase IIa, but Bayesian alternatives are becoming more widely used because they are more flexible and can easily incorporate information from prior related trials.

Phase II designs are based on statistical testing principals. Suppose p is the probability of a treatment response (measured relative to baseline at some time point t during the treatment of the patient), then one tests the null hypothesis vs. the alternative hypothesis:

$$H : p < p \text{ (e.g., } = 0.05) \text{ vs. the alternative}$$

$$A : p \geq p_1 \text{ (e.g., } = 0.25)$$

The null hypothesis states that the proportion of responses is less than or equal to some specified proportion p_0 that would not exhibit sufficient interest for further development. The alternative hypothesis states that the proportion of responses is greater than or equal to a proportion p_1 that the investigator considers clinically meaningful. If the alternative hypothesis is true, then further testing could be deemed reasonable. Of course, this decision is based on other considerations as well, such as any new information on safety. The values for p_0 and p_1 are specified in advance and depend on the results of previous trials. Typical values of p_0 are from 0.1 to 0.4, and typical values for p_1 are from $p_0 + 0.15$ to $p_0 + 0.2$, i.e., 15–20% higher than p_0. To use a Simon's two-stage design, investigators must also specify the probability of a Type I error α, the probability of rejecting the null hypothesis when it is true (declaring that the new treatment has an effect above p_0 when it actually does not), and β, the probability of accepting the null hypothesis when it is false (declaring that the new treatment has no effect above p_0 when it actually does). Note that $(1 - \beta)$ is the power of the test.

Given these values, the Simon's method will give the maximum sample size n, the stage 1 sample size

n_1, and the rejection rule at each stage. De Vita et al. (6) provides tables for Simon's two-stage design, and for example, when $\alpha = 0.05$, $\beta = 0.20$, $p_0 = 0.05$, and $p_1 = 0.25$, then $n_1 = 9$, $n = 17$, and the trial would be stopped early if there were 0 out of 9 responses. If there were 1 or more responses with 9 patients, the trial is continued, and if there are 2 or less responses among 17 patients, the null hypothesis is accepted, that is the intervention or treatment would not be of sufficient interest for further testing. Note with this design, the trial is stopped early for lack of efficacy. The Simon's design can be used to justify the sample size and for stopping early. Stopping early protects future patients from receiving inefficacious treatments.

There are some Bayesian designs that allow more flexibility. For example, suppose the maximum sample size of n patients are accrued in k cohorts of size n and that after observing the response of patients at the end of each cohort, the investigator computes the probability that the observed proportion of responses p is greater than p_1, given the responses of the observed patients as

$$\Pr[p > p_1 \mid \text{responses of patients}].$$

If this probability is small, say 0.10 or 0.20, the trial is stopped for lack of efficacy. This is very much like the Simon's design; however, a decision on lack of efficacy can be made after each cohort of patients. See Ref. 7 for additional information on Phase II trials that use Bayesian stopping rules.

If the intervention under investigation has shown some activity, a Phase IIb trial can be used to determine the extent of efficacy. This type of trial is usually comparative, since it has demonstrated prior efficacy, the study intervention will be compared to some historical control, or to some standard current treatment via a randomized design. The advantage of using historical controls over concurrent controls is the smaller number of patients required, but the disadvantages of historical controls are that the patient populations may not be comparable to those used in the current clinical trial.

Dose escalation for efficacy is often done in a Phase II, if the planned dose levels have been shown to be safe in Phase I trials. Often dose finding for efficacy and comparison of the study intervention with a standard (including placebo) for efficacy is often done in the same trial. There are many Phase IIb designs, including some Bayesian alternatives (8) and designs that use multiple outcomes (9). For example, Bryant and Day employ two responses—one for safety and one for efficacy in comparing a standard with an experimental therapy or procedure.

C. Phase III Trials

We are now at the point where we have an intervention (drug or procedure) that has been studied in a series of Phase I and Phase II trials and has demonstrated sufficient promise to be compared to the standard clinical treatment in a large randomized study. For example, Drotrecogin was investigated for safety and efficacy in several Phase I and II trials in the treatment of sepsis (10) and was further investigated in a large Phase III study, which will be described below.

Phase III trials are confirmatory where the study procedure is to be compared to the standard therapy with the goal of providing evidence that the study drug will provide substantial improvement in survival time, or in disease-free survival, or some other time-to-event endpoint such as time to response or time to hospitalization, etc. They should be designed to have a sufficient sample size to detect clinically relevant differences and are usually done in a multicenter setting. Provisions are made for interim looks by an independent Data Safety Monitoring Board (DSMB), where the trial may be stopped early for reasons of safety and/or efficacy.

An important contribution of the statistician is to provide a power analysis for the principal investigator or sponsor, whereby typically in a two-arm study, the patients are assigned at random to the group in equal numbers. A power analysis estimates the number of patients to be used in each arm of the study. The main endpoint must be chosen with care because it will be used for the sample size calculations and for the analysis of the data at the end of the trial. Drop out rates in both arms of the study should be taken into account in the sample size calculations as well as what statistical test (e.g., the log-rank) will be employed to test for differences in the major endpoint. The design might include a group sequential monitoring procedure (11,12) for early stopping.

III. CLINICAL TRIALS IN ANESTHESIOLOGY AND CRITICAL CARE

Three trials have been chosen to illustrate the ideas in designing a clinical study. The first is a Phase I study (13) of a compound, which does not reverse analgesia in the postoperative recovery room, while the second is a Phase IIb investigation (10) of the effect of Drotrecogin on coagulapathy in patients with sepsis. The Phase III trial is a continuation of the efficacy of Drotrecogin in a large randomized study, where it is compared to placebo using 28-day mortality as the major endpoint. The design elements described above will be illustrated with the three studies.

A. Phase I Trial: Optimal Dose of Nalmefene for Postoperative Analgesia

Our example for a Phase I is one of the first cases where the CRM was used in an anesthesiology study. The study's primary objective was to find the MTD of Nalmefene, an opioid antagonist. The optimal dose was the highest level of Nalmefene that did not reverse the analgesic effect in postoperative patients receiving epidural fentanyl in 0.072% bupivacaine.

Patients received a single intravenous dose of 0.25, 0.50, 0.75, or 1.0 μg/kg Nalmefene, and the major endpoint was the patient-reported pain score as measured by a visual analog pain scale which ranged from 0 (no pain) to 10 (severe pain). A score of two or more integers above baseline pain scores after administration of the study agent was considered a reversal of analgesia (ROA). Patients were treated in cohorts of size 1 starting from the lowest dose, and the MTD was defined as that dose among the four where the final probability of ROA is closest to 0.20 (i.e., there is no more than a 20% chance of ROA). A dose level that had more than a 20% chance of reversal is not acceptable, and we would want to avoid higher doses. The CRM is an iterative Bayesian procedure that was described above and uses formula (1) for the logistic regression model. After each patient's baseline pain score is known, a dose is selected that is closest to the TTL = 0.20. This is done for each of the 25 patients; thus, the MTD is the dose closest to the TTL = 0.20 after the 25th patient. The results are outlined in Table 4. The MTD chosen by the CRM was 0.50 μg/kg, and the CRM repeatedly updated the probability of the ROA via the model:

$$\Pr[\text{ROA} \mid \text{dose } d, \theta] = \exp(3+\theta d)/[1+\exp(3+\theta d)]. \quad (2)$$

The parameter θ is unknown but estimated after the results of each patient becomes known, and once the parameter is estimated, the probability of a ROA is computed with formula (2) at each dose d, where $d = 0.25$, 0.50, 0.75, and 1.00. Once these four probabilities are known that dose with a corresponding probability that is nearest to 0.20 is the dose chosen for the next cohort.

Figure 2 summarizes the statistical information based on the results of all 25 patients, where at each dose a 95% credible interval is given for the probability of a DLT or ROA. There is still some uncertainty present in outcome as illustrated with overlap of the four intervals. Thus, at the chosen dose of 0.50 μg/kg, the estimated probability of an ROA ranges from 0.08 to 0.40. We see from Table 4 that the dose = 1.0 μg/kg was never selected, however the model estimates a DLT at that dose. This study illustrates a successful application of the CRM for dose finding that accurately employs the components of such a design. For example, the dose levels and the TTL were prechosen, and the dose escalation scheme, via the CRM, was all described, and defined.

Table 4 Selection of MTD

Patient	Dose	DLT (ROA)
1	0.25	No
2	0.50	No
3	0.75	Yes
4	0.25	No
5	0.50	No
6	0.50	Yes
7	0.25	No
8	0.25	No
9	0.50	No
10	0.50	No
11	0.50	No
12	0.50	No
13	0.50	No
14	0.50	No
15	0.50	No
16	0.50	No
17	0.75	No
18	0.75	Yes
19	0.50	No
20	0.50	Yes
21	0.50	No
22	0.50	No
23	0.50	Yes
24	0.50	No
25	0.50	No

Source: Ref. 13.

B. Phase II Trial: Drotrecogin in Patients with Sepsis

The main objective of this Phase IIb trial was to assess the efficacy of human activated protein C on coagulopathy in patients with severe sepsis. Major efficacy endpoints were d-Dimer, fibrinogen and platelet levels relative to baseline, while 28-day mortality was a secondary endpoint. The study also aimed to assess the safety of human activated protein C, and the major safety endpoints were incidence of serious bleeding and incidence of serious adverse events. The trial was designed as a randomized, placebo-controlled, multicenter study. Results from four previous Phase I trials showed that it was safe to administer the agent at doses up to 30 μg/kg/hr in 48 and 96-hr infusions. This was

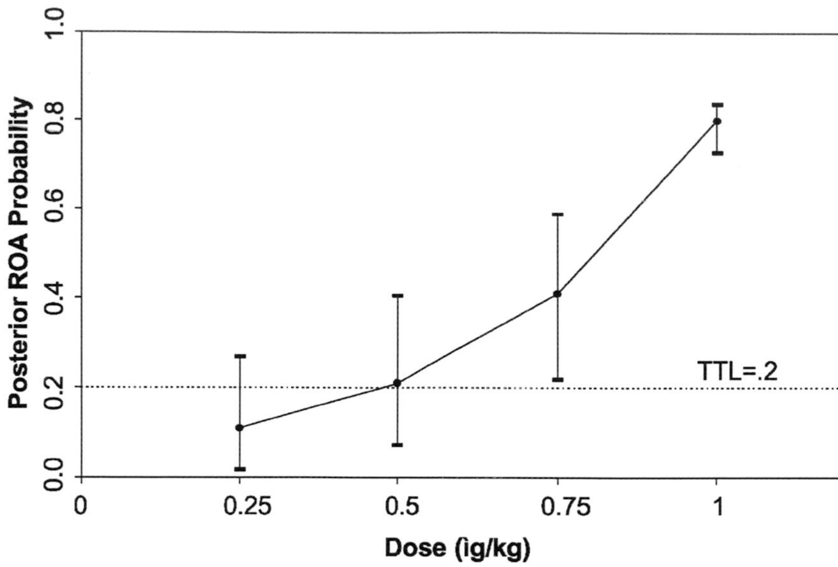

Figure 2 Phase I Results for Malmefene. *Source*: From Ref. 13.

a comparative trial, where Drotrecogin was compared to placebo at each of the dose levels in two-stages. In the first stage, there were four dose levels with 48-hr infusions, and the patients were assigned at random to either Drotrecogin or placebo in the proportion 2:1. At each dose level, 12 patients received Drotrecogin and six patients received the placebo. Because patients treated in the first stage experienced bleeding at the highest dose level, investigators omitted the highest dose level from the second stage (96-hr infusions). For each dose level in the second stage, 20 patients were randomized in a 3:1 ratio with 15 to the Drotrecogin group and five to the placebo group.

Results from this study indicated significant dose-dependent decreases in d-Dimer and IL-6 relative to baseline, but differences between fibrinogen and platelet count of the two groups were not significant. In addition, investigators found no significant differences in incidence of serious bleeding between the agent and placebo. The 28-day mortality of the study group was less (but not significantly) than that for placebo.

The use of the results from the first stage to design the second illustrates an adaptive element of this design. In addition to the adaptive element, this study design illustrates a clear randomization plan, dose finding for efficacy, and the use of multiple endpoints for safety and efficacy. Results from this clinical trial, along with the results from other Phase I and Phase II trials, generated sufficient interest to prompt a larger randomized Phase III trial.

C. Phase III Trial: Drotrecogin

As we see from the Phase IIb trial described above, Drotrecogin exhibited anti thrombotic, anti inflammatory, and profibrinolytic properties and dose-dependent reduction in the levels of markers for coagulation and inflammation for patients with severe sepsis. Based on the results of the Phase II trial described above (10), a randomized, placebo-controlled, multicenter trial for patients with severe sepsis was planned. The trial utilized 164 centers in 11 countries.

Planning for the Phase III trial included many elements from the previous Phase I and Phase II trials of Drotrecogin. The trial was designed with equal number of patients randomized to the drug study group as to the placebo control group. The study drug was administered in a 96 hr infusion at a rate of 24 μg/kg/hr. There was one major endpoint, the 28-day all cause mortality measured from the start of infusion. The trial was designed to enroll 2280 patients with two planned interim analyses by an independent monitoring board after 760 patients were enrolled in the study and again after 1520 patients were enrolled. Patients were to be followed for 28 days after the start of the infusion or until death. Baseline characteristics, including demographic information on pre-existing conditions, organ function, and markers of disease severity, infection, and hematologic and other laboratory tests were to be measured within 24 hr before the infusion began. Blood samples obtained at baseline, on days 1–7, and on days 14 and 28 were assayed for d-Dimer levels. Statistical guidelines based on and the O'Brien–Fleming spending function (11) included a suspension of enrollment if the study agent was found to be significantly more efficacious vs. placebo. The statistical section reports a plan to analyze the data with a Cochran–Mantel–Haenszel test in which groups are to be stratified on the basis of severity of disease, baseline levels of plasma protein, and 28-day mortality was to be compared between the two groups with stratified log-rank tests.

Good study design properties were followed for planning this trial, including a careful description of how to implement the randomization and how the coordinating center would interact with the various study centers. The statistical description also explained data analysis procedures and how the trial would be stopped for efficacy and lack of efficacy. Results from the study complemented those from earlier Phase I and II trials. The trial was indeed stopped at the time of the second interim analysis with data from 1520 patients according to the statistical guidelines in the protocol. Recruitment of patients was suspended because the differences in mortality rates exceeded the guidelines set for stopping the trial. For the major endpoint of 28-day survival, 259 of 840 patients (30.8%) in the placebo group had died, while 210 of 850 patients (24.7%) in the Drotrecogin group had died. This 6% increase in 28-day survival was more than would be expected by chance alone ($p = 0.005$ via log-rank test in the stratified analysis.); therefore, the trial was stopped early. Levels of d-Dimer and Il-6 were significantly lower in Drotrecogin patients vs. placebo patients on days 1 and 7 after start of infusion. The incidence of serious bleeding events was higher ($p = 0.06$) in the study group at 3.5% vs. 2% for placebo; however the incidence of thrombotic events had similar rates in the two groups. The randomization produced similar baseline characteristics for demographic and laboratory responses. Overall, the conclusion from the study was that treatment with Drotrecogin significantly reduces mortality in patients with severe sepsis but may also be associated with increased bleeding risk. Treatment with human activated protein C is now standard for patients with sepsis.

IV. CONCLUSIONS

This chapter has introduced important statistical ideas for the design of Phase I, II, and III trials in anesthesiology and critical care. The 3 + 3 and Bayesian CRM designs were introduced and the estimation of the MTD was explained. Such designs are primarily concerned with safety, but early evidence of efficacy is important to assess. The key ideas of MTD, DLT, and TTL were defined and their use in dose escalation was explained. The CRM design was illustrated with an example in anesthesiology, where the MTD of Nalmefene was selected.

Two types of Phase II trials were introduced, including Phase IIa trials, which are appropriate when previous Phase I trials reveal little information on efficacy, and Phase IIb trials, which are appropriate for estimating the extent of efficacy when some evidence of efficacy has been demonstrated in earlier trials. The relevance of the Phase IIb design was shown in the development of Drotrecogin, where in previous Phase I and II trials, the agent was shown to be safe and showed signs of efficacy. A randomized trial was planned in two-stages, where at the first stage the infusion time was 48 hr, and in the second it was 96 hr. Trial results showed that Drotrecogin could ameliorate coagulopathy and could lower 28-day mortality and that the 24 μg/kg/hr for 96 hr was the optimal infusion level for efficacy. Investigators incorporated these settings into the Phase III trial, which determined that the study agent was safe and efficacious for treating patients with severe sepsis (14).

Statistical ideas are essential in the design, implementation, and analysis of clinical trials, and their importance has been stressed in this article. The Biostatistics Department of MD Anderson has developed and is developing innovative ways to plan for Phase I and Phase II studies. Much of this development has been Bayesian. For example, the Bayesian approach has been used for the design of Phase I trials by Thall (5) using the so-called modified CRM and for stopping early (7) using multiple endpoints for safety and efficacy. In addition, Berry (15) has employed the Bayesian approach for using adaptive randomization methods to allocate two interventions to patients in Phase IIb and Phase III trials.

The interaction between clinicians and statisticians has been beneficial to both parties.

ACKNOWLEDGMENT

My sincerest appreciation is extended to Ms. Carla Warneke for assisting me with all phases in the preparation of this chapter.

REFERENCES

1. Chow S, Liu J. Design and Analysis of Clinical Trials, Concepts and Methodologies. New York: John Wiley & Sons, 1998.

2. Crowley J. Handook of Statistics in Oncology. New York: Marcel-Dekker, 2001.
3. Lee J. Design and Statistical Considerations for Phase I Cancer Clinical Trials. Unpublished Manuscript, Department of Biostatistics, University of Texas MD Anderson Cancer Center, Houston, TX, 2003.
4. O'Quigley J, Pepe M, Fisher I. Continual reassessment method: a pratical design for Phase I clinical trials in cancer. Biometrics 1990; 46:33–48.
5. Thall PF, Simon R, Estey I. New statistical strategies for monitoring safety and efficacy in single-arm clinical trials. J. Clin Oncol 1996; 14:296–303.
6. DeVita V, Hellman S, Rosenberg S. Cancer, Principals & Pactice of Oncology. 5th ed. New York: Lippincott, Williams, and Wilkins, 1997.
7. Thall PF, Simon R. Recent developments in the design of Phase II clinical trials. In: Thall P, ed. Advances in the Design and Analysis of Clinical Trials. Norwell, Mass, Kluwer, 1995:49–61.
8. Thall P, Simon R. Practical Bayesian guidelines for Phase IIb clinical trials. Biometrics 50:337–349.
9. Bryant J, Day R. Incorporating toxicity considerations into the design of two Phase II clinical trials. Biometrics 1995; 51:1372–1383.
10. Bernard GR, Wesley E, Wright TJ, Fraiz J, Stasek JE, Russell JA, Mayers I, Rosenfield BA, Morris PE, Yan SB, Helterbrand JD. Safety and dose relationship of recombinant human activated protein C for coagulopathy in severe sepsis. Crit Med 2001; 29:2051–2059.
11. O'Brien PC, Fleming TR. A multiple testing procedure for clinical trials. Biometrics 1979; 35:549–556.
12. Lan KKG, DeMets DL. Discrete sequential boundries for clinical trials. Biometrics 1983; 70:659–663.
13. Dougherty TB, Porche VH, Thall PF. Maximum tolerated dose of Nalmefene in patients receiving epidural fentanyl and dilute bupivacaine for postoperative analgesia. Anesthesiology 2000; 92:1010–1016.
14. Bernard GR et al. Efficacy and safety of recombinant human activated protein C for severe sepsis. N E J Med 2001; 344:699–709.
15. Berry D. Adaptive assignment versus balanced randomization in clinical trials: a decision analysis. Statist Med 1995; 14:231–246.

11

Clinical Trials in Oncology: Ethical Issues

MARTIN L. SMITH

Department of Critical Care, The University of Texas M.D. Anderson Cancer Center, Houston, Texas, U.S.A.

ANNE L. FLAMM

The Clinical Ethics Service, The University of Texas M.D. Anderson Cancer Center, Houston, Texas, U.S.A.

TIMOTHY M. PAWLIK

Department of Surgical Oncology, The University of Texas M.D. Anderson Cancer Center, Houston, Texas, U.S.A.

I. INTRODUCTION

Clinical research in perioperative cancer medicine can have unique challenges, primarily related to the compromised nature of the research participants. In presurgical settings where patients are more likely to be awake and alert, they are often weak, dependent, distressed, and afraid. These circumstances may make prospective research subjects increasingly suggestible and dependent upon medical advice and influence. The same can be said about many cancer patients who seek pain control—they are vulnerable and their abilities to make decisions may be compromised by significant adjustment disorders, clinical depression, delirium, or desperation for pain relief. Finally, most patients under the care of critical care physicians are in an intensive care unit (ICU), have suffered sudden catastrophic illness or injury, or have acute medical needs postoperatively and are physiologically compromised with at least single organ failure. Whether their critical care needs result from a severe or terminal illness, these patients usually have diminished or absent decisional capacity for providing informed consent. With these kinds of clinical circumstances in mind, perioperative cancer researchers must design and carry out studies that conform to standard ethical principles and guidelines for research. Because much of this research will take place in hospitals, the research will likely undergo ethical review by an independent institutional review board (IRB). To prevent abuse of human subjects, federal regulations mandate IRB review of all research conducted at institutions receiving federal funds. However, investigators' knowledge about ethical issues and principles in research constitutes an important additional mechanism and safeguard for protecting the welfare of research subjects.

This chapter highlights ethical issues encountered by cancer medicine researchers (i.e., study design, research using terminally ill patients, use of placebos, conflicts of interest). The chapter also summarizes significant historical events, research abuses, and regulations as a context for identifying ethical principles and frameworks for handling the issues to be discussed.

II. HISTORICAL BACKGROUND

Moral and medical controversies over the use of human subjects in clinical research is a relatively new phenomenon in the history of medicine. Prior to World War II, medical research tended to be small scale and driven primarily by specific therapeutic motives. During this period, little attention was given either to research itself or to the accompanying ethical issues. A number of dramatic changes occurred around the time of World War II, which, to a large degree, initiated the modern debate about research in general and the use of human subjects in clinical research in particular. During and immediately after the war, clinical research became a large-scale, highly organized, and well-funded effort harnessed to military objectives and national interests. The problems with using human subjects in clinical research were spectacularly displayed in the gruesome atrocities perpetrated by Nazi physicians and scientists and, to a lesser degree, by some research endeavors carried out in the U.S.A. (1,2). Since that time, local and national regulations have been promulgated and IRBs routinely scrutinize research protocols in most hospitals and research centers. Nevertheless, many ethical issues and controversies surrounding clinical trials remain. Despite universal disapproval of Nazi-style experimentation, a lack of consensus still exists about many aspects of using human subjects in clinical trials. To begin to address the complexity surrounding clinical research ethics, the historical context that shapes current debates must be reviewed.

Human experimentation has always been a part of medicine. The practice of medicine, especially before the 20th century, was unpredictable and unreliable. When faced with an ailing patient, physicians chose from among various treatment options, many of which had not been validated or tested by the "scientific method." Treatment represented a good-will attempt to aid the patient despite uncertainty.

Notwithstanding immense technological advances, inherent ambiguity in therapeutic and research medicine persists. Faced with unavoidable uncertainty not only in clinical trials, but also in clinical practice, two aspects of the patient–physician relationship make it morally acceptable to proceed: (i) the patient has given consent and (ii) the "therapeutic experiment" is administered with the intent of benefit (e.g., relief of suffering, potential cure, extension of life) for research participants or future patients. The basis for this therapeutic relationship springs from antiquity and is articulated in the Hippocratic Oath. The Oath, in addition to binding physicians to "do no harm," has also been argued to prohibit experiments, if reasonable probability exists that death or disabling injury of research subjects will occur. Interpreted in this way, the Hippocratic Oath outlines not only the therapeutic relationship, but also the terms and bounds of good research practices. The Oath acknowledges the uncertainty intrinsic to medicine, but in instructing the physician to "do no harm" and to focus unswervingly on the patient, it also provides a moral grounding to guide clinical research.

An important contemporary document that has shaped the way clinical research is carried out is the Nuremberg Code (3). The Code was formulated in 1947 by American judges sitting in judgment of Nazi physicians accused of conducting murderous and torturous human experiments in German concentration camps. At the Nuremberg trial, the physicians were accused of using the most vulnerable populations—institutionalized children, the mentally retarded, and prisoners—in human experimentation without their consent. Today, the Nuremberg Code stands as a fundamental document for the ethical use of human subjects in clinical research.

The Nuremberg Code outlines research principles deemed necessary for the moral and humane use of human beings in experimental research, particularly the procurement of voluntary informed consent as an "absolutely essential" condition. According to the Code, a physician should never do anything to a patient or subject that is inherently coercive, and no procedure may be performed without obtaining the patient's full consent. The Code also defines specific criteria by which the content of the experiment can be judged to be morally justifiable. These criteria include that the experiment yields fruitful results, not be random in nature, but be based on animal studies and avoid all unnecessary suffering and injury.

Following Nuremberg, additional attempts were made to codify ethical and moral criteria of human experimentation. The most prominent was the World Medical Association's 1964 Declaration of Helsinki (most recently revised in 2002) (4). Although the Declaration clearly acknowledges and is grounded on the Nuremberg Code, the Helsinki Declaration attempts to have peer review supplement, and even supplant, informed consent as a central principle. Although the Nuremberg Code focused more on the human rights of research subjects, the Declaration of

Helsinki centers more on the importance of the ethical design and content of the clinical research. Despite these differences, the major philosophical principles and norms grounding the declarations are the same. As noted in the last sentence of the Helsinki Declaration, "in research . . . the interests of science and society should never take precedence over considerations related to the well being of the subject" (4).

The history of human experimentation in the United States has also had a number of dramatic defining moments (5,6) that have shaped the ethical debate, as well as policy regulating human experimentation and clinical research. Perhaps, the most controversial study to impact the ethical landscape was the Tuskegee syphilis experiment (7).

In 1932, the U.S. Public Health Service initiated an experiment in Macon County, Alabama, to determine the natural course of untreated, latent syphilis in black males. The researchers recruited syphilitic men by telling the subjects that they would be treated for "bad blood." When penicillin became widely available in the early 1950s as the preferred treatment for syphilis, the men did not receive treatment. Moreover, a federal oversight committee repeatedly decided to continue the study and even on occasion sought to prevent treatment. Not until 1972 was the experiment brought to a halt, and in August of that year the committee issued a "Final Report" concluding that the study was "ethically unjustified" (8). In criticizing the Tuskegee study, the Final Report made the distinction between "submitting voluntarily" and "informed consent." The Report emphasized that although the participants may have been "voluntarily" participating with researchers, this did not signify that they provided informed consent. The investigatory panel held that the criterion of informed consent had not been upheld, and that the experiment was both ethically impermissible and against the spirit of the Nuremberg Code and the Helsinki Declaration (9). By focusing on informed consent, the Final Report made clear that personal autonomy over the important decisions in one's life and the right to attempt to realize one's own value-ordering take precedence over the demands of scientific advancement.

In response to Tuskegee and other ethical lapses in American scientific research, the National Commission for the Protection of Human Subjects of Biomedical and Behavioral Research issued the Belmont Report in April of 1979 (10). The Belmont Report provides "an analytical framework that will guide the resolution of ethical problems arising from research involving human subjects" (10). To do this, the Report posits three general comprehensive principles that are relevant to research involving human subjects: (i) respect for persons, (ii) beneficence, and (iii) justice. Similar to earlier international codes, the Belmont Report emphasizes that individuals must be treated as autonomous agents whose opinions and choices are critical in the decision-making process. Those individuals not capable of self-determination should be afforded protection, dependent upon the involved risk of harm and the likelihood of benefit. Moreover, the principle of beneficence dictates that researchers and physicians act in a manner commensurate with securing the well being of their subjects. Meanwhile, justice requires researchers to avoid imposing undue burdens, as well as providing benefits to those persons who are duly entitled by virtue of the patient–physician relationship. The Report affirms that these principles obligate researchers to pay particular attention to informed consent, risk–benefit assessment, and the selection of research subjects.

III. THE DOCTRINE AND PROCESS OF INFORMED CONSENT

The doctrine of informed consent has provided the foundation for ethical and legal discourse about clinical research. Before the 20th century, the medical profession as a whole was largely motivated by beneficent obligations, i.e., seek for the patient the greater balance of good over harm. However, various legal cases early in the 20th century challenged beneficence as the sole basis for physicians' obligations to patients. In 1914, Judge Cardozo wrote a landmark opinion that legally defined simple consent (11). Cardozo noted that "every human being of adult years and sound mind has a right to determine what shall be done with his body." This case was the first in a long series of legal opinions that shifted the medical–ethical paradigm from one of simple beneficence to one in which respect for patient autonomy was at least equally important.

The ethical cornerstone of informed consent is that patients exercising autonomy should be able to make value-laden decisions that bear on their lives. Physicians typically do not know the true interests and values of their patients, as patients know them. Only patients are aware of their own value ordering related to health, prolongation of life, and other goods in their lives. Given this, the paternalistic authority to dictate clinical care or enroll subjects in research without consent is unjustified. Paternalism ignores patients as ethical and moral agents who have fundamental rights to participate in shaping the course of their own lives. According to Goldman (12), "personal autonomy over important decisions in one's life, the ability to attempt to realize one's own value ordering, is indeed so important that normally no amount of other goods, pleasures, or avoidances of personal evils can take precedence." In other words, regardless of any utilitarian calculation, self-determination is inherently valuable. Autonomous-informed decisions express the inherent worth and inviolability of the individual. By participating in the decision-making process, patients and research subjects actualize themselves as persons and demonstrate that they are not objects to be acted upon. Therefore, autonomy is the foundation of informed consent, which in turn acts as the bedrock for a patient's or subject's role in decision-making.

As implied in the term, informed consent has two parts: (i) disclosure (information) and (ii) authorization (consent). Before disclosure of information can ethically occur, specific prerequisites must be satisfied. Patients must be (i) competent, or have the decisional capacity, to make autonomous decisions regarding the issues before them and (ii) they must be acting voluntarily (13).

The concept of competence is difficult to define. Taken literally, the word means "the ability to perform a task" (14). Regarding medical and research-related decision making, the term is best understood as specifying a set of cognitive skills for a limited range of decision making (i.e., competent to make decision X), rather than as a broad generalization (i.e., competent to manage every aspect of life). Avording to Beauchamp and Childress (15), "patients or subjects are competent to make a decision if they have the capacity to understand the material information, to make a judgment about the information in light of their values, to intend a certain outcome, and to communicate freely their wishes to care givers or investigators." Patients or subjects unable to demonstrate these skills are incompetent with respect to the specific clinical or research question at hand.

When subjects are deemed incompetent, surrogate models of decision making should be employed. One such model is substituted judgment. In this model, a surrogate attempts to determine what the incompetent patient would have decided had the patient been able to choose. This can only be employed if the patient or subject was at one time capable of developing preferences and values and left reliable evidence of those attitudes concerning their current medical condition (16). If substituted judgment is not possible, then the best interest standard should be used. The best interest standard aims to promote the good of the individual as viewed by the shared values of society, i.e., to maximize benefits and minimize harms. Factors such as the avoidance of death, relief of pain and suffering, preservation or restoration of functioning, and quality and extent of life are usually taken into account (17).

Critical care investigators may also encounter the need for deferred consent, a technique designed for situations in which the tested therapy must be administered promptly in order to be effective, yet neither the subject nor a legal surrogate is capable of or available for providing consent. For example, in emergency situations, families would be informed upon admission to the ICU that the patient would be enrolled in a research study and they would be asked to provide written consent post facto within 48 hrs. Obtaining proxy consent for research in emergency contexts is addressed by regulations of the Food and Drug Administration (FDA) (18) and may also be governed by state law.

Another situation necessitating consideration of surrogate decision making involves the pediatric population. Depending on age, level of maturity, and degree of insight, children may be capable of participating in medical decision making. Recognizing this, the American Academy of Pediatrics (AAP) has affirmed that "patients should participate in decision making commensurate with their development; they should provide assent to care whenever reasonable" (19). The AAP distinguishes informed consent (which some adolescents can provide by virtue of having appropriate decisional capacity or by legal empowerment), informed permission (from parents, guardians, or other surrogates), and a child's assent (an expression of a patient's willingness to accept proposed treatment). The AAP notes that there may be clinical situations in which persistent refusal to assent (i.e., dissent) can be ethically binding. "This seems most obvious in the context of research (particularly that which has no potential to directly benefit the patient)" (19).

In addition to being competent, patients and subjects must be free from undo forms of influence; i.e., they must be free to act voluntarily. An act can only be voluntary if it is not made under coercive pressure. Although overt coercion may be infrequent in clinical and research settings, more subtle forms of manipulation can occur (20) such as lying, exaggeration, or withholding information. All of these erode patient–physician trust and co-operation and exploit the physician's therapeutic privileged position in the fiduciary relationship. Physicians and researchers must be cognizant of Eliot Freidson's observation that "clients are more often bullied than informed into consent" (21) and do their best to minimize such pressure. Practical steps for safeguarding voluntariness include full disclosure of available alternatives and making clear to subjects that they can withdraw from the research at any time.

Disclosure of information represents another central tenet of informed consent. Delivering understandable information allows patients to have a basis for rational, informed decision making. The physician or researcher acts as the professional expert obligated to provide opinions, recommendations, and core data. The manner, quality, and extent of physician and researcher disclosure have been a center of controversy in medical ethics and civil law (22). Two standards of adequacy have emerged.

The initial standard for disclosure of medical information was the "professional standard," whereby adequate disclosure is determined by a professional community's customary practices. This standard directs physicians to behave as other physicians in their specialty behave, disclosing amounts, and kinds of information that other physicians in similar practices would. Ethicists, as well as legal commentators, have criticized this standard because it fails to inform physicians about the end toward which disclosure is aimed. By telling the physicians to behave as other physicians, the standard lacks an independently scrutinized criterion for disclosure.

The second standard of disclosure to emerge was the "reasonable person standard." Under this standard, physicians are obligated to disclose facts or descriptions that a reasonable person would consider material in deciding whether to refuse or consent to the proposed intervention or research. Physicians within this standard should also offer their professional recommendations and the purposes for seeking consent. The reasonable person standard more adequately respects patient's autonomy and the desired outcome of the informed consent process.

In general, informed consent needs to be considered a dynamic process rather than a static, one-time recitation of potential risks or the signing of a consent form. With a similar emphasis on process, Katz (23) envisioned true informed consent as a searching conversation between patient and physician. Refining this concept, Brody (24) has proposed a "transparency standard." In this model, disclosure is adequate neither based on adherence to existing standards of other practitioners nor based on a hypothetical reasonable person, but rather when the physician's basic thinking has been rendered transparent to the patient or research subject. Informed consent here entails physicians and researchers sharing their thinking processes with patients, encouraging and answering questions, and facilitating the level of participation in decision making that patients wish. The emphasis in this model is not simply on the listing of the nature, purpose, risks, benefits, and alternatives for a specific research proposal, but more importantly on the active engagement of the patient or subject in a deliberative thought process.

The second part of "informed consent" in research is the actual consent or authorization that the subject gives after considering the information received. Subjects need to share an understanding with professionals about the terms of the authorization before proceeding. Informed consent represents a contract with essential features permitting the performance of specific procedures or therapeutic interventions. The authorization takes the form of a written consent, except on the rare occasion when an IRB waives this requirement. The acquisition of consent should only occur when appropriate time has been allowed for adequate understanding of the information disclosed. The informed consent process can be lengthy, requiring significant time and effort. However, this time is crucial because the informed consent experience can be a turning point in shaping the patient–physician/researcher relationship. A negative experience can be disastrous for patients, engendering distrust, suspicion, and alienation. In contrast, a positive informed consent process has the ability to cultivate an environment where both the welfare of the patient or subject and the scientific integrity of the research can be optimized.

IV. STUDY DESIGN, SUBJECT SELECTION, AND MONITORING

Justification for clinical research with human subjects derives from the basic principle that anticipated benefits of conducting research must outweigh risks to subjects. Conducting ethical research is inherently challenging, because virtually all benefits are anticipatory and contingent, whereas some of the burdens are immediate (25). Thus, the ethical justification for engaging in research cannot depend solely on the usefulness of the results. Nor can the justification rely singularly on a conscientious and detailed informed consent process, although, in this chapter, informed consent is crucial. Rather, a study's purpose and design must undergo scrutiny at the outset before investigators can conclude that imposing even minimal risk on subjects is ethically permissible.

As a starting point, for clinical research to be ethical, it must have social or scientific value. "Clinical research is a practical endeavor whose purpose is to generate new therapies in the service of improved patient care" (26). A study must derive from clinical equipoise, i.e., there must be "an honest, professional disagreement among expert clinicians about the preferred treatment" (27), and the trial must be designed in a way that its successful completion will resolve the dispute. The practicability of not only completing the trial, but also implementing its results should be considered at the outset. For example, embarking on a trial that is unlikely to enroll sufficient subjects, or that tests an intervention that will not realistically be implemented even if proven to be effective, would be ethically inappropriate. In addition to skewing the balance toward disproportionate risk, engaging human subjects in poorly designed or trivial projects diverts limited resources from more worthy social and scientific pursuits, violating the principle of justice.

Even, socially valuable research can be unethical if conducted poorly. Ethical research requires scientific validity, i.e., clear scientific objectives, sufficient power to test the objectives definitively, rigorous methodology, and careful and accurate data collection and analysis. The gold standard in trial design, the randomized clinical trial (RCT), contains four elements aimed at enhancing scientific validity: (i) the trial is "controlled," so that one segment of the subject population receives a tested therapy while another receives either an existing standard therapy or no therapy; (ii) the significance of the results is established through statistical analysis; (iii) when feasible, "double-blinding" occurs, in which both investigator and subject are unaware, who received experimental therapy vs. the control until the study is concluded; and (iv) the trial is randomized, i.e., the therapies being compared are allocated among the subjects by chance (25). These components offer some protection against both statistical bias (the tendency of an estimate to deviate in one direction from a true value) and investigators' and subjects' potential partiality.

Although the scientific value of the RCT provides the strongest ethical justification for its use, the RCT also raises its own set of ethical problems. In general, prospective subjects of RCTs should be informed that their treatment arm will be chosen by chance. Historically, investigators have questioned whether consent to randomization inhibits subject recruitment, although other approaches (e.g., prerandomization, blinded randomization) also incur ethical criticism and have not clearly improved recruitment rates (25).

In addition to trial design, considerations of risk–benefit balance and justice raise their own set of ethical concerns. Critical care research likely avoids many ethical concerns related to initial recruitment methods, because the available population is generally limited by the boundaries of the ICU. For example, critical care research does not ordinarily threaten to impose disproportionate harm on healthy volunteers. However, selecting individual subjects from among the critical care population can pose other kinds of ethical challenges.

Historically, some of the most egregious reports of unethical research involved the abuse of institutionalized populations. Critical care and perioperative research runs a heightened risk of relying on a similar captive and vulnerable population, although current standards of informed consent would likely preclude abuses comparable to those that occurred at, for example, the Jewish Chronic Disease Hospital in Brooklyn and New York's Willowbrook State Hospital (28). The severity of patients' illnesses and their compromised or absent decisional capacity also exacerbate their vulnerability. Thus, research in these environments has the potential for exploitation of human subjects, and investigators conducting the research and IRBs approving such research in this setting assume even greater responsibility to minimize this possibility.

Fairness requires that the scientific goals of a study, not factors unrelated to the purpose of the research, govern participant selection. Investigators should be cautious about relying on the ICU or post-anesthesia-care-unit population because they are convenient or available; rather, they should be selected for research proposals based on their exhibiting clinical characteristics that other patients do not. Moreover, investigators should be aware of the inverse relationship between eligibility criteria and the applicability of results: as a study population becomes more homogeneous, generalizability of the study to a broader clinical population decreases (26). For example, enrolling patients based on narrowly-drawn inclusion criteria that select only ICU patients with a higher performance status may bias the results and limit the applicability of study results to the general critical care population.

Reciprocally, patients should not be excluded from the opportunity to participate in research without a scientific reason or increased susceptibility to risk that justifies their exclusion. Although performance status or other clinical traits might justify exclusion of perioperative or critical care patients from some trials, the population may deserve particular consideration for research in, for example, modalities to reverse organ failure, palliative care, or pain management. The fact that ICU patients are a severely ill "captive population" mandates caution in using them in research, but developing trials directed toward improving their welfare advances the widely held view that groups and individuals who bear the risks and burdens of research should obtain its benefits (29).

A favorable risk–benefit ratio and respect for research subjects must be sustained throughout a trial. Investigators must continually search for ways to minimize risk and maximize benefit as the trial progresses, and the research protocol should reflect this goal. Difficult dilemmas relating to the management of early data as the trial progresses can sometimes arise. Whether and how to assess preliminary data and trends, including adverse events, and whether and how to communicate these to subjects pose difficult benefit–burden analyses. Information about previous participants' experiences may be significant for later candidates' decision making. Trends identified before statistical certainty regarding causation can be attained, particularly those implicating patient's safety, may support investigators' decisions to amend protocols. Simultaneously, however, disclosing preliminary data to investigators and subjects threatens the integrity and even the continuation of the research. To mediate among these competing concerns, independent Data Safety Monitoring Boards (DSMBs) should monitor developing data trends to determine whether a study should be discontinued or its procedures modified. Regardless of whether a trial is subject to review by a DSMB, investigators' research plans should provide for sufficient monitoring to identify circumstances that would require study modification and even early termination.

V. RESEARCH ON TERMINALLY ILL PATIENTS

The U.S. Code of Federal Regulations governing human research recognizes the need for additional protections for vulnerable research populations such as pregnant women, prisoners, and children (30). In anesthesiology, critical care, and pain control, patients with terminal illnesses should be included as vulnerable populations who require special protection against violation of their rights and exposure to undue risks and burdens. Outside of many palliation and symptom-control studies (e.g., for pain, nausea, constipation, anorexia), terminally ill patients generally will not derive direct benefit from the research in which they participate. Burden on research subjects at the end of life must also be carefully weighed, with special attention to the time required for research participation; for the terminally ill, time is a precious commodity that must be carefully protected (31). Nevertheless, if improvements in the treatment and care of these populations is to occur, research using terminally ill patients must be permitted but with adequate safeguards to ensure the ethical quality of the research.

Physiologically, this patient population is in a dynamic state. Bruera (32) noted that the baseline for any studies is rarely stable, because the nature and intensity of symptoms and responses to treatment are changing continuously. These characteristics of many terminally ill patients make study design and application of results more difficult.

Cognitive and affective impairments at the end of life compound clinical researchers' challenges when designing studies that will enroll terminally ill patients. Patients' decisional capacity can be compromised by the disease itself (e.g., cerebral tumor or brain metastasis), or by delirium and depression, or by drug induction, and can vary over time. Assessment of decisional capacity may be necessary (33). If potential research subjects do not demonstrate requisite skills for decision making, surrogates able to provide substituted judgments (as described earlier) should be identified. If subjects are unable to participate fully in the process of informed consent, yet they have cognitive abilities to participate in some manner, their assent to research should be solicited and their dissent should generally be honored, similar to that described earlier for children.

Because of limited numbers of dying patients who can also be research subjects, collaborative multicenter trials may be necessary. This strategy may be able to prevent problems of inadequate sample size and underpowered studies, to permit subgroup analysis of subjects, and thus to promote studies' validity, value, generalizability, and completion within a reasonable period of time (34). For descriptive, data-gathering studies that are likely to identify specific and valuable patient management information (e.g., the presence of unrecognized or untreated pain), study designs should direct that such information be provided to subjects' primary clinicians. If, within a study's design, investigators establish that some subjects benefit from a particular study medication, allowance for an open label extension of the drug's use for these subjects can increase a study's potential benefits for participants.

Placebo-controlled studies using terminally ill patients are not necessarily unethical, but they should be subjected to the same assessment noted in the following discussion on placebo controls. Specifically, for pain management studies, ethical support for placebo use is strengthened when subjects receive a placebo combined with a standard treatment, or when a crossover design is used, or if the study design allows subjects to receive "rescue" pain medication when breakthrough pain is reported (34).

Finally, clinical researchers should be attentive to research subjects' motives for volunteering for studies. For many patients, research studies at the end of life can provide altruistic opportunities to contribute to the well being of others and to derive meaning from their terminal illnesses and suffering. However, others may feel obligated to enroll in research as a way of paying back their professional caregivers, especially if patients have received quality care and relief from severe symptoms in a supportive environment.

VI. PLACEBO CONTROLS

Despite longstanding use in RCTs, the placebo control has historically been the target of ethical challenge. For thousands of years, physicians have known that people who feel ill often will feel better after taking medication. Physicians capitalized on this knowledge by treating patients with placebos, pharmacologically inert substances (often sugar pills or saline injections). The relief of symptoms engendered by placebo administration is called the placebo effect. The use of placebos in medical treatment outside of an RCT has essentially been ruled out by the doctrine of informed consent, which condemns deception in the physician–patient relationship.

Ethical issues surrounding the use of the placebo control in research are distinct from the use of placebo as medical treatment. In a typical double-blinded RCT with placebo control, participants are told that they might receive an inert substance. If the trial is "double-blinded," they are also told that the physician–investigator is similarly unaware to which intervention arm the participant will be randomized. By making the study double-blinded, the trials are designed to minimize the placebo effect.

The pre-eminent rationale for the use of placebo controls remains their scientific value. Proponents assert that placebo controls are the simplest, clearest, and most efficient benchmark against which to measure a new therapy (35). However, critics argue that the clinically relevant question is not whether a new agent or procedure is better than nothing, but whether the trial intervention is better than a standard treatment, if one exists; pursuant to the ethical principle of respect for persons, subordinating the rights of patients to receive approved and available therapy to society's goal of advancing medical knowledge is ethically impermissible (35). Apparent disparity between FDA guidelines, which generally promote placebo-controlled testing, and the Declaration of Helsinki, which now asserts that placebo controls should only be used in the absence of existing proven therapy (4) reflects ongoing controversy related to placebo use in research.

Perioperative research, which often includes new devices and procedures, is particularly susceptible to placebo-related ethical challenge. A recent controversial "sham" surgical trial illustrates both the harms and the advantages of placebo-controlled trials. The trial involved surgical implantation of fetal cells in the brains of patients with Parkinson's disease vs. "sham" surgery as a control. Results of the study failed to demonstrate any improvement in Parkinson symptoms secondary to the implantation of fetal cells (36). Therefore, this placebo-controlled trial successfully established the (in)efficacy of the tested intervention and, in doing so, illuminated the danger and cost of adopting new procedures, before safety and efficacy had been reliably assessed. Moreover, the use of a placebo arm enabled this small trial to obtain sufficient power. Finally, the trial design minimized harm by debriefing participants after the blinding was broken. However, the placebo-controlled sham surgery inarguably exposed participants to harm and risk. Investigators also undertook great efforts to maximize the deception by actively misleading participants (e.g., asking if they were ready for the experimental procedure, boring holes in their heads, administering general anesthesia, and imitating the sounds of the "real" procedure).

In summary, placebo-controlled trials are not inherently unethical, but their justification requires at least five additional assessments and actions: (i) a determination that the placebo control is methodologically necessary to produce meaningful results; (ii) minimization of risks related to the placebo control; (iii) assessment that risk of the placebo control does not exceed a reasonable threshold of acceptable risk; (iv) the value of knowledge to be gained justifies the risk; and (v) disclosure of the use of the placebo control and the participant's consent thereto (37). Recommendations from the Council on Ethical and Judicial Affairs of the American Medical Association also note that placebo-control use is not justified when testing the effectiveness of an innovative surgical technique that represents a minor modification of an existing surgical procedure (38).

VII. CONFLICTS OF INTEREST

In a conflict of interest, obligations to a specific person, group, or enterprise conflict with self-interests (39). More comprehensively and explicitly, a conflict of interest exists "when an individual exploits, or appears to exploit, his or her position for personal gain or for the profit of a member of his or her immediate family or household ... (or) ... the undue use of a position or exercise of power to influence a decision for personal gain" (40).

Conflicts of interest can be distinguished from conflicts of commitment (41) (e.g., how much of a researcher's time must also be devoted to clinical service or teaching), conflicts of effort (40) (e.g., advisory board service that interferes with a clinical researcher's assigned duties for academic service), conflicts of conscience (40) (e.g., a scientist who opposes abortion and the use of fetal tissue and who is asked to review a grant application utilizing fetal tissue), and conflicts in scientific methodology (e.g., disagreement among coinvestigators about a particular research technique). Conflicts of interest can be financial (42) or non financial (43), actual or perceived, and individual or institutional. Conflicts of interest can occur during all stages of the research process (e.g., application for funding, recruitment of subjects, the informed consent process, the reporting of results).

There is nothing inherently unethical about a conflict of interest. In fact, they occur in all professions and in almost all spheres of life. Rather, the primary ethical determinant is how one handles a conflict of interest. Nevertheless, conflicts of interest for individual clinical investigators and academic institutions have come under special and significant scrutiny. At stake are scientific objectivity and integrity, the welfare and safety of research participants, and the public's trust in and support of research and science.

Financial relationships creating conflicts of interest for clinical researchers include consulting fees, salaried service on scientific advisory boards, ownership or options for equity and stocks, royalties from intellectual property rights and patents, honoraria for lectures, fees for expert testimony, and fees for successful recruitment of research subjects. Nonfinancial self-interests include job security, prestige and fame, academic promotion, publications, power and authority, personal sense of accomplishment, and increased research space and support.

The 1980 Bayh-Dole Act (44) was a water-shed legislative event that created new entrepreneurial and commercial opportunities, as well as new risks for conflicts of interest, for clinical researchers and academic institutions regarding financial incentives connected to research. In response to a perceived inefficient transfer of new technology to public use, the Act allowed federal contractors and nonprofit organizations (including universities) that make patentable discoveries with federal funding to retain property rights to inventions and subsequent patents. Further, institutions and researchers are allowed to share in a portion of the resulting income. This act, subsequent amendments, and other legislation in the 1980s radically changed and restructured the goals, conduct, and relationships among universities, private industries, and researchers (41). Between 1980 and 2001, at least 2900 companies were formed that were built around an innovation licensed by researchers at academic institutions (45). Researchers and universities, via contractual partnerships with business corporations and companies, have new sources of revenue for research, university infrastructure, discretionary funds, and personal gain. In 1999, the licensing of 417 new products at North American academic and nonprofit institutions generated more than $40 billion in goods and services and funded more than 270,000 jobs (46).

Clinical researchers and academic institutions do not have a uniform, comprehensive set of guidelines and regulations for identifying, managing, reducing, or eliminating conflicts of interest. Policies and procedures vary widely and are evolving with no "best practices" delineated (47). The U.S. Public Health Service (PHS) of the Department of Health and Human Services has established requirements for disclosure of financial conflicts of interest for participants in PHS-funded research (48). Public Health Service regulations permit management of conflicts of interest via internal institutional policies and conflict of interest committees (COICs). The FDA has its own set of regulations for financial disclosures, retrospectively, when an FDA application is filed for approval of a drug, device, or biologic product (49).

The Association of American Universities (AAU) (50) and the American Association of Medical Colleges (AAMC) (51) each have published recommendations for individual and institutional conflicts of interest. Common themes found in these two sets of recommendations include researchers' annual disclosures of their financial interests to internal COICs, with an attentive and consistent review of such disclosures by these committees, and a monetary threshold (e.g., $10,000) deemed significant enough for financial disclosures.

The AAU and AAMC guidelines have also begun to address institutional conflicts of interest, with the AAU document identifying a series of institutional financial relationships that can affect or appear to affect scientific objectivity and human subject protections (e.g., an institution having ownership interest or an entitlement to equity of ≥$100,000 in a publicly traded sponsor of clinical research at the institution). In March 2003, the U.S. Office of Public Health and Science (Department of Health and Human Services) published a "draft guidance document" that recommended the extension of the role of COICs to address institutional financial interests in research and the establishment of clear channels of communication between COICs and IRBs (52). The American Society of Clinical Oncology (ASCO), in 2003, also published a revised conflict of interest policy for its 20,000 members. The policy requires clinical cancer researchers seeking to publish or present trial outcomes to disclose virtually all financial ties with trial sponsors and restricts the financial interests of principle investigators and other clinical trial leaders (e.g., members of DSMBs) (53).

In managing conflicts of interest, disclosure of a conflict is a necessary (but insufficient) condition. At a minimum, subjects should be informed via the written consent form that an institution or some of its researchers have a financial stake in a specific investigational drug's development. Similarly, authors of manuscripts should disclose to potential publishers' any financial ties with companies that make products discussed in the submitted manuscript. At the same time, a researcher with a financial interest in an investigational drug or device should not be the principle investigator for a research protocol involving that drug or device.

Additional safeguards for managing, reducing, or eliminating conflicts of interest include (i) monitoring and review of conflicts of interest by specially designated COICs, knowledgeable about current regulations and guidelines; (ii) clear lines of communication between COICs and IRBs concerning specific protocols deemed problematic, because investigators have financial interests in the research; (iii) strict adherence by researchers to IRB-approved protocols, including elements such as inclusion/exclusion criteria, reporting of adverse events, data collection, and analysis; (iv) individual researcher and institutional divestiture of significant financial interests; (v) creation of research oversight committees of disinterested scientists who can review and certify the integrity of the research; and (vi) in instances of significant conflicts of interest, disqualification from participation in funded research.

As more and more clinical research moves from academic medical centers into community and private physician practices, the monitoring of conflicts of interests may become more challenging and problematic. Ultimately, an ever-expanding and increasingly specific list of regulations and guidelines cannot replace personal and institutional integrity. Researchers and their institutions must be committed to openness and honesty, scientific objectivity, and the welfare and safety of human research subjects. These commitments must be placed ahead of financial gain.

VIII. CONCLUSION

As scientific discoveries develop, as research regulations change, and as increasing numbers of researchers face new challenges in areas such as study design, subject recruitment, and funding, there will be an ever-expanding list of ethical issues to which clinical researchers must be attentive. In this chapter, the discussion was limited to foundational principles and concepts. Clinical researchers, as part of their obligation and commitment to cultivate scientific expertise and skills through continuing education, should strive to expand on this base of knowledge to increase their awareness of and abilities to address ethical issues.

Direct assistance for ethical questions related to specific protocol design and development is available from IRB members, ethics consultants, and healthcare ethics committees. Continuous educational opportunities in clinical research ethics are widely available and include national/regional conferences, expanding body of peer-reviewed literature, computer websites, and training programs dedicated to the ethics of clinical research.

REFERENCES

1. Caplan A. When Medicine Went Mad: Bioethics and the Holocaust. Totawa, NJ: Humana Press, 1992.
2. Rothman DJ. Were Tuskegee and Willowbrook 'studies in nature'? The Hastings Center Report 1982; 12:5–7.
3. The Nuremberg Code. Trials of War Criminals before the Nuremberg Military Tribunals under Control Council Law No. 10: Nuremberg; Washington: U.S. GPO, n.d., (2) Oct. 1946–Apr. 1949, 181–182.
4. World Medical Association. World Medical Association Declaration of Helsinki: ethical principles for medical research involving human subjects. J Postgrad Med 2002; 48:206–208.
5. Rothman DJ. Research ethics at Tuskegee and Willowbrook. Am J Med 1984; 77:A49.
6. Final Report of the Advisory Committee on Human Radiation Experiments. New York: Oxford University Press, 1996.
7. Jones J. Bad Blood: The Tuskegee Syphilis Experiment: A Tragedy of Race and Medicine. New York: Free Press, 1993.
8. Department of Health, Education, and Welfare (United States). Final Report of the Tuskegee Syphilis Study Ad Hoc Advisory Panel. Washington, DC: GPO, 1973.
9. Brandt AM. Racism and research: the case of the Tuskegee syphilis study. The Hastings Center Report 1978; 8:21–29.
10. U.S. Department of Health, Education and Welfare. Protection of human subjects: Belmont Report—ethical principles and guidelines for the protection of human subjects of research. Fed Registr. 1979; 44:23192–23197.
11. Schlendorff V. Society of New York Hospital, 211 N.Y. 125, 126, 105 N.E. 92, 93 (1914).
12. Goldman A. The refutation of medical paternalism. In: Arras J, Steinbock B, eds. Ethical Issues in Modern Medicine. Mountain View, California: Mayfield Publishing Co, 1999:66.
13. Beauchamp TL, Childress JF. Principles of Biomedical Ethics. 5th ed. New York: Oxford University Press, 2001:80.
14. Welie JV, Welie SP. Patient decision making competence: outlines of a conceptual analysis. Med Health Care Philos 2001; 4:127–138.

15. Beauchamp TL, Childress JF. Principles of Biomedical Ethics. 5th ed. New York: Oxford University Press, 2001:71.
16. President's Commission for the Study of Ethical Problems in Medicine and Biomedical and Behavioral Research. Deciding to forego life-sustaining treatment: ethical, medical, and legal issues in treatment decisions. Patients who Lack Decision-Making Capacity. Washington, DC: GPO; 1983:121–170.
17. Nyman DJ, Sprung CL. End-of-life decision making in the intensive care unit. Int Care Med 2000; 26: 1414–1420.
18. 21 Code of Federal Regulations, Subpart B, 50.23.
19. American Academy of Pediatrics. Informed consent, parental permission, and assent in pediatric practice. Pediatrics 1995; 95:314–317.
20. Nelson RM, Merz JF. Voluntariness of informed consent: an empirical and conceptual review. Med Care 2002; 40(Suppl 9):V69–V80.
21. Freidson E. The Profession of Medicine. New York: Dodd, Mead & Co., 1970:376.
22. Morin K. The standard of disclosure in human subject experimentation. J Leg Med 1998; 19:157–221.
23. Katz J. Informed consent—must it remain a fairy tale? J Contemp Health Law Policy 1994; 10:69–91.
24. Brody H. Transparency: informed consent in primary care. Hastings Cent Rep 1989; 19:5–9.
25. Levine RJ. Ethics and Regulation of Clinical Research. 2d ed. New Haven: Yale University Press, 1988.
26. Crouch RA. Eligibility, extrapolation and equipoise: unlearned lessons in the ethical analysis of clinical research. IRB: Ethics Hum Res 2001; 23:6–9.
27. Freedman B. Equipoise and the ethics of clinical research. N Engl J Med 1987; 317:141–145.
28. Jonson AR. The Birth of Bioethics. New York: Oxford University Press, 1998:143,153–154.
29. Emanuel EJ, Wendler D, Grady C. What makes clinical research ethical? J Am Med Assoc 2000; 283(20): 2701–2711.
30. 45 Code of Federal Regulations 46, Subparts B, C, D.
31. Ferrell BR, Grant M. Nursing research. In: Ferrell BR, Coyle N, eds. Textbook of Palliative Nursing. New York: Oxford University Press, 2001:701–709.
32. Bruera E. Research into symptoms other than pain. In: Doyle D, Hanks GWC, MacDonald N, eds. Oxford Textbook of Palliative Medicine. 2d ed. New York: Oxford University Press, 1998:179–185.
33. Grisso T, Appelbaum PS. Assessing Competence to Consent to Treatment, A Guide for Physicians and Other Health Profesisonals. New York: Oxford University Press, 1998.
34. Casarett DJ. Research ethics. In: Berger AM, Portenoy RK, Weissman DE, eds. Principles and Practice of Palliative Care and Supportive Oncology. Philadelphia: Lippincott Williams and Wilkins, 2002:1131–1140.
35. Emanuel EJ, Miller FG. The ethics of placebo-controlled trials—a middle ground. N Engl J Med 2001; 345:915–919.
36. Freed CR, Green PE, Breeze RE, Tsai W, DuMouchel W, Kao R, Dillon S, Winfield H, Culver S, Trojanowski JQ, Eidelberg D, Fahn S. Transplantation of embryonic dopamine neurons for severe Parkinson's disease. N Engl J Med 2001; 344:710–719.
37. Horng S, Miller FG. Ethical framework for the use of sham procedures in clinical trials. Crit Care Med 2003; 31(Suppl 3):S126–S130.
38. Tenery R, Rakatansky H, Riddick FA, Goldrich MS, Morse LJ, O'Bannon JM, Ray P, Smalley S, Weiss M, Kao A, Morin K, Maixner A, Seiden S. Surgical 'placebo' controls. Ann Surg 2002; 235:303–307.
39. Morreim EH. Conflict of interest. In: Reich WT, ed. Encyclopedia of Bioethics. Revised ed. New York: Simon and Schuster Macmillan, 1995:459–465.
40. Bradley SG. Managing conflicting interests. In: Macrina FL, ed. Scientific Inquiry, An Introductory Text with Cases. 2d ed. Washington, DC: ASM Press, 2000: 131–156.
41. Bulger RE. The scientist and industry, conflicts of interest and conflicts of commitment. In: Bulger RE, Heitman E, Reiser SJ, eds. The Ethical Dimensions of the Biological and Health Sciences. 2nd ed. New York: Cambridge University Press, 2002:281–289.
42. Bekelman JE, Li Y, Gross CP. Scope and impact of financial conflicts of interest in biomedical research. J Am Med Assoc 2003; 289:454–465.
43. Levinsky NG. Nonfinancial conflicts of interest in research. N Engl J Med 2002; 347:759–761.
44. Pub. L. No. 96–517, USC, Dec 12, 1980.
45. Kelch RP. Maintaining the public trust in clinical research. N Engl J Med 2002; 346:285–287.
46. Association of University Technology Managers' Licensing Survey, FY 1999. A Survey Summary of Technology Licensing (and Related) Performance for U.S. and Canadian Academic and Nonprofit Institutions, and Patent Management Forms. Northbrook, Ill: Association of University Technology Mangers, 2000.
47. Lo B, Wolf LE, Berkeley A. Conflict-of-interest policies for investigators in clinical trials. N Engl J Med 2000; 343:1616–1620.
48. 42 Code of Federal Regulations 50, subpart F, 2000.
49. 21 Code of Federal Regulations 54.
50. Task Force on Research Accountability. Report on Individual and Institutional Financial Conflict of Interest. Washington, DC: The Association of American Universities, 2001.
51. Task Force on Financial Conflicts of Interest in Clinical Research. Protecting Subjects, Preserving Trust, Promoting Progress—Policy and Guidelines for the Oversight of Individual Financial Interests in Human Subjects Research. Washington, DC: American Association of Medical Colleges, 2001.
52. Federal Register, Vol. 68, No. 61, March 31, 2003.
53. American Society of Clinical Oncology. Revised conflict of interest policy. J Clin Oncol 2003; 21: 2394–2396.

12

General Principles of Perioperative Medicine: Surgical and Medical Perspectives

GREGORY H. BOTZ

Department of Critical Care, The University of Texas M.D. Anderson Cancer Center, Houston, Texas, U.S.A.

ZDRAVKA ZAFIROVA

Department of Anesthesia and Critical Care, University of Chicago, Chicago, Illinois, U.S.A.

I. INTRODUCTION

The perioperative management of patients with cancer is often challenging due to the complicated nature of neoplastic disease. One must consider the nature and extent of the malignancy, as well as the consequences of cancer therapy and other comorbidities. By virtue of its disordered or often uncontrolled growth, cancer can permeate natural tissue planes leading to anatomic aberration, and can generate metabolic products leading to local or systemic physiologic consequences. Antineoplastic therapy can have undesirable physiologic consequences as well. Chemotherapeutic agents can have direct organ system toxicities, including cardiorespiratory (anthracycline cardiomyopathy and bleomycin lung fibrosis) and hematopoietic compromise (leukopenia, anemia, and thrombocytopenia). Radiation therapy can lead to adverse changes in surrounding tissues, including an increased risk for secondary malignancy. A multidisciplinary approach to the evaluation and management of cancer patients in the perioperative period is most effective; co-ordination and co-operation between caregivers is essential. Comprehensive review of the care for cancer patients can be found in this and other medical texts. This chapter outlines some general principles.

II. PRINCIPLES OF MEDICAL MANAGEMENT IN THE PERIOPERATIVE PERIOD

Medical evaluation of the cancer patient involves a detailed assessment, including type of malignancy, stage and grade, location and spread, and the characteristics of any associated symptoms. Particular attention should be paid to organ system involvement and any consequent dysfunction or disruption of homeostasis. Prior cancer therapy including chemotherapy, radiation, surgery, bone marrow transplantation, and their potential complications are important aspects of medical history assessment (1,2). Noncancer-related comorbid conditions need to be evaluated as well and included in the overall assessment of these patients. Symptoms attributed to malignancy or its treatment may, in fact, represent comorbid diseases.

A. Cardiovascular System

Involvement of the heart by either primary malignancy or metastatic disease has important implications. Primary cardiac tumors are rare; metastatic involvement is more frequent and can occur with many disseminated malignancies. Mediastinal masses can compress the large airways, the heart, and the great vessels. Lymphoma and metastatic tumors are the most common causes of mediastinal malignancy (3). Those malignancies frequently associated with cardiac spread are lung, breast, lymphoma, leukemia, and melanoma. The pericardium and myocardium are most frequently affected, although all parts are susceptible. Often, cardiac malignancy is silent. Pericardial involvement can present clinically as pericardial effusion and tamponade, pericarditis, and arrhythmias (4). Myocardial syndromes can include arrhythmias and conduction abnormalities, myocardial infarction and congestive heart failure. Valvular involvement, thromboembolic complications, and obstruction of the cardiac chambers and great vessels may also be seen with malignancy. Metastatic renal cell carcinoma can extend from the renal veins to the inferior vena cava including extension to intracardiac structures (5). The onset of cardiac dysfunction in cancer patients warrants evaluation for malignant involvement. Pre-existing cardiovascular disease in cancer patient should be evaluated and optimized. The effects of radiation therapy and chemotherapeutic agents such as anthracyclines with cardiotoxic properties should be considered (6,7). Vascular complications may arise from direct cancer involvement, drug extravasations, and venous access difficulties (8–10). Thorough evaluation of cardiovascular compromise, appropriate monitoring, and therapeutic interventions are paramount. Postoperative cardiac dysfunction may reflect limited cardiac reserve in the face of the surgical stress response (11).

B. Pulmonary System

Respiratory dysfunction is a frequent cause of morbidity and mortality in cancer patients. Carcinoma of the lung is the second most common malignancy in United States and is the leading cause of cancer deaths in men and women (12). Lung involvement with primary tumor or metastasis can manifest as pulmonary nodules, interstitial infiltrates, pleural effusion, pneumothorax, or atelectasis (13,14). Fistula formation, bronchial rupture, or erosion into pulmonary vasculature may complicate neoplasms and their treatment. Pulmonary infections can represent formidable diagnostic and therapeutic challenge. Radiotherapy and a variety of antineoplastic agents such as bleomycin, busulfan, carmustine, methotrexate, mitomycin, procarbazine, melphalan, chlorambucil, and cyclophosphamide have been implicated as pulmonary toxins (15). Comprehensive assessment of the pulmonary system with clinical evaluation, augmented with pulmonary function tests and pulmonary imaging, is essential. Recognition of comorbid pulmonary diseases, including atypical presentations, multiple comorbidities, and unusual diagnoses may present. Immune compromise may favor development of rare pulmonary infections not commonly seen in the immunocompetent host. Appropriate monitoring, adjustment in therapy, and use of lung protection strategies in the perioperative period can decrease attributable pulmonary morbidity and mortality.

C. Gastrointestinal Tract

Involvement of the gastrointestinal tract by primary and metastatic neoplasms can result in a variety of clinical presentations (16). Emergencies such as bowel obstruction, perforation, ischemia, and gastrointestinal bleeding are among the most challenging in medicine. Hepatic and pancreatic dysfunction can result in significant morbidity and mortality (17). Consequences of toxicity with radiotherapy and chemotherapy such as nausea, vomiting, xerostomia, mucositis, diarrhea, bleeding, and hepatotoxicity can be refractory to standard therapy and require complex management.

D. Genitourinary Tract

Neoplastic diseases can involve the genitourinary tract directly or indirectly due to effects of tumor biology. The consequences of cancer therapy can also affect genitourinary function (18,19). Examples include renal dysfunction secondary to tumor lysis syndrome, ureteral obstruction by pelvic masses, and acute tubular necrosis associated with many chemotherapy and antimicrobial agents. The resulting anatomic and physiologic dysfunction can be an important cause of short-term and long-term morbidity and mortality. Renal protection strategies should be considered an essential component of the therapeutic regimen.

E. Endocrine and Metabolic Function

Homeostatic disturbances involving metabolic, electrolyte, and acid-base balance may reflect the effects of direct or metastatic tumor involvement as well as humoral factors due to hormone production by endocrine neoplasm or paraneoplastic syndromes (9,20,21). Malnutrition in cancer patients is common and can be multifactorial; various abnormalities in carbohydrate, protein, lipid, and energy metabolisms may be present. Cancer therapy can contribute to further derangements. This homeostatic dysfunction can be multifaceted and profound; management can be challenging. Collaboration between involved providers is essential. Often, complex therapeutic strategies are needed for restoration of acid-base and electrolyte balance, and nutritional support.

F. Hematopoietic System

Hematopoietic disorders are present in almost all cancer patients at some point during the course of their disease (22–24). Bone marrow dysfunction with anemia, granulocytopenia, thrombocytopenia, and coagulation abnormalities are among the common manifestations of malignancy. Erythrocytosis, thrombocytosis, and leukocytosis can also occur. The etiology includes a wide range of hematopoietic and nonhematopoietic cancers and their therapy. Hypercoagulability is also common in malignancy (25). The mechanisms of these abnormalities are varied and frequently multifactorial. Hematopoietic dysfunction is associated with significant morbidity and mortality in cancer patients. Identification of correctable causes and appropriate therapy including replacement of blood elements, bone marrow stem-cell stimulation and maintenance of coagulation homeostasis improve patient survival.

G. Central Nervous System

The incidence of neurological dysfunction in patients with cancer is reported to be approximately 25%. Neurological complications can arise from direct invasion of primary or metastatic neoplasm or as a result of metabolic dysfunction, infection, paraneoplastic syndromes, cerebrovascular disorder, or complication of therapy. Many regions of the nervous system can be involved, and presentation can include visual disturbances, lateralizing signs, headaches, altered mental status, gait disorders, and bulbar and peripheral neuropathies (26,27). Intracranial hypertension, hemorrhage, and seizures can present as therapeutic emergencies. Early recognition and treatment of neurological complications is essential and may prevent further progression. Symptom control and prevention of irreversible neurological injury are the primary focus. Neuropsychiatric disorders such as depression, anxiety, and delirium are not uncommon in the setting of malignant disease (28). Appropriate multimodal therapy including pharmacological therapy, psychotherapy, and social support should coincide with treatment of the malignancy.

H. Immune System, Transplant, and Secondary Malignancy

Immune system disturbances are frequently associated with neoplastic diseases and their therapies. As a result of these disturbances, cancer patients are more susceptible to infections, often with more severe clinical presentation. Infections with unusual pathogens like fungus, parasites, virus, and unusual bacteria are not uncommon (29,30). Organ transplantation and bone marrow transplantation, in particular, present unique challenges in the management of the recipients (31,32). Restoration or modulation of immune function, and early and aggressive treatment of infections are important factors in reduction of infectious morbidity and mortality. Long-term risk of secondary malignancy in cancer survivors should be considered in patients with history of malignancy, especially following radiation therapy (33).

I. Other Systems

Musculoskeletal and cutaneous manifestations of primary and metastatic malignancy are not uncommon causes of morbidity (34,35). Skin eruptions, pigmentation abnormalities, nail problems, radiation recall, alopecia, and skeletal complications can result from chemotherapy and radiation therapy.

III. PERIOPERATIVE MANAGEMENT

Surgical intervention is often required in the treatment of malignancy. The indication for such intervention can include the need for tissue diagnosis, curative tumor excision, debulking, palliation, symptom relief, and intraoperative chemotherapy and radiation. The timing, urgency, and the extent and duration of the surgery have important implications for the perioperative management of these patients. Patients requiring emergency procedures are more likely to present with uncorrected metabolic dysfunction related to the malignancy and its therapy. Physiologic derangements from other comorbid conditions can compound the risks of perioperative morbidity (36).

A. Preoperative Evaluation

Evaluation of a patient presenting for surgery should consist of general medical history and physical examination, and a specific history related to their malignancy (Table 1). The physical examination should include a systematic assessment of all organ systems with particular attention to signs of malignancy-associated

Table 1 Preoperative Evaluation of Patient with Malignancy

Cancer-related history
General medical and surgical history Cancer history • Type of malignancy • Primary location and extent • Systemic spread • Time of diagnosis • Disease progression, relapse, recurrence • Symptoms related to the malignancy • Previous therapy—chemotherapy, radiation therapy, surgery • Results from the therapy and complications • Secondary malignancy

dysfunction. Laboratory and imaging studies should be based on the findings from the history and the physical examination. Integration of these findings will assist in diagnosis and staging, perioperative risk stratification, and perioperative management. The preoperative assessment is the foundation for important perioperative considerations reviewed here.

B. Perioperative Monitoring

The standards for basic anesthetic monitoring adopted by the American Society of Anesthesiologists should be applied. Additional monitoring could be indicated to maintain physiologic homeostasis or to provide early warning of worsening organ system function and to direct appropriate interventions. The benefits of selected monitors should be weighed against the inherent risks.

C. Airway

Cancer patients with tumors involving the head, neck, and mediastinum, may present with established or potential airway compromise. Perioperative airway management can be very challenging (37–39). Assessment of the airway by physical examination and appropriate imaging is of paramount importance. Patients with relatively large tumors may be asymptomatic. Attention to preoperative imaging studies may identify anatomical changes that can cause airway compromise with the induction of anesthesia or the use of positive pressure ventilation. Anticipated difficult airway issues require appropriate planning and preparation for management; alternative strategies should be planned as well. Unanticipated difficult airway management is also possible. Consideration of the available alternative strategies is likely more important in this setting. The airway may need to be secured preoperatively in patients with significant compromise. Elective tracheostomy should be considered in patients at high risk for perioperative airway compromise. Postoperative airway compromise can result from edema or hematoma in the laryngeal or cervical tissues. Head elevation and perioperative steroid administration may reduce the effects of edema formation. Prolonged endotracheal intubation is often prudent until airway patency is assured.

D. Pulmonary Function

The presence and the severity of pulmonary disease should be addressed by careful preoperative evaluation. Pulmonary dysfunction should be identified and any reversible component optimized. The intraoperative monitoring of respiratory function and anticipation of the need for postoperative ventilatory support are important considerations in patients with lung involvement. Lung protective strategies should be utilized when planning intraoperative and postoperative ventilation. For instance, the use of lower tidal volume ventilation and the maintenance of functional residual capacity with positive end expiratory pressure may reduce attributable pulmonary morbidity (40). Prior therapy with bleomycin or signs of lung toxicity may warrant ventilation with low inspired oxygen concentration.

E. Cardiovascular Function

Cardiac dysfunction resulting from malignancy, antineoplastic therapy, and pre-existing cardiovascular disease can complicate the management of cancer patients (41). Chronic or late onset cardiomyopathy following anthracycline chemotherapy may be insidious (42). Preoperative evaluation and optimization, followed by the use of appropriate intraoperative monitoring may avoid additional cardiovascular compromise. An anesthetic technique tailored to preservation of cardiac function may as well mitigate worsening cardiovascular function. Continuation or institution of additional appropriate cardiovascular monitoring in the postoperative course is essential.

F. Renal, Hepatic, and Metabolic Function

Renal and hepatic dysfunction should be assessed and optimized, as able, prior to surgical intervention. Perioperative renal or hepatic failure still carries significant mortality. The extent of dysfunction of these organ systems needs to be carefully evaluated and their effects on the perioperative management anticipated. Emphasis should be placed on utilizing organ protective strategies; avoid anesthetic and surgical techniques that may contribute to hypoperfusion or organ toxicity.

G. Fluids/Electrolytes/Blood Products

Preservation of fluid and electrolyte balance through appropriate replacement and maintenance is vital in the management of cancer patients. Preoperative assessment of fluid status may unveil symptoms and signs of fluid deficit or overload. Hematologic cytopenia and coagulopathy are common complications in cancer patients. This may result from bone marrow or hepatic dysfunction from tumor invasion or suppression from chemotherapy and/or radiation. Perioperative blood component therapy should be guided by clinical judgment considering the benefits and risks of such therapy (43,44). Intravascular access with its inherent risks can be challenging in the cancer patient (45).

H. Nutritional Management

Malnutrition in cancer patients has multiple etiologies and may contribute in various aspects to their morbidity. The assessment of the preoperative nutritional status and the planning for perioperative support merit careful attention (46).

I. Thrombosis Complications and Prophylaxis

Patients with cancer undergoing surgery are at particularly high risk for postoperative thrombotic complications (47). The incidence of these complications is related to the type of cancer, therapy, and the type of surgery. Perioperative thromboprophylaxis is a critical aspect of the care of theses patients (48).

J. Infection Prophylaxis

Infections in patients with malignancy remain one of the most serious complications (49). Relative or absolute immune suppression increases the risk for perioperative infection, especially from skin and gut flora, and opportunistic organisms. Appropriate antimicrobial prophylaxis should be started prior to surgical incision and continued into the early postoperative period in accordance with suggested perioperative regimen. The importance of infection prevention, and early diagnosis and treatment cannot be overemphasized in these patients.

K. Pain Management

Chronic cancer pain and its management often confound the effective perioperative management of acute pain. Drug tolerance and disordered nociception present therapeutic challenges in cancer patients. A comprehensive strategy should be formulated for acute perioperative pain management to include consideration of the chronic pain states that can be debilitating in cancer patients (50). Appropriate maintenance of chronic pain medications with additional coverage for incidental postoperative pain offers the best opportunity to achieve adequate pain control.

L. Wound Healing

Impaired wound healing in cancer patients is often multifactorial. Chemotherapeutic drugs and steroids can impair normal inflammatory processes inherent to wound healing. Adequate time for recovery of immune function following neoadjuvant chemotherapy reduces the effects on wound repair (37). Endocrine disorders such as hyperglycemia can also interfere with healing.

M. Postoperative Care Planning

Planning for the postoperative care of cancer patients requires recognition of the complex nature of their medical problems and should utilize a multidisciplinary approach. Comprehensive assessment of the needs of these patients should guide the need for care in a monitored unit or intensive care unit, appropriate ventilation and hemodynamic support, renal replacement, and other specialized monitoring.

REFERENCES

1. Pisters KMW, Rivera MP, Kris MG. Acute toxicities of cancer therapy. In: Groeger J, ed. Critical Care of the Cancer Patient. Mosby Year Book, Inc., 1991:1–12.
2. Hansen SW. Late effects after treatment for germ-cell cancer with cisplatin, vinblastine, and bleomycin. Danish Med Bull 1992; 39:391–399.
3. Pullerits J, Holzman R. Anaesthesia for patients with mediastinal masses. Can J Anaesth 1989; 36:681–688.
4. Swanepoel E, Apffelstaedt JP. Malignant pericardial effusion in breast cancer: terminal event or treatable complication? J Surg Oncol 1997; 64:308–311.
5. Russo P. Renal cell carcinoma: presentation, staging, and surgical treatment. Semin Oncol 2000; 27:160–176.
6. Von Hoff DD, Rozencweig M, Piccart M. The cardiotoxicity of anticancer drugs. Semin Oncol 1982; 9:23–33.
7. Steinherz LJ, Steinherz PG, Tan CT, Heller G, Murphy ML. Cardiac toxicity 4 to 20 years after completing anthracycline therapy. J Am Med Assoc 1991; 266: 1672–1677.
8. Doll DC, List AF, Greco FA, Hainsworth JD, Hande KR, Johnson DH. Acute vascular ischemic events after cisplatin-based combination chemotherapy for germ-cell tumors of the testis. Ann Intern Med 1986; 105:48–51.

9. Escalante CP, Manzullo E, Gollamudi SV, Bonin SR. Oncologic emergencies and paraneoplastic syndromes. In: Pazdur R, Cola LR, Hoskins WJ, Wagman LD, eds. Cancer Management: A Multidisciplinary Approach. Melville, NY: PRR, Inc., 2001:835–858.
10. Fisher DC, Sherril GB, Hussein A, Rubin P, Vredenburgh JJ, Elkordy M, Ross M, Petros W, Peters WP. Thrombotic microangiopathy as a complication of high-dose chemotherapy for breast cancer. Bone Marrow Transplant 1996; 18:193–198.
11. Kehlet H. The surgical stress response: should it be prevented? Can J Surg 1991; 34:565–567.
12. Weir HK, Thun MJ, Hankey BF, Ries LA, Howe HL, Wingo PA, Jemal A, Ward E, Anderson RN, Edwards BK. Annual report to the nation on the status of cancer, 1975–2000, featuring the uses of surveillance data for cancer prevention and control. J Natl Cancer Inst 2003; 95:1276–1299.
13. White P. Evaluation of pulmonary infiltrates in critically ill patients with cancer and marrow transplant. Crit Care Clin 2001; 17:647–670.
14. Stathopoulos GP, Dourakis SP, Perdicaris G, Promponas IE. Pleural effusion and pulmonary injury as an unusual complication to chemotherapy in non-small cell lung cancer patients. Oncol Rep 2000; 7:1311–1315.
15. Klein DS, Wilds PR. Pulmonary toxicity of antineoplastic agents: anaesthetic and postoperative implications. Can Anaesth Soc J 1983; 30:399–405.
16. Smith FE. Selected gastrointestinal difficulties in neoplastic disease. In: Smith FE, Lane M, eds. Medical Complications of Malignancy. John Wiley & Sons, Inc., 1984:73–90.
17. DeLeve LD. Hepatic venoocclusive disease: a major complication of hematopoietic stem cell transplantation in cancer patients. Tumori 2001; 87:S27–S29.
18. Zubler MA. Genitourinary complications of cancer. In: Smith FE, Lane M, eds. Medical Complications of Malignancy. John Wiley & Sons, Inc., 1984:45–72.
19. Fujikawa K, Yamamichi F, Nonomura M, Soeda A, Takeuchi H. Spontaneous rupture of the urinary bladder is not a rare complication of radiotherapy for cervical cancer: report of six cases. Gynecol Oncol 1999; 73:439–442.
20. Flombaum C. Electrolyte and renal abnormalities. In: Groeger J, ed. Critical Care of the Cancer Patient. Mosby Year Book, Inc., 1991:140–164.
21. Garzotto M, Beer T. Syndrome of inappropriate antidiuretic hormone secretion: a rare complication of prostate cancer. J Urol 2001; 166:1386.
22. Lynch EC. Disorders of erythrocytes. In: Smith FE, Lane M, eds. Medical Complications of Malignancy. John Wiley & Sons, Inc., 1984:161–206.
23. Alfrey CP, White MR, Zelnick PW. Abnormalities of white blood cells, platelets and hemostasis. In: Smith FE, Lane M, eds. Medical Complications of Malignancy. John Wiley & Sons, Inc., 1984:207–217.
24. Demetri GD, Vadhan-Raj S. Hematopoietic growth factors. In: Pazdur R, Cola LR, Hoskins WJ, Wagman LD, eds. Cancer Management: A Multidisciplinary Approach. Melville, NY: PRR, Inc., 2001:751–764.
25. Glassman AB. Hemostatic abnormalities associated with cancer and its therapy. Ann Clin Lab Sci 1997; 27:391–395.
26. Almeras C, Soussi N, Molko N, Azoulay-Cayla A, Richard F, Chartier-Kastler EJ. Paraneoplastic limbic encephalitis, a complication of the testicular cancer. Urology 2001; 58:105.
27. Liaw CC, Wang HM, Wang CH, Yang TS, Chen JS, Chang HK, Lin YC, Liaw SJ, Yeh CT. Risk of transient hyperammonemic encephalopathy in cancer patients who received continuous infusion of 5-fluorouracil with the complication of dehydration and infection. Anticancer Drugs 1999; 10:275–281.
28. Valentine A. Depression, anxiety and delirium. In: Pazdur R, Cola LR, Hoskins WJ, Wagman LD, eds. Cancer Management: A Multidisciplinary Approach. Melville, NY: PRR, Inc., 2001:765–778.
29. Ito J. Infectious complications. In: Pazdur R, Cola LR, Hoskins WJ, Wagman LD, eds. Cancer Management: A Multidisciplinary Approach. Melville, NY: PRR, Inc., 2001:859–887.
30. Brown AE. Neutropenia, fever and infection. Am J Med 1984; 76:421–428.
31. Meyers JD. Infection in bone marrow transplant recipients. Am J Med 1986; 81(suppl 1A):27–38.
32. Forman SJ. Hematopoietic cell transplantation. In: Pazdur R, Cola LR, Hoskins WJ, Wagman LD, eds. Cancer Management: A Multidisciplinary Approach. Melville, NY: PRR, Inc., 2001:701–714.
33. Patel SG, See AC, Williamson PA, Archer DJ, Evans PH. Radiation induced sarcoma of the head and neck. Head Neck 1999; 21:346–354.
34. Lynch GR. The skeletal system in malignancy. In: Smith FE, Lane M, eds. Medical Complications of Malignancy. John Wiley & Sons, Inc., 1984:91–105.
35. Levien MG. Osteonecrosis as a complication of treating acute lymphoblastic leukemia in children: a report from the Children's Cancer Group. Clin Pediatr 2002; 41: 63–64.
36. Kross R. Perioperative considerations. In: Groeger J, ed. Critical Care of the Cancer Patient. Mosby Year Book, Inc., 1991:320–333.
37. Lefor AT. Perioperative management of patient with cancer. Chest 1999; 115:165S–171S.
38. Gou MH, Liu XY, Gou YS. Anterior mediastinal masses: an anaesthetic challenge. Anaesthesia 1999; 54: 670–674.
39. Wessler MC. Management of complications resulting from laryngeal cancer treatment. Otolaryngol Clin N Am 1997; 30:269–278.
40. Brower RG, Rubenfeld GD. Lung-protective ventilation strategies in acute lung injury. Crit Care Med 2003; 31:S312–S316.

41. Sekine Y, Kesler KA, Behnia M, Brooks-Brunn J, Skeine E, Brown J. COPD may increase the incidence of refractory supraventricular arrhythmias following pulmonary resection for non-small cell lung cancer. Chest 2001; 120:1783–1790.
42. Shan K, Lincoff AM, Young JB. Anthracycline-induced cardiotoxicity. Ann Intern Med 1996; 125:47–58.
43. Van de Watering LMG, Brand A, Houbiers JGA, Kranenbarg WMK, Hermans J, van de Velde CJ. Perioperative blood transfusion with or without allogenic leucocytes, relate to survival, not to cancer recurrence. Br J Surg 2001; 88:267–272.
44. Blumberg N, Heal JM. Transfusion and host defenses against cancer recurrence and infection. Transfusion 1989; 29:236–245.
45. Walshe LJ, Malak SF, Eagan J, Sepkowitz KA. Complication rates among cancer patients with peripherally inserted central catheters. J Clin Oncol 2002; 20: 3276–3281.
46. Torosian MH. Nutrition and cancer. In: Bland KI, Daly JM, Karakousis CP, eds. Surgical Oncology Contemporary Principle and Practice. McGraw-Hill, 2001:473–479.
47. Casillas S, Nicholson J. Aortic thrombosis after low anterior resection for rectal cancer: report of a case. Dis Colon Rectum 2002; 45:829–832.
48. Rasmussen MS. Preventing thromboembolic complications in cancer patients after surgery: a role for prolonged thromboprophylaxis. Cancer Treat Rev 2002; 28:141–144.
49. Pursell KJ, Telzak EE. Infectious complications of neoplastic disease in the intensive care unit. In: Groeger J, ed. Critical Care of the Cancer Patient. Mosby Year Book, Inc., 1991:40–63.
50. Weinstein SM, Anderson PR, Yasko AW, Driver L. Pain management. In: Pazdur R, Cola LR, Hoskins WJ, Wagman LD, eds. Cancer Management: A Multidisciplinary Approach. Melville, NY: PRR, Inc., 2001: 715–737.

13

The Stress Response and Immunomodulation

A. C. CARR and GEORGE M. HALL

Department of Anaesthesia and Intensive Care Medicine, St. George's Hospital Medical School, London, U.K.

I. BACKGROUND

A stressor is a force or event that threatens to bring disequilibrium to the system it acts upon. In 1932, the Scotsman, Sir David Cuthbertson commenced a series of studies assessing calcium metabolism following long bone fractures (an example of a stressor). Compared with noninjured controls, he found that nitrogen, potassium, and creatinine excretion were significantly higher in injured patients. Furthermore, they were disproportionately greater than could be accounted for by traumatic tissue damage alone. He concluded that there was a systemic reaction to lower limb injuries with a breakdown of healthy skeletal muscle as part of this reaction (1).

Cuthbertson's work introduced the concepts of metabolic ebb and flow following injury. During the first 24 hr, an "ebb phase" occurred and readily available body energy stores were mobilized. This was followed by a "flow" phase with an initial catabolic period involving the breakdown of energy stores such as muscle and fat and a later anabolic period with recovery from the tissue injury and restoration of body fuel stores. These metabolic changes allow animals to survive periods of relative food deprivation following injury. By breaking down body tissues, they mobilize substrates until their injuries heal sufficiently to allow resumption of normal food gathering activities. Thus, the stress response to injury is a series of physiological changes intended to minimize the harmful effects of a stressor and ensure survival of the organism.

Ebb and flow as described by Cuthbertson are usually only found in under-resuscitated, trauma patients. During the 1950s, the stress response was further elucidated with the demonstration of rises in corticosteroid and catecholamine hormones following injury. This model remains highly applicable to most surgical patients. A neuronally conducted signal from the site of injury alters hypothalamic function which in turn activates the cortico-adrenal response. Prevention of the afferent input by neuronal transection (2) or disruption of normal hypothalamic function (3) negates the cortico-adrenal response. Additionally, activation of the sympathetic nervous system occurs and the resultant excess of catecholamines (4) together with cortisol results in a hypermetabolic state.

It is now recognized that the classical stress response model is overly simplistic. Complex metabolic and immunological changes occur following even minor elective surgical interventions and the evolutionary advantage in such circumstances is not always apparent. Research has been undertaken to characterize the effects of the stress response, identify the mediators, and introduce counter-measures to minimize the response. This chapter describes what is currently understood of the stress response to tissue injury and the associated changes that occur in the immune system, and how clinical practice may impact upon these physiological changes to the benefit or detriment of patients.

II. THE STRESS RESPONSE AND IMMUNOMODULATION

The metabolic and immunological changes that follow tissue injury are consequent to neuronal, endocrine, paracrine, autocrine, and inflammatory responses to tissue injury.

III. THE NEUROENDOCRINE STRESS RESPONSE AND SURGERY

Following surgical intervention, afferent sensory neuronal impulses are transmitted from the site of injury via the spinal cord and medulla to the hypothalamus. Stimulation of the hypothalamus causes both activation of the sympathetic nervous system and altered secretion of pituitary hormones. These changes and their subsequent effects are summarized in Fig. 1.

A. Corticotrophin Releasing Hormone

Corticotrophin releasing hormone (CRH) is a 41 amino acid neuropeptide (5) synthesized in the hypothalamus and also peripherally at sites of chronic inflammation (6). In addition to stimulating the release of adrenocorticotrophic hormone from the anterior pituitary and thus having secondary metabolic, immune, and largely anti-inflammatory modulating roles via the hypothalamic–pituitary–adrenal axis (see below), it also has direct immunomodulatory, pro-inflammatory roles. The latter may be mediated through the actions of peripherally released CRH (7); these include mast cell degranulation, increased vascular permeability (8), stimulation of leucocyte proliferation and cytokine release (7). Whether centrally released CRH has any pro-inflammatory role is unclear. Research in mice has suggested that CRH and endogenous catecholamines work independently, but synergistically, as pro-inflammatory mediators at the site of tissue injury and their pro-inflammatory effects may be modulated by the simultaneous release of glucocorticoids (9).

B. Pro-opiomelanocortin, Adrenocorticotrophic Hormone (ACTH) and β-Endorphin

Pro-opiomelanocortin is synthesized both within the hypothalamus and pituitary. It is primarily pituitary pro-opiomelanocortin which has been studied in the context of the stress response. Post-translationally, this pro-hormone is cleaved to generate a 39 amino acid peptide, ACTH; a 31 amino acid opioid peptide, β-endorphin; and α-, β-, and γ-melanocyte stimulating hormones (10).

ACTH release is under the influence of hypothalamic derived CRH which is itself regulated by afferent neural signals, cytokines such as interleukin-1 (IL-1) (11) and feedback control by both ACTH and CRH. ACTH concentrations in the blood rise within minutes of commencing surgery and act directly on the adrenal cortex stimulating release of cortisol and, to a lesser extent, aldosterone. The normal negative feedback of blood cortisol on ACTH release is temporarily lost resulting in high concentrations of both hormones. However, the concentration of ACTH returns to preoperative values within 6–8 hr of surgery whereas that of cortisol may remain elevated for several days (12).

In addition to their metabolic effects, ACTH and β-endorphin also have immunomodulatory effects. Lymphocytes and macrophages can express ACTH

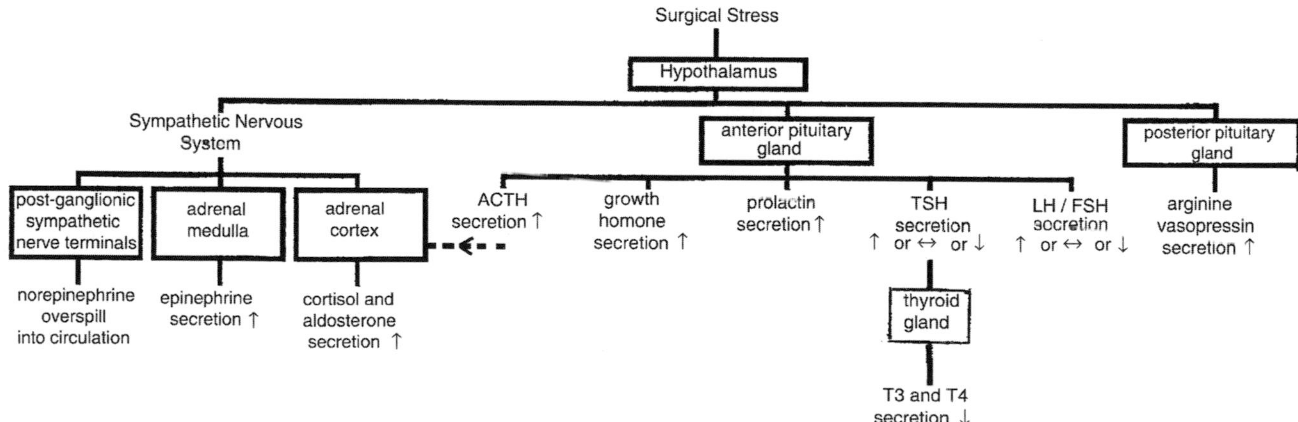

Figure 1 A simplified overview of the neuroendocrine response to surgical stress.

and opioid receptors. Beta-endorphin concentrations have been positively correlated with natural killer (NK) cell activity in patients with (13) and without (14) cancer but a relationship between β-endorphin and outcome following surgery has yet to be defined. Pro-opiomelanocortin itself is synthesized in certain cells of the immune system and immunoregulation may involve local, immunocyte-produced and pituitary-derived ACTH, and β-endorphin (15).

C. Cortisol

The peak concentration of cortisol occurs around 4–8 hr following the commencement of surgery and is dependent on the severity of surgical injury (16), appropriate functioning of the adrenal cortex, and the anesthetic techniques used (see later). In contrast to ACTH, the levels of cortisol may remain elevated for several days (12). The metabolic effects induce hyperglycemia with stimulation of glycogenolysis, lipolysis, protein breakdown, and hepatic gluconeogenesis (17) and simultaneous inhibition of peripheral glucose uptake by adipose tissue. Additionally, cortisol is necessary for catecholamines and angiotensin II to exert their normal actions upon the vasculature.

Immunologically, cortisol suppresses cell-mediated immunity. It induces T-cell progenitor-cell apoptosis and in models of endotoxaemic stress increases production of IL-10 (18) which suppress T_H1 cells (the class of T-helper cells which favor a cytotoxic rather than humoral immune response). Additionally, cortisol exerts potent anti-inflammatory effects.

The effects of cortisol on metabolism and immune function are summarized in Table 1.

D. Epinephrine and Norepinephrine

Epinephrine and norepinephrine concentrations rise rapidly following the commencement of surgery. Epinephrine is released from the adrenal medulla and norepinephrine "spills over" into the plasma following increased release from adrenergic nerve terminals. This results from reflex stimulation of the sympathetic nervous system and can be attenuated by afferent neural blockade of the operative site.

Table 1 Outline of the Metabolic, Anti-inflammatory, and Immunomodulatory Effects of Cortisol

Metabolic effects	Insulin resistance
	Reduced insulin production
	Increased glucagon production
	Increased hepatic gluconeogenesis
	Increased glycogenolysis
	Increased protein catabolism with increased circulating amino acids
	Increased lipolysis with increased free fatty acids and triglycerides
	Increased conversion of lactate to glycogen
	Increased sodium and water retention
	Up-regulation of catecholamine and angiotensin II receptors
Anti-inflammatory effects	Reduced circulating soluble phospholipase A_2
	Increased synthesis of lipocortins (phospholipase inhibitors)
	Reduced production of inducible cyclo-oxygenase II
	Reduced production of arachidonic acid and eicosanoids
	Reduced production of leukotrienes and prostacylcin E_1 and E_2
Immunomodulatory effects	T-cell progenitor apoptosis
	Inhibition of T-cell proliferation
	Inhibition of T_H1 and relative sparing of T_H2 helper-cell populations with suppression of cell-mediated immunity and relative preservation of humoral immune functions
	Inhibition of cell-mediated immunocytes with
	Inhibition of macrophage phagocytosis
	Inhibition of natural killer cells
	Inhibition of cytotoxic T-cells
	Altered cytokine production with tendency to reduced IL-1, IL-2, and IL-6 (pro-inflammatory interleukin) production and increased IL-10 (anti-inflammatory) production. The exact pattern of cytokine production is modified by actual cortisol concentration, the chronicity of the cortisol elevation and by other endocrine and cytokine responses to the stressor

Epinephrine and norepinephrine increase blood glucose values by stimulation of hepatic gluconeogenesis as well as glycogenolysis, lipolysis, and protein breakdown. They have antagonistic effects to those of insulin.

The sympathetic nervous system has direct effects on the immune system through its innervation of the spleen, thymus and lymph nodes and indirect effects via the actions of circulating catecholamines on immunocyte adrenoreceptors. Systemic effects are largely, but not exclusively (9) anti-inflammatory and include reduced production of pro-inflammatory cytokines such as IL-12 and TNFα and increased production of anti-inflammatory cytokines such as IL-10. This leads to a depression of cell-mediated immunity with reduced T-cell responsiveness to interleukin-2 (a T-cell stimulant) and reduced NK cell activity. In an experimental animal model, stress caused a reduction in NK cell-mediated immunity that was mediated by catecholamines, predisposed to increased tumor metastases and was reversible by sympathetic blockade (19).

E. Prolactin

Prolactin is a protein of 199 amino acids produced by anterior pituitary lactotroph cells. It is structurally related to growth hormone granulocyte-macrophage colony stimulating factor (GM-CSF) and interleukins (IL-2–IL-7) (20). Its concentration rises in response to the stress of surgery. In contrast to the other pituitary hormones, it is under dopaminergic inhibitory control by the hypothalamus which suppresses both its production and release. Additionally, it can be produced in T-lymphocytes (21). Although there is no obvious metabolic role for prolactin in the perioperative stress response, immunological roles have been documented in both human and animal studies.

In in vitro studies, prolactin has been shown to be a necessary comitogen in the induction of human T- and B-lymphocyte proliferation (22). Dopamine infusions reduce prolactin concentrations in critically ill patients and the responsiveness of mitogen-induced T-cell proliferation in these patients (23,24). It may also be a necessary comitogen for NK cells (25) and macrophages (26). Furthermore, prolactin appears to serve protective functions for T-cell progenitor cells against corticosteroid-induced apoptosis (27). A rise in glucocorticoid concentration can lead to immunosuppression via induction of T-cell progenitor population apoptosis. However, both in vitro (28) and in vivo (29) studies have demonstrated that prolactin can prevent apoptosis. This may be particularly important during stress-induced cortisol secretion. Although the normal development of the immune system in knock-out mice lacking a functional prolactin gene (30) led to claims that prolactin was unimportant immunologically, it is now apparent that if the knock-out mouse is stressed, prolactin does indeed have an immunomodulatory role (31). The clinical relevance of prolactin secretion to outcome following surgery is unknown.

F. Growth Hormone

Growth hormone or somatotrophin (GH) is a protein secreted from the anterior pituitary under the influence of growth hormone releasing hormone (GHRH) from the hypothalamus. Release is increased by surgical stress. Additionally, GH can be produced by cells of the immune system (32). It has a multitude of metabolic effects including stimulation of protein synthesis, lipolysis, glycogenolysis, and inhibition of peripheral glucose uptake.

Many of the actions of GH are mediated via insulin-like growth factors (IGF) which are synthesized in the liver in response to GH stimulation; IGF-1 exerts the greatest effect. There are several binding proteins which can sequestrate IGF-1 and the ratio of IGF-1/IGFBP-1 is used to assess the availability of bioactive peptide (33); IGF-1 can only exert an anabolic effect in its unbound form. Following surgery, the concentration of IGFBP-1 increases (34), whilst that of IGF-1 decreases or remains constant despite the rise in GH levels consequent to the neuro-endocrine stress response. This hepatic resistance to GH may be secondary to cytokine stimulation. Whatever the reason, the availability of active IGF-1 is decreased and the patient predisposed to protein catabolism. Insulin reduces the production of IGFBP-1 and thus increases the availability of active IGF-1 (34) and this may contribute to the anabolic effects claimed for high-dose insulin in the treatment of catabolic states.

Immunological roles have also been claimed for GH. In animal models, it stimulates proliferation of activated T-lymphocytes (35), and is necessary for normal functioning of NK cells and the phagocytic and cytotoxic activities of neutrophils and macrophages (36). It appears to have both anti-apoptotic and proliferative effects. Furthermore, under conditions of stress, GH may protect against cortisol-mediated immunosuppression by acting upon receptors expressed by lymphocytes (32). This effect may be autocrine, paracrine, or endocrine, depending upon the source of the GH mediating it.

G. Thyroid Stimulating Hormone

Concentrations of thyroid stimulating hormone (TSH) fall during the first few hours of surgery and then return to preoperative values. Simultaneously, concentrations of both active and bound T_3 fall and unlike TSH concentrations, they remain low for several days postoperatively. It is postulated that this protracted decrease may be secondary to the inhibitory effects of cortisol on T_3 secretion (37). Thyroid stimulating hormone may also have an immunomodulatory role as lymphocytes exposed to thyroid hormone releasing hormone in vitro can release TSH, suggesting an autocrine or paracrine role for it in lymphocyte function (38).

H. LH/FSH

The metabolic and imunomodulatory effects of LH, FSH, testosterone, oestrogen, and progesterone in the peri-operative period have not been well characterized.

Circulating testosterone in males and oestrogen in females decreases during surgery and remains low for several days (39,40). As testosterone and oestrogen tend to be immunosuppressive in their effects (41), this prolonged decrease may enhance immune function.

IV. INSULIN RESISTANCE

A characteristic of the neuroendocrine response is the development of hyperglycemia and insulin resistance in the peri-operative period. The resistance to insulin may be hepatic or peripheral; the latter usually predominates. In hepatic insulin resistance, normal or raised insulin concentrations fail to inhibit hepatic gluconeogenesis. In peripheral insulin resistance, normal or supranormal insulin concentrations fail to stimulate glucose uptake into the peripheral tissues, especially skeletal muscle. Following upper abdominal surgery, the sensitivity of peripheral tissues to insulin may decrease by 50% or more and can take up to three weeks to recover (42).

Insulin is a potent anabolic hormone secreted in response to a high circulating blood glucose. It normally suppresses hepatic gluconeogenesis and stimulates uptake of glucose in insulin-sensitive tissues such as skeletal muscle, and inhibits lipolysis and protein catabolism (including skeletal muscle) (43). The development of insulin resistance results in hyperglycemia, high circulating free fatty acids and urea values, together with a negative nitrogen balance (44).

It is often assumed that hyperglycemia after injury results from the acute rise in circulating catecholamines, cortisol, glucagons, and GH. Whereas these hormones have a key role in the early phase of the hyperglycemic response (45–49), the duration of insulin resistance and persistent hyperglycemia postoperatively usually exceeds that of the classical catabolic hormones.

Cytokines may have a role in promoting insulin resistance postoperatively. The onset of insulin resistance can parallel increasing plasma IL-6 concentrations (50), but causality has not been established. Correlation has also been established between the development of insulin resistance and increasing magnitude of surgery, duration of surgery and peri-operative blood loss (51). Furthermore, preoperative fasting and immobilization have been implicated in facilitating insulin resistance and preoperative administration of oral (52) or intravenous (53) carbohydrate solutions reduces postoperative insulin resistance. Features and association of insulin resistance are summarized in Table 2.

Table 2 Features and Associations of Postoperative Insulin Resistance

Postoperative insulin resistance is INCREASED by:	Postoperative insulin resistance is REDUCED by:	Postoperative insulin resistance is ASSOCIATED with:	Postoperative insulin resistance is NOT ASSOCIATED with:
Increasing duration of surgery	Laparoscopic rather than open surgery	Increased protein catabolism and muscle loss	Age
Increasing magnitude of surgery	Preoperative glucose infusions	Increased lipolysis with raised circulating free fatty acids	Body weight
Increasing magnitude of blood loss		Increased gluconeogenesis	
Preoperative fasting		Increased duration of hospital stay	
Postoperative hypocaloric intake			
Immobilization >24 hr postoperatively			

V. THE CYTOKINE AND ACUTE PHASE RESPONSES

In addition to the neurohumoral response to tissue injury, there is a separate and distinct local inflammatory response in the injured tissue. This response leads to systemic sequalae via the movement of local mediators into the systemic circulation.

A. Cytokines

Cytokines are a heterogenous group of soluble, low molecular weight polypeptides, and glycoproteins that act as chemical messengers between cells. Their functions are diverse and include cell growth, cell differentiation, inflammation, tissue repair, and regulation of the immune response. The majority of cytokines have multiple sources, in terms of cell types which produce and release them, as well as multiple target cells upon which a single cytokine may act.

Currently more than 200 cytokines have been identified. For convenience, certain cytokines may be classified as pro-inflammatory such as tumor necrosis factor α (TNFα) interleukin-1 (IL-1), interleukin-6 (IL-6) and interleukin-8 (IL-8) or anti-inflammatory such as interleukin-10 (IL-10), IL-1 receptor antagonist (IL-1 ra) and soluble TNF receptors (TNF-srI) also known as TNF binding proteins. Cytokines have high affinity for their receptors and relatively low occupancies can induce biological responses. These actions are usually autocrine or paracrine. However, with sufficient concentrations in the blood, endocrine effects may also occur.

At the time of incison and with subsequent trauma, local cell damage and lysis lead to activation of monocytes and macrophages with release of cytokines such as IL-1 and TNFα. These act upon endothelial cells and fibroblasts causing release of IL-6 and IL-8 (54). Other pro-inflammatory mediators such as prostaglandin E_2 are also released.

Production of cytokines is tightly regulated; in health only anti-inflammatory cytokines are measurable in appreciable concentrations in plasma. Pro-inflammatory cytokines generally have a short half-life (55) (0–20 min) and, in health, spillover into the systemic circulation is minimized by both the circulating anti-inflammatory cytokines and endothelial expressed glycosaminoglycans which bind and hold the cytokines close to their site of release.

The most widely studied cytokines in surgical stress are TNFα, IL-1, and IL-6. These molecules are key mediators of the innate immune response and are released from damaged epithelia, activated macrophages and leucocytes at the site of tissue trauma. Of these, TNFα and IL-1 are responsible for the nonhepatic acute phase responses of tachycardia and fever (56) and IL-6 is the major stimulant of the hepatic acute phase response, regulating the synthesis and release of the acute phase proteins (57). Additionally, these three cytokines also play a role in modulating adaptive immune responses, potentiating the transformation of naive T-helper cells into T_H1 cells. This favors a cellular, phagocytic, immuno-inflammatory response over a humoral, antibody mediated one. However, cortisol and the cytokines IL-4 and IL-10 secreted by T-suppressor cells, one of the few subsets of T-cells to increase in response to surgical stress, oppose these changes and simultaneously stimulate a T_H2 response favoring a humoral immune response (12).

Interleukin-6 is an early marker of tissue damage. Its circulating concentration rises to measurable values within 30–60 min of the commencement of surgery and, following major surgery, attains peak values at around 24 hr. The maximal concentration is proportional to the severity of the surgery (58), the duration of surgery (59), and the blood loss during surgery (59) and concentrations may remain elevated for several days postoperatively.

B. The Acute Phase Response

The acute phase response refers to the systemic changes that occur in an organism distant to the site of injury or inflammation and mediated through the action of cytokines and neuro-humoral changes (60). Although called the acute phase response, the systemic changes may be persistent and may also accompany chronic disease. The response involves changes in behavior, metabolism, biochemistry, and physiology as well as in plasma protein concentrations.

An acute phase protein is one whose plasma concentration rises or falls by at least 25% of the baseline value following the onset of an inflammatory disorder (61). The change in concentration is usually attributable to an alteration in the hepatic synthesis. The proteins act as inflammatory mediators, anti-proteinases and aid in tissue repair. One example is C-reactive protein (CRP) which binds to phospholipids within damaged cells and thereafter can both activate complement and bind to phagocytic cells resulting in the destruction of the damaged cell. Another example is immunosuppressive acidic protein (IAP). The mechanisms of IAP-mediated immunosuppression remain unresolved but it is known to rise during both the acute phase response and with tumor progression in certain malignancies where its production may correlate inversely with prognosis (62).

Table 3 Features of the Acute Phase Response

Acute phase proteins	↑ Complement C_3 and C_4
	↑ Transport and storage proteins
	Ceruloplasmin
	Ferritin
	↑ Coagulation proteins
	Fibrinogen
	Plasminogen
	Protein S
	↑ Inflammatory proteins
	CRP
	Soluble phospholipase A_2
	Granulocyte-colony stimulating factor
	↓ Concentration of
	Albumin
	Transferrin
	Insulin-like growth factor-1
CNS changes	Fever
	Anorexia
	Malaise
	Sleep disturbance
Endocrine changes	↑ CRH and ACTH secretion
	↑ Catecholamine secretion
	↑ Arginine vasopressin secretion
Metabolic changes	Protein catabolism with muscle wasting
	Lipolysis with loss of adipose tissue
	Changes in concentration of divalent cations
	↑ Copper
	↓ Zinc
	↓ Iron

source: From Ref. 60.

The purpose of the acute phase response is assumed to be the facilitation of the survival of the patient following exposure to a stressor. However, there are multiple facets to the response and it is not clear that all are beneficial in the setting of elective surgery. The features of the response are listed in Table 3.

VI. CELL-MEDIATED IMMUNITY

It has been recognized for over a decade that patients' immunocytes, especially those providing cell-mediated immune functions, can recognize and destroy autologous tumor cells (63). In order for this to occur, there must be sufficient differentiation from normal in the tumor cell to render it immunogenic and there must be normal functioning of cell-mediated immunity. However, tumor cells themselves may evolve; immunocyte-mediated tumor cell destruction can lead to the survival of only those cells which are least immunogenic such that the tumor then escapes immune control. It is thought that single cells moving into lymphocytes and blood vessels, and microdeposits of tumor out with the primary site, remain more susceptible to cell-mediated immunity than their primary counterparts and a variety of reasons for this have been described (64). Thus, whilst large primary tumors have clearly, by their existence, demonstrated escape from immune regulation, metastatic disease, at least in the early phases, may well be subject to immune control.

The importance of cell-mediated immunity in controlling micrometastatic disease is demonstrated in patients with organ transplants who receive immunosuppressive drugs. Although the rate of common de novo solid tumors is not significantly increased (65), there is an increased frequency of recurrence of previous tumors in patients believed disease free and a significantly higher rate of metastases in patients with active cancers (66). In animal studies, cytotoxic T-cells (CTC), natural killer (NK) cells, dendritic cells, and T-helper (T_H) cells have all been demonstrated to have a role in the reduction of tumor metastases. In human studies, efficacy of cell-mediated immunity at the time of tumor diagnosis has been found to be an independent predictor of disease-free survival (67).

In patients, intra-operative and postoperative suppression of cellular immunity occurs almost immediately. There are reductions in populations of T_H-inducer cells, CTC, NK cells and increases in populations of T-suppressor cells which secrete IL-4 and IL-10 which further suppress T_H1 cells and cell-mediated immunity. In comparison, T_H2 cells are relatively spared and the immunologic balance systemically shifts towards antibody-mediated, humoral immune function (12). It is possible that high levels of IL-6 and other inflammatory cytokines may preserve cell-mediated immunity at the site of injury. However, studies in animals have suggested that depression of cell-mediated immunity may predispose to both metastatic seeding (68) and an increase in tumor growth at the surgical site (69).

VII. MODULATING THE STRESS RESPONSE: WHY BOTHER?

Whereas knowledge of the metabolic and immunologic perturbations and responses to surgical trauma is of scientific interest, it has been argued that these represent complex evolutionary responses designed to increase survival after injury and as such, are best left undisturbed. Whereas there is some logic in these arguments, they ignore the fact that evolutionary responses to injury did not develop in anticipation of elective interventional surgical trauma with the benefits of techniques such as fluid resuscitation, ventilatory, renal and nutritional support. The use of such measures is proven to reduce morbidity and mortality in the peri-operative period. Attention has now turned to modulating the stress response per se rather than merely supporting the patient during the physiological upset associated with surgery. The challenge is to attenuate those aspects of the response which are believed potentially injurious to the patient such as the development of insulin resistance, the catecholamine surge, the catabolic state, and the suppression of cell-mediated immunity, whilst minimizing the risks of harming the patient through altering normal homeostatic mechanisms which allow thermoregulation, cardiovascular stability, and rapid wound healing.

VIII. ANESTHETIC AND CRITICAL CARE PERSPECTIVES

A. Feeding, Fasting, Insulin, Glycemic Control, and Immunonutrition in the Perioperative Period

The severity of postoperative insulin resistance has been found to correlate with duration of hospital stay in different types of surgery (51). Providing either oral or intravenous carbohydrates before surgery was found to reduce postoperative insulin resistance and continuation of carbohydrate intra-operatively also decreased the stress hormone response. This group also showed reductions in morbidity and mortality, and in the hormonal stress response, following exposure to hemorrhagic and endotoxaemic stressors in animals fed up to the time of injury rather than fasted for 24 hr.

In contrast, work in critically ill patients has demonstrated that use of insulin therapy to maintain blood glucose concentrations 80–110 mg/dL (4.4–6.1 mmol/L) led to a reduction in mortality of 42% during intensive care stay and an over-all reduction of in-hospital mortality of 34% when compared with patients whose blood glucose concentration was allowed to rise to 215 mg/dL (11.9 mmol/L) before insulin treatment was commenced (70). The patients with tight glycemic control also had lower morbidity with a reduction in blood stream infections, prolonged inflammation, acute renal failure requiring renal replacement therapy, critical illness polyneuropathy, and requirement for blood transfusion. Except for the reduction in acute renal failure requiring renal replacement therapy, these beneficial effects were attributed to good glycemic control and not the quantity of insulin administered (71). However, in a further analysis of the same study, it was found that the group receiving intensive insulin therapy also showed a significant reduction in acute phase response as assessed by CRP and mannose-binding lectin concentrations suggesting that an anti-inflammatory effect of the insulin itself may have contributed to the beneficial effects (72).

As well as carbohydrate drinks or infusions, studies have been undertaken to assess the benefits of preoperative and postoperative nutritional supplements by both parenteral and enteral routes on morbidity and mortality in the peri-operative period. In one major study assessing the use of peri-operative total parenteral nutrition (TPN), benefit was confined to those patients who had >15% body weight loss preoperatively and in the remainder of patients led to increased complications (73). However, in a more recent study of malnourished patients (>10% loss in usual body weight) with gastro-intestinal malignancy, the use of pre- and postoperative TPN was associated with significant reductions in both morbidity and mortality (74). Further studies are required to resolve the question whether only malnourished patients with malignancy benefit from TPN.

Studies assessing nutrition in cancer patients suggest a reduction in infectious complications, protein catabolism, and inflammatory markers with preoperative or early postoperative feeding. Enteral feeding may be superior to parenteral feeding in reducing the stress responses to surgery (75). The use of supplements to improve immunocyte function is thought to improve outcomes in postsurgical patients with malignancy but controversy exists on their use in critically ill patients. Recent reviews of TPN (76), enteral (77), immunonutrition (78) and nutrition in patients with cancer (79) cover these topics more comprehensively.

B. Sedative and Anesthetic Drugs

Benzodiazepines are increasingly recognized as having immunomodulatory actions mediated via the central nervous system (80). Although few clincial studies have been performed, there are some data to suggest that cytokine release in response to surgical stress may be reduced by midazolam (81).

Midazolam administered as a bolus followed by infusion has also been shown to reduce cortisol and insulin secretion during upper abdominal surgery (82) and to attenuate the epinephrine increase associated with minor surgery (83). The effect of midazolam on cortisol appears to be centrally mediated; patients receiving midazolam demonstrated no rise in ACTH or β-endorphin values with surgical stress and exogenously administered ACTH resulted in an appropriate incremental rise in cortisol concentration (83). In healthy volunteers, 20 mg of temazepam attenuated the peak ACTH and cortisol concentrations found in response to a bolus of intravenous corticorphin releasing hormone (84). However, studies assessing the effects of benzodiazepine as premedication have failed to demonstrate a consistent modulation of peri-operative pituitary–adrenal function (85,86).

Etomidate, a carboxylated imidazole, is an anesthetic induction agent formerly used as a sedative in intensive care units. Its use as a sedative in critically ill patients was found to be associated with a threefold increase in mortality (87,88). This increased mortality was subsequently attributed to a metabolic effect of etomidate; it reversibly inhibits 11-β-hydroxylase and cholestrol side-chain-cleavage enzyme (89), inhibiting the synthesis of cortisol and aldosterone in the adrenal cortex. Even a single induction dose may inhibit steroidogenisis in critically ill patients for 24 hr (90) and in surgical patients for 6–12 hr (91).

C. Regional Anesthesia

Epidural and spinal analgesia have been shown to modulate both the neuro-endocrine stress response and cellular immunity in the peri-operative period. With extensive preoperative epidural blockade corresponding to dermatomal segments from T_4 to S_5, somatic and autonomic afferent input from operative sites in the lower body is abolished and efferent output to the adrenal medulla and liver attenuated.

One facet of using neuraxial blockade to reduce the stress response is modulation of the hyperglycemic response. Epidural blockade during abdominal surgery in fasting patients attenuates the increase in circulating glucose (92). However, despite this, epidural analgesia does not prevent protein catabolism during the acute phase of surgery in either fasting patients (93) or those receiving i.v. glucose infusions (94).

Whereas no clinical studies have been undertaken assessing the effects of neuraxial blockade upon the incidence of tumor recurrence or metastases following surgery, animal work has suggested that there may be a significant reduction in the metastases-promoting effect of surgery when spinal analgesia is used concomitantly with general anesthesia (95). Unexpectedly, the data also suggested that spinal blockade depressed NK cell function even further than general anesthesia and surgery combined (95). This finding has been mirrored in human data associating a transient but significant reduction in NK cell and cytotoxic T-cell function in patients receiving epidural analgesia (96). The transience of the depressed function in the human study may have been related to the small dose of local anesthetic used allowing any drug effect to wear off during the period of the study. If the animal data suggesting a reduction in tumor metastases with spinal analgesia hold true in human subjects, it is possible that the reduction of the neuro-endocrine stress response to surgery is of greater immunomodulatory value than the transient reduction in cytotoxic immunity associated with central neuraxial blockade.

A meta-analysis of 141 trials including 9559 patients demonstrated a reduction in mortality of around 30% in the group of patients randomized to receive either spinal or epidural analgesia (with or without concomitant general anesthesia) (97). Neuraxial blockade reduced the risk of developing deep venous thrombosis by 44%, pulmonary embolism by 55%, pneumonia by 39%, and the need for blood transfusion by 50%. Unfortunately, it is difficult to know whether the benefits are solely attributable to neuraxial blockade or may be due in part to the avoidance of general anesthesia, in 56% of the trials, neuraxial blockade was given without concomitant general anesthesia. Furthermore, in trials where general anesthesia was administered to the neuraxial blockade group, differences existed in induction agents, inhalational agents, and opioids used. These may have been confounding factors.

There was no difference in reduction in mortality between spinal and epidural neuraxial blockade, although there was a greater reduction in the incidence of pneumonia in patients receiving thoracic epidural compared with lumbar epidural or spinal analgesia.

D. Beta-Adrenoceptor Blocking Drugs and Steroids

Beta-adrenoceptor blocking drugs are used to prevent the effects of the catecholamine "surge" during surgical stimulation and steroids may be prescribed to reduce cytokine production.

The increase in circulating catecholamines associated with surgery may be harmful in all, or certain subgroups of, patients. In addition to immunomodulatory effects and facilitation of insulin resistance and thus protein catabolism, catecholamines increase cardiac workload and oxygen consumption. In children with burns, the use of β-blockers is associated with decreases in oxygen consumption and protein catabolism (98). In patients with cardiac disease undergoing noncardiac surgery, a significant reduction in postoperative cardiac morbidity and mortality has been reported (99,100) although these findings have not always been replicated (101,102).

In patients with oesophageal cancer, both retrospective (103) and randomized prospective (104) studies have suggested that preoperative corticosteroids may attenuate postoperative pro-inflammatory cytokine responses and the incidence of organ failure. The retrospective study reported reductions in anastomotic leakage, duration of hospital stay, and major morbidity in the corticosteroid-treated patients. The randomized prospective study demonstrated a reduction in the incidence of organ failure and duration of postoperative ventilation, but failed to demonstrate any difference in long-term survival. Increased concentrations of anti-inflammatory IL-10 and reduced concentrations of pro-inflammatory IL-6 and IL-8 were reported following corticosteroid administration, corroborating results of earlier studies undertaken in human volunteers (105).

E. Analgesic Drugs

Opioids used in high doses are known to attenuate the neuroendocrine stress response during both cardiac surgery (pre-bypass) (106) and lower abdominal surgery (107). However, opioids also have potentially adverse immunomodulatory effects (108). Morphine has been shown to suppress NK cytotoxicity in healthy volunteers (109) and also to induce the expression of Fas (CD95) on human lymphocytes, potentially priming them for apoptosis (110). Endogenous opioids, released in higher quantities during the stress response, have pro-apoptotic effects on human neutrophils in vitro (111) and it is possible that exogenously administered opioids may have similar effects.

Clinically, these immunomodulatory effects may contribute to the increased susceptibility of heroin abusers to infectious diseases (112). In humans, morphine 10 mg, unlike tramadol 100 mg, was associated with a reduction of mitogen-induced T-cell proliferation two hours postoperatively (113). Whereas this single dose of morphine produced no significant decrease in NK cytotoxicity, tramadol actually enhanced NK cytotoxicity. This is in keeping with animal work which suggests that tramadol can act as an immunostimulant (114) and that it can reduce the incidence of tumor metastases attributed to surgically induced immunosuppression (115).

Nonsteroidal anti-inflammatory drugs (NSAIDs) also have immunomodulatory effects. In an animal model, prostaglandin antagonists alone (116) or in combination with β-blockers (117) have been associated with a reduction in surgically promoted tumor metastases. This may be due to a reduction in the production of prostaglandin E2, a suppressor of cell-mediated immunity (118).

F. Intraoperative Normothermia

Both general and regional anesthesia reduce the normal thermoregulatory mechanisms (119) and in the relative cold of an operating theatre, hypothermia can rapidly ensue. Hypothermia stimulates the stress response and causes elevations in circulating catecholamines and possibly glucocorticoids (120). It has been associated with an increase in postoperative wound infections, cardiac arrhythmias, and protein catabolism (119). The increase in wound infections may result from the immunomodulatory roles of mild hypothermia; mitogen-induced lymphocyte proliferation and concentrations of IL-1 and IL-2, but not IL-6 or TNFα, are reduced (121).

IX. SURGICAL PERSPECTIVES

A. Surgical Technique

Different surgical approaches to the same operative site result in variable degrees of tissue injury. This is exemplified in the comparison of open and laparoscopic abdominal surgical procedures. Laparoscopic surgery has been associated with a shorter hospital stay, a lower incidence of postoperative complications, earlier mobilization and a reduced duration of postoperative ileus (122). Nevertheless, it has been suggested that these benefits may be attributable to altered peri-operative care regimens associated with laparoscopic surgery rather than the surgical technique itself.

In general, laparoscopic abdominal surgery is associated with lower concentrations of cytokines, inflammatory markers, acute phase proteins, and less immunosuppression than the comparable open procedures (123). The neuro-endocrine response is not decreased to the same extent indicating similar stimulation of visceral afferent fiber activity. Nonetheless, some earlier studies found no diminution in the stress response using a laparoscopic approach (124,125).

As well as peri-operative care, other factors may confound the comparison of the stress and immunological responses attributed to open and laparoscopic techniques for surgery. The use of different gases within the peritoneal cavity to facilitate laparoscopy may lead to effects of the gas itself. Helium and carbon dioxide (CO_2) together with abdominal wall lifting alter abdominal wall oxygenation and cellular pH in the peritoneal cavity. This leads to differing effects on essential cell functions (126) and may influence immune and cytokine responses.

The immunological effects of laparoscopic surgery and open surgery on tumor progression differ. In an animal model of intra-abdominal tumor, laparoscopic surgery with CO_2 peritoneal insufflation showed an increased trend towards the development of lung metastases compared with the open laparotomy group (127). However, no difference in tumor growth or metastases to other organs was demonstrated and in a separate study laparotomy was associated with more lung metastases than CO_2 pneumoperitoneum (127). In a human study of laparoscopy vs. laparotomy for resection of rectal tumors, a trend to reduced local recurrence and distant metastases was reported with the laparoscopic technique (128). However, port-site metastases at the points of trochar insertion through the abdominal wall continue to be reported and are cited as a reason for avoiding laparoscopic tumor resections by many surgeons.

Large well-designed randomized studies of laparoscopic vs. open intra-abdominal tumor resections are needed before a firm conclusion can be reached regarding the metabolic and immune consequences of each technique.

B. Blood Transfusion

In 1973, Opelz et al. (129) reported that renal allograft survival was increased in the recipients of allogenic blood transfusions. A benefit persists even in patients receiving concomitant modern immunosuppressive therapies (130). This indicates a convincing immunosuppressive effect of blood transfusions, a phenomenon known as transfusion-associated immunomodulation (TRIM). Subsequent to Opelz's work, many studies have been undertaken to assess whether TRIM may lead to an increase in tumor recurrence, metastatic burden, and infection following surgery. Work has also been undertaken in critically ill patients suggesting an adverse effect of blood transfusions on morbidity and mortality (131).

There is reasonable evidence to suggest an association between allogenic blood transfusion and postoperative infection rate (132). However, the evidence associating tumor recurrence and allogenic blood transfusion is less clear; some retrospective observational studies suggest a link, whilst others, and the few randomized controlled studies available, refute one. Furthermore, linkage does not imply causality and may merely indicate that sicker patients with more advanced disease, who are more likely to develop tumor recurrence, are also more likely to receive a peri-operative blood transfusion. The available evidence suggests that a significant proportion of the TRIM effect is a result of the buffy coat and leucocytes in blood. Internationally, the trend is towards the use of buffy-coat poor, leucodeplete blood products; benefits have already been attributed to this in a retrospective comparative study (133). The current controversies and understanding of blood transfusion and its immunomodulatory effects have been concisely summarized in a recent review article by Blajchman (134).

REFERENCES

1. Cuthbertson DP. Observations on the disturbance of metabolism produced by injuries to the limbs. Q J Med 1932; 1:233–246.
2. Egdahl RH. Pituitary–adrenal response following injury to the isolated leg. Surgery 1959; 46:9–21.
3. Hume DM. The neuro-endocrine response to injury: present status of the problem. Ann Surg 1953; 138: 548–557.
4. Goodall M, Stone C, Haynes BW Jr. Urinary output of adrenaline and noradrenaline in severe thermal burns. Ann Surg 1957; 145:479–487.
5. Turnbull AV, Rivier C. Corticotropin-releasing factor (CRF) and endocrine responses to stress: CRF receptors, binding protein, and related peptides. Proc Soc Exp Biol Med 1997; 215:1–10.
6. Crofford LJ, Sano H, Karalis K, Friedman TC, Epps HR, Remmers EF, Mathern P, Chrousos GP, Wilder RL. Corticotropin-releasing hormone in synovial fluids and tissues of patients with rheumatoid arthritis and osteoarthritis. J Immunol 1993; 151: 1587–1596.
7. Karalis K, Muglia LJ, Bae D, Hilderbrand H, Majzoub JA. CRH and the immune system. J Neuroimmunol 1997; 72:131–136.
8. Theoharides TC, Singh LK, Boucher W, Pang X, Letourneau R, Webster E, Chrousos G. Corticotropin-releasing hormone induces skin mast cell degranulation and increased vascular permeability, a possible explanation for its proinflammatory effects. Endocrinology 1998; 139:403–413.
9. Karalis KP, Kontopoulos E, Muglia LJ, Majzoub JA. Corticotropin-releasing hormone deficiency unmasks the proinflammatory effect of epinephrine. Proc Natl Acad Sci USA 1999; 96:7093–7097.
10. Castro MG, Morrison E. Post-translational processing of proopiomelanocortin in the pituitary and in the brain. Crit Rev Neurobiol 1997; 11:35–57.
11. Borsody MK, Weiss JM. Alteration of locus coeruleus neuronal activity by interleukin-1 and the involvement of endogenous corticotropin-releasing hormone. Neuroimmunomodulation 2002–2003; 10:101–121.
12. Ogawa K, Hirai M, Katsube T, Murayama M, Hamaguchi K, Shimakawa T, Naritake Y, Hosokawa T, Kajiwara T. Suppression of cellular immunity by surgical stress. Surgery 2000; 127:329–336.
13. Heiny BM, Albrecht V, Beuth J. Correlation of immune cell activities and beta-endorphin release in breast carcinoma patients treated with galactose-

specific lectin standardized mistletoe extract. Anticancer Res 1998; 18:583–586.
14. Darko DF, Irwin MR, Risch SC, Gillin JC. Plasma beta-endorphin and natural killer cell activity in major depression: a preliminary study. Psychiatry Res 1992; 43:111–119.
15. Blalock JE. Proopiomelanocortin and the immune-neuroendocrine connection. Ann NY Acad Sci 1999; 885:161–172.
16. Nicholson G, Hall GM, Burrin JM. Peri-operative steroid supplementation. Anaesthesia 1998; 53:1091–1104.
17. Pilkis SJ, Granner DK. Molecular physiology of the regulation of hepatic gluconeogenesis and glycolysis. Annu Rev Physiol 1992; 54:885–909.
18. Van der Poll T, Barber AE, Coyle SM, Lowry SF. Hypercortisolemia increases plasma interleukin-10 concentrations during human endotoxemia—a clinical research center study. J Clin Endocrinol Metab 1996; 81:3604–3606.
19. Ben-Eliyahu S, Shakhar G, Page GG, Stefanski V, Shakhar K. Suppression of NK cell activity and of resistance to metastasis by stress: a role for adrenal catecholamines and beta-adrenoceptors. Neuroimmunomodulation 2000; 8:154–164.
20. Bazan JF. Haematopoietic receptors and helical cytokines. Immunol Today 1990; 11:350–354.
21. Pellegrini I, Lebrun J-J, Ali S, Kelly PA. Expression of prolactin and its receptor in human lymphoid cells. Mol Endocrinol 1992; 6:1023–1031.
22. Clevenger CV, Russell DH, Appasamy PM, Prystowsky MB. Regulation of IL-2 driven T-lymphocyte proliferation by prolactin 1990. Proc Natl Acad Sci 1990; 87:6460–6464.
23. Bailey AR, Burchett KR. Effect of low-dose dopamine on serum concentrations of prolactin in critically ill patients. Br J Anaesth 1997; 78:97–99.
24. Devin SS, Miller A, Herndon BL, O'Toole L, Reisz G. Effects of dopamine on T-lymphocyte proliferative responses and serum prolactin concentrations in critically ill patients. Crit Care Med 1992; 20:1644–1649.
25. Matera L, Cesano A, Bellone G, Oberholtzer E. Modulatory effect of prolactin on the resting and mitogen-induced activity of T, B and NK lymphocytes. Brain Behav Immun 1992; 6:409–417.
26. Bernton EW, Meltzer MS, Holaday JW. Suppression of macrophage activation and T-lymphocyte function in hypoprolactinaemic mice. Science 1988; 239:401–404.
27. Cidlowski JA, King KL, Evans-Storms RB, Montague JW, Bortner CD, Hughes FM Jr. The biochemistry and molecular biology of glucocorticoid-induced apoptosis in the immune system. Recent Prog Horm Res 1996; 51:457–490.
28. Witorsch RJ, Day EB, LaVoie HA, Hashemi N, Taylor JK. Comparison of glucocorticoid-induced effects in prolactin-dependent and autonomous rat Nb2 lymphoma cells. Proc Soc Exp Biol Med 1993 Sep; 203:454–460.
29. Krishnan N, Thellin O, Buckley DJ, Horseman ND, Buckley AR. Prolactin suppresses glucocorticoid-induced thymocyte apoptosis in vivo. Endocrinology 2003; 144:2102–2110.
30. Horseman ND, Zhao W, Montecino-Rodriguez E, Tanaka M, Nakashima K, Engle SJ, Smith F, Markoff E, Dorshkind K. Defective mammopoiesis, but normal hematopoiesis, in mice with a targeted disruption of the prolactin gene. EMBO J 1997 1; 16:6926–6935.
31. Dugan AL, Thellin O, Buckley DJ, Buckley AR, Ogle CK, Horseman ND. Effects of prolactin deficiency on myelopoiesis and splenic T lymphocyte proliferation in thermally injured mice. Endocrinology 2002; 143: 4147–4151.
32. Jeay S, Sonenshein GE, Postel-Vinay MC, Kelly PA, Baixeras E. Growth hormone can act as a cytokine controlling survival and proliferation of immune cells: new insights into signaling pathways. Mol Cell Endocrinol 2002; 188:1–7.
33. Brismar K, Hall K. Clinical applications of IGFBP-1 and its regulation. Growth Regul 1993; 3:98–100.
34. Nygren JO, Thorell A, Soop M, Efendic S, Brismar K, Karpe F, Nair KS, Ljungqvist O. Perioperative insulin and glucose infusion maintains normal insulin sensitivity after surgery. Am J Physiol 1998; 275:E140–E148.
35. Postel-Vinay MC, de Mello Coelho V, Gagnerault MC, Dardenne M. Growth hormone stimulates the proliferation of activated mouse T lymphocytes. Endocrinology 1997; 138:1816–1820.
36. Auernhammer CJ, Strasburger CJ. Effects of growth hormone and insulin-like growth factor I on the immune system. Eur J Endocrinol 1995; 133:635–645.
37. Desborough JP. The stress response to trauma and surgery. Br J Anaesth 2000; 85:109–117.
38. Kruger TE, Smith LR, Harbour DV, Blalock JE. Thyrotropin: an endogenous regulator of the in vitro immune response. J Immunol 1989 Feb l; 142:744–747.
39. Wang C, Chang V, Yeung RT. Effects of surgical stress on pituitary testicular function. Clin Endocrinol 1978; 9:255–266.
40. Woolf PD, Hamill RW, McDonald JV, Lee LA, Kelly M. Transient hypogonadotropic hypogonadism caused by critical illness. J Clin Endocrinol Metab 1985; 60:444–450.
41. Grossman CJ. Interactions between the gonadal steroids and the immune system. Science 1985; 227: 257–261.
42. Thorell A, Ljungqvist O, Efendic S, Gutniak M, Haggmark T. Insulin resistance after abdominal surgery. Br J Surg 1994; 81:59–63.
43. Nair KS, Adey D, Charlton M, Lijungqvist O. Protein metabolism in diabetes mellitus. Diab Nutr Metab 1995; 8:113–122.
44. Frayn KN. Hormonal control of metabolism in trauma and sepsis. Clin Endocrinol 1986; 24:577–599.
45. Uchida A, Asoh T, Shirasaka C, Tsuji H. Effect of epidural analgesia on postoperative insulin resistance

as evaluated by insulin clamp technique. Br J Surg 1988; 75:557–562.
46. Bessey PQ, Watters JM, Aoki TT, Wilmore DW. Combined hormonal infusion simulates the metabolic response to injury. Ann Surg 1984; 200:264–281.
47. Deibert DC, DeFronzo RA. Epinephrine-induced insulin resistance in man. J Clin Invest 1980; 65: 717–721.
48. Rizza RA, Mandarino LJ, Gerich JE. Cortisol-induced insulin resistance in man: impaired suppression of glucose production and stimulation of glucose utilization due to a postreceptor detect of insulin action. J Clin Endocrinol Metab 1982; 54:131–138.
49. Rizza RA, Mandarino LJ, Gerich JE. Effects of growth hormone on insulin action in man. Mechanisms of insulin resistance, impaired suppression of glucose production, and impaired stimulation of glucose utilization. Diabetes 1982; 31:663–669.
50. Thorell A, Essen P, Andersson B, Ljungqvist O. Postoperative insulin resistance and circulating concentrations of stress hormones and cytokines. Clin Nutr 1996; 15:75–79.
51. Thorell A, Nygren J, Ljungqvist O. Insulin resistance: a marker of surgical stress. Curr Opin Clin Nutr Metab Care 1999; 2:69–78.
52. Nygren J, Soop M, Thorell A, Efendic S, Nair KS, Ljungqvist O. Preoperative oral carbohydrate administration reduces postoperative insulin resistance. Clin Nutr 1998; 17:65–71.
53. Ljungqvist O, Thorell A, Gutniak M, Haggmark T, Efendic S. Glucose infusion instead of preoperative fasting reduces postoperative insulin resistance. J Am Coll Surg 1994; 178:329–336.
54. Elias JA, Lentz V. IL-1 and tumor necrosis factor synergistically stimulate fibroblast IL-6 production and stabilize IL-6 messenger RNA. J Immunol 1990; 145:161–166.
55. Bocci V. Interleukins. Clinical pharmacokinetics and practical implications. Clin Pharmacokinet 1991; 21:274–284.
56. Pullicino EA, Carli F, Poole S, Rafferty B, Malik ST, Elia M. The relationship between circulating concentrations of interleukin-6 (IL-6), tumor necrosis factor (TNF) and the acute phase response to elective surgery and accidental injury. Lymphokine Res 1990; 9:231–238.
57. Baumann H, Gauldie J. Regulation of hepatic acute phase plasma protein genes by hepatocyte stimulating factors and other mediators of inflammation. Mil Biol Med 1990; 7:147–159.
58. Cruickshank AM, Fraser WD, Burns HJG, Shenkin A. Response of serum interleukin-6 in patients undergoing elective surgery of varying severity. Clin Sci 1990; 79:161–165.
59. Ohzato H, Yoshizaki K, Nishimoto N, Ogata A Tagoh H, Monden M, Gotoh M, Kishimoto T, Mori T Interleukin-6 as a new indicator of inflammatory status: detection of serum levels of interleukin-6 and C-reactive protein after surgery. Surgery 1992; 111: 201–209.
60. Gabay C, Kushner I. Acute-phase proteins and other systemic responses to inflammation. N Engl J Med 1999; 340:448–454.
61. Morley JJ, Kushner I. Serum C-reactive protein levels in disease. Ann NY Acad Sci 1982; 389:406–418.
62. Takeuchi H, Maehara Y, Tokunaga E, Koga T, Kakeji Y, Sugimachi K. Prognostic value of preoperative immunosuppressive acidic protein levels in patients with gastric carcinoma. Hepatogastroenterology 2003; 50:289–292.
63. Uchida A, Kariya Y, Okamoto N, Sugie K, Fujimoto T, Yagita M. Prediction of postoperative clinical course by autologous tumour-killing activity in lung cancer patients. J Natl Cancer Inst 1990; 82:1697–1701.
64. Pantel K, Cote RJ, Fodstad O. Detection and clinical importance of micrometastatic disease. J Natl Cancer Inst 1999; 91:1113–1124.
65. Penn I. Posttransplant malignancies. Transplant Proc 1999; 31:1260–1262.
66. Detry O, Honore P, Meurisse M, Jacquet N. Cancer in transplant recipients. Transplant Proc 2000; 31:127.
67. McCoy JL, Rucker R, Petros JA. Cell-mediated immunity to tumour-associated antigens is a better indicator of survival in early stage breast cancer than stage, grade or lymph node status. Breast Cancer Res Treat 2000; 60:227–234.
68. Yakar I, Melamed R, Shakhar G, Shakhar K, Rosenne E, Abudarham N, Page GG, Ben-Eliyahu S. Prostaglandin e(2) suppresses NK activity in vivo and promotes postoperative tumor metastasis in rats. Ann Surg Oncol 2003; 10:469–479.
69. Eggermont AM, Steller EP, Marquet RL, Jeekel J, Sugarbaker PH. Local regional promotion of tumor growth after abdominal surgery is dominant over immunotherapy with interleukin-2 and lymphokine activated killer cells. Cancer Detect Prev 1988; 12:421–429.
70. Van den Berghe G, Wouters P, Weekers F, Verwaest C, Bruyninckx F, Schetz M, Vlasselaers D, Ferdinande P, Lauwers P, Bouillon R. Intensive insulin therapy in the critically ill patients. N Engl J Med 2001; 345: 1359–1367.
71. Van den Berghe G, Wouters PJ, Bouillon R, Weekers F, Verwaest C, Schetz M, Vlasselaers D, Ferdinande P, Lauwers P. Outcome benefit of intensive insulin therapy in the critically ill: insulin dose versus glycemic control. Grit Care Med 2003; 31:359–366.
72. Hansen TK, Thiel S, Wouters PJ, Christiansen JS, Van den Berghe G. Intensive insulin therapy exerts antiinflammatory effects in critically ill patients and counteracts the adverse effect of low mannose-binding lectin levels. J Clin Endocrinol Metab 2003; 88:1082–1088.
73. The Veterans Affairs Total Parenteral Nutrition Cooperative Study Group Perioperative total parenteral nutrition in surgical patients. N Engl J Med 1999; 325:525–532.

74. Bozzetti F, Gavazzi C, Miceli R, Rossi N, Mariani L, Cozzaglio L, Bonfanti G, Piacenza S. Perioperative total parenteral nutrition in malnourished, gastrointestinal cancer patients: a randomized, clinical trial. J Parenteral Enteral Nutr 2000; 24:7–14.
75. Takagi K, Yamamori H, Toyoda Y, Nakajima N, Tashiro T. Modulating effects of the feeding route on stress response and endotoxin translocation in severely stressed patients receiving thoracic esophagectomy. Nutrition 2000; 16:355–360.
76. Jeejeebhoy KN. Enteral and parenteral nutrition: evidence-based approach. Proc Nutr Soc 2001; 60: 399–402.
77. Wray CJ, Mammen JM, Hasselgren PO. Catabolic response to stress and potential benefits of nutrition support. Nutrition 2002; 18:971–977.
78. McCowen KC, Bistrian BR. Immunonutrition: problematic or problem solving? Am J Clin Nutr 2003; 77: 764–770
79. Bozzetti F, Gavazzi C, Mariani L, Crippa F. Artificial nutrition in cancer patients: which route, what composition. World J Surg 1999; 23:577–583.
80. Covelli V, Maffione AB, Nacci C, Tato E, Jirillo E. Stress, neuropsychiatric disorders and immunological effects exerted by benzodiazepines. Immunopharmacol Immunotoxicol 1998; 20:199–209.
81. Taupin V, Jayais P, Descamps-Latscha B, Cazalaa JB, Barrier G, Bach JF, Zavala F. Benzodiazepine anesthesia in humans modulates the interleukin-1 beta, tumor necrosis factor-alpha and interleukin-6 responses of blood monocytes. J Neuroimmunol 1991; 35:13–19.
82. Desborough JP, Hall GM, Hart GR, Burrin JM. Midazolam modifies pancreatic and anterior pituitary hormone secretion during upper abdominal surgery. Br J Anaesth 1991; 67:390–396.
83. Crozier TA, Beck D, Schlaeger M, Wuttke W, Kettler D. Endocrinological changes following etomidate, midazolam, or methohexital for minor surgery. Anesthesiology 1987; 66:628–635.
84. Korbonits M, Trainer PJ, Edwards R, Besser GM, Grossman AB. Benzodiazepines attenuate the pituitary–adrenal responses to corticotrophin-releasing hormone in healthy volunteers, but not in patients with Cushing's syndrome. Clin Endocrinol 1995; 43: 29–35.
85. Lindahl SG, Charlton AJ, Hatch DJ, Norden NE. Endocrine response to surgery in children after premedication with midazolam or papaveretum. Eur J Anaesthesiol 1985; 2:369–377.
86. Rodriguez-Huertas F, Carrasco MS, Garcia-Baquero A, Coq FD, Freire J. Changes in plasma cortisol and ACTH caused by diazepam, bromazepam, triazolam, and alprazolam in oral premedication [Spanish]. Revista Espanola de Anestesiologia y Reanimacion 1992; 39:145–148.
87. Watt I, Ledingham IM. Mortality amongst multiple trauma patients admitted to an intensive therapy unit. Anaesthesia 1984 Oct; 39:973–981.
88. Ledingham IM, Watt I. Influence of sedation on mortality in critically ill multiple trauma patients. Lancet 1983; 1:1270.
89. Wagner RL, White PF, Kan PB, Rosenthal MH, Feldman D. Inhibition of adrenal steroidogenesis by the anesthetic etomidate. N Engl J Med 1984; 310: 1415–1421.
90. Absalom A, Pledger D, Kong A. Adrenocortical function in critically ill patients 24 hr after a single dose of etomidate. Anaesthesia 1999; 54:861–867.
91. Wagner RL, White PF. Etomidate inhibits adrencortical function in surgical patients. Anesthesiology 1984; 61:647–651.
92. Please Refs. details.
93. Lattermann R, Carli F, Wykes L, Schricker T. Epidural blockade modifies perioperative glucose production without affecting protein catabolism. Anesthe siology 2002; 97:374–381.
94. Lattermann R, Carli F, Wykes L, Schricker T. Perioperative glucose infusion and the catabolic response to surgery: the effect of epidural block. Anesth Analg 2003; 96:555–562.
95. Bar-Yosef S, Melamed R, Page GG, Shakhar G, Shakhar K, Ben-Eliyahu S. Attenuation of the tumor-promoting effect of surgery by spinal blockade in rats. Anesthesiology 2001; 94:1066–1073.
96. Yokoyama M, Itano Y, Mizobuchi S, Nakatsuka H, Kaku R, Takashima T, Hirakawa M. The effects of epidural block on the distribution of lymphocyte subsets and natural-killer cell activity in patients with and without pain. Anesth Analg 2001; 92: 463–469.
97. Rodgers A, Walker N, Schug S, McKee A, Kehlet H, van Zundert A, Sage D, Futter M, Saville G, Clark T, MacMahon S. Reduction of postoperative mortality and morbidity with epidural or spinal anaesthesia: results from overview of randomised trials. BMJ 2000; 321:1493–1498.
98. Herndon DN, Hart DW, Wolf SE, Chinkes DL, Wolfe RR. Reversal of catabolism by beta-blockade after severe burns. N Engl J Med, 2001; 345: 1223–1229.
99. Poldermans D, Boersma E, Bax JJ, Thomson IR, van de Ven LL, Blankensteijn JD, Baars HF, Yo TI, Trocino G, Vigna C, Roelandt JR, van Urk H. The effect of bisoprolol on perioperative mortality and myocardial infarction in high-risk patients undergoing vascular surgery. N Engl J Med 1999; 341: 1789–1794.
100. Mangano DT, Layug EL, Wallace A, Tateo I. Effect of atenolol on mortality and cardiovascular morbidity after noncardiac surgery. N Engl J Med 1996; 335: 1713–1720.
101. Urban MK, Markowitz SM, Gordon MA, Urquhart BL, Kligfield P. Postoperative prophylactic administration of β-adrenergic blockers in patients at risk for myocardial ischaemia. Anesth Analg 2000; 90: 1257–1261.

102. Howell SJ, Foex P. Perioperative β-blockade: a useful treatment that should be greeted with cautious enthusiasm. Br J Anaesth 2001; 86:161–164.
103. Shimada H, Ochiai T, Okazumi S, Matsubara H, Nabeya Y, Miyazawa Y, Arima M, Funami Y, Hayashi H, Takeda A, Gunji Y, Suzuki T, Kobayashi S. Clinical benefits of steroid therapy in patients with oesophageal cancer. Surgery 2000; 128:791–798.
104. Sato N, Koeda K, Ikeda K, Kimura Y, Aoki K, Iwaya T, Akiyama Y, Ishida K, Saito K, Endo S. Randomized study of the benefits of preoperative corticosteroid administration on postoperative morbidity and cytokine response in patients undergoing surgery for oesophageal cancer. Ann Surg 2002; 236:184–190.
105. Van der Poll T, Barber AE, Coyle SM, Lowry SF. Hypercortisolemia increase plasma interleukin-10 concentrations during human endotoxaemia—a clinical research centre study. J Clin Endocrinol Metab 1996; 81:3604–3606.
106. Desborough JP, Hall GM. Modification of the hormonal and metabolic response to surgery by narcotics and general anaesthesia. Clin Anesthesiol 1989; 3:317–334.
107. Lacoumenta S, Yeo TH, Burrin JM, Bloom SR, Paterson JL, Hall GM. Fentanyl and the β-endorphin, ACTH and glycoregulatory hormonal response to surgery. Br J Anaesth 1987; 59:713–720.
108. Carr DJJ, Rogers TJ, Weber RJ. The relevance of opioids and opioid receptors on immunocompetence and immune homeostasis. Proc Soc Exp Biol Med 1996; 213:248–257.
109. Yeager MP, Colacchio T, Yu CT, Hildebrandt L, Howell AL, Weiss J, Guyre PM. Morphine inhibits spontaneous and cytokine-enhanced natural killer cell cytotoxicity in volunteers. Anesthesiology 1995; 83:500–508.
110. Yin D, Mufson A, Wang R, Shi Y. Fas-mediated cell death promoted by opioids. Nature 1999; 397:218.
111. Sulowska Z, Majewska E, Krawczyk K, Klink M, Tchorzewski H. Influences of opioid peptides on human neutrophil apoptosis and activation in vitro. Mediators Inflamm 2002; 11:245–250.
112. Brown SM, Stimmel B, Taub RN. Immunologic dysfunction in heroin addicts. Arch Intern Med 1974; 134:1001–1006.
113. Sacerdote P, Bainchi M, Gaspani L, Manfredi B, Maucione A, Terno G, Ammatuna M, Panerai A. The effects of tramadol and morphine on immune responses and pain after surgery in cancer patients. Anesth Analg 2000:1411–1414.
114. Sacerdote P, Bianchi M, Manfredi B, Panerai AE. Effects of tramadol on immune responses and nociceptive thresholds in mice. Pain 1997; 72:325–330.
115. Gaspani L, Bianchi M, Limiroli E, Panerai AE, Sacerdote P. The analgesic drug tramadol prevents the effect of surgery on natural killer cell activity and metastatic colonization in rats. J Neuroimmunol 2002; 129:18–24.
116. Colacchio TA, Yeager MP, Hildebrandt LW. Perioperative immunomodulation in cancer surgery. Am J Surg 1994; 167:174–179.
117. Rosenne E, Melamed R, Abudarham N, Ben-Eliyahu S. Attenuation of the immunosuppressive and metastasis-promoting effect of surgery by the combined use of B-adrenergic and prostaglandin antagonists [abstr]. Brain Behav Immun 2001; 15:180.
118. Ben-Eliyahu S. The promotion of tumour metastasis by surgery and stress: immunological basis and implications for psychoneuroimmunology. Brain Behav Immun 2003; 17:S27–S36.
119. Sessler DI. Mild perioperative hypothermia. N Engl J Med 1997; 336:1730–1737.
120. Frank SM, Higgins MS, Breslow MJ, Fleisher LA, Gorman RB, Sitzmann JV, Raff H, Beattie C. The catecholamine, cortisol, and hemodynamic responses to mild perioperative hypothermia. A randomized clinical trial. Anesthesiology 1995; 82:83–93.
121. Beilin B, Shavit Y, Razumovsky J, Wolloch Y, Zeidel A, Bessler H. Effects of mild perioperative hypothermia on cellular immune responses. Anesthesiology 1998; 89: 1133–1140.
122. Champault GG, Barrat C, Raselli R, Elizalde A, Catheline JM. Laparoscopic versus open surgery for colorectal carcinoma: a prospective clinical trial involving 157 cases with a mean follow-up of 5 years. Surg Laparosc Endosc Percutan Tech 2002; 12:88–95.
123. Nishiguchi K, Okuda J, Toyoda M, Tanaka K, Tanigawa N. Comparative evaluation of surgical stress of laparoscopic and open surgeries for colorectal carcinoma. Dis Colon Rectum 2001; 44:223–230.
124. McMahon AJ, O'Dwyer PJ, Cruikshank AM, McMillan DC, O'Reilly DS, Lowe GD, Rumley A, Logan RW, Baxter JN. Comparison of metabolic responses to laparoscopic and minilaparotomy cholecystectomy. Br J Surg 1993; 80:1255–1258.
125. Stage JG, Schulze S, Moller P, Overgaard H, Andersen M, Rebsdorf-Pedersen VB, Nielsen HJ. Prospective randomized study of laparoscopic versus open colonic resection for adenocarcinoma. Br J Surg 1997; 84:391–396.
126. Wildbrett P, Oh A, Naundorf D, Volk T, Jacobi CA. Impact of laparoscopic gases on peritoneal microenvironment and essential parameters of cell function. Surg Endosc 2003; 17:78–82.
127. Wildbrett P, Oh A, Carter JJ, Schuster H, Bessler M, Jaboci CA, Whelan RL. Increased rates of pulmonary metastases following sham laparotomy compared to CO_2 pneumoperitoneum and the inhibition of metastases utilizing perioperative immunomodulation and a tumor vaccine. Surg Endosc 2002; 16:1162–1169.
128. Lezoche E, Feliciotti F, Paganini AM, Guerrieri M, De Sanctis A, Campagnacci R, D'Ambrosio G. Results of laparoscopic versus open resections for non-early rectal cancer in patients with a minimum

follow-up of four years. Hepatogastroenterology 2002; 49:1185–1190.
129. Opelz G, Sengar DP, Mickey MR, Terasaki PI. Effect of blood transfusions on subsequent kidney transplants. Transplant Proc 1973; 5:253–259.
130. Opelz G, Vanrenterghem Y, Kirste G, Gray DW, Horsburgh T, Lachance JG, Largiader F, Lange H, Vujaklija-Stipanovic K, Alvarez-Grande J, Schott W, Hoyer J, Schnuelle P, Descoeudres C, Ruder H, Wujciak T, Schwarz V. Prospective evaluation of pretransplant blood transfusions in cadaver kidney recipients. Transplantation 1997; 63:964–967.
131. Hebert PC, Wells G, Blajchman MA, Marshall J, Martin C, Pagliarello G, Tweeddale M, Schweitzer I, Yetisir E. A multicenter, randomized, controlled clinical trial of transfusion requirements in critical care. Transfusion Requirements in Critical Care Investigators, Canadian Critical Care Trials Group. N Engl J Med 1999; 340:409–417.
132. Vamvakas EC, Blajchman MA. Deleterious clinical effects of transfusion associated immunomodulation: fact or fiction? Blood 2001; 97:1180–1195.
133. Hebert PC, Fergusson D, Blajchman MA, Wells GA, Kmetic A, Coyle D, Heddle N, Germain M, Goldman M, Toye B, Schweitzer I, vanWalraven C, Devine D, Sher GD. Leukoreduction Study Investigators. Clinical outcomes following institution of the Canadian universal leukoreduction program for red blood cell transfusions. JAMA 2003; 289:1941–1949.
134. Blajchman MA. Immunomodulation and blood transfusion. Am J Therap 2002; 9:389–395.

14

Inflammation, Coagulation, and Endothelial Dysfunction: Implications in Perioperative Care

RAVI TANEJA

Department of Anesthesia and Perioperative Medicine, London Health Sciences Centre, University of Western Ontario, London, Ontario, Canada

DAVY C. H. CHENG

Department of Anesthesia and Perioperative Medicine, London Health Sciences Centre, St. Joseph's Health Care, University of Western Ontario, London, Ontario, Canada

I. INTRODUCTION

The perioperative care of an oncology patient involves consideration of various complex issues. Besides having to confront a host of social and emotional aspects, the patient often faces a torrent of investigations and interventions in the hospital leading up to the perioperative period. It is the prime responsibility of the health care team to optimize organ function and aim for physiological homeostasis in an attempt to improve postoperative outcome.

A variety of factors may affect the ability of the patient to elicit appropriate immune responses in the perioperative period (Table 1). The process and significance of the host response to various perioperative insults is still poorly understood. However, the last two decades of research into inflammatory responses to surgery and critical illness have not only shed light on pertinent cellular and biological mechanisms but also have been portal to many a new paradigm. Most of our current understanding of these complex issues arises from lessons learnt in critical care, and this section reviews these and the possible therapies that may be of benefit to patients in the perioperative period.

II. INFLAMMATION

> The literature on inflammation is infinite, its complete utilization can only confuse, not assist.
>
> —*Vogen, 1842*

During good health, homeostasis is maintained in the face of a constantly changing external environment. Injurious stimuli evoke various responses in host tissues—inflammation, neoplasia, and even cellular regeneration. Inflammation, in particular, is fundamental to the survival of an organism not only for defense against a noxious stimulus like infection or tissue injury but also as a mechanism to repair damaged tissues. The process is characterized by local release of vasoactive mediators that facilitates influx of cells of the adaptive innate immune system, in particular, macrophages and polymorphonuclear cells. The inflammatory microenvironment, fuelled by an

Table 1 Factors Influencing Altered Immune Responses in the Perioperative Period in the Oncology Patient

Preoperative	Intraoperative	Postoperative
Immunosuppression	Stress response to surgery	Primed immune system
Chemotherapy	Tissue injury	Organ dysfunction
Radiotherapy	Endothelial dysfunction	Mechanical ventilation
Neutropenia	Blood loss + associated blood transfusion	Infections
	Hypothermia	Malnutrition
Infections	Coagulopathy	Lack of enteral nutrition
Bacterial, viral, fungal	Effects of anesthetic drugs	Idiopathic
	Inadequate oxygen delivery	Excessive inflammation
	Inadequate oxygen uptake	Immunosuppression/paralysis
Malnutrition	Genetic	Immunosuppressive drugs
Hypovolemia		ARDS/MODS
Inadequate intake		Genetic
Excess losses		
Concurrent disease		
Genetic		

agglomeration of pro- and anti-inflammatory cytokines, not only promotes phagocytosis of invading organisms but also tissue repair. Finally, the interaction of host phagocytic cells and invading microorganisms triggers a yet poorly understood sequence of events that results in termination of the acute nonspecific inflammatory response.

Whilst defects in the co-ordinated expression of inflammatory response render the host vulnerable to infection, acute inflammation may also result in significant local tissue injury (1,2). Host phagocytic cells (predominantly neutrophils and macrophages) and their soluble products play a central role in both containment of the insult and the ensuing tissue injury (2). Ample experimental data implicate the neutrophil in the injury to organs such as the lung (3,4), liver (5), intestine (6), and kidney (7) and the increased vascular permeability that accompanies acute inflammation (8). The critical role of neutrophil activation in sepsis is underlined by studies in mice with targeted deletion of Src-family kinases (*hck* and *fgr*) resulting in defects of PMN adhesion: despite high levels of proinflammatory cytokines TNF-α and IL-1β, the knock out mice have increased survival following endotoxin challenge, and show little of the liver or kidney injury seen in wild type animals (7). Therefore, termination of an inflammatory response may be as important to the host as is its activation in the first place.

The most compelling reason for exaggerated inflammatory responses to achieve notoriety in modern medicine has been their association with the multiple organ dysfunction syndrome (MODS). For a full understanding of MODS, the most formidable sequel of systemic inflammation, it would be imperative to go over its evolution in perioperative and critical care medicine.

A. MODS—A Historical Perspective and Current Concepts

Early in the last century, physiological dysfunction of any organ system was a terminal event. Remote organ failure was probably first encountered during World War II, when resuscitation from hypovolemic shock was followed by renal and hepatic dysfunction. The 1960s provided frequent reports of organ failure remote from the site of surgery (9–11), trauma (12,13), and overwhelming infection (14–16). It was only with the development of intensive care units that the perception of organ failure secondary to acute illness came to light. Although overwhelming infection seemed to be the most common characteristic of sequential/progressive organ failure, it was soon brought about that the characteristic clinical findings in sepsis (fever, leukocytosis, and hyperdynamic shock) could manifest without demonstrable infection. Further validation of this concept came from reports that it was the presence of a septic response (17) and organ failure (18,19) rather than mere infection, which influenced outcome from critical illness. A variety of host mechanisms for multiple organ failure were illustrated and these included the gastrointestinal tract and translocation of endotoxin as well as humoral mediators like interleukins-1, 6, and 10, TNF, prostaglandins, activated complement, growth hormone, and oxygen radicals.

Multiple organ dysfunction syndrome is the leading cause of morbidity and mortality in the contemporary ICU. It presents as a progressive derangement of organ systems not originally involved in the disease and may occur as a sequel to infection, ischemia, tissue injury, and acute inflammation—all processes associated with the incongruous host immune responses (5–11). A myriad of cellular and biological abnormalities have been identified in patients with MODS and their very number have made it difficult, if not impractical, to identify a single process as a common pathophysiological basis of this complex disorder (Table 2). Moreover, critically ill patients in the ICU, who seem to be the unrivaled recipients of the systemic inflammatory response, represent a heterogeneous group of patients and commonly have diseases that cause direct organ injury. Although presence of infection commonly heralds an inflammatory response, it is not yet proven if it is the infection per se or the host response to it that is responsible for the clinical manifestations at the bedside. Moreover, infections can be identified in only up to 40% patients with MODS leading us to dispute its precise role in the pathogenesis of this syndrome. Techniques such as selective decontamination of the digestive tract (SDD) show a striking reduction in the rates of infection such as pneumonia and wound infection but a much more modest reduction in mortality (20,21). Infections such as pneumonia and peritonitis are frequent causes of MODS but successful treatment of either does not seem to alter outcome.

Both epidemiological (16,17,22–25) and mechanistic studies (26–28) support the hypothesis that systemic inflammation leads to organ dysfunction. Consistent with the model of MODS as the result of excessive inflammation, organ dysfunction in the experimental animal can be induced by the administration of proinflammatory cytokines (29,30), activation of inflammatory cells, particularly neutrophils and macrophages (3,31–34), alterations in regulatory T cell populations (35), or targeted deletion of counterinflammatory genes such as transforming growth factor-β (TGF-β) (36). There are literally hundreds, if not thousands, of physiological abnormalities, changes in levels of biochemical markers, and abnormalities of cellular morphology or function that have been identified in critically ill patients with MODS. Many of these have been proposed to be useful markers of the presence, severity, or course of sepsis and have been evaluated to ascertain their association with clinically relevant outcomes. However, although it is readily demonstrable that most correlate with an increased risk of mortality in sepsis, it is much less clear how we should interpret them, what specifically we are trying to measure, and what the properties of a valid marker should be.

Lipopolysaccharide or endotoxin levels have been shown to be consistently elevated in both human and animal models of sepsis; however, all clinical trials with antiendotoxin therapies have failed (37). Nitric oxide, the endothelial derived releasing factor, is responsible for vasodilatation in severe sepsis and its levels correlate with elevated endotoxin and organ failure scores (38,39): its modulation by selective NOS inhibitors has been disappointing (40,41). Interleukin-1β and TNF-α have been implicated in the inflammatory response (42–44) but effects of their antagonism have been merely modest (45–50). Whilst a detailed description of rationale for failure of these immunomodulatory therapies is beyond the scope of this text, many hypotheses have been proposed—ineffective drugs, inadequate doses of drugs, lack of comparable inclusion criteria, heterogeneous patient population, and limited insight into pathophysiology.

Table 2 Conceptual Models of Multiple Organ Dysfunction Syndrome

Pathological process	Manifestations	Therapeutic interventions
Uncontrolled infection	Persistent infection, nosocomial infections, endotoxemia	Aggressive use of antibiotics, source control measures
Systemic inflammation	Cytokinemia (particularly IL-6, TNF), leukocytosis, increased capillary permeability	Neutralization of specific cytokines (IL-1β, TNF, PAF)
Immune paralysis	Increased anti-inflammatory (TH2) response, anergy, loss of macrophage expression of MHC class II, apoptosis induced loss of CD4 T, B, dendritic cells	G-CSF, interferon
Tissue hypoxemia	Increased lactate	Augmentation of DO_2
Microvascular coagulopathy, endothelial activation	Increased procoagulant activity, increased thrombomodulin, decreased APC	Increase anticoagulant mechanisms (APC, TFPI, antithrombin III)
Gut–liver axis	Increased infection with gut organisms, endotoxemia, Kupffer cell activation	Enteral feeding, selective decontamination of the digestive tract

Source: From Ref. 155.

B. SIRS—A Unifying Concept?

One of the most challenging issues has been to identify those patients who may be manifesting systemic effects of inflammation at the bedside. The cardinal signs of local inflammation are calor (heat), rubor (redness), dolor (pain) tumor (swelling), and functio laesa (loss of function). The extent of inflammation is intuitively a reflection of both the inciting stimulus and the host response to it. Extension of a localized process would be expected to have systemic effects like pyrexia, malaise, myalgia, increased production of leukocytes, and other acute phase proteins. Early recognition would allow a rational basis for the development of novel approaches to anti-inflammatory therapy that may help limit the deleterious sequelae of acute inflammation. It is with this rationale that the American College of Chest Physicians and the Society of Critical Care Medicine coined a term "systemic inflammatory response syndrome (SIRS)" in 1992 (51). The need for such a definition arose from the recognition that the clinical manifestations of infection were frequently encountered in the ICU but were not specific for it. Thus, SIRS was thought to represent the clinical manifestations of inflammation and was proposed as a concept and not a diagnosis on which to base therapy.

Although meant for both clinicians and investigators alike, both the terminology and the philosophy have been disputed over the years (52–54). Few epidemiological studies (55–58) have been able to substantiate the concept with conclusive evidence. None of the studies have been able to relate biological changes in patients with SIRS, thus failing to emphasize that SIRS does indeed reflect a host response to inflammation. As an entity, when applied to patients with possible infection or inflammation, it remains overly sensitive and very poorly specific. The concept of SIRS has achieved notoriety only while receiving criticism; nonetheless, it inscribed an era by raising awareness to noninfectious causes of MODS. Inflammation, in its most severe life threatening form, is certainly thought to present the same clinical features as classic gram-negative bacteremia. It is this latter manifestation of a "high cardiac output/low systemic vascular resistance state" that the clinician intensivist often identifies as a *systemic inflammatory response* (Fig. 1). Therapeutic management at this stage remains entirely supportive; restoration of organ perfusion and source control of infection remain prime therapeutic objectives.

The archetypal doctrine that inflammation is a "double-edged sword" has stood the test of time. While its critical role in wound healing cannot be denied, the dogma of disproportionate inflammatory responses and their modulation remains intriguing. Diagnostic markers and prognostic measures play a critical role in clinical research to facilitate an understanding of pathophysiology and to facilitate therapeutic decisions in all areas of medicine. In systemic inflammation, as it presents at the bedside, the problem has been an excess of potential markers and a lack of a systematic approach to evaluating their potential utility.

III. COAGULATION

Until recently, most derogatory effects of systemic inflammation were presumed to reflect an uncontrolled and extensive release of proinflammatory mediators and aberrations in coagulation were thought of as epiphenomena intertwined in its complex networks. However, in this rapidly evolving field, it has now emerged that coagulopathy and endothelial dysfunction are inextricably linked with inflammation. Traditionally, the coagulation cascade was divided into the intrinsic, extrinsic, and common pathways (Fig. 2a). The intrinsic pathway was activated after exposure of blood to negatively charged surfaces leading to recruitment of factors XI, IX, platelet factor 3, factor VIIIa, and calcium. Exposure of blood to membrane bound tissue factor, on the other hand, initiated the extrinsic pathway through factor VIIa. The common pathway, beginning with the activation of factor X, proceeded to convert prothrombin (factor II) to thrombin (factor IIa) and then fibrinogen to fibrin. Based on this schema, all individual components of the clotting cascade are distinctive in their function and any aberration in any one of these systems would lead to coagulopathy. Nevertheless, research in the 1990s has shown this was not the case—the extrinsic system seems to "initiate" the coagulation cascade and the intrinsic system functions effectively to "amplify" that response.

Under normal conditions, tissue factor (TF), a transmembrane protein, is not exposed to peripheral blood or endothelial cells. Disruption of endothelium or challenge with endotoxin/cytokines (59) stimulates monocytes and leukocyte derived microparticles to express TF (60,61). Tissue factor activates factor VII and IX (Fig. 2b), which in turn catalyzes activation of factor X and then thrombin. Once formed, thrombin activates factors V, VIII, and IX in the intrinsic pathway (Fig. 2c), thus increasing its own formation in a positive feedback loop. Under physiological conditions, tissue factor pathway inhibitor (TFPI) tightly regulates TF pathway activation (62). Even though TFPI rapidly inactivates factor TF/VII/thrombin induced coagulation via the extrinsic pathway, the briefest of TF induced thrombin activation is enough for

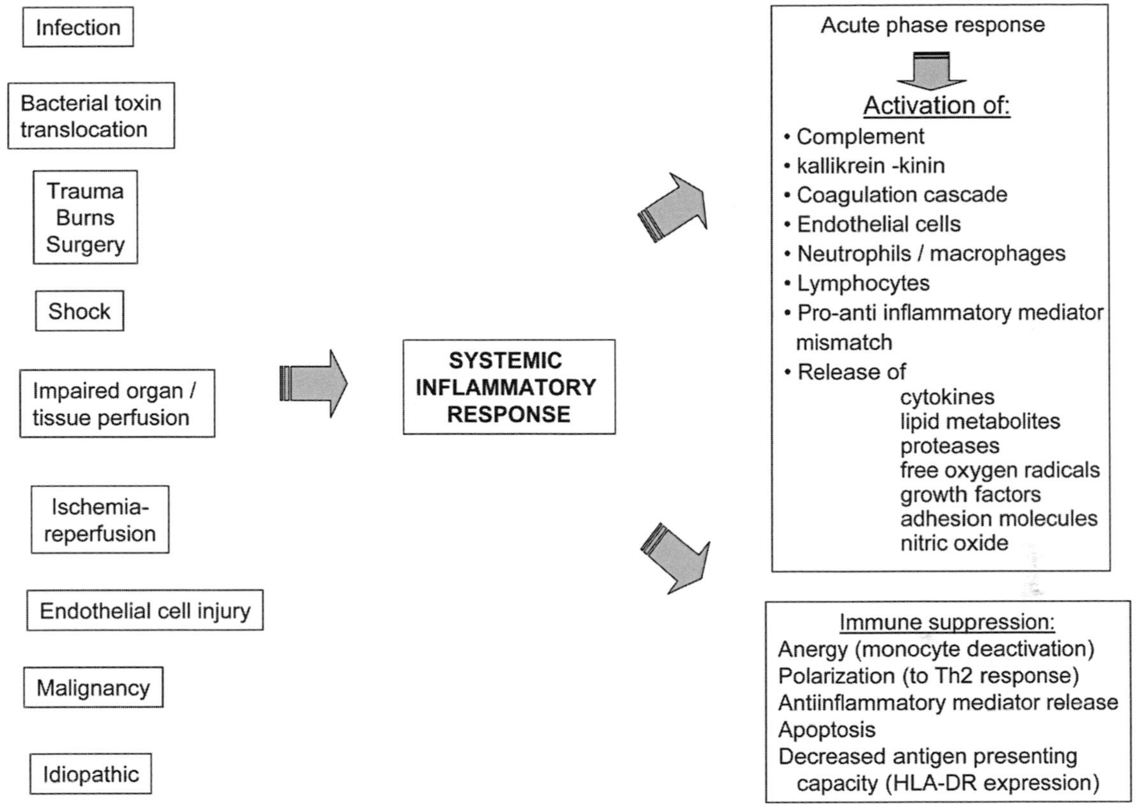

Figure 1 Schematic representation of etiological and biological manifestations of a systemic inflammatory response.

amplifying the procoagulant process through the intrinsic pathway.

Central to the coagulation cascade is thrombin, with its diverse biological influences (63): (1) it is mitogenic for fibroblasts and macrophages; (2) it triggers platelet activation with concomitant release of vasoactive substances and growth factors; (3) it activates endothelial cell responses like factor VIII and platelet activating factor (PAF) release; (4) it propagates inflammatory responses by increasing endothelial cell P-selectin expression and increasing monocyte chemotaxis and adhesion; and (5) it manifests both pro- and anticoagulant effects by enhancing and inhibiting its own effects (vide infra).

A. Regulatory Mechanisms and Interactions with Inflammation

Thrombin formation is maintained at low levels and restricted to wound sites through a series of tightly regulated anticoagulant systems. The procoagulant actions of thrombin are kept in fine balance by the three principal anticoagulant systems (Fig. 2d). Antithrombin III (a serine protease inhibitor) inhibits the common pathway (factor Xa and IIa activation), intrinsic (factor XIIa, XIa, and IXa) (64) and complexes with TFPI to inhibit the extrinsic pathway (65). Tissue factor pathway inhibitor is produced by endothelial cells and monocytes and inhibits activated factor X and the factor VIIa/TF complex in the extrinsic pathway. By far the most distinct anticoagulant system in the last few years has been the thrombomodulin/protein C pathway. This pathway is initiated when thrombin binds to an endothelial cell surface protein, thrombomodulin (TM) (66,67). The reaction acts as a switch to convert the procoagulant thrombin to an anticoagulant by proteolizing protein C to activated protein C (APC). Once bound to TM, the thrombin can no longer catalyze fibrin formation, platelet and factor XIII activation (68). The APC, in concert with protein S, promotes fibrinolysis by inactivating factors Va and VIIIa and thus limits downstream production (69).

Inflammation leads to a procoagulant state: proinflammatory cytokines (24,70,71) increase expression of TF and inhibit the expression of endothelial protein C receptor (72) and TM (73) on the endothelium. Increased levels of C4 binding protein (an acute phase protein) in sepsis may cause a relative deficiency of protein S thereby predisposing to an increased procoagulant response (74). Neutrophils, in the presence of TNF-α, induce the release of TM from the endothelial

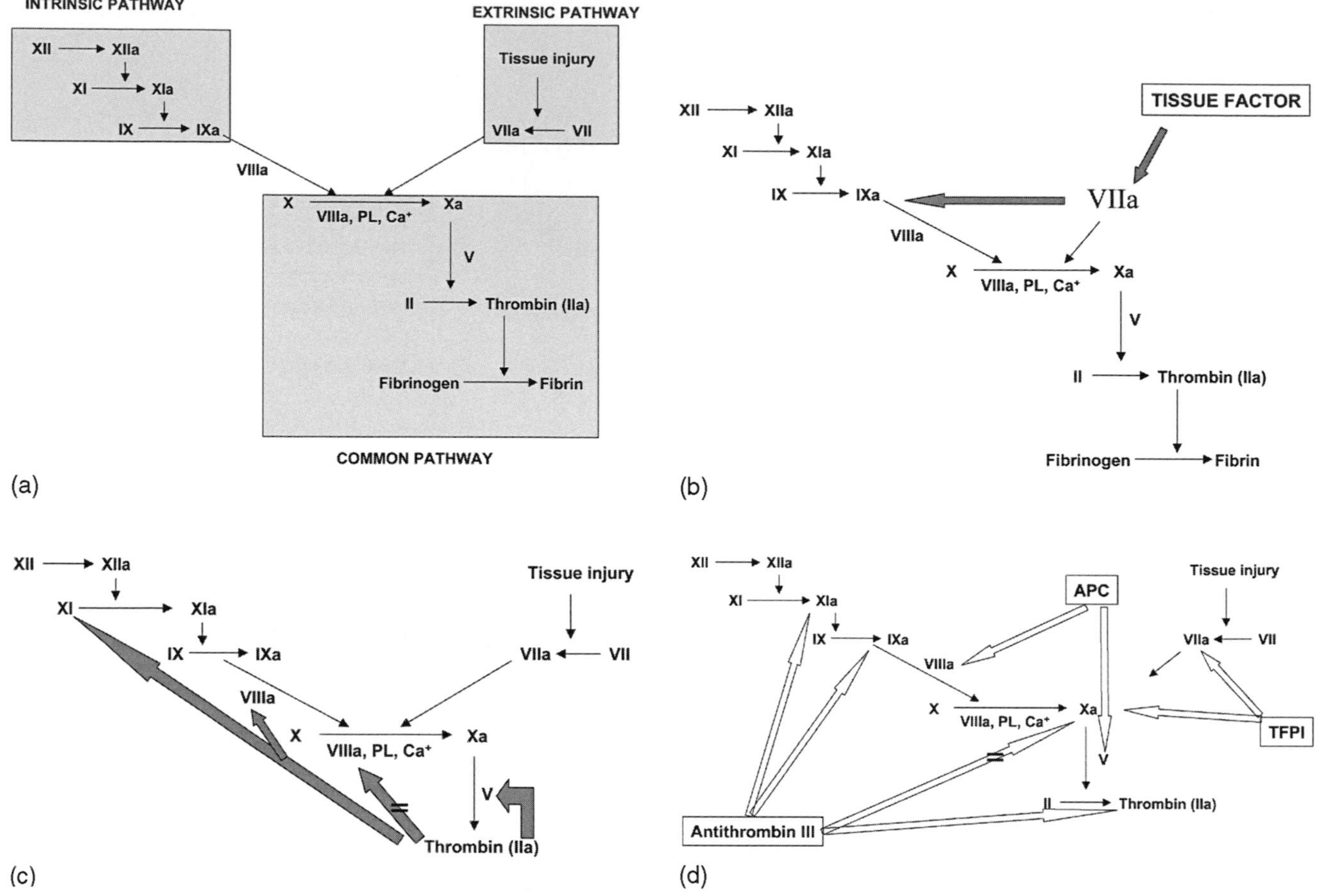

Figure 2 (a) The classic coagulation cascade. (b) The revised pathway. Tissue factor induced activation of the extrinsic pathway "initiates" the process and "amplifies" the procoagulant signal through the intrinsic pathway; once formed, thrombin acts in a positive feedback loop (c). (d) The regulatory anticoagulant mechanisms (see the text for details). ▬▶= activation; ▭▷= inhibition.

surface (75) and reduced levels of protein C are commonly found in patients with sepsis and MODS (76,77). To add to the complexity of the paradigm, induction of clotting heralds a proinflammatory response: thrombin induces P- and E-selectin, PAF, and PMN–endothelial interactions (vide supra), reduced protein C levels effect cytokine release and neutrophil adherence (78), and reduced antithrombin III results in loss of prostacyclin synthesis and increased leukocyte adherence (79,80).

For the critically ill patient, the biological pathways of inflammation and coagulation are intimately interrelated. Inflammation propagates coagulation and a procoagulant response in turn has the potential to amplify proinflammatory signals and augment tissue injury. Microvascular thrombosis has the potential for microembolization, redistribution of flow, intravascular pooling, arterio-venous shunting, tissue hypoxia, and eventually organ dysfunction.

IV. ENDOTHELIAL DYSFUNCTION: A *CHEF D'OEUVRE PAR EXCELLENCE*

The innermost layer of blood vessels, intima, lines the vessel lumen and is in direct contact with the blood. It is composed of endothelial cells supported by extracellular matrix and loose connective tissue. The endothelial cells are 0.2–0.3 μm thick, and are cobblestoned in a single layer of squamous epithelium, with intercellular clefts between them. The endothelium is far from an inert lining of the blood vessels and under normal physiological conditions, endothelial cells play a crucial role in maintaining homeostasis:

- Inhibition of coagulation via expression of TM (81), potentiation of antithrombin III and TFPI by cell surface proteoglycans (82,83), and synthesis of tissue plasminogen activator (tPA).
- Formation of prostacyclin, which inhibits platelet aggregation (84).

- NO synthesis that modulates vascular smooth muscle relaxation (85), TF (86), and cytokine gene expression (87).
- Expression of adhesion molecules, recruitment of leukocytes, and facilitating transmigration to prerequisite sites (88–90).

Various forms of endothelial cell impairment (91) may occur even though these terms have been used synonymously in the literature. Endothelial *injury* refers to microscopically visible endothelial cell damage or defects in continuity of cell lining. Endothelial *dysfunction*, on the other hand, occurs when there is decreased endothelial—dependent NO and constitutive nitric oxide synthase (cNOS) release, a state distinctly induced by inflammatory mediators such as bradykinin, histamine, and thrombin (92). Tumor necrosis factor-alpha can increase NO production by stimulating the iNOS pathway in a calcium independent manner (93) and the resultant drop in blood pressure is well documented in sepsis and MODS (94). The most well accepted function of the endothelium has been to act as a portal for the leukocytes to migrate to various body tissues. The process comprises three distinct steps: rolling, adhesion, and transmigration (extravasation), and each of these is facilitated by interaction of complementary molecules present on both leukocytes and endothelium (95). An increased expression or release of these endothelial adhesion molecules results from endothelial *activation*.

A multitude of factors may influence this fine balance of homeostasis. Tumor necrosis factor can induce endothelial cell apoptosis (96) and it is well accepted that activated neutrophils can cause endothelial damage via production of elastase and oxygen free radicals (97,98). Intracellular adhesion molecule-1 levels are raised in sepsis and correlate with the degree of MODS (99) and ischemia–reperfusion models of ICAM-1 knockout mice have decreased incidence of organ injury (100) and death (101). While quiescent endothelium asserts anticoagulant properties, activation of inflammation induced TF release is associated with decreased membrane bound TM and release of inactive TM in the blood. Circulating TM antigen is, therefore, a marker for endothelial injury and its levels are prognostic for organ dysfunction and death (102). Activated protein C, produced via activation of thrombin–thrombomodulin complex blocks p53-mediated apoptosis in ischemic human brain endothelium and is proposed to be neuroprotective (103). A recent study in post-trauma patients has shown that the incidence of ARDS and MODS is higher in those patients who develop DIC and DIC scores show good correlations with peak levels of sICAM-1, sVCAM-1, neutrophil elastase, and sThrombomodulin (104).

The size and extent of vascular endothelium in the human body is simply enormous. The endothelial lining of the vascular tree is heterogeneous in both structural and functional aspects. The endothelial cells vary in different sites of the body with respect to production of surface binding glycoproteins, protein expression, fibroblast growth factor (FGF), and the vascular endothelial growth factor (VEGF) (105,106). Functionally, TFPI (107) is most abundant in the microvascular endothelium and TM (108) is expressed in all vascular beds except that of the brain. Knockout mice with severely reduced capacity to generate APC exhibit increased thrombosis in specific organs (109). Both the intact and activated endothelium have organ specific expression of adhesion molecules in vivo and this again highlights diverse phenotype and raises awareness of complex host response in critical illness (110). It will indeed be crucial to determine if any specific patterns of host response to inflammation exist and relate to morbidity and mortality (111,112).

V. THERAPEUTIC INTERVENTIONS

The greatest challenge in the management of any disease in modern medicine would be an admissible diagnosis and nowhere else has this been more pertinent than for the patient with an altered immune response. As physicians tending for the acutely ill patient in the perioperative period, we cannot yet revel in our ability to recognize the consequences of a host immune response, let alone in our exploits to modulate it. Most therapeutic strategies in use today have been revolved around preserving physiological homeostasis while the initial insult and its crippling effects recede. While there may be enough evidence for augmenting a host response in chemotherapy induced neutropenia, no such "magic bullets" exist in the critically ill patient. Few clinical trials in the field of severe sepsis and MODS have been unequivocal in the last decade and they indeed reflect translation of research from bench to bedside. We feel it is appropriate to highlight recent Level 1 evidence here as it applies to MODS patients in the adult intensive care unit.

A. Activated Protein C

Patients with severe sepsis were enrolled in a double-blind placebo-controlled multicentre trial and recombinant human APC was associated with an absolute reduction of 6.1% in all cause 28-day mortality ($p = 0.005$) (113). The trial represents a milestone in adult critical care medicine and has been scrutinized ubiquitously. It brings forth many compelling questions—what are the effects of this drug in less seriously ill patients with lower APACHE scores (currently under investigation) and why is this antithrombin drug effective while its contemporaries (AT III, TFPI, and PAF receptor antagonists) are not (114–116). A major risk with APC is the incidence of hemorrhage (3.5%). Although, in the clinical trial, the study drug was stopped 1 hr prior to and up to 12 hr post-major surgery, use of this drug during the perioperative period or in patients who have been on any anticoagulant has not yet been well defined. Much has to be learnt about the use of APC and for now although its biological activity is associated with lower levels of IL-6 and d-dimers, it should not be used when there is an associated coagulopathy or marked thrombocytopenia (platelets $< 30{,}000$) (117,118).

Decreased protein C levels in patients with septic shock are associated with a poor outcome. An intriguing development has been the discovery of factor V Leiden mutation that makes the activated form of factor V relatively resistant to degradation by APC. This, in turn, causes resistance to APC (119–121). Recent studies suggest that factor V Leiden mutation is associated with an increased risk of venous thromboembolism, a common occurrence in cancer patients (122). Whether these patients are more susceptible to the development of MODS in the perioperative period is not yet known, but it is quite likely that phenotypical evaluation of such inherited disorders will need to be established in order to make progress in perioperative care.

B. Oxygen Delivery

The concept of supranormal oxygen delivery came into vogue in the late 1980s when it was noted that physiological patterns of high-risk postoperative patients were significantly better in survivors as compared to nonsurvivors. It was deemed that the observed increases in cardiac indices and $\dot{D}_{O2}$ seen in survivors were compensatory responses to improve tissue oxygenation that could be reflected in the pattern of oxygen consumption (123). These supranormal values achieved in survivors then provided objective therapeutic goals for critically ill patients in the perioperative period with good results (124,125). Although augmentation of supranormal $\dot{D}_{O2}$ via vasoactive drugs, fluids or blood transfusions in sepsis has not resolved outcome issues in intensive care, maintenance of $\dot{D}_{o2}$ at supranormal levels may be associated with better outcome in high-risk surgical patients (126,127).

C. Optimal Fluid Management

A recent Cochrane review (128) has concluded that invasive methods of fluid optimization during surgery for proximal femoral fractures may shorten hospital stay, but its effects on longer-term outcomes are uncertain. Although many techniques of invasive monitoring and optimization have been described, it is not yet entirely clear whether it is the fluids, inotropes (like dobutamine), or intensive monitoring that confers greatest benefit. The transfusion requirements in critical care (TRICC) trial (129) quite dramatically suggested that critically ill patients have a significantly worse prognosis if they are managed with a liberal transfusion strategy to maintain a hemoglobin level of 10–12 gm/dL. Patients in the restricted transfusion group (Hb 7–9 gm/dL) had a significantly lower hospital mortality; this was particularly pronounced in patients who were younger (<55 years) and less acutely ill (APACHE II score ≤ 20) but not amongst those who had significant cardiac disease. Ironically, the higher mortality in the liberal transfusion group was associated with adverse cardiac events like pulmonary edema and myocardial infarction, although not in the 48 hr preceding death.

While the threshold for red blood cell transfusions has consistently fallen both in the OR and ICU in the last few years, a liberal fluid transfusion policy has assumed an ever-important role during perioperative care. Most intensivists now resort to fluids (crystalloids or colloids) during resuscitation in the perioperative period, in an effort to maintain peripheral perfusion and minimize derangements in pH, base deficits, and lactate concentrations. A recent study by Rivers et al. (130) demonstrates that early aggressive therapy that optimized cardiac preload, contractility, and afterload improves outcome in severe sepsis and septic shock. Probably, the most valuable lesson from the study is "early" goal directed therapy. Not only do prompt therapeutic interventions seem crucial, institution of simple guidelines for fluid management does also hold promise in management of such patients.

D. Corticosteroids

High-dose steroids in septic shock were dismissed more than 10 years ago, when it was shown that their administration was associated with increased mortality (131). However, recent work by Annane et al. (132) suggests that such patients may have adrenocortical insufficiency and that low-dose hydrocortisone and fludrocortisone were safe and associated with decreased vasopressor requirement and improved survival. An intriguing finding in the study was association of corticosteroids with increased mortality in those patients who did not manifest adrenocortical suppression. Although low-dose steroids seem to be gaining a stronghold in the therapeutic armamentarium against septic shock, much needs to be done to better delineate the role of steroids in systemic inflammation.

E. Insulin Therapy

Hyperglycemia, common during the perioperative period, has often been ascribed to stress response. A recent randomized, controlled study (133) conducted on mechanically ventilated patients has suggested that maintenance of blood glucose levels (at 80–110 mg/dL or 4.4–6.1 mmol/L) is beneficial in comparison to conventional blood glucose management (180–200 mg/dL or 10–11.1 mmol/L). The authors found that intensive insulin therapy was associated with decreased mortality, bacteremia, and organ dysfunction, albeit in a surgical patient population. It was proposed that hyperglycemia per se was associated with impaired neutrophil and monocyte function (134–136) and axonal dysfunction and degeneration. Insulin may have direct anabolic effects on respiratory muscles (137), and thus may have a role in preventing critical illness polyneuropathy although it seems to be the glycemic status rather than the insulin that may be important (138). The study highlights the importance of simple and economical measures of improving outcome in ventilated patients in a surgical ICU setting. It is yet to be seen if such benefits extend to nonsurgical patients and if there is a role for pursuing normoglycemia rigorously during the intraoperative period.

F. Lung Protective Strategy

This hallmark multicentre randomized trial compared traditional ventilation (tidal volumes 12 mL/kg and a plateau pressure $\leq$50 cm H_2O) with low tidal volumes (6 mL/kg; plateau pressures $\leq$30 cm H_2O) in ARDS patients (139). In spite of higher requirements of PEEP and resulting lower P/F ratios, low tidal volume strategy was associated with lower mortality, increased ventilator free days, and lower IL-6 levels.

It is now generally accepted that we should try to prevent excess lung stretch in ALI (acute lung injury) or ARDS and use tidal volumes in the range of 6–8 ml per predicted body weight. Whether this has implications intraoperatively in preventing ALI/ ARDS is not yet known. New therapies like high frequency oscillatory ventilation (HFOV) (140) may hold promise in patients with ALI or ARDS.

VI. INFLAMMATION AND CARCINOGENESIS

Inflammation may have complex interactions with tumor formation and development. Infections with *Helicobacter pylori* have been linked with adenocarcinoma of the stomach. Although the precise mechanism is not understood, it is hypothesized that *H. pylori* results in a chronic inflammatory response through activated macrophages that help form nitrosamines from nitrates. Similarly, for mechanisms that are again poorly understood, hepatitis B and C viruses have been implicated in hepatocellular carcinoma; Epstein–Barr virus in Burkitt's lymphoma and human papilloma viruses appear to be chief etiological agents in cervical cancer. Chronic irritation due to ill fitting dentures is well known to lead to oral cancers and mutant *ras* transgenic develop squamous papillomas at sites of injury (141).

Chemical irritants such as phorbol esters cause cellular proliferation and increased production of reactive oxygen species by many cell types, with resulting oxidative DNA damage and structural anomalies in protein/lipid structure that may promote carcinogenesis. DNA damage may occur under normal physiological conditions as well; normally these cells would undergo repair or apoptosis to prevent further propagation, processes that may be impaired in the inflammatory milieu. Leukocytes may contribute to tumor angiogenesis (142,143) and prevention of their infiltration by IL-10 may prevent tumor growth (144). In fact, macrophages may produce angiogenic factors such as FGF, VEGF, TGF-β, and prostaglandins. Depletion of granulocytes in mice with a granulocyte specific antibody inhibits the growth rate of transplanted progressor tumors (145,146) and there is suggestion that granulocytosis can correlate with increased growth of lung metastases (147) in animal models.

On the contrary, macrophages can also secrete antiangiogenic factors like thrombospondin, TNF-α, and IL-12 (148). Neutrophils, in particular, possess antitumor activity and under experimental conditions (149–151). It is well accepted that instillation of Bacille Calmette–Guérin (BCG) into the bladder cavity is effective in reducing recurrence in invasive bladder carcinoma presumably due to activation of a local inflammatory response (152). Tumor cells engineered to produce large amounts of G-CSF, IL-2, or IL-4 exhibit significant growth inhibition and those transfected to produce IL-10 fail to grow in vivo in mice with severe immune combined deficiency (153). Cytokines such as TNF, IFN-γ, G-CSF, and interleukins 2, 4, 6, and 12 may have powerful antitumor effects as well (154).

Thus, inflammatory cells may have contrasting effects on malignant transformation in the human body. The inflammatory response may induce tumor growth as well as help inhibit its progression. While the intricate role of innate immune cells in tumor tissue remains unknown, its relevance to inflammatory responses in the individual oncology patient is far from been resolved.

VII. CONCLUSION

Inflammation is an enormously complex process and its mediators allow for a number of biological processes that constitute a host response to severe infection or tissue injury. Until recently, it was hypothesized that development of multiple organ dysfunction was a consequence of exaggerated immune responses. It now seems quite certain that altered coagulation in critically ill patients may play a critical role in pathogenesis of this disorder. The extent to which these inflammatory–coagulation pathways may be affected uniquely in the oncology patient is not yet known.

Management of patients with multiple organ dysfunction remains largely supportive. Besides the evidence for APC in critically ill patients with severe sepsis, the role for immune modulation is yet to be validated. Perioperative management of the oncologic patient may include hemodynamic optimization with fluids and judicious use of packed red cell transfusions. Prompt treatment of hypovolemia and peripheral perfusion should remain prime therapeutic objectives. Postoperatively, establishment of early enteral nutrition and prompt treatment of infections may be beneficial.

REFERENCES

1. Weiss SJ. Tissue destruction by neutrophils. N Engl J Med 1989; 320:365–376.
2. Smith JA. Neutrophils, host defense, and inflammation: a double-edged sword. J Leukoc Biol 1994; 56: 672–686.
3. Movat HZ, Cybulsky MI, Colditz IG, Chan MK, Dinarello CA. Acute inflammation in gram-negative infection: endotoxin, interleukin 1, tumor necrosis factor, and neutrophils. Fed Proc 1987; 46:97–104.
4. Steinberg KP, Milberg JA, Martin TR, Maunder RJ, Cockrill BA, Hudson LD. Evolution of bronchoalveolar cell populations in the adult respiratory distress syndrome. Am J Respir Crit Care Med 1994; 150: 113–122.
5. Ho JS, Buchweitz JP, Roth RA, Ganey PE. Identification of factors from rat neutrophils responsible for cytotoxicity to isolated hepatocytes. J Leukoc Biol 1996; 59:716–724.
6. Kubes P, Hunter J, Granger DN. Ischemia/reperfusion-induced feline intestinal dysfunction: importance of granulocyte recruitment. Gastroenterology 1992; 103:807–812.
7. Lowell CA, Berton G. Resistance to endotoxic shock and reduced neutrophil migration in mice deficient for the Src-family kinases Hck and Fgr. Proc Natl Acad Sci USA 1998; 95:7580–7584.
8. Sugahara K, Cott GR, Parsons PE, Mason RJ, Sandhaus RA, Henson PM. Epithelial permeability produced by phagocytosing neutrophils in vitro. Am Rev Respir Dis 1986; 133:875–881.
9. MacLean LD, Mulligan WG, McLean AP, Duff JH. Patterns of septic shock in man—a detailed study of 56 patients. Ann Surg 1967; 166:543–562.
10. Ashbaugh DG, Bigelow DB, Petty TL, Levine BE. Acute respiratory distress in adults. Lancet 1967; 2: 319–323.
11. Bigelow DB, Petty TL, Ashbaugh DG, Levine BE, Nett LM, Tyler SW. Acute respiratory failure. Experiences of a respiratory care unit. Med Clin North Am 1967; 51:323–340.
12. Moore FD. Shock and sepsis: some historical perspectives. Surg Clin North Am 1969; 49:481–487.
13. Tilney NL, Bailey GL, Morgan AP. Sequential system failure after rupture of abdominal aortic aneurysms: an unsolved problem in postoperative care. Ann Surg 1973; 178:117–122.
14. Fry DE, Pearlstein L, Fulton RL, Polk HCJ. Multiple system organ failure. The role of uncontrolled infection. Arch Surg 1980; 115:136–140.
15. Polk HCJ, Shields CL. Remote organ failure: a valid sign of occult intra-abdominal infection. Surgery 1977; 81:310–313.
16. Goris RJ, te BT, Nuytinck JK, Gimbrere JS. Multiple-organ failure Generalized autodestructive inflammation? Arch Surg 1985; 120:1109–1115.
17. Marshall J, Sweeney D. Microbial infection and the septic response in critical surgical illness. Sepsis, not infection, determines outcome. Arch Surg 1990; 125:17–22.
18. Poole GV, Muakkassa FF, Griswold JA. The role of infection in outcome of multiple organ failure. Am Surg 1993; 59:727–732.
19. Poole GV, Griswold JA, Muakkassa FF. Sepsis and infection in the intensive care unit: are they related? Am Surg 1993; 59:60–64.
20. Liberati A, D'Amico R, Pifferi S, Leonetti C, Torri V, Brazzi L, Tinazzi A. Antibiotics for preventing respiratory tract infections in adults receiving intensive care. Cochrane Database Syst Rev 2000; 4:CD000022.
21. D'Amico R, Pifferi S, Leonetti C, Torri V, Tinazzi A, Liberati A. Effectiveness of antibiotic prophylaxis in critically ill adult patients: systematic review of randomised controlled trials. Br Med J 1998; 316:1275–1285.

22. Tran DD, Cuesta MA, Van Leeuwen PA, Nauta JJ, Wesdorp RI. Risk factors for multiple organ system failure and death in critically injured patients. Surgery 1993; 114:21–30.
23. Borrelli E, Roux-Lombard P, Grau GE, Girardin E, Ricou B, Dayer J, Suter PM. Plasma concentrations of cytokines, their soluble receptors, and antioxidant vitamins can predict the development of multiple organ failure in patients at risk. Crit Care Med 1996; 24:392–397.
24. Gando S, Nakanishi Y, Tedo I. Cytokines and plasminogen activator inhibitor-1 in posttrauma disseminated intravascular coagulation: relationship to multiple organ dysfunction syndrome. Crit Care Med 1995; 23:1835–1842.
25. Roumen RM, Redl H, Schlag G, Zilow G, Sandtner W, Koller W, Hendriks T, Goris RJ. Inflammatory mediators in relation to the development of multiple organ failure in patients after severe blunt trauma. Crit Care Med 1995; 23:474–480.
26. Mallick AA, Ishizaka A, Stephens KE, Hatherill JR, Tazelaar HD, Raffin TA. Multiple organ damage caused by tumor necrosis factor and prevented by prior neutrophil depletion. Chest 1989; 95:1114–1120.
27. Jansen MJ, Hendriks T, Vogels MT, van der Meer JW, Goris RJ. Inflammatory cytokines in an experimental model for the multiple organ dysfunction syndrome. Crit Care Med 1996; 24:1196–1202.
28. Nuytinck JK, Goris RJ, Weerts JG, Schillings PH, Stekhoven JH. Acute generalized microvascular injury by activated complement and hypoxia: the basis of the adult respiratory distress syndrome and multiple organ failure? Br J Exp Pathol 1986; 67:537–548.
29. Tracey KJ, Fong Y, Hesse DG, Manogue KR, Lee AT, Kuo GC, Lowry SF, Cerami A. Anti-cachectin/TNF monoclonal antibodies prevent septic shock during lethal bacteraemia. Nature 1987; 330:662–664.
30. Okusawa S, Gelfand JA, Ikejima T, Connolly RJ, Dinarello CA. Interleukin 1 induces a shock-like state in rabbits. Synergism with tumor necrosis factor and the effect of cyclooxygenase inhibition. J Clin Invest 1988; 81:1162–1172.
31. Stephens KE, Ishizaka A, Wu ZH, Larrick JW, Raffin TA. Granulocyte depletion prevents tumor necrosis factor-mediated acute lung injury in guinea pigs. Am Rev Respir Dis 1988; 138:1300–1307.
32. Heflin ACJ, Brigham KL. Prevention by granulocyte depletion of increased vascular permeability of sheep lung following endotoxemia. J Clin Invest 1981; 68:1253–1260.
33. Iimuro Y, Yamamoto M, Kohno H, Itakura J, Fujii H, Matsumoto Y. Blockade of liver macrophages by gadolinium chloride reduces lethality in endotoxemic rats—analysis of mechanisms of lethality in endotoxemia. J Leukoc Biol 1994; 55:723–728.
34. Nieuwenhuijzen GA, Haskel Y, Lu Q, Berg RD, van Rooijen N, Goris RJ, Deitch EA. Macrophage elimination increases bacterial translocation and gut-origin septicemia but attenuates symptoms and mortality rate in a model of systemic inflammation. Ann Surg 1993; 218:791–799.
35. Powrie F, Correa-Oliveira R, Mauze S, Coffman RL. Regulatory interactions between CD45RB high and CD45RB low CD4+ T cells are important for the balance between protective and pathogenic cell-mediated immunity. J Exp Med 1994; 179:589–600.
36. Shull MM, Ormsby I, Kier AB, Pawlowski S, Diebold RJ, Yin M, Allen R, Sidman C, Proetzel G, Calvin D. Targeted disruption of the mouse transforming growth factor-beta 1 gene results in multifocal inflammatory disease. Nature 1992; 359:693–699.
37. Natanson C, Hoffman WD, Suffredini AF, Eichacker PQ, Danner RL. Selected treatment strategies for septic shock based on proposed mechanisms of pathogenesis. Ann Intern Med 1994; 120:771–783.
38. Gomez-Jimenez J, Salgado A, Mourelle M, Martin MC, Segura RM, Peracaula R, Moncada S. L-arginine: nitric oxide pathway in endotoxemia and human septic shock. Crit Care Med 1995; 23:253–258.
39. Groeneveld PH, Kwappenberg KM, Langermans JA, Nibbering PH, Curtis L. Nitric oxide (NO) production correlates with renal insufficiency and multiple organ dysfunction syndrome in severe sepsis. Intensive Care Med 1996; 22:1197–1202.
40. Cobb JP. Use of nitric oxide synthase inhibitors to treat septic shock: the light has changed from yellow to red. Crit Care Med 1999; 27:855–856.
41. Grover R, Zaccardelli D, Colice G, Guntupalli K, Watson D, Vincent JL. An open-label dose escalation study of the nitric oxide synthase inhibitor, *N*(G)-methyl-L-arginine hydrochloride (546C88), in patients with septic shock. Glaxo Wellcome International Septic Shock Study Group. Crit Care Med 1999; 27:913–922.
42. Starnes HFJ, Warren RS, Jeevanandam M, Gabrilove JL, Larchian W, Oettgen HF, Brennan MF. Tumor necrosis factor and the acute metabolic response to tissue injury in man. J Clin Invest 1988; 82:1321–1325.
43. Michie HR, Spriggs DR, Manogue KR, Sherman ML, Revhaug A, O'Dwyer ST, Arthur K, Dinarello CA, Cerami A, Wolff SM. Tumor necrosis factor and endotoxin induce similar metabolic responses in human beings. Surgery 1988; 104:280–286.
44. Morimoto A, Sakata Y, Watanabe T, Murakami N. Characteristics of fever and acute-phase response induced in rabbits by IL-1 and TNF. Am J Physiol 1989; 256:R35–R41.
45. Reinhart K, Wiegand-Lohnert C, Grimminger F, Kaul M, Withington S, Treacher D, Eckart J, Willatts S, Bouza C, Krausch D, Stockenhuber F, Eiselstein J, Daum L, Kempeni J. Assessment of the safety and efficacy of the monoclonal anti-tumor necrosis factor antibody-fragment, MAK 195F, in patients with sepsis and septic shock: a multicenter, randomized, placebo-controlled, dose-ranging study. Crit Care Med 1996; 24:733–742.

46. Opal SM, Fisher CJJ, Dhainaut JF, Vincent JL, Brase R, Lowry SF, Sadoff JC, Slotman GJ, Levy H, Balk RA, Shelly MP, Pribble JP, LaBrecque JF, Lookabaugh J, Donovan H, Dubin H, Baughman R, Norman J, DeMaria E, Matzel K, Abraham E, Seneff M. Confirmatory interleukin-1 receptor antagonist trial in severe sepsis: a phase III, randomized, double-blind, placebo-controlled, multicenter trial. The Interleukin-1 Receptor Antagonist Sepsis Investigator Group. Crit Care Med 1997; 25:1115–1124.
47. Dhainaut JF, Vincent JL, Richard C, Lejeune P, Martin C, Fierobe L, Stephens S, Ney UM, Sopwith M. CDP571, a humanized antibody to human tumor necrosis factor-alpha: safety, pharmacokinetics, immune response, and influence of the antibody on cytokine concentrations in patients with septic shock. CPD571 Sepsis Study Group. Crit Care Med 1995; 23:1461–1469.
48. Fisher CJJ, Agosti JM, Opal SM, Lowry SF, Balk RA, Sadoff JC, Abraham E, Schein RM, Benjamin E. Treatment of septic shock with the tumor necrosis factor receptor: Fc fusion protein The Soluble TNF Receptor Sepsis Study Group. N Engl J Med 1996; 334:1697–1702.
49. Abraham E, Matthay MA, Dinarello CA, Vincent JL, Cohen J, Opal SM, Glauser M, Parsons P, Fisher CJJ, Repine JE. Consensus conference definitions for sepsis, septic shock, acute lung injury, and acute respiratory distress syndrome: time for a reevaluation. Crit Care Med 2000; 28:232–235.
50. Fisher CJJ, Dhainaut JF, Opal SM, Pribble JP, Balk RA, Slotman GJ, Iberti TJ, Rackow EC, Shapiro MJ, Greenman RL. Recombinant human interleukin 1 receptor antagonist in the treatment of patients with sepsis syndrome. Results from a randomized, double-blind, placebo-controlled trial. Phase III rhIL-1ra Sepsis Syndrome Study Group. JAMA 1994; 271: 1836–1843.
51. Bone RC, Sibbald WJ, Sprung CL. The ACCP–SCCM consensus conference on sepsis and organ failure. Chest 1992; 101:1481–1483.
52. Vincent JL. Dear SIRS, I'm sorry to say that I don't like you. Crit Care Med 1997; 25:372–374.
53. Dellinger RP, Bone RC. To SIRS with love. Crit Care Med 1998; 26:178–179.
54. Marshall J. Both the disposition and the means of cure: "Severe SIRS," "sterile shock," and the ongoing challenge of description. Crit Care Med 1997; 25:1765–1766.
55. Pittet D, Rangel-Frausto S, Li N, Tarara D, Costigan M, Rempe L, Jebson, Wenzel RP. Systemic inflammatory response syndrome, sepsis, severe sepsis and septic shock: incidence, morbidities and outcomes in surgical ICU patients. Intensive Care Med 1995; 21:302–309.
56. Rangel-Frausto MS, Pittet D, Hwang T, Woolson RF, Wenzel RP. The dynamics of disease progression in sepsis: Markov modeling describing the natural history and the likely impact of effective antisepsis agents. Clin Infect Dis 1998; 27:185–190.
57. Brun-Buisson C, Doyon F, Carlet J, Dellamonica P, Gouin F, Lepoutre A, Mercier JC, Offenstadt G, Regnier B. Incidence, risk factors, and outcome of severe sepsis and septic shock in adults. A multicenter prospective study in intensive care units. French ICU Group for Severe Sepsis. JAMA 1995; 274: 968–974.
58. Salvo I, de Cian W, Musicco M, Langer M, Piadena R, Wolfler A, Montani C, Magni E. The Italian SEPSIS study: preliminary results on the incidence and evolution of SIRS, sepsis, severe sepsis and septic shock. Intensive Care Med 1995; 21(suppl 2): S244–S249.
59. Menges T, Hermans PW, Little SG, Langefeld T, Boning O, Engel J, Sluijter M, de Groot R, Hempelmann G. Plasminogen-activator-inhibitor-1 4G/5G promoter polymorphism and prognosis of severely injured patients. Lancet 2001; 357:1096–1097.
60. Giesen PL, Rauch U, Bohrmann B, Kling D, Roque M, Fallon JT, Badimon JJ, Himber J, Riederer MA, Nemerson Y. Blood-borne tissue factor: another view of thrombosis. Proc Natl Acad Sci USA 1999; 96: 2311–2315.
61. Rauch U, Bonderman D, Bohrmann B, Badimon JJ, Himber J, Riederer MA, Nemerson Y. Transfer of tissue factor from leukocytes to platelets is mediated by CD15 and tissue factor. Blood 2000; 96:170–175.
62. Sandset PM. Tissue factor pathway inhibitor (TFPI)—an update. Haemostasis 1996; 26(suppl 4): 154–165.
63. Esmon CT. Cell mediated events that control blood coagulation and vascular injury. Annu Rev Cell Biol 1993; 9:1–26.
64. Mammen EF. Antithrombin: its physiological importance and role in DIC. Semin Thromb Hemost 1998; 24:19–25.
65. Jesty J, Lorenz A, Rodriguez J, Wun TC. Initiation of the tissue factor pathway of coagulation in the presence of heparin: control by antithrombin III and tissue factor pathway inhibitor. Blood 1996; 87: 2301–2307.
66. Sadler JE. Thrombomodulin structure and function. Thromb Haemost 1997; 78:392–395.
67. Esmon C. The protein C pathway. Crit Care Med 2000; 28:S44–S48.
68. Esmon CT. The roles of protein C and thrombomodulin in the regulation of blood coagulation. J Biol Chem 1989; 264:4743–4746.
69. Hanson SR, Griffin JH, Harker LA, Kelly AB, Esmon CT, Gruber A. Antithrombotic effects of thrombin-induced activation of endogenous protein C in primates. J Clin Invest 1993; 92:2003–2012.
70. Gando S, Kameue T, Nanzaki S, Nakanishi Y. Disseminated intravascular coagulation is a frequent complication of systemic inflammatory response syndrome. Thromb Haemost 1996; 75:224–228.

71. Levi M, Ten Cate H. Disseminated intravascular coagulation. N Engl J Med 1999; 341:586–592.
72. Fukudome K, Esmon CT. Identification, cloning, and regulation of a novel endothelial cell protein C/ activated protein C receptor. J Biol Chem 1994; 269: 26486–26491.
73. Conway EM, Rosenberg RD. Tumor necrosis factor suppresses transcription of the thrombomodulin gene in endothelial cells. Mol Cell Biol 1988; 8: 5588–5592.
74. Fourrier F, Chopin C, Goudemand J, Hendrycx S, Caron C, Rime A, Marey A, Lestavel P. Septic shock, multiple organ failure, and disseminated intravascular coagulation. Compared patterns of antithrombin III, protein C, and protein S deficiencies. Chest 1992; 101:816–823.
75. Boehme MW, Deng Y, Raeth U, Bierhaus A, Ziegler R, Stremmel W, Nawroth PP. Release of thrombomodulin from endothelial cells by concerted action of TNF-alpha and neutrophils: in vivo and in vitro studies. Immunology 1996; 87:134–140.
76. Lorente JA, Garcia-Frade LJ, Landin L, de Pablo R, Torrado C, Renes E, Garcia-Avello A. Time course of hemostatic abnormalities in sepsis and its relation to outcome. Chest 1993; 103:1536–1542.
77. Powars D, Larsen R, Johnson J, Hulbert T, Sun T, Patch MJ, Francis R, Chan L. Epidemic meningococcemia and purpura fulminans with induced protein C deficiency. Clin Infect Dis 1993; 17:254–261.
78. Murakami K, Okajima K, Uchiba M, Johno M, Nakagaki T, Okabe H, Takatsuki K. Activated protein C attenuates endotoxin-induced pulmonary vascular injury by inhibiting activated leukocytes in rats. Blood 1996; 87:642–647.
79. Yamauchi T, Umeda F, Inoguchi T, Nawata H. Antithrombin III stimulates prostacyclin production by cultured aortic endothelial cells. Biochem Biophys Res Commun 1989; 163:1404–1411.
80. Ostrovsky L, Woodman RC, Payne D, Teoh D, Kubes P. Antithrombin III prevents and rapidly reverses leukocyte recruitment in ischemia/reperfusion. Circulation 1997; 96:2302–2310.
81. Esmon CT. Thrombomodulin as a model of molecular mechanisms that modulate protease specificity and function at the vessel surface. FASEB J 1995; 9:946–955.
82. Iversen N, Sandset PM, Abildgaard U, Torjesen PA. Binding of tissue factor pathway inhibitor to cultured endothelial cells-influence of glycosaminoglycans. Thromb Res 1996; 84:267–278.
83. Mertens G, Cassiman JJ, Van den Berghe H, Vermylen J, David G. Cell surface heparan sulfate proteoglycans from human vascular endothelial cells. Core protein characterization and antithrombin III binding properties. J Biol Chem 1992; 267:20435–20443.
84. Murata T, Ushikubi F, Matsuoka T, Hirata M, Yamasaki A, Sugimoto Y, Ichikawa A, Aze Y, Tanaka T, Yoshida N, Ueno A, Oh-ishi S, Narumiya S. Altered pain perception and inflammatory response in mice lacking prostacyclin receptor. Nature 1997; 388: 678–682.
85. Rees DD, Palmer RM, Moncada S. Role of endothelium-derived nitric oxide in the regulation of blood pressure. Proc Natl Acad Sci USA 1989; 86: 3375–3378.
86. Yang Y, Loscalzo J. Regulation of tissue factor expression in human microvascular endothelial cells by nitric oxide. Circulation 2000; 101:2144–2148.
87. Papapetropoulos A, Piccardoni P, Cirino G, Bucci M, Sorrentino R, Cicala C, Johnson K, Zachariou V, Sessa WC, Altieri DC. Hypotension and inflammatory cytokine gene expression triggered by factor Xa–nitric oxide signaling. Proc Natl Acad Sci USA 1998; 95:4738–4742.
88. Gardinali M, Borrelli E, Chiara O, Lundberg C, Padalino P, Conciato L, Cafaro C, Lazzi S, Luzi P, Giomarelli PP, Agostoni A. Inhibition of CD11–CD18 complex prevents acute lung injury and reduces mortality after peritonitis in rabbits. Am J Respir Crit Care Med 2000; 161:1022–1029.
89. Kuebler WM, Borges J, Sckell A, Kuhnle GE, Bergh K, Messmer K, Goetz AE. Role of L-selectin in leukocyte sequestration in lung capillaries in a rabbit model of endotoxemia. Am J Respir Crit Care Med 2000; 161:36–43.
90. Varani J, Ward PA. Mechanisms of endothelial cell injury in acute inflammation. Shock 1994; 2:311–319.
91. Stefanec T. Endothelial apoptosis: could it have a role in the pathogenesis and treatment of disease? Chest 2000; 117:841–854.
92. Moncada S, Higgs A. The L-arginine-nitric oxide pathway. N Engl J Med 1993; 329:2002–2012.
93. Marsden PA, Schappert KT, Chen HS, Flowers M, Sundell CL, Wilcox JN, Lamas S, Michel T. Molecular cloning and characterization of human endothelial nitric oxide synthase. FEBS Lett 1992; 307:287–293.
94. Gross SS, Kilbourn RG, Griffith OW. NO in septic shock: good, bad or ugly? Learning from iNOS knockouts. Trends Microbiol 1996; 4:47–49.
95. Springer TA. Traffic signals on endothelium for lymphocyte recirculation and leukocyte emigration. Annu Rev Physiol 1995; 57:827–872.
96. Deshpande SS, Angkeow P, Huang J, Ozaki M, Irani K. Rac1 inhibits TNF-alpha-induced endothelial cell apoptosis: dual regulation by reactive oxygen species. FASEB J 2000; 14:1705–1714.
97. Weiss SJ, Young J, LoBuglio AF, Slivka A, Nimeh NF. Role of hydrogen peroxide in neutrophil-mediated destruction of cultured endothelial cells. J Clin Invest 1981; 68:714–721.
98. Harlan JM. Leukocyte–endothelial interactions. Blood 1985; 65:513–525.
99. Sessler CN, Windsor AC, Schwartz M, Watson L, Fisher BJ, Sugerman HJ, Fowler AA. Circulating ICAM-1 is increased in septic shock. Am J Respir Crit Care Med 1995; 151:1420–1427.

100. Kelly KJ, Williams WWJ, Colvin RB, Meehan SM, Springer TA, Gutierrez-Ramos JC, Bonventre JV. Intercellular adhesion molecule-1-deficient mice are protected against ischemic renal injury. J Clin Invest 1996; 97:1056–1063.
101. Xu H, Gonzalo JA, St Pierre Y, Williams IR, Kupper TS, Cotran RS, Springer TA, Gutierrez-Ramos JC. Leukocytosis and resistance to septic shock in intercellular adhesion molecule 1-deficient mice. J Exp Med 1994; 180:95–109.
102. Krafte-Jacobs B, Brilli R. Increased circulating thrombomodulin in children with septic shock. Crit Care Med 1998; 26:933–938.
103. Cheng T, Liu D, Griffin JH, Fernandez JA, Castellino F, Rosen ED, Fukudome K, Zlokovic BV. Activated protein C blocks p53-mediated apoptosis in ischemic human brain endothelium and is neuroprotective. Nat Med 2003; 9:338–342.
104. Gando S, Kameue T, Matsuda N, Hayakawa M, Ishitani T, Morimoto Y, Kemmotsu O. Combined activation of coagulation and inflammation has an important role in multiple organ dysfunction and poor outcome after severe trauma. Thromb Haemost 2002; 88:943–949.
105. LeCouter J, Kowalski J, Foster J, Hass P, Zhang Z, Dillard-Telm L, Frantz G, Rangell L, DeGuzman L, Keller GA, Peale F, Gurney A, Hillan KJ, Ferrara N. Identification of an angiogenic mitogen selective for endocrine gland endothelium. Nature 2001; 412:877–884.
106. Allen BL, Filla MS, Rapraeger AC. Role of heparan sulfate as a tissue-specific regulator of FGF-4 and FGF receptor recognition. J Cell Biol 2001; 155:845–858.
107. Osterud B, Bajaj MS, Bajaj SP. Sites of tissue factor pathway inhibitor (TFPI) and tissue factor expression under physiologic and pathologic conditions. On behalf of the Subcommittee on Tissue factor Pathway Inhibitor (TFPI) of the Scientific and Standardization Committee of the ISTH. Thromb Haemost 1995; 73:873–875.
108. Ishii H, Salem HH, Bell CE, Laposata EA, Majerus PW. Thrombomodulin, an endothelial anticoagulant protein, is absent from the human brain. Blood 1986; 67:362–365.
109. Weiler-Guettler H, Christie PD, Beeler DL, Healy AM, Hancock WW, Rayburn H, Edelberg JM, Rosenberg RD. A targeted point mutation in thrombomodulin generates viable mice with a prethrombotic state. J Clin Invest 1998; 101:1983–1991.
110. Chinnaiyan AM, Huber-Lang M, Kumar-Sinha C, Barrette TR, Shankar-Sinha S, Sarma VJ, Padgaonkar VA, Ward PA. Molecular signatures of sepsis: multiorgan gene expression profiles of systemic inflammation. Am J Pathol 2001; 159:1199–1209.
111. Aird WC. Endothelial cell heterogeneity. Crit Care Med 2003; 31:S221–S230.
112. Aird WC. Endothelial cell dynamics and complexity theory. Crit Care Med 2002; 30:S180–S185.
113. Bernard GR, Vincent JL, Laterre PF, LaRosa SP, Dhainaut JF, Lopez-Rodriguez A, Steingrub JS, Garber GE, Helterbrand JD, Ely EW, Fisher CJJ. Efficacy and safety of recombinant human activated protein C for severe sepsis. N Engl J Med 2001; 344: 699–709.
114. Warren BL, Eid A, Singer P, Pillay SS, Carl P, Novak I, Chalupa P, Atherstone A, Penzes I, Kubler A, Knaub S, Keinecke HO, Heinrichs H, Schindel F, Juers M, Bone RC, Opal SM. Caring for the critically ill patient. High-dose antithrombin III in severe sepsis: a randomized controlled trial. JAMA 2001; 286: 1869–1878.
115. Abraham E, Reinhart K, Svoboda P, Seibert A, Olthoff D, Dal Nogare A, Postier R, Hempelmann G, Butler T, Martin E, Zwingelstein C, Percell S, Shu V, Leighton A, Creasey AA. Assessment of the safety of recombinant tissue factor pathway inhibitor in patients with severe sepsis: a multicenter, randomized, placebo-controlled, single-blind, dose escalation study. Crit Care Med 2001; 29:2081–2089.
116. Dhainaut JF, Tenaillon A, Hemmer M, Damas P, Le Tulzo Y, Radermacher P, Schaller MD, Sollet JP, Wolff M, Holzapfel L, Zeni F, Vedrinne JM, de Vathaire F, Gourlay ML, Guinot P, Mira JP. Confirmatory platelet-activating factor receptor antagonist trial in patients with severe gram-negative bacterial sepsis: a phase III, randomized, double-blind, placebo-controlled, multicenter trial. BN 52021 Sepsis Investigator Group. Crit Care Med 1998; 26: 1963–1971.
117. Siegel JP. Assessing the use of activated protein C in the treatment of severe sepsis. N Engl J Med 2002; 347:1030–1034.
118. Warren HS, Suffredini AF, Eichacker PQ, Munford RS. Risks and benefits of activated protein C treatment for severe sepsis. N Engl J Med 2002; 347:1027–1030.
119. Rodeghiero F, Tosetto A. Activated protein C resistance and factor V Leiden mutation are independent risk factors for venous thromboembolism. Ann Intern Med 1999; 130:643–650.
120. Folsom AR, Cushman M, Tsai MY, Aleksic N, Heckbert SR, Boland LL, Tsai AW, Yanez ND, Rosamond WD. A prospective study of venous thromboembolism in relation to factor V Leiden and related factors. Blood 2002; 99:2720–2725.
121. Price DT, Ridker PM. Factor V Leiden mutation and the risks for thromboembolic disease: a clinical perspective. Ann Intern Med 1997; 127:895–903.
122. Haim N, Lanir N, Hoffman R, Haim A, Tsalik M, Brenner B. Acquired activated protein C resistance is common in cancer patients and is associated with venous thromboembolism. Am J Med 2001; 110:91–96.
123. Shoemaker WC, Patil R, Appel PL, Kram HB. Hemodynamic and oxygen transport patterns for outcome prediction, therapeutic goals, and clinical algorithms to improve outcome. Feasibility of artificial intelli-

gence to customize algorithms. Chest 1992; 102: 617S–625S.
124. Fleming A, Bishop M, Shoemaker W, Appel P, Sufficool W, Kuvhenguwha A, Kennedy F, Wo CJ. Prospective trial of supranormal values as goals of resuscitation in severe trauma. Arch Surg 1992; 127:1175–1179.
125. Shoemaker WC, Appel PL, Kram HB. Role of oxygen debt in the development of organ failure sepsis, and death in high-risk surgical patients. Chest 1992; 102:208–215.
126. Sinclair S, James S, Singer M. Intraoperative intravascular volume optimisation and length of hospital stay after repair of proximal femoral fracture: randomised controlled trial. Br Med J 1997; 315:909–912.
127. Wilson J, Woods I, Fawcett J, Whall R, Dibb W, Morris C, McManus E. Reducing the risk of major elective surgery: randomised controlled trial of preoperative optimisation of oxygen delivery. Br Med J 1999; 318:1099–1103.
128. Price J, Sear J, Venn R. Perioperative fluid volume optimization following proximal femoral fracture. Cochrane Database Syst Rev 2002; 1:CD003004.
129. Hebert PC, Wells G, Blajchman MA, Marshall J, Martin C, Pagliarello G, Tweeddale M, Schweitzer I, Yetisir E. A multicenter, randomized, controlled clinical trial of transfusion requirements in critical care. Transfusion Requirements in Critical Care Investigators, Canadian Critical Care Trials Group. N Engl J Med 1999; 340:409–417.
130. Rivers E, Nguyen B, Havstad S, Ressler J, Muzzin A, Knoblich B, Peterson E, Tomlanovich M. Early goal-directed therapy in the treatment of severe sepsis and septic shock. N Engl J Med 2001; 345:1368–1377.
131. Bone RC, Fisher CJJ, Clemmer TP, Slotman GJ, Metz CA, Balk RA. A controlled clinical trial of high-dose methylprednisolone in the treatment of severe sepsis and septic shock. N Engl J Med 1987; 317: 653–658.
132. Annane D, Sebille V, Charpentier C, Bollaert PE, Francois B, Korach JM, Capellier G, Cohen Y, Azoulay E, Troche G, Chaumet-Riffaut P, Bellissant E. Effect of treatment with low doses of hydrocortisone and fludrocortisone on mortality in patients with septic shock. JAMA 2002; 288:862–871.
133. Van den Berghe G, Wouters P, Weekers F, Verwaest C, Bruyninckx F, Schetz M, Vlasselaers D, Ferdinande P, Lauwers P, Bouillon R. Intensive insulin therapy in the critically ill patients. N Engl J Med 2001; 345: 1359–1367.
134. Losser MR, Bernard C, Beaudeux JL, Pison C, Payen D. Glucose modulates hemodynamic, metabolic, and inflammatory responses to lipopolysaccharide in rabbits. J Appl Physiol 1997; 83:1566–1574.
135. Rassias AJ, Marrin CA, Arruda J, Whalen PK, Beach M, Yeager MP. Insulin infusion improves neutrophil function in diabetic cardiac surgery patients. Anesth Analg 1999; 88:1011–1016.
136. Geerlings SE, Hoepelman AI. Immune dysfunction in patients with diabetes mellitus (DM). FEMS Immunol Med Microbiol 1999; 26:259–265.
137. Sidenius P. The axonopathy of diabetic neuropathy. Diabetes 1982; 31:356–363.
138. Van den Berghe G, Wouters PJ, Bouillon R, Weekers F, Verwaest C, Schetz M, Vlasselaers D, Ferdinande P, Lauwers P. Outcome benefit of intensive insulin therapy in the critically ill: insulin dose versus glycemic control. Crit Care Med 2003; 31:359–366.
139. Ventilation with lower tidal volumes as compared with traditional tidal volumes for acute lung injury and the acute respiratory distress syndrome. The Acute Respiratory Distress Syndrome Network. N Engl J Med 2000; 342:1301–1308.
140. Derdak S, Mehta S, Stewart TE, Smith T, Rogers M, Buchman TG, Carlin B, Lowson S, Granton J. High-frequency oscillatory ventilation for acute respiratory distress syndrome in adults: a randomized, controlled trial. Am J Respir Crit Care Med 2002; 166:801–808.
141. Leder A, Kuo A, Cardiff RD, Sinn E, Leder P. v-Ha-ras transgene abrogates the initiation step in mouse skin tumorigenesis: effects of phorbol esters and retinoic acid. Proc Natl Acad Sci USA 1990; 87: 9178–9182.
142. Sunderkotter C, Steinbrink K, Goebeler M, Bhardwaj R, Sorg C. Macrophages and angiogenesis. J Leukoc Biol 1994; 55:410–422.
143. Ono M, Torisu H, Fukushi J, Nishie A, Kuwano M. Biological implications of macrophage infiltration in human tumor angiogenesis. Cancer Chemother Pharmacol 1999;(suppl 43):S69–S71.
144. Bogdan C, Vodovotz Y, Nathan C. Macrophage deactivation by interleukin 10. J Exp Med 1991; 174: 1549–1555.
145. Pekarek LA, Starr BA, Toledano AY, Schreiber H. Inhibition of tumor growth by elimination of granulocytes. J Exp Med 1995; 181:435–440.
146. Seung LP, Seung SK, Schreiber H. Antigenic cancer cells that escape immune destruction are stimulated by host cells. Cancer Res 1995; 55:5094–5100.
147. Ishikawa M, Koga Y, Hosokawa M, Kobayashi H. Augmentation of B16 melanoma lung colony formation in C57BL/6 mice having marked granulocytosis. Int J Cancer 1986; 37:919–924.
148. Seljelid R, Busund LT. The biology of macrophages: II. Inflammation and tumors. Eur J Haematol 1994; 52:1–12.
149. Dallegri F, Ottonello L. Neutrophil-mediated cytotoxicity against tumour cells: state of art. Arch Immunol Ther Exp (Warsz) 1992; 40:39–42.
150. Colombo MP, Lombardi L, Stoppacciaro A, Melani C, Parenza M, Bottazzi B, Parmiani G. Granulocyte colony-stimulating factor (G-CSF) gene transduction in murine adenocarcinoma drives neutrophil-mediated tumor inhibition in vivo. Neutrophils discriminate between G-CSF-producing and G-CSF-nonproducing tumor cells. J Immunol 1992; 149:113–119.

151. Noffz G, Qin Z, Kopf M, Blankenstein T. Neutrophils but not eosinophils are involved in growth suppression of IL-4-secreting tumors. J Immunol 1998; 160: 345–350.
152. Morales A, Eidinger D, Bruce AW. Intracavitary Bacillus Calmette–Guérin in the treatment of superficial bladder tumors. 1976. J Urol 2002; 167: 891–893.
153. Richter G, Kruger-Krasagakes S, Hein G, Huls C, Schmitt E, Diamantstein T, Blankenstein T. Interleukin 10 transfected into Chinese hamster ovary cells prevents tumor growth and macrophage infiltration. Cancer Res 1993; 53:4134–4137.
154. Blankenstein T, Cayeux S, Qin Z. Genetic approaches to cancer immunotherapy. Rev Physiol Biochem Pharmacol 1996; 129:1–49.
155. Marshall JC. Inflammation, coagulopathy, and the pathogenesis of multiple organ dysfunction syndrome. Crit Care Med 2001; 29:S99–S106.

SUGGESTED READINGS

Deitch EA, Vincent JL, Windsor A. Sepsis and Multiple Organ Dysfunction. A multidisciplinary approach. London: W.B. Saunders, 2002.

The Margaux Conference on Critical Illness. Sepsis: interface between inflammation, coagulation and the endothelium. Crit Care Med 2001; 29(suppl 7).

The Margaux Conference on Critical Illness. Activation of coagulation system in critical illnesses. Crit Care Med 2000; 28(suppl 9).

15

Perioperative Care of the Immunocompromised Patient

SANDRA L. PEAKE and DHAVAL R. GHELANI

Department of Intensive Care Medicine, The Queen Elizabeth Hospital, Woodville, Adelaide, South Australia, Australia

I. INTRODUCTION

The host immune response to an infectious agent or other foreign material involves both natural or innate response and adaptive response. The innate response [mediated by natural killer (NK) cells and phagocytic cells] is rapid and nonspecific and is not enhanced following repeated antigen exposure. In contrast, the adaptive response (mediated by specific T and B cells) is specific for a particular antigen and is improved upon successive exposure to the antigen. Any defect in either the innate or the adaptive response (congenital or acquired) may lead to an increased susceptibility to infection.

Acquired immunosuppression may be associated with a number of conditions including (i) infections, such as human immunodeficiency virus (HIV); (ii) diseases such as diabetes, autoimmune disorders, and malignancies; and (iii) drugs such as steroids, cancer chemotherapeutic agents, and immune-suppressing drugs used in the prevention of transplant organ rejection. The numerous mechanisms underlying the pathogenesis of immunosuppression in the various conditions are beyond the scope of this chapter, and only immunosuppression associated with cancer will be discussed further.

II. IMMUNOSUPPRESSION ASSOCIATED WITH CANCER

Cancer-associated immunosuppression may be related to the immunomodulatory effects of both the underlying neoplasm and the various therapies (chemotherapeutic agents, radiation, surgery) used to treat the tumor. Importantly, the widespread use of hematopoietic cytokines and growth factors means that many patients now receive significantly greater doses of chemotherapy at shorter intervals, resulting in an increased risk of prolonged and severe immunodeficiency (1); albeit the quantitative immune dysfunction associated with chemotherapy is poorly defined and lacks clinical correlation (2). Finally, elderly cancer patients often have multiple comorbidities that increase the risk of immunosuppression.

The harmful effects of cancer and associated therapies on epithelial and mucous membranes and cellular immune functions are:

1. Loss of integrity of the skin and epithelial lining of the intestinal, respiratory, and urinary tracts (predisposes to bacterial and yeast infections until epithelial integrity is restored).
2. Defective production of mucous with secretory IgA.

3. Altered resident phagocytic cell and lymphocyte function (affected by both preparatory chemotherapy and radiation) (3).
4. Neutropenia (common after chemotherapy, but rapid recovery after treatment is completed).
5. Impaired migration and chemotaxis of granulocytes with decreased superoxide production (more common after stem cell transplantation, especially with steroid-containing chemotherapy regimens).
6. Impaired B-lymphocyte function. Reduced absolute B-cell numbers, and immunoglobulin (Ig) levels occur with both acute lymphocytic leukemia and solid tumors (4). Patients with multiple myeloma also have defective Ig function, and 30% of chemotherapy patients have Ig subclass abnormalities in the first year post-treatment (5). However, the precise clinical significance of chemotherapy-associated B-cell impairment is uncertain, and abnormalities usually normalize within 3–6 months post-treatment.
7. Impaired T-lymphocyte function. T-cell function (as determined by response to mitogen stimulation) has been reported to be low early postchemotherapy but normal at one year (5). Furthermore, of all the immune parameters affected, the recovery of T-cell function is the most protracted, especially with advancing age. Significantly, CD8+ cells (which recover in a thymus-independent fashion) recover faster than CD4+ cells (which recover in a thymus-dependent fashion), leading to an inverted CD4/CD8 ratio and an increased risk of opportunistic infections (2).

In summary, cancer patients may have prolonged impairment of immune function, even after the completion of chemotherapy. This impairment has important consequences for patients undergoing surgery, and such knowledge is important in order to optimize perioperative management and improve clinical outcomes.

III. ANESTHETIC PERSPECTIVES

A. Preoperative Assessment

The assessment of any patient with malignancy should include a thorough preoperative history and physical examination targeted at identifying any problems related to (i) the tumor itself (anatomical and physiological effects), (ii) immunosuppression secondary to radiation and chemotherapy, (iii) organ-specific side effects of the various chemotherapy agents, and (iv) comorbid conditions.

Laboratory studies should include a complete blood count, serum electrolytes, liver function tests, and coagulation profile. A chest radiograph and 12-lead electrocardiograph are also necessary (6). Pulmonary function tests including arterial blood gases, spirometry, lung computerized tomography (CT), and carbon monoxide diffusing capacity should be considered in specific patients. These tests will help both the surgeon and anesthesiologist to anticipate pulmonary complications and the need for postoperative mechanical ventilation.

A list of chemotherapeutic agents administered, as well as their timing of administration, is also essential to determine cumulative toxicity. For example, bleomycin has significant effects on the lungs and symptoms such as nonproductive cough, dyspnea, fever, and tachypnea should be ascertained. Patients receiving doxorubicin or daunorubicin should be evaluated for possible drug-related cardiotoxicity. Any suspicion of congestive cardiac failure (or associated ischemic heart disease) should be further evaluated (7).

Finally, the production of any or all blood cells and clotting factors may be impaired and close cooperation between surgeon, anesthesiologist, and hematologist is essential for optimal management and maximal safety.

B. Anesthesia

Many anesthetic and intensive care drugs are immunomodulatory and stimulate the release of pro- and anti-inflammatory mediators. In postoperative patients, the risk of immunosuppression is further compounded by the immunomodulatory effects of surgery. Therefore, the desired aim in anesthetic delivery is to maintain homeostatic balance between the various inflammatory mediators and achieve a minimal degree of immune alteration.

1. Premedication

Usual premedication is generally appropriate and, unless contraindicated, regular medications should be continued.

2. Monitoring

Electrocardiograph, noninvasive arterial pressure, pulse oximetry, and end-tidal carbon dioxide monitoring are usually sufficient (8). An indwelling urinary catheter may also be required for prolonged procedures or if kidney function is compromised. To avoid infection, invasive monitoring should be limited.

However, central venous and arterial catheters may be necessary when massive bleeding or hemodynamic instability is anticipated. They may also be required when there is evidence of renal, respiratory, or cardiac compromise (8). The use of antiseptic impregnated catheters may significantly reduce the incidence of catheter colonization and infection in immunocompromised patients (9). Additional sterility measures are not usually necessary.

3. Airway Control

Intubation is potentially difficult in some cancer patients and risk of aspiration may be increased, especially in diabetic patients with autonomic neuropathy (10). Mucosal damage and stomatitis may be present after bone marrow transplantation (11), and awake fibre optic intubations should be considered for patients with head and neck tumors.

Because of the risk of nosocomial infection, oral intubation is preferable to nasal intubation (12) and humidification of airway gases will prevent drying of secretions (13). Current heat and moisture exchange filters also act as bacterial filters. Prolonged mechanical ventilation increases the risk of ventilator-associated pneumonia, and early extubation is prudent (14,15).

4. Local Anesthetics

Local anesthetic agents can have important effects on immune function. Lignocaine and bupivacaine both modulate in vitro lipopolysaccharide-mediated interleukin (IL) -1β release from human mononuclear cells and depress neutrophil chemotaxis and phagocytosis (16). They also inhibit mitogen-induced lymphocyte proliferation (17) and immunoglobulin synthesis (18), although NK cell cytotoxicity is not suppressed by bupivacaine (19). Cortisol response to epidural anesthesia is also reduced. The use, wherever possible, of local anesthesia may, therefore, attenuate both the acute stress response and perioperative immunomodulation.

5. Regional Anesthesia

Regional anesthesia is thought to reduce anesthetic-related postoperative immunosuppression. Extradural anesthesia has been shown to improve CD4+-lymphocyte response during gastrectomy (20) and to not suppress NK cell activity during abdominal hysterectomy (19). Monocyte-mediated lysis of tumor target cells is also greater in patients undergoing hip arthroplasty receiving regional anesthesia (21). However, the potential beneficial effects of regional anesthesia on outcome in immunocompromised patients require further evaluation.

6. Inhalation Anesthetics

There is limited data on the immunomodulatory effects of volatile anesthetic agents. Clinical concentrations of nitrous oxide, halothane, and enflurane transiently depress in vitro NK cell activity. However, 1 hr after anesthetic withdrawal, activity returns to normal (22). Halothane and enflurane also depress in vitro neutrophil chemotaxis at one MAC (23), and isoflurane inhibits tumor necrosis factor-α (TNF-α) and IL-1 secretion from stimulated lymphocytes (unknown mechanism) (24). Clinically, however, there is little evidence to support the use of one volatile anesthetic agent over another.

7. Intravenous Anesthetics

There are limited in vivo or controlled clinical studies comparing intravenous anesthetic agents. However, in vitro, propofol exerts a number of immunomodulatory effects including (a) inhibition of mitogen-provoked lymphocyte proliferation in critically ill surgical patients, but not healthy subjects (25); (b) increased TNF-α, IL-1β, IL-6, and interferon-γ (IFN-γ) production (26); (c) inhibition of neutrophil chemotaxis and respiratory burst activity (27–29); and (d) decreased total T-cell numbers and increased T-helper cell numbers (30). Significantly, some of the immunosuppressive effects of propofol may relate to the intralipid solvent.

Thiopentone also decreases neutrophil chemotaxis (31) and respiratory burst activity (29) and inhibits IFN-γ and IL-2 (32) release. Clinically, long-term, high-dose infusion has been associated with an increased risk of bacterial pneumonia (33). Etomidate inhibits basal cortisol production, abolishes the stress response, and increases mortality from wound infection in trauma patients admitted to intensive care (34).

8. Opioids

Intra- and postoperatively, high-dose fentanyl and morphine suppress NK cell activity, and inhibition persists for 24–48 hr (35,36). Other in vitro immunomodulatory effects of opioids include (a) down regulation of human class II (HLA-DR) expression (37); (b) increased TNF-α and IL-8 levels; (c) decreased IL-6 and IFN-γ levels (38,39); and (d) increased anti-inflammatory cytokine levels (IL-10, IL-1 receptor antagonist, TNF-soluble receptor). Although chronic morphine administration has also been shown to be immunosuppressive in preclinical animal models (40), the clinical importance of long-term opioid administration on intensive care outcome is unclear.

9. Benzodiazepines

Midazolam, the most commonly used benzodiazepine, attenuates postsurgical adrenocorticotropin hormone increase and inhibits mouse mast cell proliferation and subsequent TNF-α release (41). Prolonged (>48 hr) infusion also suppresses proinflammatory (TNF-α, IL-1β, IL-6,) and anti-inflammatory (IL-8) cytokine production (42). However, there are no significant effects on neutrophil function, and long- term use in intensive care may be less harmful than propofol (42).

In summary, although various anesthetic agents and techniques would appear to have important effects on immune function, clinical significance is not well established. Available evidence suggests that anesthetic agents have short-term, but reversible, effects on host defense mechanisms, and there is no direct evidence to suggest that one anesthetic technique is uniformly associated with a higher postsurgical infection rate or increased incidence of tumor metastases. The immunosuppressive properties of drugs appear to be more pertinent in the intensive care environment where they are used for prolonged periods.

IV. INTENSIVE CARE PERSPECTIVES

Increasing numbers of immunocompromised cancer patients are being admitted to ICU. Major indications for admission include (i) postexcision of cancer and/or postoperative complications; (ii) infectious complications secondary to immunosuppression; (iii) noninfectious complications secondary to cancer or immunosuppression; and (iv) associated comorbid conditions.

Hospital mortality in immunocompromised patients admitted to ICU is 20–95% (depending on the subgroup studied) (43–45). In contrast, mortality in patients without cancer is 10–47% (46). Morbidity is also higher in immunocompromised patients with prolonged length of ventilation and increased ICU and hospital lengths of stay. Optimal ICU management should be directed towards providing adequate nutritional support to prevent malnutrition, preventing and promptly treating infections, and preventing further immune suppression.

A. Nutritional Support

Immunocompromised patients are frequently malnourished due to the effects of both the tumor itself and the effects of surgery, radiation therapy, and chemotherapy. Nutritional depletion is associated with the following conditions:

- Intolerance to surgery, radiotherapy, and chemotherapy
- Impaired tissue repair and poor wound healing, leading to an increased risk of wound complications and anastomotic dehiscence
- Impaired cellular and humoral immunity
- Increased risk of postoperative infections
- Increased ICU morbidity and mortality

Desirable goals of nutritional support include minimizing the metabolic effects of starvation, preventing specific nutrient deficiencies, and supporting the acute inflammatory response until the hypermetabolic phase has resolved and healing has begun.

Immunocompromised patients do not have greater or more specific nutritional requirements than nonimmunocompromised patients. The initial nutritional regimen should, therefore, provide 25–30 kcal/kg per day and include the following.

1. Carbohydrates (60–70% of nonprotein calories). Complications related to glucose administration include hyperglycemia, hyperosmolar states, increased carbon dioxide production, and hepatic steatosis.
2. Fats (25–30% of nonprotein calories). Parenteral lipid side effects include hyperlipidemia, cytokine release, impaired immunity, hypoxemia (reduced diffusing capacity), and ventilation/perfusion abnormalities.
3. Protein (1.2–2 g/kg per day). Excessive protein supplementation may worsen azotemia in patients with renal insufficiency and encephalopathy in patients with hepatic failure.
4. Fluid and electrolytes to maintain fluid balance and normal serum electrolyte levels.
5. Vitamins and trace elements as per recommended daily allowance.

Enteral nutrition is generally the preferred form of support in the critically ill. It is administered easily, promotes mucosal growth and development, and helps maintain the gastrointestinal barrier. Infectious complications are reduced with enteral, compared to parenteral, nutrition (47,48). However, a consistent reduction in mortality has not been demonstrated.

In patients unsuited to oral or enteral nutrition, total parenteral nutrition (TPN) is an important alternative. Randomized, controlled trials have shown little clinical benefit from TPN in well-nourished or mildly malnourished patients with cancer undergoing chemotherapy, radiotherapy, or surgery. However, in severely malnourished patients undergoing major elective surgery (including cancer surgery) and in bone marrow transplant (BMT) recipients undergoing intensive anticancer therapy, TPN has been shown to improve clinical outcomes (49,50). It is recommended that TPN be given to malnourished patients with gastrointestinal cancer for 7–10 days before surgery to decrease postoperative complications. Total parenteral nutrition should also be administered postoperatively to any cancer patient unable to eat for >7 days (51).

B. Immunonutrition

When ingested in excess of normal daily requirements, certain key nutrients are believed to modulate various inflammatory, metabolic, and immune processes (52) (Table 1). Numerous studies have evaluated the role of single nutrients or a combination of nutrients on various clinical outcomes in critically ill surgical patients (including those with cancer) and BMT patients. Although ICU and hospital length of stay are reduced, a consistent reduction in mortality has not been demonstrated (53–55). Routine use of immunonutrients in immunocompromised patients cannot, therefore, be recommended at the present time.

C. Infections

Infections are the major cause of death in patients with hematological malignancies and the major cause of morbidity and mortality in patients with solid tumors or transplants, accounting for 75% of deaths (56–59). The presence of polymicrobial infections, multiorgan dissemination, and septic shock further increases the risk of death (60,61). Early recognition and prompt institution of empirical antimicrobial therapy is essential (62) and requires knowledge of the recognized association between certain infections and patient's immunocompetence. Table 2 lists the immune defects present in various malignancies and the commonly associated pathogens.

1. Organisms

The predominant organisms are generally gram-negative bacilli (e.g., *Pseudomonas aeruginosa*, *Escherichia coli*, and *Enterobacter* species) and gram-positive cocci (e.g., *Staphylococcus aureus*, including methicil-

Table 1 Immunomodulatory Effects of Nutrients

Nutrient	Effects
L-Arginine	Reduces nitrogen excretion and improves balance
	Enhances wound healing and collagen deposition
	Enhances splenocyte and thymocyte response to collagen
	Enhances NK and lymphokine-activated killer cell cytotoxicity
	Increases lymphocyte response to mitogens
	Increases CD4+ lymphocyte count
	Increases macrophage antitumor cytotoxic mechanisms
	Increases tumor cell proliferation/metabolism (increases chemotherapy response)
L-Glutamine	Improves nitrogen balance
	Increases gut mucosal growth/repair post-TPN, chemotherapy, irradiation sepsis, colitis
	Important lymphocyte and macrophage fuel substrate
	Enhances in vitro bacterial killing by neutrophils and monocytes
	Increases T-cell DNA synthesis
	Modulates tumor cell metabolism
	Increases postoperative blood lymphocyte levels
	Upregulates neutrophil and monocyte intracellular reactive O_2 species generation
Essential fatty acids	Increase PGE_3 production (less immunosuppressive than PGE_2)
	Reduce circulating IL-1β, IL-2, and IL-6 levels
	Inhibit in vitro T-cell response to mitogens
	Increase tumor cell death and reduces tumor size
	Enhance chemotherapy-induced cytotoxic effect on tumor cells
RNA and synthetic polyribonucleotides	Increase T lymphocyte number and function
	Enhance delayed-type hypersensitivity reactions
	Increase T suppressor cell activity
	Increase IL-1β, IL-2, IL-6, TNF-α, and IFN-β release
	Augment NK cell cytotoxicity

Abbrevations: TPN, total parenteral nutrition; DNA, deoxyribonucleic acid; O_2, oxygen; PG, prostaglandin.

Table 2 Cancer-Related Immune Defects and Common Microbial Pathogens

Immune defect	Associated conditions	Common pathogens
Defective phagocytosis and neutropenia (absolute count $<1000/\mu$L)	Acute leukemias Lymphomas Metastatic solid tumors Cytotoxic chemotherapy	*Candida* species *Aspergillus* species *Staphylococci species* *Streptococcus* species *Pseudomonas aeruginosa* Enterobacteriaceae *Enterococcus* species HSV types 1 and 2
Altered B-lymphocyte function and antibody production	Chronic lymphocytic leukemia Multiple myeloma Lymphomas Allogeneic BMT Splenectomy Graft-vs.-host disease	*Streptococcus pneumoniae* *Hemophilus influenzae* *Neisseria menigitidis* *Pseudomonas aeruginosa* *Giardia lamblia* Varicella-zoster virus *Salmonella* species *Escherichia coli*
Impaired cell-mediated immunity	Hodgkin's disease Non-Hodgkin's lymphomas Hairy cell leukemia Adult T-cell leukemia Antirejection drugs Long-term corticosteroids HIV infection	*Listeria monocytogens* *Salmonella* species *Nocardia asteroids* complex Mycobacteria *Legionella* species *Candida* species *Cryptococcus neoformans* *Pneumocystis carini* *Aspergillus* *Toxoplasma gondii* *Cryptosporidium* species Cytomegalo virus HSV Varicella-zoster virus
Breach in skin/mucous membrane	Cytotoxic chemotherapy Venipuncture site Finger pricks Lumbar punctures Indwelling urinary catheters Central/venous arterial catheters Intubation/mechanical ventilation Endoscopy	*Staphylococci* species *Streptococci* species *Pseudomonas aeruginosa* Enterobacteriaceae *Corynebacterium* *Candida* species *Aspergillus* species Varicella zoster HSV types 1 and 2

Note: HSV, herpes simplex virus; HIV, human immunodeficiency virus.

lin-resistant *S. aureus* (MRSA), coagulase-negative staphylococci, and various streptococci). Increasing antibiotic use and neutropenia increase susceptibility to fungal infections. *Pneumocystis carinii* and cytomegalovirus infections are also common in patients with impaired cell-mediated immunity.

2. *Sites of Infection*

The commonest sites of serious infection in the immunocompromised host are generally the lungs, mucosal surfaces (including oral and perirectal areas), and the bloodstream. Bacteremia and fungemia commonly occur without a documented source. Continued vigilance combined with a thorough history and physical examination and regular laboratory studies are essential to early diagnosis.

Necrotic skin lesions (e.g., ecthyma gangrenosum) due to bacteria, such as *Pseudomonas aeruginosa* and *Aeromonas hydrophila*, or fungi can develop. The surgical site may become infected, and the mouth, sinuses, and teeth are all potential sites of infection. Herpes simplex virus often causes mucous membrane lesions, and anaerobic necrotizing gingivostomatitis may occur in neutropenic patients. Perianal lesions are common in patients with acute leukemia. Other gastrointestinal infections include anorectal cellulitis, fasciitis and abscesses, necrotizing enterocolitis, and pseudomembranous colitis. Unusually, severe and prolonged viral gastroenteritis caused by adenovirus, rotavirus, and coxsackie virus has also been observed in BMT recipients. Genitourinary tract infections are common, especially in the elderly, if an indwelling urinary catheter is in situ and when pelvic tumor causes urethral obstruction. Central nervous system infections are uncommon, except for cryptococcal or *Listeria* species meningitis in patients with impaired cell-mediated immunity. Finally, immunocompromised patients in ICU are at increased risk of developing a nosocomial infection including ventilator-associated pneumonia and catheter-related blood stream infections.

3. *Investigations*

Evaluation of the acutely ill, febrile, immunocompromised patient should include the following:

- Full blood count, liver and renal chemistries, coagulation profile
- Peripheral blood and urine cultures
- Sputum cultures (if pulmonary disease is suspected)
- Swab, aspiration, or biopsy of suspected skin, mucous membrane, wound or other lesions for culture and pathologic examination
- Intravenous catheter cultures (semiquantitative),if catheter removed
- Chest radiograph

Additional tests such as mannose-binding protein and TNF-α and IFN-β levels are experimental and have been found to be noncontributory in the early diagnosis of infection in neutropenic patients with sepsis-like syndrome (63). C-reactive protein has also not been shown to be useful. Recently, increased IL-6 and IL-8 levels have been reported to be associated with a higher probability of infection, although large prospective trials are needed to validate their clinical application (64,65).

Specific infections due to organisms such as *P. carinii* and toxoplasma are best diagnosed by direct histological examination. Mycobacterial and viral infections require special culture techniques; specimens can be obtained by gastrointestinal endoscopy, bronchoscopy, or surgery. Computerized tomography, magnetic resonance imaging, and nuclear medicine scans (e.g., gallium-67 scan to detect *P. carinii* pneumonia) may be required to assess localized symptoms and signs.

4. *Antimicrobial Therapy*

Early intervention with a combination of broad-spectrum antibiotics is recommended in immunocompromised patients with sepsis. The choice of antibacterial agents usually includes a glycopeptide plus an aminoglycoside (gentamicin or tobramycin) plus either a third- or fourth-generation cephalosporin (ceftazidime or cefepime), a fluoroquinolone (ciprofloxacin or levofloxacin) or a carbapenem (imipenem or meropenem) (66). An excellent response rate (91%) to early, empirical triple-antibiotic therapy has been observed in high-risk neutropenic transplant recipients (67). In choosing an appropriate empirical antimicrobial regimen, institutional patterns of microbial resistance should be considered. Vancomycin may be used to treat *S. aureus*, especially in centers with a high prevalence of MRSA. The addition of an antifungal agent should be considered if *C. fungemia* is suspected or if fever is prolonged (>7 days), despite triple antibiotics. Amphotericin is usually the initial agent of choice for patients with severe sepsis or septic shock.

Trimethoprim-sulfamethoxazole with an aminoglycoside is needed to treat *Stenotrophomonas maltophilia*, and the newer fluoroquinolones plus an aminoglycoside may be required if an *Aeromonas* or *Plesiomonas* biliary tract infection is suspected (granulocytopenic patients).

There is an increasing pattern of antibiotic resistance emerging under broad-spectrum antimicrobial selection pressure in the immunocompromised host (68). Increased induction of extended spectrum β-lactamases has led to high-level resistance among gram-negative bacilli to cefoperazone and ceftazidime (69). Infections with vancomycin-resistant enterococci (VRE) have also increased, especially in the ICU. Alternative therapies include linezolid, quinopristin/dalfopristin, and a combination of doxycycline and chloramphenicol (70).

5. *Adjuvant Cytokine and Immune Therapy*

Granulocyte-macrophage colony-stimulating factor (CSF) and granulocyte-CSF administration are associated with an increased number and function (antibody-dependent cellular cytotoxicity, bacterial killing) of circulating neutrophils. However, myeloid growth factors are most beneficial when used prophylactically in neutropenic cancer patients. Mortality is not decreased when these are used in the treatment of infections, and antibiotics are still the mainstay of treatment (71). The American Society of Clinical Oncology guidelines (72) recommends the use of CSFs to reduce the likelihood of febrile neutropenia when the expected incidence is >40% and when severe febrile neutropenia has been documented following previous chemotherapy. The concomitant use of CSFs and antibiotics at the onset of a neutropenic fever should be reserved for patients with a high risk of infectious complications, including patients with myelodysplastic syndromes. The use of myeloid growth factors for the non-neutropenic, critically ill, infected cancer patient is of no proven benefit (71).

Recombinant human activated protein C (APC) is a potent anti-inflammatory and antithrombotic agent that has been reported to improve organ perfusion in patients with severe sepsis and septic shock (73). Owing to the increased risk of bleeding, APC should be used with caution in patients with a high-risk of severe hemorrhage, e.g., profound thrombocytopenia, coagulopathy, ulcerative lesions in the gastrointestinal tract.

6. *Supportive Therapy*

- Treatment of hypotension with optimal fluid resuscitation and vasoactive agents.
- Timely mechanical ventilation. Noninvasive ventilation in immunosuppressed patients with fever, pulmonary infiltrates, and respiratory failure is associated with reduced need for endotracheal intubation and decreased morbidity and mortality (74).
- Judicious sedation to prevent anxiety and agitation. Prolonged sedation with propofol should be avoided (42).
- Stress ulcer prophylaxis with H_2-receptor antagonists or proton pump inhibitors.
- Deep venous thrombosis prophylaxis with unfractionated heparin, low molecular weight heparin, or venous-compression devices.
- An appropriate nutritional regimen.
- Maintenance of skin integrity with air mattresses, positioning, etc.

D. Specific Conditions

1. *Necrotizing Enterocolitis (Typhlitis)*

Necrotizing enterocolitis usually affects patients with leukemia, solid tumors, BMT, and high-dose chemotherapy especially etoposide and cytosine arabinoside (75–77). It is characterized by full-thickness necrosis of the intestine, especially the caecum and ascending colon and is thought to arise from loss of integrity of the colonic mucosa secondary to either leukemic infiltration or a direct cytotoxic effect of chemotherapy. Enteric bacteria and fungal pathogens are then able to translocate through the bowel wall to cause bacteremia and sepsis (78).

Most patients present with fever, abdominal pain, nausea, vomiting, and diarrhoea. Typical signs of an acute abdomen are often absent or blunted by immunosuppression. Plain abdominal radiographs are usually nonspecific but may show *Pneumatosis coli*. Abdominal CT scanning (investigation of choice) shows bowel-wall thickening, dilated bowel loops, speculations, and inflammation of the pericolic fat and pneumatosis intestinalis. The differential diagnosis should include appendicitis, intramesenteric hemorrhage, ischemic colitis, and *Clostridium difficile* enterocolitis.

Medical management is usually successful, especially if immunosuppressive medication can be safely discontinued and the neutrophil count is rising. Treatment consists of nasogastric decompression, bowel rest, intravenous fluids, and broad-spectrum antibiotics. A recommended antibiotic regimen includes vancomycin, aminoglycoside, carbapenem, metronidazole, and amphotericin B (79). Granulocyte-CSF has been shown to improve outcome (80). Indications for surgery include bowel necrosis, acute perforation, toxic megacolon, and peritonitis.

2. *Hepatosplenic Candidiasis*

Hepatosplenic candidiasis (or chronic disseminated candidiasis) commonly occurs in leukemic patients with chemotherapy-induced neutropenia or following blood or marrow transplantation. Risk factors include prolonged granulocytopenia, parenteral nutrition, *Candida* colonization of oropharynx and urine, corticosteroid therapy, and advancing multiorgan dysfunction (81). Clinical findings include fever and elevated serum alkaline phosphatase. Computerized tomography scan usually reveals multiple embolic lesions in the liver and spleen. Various antifungal drugs, including amphotericin B and fluconazole, have been prescribed with varying results. Lipid-based amphotericin formulations and newer antifungals such as voriconazole, posaconazole, and caspofungin have been found to be useful. Recovery is slow (defervescence may take up to 2 weeks) and may need prolonged antifungal therapy (82). Prognosis remains poor in the setting of persistent neutropenia (81).

E. Preventing Nosocomial Infections

Immunosuppressed patients in ICU generally have multiple invasive vascular catheters and monitoring devices, which predispose them to a higher risk of nosocomial infection. Although the majority of infection control measures have not been specifically studied in immunocompromised patients, the general principles remain valid.

1. General Preventive Measures

Routine hand washing before and after patient contact remains the single most important infection-control measure (83,84). Other measures such as the use of gloves, masks, and gowns should be routine for patients with resistant organisms such as MRSA and VRE. Isolation precautions and/or cohorting to prevent transmission should also be considered. Protective isolation measures, including filtrated, positive pressure ventilation, may be used in BMT recipients and patients with profound neutropenia (85).

2. Selective Digestive Decontamination

Colonization of the oropharyngeal and gastrointestinal tract with endogenous flora usually precedes the development of nosocomial infections. The aim of selective digestive decontamination (SDD) is to prevent the overgrowth of potentially pathogenic gram-negative bacteria and yeast with the use of oral, nonabsorbable antibiotics that preserve endogenous anaerobic flora (86). There are usually three aspects to SDD:

- Oral nonabsorbable antibiotics (polymystin E or colistin sulphate plus an aminoglycoside) and an antifungal agent (amphotericin B or nystatin)
- A third generation cephalosporin (ceftriaxone or cefotaxime) intravenously for the first 3 days to eradicate previously colonized bacteria and prevent early infection
- Regular microbiological surveillance samples from throat, rectum, stomach, and trachea to monitor compliance and efficacy of SDD, to distinguish exogenous (without previous carriage) from endogenous infections, and to detect antimicrobial resistance

Although randomized, controlled studies have reported that SDD prevents late-onset nosocomial infections in selected patient subgroups (87,88), recent meta-analyses have been conflicting (87,89). However, SDD may have a place in carefully selected groups of high-risk patients such as solid organ transplant recipients, patients with prolonged (>2 weeks) neutropenia and multiple traumas, in whom its efficacy and cost effectiveness have been established (87,90,91).

3. Systemic Antimicrobial Prophylaxis

Various antibiotics (fluoroquinolones), antifungals (fluconazole), and antivirals (acyclovir, ganciclovir) have been prophylactically administered in patients with leukemia, neutropenia, and BMT recipients. Although the incidence of infection is favorably affected by these regimens, there has been no proven benefit on morbidity or mortality. Moreover, the widespread use of antimicrobial prophylaxis to prevent nosocomial infections in the immunocompromised patients may lead to the development of resistant bacterial strains and cannot be recommended.

4. Measures to Prevent Specific Infections

In addition to the earlier-mentioned measures, various specific measures to prevent the development of nosocomial blood stream, urinary tract infection, and ventilator-associated pneumonia are listed in Table 3.

V. SURGICAL PERSPECTIVES

Surgical issues for the immunocompromised patients relate to the curative or palliative resection of the tumor, the treatment of cancer-specific problems, the need for access (e.g. intravenous, airway, feeding), and the evaluation of noncancer-related conditions.

A. Surgery and Immunity

Surgery has profound effects on the immune system in the postoperative period, potentially activating latent viral infections and suppressing both cellular and humoral immune function (92). Although minor surgery is less immunomodulatory than major surgery, it may take up to 8 days, before surgery-induced immune alterations return to normal. Some of the specific immune suppressive effects of surgery include (93) the following:

- Decreased delayed hypersensitivity response
- Reduced macrophage phagocytic activity and antigen presentation
- Decreased IL-1, IL-2, and IL-6 release
- Reduced NK cell activity
- Increased TNF-α production
- Reduced helper-T cells, suppressor cells, and NK cells

The mechanisms underlying these immunomodulatory effects are unclear but are hypothesized to include the presence of a circulating immunosuppressive polypeptide associated with surgery and trauma (94) and the activation of the sympathetic nervous system and hypothalamic–pituitary axis due to pain and local tissue damage, leading to the release of neuroendocrine mediators (corticosteroids and catecholamines) (95).

B. Wound Healing

Activated macrophages play an important role in removing debris from the healing wound by triggering the

Table 3 Recommended Preventive Measures for Specific Infections

Urinary tract infections
Avoid and/or minimize IDUC use
Aseptic IDUC insertion and maintenance of closed drainage systems
Silver-alloy catheters
Catheter-related blood stream infections
Avoid prolonged CVC insertion
Alcohol-based (70%) skin solution with chlorhexidine gluconate (0.5%)
Systematic promotion of subclavian site for central venous catheters
Antibiotic-coated central venous catheters (e.g., chlorhexidine/silver sulfadiazine)
Replacement of administration sets and devices at 72 hr intervals
Replacement of CVC if evidence of local skin punctures site infection
Removal of CVC if clinical sepsis is unexplained by another potential source
Promotion of standard precautions including strict hand hygiene
Ventilator-associated pneumonia
Nonpharmacologic measures
Use of noninvasive ventilation where possible
Removal of nasogastric or endotracheal tube as soon as clinically feasible
Avoidance of unnecessary reintubation
Provision of adequate nutritional support
Avoidance of gastric over-distension
Scheduled drainage of condensate from ventilator circuits
Continuous subglottic suction of secretions above the tracheal cuff
Maintenance of adequate pressure in endotracheal tube
Humidification with heat and moisture exchanger
Promotion of standard precautions including hand hygiene
Pharmacologic measures
Avoidance of unnecessary antibiotics
Antibiotic class rotation
Limitation of stress ulcer prophylaxis to high-risk patients
G-CSF and antibiotics for neutropenic fever
Selective digestive decontamination in high-risk groups
Pneumococcal and influenza vaccination to high-risk groups
Nosocomial sinusitis
Avoidance of nasotracheal intubation
Scrupulous oral hygiene for patients receiving mechanical ventilation
Use of fine bore nasogastric tubes
Surgical site infections
Avoidance of perioperative hypothermia
Prophylactic perioperative antibiotics as short as possible
Clostridium difficile diarrhoea
Promotion of hand hygiene measures
Barrier precautions for infected patients
Reduction of environmental contamination by cleansing and disinfection
Antibiotic restriction policies

Abbrevations: IDUC, indwelling urinary catheter; CVC, central venous catheter.

immune response, releasing inflammatory mediators, stimulating B-cell and T-cell activity, and attracting fibroblasts to the wound site. Deficient immune mechanisms lead to an increased incidence of wound complications and delayed wound healing. Chemotherapy-associated neutropenia can also interfere with the early phases of wound healing, although, clinically, the adverse effects of chemotherapeutic agents on wound healing (except for corticosteroids) are not well documented.

C. Preoperative Management

General supportive measures (including appropriate fluid resuscitation and correction of electrolytes) should be undertaken. Control of underlying disease is important. For transplant recipients, it may be necessary to reduce the dosage of immunosuppressive agents. Increased steroid dosage may be necessary for patients receiving prolonged corticosteroid therapy.

D. Intraoperative Management

Surgery should be avoided, unless essential. Meticulous surgical technique will help to prevent infected hematoma and leaking anastomoses. The role of specific antimicrobial prophylaxis in immunocompromised patients is controversial, and appropriate antibiotics should be used to cover perioperative bacteremia. Antibiotics should be given no more than 30 min before the skin is incised and continued for no longer than 24 hr after surgery.

E. Postoperative Management

There should be minimal handling of the wound and drains, and catheters and vascular access devices removed at the earliest opportunity. Total parenteral nutrition may be needed for patients with prolonged postoperative ileus. Tunnelled central venous catheters may be needed for long-term nutrition in some patients. Regular examination and appropriate investigations should be carried out to detect any nosocomial infections in the postoperative period.

F. Temperature Regulation

Mild perioperative hypothermia (2°C below core temperature) due to anesthetic-induced impairment of thermoregulation, exposure to cold, and altered distribution of body heat is common during surgery. Hypothermia increases susceptibility to perioperative wound infections by (i) causing vasoconstriction, reducing oxygen tension in the tissues, and lowering resistance to infections; (ii) impairing granulocyte phagocytosis and chemotaxis; (iii) reducing macrophage mobility; and (iv) reducing antibody production. Although there are no studies specifically evaluating perioperative temperature control in immunocompromised patients, maintaining normothermia is desirable.

VI. CONCLUSIONS

Advances in cancer treatment have resulted in an increasing number of immunocompromised patients presenting for surgery and intensive care admission. Various anesthetic agents have important effects on immune function. No individual anesthetic technique has been proven to have a significant clinical advantage in immunocompromised patients, although regional anesthesia has some postulated benefits. Intensive care management of these patients includes provision of adequate nutritional support, noninvasive ventilation, early extubation, and early recognition of infection with prompt institution of broad-spectrum antibiotics. Presently, immunonutrients do not seem to have major clinical benefit. Drugs commonly used in intensive care may have important effects on immune system.

REFERENCES

1. Mackall CL, Fleisher TA. Lymphocyte depletion during treatment with intensive chemotherapy for cancer. Blood 1994; 84:2221–2226.
2. Yaniv I, Danon YL. Immune reconstitution after chemotherapy for malignant solid tumours in children. Pediatr Hematol Oncol 1994; 11:1–6.
3. Udit NV, Mazumdar A. Immune reconstitution following bone marrow transplantation. Cancer Immunol Immunother 1993; 37:351–355.
4. Alanko S, Pelliniemi T. Recovery of blood B-lymphocytes and serum immunoglobulins after chemotherapy for childhood acute lymphoblastic leukemia. Cancer 1992; 1481–1486.
5. Mustafa MM, Buchanan GR. Immune recovery in children with malignancy after cessation of chemotherapy. J Pediatr Hematol Oncol 1998; 20:451–457.
6. Mathes DD, Bogdonff DL. Preoperative evaluation of the cancer patient. In: Lefor AT, ed. Surgical Problems Affecting Patient with Cancer. Philadelphia: Lippincott–Rave, 1996:273–304.
7. Billingham ME, Mason JW, Bristow MR. Anthracycline cardiomyopathy monitored by morphologic changes. Cancer Treat Rep 1978; 62:865–872.
8. Shaw IH, Kirk AJB, Conacher ID. Anaesthesia for patients with transplanted hearts and lungs undergoing non-cardiac surgery. Br J Anaesth 1991; 67:772–778.
9. George SJ, Vuddamalay P, Boscoe MJ. Antiseptic-impregnated central venous catheters reduce the incidence of bacterial colonisation and associated infection in immunocompromised transplant patients. Eur J Anaesthesiol 1997; 14:428–431.
10. Reissell E, Orko R, Manuksela E-L, Lindgren L. Predictability of difficult laryngoscopy in patients with long-term diabetes mellitus. Anaesthesia 1990; 45:1024–1027.
11. Ruutu T. Bone marrow transplantation. Ann Chir Gynaecol 1997; 86:127–137.
12. Sharpe MD. Anesthesia and the transplanted patient. Can J Anaesth 1996; 43:R89–R93.
13. Boscoe M. Anesthesia for patients with transplanted heart and lungs. Int Anesthesiol Clin 1995; 33:21–44.
14. Ettinger NA, Trulock EP. Pulmonary considerations of organ transplantation Part I. Am Rev Respir Dis 1991; 143:1386–1405.
15. Haddow GTR, Brock-Utne JG. A non-thoracic operation for a patient with single transplantation. Acta Anaesthesiol Scand 1999; 43:960–963.
16. Ramus GV, Cesano L, Barbalonga A. Different concentrations of local anaesthetics have different modes of action on human lymphocytes. Agents Actions 1983; 13:333–341.
17. Sinciair R, Eriksson AS, Gretzer G, Cassuto J, Thomsen P. Inhibitory effects of amide local anaesthetics on stimulus-induced human leucocyte metabolic activation. LTB4 release and ZL-1 secretion in vitro. Acta Anaesthesiol Scand. 1983; 37:159–165.
18. Salo M. Effects of lignocaine and bupivacaine on immunoglobulin synthesis in vitro. Eur J Anaesthesiol 1990; 7:133–135.
19. Tonneson E, Wahlgreen C. Influence of extradural and general anaesthesia on natural killer cell activity and lymphocyte subpopulations in patients undergoing hysterectomy. Br J Anaesth 1998; 73:315–317.
20. Hashimoto T, Hashimoto S, Hon Y. Epidural anaesthesia blocks changes in peripheral lymphocyte subpopulation gastrectomy for stomach cancer. Acta Anaesthesiol Scand 1995; 39:294–298.
21. Hole A, Unsgaard G, Bseink H. Monocyte functions are depressed during and after surgery under general anaesthesia but not under epidural anaesthesia. Acta Anaesthesiol Scand 1982; 26:301–307.
22. Woods GM, Griffiths DM. Reversible inhibition of NK cell activity by volatile anaesthetic agents in vitro. Br J Anaesth 1986; 58:53–59.
23. Moudgil GC, Forest JB. Comparative effects of volatile anaesthetic agents and N_2O on human leucocyte chemotaxis in vitro. Can Anaesth Soc J 1984; 31:631–637.
24. Rossano F, Tufano R, Cipollaro de L'Ero. Anaesthetic agents induce human mononuclear leucocytes to release cytokines. Immunopharmacol Immunotoxicol 1992; 14:439–450.
25. Pirttikangas C-O, Pertilla J, Salo M. Propofol emulsion reduces proliferative responses of lymphocytes

from intensive care patients. Intensive Care Med 1993; 19:299–302.
26. Larsen B, Hoff G, Wilhelm W, Buchinger H, Wanner G, Bauer M. Effect of intravenous anaesthetics on spontaneous and endotoxin stimulated cytokine response in cultured human whole blood. Anaesthesiology 1998; 89:1218–1222.
27. Jensen AG, Dahlgaeen C, Entrei C. Propofol decreases random and chemotactic stimulated locomotion of human neutrophils in vitro. Br J Anaesth 1993; 70:99–100.
28. O'Donnell NG, McSharry V, Wilkinson PC, Asbury AJ. Comparison of the inhibitory effects of propofol, thiopentone and midazolam on neutrophil polarisation in vitro in the presence or absence of human serum albumin. Br J Anaesth 1992; 69:70–74.
29. Heine J, Leuuer K, Scheinichen D, Ansenier L, Taeger K, Piepenbrock S. Flow cytometry evaluation of the in vitro influence of IV anaesthetics in respiratory burst of neutrophils. Br J Anaesth 1996; 77: 387–390.
30. Salo M, Pirttikangas C-O, Pulkki K. Effects of propofol emulsion and thiopentone on T1 helper cell type 1/type 2 balance in vitro. Anaesthesia 1997; 52: 341–344.
31. Heller A, Heller S, Belacrkken SA, Urbanschek R, Koch T. Effects of intravenous anaesthetics in bacterial elimination in human blood in vitro. Acta Anaesthesiol Scand 1998; 42:518–526.
32. Correa-Sales C, Tosta CE, Rizzo W. The effects of anaesthesia with thiopentone on T lymphocyte responses to antigen and mitogens in vivo and in vitro. Int J Immunopharmacol 1997; 192:117–128.
33. Braun SR, Lain AB, Clark KL. Role of corticosteroids in the development of pneumonia in mechanically ventilated head trauma victims. Crit Care Med 1986; 14:198–201.
34. Watt I, Ledingham I. Mortality amongst multiple trauma patients admitted to an intensive therapy unit. Anaesthesia 1984; 39:973–981.
35. Beilin B, Shant Y, Hart J. Effects of anaesthesia based on large vs. small doses of fentanyl on NK cell cytotoxicity in the perioperative period. Anaesth Analg 1996; 82:492–497.
36. Yeager MP, Colacehio T, Yu CT. Morphine inhibits spontaneous and cytokine enhanced NK cell cytotoxicity in volunteers. Anaesthesiology 1995; 83:50–58.
37. McBride WI, Armstrong WA, Crockford AD. Selective reduction in leucocyte antigen expression after high dose fentanyl administration at cardiac surgery. Br J Anaesth 1994; 73:717–718.
38. Morgan EL. Regulation of human B lymphocyte activation by opioid peptide hormones. Inhibition of IgG production by opioid receptor class (mu-, kappa- and delta-) selective antagonists. J Neuroimmunol 1996; 65:21–30.
39. Nair MP, Schwarts SA, Polasani R, Hou J, Sweet A, Chadna KC. Immunoregulatory effects of morphine on human lymphocytes. Clin Diagn Lab Immunol 1997; 4:127–132.
40. Di Francesco P, Gazino R, Casalinuovo IA, Palamaro AT, Favalli C, Graci E. Antifungal and immunoadjuvant properties of fluconazole in mice immunosuppressed with morphine. Chemotherapy 1997; 43:198–203.
41. Bidri M, Royer B, Averlant G, Bismuth G, Guillosson JJ, Aroa M. Inhibition of mouse mast cell proliferation and pro-inflammatory mediator release by benzodiazepines. Immunopharmacology 1999; 43:75–86.
42. Helmy SA, Al-Attiyah RJ. The immunomodulatary effects of prolonged intravenous infusion of propofol versus midazolam in critically ill surgical patients. Anaesthesia 2001; 56:4–8.
43. Afessa B, Tefferi A, Hoagland HC. Outcome of recipients of BMT who require ICU support. Mayo Clin Proc. 1992; 67:117–122.
44. Groeger JS, White P Jr, Nierman DM. Multicentre outcome of cancer patients admitted to the ICU. A probability of mortality model. J Clin Oncol 1998; 16: 761–770.
45. Hauser MJ, Tosak J, Baler H. Survival of patients with cancer in a medical critical care unit. Arch Intern Med 1982; 142:527–529.
46. Dragsted L, Qrist J. Outcome from intensive care. A 5-year study of 1308 patients: methodology and patient population. Eur J Anaesthesiol 1989; 6:23–27.
47. Moore FA, Feliciano DV, Andrassy RJ. Early enteral feeding compared with parenteral reduces postoperative septic complications. The results of a meta-analysis. Ann Surg 1991; 216:172–183.
48. Kudsk KA, Croce MA, Fabian TC, Tolley EA, Poret HA, Kuhl MR, Brown RO. Enteral versus parenteral feeding: effects on septic morbidity after blunt and penetration abdominal trauma. Ann Surg 1992; 215:503–513.
49. Rivadeneira DE, Evoy D, Fahey TJ, et al. Nutritional support of the cancer patient. Cancer J Clin 1998; 48: 69–80.
50. Scouba WW. Nutritional support. N Engl J Med 1997; 336:41–48.
51. Klein S, Kinney J, Jeejeeboy K. Nutritional support in clinical practice. Review of published data and recommendation for future research directions. Am J Clin Nutr 1997; 66:683–706.
52. Heys SD, Gough DB, Khan L, Eremin O. Nutritional pharmacology and malignant disease: a therapeutic modality in patients with cancer? Br J Surg 1996; 83:608–619.
53. Heys SD, Walker LG, Smith I, Eremin O. Enteral nutritional supplementation with key nutrients in patients with critical illness and cancer: a meta-analysis of randomised controlled clinical trials. Ann Surg 1999; 229:467–477.
54. Wilmore DG. The effect of Glutamine supplementation in patients following elective surgery and accidental surgery. J Nutr 2001; 131:2543S–2584S.

55. Ziegler TR. Glutamine supplementation in cancer patients receiving BMT and high dose chemotherapy. J Nutr 2001; 131:2578S–2584S.
56. Winston DJ, Emmanouilides C, Busuttil RW. Infection in liver transplant recipients. Clin Infect Dis 1995; 21:1077–1089.
57. Chang HY, Rodriguez V, Narboni G, Bodey GP, Luna MA, Freireich EJ. Causes of death in adults with acute leukemia. Medicine (Baltimore) 1976; 55:259–268.
58. Sable CA, Donowitz GR. Infections in BMT recipients. Clin Infect Dis 1994; 18:273–281.
59. Masur H, Cheigh JS, Stubenbord WT. Infection following renal transplantation: a changing pattern. Rev Infect Dis 1982; 4:1208–1219.
60. Bone RC. The pathogenesis of sepsis. Ann Intern Med 1991; 115:457–469.
61. Parillo JE. The pathogenetic mechanisms of septic shock. N Engl J Med 1993; 328:1471–1478.
62. Bryan CS, Reynolds KL, Brenner ER. Analysis of 1186 episodes of gram-negative bacteremia in a non-university hospital. The effects of antimicrobial therapy. Rev Infect Med 1983; 5:629–638.
63. Engel A, Mack E, Kern P, Kern WV. An analysis of IL-8, IL-6 and CRP serum concentrations to predict fever, gram-negative bacteremia and complicated infection in neutropenic patients. Infection 1998; 26:213–221.
64. De Bont ES, Vellenga E, Swaanenburg JL, Fiddler V, Viser-vaan Brummen PJ, Kamps WA. Plasma IL-8 and IL-6 levels can be used to define a group with low risk of septicemia among cancer patients with fever and neutropenia. Br J Haematol 1999; 107:375–380.
65. Lehrnbecher T, Venzon D, de Hass M, Channock SJ, Kuhl J. Assessment of measuring circulating levels of IL-6, IL-8, CRP, soluble Fc gamma receptor type III and mannose-binding protein in febrile children with cancer and neutropenia. Clin Infect Dis 1999; 29:414–419.
66. Hughes WT, Armstrong D, Bodey G, Feld R, Mandell GL, Meyers JD, Pizzo PA, Schimpff SC, Shenep JL, Wade JC. From the infectious Diseases Society of America. Guidelines for the use of antimicrobial agents in neutropenic patients with unexplained fever. J Infect Dis 1990; 161:381–396.
67. Bosi A, Laszlo D, Bacci S, Fanci R, Guidi S, Saccardi R, Vannucchi AM, Rossi-Ferrini P. An open evaluation of triple antibiotic therapy including vancomycin for febrile BMT recipients with severe neutropenia. J Chemother 1999; 11:287–292.
68. Wilson APR. Emerging antimicrobial resistance in the surgical compromised host. J Chemother 1999; 11: 518–523.
69. Rolston KV, Elting L, Waguespack S, Ho DH, LeBlanc B, Bodey GP. Survey of antibiotic susceptibility among gram-negative bacilli at a cancer center. Chemotherapy 1996; 42:348–353.
70. McNeil SA, Clark NM, Chandrasekar PH, Kauffman CA. Successful treatment of vancomycin-resistant enterococcus faecium bacteremia with linezolid after failure of treatment with synercid (quinopristin/dalfopristin). Clin Infect Dis 2000; 30:403–404.
71. Glaspy JA. Hematologic supportive care of the critically ill cancer patients. Semin Oncol 2000; 27:375–383.
72. American Society of Clinical Oncology. Recommendations for the use of haemopoietic colony-stimulating factors: evidence based, clinical practice guidelines. J Clin Oncol 1994; 12:2471–2508.
73. Bernard GR, Vincent JL, Latere PF, LaRosa SP, Dhainaut J-F, Lopez-Rodriguez A, Steingrub JS, Garber GE, Helterbrand JD, Ely EW, Fisher CJ. Efficacy and safety of recombinant human activated protein C for severe sepsis. N Engl J Med 2001; 344: 699–709.
74. Gilles H, Gruson D, Vargas F, Valcitiono P, Gbikpi-Benissar G, Michael R, Cardinaud JP. Noninvasive ventilation in immunosuppressed patients with pulmonary infiltrates, fever and acute respiratory failure. N Engl J Med 2001; 344:481–487.
75. Baerg J, Murphy JJ, Anderson R, Maggey JF. Neutropenic enteropathy: a 10-year review. J Pediatr Surg 1999; 34:1068–1071.
76. Boggio L, Pooley R, Roth SI, Winter JN. Typhlitis complicating autologous blood stem cell transplantation for breast cancer. Bone Marrow Transplant 2000; 25:321–326.
77. Kunkel JM, Rosenthal D. Management of ileocaecal syndrome. Dis Colon Rectum 1985; 29:196–199.
78. Katz JA, Wagner ML, Goesik MV. Typhlitis: an 18-year experience and postmortem review. Cancer 1990; 65:1041–1047.
79. Wade DS, Nava HR, Douglass HO Jr. Neutropenic enterocolitis. Clinical diagnosis and treatment. Cancer 1992; 69:17–23.
80. Hanada T, Ono I, Hirano C, Kurosaki Y. Successful treatment of neutropenic enterocolitis with recombinant granulocyte stimulating factors in a child with ALL. Eur J Pediatr 1990; 149:811–812.
81. Maksymiuk AW, Thongprasert S, Hopfer R, Luna M, Fainstein V, Bodey GP. Systemic candidiasis in cancer patients. Am J Med 1984; 77:20–27.
82. Sallah S, Semelka RC, Wehbie R, Sallah W, Nguyen NP, Vos P. Systemic candidiasis in patients with acute leukaemia. Br J Haematol 1999; 106:697–701.
83. Goldman D, Larson E. Hand washing and nosocomial infection. N Engl J Med 1992; 327:120–122.
84. Voss A, Widmer AF. No time for handwashing? Handwashing versus alcoholic rub; can we afford 100% compliance? Infect Control Hosp Epidemiol 1997; 18:205–208.

85. Pizzo PA. The value of protective isolation in preventing nosocomial infections in high risk patients. Am J Med 1981; 70:631–637.
86. Heyland DK, Cook DJ, Jaeschke R, et al. Selective decontamination of the digestive tract: an overview. Chest 1994; 105:1221–1229.
87. Nathens AB, Marshall JC. Selective decontamination of the digestive tract in surgical patients: a systematic review of the evidence. Arch Surg 1999; 134:170–176.
88. Ramsay G, Van Saene RH. Selective gut decontamination in intensive care and surgical practice: where are we? World J Surg 1998; 22:164–170.
89. Kollef MH. The role of selective digestive decontamination on mortality and respiratory tract infections: a meta analysis. Chest 1994; 105:1101–1108.
90. Emre S, Sebastian A, Chodoff L, et al. Selective decontamination of the digestive tract helps prevent bacterial infections in the early postoperative period after liver transplant. Mt Sinai J Med 1999; 66:310–313.
91. Silvestri L, Mannucci F, Van Saene HK. Selective decontamination of the digestive tract: a lifesaver. J Hosp Infect 2000; 45:185–190.
92. Howard EJ, Simmons RL. Acquired immunologic deficiencies after trauma and surgical procedures. Surg Gynecol Obst 1974; 139:771–777.
93. Nelson CJ, Lysle DT. Severity, time and B-adrenergic receptor involvement in surgery-induced immune alterations. J Surg Res 1998; 80:115–122.
94. Luecken L, Lysle DT. Evidence for the involvement of B-adrenergic receptors in conditional immunomodulation. J Neuroimmunol 1992; 38:209–219.
95. Constantian MB, Menzoian JO, Nimberg RB, Schmid K, Mannick JA. Association of a circulating immunosuppressive polypeptide with operative and accidental trauma. Ann Surg 1976; 185:73–79.

SUGGESTED READINGS

Lefor AT. Perioperative management of the patient with the cancer. Chest 1999; 115:165S–171S.

McBride WT, Armstrong MA, McBride SJ. Immunomodulation: an important concept in anaesthesia. Anaesthesia 1996; 51:465–473.

Wong PW, Enriquez A, Barrera R. Nutritional support in critically ill patients with cancer. Critical Care Clin 2001; 17:743–767.

Safdar A, Armstrong D. Infectious morbidity in critically ill patients with cancer. Crit Care Clin 2001; 17:531–570.

Heys SD, Gough DB, Khan L, Eremin O. Nutritional pharmacology and malignant disease: a therapeutic modality in patients with cancer. Br J Surg 1996; 83:608–619.

16

Anesthesia for the Chronic Pain Patient

ARUN RAJAGOPAL and HEMANT N. SHAH

Section of Cancer Pain Management, Department of Anesthesiology, The University of Texas M.D. Anderson Cancer Center, Houston, Texas, U.S.A.

I. INTRODUCTION

Pain is a ubiquitous symptom that manifests in many forms, ranging from acute to chronic, simple to complex, nociceptive to neuropathic, and simple-to-treat to extremely difficult. In an attempt to develop consensus guidelines for treating pain, the International Association for the Study of Pain (IASP) developed what has become the standard definition for pain: an unpleasant sensory and emotional experience associated with actual or potential damage, or described in terms of such damage (1). From this definition, it can be readily appreciated that "sensory" and "emotional," "actual," or "potential" convey the difficulty assessing such a subjective experience. There are no laboratory tests, radiographs, or other analytical studies available to define exactly *how much* pain a person experiences. To further clarify and organize pain, the IASP developed a set of terms to facilitate communication and guide appropriate treatment (2). Although the IASP did not specifically address the difference between acute and chronic pain, this distinction is relevant to the practice of anesthetizing a "chronic pain" patient.

The principal differences between acute and chronic pain lie in the differences in time until the reasonably expected period of healing has passed. Acute pain is generally of sudden onset and is, for the most part, associated with readily identifiable injury to body tissues. Chronic pain may or may not originate with tissue injury but generally extends for a long period of time and attempts to identify ongoing tissue injury are less successful. The presence or extent of pain, as reported by the patient, may be out of proportion to the actual tissue injury present. Patients experiencing chronic pain often continue to seek treatment and long-term treatment may or may not be effective. The chronic nature of the typical "chronic pain" patient has led some investigators to suggest an affective component to the pain experience (2). Because the brain is modified by experience, perhaps the method in which the brain processes noxious input is affected. As such, chronic pain patients may indeed experience more "pain" than otherwise healthy individuals.

For the purposes of our discussion on anesthetizing the chronic pain patient, the term "pain" is too broad. The experience of "pain" may include *nociception* (activation of specialized nerve receptors from ongoing tissue damage), *perception* (the brain's interpretation of incoming signals), and *expression* (the patient's report, either verbally or by other means). Complicating this experience further, especially in the chronic pain patient, may be *fatigue*, *depression*, *anxiety*, or *somatization* (the conversion of an emotional experience into a bodily symptom). These factors can amplify the presentation of pain by increasing the perception and expression of pain in the absence of ongoing tissue damage.

The practice of anesthetizing a patient is a simple exercise in blocking the patient's ability to experience an "acute," purely "nociceptive" stimulus. However, for the chronic pain patient, the preexisting issues discussed above may make this a challenging exercise. In this chapter, the pertinent issues in preoperative assessment, intraoperative management, and postoperative care will be discussed. Postoperative care in the intensive care setting will also be discussed, especially as it relates to guidelines for extubation and ongoing management.

II. IMPLICATIONS FOR THE ANESTHESIOLOGIST

In 1992, the agency for Health Care Policy and Research (AHCPR) released guidelines titled "Acute Pain management: Operative or Medical Procedures and Trauma." The Joint Commission on Accreditation of Healthcare Organization (JCAHO) instituted new pain management standards for 2001 (3). These standards mandate that hospital and clinic staff ensure comprehensive pain assessment and management in all patients treated in those facilities. The American Pain Society has created a slogan calling pain "the fifth vital sign" (4). With this increasing attention to pain management, more patients are consuming opioids on a long-term basis. There is a growing trend toward using these agents in patients with chronic nonmalignant pain (5–7). Thus, it is likely that anesthesiologists will see increasing numbers of patients who are on chronic opioid therapy. Chronic pain patients who are opioid-tolerant pose unique challenges in the perioperative period.

Any patient with chronic pain can be difficult to manage when acute pain is superimposed on the chronic pain condition. These patients may experience a heightened perception of pain with greater difficulty in managing this pain. Furthermore, the chronic use of opioids may limit the effectiveness of opioids in the intra- and postoperative period. Finally, a small subset of chronic pain patients may be using opioids for illegitimate reasons. These patients may be reluctant to discuss their social habits during a preoperative visit. Thus, greater difficulty may be expected in the perioperative management of illicit drug users who require surgery.

III. BASIC DEFINITIONS

The following definitions should be familiar to all clinicians who are managing a chronic pain patient undergoing a surgical procedure (2,8).

Morphine-equivalent daily dose (MEDD): It is the patient's daily dose of chronic opioid medication, standardized to its equivalent daily dose of oral morphine. For example, a patient consuming oxycodone 100 mg per os daily would have an MEDD of 150. A patient consuming morphine sulfate 200 mg per os daily would have an MEDD of 200 (see Tables 1 and 2).

Nociceptive pain: It is associated with ongoing tissue damage. Nociceptive pain is classified into *somatic and visceral pain*. Somatic pain is from activation of cutaneous and deep tissue nociceptors. It is usually throbbing and well localized. Visceral pain is activation of nociceptors from stretching and/or inflammation of visceral organs. It is usually an aching, pressure-like pain and is poorly localized. Nociceptive pain usually responds to opioids.

Neuropathic pain: It is described as burning or lancinating. It may have an electric, shock-like quality. It is usually caused by damage to nerve or nerve plexi by surgery, radiation, tumors, or traumatic events.

Table 1 Opioid Conversion Table

Opioid	From IV opioids to IV morphine	From same IV opioid to oral opioid	From oral opioid to oral morphine	From oral morphine to oral opioid
Morphine	1.0	3.0	1.0	1.0
Hydromorphone	5.0	3.0	5.0	0.2
Meperidine	0.13	3.0	0.1	10.0
Oxycodone	—	—	1.5	0.7
Hydrocodone	—	—	0.15	7.0
Methadone[a]	—	1.0	1.0	0.1
Codeine	—	—	0.15	7.0

[a] The conversion factors between methadone and other opioids shown above are valid only in opioid-naïve patients. Methadone may be 10–15 times more potent than other opioids at higher doses. Thus, caution must be exercised in opioid-tolerant patients.

Table 2 Conversion Table for Transdermal Fentanyl

IV morphine (mg/24 hr)	Fentanyl equivalent (mcg/hr)
8–22	25
23–37	50
38–52	75
53–67	100
68–82	125
83–97	150

To determine the 24-hr morphine equivalent dose requirement, select the mcg/hr dose according to the ranges listed above. For dosage requirement > 100 mcg/hr, multiple patches can be used (patch duration = 72 hr). To titrate the dose effectively, prescribe a dose of morphine or other opioids as needed, especially during the first 12 hr. The patch will take 18 hr to achieve the peak dose. Increase the dose based on the additional amount of opioids required during the 72-hr period.
Rule of thumb: 25 mcg/hr patch = 60 mg oral morphine daily.

Neuropathic pain does not respond as well to opioids; thus, higher doses are generally required (9).

Tolerance: It is a pharmacologic property of many opioids (and other drug) defined as less susceptibility to the effects of the drug as a consequence of its prior administration. Clinically, in relation to the treatment of pain with opioids, tolerance is manifested as a pattern of increasing dose requirements to maintain a given level of analgesia. Special caution is needed in dealing with "incomplete cross-tolerance" seen in patients with cancer pain when one opioid is replaced with another (10).

Physical dependence: It is characterized by the occurrence of an abstinence syndrome after abrupt discontinuation of the drug or administration of an antagonist.

Addiction: The labels of pharmacologic tolerance and physical dependence do not imply the aberrant psychologic state or behaviors of the addicted patient. Addiction is a chronic disorder characterized by the compulsive use of a substance resulting in physical, psychological, or social harm to the user and continued use despite that harm.

IV. PREANESTHETIC EVALUATION

In addition to the standard preoperative assessment for all patients, the preanesthetic evaluation for the chronic pain patient begins with an assessment of the MEDD. Chronic pain patients often consume opioids and adjuvants on a daily basis and many of these medications are known to affect anesthetic requirements (i.e., minimum alveolar concentration or MAC) (Table 3). Although a general evaluation of chronic pain patients includes many other factors (Table 4), the relevant points to consider for a preanesthetic evaluation are the type of pain syndrome and possible effect on other bodily systems, and the pharmacologic medications consumed.

A. Preanesthetic Guidelines (Fig. 1)

Know the MEDD: Calculating the MEDD allows the clinician to safely guide intraoperative and postoperative analgesia. There is no "standard" or routine dose of preoperative analgesia. Each patient's needs are different and an awareness of the MEDD will prevent a patient from experiencing too much pain from inadequate analgesia.

Know the pain syndrome: Certain pain syndromes can affect the patient's response to analgesics. For example, patients with neuropathic pain syndromes such as Complex Regional Pain Syndrome Types I or II (CRPS I or II, formerly known as RSD or causalgia, respectively), postherpetic neuralgia, or phantom limb pain may experience hyperalgesia on a chronic basis and may not respond as effectively to

Table 3 Factors Affecting Minimum Alveolar Concentration (MAC) of Inhaled Anesthetics

Factor	Increase or decrease MAC
Pharmacologic agents	
Opioids	++ Decrease at high doses + Decrease at low doses (32)
Tramadol	Decrease (33)
Nonsteroidal anti-inflammatory drugs (NSAIDs)	Decrease (34)
Lithium	Decrease
Clonidine	Decrease
Ketamine	Decrease
Benzodiazepines	Decrease
Lidocaine	Decrease
Barbiturates	Decrease
Alcohol use	
Chronic alcohol use	Increase
Acute alcohol use	Decrease
Illicit drugs	
Acute increase of central neurotransmitter levels (cocaine, ephedrine, amphetamines)	Increase
Tetrahydrocannabinol (marijuana)	Decrease

Source: From Ref. 31.

Table 4 Multidimensional Pain Assessment: Items with an (*) Are Important in Preoperative Evaluation

General	*Location and radiation of pain
	*Onset and time course of pain
	*Severity of pain, based on numerical pain scale score of 0 (least) to 10 (worst)
	*Exacerbating and relieving factors
	*Current and past pain medication regimens. Record type, dose, and dosing interval as well as duration of all opioid analgesics and adjuvant drugs
	*Other treatments in the past for pain relief
	Effectiveness of the treatment/medication
Psychological	*Cognitive status: any impairment/delirium
	*Psychological distress
	Patient's coping ability to stress
	*History of alcohol or drug addiction
	*Psychological evaluation should include information about the presence of psychological symptoms (e.g., anxiety, depression), psychiatric disorders, personality traits or states, coping mechanisms, and the meaning of the pain
	Prior treatment for anxiety, depression, or psychological problems
Social	Influence of pain on social living
	Patient's social support network
	Financial stressors
Cultural	Influence of patient's cultural traditions, customs, beliefs, and values that influence pain
Spiritual	Meaning of pain by patient
	Influence of spiritual issue on expression of pain

opioids. These patients may be consuming high-dose opioids on a chronic basis and may need higher intraoperative and postoperative doses.

Impact on airway control: Certain chronic pain syndromes, such as rheumatoid arthritis or cervical degenerative disc disease, may result in a chronically unstable cervical spine. The implications of this, in terms of airway control, may be very important, as these patients may need higher doses of preoperative medications before being able to attempt an awake airway.

Know the pharmacologic effect of chronic pain medications: Routinely stopping the newer COX-2 inhibitors (Celecoxib and Rofecoxib) is unnecessary perioperatively. These medications do not affect platelet function, in contrast to the standard nonselective anti-inflammatory medications (Ibuprofen, Naproxen, etc.) (11). Be aware of medications that may lead to withdrawal syndromes if abruptly stopped (opioids, benzodiazepines, anti-epileptics).

Consider regional anesthesia: For the chronic pain patient consuming high doses of pain medications, regional anesthesia offers significant perioperative benefit. Epidural analgesia should be considered whenever feasible, especially for surgery involving the lower extremities, trunk, and thorax. Local anesthetic admixtures may reduce the overall opioid burden, although adequate replacement is still essential to avoid withdrawal. Preliminary evidence suggests that sufentanil in combination with local anesthetics may be more effective than a morphine and local anesthetic combination (12).

Counsel the patient: Often, chronic pain patients have significant overlying anxiety and this may manifest as increased pain. Allaying the patient's fears by discussing postoperative analgesic options can also prevent the patient from developing unreasonable expectations.

V. INTRAOPERATIVE ANESTHETIC CONSIDERATIONS

The intraoperative period may be very challenging for the anesthesiologist. The amount of opioid to be used and duration of surgery needs to be taken into consideration. Underdosing a patient chronically exposed to opioids may lead to significant intraoperative pain and distress. Since the patient may be under neuromuscular blockade, the only signs may be profound hemodynamic fluctuations.

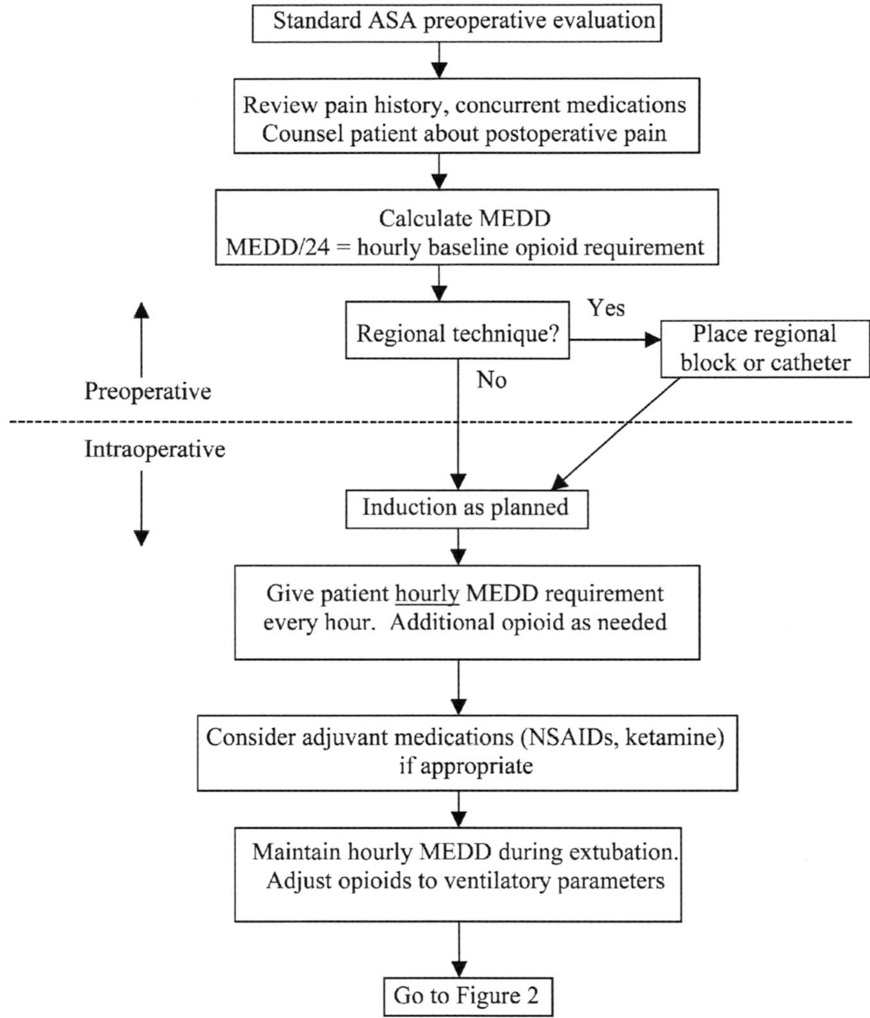

Figure 1 Preoperative and intraoperative algorithm for the chronic pain patient.

A. Intraoperative Guidelines (Fig. 1)

Although there are no previously published guidelines for anesthetizing a chronic pain patient, we recommend the following general guidelines:

(1) *Opioid management*: Use a standard equianalgesia conversion table to convert the patient's MEDD into parenteral morphine (or other suitable intravenous analgesic) equivalents per hour. Continue opioids throughout the perioperative period and titrate liberally intraoperatively, bearing in mind that tolerance is commonly present. The presence of tolerance may necessitate frequent and higher dosing. Adequate doses of opioids should be provided to replace regular use, and at least an additional 30% (or more) is required for the acute postoperative period.

(2) During induction, this group of patients may experience a greater degree of nociception which may lead to a greater degree of hemodynamic instability. If possible, the use of prophylactic lidocaine or esmolol before laryngoscopy is advisable.

(3) Intraoperative supplementation with ketamine may be associated with additional benefit as a result of its interaction with the *N*-methyl-D-aspartate receptor (13). Since ketamine has no opioid-receptor activity, it may serve as an excellent adjuvant in the perioperative period. Supplemental use of benzodiazepines may be advisable because of ketamine's psychotropic side effects.

(4) Certain groups of patient with chronic pain may have limb deformities or spastic contractures, which will need to be addressed in view of positioning and padding the pressure-sensitive areas. In addition, the length of time between development of contracture and administering anesthesia may need to be considered if succinylcholine is to be used as part of the anesthetic.

VI. POSTOPERATIVE CONSIDERATIONS

In the postoperative period, chronic pain patients can present challenges to satisfactory pain control, recovery from surgery, patient satisfaction, and optimizing hemodynamic stability. Depending on the nature of the surgical procedure, postoperative care may include a short postanesthesia care unit stay, a longer inpatient stay, or a period of time spent in the intensive care unit. For the chronic pain patient, each situation requires careful knowledge of the patient's history to provide satisfactory pain control. In the intensive care unit, careful knowledge of the patient's history, especially medication history, may mean the difference between an uneventful stay leading to a smooth extubation and a prolonged and difficult stay with problems during weaning. Because postoperative pain is primarily acute and nociceptive, differentiation between the postoperative presentation of acute and chronic pain is important. Chronic pain is not simply an extension of acute pain as an isolated entity but involves multiple other factors such as altered mechanism of nociceptive modulation and amplification of neural responses that account for the differences in clinical presentation and, more importantly, the choice of therapeutic modality (14). In the chronic pain patient, the presence of concomitant psychological distress also needs to be considered.

The aim of acute postoperative pain treatment is to eliminate nociceptive input as completely as possible and to return the patient to a premorbid functional level. A background of "chronic pain" or chronic opioid use may or may not be clinically obvious (15,16). The clinician should consider the possibility of this when the following clinical triad is seen: (a) high self-reported pain score compared with other patients having similar procedures, (b) high opioid use compared with other patients having similar procedures, and (c) a relative absence of opioid-induced side effect (17).

When postoperative pain is encountered in patients with underlying documented chronic pain, a standard approach to assessment and therapy may be inadequate. Although each patient is unique, a number of general principles involving pain assessment and treatment can be applied: (a) expect high self-reported pain scores; these are common in patient with chronic pain, (b) base treatment decisions as much as possible on objective pain and functional assessment (ability to deep breath, cough, ambulate), and (c) recognize and treat non-nociceptive sources of suffering (e.g., provide anxiolytics for anxiety). When opioids are used, continue as long as is appropriate for acute pain; avoid extended therapy if it is not appropriate for a concomitant chronic condition.

A. Postoperative Guidelines (Fig. 2)

- Maintain the patient's basal opioid requirement. Make it clear that the patient will receive basal opioid replacement unconditionally and irrespective of pain reports.
- Attempt to control incidental pain as much as possible.
- Choose a nonopioid-based approach (e.g., regional anesthesia, NSAID) to treat the acute pain whenever possible.
- Expect high subjective pain scores. Do not rely only on pain scores to guide therapy.
- Recognize that detoxification is usually not an appropriate goal in the perioperative period.
- Treat comorbid psychological symptoms such as depression, anxiety, somatization as aggressively as possible. It is appropriate to use short courses of benzodiazepines in this setting.
- Respiratory depression is rarely seen in patients who are opioid tolerant. Some degree of tolerance develop to analgesia and to most side effects, such as nausea, sedation, and respiratory depression (18–20). Tolerance rarely develops to constipation and most opioid-tolerant patients will continue to require laxatives for chronic constipation.
- Consider withdrawal in the differential diagnosis for a patient who is agitated, complaining of excessive pain, restless, or confused.
- If a regional technique, such as an epidural catheter, is inserted, the total opioid dose should be reduced gradually by 50% the first day and by 20% per day thereafter to avoid withdrawal symptoms. Even if a patient experiences satisfactory analgesia with a regional technique, baseline opioids and other adjuvants should be maintained and gradually weaned.

The clinician should remember that just taking away acute postoperative pain does not eliminate the patient's environmental, cognitive, behavioral, emotional, biochemical, neurophysiologic, and social consequence of the chronic pain (21–23). Because of the neuroadaptive changes, the treatment of chronic pain must continue well past the presumed healing period of surgery. Therefore, patients should be referred to an ambulatory pain clinic for continued pain management by skilled clinicians.

B. Opioid Analgesics

Opioid analgesics form the cornerstone of pharmacological postoperative management for chronic pain

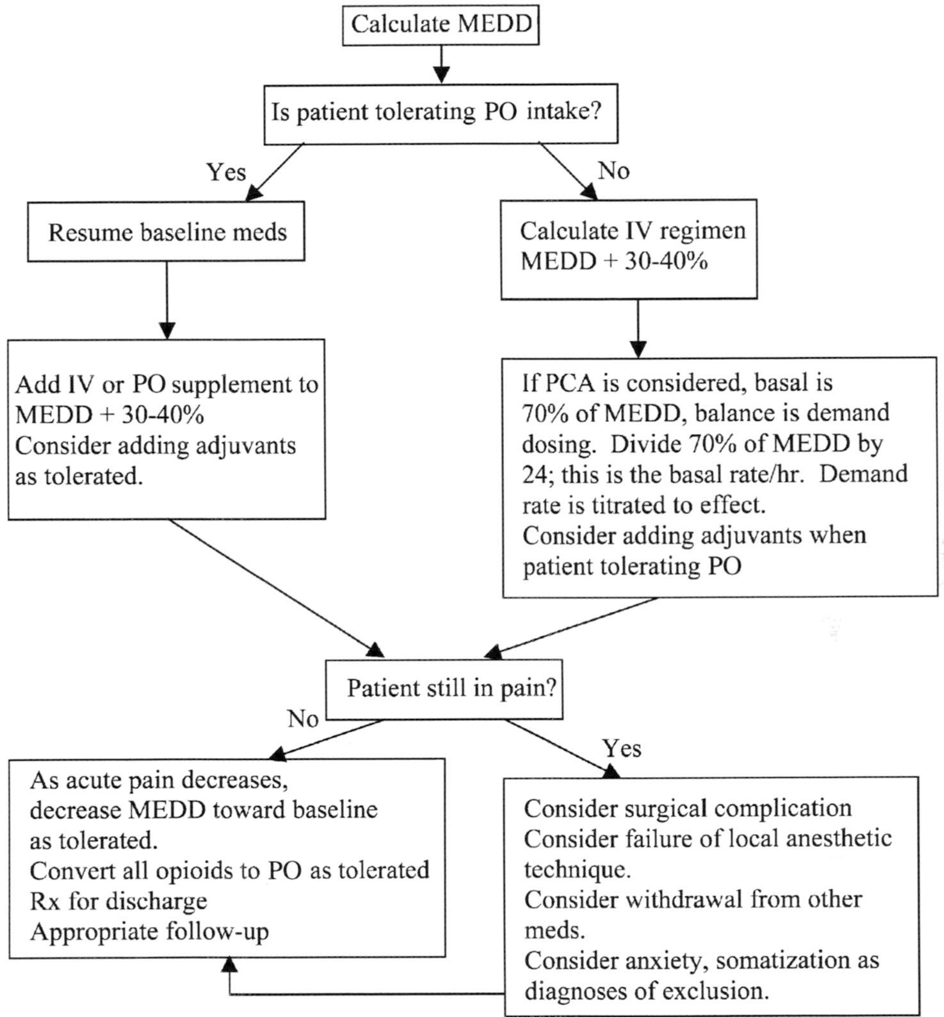

Figure 2 Postoperative pain management algorithm.

patients. For opioid-naïve patients, adjusting opioids and adjuvants as needed may be sufficient, until adverse side effects develop. For opioid-tolerant patients, stricter guidelines should be followed if opioid analgesics are prescribed as a supplement to their baseline medication in the postoperative period (24). The immediate goal is to resume or maintain the preoperative regimen as quickly as possible. A reasonable target for the desired MEDD should be a starting regimen that is 20–30% higher than the baseline MEDD. Start 70% of the total MEDD as long-acting medication and the rest as breakthrough medication. Although starting the long-acting regimen at only 70% of the baseline regimen may leave the patient slightly underdosed, this practice allows for differences in cross-tolerances of different opioids and safely minimizes the risk of overdosage. The clinician should provide an adequate breakthrough dose to allow the patient to self-medicate to the desired analgesic effect. Special precautions should be taken with elderly patients. Elderly patients should be started with only 50% as basal and the rest as breakthrough medication to prevent the risk of sedation and overdosage.

Occasionally, patients may develop unpleasant side effects with inadequate analgesia. After optimizing adjuvant medications to minimize side effects, an opioid rotation may be indicated. The rationale for opioid rotation is based on the premise that different opioids have differences in receptor activity (25,26), differences in cross-tolerances between opioid, different intrinsic efficacies, and different metabolites. As such, an opioid rotation may result in increased analgesia with fewer side effects. Because opioid conversion tables vary widely and patient response cannot be predicted, patients should be observed closely after an opioid conversion. Opioids can be weaned gradually toward preoperative doses as surgical pain resolves.

C. Adjuvant Medications

Adjuvant drugs, such as ketorolac, ketamine, metoclopramide, stool softeners, anti-epileptics, and intravenous lidocaine, should be used as supplements as required. Many side effects are seen with opioids, including constipation, nausea, and pruritus. All of these symptoms can be easily treated by the addition of stool softeners for constipation, anti-emetics for nausea, or by changing opioids. If the surgery involves the disruption of nervous tissue, a low-dose intravenous lidocaine infusion may be a helpful supplement until acute pain has subsided (27). If the patient's pain is predominantly neuropathic, a trial of gabapentin (or other suitable anti-epileptic) may be tried.

D. Patient-Controlled Analgesia (PCA)

There is varying consensus about the use of IV PCA in this group of patients. Some anesthesiologists or pain physicians believe that IV PCA probably should not be used for the purpose of providing baseline preoperative opioid medication. However, for patients who cannot tolerate oral intake in the immediate postoperative period, the PCA is a valuable adjunct method for administering opioids. Guidelines are shown in Fig. 2 and in the clinical examples shown in Sec. VIII.

VII. INTENSIVE CARE ISSUES

The two predominant issues in the intensive care unit for the chronic pain patient are adequate analgesia and prevention of withdrawal. Multiple studies have shown that provision of adequate analgesia improves ventilatory function and leads to smooth extubation (28–30). These studies looked at the "acute pain" situation in, presumably, opioid-naïve patients. For opioid-tolerant chronic pain patients, the possibility of respiratory depression affecting extubation is even more remote. Historically, the fear of respiratory depression from opioids has sometimes led to the practice of withholding opioids prior to extubation. Although there are no published guidelines for managing analgesia and extubation in the chronic pain patients, the guidelines shown below should ensure adequate analgesia and a relatively uneventful extubaion.

Withdrawal from benzodiazepines, opioids, alcohol, or other drugs remains a strong possibility in chronic pain patients and the clinician should keep this in mind if a patient becomes agitated, restless, hyperdynamic, or confused.

A. ICU Management

- Maintain analgesia at the patient's baseline MEDD plus an additional 30–40%, depending on the severity of the operative procedure.
- Maintain other routine preoperative medications if possible.
- If patient has a history of alcoholism, consider alcohol withdrawal syndrome if the patient shows signs of autonomic excitability (tachycardia, tremors, restlessness, agitation). Treatment is by intravenous supplementation of multiple vitamins, thiamine 50–100 mg daily for a week, folate 1 mg daily, intravenous sedation with benzodiazepines with gradual weaning over a week. Symptoms usually peak at day 2–3 and improve by day 4–5.
- Do not discontinue all opioids; respiratory depression is generally not a problem if the clinician follows guidelines in knowing the patient's MEDD and calculating additional doses as necessary.

VIII. CLINICAL EXAMPLES

A. Case 1

A 30-year-old man with chronic lymphocytic leukemia presents with acute appendicitis for an emergency exploratory laparotomy. His past medical history is significant for chronic back pain, depression, anxiety, and illicit drug use. He maintains he is "clean" from an illicit drug use perspective. His cancer is currently in remission but he has chronic arthralgias from his chemotherapy. He is currently taking oxycontin 60 mg per os twice daily and oxycodone 40 mg per os daily for breakthrough pain. He is also on lorazepam at an unspecified dose for anxiety. He has been on these medications for over a year.

1. *Preoperative Assessment*

- Calculate the MEDD: 240.
- Consider his chronic benzodiazepine use.
- Recent drug use? Consider toxicology screen.
- History of alcohol use?
- Note that this patient will have an increased MAC based on his opioid and benzodiazepine use and possible alcohol use.
- The acuity of the diagnosis precludes use of any regional anesthetic technique.

2. *Intraoperative Management*

- Assuming he will remain NPO in the postoperative period, he will need an MEDD of at least

240 and an additional 30% over the next 24 hours. His increased MEDD will be approximately 310–320. In the operating room, he will need his baseline MEDD divided by 24 to be given hourly (approximately 10 mg oral morphine equivalent) during his procedure plus an additional dose (usually 30–40%) to cover surgical nociception.
- Consider using intravenous hydromorphone or morphine in the operating room to approximate 70% of his basal requirements and then titrate short-acting opioids (e.g., fentanyl or sufentanil) to desired analgesic and hemodynamic effect.

3. Postoperative Management

- Maintain postoperative analgesia with at least 70% of his basal requirement to be given around-the-clock with frequent "breakthrough" dosing for his additional postoperative requirements.
- Patient may need short course of intravenous benzodiazepines to prevent withdrawal.
- If the patient continues to report poor analgesia, first consider complications of surgery. Then, consider certain other factors (hyperalgesia, anxiety, somatization) that may play a role. These factors are only considered as "diagnoses of exclusion" after increased nociception as a consequence of surgery is thoroughly evaluated.
- Consider withdrawal as a possible etiology if the patient becomes agitated, confused, or hyperdynamic.

B. Case 2

A 58-year-old woman with a history of fibromyalgia and "panic attacks" presents to the operating room for a left upper lobectomy for nonsmall cell adenocarcinoma of the lung. She is extremely anxious and tearful during the preoperative interview. She has been on a transdermal fentanyl patch for many years for her fibromyalgia and her current patch strength is 125 mcg/hr. She is also consuming lorazepam at 4 mg per os daily for anxiety.

1. Preoperative Assessment

- Calculate MEDD: 300.
- Consider her chronic benzodiazepine use.
- Any recent drug use? Consider toxicology screen.
- History of alcohol use?
- Note that this patient will have an increased MAC based on her opioid and benzodiazepine use and possible alcohol use.
- Regional anesthesia is strongly indicated unless there are contraindications. An epidural catheter will significantly reduce the postoperative opioid burden.

2. Intraoperative Management

- Assuming she will remain NPO in the postoperative period, she will need an MEDD of at least 300 and an additional 30% over the next 24 hours. Her increased MEDD will be approximately 390. She may actually need more than this because of the painful nature of this procedure. In the operating room, she will need her basline MEDD divided by 24 (approximately 12.5 mg oral morphine equivalent) to be given hourly plus an additional 30–40% to cover surgical nociception.
- Consider using the epidural catheter with a local anesthetic/opioid combination intraoperatively.
- Titrate short-acting opioids (e.g., fentanyl or sufentanil) to desired analgesic and hemodynamic effect. Even if the epidural is working satisfactorily, patient will need at least half of her baseline MEDD to avoid postoperative withdrawal.

3. Postoperative Management

- Maintain postoperative analgesia with at least 70% of her basal requirement to be given around-the-clock with frequent "breakthrough" dosing for her additional postoperative requirements. This may be delivered via the epidural as a "patient-controlled epidural."
- Patient may need short course of intravenous benzodiazepines to prevent withdrawal.
- If patient continues to report poor analgesia, first consider complications of surgery or failure of the epidural. Then, consider certain other factors (hyperalgesia, anxiety, somatization) that may play a role. These factors are only considered as "diagnoses of exclusion" after increased nociception as a consequence of surgery or catheter failure is thoroughly evaluated.
- Consider withdrawal as a possible etiology if the patient becomes agitated, confused, or hyperdynamic.
- If patient is intubated in the ICU postoperatively, maintain analgesia as calculated above during the weaning process off the ventilator.

Table 5 Perioperative "Pearls" for the Practitioner

Always know the MEDD
Use the MEDD as a guide for perioperative analgesic dosing
Do not forget to counsel the patient about expectations in the postoperative period
Consider a regional anesthetic technique if possible
Respiratory depression is rare in opioid-tolerant patients
Chronic pain patients may experience more pain
Chronic pain patients may have significant levels of depression, anxiety, and somatization
Consider withdrawal for postoperative patients who may be restless, agitated, or confused
Restart baseline medications as soon as possible

IX. CONCLUSIONS

The chronic pain patient may present many challenges to the clinician in the perioperative period. Since the presentation of "chronic pain" is quite different from "acute pain," it is incumbent on the clinician to follow basic guidelines in assessing and treating the patient's pain. A few chronic pain "pearls" are shown in Table 5 and should be kept in mind to minimize pain and distress to the chronic pain patient.

REFERENCES

1. Merskey H, Bugduk N. Classification of Chronic Pain. Descriptions of Chronic Pain Syndromes and Definitions of Pain Terms. 2nd ed. Seattle, WA: IASP Press, 1994.
2. Turk DC, Okifuji A. Pain terms and taxonomies of pain. In: Loeser JD, ed. Bonica's Management of Pain. 3rd ed. Philadelphia: Lippincott Williams & Wilkins, 2001:18.
3. Joint Commission on Accreditation of Healthcare Organizations. Pain Management standards 2001. Available at: http//www.jcaho.com/standard/stds 2001_mpfrm.html. Accessed August 14, 2001.
4. Jackson M. Pain: The Fifth Vital Sign. New York: Crown Publishers, 2002.
5. Management of Cancer Pain. Rockville, MD: U.S. Dept of Health and Human Services, Agency for Health Care Policy and Research, 1994. AHCPR Publication 94–0592.
6. Coombs DW, Saunders RL, Gaylor MS. Relief of continuous chronic pain by intraspinal narcotics infusion via an implanted reservoir. JAMA 1983; 250:2336–2339.
7. Penn RD, Paice JA. Chronic Intrathecal morphine for intractable pain. J Neurosurg 1987; 67:182–186.
8. Ready LB. Acute postoperative pain. In: Cucchiara RF, Miller ED, Gerald Reves J, Roizen MF, Savarese JJ, eds. Anesthesia. Philadelphia: Churchill Livingstone-Harcourt Brace & Co., 2000:2323–2350.
9. Rowbotham MC, Twilling L, Davies PS, Reisner L, Taylor K, Mohr D. Oral opioid therapy for chronic peripheral and central neuropathic pain. N Engl J Med 2003; 348:1223–1232.
10. Crews JC, Sweeney NJ, Denson DD. Clinical efficacy of methadone in patients refractory to other mu-opioid receptor agonist analgesics for management of terminal cancer pain: case presentation and discussion of incomplete cross-tolerance among opioid agonist analgesics. Cancer 1993; 72:2266–2272.
11. Leese PT, Hubbard RC, Karim A. Effects of Celecoxib, a novel cyclooxigenase-2 inhibitor, on platelet function in healthy adults: a randomized controlled trail. J Clin Pharmacol 2000; 40:124–132.
12. De Leon-Casasola OA, Myers DP, Donaparthi S. A comparison of post-operative epidural analgesia between chronic cancer patients taking high doses of oral opioid and opioid-naïve patients. Anesth Analg 1993; 76: 302–307.
13. Herman BH, Vocci F, Bridge P. The effects of NMDA receptor antagonist and nitric oxide synthase inhibitors on opioid tolerance and withdrawal. Medication development issues for opiate addiction. Neuropsychopharmacology 1995; 13:269–293.
14. Lubenow TB, Ivankovich AD, Mccarthy RJ. Management of acute post-operative pain. In: Barash PG, Cullen BK, Stoelting RK, eds. Clinical Anesthesia. Philadelphia: Lippincott, 2001:1403–1434.
15. Ready LB, Hare B. Drug problem in chronic pain patients. Anesthesiol Rev 1979; 6:28.
16. Turner JA, Calsyn DA, Fordyce WE. Drug utilization pattern in chronic pain patients. Pain 1982; 12:357–363.
17. Rapp SE, Ready LB, Nessly ML. Acute pain management in patients with prior opioid consumption: a case-controlled retrospective study. Pain 1995; 61:195–201.
18. Auld AW, Maki-Jokela A, Murdoch DM. Intraspinal narcotic analgesia in the treatment of chronic pain. Spine 1985; 10:777–781.
19. Twycross RG. Choice of strong analgesic in terminal cancer: dia-morphine or morphine? Pain 1977; 3: 93–104.
20. Cox BM. Molecular and cellular mechanisms in opioid tolerance. In: Towards a New Pharmacology of Pain. Chichester, UK: John Wiley and Sons Ltd, 1991:137.
21. Haddox JD, Bonica JJ. Evolution of the specialty of pain medicine and the multidisciplinary approach to pain. In: Cousin MJ, Bridenbaugh PO, eds. Neural Blockade in Clinical Anesthesia and Management of Pain 3rd ed. Philadelphia: Lippincott-Raven, 1998:113.
22. Ready LB, Laird D. The interface between acute and chronic pain. In: Ashburn MA, Rice LJ, eds. The Management of Pain. New York: Churchill Livingstone, 1998:613.
23. Murphy TM. Chronic pain. In: Miller RD, ed. Anesthesia. 4th ed. New York: Churchill Livingstone, 1994:2345.

24. Clinical Practice Guidelines Number 1: Acute Pain Management: Operative or Medical Procedures and Trauma. Rockville, MD: U.S. Dept of Health and Human Services, Agency for health Care Policy and Research, 1992. AHCPR Publication 92–0032.
25. Mercadante S. Opioid rotation for cancer pain: rationale and clinical aspects. Cancer 1999; 86:1856–1866.
26. Switzer ND, Rajagopal A. Cancer Pain Emergencies. In: Yeung SJ, Escalante C, eds. Holland-Frei Oncologic Emergencies 2002:355–368.
27. Cassuto J, Wallin G, Hogstrom S. Inhibition of postoperative pain by continuous low-dose intravenous infusion of lidocaine. Anesth Analg 1985; 64:971–974.
28. Renaud KL. Cardiovascular surgery patients' respiratory responses to morphine before extubation. Pain Manag Nurs 2002; 2:53–60.
29. Bowler I, Djaiani G, Abel R, Pugh S, Dunne J, Hall J. A combination of intrathecal morphine and remifentanil anesthesia for fast-track cardiac anesthesia and surgery. J Cardiothorac Vasc Anesth 2002; 16: 709–714.
30. Kahn L, Baxter FJ, Dauphin A, Goldsmith C, Jackson PA, McChesney J, Miller JD, Takeuchi HL, Young JE. A comparison of thoracic and lumbar epidural techniques for post-thoracoabdominal esophagectomy analgesia. Can J Anaesth 1999; 46:415–422.
31. Stevens WC, Kingston HGG. Inhalation anesthesia. Barash PG, Cullen BF, Stoelting RK In: Clinical Anesthesia. 2nd Philadelphia: JB Lippincott Co., 1992:443.
32. Ilkiw JE, Pascoe PJ, Tripp LD. Effects of morphine, butorphanol, buprenorphine, and U50488H on the minimum alveolar concentration of isoflurane in cats. Am J Vet Res 2002; 63:1198–1202.
33. de Wolff MH, Leather HA, Wouters PF. Effects of tramadol on minimum alveolar concentration (MAC) of isoflurane in rats. Br J Anaesth 1999; 83:780–783.
34. Gomez de Segura IA, Criado AB, Santos M, Tendillo FJ. Aspirin synergistically potentiates isoflurane minimum alveolar concentration reductionproduced by morphine in the rat. Anesthesiology 1998; 89:1489–1494.

SUGGESTED READINGS

ASA Task Force on Pain management, Practice Guidelines for Chronic Pain Management. Anesthesiology 1997; 86:995–1004.

Elsayem A, Driver L, Bruera E. The M. D. Anderson Symptom Control and Palliative Care Handbook. 2nd ed. Houston: UT-Houston Health Science Center Press, 2002.

Jacobson L, Mariano AJ. General considerations of chronic pain. In: Loeser JD, ed. Bonica's Management of Pain. 3rd ed. Philadelphia: Lippincott Williams & Wilkins, 2001.

Turk DC, Okifuji A. Pain terms and taxonomies of pain. In: Loeser JD, ed. Bonica's Management of Pain. 3rd ed. Philadelphia: Lippincott Williams & Wilkins, 2001.

17

Preoperative Anesthesia Evaluation

TAYAB R. ANDRABI

Department of Anesthesiology, The University of Texas M.D. Anderson Cancer Center, Houston, Texas, U.S.A.

MARC A. ROZNER

Departments of Anesthesiology and Cardiology, The University of Texas M.D. Anderson Cancer Center, Houston, Texas, U.S.A.

I. INTRODUCTION/BACKGROUND

Preoperative anesthesia evaluation and risk assessment have become an integral part of the anesthetic management of a patient about to undergo a surgical procedure. At the University of Texas M.D. Anderson Cancer Center, the Preoperative Consultation Center is the last stop for the patient on their journey to any procedure that will require an anesthetic. Although this type of consultative service is common in anesthesiology, few of our patients receive their primary care at our institution. Many of these patients have no institutional physician other than their surgeon, and the patients bring records related to their cancer but not their other medical problems. Because our patients frequently have other diseases in addition to cancer, the preoperative anesthesiologist is charged with reviewing the medical history, performing a limited physical examination, determining whether comorbid diseases have been addressed satisfactorily, and arranging appropriate tests and consultations where indicated. For 10–15% of our preoperative patients, the clinic anesthesiologist orders additional consultative testing.

In 1846, four years after Crawford Long publicly demonstrated the use of ether anesthetic, the field of surgical anesthesia became accepted by the medical profession and the general public. This new specialty was viewed as an innovative step in the management of surgical patients, and with the development of this specialty came studies of complications and untoward events associated with the use of anesthetic agents. Since then, efforts to improve anesthetic (and therefore surgical) safety have included the following: (1) advances in anesthetic pharmacology, (2) better understanding of the pharmacokinetics and pharmacodynamics of anesthetic agents, (3) development and use of "smart" monitoring devices, (4) improved training of personnel, and (5) reliable, automated drug delivery systems.

For many years, anesthesiologists have been asked to assist in the assignment of risk for an operative procedure. This practice appears to have been "codified" in 1941 with the development of the New York Society of Anesthesiologists physical status scale, first published by Saklad (1). Although the physical status score of the American Society of Anesthesiologists (ASA PS) (see Table 1) has been modified a few times and is sometimes

Table 1 The ASA Physical Status Classification System

P1	A normal healthy patient
P2	A patient with mild systemic disease
P3	A patient with severe systemic disease
P4	A patient with severe systemic disease that is a constant threat to life
P5	A moribund patient who is not expected to survive without the operation
P6	A declared brain-dead patient whose organs are being removed for donor purposes

Source: From Ref. 2.

used by nonanesthesiologists (2–4), the ASA PS scale is fundamentally static and global in nature. It takes into account a large number of factors, many of which are subtle, and most of which are known only to anesthesiologists. The ASA PS offers little guidance for identifying or modifying individual risk factors for the perioperative period. Nevertheless, it serves the specialty well, as documented by Vacanti et al. (5).

The ASA PS score has not, however, been validated for the cancer patient, and it does not take into account their cancer comorbidities, the physiological issues surrounding chemotherapeutic and radiation exposures, or the complexity of the surgery that will result. For example, multiple previous abdominal surgeries (6) or cancer therapy (7) can lead to the formation of adhesions, which might increase the operative time of abdominal surgery, exacerbate bowel swelling, and increase intraoperative fluid requirements. All of these issues might lead to increased postoperative problems. Also, not well studied are the effects of noncancer comorbid diseases (e.g., coronary artery disease, cardiomyopathy, brittle diabetes, etc.) on the outcomes from cancer therapy, whether surgical or medical. This issue is discussed in a paper by Adachi et al. (8), wherein they describe a case–control study of overweight patients with gastric cancer who have a higher incidence of hypertension and diabetes, longer operative times, and a higher incidence of cancer recurrence and death.

Therefore, at our Preoperative Consultation Center, we examine the patient's comorbidities, attempt modification of the identified risk factors to optimize the patient's medical condition within a reasonable timeframe, and sometimes discuss modifying the patient's treatment plan with the patient's other providers. Frequently at our institution, all of these activities take place within 2–3 days of initial presentation and the patient undergoes surgery shortly thereafter. Many of the patients who present to M.D. Anderson Cancer Center for a second opinion enter the operating room within a day or two of their initial visit.

More than 95% of our patients have a malignant or premalignant condition as their primary problem (our Plastic and Reconstructive Surgery Department physicians operate on some noncancer patients, our Pediatric and Neurosurgery Departments follow patients with neurofibromatosis, and patients who have had prior treatment at M.D. Anderson Cancer Center return for surgery of such nonmalignant conditions such as cholecystectomy or eye surgery). Prior treatments for malignancy—whether surgical, chemotherapeutic, or radiotherapeutic—can affect a patient's response to anesthesia and surgery. Additionally, certain tumors can cause physiological disturbances by virtue of their secretory potentials, paraneoplastic syndromes, or because of simple mass effect (e.g., increased intracranial pressure from a space-occupying mass). Adverse effects due to secretory products include: "tumor fever" from cytokine release (9), hypotension and bronchospasm from metastatic carcinoid tumors (10), and hypermetabolic syndromes from thyroid cancers (11) or pheochromocytoma (12). Adverse effects of paraneoplastic syndromes include: Eaton–Lambert syndrome (13), cancer-associated retinopathy (14), hypercalcemia of malignancy syndrome (15), and complex regional pain syndromes (16).

Activity in most preoperative clinics is revenue-negative, i.e., patients are not charged either a professional or technical fee for this evaluation. Traditionally, hospitals and practices have written off the costs associated with a preanesthesia evaluation by a member of the anesthesiology team prior to the day of surgery because of the belief that these evaluations reduced or eliminated day-of-surgery delays and cancellations. However, Stanford University, as well as the University of Florida, have charged "facility fees" for these services since 2000 (17).

In July 2001, we obtained permission from the Centers for Medicare and Medicaid Services (CMS) to render both professional and technical charges for our preoperative evaluations, as most of these evaluations are performed in lieu of perioperative management by an internist or other medical specialist outside the field of anesthesiology. Currently, our professional and technical billings from the Preoperative Consultation Center exceed our cost of operation. Additionally, our compliance with billing initiatives from CMS, commercial payers, and our own institutional rules has been substantially enhanced by the development and deployment of an electronic medical record system in the Preoperative Consultation Center (Picis Corp., MA).

II. GOALS OF PREOPERATIVE EVALUATION

The evaluation and preoperative preparation of the cancer patient must balance the urgency of operative intervention with the need to treat an intercurrent medical problem that will clearly affect the patient's perioperative course (18). After all, the patient with pancreatic cancer who has a mean life expectancy of 12 months would not benefit from a Whipple operation (pancreatectomy) if she or he suffers a preventable perioperative myocardial infarction and expires shortly after the surgery. Thus, the goals of our preoperative anesthesia assessment are similar to those in any preoperative clinic and often include extensive discussions with other physicians who will care for the patient.

The goals at our preoperative anesthesia assessment are as follows:

1. Obtain pertinent information about the patient's medical and social history and relevant records and tests, perform a physical exam according to anesthesia needs, determine if further testing or consultation is required, assign risk (ASA PS Classification), and take steps to modify risks where possible.
2. Discuss significant abnormal findings likely to increase the patient's perioperative risk with the patient's surgeon and, if need be, an oncologist, cardiologist, internist, or neurologist. Occasionally, surgery is planned in the pregnant patient, necessitating inclusion of an obstetrician.
3. Educate the patient (and his or her family) about the various forms of anesthetics that could be utilized in their case, the benefits and risks of these choices, and the reasons for choosing one over the other. For example, nearly every patient undergoing an open lung procedure at M.D. Anderson Cancer Center will receive thoracic epidural postoperative analgesia, and this modality is described in detail to the patient during the preoperative visit.
4. Prepare the patient (and his or her family) for entrance into the operating environment by explaining the equipment used, the personnel expected to be present, and the reasons that surgery might take longer than scheduled. For the patient with significant comorbidity, discussions of possible adverse events, ICU admission, and palliative measures that might be needed also take place.
5. Obtain oral consent to administer an anesthetic from the patient or guardian.
6. Ensure that the minimum guidelines for laboratory screening (see Table 2) and testing (see Table 3) have been met.
7. Determine whether a woman of childbearing age, who has not been surgically sterilized, will need a pregnancy test. Although denial of pregnancy to the 20th week of gestation occurs in 1 out of 475 deliveries (19), most preoperative anesthesiologists accept and document an immediate denial to the question "Is there any chance that you could be pregnant?" without laboratory testing. For the patient who cannot provide this assurance, a beta-HCG blood assay is ordered. Although routine testing has been advocated by some clinicians (20), it can lead to inappropriate surgical delays (21). There is also a small risk (1 per 1000–10,000 tests) of false-positive tests (22,23), which might be increased in the setting of some malignancies* (24).
8. Document the visit in a form acceptable to both our institutional needs and any governmental or commercial payer.
9. Provide guidance for the day-of-surgery use of ambulatory drugs. Currently, we ask patients to refrain from taking oral and injectable hypoglycemic agents, angiotensin-converting enzyme inhibiting drugs, and angiotensin receptor antagonists. We also ask patients to hold their insulin glargine (Lantus®) on the night prior to surgery. If the patient is to undergo

Table 2 Preoperative Screening Guidelines at M.D. Anderson Cancer Center

Test	Application
CBC	Any surgery with a risk of major bleeding or if previous CBC values are older than 1 year
BUN/Cr	Any operation involving the kidneys, ureters, bladder, or urethra. Values are acceptable for 3 months in the absence of changes in clinical condition or treatment regimens
EKG	Any male patient 45 years of age or older or any female patient 50 years of age or older; within 1 year of surgery or as indicated by medical history
T&S	Any surgery with a risk of major bleeding (e.g., any body cavity entrance, all open intracranial neurosurgery, significant sarcoma mass excision)

CBC, complete blood count (hematological) to include white blood cell count, hemoglobin, and platelet determinations; BUN/Cr, determination of the blood urea nitrogen level and the creatinine concentration; EKG, standard 12-lead electrocardiogram; T&S, a type and screen to include blood type and Rh determination as well as a Coombs' indirect test.

*Management of a positive beta-HCG pregnancy test includes the possible delay of the case due to the need for repeat testing to ensure a rising titer. Although we rarely test our patients for pregnancy, we have had one false-positive test result in the past five years.

Table 3 Preoperative Diagnostic Testing Guidelines at M.D. Anderson Cancer Center

Test	Application
Electrolytes, BUN/Cr	Hypertension Diuretic use Digitalis Bowel obstruction History of renal dysfunction Diabetes Values up to 6 months old are acceptable in the absence of changes in clinical condition or chemotherapeutic treatment regimens
Glucose	Reasonable evidence that the glucose is <300 mg/dL at the time of the surgery in the diabetic patient or the patient undergoing steroid therapy
Coagulation studies	Prothrombin (PT) and activate partial thromboplastin time (aPTT) studies are indicated for the patient on anticoagulant medicine or for the patient with a history of coagulation problems
Platelet aggregation study	Clopridogel (Plavix®) use within 5 days of surgery
EKG	History of coronary artery disease or congestive heart failure (unless there is a documented EKG within the prior 6 months and no new symptomatology) Significant risk factors for perioperative ischemia such as hypertension and diabetes mellitus Abnormal physical exam suggesting cardiac abnormalities
Chest x-ray	Signs or symptoms of active pulmonary disease

a procedure requiring NPO status the day prior to surgery (e.g., embolization to reduce bleeding), we hold insulin glargine for two nights. When a patient has been taking clopridogel (Plavix®), we ascertain 5 days of avoidance prior to surgery or schedule a platelet aggregation test for the day of surgery.

As in most other preoperative centers, any patient presenting to the Preoperative Consultation Center is asked to complete a questionnaire, which includes a review of systems and surgical and medical history items. Items on our preoperative questionnaire that are not typically found on those at other centers include information about chemotherapy, radiation therapy, specialized cardiac testing (i.e., stress tests, echocardiography, coronary angiography), and implanted devices (cardiac pacemakers and defibrillators).

III. CHEMOTHERAPY AND RADIATION THERAPY

Many patients with cancer have undergone chemotherapy, radiation therapy, or both during their cancer treatment, yet there are few studies that can be used to guide preoperative evaluation, anesthetic choice, or anesthetic management in these patients. Nevertheless, there are clear relationships between particular types of chemotherapy or radiation therapy and certain physiological derangements. The more commonly used chemotherapeutic drugs, as well as those agents that are associated with significant cardiopulmonary morbidity, will be discussed.

A. Chemotherapy

1. Anthracyclines

The anthracycline class of chemotherapeutic agents includes daunorubicin (Cerubidine®), doxorubicin (Adriamycin®), and epirubicin (Ellence®). These agents are used in patients who have breast cancer, sarcoma, leukemia, or lymphoma (Table 4). Most anesthesiologists understand that these agents produce cardiotoxic effects that manifest as decreased cardiac performance. Administration by continuous infusion seems to be better tolerated and less likely to produce cardiomyopathy than administration by bolus. Preexisting cardiac disease, concomitant administration of other chemotherapeutic agents [particularly cyclophosphamide (Cytoxan®), paclitaxel (Taxol®), and trastuzumab (Herceptin®)], chest irradiation, and extremes of age when exposed to the drug seem to increase the likelihood of developing cardiomyopathy. The risk of cardiomyopathy increases greatly above a total dose of 550 mg/m^2 for both daunorubicin and doxorubicin, and 900 mg/m^2 for epirubicin (25–27).

At our institution, most of the anesthesiologists have stopped requiring a determination of left ventricular ejection fraction prior to delivering an anesthetic in a functionally intact patient. For the patient with chemotherapy-induced cardiomyopathy (history of heart failure, inability to climb two flights of stairs, or other unexplained dyspnea on exertion), a cardiology evaluation seems prudent. These patients seem to improve on regimens such as beta blockers, angiotensin-converting enzyme inhibitors, diuretics,

Table 4 Anthracycline Chemotherapy Agents

Agent	FDA-labeled uses	Nonlabeled Uses
Daunorubicin (Cerubidine)	Acute leukemia (lymphocytic, nonlymphocytic)	Chronic myelogenous leukemia Non-Hodgkin's lymphoma Psoriasis
Doxorubicin (Adriamycin)	Bladder cancer Breast cancer Gastric cancer Leukemias (acute lymphoblastic, acute nonlymphocytic) Lung cancer, small-cell Lymphoma (Hodgkin's, non-Hodgkin's) Neuroblastoma Ovarian cancer Sarcomas Thyroid cancer Wilms' tumor	Endometrial cancer Islet cell cancer Multiple myeloma
Epirubicin (Ellence)	Breast cancer	Bladder cancer Endometrial cancer Lung cancer Nasopharyngeal carcinoma Ovarian cancer Soft tissue sarcomas

and cardiac pacing (28). Whether delaying elective surgery to institute these therapies will improve perioperative outcome is currently under investigation at our hospital.

2. *Taxanes*

Paclitaxel (Taxol) and docetaxel (Taxotere®) are used to treat breast, lung, and ovarian cancer. Both of these drugs have been associated with cardiomyopathy, peripheral neuropathy, seizures, nephropathy, and pulmonary toxicity. Docetaxel is associated with ocular canalicular stenosis (29), which might increase the probability of eye injury during a subsequent anesthetic. Paclitaxel (but not docetaxel) has been associated with bradycardia (26). Currently, there are no published treatment recommendations to reduce the toxicity of these drugs.

3. *Bleomycin*

Bleomycin (Blenoxane®) is used to treat testicular and germ cell cancers, lymphoma (both Hodgkin's and non-Hodgkin's), squamous cell carcinoma (e.g., of the head and neck, penis, cervix, and vulva) and malignant pleural effusions. Its use is complicated primarily by pulmonary toxic effects, which include interstitial pneumonitis and pulmonary fibrosis (25). In his review, Mathes (30) states that the incidence of pulmonary toxic effects increases with a total Bleomycin dose >450 U, creatinine clearance <35 ml/min, concurrent cyclophosphamide use, or a history of chest irradiation. Although perioperative oxygen restriction has been advocated to reduce postoperative pulmonary morbidity, Donat and Levy (31) found that intravenous fluid management, including transfusion, appears to be the most significant factor affecting postoperative pulmonary morbidity and overall clinical outcome, regardless of oxygen administration.

4. *5-Fluorouracil*

5-fluorouracil (5-FU, Adrucil®, Effudex®, and Fluoroplex®), which is used to treat a variety of cancers (Table 5), has the potential to induce myocardial ischemia, with or without progression to myocardial infarction. Ischemic events are more frequent when 5-FU is administered with cisplatin (26). These events are believed to be related to coronary spasm (32), and electrocardiographic changes as well as chest pain can be observed in patients with normal coronary artery anatomy during the administration of 5-FU (33). In our Preoperative Consultation Center, we refer any patient with a history of chest pain during 5-FU administration to the cardiology department, as many of these patients have underlying coronary artery disease (34).

Capecitabine (Xeloda®) is an oral, prodrug formulation of 5-FU. Because conversion of the drug from

Table 5 Therapeutic Uses for 5-Fluorouracil

FDA-labeled uses	Nonlabeled uses
Actinic/solar keratoses	Cervical cancer
Basal cell carcinoma, superficial	Condyloma acuminata
Breast cancer	Glaucoma
Colorectal cancer	Head/neck cancer
Pancreatic cancer	Liver cancer
Stomach cancer	

the inactive form to the active form takes place mainly in cancer cells, the toxicity profile of capecitabine is believed to be lower than that of 5-FU (35). Nevertheless, capecitabine use has reportedly produced myocardial ischemia and infarction, presumably by mechanisms similar to that of 5-FU (25).

5. *Platins*

Cisplatin (Platinol®) and carboplatin (Paraplatin®) are alkylating agents that are used individually as well as in combination with other chemotherapy agents for a large number of malignancies (Table 6) (25,36). Cisplatin-induced nephrotoxicity is dose-related and cumulative. It represents the major dose-limiting toxicity of cisplatin, occurring in 28–36% of patients after a single 50 mg/m^2 dose manifested by elevations in blood urea nitrogen, creatinine, and serum uric acid levels. Magnesium wasting and hypomagnesemia can be found in a significant number of patients receiving cisplatin. Carboplatin is believed to be less nephrotoxic than cisplatin owing to its greater water solubility (37).

Table 6 Therapeutic Uses for Platin Antineoplastic Agents

Agent	FDA-labeled uses	Nonlabeled uses
Cisplatin (Platinol)	Bladder cancer, advanced Ovarian cancer, metastatic Testicular cancer, metastatic	Breast cancer Cervical cancer Endometrial cancer Gastric cancer Head/neck cancer Lung cancer Lymphoma, non-Hodgkin's Melanoma
Carboplatin (Paraplatin)	Ovarian cancer	Bladder cancer Brain cancer Breast cancer Cervical cancer Endometrial cancer Head/neck cancers Leukemia Lung cancer Neuroblastoma Testicular cancer

The preoperative evaluation and preparation of a patient who has been exposed to the platins includes an electrolyte determination, probably including a magnesium level, to ascertain the degree of renal insult. Prolonged Q–T intervals as well as rapid atrial fibrillation have been described after cisplatin infusion (38), and renal impairment in the presence of antifungal therapy (a common occurrence at our hospital) can produce prolonged Q–T intervals and cardiac arrhythmias (39).

6. *Thalidomide*

Thalidomide (Thalomid®) currently has no labeled indications from the U.S. Food and Drug Administration in cancer treatment. At our institution, it is being used in clinical trials for astrocytoma, glioma, metastatic renal cell cancer, multiple myeloma, lymphoma, endometrial cancer, prostate cancer, hepatocellular cancer, and some head and neck cancers. Possible antitumor mechanisms of action of thalidomide involve the inhibition of angiogenesis, cytokine-mediated pathways, modulation of adhesion molecules, inhibition of cyclo-oxygenase-2, and stimulation of immune response (40). Thalidomide appears to cause sinus bradycardia in a small number of patients (41–43), and some patients at our institution have undergone permanent pacemaker implantation as a result of their thalidomide therapy. Other adverse events most frequently associated with thalidomide administration include somnolence, fatigue, peripheral neuropathy, and thromboembolism (44).

7. *Imatinib Mesylate (Gleevec®)*

Imatinib mesylate is an exciting new agent designed to treat chronic myelogenous leukemia (45,46) and gastrointestinal stromal-cell tumors (47). Our institution has several protocols investigating the use of imatinib mesylate in other cancers as well. Over the past two years, we have observed a few cases of congestive heart failure in patients who have received imatinib mesylate, and coronary artery angiography in two of these patients failed to identify any hemodynamically significant lesions. Although the relationship between imatinib mesylate and congestive heart failure has not been established, one report has suggested that imatinib mesylate treatment for chronic myelogenous leukemia predisposes certain patients to congestive heart failure (48).

B. Radiation Therapy

Radiation therapy is an integral part of cancer management, and it is often combined with chemotherapy and surgery. Many of our patients undergo staged preoperative chemoradiation 4–6 weeks prior to definitive surgery. There are two specific issues related to radiation therapy that deserve attention in any preoperative evaluation.

Radiation to the head and neck area can produce both trismus and limited neck extension. After radiation to the head and neck area, some patients who continue to demonstrate a normal airway on physical examination will become difficult to intubate in the operating room. Thus, alternatives to direct laryngoscopy must be readily available for use in these patients. At our institution, many of these patients undergo elective fiber-optic intubation or intubation via the Fastrach® laryngeal mask airway (49).

The second issue is damage to the myocardium or coronary arteries from radiation delivered to the chest. The potential adverse effects of mediastinal irradiation are numerous and include coronary artery disease, pericarditis, cardiomyopathy, valvular disease, and conduction abnormalities (50). A significantly higher risk of death due to ischemic heart disease has been reported for patients treated with radiation therapy to the chest for Hodgkin's disease and breast cancer (51), although not all investigators agree that breast irradiation leads to increased heart disease (52). Damage to the endothelial cells in the coronary arteries has been proposed as one mechanism for heart disease after chest irradiation. Factors affecting the extent of coronary artery perfusion defects in radiation-induced coronary artery disease include the percentage of the left ventricle irradiated, concurrent hormonal treatment, and a history of hypercholesterolemia (53). The risk from radiation increases when radiation therapy is combined with doxorubicin, because there appears to be a synergistic toxic effect on the myocardium (51). According to the cardiologists at our institution, concomitant use of any anthracycline chemotherapeutic agent or mitoxantrone during the course of radiation therapy will produce this synergistic effect.

The assessment of heart disease in a patient who has undergone radiation therapy begins with an evaluation of their functional status (see the next section). It can include stress-myocardial perfusion tests, echocardiography to evaluate pericardial or valvular disease, and echocardiography or multigated acquisition uptake (MUGA) scans to evaluate myocardial performance when indicated.

IV. THE CANCER PATIENT WITH HEART DISEASE

As improved anesthetic agents and techniques have reduced the complication rate of anesthesia, predicting and preventing perioperative morbidity and mortality due to cardiac disease has become the Holy Grail for many anesthesiologists, internists, and cardiologists. One of the earliest publications to assign levels of risk from cardiac disease in surgical patients is the paper published by Goldman et al. (54) in 1977; it is likely that every anesthesiologist, internist, cardiologist, and surgeon who is interested in the classification of perioperative risk has read this paper many times.

Currently, the "working document" for preoperative evaluation of the cardiac patient for noncardiac surgery is the publication from the American College of Cardiology/American Heart Association (ACC/ AHA), first published in 1996 (55) and revised and republished in 2002 (56). The complete summary is available on the ACC website, and the document has been shortened and summarized into a number of other publications (57,58). These guidelines have been endorsed by the Society of Cardiovascular Anesthesiologists (59) and the American Academy of Family Practice (60). Both of these groups endorsed the 1996 guidelines as well.

Despite these well-accepted guidelines, much of medical practice is based on "usual and customary behavior," and using guidelines to change this physician practice remains difficult (61,62). Even though our institution has endorsed the ACC/AHA guidelines, we continue to find patients who, according to the guidelines, should have undergone additional testing prior to arriving at our Preoperative Consultation Center. We also find patients who have undergone some sort of cardiac evaluation (stress testing, echocardiography, coronary angiography, or percutaneous coronary intervention), even though they did not meet the guideline criteria for such testing and intervention. Each of these scenarios is complicated by financial and medical issues that are beyond the scope of this document. It is important to keep in mind, however, that every medical test has a potential downside—a point of particular significance to the patient with an unfavorable stress test result who has a stroke during the follow-up, clean cardiac catheterization. In their guideline update for exercise testing, the ACC/AHA quotes a rate for myocardial infarction or death as a result of exercise stress testing of 1 per 2500 tests (63). In their review of exercise testing, Chou and Knilans (64) cite a variety of studies suggesting that for every 10,000 exercise tests, there is at least one death and three nonfatal complications requiring hospitalization.

1. Cardiac Stress Testing

A cardiac stress test can be envisioned as a two-part procedure. In the first part, some sort of activity or drug is used to either increase the heart rate (i.e., cause the heart to need more oxygen) or identify impediments to coronary blood flow by dilating the coronary vascular bed to induce blood flow redistribution. The second part of the stress test is the determination of ischemia secondary to the stressor. The following are important points to remember:

1. Heart rate is the principle determinant of myocardial oxygen demand.
2. Unlike most other tissues in the body, the heart extracts nearly all the oxygen from the blood that passes through the myocardium (i.e., there is little or no reserve when compared to the ability of other vascular beds to increase oxygen extraction).
3. The only way to meet an increased oxygen demand by the myocardium is to increase oxygen delivery, which depends upon cardiac output (stroke volume and heart rate), hemoglobin concentration, oxygen saturation, and PaO_2 (PaO_2 has increasing importance as the hemoglobin concentration becomes reduced).

In tests that increase the heart rate in order to provoke myocardial ischemia, a maximum heart rate for age (MHRA, which is defined as 220−age) and a target heart rate (80% MHRA) should be calculated. Any heart rate stress test that does not achieve at least 80% MHRA is inadequate for the conclusion of "no inducible ischemia."

Cardiac stressors are shown in Table 7. The most common and most studied stressor is the Bruce Protocol (Table 8) for a treadmill exercise stress test. In the Bruce Protocol, a patient begins walking on treadmill at 1.7 mph (2.5 ft/sec) at an incline of 10%. Every 3 min, the treadmill speed is increased by a predetermined amount, and the treadmill incline is increased 2%. Each of these Bruce stages has a known amount of oxygen work associated with it, and most cardiologists will report the maximum oxygen demand attained during the test. Oxygen demand is reported as the metabolic oxygen equivalent (MET) of 3.5 ml O_2/min/kg (one MET is considered the awake, resting oxygen demand). There is good correlation between New York Heart Association functional status and workload METs (Table 9).

In some stress tests, drugs are used to increase heart rate (e.g., dobutamine with or without atropine) or alter coronary blood flow by decreasing the resistance of the coronary bed (e.g., adenosine or dipyridamole). For tests using dobutamine, the target heart rate remains the MHRA. In tests using a vasodilator, heart rate is rarely affected. Instead, the vasodilator is used as an to attempt to identify significant epicardial artery obstructions by inducing blood flow alterations related to changes in vascular bed resistance. For example, prior to the administration of a vasodilator, myocardium distal to an obstruction might be adequately perfused due to high vascular resistance in other beds. Upon dilation of these other beds, though, these areas might undergo a significant perfusion defect (called coronary steal), which can be identified by nuclear scan (65).

Common modalities for evaluating myocardial ischemia in the setting of a stress test are shown in Table 10. For a treadmill (or other exercise) test, the most common and easiest-to-use evaluation for ischemia is surface electrocardiography. This modality can be used for ischemic evaluation only in the patient with normal resting electrocardiogram without bundle-branch block, abnormal ST segments, abnormal T-wave morphology, or ventricular pacing artifacts. Other evaluation modalities include echocardiography and nuclear imaging. Figure 1 shows the guidelines that we use at M.D. Anderson for ordering a stress test with imaging.

Table 7 Cardiac Stress Test "Stressors"

Exercise protocols	Bruce Protocol (treadmill)—1.7 mph, 10% incline at start, increases speed and incline every 3 min
	Modified Bruce Protocol (treadmill)—no incline at start, progresses to 10% at 1.5 min, then becomes the same as Bruce Protocol
	Naughton Protocol (treadmill)—2–3.4 mph, 2 min stages, low workload differential each stage
	McHenry Protocol (treadmill)—2–3.3 mph, 3 min stages, 3–21% grade
	Balke Protocol (treadmill)—3.3 mph, 1 min stages, incline increases 1% each stage
	Bicycle Ergometer
	Arm Grip Test
Pharmacological protocols	Dobutamine (heart rate test)—difficult if patient on beta blocker
	Adenosine (vasodilator)—sometimes contraindicated in a patient with pulmonary disease
	Dipyridamole (vasodilator, precursor substance to adenosine)

Table 8 Bruce Protocol

Stage	Speed (mph)	Grade (%)	Duration (min)	METs	Total time (min)
1	1.7	10	3	4	3
2	2.5	12	3	7	6
3	3.4	14	3	9	9
4	4.2	16	3	14	12
5	5.0	18	3	16	15
6	5.5	20	3	20	18

Source: Adapted from Ref. 67.

The reporting of stress testing has not been standardized, and shortcuts in reporting frequently are taken. The scribbled note "normal stress test, cleared for surgery" on a prescription pad from any consultant is inadequate and should not be accepted. At a minimum, every stress test report should include:

- Indication for testing
- Type of test and evaluation
- Duration of exercise, if exercise was used
- Heart rate achieved and percentage of MHRA (if heart rate tests)
- Reason for stopping the test
- Patient symptoms during the test
- Interpretation of test
- Ejection fraction, wall motion, and heart volumes (nuclear or echo study)
- Follow-up recommendations guided by the test results

As with any test, stress testing can yield both false-negative (i.e., the test was interpreted as normal but the patient has coronary artery disease) and false-positive (i.e., the test was positive for coronary artery disease but the patient has none) results. In a Bruce Protocol exercise test, if 80% MHRA is achieved and the patient exercises more than 6 min (into stage 3), the incidence of false-negative results is low. In fact, the longer a patient exercises on the Bruce Protocol, the lower the incidence of a false-negative result. Any patient who cannot exercise sufficiently (i.e., the patient achieves >80% MHRA before 5 min) should be evaluated for cardiomyopathy prior to an elective case. Women have higher false-positive exercise treadmill test results compared to men when evaluated only by electrocardiography, and some sources report this rate to exceed 60% (66). Other factors commonly associated with common causes of a false-positive stress test result include severe anemia, left ventricular hypertrophy, hypertension, hypokalemia, and antiarrhythmic drug use (e.g., digoxin, quinidine, and procainamide) (64,67). For tests utilizing nuclear perfusion scans, certain areas of the heart (especially the inferior wall) and patients with certain characteristics (e.g., large, pendulous breasts, morbid obesity, diabetes) often have "thinned" nuclear uptake without hemodynamically significant coronary artery lesions.

Contraindications to exercise testing generally include poor exercise conditioning (debilitation), lower extremity peripheral vascular disease, severe hypertension, and significant valvular stenosis. In general, if a stress test is indicated to rule coronary artery disease, one can identify a suitable testing modality based upon patient characteristics. Alternatively, in the absence of any contraindication to an intravenous contrast agent (primarily renal insufficiency or a history of anaphylaxis), one can, if need be, proceed directly to coronary angiography.

It is important to remember that, most of the time, stress testing will identify the patient with a hemodynamically significant (>70%) stenosis in an epicardial vessel. Small vessel disease (like that present in diabetes), left ventricular hypertrophy, elevated left ventricular end diastolic pressure, or an epicardial vessel stenosis less than 70% can produce positive stress test results without a positive finding at angiography. Thus, the patient with an "abnormal" stress test but a coronary angiogram without any lesion amenable to intervention should be considered at higher risk than the patient with a normal stress test, especially in the presence of multiple risk factors for coronary artery disease (e.g., male sex, advanced age, family history of coronary artery disease, history of hypertension, presence of diabetes, sedentary lifestyle, and diabetes).

Table 9 Relationship Between New York Heart Association Functional Classification and METs

NYHA functional class	Limitation(s)	METs workload on stress test
I	No limitation	>7
II	Mild dyspnea on exertion	4–7
III	Significant dyspnea on exertion	2–3
IV	Dyspnea with activities of daily living	1

Abbreviations: NYHA, New York Heart Association; METs, metabolic equivalent (3.5 ml oxygen uptake/kg body mass/minute).

Table 10 Cardiac Stress Evaluation Modalities

Surface electrocardiography
Echocardiography
Transthoracic
Transesophageal
Nuclear imaging studies—agents
Thallium
Tetrafosmin (Myoview®)
Sestamibi (Cardiolyte®)

Finally, the patient with any epicardial vessel lesion in the 50–70% occlusive range could have atherosclerotic plaques, which can rupture under stress. These patients rarely have significant collateral circulation; thus, they are more likely to present with sudden death as their evidence of plaque rupture.

2. Indications for Stress Testing

At the M.D. Anderson Preoperative Consultation Center, we have adopted the ACC/AHA guidelines as minimal criteria for the referral of patients for stress testing (56). These criteria take into account patient risk factors (Table 11), patient functional status, and operative risk factors (Table 12) in an effort to predict which patients should undergo preoperative, noninvasive cardiac stress testing.

These guidelines are based on expert opinion and have not been subjected to rigorous, peer-reviewed investigation. However, a recent report suggests that the use of these guidelines reduces testing and the costs associated with preoperative evaluation without increasing the complication rate (68). On the other hand, another report suggests that the criteria used in these guidelines for selecting patients for noninvasive cardiac stress testing are too broad and lead to increased testing without benefit (69). The most complicated issues relating to these guidelines that we face at M.D. Anderson include the following:

1. The patient with previous exposure to cardiotoxic chemotherapy, as these patients can be markedly deconditioned and have cardiomyopathy unrelated to coronary artery disease. As a result, we classify these patients as being in the "intermediate risk" category for the purpose of using the ACC guidelines.
2. The patient who has undergone chest wall (mediastinal or breast) irradiation, as this treatment can accelerate the development of coronary artery disease (see the section on Radiation Therapy).
3. The patient with recently discovered diabetes but no evidence of end-organ involvement who is scheduled for a "high risk" operation.
4. The patient with recently discovered renal insufficiency who is scheduled for a "high risk" operation.

In an effort to produce uniform results in the Preoperative Consultation Center and the Cardiology Clinic, we have added "history of cardiotoxic

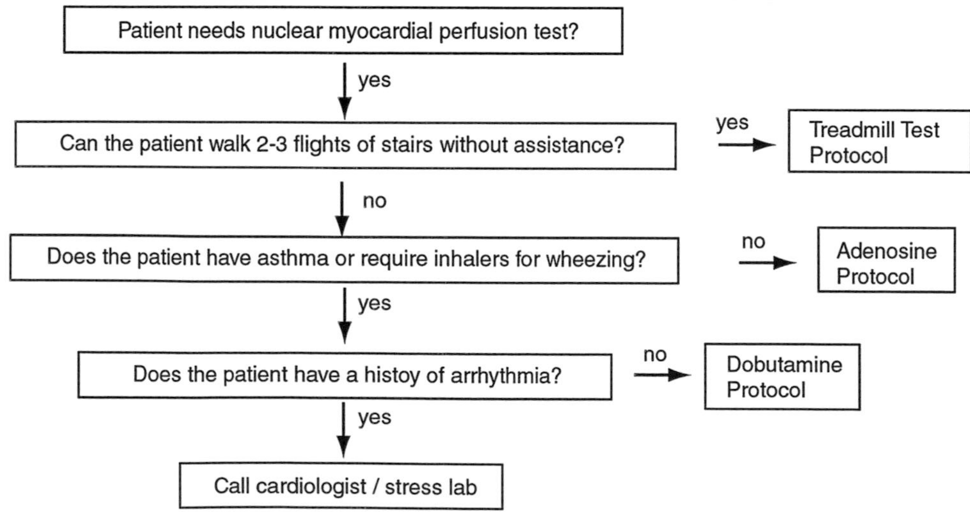

Figure 1 The nuclear imaging stress test decision tree. When ordering a nuclear-imaged stress test, the anesthesiologist must decide which exercise protocol to employ. This decision tree facilitates the decision process and reduces calls to the cardiologist and the stress lab.

Table 11 Patient Risk Assignments at M.D. Anderson Cancer Center[a]

High risk	Intermediate risk	Minimal risk
Decompensated CHF	Compensated CHF	Advanced age (>70 years)
Unstable coronary syndromes	Prior CHF	Low functional capacity
Recent MI (<30 days)	Stable CAD	Uncontrolled hypertension (except in endocrine tumor where considered intermediate risk)
Unstable angina	Post-CABG	Cerebrovascular disease
Large "area of risk" by noninvasive study	Post-PCI	Abnormal EKG
Significant arrhythmia	Stable angina	Nonsinus cardiac rhythm
High-grade A-V block	Prior MI	
Ventricular arrhythmias with concomitant heart disease	Diabetes	
Uncontrolled ventricular rate in supraventricular arrhythmia	Renal insufficiency	
Severe valvular disease	History of cardiotoxic chemotherapy	
	History of chest wall irradiation	

[a] Criteria have been adapted from the ACC/AHA guideline update for perioperative cardiovascular evaluation for noncardiac surgery (56) for use at the Preoperative Consultation Center at The University of Texas M.D. Anderson Cancer Center.
Abbreviations: CABG, coronary artery bypass grafting; CAD, coronary artery disease; CHF, congestive heart failure; EKG, electrocardiogram; MI, myocardial infarction; PCI, percutaneous coronary artery intervention (either simple angioplasty or stent placement).

chemotherapy" as well as "history of chest wall irradiation" to the list of intermediate patient risk factors (see Table 11). Thus, patients who have undergone cardiotoxic chemotherapy or chest wall irradiation are more likely to undergo noninvasive stress testing, but only when their functional status has been impaired or when they are scheduled for a significant operative procedure. Additionally, we classify any patient with diabetes or renal insufficiency, regardless of the duration of the problem, as "intermediate risk" for the purpose of risk-stratification and the need for additional noninvasive cardiac testing.

3. *Preoperative Coronary Artery Intervention*

While the determination of epicardial disease utilizing some form of cardiac stress test seems relatively straight-forward, the treatment of patients with a variety of lesions is not. In a survey of preoperative practitioners. Pierpont et al. found considerable disagreement regarding the use of medical management, percutaneous coronary intervention, and coronary artery bypass grafting in those patients (70). However, a recent randomized study sheds considerable light on this issue. In a multicenter study involving 462 Veteran's Adminstration patients with significant angiographic epicardial lesions (but without unstable coronary disease, left main lesions, significant cardiomyopathy, or aortic stenosis) scheduled for abdominal or infrainguinal vascular surgery, McFalls et al. randomized patients to percutaneous intervention coronary artery bypass grafting surgery, or medical management prior to surgery (71). They found no difference in the 30 day rate for myocardial infarction (12% intervention group vs 14% medical management group, $P = 0.37$), and no difference in mortality at 32 months post surgery (22% intervention group vs 23% medical management group, $P = 0.92$). They did find, though

Table 12 Surgical Risk Assignments at M.D. Anderson Cancer Center[a]

High risk	Intermediate risk	Minimal risk
Emergent surgery	Intraperitoneal surgery	Endoscopic procedures
Long surgery (>6 hr)	Intrathoracic surgery	Superficial procedures
Expected blood loss >25% blood volume	Head/neck surgery	Breast surgery
Large fluid shift expected	Carotid surgery	Wide local excision
Aortic or other major vascular surgery	Orthopedic surgery	Tandem and ovoid insertion
Peripheral vascular surgery	Radical prostate surgery	Cervical procedures
	Pelvic tumor-reductive surgery	Brain biopsy
	Free-flap reconstruction	Nonreconstructive eye surgery

[a] Criteria have been adapted from the ACC/AHA guideline update for perioperative cardiovascular evaluation for noncardiac surgery (56) for use at the Preoperative Consultation Center at The University of Texas M.D. Anderson Cancer Center.

that the vascular surgical event was significantly delayed owing to the intervention when compared to the medical management group, (54 days vs. 18 days to surgery from study entry, $P < 0.001$). They also noted 10 deaths in the intervention group and 1 death in the medical management group after randomization but prior to the vascular surgery, as well as 21 patients originally assigned to medical management who underwent a coronary artery intervention procedure during the study follow-up period.

Noting that no survival benefit accrued to those patients with a preoperative coronary artery intervention. Mosoussi and Eagle wrote in an editorial that providing expert medical perioperative care (beta blockade with bisoprolol (72), atenolol (73) or and administration of statin drugs (74)) is superior and less costly that coronary artery intervention for these patients.

This issue is far from settled. An increasing number of retrospective studies suggest that statins reduce perioperative mortality following major cardiac, vascular, and noncardiac surgery (74,75). Statin therapy is further associated with a long-term reduction in all cause and cardiovascular mortality following successful abdominal aortic surgery, independent of other pharmacologic therapy (76). This survival benefit is increasingly attributed to the pleiotropic effects (anti-inflammatory effects, improved endothelial function and coagulation) of statins, which appear to be independent of their cholestrol lowering and atherosclerotic plaque stabilizing effects. Whether or not cancer patients, or all patients with atherosclerotic risks, who undergo surgery should be started on statin therapy has not been addressed.

4. *Echocardiographic Evaluation*

According to ACC guidelines, the routine use of echocardiography to determine ejection fraction should be avoided (56). Nevertheless, many anesthesiologists continue to order echocardiograms or MUGA scans in the setting of exposure to cardiotoxic chemotherapy, especially from the anthracycline class. In the Preoperative Consultation Center, we attempt to discourage such testing in the patient with adequate functional status, a normal cardiac exam, and no history of cardiomyopathy.

For the patient who might have a cardiomyopathy, hematological screening for elevated levels of B-type natriuretic peptide (BNP) might be more efficient than referring the patient for echocardiography or radionuclide testing (77,78). B-type natriuretic peptide testing is currently under intense evaluation to determine its usefulness in rapid detection of heart failure as well as in guiding therapy (79,80). At present, however, no studies have examined the sensitivity and specificity of this test in the postchemotherapeutic patient.

V. THE CANCER PATIENT WITH AN IMPLANTED CARDIAC GENERATOR

As noted above, improvements in surgical techniques, anesthetic care, and the management of comorbid diseases has increased the number of patients with cancer on whom surgeons are willing to operate. This willingness extends to patients with implanted cardiac devices as well. At the Preoperative Consultation Center, we have about 130 visits per year from patients with traditional pacemakers, and we see about 35 patients per year who have an implanted defibrillator. Thus, approximately 1% of all the patients seen in the center have an implanted cardiac device. This frequency is similar to that reported in another academic, tertiary care medical center (81).

In our patient population, indications for implantation of a pulse generator include traditional reasons such as bradycardia and diseases of the atrioventricular node. Also, about 15% of our patients have a cardiac device because of a complication of their cancer or cancer therapy [e.g., thalidomide can produce symptomatic bradycardia (42,43), epirubicin has been reported to cause sino-atrial block (82), and anthracyclines can produce myocardial failure (83)]. Changes in implant indications for traditional pacemakers, defibrillators, antiatrial fibrillation devices, and biventricular devices will likely increase the number of cancer patients who have an implanted device (84–87). For example, our institution is evaluating the implantation of biventricular pacing devices in patients who develop dilated cardiomyopathy as a result of their cancer or cancer therapy.

Few studies have evaluated perioperative outcomes in patients with a cardiac device. In an abstract reporting prospectively obtained data, Samain et al. (88) found that 12 of 73 patients with an implanted pacemaker suffered a cardiac event (myocardial infarction or congestive heart failure) or cardiac death during their postsurgical hospitalization. Trankina et al. (81), using a retrospective chart review, found that 32 of 169 patients (19%) had some type of change to their pacemaker status after surgery, most likely related to the use of an electrosurgical cautery unit. For the period of January 1, 2000 to December 31, 2001, we retrospectively reviewed the charts of patients with implanted cardiac devices who had been seen prior to their anesthetic at the Preoperative Consultation Center (89). At the first visit to the center (some patients were seen more than once), we found that 33% of our 172 patients with pacemakers had not had an appropriate, timely visit to their cardiologist prior to their presentation for surgery, as is recommended by the North American Society of

Pacing and Electrophysiology (90), and 43% of our 143 patients 65 years old or older failed to meet Medicare guidelines for pacemaker follow-up care (91). More important, a comprehensive evaluation of each pacemaker in the Preoperative Consultation Center revealed a pacemaker problem in 16% (27 patients) of first-visit patients. In one third of these problems (nine patients), a pacemaker replacement for battery depletion was needed prior to the patient's elective procedure, and four of these nine patients who had a note from a cardiologist indicating that the patient was "cleared for anesthesia and surgery." Likewise, there was a "cleared for surgery" note from an internal medicine specialist in three of the nine patients.

Whether these data are unique to cancer patients or are applicable to all presurgical patients remains unknown. Also, we have not evaluated any relationship between chemotherapy and pacemaker behavior, but there is one report of a pacing threshold increase in the setting of chemotherapy (92).

For the same period, we had 45 patients with implanted defibrillators. Review of our data (unpublished) shows that 15 had not undergone an in-office comprehensive evaluation within the past 4 months, which is the maximum recommended period for follow-up. We have also found two devices that were in need of replacement for battery depletion or prolonged charge time.

For the two years noted, we had no documented perioperative myocardial infarctions or cardiac-related deaths within 30 days of the procedure in any patient with an implanted cardiac generator, although we did not routinely measure troponins, as was done by Samain et al. (88). Whether our 30-day cardiac morbity and mortality rate during this period was affected by pre- and postoperative checking of the devices cannot be determined, but it is interesting to note that the American College of Cardiology has since published a recommendation that all implanted cardiac devices be comprehensively evaluated both before and after surgery, especially when an electrosurgical unit has been used (56). Although there are no agreed reprogramming guidelines for the pacemaker patient undergoing surgery, the Guidant Corporation recommends increasing the pacing energy for their devices manufactured from 1987 to 2002 in any setting where "electrosurgical cautery" would be used (93).

Therapeutic radiation can also cause problems with implanted cardiac devices. The pacemaker manufacturers recommend shielding the device, calculating the delivered radiation dose, and relocating the device (a surgical procedure) out of the radiation field where necessary. In his review, Last states that generator outcome following radiation therapy cannot be predicted in a consistent manner, which is similar to the behavior of these devices in the operating room with electrosurgical cautery. He does state that review of the literature suggests that no significant failure of a generator has been observed at doses less than 10 Gy, and he recommends that a pacemaker be regarded as a critical structure with a tolerance dose of 2 Gy (94). Interestingly, Guidant recommends that its newest pacing device (called Insignia®) be checked after any therapeutic radiation administration, regardless of the proximity of the radiation to the device (95). Currently, neither Medtronic nor St. Jude Cardiac Rhythm Management has specific programming or testing recommendations in the setting of electrosurgical cautery use or therapeutic radiation.

VI. SUMMARY

The preoperative evaluation of a patient with cancer must take into account the severity of their cancer disease, chemotherapeutic exposure, radiation exposure, and comorbid nonmalignant diseases. In addition, many cancer operations are part of a staged intervention in these patients; that is, the surgery needs to be performed in a timely manner to complement the chemotherapy or radiation therapy. In the cancer patient, the discovery of untreated comorbid disease must lead to a discussion between the patient's oncologist, surgeon, and specialist who will be treating the comorbidity. In such a setting, it is not appropriate to proceed to the operating room without such a discussion, nor is it appropriate to delay any case without speaking to the patient's other caregivers. The goal of every physician should be to achieve the best outcome with the lowest risk (89). Although anesthesiologists prefer to anesthetize patients only after any coexisting medical conditions have been successfully mitigated, some cancer operations, while not true emergencies, cannot wait for interventions that could delay surgery and allow the cancer to spread.

REFERENCES

1. Saklad M. Grading of patients for surgical procedures. Anesthesia 1941; 2:281–284.
2. ASA physical status classification system, American Society of Anesthesiologists. Available at: http://www.asahq.org/clinical/physicalstatus.htm. Accessed August 10, 2003.
3. Culver DH, Horan TC, Gaynes RP, et al. Surgical wound infection rates by wound class, operative procedure, and patient risk index. National Nosocomial

Infections Surveillance System. Am J Med 1991; 91(3B):152S–157S.
4. Goldmann DA, Weinstein RA, Wenzel RP, et al. Strategies to prevent and control the emergence and spread of antimicrobial-resistant microorganisms in hospitals. A challenge to hospital leadership. JAMA 1996; 275(3):234–240.
5. Vacanti CJ, VanHouten RJ, Hill RC. A statistical analysis of the relationship of physical status to postoperative mortality in 68,388 cases. Anesth Analg 1970; 49(4):564–566.
6. Scott-Coombes D, Whawell S, Vipond MN, Thompson J. Human intraperitoneal fibrinolytic response to elective surgery. Br J Surg 1995; 82(3):414–417.
7. Adachi W, Koike S, Rafique M, et al. Preoperative intraperitoneal chemotherapy for gastric cancer, with special reference to delayed peritoneal complications. Surg Today 1995; 25(5):396–403.
8. Adachi W, Kobayashi M, Koike S, et al. The influence of excess body weight on the surgical treatment of patients with gastric cancer. Surg Today 1995; 25(11):939–945.
9. Liaw CC, Chen JS, Wang CH, Chang HK, Huang JS. Tumor fever in patients with nasopharyngeal carcinoma: clinical experience of 67 patients. Am J Clin Oncol 1998; 21(4):422–425.
10. Kinney MA, Warner ME, Nagorney DM, et al. Perianaesthetic risks and outcomes of abdominal surgery for metastatic carcinoid tumours. Br J Anaesth 2001; 87(3):447–452.
11. Zanella A. Noninfective complications of blood transfusions. Tumori 2001; 87(2):S20–S23.
12. Plouin PF, Duclos JM, Soppelsa F, Boublil G, Chatellier G. Factors associated with perioperative morbidity and mortality in patients with pheochromocytoma: analysis of 165 operations at a single center. J Clin Endocrinol Metab 2001; 86(4):1480–1486.
13. Lin JT, Lachmann E. Lambert–Eaton myasthenic syndrome: a case report and review of the literature. J Womens Health (Larchmt) 2002; 11(10):849–855.
14. Ohguro H, Nakazawa M. Pathological roles of recoverin in cancer-associated retinopathy. Adv Exp Med Biol 2002; 514:109–124.
15. Hurtado J, Esbrit P. Treatment of malignant hypercalcaemia. Expert Opin Pharmacother 2002; 3(5):521–527.
16. Mekhail N, Kapural L. Complex regional pain syndrome type I in cancer patients. Curr Rev Pain 2000; 4(3):227–233.
17. Gibby GL. How preoperative assessment programs can be justified financially to hospital administrators. Int Anesthesiol Clin 2002; 40(2):17–30.
18. Ewer MS. Specialists must communicate in complex cases. Intern Med World Rep 2001; 16(5):17.
19. Wessel J, Endrikat J, Buscher U. Frequency of denial of pregnancy: results and epidemiological significance of a 1-year prospective study in Berlin. Acta Obstet Gynecol Scand 2002; 81(11):1021–1027.
20. Wheeler M, Cote CJ. Preoperative pregnancy testing in a tertiary care children's hospital: a medico-legal conundrum. J Clin Anesth 1999; 11(1):56–63.
21. Manley S, de Kelaita G, Joseph NJ, Salem MR, Heyman HJ. Preoperative pregnancy testing in ambulatory surgery. Incidence and impact of positive results. Anesthesiology 1995; 83(4):690–693.
22. ACOG. Committee opinion: number 278, November 2002. Avoiding inappropriate clinical decisions based on false-positive human chorionic gonadotropin test results. Obstet Gynecol 2002; 100(5 Pt 1):1057–1059.
23. Esfandiari N, Goldberg JM. Heterophile antibody blocking agent to confirm false positive serum human chorionic gonadotropin assay. Obstet Gynecol 2003; 101(5 Pt 2):1144–1146.
24. Bussar-Maatz R, Weissbach L, Dahlmann N, Mann K. The "false positive" tumor marker in malignant testicular tumor. Urologe A 1993; 32(3):177–182.
25. Micromedix(R) Healthcare Series. Vol. 117. Greenwood Village, CO: Thompson Micromedix, 2003.
26. Ewer MS, Benjamin RS. Cardiac complications. In: Bast RC, Kufe DW, Pollock RE, Weichselbaum RR, Holland JF, Frei E, eds. Cancer Medicine. London: B.C. Decker, 2000:2324–2339.
27. Zambetti M, Moliterni A, Materazzo C, et al. Long-term cardiac sequelae in operable breast cancer patients given adjuvant chemotherapy with or without doxorubicin and breast irradiation. J Clin Oncol 2001; 19(1):37–43.
28. Keefe DL. Anthracycline-induced cardiomyopathy. Semin Oncol 2001; 28(4 suppl 12):2–7.
29. Esmaeli B, Valero V, Ahmadi MA, Booser D. Canalicular stenosis secondary to docetaxel (taxotere): a newly recognized side effect. Ophthalmology 2001; 108(5): 994–995.
30. Mathes DD. Bleomycin and hyperoxia exposure in the operating room. Anesth Analg 1995; 81(3):624–629.
31. Donat SM, Levy DA. Bleomycin associated pulmonary toxicity: is perioperative oxygen restriction necessary? J Urol 1998; 160(4):1347–1352.
32. Keefe DL. Cardiovascular emergencies in the cancer patient. Semin Oncol 2000; 27(3):244–255.
33. Akpek G, Hartshorn KL. Failure of oral nitrate and calcium channel blocker therapy to prevent 5-fluor ouracil-related myocardial ischemia: a case report. Cancer Chemother Pharmacol 1999; 43(2):157–161.
34. Anand AJ. Fluorouracil cardiotoxicity. Ann Pharmacother 1994; 28(3):374–378.
35. Kaklamani VG, Gradishar WJ. Role of capecitabine (Xeloda) in breast cancer. Expert Rev Anticancer Ther 2003; 3(2):137–144.
36. Fischer DS, Knobf MT, Durivage HJ. The Cancer Chemotherapy Handbook. 5th ed. St. Louis, MO: Mosby, 1997.
37. Kintzel PE. Anticancer drug-induced kidney disorders. Drug Saf 2001; 24(1):19–38.
38. Tassinari D, Sartori S, Drudi G, et al. Cardiac arrhythmias after cisplatin infusion: three case reports and a review of the literature. Ann Oncol 1997; 8(12): 1263–1267.

39. Albengres E, Le Louet H, Tillement JP. Systemic antifungal agents. Drug interactions of clinical significance. Drug Saf 1998; 18(2):83–97.
40. Fanelli M, Sarmiento R, Gattuso D, et al. Thalidomide: a new anticancer drug? Expert Opin Investig Drugs 2003; 12(7):1211–1225.
41. Kaur A, Yu SS, Lee AJ, Chiao TB. Thalidomide-induced sinus bradycardia. Ann Pharmacother 2003; 37(7–8):1040–1043.
42. Singhal S, Mehta J. Thalidomide in cancer: potential uses and limitations. BioDrugs 2001; 15(3):163–172.
43. Rajkumar SV, Gertz MA, Lacy MQ, et al. Thalidomide as initial therapy for early-stage myeloma. Leukemia 2003; 17(4):775–779.
44. Matthews SJ, McCoy C. Thalidomide: a review of approved and investigational uses. Clin Ther 2003; 25(2):342–395.
45. Feig SA. Designer drugs: new directed therapies for cancer. Int J Hematol 2002; 76(suppl 2):281–283.
46. Tallman MS. Advancing the treatment of hematologic malignancies through the development of targeted interventions. Semin Hematol 2002; 39(4 suppl 3):1–5.
47. Eisenberg BL, von Mehren M. Pharmacotherapy of gastrointestinal stromal tumours. Expert Opin Pharmacother 2003; 4(6):869–874.
48. Sohn SK, Kim JG, Kim DH, Lee KB. Cardiac morbidity in advanced chronic myelogenous leukaemia patients treated by successive allogeneic stem cell transplantation with busulphan/cyclophosphamide conditioning after imatinib mesylate administration. Br J Haematol 2003; 121(3):469–472.
49. Ferson DZ, Rosenblatt WH, Johansen MJ, Osborn I, Ovassapian A. Use of the intubating LMA Fastrach in 254 patients with difficult-to-manage airways. Anesthesiology 2001; 95(5):1175–1181.
50. Adams MJ, Hardenbergh PH, Constine LS, Lipshultz SE. Radiation-associated cardiovascular disease. Crit Rev Oncol Hematol 2003; 45(1):55–75.
51. Basavaraju SR, Easterly CE. Pathophysiological effects of radiation on atherosclerosis development and progression, and the incidence of cardiovascular complications. Med Phys 2002; 29(10):2391–2403.
52. Vallis KA, Pintilie M, Chong N, et al. Assessment of coronary heart disease morbidity and mortality after radiation therapy for early breast cancer. J Clin Oncol 2002; 20(4):1036–1042.
53. Lind PA, Pagnanelli R, Marks LB, et al. Myocardial perfusion changes in patients irradiated for left-sided breast cancer and correlation with coronary artery distribution. Int J Radiat Oncol Biol Phys 2003; 55(4): 914–920.
54. Goldman L, Caldera DL, Nussbaum SR, et al. Multifactorial index of cardiac risk in noncardiac surgical procedures. N Engl J Med 1977; 297(16):845–850.
55. Eagle KA, Brundage BH, Chaitman BR, et al. Guidelines for perioperative cardiovascular evaluation for noncardiac surgery. Report of the American College of Cardiology/American Heart Association Task Force on Practice Guidelines. Committee on Perioperative Cardiovascular Evaluation for Noncardiac Surgery. Circulation 1996; 93(6):1278–1317.
56. Eagle KA, Berger PB, Caulkins H, et al. ACC/AHA guideline update for perioperative cardiovascular evaluation for noncardiac surgery. Published January, 2002. Available at: http://www.acc.org/clinical/guidelines/perio/update/pdf/perio_update.pdf. Accessed August 12, 2003.
57. Eagle KA, Berger PB, Calkins H, et al. ACC/AHA guideline update for perioperative cardiovascular evaluation for noncardiac surgery—executive summary. A report of the American College of Cardiology/ American Heart Association Task Force on Practice Guidelines (Committee to Update the 1996 Guidelines on Perioperative Cardiovascular Evaluation for Noncardiac Surgery). Circulation 2002; 105(10):1257–1267.
58. Eagle K, Berger P, Caulkins H, et al. ACC/AHA guideline update for perioperative cardiovascular evaluation for noncardiac surgery—executive summary. J Am Coll Cardiol 2002; 39:543–553.
59. Eagle KA, Berger PB, Calkins H, et al. ACC/AHA Guideline update for perioperative cardiovascular evaluation for noncardiac surgery—executive summary. A report of the American College of Cardiology/ American Heart Association Task Force on Practice Guidelines (Committee to Update the 1996 Guidelines on Perioperative Cardiovascular Evaluation for Noncardiac Surgery). Anesth Analg 2002; 94(5): 1052–1064.
60. Mukherjee D, Eagle KA. A common sense approach to perioperative evaluation. Am Fam Physician 2002; 66(10):1824–1826.
61. McGlynn EA, Asch SM, Adams J, et al. The quality of health care delivered to adults in the United States. N Engl J Med 2003; 348(26):2635–2645.
62. Justice AC, Covinsky KE, Berlin JA. Assessing the generalizability of prognostic information. Ann Intern Med 1999; 130(6):515–524.
63. Gibbons RJ, Bricker JT, Chaitman BR, et al. ACC/ AHA 2002 guideline update for exercise testing. Published 2002. Available at: http://www.acc.org/clini-/clinical/guidelines/exercise/exercise_clean.pdf. Accessed January 3, 2003.
64. Chou TC, Knilans TK. Electrocardiography in Clinical Practice. 4th ed. Philadelphia: W.B. Saunders Company, 1996.
65. McLaughlin DP, Beller GA, Linden J, et al. Hemodynamic and metabolic correlates of dipyridamole-induced myocardial thallium-201 perfusion abnormalities in multivessel coronary artery disease. Am J Cardiol 1994; 73(16):1159–1164.
66. Sketch MH, Mohiuddin SM, Lynch JD, Zencka AE, Runco V. Significant sex differences in the correlation of electrocardiographic exercise testing and coronary arteriograms. Am J Cardiol 1975; 36(2):169–173.

67. Kligfield P. ST segment analysis in exercise stress testing. In: Zareba W, Maison-Blanche P, Locati EH, eds. Noninvasive Electrocardiology in Clinical Practice. Armonk, NY: Futura Publishing Company, 2001:227–256.
68. Froehlich JB, Karavite D, Russman PL, et al. American College of Cardiology/American Heart Association preoperative assessment guidelines reduce resource utilization before aortic surgery. J Vasc Surg 2002; 36(4):758–763.
69. Morgan PB, Panomitros GE, Nelson AC, Smith DF, Solanki DR, Zornow MH. Low utility of dobutamine stress echocardiograms in the preoperative evaluation of patients scheduled for noncardiac surgery. Anesth Analg 2002; 95(3):512–516.
70. Pierpont GL, Mortiz TE, Goldman S, et al. Disparate opinions regarding indications for coronary artery revasularization before elective vascular surgery. Am J Cardiol 2004; 94(9):1124–1128.
71. McFalls EO, Ward HB, Moritz TE, et al. Coronary-artery revascularization before elective major vascular surgery. N Engl J Med 2004; 351(27):2795–2804.
72. Poldermans D, Boersma E, Bax JJ, et al. The effect of bisoprolol on perioperative mortality and myocardial infarction in high-risk patients undergoing vascular surgery. Dutch Echocardiographic Cardiac Risk Evaluation Applying Stress Echocardiography Study Group. N Engl J Med 1999; 341(24):1789–1794.
73. Mangano DT, Layug EL, Wallace A, Tateo I. Effect of atenolol on mortality and cardiovascular morbidity after noncardiac surgery. Multicenter Study of Perioperative Ischemia Research Group. N Engl J Med 1996; 335(23):1713–1720.
74. Poldermans D, Bax JJ, Kertai MD, et al. Statins are associated with a reduced incidence of perioperative mortality in patients undergoing major noncardiac vascular surgery. Circulation 2003; 107(14):1848–1851.
75. Lindenauer PK, Pekow P, Wang K, Gutierrez B, Benjamin EM. Lipid-lowering therapy andin-hospital mortality following major noncardiac surgery. JAMA 2004; 291(17):2092–2099.
76. Kertai MD, Boersma E, Westerhout CM, et al. Association between long-term statin use and mortality after successful abdominal aortic aneurysm surgery. Am J Med 2004; 116(2):96–103.
77. Silver MA, Pisano C. High incidence of elevated B-type natriuretic peptide levels and risk factors for heart failure in an unselected at-risk population (stage A): implications for heart failure screening programs. Congest Heart Fail 2003; 9(3):127–132.
78. Maisel A. B-type natriuretic peptide levels: a potential novel "white count" for congestive heart failure. J Card Fail 2001; 7(2):183–193.
79. Hobbs RE. Using BNP to diagnose, manage, and treat heart failure. Cleve Clin J Med 2003; 70(4):333–336.
80. McCullough PA, Nowak RM, McCord J, et al. B-type natriuretic peptide and clinical judgment in emergency diagnosis of heart failure: analysis from Breathing Not Properly (BNP) Multinational Study. Circulation 2002; 106(4):416–422.
81. Trankina MF, Black S, Gibby G. Pacemakers: perioperative evaluation, management and complications. Anesthesiology 2000; 9:A1193.
82. Okamoto T, Ogata J, Minami K. Sino-atrial block during anesthesia in a patient with breast cancer being treated with the anticancer drug epirubicin. Anesth Analg 2003; 97(1):19–20.
83. Steinherz LJ, Steinherz PG, Tan C. Cardiac failure and dysrhythmias 6–19 years after anthracycline therapy: a series of 15 patients. Med Pediatr Oncol 1995; 24(6): 352–361.
84. Hayes DL. Evolving indications for permanent pacing. Am J Cardiol 1999; 83(5B):161D–165D.
85. Prystowsky EN, Nisam S. Prophylactic implantable cardioverter defibrillator trials: MUSTT, MADIT, and beyond. Multicenter Unsustained Tachycardia Trial. Multicenter Automatic Defibrillator Implantation Trial. Am J Cardiol 2000; 86(11):1214–1215.
86. Bristow MR, Feldman AM, Saxon LA. Heart failure management using implantable devices for ventricular resynchronization: comparison of Medical Therapy, Pacing, and Defibrillation in Chronic Heart Failure (COMPANION) trial. COMPANION Steering Committee and COMPANION Clinical Investigators. J Card Fail 2000; 6(3):276–285.
87. Pinski SL. Continuing progress in the treatment of severe congestive heart failure. JAMA 2003; 289(6):754–756.
88. Samain E, Schauveliege F, Henry C, Marty J. Outcome in patients with a cardiac pacemaker undergoing noncardiac surgery. Anesthesiology 2001; 95:A142.
89. Rozner MA, Nguyen AD. Unexpected pacing threshold changes during non-implant surgery. Anesthesiology 2002; 96:A1070.
90. Bernstein AD, Irwin ME, Parsonnet V, et al. Report of the NASPE Policy Conference on antibradycardia pacemaker follow-up: effectiveness, needs, and resources. North American Society of Pacing and Electrophysiology. Pacing Clin Electrophysiol 1994; 17(11 Pt 1):1714–1729.
91. Medicare: cardiac pacemaker evaluation services. Effective Oct 1, 1984. Coverage Issues Manual, CMS Publication No. 6: Section 50–1, 1984.
92. Wilke A, Hesse H, Gorg C, Maisch B. Elevation of the pacing threshold: a side effect in a patient with pacemaker undergoing therapy with doxorubicin and vincristine. Oncology 1999; 56(2):110–111.
93. Pacemaker System Guide for the Discovery Series Pacemakers. St. Paul, MN: Guidant Corporation, 1998.
94. Last A. Radiotherapy in patients with cardiac pacemakers. Br J Radiol 1998; 71(841):4–10.
95. Pacemaker System Guide for the Insignia Series Pacemakers. St Paul, MN: Guidant Corporation, 2002.

18

Perioperative Management of Brain Tumors

RASHMI N. MULLER

Department of Anesthesiology, University of Texas Medical Branch, Galveston, Texas, U.S.A.

I. BACKGROUND

Craniotomies have been performed on humans since prehistoric times in several cultures throughout the world. Skulls from as long ago as the late. Paleolithic period show evidence of trephination with some apparently even having undergone "redo surgery" (1). While the purpose of these procedures can only be guessed, the first resection of a brain tumor more recently was performed by Rickman Godlee in London, England in 1884 (2). Although the patient did not survive for more than a month, the resection did result in diagnosis of the lesion. Modern neurosurgery and neuroanesthesia have benefited from numerous advances such as sophisticated diagnostic and neurophysiologic monitoring techniques, improved knowledge of neuropathophysiology and the interactions of various anesthetics with the brain, and surgical breakthroughs such as the operating microscope, image-guided neuronavigation systems, and ultrasonic aspirators (3). Over the last one to two decades, in particular, these developments have improved surgical outcome (4). The anesthesiologist makes a vital contribution to the successful perioperative care of patients with brain tumors. This chapter discusses the perioperative anesthetic management of such patients with some surgical perspectives.

II. INTRACRANIAL DYNAMICS AND THE EFFECTS OF ANESTHETICS

Anesthetic management of patients with brain tumors revolves around the consideration of a few key concepts namely, cerebral blood flow (CBF), cerebral metabolism, and intracranial pressure (ICP). These are briefly addressed below.

Cerebral function and vitality are dependent on a continuous supply of oxygen and glucose which in turn depends on the CBF. The human brain comprises 2% of the total body weight while its blood flow is approximately 20% of the cardiac output. Average CBF is 50 mL/100 g/min and varies regionally from 20 to 80 mL/100 g/min. This proportionally high blood flow is necessary due to the high metabolic rate of the brain. Neurons use primarily oxygen and glucose as substrates for energy production by oxidative phosphorylation. (During starvation, ketones are also utilized for energy production.) The cerebral metabolic rate for oxygen ($CMRO_2$) is 3–5 mL/100 g/min, while the cerebral metabolic rate for glucose consumption is 5.5 mg/100 g/min (5). Cellular processes that consume energy are the creation and maintenance of ionic gradients across cell membranes (including depolarization and repolarization), synthesis of neurotransmitters, and the metabolism of proteins, lipids, and carbohydrates (6).

Anaerobic metabolism is an ineffective means of energy production in the brain and is tolerated poorly. If the oxygen supply is interrupted, consciousness is lost within a few seconds (6). Eventually, anoxic neurons undergo cell death by necrosis and apoptosis. Below a CBF of 15–20 mL/100 g/min, the electroencephalogram (EEG), which reflects the electrophysiological activity of the brain, is isoelectric. Irreversible brain damage occurs at CBF of 10 mL/100 g/min.

A. Cerebral Blood Flow

Several elements influence CBF. Factors that may change CBF are the metabolic rate of the brain, arterial carbon dioxide and oxygen levels, arterial blood pressure, intracranial pressure, temperature, and the viscosity of blood, drugs, and neurogenic factors. In general, changes in CBF are assumed to correlate with similar changes in cerebral blood volume (CBV), but this may not always be the case.

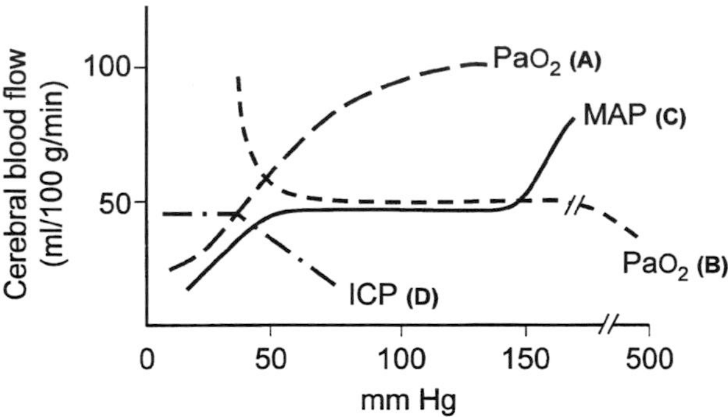

Figure 1 (A) Effect of $PaCO_2$ on CBF. There is a linear relationship between $PaCO_2$ (20 to 80 mm Hg) and CBF. (B) Effect of PaO_2 on CBF. Below a PaO_2 of 50 mmHg, CBF increases markedly. (C) CBF autoregulation: for MAP between 50 and 150mm Hg, CBF is maintained at 50 ml/100 g/min. (D) Effect of ICP on CBF: as ICP rises, CBF is compromised. *Source*: From Ref. 174, with permisson from Elsevier.

1. *Metabolism*

Cerebral blood flow is normally coupled to $CMRO_2$ at a ratio of 15:1 (7). When the metabolic rate increases in an area of the brain, the local CBF is also augmented. Various factors at the cellular level are implicated in this coupling of blood flow and metabolism, including calcium, nitric oxide, prostaglandins, potassium, and hydrogen concentration in the extracellular fluid (ECF) of the brain. Seizures, pain, and arousal states cause a large increase in CBF. Surgical stimulation itself increases CBF as measured by the velocity of blood flow in the middle cerebral artery during 1 and 2 MAC isoflurane anesthesia and maintenance of systemic arterial blood pressure (8). Inhaled anesthetics lower $CMRO_2$ and increase CBF. Most intravenous anesthetics decrease both $CMRO_2$ and CBF.

2. *Carbon Dioxide*

Between arterial partial pressures of carbon dioxide ($PaCO_2$) of 20–80 mmHg, CBF changes 1–2 mL/100 g/min for every 1 mmHg change in $PaCO_2$ [Fig. 1(A)] (9). At a $PaCO_2$ of 20–25 mmHg, the CBF is reduced by approximately 50%. Metabolic acidosis or alkalosis have no direct effects on CBF. Carbon dioxide, but not the bicarbonate ion, can diffuse easily across the blood–brain barrier (10). Subsequent changes in the local hydrogen ion concentration and extracellular pH effect changes in blood flow by relaxation of cerebral arterioles. Intracellular calcium fluxes appear to be the final step mediating changes in vascular diameter. Nitric oxide, cGMP, and potassium have been implicated in $PaCO_2$-mediated CBF alterations. In neonates, prostanoids play a role in this process (11).

With sustained hyperventilation, CBF returns to baseline after 6–30 hr (12). This occurs due to active transport of bicarbonate and hydrogen ions from the cerebrospinal fluid (CSF) by the choroid plexus, with subsequent normalization of the pH of the ECF of the brain (10). Thereafter abrupt cessation of hyperventilation is perceived by the brain as relative hypercarbia and results in CSF acidosis and vasodilatation. Therefore, after hyperventilation for a given period, normoventilation should be reintroduced gradually to avoid a "rebound" increase in CBF and ICP. Rapid normalization of carbon dioxide may also result in reperfusion injury (13).

The CO_2 reactivity of CBF varies depending on the baseline CBF, cerebral perfusion pressure (CPP), and the background effects of any drugs (pure vasodilators, anesthetics) that may have been administered (9). In awake, nonanesthetized patients, elevated catecholamines augment the $CMRO_2$ and produce a greater rise in CBF with hypercapnia.

Vessels in normal areas of the brain dilate in response to high blood levels of carbon dioxide while those in ischemic areas may already be maximally dilated and unable to dilate further. This phenomenon can shunt blood away from injured areas to normal regions of the brain and is described as steal. Vasoconstriction in normal areas of the brain and the diversion of blood to ischemic regions during hypocapnia is termed as reverse steal. The clinical importance of these phenomena is unclear.

Intraoperative hyperventilation is useful for rapidly controlling ICP, offsetting the effect of volatile agents and for improving surgical exposure (9). Although hyperventilation and respiratory alkalosis are widely used in neurosurgical patients, hypocapnia is not benign. Besides the complications of abruptly terminating hyperventilation, deleterious effects of hypocapnia include decreased oxygen delivery due to local cerebral ischemia, decreased oxygen unloading from hemoglobin due to a left shift of the oxygen–hemoglobin dissociation curve, and increased neuronal excitability which may augment oxygen demand at the cellular level (13). Data from head-injured patients indicates that acute hyperventilation below a $PaCO_2$ of 25 mmHg may be accompanied by regional ischemia (14). Reduced CBF was associated with a poor outcome in these patients. Adverse pulmonary effects of hypocapnia include bronchoconstriction, the attenuation of hypoxic pulmonary vasoconstriction and increased intrapulmonary shunting (13). Accordingly, mild-to-moderate hyperventilation should be employed only when there is a definite indication and continued for a limited period of time. Resumption of normocapnia is best performed gradually.

3. Oxygen

Below an arterial partial pressure of oxygen (PaO_2) of 50 mmHg, CBF is markedly increased [Fig. 1(B)] (15). Above 300 mmHg, there is a slight decrease in CBF. Between 50 and 300 mmHg, changes in PaO_2 have little effect on the CBF. A lower oxygen content in the blood due to anemia produces a rise in CBF (16).

4. Arterial Pressure

Cerebral blood flow is maintained at a constant rate over a range of systemic mean arterial pressure or CPP by means of vasoconstriction or vasodilation. [Fig. 1(C)]. Some argue that the lower limit of this autoregulation may be closer to an MAP of 70 mmHg in humans, rather than 50 mmHg as often cited (15). The higher limit of autoregulation is believed to be an MAP of 150 mmHg. As the MAP or CPP rises, cerebral arterioles constrict to preserve a constant CBF. Conversely, hypotension triggers intracranial vasodilation. Beyond the limits of autoregulation, blood flows to the brain in a passive pressure-dependent manner. This myogenic autoregulatory response of arterioles takes place within 1–3 min. During this time period, sudden changes in blood pressure are directly transmitted to the cerebral circulation. Autoregulation is regionally abolished by several pathological processes including trauma, tumors, hypoxia, drugs, and infection. Such areas of the brain are vulnerable to ischemia with arterial hypotension and to hyperemia, bleeding, or edema formation with hypertension.

While autoregulation may be impaired in areas of severe CNS injury, it is usually grossly intact. The vasodilatory cascade describes rises in CBF due to a low CPP and resultant vasodilation (16). Intracranial hypertension due to increased CBV compromises the CPP further. As CPP is lowered, the smooth muscle in the arterioles relaxes further augmenting CBF. This further increases the ICP which in turn reduces the CPP even more. Unless CPP is improved, this cycle continues until maximal vasodilatation is produced. Hypotension, hypoxia, venous obstruction, and hypercapnia are among the factors that can trigger this vasodilatory cascade in susceptible patients. Restoration of the CPP abolishes ICP waves and lowers the ICP. Cerebral perfusion pressure above 70–80 Torr may be optimal in neurosurgical patients with neoplastic or traumatic CNS injury. The autoregulatory curve is shifted to the right in patients with chronic hypertension (17). These patients require a higher MAP for optimal cerebral perfusion.

5. Viscosity

The viscosity of blood is largely determined by the hematocrit. Significant changes in CBF due to viscosity occur outside the usual range of hematocrit values seen clinically (33–45%) (18). Increased CBF due to anemia occurs at the cost of the oxygen-carrying capacity. The ideal hematocrit for optimal delivery of oxygen to the brain in the presence of focal cerebral ischemia may be 30–34% (19).

6. Temperature

Hyperthermia (37–42°C) increases $CMRO_2$ and CBF and may worsen cerebral edema (20). Hypothermia decreases $CMRO_2$ by its effects on electrophysiological activities and basal cellular ("housekeeping") functions, with continued effects on metabolism after burst suppression of the EEG has been achieved. There is a definite benefit due to mild hypothermia (31–34°C) in laboratory animals undergoing various cerebral insults including global and focal ischemia. These beneficial effects are due to cellular and biochemical effects rather than the reduction in $CMRO_2$ which is minimal during mild hypothermia (21). Mild hypothermia may be neuroprotective in surgical patients, while avoiding some of the complications of deep hypothermia (coagulopathy, wound infection, delayed emergence, and cardiac arrhythmias). However, there is no evidence to date demonstrating improved outcome due to hypothermia in patients undergoing brain tumor resection.

Furthermore, increases in oxygen consumption due to shivering during emergence from anesthesia may render patients vulnerable to myocardial ischemia.

7. Neurogenic Factors

Neurogenic factors may be involved in regulation of CBF but their clinical significance in humans is unclear.

B. Intracranial Pressure

1. General Considerations

The Monroe–Kellie doctrine describes the homeostasis of intracranial volume and pressure (22). The cranium is a rigid vault which primarily contains brain, blood, and cerebrospinal fluid. The normal volumes of each of these components are as follows: brain—1400 mL; blood—150 mL; and CSF—150 mL. The normal ICP is 3–15 mmHg. An increase in brain volume due to a small intracranial lesion is initially accommodated by a compensatory reduction in other compartments (Fig. 2). The intracranial venous, capillary, and CSF compartments contract. Cerebrospinal fluid is displaced into the spinal subarachnoid space and there is reduced formation and enhanced absorption of CSF. Normal brain parenchyma may be compressed by the space-occupying lesion. All these processes accommodate the slow-growing lesion without drastic changes in the ICP and contribute to the initial preservation of intracranial compliance. (Strictly speaking, changes in pressure due to changes in volume should be described as elastance. However, this relationship is commonly labeled as compliance—which is defined as changes in volume secondary to changes in pressure—in the neuroanesthesia literature.)

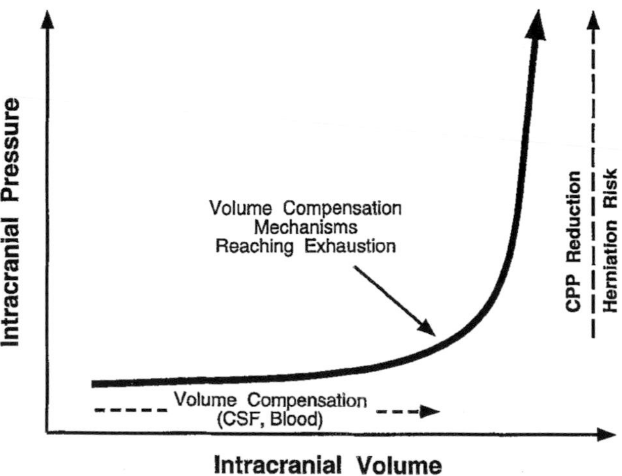

Figure 2 The intracranial pressure–volume relationship. The horizontal portion of the curve indicates that there is initially some latitude for compensation in the face of an expanding intracranial lesion. That compensation is accomplished largely by displacement of CSF and venous blood from intracranial to extracranial spaces. Once the compensatory latitudes are exhausted, small increments in volume result in large increases in ICP, with the associated hazards of either herniation and/or decreased CPP resulting in ischemia. *Source*: From Ref. 131, with permission from Elsevier.

Slowly growing, supratentorial tumors may become quite large without significant clinical signs. As the lesion grows further and overwhelms compensatory mechanisms, the ICP begins to rise dramatically (22). At this point, small increases in intracranial volume lead to steep rises in ICP (Fig. 2). Rapidly growing lesions and lesions in more confined areas, such as in the posterior fossa, quickly exhaust the compensatory processes. These tumors cause critically high ICP much earlier than tumors in less restricted regions of the brain. Obstructive hydrocephalus will prevent the displacement of CSF into the subarachnoid compartment and accelerate the rate of rise of ICP. Peritumoral edema as well as hemorrhage and necrosis add to the intracranial volume.

Increased ICP can cause ischemia of the brain due to decreased CPP. Cerebral perfusion pressure is defined as the mean arterial pressure minus the outflow pressure (ICP or CVP: whichever is higher). When ICP rises, perfusion to the brain is compromised [Fig. 1(D)]. Hypertension may occur in an attempt to preserve perfusion to the vital centers in the brainstem. Cushing's triad (23) describes such hypertension, accompanying reflex bradycardia, and respiratory abnormalities, all of which occur due to dangerously high ICP. Occasionally, systemic hypertension without bradycardia may be a warning of significantly elevated ICP and should prompt the clinician to identify and treat intracranial hypertension. Other signs of high ICP are nausea, vomiting, headache, mental status changes, nuchal rigidity, papilledema, sixth nerve palsy, and other focal neurological deficits.

During progressive intracranial hypertension, pathologic pressure waves can be seen on ICP recordings (16,24). The vasodilatory cascade and reduced CPP have been used to explain the generation of these waves. Plateau waves or Lundberg A waves which may have amplitudes as high as 50–100 mmHg coincide with increases in regional CBV, reduced CBF and CPP (25,26). Lundberg B waves are of lesser amplitude and less ominous but also mark abnormal intracranial compliance. Lundberg C are believed to be harmless waves reflecting fluctuations of systemic arterial pressure. Restoration of the CPP eliminates these CSF pressure waves (16). Ultimately, unchecked intracranial

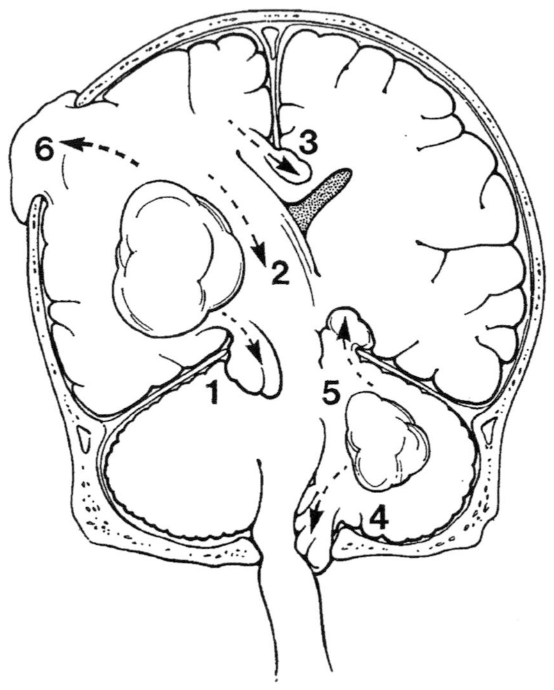

Figure 3 Sites of brain herniation. (1) Transtentorial herniation. (2) Central transtentorial herniation. (3) Subfalcine herniation. (4) Tonsillar herniation. (5) Upward transtentorial herniation. (6) Extracalvarial herniation. *Source*: From Ref. 27.

hypertension results in herniation at one or more of several sites (Fig. 3).

2. *Herniation Syndromes*

Displacement of the brain from the supratentorial into the infratentorial compartment across the tentorium is termed transtentorial herniation. Clinical signs are a decrease in the level of consciousness, dilated, nonreactive pupils, decorticate or decerebrate posturing, and respiratory abnormalities (27). Death may result from respiratory arrest.

Displacement of the cerebral hemisphere within the supratentorial compartment beneath the falx and across the midline is described as subfalcine or cingulate herniation. This occurs most often due to a frontal or parietal mass lesion. Compression of the anterior cerebral arteries by the displaced brain can produce motor or sensory deficits in the legs (28). Effacement and lateral shift of the third ventricle can be seen radiologically. Coma with asymmetric posturing (contralateral more than ipsilateral) may occur (26).

Lateral transtentorial herniation which occurs due to temporal mass lesions is termed "uncal herniation." The uncus, which is the anterior medial portion of the temporal lobe, is shifted down against the tentorial edge. Ipsilateral third nerve palsy may occur along with contralateral posturing. Anisocoria or unilateral pupillary dilation may be an early warning of this process (28).

Tonsillar herniation is the displacement of the cerebellar tonsils through the foramen magnum. The tonsils compress the medulla and press down on the upper cervical cord (27). Sudden death due to respiratory arrest or cardiac arrhythmias can occur. Vomiting, aspiration, coma, loss of postural sensibility, and spasticity with an extensor plantar response are other manifestations of cerebellar herniation.

Upward transtentorial herniation of the infratentorial contents occurs rarely. The midbrain is compressed against the clivus by the ascending cerebellum. Signs of brainstem dysfunction followed by signs of midbrain injury may develop. This phenomenon can be precipitated by excessive CSF drainage or following craniotomy for posterior fossa masses. It has been described mainly in association with cerebellar space-occupying lesions or hydrocephalic dilatation of the fourth ventricle (29). More rarely, it may occur with brainstem tumors.

C. Effects of Anesthetics and Muscle Relaxants

The effects of anesthetics on CBV and metabolism are complex. Following is a brief discussion of these and other considerations during the perioperative use of anesthetic agents.

1. *Volatile Agents*

All volatile anesthetics decrease cerebral metabolism and increase CBF in a dose-dependent fashion. The increase in CBF occurs by direct vasodilation. Regional coupling of flow and metabolism is preserved when volatile anesthetics are used but there is an overall "resetting" of the relationship between flow and metabolism (30). Increases in CBF and ICP are more marked when volatile agents are used along with nitrous oxide. The effect of volatile agents on CBF also depends on the CPP. With systemic hypotension and decreased CPP, the rise in CBF is less marked (31). Reactivity of blood vessels to carbon dioxide is maintained by clinically used concentrations of volatile agents (32,33). High concentrations of volatile agents impair CO_2 reactivity and CBF autoregulation.

Among volatile agents, $CMRO_2$ is reduced maximally by isoflurane, desflurane, and sevoflurane. Cerebral vasodilation has been reported to be most pronounced with halothane (34,35) followed by enflurane, with lesser increases in CBF due to isoflurane, sevoflurane, and desflurane (36). Brain surface protrusion into a craniotomy site was reported to be more with halothane as compared to isoflurane or enflurane (37). Subsequently, it was observed that increases in CBF with halothane occur more in the neocortex, while the vasodilatory effect of isoflurane is more pronounced in subcortical regions (38). These regional differences in CBF may explain at least some of the observations of a greater increase in CBF with halothane, as most of the previous experiments measured cortical blood flow. There may be little difference in global CBF increases between halothane and isoflurane.

Increases in CBF with halothane can be minimized by hyperventilation begun prior to the use of the agent, by the use of barbiturates along with halothane and by limiting the concentration of halothane to less than 1 MAC. Increased CBF due to isoflurane is attenuated by hyperventilation begun simultaneously with the use of the agent (39,40) and by concomitant barbiturate use. Isoflurane (2 MAC), but not halothane, causes burst suppression of the EEG. After this, there is no further decrease in $CMRO_2$ with increasing concentrations of isoflurane up to 4 MAC.

Enflurane can cause epileptiform spike-and-wave activity on the EEG, which is enhanced by hypocapnia and auditory stimuli (41). Hence, enflurane is generally not used in neurosurgical patients. The effects of sevoflurane on $CMRO_2$ and CBF are similar to those of isoflurane (41). Sevoflurane has been very useful for inhalational induction of anesthesia in pediatric patients with preserved intracranial compliance. However, epileptiform activity due to high doses of sevoflurane, such as those used for inhalational induction, has been described (42,43). There have been theoretical concerns regarding nephrotoxicity due to fluoride ion production during the biotransformation of sevoflurane. Additionally, degradation of sevoflurane by carbon dioxide absorbents, particularly during the use of low fresh gas flows, can produce compound **A**. Compound **A** is responsible for renal toxicity when administered in large doses to rats. Hence, sevoflurane may not be ideal for long neurosurgical cases (44).

In patients with supratentorial masses, 1 MAC desflurane, but not 1 MAC isoflurane, was reported to increase CSF pressure in spite of hyperventilation (45). However, more recently, it was found that during craniotomy for tumor resection, desflurane did not increase ICP in normocapnic patients with absence of preoperative midline shift on computed tomography (CT) scan (46). One advantage of desflurane and sevoflurane over isoflurane is that these agents are less soluble in the blood, and therefore may facilitate faster recovery and neurologic assessment after neurosurgical cases of long duration (47).

Volatile agents have varying effects on the absorption and production of CSF (48–50). Changes in CSF dynamics are most likely of minimal relevance even during the most prolonged surgical procedure.

Volatile agents are safe to use in low concentrations in neurosurgical patients, with concomitant mild hyperventilation, and when intracranial compliance is preserved or only mildly decreased (51). Among volatile agents, isoflurane is most widely used for neuroanesthesia.

2. *Nitrous Oxide*

Nitrous oxide causes cerebral stimulation and direct vasodilation resulting in increased $CMRO_2$ and CBF in humans and other species (52–55). Its effects are usually attenuated by active regulatory mechanisms in the healthy brain (56), hyperventilation (57) and the simultaneous use of anesthetics (intravenous more than volatile). Advantages of nitrous oxide are its speed of elimination and the lower concentration of volatile agents needed when nitrous oxide is used. In situations of grossly impaired cerebral autoregulation or intracranial compliance, nitrous oxide is contraindicated.

3. *Intravenous Anesthetics*

Most intravenous anesthetics—with the exception of ketamine—lower CBF by reduction of cerebral metabolism. In general, reactivity to carbon dioxide as well as autoregulation are preserved during the administration of intravenous anesthetics (58,59).

Barbiturates

Barbiturates have been investigated for neuroprotective properties since the 1960s. Barbiturates reduce $CMRO_2$ in increasing doses until burst suppression of the EEG is achieved (60,61). Subsequent doses do not affect the $CMRO_2$ further. Barbiturates have been used for neuroprotection in cases of focal cerebral ischemia but are ineffective in global cerebral ischemia. In patients with intractable intracranial hypertension, barbiturates may be administered to the point of isoelectricity of the EEG. Phenobarbital is usually used for this purpose. However, even in focal ischemia, the benefit from barbiturates may be small (21). Large doses of barbiturates cause hypotension, myocardial depression, and prolonged sedation, all of which complicate the management of neurosurgical patients.

Propofol

Propofol produces a dose-dependent reduction in $CMRO_2$ and CBF. There is no further effect on metabolism after burst suppression of the EEG is achieved. Contradictory data exist on the effect of propofol on cerebral vascular reactivity to CO_2. Some have reported that CBF and CBV are not responsive to hyperventilation during the use of propofol (while remaining responsive to hyperventilation during the administration of isoflurane) in patients with brain tumors (62). This discrepancy may be due to the high degree of vasoconstriction caused by propofol alone, with minimal additional effect due to superimposed hyperventilation. The strong antiemetic effect of propofol is useful in neurosurgical patients. As an induction agent, propofol should be administered carefully to avoid significant systemic hypotension and a decrease in CPP. Propofol can very rarely cause seizures and ophistotonus. Prolonged infusions of propofol have been reported to cause unexplained lactic acidosis, bradyarrhythmias, cardiac failure, and death in critically ill, mechanically ventilated children (63).

Etomidate

Etomidate decreases $CMRO_2$ and CBF. There is less cardiovascular depression with etomidate as compared to barbiturates. Etomidate may aggravate focal cerebral ischemia (64,65) and therefore its use in neuroanesthesia has been questioned (66). Other side effects associated with etomidate are adrenocortical suppression (which is unlikely to be a problem in patients scheduled for brain tumor resection as they receive perioperative steroids) and myoclonus.

Ketamine

Ketamine is generally avoided in patients with intracranial tumors as it can increase $CMRO_2$, CBF, and ICP (67,68). Delirium and hallucinations can occur, as ketamine is a phencyclidine derivative. Ketamine has the ability to produce delirium and hallucinations. When used along with other anesthetics and hyperventilation, the effects of ketamine on ICP and CBF may be attenuated (69). Features of ketamine that may be occasionally of benefit are its bioavailability when administered intramuscularly, bronchodilation, lack of respiratory depression, and its sympathomimetic effect on blood pressure (44).

Opioids

Opioids have minimal effect on CBF and metabolism. Although there have been reports of increased ICP with sufentanil and alfentanil (70,71), this was most likely due to reflex cerebral vasodilation as a consequence of systemic hypotension. Low doses of narcotics blunt the circulatory response to tracheal intubation, do not delay recovery and are useful adjuncts to low-dose volatile agents and nitrous oxide for the maintenance of anesthesia (72,73). Remifentanil is particularly advantageous in neuroanesthesia due to its rapid elimination by plasma esterases (74). Doses of narcotics much higher than those usually used clinically may cause epileptoid activity (75). Normeperidine, a metabolite of meperidine which accumulates in patients with renal failure, can cause seizures. Naloxone, an opioid antagonist, when administered injudiciously in large boluses can increase CBF and $CMRO_2$. Smaller doses of naloxone may be safely titrated in narcotized patients (44).

Benzodiazepines

Commonly used benzodiazepines such as midazolam, diazepam, and lorazepam cause small dose-related decreases in CBF and $CMRO_2$ and do not significantly affect ICP (76,77). When flumazenil, a competitive receptor antagonist, is used to reverse a high dose of midazolam, a marked increase in CBF and ICP may result.

4. Overview of Anesthetics for Tumor Resection

In clinical practice, the choice of anesthetics appears to have little effect on the short-term outcome after craniotomies (78). Most anesthesiologists avoid ketamine, enflurane, and high doses of halothane for craniotomies. Sub-MAC concentrations of isoflurane with or without nitrous oxide are commonly employed. Induction agents that are most often used are sodium thiopental and propofol. As most intravenous anesthetics decrease CBF and $CMRO_2$, operating conditions for brain surgery can be predicted to be better with a total intravenous technique. A recent investigation comparing different anesthetics for supratentorial craniotomy for tumor resection was conducted in patients with preserved intracranial compliance. Patients anesthetized with propofol/fentanyl had lower subdural ICP (which correlates with dural tension) as estimated by neurosurgeons (79). The degree of cerebral swelling was less pronounced and CPP was found to be higher in patients anesthetized with propofol compared with isoflurane/fentanyl or sevoflurane/fentanyl. The mixed venous oxygen saturation was also significantly higher and the arteriovenous oxygen content difference significantly lower in patients receiving isoflurane and sevoflurane compared to those receiving propofol. This may reflect higher CBF with the use of volatile agents. In patients with severe preoperative derangement of intracranial compliance or those who develop a swollen brain intraoperatively, nitrous oxide and volatile agents should be avoided in favor of a totally intravenous technique.

5. *Muscle Relaxants*

Succinylcholine can cause rises in ICP due to afferent activity from the muscle spindle apparatus causing cerebral stimulation (80). A prior defasciculating dose of vecuronium or metocurine is effective in preventing this increase in ICP (81). Concomitant hyperventilation and the administration of thiopental also attenuates the intracranial hypertension caused by succinylcholine (82). Succinylcholine is the drug of choice in rapid sequence induction and endotracheal intubation due to its unmatched speed of onset and short duration of action. Patients with hemiparesis or paraplegia have proliferation of extrajunctional receptors. Succinylcholine can produce dangerous hyperkalemia in these patients and should be avoided.

Among the nondepolarizing muscle relaxants, cisatracurium, vecuronium, rocuronium, and pancuronium are commonly used. These muscle relaxants have no effect on ICP (83,84). Pancuronium is vagolytic and can cause hypertension and tachycardia, which is undesirable in many patients (85). High-dose rocuronium (0.9–1.2 mg/kg) may be used for a fast onset of muscle relaxation when succinylcholine is contraindicated. It should be remembered that the duration of action of rocuronium is approximately an hour at this dose. Histamine release due to atracurium, mivacurium, and D-tubocurarine can cause vasodilatation and consequent increases in ICP (86). Cerebral stimulation and seizures may result from the effects of laudanosine, a metabolite of atracurium.

Long-acting nondepolarizing muscle relaxants, like pancuronium, should be used cautiously as residual neuromuscular weakness can persist in the PACU even after the administration of antagonists. Even after a single dose of muscle relaxant of intermediate duration, residual paralysis was common more than 2 hr later, in the absence of pharmacological reversal (87). Clinical tests and manual assessment of fade of train-of-four ratio have poor sensitivity for the detection of the residual paralysis. Accordingly, when muscle relaxants of intermediate duration are used, and extubation is planned at the end of the case, the administration of an antagonist (such as neostigmine) is recommended.

Patients receiving chronic treatment with phenytoin and carbamazepine are resistant to the effects of nondepolarizing muscle relaxants with the exception of atracurium and *cis*-atracurium (88–90). The mechanism of this resistance appears to be enhanced prejunctional release of acetylcholine and higher postjunctional sensitivity to acetylcholine. These patients need larger doses of nondepolarizing agents. Acute administration of antiepileptics can potentiate neuromuscular blockade by nondepolarizing agents.

D. Drugs Used to Treat Intracranial Hypertension

Steroids, mannitol, furosemide, and hypertonic saline are often used for the control of intracranial hypertension in patients with brain tumors.

1. *Steroids*

Vasogenic edema occurs in the vicinity of brain tumors (see Fig. 4) due to local disruption of the BBB and increased permeability of capillaries (24). Systemic hypertension facilitates the formation of vasogenic edema (91). Most patients with brain tumors receive steroids for the control of cerebral edema. Steroids may dramatically improve neurologic status in these patients. Dexamethasone is preferred because of its lack of mineralocorticoid activity. Intravenous loading doses of 8–32 mg are administered beginning at least 48 hr before surgery, followed by 16 mg/day in divided doses. Maximum benefit is seen in 48–72 hr following the first dose.

Mechanisms whereby steroids may help reduce cerebral edema include the stabilization of the cerebral endothelial cell membrane, reduced plasma filtration across the endothelium, decreased release of free radicals, prostaglandins, and fatty acids, effects on lysosomal activity, improved water and electrolyte excretion, and improved glucose utilization. In patients with brain tumors, magnetic resonance imaging (MRI), performed 1–6 hr after the administration of dexamethasone, confirmed acute reversal of blood–tumor barrier permeability and reduced regional CBV (92). Positron emission tomography (PET) similarly showed decreased CBF, CBV, and increased fractional extraction of oxygen throughout the brain after dexamethasone treatment in patients with brain tumors (93). Thus, acute changes in CBV in the peritumoral gray matter may be the primary source of the immediate clinical improvement seen after the administration of dexamethasone.

Besides symptomatic relief, steroids may improve operating conditions, and help predict which patients will benefit from extensive resection. Patients who do not respond to treatment with dexamethasone may have irreversible tumor infiltration as opposed to reversible compression of brain tissue by tumor mass

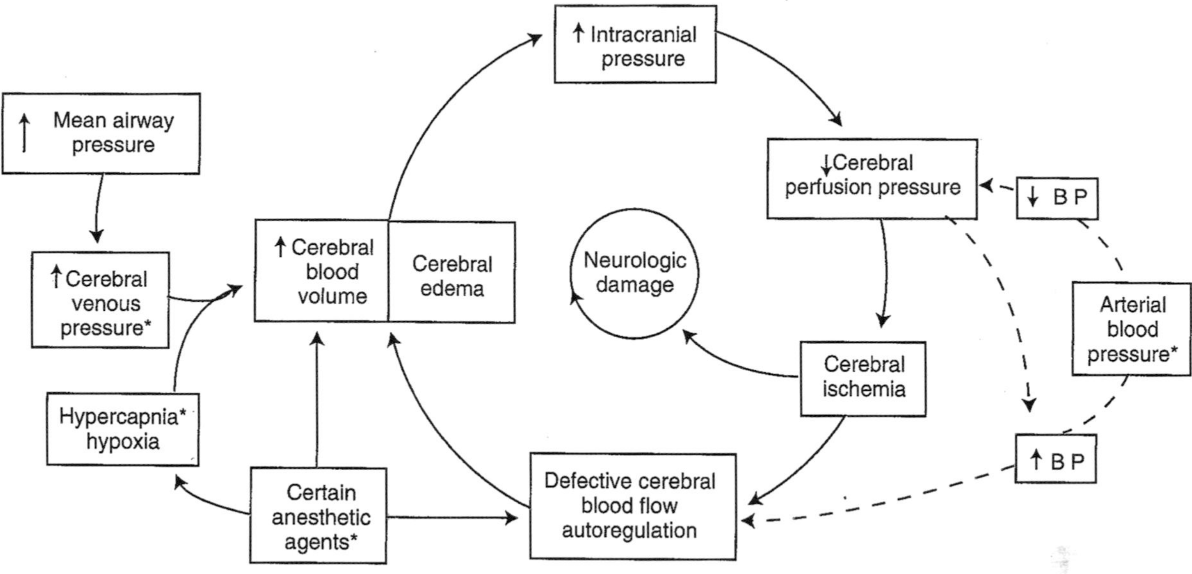

Figure 4 The pathophysiology of intracranial hypertension. Those elements that are potentially under the control of the anesthesiologist are indicated by asterisks (*). BP, blood pressure. *Source*: From Ref. 131, with permission from Elsevier.

(94). Patients with marked improvement due to steroids often show a similar and sustained benefit with extensive surgical resection. For primary central nervous system lymphomas (PCNSLs), corticosteroids can cause regression or even total disappearance of lesions within days. Hence, if PCNSL is suspected by imaging, corticosteroids should be withheld until a biopsy is performed.

Complications of long-term steroid use include hyperglycemia, gastrointestinal ulceration and bleeding, immunosuppression, electrolyte changes, steroid myopathy, osteoporosis, and psychosis. Patients with brain tumors receiving steroids may be at increased risk of developing *Pneumocystis carinii pneumonia* (95,96). The presentation can be subtle and clinicians should have a high index of suspicion, especially in patients who receive prolonged therapy with corticosteroids. Trimethoprim–sulfamethoxazole is an effective prophylactic agent against *Pneumocystis carinii pneumonia* (96).

2. *Osmotherapy*

As mentioned above, intracranial tumors are usually associated with vasogenic edema which occurs in the extracellular space of the brain. While the movement of water across the capillaries of peripheral tissues into the extracellular tissue depends on the plasma oncotic gradient, movement of water across the BBB into the extracellular compartment occurs due to the osmolar gradient between plasma and the ECF of the brain (97). Free water moves across the BBB from the hypo-osmolar towards the more hyperosmolar compartment. Hypo-osmolarity of plasma facilitates the development or worsening of existing cerebral edema. Conversely, in the presence of an intact BBB, hyperosmolar solutions (mannitol or hypertonic saline) can reduce brain water. If the BBB is disrupted in some regions of the brain, hyperosmolar agents reduce cerebral edema by drawing fluid across other areas of the brain where the BBB is intact. Hyperosmolar agents may actually worsen cerebral edema locally at the regions with disrupted BBB.

Mannitol

Mannitol (0.25–1 g/kg) is generally administered before dural opening to reduce cerebral edema and improve operating conditions (98). Additional doses of mannitol may also be administered during tumor resection and following surgery as therapy for intracranial hypertension. An upper limit of serum osmolarity of 320–330 mosm/L is generally accepted when hyperosmolar therapy is employed. Mannitol is effective within 10 min of administration and lasts for approximately 2 hr. A positive blood–CSF osmotic gradient is created across the intact BBB (99). Free water is subsequently drawn from the brain into the vascular compartment. The rheology of blood is improved by mannitol and cerebral arteriolar vasoconstriction may also result. Mannitol can exacerbate cerebral edema in regions of disrupted BBB by crossing into the brain and drawing free water from plasma into the ECF of the brain. The sudden initial increase in plasma osmolality and vasodilatation due to mannitol can cause transiently high ICP and low systemic blood pressure (100). Hypokalemia and hyponatremia can occur with the use of mannitol. Cardiac output and pulmonary capillary wedge pressure are significantly increased (99). This drug is best avoided in patients at risk for left ventricular dysfunction as the increased intravascular volume may precipitate left ventricular volume overload and failure.

Furosemide

Furosemide (0.7–1 mg/kg), a distal-loop diuretic, is frequently used together with mannitol to reduce cerebral edema. The diuresis caused by furosemide diminishes CSF production and improves cellular water transport. Together with mannitol, synergism is evident: a greater and more sustained effect on the osmotic gradient across the BBB and ICP occurs than with either drug alone (101). Injudicious use of furosemide along with mannitol can result in severe hypovolemia and electrolyte disturbances.

Hypertonic Saline

Hypertonic saline (2.5 mL/kg of 7.5% saline over a 15-min period) may be as effective as 20% mannitol (0.5 g/kg over 15 min) in reducing brain bulk and lumbar CSF pressure in patients undergoing elective supratentorial surgery (102). Alternatively, 3% hypertonic saline may be administered (75–150 mL/hr) for the rapid reduction of ICP in patients with brain tumors (103). Transient hypernatremia following the infusion of hypertonic saline mandates caution in the administration of chronic or multiple doses of this solution (104).

E. Altered Intracranial Compliance and Surgical Concerns

In patients with intracranial pathology, clinical concerns include the development of cerebral ischemia, edema, bleeding, and/or herniation. Patients undergoing craniotomy for brain tumors may have areas of the brain which are underperfused due to local pressure from the tumor mass, or due to pressure under retractors. Low MAP or CPP can further jeopardize these areas of the brain. When the CBF increases, CBV and the brain bulk are usually augmented. This can lead to intracranial hypertension before craniotomy and difficult operating conditions due to bulging of the brain or a "tight brain" after dural opening. The brain may herniate through the craniotomy site. Marked elevations in CPP can cause hyperemia of the brain and predispose to intracranial hemorrhage. After craniotomy, the CPP is primarily dependent on the MAP as the ICP is zero. When the cranium is open to ambient atmospheric pressure, changes in systemic venous pressure can produce changes in the volume of the brain (105). Anesthesiologists can perform several maneuvers to improve operating conditions (Fig. 5). These include hyperventilation, the reduction of $CMRO_2$ by various means, and the control of excessive rises in intrathoracic pressure and systemic venous pressure. Additionally, the anesthesiologist can optimize the patient's position to improve venous drainage, administer vasoconstricting drugs, and discontinue vasodilators such as volatile agents, nitrous oxide, sodium nitroprusside, nitroglycerin, or calcium-channel blockers.

III. EPIDEMIOLOGY OF BRAIN TUMORS

The incidence of primary brain tumors in the United States is 11–12 per 100,000 person-years (106). In 1999, primary brain tumors were the cause of death in approximately 13,100 people (107). Additionally, more than 100,000 patients die per year with symptomatic intracranial metastases. Meningiomas and gliomas are the most frequently occurring primary brain tumors with an incidence of 24% and 22.6%, respectively (106). The average age of onset for primary brain tumors is 53 years. The incidence of most brain tumors rises with age; this is especially the case for meningiomas. Neuroepithelial tumors are more common among men, while meningeal tumors are more likely to occur in women. In children, primary brain tumors are the second leading cause of mortality after leukemias, are the most common solid tumor, and comprise 16% of all childhood tumors (108). The most common pediatric tumors are embryonal tumors (medulloblastomas), pilocytic astrocytomas, other varieties of astrocytomas, and malignant gliomas (106,109).

IV. PRESENTATION OF PATIENTS WITH BRAIN TUMORS

The initial presentation depends on the location of the tumor and the rate of growth. Most brain tumors are located in the supratentorial compartment. Primary tumors constitute approximately 60% of all supratentorial tumors; 40% are metastases from other sites. The majority of primary pediatric brain tumors arise in the infratentorial compartment (108). In adults over the age of 20 years, most posterior fossa tumors, particularly single lesions, are metastatic in origin.

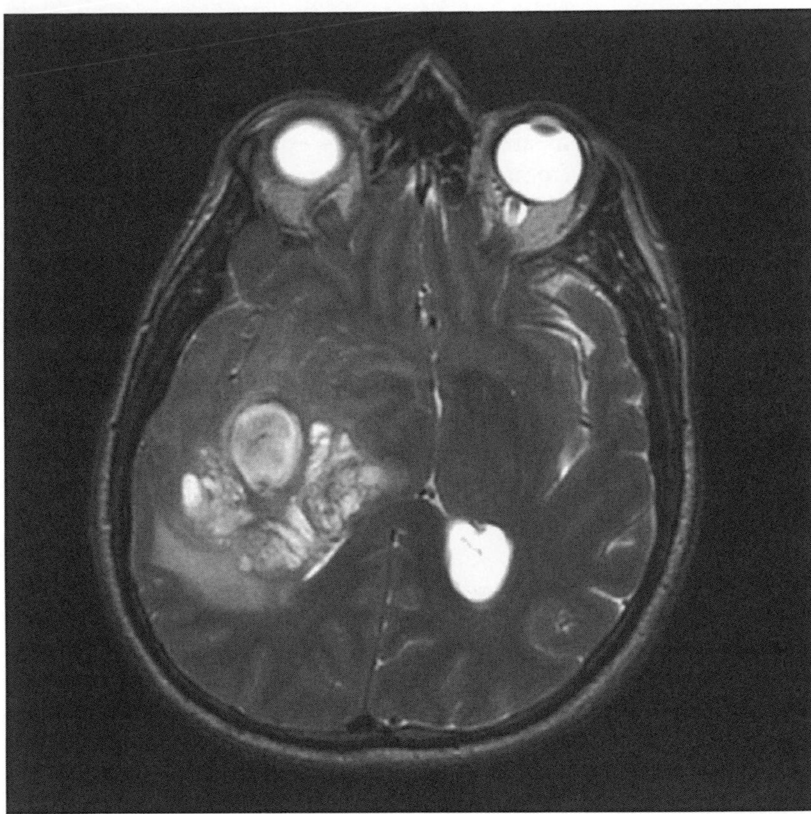

Figure 5 Glioblastoma multiforme. Axial MRI after gadolinium contrast showing a large heterogeneous tumor in the right temporal lobe. Note the multiple areas of cystic necrosis with ring enhancement and extensive surrounding edema. A mass effect with midline shift to the left and venticular effacement is seen

Patients with supratentorial lesions commonly present with seizures, focal neurologic deficits, and signs of intracranial hypertension. Seizures may occur in 15–95% of patients depending on the type of tumor (107). Rapidly growing lesions and those located in the cortex are most prone to cause seizures. Approximately 59% of patients present with postural headaches. Headaches may occur due to generalized intracranial hypertension, due to local tumor effects such as traction on blood vessels, or as a result of diplopia or blurry vision. Other signs and symptoms of intracranial hypertension have been discussed in a preceding section.

Focal signs depend on the location of the tumor (27). Tumors in the frontal lobes may cause motor weakness, personality, or cognitive changes. Involvement of Broca's area may give rise to motor aphasia. Tumors located in the parietal area may cause changes in body and object perception as well as language deficits. Patients with occipital lobe tumors may present with visual deficits, typically contralateral homonymous hemianopsia. Lesions in the temporal lobes can produce language deficits, visual field deficits, or complex partial seizures. Posterior fossa tumors may cause ataxia due to cerebellar involvement or hydrocephalus due to involvement of the fourth ventricle. Brain stem lesions are likely to produce cranial nerve (CN) deficits. Patients with tumors in the posterior fossa usually develop clinical signs and symptoms early compared with patients who have supratentorial tumors. "Cerebellar fits"—posturing as a result of pyramidal tract compression—may occur. Rapidly growing tumors in the posterior fossa can cause critical cardiorespiratory embarrassment as well as herniation of the brain through the foramen magnum. Patients who have pituitary tumors present with endocrine changes, hypopituitarism, or focal effects such as visual changes. Tumors may be a part of familial syndromes such as multiple endocrine neoplastic syndrome, tuberous sclerosis, and neurofibromatosis.

Some characteristics of the more common types of brain tumors are discussed below.

A. Astrocytomas

Astrocytes are the major structural components of the brain and the BBB. Astrocytomas are the most common type of primary brain tumors. Astrocytomas can be classified as low-grade astrocytoma, anaplastic astrocytoma, or glioblastoma multiforme (GBM). Additional variants of astrocytomas exist.

In adults, most low-grade astrocytomas are supratentorial and frequently involve the frontal lobe. Patients may present with seizures, headaches, visual, and motor deficits. In children, astrocytomas occur in the cerebellum. Patients develop cerebellar signs, signs of obstructive hydrocephalus and raised ICP. Astrocytic tumors may very rarely metastasize to the lungs, bone, and lymph nodes.

Although radical surgery for low-grade gliomas is a topic of controversy, aggressive resection is generally believed to be associated with improved survival for most astrocytic tumors (110). Intraoperative imaging and mapping techniques enable larger resections to be performed with a higher margin of safety (110,111). However, as gliomas are highly infiltrative, tumor cells extend beyond the areas seen on MRI and the most radical resection may not be curative. In spite of advances in the field, the overall prognosis for high-grade gliomas remains bleak. Young patients and patients who have seizures and no fixed neurological deficits generally have a better outcome (112). Recurrence at the primary site of tumor following resection is the most common cause of mortality in patients with astrocytic tumors. In patients with tumor recrudescence, reoperation is often performed if the tumor mass is limited and if there was good response to the initial operation.

Astrocytomas may occur in the brainstem in the pediatric population. Overall, brain stem tumors have a poor prognosis. While the removal of well-defined low-grade brain stem tumors may improve survival, the resection of more diffuse tumors is fraught with risk and has no advantage in prolonging life. Stereotactic biopsy may be performed for diagnosis, although radiological diagnosis may be safer in these patients.

Pilocytic astrocytomas often involve the hypothalamus and optic pathways in adults and the cerebellum in children. Pilocytic astrocytomas have a favorable prognosis with a 20-year survival of approximately 80%. Resection may be curative for these tumors.

Low-grade astrocytomas have a less favorable prognosis and may undergo malignant progression particularly in patients who have undergone subtotal resection (112).

Anaplastic astrocytomas have a higher mitotic index than low-grade gliomas and may be confused histologically and radiologically with GBM, which has a worse prognosis. The histologic features of GBM are endovascular proliferation and necrosis. Median survival for anaplastic astrocytomas is 15–28 months.

Glioblastoma multiforme (see Fig. 4) is the commonest primary malignant tumor in adults and is associated with the highest mortality. Patients are frequently in their fifth or sixth decade of life. Median life expectancy is 12 months while the 5-year survival rate is only approximately 3% (110,113).

Gliomatosis cerebri consists of large, multifocal, proliferative glial tumors usually occurring in the cerebral hemispheres. Patients with GBM tend to develop severe intracranial hypertension and have an extremely poor prognosis. Corticosteroids may be administered for palliation (112).

B. Oligodendrogliomas

Oligodendrocytes form the myelin sheath in the central nervous system. Oligodendrogliomas tend to occur in middle-aged patients and involve the frontal and temporal lobes. A "fried egg" appearance on histology is characteristic of these tumors. Median survival is approximately 60% for 5 years (113). Aggressive surgical resection leads to improved survival. Postoperative radiation and chemotherapy may also be considered.

C. Ependymomas

Ependymocytes line the ventricular system of the brain. Ependymomas frequently arise intraventricularly in the posterior fossa in children. Patients present with signs of obstructive hydrocephalus. Histologically, perivascular pseudorosettes are a characteristic of ependymomas. Ependymomas can metastasize through CSF seeding. Surgical resection and postoperative radiation are the main treatment for these patients, although the role of chemotherapy is being re-evaluated due to the complications of cranial radiation in children (112). The 5-year survival rate is approximately 65% (113).

D. Meningiomas

Meningiomas are extra-axial, slow-growing tumors arising from arachnoidal cells. A histologic characteristic of these tumors is the presence of psammoma bodies. Most meningiomas occur parasagittally or along the falx, along the sphenoid bone, or over the cerebral convexity. If total resection is performed, a complete cure may result. Recurrence after excision may be related to the degree of resection (4,114). On the other hand, benign-appearing meningiomas may be observed without immediate surgery. In some patients, enlarging meningeal tumors did not produce symptoms during periods ranging from 6 months to 15 years (4,115). During surgery, there is a potential for significant blood loss as these tumors can be very vascular. Preoperative embolization may help reduce blood loss and enable more complete resection of the tumor. Average 5-year survival is about 90% in these patients (113).

E. Medulloblastomas

Medulloblastomas are the most common tumors that arise from primitive neuroectodermal tissue. They tend to occur in children and involve the cerebellum. Patients present with hydrocephalus and signs of raised ICP. Extracranial metastases and CSF dissemination may occur, with secondary tumor occurring in bone. Complete resection and postoperative radiation are the treatment of choice. The 5-year survival rate is 55% in patients with medulloblastomas (113).

F. Pineal Gland Tumors

Tumors of the pineal gland may be of diverse cell types, including primary parenchymal tumors, germ cell tumors, and glial tumors, and occur more frequently in children. Patients may present with hydrocephalus, cerebellar signs, and hypothalamic disturbances. Symptoms such as headache, nausea and vomiting, ataxia, papilledema, and paresis of upward gaze (Parinaud's syndrome) are a characteristic presentation (112). The pineal gland is located outside of but may be approached through the posterior cranial fossa. Access to pineal gland tumors is achieved either through the supracerebellar infratentorial approach in the sitting position or through a bioccipital craniotomy in the sea lion position (hyperextension of the upper body).

G. Primary CNS Lymphoma

Primary central nervous system lymphoma is a B-cell lymphoma which usually occurs in the frontal lobes and sometimes in the cerebellum. Surgery does not improve survival and accordingly is used only for diagnostic purposes. Radiation is the treatment of choice, although chemotherapy has been a recent focus of treatment in these patients (116). Glucocorticoids are administered for the relief of symptoms.

H. Schwannomas

Schwann cells form the myelin sheath of the peripheral nerves. Acoustic neuromas are schwannomas which arise from the superior vestibular division of CN VIII. Patients are most often elderly present with hearing loss, tinnitus, disequilibrium and facial nerve palsy. Schwannomas, particularly if bilateral, may be associated with neurofibromatosis Type 2. Treatment consists of expectant management, surgery, and/or radiation. Surgical approaches to the tumor are suboccipital through the posterior fossa, translabyrinthine, or extradural subtemporal. The suboccipital approach has the best chance of preservation of hearing, and the facial nerve.

I. Cerebral Metastases

Metastatic brain tumors are the most common type of intracranial tumor. At autopsy, 25% of patients with cancer have intracranial metastases. Primary sites of metastatic tumors are most often the lung, breast, skin, colon, or kidney in adults. Of these, the lung and breast comprise more than 50% of the primary sites of metastases to the brain. Most solitary lesions are in the cerebral hemispheres. In adults, a solitary lesion in the cerebellum is most likely to be metastatic in origin. Primary solid tumors in children are frequently sarcomas or germ cell tumors (117). Patients with a single intracranial lesion may be offered surgery if the mass is accessible, systemic cancer is limited and survival for longer than 2 months is expected (118,119). Although controversial, the resection of multiple metastases may improve survival and confer a prognosis similar to that of patients undergoing surgery for a single metastatic lesion (119).

V. DIAGNOSIS

Currently, the cornerstone in the management of most patients with brain tumors is obtaining an accurate histological diagnosis. Preliminary diagnosis and grading of brain tumors is most commonly accomplished by CT or MRI. Magnetic resonance imaging is superior to CT in detection of both tumor presence and spread as it provides excellent tissue contrast and is impervious to beam-hardening bone artifact (120). Small lesions and lesions in areas such as the temporal lobes (see Fig. 4), pineal gland, pituitary area, and posterior fossa can be evaluated in detail with MRI. Computed tomography is apt to fail under these circumstances. The ability to image directly in multiple planes by MRI allows differentiation between intra- and extra-axial tumors. A normal contrast-enhanced MRI essentially rules out chances of a brain tumor (107). Computed tomography scans are preferred in emergent circumstances and when contraindications to the use of MRI exist.

One major drawback of MRI is its occasional lack of specificity. Infarcts, abscesses, demyelinating lesions, and radiation necrosis can all be mistaken for brain tumors (120). In some of these circumstances, PET or magnetic resonance spectroscopy (MRS) provides more information, including blood flow and the metabolic state of the lesion (121). Vascular tumors can be well delineated by cerebral angiography. Cerebral angiography may additionally predict the likelihood of excessive blood loss during the resection of vascular tumors. Embolization of very vascular tumors during angiography is often carried out as an adjunct to surgical rescction.

VI. SURGICAL PRINCIPLES

Surgery for brain tumors may be performed for the relief of symptoms or in order to obtain a histological sample for diagnosis. Symptoms may be general or focal due to mass effect and/or edema. Some types of tumors, even if small in size, are especially susceptible to edema formation. Radiation necrosis of gliomas often results in severe edema which is refractory to treatment except by resection of the dead tissue (122). Seizures that are refractory to medical therapy may be relieved by surgery (123). Tumors may act as seizure foci in the brain or they may activate seizure foci in the surrounding or distant brain tissue. Intraoperative EEG can ensure that all significant seizure foci are resected and may improve seizure control after surgery (123). The anticonvulsant effects of most intravenous and volatile anesthetic agents should be kept in mind during such surgery. Methohexital may be administered for improved detection of epileptic foci (66).

Surgery may additionally be performed for the reduction of tumor mass, and for the delivery and improved efficacy of adjuvant therapy. In other instances, resection of the lesion may be performed to prolong survival. Surgical intervention may be deferred for selected tumors (110). A large proportion of brainstem tumors carry a high risk of morbidity and mortality with invasive intervention and are managed by nonsurgical means. For primary malignant tumors in other locations, most studies show improved long-term survival with extensive resection. Occasionally, surgery is curative, although more often it improves the duration and quality of life without conferring a complete cure. Surgery may also lessen the patient's dependency on steroids (110).

The extent of resection depends on the location of the tumor, the grade and histologic type of tumor, and the clinical status of the patient (94). Patient factors such as age, life expectancy, comorbidities, and neurological status impact the surgeon's decision to operate (4). The Karnofsky Performance Scale (27,124) is often used to assess functional capacity in patients with brain tumors. This scale ranges from 0 (dead) to 100 (completely normal). A score of higher than 70 on this scale indicates an ambulatory patient who is independent in self-care activities. This level of function is often used to justify aggressive surgical resection. In such cases, the aim of the surgery is to excise as much of the tumor as possible, while causing minimal new neurologic deficits.

The safety of aggressive treatment may be facilitated by intraoperative cortical mapping of areas of the eloquent cortex and subcortical white matter (110,111). Other means of limiting neurological injury during resection are the intraoperative use of imaging systems and "awake craniotomies" with conscious, communicative patients serving as primary monitors of neurological function. Neuronavigation permits detailed delineation of tumors pre- and intraoperatively. More complete tumor resection was reported with the use of neuronavigation in patients with glioblastomas (125).

A. Craniotomy and Tumor Resection

What follows is a very basic outline of the procedure of supratentorial tumor resection (2). After a sterile preparation, a skin incision is made and the skin and muscle flap reflected. A craniotomy is then performed using a high-speed drill. The dura is separated from the bone flap, incised and reflected to expose the brain. Electrocautery and incision of the cortical matter provides initial access to the tumor. Further exposure is obtained by division of the gray and white brain matter using bipolar electrocautery forceps. The lesion is removed by debulking its mass from the center outward or by delineating the margins of the tumor and removing it either en-bloc or piecemeal. After achieving adequate hemostasis, the dura is closed and the bone flap replaced with wires or plates. If the bone flap has been damaged by surgery or tumor, a cranioplasty may be created. After closure of superficial layers, the dressing is applied to the head.

B. Stereotactic Brain Biopsy

A stereotactic brain biopsy is commonly performed for the retrieval of tissue for diagnosis. Stereotactic biopsies are especially ideal if no further surgical therapy is anticipated. This may be the case for tumors which are very responsive to radiation and chemotherapy, or if the location renders surgical resection dangerous (e.g., lesions in the brainstem or thalamus, or bifrontal gliomas) (2). Pineal or suprasellar tumors may more amenable to endoscopic or open excision, rather than a stereotactic procedure. Lesions that are smaller than 5 mm in diameter are also unsuitable for stereotactic procedures due to technical reasons.

During a stereotactic biopsy, the stereotactic frame is affixed to the patient's head under local anesthesia (2). Pins anchor the frame to the frontal and parietal areas of the skull. Computed tomography or MRI is performed after a fiducial device is affixed to the frame, and the target tissue is selected in the brain. The fiducial device is then replaced by an arc which helps guide the biopsy needle to the target. For the biopsy itself, a small skin incision and a burr hole in the skull are made under local anesthesia, and the needle is advanced to the target. A small piece of the tissue is biopsied and frozen for histologic examination. If the sample appears adequate, the incision is closed and the frame removed.

Stereotactic biopsies are generally tolerated well by patients. Complications include bleeding, seizures, and postoperative neurologic deficits due to infection or edema. The type of tumor and the location may increase risk of complications. For example, some tumors such as pinealoblastomas and lymphomas are more likely to hemorrhage after the biopsy. Patients with tumors in the eloquent cortex or the brain stem may have a higher incidence of postoperative deficits due to edema or hemorrhage (2). The rate of obtaining a diagnosis from a stereotactic biopsy is more than 95% (126). An important drawback of stereotactic brain biopsies is that the tissue harvested may not be representative of the whole tumor. This may lead to a lower grading of the tumor than that obtained by resection of the tumor.

VII. PREOPERATIVE CONSIDERATIONS

A. General Considerations

As for any other patient presenting for surgery, the preoperative evaluation for patients with brain tumors includes a directed history and physical examination. The neurological examination must be documented in the preoperative note by the anesthesiologist. This examination focuses mainly on the mental status, and the presence of focal neurologic deficits, seizures, and raised ICP. The Glasgow Coma Scale (Table 1) is a convenient way to quantify some aspects of the neurological status (127).

A review of CT or MRI images should be performed. Ventricular effacement, basal cisternal compression, or a midline shift of greater than 10 mm indicates raised ICP. During surgery, patients with extensive brain edema surrounding tumors are at risk for developing intracranial hypertension prior to dural opening. These patients should undergo a particularly careful conduct of anesthesia. Pneumocephalus may be present in a patients who have undergone prior craniotomies and may influence the decision to use nitrous oxide intraoperatively (129). The location of the tumor should alert the anesthesiologist to anticipate perioperative problems. The anesthesiologist should also have an appreciation of the surgeon's perspective on the procedure, including intraoperative positioning, the anticipated extent of resection, and the probable histological diagnosis.

Table 1 Glasgow Coma Scale

Category	Score
Eye opening	
Spontaneous	4
To speech	3
To pain	2
Nil	1
Best motor response	
To verbal commands	
Obeys	6
To pain	
Localizes	5
Withdrawals	4
Decorticate flexion	3
Extensor response	2
Nil	1
Best verbal response	
Oriented	5
Confused conversation	4
Inappropriate words	3
Incomprehensible sounds	2
Nil	1

The presence of cardiac, pulmonary, and renal disease and coagulopathy should be evaluated and every effort made to optimize these and any other coexisting conditions prior to elective surgery. Preoperative medications must be noted including chemotherapeutic drugs. Patients frequently receive steroids, anticonvulsants, and diuretics. Steroids may cause hypertension, hypervolemia, and hyperglycemia.

Antiepileptics such as phenytoin, carbamazepine, phenobarbital, and valproic acid are used for prophylaxis against seizures in patients with supratentorial tumors. Phenytoin is the most widely used anticonvulsant as it can be given parenterally, and has a low incidence of side effects (130). Phenytoin is administered as an initial loading dose of 15–18 mg/kg body weight, followed by 5 mg/kg/day. Side effects include mild mental status changes, Steven Johnson syndrome, fever, rash, blood dyscrasias, and gingival hyperplasia. The drug level of phenytoin in the serum requires close monitoring due to the effect of this drug on its own metabolism. Phenytoin also induces hepatic metabolism of dexamethasone and decreases its half-life (96). Carbamazepine cannot be administered parenterally. Side effects of phenobarbital include sedation and shoulder-hand syndrome. Valproic acid may cause thrombocytopenia, hepatotoxicity, and pancreatitis.

Dehydration, hypovolemia, and electrolyte changes due to diuretics, or vomiting may be present. Hypovolemia may need correction prior to induction in order to maintain CPP. If the tumor is vascular (e.g., meningioma) or lies near large vessels, crossmatched blood should be available. Further directed investigations should be performed based on the history and physical examination. Additional workup will be necessary for patients with familial syndromes, paraneoplastic syndromes, or pituitary tumors.

B. Premedication

A reassuring visit with the anesthesiologist may suffice to allay a majority of the patient's anxieties. In patients with a preserved level of consciousness, anxiolytics (midazolam 1–2 mg) or analgesics (fentanyl 25–150 μg or sufentanil 5–20 μg) may be administered in titrated doses. An anesthesiologist should remain in attendance with the patient at all times following the administration of sedatives. If concerns regarding high ICP exist, sedation should be withheld. Respiratory depression is especially detrimental in patients with intracranial pathology. Additionally, neurologic deterioration may be masked by the effect of sedatives. Other premedications are administered as indicated. Patients often receive antiemetic agents, histamine-2 receptor blockers, and antistaphylococcal coverage with vancomycin.

VIII. INTRAOPERATIVE MANAGEMENT

A. Monitoring

Some of the standard monitors anesthesiologists employ assume special significance in neurosurgical patients. Capnography aids the anesthesiologist in the management of arterial carbon dioxide and manipulation of CBF. Hemodynamic monitoring and electrocardiography can assist in the detection of stimulation of cardiovascular centers in the brain stem. Furthermore, capnography and cardiovascular monitors are important monitors in the event of an air embolism. Attentive monitoring of the body temperature is worthwhile in patients undergoing craniotomies, while the administration of diuretics and the occasional development of diabetes insipidus (DI) render close monitoring of urine output especially significant in these patients.

In patients with relatively preserved intracranial compliance, arterial cannulation (most commonly, radial arterial) is performed after the induction of general anesthesia. Otherwise, it is carried out prior to induction. Beat-to-beat blood pressure measurement is crucial in the maintenance of tight control of ICP and CPP. The transducer is usually zeroed at the level of the ear which corresponds to the circle of Willis. The arterial catheter is also useful for the sampling of blood for gas and electrolyte measurements. A baseline arterial carbon dioxide measurement can help determine whether a significant gradient exists between the end-expired and arterial carbon dioxide concentration, and guide hyperventilation therapy.

Central venous cannulation is performed if there is significant risk of the occurrence of either air embolism or major intraoperative hemorrhage. A central venous catheter (CVC) can also assist in intraoperative fluid management, particularly when diuretics are used and during long procedures. Additionally, poor venous access or systemic disease influences the need for a CVC. A double or triple lumen CVC may be safely placed in the internal jugular vein. Care must be taken to avoid producing a large hematoma in the neck. Larger venous cannulae (such as a 7 French catheter) are best placed in sites other than the neck in order to avoid interference with venous drainage from the brain. Subclavian vein catheterization may be more comfortable for the patient in the postoperative period. Attempts to insert a catheter in the subclavian vein can be complicated by the formation of a pneumothorax. Intraoperative increases in peak expiratory pressures should alert the anesthesiologist to this possibility. The antecubital route for the insertion of a CVC is popular among many neuroanesthesiologists. Pulmonary arterial catheterization for neurosurgical cases is generally limited to patients with moderate-to-severe cardiac dysfunction.

Routine preoperative invasive ICP monitoring is no longer performed as radiological images in conjunction with the clinical examination provide valuable information concerning intracranial dynamics. This information is critical in managing the induction of anesthesia. Once the dura is opened, visual assessment of cerebral bulk can help guide anesthetic management (131).

Neuromuscular monitoring is performed intraoperatively and should be carried out on nonhemiplegic extremities. Hemiplegic muscles are resistant to nondepolarizing muscle relaxants and will mislead the anesthesiologist seeking to estimate the state of neuromuscular blockade (132).

Intraoperative monitoring of somatosensory evoked potentials (SSEPs) is performed to localize the somatosensory cortex prior to resection. The continuous monitoring of SSEPs has recently been described as a means for real-time assessment of cortical function during resection under general anesthesia (133). Somatosensory evoked potentials may also be monitored during the excision of brainstem lesions. Cortical blood flows below 20 mL/min/100 g produce changes in SSEPs (134). As a general guideline, an amplitude reduction of 50% or a latency increase of 10% is considered significant.

Anesthetic agents can have significant effects on cortical SSEPs. When SSEPs are being monitored, the effects of drugs and physiological changes on SSEPs should be appreciated. Hypothermia, hypoxia, hypotension, anemia, hypoglycemia, and alterations in serum sodium and potassium influence SSEPs. Nitrous oxide reduces the amplitude and has no effect on the latency of SSEPs. A dose-related increase in latency and a reduction in the amplitude of cortical SSEPs are produced by volatile agents. If necessary, the dose of the inhalational agent should be reduced to less than 0.5 MAC. Opioids cause a mild depression of amplitude and an increase in latency of cortical responses at doses producing sedation (134). Etomidate and ketamine can enhance cortical SSEPs. Propofol may produce depression of the amplitude of cortical SSEPs but rapid recovery results when the infusion is stopped (134). Sudden changes in anesthetic depth must be avoided at critical junctures in the surgery.

Additional monitoring during tumor resection may include cranial nerve monitoring for posterior fossa surgeries, precordial Doppler monitoring if there is a significant risk of venous air embolism (VAE), the monitoring of brainstem acoustic evoked potentials for the resection of acoustic neuromas, and visual evoked responses during the excision of parasellar tumors. The administration of muscle relaxants is usually avoided during cranial nerve monitoring.

B. Positioning

Some commonly used positions of the patient during the resection of brain tumors are described below.

1. Supine Position

The supine position with the head mildly elevated is employed for surgery anterior to the coronal suture (28). Some approaches which are frequently used in the supine patient are the pterional, frontal, and parasagittal approaches. The pterional approach is suitable for access to the anterior and medial parts of the temporal lobe, the parasellar and suprasellar space, and the upper portion of the clivus. Figure 6 depicts the pterional and frontal approaches, and the usual operating room layout for these procedures. For the pterional approach, an incision is made posterior and lateral to the frontal area, just behind the hairline, to end anterior to the tragus of the ear, at the level of the zygomatic arch [Fig. 6(A)]. The frontal approach provides access to the frontal lobes, the anterior horn of the lateral ventricle, and the foramen of Munro (28). The incision is made just behind the hairline parallel to the coronal suture [Fig. 6(B)]. With the ideal operating room layout, the anesthesiologist has access to the airway and arterial and venous lines and the surgeon has optimal exposure of the surgical field, while the scrub nurse can hand instruments to the surgeon in an unimpeded way.

The supine position with the head maximally turned to the side may sometimes be utilized for infratentorial surgery, but carries the risk of venous obstruction in the neck (135). Moreover, positioning may be difficult in a patient with a spondylotic spine.

2. Sitting Position

The sitting position (Fig. 7) is convenient for surgical exposure of posterior fossa tumors and the upper cervical spinal cord. It is ideal for operating on midline or fourth ventricular lesions and lesions at the cerebello-pontine angle (135). This position is also optimal for accessing the pineal gland via the supracerebellar infratentorial approach. In fact, many neurosurgeons believe that resection of pineal gland tumors is the only remaining indication for a sitting craniotomy (131).

Besides optimal surgical access, there are several advantages of the sitting position. There is less blood loss, better CSF and venous drainage (provided extreme flexion of the neck is avoided), and ease of ventilation (136). Improved access to the airway and extremities and good intraoperative visibility of the face (useful for facial nerve monitoring) are other benefits of operating on the sitting patient. A number of complications are associated with the sitting position, including VAE, pneumocephalus, and cardiovascular changes (136). Peripheral venous pooling, hypotension, decreased cardiac output, increased systemic vascular resistance, and elevated pulmonary vascular resistance can occur when the patient is in the traditional sitting position. Peripheral nerve injuries (ulnar, sciatic, and common peroneal) and quadriplegia have also been reported following surgery with the patient in the sitting position. Careful padding of the extremities and prevention of extreme flexion at the hip may reduce the risk of neuropathy in these patients. Cervical cord injury in the sitting position is more likely in

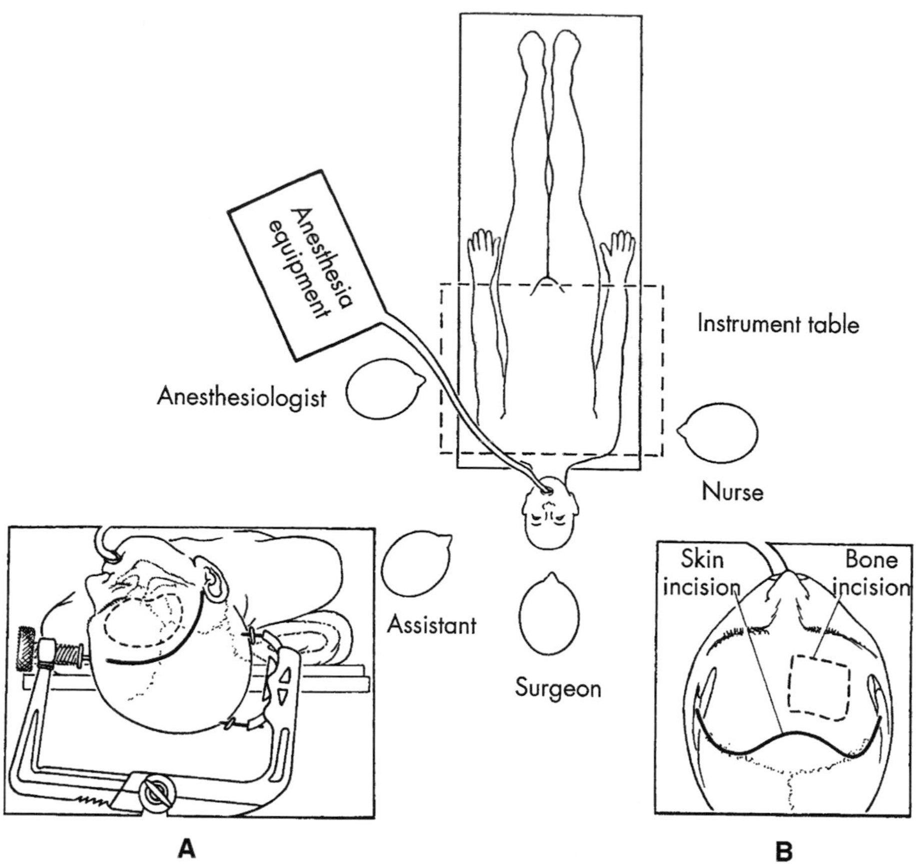

Figure 6 Two commonly used surgical approaches for the removal of mass lesions in the anterior and temporal cranial fossae in the supine patient. For lesions at the tip of the temporal lobe and along the sphenoid wing and for transcranial exposure of the region of the sella and parasellar area, the pterional approach (A) with the head turned to one side is used, whereas for lesions in the frontal lobes and at the base of the anterior fossa, frontal craniotomy (B) with the head straight up is performed. One configuration for the distribution of operating room personnel and equipment is shown. In (A) and (B), the sites of skin incision (bold line) and craniotomy (dashed line) are indicated. *Source*: From Ref. 28, with permission from Elsevier.

elderly patients with degenerative disease of the spine. Hypotension and anemia will exacerbate spinal cord ischemia. Extreme flexion of the head against the chest, especially with an endotracheal tube and an oral airway in place, can compress the base of the tongue causing obstruction of venous drainage. As a result, macroglossia, necrosis of the tongue, or massive swelling of the head and neck can occur (137–139). Supratentorial intracerebral hemorrhage in the subcortical white matter has been reported as a rare complication of the sitting position (140,141).

In a study of 579 posterior fossa craniotomies—333 sitting and 246 horizontal—the incidence of hypotension was found to be similar between the two groups (142,143). Venous air embolism occurred more frequently (45%) in the patients who underwent surgery in the sitting position compared to those who were horizontal (12%). Additionally, the need for blood transfusion was greater in the horizontal position with 13% vs. 3% of patients requiring more than two units of blood.

The sitting position may be somewhat hazardous in patients with an open ventriculoatrial shunt, patients who experience cerebral ischemia when upright, and those who have right-to-left cardiac shunts or a patent foramen ovale (PFO) (143). Patients with a PFO have a higher chance of developing paradoxical air embolism (PAE) should VAE occur. Markedly hypovolemic patients have a greater risk of VAE in the sitting position. Severe hydrocephalus may predispose to the formation of pneumocephalus and subdural hemorrhage in this position (144).

When the patient is sitting intraoperatively, the positioning should be meticulously checked to avoid some of the above-mentioned problems. A true sitting position is no longer used. Rather, a modified sitting position is employed where the back is raised approximately 60° and there is flexion at the hips and knees

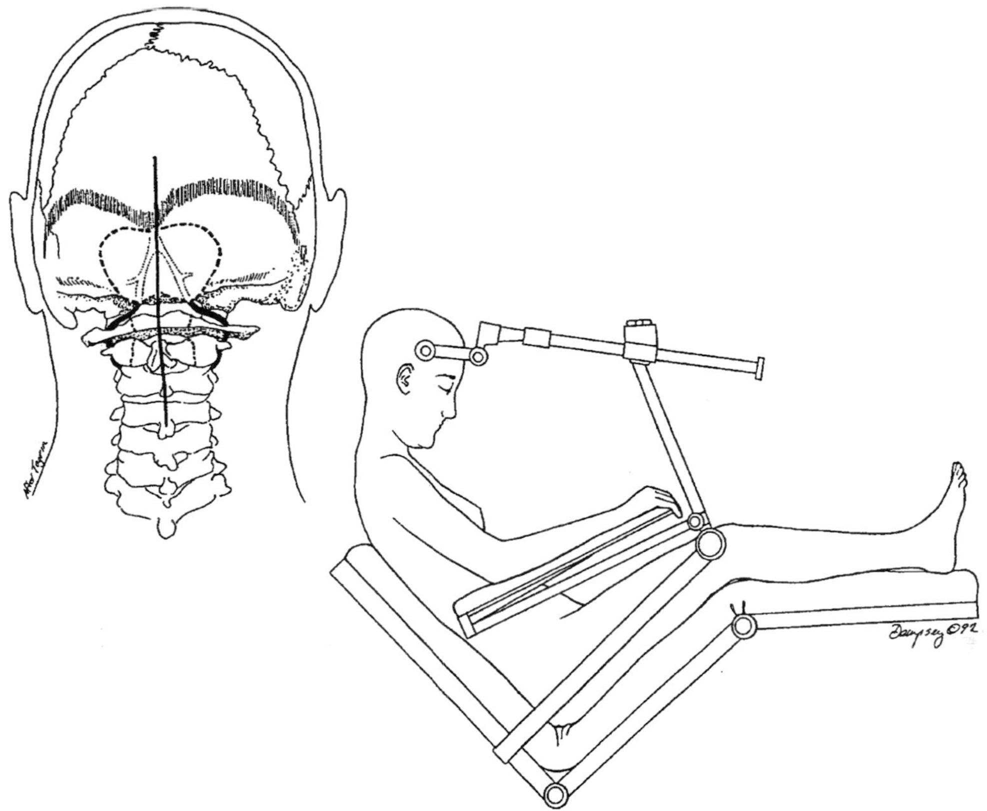

Figure 7 The sitting position provides access to the posterior fossa and the upper cervical cord. The head-holder is attached to the table such that the head and trunk always move together as a unit. This precaution will prevent serious injury to the patient if the back of the table is lowered quickly in an emergency. Excessive flexion and rotation of the neck is avoided. The hips and knees are moderately flexed. The commonest surgical approach to the posterior fossa is the suboccipital one, which allows exposure of the vermis and cerebellar hemispheres with a midline incision (shown) or exposure of the cerebellum and the pontocerebellar angle through a lateral incision (not shown). *Source*: From Ref. 135, with permission from Elsevier.

(144). The arms may be crossed across the chest and the extremities padded to prevent neuropraxias. The use of compression stockings decreases venous pooling in the legs. Extreme flexion and rotation of the neck should be avoided. Large oral airways may interfere with venous drainage. There should be a distance of at least 4–5 cm between the chin and the chest. A reinforced endotracheal tube is often used to prevent kinking of the tube during surgical manipulation. The head-holder is attached to the table such that the head and upper body can move as one unit enabling the operating team to rapidly and safely reposition the patient supine in the event of an emergency (Fig. 7).

3. *Prone Position*

The prone position (Fig. 8) is useful for surgical access to posterior fossa tumors including lesions that are close to the midline (135). The incidence of VAE is lower (approximately 12%) during craniotomy in the prone position. Some complications associated with the prone position include blindness, facial edema, and difficulty with ventilation as a result of restricted excursion of the chest. Blindness can occur due to retinal ischemia as a result of pressure on the globes, compounded by concomitant anemia and hypotension. Accordingly, care must be taken intraoperatively to prevent pressure on the eyes and to correct excessive anemia and hypotension. Other pressure points such as the abdomen, chin, breasts, elbows, knees, and the genitals should also be protected.

4. *Lateral Position*

The lateral position provides access to the cerebellopontine angle, cerebellum, and infracerebellar region (135). Once again, proper positioning should emphasize the protection of pressure points (such as the lower shoulder). The fibula of the dependent leg is meticulously padded in order to prevent injury to the common peroneal nerve. An infra-axillary roll protects the neurovascular bundle in the axilla. When

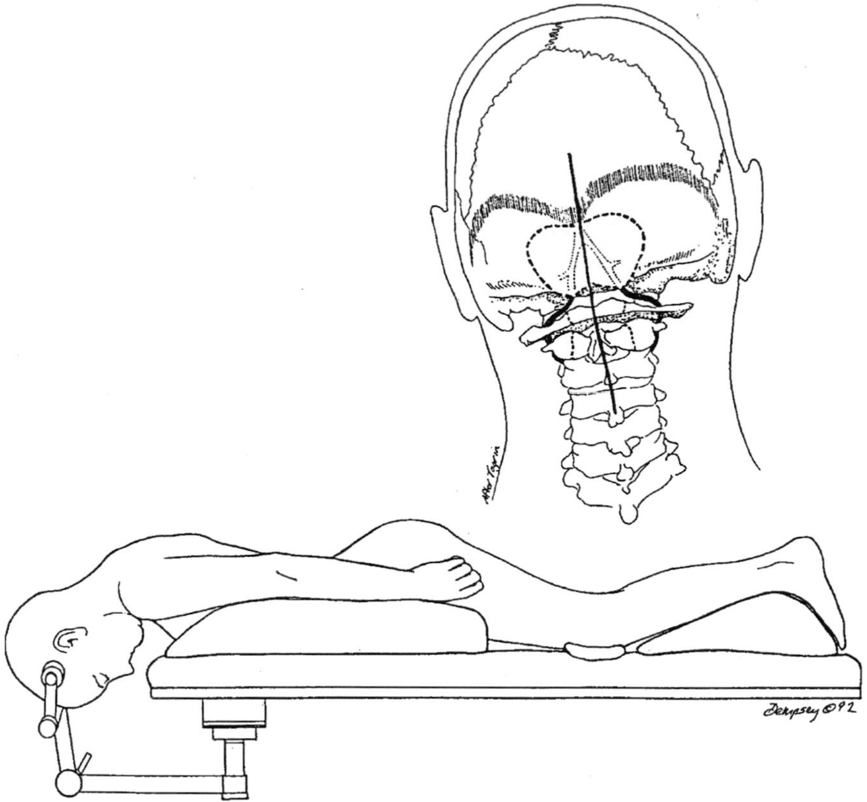

Figure 8 In the prone position, the head is slightly flexed and held in position with a skull-fixation device. This opens the space between the foramen magnum and the atlas and makes it easier to view the supracerebellar space (as needed for pineal tumors). The pressure points are protected with appropriate padding. *Source*: From Ref. 135, with permission from Elsevier.

accessing the cerebellopontine angle in the lateral position, a hasty dissection may result in torrential bleeding from the superior petrosal venous sinus (135).

5. Park-Bench or Semiprone Position

The park-bench position is useful in emergent situations for gaining quick access to the cerebellum (135). In this position, the patient appears to be midway between the prone and lateral position, with the face turned downwards and the ipsilateral shoulder moved out of the surgeon's way. It is important to avoid excessive rotation of the neck which may result in venus obstruction.

C. Intraoperative Management of Anesthesia

1. Goals of Intraoperative Management

The goals of intraoperative management for supratentorial tumors are the avoidance of high ICP, maintenance of CPP, facilitation of optimal surgical conditions in the brain, and the provision of a smooth, timely emergence. Specific considerations, such as the potential for significant blood loss, depend on the characteristics (size, type, and location) of the tumor.

2. Induction of Anesthesia

During induction, CPP is maintained by the control of systemic arterial pressure and the avoidance of hypercarbia and hypoxia. After the application of standard monitors and preoxygenation, anesthesia is frequently induced with sodium thiopental (3–5 mg/kg) or propofol (1–3 mg/kg). An opioid, such as fentanyl (3–5 μg/kg) is also frequently administered. Succinylcholine may be used if indicated. A priming dose of a nondepolarizing muscle relaxant can assist in the prevention of fasciculations and intracranial hypertension due to succinylcholine (80). If the use of succinylcholine is not indicated, a nondepo larizing muscle relaxant is administered and mask ventilation continued until optimal conditions for endotracheal intubation are achieved. Laryngoscopy and intubation can cause sharp increases in ICP and CBF (145). An additional dose of thiopental can ensure adequate depth of anesthesia and prevent ICP increases due to the intubation (146). Intravenous, but not laryngotracheal, lidocaine attenuates the increase in ICP due to laryngoscopy and intubation (147). The hemodynamic response to intubation can also be controlled by small doses of opioids. Labetalol, esmolol, or sodium nitroprusside are other drugs that ablate the hypertensive response to intubation. Sodium nitroprusside or nitroglycerin should be used with caution in patients with poor intracranial compliance as these agents are vasodilators and can increase CBV and ICP (148,149). Limiting the duration of laryngoscopy will reduce hypertension and tachycardia due to laryngoscopy.

3. *Maintenance of Anesthesia*

Adequate oxygenation and ventilation must be maintained at all times. Hyperventilation may be instituted if indicated, with a target $PaCO_2$ of between 30 and 35 mmHg. Positive end-expiratory pressure (PEEP) can increase CVP and CBV, and also affect the CPP by reducing arterial blood pressure (105). Accordingly, in patients with deranged intracranial compliance, high levels of PEEP must be applied with close attention to the hemodynamic and neurological consequences.

Maintenance of anesthesia is usually performed by the administration of an infusion of propofol (50–300 μg/kg/min) or sub-MAC doses of isoflurane along with an opioid infusion (74,78,150,151). Nitrous oxide can be used safely for most craniotomies. However, it should be discontinued if good operating conditions of the brain cannot be achieved.

Profound neuromuscular blockade is generally maintained throughout the procedure in order to prevent the deleterious effects of patient movement. Prior to craniotomy, a straining patient may develop elevated intrathoracic pressure which will result in high CVP and ICP. After dural opening, increases in intrathoracic pressure will lead to increased CBV and bulging of the brain. Severe injury to the cervical spine may result due to violent patient motion with the head secured in pins. Additionally, uncontrolled surgical instruments may inflict brain injury during patient movement.

Placement of the pin head-holder for the skull is a very painful stimulus and can trigger severe hypertension and tachycardia. This should be anticipated and prevented by the administration of small boluses of thiopental, propofol, or opioid. Short-acting opioids like remifentanil, fentanyl, and sufentanyl are particularly well suited for this purpose (152). Preoperatively administered oral clonidine also reduces hemodynamic responses to the pin head-holder during craniotomy (153). The injection of local anesthetics at the site provides additional analgesia during pinning.

4. *Facilitation of Venous Drainage*

Excessive rotation or flexion of the neck or constricting neck collars may interfere with venous outflow and elevate ICP (154,155). Head elevation and the alleviation of constriction of neck veins are simple and highly effective maneuvers that facilitate venous drainage from the brain thereby reducing ICP (156). Head elevation to 30° is frequently performed in neurosurgical patients. Some have argued that this position is associated with a corresponding reduction in CPP and precipitates an increase in ICP in a subset of patients (157). These authors suggested that CPP is optimal when the patient is horizontal (although the ICP is also higher in this position). However, a subsequent investigation in head-injured patients demonstrated that head elevation to 30° was safe and significantly reduced ICP in the majority of patients without reducing CPP or CBF (158).

5. *Intraoperative Fluid Management*

Intraoperative fluid management is tailored to limit the formation of cerebral edema. At the same time, excessive intravascular dehydration to the point of hypovolemia and decreased systemic blood pressure is undesirable. Both intracranial hypertension due to cerebral edema and systemic hypotension will decrease CPP and contribute to poor outcome following surgery.

In the past, severe fluid restriction creating serum hyperosmolality was often used in patients with intracranial hypertension. Even now, if there is severe brain edema, fluid restriction may be requested by some neurosurgeons. However, complete restriction of water in dogs over a period of 72 hr resulted in an 8% loss of body weight, with only a 1% decrease in cerebral water content (159,160). Thus, the validity of fluid restriction therapy to control edema formation in humans is questionable at best. Moreover, this maneuver is likely to decrease CPP by causing systemic hypotension. The current recommendation is to maintain normovolemia, and to rigorously avoid hypotension due to hypovolemia.

Replacement fluids that are commonly used are normal saline (309 mosm/L), lactated Ringer's (273 mosm/L), and 5% or 25% albumin (5% albumin–290 mosm/L). Lactated Ringer's solution is slightly hypo-osmolar compared to plasma (295 mosm/L). Large quantities of lactated Ringer's solution are not administered to neurosurgical patients so as to avoid serum hypoosmolality and the consequent exacerbation of cerebral edema. When a large volume of normal saline is administered, hyperchloremic metabolic acidosis can develop (161). Colloids such as hetastarch and dextrans are generally avoided in neurosurgical patients due to the potential for coagulopathy with these fluids. Hetastarch may cause coagulopathy only after the administration of a certain volume (20 mL/kg). Yet, the disastrous consequences of coagulopathy in neurosurgical patients lead most anesthesiologists to choose an alternative solution. Dextrans can also cause anaphylactic reactions, as well as interfere with subsequent typing and crossmatching of blood. Albumin may be administered in the perioperative period in neurosurgical patients, although use is limited due to its expense. Albumin is a reasonable alternative to iso-osmolar crystalloids when a large amount of fluid transfusion is indicated and the transfusion trigger for blood has not been reached. The use of colloids, in contrast to crystalloids, will limit the formation of peripheral edema, but not that of cerebral edema. Packed red blood cells are administered for the treatment of anemia. The hematocrit is maintained between 25% and 30% depending on the patient's condition. Other blood products are administered as specifically indicated, e.g., FFP and platelet transfusions are used to treat coagulopathies.

During craniotomy for tumor resection, regions of the brain are likely to be underperfused due to local pressure from surgical retractors, pressure from the tumor, or from peritumoral edema. While global cerebral ischemia appears to be conclusively worsened by even mild hyperglycemia, reports of outcome following focal cerebral ischemia are conflicting, with both adverse and beneficial effects being reported (159). However, the general consensus is to maintain normoglycemia during intracranial operations. Solutions containing dextrose are not recommended unless the patient is hypoglycemic. Although insulin should be administered to control hyperglycemia, it is unclear whether the administration of insulin to hyperglycemic patients may actually worsen outcome due to the resultant intracellular hyperglycemia (159).

6. *Lowering the ICP Intraoperatively—Checklist*

Intraoperatively, the development of a "tight" brain and difficult surgical operating conditions mandates a systematic approach in an attempt to improve the situation. The bulging brain may be "relaxed" by the following means.

Ventilation and Hemodynamics

Adequate oxygenation should be ensured. The patient may be hyperventilated to a $PaCO_2$ of 30–35 mmHg. Further hyperventilation should be performed judiciously, if necessary. "Bucking" and straining of the patient are associated with increases in CBF and ICP (162). High peak pressures should be corrected (treat bronchospasm or pneumothorax, administer additional muscle relaxant, rectify a kinked or clogged endotracheal tube, lower PEEP, etc.). Systemic blood pressure should be rigorously maintained. Mild hypertension may be beneficial by causing cerebral vasoconstriction and interrupting the cerebral vasodilatory cascade.

Position

The patient's positioning should be checked. As discussed previously, a slight head-up position without obstruction of venous drainage is optimal.

Drugs and Anesthetics

The anesthetic depth should be increased, if indicated. It may be necessary to discontinue nitrous oxide and volatile agents and switch to a completely intravenous anesthetic regimen. Other vasodilators such as sodium nitroprusside or nitroglycerin may need to be discontinued. One should consider administering an additional dose of diuretics (mannitol, furosemide, and hypertonic saline).

CSF Drainage

The surgeons may perform CSF drainage if a "tight" brain persists. Cerebrospinal fluid is often drained through a needle inserted into a lateral ventricle. Lumbar drainage may be performed only if there is no danger of precipitating herniation of the brain and is best performed after opening of the dura.

Temperature

If the patient's temperature is high, it should be lowered. Mild hypothermia may be beneficial.

Barbiturates

If no improvement has resulted after performing the above-mentioned maneuvers, barbiturates may be considered for metabolic suppression. Bolus doses of thiopental (1.5–3 mg/kg) or an infusion of pentobarbital (10 mg/kg bolus followed by 1.5 mg/kg/hr) may be administered (163). There must be agreement between the surgeon and anesthesiologist before this step is taken as prolonged postoperative sedation will ensue. Systemic blood pressures will require support as large doses of barbiturates produce myocardial depression and systemic hypotension. Electroencephalogram monitoring is performed in these patients.

Surgical Decompression

The removal of a collection of intracranial blood or in extreme circumstances, a partial lobectomy may be undertaken by the surgeons in an attempt to control ICP.

D. Local Anesthesia for Tumor Resection or Biopsy

Lesions which are in close proximity to the eloquent cortex of the brain are frequently resected during a craniotomy performed under monitored anesthesia care. The awake patient facilitates intraoperative neurological testing and enables the surgeons to perform a more aggressive tumor resection, while inflicting minimal neurological disability. Most patients appear to tolerate the procedure well under conscious sedation. It is essential to have cooperative and motivated patients; children and uncooperative adult patients are not candidates for conscious sedation. Extensive preoperative briefing of the patient is necessary—patients should know what to expect during the procedure. Preoperative evaluation and anesthetic preparation should be performed as for the administration of general anesthesia for craniotomy. Close intraoperative communication and co-operation between the surgeon, patient, the anesthesiologist, and other operating room personnel is vital.

A combination of local anesthesia and intravenous sedation is often used for these procedures. The patient should be made comfortable enough to tolerate the procedure which may be long. Excessive sedation is avoided to prevent respiratory depression or loss of the patient's ability to communicate. The application of the three-point head-holder for a craniotomy can be performed under sedation with propofol and local anesthesia. Additionally, nerve blocks (supraorbital, temporal, and occipital) for the scalp can be performed along with infiltration of the temporalis muscle. Various techniques for sedation for awake craniotomy have been described including neurolept anesthesia with fentanyl, sufentanil or alfentanil, and droperidol (164,165), various combinations of midazolam, fentanyl, sufentanil, alfentanil and/or propofol (166,167), and patient-controlled administration of propofol (164). Sufentanil and alfentanil do not confer any advantage over fentanyl when used with droperidol for awake craniotomy (165).

"Asleep–awake–asleep" techniques have also been used successfully for resection of brain tumors. In one such technique, propofol and remifentanil infusions are administered and an LMA is inserted (168). Ventilation is controlled until exposure of the lesion is achieved. At this point, the remifentanil infusion is reduced until the patient begins to breathe spontaneously. The LMA is then extracted and the propofol infusion discontinued. A low-dose remifentanil infusion is continued for conscious sedation. When the resection is complete, the LMA is reinserted and the patient is reanesthetized. Other variations of the asleep–awake–asleep technique for procedures requiring intraoperative language mapping have been described (169).

Awake craniotomy as a routine approach to the resection of intra-axial supratentorial tumors, regardless of the involvement of the eloquent cortex, has been advocated as a practical and effective alternative to craniotomy under general anesthesia. Two hundred patients who had a variety of supratentorial tumors underwent awake craniotomy and participated in a prospective study (170). Awake craniotomy permitted intraoperative brain mapping, required less invasive monitoring, and resulted in considerable reduction in resource utilization such as reduced ICU and hospital stay in these patients.

Complications of awake craniotomy include respiratory depression in a patient with an uncontrolled airway which is often not promptly accessible to the anesthesiologist and neurologic problems such as bleeding, vasospasm, ischemia, intracranial hypertension, and seizures. Discomfort, pain, and intraoperative nausea and vomiting triggered by traction on blood vessels or the dura may also occur (164).

Stereotactic surgical procedures may also be performed under local anesthesia. If the patient in the stereotactic head frame needs induction of general anesthesia during the procedure, airway management may be a challenge. The anesthesiologist should have a plan prepared for such a contingency. Endotracheal intubation under fiberoptic guidance or the use of an LMA may be necessary, as the airway is frequently inaccessible for direct laryngoscopy. In emergencies, the team should be prepared to remove the head ring, if necessary. Newer CT head rings may provide better access to the airway.

IX. EMERGENCE

After a craniotomy, the decision to extubate the patient in the operating room should be reached in agreement with the surgical team. Emergence should be smooth with an emphasis on control of hypertension, straining, and coughing. To this end, narcotics may be administered in sufficient doses throughout the case while allowing the return of spontaneous ventilation. If remifentanil is used, it should be continued until the head dressing is complete and adequate analgesia ensured prior to its discontinuation (74,151). Intravenous morphine (0.1 mg/kg) and rectal acetaminophen (30 mg/kg) work well in conjunction with the injection of local anesthetic at the incision site by the surgeon. Acetaminophen is avoided in patients with liver disease.

Reversal of neuromuscular relaxation should be performed only after the complete application of the dressing in order to prevent coughing on the endotracheal tube during manipulation of the head. Lidocaine (1.5 mg/kg) suppresses coughing and gagging on the endotracheal tube during emergence. Nitrous oxide and propofol are frequently used towards the end of craniotomies after the discontinuation of volatile agents. The substitution of isoflurane at dural closure by a propofol infusion does not result in earlier recovery and return of cognition than the intraoperative use of isoflurane alone (171).

Meticulous control of the blood pressure is necessary in order to prevent cerebral edema or intracranial hemorrhage. Sympathetic overactivity contributes to cerebral hyperemia during emergence from craniotomy (172). Intravenous boluses of labetalol (10 mg increments) or an esmolol infusion (0.3 mg/kg/min) are useful for this purpose (172). Other agents that may be used include sodium nitroprusside and nicardipine with the caveat that they may increase CBF due to vasodilatation. In the presence of altered intracranial compliance, a slow infusion of nitroprusside, along with hyperventilation, may have a milder effect on ICP than if it were administered as a rapid bolus (173).

Patients who were obtunded preoperatively or those who had a difficult intraoperative surgical course predisposing them to brain edema are best left intubated and anesthetized at the end of the procedure. Patients who had surgery lasting for more than 6 hr, repeat surgery, major glioblastoma surgery, or surgery near the brain stem should also remain intubated (174). It is important to ascertain the return of adequate respiration and airway reflexes prior to extubation after posterior fossa surgery. Injury to CNs IX, X, XII during the surgery will jeopardize airway patency and the ability to protect against aspiration. Additionally, edema due to retraction can affect the respiratory centers. It is prudent to continue postoperative ventilation in such patients.

The commonly held belief is that patients experience less pain after craniotomy than after other major surgery. Indeed, in a retrospective investigation, neurosurgical patients reported less pain and required less opioid analgesia than patients undergoing other procedures such as major facial surgery or lumbar laminectomy (175). The perception of less pain may be due to the site of the surgery or altered processing of nociception in this subset of surgical patients. Patients who undergo frontal, subfrontal, and temporal surgical approaches report higher pain scores postoperatively than patients who undergo craniotomies at other sites. Others have challenged the theory that patients have less pain after craniotomy, with more than 50% of surveyed British neuroanesthesiologists expressing their belief that postoperative neurosurgical pain is undertreated (176). Besides opioids and acetaminophen, scalp nerve blocks with ropivacaine after skin closure, and before awakening, may decrease the severity of pain for a period of 48 hr after supratentorial craniotomy (177). In one investigation, when the scalp was infiltrated with 0.25% bupivacaine and 1:200,000 epinephrine at pin sites before skeletal fixation, and at the site of incision, postoperative pain was reduced and some intraoperative hemodynamic responses were blunted; these blocks were performed at the start and repeated at the conclusion of the craniotomy (178).

Sedation and analgesia in neurosurgical patients can be tricky. Obviously, careful attention must be directed to the respiratory and sedative effects of opioids. A sympathomimetic state due to pain and discomfort may increase the risk of bleeding from freshly operated sites in the brain and cause intracranial hypertension in areas with impaired autoregulation. On the other hand, excessive or prolonged sedation may interfere with serial neurological examinations and mask significant neurological deterioration. Short-acting sedatives such as propofol, midazolam, and analgesics like morphine, fentanyl, and sufentanil have all been used successfully. Codeine is commonly prescribed by neurosurgeons for analgesia since it does not cause excessive sedation and has potent antitussive effects; however, it is a weak analgesic agent.

X. POSTOPERATIVE CONSIDERATIONS AFTER CRANIOTOMY

A. Hemorrhage

Postoperatively, an intracranial hematoma frequently presents clinically as delayed emergence. A postoperative hematoma usually occurs at the freshly operated site, and most frequently, within 6 hr of surgery (179). Intracranial bleeding may sometimes manifest as clinical deterioration after more than 24 hr following surgery. Changes in mental status may be more pronounced due to edema formation around the hematoma. Hypertension and coagulopathy are risk factors for the development of intracranial bleeding. Meticulous surgical hemostasis, a smooth emergence from anesthesia and prompt treatment of systemic arterial hypertension may decrease the incidence of such bleeding. Close postoperative neurologic monitoring with prompt radiological imaging in the event of deterioration will aid in rapid detection of this serious complication. It has been suggested that patients who regain preoperative neurological status by 6 hr following biopsy or elective supratentorial surgery, barring any other complications, may be safely transferred from an intensive care unit to a neurosurgical ward for observation (179). After supratentorial craniotomy, there are rare reports of cerebellar hemorrhage (180). This complication is associated with significant morbidity and has a mortality rate of 25%.

B. Delayed Emergence

Nonsurgical causes of delayed emergence include sedation and/or immobility due to residual anesthetics or neuromuscular blocking agents, metabolic and electrolyte abnormalities—notably hypoglycemia, hyper- or hyponatremia, and hypothermia. Delayed emergence directly related to the surgery may occur as a result of intracranial hypertension due to bleeding, hydrocephalus, cerebral edema, or pneumocephalus.

Pneumocephalus is common after craniotomies performed with head elevation and dural opening (144). In fact, all patients have some amount of pneumocephalus in the first 2 days following supratentorial craniotomy (129). However, clinical problems due to pneumocephalus are infrequent. Occasionally, a tension pneumocephalus develops and can enlarge due to nitrous oxide use. Delayed emergence or a decreased level of consciousness following the surgery will result. Plain x-rays or a CT scan aid in the diagnosis. Intraoperatively, the presence of a pneumocephalus may be heralded by loss of SSEPs (181). Once detected, if the administration of 100% oxygen and supine positioning of the patient does not improve the patient's condition, a burr hole can be easily performed (182).

C. Seizures

Seizures should be managed immediately, as they may precipitate intracranial bleeding, aspiration, hypoxia, and hypercarbia. Prompt airway management and adequate ventilation should be provided. Termination of the seizure with benzodiazepines, or barbiturates, and the administration of a loading dose of an anticonvulsant such as phenytoin may be necessary. A postoperative neurosurgical patient who has a decreased level of consciousness following a seizure should undergo CT scanning of the brain to screen for an intracranial hematoma (182).

D. Volume Status and Electrolyte Abnormalities

Postoperatively, patients can be hypovolemic due to diuretics, vomiting, or intraoperative hemorrhage. Electrolyte abnormalities may occur as an effect of diuretics, mannitol, or due to disturbances of sodium homeostasis. Urine volume and specific gravity should be carefully monitored. Patients with DI have an increased output of hypo-osmolar urine along with serum hyperosmolarity. Diabetes insipidus is particularly common after pituitary surgery and occurs on the sixth or seventh postoperative day (183). Fluid replacement using half-normal saline (hourly maintenance, combined with two-thirds of the previous hour's urine output) should be performed (131). Intravenous or intramuscular aqueous vasopressin (5–10 units), intranasal desmopressin (5–20 μg every 12–24 hr), or subcutaneous desmopressin (4 μg) may be used to treat diabetes insipidus (159). Rarely, DI may be permanent following pituitary surgery.

Syndrome of inappropriate ADH secretion (SIADH) may produce hyponatremia in neurosurgical patients. The diagnosis of SIADH is made after excluding other causes of hyponatremia such as hypovolemia. The collecting tubules of the kidneys absorb excessive water producing an increase in total body water and hypo-osmolarity of serum. Hyperosmolar urine and normal adrenal function are additional features of this syndrome. Free water restriction and furosemide administration may be used to manage SIADH. Severe cases (symptomatic patient, serum sodium less than 115–120 meq/L) may require the transfusion of 3% saline at the rate of 1–2 mL/kg/hr. More rapid correction of hyponatremia can trigger central pontine myelinolysis which is a devastating complication.

E. Postoperative Nausea and Vomiting

Postoperative nausea and vomiting (PONV) occurs frequently after craniotomy. First, it should be ascertained that the PONV is not a manifestation of increased ICP due to bleeding, hydrocephalus, or cerebral edema. Postoperative nausea and vomiting should then be rapidly treated as it can precipitate severe intracranial hypertension and hemorrhage as well as predispose to pulmonary aspiration. Persistent PONV may also cause hypovolemia and electrolyte abnormalities. The incidence of PONV is greater in patients who undergo infratentorial surgery, and young and female patients. Although some report increased incidence of PONV with general anesthesia rather than awake craniotomy (184), others have found no influence of the anesthetic technique, duration, and perioperative opioid use on PONV (185).

Effective intravenous antiemetics for PONV after craniotomy include ondansetron (4 mg), tropisetron (2 mg), droperidol (0.625 mg), and promethazine (12.5–25 mg) (186,187). In a comparison between droperidol and ondansetron, droperidol emerged as the superior treatment for PONV after craniotomy for supratentorial surgery. Although both droperidol and ondansetron administered at skin closure prevented nausea after craniotomy, only droperidol, and not ondansetron, significantly reduced emesis after craniotomy. This dose of droperidol (0.625 mg) was not excessively sedating (186). However, recent Food and Drug Administration warnings regarding the use of droperidol and its adverse cardiac effects may decrease its popularity among anesthesiologists.

F. Venous Thromboembolism

Venous thromboembolism is the most frequent complication following craniotomy for tumor resection (188). Rapid postoperative mobilization, the perioperative use of compression stockings and intermittent pneumatic compression hose in patients with brain tumors decrease the incidence of DVT in these patients (188). Prophylactic use of perioperative subcutaneous heparin (5000 units every 12 hr) or enoxaparin (40 mg/day) in combination with the use of graduated compression stockings, intermittent pneumatic compression and surveillance ultrasonography may be safe and more efficacious in decreasing the incidence of symptomatic venous thromboembolism after craniotomy for tumor resection (189,190). Still, concern about the potential for intracranial hemorrhage precludes the widespread use of pharmacological methods of prophylaxis for deep venous thrombosis in these patients.

G. Gastrointestinal Hemorrhage

Gastrointestinal ulceration and bleeding is likely in patients after craniotomy for tumor resection, particularly as almost all these patients are on corticosteroids. Patients who are in a coma preoperatively, are over 60 years old, have central nervous system infection, develop SIADH, or undergo more than one surgical procedure are at an especially high risk (130,191). Histamine-2 receptor blockers or H^+ pump blockers should be administered to lower this risk.

H. ICP Monitoring

Intracranial hypertension after elective intracranial surgery is more likely in patients after surgery lasting for over 6 hr, a repeat craniotomy, and glioblastoma resection (192). Some of these patients and others who are prone to hydrocephalus and cerebral swelling may be candidates for ICP monitoring. Intracranial pressure monitoring also aids in the management of comatose patients, as they have abnormal intracranial compliance that makes it difficult to monitor neurological status without radiological means. Patients who have had posterior fossa tumor resection may need ICP monitoring. It should be remembered that supratentorial ICP monitoring does not always correlate with the pressure in the infratentorial compartment, particularly in the early postoperative period following posterior fossa surgery (193). Complications of direct ICP monitoring and therapeutic drainage from the posterior fossa include CSF leak, cranial nerve palsies, and brain-stem irritation.

Intracranial pressure monitoring systems include intraventricular or subdural catheters, subarachnoid bolts, and parenchymal, subdural, or epidural transducers. Postoperative ICP monitoring for uncomplicated craniotomy cases may be accomplished by the use of a subdural catheter (194). Subdural catheters are easy to place, safe, and accurate for ICP monitoring but do not permit the withdrawal of CSF (130). Patients with obstruction of the ventricular system are best managed with an intraventricular catheter (194). A catheter placed in the lateral ventricle is the gold standard for the diagnosis and management of elevated ICP. The benefit of a ventriculostomy is the ability to diagnose as well as treat intracranial hypertension. Patients who have massive edema of the brain and slit-like ventricles may be managed by a means of a subarachnoid bolt, or a parenchymal, sub- or epidural transducer.

Complications of ICP monitoring include infection, brain injury and hemorrhage, and poor therapy based on inaccurate data such as may be obtained from occluded intraventricular and subdural catheters, obstructed subarachnoid bolts, or malfunctioning external transducers (194). The waveform of the CSF pulse should be inspected for damping which will alert one to the presence of an obstruction. Risk factors for the development of infection due to ICP monitoring devices include the duration of monitoring (increased risk after 5 days), the patient's age, disease, the consistency of maintaining a closed system, and the environment in which the monitor was inserted as well as the type of device (195). Gram-positive antibiotic coverage (vancomycin, oxacillin) and careful handling of the system to prevent contamination can reduce the incidence of infections (130). Most neurosurgeons retain the monitoring systems only for 72 hours.

I. Treatment of Elevated ICP in the Intensive Care Unit

The management of intracranial hypertension in the intensive care unit is similar to the intraoperative management of high ICP (26). Some additional considerations for patients in the ICU follow. Early imaging of the brain should be considered so that new or enlarging lesions are not missed. If the patient was extubated after surgery, reintubation may be necessary in order to avoid hypoxia and hypercarbia, and to protect against aspiration. Mechanical ventilation will facilitate hyperventilation for discrete periods in an effort to decrease the ICP. Agitated and anxious patients with intracranial hypertension should be sedated, after ensuring that they are adequately oxygenated and ventilated, and have no new intracranial lesion. The combination of a short-acting sedative like propofol (0.6–6 mg/kg/hr) or midazolam (0.05–0.1 mg/kg/hr) combined with an opioid, e.g., morphine sulfate (2–5 mg) intravenously every 1–4 hr, fentanyl (0.5–3.0 μg/kg/hr) or sufentanil (0.1–0.6 μg/kg/hr), is effective (26). These medications should be stopped for frequent neurological examinations.

XI. INFRATENTORIAL SURGERY

There are special considerations for tumor resection in the posterior fossa due to the unique anatomical features of this region. The posterior fossa is a rigid area containing vital structures (the brainstem, cerebellum, and cranial nerves) densely packed within its confines. The effluence of CSF occurs within the posterior fossa through the aqueduct of Sylvius into the fourth ventricle and through the foramen of Magendie and Luschka into the basal cisterns. Infratentorial masses or edema can produce obstruction within this pathway resulting in secondary hydrocephalus. The large venous sinuses (the torcula, superior petrosal sinuses, transverse sinus, and sigmoid sinus) present throughout this compartment assume special significance during the sitting position by increasing the risk of air embolism (144).

Specific complications of posterior fossa surgery are hemodynamic and cardiac rhythm disturbances, and cranial nerve injury causing an inability to maintain a patent airway. Cerebellar mutism may occur postoperatively in children following division of the inferior vermis while accessing a midline posterior fossa tumor (112). This usually resolves after a few months. Venous air embolism may occur during posterior fossa surgery in the sitting position. Other complications related to the sitting position have been addressed previously.

A. Hemodynamic Changes

Lower cranial nerve nuclei, cardiovascular centers, and respiratory centers are located in close proximity in the brainstem. Injury to these structures may occur during procedures involving dissection of the floor of the fourth ventricle. Cranial nerves IX, X, XII are also in jeopardy during surgery at the cerebellopontine angle. In the past, resection of posterior fossa tumors was carried out in a spontaneously breathing patient. Then, intraoperative disturbances of respiration played an important role in signaling injury to the lower cranial nerve nuclei and respiratory centers in the brain stem. Controlled ventilation is now almost always performed, and cardiovascular abnormalities such as hypertension and tachycardia, hypotension or hypertension and bradycardia, sinus arrhythmia and ventricular arrhythmias may warn of impending brain stem injury (196).

If arrhythmias or sudden changes in arterial blood pressure or heart rate occur during procedures performed at the brain stem, the surgeon should be immediately warned. Additionally, if such disturbances are noted intraoperatively, extubation should be performed only after adequate return of respiration and upper airway protective reflexes is observed (196).

B. Venous Air Embolism

The spontaneous entry of air into the venous circulation during surgery depends on the magnitude of the negative gradient between the exposed vein and the right side of the heart (197). Although VAE can occur during many non-neurosurgical operations, sitting craniotomies are most notoriously associated with VAE. Elevation of the operative site above the heart results in subatmospheric pressure in the noncollapsible dural sinuses and increases the negative gravitational gradient, predisposing to the venous entrainment of air. The incidence of VAE is as high as 76% in patients undergoing craniotomy in the sitting position as estimated by transesophageal echocardiography (TEE) (198). When precordial Doppler was used as a monitor, 40% of patients in the sitting position and 12% in other positions were found to develop VAE (142). Air embolism may also occur during the resection of supratentorial tumors located adjacent to the posterior half of the sagittal sinus (131). Pin head-holder placement and burr holes have been rarely associated with the development of VAE (199).

1. Pathophysiology

Factors modifying the entrainment of air include the position of the patient, the depth of ventilation, the volume and rate of air entering the venous system, and the central venous pressure (200). Spontaneous ventilation (which is rare nowadays in the context of infratentorial surgery) and a low central venous pressure (e.g., due to hypovolemia) each produce an increased gradient between the open cranial veins and the heart, predisposing to air embolism. The use of intraoperative PEEP can predispose to a PAE by augmenting the pressure gradient between the right and the left heart. Nitrous oxide (50%) does not increase either the incidence or the severity of VAE provided that it is discontinued immediately upon the detection of VAE by Doppler (201).

The cardiovascular response to VAE varies depending on whether the air is entrained in a single large bolus or as a continuous infusion of gas (200). When a significant amount of air is slowly entrained into the venous system, it passes into the lungs and impairs blood flow distal to the pulmonary artery (PA) causing a progressive increase in central venous and pulmonary arterial pressure. This leads to decreased systemic vascular resistance and compensatory tachycardia. Increased dead space, V/Q mismatch, pulmonary edema, hypoxia, and hypercarbia may occur. Peak airway pressures may be elevated due to bronchoconstriction.

Rapid entrainment of a large amount of air may cause an air lock to form in the right heart, leading to acute right ventricular failure, arrhythmias, myocardial ischemia, and total cardiovascular collapse. Children frequently have more severe hemodynamic complications from VAE (202).

A PAE may gain entry into the left heart through a PFO (patent foramen ovale) and enters the systemic circulation. Severe consequences such as cardiac or cerebral ischemia may ensue following a PAE. The patient may manifest new postoperative neurological deficits. Preoperative echocardiography can be performed to identify PFO and detect right-to-left shunting in patients. However, the incidence of PFO as detected by preoperative echocardiography was much lower than expected in some reports (143). Furthermore, the risk of PAE still exists if a PFO has not been detected by echocardiography. Thus the role of preoperative echocardiography as a screening tool for this purpose is limited.

2. Monitoring for VAE

Transesophageal Echocardiography

Transesophageal echocardiography is the most sensitive monitor for the detection of air embolism and can also aid in the detection of a PFO (Fig. 9). However, TEE is invasive and requires the constant attention of an expert for its use and interpretation.

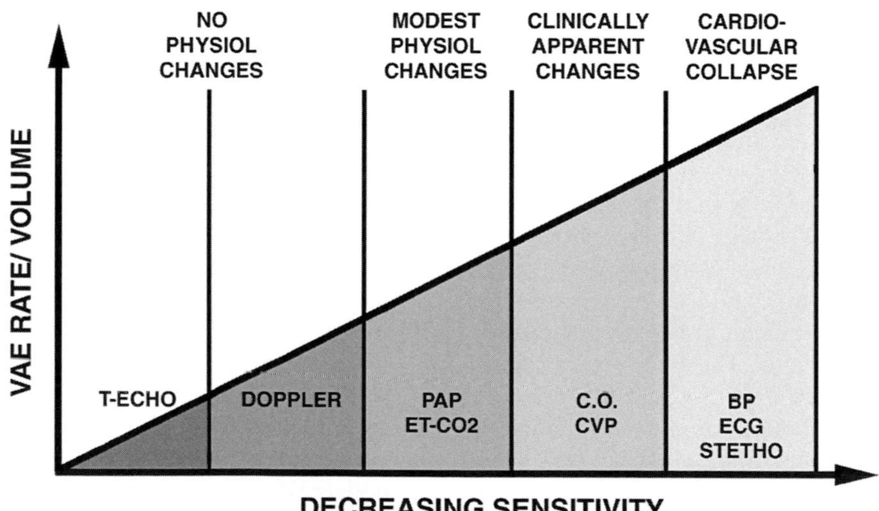

Figure 9 The relative sensitivity of various monitors to the occurrence of VAE. BP, blood pressure; CO, cardiac output; CVP, central venous pressure; ECG, electrocardiogram; ET-CO_2, end-tidal carbon dioxide; PAP, pulmonary artery pressure; physiol, physiological; stetho, stethoscope (auscultation); T-Echo, transesophageal echocardiography. *Source*: From Ref. 131, with permission from Elsevier.

Precordial Doppler Ultrasound

Precordial cardiac auscultation by means of Doppler ultrasound is the next sensitive diagnostic method for the detection of VAE (197,203). Air embolism can be detected by Doppler ultrasound before pathophysiologic changes occur (Fig. 9) (203). Although it is sometimes criticized as being too sensitive, Doppler monitoring is useful as it is easy to employ. Precordial Doppler monitoring is frequently used along with end-expired carbon dioxide measurement when the risk of occurrence of VAE is deemed high. Proper placement over the right heart (third to sixth right parasternal intercostal space) can be verified by injecting agitated saline or 0.25–0.5 mL of air through the CVC (197). A characteristic "chirping" sound should be heard.

Capnography

A decreased end-tidal carbon dioxide concentration is suggestive of VAE. Capnography is a useful and practical monitor that is always available in modern anesthetic practice. Rapid respiratory rates in spontaneously breathing patients, low cardiac output, and chronic obstructive pulmonary disease affect the sensitivity of this monitor (204).

Right Atrial Catheter

Right artial catheterization allows detection of an elevated CVP; a high CVP is a nonspecific sign of VAE. Furthermore, a significant benefit of a right atrial catheterization is the ability to aspirate air from the heart. Optimal aspiration of air occurs when the tip is positioned 2 cm below the right atrial-superior vena caval junction for a multiorificed catheter, and 3 cm above this junction for a single-orificed catheter (205). Aspiration of air from the middle right atrium is poor with either type of catheter. Intravascular electrocardiography can assist in placement of the CVC. A negative P wave on the EKG is indicative of placement at or just below the SA node. When the tip of the electrolyte-filled catheter is in the middle of the right atrium, the P wave on the EKG becomes biphasic.

Pulmonary Artery Catheter

A PA catheter is a nonspecific monitor and indicates pulmonary hypertension due to VAE. It is difficult to aspirate air through a PA catheter.

Cardiovascular Signs

As discussed previously, the patient may initially be tachycardic and hypertensive and subsequently develop hypotension, arrhythmias and frank CV collapse. The characteristic mill-wheel murmur is a late sign of VAE.

Somatosensory Evoked Potentials

Although monitoring of SSEPs is not usually performed solely for the detection of VAE, evoked potentials may correlate with neurological outcome after a cerebral air embolism (206).

3. *Treatment of VAE*

The surgeons must be informed immediately if there is suspicion regarding the occurrence of VAE. The field is flooded with saline and open bone sealed with wax to prevent more air from entering the venous sinuses. Nitrous oxide should be discontinued and 100% oxygen administered. An attempt should be made to aspirate air from the heart through the CVC. Hemodynamic support is provided as indicated and the sitting patient placed supine as soon as possible. The left lateral decubitus position has been advocated to decrease passage of air through the pulmonary circulation. However, cardiopulmonary resuscitation is most effective and easier to perform in the supine position. Compression of the jugular veins to increase venous pressure and prevent further entrainment of air has also been suggested. It should be borne in mind that this maneuver can decrease cerebral venous outflow and increase CBV, and carries the risk of concomitant carotid artery compression. It is also difficult to aspirate air from the CVC during compression of the neck veins. Positive end-expiratory pressure should be discontinued or lowered in order to avoid the occurrence of PAE.

Postoperatively, the patient may need supplemental oxygen. Close neurologic and cardiac monitoring, arterial blood gas measurements and chest radiography should be performed. Hyperbaric oxygen therapy may be beneficial in the treatment of cerebral air embolism (207).

XII. VENTRICULOPERITONEAL SHUNTING

Ventriculoperitoneal shunting is performed for the relief of obstructive hydrocephalus which may be caused by posterior fossa tumors near the ventricular system. These procedures are brief, and can be performed under MAC with standard monitors. Patients exprience minimal postoperative pain. Intraoperatively, overly aggressive hyperventilation may lead to collapse of the ventricles which makes the procedure difficult to perform (116). Relief of high ICP at the time of the initial cannulation may cause sudden hypotension. Patients are placed supine following the procedure to prevent excessive CSF drainage.

XIII. SURGERY FOR PITUITARY TUMORS

It is important to remember the regional anatomy of the pituitary gland as one can then predict perioperative complications. The pituitary is encased in the sella turcica of the sphenoid bone and is connected to the hypothalamus by the pituitary stalk that traverses through the diaphragma sellae. Anterosuperior to the pituitary is the optic chiasma which is the confluence of the two optic nerves and which continues posteriorly as the optic tracts. The cavernous sinus contains the internal carotid artery, CNs III, IV, and VI, and the ophthalmic and maxillary divisions of CN V and is situated along the lateral walls of the sella turcica, extending posteriorly into the petrosal sinuses.

A. Presentation of Patients with Pituitary Tumors

Pituitary tumors can present with manifestations due to syndromes of hormone excess, hypofunction of the gland, or with symptoms due to local pressure or invasion by the tumor.

The anterior pituitary secretes six hormones: thyroid-stimulating hormone (TSH), adrenocorticotrophic hormone (ACTH), luteinizing hormone (LH), follicle-stimulating hormone (FSH), and prolactin and growth hormone (GH). The posterior pituitary secretes oxytocin and vasopressin (Table 2).

Pituitary adenomas are the most common type of pituitary tumors. Secretory adenomas are infrequent and secrete prolactin, ACTH, GH, or rarely TSH. Patients may present with Cushing's disease due to ACTH and cortisol excess. Hypersecretion of GH before puberty causes gigantism, and acromegaly after puberty and epiphyseal union. Patients rarely develop imbalances of TSH secretion. Hypopituitarism may occur. Mass effect of the tumor may cause visual disturbances: the commonest is bitemporal heteronymous hemianopsia. Other visual field defects or oculomotor palsy may occur. Stretching of the diaphragma sella by the tumor may cause headaches. Large pituitary tumors can produce hypothalamic dysfunction. Patients with pituitary apoplexy may present emergently for surgery.

The treatment of choice for symptomatic adenomas is excision of the lesions with or without postoperative radiotherapy to prevent recurrence. Most adenomas can be resected through the transsphenoidal approach. Contraindications to the transsphenoidal approach include extensive lateral tumor herniating into the middle fossa with minimal midline mass, ectatic carotid arteries at risk of injury by the transsphenoidal approach, and acute sinusitis (208). A transcranial approach may be preferred in some of these cases.

B. Preoperative Evaluation

In patients with pituitary tumors, the preoperative evaluation should focus on any abnormalities related to the endocrine system and signs of pituitary hypofunction. The radiologic images must be reviewed to determine whether the tumor is confined to the sella turcica or extends into the suprasellar region.

Prolactinomas are the most frequently occurring secretory adenomas. Patients may develop galactorrhea and hypogonadism. Acromegaly manifests as overgrowth of bony and soft tissue. The main concerns for the anesthesiologist are the airway, pulmonary, and cardiovascular system. The patient usually has hypertrophy of the facial bones and soft tissue. Laryngeal stenosis, fixed vocal cords, recurrent laryngeal nerve palsy, and chondrocalcinosis of the larynx can occur (209). Mask ventilation, laryngoscopy, and tracheal intubation can be challenging in these patients and fiberoptic-assisted intubation may be necessary. These patients may also have obstructive sleep apnea. Left ventricular hypertrophy, cardiomyopathy, hypertension, and diabetes mellitus may be present. A thorough cardiac evaluation should be performed in these patients.

Patients with Cushing's disease may present with hyperglycemia, hypokalemia, water and sodium retention, metabolic alkalosis, moon facies, obesity, and a characteristic "buffalo hump" that may complicate mask ventilation and intubation. There is an increased incidence of hypertension, coronary artery disease, and left ventricular hypertrophy in these patients. Besides the history and physical examination, additional tests include an electrocardiogram and an echocardiogram, if indicated. Laboratory studies should assess serum electrolytes (sodium and potassium) and glucose. Perioperative stress dose steroids may be administered in these patients, if adrenal insufficiency is present.

Thyroid-stimulating hormone levels should be checked and further tests including a full thyroid hormone panel and an EKG obtained if indicated. Hyperthyroid patients can develop tachycardia and cardiac arrhythmias, and are at risk for a thyroid storm with hyperpyrexia, heart failure, delirium, and coma. Patients with hyperthyroidism should undergo preoperative control with antithyroid drugs such as propylthiouracil. Hypothyroidism may manifest as cardiac dysfunction, pericardial effusions, hypothermia, hyponatremia, and increased sensitivity to sedatives.

Table 2 Pituitary Adenomas

	Normal function				Pituitary adenoma
	Pituitary		Endorgan		Adenoma
Hypothalamus	Pituitary cell	Pituitary hormone	Organ/hormone	Primary functions	Tumor/clinical syndrome
Releasing factors					
Corticotropin-releasing hormone (CRH)	Corticotroph	Adrenocorticotropin (corticotropin, ACTH)	Adrenals; cortisol	General metabolism; required for physiologic adaptation to stress	ACTH-secreting adenoma (corticotropinoma); Cushing's disease
	Thyrotroph	Thyroid-stimulating hormone (TSH)	Thyroid; thyroid hormones (T_3, T_4)	General metabolism; influences pace of metabolism	TSH-secreting adenoma (thyrotropinoma); hyperthyroidism
Gonadotropin-releasing hormone (GnRH)	Gonadotroph	Follicle-stimulating hormone (FSH)	Ovaries; estradiol progesteron	Required for normal female sexual development and fertility	FSH-secreting adenoma; endocrine-inactive macroadenoma
		Luteinizing hormone (LH)	Testes; testosterone	Required for normal male sexual development and fertility	LH-secreting adenoma; endocrine-inactive macroadenoma
Growth hormone-releasing hormone (GHRH)	Somatotroph	Growth hormone (somatotropin, GH)	Liver and other tissues; somatomedin (insulin-like growth factor-I) (IGF-1)	Growth, glucose regulation	GH-secreting adenoma (somatotropinoma); acromegaly (in children, gigantism)
Inhibiting factors					
Dopamine (PIF)	Lactotroph	Prolactin (PRL)	Breast; gonads	Lactation	PRL-secreting adenoma (prolactinoma); amenorrhea–galactorrhea
Somatostatin	Somatotroph	Growth hormone (GH)	Liver and other tissues; somatomedin (insulin-like growth factor-I) (IGF-I)	Growth, glucose regulation	None

Source: From Ref. 28, with permission from Elsevier.

Patients with severe hypothyroidism should receive hormone replacement therapy before elective surgery.

Hypopituitarism causing adrenal insufficiency may manifest as orthostatic hypotension, volume depletion, and various electrolyte disturbances, including hyponatremia, hyperkalemia, and hypoglycemia. Intravascular volume status should be estimated by blood pressure and heart rate determinations in supine and standing positions (209). Patients may need corticosteroid replacement therapy.

Typed and crossmatched blood should be available for patients undergoing pituitary surgery as massive hemorrhage can occur due to the proximity of the internal carotid artery in the cavernous sinus.

C. Intraoperative Management

The patient is often in a head-up position to facilitate venous drainage. If the position is more than 15° above the horizontal, a right atrial catheter and a precordial Doppler should be placed. A straight reinforced or oral RAE endotracheal tube may be used in these patients. An esophageal stethoscope is frequently employed as the head and upper body are not immediately accessible to the anesthesiologist during the procedure. The posterior hypopharynx is packed with moist gauze to prevent blood trickling into the stomach or trachea. The nasal septal and sublabial routes are used for surgical access. Epinephrine and cocaine are frequently injected submucosally by the surgeons to achieve a bloodless field and may cause dysrhythmias. Total spinal anesthesia during local anesthesia of the nasal mucosa has been reported (210).

The surgeons may request hypocapnia to reduce brain volume and prevent the bulging of the arachnoid membrane into the sella. If the arachnoid membrane is incised, persistent CSF leaks and meningitis may result. On the contrary, if there is suprasellar extension of the mass, normocapnia, hypercapnia, or a Valsalva maneuver may be requested in order to draw the mass into the sella for resection (131). Air or saline may be injected through a lumbar subarachnoid catheter to outline suprasellar lesions by C-arm fluoroscopy (Fig. 10). Nitrous oxide should not be used if air is injected. The anesthesiologist may be asked to perform a Valsalva maneuver again prior to closure of the surgical incision to assess the integrity of the graft. During the procedure, the anesthesiologist should be prepared for massive intraoperative bleeding which may be impossible to control. At the end of the surgery, the nose is packed. The airway is gently but thoroughly suctioned prior to extubation. During emergence, coughing and bucking should be avoided. If the patient coughs excessively, the arachnoid membrane may be reopened, increasing the risk of infection. The surgeons may place a lumbar CSF drain to prevent persistent postoperative CSF leakage (208).

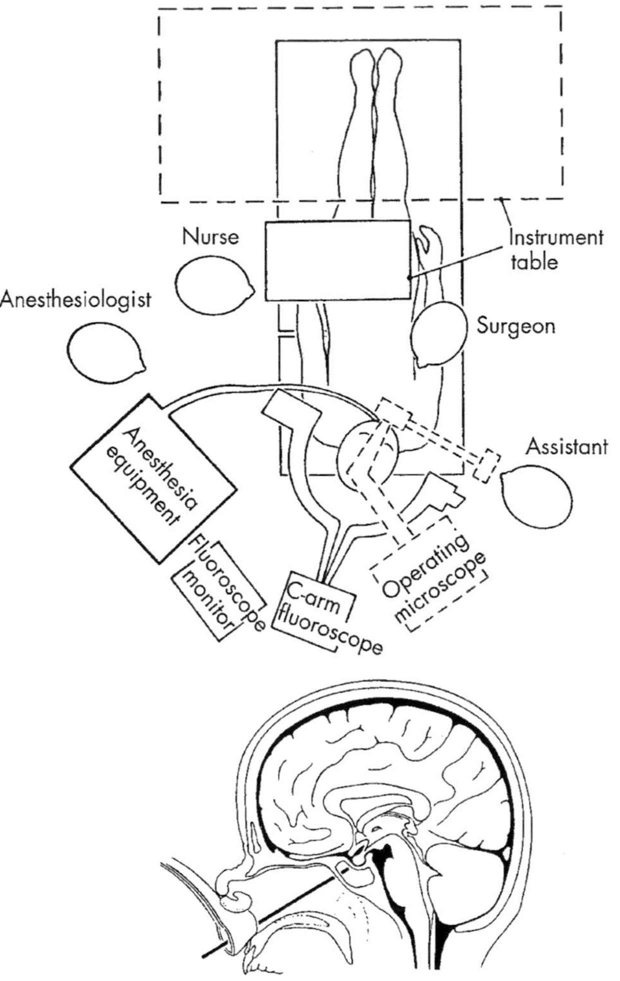

Figure 10 Transsphenoidal pituitary surgery uses lateral imaging of the skull with C-arm fluoroscopy to guide the intraoperative route to the sella turcica. The positioning of personnel shown here provides optimal ease of interaction between the scrub nurse and surgeon and still permits the anesthesiologist access to the patient. The midsagittal route of approach is shown in the lower portion of the figure. *Source*: From Ref. 28, with permission from Elsevier.

D. Postoperative Management after Hypophysectomy

Besides the general care of postoperative neurosurgical patients, there are some specific concerns in these patients following surgery. Postoperatively, patients continue to receive glucocorticoids, especially if low cortisol levels were present preoperatively. Hypothalamic injury is the major cause of death due to surgery in these patients (183). Delayed morbidity occurs due to CSF leaks and meningitis or vascular injury.

Serial visual field testing is performed in the PACU and ICU to follow recovery and assess visual function. Both the transfrontal and transsphenoidal approaches are associated with good visual recovery (208). Improvement in visual symptoms may continue up to a year postoperatively. New visual deficits in the postoperative period can be a sign of intracranial bleeding and necessitate emergent CT scanning and surgical re-exploration. Extraocular muscle function can also be impaired postoperatively due to cranial nerve injury sustained during surgery. Diabetes insipidus or SIADH may occur. The management of these complications has been discussed in a preceding section. Other complications of pituitary surgery include stroke, nasal or sinus problems, and transient psychosis (183).

XIV. EMERGENCY CRANIOTOMY FOR BRAIN TUMORS

Patients with tumors who present for emergency surgery may have acute hydrocephalus or impending brain herniation (211). A quick assessment of the neurological status, the airway and hemodynamics should be performed. These patients have significantly raised ICP and a decreased level of consciousness. The anesthesiologist's major concern is to expeditiously secure the airway and enable the surgeons to proceed with decompression promptly (66). During endotracheal intubation, it is critical to maintain CPP and minimize increases in ICP. Minimal sedatives are needed. A muscle relaxant should be administered to prevent an increase in ICP with coughing, direct laryngoscopy, and tracheal intubation (145,211). Intraoperatively, these are the patients in whom nitrous oxide, volatile agents, and other vasodilators should be avoided. Mild-to-moderate hyperventilation will aid in the control of ICP.

ACKNOWLEDGMENTS

I would like to thank: Martin Müller, M.D., for his review of this chapter and thoughtful suggestions; Christy B. Perry, Christopher J. Kicklighter, B.A., and Isela Ramos for their expert editorial assistance; Erik Haupt, M.D., and Gregory Chaljub, M.D., for providing the photograph of the MRI.

REFERENCES

1. Frost EA. History of neuroanesthesia. In: Albin MS, ed. Textbook of Neuroanesthesia with Neurosurgical and Neuroscience Perspectives. New York: McGraw-Hill Companies, 1997:1–20.
2. Barker FGI, Sztramski P. Surgery for brain tumors. In: Prados M, ed. Brain Cancer. Hamilton, Ont.: BC Decker, 2002:238–261.
3. Liu CY, Apuzzo ML. The genesis of neurosurgery and the evolution of the neurosurgical operative environment: part I—prehistory to 2003. Neurosurgery 2003; 52(1):3–19.
4. McDermott MW, Quinones-Hinojosa A, Bollen AW, Larson DA, Prados M. Meningiomas. In: Prados M, ed. Brain Cancer. Hamilton, Ont.: BC Decker, 2002:333–364.
5. Siesjo BK. Cerebral circulation and metabolism. J Neurosurg 1984; 60(5):883–908.
6. Lassen NA. Cerebral blood flow and oxygen consumption in man. Physiol Rev 1959; 39:183–238.
7. Black S, Michenfelder JD. Cerebral blood flow and metabolism. In: Cucchiara RF, Black S, Michenfelder JD, eds. Clinical Neuroanesthesia. New York: Churchill Livingstone, 1998:1–40.
8. von Knobelsdorff G, Kusagaya H, Werner C, Kochs E, Esch J. The effects of surgical stimulation on intracranial hemodynamics. J Neurosurg Anesthesiol 1996; 8(1):9–14.
9. Brian JE Jr. Carbon dioxide and the cerebral circulation. Anesthesiology 1998; 88(5):1365–1386.
10. Koehler RC, Traystman RJ. Bicarbonate ion modulation of cerebral blood flow during hypoxia and hypercapnia. Am J Physiol 1982; 243(1):H33–H40.
11. Armstead WM, Zuckerman SL, Shibata M, Parfenova H, Leffler CW. Different pial arteriolar responses to acetylcholine in the newborn and juvenile pig. J Cereb Blood Flow Metab 1994; 14(6):1088–1095.
12. Christensen MS, Brodersen P, Olesen J, Paulson OB. Cerebral apoplexy (stroke) treated with or without prolonged artificial hyperventilation. 2. Cerebrospinal fluid acid-base balance and intracranial pressure. Stroke 1973; 4(4):620–631.
13. Laffey JG, Kavanagh BP. Hypocapnia. N Engl J Med 2002; 347(1):43–53.
14. Cold GE. Does acute hyperventilation provoke cerebral oligaemia in comatose patients after acute head injury? Acta Neurochir (Wien) 1989; 96(3–4):100–106.
15. Drummond JC. The lower limit of autoregulation: time to revise our thinking? Anesthesiology 1997; 86(6):1431–1433.
16. Rosner MJ. The vasodilatory cascade and intracranial pressure. In: Miller JD, Teasdale GM, Rowan JO, Galbraith SL, Mendelow AD, eds. Intracranial Pressure. Berlin Heidelberg: Springer-Verlag, 1986.
17. Strandgaard S, Olesen J, Skinhoj E, Lassen NA. Autoregulation of brain circulation in severe arterial hypertension. Br Med J 1973; 1(5852):507–510.

18. Drummond JC, Patel PM. Cerebral physiology and the effects of anesthetics and techniques. In: Miller RD, ed. Anesthesia. Philadelphia: Churchill Livingstone, 2000:695–734.
19. Lee SH, Heros RC, Mullan JC, Korosue K. Optimum degree of hemodilution for brain protection in a canine model of focal cerebral ischemia. J Neurosurg 1994; 80(3):469–475.
20. Clasen RA, Pandolfi S, Laing I, Casey D Jr. Experimental study of relation of fever to cerebral edema. J Neurosurg 1974; 41(5):576–581.
21. Warner DS. Effects of anesthetic agents and temperature on the injured brain. In: Albin MS, ed. Textbook of Neuroanesthesia with Neurosurgical and Neuroscience Perspectives. New York: McGraw-Hill, 1997:595–611.
22. Shapiro HM. Intracranial hypertension: therapeutic and anesthetic considerations. Anesthesiology 1975; 43(4):445–471.
23. Cushing H. Concerning a definite regulatory mechanism of the vasomotor center which controls blood pressure during cerebral compression. Johns Hopkins Med J 1901; 12:290–292.
24. Fishman RA. Brain edema. N Engl J Med 1975; 293(14):706–711.
25. Risberg J, Lundberg N, Ingvar DH. Regional cerebral blood volume during acute transient rises of the intracranial pressure (plateau waves). J Neurosurg 1969; 31(3):303–310.
26. Mayer SA, Chong JY. Critical care management of increased intracranial pressure. J Intensive Care Med 2002; 17:55–67.
27. Rajaraman V, Jackson CH, Branch CL Jr, Petrozza PH. Supratentorial and pituitary surgery. In: Albin MS, ed. Textbook of Neuroanesthesia with Neurosurgical and Neuroscience Perspectives. New York: McGraw-Hill, 1997:931–970.
28. O'Rourke DK, Oldfield EH. Supratentorial masses: surgical considerations. In: Cottrell JE, Smith DS, eds. Anesthesia and Neurosurgery. 4th ed. St Louis, MO: Mosby, 2001:275–295.
29. Spiegelmann R, Hadani M, Ram Z, Faibel M, Shacked I. Upward transtentorial herniation: a complication of postoperative edema at the cervicomedullary junction. Neurosurgery 1989; 24(2):284–288.
30. Hansen TD, Warner DS, Todd MM, Vust LJ. The role of cerebral metabolism in determining the local cerebral blood flow effects of volatile anesthetics: evidence for persistent flow–metabolism coupling. J Cereb Blood Flow Metab 1989; 9(3):323–328.
31. Artru AA. Partial preservation of cerebral vascular responsiveness to hypocapnia during isoflurane-induced hypotension in dogs. Anesth Analg 1986; 65(6):660–666.
32. McPherson RW, Traystman RJ. Effects of isoflurane on cerebral autoregulation in dogs. Anesthesiology 1988; 69(4):493–499.
33. Drummond JC, Todd MM. The response of the feline cerebral circulation to $PaCO_2$ during anesthesia with isoflurane and halothane and during sedation with nitrous oxide. Anesthesiology 1985; 62(3):268–273.
34. Todd MM, Drummond JC. A comparison of the cerebrovascular and metabolic effects of halothane and isoflurane in the cat. Anesthesiology 1984; 60(4): 276–282.
35. Algotsson L, Messeter K, Nordstrom CH, Ryding E. Cerebral blood flow and oxygen consumption during isoflurane and halothane anesthesia in man. Acta Anaesthesiol Scand 1988; 32(1):15–20.
36. Artru AA. Relationship between cerebral blood volume and CSF pressure during anesthesia with isoflurane or fentanyl in dogs. Anesthesiology 1984; 60(6):575–579.
37. Drummond JC, Todd MM, Toutant SM, Shapiro HM. Brain surface protrusion during enflurane, halothane, and isoflurane anesthesia in cats. Anesthesiology 1983; 59(4):288–293.
38. Hansen TD, Warner DS, Todd MM, Vust LJ, Trawick DC. Distribution of cerebral blood flow during halothane versus isoflurane anesthesia in rats. Anesthesiology 1988; 69(3):332–337.
39. Adams RW, Cucchiara RF, Gronert GA, Messick JM, Michenfelder JD. Isoflurane and cerebrospinal fluid pressure in neurosurgical patients. Anesthesiology 1981; 54(2):97–99.
40. Gordon E, Lagerkranser M, Rudehill A, von Holst H. The effect of isoflurane on cerebrospinal fluid pressure in patients undergoing neurosurgery. Acta Anaesthesiol Scand 1988; 32(2):108–112.
41. Scheller MS, Nakakimura K, Fleischer JE, Zornow MH. Cerebral effects of sevoflurane in the dog: comparison with isoflurane and enflurane. Br J Anaesth 1990; 65(3):388–392.
42. Yli-Hankala A, Vakkuri A, Sarkela M, Lindgren L, Korttila K, Jantti V. Epileptiform electroencephalogram during mask induction of anesthesia with sevoflurane. Anesthesiology 1999; 91(6):1596–1603.
43. Watts AD, Herrick IA, McLachlan RS, Craen RA, Gelb AW. The effect of sevoflurane and isoflurane anesthesia on interictal spike activity among patients with refractory epilepsy. Anesth Analg 1999; 89(5):1275–1281.
44. Carras D, Farrell S, Todd MM. Neuroanesthesia. In: Grossman RG, Loftus CM, eds. Principles of Neurosurgery. Philadelphia: Lippincott-Raven, 1999:15–30.
45. Muzzi DA, Losasso TJ, Dietz NM, Faust RJ, Cucchiara RF, Milde LN. The effect of desflurane and isoflurane on cerebrospinal fluid pressure in humans with supratentorial mass lesions. Anesthesiology 1992; 76(5):720–724.
46. Fraga M, Rama-Maceiras P, Rodino S, Aymerich H, Pose P, Belda J. The effects of isoflurane and desflurane on intracranial pressure, cerebral perfusion pressure, and cerebral arteriovenous oxygen content difference in normocapnic patients with supratentorial brain tumors. Anesthesiology 2003; 98(5):1085–1090.

47. Gauthier A, Girard F, Boudreault D, Ruel M, Todorov A. Sevoflurane provides faster recovery and postoperative neurological assessment than isoflurane in long-duration neurosurgical cases [table]. Anesth Analg 2002; 95(5):1384–1388.
48. Artru AA. Rate of cerebrospinal fluid formation, resistance to reabsorption of cerebrospinal fluid, brain tissue water content, and electroencephalogram during desflurane anesthesia in dogs. J Neurosurg Anesthesiol 1993; 5(3):178–186.
49. Artru AA. Effects of enflurane and isoflurane on resistance to reabsorption of cerebrospinal fluid in dogs. Anesthesiology 1984; 61(5):529–533.
50. Artru AA. Isoflurane does not increase the rate of CSF production in the dog. Anesthesiology 1984; 60(3): 193–197.
51. Madsen JB, Cold GE, Hansen ES, Bardrum B. The effect of isoflurane on cerebral blood flow and metabolism in humans during craniotomy for small supratentorial cerebral tumors. Anesthesiology 1987; 66(3): 332–336.
52. Pelligrino DA, Miletich DJ, Hoffman WE, Albrecht RF. Nitrous oxide markedly increases cerebral cortical metabolic rate and blood flow in the goat. Anesthesiology 1984; 60(5):405–412.
53. Reasoner DK, Warner DS, Todd MM, McAllister A. Effects of nitrous oxide on cerebral metabolic rate in rats anaesthetized with isoflurane. Br J Anaesth 1990; 65(2):210–215.
54. Algotsson L, Messeter K, Rosen I, Holmin T. Effects of nitrous oxide on cerebral haemodynamics and metabolism during isoflurane anaesthesia in man. Acta Anaesthesiol Scand 1992; 36(1):46–52.
55. Matta BF, Lam AM. Nitrous oxide increases cerebral blood flow velocity during pharmacologically induced EEG silence in humans. J Neurosurg Anesthesiol 1995; 7(2):89–93.
56. Field LM, Dorrance DE, Krzeminska EK, Barsoum LZ. Effect of nitrous oxide on cerebral blood flow in normal humans. Br J Anaesth 1993; 70(2):154–159.
57. Hormann C, Schmidauer C, Kolbitsch C, Kofler A, Benzer A. Effects of normo- and hypocapnic nitrous-oxide-inhalation on cerebral blood flow velocity in patients with brain tumors. J Neurosurg Anesthesiol 1997; 9(2):141–145.
58. Pierce EC Jr, Lambertsen CJ, Deutsch S, Chase PE, Linde HW, Dripps RD, et al. Cerebral circulation and metabolism during thiopental anesthesia and hyper-ventilation in man. J Clin Invest 1962; 41: 1664–1671.
59. Fox J, Gelb AW, Enns J, Murkin JM, Farrar JK, Manninen PH. The responsiveness of cerebral blood flow to changes in arterial carbon dioxide is maintained during propofol–nitrous oxide anesthesia in humans. Anesthesiology 1992; 77(3):453–456.
60. Nilsson L, Siesjo BK. The effect of phenobarbitone anaesthesia on blood flow and oxygen consumption in the rat brain. Acta Anaesthesiol Scand Suppl 1975; 57:18–24.
61. Newberg LA, Milde JH, Michenfelder JD. The cerebral metabolic effects of isoflurane at and above concentrations that suppress cortical electrical activity. Anesthesiology 1983; 59(1):23–28.
62. Cenic A, Craen RA, Lee TY, Gelb AW. Cerebral blood volume and blood flow responses to hyperventilation in brain tumors during isoflurane or propofol anesthesia. Anesth Analg 2002; 94(3):661–666.
63. Bray RJ. Propofol infusion syndrome in children. Paediatr Anaesth 1998; 8(6):491–499.
64. Drummond JC, Cole DJ, Patel PM, Reynolds LW. Focal cerebral ischemia during anesthesia with etomidate, isoflurane, or thiopental: a comparison of the extent of cerebral injury. Neurosurgery 1995; 37(4):742–748.
65. Hoffman WE, Charbel FT, Edelman G, Misra M, Ausman JI. Comparison of the effect of etomidate and desflurane on brain tissue gases and pH during prolonged middle cerebral artery occlusion. Anesthesiology 1998; 88(5):1188–1194.
66. Warner DS. Anesthesia for craniotomy. IARS 2003 Review Course Lectures 2003:107–113.
67. Takeshita H, Okuda Y, Sari A. The effects of ketamine on cerebral circulation and metabolism in man. Anesthesiology 1972; 36(1):69–75.
68. Shaprio HM, Wyte SR, Harris AB. Ketamine anaesthesia in patients with intracranial pathology. Br J Anaesth 1972; 44(11):1200–1204.
69. Mayberg TS, Lam AM, Matta BF, Domino KB, Winn HR. Ketamine does not increase cerebral blood flow velocity or intracranial pressure during isoflurane/nitrous oxide anesthesia in patients undergoing craniotomy. Anesth Analg 1995; 81(1):84–89.
70. Milde LN, Milde JH, Gallagher WJ. Effects of sufentanil on cerebral circulation and metabolism in dogs. Anesth Analg 1990; 70(2):138–146.
71. Marx W, Shah N, Long C, Arbit E, Galicich J, Mascott C, et al. Sufentanil, alfentanil, and fentanyl: impact on cerebrospinal fluid pressure in patients with brain tumors. J Neurosurg Anesth 1989; 1:3–7.
72. Martin DE, Rosenberg H, Aukburg SJ, Bartkowski RR, Edwards MW Jr, Greenhow DE, et al. Low-dose fentanyl blunts circulatory responses to tracheal intubation. Anesth Analg 1982; 61(8):680–684.
73. Bristow A, Shalev D, Rice B, Lipton JM, Giesecke AH Jr. Low-dose synthetic narcotic infusions for cerebral relaxation during craniotomies. Anesth Analg 1987; 66(5):413–416.
74. Guy J, Hindman BJ, Baker KZ, Borel CO, Maktabi M, Ostapkovich N, et al. Comparison of remifentanil and fentanyl in patients undergoing craniotomy for supratentorial space-occupying lesions. Anesthesiology 1997; 86(3):514–524.
75. Tommasino C, Maekawa T, Shapiro HM, Keifer-Goodman J, Kohlenberger RW. Fentanyl-induced

seizures activate subcortical brain metabolism. Anesthesiology 1984; 60(4):283–290.
76. Hoffman WE, Miletich DJ, Albrecht RF. The effects of midazolam on cerebral blood flow and oxygen consumption and its interaction with nitrous oxide. Anesth Analg 1986; 65(7):729–733.
77. Giffin JP, Cottrell JE, Shwiry B, Hartung J, Epstein J, Lim K. Intracranial pressure, mean arterial pressure, and heart rate following midazolam or thiopental in humans with brain tumors. Anesthesiology 1984; 60(5):491–494.
78. Todd MM, Warner DS, Sokoll MD, Maktabi MA, Hindman BJ, Scamman FL, et al. A prospective, comparative trial of three anesthetics for elective supratentorial craniotomy. Propofol/fentanyl, isoflurane/nitrous oxide, and fentanyl/nitrous oxide. Anesthesiology 1993; 78(6):1005–1020..
79. Petersen KD, Landsfeldt U, Cold GE, Petersen CB, Mau S, Hauerberg J, et al. Intracranial pressure and cerebral hemodynamic in patients with cerebral tumors: a randomized prospective study of patients subjected to craniotomy in propofol–fentanyl, isoflurane–fentanyl, or sevoflurane–fentanyl anesthesia. Anesthesiology 2003; 98(2):329–336.
80. Minton MD, Grosslight K, Stirt JA, Bedford RF. Increases in intracranial pressure from succinylcholine: prevention by prior nondepolarizing blockade. Anesthesiology 1986; 65(2):165–169.
81. Stirt JA, Grosslight KR, Bedford RF, Vollmer D. "Defasciculation" with metocurine prevents succinylcholine-induced increases in intracranial pressure. Anesthesiology 1987; 67(1):50–53.
82. Marsh ML, Dunlop BJ, Shapiro HM, Gagnon RL, Rockoff MA. Succinylcholine-induced intracranial pressure effects in neurosurgical patients [abstr]. Anesth Analg 1980; 67:550–551.
83. Stirt JA, Maggio W, Haworth C, Minton MD, Bedford RF. Vecuronium: effect on intracranial pressure and hemodynamics in neurosurgical patients. Anesthesiology 1987; 67(4):570–573.
84. Lanier WL, Milde JH, Michenfelder JD. The cerebral effects of pancuronium and atracurium in halothane-anesthetized dogs. Anesthesiology 1985; 63(6): 589–597.
85. Stoelting RK. The hemodynamic effects of pancuronium and D-tubocurarine in anesthetized patients. Anesthesiology 1972; 36(6):612–615.
86. Basta SJ, Savarese JJ, Ali HH, Moss J, Gionfriddo M. Histamine-releasing potencies of atracurium, dimethyl tubocurarine and tubocurarine. Br J Anaesth 1983; 55(suppl 1):105S–106S.
87. Debaene B, Plaud B, Dilly MP, Donati F. Residual paralysis in the PACU after a single intubating dose of nondepolarizing muscle relaxant with an intermediate duration of action. Anesthesiology 2003; 98(5):1042–1048.
88. Gray HS, Slater RM, Pollard BJ. The effect of acutely administered phenytoin on vecuronium-induced neuromuscular blockade. Anaesthesia 1989; 44(5):379–381.
89. Ornstein E, Matteo RS, Schwartz AE, Silverberg PA, Young WL, Diaz J. The effect of phenytoin on the magnitude and duration of neuromuscular block following atracurium or vecuronium. Anesthesiology 1987; 67(2):191–196.
90. Ornstein E, Matteo RS, Young WL, Diaz J. Resistance to metocurine-induced neuromuscular blockade in patients receiving phenytoin. Anesthesiology 1985; 63(3):294–298.
91. Durward QJ, Del Maestro RF, Amacher AL, Farrar JK. The influence of systemic arterial pressure and intracranial pressure on the development of cerebral vasogenic edema. J Neurosurg 1983; 59(5):803–809.
92. Ostergaard L, Hochberg FH, Rabinov JD, Sorensen AG, Lev M, Kim L, et al. Early changes measured by magnetic resonance imaging in cerebral blood flow, blood volume, and blood–brain barrier permeability following dexamethasone treatment in patients with brain tumors. J Neurosurg 1999; 90(2):300–305.
93. Leenders KL, Beaney RP, Brooks DJ, Lammertsma AA, Heather JD, McKenzie CG. Dexamethasone treatment of brain tumor patients: effects on regional cerebral blood flow, blood volume, and oxygen utilization. Neurology 1985; 35(11):1610–1616.
94. Macarthur DC, Buxton N. The management of brain tumours. J R Coll Surg Edinb 2001; 46(6):341–348.
95. Schiff D. *Pneumocystis pneumonia* in brain tumor patients: risk factors and clinical features. J Neurooncol 1996; 27(3):235–240.
96. Wen PY, Marks PW. Medical management of patients with brain tumors. Curr Opin Oncol 2002; 14(3): 299–307.
97. Zornow MH, Todd MM, Moore SS. The acute cerebral effects of changes in plasma osmolality and oncotic pressure. Anesthesiology 1987; 67(6):936–941.
98. Wise BL, Chater N. Effect of mannitol on cerebrospinal fluid pressure. The actions of hypertonic mannitol solutions and of urea compared. Arch Neurol 1961; 4:200–202.
99. Rudehill A, Gordon E, Ohman G, Lindqvist C, Andersson P. Pharmacokinetics and effects of mannitol on hemodynamics, blood and cerebrospinal fluid electrolytes, and osmolality during intracranial surgery. J Neurosurg Anesthesiol 1993; 5(1):4–12.
100. Cottrell JE, Robustelli A, Post K, Turndorf H. Furosemide- and mannitol-induced changes in intracranial pressure and serum osmolality and electrolytes. Anesthesiology 1977; 47(1):28–30.
101. Pollay M, Fullenwider C, Roberts PA, Stevens FA. Effect of mannitol and furosemide on blood–brain osmotic gradient and intracranial pressure. J Neurosurg 1983; 59(6):945–950.
102. Gemma M, Cozzi S, Tommasino C, Mungo M, Calvi MR, Cipriani A, et al. 7.5% Hypertonic saline versus 20% mannitol during elective neurosurgical

supratentorial procedures. J Neurosurg Anesthesiol 1997; 9(4):329–334..

103. Qureshi AI, Suarez JI, Bhardwaj A, Mirski M, Schnitzer MS, Hanley DF, et al. Use of hypertonic (3%) saline/acetate infusion in the treatment of cerebral edema: effect on intracranial pressure and lateral displacement of the brain. Crit Care Med 1998; 26(3): 440–446.
104. Shackford SR, Fortlage DA, Peters RM, Hollingsworth-Fridlund P, Sise MJ. Serum osmolar and electrolyte changes associated with large infusions of hypertonic sodium lactate for intravascular volume expansion of patients undergoing aortic reconstruction. Surg Gynecol Obstet 1987; 164(2):127–136.
105. Lofgren J. Editorial: airway pressure—neurosurgical aspects. Anesthesiology 1976; 45(3):269–272.
106. Surawicz TS, McCarthy BJ, Kupelian V, Jukich PJ, Bruner JM, Davis FG. Descriptive epidemiology of primary brain and CNS tumors: results from the Central Brain Tumor Registry of the United States, 1990–1994. Neurooncology 1999; 1(1):14–25.
107. DeAngelis LM. Brain tumors. N Engl J Med 2001; 344(2):114–123.
108. Sklar CA. Childhood brain tumors. J Pediatr Endocrinol Metab 2002; 15(suppl 2):669–673.
109. Reddy AT. Advances in biology and treatment of childhood brain tumors. Curr Neurol Neurosci Rep 2001; 1(2):137–143.
110. Burton E, Prados M. Management of primary malignant brain tumors in adults. In: Prados M, ed. Brain Cancer. Hamilton, Ont.: BC Decker, 2002:262–278.
111. Matz PG, Cobbs C, Berger MS. Intraoperative cortical mapping as a guide to the surgical resection of gliomas. J Neurooncol 1999; 42(3):233–245.
112. Feigenbaum F, Manz HJ, Platenberg LC, Martuza RL. Primary intrinsic tumors of the brain. In: Grossman RG, Loftus CM, eds. Principles of Neurosurgery. Philadelphia: Lippincott-Raven, 1999: 469–520.
113. Davis FG, McCarthy BJ, Freels S, Kupelian V, Bondy ML. The conditional probability of survival of patients with primary malignant brain tumors: surveillance, epidemiology, and end results (SEER) data. Cancer 1999; 85(2):485–491.
114. Simpson D. The recurrence of intracranial meningiomas after surgical treatment. J Neurochem 1957; 20(1): 22–39.
115. Olivero WC, Lister JR, Elwood PW. The natural history and growth rate of asymptomatic meningiomas: a review of 60 patients. J Neurosurg 1995; 83(2): 222–224.
116. DeAngelis LM. Primary central nervous system lymphomas. Curr Treat Options Oncol 2001; 2(4):309–318.
117. Graus F, Walker RW, Allen JC. Brain metastases in children. J Pediatr 1983; 103(4):558–561.
118. Patchell RA, Tibbs PA, Walsh JW, Dempsey RJ, Maruyama Y, Kryscio RJ, et al. A randomized trial of surgery in the treatment of single metastases to the brain. N Engl J Med 1990; 322(8):494–500.
119. Bindal RK, Sawaya R, Leavens ME, Lee JJ. Surgical treatment of multiple brain metastases. J Neurosurg 1993; 79(2):210–216.
120. Chin CT, Dillon WP. Magnetic resonance imaging of central nervous system tumors. In: Prados M, ed. Brain Cancer. Hamilton, Ont.: BC Decker, 2002: 104–128.
121. Preul MC, Caramanos Z, Collins DL, Villemure JG, Leblanc R, Olivier A, et al. Accurate, noninvasive diagnosis of human brain tumors by using proton magnetic resonance spectroscopy. Nat Med 1996; 2(3):323–325.
122. Gutin PH. Treatment of radiation necrosis of the brain. In: Gutin PH, Leibel SAS, eds. Radiation Injury to the Nervous System. New York: Raven Press, 1991:271–282.
123. Berger MS, Ghatan S, Haglund MM, Dobbins J, Ojemann GA. Low-grade gliomas associated with intractable epilepsy: seizure outcome utilizing electrocorticography during tumor resection. J Neurosurg 1993; 79(1):62–69.
124. Karnofsky D. Triethylene melamine in the treatment of neoplastic disease. Arch Intern Med 1951; 87: 477–516.
125. Wirtz CR, Albert FK, Schwaderer M, Heuer C, Staubert A, Tronnier VM, et al. The benefit of neuronavigation for neurosurgery analyzed by its impact on glioblastoma surgery. Neurol Res 2000; 22(4):354–360.
126. Krieger MD, Chandrasoma PT, Zee CS, Apuzzo ML. Role of stereotactic biopsy in the diagnosis and management of brain tumors. Semin Surg Oncol 1998; 14(1):13–25.
127. Teasdale G, Jennett B. Assessment of coma and impaired consciousness. A practical scale. Lancet 1974; 2(7872):81–84.
128. Bedford RF, Morris L, Jane JA. Intracranial hypertension during surgery for supratentorial tumor: correlation with preoperative computed tomography scans. Anesth Analg 1982; 61(5):430–433.
129. Reasoner DK, Todd MM, Scamman FL, Warner DS. The incidence of pneumocephalus after supratentorial craniotomy. Observations on the disappearance of intracranial air. Anesthesiology 1994; 80(5):1008–1012.
130. Andrews BT. General management and intensive care of the neurosurgical patient. In: Grossman RG, Loftus CM, eds. Principles of Neurosurgery. Philadelphia: Lippincott-Raven, 1999:3–14.
131. Drummond JC, Patel PM. Neurosurgical anesthesia. In: Miller RD, ed. Anesthesia. 5th ed. Vol. 2. Philadelphia: Churchill Livingstone, 2000:1895–1933.
132. Moorthy SS, Hilgenberg JC. Resistance to nondepolarizing muscle relaxants in paretic upper extremities of patients with residual hemiplegia. Anesth Analg 1980; 59(8):624–627.
133. Grant GA, Farrell D, Silbergeld DL. Continuous somatosensory evoked potential monitoring during

brain tumor resection. Report of four cases and review of the literature. J Neurosurg 2002; 97(3):709–713.

134. Sloan TB. Evoked potentials. In: Cottrell JE, Smith DS, eds. Anesthesia and Neurosurgery. St. Louis, MO: Mosby, 2001:183–200.

135. Patel SJ, Wen DYK, Haines SJ. Posterior fossa: surgical considerations. In: Cottrell JE, Smith DS, eds. Anesthesia and Neurosurgery. 4th ed. St Louis, MO: Mosby, 2001:319–333.

136. Miller RA. Neurosurgical anesthesia in the sitting position. A report of experience with 110 patients using controlled or spontaneous ventilation. Br J Anaesth 1972; 44:495–505.

137. Ellis SC, Bryan-Brown CW, Hyderally H. Massive swelling of the head and neck. Anesthesiology 1975; 42(1):102–103.

138. Teeple E, Maroon J, Rueger R. Hemimacroglossia and unilateral ischemic necrosis of the tongue in a long-duration neurosurgical procedure. Anesthesiology 1986; 64(6):845–846.

139. McAllister RG. Macroglossia—a positional complication. Anesthesiology 1974; 40(2):199–200.

140. Haines SJ, Maroon JC, Jannetta PJ. Supratentorial intracerebral hemorrhage following posterior fossa surgery. J Neurosurg 1978; 49(6):881–886.

141. Seiler RW, Zurbrugg HR. Supratentorial intracerebral hemorrhage after posterior fossa operation. Neurosurgery 1986; 18(4):472–474.

142. Black S, Ockert DB, Oliver WC Jr, Cucchiara RF. Outcome following posterior fossa craniectomy in patients in the sitting or horizontal positions. Anesthesiology 1988; 69(1):49–56.

143. Black S, Cucchiara RF. Tumor surgery. In: Cucchiara RF, Black S, Michenfelder JD, eds. Clinical Neuroanesthesia. New York: Churchill Livingstone, 1998:343–366.

144. Porter SS, Sanan A, Rengachary SS. Surgery and anesthesia of the posterior fossa. In: Albin MS, ed. Textbook of Neuroanesthesia with Neurosurgical and Neuroscience Perspectives. New York: McGraw-Hill, 1997:971–1008.

145. Burney RG, Winn R. Increased cerebrospinal fluid pressure during laryngoscopy and intubation for induction of anesthesia. Anesth Analg 1975; 54(5): 687–690.

146. Unni VK, Johnston RA, Young HS, McBride RJ. Prevention of intracranial hypertension during laryngoscopy and endotracheal intubation. Use of a second dose of thiopentone. Br J Anaesth 1984; 56(11): 1219–1223.

147. Hamill JF, Bedford RF, Weaver DC, Colohan AR. Lidocaine before endotracheal intubation: intravenous or laryngotracheal? Anesthesiology 1981; 55(5):578–581

148. Cottrell JE, Patel K, Turndorf H, Ransohoff J. Intracranial pressure changes induced by sodium nitroprusside in patients with intracranial mass lesions. J Neurosurg 1978; 48(3):329–331.

149. Ghani GA, Sung YF, Weinstein MS, Tindall GT, Fleischer AS. Effects of intravenous nitroglycerin on the intracranial pressure and volume pressure response. J Neurosurg 1983; 58(4):562–565.

150. Van Hemelrijck J, Van Aken H, Merckx L, Mulier J. Anesthesia for craniotomy: total intravenous anesthesia with propofol and alfentanil compared to anesthesia with thiopental sodium, isoflurane, fentanyl, and nitrous oxide. J Clin Anesth 1991; 3(2):131–136.

151. Gerlach K, Uhlig T, Huppe M, Nowak G, Schmitz A, Saager L, et al. Remifentanil–propofol versus sufentanil–propofol anaesthesia for supratentorial craniotomy: a randomized trial. Eur J Anaesthesiol 2003; 20(10):813–820..

152. Jamali S, Archer D, Ravussin P, Bonnafous M, David P, Ecoffey C. The effect of skull-pin insertion on cerebrospinal fluid pressure and cerebral perfusion pressure: influence of sufentanil and fentanyl. Anesth Analg 1997; 84(6):1292–1296.

153. Costello TG, Cormack JR. Clonidine premedication decreases hemodynamic responses to pin head-holder application during craniotomy. Anesth Analg 1998; 86(5):1001–1004.

154. Lipe HP, Mitchell PH. Positioning the patient with intracranial hypertension: how turning and head rotation affect the internal jugular vein. Heart Lung 1980; 9(6):1031–1037.

155. Hung OR, Hare GM, Brien S. Head elevation reduces head-rotation associated increased ICP in patients with intracranial tumours. Can J Anaesth 2000; 47(5):415–420.

156. Iwabuchi T, Sobata E, Suzuki M, Suzuki S, Yamashita M. Dural sinus pressure as related to neurosurgical positions. Neurosurgery 1983; 12(2):203–207.

157. Rosner MJ, Coley IB. Cerebral perfusion pressure, intracranial pressure, and head elevation. J Neurosurg 1986; 65(5):636–641.

158. Feldman Z, Kanter MJ, Robertson CS, Contant CF, Hayes C, Sheinberg MA, et al. Effect of head elevation on intracranial pressure, cerebral perfusion pressure, and cerebral blood flow in head-injured patients. J Neurosurg 1992; 76(2):207–211.

159. Zornow MH, Scheller MS. Intraoperative fluid management. In: Cottrell JE, Smith DS, eds. Anesthesia and Neurosurgery. St Louis, MO: Mosby, 2001:237–249.

160. Jelsma LF, McQueen JD. Effect of experimental water restriction on brain water. J Neurosurg 1967; 26(1): 35–40.

161. Prough DS, Bidani A. Hyperchloremic metabolic acidosis is a predictable consequence of intraoperative infusion of 0.9% saline. Anesthesiology 1999; 90(5): 1247–1249.

162. Greenfield JC Jr, Rembert JC, Tindall GT. Transient changes in cerebral vascular resistance during the Valsalva maneuver in man. Stroke 1984; 15(1): 76–79.

163. Shapiro HM, Galindo A, Wyte SR, Harris AB. Rapid intraoperative reduction of intracranial pressure with thiopentone. Br J Anaesth 1973; 45(10):1057–1062.
164. Herrick IA, Craen RA, Gelb AW, Miller LA, Kubu CS, Girvin JP, et al. Propofol sedation during awake craniotomy for seizures: patient-controlled administration versus neurolept analgesia. Anesth Analg 1997; 84(6):1285–1291.
165. Gignac E, Manninen PH, Gelb AW. Comparison of fentanyl, sufentanil and alfentanil during awake craniotomy for epilepsy. Can J Anaesth 1993; 40(5 Pt 1):421–424.
166. Blanshard HJ, Chung F, Manninen PH, Taylor MD, Bernstein M. Awake craniotomy for removal of intracranial tumor: considerations for early discharge. Anesth Analg 2001; 92(1):89–94.
167. Danks RA, Rogers M, Aglio LS, Gugino LD, Black PM. Patient tolerance of craniotomy performed with the patient under local anesthesia and monitored conscious sedation. Neurosurgery 1998; 42(1):28–34.
168. Sarang A, Dinsmore J. Anaesthesia for awake craniotomy—evolution of a technique that facilitates awake neurological testing. Br J Anaesth 2003; 90(2): 161–165.
169. Huncke K, Van de WB, Fried I, Rubinstein EH. The asleep–awake–asleep anesthetic technique for intraoperative language mapping. Neurosurgery 1998; 42(6): 1312–1316.
170. Taylor MD, Bernstein M. Awake craniotomy with brain mapping as the routine surgical approach to treating patients with supratentorial intraaxial tumors: a prospective trial of 200 cases. J Neurosurg 1999; 90(1):35–41.
171. Talke P, Caldwell JE, Brown R, Dodson B, Howley J, Richardson CA. A comparison of three anesthetic techniques in patients undergoing craniotomy for supratentorial intracranial surgery [table]. Anesth Analg 2002; 95(2):430–435.
172. Grillo P, Bruder N, Auquier P, Pellissier D, Gouin F. Esmolol blunts the cerebral blood flow velocity increase during emergence from anesthesia in neurosurgical patients [table]. Anesth Analg 2003; 96(4):1145–1149.
173. Marsh ML, Aidinis SJ, Naughton KV, Marshall LF, Shapiro HM. The technique of nitroprusside administration modifies the intracranial pressure response. Anesthesiology 1979; 51(6):538–541.
174. Ravussin P, Wilder-Smith OHG. Supratentorial masses: anesthetic considerations. In: Cottrell JE, Smith DS, eds. Anesthesia and Neurosurgery. 4th ed. St. Louis, MO: Mosby, 2001:297–317.
175. Dunbar PJ, Visco E, Lam AM. Craniotomy procedures are associated with less analgesic requirements than other surgical procedures. Anesth Analg 1999; 88(2):335–340.
176. Stoneham MD, Walters FJ. Post-operative analgesia for craniotomy patients: current attitudes among neuroanaesthetists. Eur J Anaesthesiol 1995; 12(6): 571–575.
177. Nguyen A, Girard F, Boudreault D, Fugere F, Ruel M, Moumdjian R, et al. Scalp nerve blocks decrease the severity of pain after craniotomy. Anesth Analg 2001; 93(5):1272–1276.
178. Bloomfield EL, Schubert A, Secic M, Barnett G, Shutway F, Ebrahim ZY. The influence of scalp infiltration with bupivacaine on hemodynamics and postoperative pain in adult patients undergoing craniotomy. Anesth Analg 1998; 87(3):579–582.
179. Taylor WA, Thomas NW, Wellings JA, Bell BA. Timing of postoperative intracranial hematoma development and implications for the best use of neurosurgical intensive care. J Neurosurg 1995; 82(1):48–50.
180. Marquardt G, Setzer M, Schick U, Seifert V. Cerebellar hemorrhage after supratentorial craniotomy. Surg Neurol 2002; 57(4):241–251.
181. Schubert A, Zornow MH, Drummond JC, Luerssen TG. Loss of cortical evoked responses due to intracranial gas during posterior fossa craniectomy in the seated position. Anesth Analg 1986; 65(2):203–206.
182. Petrozza PH, Prough DS. Postoperative and intensive care. In: Cottrell JE, Smith DS, eds. Anesthesia and Neurosurgery. St. Louis, MO: Mosby, 2001:623–661.
183. Ciric I, Ragin A, Baumgartner C, Pierce D. Complications of transsphenoidal surgery: results of a national survey, review of the literature, and personal experience. Neurosurgery 1997; 40(2):225–236.
184. Manninen PH, Tan TK. Postoperative nausea and vomiting after craniotomy for tumor surgery: a comparison between awake craniotomy and general anesthesia. J Clin Anesth 2002; 14(4):279–283.
185. Fabling JM, Gan TJ, Guy J, Borel CO, el Moalem HE, Warner DS. Postoperative nausea and vomiting. A retrospective analysis in patients undergoing elective craniotomy. J Neurosurg Anesthesiol 1997; 9(4): 308–312.
186. Fabling JM, Gan TJ, el Moalem HE, Warner DS, Borel CO. A randomized, double-blinded comparison of ondansetron, droperidol, and placebo for prevention of postoperative nausea and vomiting after supratentorial craniotomy. Anesth Analg 2000; 91(2):358–361.
187. Madenoglu H, Yildiz K, Dogru K, Kurtsoy A, Guler G, Boyaci A. Randomized, double-blinded comparison of tropisetron and placebo for prevention of postoperative nausea and vomiting after supratentorial craniotomy. J Neurosurg Anesthesiol 2003; 15(2):82–86.
188. Hamilton MG, Hull RD, Pineo GF. Venous thromboembolism in neurosurgery and neurology patients: a review. Neurosurgery 1994; 34(2):280–296.
189. Macdonald RL, Amidei C, Lin G, Munshi I, Baron J, Weir BK, et al. Safety of perioperative subcutaneous heparin for prophylaxis of venous thromboembolism in patients undergoing craniotomy. Neurosurgery 1999; 45(2):245–251.
190. Goldhaber SZ, Dunn K, Gerhard-Herman M, Park JK, Black PM. Low rate of venous thromboembolism

after craniotomy for brain tumor using multimodality prophylaxis. Chest 2002; 122(6):1933–1937.

191. Chan KH, Lai EC, Tuen H, Ngan JH, Mok F, Fan YW, et al. Prospective double-blind placebo-controlled randomized trial on the use of ranitidine in preventing postoperative gastroduodenal complications in high-risk neurosurgical patients. J Neurosurg 1995; 82(3):413–417.
192. Constantini S, Cotev S, Rappaport ZH, Pomeranz S, Shalit MN. Intracranial pressure monitoring after elective intracranial surgery. A retrospective study of 514 consecutive patients. J Neurosurg 1988; 69(4): 540–544.
193. Rosenwasser RH, Kleiner LI, Krzeminski JP, Buchheit WA. Intracranial pressure monitoring in the posterior fossa: a preliminary report. J Neurosurg 1989; 71(4):503–505.
194. Silverberg GD. Intracranial pressure monitoring. In: Wilkins RHRSS, ed. Neurosurgery. New York: McGraw-Hill, 1996:185–191.
195. Mayhall CG, Archer NH, Lamb VA, Spadora AC, Baggett JW, Ward JD, et al. Ventriculostomy-related infections. A prospective epidemiologic study. N Engl J Med 1984; 310(9):553–559.
196. Drummond JC, Todd MM. Acute sinus arrhythmia during surgery in the fourth ventricle: an indicator of brain-stem irritation. Anesthesiology 1984; 60(3): 232–235.
197. Albin MS, Carroll RG, Maroon JC. Clinical considerations concerning detection of venous air embolism. Neurosurgery 1978; 3(3):380–384.
198. Papadopoulos G, Kuhly P, Brock M, Rudolph KH, Link J, Eyrich K. Venous and paradoxical air embolism in the sitting position. A prospective study with transesophageal echocardiography. Acta Neurochir (Wien) 1994; 126(2–4):140–143.
199. Cabezudo JM, Gilsanz F, Vaquero J, Areitio E, Martinez R. Air embolism from wounds from a pin-type head-holder as a complication of posterior fossa surgery in the sitting position. Case report. J Neurosurg 1981; 55(1):147–148.
200. Albin MS. Air embolism. In: Albin MS, ed. Textbook of Neuroanesthesia with Neurosurgical and Neuroscience Perspectives. New York: McGraw-Hill, 1997: 1009–1025.
201. Losasso TJ, Muzzi DA, Dietz NM, Cucchiara RF. Fifty percent nitrous oxide does not increase the risk of venous air embolism in neurosurgical patients operated upon in the sitting position. Anesthesiology 1992; 77(1):21–30.
202. Matjasko J, Petrozza P, Cohen M, Steinberg P. Anesthesia and surgery in the seated position: analysis of 554 cases. Neurosurgery 1985; 17(5):695–702.
203. Maroon JC, Albin MS. Air embolism diagnosed by Doppler ultrasound. Anesth Analg 1974; 53(3): 399–402.
204. Smith DS, Osborn I, Adams RW. Posterior fossa: anesthetic considerations. In: Cottrell JE, Smith DS, eds. Anesthesia and Neurosurgery. St. Louis, MO: Mosby, 2001:335–351.
205. Bunegin L, Albin MS, Helsel PE, Hoffman A, Hung TK. Positioning the right atrial catheter: a model for reappraisal. Anesthesiology 1981; 55(4):343–348.
206. Reasoner DK, Dexter F, Hindman BJ, Subieta A, Todd MM. Somatosensory evoked potentials correlate with neurological outcome in rabbits undergoing cerebral air embolism. Stroke 1996; 27(10):1859–1864.
207. Dutka AJ. A review of the pathophysiology and potential application of experimental therapies for cerebral ischemia to the treatment of cerebral arterial gas embolism. Undersea Biomed Res 1985; 12(4):403–421.
208. Couldwell WT, Simard MF, Weiss MH. Pituitary tumors. In: Grossman RG, Loftus CM, eds. Principles of Neurosurgery. Philadelphia: Lippincott-Raven, 1999:533–556.
209. Culley DJ, Crosby G. Central nervous system disorders. In: Sweitzer B, ed. Handbook of Preoperative Assessment and Management. Philadelphia: Lippincott Williams & Wilkins, 2000:255–275.
210. Hill JN, Gershon NI, Gargiulo PO. Total spinal blockade during local anesthesia of the nasal passages. Anesthesiology 1983; 59(2):144–146.
211. Domino KB. Care of the acutely unstable patient. In: Cottrell JE, Smith DS, eds. Anesthesia and Neurosurgery. St. Louis, MO: Mosby, 2001:251–274.

19

Perioperative Management of Spinal Tumors

ROBERT J. BOHINSKI
Department of Neurosurgery, The University of Cincinnati College of Medicine and The Mayfield Clinic and Spine Institute, Cincinnati, Ohio, U.S.A.

LAURENCE D. RHINES
Department of Neurosurgery, The University of Texas M.D. Anderson Cancer Center, Houston, Texas, U.S.A.

ZIYA GOKASLAN
Department of Neurosurgery, Johns Hopkins University, Baltimore, Maryland, U.S.A.

Patients with cancer of the spine present many challenges to the surgeon, anesthesiologist, and critical care physician. Cancer affecting the spine may result in neurologic dysfunction and/or spinal instability that significantly impact the perioperative management of these patients. Airway management is made more difficult by the limited range of motion mandated in patients with cervical spine instability. Transfer and positioning of patients is more complicated when spinal segments are deemed unstable. If spinal cord or nerve root function is at risk during surgery, then neurophysiologic monitoring may be necessary, adding to the special requirements of anesthetic management and the overall complexity of patient monitoring.

Involvement of the spine with tumor can be extensive with significant extension into paraspinal tissues and body cavities such as the thorax, abdomen, and pelvis (Fig. 1). Surgical approaches to the spine are highly varied and depend upon the level of involvement and the extent of disease. Transoral/transmadibular, anterior cervical, transsternal, transthoracic, transabdominal, retroperitoneal, dorsal, and combined approaches, all pose unique perioperative challenges. The hypervascularity of many spinal tumors combined with the extensive dissection required to remove them and the complex reconstructive procedures that follow often results in extensive blood loss. Operative time may exceed 10 hr and in some cases a staged approach is used when surgery is expected to require two full days. The successful completion of complex spine tumor surgery depends upon the patient's ability to tolerate enormous physiologic stresses. Patients must be properly selected and be in optimal medical condition prior to surgery if uncomplicated intraoperative and postoperative courses are to be realized.

I. HISTORY AND PHYSICAL EXAMINATION

The purpose of the preoperative evaluation is to identify patient factors that affect surgical risk and thereby reduce perioperative morbidity and mortality.

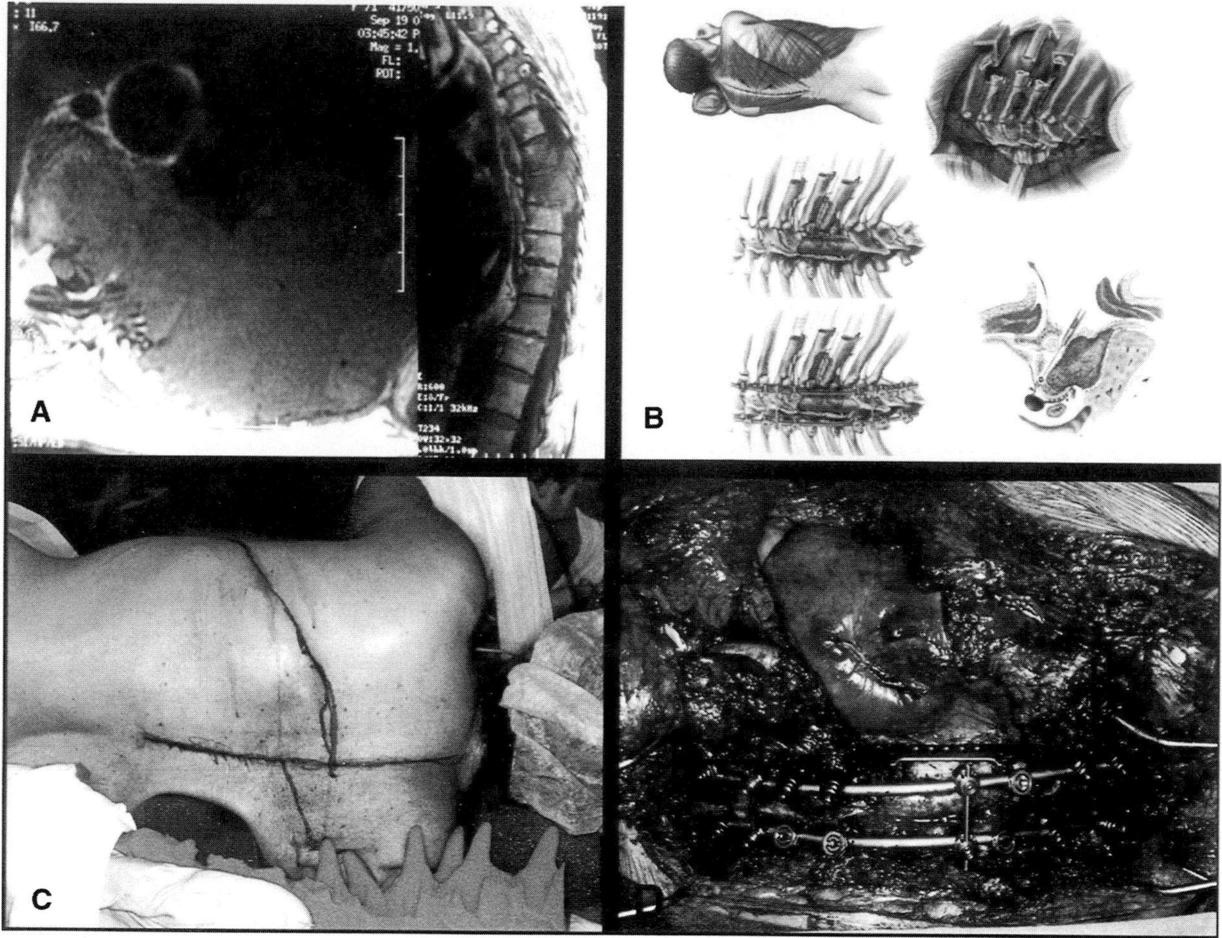

Figure 1 (A) Axial and sagittal T1-weighted MRI image of the thoracic spine in a patient with nonsmall cell lung cancer. The tumor originates in the lung and extends directly into the chest wall, spine, and paraspinal soft tissues. (B) Artist's depiction of the combined anterior/posterior approach to the spine. The patient is placed in the lateral position and a combined thoracotomy incision and posterior midline spinal incision is used to gain simultaneous access to the intrathoracic compartment and the posterior spine. (C) Intraoperative photograph of the aforementioned patient prior to draping. Patient is in lateral decubitus postion with the left side up. The head is cushioned so that the neck is in neutral position. Note the axillary roll beneath the right chest. The thoracotomy incision and midline spine incision meet at a 90° angle. (D) Intraoperative photograph after tumor resection, spinal reconstruction, and stabilization. The spine is visualized from posteriorly as well as through the chest. Note that the diseased portion of the lung has been resected and the chest wall has been removed. The thecal sac has been completely decompressed. Anterior and posterior spinal stabilization has been placed.

A thorough preoperative evaluation often uncovers patient health problems that require attention prior to the proposed surgery or that may alter the perioperative care. A complete history and physical should be obtained, including the history of the present illness, past medical history, and past surgical/medical treatment history. The history and physical alone should provide all the information needed to guide further testing or treatment prior to surgery. A good perioperative/ anesthetic plan relies heavily on the quality of this information. Although all organ systems are important to the success of an operation, the status of the cardiovascular, pulmonary, and neurologic systems will have a major impact on patient management and outcome. If cardiac or pulmonary disease is suspected, then consultation with specialists in these areas is mandatory as specialized care in the perioperative period will likely be necessary.

II. PATIENT POSITIONING

Surgery on the spine spans a wide spectrum of interventions. Surgery may involve interventions that are transoral, transmandibular, anterior cervical, transthoracic, transabdominal, or transpelvic. The patient may be positioned supine, prone, lateral, or sitting, and the position of the patient may need to be changed during surgery.

Essentially all patients undergoing spine surgery for treatment of a spinal neoplasm will be under general anesthesia. One exception would be the treatment of some pathologic fractures with either vertebroplasty or kyphoplasty (1). Inherent to inducing general endotracheal anesthesia comes the task of safely intubating the patient who may have cervical spine instability. Patients with cervical spine instability require awake, fiberoptic intubation. Patients are given a topical anesthetic and the endotracheal tube is placed under direct fiberoptic visualization while maintaining the neck in a neutral position. The patient's motor exam is carefully monitored during awake intubation. If any change in the exam is noted, then interventions are either stopped or reversed.

Prone procedures make immediate or emergency access to the airway problematic. Endotracheal tubes and vascular access lines should be tightly secured prior to patient positioning. In case of airway compromise, a gurney should always be kept nearby so that the patient could be turned supine for emergent airway management. The prone position can also lead to an increase in intra-abdominal and intrathoracic pressure. As a consequence, there is increased ventilatory pressures and decreased cardiac stroke volume. The increased abdominal pressures also increase venous pressures, which lead to increased blood loss. For these reasons, patients should be positioned on a Jackson table, four-poster frame, or equivalent device that allows the abdomen to hang freely (Fig. 2). When placing the patient in the prone position, care must be taken to support the head with the neck in a neutral position, while avoiding direct pressure on the eyes. Appropriate padding at the elbows, knees, and feet will prevent nerve and soft-tissue injury. Note that the arms are positioned with enough padding so that they do not hang, and the shoulders are abducted no more than 90° in order to avoid brachial plexus stretch. For upper thoracic and cervical procedures, the head may be fixed in a Mayfield skull clamp, and the arms may be tucked to allow the surgeon unimpeded access to the surgical site. Again, padding of the elbows, wrists, and hands is crucial to decrease the risk of nerve/soft-tissue injury.

The sitting position is an alternative to the prone position for posterior cervical procedures (Fig. 3). The main advantage of this approach is less blood loss from the lower venous pressures associated with an upright position. The main disadvantage is the potential for venous air embolism. Intraoperative monitoring for air embolism is mandatory and a central venous catheter that may be used to aspirate an air embolism should be placed preoperatively.

Patients are positioned supine for anterior cervical, transsternal, and midline transabdominal/pelvic procedures. The anterior cervical approach requires that the patient's arms be tucked at their side, limiting the anesthesiologist's access to intravenous lines and monitoring equipment. Airway interventions are impeded by the proximity of the surgical field to the endotracheal tube. The lower thoracic, lumbar, and sacral spine may be accessed in a supine position. Inherent in this approach are the anesthetic risks that accompany the increased fluid requirements that accompany intra-abdominal surgery, and the surgeon's need to retract on visceral organs, aorta, and vena cava. Excessive retraction on the intra-abdominal and intrapelvic great vessels (aorta, vena cava, iliac arteries and veins) can adversely affect circulation to the lower extremities. We have employed frequent pedal pulse checks or continuous pulse oximetry on the bilateral great toes to monitor lower extremity perfusion during lengthy procedures.

The lateral position is used to approach the anterior aspects of the thoracic or lumbar spine or when access to both the anterior and posterior spine is desired. Proper positioning is shown in Fig. 4. The lateral position is inherently unstable so steps must be taken to secure the patient. A bean bag combined with a strap over the hips is usually sufficient. The head is cushioned with the neck in neutral position and the arms are placed at an angle of 90° with respect to the torso so as not to stretch the brachial plexus. The elbows are padded to protect the ulnar nerves. An axillary roll must be placed to protect the neurovascular structures in the axilla from injury. Lastly, the hips and knees are flexed and cushions are placed under the fibular head of the lower leg and between the legs. A double-lumen endotracheal tube allows selective ventilation of the dependent lung so that the nondependent lung can be easily retracted from the surgical field. During intrathoracic or intra-abdominal approaches, sudden hypotension without bleeding may occur. In most cases, this is related to decreased blood return to the right side of the heart. The common causes are retractors placed on the inferior vena cava. The solution is to remove the retractors, especially those retracting the inferior vena cava, liver, or spleen and to wait for the blood pressure to normalize. Failure of the blood pressure to normalize after removal of retractors should raise suspicion for myocardial ischemia, pulmonary embolism, or collapsed lung.

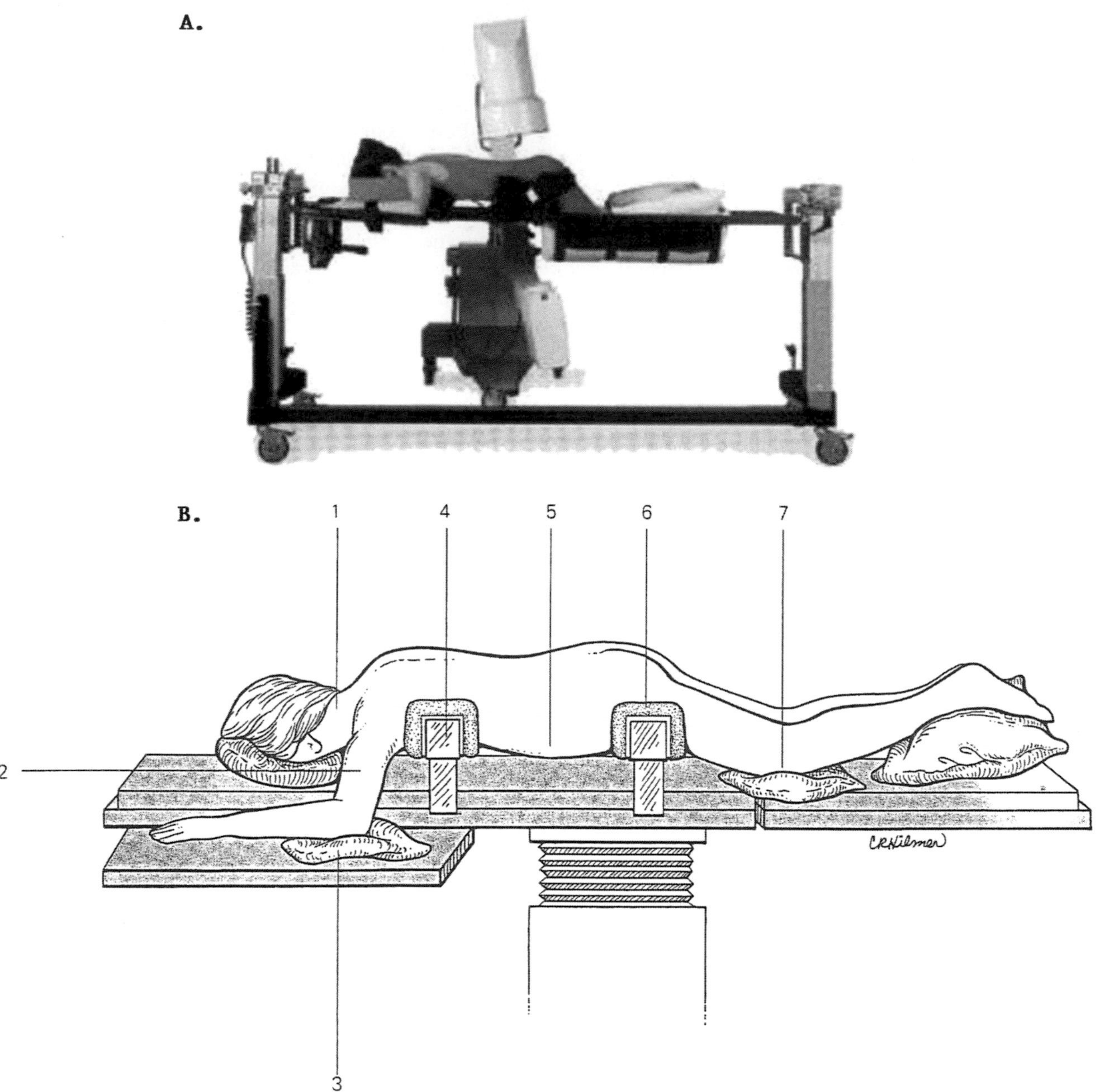

A prone position utilizing a four poster frame.

1. The neck is in a neutral position and not hyperextended.
2. The arms are positioned at 90° or less of adduction and slightly hanging down.
3. The ulnar nerves are padded.
4. The proximal pads will support the chest just distal to the axilla and slightly lateral to the nipple line.
5. This position allows the abdomen to hang free.
6. The distal pads are against the proximal thighs just distal to the iliac crests.
7. The hips and knees are flexed slightly.

Figure 2 (A) Photograph of a volunteer positioned prone on the Jackson spinal surgery table. (B) Artist's depiction of a patient positioned prone on a four poster frame. *Source*: From Refs. 2 and 3.

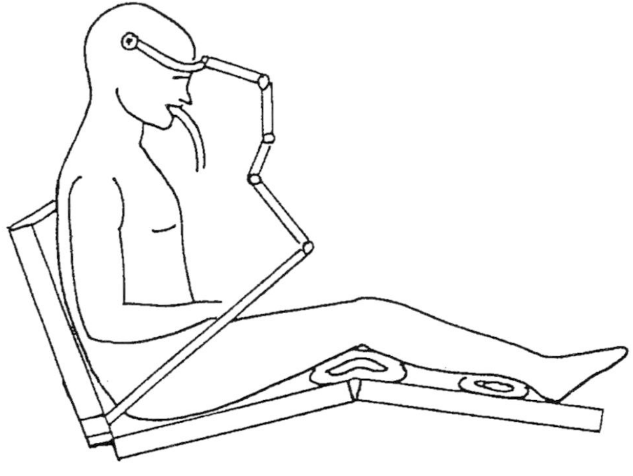

Figure 3 Artist's depiction of a patient placed in the sitting position. *Source*: From Ref. 4.

III. INTRAOPERATIVE NEUROLOGIC MONITORING

In many spinal procedures, it is beneficial to be able to monitor neurologic function during the operation. Intraoperative monitoring of neurologic function allows the surgeon to work around vital neural elements with some degree of confidence that the required surgical manipulations are not harmful. If monitoring suggests that neural elements are being affected by the surgery, then the surgeon can change his technique or reverse previous maneuvers. This presents the anesthesiologist with unique anesthetic concerns. Nonparalytic anesthesia can result in patient movement if there is a mismatch between the level of anesthesia and the level of surgical stimulation. A greater degree of vigilance is thus required by the anesthesiologist in order to maintain a quiet surgical field.

Somatosensory evoked potentials (SSEPs) are the electrophysiologic responses of the central nervous system to the stimulation of a peripheral nerve. Most commonly, the response to peripheral nerve

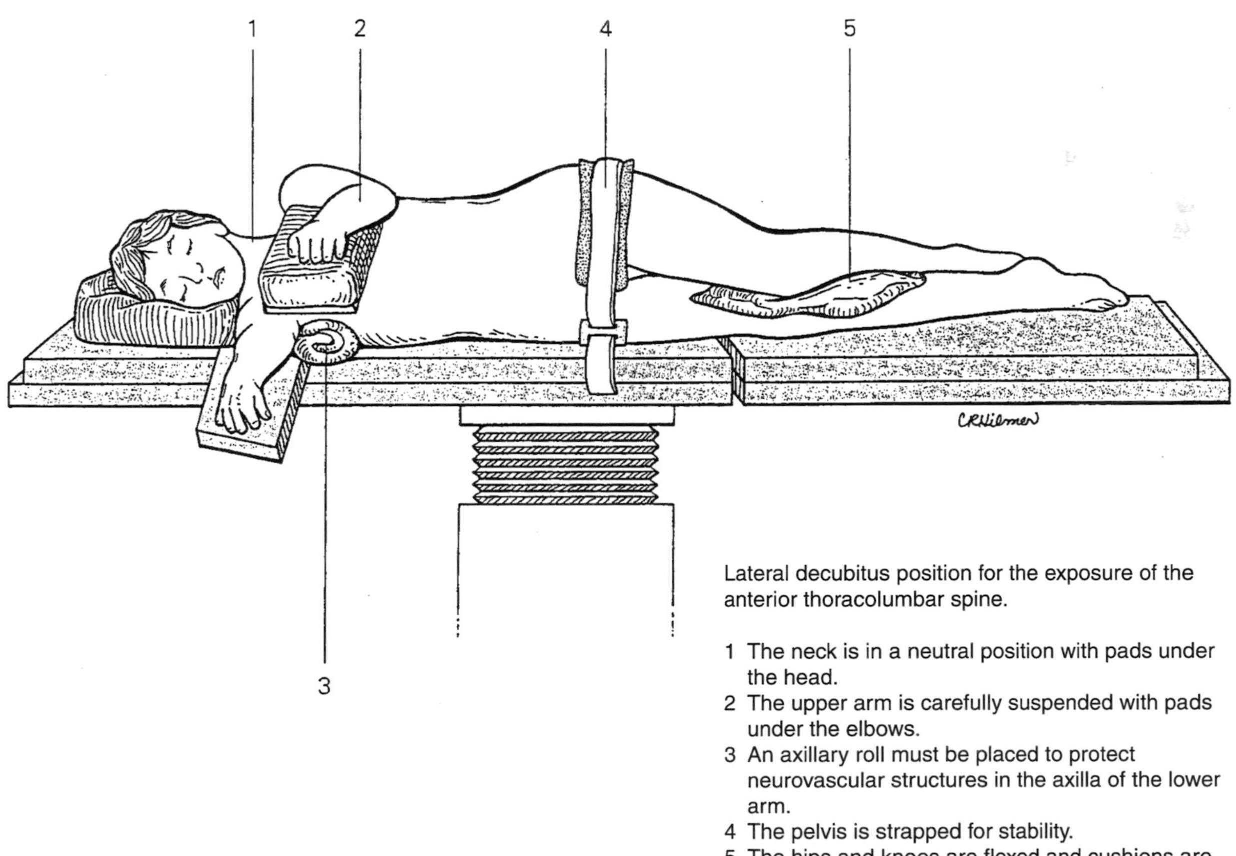

Figure 4 Artist's depiction of a patient in the lateral decubitus position. *Source*: From Ref. 5.

stimulation is monitored at the level of the cerebral cortex. Peripheral nerves that are commonly used for stimulation are the tibial, peroneal, and median. The usefulness of SSEPs lies in their ability to demonstrate the functional integrity of neural pathways in an anesthetized patient. Numerous cases have been reported wherein early recognition of changes in SSEPs have changed the surgeon's technique and apparently prevented neurologic injury (6–8). In the operating room, baseline SSEPs are obtained after the induction of anesthesia. Serial recordings are then obtained throughout the surgery and compared to the baseline. Physiologic changes may alter the quality of SSEP recordings. These changes include hypotension, hypothermia, anemia, hypoxia, and changes in pCO_2. Changes in the depth of anesthesia can also alter SSEP recordings. Every effort should be made to avoid fluctuations in inhaled gas concentration and bolus injection of hypnotic agents during the period of surgery that is deemed most at risk for neurologic injury (e.g., during decompression and placement of spinal instrumentation). In general, inhaled agents will affect SSEP monitoring more so than intravenous agents. An anesthetic technique that relies on the use of a narcotic agent will generally result in the least amount of interference with SSEPs.

Motor evoked potentials (MEPs) monitor the integrity of motor pathways. The MEPs are a measure of the response of peripheral motor nerves and the muscles they supply to stimulation centrally. When SSEPs and MEPs are used together, information about the integrity of both sensory and motor pathways is possible in the anesthetized patient. The MEPs are very sensitive to anesthetic agents. In particular, isoflurane and propofol both cause significant depression of MEPs. Most authors recommend a fentanyl/nitrous oxide technique supplemented with a continuous etomidate infusion (9).

Latency increase of 10% and an amplitude drop of more than 50% in SSEPs are warning signs that spinal cord function may be compromised (4,10). If worrisome monitoring changes are encountered, then the precise time that they occurred should be noted and correlated with any particular event such as spinal cord retraction or pedicle screw placement. The surgeon should immediately consider releasing retraction, removing implants, or reversing any corrective reduction that has been made. Correction of hypotension, hypothermia, hypoxia, and other adverse anesthetic events should also be performed rapidly. Halothane is one inhaled anesthetic that should not be used in conjunction with SSEP monitoring due to its negative effect on evoked potentials; however, a low concentration of isoflurane can often be used during SSEP monitoring.

IV. POSTOPERATIVE NEUROLOGIC MONITORING

Every attempt should be made to awaken the patient for neurologic assessment prior to leaving the operating room. Patients not suitable for extubation should still be allowed to awaken for neurologic exam prior to leaving the operating room. If the patient demonstrates a neurologic deficit, then a CT myelogram through the operated levels should be obtained immediately to rule out the possibility of malpositioned instrumentation or wound hematoma. If myelography is not readily available, then a plain CT exam may suffice. A CT study will prevent the surgeon from having to remove all the implanted hardware. If a mass lesion has not been identified and the cord has been lengthened or stretched by a reduction maneuver, then the maneuver should be reversed, returning the cord to its preoperative morphology. Every attempt should be made to maintain fixation, since spinal instability may lead to further problems.

Following major reconstructive surgery for spine tumors, patients should be observed in the intensive care unit for 24–48 hr. Neurologic examination is performed every 1 hr. Motor power in all four extremities and sensory exam are most important to check. Rarely, patients will have a delayed onset of neurologic deficit. In these cases, hypotension and spinal cord ischemia may be the culprit. The immediate response to a delayed postoperative deficit should be to aggressively treat any hypotension if present and to then obtain a CT scan of the operated site to rule out the development of a hematoma or instrumentation failure. If CT myelography is obtained, then cerebrospinal fluid (CSF) should be removed prior to instillation of the intrathecal contrast to avoid the potential for increasing extramural spinal cord pressure, which could further compromise spinal cord perfusion. A lumbar drain may be left in place to divert CSF and reduce extramural spinal cord pressure for up to 72 hr if spinal cord ischemia is suspected (11). Sacrifice of thoracic nerve roots and corresponding radicular arteries during tumor removal has the potential to cause relative spinal cord ischemia. In case of nerve root/radicular artery sacrifice, intraoperative and postoperative hypotension should be avoided and reversed aggressively if encountered.

V. COAGULATION ABNORMALITIES/ BLOOD LOSS

Spinal procedures may result in substantial blood loss. Excessive bleeding at the surgical site increases the chances of wound infection and poor wound healing.

The heart and lungs are also stressed by the large volume shifts. Every attempt should be made to identify patients at risk for excessive intraoperative bleeding. In addition to verifying the prothrombin time and partial thromboplastin time, one should consider checking platelet function directly by obtaining a bleeding time. Patients undergoing chemotherapy may have low platelet counts or altered platelet function. Nonsteroidal anti-inflammatory drugs also impair platelet function and should be stopped at least one week prior to a major spinal procedure.

Certain types of tumors are particularly hypervascular and may produce significant blood loss during resection. Renal cell carcinoma, thyroid carcinoma, myeloma, and some sarcomas can be highly vascularized. Preoperative intravascular embolization can drastically reduce the blood supply to these tumors, there by decreasing the blood loss during resection.

Surgical technique plays an important role in blood loss. Injecting the skin with a 1:100,000 solution containing epinephrine can dramatically reduce the amount of blood lost during the creation of a long surgical incision. If used, it is extremely important to alert the anesthesiologist, as significant hyperdynamic effects can occur if inadvertently injected directly into an artery or vein. This technique will also limit the excessive use of cautery on the skin. Meticulous attention should be payed to hemostasis and to dissection in avascular planes. Anterior spinal surgery often results in less blood loss than the classic posterior approach and may, therefore, affect surgical decision making in certain cases. In most cases, maintaining a mean arterial pressure around 65–70 mm Hg is recommended to reduce bleeding. If generalized bleeding is more than expected, then the position of the patient should be checked. The patient may be malpositioned with increased pressure on the abdominal viscera, resulting in high venous pressure. By leaving the abdomen free in the prone position, there is decreased inferior vena cava pressure and thus decreased venous plexus filling around the spine (12–14).

Antifibrinolytic agents are also an effective means of reducing blood loss, particularly when microvascular oozing from a large open wound is the problem. Aprotonin is a serine protease inhibitor, but the exact mechanism by which it improves hemostasis is unknown. Lentschener et al. (15,16) reported that aprotonin reduced blood loss and transfusion requirements during posterior fusion of the lumbar spine. Epsilon amino-caproic acid (EACA—Amicar) also has a reported benefit in reducing blood loss in patients undergoing spine surgery (17). However, not all studies confirm the efficacy of either amicar or aprotonin (18). Although intraoperative blood salvage is another technique used to avoid or minimize the need for homologous transfusion, its use in the presence of tumor cells is controversial.

The suspicion of a hypocoagulable state or disseminated intravascular coagulation (DIC) is heralded by the presence of diffuse oozing without the formation of blood clots. This usually happens in the context of prolonged surgery and excessive bleeding with massive transfusion of blood products (more than one blood volume). The DIC is confirmed by elevated prothrombin and partial thromboplastin times, low platelet count, and elevated fibrin split products. Treatment of DIC is facilitated by early recognition and transfusion of fresh frozen plasma, cryoprecipitate, platelets, and red blood cells. DIC is best prevented by good surgical technique that minimizes blood loss and by the staging of procedures that will require obligatory high blood loss and extended operative time.

VI. ANTIBIOTIC PROPHYLAXIS

Postoperative wound infections following spine surgery occur with varying incidence depending on the type of surgery performed. For simple lumbar discectomy, the incidence is approximately 1%, whereas for complex posterior instrumented fusion the incidence is between 3% and 8% (19–21). Malnourished and immuno-compromised individuals are at increased risk for developing postoperative wound infection. Prophylactic antibiotic therapy has been shown to reduce the incidence of infection after spinal surgery (22). Antibiotic prophylaxis reduces infection rates by 50–70% compared with baseline rates (22). The optimal choice of antibiotic prophylaxis is based on the most likely organism to be involved in the infection for the type of surgery being performed. In most clean spine cases, resident gram-positive skin flora such as *Staphylococcus aureus* and *S. epidermidis* are anticipated. Given their safety, antimicrobial spectra, low incidence of side effects, and pharmacokinetic profile, first generation cephalosporins are the preferred choice of antibiotic prophylaxis. Cefazolin, in particular, has become the primary choice in clean surgical procedures (23).

In order for antibiotic prophylaxis to be effective, it is critical to administer the drug at a time prior to the skin incision such that the optimal tissue concentration is present when the skin incision is actually made. In general, complete administration of antibiotic prior to but within 2 hr of skin incision is most effective (24). In addition, adequate antibiotic levels should be maintained throughout the duration of the procedure by timed redosing (23). Continued postoperative dosing for up to 72 hr after surgery has been employed but is no more effective than a single preoperative dose and it will lead to the proliferation of resistant strains of bacteria (25). Although vancomycin is more effective than first generation cephalosporins against gram-positive organisms, use of vancomycin should be limited because of its increased potential for toxicity, cost, and development of resistance (26). Vancomycin, however, is a reasonable alternative to cefazolin in patients with penicillin/cephalosporin allergy.

VII. MALNUTRITION

Patients undergoing major spine surgery are at significant risk of malnutrition postoperatively (27). Extensive surgical wounds significantly increase caloric requirements and optimal wound healing depends on adequately meeting these needs. A normal active adult may require between 2500 and 3000 calories/day, whereas the surgical patient may need as much as 6000 calories/day (28,29). Two of the most common complications following major reconstructive spine surgery are infection and wound healing problems, and malnutrition may play a significant role in this.

Many patients requiring surgery for spine tumors may already be malnourished prior to surgery (29–31). A postoperative ileus, lasting 2–5 days, is often present after major spinal surgery, particularly after anterior approaches to the spine. For these reasons, consideration should be given to aggressive enteral or total parenteral nutrition before and after surgery. Patients should not be allowed to maintain a catabolic state in the immediate postoperative period. For patients who cannot tolerate adequate oral intake on the first or second postoperative day, then a nasogastric feeding tube should be placed and tube feeds given at caloric goal. For patients undergoing anterior and posterior surgery in a staged fashion, it is probably best to place a central venous line preoperatively and to start total parenteral nutrition immediately after surgery (32,33). Because depletion of nutritional parameters appears to correlate with an increased incidence of wound complications, the maintenance of adequate nutrition may result in a decrease in these complications (29–31,34).

VIII. PREVENTION OF THROMBOEMBOLISM

Venous thromboembolism remains a significant cause of morbidity and mortality in surgical patients. In adult patients undergoing major reconstructive spine surgery, the incidence of deep venous thrombosis has been reported to vary from 0.3% to 25% using Doppler imaging techniques as a screening tool (35–38). Patients with spinal cord injury are known to have a significant incidence of pulmonary embolus (39). Immobilization increases the incidence of deep vein thrombosis. In one study, the incidence of symptomatic pulmonary embolism following anterior/posterior spine surgery was 6% (40). Factors that may contribute to the development of deep vein thrombosis in postoperative spine patients include prolonged immobilization, extended operative times, and prone positioning that may lead to compression of femoral veins. Also, despite modern internal fixation methods, patients may be slow to mobilize after major spine surgery because of postoperative pain and critical care needs.

Unfortunately, the true incidence of thromboembolic complications in spine surgery patients remains unknown, and the need for postoperative prophylaxis is not yet widely accepted. Use of intermittent compression boots appears to provide a reasonable level of primary prevention (41). One study, however, found an unacceptably high rate of symptomatic pulmonary embolism (6%) in patients undergoing anterior and posterior spine surgery treated with compression boots alone (40).

Hesitancy to use prophylactic pharmacologic anticoagulation in spine surgery patients is due to the theoretic risk of bleeding complications, which may result in epidural hematoma and spinal cord/cauda equina compression. Currently, limited evidence suggests that bleeding complications associated with the use of low molecular weight heparin are not significant in patients felt to be at greatest risk—those undergoing craniotomy (42). Also, the combination of compression stockings plus treatment with low dose heparin decreases the incidence of symptomatic deep vein thrombosis (43). Limited reporting indicates that the use of low molecular weight heparin is safe and effective in preventing deep vein thrombosis and its complications in patients undergoing spine surgery (44). Based on the available evidence, some feel that it is safe and effective to treat postoperative spine patients with compression boots and subcutaneous enoxaparin, 30 mg every 12 hr. Enoxaparin may be given just prior to surgery or started the morning after surgery.

IX. PAIN CONTROL

Patients undergoing major reconstructive spine surgery after tumor resection are at high risk for experiencing significant postoperative pain as a result of the extent of surgery that has been performed often involving extensive muscle dissection both anteriorly over the abdomen and thorax and dorsally over the paraspinal support muscles. Poorly controlled pain has a major impact on the development of other postoperative complications, as the patient's ability to cough, breathe, ambulate, and participate actively in their postoperative recovery will be extremely limited if pain is severe. Immediate and long-term patient outcome may be improved as a result of optimized postoperative analgesia (45,46). Adequate postoperative pain control is increasingly recognized as an integral part of perioperative patient management. For the spinal surgery patient in particular, pain control will likely play a major role in postoperative care. The use of patient-controlled analgesia, local anesthetic during wound closure, intercostal blocks, and epidural or intrathecal injections have all been successful in controlling postoperative pain and improving patient outcome and satisfaction. Patient-controlled analgesia is an excellent alternative to traditional nurse-administered bolus injections of opiod. Patient-controlled analgesia allows the patient to anticipate painful stimuli such as ambulation and dressing changes and to conveniently self-administer medication prior to an escalation in pain responses (45). The availability of a specialized "pain service" that relies on the expertise of uniquely trained anesthesiologists and nurses has greatly enhanced the efficacy of postoperative pain management (46,47).

REFERENCES

1. Fourney DR, Schomer DF, Nader R, Chlan-Fourney J, Suki D, Ahrar K, Rhines LD, Gokaslan ZL. Percutaneous vertebroplasty and kyphoplasty for painful vertebral body fractures in cancer patients. J Neurosurg 2003; 98:21–30.
2. Branch CL. Operative positioning and retraction. In: Benzel EC, ed. Surgical Exposure of the Spine: An Extensile Approach Park Ridge, IL: American Association of Neurological Surgens, 1995: 154.
3. An HS, Botte MJ, Byrna T, Garfin SR. Patient positioning and application of tongs and halo. In: An Atlas of Surgery of the Spine. Philadelphia: Lippincot-Raven Publishers, 1998: 3.
4. Zileli M, Benxel EC, Alberstone CD. Surgical incision, positioning, and retraction.In: Spine Surgery: Techniques, Complication Avoidance and Management.New York: Churchill Livingstone, 1999: 1162.
5. An HS, Botte MJ, Byrna T, Garfin SR. Patient positioning and application of tongs and halo. In: An Atlas of Surgery to the Spine. Philadelphia: Lippincott-Raven Publishers, 1998: 4.
6. Apel DM, Marrero G, King J, Tolo VT, Bassett GS. Avoiding paraplegia during anterior spinal surgery. The role of somatosensory evoked potential monitoring with temporary occlusion of segmental spinal arteries. Spine 1991; 16:S365–S370.
7. Bieber E, Tolo V, Uematsu S. Spinal cord monitoring during posterior spinal instrumentation and fusion. Clin Orthop 1988; 121–124.
8. Owen JH. The application of intraoperative monitoring during surgery for spinal deformity. Spine 1999; 24:2649–2662.
9. Ubags LH, Kalkman CJ, Been HD, Porsius M, Drummond JC. The use of ketamine or etomidate to supplement sufentanil/N_2O anesthesia does not disrupt monitoring of myogenic transcranial motor evoked responses. J Neurosurg Anesthesiol 1997; 9:228–233.
10. Potenza V, Weinstein SL, Neyt JG. Dysfunction of the spinal cord during spinal arthrodesis for scoliosis: recommendations for early detection and treatment. A case report. J Bone Joint Surg Am 1998; 80: 1679–1683.
11. Ackerman LL, Traynelis VC. Treatment of delayed-onset neurological deficit after aortic surgery with lumbar cerebrospinal fluid drainage. Neurosurgery 2002; 51:1414–1421, discussion 1412–1421.
12. Lee TC, Yang LC, Chen HJ. Effect of patient position and hypotensive anesthesia on inferior vena caval pressure. Spine 1998; 23:941–947, discussion 947–948.
13. Nuttall GA, Horlocker TT, Santrach PJ, Oliver WC Jr, Dekutoski MB, Bryant S. Predictors of blood transfusions in spinal instrumentation and fusion surgery. Spine 2000; 25:596–601.
14. Relton JE, Hall JE. An operation frame for spinal fusion. A new apparatus designed to reduce haemorrhage during operation. J Bone Joint Surg Br 1967; 49:327–332.
15. Lentschener C, Cottin P, Bouaziz H, Mercier FJ, Wolf M, Aljabi Y, Boyer-Neumann C, Benhamou D. Reduction of blood loss and transfusion requirement by aprotinin in posterior lumbar spine fusion. Anesth Analg 1999; 89:590–597.
16. Urban MK, Beckman J, Gordon M, Urquhart B, Boachie-Adjei O. The efficacy of antifibrinolytics in the reduction of blood loss during complex adult reconstructive spine surgery. Spine 2001; 26:1152–1156.
17. Florentino-Pineda I, Blakemore LC, Thompson GH, Poe-Kochert C, Adler P, Tripi P. The effect of epsilon-aminocaproic acid on perioperative blood loss in patients with idiopathic scoliosis undergoing posterior spinal fusion: a preliminary prospective study. Spine 2001; 26:1147–1151.
18. Amar D, Grant FM, Zhang H, Boland PJ, Leung DH, Healey JA. Antifibrinolytic therapy and perioperative blood loss in cancer patients undergoing major orthopedic surgery. Anesthesiology 2003; 98:337–342.
19. Abbey DM, Turner DM, Warson JS, Wirt TC, Scalley RD. Treatment of postoperative wound infections following spinal fusion with instrumentation. J Spinal Disord 1995; 8:278–283.
20. Levi AD, Dickman CA, Sonntag VK. Management of postoperative infections after spinal instrumentation. J Neurosurg 1997; 86:975–980.

21. Massie JB, Heller JG, Abitbol JJ, McPherson D, Garfin SR. Postoperative posterior spinal wound infections. Clin Orthop 1992:99–108.
22. Barker FG II. Efficacy of prophylactic antibiotic therapy in spinal surgery: a meta-analysis. Neurosurgery 2002; 51:391–400, discussion 391–400.
23. Huang RP, Thompson GH. Antibiotic therapy in spine surgery. In: DeWald RL, Arlet V, Carl AL, O'Brien MF, eds. Spinal Deformities: The Comprehensive Text. New York: Thieme, 2003:188–194.
24. Classen DC, Evans RS, Pestotnik SL, Horn SD, Menlove RL, Burke JP. The timing of prophylactic administration of antibiotics and the risk of surgical-wound infection. N Engl J Med 1992; 326:281–286.
25. Kernodle DS, Barg NL, Kaiser AB. Low-level colonization of hospitalized patients with methicillin-resistant coagulase-negative staphylococci and emergence of the organisms during surgical antimicrobial prophylaxis. Antimicrob Agents Chemother 1988; 32: 202–208.
26. Janning SW, Rybak MJ. Antimicrobial prophylaxis in surgery. In: DiPiro JT, Talbert RL, Yee GC, Matzke GR, Wells BG, Posey LM, eds. Pharmacotherapy: A Pathophysiologic Approach. Stamford: Appleton & Lange, 1999:1888–1889.
27. Mandelbaum BR, Tolo VT, McAfee PC, Burest P. Nutritional deficiencies after staged anterior and posterior spinal reconstructive surgery. Clin Orthop 1988; 5–11.
28. Blackburn GL, Bistrian BR, Maini BS, Schlamm HT, Smith MF. Nutritional and metabolic assessment of the hospitalized patient. JPEN J Parenter Enteral Nutr 1977; 1:11–22.
29. McPhee IB, Williams RP, Swanson CE. Factors influencing wound healing after surgery for metastatic disease of the spine. Spine 1998; 23:726–732, discussion 723–732.
30. Daly JM, Redmond HP, Gallagher H. Perioperative nutrition in cancer patients. JPEN J Parenter Enteral Nutr 1992; 16:100S–105S.
31. Schlag P, Decker-Baumann C. Strategies and needs for nutritional support in cancer surgery. Recent Results Cancer Res 1991; 121:233–248.
32. Hu SS, Fontaine F, Kelly B, Bradford DS. Nutritional depletion in staged spinal reconstructive surgery. The effect of total parenteral nutrition. Spine 1998; 23: 1401–1405.
33. Lapp MA, Bridwell KH, Lenke LG, Baldus C, Blanke K, Iffrig TM. Prospective randomization of parenteral hyperalimentation for long fusions with spinal deformity: its effect on complications and recovery from postoperative malnutrition. Spine 2001; 26:809–817, discussion 817.
34. Stambough JL, Beringer D. Postoperative wound infections complicating adult spine surgery. J Spinal Disord 1992; 5:277–285.
35. Prevention of venous thrombosis and pulmonary embolism. NIH Consensus Development. JAMA 1986; 256:744–749.
36. Rokito SE, Schwartz MC, Neuwirth MG. Deep vein thrombosis after major reconstructive spinal surgery. Spine 1996; 21:853–858; discussion 859.
37. Smith MD, Bressler EL, Lonstein JE, Winter R, Pinto MR, Denis F. Deep venous thrombosis and pulmonary embolism after major reconstructive operations on the spine. A prospective analysis of 317 patients. J Bone Joint Surg Am 1994; 76:980–985.
38. West JL III, Anderson LD. Incidence of deep vein thrombosis in major adult spinal surgery. Spine 1992; 17:S254–S257.
39. Waring WP, Karunas RS. Acute spinal cord injuries and the incidence of clinically occurring thromboembolic disease. Paraplegia 1991; 29:8–16.
40. Dearborn JT, Hu SS, Tribus CB, Bradford DS. Thromboembolic complications after major thoracolumbar spine surgery. Spine 1999; 24:1471–1476.
41. Ferree BA, Wright AM. Deep venous thrombosis following posterior lumbar spinal surgery. Spine 1993; 18:1079–1082.
42. Iorio A, Agnelli G. Low-molecular-weight and unfractionated heparin for prevention of venous thromboembolism in neurosurgery: a meta-analysis. Arch Intern Med 2000; 160:2327–2332.
43. Agnelli G, Piovella F, Buoncristiani P, Severi P, Pini M, D'Angelo A, Beltrametti C, Damiani M, Andrioli GC, Pugliese R, Iorio A, Brambilla G. Enoxaparin plus compression stockings compared with compression stockings alone in the prevention of venous thromboembolism after elective neurosurgery. N Engl J Med 1998; 339:80–85.
44. Voth D, Schwarz M, Hahn K, Dei-Anang K, Al Butmeh S, Wolf H. Prevention of deep vein thrombosis in neurosurgical patients: a prospective double-blind comparison of two prophylactic regimen. Neurosurg Rev 1992; 15:289–294.
45. Gottschalk A, Wu CL, Ochroch EA. Current treatment options for acute pain. Expert Opin Pharmacother 2002; 3:1599–1611.
46. Sherwood GD, McNeill JA, Starck PL, Disnard G. Changing acute pain management outcomes in surgical patients. AORN J 2003; 77:374, 377–380, 384–390 passim.
47. Breivik H. How to implement an acute pain service. Best Pract Res Clin Anaesthesiol 2002; 16:527–547.

20

Perioperative Care of Patients with Head and Neck Cancer

ANDREW MacLACHLAN and DAVID FERSON

Department of Anesthesiology, The University of Texas M.D. Anderson Cancer Center, Houston, Texas, U.S.A.

KRISTEN PYTYNIA and ED DIAZ

Department of Head and Neck Surgery, The University of Texas M.D. Anderson Cancer Center, Houston, Texas, U.S.A.

N. NGUYEN

Shriners Orthopedic Hospital, Houston, Texas, U.S.A.

W. BOTNICK

Perioperative Services, The University of Texas M.D. Anderson Cancer Center, Houston, Texas, U.S.A.

I. INTRODUCTION

Patients with cancer of the head and neck are generally challenging to manage (1). They frequently have comorbidities resulting from chronic smoking combined with alcohol abuse. In addition, neoplastic processes often produce anatomical changes in the patient's airway that require specialized techniques of tracheal intubation (2). Moreover, during oncologic surgery, it is essential for the surgeon and anesthesiologist to share access to the patient's airway and work, collaboratively to ensure patient safety, and success of the procedure.

This chapter will address the medical and surgical issues specific to patients with head and neck malignancies. We will present the preoperative evaluation from both the surgical and anesthetic perspective and illustrate the importance of a meticulously thorough evaluation of the patient prior to surgery. Intraoperative planning and management are developed directly from the preoperative evaluation and clinical findings; however, different surgical procedures have their own idiosyncrasies and require special consideration. Therefore, the section on intraoperative management will include a discussion of the most common head and neck cancer procedures from both the surgical and anesthetic perspective. Just as intraoperative planning reflects the preoperative evaluation, postoperative care is an extension of the intraoperative management of the patient. In the immediate postoperative period, some issues may require special attention and monitoring in the Surgical Intensive Care Unit (SICU). Consequently, the section on postoperative care will address the concerns of head and neck surgery from the intensivist's point of view.

This chapter was prepared with input from surgeons, anesthesiologists, and intensivists with expertise in the perioperative management of patients with head and neck cancers. We hope to provide our readers with concise, practical information, and guidance that will help them to understand the nuances of perioperative care in the clinical management of these patients.

II. PREOPERATIVE EVALUATION

Although head and neck cancer is the fifth most common cancer worldwide, it is relatively uncommon in the United States (3). The vast majority of head and neck cancers are squamous cell carcinomas, and more than 90% of these are related to tobacco and alcohol exposure (4). Chronic smoking and alcohol abuse can also lead to chronic obstructive pulmonary disease, coronary artery disease, liver damage, and malnutrition. Such comorbidities are critical in determining what type of treatment is appropriate for a patient during the preoperative period (5,6).

A. Surgical Perspective

Squamous cell carcinoma of the head and neck (SCCHN) is classified according to the American Joint Committee on Cancer guidelines. The staging and treatment of SCCHN is complicated. One of the most comprehensive staging and treatment guidelines for head and neck cancer has been developed by the National Comprehensive Cancer Network (NCCN). A full discussion of the NCCN guidelines exceeds the scope of this chapter, but the reader is encouraged to visit the NCCN website (www.nccn.org) for clinical guidelines for the diagnosis, staging, and treatment of head and neck cancer. Based on the initial evaluation of the patient, the surgeon usually orders radiological studies of the neck, such as plain radiography, computed tomography (CT), and magnetic resonance imaging (MRI), to determine the anatomical location, size, and extent of invasion of the tumor (7,8). Regional and distant metastases to draining lymph nodes are the primary staging factors for head and neck cancer. Although radiological studies are instrumental in the initial diagnosis and staging of head and neck tumors, diagnosis and final staging in patients with SCCHN ultimately require tissue biopsy to accurately define the primary site and rule out other primary lesions. Treatment for SCCHN usually consists of surgery followed by radiation therapy, depending on the site of the disease; however, aggressive disease may require a combination of surgery, radiation therapy, and chemotherapy (9).

A dental evaluation is of prime importance prior to radiation therapy, and extractions may be required to prevent systemic infections in patients with gum and dental disease. Dental extractions are usually performed while the patient is under anesthesia for examination and biopsy.

The main subsites of SCCHN are anatomically divided into the oral cavity, oropharynx, larynx, hypopharynx, and nasopharynx. Forty-five percent of all SCCHN lesions are in the oral cavity, followed by laryngeal lesions (30%), oro- and hypopharyngeal lesions (16%), and nasopharyngeal lesions (11%) (10).

The oral cavity includes the tongue, floor of the mouth, buccal mucosa, gingiva, and hard palate. The oral cavity is easily accessible, and wide resections can be achieved with minimal loss of function. Consequently, most oral cavity cancers are treated with surgery. The incidence of occult nodal metastasis in oral cavity cancers is 30–70%, depending on the specific site and size of the primary lesion. Therefore, resection of the primary tumor frequently includes neck dissection. Resection of large oral cavity lesions may require tracheostomy for postoperative control of the airway.

Early stage laryngeal lesions may be treated with either radiation therapy or organ-preservation surgery (partial laryngectomy). Patients undergoing partial laryngectomy must be prepared for a temporary tracheostomy to avoid airway-related problems in the immediate postoperative period. If a laryngeal lesion cannot be completely removed by a partial laryngectomy, a total laryngectomy may be necessary. Advanced laryngeal lesions require a total laryngectomy or, alternatively, radiation therapy and chemotherapy to preserve a functional larynx (11).

Oropharyngeal sites include the soft palate, tonsils, and base of the tongue. Accordingly, the majority of oropharyngeal lesions are treated primarily with radiation therapy and chemotherapy to avoid the significant functional losses associated with surgery. Nasopharyngeal tumors also are most commonly treated with chemotherapy and radiation therapy (9).

Complications of radiation therapy and chemotherapy that may compromise the airway and lead to a temporary or long-term tracheostomy include immediate and long-term tissue changes such as severe edema and scarring. Tracheostomy may be planned before treatment begins or, if serious airway complications arise during therapy, performed emergently. The surgical salvage of patients for whom chemotherapy and radiation therapy fails is complex and challenging because of tissue changes and the potential need for more radical surgery. Some patients who have a good response to radiation therapy at the primary site require salvage neck dissection because of persistent disease in the neck.

Large defects may require multiple surgical procedures performed by surgeons from several other surgical disciplines, including plastic surgery, orthopedic surgery, oral surgery, and neurosurgery. For example, patients undergoing reconstruction of mandibular defects may require an osseocutaneous flap, such as an iliac crest, or a fibular or scapular flap, while patients requiring soft-tissue closure may undergo a radial forearm, rectus abdominus, or lateral thigh flap procedure. Occasionally, the jejunal free flap is used for closure of extensive pharyngeal wounds (12). Anesthesia should be adjusted to manage such procedures (see the chapter on perioperative care for reconstructive surgery).

B. Anesthetic Perspective

In addition to a routine preanesthetic evaluation, patients with head and neck cancer usually require an assessment of organ systems affected by smoking and alcohol abuse. Specialized pulmonary and cardiovascular testing may be indicated in the preanesthetic evaluation of these patients. Cardiovascular testing can detect coronary disease, peripheral vasculopathy, and possible alcoholic cardiomyopathy. The results of these tests help the anesthesiologist to evaluate the patient's functional reserve and plan for any special intraoperative monitoring (e.g., measuring central venous pressure or hemodynamic monitoring with a pulmonary artery catheter) to guide, if necessary, intraoperative therapies. If significant pathology is diagnosed by the preoperative testing, the anesthesiologist must discuss the results with the surgeon to determine whether the patient will be able to tolerate surgery (13). Preoperative laboratory tests in patients with head and neck cancer also may reveal evidence of anemia, coagulopathy, electrolyte abnormalities, and acid–base disturbances that may require treatment before or during surgery. Many patients will have a history of alcohol abuse that changes their intraoperative anesthetic requirements and calls for careful monitoring for delirium tremens (DT) in the early postoperative period.

One of the most important functions of an anesthesiologist is to secure and maintain the patent airway. In patients with head and neck cancers, the presence of the tumor may significantly alter airway anatomy and patency (2). Consequently, careful evaluation of the airway is an essential part of the preoperative assessment. However, routine airway examination, which includes determination of Mallampati class (14,15), may not be sufficient because pathological processes can significantly distort the periglottic anatomy. Therefore, it is important to also obtain from the surgeons the findings from indirect laryngoscopy or nasal fiberoscopy performed in the clinic and to review preoperative imaging studies with the head and neck radiologist. CT scans and MRI studies contain valuable information about the bones and soft tissues of the neck and, with the use of modern three-dimensional reconstruction techniques, additional images may provide decisive information concerning the feasibility of tracheal intubation (16). Also, radiologists can provide anesthesiologists with images derived from software programs that permit "virtual fiberoptic intubation" (17). Combining information from physical examination with the radiological findings is essential for developing an effective, safe, and comfortable strategy to secure the patient's airway. However, many patients with neoplastic tumors of the upper aerodigestive tract will have severe anatomical distortion, which may make intubation difficult or impossible. These patients will frequently require temporary or permanent tracheostomy under local anesthesia at the beginning of surgery.

Once the decision is made to proceed with surgery, clear communication between the surgeon and anesthesiologist is essential to coordinate the surgical and anesthetic plans. This conversation benefits the patient by clarifying important issues that are not readily apparent from a review of the patient's chart alone.

III. INTRAOPERATIVE MANAGEMENT

This part of the chapter focuses on the most common procedures for patients with head and neck cancer presented from both the surgical and anesthetic perspective.

A. Neck Dissection: Functional, Radical, and Modified Radical

Neck dissections are rarely performed as isolated surgical procedures; rather, they are usually combined with resection of the primary lesion, which may arise from any part of the oropharynx or larynx (18). The typical preoperative diagnosis is cancer of the mouth, oropharynx, or tonsils, with suspected or documented spread to the cervical lymph nodes.

All neck dissections are performed with the patient in the supine position. The duration of surgery ranges from 1.5 to 3 hr; however, if the neck dissection is performed with primary resection and reconstruction, the surgery will take from 3 to 6 hr. Blood loss during neck dissection is usually limited to 150–200 mL. However, in patients who have undergone radiation therapy, the blood loss can easily double. If the primary lesion is also resected, the blood loss may increase from 400 to 700 mL and up to 1200 mL with concurrent flap reconstruction (9). Although sudden, unexpected blood loss is rare during neck dissection, it can occur if the internal jugular vein is transected. Therefore, anesthesiologists must always be prepared to rapidly administer fluids and blood products.

1. *Functional Neck Dissection*

A functional neck dissection involves a complete cervical lymphadenectomy with preservation of neck structures such as the sternocleidomastoid muscle and internal jugular vein.

2. *Radical Neck Dissection*

A radical neck dissection consists of a complete cervical lymphadenectomy with resection of the internal jugular vein, sternocleidomastoid muscle, and accessory nerve (cranial nerve XI).

Composite resection, also known as the "commando procedure," is a variant of radical neck dissection that consists of a partial mandibulectomy with or without a partial glossectomy. The goal of this procedure is to minimize the risk of local or systemic metastasis by resecting the neck specimen in continuity with the primary lesion. A tracheostomy is almost always performed as part of the composite resection.

3. *Modified Radical Neck Dissection*

A modified radical neck dissection falls between a functional neck dissection and radical neck dissection and includes a supraomohyoid neck dissection, posterior neck dissection, and anterior neck dissection in combination with other procedures.

Radical neck dissections were once standard therapy in all patients requiring a neck dissection, but research by Byers et al. (11) has shown that oncological control can be achieved with a modified approach. At present, the most common types of neck dissection are the modified radical neck dissection, which includes cervical lymph nodes levels 1–5 but spares the internal jugular vein, sternocleidomastoid muscle, accessory nerve, and selective neck dissections, which also spare the internal jugular vein, sternocleidomastoid muscle, and accessory nerve but do not include all of levels 1–5.

B. Laryngectomy

Laryngectomy is most frequently performed in patients with cancer of the larynx. Chronic and intractable aspirations are the most common nononcologic indications for laryngectomy. The usual blood loss from a total laryngectomy ranges from 200 to 300 mL. However, if this procedure is combined with a neck dissection, as well as pharyngectomy and flap reconstruction, the blood loss may increase to 700 and 1200 mL, respectively. Sudden, large losses of blood generally do not occur during laryngectomy procedures, and blood transfusions are usually not required. Laryngectomy includes the following group of surgical procedures: total laryngectomy, supraglottic laryngectomy, hemilaryngectomy, and near-total laryngectomy.

1. *Total Laryngectomy*

A total laryngectomy consists of removal of the larynx with vallecula and, if necessary, the posterior third of the tongue. With the patient in the supine position, a tracheostomy is usually performed, and airway is secured with a flexible reinforced anode tube sutured to the patient's chest. Following the tracheostomy, an apron flap incision is made from the hyoid bone to the clavicle to provide exposure in the subplatysmal plane. The strap muscles are then divided inferiorly, and hyoid bone is skeletonized. The thyroid gland is then resected away from the trachea, unless the surgery includes partial or total thyroidectomy. Once this is achieved, the larynx is transected above the hyoid bone and removed. The pharynx is closed in a T-shaped fashion, and trachea is pulled to the skin to create an end-tracheostomy, thus eliminating the need for a tracheostomy tube.

2. *Supraglottic Laryngectomy*

This procedure, which requires a mandatory temporary tracheostomy, involves the resection of the larynx from the ventricle to the base of the tongue, thus leaving the true vocal cords intact to preserve speech. The initial phase of this procedure is similar to that of a total laryngectomy, but the strap muscles are preserved. After the thyroid cartilage is exposed, the subperichondral flaps are lifted off the thyroid lamina so they can be used for reconstruction during the latter phase of the surgery. The thyroid cartilage is cut in the midportion just above the true vocal cords with either a scalpel or surgical saw. The excision is completed at the base of the tongue so that the final specimen includes the false vocal cords, supraglottic larynx, epiglottis, and a portion of the tongue. The wound is closed by approximating the thyroid perichondrium to the base of the tongue and using the strap muscles, which are also sutured to the base of the tongue.

3. Hemilaryngectomy

A hemilaryngectomy, also frequently referred to as a vertical laryngectomy, involves the removal of a unilateral true and false vocal cord, while leaving intact the epiglottis as well as the true and false vocal cord on the contralateral side to preserve laryngeal function. The surgical exposure during hemilaryngectomy is similar to that during a supraglottic laryngectomy, with the exception that the hemilaryngectomy is limited to only half of the larynx. After the subperichondral flap is raised, cuts are made on the ipsilateral thyroid cartilage using either a scalpel or surgical saw. The anterior commissure is then divided using Pott's scissors. After resection is completed, vocal cord reconstruction is accomplished using the sternocleidomastoid muscle. A temporary tracheostomy procedure is required during a hemilaryngectomy to facilitate intraoperative and postoperative airway management.

4. Near-Total Laryngectomy

A near-total laryngectomy is a surgical technique that includes removal of the entire larynx with the exception of one arytenoid, which is used to construct a phonatory shunt for speaking. A temporary or permanent tracheostomy is always performed during a near-total laryngectomy. Also, this procedure is usually combined with a radical or functional neck dissection and with a partial or total pharyngectomy. A total pharyngectomy requires flap reconstruction, which is usually performed by a plastic surgeon.

C. Glossectomy

A partial or total glossectomy is indicated when the neoplastic lesion involves the tongue or adjacent structures such as the alveolus or floor of the mouth. A glossectomy is also performed in combination with other head and neck surgeries such as neck dissection, mandibulectomy, and occasionally, total laryngectomy. The lesion is resected via the oral approach using electrocautery, and primary closure of the wound is usually possible. Depending on the extent of surgical resection and location of the lesion, a short-term tracheostomy may be required to prevent airway obstruction resulting from soft-tissue edema. However, if tracheostomy is not performed, a short course of steroid therapy is administered to the patient in the immediate postoperative period to rapidly decrease tissue swelling. After the surgery, the patient remains intubated for 24–48 hr. Blood loss during partial and total glossectomy ranges from 50 to 100 mL and 200 to 400 mL, respectively.

D. Anesthetic Perspective

Anesthetic considerations during surgery for head and neck cancer include managing the patient's airway, monitoring the patient's hemodynamic status, intraoperatively monitoring the nerves controlling the function of the larynx, and minimizing the risk of fire during laser surgery.

1. Maintaining the Patent Airway

Airway management is one of the most challenging anesthetic tasks in patients undergoing surgery for head and neck cancer, which frequently invades and distorts the airway. This management requires not only careful preparation but also a clear and well-defined plan, which should include communication with the surgeon regarding performing a tracheostomy under local anesthesia in the event that intubation proves to be difficult or impossible. With the airway techniques now available for use in patients with difficult-to-manage airways, however, a modern anesthesiologist should be able to manage most of these patients successfully without resorting to an emergency tracheostomy.

An important step in developing a systematic approach to airway management was the introduction in 1993 of the Difficult Airway Algorithm (DAA) (19). The algorithm, developed by the Task Force on Management of the Difficult Airway from the American Society of Anesthesiologists (ASA), was quickly incorporated into clinical practice in the United States and abroad. The popularity and clinical relevance of this algorithm is due to the fact that it originated from an evidence-based review of the medical literature, the opinions of consultants selected by the Task Force, and a consensus of the community of practitioners likely to be affected. The algorithm provides an organized, clinically useful, and nonrestrictive framework for practitioners caring for patients with difficult-to-manage airways. Recently, the DAA was updated to reflect findings from evidence-based reviews of the medical literature pertinent to airway management (20). Because the DAA offers only a framework for developing an organized clinical plan for patients with difficult-to-manage airways, clinicians should always use their best judgment and the techniques that they are most familiar with to ensure the best outcomes and most comfort for their patients.

Head and neck cancer patients represent only a subset of the patients with difficult-to-manage airways.

However, they frequently present a challenge to even the most experienced clinicians, due to anatomical distortions of the airway caused by the neoplastic process or previous surgical interventions and radiation therapy. Based on the preoperative evaluation of the patient, a review of their radiological studies, and consultation with the surgeon, an anesthesiologist can determine whether intubation will be feasible or whether tracheostomy under local anesthesia will be required. However, if uncertainty exists as to whether the intubation will be possible, appropriate arrangements should be made in advance regarding tracheostomy under local anesthesia if intubation attempts fail. In our clinical practice at The University of Texas M.D. Anderson Cancer Center, the technique of choice for patients with airways distorted by cancer is an awake intubation with the aid of a fiberoptic bronchoscope (FOB). An important step in achieving a successful awake FOB intubation is careful preparation of the patient. This consists of a complete but concise explanation of the technique in a manner that can be easily understood by the patient. Also, it is important to state that an awake FOB intubation is necessary for the patient's safety and to reassure the patient that sedation and topical anesthesia will be used to provide comfort during intubation. To decrease mucous secretions in the airway and to achieve more effective topical anesthesia, 0.2–0.4 mg of glycopyrolate is given intravenously to the patient 20–30 min before fiberoptic intubation. The technical aspects of performing FOB intubation have been extensively described by Ovassapian (21), who is considered to have the most experience with the FOB of any anesthesiologist in the United States; therefore, for a detailed discussion, we refer the reader to his publication.

In our clinical practice at M.D. Anderson Cancer Center, we find Ovassapian's technique of topical anesthesia to the airway using 2–4% lidocaine very useful, especially because nerve blocks may be ineffective in patients with head and neck cancers because of an altered anatomy. Unless a partial upper airway obstruction is manifested clinically by stridor and difficulty breathing, all patients undergoing fiberoptic intubation at M.D. Anderson receive midazolam with small incremental doses of sufentanil intravenously, to attain the desired level of sedation in the operating room. This allows patients to feel relaxed and comfortable, yet able to breathe and maintain their airways spontaneously. Patients with an obstruction that blocks 50% or more of their airway, who usually present to the operating room with stridor and difficulty breathing, receive no sedation at all or very small doses of midazolam alone. Recently, we began using intravenous dexmetetomidine (dose range: 0.2–0.7 μg per kg per min) to sedate patients with head and neck cancers. Dexmetetomidine has excellent sedating and analgesic properties but is completely devoid of any negative effects on respiration. Although controlled studies are needed to define the role of dexmetetomidine for sedation during awake FOB, we find it very useful in patients with partial airway obstruction.

Another useful tool for patients with difficult-to-manage airways is the laryngeal mask airway (LMA). The LMA is very effective in providing ventilation and oxygenation to patients who after induction of general anesthesia are difficult to intubate using conventional laryngoscopy and difficult to ventilate using a face mask (22,23). In these patients, the LMA is frequently lifesaving, and it is now recommended in all pathways of the DAA because it allows for ventilation to be easily established and can then be used as a conduit for endotracheal intubation. An FOB is frequently used to ensure the atraumatic and successful placement of the tracheal tube through the LMA (22,23). In patients with head and neck cancer and associated supraglottic pathology, elective use of the LMA is controversial and may be contraindicated (24). However, as our experience at M.D. Anderson indicates, the LMA can be a useful tool during emergency situations, even in the face of existing supraglottic pathology.

If tracheal intubation is difficult or if tracheostomy is a part of the elective surgical plan, then the procedure is performed in the operating room under local anesthesia with or without sedation. Once the tracheostomy is completed, general anesthesia can be quickly induced to ensure the patient's comfort during the rest of the surgery.

2. *Hemodynamic Monitoring*

In addition to managing the airway, anesthesiologists perform several other tasks during surgery. For example, using different classes of medications and routes of administration, anesthesiologists provide analgesia and amnesia to the patient and a motionless surgical field. Because all anesthetic agents have a significant impact on a patient's physiological functions, anesthesiologists must monitor the patient very closely during the course of surgery and anesthesia. Monitoring also provides information regarding the need for therapeutic interventions and assesses the effects of these interventions on the physiological homeostasis of the patient. The selection of intraoperative monitoring modalities is usually based on the preoperative assessment of the patient's physical condition. Arterial lines and central venous or pulmonary artery catheters are frequently used in patients with cardiovascular pathologies to closely monitor the patient's hemodynamic condition. To avoid interference with the surgical field of the neck, central venous catheters are usually inserted via the subclavian, basilic, or femoral veins. However, if reconstruction is planned at the same time as the head and neck surgery, the anesthesiologist must communicate with the plastic surgeon regarding the planned donor site, which may limit the sites available for placement of the central venous line. Specifically, the use of a pectoralis myocutanous flap would preclude the insertion of the catheter via an ipsilateral subclavian vein; the femoral vein should be avoided if the surgeon is planning an iliac crest, rectus flap, or anterior thigh flap. The large-bore central venous catheters are also very useful for treating sudden, and usually unexpected, blood loss during surgery with the rapid infusion of intravenous fluids and blood products.

3. *Functional Surgical Monitoring*

Special requirements during head and neck surgery for monitoring the integrity of nerves controlling the function of pharyngeal and laryngeal muscles must be communicated clearly by the surgeons to the anesthesiologist, who must then use a special endotracheal tube (i.e., NIM-2 XL EMG Endotrachel Tube, Xomed, Jacksonville, FL) from the outset of surgery. Also, certain medications (i.e., muscle relaxants) that are routinely administered by anesthesiologists can significantly affect the ability to monitor the functional status of the nerve bundles. Therefore, the anesthesiologist must adjust the dose of muscle relaxants to provide optimal conditions for intraoperative monitoring of functional neuronal integrity.

4. *Special Requirements During Laser Surgery*

LASER is an acronym for Light Amplification by Stimulated Emission of Radiation. Different types of lasers have unique medical applications. The CO_2 laser is used almost exclusively during microlaryngeal surgery, while the neodymium-yttrium-aluminum-garnet (Nd:YAG) laser is used to debulk airway tumors. Although lasers offer distinct advantages to the surgeon, such as precise cutting, decreased tissue edema, and reduced bleeding, there are also serious hazards associated with laser use. The most serious of these is the risk of fire. Other risks associated with laser use include eye injury, inhalation of smoke and infectious viral particles, and skin burns. The risk of accidents caused by lasers can be minimized by implementing safety rules and using protective gear. All personnel in the operating room must wear goggles appropriate for the wavelength of the laser beam in use: orange for an argon laser; green for a Nd:YAG laser; and orange/red for a potassium-titanyl phosphate laser. The patient's eyes should be protected with wet gauze or a towel. In addition, special micro-pore face masks should be worn by the operating room personnel to prevent inhalation of infectious particles such as viral DNA, and warning signs should be posted outside the operating room in which the laser is being used.

Fire in the airway, caused by the ignition of the endotracheal tube, is the most serious complication of laser surgery (25–27). The blowtorch-like flame produced by the propagation of the fire along the oxygen-enriched environment inside the endotracheal tube can cause life-threatening injury to the patient. Several endotracheal tubes have been designed to reduce the risk of fire including the Xomed Treace Laser Shield II (Xomed, Jacksonville, FL), the Fome-Cuf (Bivona Inc., Gary, IN), and the Laser-Flex (Mallinckrodt Medical Inc., St. Louis, MO). However, even when a special endotracheal tube is used and the patient is ventilated with gas mixture containing low concentration of oxygen, there is no guarantee that the risk of fire is eliminated (28,29). Therefore, the anesthesiologist must be familiar with and practice the response algorithm for airway fire during laser surgery: (1) first disconnect the oxygen source at the Y piece and immediately remove the burning objects from the airway; (2) if the fire is smoldering, irrigate the site with water; and (3) ventilate the patient using a face mask or reintubate and ventilate with as lowest fraction of inspired oxygen possible (30). Once these steps are accomplished, one needs to evaluate the extent of injury using fiberoptic bronchoscopy and laryngoscopy and institute appropriate therapies.

IV. POSTOPERATIVE CARE

Taking into consideration the length and extent of the procedure as well as the patient's intraoperative course, the anesthesiologist and surgeon should determine where to admit the patient after surgery.

Most patients with head and neck cancers who have undergone surgery at M.D. Anderson are cared for on the hospital ward or in a "step-down unit," and few require admission to the SICU. This mirrors the medical practices in other major cancer centers in the United States (31,32). As reported by Downey et al. (33), at Memorial Sloan-Kettering Cancer Center, only 1.5% of the patients undergoing head and neck surgical procedures were admitted to the ICU postoperatively. Specifically, the ICU admissions were mainly required to manage respiratory (38%) or cardiac (31%) complications, while 19% of patients had wound-related problems (33). Identifying patients, before surgery, who may need ICU care or who are at high risk for postoperative complications is important because it allows for planning optimization and timely intervention.

A. Respiratory Complications

Respiratory complications are the primary source of higher morbidity and cost associated, head and neck surgery. Patients who continue to smoke prior to surgery have higher incidences of postoperative pneumonia and acute respiratory distress syndrome and are frequently difficult to wean from the ventilator. A study by McCulloch et al. (34) showed that 85% of the respiratory complications after head and neck surgery resulted from pneumonia; the respiratory complication rate in smokers was 15%, compared with 0% in patients who had quit smoking or had never smoked. The management of pulmonary complications usually consists of administering intravenous antibiotics and providing respiratory support with a ventilator and vigorous pulmonary toilet.

B. Airway Complications

Tracheostomy is commonly performed in head and neck surgery. About 32% of head and neck cancer patients had a tracheostomy in a study by Halfpenny and McGurk (35), and 8% of patients with tracheostomies had complications. Early complications (within the first week) include hemorrhage, obstructed tracheostomy, tracheitis, and displaced tracheostomy tube. Late complications include tracheocutaneous fistula, tracheoesophageal fistula, tracheal stenosis, erosion into the esophagus, erosion into the brachiocephalic artery, and stomal recurrence. The management of early complications includes suturing the tracheostomy tube into its proper position, humidification, suctioning, and close monitoring for any obstruction or displacement of the tracheostomy tube. Late complications are managed with additional surgery.

C. Swallowing Problems and Aspiration

Patients with head and neck cancer are at high risk for aspiration, and those who have had a subtotal or total glossectomy are at the highest risk (34). Prevention is the key to managing aspiration; early swallowing studies can identify potentially dangerous aspiration (36). If an aspiration has occurred, fiberoptic bronchoscopy is used to suction and remove any food particles; this is followed by supportive care, including intubation and ventilation, if necessary.

D. Cardiovascular Complications

Patients with head and neck cancers also are at risk for perioperative cardiovascular complications due to the effects of chronic smoking. Factors that increase the risk of perioperative cardiac events in patients with head and neck cancers are myocardial infarction less than 6 months prior to surgery, unstable angina, emergency surgery, history of congestive heart failure, and nonsinus rhythm (37). Although head and neck cancer surgery is an intermediate-risk surgery, the risk of myocardial infarction in patients undergoing head and neck cancer surgery, with or without microvascular reconstruction, ranges between 2% and 3.6%, and patients who have a perioperative myocardial infarction have a mortality rate of 28%, which is higher than that in other types of surgery (38). Therefore, the careful cardiac evaluation of patients scheduled for head and neck cancer surgery is of paramount importance in determining postoperative monitoring and management.

E. Prolonged QT Syndrome After Right Radical Neck Dissection

In 1983, Otten et al. (39) reported prolonged QT syndrome with subsequent cardiac arrest in a patient undergoing right radical neck dissection. The postulated mechanism for prolonged QT syndrome is disruption of sympathetic neural transmission by elevation of carotid sheath structures and the sympathetic chain during surgery. Also, as reported by Strickland et al. (40), in patients with pre-existing prolonged QT syndrome, a decrease in sympathetic activity on the right side may lead to ventricular fibrillation. The management of this complication consists of stopping the surgical stimulation and instituting appropriate treatment for cardiac dysrhythmias.

F. Wound-Related Complications

de Melo et al. (41) reported that patients with oral cancer who had bilateral neck dissections and APACHE II, score higher than 10 were at risk for postoperative surgical complications and prolonged hospital stays. Specifically, simultaneous bilateral neck dissections were associated with a 60% rate of postoperative complications and carried a mortality rate of 2.7% (42). Other factors, such as tobacco use, age greater than 55 years, a prolonged operation with the involvement of multiple surgeons, and the administration of more than 7 L of crystalloid during the procedure, were associated with an increased rate of flap complications and wound infections, which can occur in up to 42% of head and neck surgical patients (43,44). Prior chemotherapy and hypothyroidism increase the risk of postoperative wound infections, and the perioperative use of parenteral antibiotics did not appear to significantly lower the infection rates (44,45). However, aggressive wound care and the early treatment of infections using antibiotics that target specific bacteria from wound cultures may improve outcomes.

G. Problems Related to Alcohol Abuse

A study by Weinfeld et al. (46) reported a 12% incidence of alcohol withdrawal syndrome (AWS) in patients with head and neck cancer. The clinical diagnosis and treatment of AWS is important; if alcohol withdrawal is not recognized, it can progress to DT. The mortality rate in patients treated for DT is 2–4%, whereas untreated DT has a mortality rate of up to 20% (47). The clinical signs of mild AWS include coarse tremor, nausea, malaise, anxiety, mood changes, headache, sleep–wake disturbances, and mild hyperautonomia (tachycardia, diaphoresis, papillary dilatation, urinary incontinence, and hypertension) in the first 24–48 hours after the surgery. The clinical signs of major AWS are the same as those for mild AWS, with the addition of fever, disorientation, hallucinations, and seizures, usually occurring in the first 5 days after abstinence. Five percent of patients with AWS will eventually develop DT; moreover, one-third of patients who have a withdrawal seizure will have DT. The clinical manifestations of DT include inattention, disorganized mentation, an altered level of consciousness, sleep disturbance, psychomotor retardation, hallucinations, seizures, and profound autonomic hyperactivity. Delirium tremens can cause circulatory collapse, coma, and death from cardiac arrhythmias and respiratory failure. The management of AWS and DT includes correcting the electrolyte levels, maintaining a sleep–wake cycle, and administering thiamine, folic acid, multivitamin therapy, magnesium, and benzodiazepines.

H. Hypertension

Risk factors for postoperative hypertension include preoperative hypertension, alcohol abuse, radical neck dissection, and previous postoperative hypertension from neck dissection on the contralateral side (48,49). Nicardipine is an effective antihypertensive agent for the control of postoperative hypertension. Careful titration of antihypertensive agents is required because hypotension may lead to hypoperfusion and have devastating consequences in patients with surgical flaps (43).

I. Fluid and Electrolyte Abnormalities

Syndrome of inappropriate antidiuretic hormone production (SIADH) can occur in up to 3% of head and neck cancer patients (50). Often, this paraneoplastic syndrome is the result of squamous cell carcinomas of the oral cavity. Other risk factors include neck dissection and preoperative radiation therapy (51). The management of SIADH includes restricting fluid intake between 800 and 1000 mL per 24 hr and treating the underlying cause (e.g., hypothyroidism can be treated with thyroxine).

J. Problems Related to Nerve Injury

Nerve injuries may also occur during head and neck surgery. Recurrent laryngeal nerve injury and carotid body denervation have pulmonary implications. Recurrent laryngeal nerve injury occurs in 2% of thyroid surgery cases (52) and is transient in 1–2% of these cases (53). The recurrent laryngeal nerve innervates abductors and adductors of the vocal cords. Partial or total injury to this nerve can cause airway obstruction, which is managed with intubation. Bilateral neck dissection can denervate the carotid body, which leads to the loss of the hypoxic ventilatory response (54). There is no treatment for this loss, and the patient's ventilatory drive is dependent on maintaining eucapnia.

V. CONCLUSION

Patients with head and neck cancer have unique problems from an anesthetic, surgical, and intensive care perspective. From an anesthetic perspective, caring for head and neck cancer patients requires managing difficult or compromised airways and, often, sharing access to the airway with the surgical team. Surgeons must determine when surgery is appropriate and ensure that the airway is maintained during and after the procedure. Also, the surgeons must exercise care and handle friable tissue after chemotherapy and fibrosed tissue after radiation therapy without sacrificing nerves unless necessary. Postoperatively, cardiopulmonary problems, airway complications, nerve damage, infections, and AWS must be identified and managed appropriately.

REFERENCES

1. Dougherty TB, Nguyen DT. Anesthetic management of the patient scheduled for head and neck surgery. J Clin Anesth 1994; 6:74–82.

2. Jensen NF, Benumof J. The difficult airway in head and neck tumor surgery. Anesth Clin North Am 1993; 11:475.
3. Jemal A, Murray T, Samuels A, Ghafoor A, Ward E, Thun MJ. Cancer statistics, 2003. CA Cancer J Clin 2003; 53(1):5–26.
4. Blot WJ, McLaughlin JK, Winn DM, et al. Smoking and drinking in relation to oral and pharyngeal cancer. Cancer Res 1988; 48(11):3282–3287.
5. Hall SF, Groome PA, Rothwell D. The impact of comorbidity on the survival of patients with squamous cell carcinoma of the head and neck. Head Neck 2000; 22(4):317–322.
6. MacComb WS. Mortality from radical neck dissection. Am J Surg 1968; 115:352–354.
7. Hoover LA, Wortham DG, Lufkin RB, Hanafee WN. Magnetic resonance imaging of the larynx and tongue base: clinical applications. Otolaryngol Head Neck Surg 1987; 97:245–256.
8. Phelps PD. Carcinoma of the larynx—the role of imaging in staging and pre-treatment assessments. Clin Radiol 1992; 46:77–83.
9. Diaz EM Jr, Sturgis EM, Laramore GE, Sabichi AL, Lippman SM, Clayman G. Neoplasms of the head and neck. In: Holland and Frei, eds. Cancer Medicine. 6th ed. London: BC Decker, 2003.
10. Parkin DM, Bray F, Ferlay J, Pisani P. Estimating the world cancer burden: Globocan 2000. Int J Cancer 2001; 94(2):153–156.
11. Byers RM, Wolf PF, Ballantyne AJ. Rationale for elective modified neck dissection. Head Neck Surg 1988; 10(3):160–167.
12. Schusterman MA, Miller MJ, Reece GP, Kroll SS, Marchi M, Goepfert H. A single center's experience with 308 free flaps for repair of head and neck cancer defects. Plas Reconst Surg 1994; 93:472.
13. Goldman L, Caldera DL, Nussbaum SB, et al. Multifactorial index of cardiac risk in noncardiac surgical procedures. N Engl J Med 1977; 297:843.
14. Mallampati SR, Gatt SP, Gugino LD, et al. A clinical sign to predict difficult tracheal intubation: a prospective study. Can Anaesth Soc J 1985; 32:429–434.
15. Samsoon GLT, Young JRB. Difficult tracheal intubation: a retrospective study. Anaesthesia 1987; 42: 487–490.
16. Giron J, Joffre P, Serres-Cousine O, Castan P, Senac JP. Magnetic resonance imaging of the larynx. Its contribution compared to X-ray computed tomography in the pretherapeutic evaluation of cancers of the larynx. Apropos of 90 surgical cases. Ann Radiol 1990; 98: 55–58.
17. Charlin B, Brazeau-Lamontagne L, Guerrier B, Leduc C. Assessment of laryngeal cancer: CT scan versus endoscopy. J Otolaryngol 1989; 18:283–288.
18. Reed GF, Rabuzzi DD. Neck dissection. Otolaryngol Clin North Am 1969; 2:247–263.
19. Caplan RA, Benumoff JL, Berry FA, Blitt CA, Bode RH, Cheney FW, Connis RT, Guidry OR, Ovassapian A. Practice guidelines for management of the difficult airway: a report by the ASA Task Force on Management of the Difficult Airway. Anesthesiology 1993; 78:597–602.
20. Practice guidelines for management of difficult airway: an updated report by the American Society of Anesthesiologists Task Force on Management of the Difficult Airway. Anesthesiology 2003; 98:1269–1277.
21. Ovassapian A. Topical anesthesia of the airway. In: Ovassapian A, ed. Fiberoptic Endoscopy and the Difficult Airway. 2nd ed. Philadelphia: Lippincott-Raven, 1996:47–61.
22. Brain AIJ. The laryngeal mask airway—a possible new solution to airway problems in the emergency situation. Arch Emerg Med 1984; 1:229–232.
23. Silk JM, Hill HM, Calder I. Difficult intubation and the laryngeal mask. Eur J Anaesthesiol 1991; 4:47–51.
24. Giraud O, Bourgain JL, Marandas P, et al. Limits of laryngeal mask airway in patients after cervical or oral radiotherapy. Can J Anaesth 1997; 44:1237–1241.
25. Snow JC, Norton ML, Saluja TS, et al. Fire hazard during CO_2 laser microsurgery on larynx and trachea. Anesth Analg 1976; 55:146.
26. Burgess GE, LeJeune FE. Endotracheal tube ignition during laser surgery of the larynx. Arch Otolaryngol 1979; 85:71.
27. Cozine K, Rosenbaum LM, Askenazi J, et al. Laser-induced endotracheal tube fire. Anesthesiology 1981; 55:583.
28. Sosis MB, Heller S. A comparison of special endotracheal tubes for use with the CO_2 laser. Anesthesiology 1988; 69:A251.
29. Sosis MB. Airway fire during CO_2 laser surgery using a Xomed laser endotracheal tube. Anesthesiology 1990; 72:747.
30. Pashayan AG. Anesthesia for laser surgery. ASA Refresher Courses in Anesthesiology. Philadelphia: JB Lippincott, 1995:276.
31. Strauss M, Bellian K. Otolaryngology care unit: a safe and cost-reducing way to deliver quality care. Laryngoscope 1999; 109:1428–1432.
32. Garantziotis S, Kyrmizakis DE, Liolios AD. Critical care of the head and neck patient. Crit Care Clin 2003; 19(1):73–90.
33. Downey RJ, Friedlander P, Groeger J, et al. Critical care for the severely ill head and neck patient. Crit Care Med 1999; 27(1):95–97.
34. McCulloch TM, Jensen NF, Girod DA, et al. Risk factors for pulmonary complications in the postoperative head and neck surgery patient. Head Neck 1997; 19(5):372–377.
35. Halfpenny W, McGurk M. Analysis of tracheostomy-associated morbidity after operations for head and neck cancer. Br J Oral Maxillofac Surg 2000; 38(5):509–512.
36. Eibling DE, Carrau RL. Detection, evaluation, and management of aspiration in rehabilitation hospitals: role of the otolaryngologist—head and neck surgeon. J Otolaryngol 2001; 30(4):235–241.

37. Chiang S, Cohen B, Blackwell K. Myocardial infarction after microvascular head and neck reconstruction. Laryngoscope 2002; 112(10):1849–1852.
38. Bhattacharyya N, Fried MP. Benchmarks for mortality, morbidity, and length of stay for head and neck surgical procedures. Arch Otolaryngol Head Neck Surg 2001; 127:127–132.
39. Otten JC, Pottecher T, Bronner G, et al. Prolongation of the Q–T interval and sudden cardiac arrest following right radical neck dissection. Anesthesiology 1983; 59:358.
40. Strickland RA, Stanton MS, Olsen KD. Case report—prolonged QT syndrome: perioperative management. Mayo Clin Proc 1993; 68:1016–1020.
41. de Melo GM, Ribeiro KC, Kowalski LP, et al. Risk factors for postoperative complications in oral cancer and their prognostic implications. Arch Otolaryngol Head Neck Surg 2001; 127:828–833.
42. Magrin J, Kowalski L. Bilateral radical neck dissection: results in 193 cases. J Surg Oncol 2000; 75:232–240.
43. Haughey BH, Wilson E, Kluwe L, et al. Free flap reconstruction of the head and neck: analysis of 241 cases. Otolaryngol Head Neck Surg 2001; 125: 10–17.
44. Penel N, Lefebvre D, Fournier C, et al. Risk factors for wound infection in head and neck cancer surgery: a prospective study. Head Neck 2001; 23:447–455.
45. Gal RL, Gal TJ, Klotch DW, et al. Risk factors associated with hypothyroidism after laryngectomy. Otolaryngol Head Neck Surg 2000; 123:211–217.
46. Weinfeld AB, Davison SP, Mason AC, et al. Management of alcohol withdrawal in microvascular head and neck reconstruction. J Reconstr Microsurg 2000; 16:201–206.
47. Alvi A, Gonzalez RM. Management of delirium tremens on the head and neck service. Am J Otolaryngol 1995; 16:224–231.
48. Celikkanat S, Akyol MU, Koc C, et al. Postoperative hypertension after radical neck dissection. Otolaryngol Head Neck Surg 1997; 117:91–92.
49. Koc C, Ensari S, Kaymakci M, et al. Postoperative hypertension effect of carotid sinus denervation. Otolaryngol Head Neck Surg 1999; 121:150–152.
50. Ferlito A, Rinaldo A, Devaney KO. Syndrome of inappropriate antidiuretic hormone secretion associated with head neck cancers: review of the literature. Ann Otol Rhinol Laryngol 1997; 106:878–883.
51. Sorensen JB, Andersen MK, Hansen HH. Syndrome of in appropriate secretion of antidiuretic hormone (SIADH) in malignant disease. J Intern Med 1995; 238:97–110.
52. Kasemsuwan L, Nubthuenetr S. Recurrent laryngeal nerve paralysis: a complication of thyroidectomy. J Otolaryngol 1997; 26:365–367.
53. Lo CY, Kwok KF, Yuen PW. A prospective evaluation of recurrent laryngeal nerve paralysis during thyroidectomy. Arch Surg 2000; 135:204–207.
54. Moorthy SS, Sullivan TY, Fallon JH, et al. Loss of hypoxic ventilatory response following bilateral neck dissection. Anesth Analg 1993; 76:791–794.

21

Perioperative Care for Thoracic Neoplasms in Acute Cancer Medicine

JAY B. BRODSKY, JOHN L. CHOW, and JESSICA S. DONINGTON

Departments of Anesthesia and Cardiothoracic Surgery, Stanford University School of Medicine, Stanford, California, U.S.A.

I. INTRODUCTION

Lung cancer is one of the leading causes of death in the United States. Surgical resection, often combined with chemo- and/or radiation therapy, is an important part of the treatment of this disease. In order to provide optimal care for the surgical patient, each member of the health care team must understand the needs and concerns of their colleagues. This chapter reviews the clinical perspectives of the anesthesiologist, surgeon, and critical care physician in managing the patient with an intrathoracic neoplasm.

II. ANESTHESIA PERSPECTIVES

Anesthetic considerations for the patient with a thoracic neoplasm are similar to those for any patient undergoing an intrathoracic procedure. The lungs must be isolated and selectively ventilated, the patient must tolerate one-lung ventilation (OLV), and postoperative analgesia must be adequate. Patients with pulmonary or esophageal cancer have additional factors that must be considered. These can include poor preoperative pulmonary function, generalized debility, the metabolic effects from paraneoplastic syndromes, mass effects from the tumor, and the complications of radiation and chemotherapy.

A. Preoperative Evaluation and Testing

Both the anesthesiologist and surgeon must completely assess the patient preoperatively, with attention directed to the nature and extent of cardiopulmonary disease. Pertinent information is obtained from the medical history, physical examination, diagnostic imaging studies, and pulmonary function tests (PFTs) (1,2).

All chest-imaging studies (radiography (CXR), computed tomography (CT), magnetic resonance imaging (MRI) studies) should be reviewed for evidence of the disease process, airway deviation and obstruction, and to help select an appropriate airway tube (3–5).

Standard spirometry can assess general pulmonary function, help predict risk, and demonstrate evidence of pharmacologic reversible bronchospasm (6–11). Predicted postoperative diffusing capacity (DLCO) is a strong predictor of risk from lung resection (12,13).

Ventilation–perfusion scintigraphy (V/Q scan) can help predict how well pulmonary resection will be tolerated, since excision of nonfunctioning lung will have minimal effects on postoperative pulmonary function (14–16). A dynamic flow-volume loop study will give information as to the site (extra- vs. intrathoracic) and type of tracheal or bronchial obstruction (17,18).

Positron emission tomography (PET) is a sensitive method of detecting and staging thoracic malignancy (19–21). Since up to 50% of surgery for nonsmall cell lung cancer is not curative, a PET scan positive for extrathoracic metastasis may help avoid an unnecessary operation (22,23).

Other important preoperative preparations, including the treatment of active pulmonary infection with appropriate antibiotics, minimizing airway reactivity with bronchodilators and steroids, and cessation of smoking, all reduce postoperative pulmonary complications (24–27).

B. Premedication

Sedative premedication should be avoided. Anticholinergic agents can be given to reduce excessive airway secretions. Gastroesophageal reflux can be reduced with an H_2-receptor blocker (28).

Increased sympathetic activity may play a role in cardiovascular complications. Preoperative betablockade stabilizes heart rate and cardiac index and decreases intraoperative oxygen consumption (29). The use of selective beta-1 blockers may minimize exacerbation of airway reactivity in COPD patients.

C. Monitoring

Noninvasive pulse oximetry (S_pO_2) and capnography accurately monitor oxygenation and ventilation (30,31). An indwelling arterial line is helpful, but not always needed. Real-time assessment of arterial oxygen tension (P_aO_2) and mixed venous oxygen saturation (S_vO_2) is possible with continuous intravascular monitors (32–34). Perioperative pulmonary artery (PA) catheterization may not offer additional intraoperative benefit, even for patients with significant preoperative cardiac dysfunction (35). Central venous pressure (CVP) and PA pressure measurements are useful for postoperative fluid management.

Transesophageal echocardiography (TEE) during pulmonary resection helps identify the etiology of hemodynamic instability and guide appropriate interventions (36). TEE may identify patients with cardiac disease undergoing pneumonectomy at risk for postoperative right ventricular failure (37). TEE can demonstrate tumor in the pulmonary veins and help diagnose tumor embolism during thoracotomy (38).

D. Choice of Anesthetic

General anesthesia normally increases airway resistance, changes which are further increased if the bronchus is obstructed (39,40). These effects can be partially alleviated with the inhalational anesthetics halothane, enflurane, isoflurane, and sevoflurane, which are direct bronchodilators (41). Desflurane is an airway irritant and can potentially increase airway resistance.

Anesthetic drugs that release histamine can produce bronchospasm, and must be used with caution in patients with reactive airway disease. Among the opioids, morphine and meperidine release histamine, whereas fentanyl, remifentanil, alfentanil, and sufentanil do not (42,43). Methohexital, etomidate and propofol, and the muscle relaxants succinylcholine, *cis*-atracurium, pancuronium, vecuronium, and rocuronium do not cause significant histamine release (44–46). Ketamine can be considered for induction of the hemodynamically unstable thoracotomy patient. It has a rapid onset of action, is a direct bronchodilator, and maintains cardiovascular stability (47,48). Ketamine offers no advantages for routine thoracotomy (49).

The hypoxic pulmonary vasoconstriction (HPV) reflex matches pulmonary perfusion to ventilation by redistributing cardiac output from poorly ventilated hypoxic areas to better oxygenated regions (50,51). Experimentally, all intravenous drugs (barbiturates, benzodiazepines, droperidol, ketamine, propofol, opioids) maintain HPV (52–54), and all inhalational anesthetics inhibit HPV (55–60). Clinically, during OLV there are no significant differences between a total intravenous anesthetic (TIVA) technique, which spares the HPV response and an inhalational anesthetic technique, which may depress HPV (61–63). Likewise, there are no differences between the inhalational anesthetic agents themselves (64–68).

Nitrous oxide produces a small inhibition of HPV (69,70). Nitrous oxide expands air-containing spaces (such as a pneumothorax or blebs) and dilutes the amount of oxygen that can be delivered, and should not be used during OLV.

Vasoconstrictors (e.g., epinephrine, phenylephrine) preferentially constrict vessels perfusing normoxic lung segments increasing pulmonary vascular resistance (PVR) in the ventilated lung, resulting in increased blood flow to the collapsed lung, with further V/Q mismatch and lowering P_aO_2 (71,72). Clinical experience, however, suggests that P_aO_2 is improved when vasoconstrictors are used to correct hypotension. It may be that improved perfusion results in increased West's zone one within the dependent lung. Vasodilator drugs (e.g., nitroprusside, nitroglycerin) blunt

HPV, increase blood flow to the nonventilated lung and also lower P_aO_2 (73–75).

E. Isolation of the Lungs

Surgical exposure during intrathoracic procedures is improved by selective lung collapse. Any balloon-tipped catheter (Fogarty® embolectomy catheter, PA catheter, Foley catheter) can be used as a bronchial blocker (BB) (76–80). A new catheter (WEB catheter, Cook Critical Care, Bloomington, IN) is specifically designed for bronchial blockade (81,82). It has a wire snare that couples to a fiberoptic bronchoscope (FOB) for blocker placement under direct visual guidance. Bronchial blockade can also be accomplished with the Univent tube (Fuji Systems Corp., Tokyo, Japan), which is a large endotracheal tube (ETT) that incorporates a movable balloon-tipped BB within the main body of the tube (83–87).

Double lumen tubes (DLTs) are, however, the safest and simplest means of achieving OLV (88–90). The lungs can be isolated and protected from each other, and either lung can be intentionally collapsed while ventilation to the other lung continues uninterrupted. Correct positioning of double lumen tubes can be determined through auscultation, however, inspection using a pediatric fibreoptic bronchoscope is rapid and more reliable and therefore recommended. Placement of a left-sided double lumen tube is preferred since left-sided anatomic characteristics (longer bronchus intermedius and absence of early take off of the upper lobe bronchus) are more favorable and thus prevent collapse of the upper lobe. Left-sided double lumen tube placement should suffice for most thoracic procedures; however, care should be taken when a left-sided lobectomy with bronchial sleeve resection or left-sided pneumonectomy is performed. A discussion with the surgeon as to his preference for these latter cases is recommended.

F. Anesthetic Technique

A general anesthesia (inhalational or TIVA) technique is usually combined with epidural anesthesia (91). Local anesthetics, administered at either the lumbar or thoracic epidural level, reduce the amount of opioid or inhalation agent needed during surgery. If cardiac output and blood pressure are maintained, oxygenation during OLV is not affected (92). Epidural opioids are added for postoperative pain management.

Advantages of this "combined" technique include significantly lower postoperative pain scores, reduced incidence of postoperative nausea and vomiting, improved postoperative ventilation, and shorter hospital stays (93). With adequate pain control, epidural anesthesia suppresses perioperative hormonal, metabolic, and physiologic stress responses (94,95).

G. Oxygenation During One-Lung Ventilation

In the lateral decubitus position during OLV, the operated lung continues to be perfused ("shunt") but not ventilated (96). The abdominal contents push the diaphragm cephalad producing low V/Q areas in the dependent, ventilated lung. When changing from two-lung to OLV, tidal volume is left unchanged. Larger tidal volumes (10–12 mL/kg) with zero positive end-expiratory pressure (PEEP) recruit dependent lung alveoli (97). When combined with a F_iO_2 of 1.0, a satisfactory P_aO_2 is usually achieved during OLV.

Since all ventilation is delivered to one lung, peak inspiratory pressure is increased (98). Although inflammatory mediator release seems unchanged when comparing large and small tidal volume ventilation strategies intraoperatively, small tidal volume ventilation strategies have been shown to reduce mortality in critically ill patients with acute respiratory distress syndrome (ARDSNet Trial). Although it is not at all clear if it is the reduction in tidal volume, the reduction in plateau airway pressure, or increased intrinsic PEEP that is responsible for this survival benefit in patients with ARDS, it seems prudent to adapt ventilation strategies during OLV. Instantaneous breath-to-breath analysis to adjust ventilatory patterns (adaptive lung ventilation) has been recommended to minimize the risk of barotraumas (99). Pressure-controlled ventilation is another alternative to volume-controlled ventilation (100,101).

H. Treatment of Hypoxemia During OLV

Hypoxemia during OLV is relatively uncommon. It can be due to luminal obstruction (by blood or secretions), bronchospasm, underventilation and/or hypoperfusion of the dependent lung, an increase in shunt, and airway tube malposition. Initial treatment approaches involve suctioning the tube, use of a bronchodilator, reconfirming DLT position, and even return to two-lung ventilation.

Positive PEEP [5–10 cm H_2O] applied to the ventilated lung can recruit collapsed alveoli (102). If alveolar pressure fails to decrease to atmospheric pressure at the end of expiration, intrinsic-PEEP ($PEEP_i$) will be generated (103,104). Application of external PEEP may be therapeutic in patients who do not generate a significant amount of $PEEP_i$ (105). PEEP applied to the ventilated lung can, however, decrease cardiac output and increase dependent lung PVR, which increases shunt and worsens hypoxemia (106). A PEEP 'search' protocol is recommended, whereby the optimal PEEP is sought.

A single-breath will partially re-expand the collapsed lung correcting hypoxemia temporarily (107). Insufflation of the nonventilated lung with 100% oxygen by continuous positive airway pressure (CPAP) (5–10 cm H_2O) maintains alveoli patency and oxygenates shunted blood (108–110). CPAP is only effective when the bronchial tree is intact, since airway distention must be maintained. During procedures for bronchopleural fistula (BPF), airway sleeve resection, or if the bronchus is completely obstructed, CPAP will not be helpful. The use of CPAP during video-assisted thoracoscopy surgery (VATS) is limited since any lung distention will compromise surgical exposure.

I. Modulating the Pulmonary Circulation

Selective infusion (via a PA catheter) of a vasoconstrictor into the PA of the nonventilated lung will decrease shunt and increase P_aO_2 (111). Infusion of a vasodilator into the PA of the ventilated lung will decrease shunt and improve oxygenation (112).

Although the potent vascular smooth muscle vasodilator inhaled nitric oxide ($_i$NO) has been administered to directly increase blood flow to the PA of the ventilated lung (113–117), little if any benefit occurs for most patients during OLV (118). The effects of $_i$NO are directly proportional to the degree of PVR present (119), and the majority of patients undergoing pulmonary resection have normal or slightly elevated PVR. For patients with normal PVR, shunt remains relatively unchanged (120,121). The combination of a vasoconstrictor (e.g., phenylephrine, almitrine bismesylate) to reduce total pulmonary perfusion, and $_i$NO to increase blood flow to the ventilated lung has had some success during OLV (122–128).

J. Intraoperative Fluid Management

Pulmonary edema after thoracotomy can be due to many causes including cardiac failure, aspiration, and/or fluid overload. A specific entity, postpneumonectomy pulmonary edema can occur in patients undergoing pneumonectomy or lobectomy (129,130) (see Critical Care Perspectives section). Although positive fluid balance has not been demonstrated as the cause (131–134), as a rule fluid restriction is practiced during pulmonary resection (135–137) and a vasopressor, rather than intravenous fluid, is preferred to correct hypotension.

K. Radiation and Chemotherapy

Small cell lung cancer is primarily managed with systemic chemotherapy and radiation. Surgical resection, although controversial, is optional for peripheral (Stage 1) small cell cancers, followed by postoperative systemic chemotherapy (138) and often prophylactic cranial irradiation (141,142). Chemotherapy and radiation are used for palliation of patients with advanced disease.

Localized (Stage I, II) nonsmall cell lung cancer is primarily treated with surgical resection, unless patients are considered poor candidates for surgery because of impaired pulmonary function, medical comorbidities, or the patient's decision not to undergo surgery (139, 140). Prophylactic cranial irradiation is controversial at this time.

Patients with stage IIIA usually also undergo surgical resection. Patients with localized IIIB (T4 N0) lesion, e.g., vertebral invasion, invasion of great vessels, carinal invasion, etc. may have surgical resection with excellent survival. This, however, is not the case for Stage III patients with malignant pleural effusion or N3 nodal disease. Patients with stage III usually also have preoperative chemotherapy (also known as induction or neoadjuvant chemotherapy) and are often treated with postoperative radiation.

Patients with stage IV disease are usually treated with systemic chemotherapy and radiation added for palliative reasons e.g., vertebral involvement, chest wall invasion, and bronchial obstruction, etc.

Recent studies indicate that postoperative chemotherapy may result in a small improvement in survival for Stage I, II, and IIIA patients. Although not considered standard of care, some institutions offer patients with Stage II and IIIA postoperative chemotherapy.

Postoperative radiation is given for microscopic positive margins, and for unsuspected N2 (mediastinal) disease found at surgery. In the latter case, it improves local control but not overall survival since N2 positivity is considered a marker for systemic disease.

The complications of radiation treatment for esophageal and lung cancers include pneumonitis and mediastinal fibrosis, cardiomyopathy with cardiac valvular dysfunction pericarditis, myelitis, and increased bleeding during surgery (143–145).

Physicians caring for these patients should be aware of side effects of chemotherapeutic agents, like the antibiotic adriamycin can cause dose-related cardiomyopathy with arrhythmias, ECG changes and cardiac failure and also of interaction with anesthetic agents or drugs. For example, a F_iO_2 of 1.0 is routinely used during OLV and this may have clinical relevance for patients exposed to certain agents (e.g., bleomycin, nitrofurantoin, amiodarone, mitomycin-C) that have been associated with pulmonary oxygen toxicity. In these patients, F_iO_2 is diluted with air to the minimum concentration needed to maintain adequate oxygenation (146).

Chemotherapeutic regimens are constantly changing, so side effects and complications must be reviewed prior to surgery (147–149). Agents are being developed that selectively target cancer cells at the molecular, biochemical, and genetic level to minimize toxic effects on normal tissues. Molecularly targeted approaches for lung cancer include epidermal growth factor receptor inhibitors, antiangiogenic agents, inhibitors of biologically important enzymes (e.g., matrix metalloproteinases, farnesyltransferase), gene therapy, and cell cycle disruptors (150). Current chemotherapeutic regimens, however, usually consist of a combination of a platinum-based agent (cisplatin [Europe] or carboplatin [America]) combined with a second agent (Etopiside or Vinblastin [Europe] or Taxane (paclitaxil or doxetaxol) [America]) as first line therapy.

III. INTRATHORACIC MALIGNANCIES

A. Lung Cancer

Presenting symptoms vary according to tumor size, location, and stage. A patient may be asymptomatic with early tumors. Tumors involving the airway can cause shortness of breath, cough, wheezing, or hemoptysis. Invasion of the parietal pleura or chest wall can produce persistent localized chest or arm pain. Tumors can be very large at the time of surgery and produce local effects (e.g., postobstructive pneumonia, superior vena cava (SVC) syndrome, Pancoast syndrome) or systemic effects (paraneoplastic syndrome).

Primary lung tumors are divided into major groups depending on their histology (Table 1) and on their staging (Table 2). Evaluation, treatment options, and prognosis differ for each histological and staging group.

Sputum cytology generally has a low positive diagnostic yield. Percutaneous needle biopsy is a safe, accurate technique for diagnosing peripheral lung lesions larger than 1.0 cm. Bronchoscopy is used to sample hilar and endobronchial lesions.

Small cell lung cancer is primarily treated with chemotherapy and radiation. The role of surgery in the management of these patients includes diagnosis and staging by mediastinoscopy or open biopsy, and resection of Stage I tumors in conjunction with pre- and postoperative chemotherapy and possible prophylactic cranial irradiation.

Table 1 Histological Classification of Primary Lung Malignancy

Adenocarcinomas
Acinar
Papillary
Bronchoalveolar
Solid adenocarcinoma with mucin formation
Nonmucinous
Mucinous
Mixed mucinous and nonmucinous, or indeterminent
Adenocarcinoma with mixed subtypes
Well-differentiated fetal adenocarcinoma
Mucinous ("Colloid")
Mucinous cystadenocarcinoma
Signet ring adenocarcinoma
Clear cell adenocarcinoma
Squamous cell carcinoma
Papillary
Clear cell
Small cell
Basaloid
Small cell carcinoma
Combined small cell carcinoma
Large cell carcinoma
Large cell neuroendocrine carcinoma
Combined large cell neuroendocrine carcinoma
Basaloid carcinoma
Lymphoepithelioma-like carcinoma
Clear cell carcinoma
Large clear cell carcinoma with rhabdoid phenotype
Carcinoid tumors

Early, localized (Stage I, II, IIIA) nonsmall cell lung cancers (e.g., squamous cell carcinoma, adenocarcinoma, large cell carcinoma, and mixed histology tumors) are treated surgically. Survival rates after surgery depend on the stage of the cancer. Stage III patients are generally treated with preoperative chemotherapy. Recent studies suggest that postoperative chemotherapy may improve survival.

Carcinoid tumors are low-grade malignancies, which typically occur in the bronchi and trachea. It is extremely rare for an airway carcinoid to produce "carcinoid syndrome" which is caused by serotonin secretion from gut tumors with hepatic metastasis. Mesotheliomas are pleural-based tumors frequently associated with asbestos exposure and have a poor prognosis despite aggressive medical and surgical treatment. Surgical treatment is aggressive with extrapleural pneumonectomy, where the parietal pleura, lung, diaphragm, and pericardium are resected en bloc, followed by reconstruction of the pericardium and diaphragm.

Table 2 TNM Staging of Lung Carcinoma

Stage	T	N	M
0	*cis*		
Ia	1	0	0
Ib	2	0	0
IIa	1	1	0
IIb	2	1	0
	3	0	0
IIIa	3	1	0
	1–3	2	0
IIIb	4	0–2	0
	1–4	3	0
IV	any T	any N	1

T = primary tumor
cis = carcinoma in situ
T1 = tumor < 3 cm without evidence of invasion of proximal to lobar bronchus
T2 = tumor > 3 cm, visceral pleural invasion, or with a telectasis/pneumonia extending proximally to hilum
T3 = tumor invading chest wall, diaphragm, mediastinal pleura, pericardium, or within 2 cm of carina
T4 = tumor involving mediastinum, heart, great vessels, trachea, esophagus, vertebral bodies, carina; or malignant effusion
N = nodal involvement
N0 = no nodal metastasis
N1 = metastasis to peribronchial or ipsilateral hilar nodes
N2 = metastasis to ipsilateral mediastinal and/or subcarinal nodes
N3 = metastasis to contralateral mediastinal, any scalene, or supraclavicular nodes
M = distant metastasis
M0 = no distant metastasis
M1 = distant metastasis

B. Associated Syndromes

1. *Paraneoplastic Syndromes*

Lung neoplasms, particularly small cell carcinoma, are associated with a variety of paraneoplastic syndromes (151–153). These conditions are caused by tumor production of polypeptide hormones such as adrenocorticotropic hormone, or by antibodies directed against tumor antigens that cross-react with neural tissue (154).

The most frequent paraneoplastic syndrome is hyponatremia from production of antidiuretic hormone. Hypocalcemia due to a parathyroid-like factor is associated with squamous cell lung cancer. Cushing's syndrome is also common.

The Eaton–Lambert or "myasthenic syndrome" is characterized by defective neurotransmitter release of acetylcholine at autonomic neurons and presynaptic terminals of the neuromuscular junction caused by an IgG autoantibody formed against calcium channels (155,156).

Clinically, there is subacute muscular fatigability with weakness and wasting affecting the proximal parts of the limbs and trunk. A combined epidural and general anesthetic technique provides the best operating conditions and postoperative analgesia for these patients (157). Muscle relaxants must be used with caution and titrated to neuromuscular activity with careful monitoring since there is increased sensitivity to nondepolarizing agents (158).

2. *Superior Vena Cava Syndrome*

The thin-walled SVC is easily compressed by intrathoracic lymph nodes or a lung mass (159). The SVC syndrome develops from impairment of blood flow through the SVC to the right atrium. Symptoms include dyspnea and coughing, and swelling of the face, neck, conjunctiva, upper trunk, and upper extremities. Other symptoms are chest pain, dysphagia, stridor, hemoptysis, nasal stuffiness, proptosis, and nausea. Increased venous pressure causes dilation of collateral veins in the neck and chest wall.

Headache, papilledema and visual distortion, altered mentation, dizziness, syncope, stupor, and even coma can occur from edema of the central nervous system (CNS). Compression of the nerves of the superior mediastinum (vagus and phrenic) can cause hoarseness and diaphragmatic paralysis.

The SVC syndrome develops in 5–10% of patients with right-sided malignant intrathoracic mass lesions (160). The most common causes are small cell bronchogenic carcinoma (75–80%) and non-Hodgkin's lymphoma (10–15%) (161). Other primary pulmonary neoplasms associated with SVC syndrome are squamous cell carcinoma, adenocarcinoma, and large cell carcinoma.

A CT scan can provide accurate details as to the type and location of the obstruction, and can guide attempts at biopsy. If the patient has respiratory symptoms, particularly if dyspnea worsens when the patient is recumbent, a pulmonary flow-volume study should be performed.

Biopsy is obtained by bronchoscopy, from palpable cervical or supraclavicular lymph nodes, by needle biopsy of a lung or mediastinal mass using CT or ultrasound guidance, and by mediastinoscopy, mediastinotomy, or VATS (162).

Venous access in the lower limbs is preferred with SVC obstruction. Intravenous injections in the upper extremities are unpredictable since drug distribution may be slowed.

During surgery substantial blood loss can result from the abnormally high venous pressure, so cross-matched blood should be immediately available.

Balloon angioplasty, with or without stent placement, is currently used to reopen occluded vessels (163,164).

3. Pancoast Syndrome

Pancoast tumors are located in the superior pulmonary ulcus at the apex of the lung. They are characterized by pain, Horner's syndrome, bone destruction, and atrophy of the intrinsic hand muscles. A Pancoast tumor can invade lymphatics, the sympathetic chain, intercostals nerves, ribs, vertebral bodies and subclavian blood vessels. Clinical signs are caused by compression of the C_8–T_2 nerve roots of the brachial plexus (165).

The CXR may reveal a sharply defined shadow in the apex of the thorax, and destruction of the posterior portions of the first three ribs and transverse processes. The degree of brachial plexus involvement can be assessed by a MR study (166).

Treatment includes staging by mediastinoscopy, preoperative radiotherapy, followed by complete "en bloc" tumor resection (167). A neck dissection with anterior fat pad resection, with or without partial sternotomy, may be done prior to thoracotomy to free the tumor from the brachial plexus and/or subclavian vessels.

C. Esophageal Cancer

Esophageal tumors typically present as fungating, ulcerated, intraluminal lesions. They may directly invade surrounding mediastinal structures, and metastasize through the blood and lymphatic system. The trachea, main bronchi, and the aorta can also be involved. The signs and symptoms of esophageal cancer are listed in Table 3.

Surgical resection is the standard of care for Barrett's esophagus with high-grade dysplasia, and for early and locally advanced esophageal cancer (168,169).

Preoperative assessment of the patient involves evaluation of cardiopulmonary reserve, and tumor staging (Table 4). A chest radiograph may demonstrate an air–fluid level in the esophagus. Advanced disease may be associated with evidence of pneumonia, abscess, or pleural effusion. Barium contrast studies will show narrowing of the esophageal lumen. Patients routinely undergo esophagoscopy and bronchoscopy with biopsy, endoscopic ultrasound, and CT and/or PET scans preoperatively for diagnosis and staging (170–172).

Table 3 Esophageal Cancer

Symptoms at the time of diagnosis:

Symptom	Frequency (%)
Dysphagia	74.0
Weight loss	57.3
Heartburn	20.5
Odynophagia	16.6
Shortness of breath	12.1
Chronic cough	10.8
Hoarse voice	6.1
Hematemesis	5.6
Cervical adenopathy	5.5
Hemoptysis	3.6

Diagnostic or surgical evaluation:

Diagnostic procedure	Abnormal or suggestive of malignancy (%)
Esophagoscopy	89.0
CT scan primary site	71.3
Barium esophagraphy	68.9
Bronchoscopy	21.4
Chest radiograph	17.0
Laryngoscopy	16.7
CEA	15.1
Albumin	12.5
Bone scan	11.0
Alkaline phosphatase	10.8
SGOT	9.4
MRI primary site	7.8
PFT	7.1
Mediastinoscopy	4.6

Abnormal = expressed as percent of patients receiving the test.

IV. SURGICAL PERSPECTIVES

A. Preoperative Evaluation

The extent of the preoperative evaluation depends on the underlying disease, comorbidities and on the type and urgency of the proposed operation. In most situations, the surgeon will provide the anesthesiologist with a medical history and results of a physical exam and appropriate laboratory studies. There should be a mechanism for the surgeon and anesthesiologist to communicate their concerns prior to surgery, and in particular, the anesthesiologist must be completely familiar with the proposed operation and the surgeon's specific needs.

B. Preparation

Issues of antibiotic and deep venous thrombosis (DVT) prophylaxis are addressed prior to the induction of anesthesia (173,174). Prophylactic antibiotic practices are unique to each surgeon, but in general 24 hr of therapy with a first generation cephalosporin is currently indicated, with the initial dose being given by the anesthesiologist just prior to skin incision (175).

The protocol for DVT prophylaxis can also be highly variable. Thoracic surgeons are in agreement as to the importance of DVT prophylaxis for patients

Table 4 TNM Staging of Esophageal Cancer

Stage	T	N	M
Stage 0	T*cis*	N0	M0
Stage 1	T1	N0	M0
Stage IIa	T2	N0	M0
	T3	N0	M0
Stage IIb	T1	N1	M0
	T2	N1	M0
Stage III	T3	N1	M0
	T4	any N	M0
Stage IV	any T	any N	M1
Stage IVa	any T	any N	M1a
Stage IVb	any T	any N	M1b

T = primary tumor
TX = primary tumor cannot be assessed
T0 = no evidence of primary tumor
T*cis* = carcinoma in situ
T1 = tumor invades the lamina propria or submucosa
T2 = tumor invades the muscularis propria
T3 = tumor invades the periesophageal tissue
T4 = tumor invades adjacent structures
N = Regional lymph nodes
NX = regional lymph nodes cannot be assessed
N0 = no regional lymph node metastasis
N1 = regional lymph node metastasis
M = Distant metastasis
MX = distant metastasis cannot be assessed
M0 = no distant metastasis
M1a = distant metastasis—cervical nodes
M1b = other distant metastasis

with malignancy and who may be immobilized for a prolonged period postoperatively (176,177). Whether sequential compression devices, subcutaneous heparin, or both are used, therapy should be initiated prior to the induction of anesthesia for optimal effect.

C. Patient Positioning and Surgical Incisions

Commonly used incisions for thoracic procedures include the posterior–lateral thoracotomy, VATS port-sites, median sternotomy, anterior thoracotomy (often bilateral, also known as a clam-shell thoracotomy), laparotomy, and a variety of cervical approaches (178–183). The application of monitors and placement of intravenous lines will depend on the planned incision.

The majority of pulmonary procedures (e.g., posterior–lateral thoracotomy, VATS operations) are performed with the patient in the lateral decubitus position. Patients are anesthetized while still supine on an operating table that already has a beanbag or chest bolsters in place. Once anesthetized, the patient is often evaluated by flexible bronchoscopy and or esophagoscopy. A laryngeal mask airway (LMA) is suitable for this as it allows the upper airway to be evaluated. After bronchoscopy, a double lumen tube or bronchial blocker is placed and the patient rolled into the lateral position. The bed is flexed to spread the ribs on the operative side, and an axillary roll is placed on the dependent side. Appropriate padding is used to keep the head, neck, and spine in neutral alignment. The lower arm is extended on an arm board and an airplane holder or multiple pillows are used to support the upper arm. The lower leg is bent and the upper leg extended straight with supportive pillows in between. The patient is secured with the beanbag or chest bolsters, and with tape across the hip. At the end of the operation, the flex may be taken out of the bed to help facilitate incision closure, and the beanbag softened.

Occasionally, patients with large pleural effusions may decompensate when turned into the lateral decubitus position, as the effusion may distort mediastinal structures or obstruct venous return. The patient should be returned to the supine position and the effusion drained prior to positioning in the decubitus position.

Anterior thoracotomies are performed with the patient supine and tilted up with a roll or beanbag under the operative hemi-thorax.

For esophageal procedures, both arms are usually tucked in at the side. A small roll is frequently placed under the shoulder blades to extend the neck and facilitate access to structures in the neck and upper mediastinum. The head should be rotated (generally to the right) for exposure to the cervical esophagus. Ivor–Lewis and 3-field esophagectomies require the patient to be repositioned multiple times in the supine and lateral decubitus positions.

D. Procedures

Thoracic procedures and their primary postoperative complications are listed in Table 5.

1. *Fiberoptic Bronchoscopy (FOB)*

FOB is used for routine airway inspection, trans- and endobronchial biopsy, and bronchoalveolar lavage. It can be performed with the patient sedated under topical anesthesia (184–186) and as an outpatient procedure.

If general anesthesia is required an "awake" intubation using topical anesthesia, an inhalation anesthetic induction preserving spontaneous ventilation, or intravenous agents and muscle relaxants can all be

Table 5 Thoracic Surgeries and Primary Postoperative Complications

Surgery	Complications
Flexible bronchoscopy with or without biopsy	Bronchospasm, atelectasis, pneumothorax, intrapulmonary hemorrhage
Rigid bronchoscopy with or without biopsy	Aspiration, pneumothorax, tracheobronchial rupture, intrapulmonary hemorrhage, vocal cord dysfunction
Mediastinoscopy and mediastinal mass resection	Pneumothorax, intrapleural hemorrhage, recurrent laryngeal nerve injury, phrenic nerve injury, chylothorax, air embolism, tension pneumomediastinum, tracheal collapse, hemothorax
Thymectomy	Postoperative weakness, pneumothorax, recurrent laryngeal nerve injury
Video-assisted thoracoscopy Surgery (VATS)	Pneumothorax, pulmonary hemorrhage, atelectasis
Pulmonary resection: Wedge resection Lobectomy Pneumonectomy	Pneumothorax, pulmonary edema/ARDS, phrenic nerve injury, recurrent laryngeal injury, chylothorax, pulmonary hemorrhage, pulmonary torsion, arrhythmias, right heart failure, atelectasis, pneumonia, BPF, cardiac herniation, paralysis
Tracheal resection and reconstruction	Tracheobronchial disruption, recurrent laryngeal nerve injury, airway obstruction, pneumothorax
Chest wall resection	Pneumothorax, arrhythmias, intrapleural hemorrhage, flail chest
SVC decompression	Pneumothorax, airway obstruction, bronchospasm, postoperative weakness
Esophagectomy	Hypovolemia, arrhythmias, anastamotic leak

Abbreviations: ARDS, acute respiratory distress syndrome; BPF, bronchopleural fistula; SVC, superior vena cava.

employed depending on the nature of the airway disease (187).

The FOB is placed through a diaphragm connected to either an LMA or ETT.The LMA allows the trachea and vocal chords to be assessed. The bronchoscope reduces the available cross-sectional area within the tube and therefore an internal diameter of at least 8.0 mm is recommended. Suctioning during FOB will deplete fresh gas flow and ventilator bellow filling. One-hundred percent oxygen and high fresh gas flow are therefore recommended.

During bronchoscopy cardiovascular instability (hypertension, hypotension) due to "light" anesthesia, hypoxia and hypercapnia are not uncommon (188). Administering an anticholinergic, midazolam, and/or propofol will reduce the incidence of arrhythmia (189–191).

Pulmonary function usually decreases immediately following bronchoscopy (192). Other complications include laryngeal and bronchial spasm and direct airway trauma which can produce bleeding, edema, and tumor fragmentation (193,194). Coughing increases bleeding. Subcutaneous emphysema and tension pneumothorax can result from mucosal perforation or barotrauma.

2. *Rigid Bronchoscopy*

Rigid bronchoscopy is performed to evaluate hemoptysis, inspect, and mechanically dilate tracheal or bronchial strictures, for tumor debridement and removal of foreign bodies. A general anesthetic is required with the patient supine. The head and neck are extended and eyes, teeth, and gums are carefully protected.

After anesthesia is achieved, the patient's trachea is extubated and rigid bronchoscope is inserted into the posterior pharynx. The epiglottis is visualized and lifted anteriorly allowing visualization of the vocal cords. The patient is paralyzed and ventilation is controlled using one of several techniques (195,196).

Oxygen can be delivered by insufflation at a high flow (10–15 L/min) without actually ventilating the patient ("apneic oxygenation"). Although satisfactory oxygenation is achieved, carbon dioxide accumulates so apnea should not extend beyond 5 min.

The rigid bronchoscope has a viewing lens. While it is in place, oxygen and anesthetic gases can be delivered through the side-arm of the bronchoscope by intermittent ventilation. The anesthesiologist must be continuously aware of when the lens is removed to coordinate ventilation.

High fresh gas flows are used to compensate for the leak around the bronchoscope. During long procedures, carbon dioxide can accumulate predisposing the patient to arrhythmias. Intermittent hyperventilation lowers P_aCO_2 and deepens inhalation anesthesia. Use of the oxygen flush should be kept to a minimum since it bypasses the anesthetic vaporizer and dilutes the inhalational agent. Since ventilation must be interrupted whenever biopsy or suctioning is performed, a

TIVA technique is preferred since it allows continuous maintenance of anesthesia and reduces OR pollution (197).

Oxygen can also be delivered by jet ventilation using a Sanders system (198,199). Presence of the eyepiece is not necessary so continuous uninterrupted ventilation is possible.

3. *Mediastinoscopy*

Mediastinal adenopathy can be evaluated by mediastinoscopy (transcervical or transthoracic mediastinoscopy) to facilitate staging and assess whether pulmonary resection is indicated (200–203).

Transcervical mediastinoscopy can provide access to pretracheal, paratracheal, and subcarinal lymph nodes. It can be performed under local anesthesia (204,205). General anesthesia is preferred because of the risk of pneumothorax, venous air embolism, and mediastinal injury all increase if the patient moves (206).

Patients are placed in the supine position with their neck extended. They are prepped from chin to umbilicus. A short transverse cervical incision is made one finger breath above the sternal notch and the dissection is taken down to the pretracheal plane. Blunt dissection is used to carry this plane into the mediastinum.

The mediastinoscope can compress the innominate artery causing loss of the right radial pulse. In the presence of a normal ECG, this has been misinterpreted as "hypotension" and has led to inappropriate aggressive treatment (207). During mediastinoscopy, blood pressure measurements should be obtained from the left arm, while the right radial pulse is monitored by pulse oximetry (208,209). If a unilateral decrease in the right radial pulse occurs, the mediastinoscope should be repositioned. This is especially important for a patient with a history of impaired cerebral vascular circulation since carotid artery perfusion can be compromised by vascular compression.

Meticulous care is taken to distinguish lymph nodes from vascular structures prior to biopsy, but intraoperative hemorrhage can be sudden and substantial. Vascular structures at risk include the aorta, innominate artery, azygous vein, and the pulmonary arteries. Temporary packing of the wound controls most bleeding from small vessels and lymph nodes, and packing can tamponade larger vascular injuries while thoracotomy or sternotomy is performed for definitive repair.

If a large mediastinal blood vessel is torn, fluids given through an intravenous line in the arm may enter the mediastinum. In this situation, intravenous fluid should be infused in a lower extremity vein, and cardiopulmonary bypass (CPB) should be considered (210).

The complications of mediastinoscopy include tension pneumothorax, recurrent laryngeal nerve damage, air embolism, hemorrhage, acute tracheal collapse, tension pneumomediastinum, hemothorax, and chylothorax (211,212). Patients should have a CXR in the immediate postoperative period to exclude these complications.

Transthoracic mediastinoscopy (also referred to as a Chamberlain's procedure or anterior mediastinotomy) provides excellent exposure to the lymph nodes in the aortopulmonary window. The chest is entered above the left third costal cartilage and the mediastinum explored without entering the pleural space (213). Care needs to be taken to identify and avoid injury to the internal mammary artery. If the pleural space is entered, a chest tube should be inserted or the air evacuated prior to closure.

4. *Video-Assisted Thoracoscopic Surgery (VATS)*

VATS describes an operative approach rather than a specific procedure. To be used effectively, the surgeon and anesthesiologist must be willing and ready to convert to open operation when the situation dictates. Patients are generally placed in lateral position and port-site numbers and position vary depending on the procedure performed.

VATS can be an alternative to open thoracotomy to obtain pulmonary and pleural biopsies, for limited lung, esophageal and mediastinal resection, and for laser treatment of tumors (214–219). Its benefits include smaller incisions, more rapid recovery with shortened hospital stay, and less postoperative pain (220,221).

Patients range from healthy low risk to those with severe pulmonary disease. Therefore, the anesthetic technique and choice of monitors will depend on the overall status of the patient and not necessarily on the procedure.

Selective collapse of the operated lung is essential. As soon as the lungs are isolated, ventilation to the operated lung is discontinued. Insufflation of carbon dioxide into the pleural space can speed lung collapse, but can cause marked hemodynamic instability similar to a tension pneumothorax (222).

Pain after VATS is unpredictable and analgesic requirements vary greatly. Systemic opioids, NSAIDs, intercostal nerve blocks, intrapleural local anesthetics, and occasionally epidural opioids are used.

5. *Pulmonary Resection*

Pulmonary resection can be divided into anatomic and nonanatomic procedures. Anatomic techniques involve dissection, ligation, and division of the pulmonary vessels and airways as anatomic segments. A segmentectomy is the smallest anatomic operation, followed by lobectomy, bilobectomy, and pneumonectomy. Nonanatomic resections involve removal of lung tumor without regard for pulmonary anatomy. A wedge resection is an example of a nonanatomic operation.

Wedge Resection

Pulmonary wedge resections are frequently performed to evaluate and resect pulmonary nodules. If the nodule is malignant on frozen section, the procedure may be converted to a lobectomy. Therefore, preoperative evaluation is similar to lobectomy, and patients need to be counseled about the possibility of a more extensive operation.

Most benign nodules and metastatic lesions are removed by wedge resection. Open lung biopsy is a form of wedge resection. Patients with limited pulmonary reserve may undergo wedge resection as definitive treatment of their primary lung cancer.

Wedge resection is most commonly performed by a VATS approach or posterior–lateral thoracotomy, but it can also be performed through an anterior thoracotomy. A median sternotomy can be used for wedge resection of bilateral metastatic disease.

Lobectomy

Lobectomy is the approach for primary lung cancer. Preoperative assessment includes a thorough staging of the tumor (Table 2).

Patients with Stage I or II nonsmall cell tumors are generally offered surgery, unless pulmonary function or comorbid conditions pose a prohibitive risk. Patients with Stage IIIA disease can be surgical candidates following induction chemotherapy and radiation (223). Patients with Stage IIIB or IV disease are rarely offered surgery (224,225), although patients with localized stage IIIB tumors without malignant pleural effusion may undergo successful surgery.

In patients scheduled for lobectomy, an FOB is first performed to inspect airway anatomy and to determine resectability of a proximal lesion. Lobectomy is usually performed with the patient in the lateral decubitus position through a muscle-sparing or full posterior–lateral thoracotomy (226–228), but VATS techniques are gaining acceptance (229–232).

Once the operative lung is adequately deflated, bronchovascular anatomy is identified. Vascular structures are generally divided first. Hypotension and arrhythmias can occur when the hilar structures are vigorously retracted. Instability usually resolves quickly with restoration of the normal anatomic relationships. Next the bronchus is clamped and divided. Temporary reinflation of the lung is required at this stage to insure that the remaining lobes inflate properly prior to surgical division and stapling. It is recommended that the mobility of the endobronchial tube, and other devices such as a nasogastric tube (NGT) or temperature probe be checked to ensure that they are not stapled in.

The integrity of the bronchial repair must be tested after the lobe is removed but before the chest is closed. While the anesthesiologist manually applies inflation pressures incrementally up to 30–40 cm H_2O, the bronchus is inspected under water to check for air leaks. Following pneumonectomy, the integrity of the bronchial suture line is tested in a similar manner. The patient's airway should be extubated as soon as possible following surgery to reduce stress on the bronchial suture line from positive pressure ventilation.

One or two chest tubes are placed prior to closure. Placing the chest tubes to suction will increase any observed air leak in an intubated patient. To reduce leak, it is helpful to leave the tubes to water seal until the airway is extubated.

Pneumonectomy

Preoperative assessment is similar to lobectomy, with thorough tumor staging and adequate evaluation of cardiopulmonary reserve. The operation is conducted in a similar manner to a lobectomy.

Postoperative BPF is a worrisome complication, with high morbidity and mortality, and therefore special care is taken to resect and close the bronchus. The resected right bronchial stump is not as well protected by mediastinal structures as the left bronchus. Pericardial fat, pleura, intercostal muscle, and latissimus muscle can all be used as a flap to reinforce the bronchial suture line (233–237).

Chest drainage is not standard following pneumonectomy. If a chest tube is used, it is placed to a balanced drainage system, and is never placed to suction. Suction can result in significant mediastinal shift with hemodynamic compromise. If a drainage tube is not left in place, the mediastinum is usually balanced at the end of the procedure by aspirating air out of the pneumonectomy space.

6. *Tracheal Resection*

The indications for tracheal resection are primary tracheal tumors and strictures (238–240). Strictures are frequently related to prior intubation or tracheostomy. Imaging with CT or MRI to measure length, position, and caliber of the stenosis is an essential part of preoperative assessment.

Lesions of the upper and midtrachea are approached through the neck, while lesions of the lower trachea and carina are approached through the right chest. The trachea can be extensively mobilized in the anterior and posterior planes, but circumferential dissection is limited to the area of resection to avoid devascularization. When the trachea is opened, the oral ETT is pulled back into the proximal airway and a sterile armored ETT is placed across the operative field into the distal airway. Prior to completion of the anastomosis, the cross-field ETT is removed and the original ETT is advanced into place under direct vision.

Occasionally, special techniques such as Jet ventilation or CPB are required (241,242).

Neck flexion is often necessary to relieve tension on the anastomosis. A stitch is usually placed from the chin to the chest for the first several postoperative days. The patient's trachea is extubated at the end of the procedure. The need for postoperative mechanical ventilation is associated with poor outcome (243).

7. *Chest Wall Resection*

Chest wall resect is generally performed for primary chest wall tumors and for bronchogenic carcinomas extending into the chest wall. For primary lung cancers, the most important prognostic factor is not the extent of chest wall involvement, but rather the nodal staging of the tumor.

Chest wall resection for lung cancer usually involves resection of the ribs and intercostal muscle en bloc with the lobectomy specimen. The skin and overlying muscle are left intact. Small defects (two ribs or less) and posterior chest wall defects that are covered by the scapula do not usually require reconstruction. Larger defects and those not protected by the scapula frequently require mesh (Gortex or Marlex) reconstruction to re-establish the integrity of the rib cage (244,245).

Resection is the treatment of choice for most primary chest wall tumors, except for Ewing's sarcomas and rhabdomyosarcomas, which are routinely treated with preoperative chemotherapy. Resections for primary chest wall tumors involve wide local excision with en bloc resection of adjacent involved structures. A 4 cm margin around the tumor is ideal and the overlying muscle and skin are included with the specimen. This frequently creates a very large defect. Reconstruction is more complex and often requires collaboration with a plastic surgeon (246).

8. *Mediastinal Mass*

Mediastinal tumors are characterized by their location in the anterior, middle, or posterior mediastinum. Common anterior mediastinal lesions are thymic tumors, substernal goiters, lymphomas, and germ cell tumors. Lymphomas usually require only biopsy. Thymic tumors and germ cell tumors warrant resection via median sternotomy.

Preoperative evaluation for an anterior mediastinal mass includes CT scan, and in males tumor markers for germ cell neoplasms.

Anterior mediastinal masses can compress the SVC, major airways, and even the heart. Complete or partial airway obstruction from an anterior mediastinal mass can occur following patient positioning and with pharmacologic relaxation of the muscles maintaining airway patency (247,248). It is important to determine if the patient has experienced dyspnea in the supine position. Imaging studies should determine the extent of tumor mass and any involvement with surrounding structures (249). Flow-volume loops are obtained in both the upright and supine positions (250,251). A marked decrease in FEV_1 and peak expiratory flow rate in the supine position suggests the potential for airway obstruction with anesthesia. In this situation, radiation to the mass should be considered prior to surgery.

If biopsy of a mediastinal mass cannot be performed under local anesthesia, a FOB-assisted awake airway intubation followed by induction of general anesthesia is recommended. For patients with a variable intrathoracic mass, an inhalation anesthetic induction avoids the need for a muscle relaxant for intubation (252,253). A rigid bronchoscope may be needed to bypass an obstruction to ventilate the patient. Position may need to be changed from supine to lateral or even prone to relieve symptomatic airway compression.

Most middle mediastinal lesions are benign cysts, most can be removed by VATS. Larger cysts may require thoracotomy. Most posterior mediastinal masses are neurogenic tumors and are resected in a combined procedure with a neurosurgeon.

9. *Procedures for Central-Airways Obstruction*

A variety of procedures, usually performed through a bronchoscope, are used to relieve central-airways (trachea, carina, main-bronchi) obstruction (254–258).

Airway stents provide structural support for both intrinsic and extrinsic tumor obstruction (259–261), usually with immediate symptomatic relief of dyspnea (262–267).

The neodymium yttrium aluminum garnet (Nd:YAG) laser is used to resect intraluminal malignancies (268–271). To avoid combustion, F_iO_2 should never exceed 0.4, with air used in place of nitrous oxide (272–279). The laser, passed down either an FOB or rigid bronchoscope, can tunnel through a complete obstruction or widen a narrowed lumen. Coagulated tissue must then be debrided (280,281). Underlying edema formation can result in obstruction and hemorrhage hours after therapy so prophylactic steroids are often given (282,283).

Brachytherapy is the direct application of a highly localized dose of radiation to tumor. It is an effective treatment of dyspnea, hemoptysis, intractable cough, postobstructive atelectasis, and pneumonia due to airway malignancy (284–286).

Photodynamic therapy (PDT) involves the intra venous injection of a photosensitizing compound followed several days later by activation by light (287–290). Neoplastic tissue selectively takes up the photosensitizer, and during the PDT procedure a light delivered through a bronchoscope selectively targets the tumor, activates the sensitizer, and destroys tumor (291).

Other bronchoscopic procedures for airway stenosis include balloon dilation (292), application of extreme cold (cryotherapy) (293–296), and electrocautery resection (297–300).

10. Esophagectomy

Most patients undergo esophagectomy for palliation or attempted cure of esophageal cancer. The utility of preoperative chemoradiation is controversial (301,302).

Many patients have dysphagia and may present with dehydration, malnutrition, and retained food in their esophagus. The esophagus above the obstruction can be filled with food and become infected. Material may be present even after prolonged fasting. To reduce the chance of regurgitation and pulmonary aspiration prior to anesthesia, the esophagus is suctioned with a large oral or NGT.

There are several surgical approaches for esophagectomy, with the Ivor–Lewis and the transhiatal approaches being the most popular (303,304). Both are equally safe and have equivalent long-term survival rates (305).

The Ivor–Lewis operation involves two separate incisions. The procedure begins with a laparotomy with the patient supine. Once the stomach is fully mobilized, the abdomen is closed and the patient is repositioned for a right thoracotomy. Single lung ventilation is required for the transthoracic esophageal mobilization and creation of the anastomosis, which is placed in the apex of the right chest.

In the transhiatal operation, the entire procedure is performed with the patient supine using separate abdominal and cervical incisions. Thoracic esophageal mobilization is accomplished bluntly. The stomach is passed through the posterior mediastinum and anastomosed to the cervical esophagus in the left neck. The chest is not opened, obviating the need for single lung ventilation.

The stomach is preferred as the conduit for reconstruction for both types of esophagectomy operations. When the stomach is not available, a portion of the colon may be interposed between the cervical esophagus and the upper gastrointestinal tract (306).

The NGT, placed at induction of anesthesia to decompress the stomach, is pulled back into the pharynx during resection. It is reinserted into the neoesophagus under direct vision prior to completion of the anastomosis. The NGT suction is continued postoperatively until there is a return of bowel function and no evidence of anastomotic leak.

Perioperative cardiorespiratory instability is associated with postoperative respiratory failure and other complications (307–310).

V. CRITICAL CARE PERSPECTIVES

Patients with thoracic or esophageal neoplasms who are admitted to the intensive care unit (ICU) following surgery present unique clinical challenges related to their underlying respiratory, cardiovascular, gastrointestinal, hematologic, immunologic, and nutritional status. These issues are compounded by potentially life-threatening surgery-related complications that can occur in the recovery period. Since special knowledge and skills are required, a multidisciplinary approach involving intensivists, surgeons, nurses, pharmacists, nutritionists, and respiratory therapists provides optimal patient care (311–313).

A. General Considerations

1. Respiratory Management

Supplemental oxygen, through a nasal cannula or by face-mask, is usually sufficient to maintain oxygenation after most thoracic procedures. Postoperative pulmonary function can be further optimized by treatment of bronchospasm with bronchodilators, use of incentive spirometry, airway suctioning, coughing and deep breathing exercise, and early ambulation.

Patients who experience hypoxemia despite supplemental oxygen require a complete evaluation. Hypoxemia can lead to significant adverse hemodynamic and metabolic consequences that must be aggressively rectified. A Venturi mask, which allows precise control of F_iO_2, or a nonrebreather oxygen mask with 100% oxygen, should be applied. Patients with obstructive sleep apnea (OSA) and others recovering from thoracotomy should be considered for CPAP if no contraindications (e.g., patients with inability to protect the airway, postesophageal surgery) exist (314).

The use of noninvasive ventilation has been shown to decrease mortality in patients with respiratory failure following thoracic surgery (315). Reversible respiratory insufficiency (e.g., COPD exacerbation, cardiogenic pulmonary edema) can be initially managed by noninvasive mechanical ventilation (316). For patients with diminished respiratory drive compromising gas exchange, the trachea should be intubated and ventilation mechanically assisted (317). Indications, modes, complications, and weaning from mechanical ventilation are discussed in chapter Respiratory Support and Mechanical Ventilation in Sec. 3.

2. Fluid Management

Fluid management following lung resection continues to be a topic of debate. Although intraoperative fluid overload was once believed to be the cause of postpneumonectomy respiratory failure, no definitive study has confirmed this relationship (129,318).

Fluid balance of <20 mL/kg for the first 24 hr and a urine output >0.5 mL/kg/hr are acceptable as general guides for patients undergoing pulmonary resection (319). In hypovolemic patients, appropriate fluid or blood product replacement is justified to avoid end-organ injury. Hypotension due to epidural local anesthetics should be treated with a vasopressor rather than liberal fluid boluses.

Patients with esophageal cancer generally are malnourished and are hypovolemic prior to surgery. There can be significant third space fluid loss and bleeding during esophagectomy. Unlike the situation after lung resection, continuous liberal fluid replacement is required postesophagectomy.

3. Nutrient Management

Cancer patients can be immunosuppressed due to malnutrition, cytotoxic therapy, and a hypermetabolic stress state. Proper nutritional support in the perioperative period promotes wound healing and recovery (320), and may reduce postoperative morbidity and mortality (321). Early enteral feeding decreases the risk of stress ulcer formation, sepsis, and a further worsening of nutritional status (322,323).

Following thoracotomy, patients whose airways are extubated and who are capable of protecting their airway, and who are hemodynamically stable and have no evidence of ileus should be started on an oral diet. The diet is advanced as tolerated. Postesophagectomy patients should not receive oral or gastric feedings until their barium contrast study demonstrates no anastomotic leak.

Maintenance intravenous fluid therapy should be begun for patients who cannot be started on an oral diet or enteral feeding. If oral intake or tube feeding is not anticipated within 7 days after surgery, total parenteral nutrition (TPN) should be initiated early. Combination of TPN and enteral feeding can meet nutrient and caloric requirements until transition to full enteral feeding (324).

4. Pain Management

The fundamental principle in pain management is to provide adequate pain relief while minimizing the adverse effects of the medications.

Some procedures (e.g., rigid bronchoscopy, tracheal resection, mediastinoscopy) are not very painful, while others (e.g., thoracotomy) are associated with moderate to severe postoperative pain. Cancer patients with pre-existing chronic pain syndrome may experience exacerbation following surgery (325). Patients requiring prolonged ICU care may experience intense pain secondary to multifactorial etiologies requiring a multimodal analgesic regimen.

Regimens associated with the best postoperative pulmonary function are usually considered superior (326,327). In addition to spirometry and arterial blood gases, analgesia is assessed by pain scores (at rest and with movement), amount of supplemental opioid requested, length of hospital stay, and patient satisfaction (328).

Mild to moderate pain generally can be managed with opioids by patient-controlled analgesia (PCA) or by continuous or intermittent intravenous administration (329–332). PCA provides more stable plasma drug levels, greater pain relief, and better patient satisfaction (333). Potential side effects include sedation and respiratory depression, which can become exaggerated in elderly patients with limited pulmonary reserve.

Systemic opioids alone generally do not provide adequate analgesia for post-thoracotomy pain (334). Epidural analgesia with local anesthetics, an opioid, or a combination of the two provides excellent pain control with fewer side effects (335). The major factor limiting use of epidural local anesthesia is the potential for systemic hypotension.

Epidural opioid analgesia is preferred for post-thoracotomy pain since patients have better pulmonary function and are more comfortable than those receiving systemic opioids (336,337). The catheter is inserted in an awake patient at a lumbar or thoracic level, and its position is confirmed prior to surgery. Only the lumbar route should be considered if the catheter needs to be placed during surgery, as may occur when a VATS procedure is converted to an open thoracotomy.

Contraindications for epidural placement include active systemic infection and coagulopathy.

Opioids can be given either at the thoracic or lumbar level without differences in analgesic efficacy (338). Lipophilic opioids (e.g., fentanyl, sufentanil) produce a rapid onset of analgesia (339–343), while hydrophilic agents (e.g., morphine, hydromorphone) diffuse more slowly into the CSF and have a delayed onset but longer duration of action (344).

Epidural analgesia may not control the discomfort caused by a chest tube. This pain can be treated with nonsteroidal anti-inflammatory drugs (NSAIDs), intrapleural local anesthetics, or intercostal nerve blocks. Cryoanalgesia, transcutaneous electric nerve stimulation, ketamine, intercostal nerve blocks, paravertebral blocks, and intrapleural infusion of local anesthetics can each be combined with epidural analgesia (345–354).

NSAIDs, alone or as adjuncts, may improve pain relief and pulmonary function while reducing the amount and side effects of opioids (355–359). Ketorolac is particularly useful for the shoulder pain associated with lateral thoracotomy (360). Gastrointestinal bleeding and renal and platelet dysfunction are potential concerns. Establishing euvolemia prior to the use of NSAIDs may minimize renal insult (361).

Newer agents like cyclooxygenase II inhibitors (i.e., celecoxib) may produce fewer gastrointestinal side effects (362).

Chronic ICU patients with escalating systemic opioid requirements should be thoroughly evaluated for potential causes of pain, discomfort, and agitation. Reversible causes should be treated promptly. The use of rotational opioids (because of incomplete cross-tolerance) (363), anxiolytic agents (e.g., benzodiazepines), and intravenous anesthesia (e.g., propofol) should be considered. Patients with chronic pain syndrome may benefit from other adjuvant medications such as gabapentin, tricyclic antidepressants (e.g., amitriptyline), *N*-methyl-d-aspartate (NMDA) receptor antagonist (e.g., ketamine) (364–366). Short-term use of the alpha$_2$ agonist dexmedetomidine provides both analgesia and mild sedation (367,368).

5. *Chest Tube Management*

Chest tubes are used to drain pleural fluid and to maintain lung expansion. One tube is positioned in the anterior apical region to facilitate suctioning of air with the patient upright, while another tube is placed in the posterior basal region to promote fluid drainage with the patient supine. Position must be confirmed by CXR. The side ports should be located inside the pleural cavity.

The chest tube drainage system consists of three chambers. The first chamber is designed to collect and measure the volume of drained pleural fluid. The second chamber is the underwater seal system that allows air to escape from the pleural space, but prevents air reentry by means of a one-way valve (369). The last chamber is used to regulate the negative pressure [0–30 cm H_2O] generated by the suction through adjusting the depth of water filling the chamber. Continuous bubbling through the underwater seal chamber indicates persistent intrapleural air leak (370,371).

The tubing can become clotted and obstructed if not stripped periodically. An obstructed tube can result in development of a tension pneumothorax. A chest tube in place after pneumonectomy should never be placed on suction since this can result in mediastinal shift and cardiac herniation (372).

Prophylactic antibiotic coverage for gram-positive organisms should be continued as long as a chest tube is in place (373). Indications for chest tube discontinuation include full re-expansion of the lung without evidence of air leak and pleural fluid drainage < 100–150 mL/day. Persistent air leak, which prevents chest tube removal, is the major factor prolonging hospital stay after pulmonary resection (374).

6. *Prophylactic Measures*

Patients with neoplasms are at high risk for developing DVTs and acute pulmonary embolism (PE). Risk factors include a major surgical procedure, hypercoagulable state due to cancer, prolonged bed rest, and advanced age. Routine postoperative thromboprophylaxis with intermittent compression boots and low dose subcutaneous heparin (5000 units every 12 hr) is recommended (375).

Stress ulcer development in the ICU can be due to gastric ischemia and hypoperfusion (376). Although majority of ulcers are clinically silent, potentially life-threatening gastric bleeding can occur. While enteral nutritional support may reduce ulcer development, definitive clinical data are limited (377). In patients who are unable to tolerate enteral feeding, sucralfate has been shown to minimize formation of stress ulcer and hemorrhage (378). Sucralfate appears to be less effective than H_2-blockers, but it is associated with fewer side effects (e.g., nosocomial pneumonia) (379).

H_2-receptor blockers and proton-pump inhibitors are used for ulcer prophylaxis, but are expensive and interact with a large number of other medications. However, previous concern that their gastric pH neutralizing effect promoted bacterial colonization contributing to nosocomial or ventilator-associated pneumonia (VAP) is now questioned (380).

B. Specific Considerations

1. Respiratory Considerations

Bronchospasm

Patients often have pre-existing reactive airway disease. Bronchospasm can lead to air trapping, dynamic hyperinflation, impaired gas exchange, respiratory distress, and even pulmonary hypertension. Causes of increased airflow resistance in the postoperative period include inadequate preoperative optimization of bronchial reactivity, pain and anxiety, pulmonary secretions, fluid overload ("cardiac asthma"), foreign body irritation, and pneumonia.

The mainstays for treating bronchospasm are beta-agonist drugs, anticholinergic agents, and corticosteroids. Additional therapies are directed at the underlying causes of airflow limitation and include management of pain and judicious use of anxiolytics (381). Propofol (without metabisulfite) is used for anxiety, but also offers potential bronchial dilating properties (382).

Treatment of pulmonary secretions with suctioning, fluid overload with diuretics, and pulmonary infections with antibiotics, may also be required.

Beta$_2$-agonists (e.g., albuterol), alone or in combination with an anticholinergic agent, given by meter dose inhaler or nebulizer reduce acute bronchoconstriction, stabilize mast cells, and inhibit the release and effects of acetylcholine. Corticosteroids are used as adjuvant therapy to enhance the effects of beta$_2$-agonists and reduce airway inflammation and histamine release (383). Dosage should be tapered after the first 24–48 hr, or when the acute bronchospasm is controlled.

Humidifying inspired air may help reduce airway reactivity. Heliox, traditionally used for upper airway obstruction, improves gas exchange, work of breathing, and may have some benefit in early severe bronchospasm (384). Theophylline, cromolyn, and leukotriene inhibitors have no application in the acute settings.

Noninvasive ventilation or airway intubation may be required for patients with significant impairment of gas exchange. Air trapping may worsen in patients on mechanical ventilation. Extrinsic PEEP should be applied with caution. For patients with severe bronchospasm refractory to standard therapies, an epinephrine infusion, neuromuscular blockade, and use of an inhalational anesthetic (e.g., isoflurane) should be considered.

Atelectasis

Atelectasis may develop due to incomplete intraoperative lung re-expansion, bronchial obstruction by mucous or blood clots, hypoventilation, respiratory splinting, diaphragmatic dysfunction, and surgical trauma to the lung and respiratory muscles.

Clinical signs and symptoms include diminished breath sounds, crackles, cough, and CXR findings consistent with decreased lung volume (385). Fever in the early postoperative period is common, but not diagnostic. Limited atelectasis generally is well tolerated. Moderate to severe atelectasis may lead to inadequate gas exchange, reduction in FRC, and mediastinal shift toward the atelectatic hemithorax. Unresolved atelectasis can progress to pneumonia and empyema (386).

Postoperative deep breathing exercise, coughing, pulmonary toilet with suctioning, use of incentive spirometry, aerosolized bronchodilators, and early progressive ambulation are important in conjunction with effective pain relief (386). Fiberoptic bronchoscopy may be required to assist clearance of mucus plugs. For lobar or whole lung alveolar collapse, the patient should be positioned with the atelectatic lung nondependent to improve V/Q matching and facilitate mucus drainage. Pharmacologic interventions such as respiratory stimulants or mucolytic agents have not been shown to be beneficial (387). CPAP can be an effective treatment of persistent atelectasis. Severe refractory atelectasis may require tracheal intubation and mechanical ventilation.

Pneumonia

A common cause of postoperative respiratory insufficiency is pneumonia. Early administration of appropriate empirical antibiotics improves outcome (388,389)

If untreated or inadequately treated, respiratory failure, sepsis, and multiorgan dysfunction can occur (390,391). Cancer patients are at higher risks because of patient factors (e.g., immunocompromised), surgical factors (e.g., decreased pulmonary reserve after lung resection), and anesthesia factors (e.g., reduced level of consciousness from sedative or analgesia medications) (392–394). Evaluation includes CXR, sputum gram-stain and culture, and blood cultures. Four major types of pneumonia are seen after thoracic surgery.

Aspiration pneumonitis and pneumonia: Clinically significant aspiration can occur due to esophageal or gastric dysmotility, failure to isolate the lungs during thoracotomy in the lateral position (395), postoperative vocal cord dysfunction (396), decreased sensorium from medications (397), and following esophageal surgery (398).

Inhalation of regurgitated sterile gastric contents produces an acute chemical pneumonitis with clinical manifestations that include wheezing, coughing, arterial desaturation, and shortness of breath (399). Aggressive airway suctioning and tracheal intubation in patients who are unable to protect their airways are required. Empirical antibiotic treatment is only indicated in patients who are neutropenic, have small bowel obstruction or evidence of bacterial colonization of gastric contents, or who have signs and symptoms greater than 48 hr (399). Corticosteroids have no proven benefit and are not recommended (400,401).

Aspiration pneumonia can occur after inhalation of colonized naso- or oropharyngeal secretions. Patients at higher risk include those with impaired host defense, dysphagia, an incompetent gastroesophageal sphincter, gastroparesis, abnormalities of aerodigestive tract, supine positioning, nasogastric intubation, and swallowing dysfunction after recent tracheal extubation (399,402).

Common pathogens are listed in Table 6. Anaerobic organisms are rarely found. Although antibiotics are indicated, the use of anaerobic coverage is only justified in patients with periodontal disease, putrid sputum, or evidence of necrotizing pneumonia or lung abscess (399).

Community-acquired pneumonia (CAP): Pneumonia diagnosed within 48 hr after surgery is generally community acquired prior to hospitalization. Due to a depressed immune system, some patients may be asymptomatic before surgery and become symptomatic postoperatively. Patients with advanced age, with significant comorbid conditions, and those who are immunosuppressed have increased risk of poor outcome from community-acquired pneumonia (CAP). Urine legionella antigen should be checked. Antibiotic coverage reduces mortality (389,403) Table 6.

Nosocomial pneumonia (NP): Nosocomial pneumonia (NP) or hospital-acquired pneumonia develops 48–72 hr after ICU admission and is associated with a higher mortality than CAP (404). Risk factors include severe underlying disease, the use of immunosuppressive agents (e.g., corticosteroids, cytotoxic agents), and empirical broad-spectrum antibiotics, and the presence of invasive devices (e.g., ETT, CVP lines) (404,405).

Potential routes of transmission include direct inhalation of respiratory droplets, oropharyngeal or gastric aspiration, contamination by health care personnel, hematologenous spread, and gastrointestinal bacterial translocation (406). Although the predominant pathogens are bacterial, other opportunistic organisms must be considered in immunocompromised patients. Since the specific type of organisms and patterns of antibiotic resistance are a function of local hospital flora, initial use of broad-spectrum antibiotics with subsequent regimen based on culture results is recommended (404,405) Table 6.

Nonpharmacologic preventive measures include routine hand washing between patient contacts, recovering the patient in the semirecumbent position, isolation of patients with resistant organisms, and maintenance of adequate ETT cuff pressure. Rotating antibiotics on fixed intervals have been shown to be an effective means of reducing selective pressure on ICU bacterial flora (407).

Ventilator-associated pneumonia (VAP): VAP, a form of NP, usually occurs after 48–72 hr of mechanical ventilation (408). VAP can manifest as tracheobronchitis, bronchopneumonia, and bronchiolitis. Progression to lung abscess (especially with aspiration pneumonia) or empyema is possible. VAP has a very high mortality risk. Risk factors, routes of transmission, pathogens, treatment, and prevention measures are the same as those for NP (409) Table 6.

Empyema

Pleural empyema generally develops from infected pleural fluid or as a complication of pneumonia (410). Empyema in postpneumonectomy patients is often associated with a BPF, and can occur days to years following surgery (411,412). Gram-positive bacteria are usually found, but fungal and gram-negative etiologies must be considered in immunocompromised patients. The three distinct phases of empyema progression are (a) exudative (increase in leukocytes), (b) fibropurulent (fibrin formation), and (c) organizing (scarring development) (413).

Because of the high mortality, early diagnosis and treatment are important (414). Sepsis, multiorgan failure, and ARDS occur in patients unresponsive to treatment (415,416). Signs and symptoms are nonspecific and include fever, chills, weight loss, dyspnea, chest pain, and leukocytosis despite antibiotic treatment.

Effusions can be appreciated by physical examination and by CXR, ultrasound, or CCT scan. Thorocentesis will confirm pleural fluid or pus. Positive fluid gram-stain and culture results are helpful, but may not be revealing in some patients. Analysis of the pleural fluid generally demonstrates $pH < 7.2$, glucose < 40 mg/dL, and lactic dehydrogenase activity > 1000 mg/dL (417,418).

Table 6 Types, Pathogens, and Antibiotic Choices for Pneumonia

Type	Typical pathogens	Antibiotics
Aspiration pneumonitis		
Signs and symptoms >48 hr		Fluoroquinolone or 3rd generation cephalosporin
SBO, gastric content colonization, neutropenia		Fluoroquinolone or 3rd generation cephalosporin or antipseudomonal penicillin
Aspiration pneumonia		
Community acquired	*Streptococcus pneumoniae*, *Staphylococcus aureus*, *Haemophilus influenza*, enterobacteriaceae	Fluoroquinolone or 3rd generation cephalosporin
Hospital acquired	*S. aureus*, *Pseudomonas aeruginosa*, *Klebsiella pneumoniae*. Rarely anaerobes	Fluoroquinolone or 3rd generation cephalosporin with antipseudomonal activity or antipseudomonal penicillin
Severe periodontal disease, putrid sputum, or necrotizing pneumonia or lung abscess	*S. aureus*, *P. aeruginosa*, *K. pneumoniae*, *Bacteroides* spp., *Peptostreptococcus* spp., *Fusobacterium* spp. *Prevotella* spp.	Antipseudomonal penicillin or imipenem; or 3rd generation cephalosporin with antipseudomonal activity or fluoroquinolones + clindamycin or metronidazole
CAP		
In ICU patients	Typical pathogens: *S. pneumoniae*, *H. influenza*, *S. aureus*, other gram-negative rods. Atypical pathogens: *Mycoplasma pneumoniae*, *Legionella* spp., *Chlamydia pneumoniae*	3rd generation cephalosporin + fluoroquinolone or macrolide
At risk for pseudomonal infection	Same as above plus *P. aeruginosa* and other resistant gram-negative rods	Antipseudomonal penicillin + aminoglycoside + fluoroquinolone or macrolide
Nosocomial pneumonia	*S. aureus* (including MRSA), *S. pneumoniae*, *Enterococcus* spp., *P. aeruginosa*, *H. influenzae*, *Acinetobacter* spp., *K. pneumoniae*, *Escherichia coli*, *Enterobacter* spp., *Proteus* spp., anaerobes	Antipseudomonal penicillin or imipenem or 3rd generation cephalosporin with antipseudomonal activity + fluoroquinolone or aminoglycoside. Vancomycin for MRSA
VAP	Same as above	Same as above

SBO = small bowel obstruction; MRSA = methicillin-resistant *S. aureus*; example for fluoroquinolones = levofloxacin or moxifloxacin; 3rd generation cephalosporins = ceftriaxone or ceftazidime (with antipseudomonal activity); antipseudomonal penicillin = piperacillin tazobactam or cefepime; macrolides = azithromycin or clarithromycin; aminoglycosides = gentamicin; CAP = community aquired pneumonia; VAP = ventilator-associated pneumonia.

Treatment includes adequate pleural drainage and appropriate antibiotics (Table 7), debridement of necrotic tissue, lung re-expansion, and obliteration of residual pleural space (419).

Patients suspected of having BPF should have their airway inspected by FOB. If a BPF is present, a chest tube is placed. Patient with empyema secondary to BPF following pneumonectomy should be recovered in the lateral decubitus position with the operated side down. A DLT may be needed to isolate the remaining lung.

Patients with uncomplicated empyema can be treated conservatively with percutaneous catheter drainage (420). Those with loculated empyema require initial tube thoracostomy for continuous drainage, antibiotics, streptokinase (contraindicated in patients with BPF), and VATS or open procedure to break down the empyema (421).

Table 7 Pathogens and Antibiotic Choices for Empyema

Typical pathogens	Antibiotic
S. pneumoniae, *Streptococcus pyogenes*, *H. influenza*	Ceftriaxone
S. aureus	Nafcillin
Gram-negative bacilli	Ceftriaxone
Anaerobes	Clindamycin
Fungi	Fluconazole

In complicated empyema, thoracotomy for decortication, rib resection, instillation of antibiotics, and BPF closure with muscle flaps may be required (413,422). Additional lung resection and thoracoplasty are reserved for refractory cases. VATS pleurodesis has a higher success rate than thoracotomy (423,424), and/or medical management (chest tube drainage combined with streptokinase) (425).

Airway Obstruction

In the postoperative period, partial or complete upper airway obstruction can occur from a variety of causes including pre-existing OSA, oversedation, a foreign body, blood or vomitus, upper airway edema, tissue trauma from airway instrumentation, laryngospasm, inadequate reversal of neuromuscular blockade, recurrent laryngeal nerve injury, external neck compression by hematoma, or disruption of tracheal anastomosis after resection and reconstruction.

Nasopharyngeal obstruction presents with snoring while laryngeal obstruction manifests as stridor. Diminished breath sounds and paradoxical chest wall movement may be seen. Hypoxemia and hypercapnia can result. Negative pressure pulmonary edema can occur after forceful inspiration against a closed or nearly closed upper airway (426,427).

Treatment is tailored to the urgency and etiology. Supplemental oxygen should be administered. An obstruction due to OSA is managed with a naso- or oropharyngeal airway, CPAP, upright or lateral positioning, and pharmacological reversal of sedation.

Airway examination and removal of obstructive material by suctioning are required for a foreign body, blood, or vomitus. Upper airway tissue edema or inflammation is treated by head elevation and with aerosolized racemic epinephrine and steroids.

Laryngospasm is treated with jaw thrust, head tilt, and CPAP. Low dose succinylcholine and airway support by mask ventilation may be required for refractory laryngospasm until recovery of spontaneous respiration. Patients with postoperative residual muscle blockade must have the relaxant fully reversed.

Patients who are unable to protect their airway should have their trachea intubated. A neck hematoma causing airway compromise must be decompressed at the bedside with definitive repair in the operating room once airway patency is secured.

For unconscious patients, those unable to protect their airway, and for impending airway obstruction, the trachea should be intubated. Depending on the situation, intubation is achieved by awake direct laryngoscopy, FOB, or by inhalation anesthetic induction. The presence of a surgeon able to perform a tracheostomy is important if the airway cannot be easily secured by conventional techniques.

Tracheobronchial Disruption

Tracheobronchial disruption is associated with a high morbidity and mortality, especially if unrecognized. Injury can result from airway intubation, bronchoscopy, or from trauma during esophageal or thoracic surgery (428,429).

The onset of clinical manifestations may be abrupt or insidious, but can progress suddenly to acute respiratory arrest (430). Signs include dyspnea, cough, subcutaneous emphysema, and/or hemoptysis. Cardiovascular instability may result from a tension pneumothorax.

CXR or CTT is not always diagnostic. Findings such as cervical emphysema, pneumomediastinum, pneumothorax, interruption of the normal tracheal air column, air surrounding the bronchus, and obstruction in the course of an air filled bronchus should heighten the suspicion (431). Bronchoscopy by an experienced endoscopist is the most reliable means of defining the site, nature, and extent of the injury. If pneumothorax is present, a thoracostomy tube should be inserted.

The initial goal should be to preserve spontaneous ventilation with supplemental oxygen, before securing the airway. Awake tracheal intubation is preferred. A rapid sequence anesthetic induction is not recommended since the use of neuromuscular blockade could in theory result in airway collapse. Inhalation anesthetic induction in the operating room may be appropriate for hemodynamically stable patients. Intubation under direct vision using a FOB is preferred to "blind" intubation. With the latter, the ETT may inadvertently be advanced into a false passage, resulting in additional injury. For a tracheal injury, the ETT should be carefully positioned past the defect. For a bronchial injury the tube should be placed in the intact bronchus and the injured lung isolated. In situations when tracheal intubation is unsuccessful or airway compromise is imminent, emergency tracheostomy is indicated.

Patients with small tracheal tears may be managed conservatively after a brief period of airway intubation or tracheostomy (432,433). However, definitive surgical repair of the disrupted segment or tracheal reconstruction is usually required (434).

For those undergoing tracheal reconstruction, early postoperative complications include anastomotic failure, airway obstruction from tissue edema, mucus plugging, or blood clots, and rarely tracheoesophageal fistula (435). Tracheal stenosis is a late complication. The anastomosis should be examined by bronchoscopy 1–2 weeks after the operation and at regular intervals for two years.

Bronchopleural Fistula (BPF)

BPF is a complication of lung resection, with the highest incidence following pneumonectomy (436). Patients are at risk for developing empyema, with mortality as high as 25–50% (437). Acute development of BPF is primarily due to disruption of the surgical anastomosis, rupture of lung abscess, or barotraumas (438,439). Late (> 1 week) onset of BPF is due to necrosis and devascularization of the bronchial stump (438,439).

Patients often report sudden production of copious, serosanguanous sputum. Dyspnea, hemoptysis, pneumothorax, and persistent air leaks are common. The CXR findings include pneumothorax and a decreasing air–fluid level when compared to prior studies. Bronchoscopy assesses the precise location and extent of the BPF.

Conservative interventions include immediate chest tube drainage, culture of the pleural fluid, and institution of broad-spectrum antibiotics. Surgical management involves reclosure of the bronchial stump and covering the defect by transposition of vascularized muscle or omental pedicle flaps (440–442). Metallic coils and glue, placed through a FOB under local anesthesia, can be used to occlude a BPF in patients at risk for curative surgery under general anesthesia (443).

Surgical repair may be technically difficult for a BPF that occurs 10 days or later after pneumonectomy. The situation may require wide-open drainage on a long-term basis by creating a Claggett window or Eloesser flap to allow granulation and spontaneous closure (437,444,445).

Air leak can be significant in patients with a BPF requiring positive pressure ventilation. Limiting inspired pressure using pressure control ventilation helps minimize further stump disruption and may allow spontaneous fistula healing. In severe cases, independent lung ventilation using two ventilators and a DLT are required (446).

Pulmonary Edema and Acute Respiratory Distress Syndrome (ARDS)

An often fatal form of respiratory failure after lung resection (usually pneumonectomy) is noncardiogenic pulmonary edema (447). The incidence is < 5% after pneumonectomy, but with an associated mortality rate of 25–100% (448). The peak incidence occurs during the first 24–48 hr following surgery, although it can occur anytime up to postoperative day 7 (447).

The hallmark is progressive arterial hypoxemia despite supplemental oxygen, mechanical ventilation and/or forced diuresis. Signs and symptoms include respiratory distress, rales, low-grade fever, and elevated white blood cell count. The CXR may reveal diffuse interstitial infiltration, pulmonary consolidation, or frank alveolar edema. Differential diagnose includes cardiogenic pulmonary edema, pneumonia, BPF, and pulmonary thromboembolism.

Although the term "postpneumonectomy pulmonary edema" is used, this condition should correctly be termed "postpneumonectomy ARDS" since it meets the criteria of classic ARDS. Signs and symptoms include acute hypoxemia with P_aO_2 to F_iO_2 ratio < 200, CXR showing diffuse infiltration, and no evidence of left atrial hypertension (449). Findings of pulmonary capillary hyperpermeability, endovascular injury, and histological evidence of protein leakage in lung tissue are all consistent with ARDS.

Postpneumonectomy ARDS is a complex clinical entity. No unifying theory has been established to explain its etiology and pathophysiology. Fluid overload as the cause remains controversial. Pulmonary capillary permeability changes may occur from lung injury due to increased PVR (129), volutrauma or lung hyperinflation (450), and inflammatory response. Plasma transfusion-induced activation of leukocytes can lead to acute lung injury (451). Other potential factors include radiotherapy-induced pneumonitis and lymphatic blockade, disruption of lymphatic drainage, and a potential role of lung ischemia and reperfusion in modulating oxidative damage on lung parenchyma (452,453). Finally, the possible role of inflammation on deregulating the apoptotic pathway could contribute to epithelial injury and pulmonary parenchymal damage (454).

Prevention includes limiting intravenous fluid and minimizing PVR by avoiding hypoxemia, acidosis, hypercarbia, or exaggerated catecholamine release due to inadequate pain control, stress, activity, and fever. The patient should be placed supine to avoid compressing residual lung or causing mediastinal shift. Avoidance of over-inflation of the remaining lung, balanced drainage without suction by chest tube on the operative side in the first 24–48 hr, and correcting mediastinal shift by injecting 300–500 mL of air into the pleural space of the operative hemithorax are other means of attempting to prevent this complication.

Management of patients with postpneumonectomy ARDS is primarily supportive. Early institution of mechanical ventilation, antibiotics, and aggressive diuresis are paramount. Lung protective strategy using low tidal volume and higher PEEP are recommended (455). $_i$NO in selected patients may be beneficial (456). Successful management with HFV has also been reported (457). Although a small randomized, controlled trial has demonstrated benefit of steroids in the fibroproliferative phase of late ARDS (458), the role of steroids is unresolved (459).

Pneumothorax and Air Leaks

Chest tubes are placed in the operative thorax to assist in lung re-expansion and fluid drainage (460). Persistent air leak may occur due to bronchial stump disruption, BPF, inadequate underwater seal suction pressure, an occluded chest tube, or one malpositioned with the suctioning port outside the pleural cavity (461,462). Recurrent or delayed onset of pneumothorax may be due to premature thoracostomy tube removal or necrosis of the bronchial suture line from ischemia or infection. New onset pneumothorax in an intubated patient is generally due to barotrauma. CXR is diagnostic (463).

A small pneumothorax (< 10–15%) developing after removal of the chest tube can be managed without tube replacement. However, for patients on positive pressure ventilation, a chest tube is required to minimize a worsening of air leak. Expansion of the air space can cause a tension pneumopericardium (464) or pneumothorax with tracheal deviation, mediastinal shift with tension on the contralateral lung, a decrease in lung compliance, and reduction of venous return to the heart (465).

Patients experience respiratory distress, tachycardia, and hypotension (466). Since cardiorespiratory collapse can occur rapidly, early recognition (even before confirmation by CXR) and appropriate interventions can be life-saving (467). Immediate decompression with a needle in the second intercostal space in the mid clavicular line should be followed by tube thoracostomy placement in the fifth intercostal space in midaxillary line. Return of cardiorespiratory parameters is usually immediate.

Postoperative Weakness

Incomplete reversal of neuromuscular blockade is the major cause of generalized weakness in the immediate recovery period (468). Quantitative monitoring of neuromuscular recovery and appropriate reversal with an anticholinesterase agent will avoid residual paralysis and respiratory compromise (469,470).

Patients with a critical illness on corticosteroid therapy and those requiring prolonged muscle paralysis for mechanical ventilation are at risk for developing myopathy (471). Depending on the etiology, myopathy may be due to myonecrosis, muscle atrophy, and/or axonopathy (472,473). Treatment of the underlying condition, aggressive mobilization, and early discontinuation of steroids and neuromuscular blockade agents allows gradual recovery of muscle strength (474).

2. Hemodyanamic Considerations

Arrhythmia

Postoperative arrhythmias are common, especially in patients with pre-existing structural heart disease (475). Major contributing factors include electrolyte and acid–base derangement, hypoxemia, hypercapnia, myocardial ischemia, increased sympathetic outflow, fluid shifts, PE, and drug effects (476–478). Surgical factors include compression or cardiac trauma and distention of the right atrium and ventricle (479). Postoperative arrhythmias are associated with increased length of hospital stay and higher mortality (480).

Treatments are directed at the underlying causes, especially correction of electrolyte (e.g., hypokalemia, hypocalcemia, hypomagnesemia) abnormalities.

Transient premature atrial contractions and unifocal ventricular premature contractions generally do not require treatment in hemodynamically stable patients (479). Sinus tachycardia is usually due to pain, agitation, hypovolemia, agitation, fever, hypoxemia, and/or congestive heart failure. Correction of the underlying etiology should occur before a sinus tachycardia is treated pharmacologically, unless cardiac ischemia is a potential risk.

Paroxysmal supraventricular tachycardias include paroxysmal atrial tachycardia, multifocal atrial tachycardia, atrial fibrillation (AF), and atrial flutter. They can result in hemodynamic instability and should be treated with synchronized cardioversion (479). In hemodynamically stable patients, pharmacologic treatment may include adenosine, amiodarone, beta-blockade, calcium channel blockers, or digoxin (481–483).

AF is the most common post-thoracotomy arrhythmia (484). Even though most AF episodes resolve spontaneously after 24–48 hr, pharmacologic rate control is still indicated. The incidence of stoke and transient ischemic attacks increase after 48 hr (485), so anticoagulation should be considered and weighed against the potential risk of postoperative bleeding.

After 48 hr, TEE should be performed to rule out evidence of left atrial thrombus before cardioversion (486). Prophylaxis with a beta-blocker, sotalol, or amiodarone reduces the incidence of AF after thoracic surgery (487,488).

Increased sympathetic activity is a major factor causing AF after thoracotomy. Perioperative oral beta-blockade reduces its frequency without causing side effects (489). Beta-blockers should be used with caution in patients with severe reactive airway disease. The benefit of epidural anesthesia for reducing AF after lung resection is controversial (490,491).

Patients with stable monophasic ventricular tachycardia should be treated with lidocaine, procainamide, or amiodarone (479). Ventricular fibrillation or unstable ventricular tachycardia requires immediate termination by cardioversion. Biphasic waveforms may be more effective than the traditional monophasic shocks (492).

Pulmonary Hypertension and Right Heart Failure

Pulmonary hypertension due to an increase in PVR can be due to exacerbation of baseline pulmonary hypertension, hypoxemia, hypercapnia, acidosis, bronchospasm, positive pressure ventilation with extrinsic PEEP, vasoactive medication, increases in sympathetic tone, and decreases in pulmonary vascular cross-sectional area after extensive lung resection (493–495).

Pulmonary hypertension can develop gradually or acutely. In moderate to severe pulmonary hypertension, increases in right ventricular after-load can lead to right heart ischemia and failure (496,497). An increase in CVP and PAP, decrease in cardiac output, systemic hypotension, arrhythmias, and end organ failure may occur (498). Patients should be monitored with a PA catheter. ECG reveals right heart strain and axis deviation. Echocardiography will help evaluate the severity of right heart failure (499).

Treatment is directed at correcting underlying causes. Mechanical ventilation may be needed to improve gas exchange and respiratory acidosis. Bronchodilators, avoidance of vasopressors, and adequate control of pain and anxiety are important. Augmentation of preload maintains adequate cardiac output.

Pharmacologic interventions to decrease PVR and improve right ventricular outflow are critical. Nitroglycerine and nitroprusside are both systemic and pulmonary vasodilators that can reduce PVR in patients without significant ventricular dysfunction (500). Epoprostenol, a prostacyclin, is similar in activity to nitroglycerine and nitroprusside (501). Dobutamine, a catecholamine, and milrinone, a phosphodiesterase inhibitor, provide positive inotropy while decreasing PVR (500,502).

The major disadvantage of these agents is nonselective vasodilation, which can result in significant systemic hypotension compromising target-organ perfusion. Selective PA vasodilators (e.g., ${}_{i}$NO, inhaled prostacyclin (${}_{i}PGI_2$)) may improve clinical response (503–505). The effect of ${}_{i}$NO is short-lived and can result in rebound pulmonary hypertension when discontinued (506,507). Addition of the oral phosphodiesterase inhibitor sildenafil augments the pulmonary vasodilating effect of ${}_{i}$NO, even after the latter has been withdrawn (508,509).

Cardiac Herniation

A potentially catastrophic complication after intrapericardial pneumonectomy is cardiac herniation. Prolapse of the heart through the pericardial defect with subsequent torsion of the heart and great vessels can cause profound hemodynamic instability (510). Intraoperative closure of the pericardial defect reduces risk (511).

An increase in positive intrathoracic pressure in the nonoperative thorax from mechanical ventilation with high PEEP, increases in negative intrathoracic pressure on the operative thorax from chest tube suction or lateral positioning with the operative side dependent, and coughing and vomiting are potential contributing factors. Right-sided cardiac herniation can produce SVC syndrome and involvement in the inferior vena cava resulting in a reduction of venous return. Left-sided herniation may cause constriction of the atrioventricular groove, myocardial ischemia and infarction, and ventricular outflow obstruction.

Signs and symptoms may mimic those of cardiac tamponade, massive PE, or myocardial infarction (512). They include increased CVP, decreased venous return and cardiac output, profound hypotension, atrial and ventricular arrhythmias, myocardial ischemia, and cardiovascular collapse (513).

Abnormal ST-segment and T-wave changes, arrhythmias, and new axis deviation from baseline may be evident on ECG (514). CXR may reveal the silhouette of the herniated heart in the pleural cavity on the side of pneumonectomy. TEE may demonstrate the presence of teardrop sign produced by the narrowed atria and bulbous ventricles as well as hypermobility of the heart (515). Once diagnosed, immediate surgcial re-exploration with reduction of the heart into the pericardium and repair of the defect is required. Despite aggressive intervention, mortality approaches 50% (516).

Pulmonary Torsion

Pulmonary torsion after lung resection can lead to significant morbidity and mortality (517). The median time of diagnosis is day 10 (range day 2–14) after pulmonary lobectomy (518). This complication is more common following right-upper lobectomy, and is usually due to hypermobility of the remaining hilar structures following lung re-expansion. The rotational effects compromise gas exchange through the bronchus, blood flow in the pulmonary vasculature (mainly in the low pressure pulmonary venous system), and lead to venous outflow obstruction.

Patients may display fever, dyspnea, tachycardia, and hemoptysis. Pulmonary infarct, gangrene, and interstitial pulmonary edema can develop.

CXR demonstrates pulmonary infiltrates and reduced lung volume. CCT may reveal obliteration of the proximal PA and adjacent bronchus of the involved lobe. Bronchoscopy is diagnostic and demonstrates an obliterated or distorted bronchial orifice (519). Fixation of the middle lobe to the remaining lobe at the time of surgery may reduce the incidence of occurrence (520). Early recognition with prompt intervention is required to salvage lung parenchyma and to prevent hemorrhagic infarction or gangrene.

Postoperative Hemorrhage

Postoperative hemorrhage can present as intrapulmonary bleeding with hemoptysis or as intrapleural bleeding with excessive chest tube drainage (>150 mL/hr, or >500 mL for the first 24 hr after surgery) (521). Signs of hypovolemia including tachycardia, hypotension, decreased CVP, and decreased urine output may be present.

Initial interventions include supplemental oxygen, establishment of adequate intravenous access, obtaining cross-matched blood products, and restoring intravascular volume. Hemoptysis requires clearing of the airway by aggressive suctioning. In patients with significant hemoptysis, the airway should be protected with an ETT (522). Rigid bronchoscopy is better than FOB for clearing clots and identifying the site of bleeding.

For unilateral bleeding, lung isolation with a DLT or BB will protect the unaffected lung (523). The BB can tamponade the bleeding site. In emergency situations, an uncut ETT can be advanced into the uninvolved bronchus. The patient should be placed with the bleeding side dependent. Tube suctioning is important since obstruction by blood can impair gas exchange.

Significant intrapleural bleeding is an indication for surgical re-exploration, once other factors such as hypothermia or coagulopathy are corrected. Bleeding may be due to inadequate ligation of pulmonary vessels, diffuse bleeding from raw pleural surfaces, or disseminated intravascular coagulation. Patients with signs of hypovolemia despite minimal chest tube drainage may have an obstructed tube. CXR or CCT may reveal decreased lung volume and fluid accumulation on the surgical side.

Close monitoring of chest tube output and adequate resuscitation with fluid and blood products is indicated, but return to the operating room for surgical correction may be necessary (524). A hemodynamically stable patient with isolated bleeding can be treated by selective arterial embolization (525).

3. Structural Considerations

Thoracic Duct Injury and Chylothorax

Trauma to the thoracic duct during pulmonary resection or esophagectomy can result in chylothorax, the accumulation of chyle in the pleural space (526). Fluid with a high triglyceride concentration (>110 mg/dL) draining from pleural cavity is diagnostic.

Conservation management involves a fat-free diet or cessation of oral intake supplemented by TPN (527). Octreotide, a synthetic somatostatin analogue, has been used as adjunctive therapy to reduce thoracic duct flow and triglyceride levels (528,529). Since prolonged medical management of chylothorax is associated with increased mortality (530), early surgical intervention is indicated especially if chest tube drainage is >500 mL after 24 hr of conservative therapy (531). Lymphangiography will help determine location of the leak and identify appropriate candidates for surgical intervention (532). Operative choices include thoracotomy or VATS ligation of the thoracic duct, pleurodesis, decortication, or pleuroperitoneal shunt (533–535).

Neurological Dysfunction

Thoracic procedures can be complicated by neural injury (536).

Intraoperative trauma to the recurrent laryngeal nerve usually is unrecognized until the airway is extubated (537). Bilateral recurrent laryngeal nerve damage may result in complete airway obstruction requiring immediate ETT replacement or tracheostomy.

Patients who fail to wean from the ventilator without obvious reasons should have their CXR evaluated for diaphragmatic paralysis (538). Unilateral phrenic nerve damage may be evident by elevation of the ipsilateral hemidiaphragm. Diagnosis is confirmed by transcutaneous phrenic nerve conduction studies or fluoroscopic evaluation of diaphragmatic movement (539).

Patients may be asymptomatic or have significant respiratory distress if baseline respiratory reserve is limited. Prolonged mechanical ventilatory support may be required (538,539). For symptomatic patients, treatment options include diaphragmatic plication or diaphragmatic pacing (540–542).

The differential diagnosis of postoperative lower extremity paralysis includes motor blockade from epidural local anesthetics, epidural hematoma, and spinal cord ischemia or infarction (543,544). A complete neurological examination must always be performed.

Immediate discontinuation of local anesthetic epidural infusion and subsequent evaluation of motor function should occur. The patient's back should be examined and palpated for pain and induration secondary to epidural hematoma. Immediate MR of the thoracolumbar spine is indicated since an epidural hematoma requires emergency surgical decompression.

During thoracotomy, spinal cord ischemia with resultant paraplegia can occur after interruption of blood supply to the spinal branches of the intercostals arteries. Treatment options are limited once spinal cord injury occurs. Maintaining adequate spinal cord perfusion in the perioperative period may minimize development and prevent further damage once injury has occurred. Steroids may be of some benefit (545,546). For patients with established spinal cord ischemia or infarct, the placement of a spinal catheter for cerebral spinal fluid drainage to decompress spinal cord pressure is controversial (547).

Brachial plexus trauma can be resulted from sternal retraction during median sternotomy, stretching from hyperextension and excessive rotation of the upper arms during surgery, and from direct compression from extreme cephalad positioning of a chest tube (548–550).

Anastomotic Leaks

Leaks at the site of the cervical esophageal anastomosis can present with fever and a painful, swollen neck. Treatment is to open the incision and establish adequate drainage. Intrathoracic leaks are more serious, and are associated with a mortality rate as high as 50%. Immediate reoperation for leak repair is essential.

After esophagectomy, the integrity of the anastomosis is evaluated by barium contrast before instituting oral feeding. The incidence of anastomotic dehiscence after esophagectomy is approximately 12% (551), with a higher incidence after cervical anastomosis (552).

The primary etiology of anastomotic failure is poor wound healing secondary to arterial ischemia, venous congestion, gastric distention, infection, tension or compression, malnutrition, and technical difficulties during surgery (552,553). Severity is a function of the onset time, the site, the extent, and the amount of residual viable tissue. Associated mortality is high and most patients succumb to sepsis and multiorgan failure.

Clinically silent leaks, evident only on routine postoperative contrast studies, generally have low mortality and can be managed conservatively with NGT decompression, broad-spectrum antibiotics, and nutritional support. Nutritional support can be by enteral feeding through a jejunostomy tube or NGT or by TPN.

Patients with symptomatic cervical leaks can be treated with bedside open drainage and packing initially, along with broad-spectrum antibiotics and TPN support. Mortality is approximately 20% (554). Those with clinically apparent thoracic leaks have a greater risk of developing fatal infection (554). Aggressive treatment by drainage and surgical revision with a vascular pedicle is recommended in addition to antibiotics and nutrimental support. All patients who have anastomotic failure should be reassessed for healing with contrast or endoscopic studies after appropriate treatment. Stricture is a potential complication requiring periodic endoscopic dilation.

VI. CONCLUSIONS

The successful management of the patient with intrathoracic neoplastic disease requires the expertise of physicians from many disciplines. The primary care physician, oncologist, surgeon, anesthesiologist, nutritionalist, and critical care specialist must all coordinate their efforts in order to provide optimal management of the patient's disease and any associated medical comorbidities.

Following major thoracotomy for pulmonary or esophageal cancer now with modern anesthetic and surgical techniques, most patients do not require admission to an ICU. For patients with complications or medical problems who require admission to a critical care unit, advances in monitoring, ventilatory management, fluid and nutritional support, and postoperative analgesia have improved the prognosis for recovery.

REFERENCES

1. Brunelli A, Al Refai M, Monteverde M, Borri A, Salati M, Fianchini A. Stair climbing test predicts cardiopulmonary complications after lung resection. Chest 2002; 121:1106–1110.

2. Beckles MA, Spiro SG, Colice GL, Rudd RM. The physiologic evaluation of patients with lung cancer being considered for resectional surgery. Chest 2003; 123:105S–114S.
3. Brodsky JB, Macario A, Mark JB. Tracheal diameter predicts double-lumen tube size: a method for selecting left double-lumen tubes. Anesth Analg 1996; 82: 861–864.
4. Eberle B, Weiler N, Vogel N, Kauczor HU, Heinrichs W. Computed tomography-based tracheobronchial image reconstruction allows selection of the individually appropriate double-lumen tube size. J Cardiothorac Vasc Anesth 1999; 13:532–537.
5. Brodsky JB, Malott K, Angst M, Fitzmaurice BG, Kee SP, Logan L. The relationship between tracheal width and left bronchial width: implications for left-sided double-lumen tube selection. J Cardiothorac Vasc Anesth 2001; 15:216–217.
6. Pierce RJ, Copland JM, Sharpe K, Barter CE. Preoperative risk evaluation for lung cancer resection: predicted postoperative product as a predictor of surgical mortality. Am J Respir Crit Care Med 1994; 150:947–955.
7. Kearney DJ, Lee TH, Reilly JJ, DeCamp MM, Sugarbaker DJ. Assessment of operative risk in patients undergoing lung resection. Importance of predicted pulmonary function. Chest 1994; 105:753–759.
8. Zeiher BG, Gross TJ, Kern JA, Lanza LA, Peterson MW. Predicting postoperative pulmonary function in patients undergoing lung resection. Chest 1995; 108: 68–72.
9. Pate P, Tenholder MF, Griffin JP, Eastridge CE, Weiman DS. Preoperative assessment of the high-risk patient for lung resection. Ann Thorac Surg 1996; 61: 1494–1500.
10. Wang J, Olak J, Ultmann RE, Ferguson MK. Assessment of pulmonary complications after lung resection. Ann Thorac Surg 1999; 67:1444–1447.
11. Dunn WF, Scanlon PD. Preoperative pulmonary function testing for patients with lung cancer. Mayo Clin Proc 1993; 68:371–377.
12. Ferguson MK, Reeder LB, Mick R. Optimizing selection of patients for major lung resection. J Thorac Cardiovasc Surg 1995; 109:275–281.
13. Ferguson MK, Little L, Rizzo L, Popovich KJ, Glonek GF, Leff A, Manjoney D, Little AG. Diffusing capacity predicts morbidity and mortality after pulmonary resection. J Thorac Cardiovasc Surg 1988; 96:894–900.
14. Bria WF, Kanarek DJ, Kazemi H. Prediction of postoperative pulmonary function following thoracic operations. Value of ventilation–perfusion scanning. J Thorac Cardiovasc Surg 1983; 86:186–192.
15. Giordano A, Calcagni ML, Meduri G, Valente S, Galli G. Perfusion lung scintigraphy for the prediction of postlobectomy residual pulmonary function. Chest 1997; 111:1542–1547.
16. Wu MT, Pan HB, Chiang AA, Hsu HK, Chang HC, Peng NJ, Lai PH, Liang HL, Yang CF. Prediction of postoperative lung function in patients with lung cancer: comparison of quantitative CT with perfusion scintigraphy. AJR Am J Roentgenol 2002; 178: 667–672.
17. Rotman HH, Liss HP, Weg JG. Diagnosis of upper airway obstruction by pulmonary function testing. Chest 1975; 68:796–799.
18. Mohsenifar Z, Jasper AC, Koerner SK. Physiologic assessment of lung function in patients undergoing laser photoresection of tracheobronchial tumors. Chest 1988; 93:65–69.
19. Dunagan D, Chin R Jr, McCain T, Case L, Harkness B, Oaks T, Haponik E. Staging by positron emission tomography predicts survival in patients with non-small cell lung cancer. Chest 2001; 119:333–339.
20. Coleman RE. PET in lung cancer staging. Q J Nucl Med 2001; 45:231–234.
21. Kernstine KH, Mclaughlin KA, Menda Y, Rossi NP, Kahn DJ, Bushnell DL, Graham MM, Brown CK, Madsen MT. Can FDG-PET reduce the need for mediastinoscopy in potentially resectable non small cell lung cancer? Ann Thorac Surg 2002; 73:394–401.
22. Weder W, Schmid RA, Bruchhaus H, Hillinger S, von Schulthess GK, Steinert HC. Detection of extrathoracic metastases by positron emission tomography in lung cancer. Ann Thorac Surg 1998; 66:886–892.
23. van Tinteren H, Hoekstra OS, Smit EF, van den Bergh JH, Schreurs AJ, Stallaert RA, van Velthoven PC, Comans EF, Diepenhorst FW, Verboom P, van Mourik JC, Postmus PE, Boers M, Teule GJ. Effectiveness of positron emission tomography in the preoperative assessment of patients with suspected non-small-cell lung cancer: the PLUS multicentre randomised trial. Lancet 2002; 359:1388–1393.
24. Bluman LG, Mosca L, Newman N, Simon DG. Preoperative smoking habits and postoperative pulmonary complications. Chest 1998; 113:883–889.
25. Moores LK. Smoking and postoperative pulmonary complications. An evidence-based review of the recent literature. Clin Chest Med 2000; 21:139–146.
26. Vaporciyan AA, Merriman KW, Ece F, Roth JA, Smythe WR, Swisher SG, Walsh GL, Nesbitt JC, Putnam JB Jr. Incidence of major pulmonary morbidity after pneumonectomy: association with timing of smoking cessation. Ann Thorac Surg 2002; 73: 420–425.
27. Moller AM, Villebro N, Pedersen T, Tonnesen H. Effect of preoperative smoking intervention on postoperative complications: a randomised clinical trial. Lancet 2002; 359:114–117.
28. Agnew NM, Kendall JB, Akrofi M, Tran J, Soorae AS, Page R, Russell GN, Pennefather SH. Gastroesophageal reflux and tracheal aspiration in the thoracotomy position: should ranitidine premedication be routine? Anesth Analg 2002; 95:1645–1649.

29. Jakobsen CJ, Bille S, Ahlburg P, Rybro L, Pedersen KD, Rasmussen B. Preoperative metoprolol improves cardiovascular stability and reduces oxygen consumption after thoracotomy. Acta Anaesthesiol Scand 1997; 41:1324–1330.
30. Brodsky JB, Shulman MS, Swan M, Mark JBD. Pulse oximetry during one-lung ventilation. Anesthesiology 1985; 63:212–214.
31. Ishikawa S, Nakazawa K, Makita K. Progressive changes in arterial oxygenation during one-lung anaesthesia are related to the response to compression of the non-dependent lung. Br J Anaesth 2003; 90:21–26.
32. Zollinger A, Spahn DR, Singer T, Zalunardo MP, Stoehr S, Weder W, Pasch T. Accuracy and clinical performance of a continuous intra-arterial blood–gas monitoring system during thoracoscopic surgery. Br J Anaesth 1997; 79:57–52.
33. Ishikawa S, Makita K, Nakazawa K, Amaha K. Continuous intra-arterial blood gas monitoring during oesophagectomy. Can J Anaesth 1998; 45:273–276.
34. Mark JB, FitzGerald D, Fenton T, Fosberg AM, Camann W, Maffeo N, Winkelman J. Continuous arterial and venous blood gas monitoring during cardiopulmonary bypass. J Thorac Cardiovasc Surg 1991; 102:431–439.
35. Sandham JD, Hull RD, Brant RF, Knox L, Pineo GF, Doig CJ, Laporta DP, Viner S, Passerini L, Devitt H, Kirby A, Jacka M. A randomized, controlled trial of the use of pulmonary–artery catheters in high-risk surgical patients. N Engl J Med 2003; 348:5–14.
36. Wang KY, Lin CY, Kuo-Tai J, Yuan L, Chang HJ. Use of tranesophageal electrocardiography for evaluation of resectability of lung cancer. Acta Anaesthesiol Sin 1994; 32:255–260.
37. Barletta G, Del Bene MR, Palminiello A, Fantini F. Left-ventricular diastolic dysfunction during pneumonectomy—a transesophageal lectrocardiographic study. Thorac Cardiovasc Surg 1996; 44:92–96.
38. Neustein SM, Cohen E, Reich D, Kirschner P. Transoesophageal echocardiography and the intraoperative diagnosis of left atrial invasion by carcinoid tumor. Can J Anaesth 1993; 40:664–666.
39. Don H. The mechanical properties of the respiratory system during anesthesia. Int Anesthesiol Clin 1977; 15:113–136.
40. Wahba RW. Perioperative functional residual capacity. Can J Anaesth 1991; 38:938–939.
41. Hirschmann CA, Bergman NA. Factors influencing intrapulmonary airway caliber during anesthesia. Br J Anaesth 1990; 65:30–42.
42. Moss J, Rosow CE, Savarese JJ, Philbin DM, Kniffen KJ. Role of histamine in the hypotensive action of d-tubocurarine in humans. Anesthesiology 1981; 55: 19–25.
43. Egan TD. Remifentanil pharmacokinetics and pharmacodynamics. A preliminary appraisal. Clin Pharmacokinet 1995; 29:80–94.
44. Eisenkraft JB. Effects of anaesthetics on the pulmonary circulation. Br J Anaesth 1990; 65:63–78.
45. Doenicke AW, Czeslick E, Moss J, Hoernecke R. Onset time, endotracheal intubating conditions, and plasma histamine release after cisatracurium and vecuronium administration. Anesth Analg 1998; 87:434–438.
46. Naguib M, Samarkandi AH, Bakhamees HS, Magboul MA, el-Bakry AK. Histamine-release haemodynamic changes produced by rocuronium, vecuronium, mivacurium, atracurium and tubocurarine. Br J Anaesth 1995; 75:588–592.
47. Cheng EY, Mazzeo AJ, Bosnjak ZJ, Coon RL, Kampine JP. Direct relaxant effects of intravenous anesthetics on airway smooth muscle. Anesth Analg 1996; 83:162–168.
48. Weinreich AI, Silvay G, Lumb PD. Continuous ketamine infusion for one-lung anaesthesia. Can Anaesth Soc J 1980; 27:485–490.
49. Rees DI, Gaines GY III. One-lung anesthesia—a comparison of pulmonary gas exchange during anesthesia with ketamine or enflurane. Anesth Analg 1984; 63: 521–525.
50. Eisenkraft JB. Hypoxic pulmonary vasoconstriction. Curr Opin Anaesthesiol 1999; 12:43–48.
51. Domino KB, Wetstein L, Glasser SA, Lindgren L, Marshall C, Harken A, Marshall BE. Influence of mixed venous oxygen tension (PvO_2) on blood flow to atelectatic lung. Anesthesiology 1983; 59:428–434.
52. Van Keer L, Van Aken H, Vandermeersch E, Vermaut G, Lerut T. Propofol does not inhibit hypoxic pulmonary vasoconstriction in humans. J Clin Anesth 1988; 1:284–288.
53. Nakayama M, Murray PA. Ketamine preserves and propofol potentiates hypoxic pulmonary vasoconstriction compared with the conscious state in chronically instrumented dogs. Anesthesiology 1999; 91:760–771.
54. Kondo U, Kim SO, Murray PA. Propofol selectively attenuates endothelium-dependent pulmonary vasodilation in chronically instrumented dogs. Anesthesiology 2000; 93:437–446.
55. Marshall C, Lindgren L, Marshall BE. Effects of halothane, enflurane, and isoflurane on hypoxic pulmonary vasoconstriction in rat lungs in vitro. Anesthesiology 1984; 60:304–308.
56. Ishibe Y, Gui X, Uno H, Shiokawa Y, Umeda T, Suekane K. Effect of sevoflurane on hypoxic pulmonary vasoconstriction in the perfused rabbit lung. Anesthesiology 1993; 79:1348–1353.
57. Loer SA, Scheeren TW, Tarnow J. Desflurane inhibits hypoxic pulmonary vasoconstriction in isolated rabbit lungs. Anesthesiology 1995; 83:552–556.
58. Karzai W, Haberstroh J, Priebe HJ. Effects of desflurane and propofol on arterial oxygenation during one-lung ventilation in the pig. Acta Anaesthesiol Scand 1998; 42:648–652.
59. Moore PG, Nguyen DK, Reitan JA. Inhibition of nitric oxide synthesis causes systemic and pulmonary

vasoconstriction in isoflurane-anesthetized dogs. J Cardiothorac Vasc Anesth 1994; 8:310–316.
60. Lennon PF, Murray PA. Attenuated hypoxic pulmonary vasoconstriction during isoflurane anesthesia is abolished by cyclooxygenase inhibition in chronically instrument dogs. Anesthesiology 1996; 84:404–414.
61. Pilotti L, Torresini G, Crisci R, De Sanctis A, De Sanctis C. Total intravenous anesthesia in thoracotomy with one-lung ventilation. Minerva Anesthesiol 1999; 65:483–489.
62. Reid CW, Slinger PD, Lenis S. A comparison of the effects of propofol-alfentanil versus isoflurane anesthesia on arterial oxygenation during one-lung ventilation. J Cardiothorac Vasc Anesth 1996; 10:860–863.
63. Beck DH, Doepfmer UR, Sinemus C, Bloch A, Schenk MR, Kox WJ. Effects of sevoflurane and propofol on pulmonary shunt during one-lung ventilation for thoracic surgery. Br J Anaesth 2001; 86:38–43.
64. Shimizu T, Abe K, Kinouchi K, Yoshiya I. Arterial oxygenation during one lung ventilation. Can J Anaesth 1997; 44:1162–1166.
65. Abe K, Mashimo T, Yoshiya I. Arterial oxygenation and shunt fraction during one-lung ventilation: a comparison of isoflurane and sevoflurane. Anesth Analg 1998; 86:1266–1270.
66. Wang JY, Russell GN, Page RD, Jackson M, Pennefather SH. Comparison of the effects of sevoflurane and isoflurane on arterial oxygenation during one lung ventilation. Br J Anaesth 1998; 81:850–853.
67. Pagel PS, Fu JL, Damask MC, Davis RF, Samuelson PN, Howie MB, Warltier DC. Desflurane and isoflurane produce similar alterations in systemic and pulmonary hemodynamics and arterial oxygenation in patients undergoing one-lung ventilation during thoracotomy. Anesth Analg 1998; 87:800–807.
68. Wang JY, Russell GN, Page RD, Oo A, Pennefather SH. A comparison of the effects of desflurane and isoflurane on arterial oxygenation during one-lung ventilation. Anaesthesia 2000; 55:167–173.
69. Benumof JL, Wahrenbrock EA. Local effects of anesthetics on regional hypoxic pulmonary vasoconstriction. Anesthesiology 1975; 43:525–532.
70. Mathers J, Benumof JL, Wahrenbrock EA. General anesthesia and regional hypoxic pulmonary vasoconstriction. Anesthesiology 1977; 46:111–114.
71. Marin JL, Orchard C, Chakrabarti MK, Sykes MK. Depression of hypoxic pulmonary vasoconstriction in the dog by dopamine and isoprenaline. Br J Anaesth 1979; 5:303–312.
72. Furman WR, Summer WR, Kennedy TP, Sylvester JT. Comparison of the effect of dobutamine, dopamine, and isoproterenol on hypoxic pulmonary vasoconstriction in the pig. Crit Care Med 1982; 10:371–374.
73. Miller JR, Benumof JL, Trousdale FR. Combined effects of sodium nitroprusside and propranolol on hypoxic pulmonary vasoconstriction. Anesthesiology 1982; 57:267–271.
74. D'Oliveira M, Sykes MK, Chakrabarti MK, Orchard C, Keslin J. Depression of hypoxic pulmonary vasoconstriction by sodium nitroprusside and nitroglycerine. Br J Anaesth 1981; 53:11–18.
75. Porcelli RJ, Bergofsky EH. Adrenergic receptors in pulmonary vasoconstrictor responses to gaseous and humoral agents. J Appl Physiol 1973; 34:483–488.
76. Conacher ID. The urinary catheter as a bronchial blocker. Anaesthesia 1983; 38:475–477.
77. Dalens B, Labbe A, Haberer JP. Selective endobronchial blocking vs selective intubation. Anesthesiology 1982; 57:555–556.
78. Ginsberg RJ. New technique for one-lung anesthesia using an endobronchial blocker. J Cardiovasc Surg 1981; 82:542–546.
79. Oxorn D. Use of fiberoptic bronchoscope to assist placement of a Fogarty catheter as a bronchial blocker. Can J Anaesth 1987; 34:427–428.
80. Kraenzler EJ, Rice TW, Stein SL, Insler SR. Bilateral bronchial blockers for bilateral pulmonary resections in a patient with a previous laryngectomy. J Cardiothorac Vasc Anesth 1997; 11:201–202.
81. Arndt GA, Buchika S, Kranner PW, DeLessio ST. Wire-guided endobronchial blockade in a patient with a limited mouth opening. Can J Anaesth 1999; 46: 87–89.
82. Arndt GA, Kranner PW, Rusy DA, Love R. Single-lung ventilation in a critically ill patient using a fiberoptically directed wire-guided endobronchial blocker. Anesthesiology 1999; 90:1484–1486.
83. Inoue H, Shohtsua A, Ogawa J, Koides S, Kawada S. Endotracheal tube with movable blocker to prevent aspiration of intratracheal bleeding. Ann Thorac Surg 1984; 37:497–499.
84. Kamaya H, Krishna PR. New endotracheal tube (Univent tube) for selective blockade of one lung. Anesthesiology 1985; 63:342–343.
85. Karwande SV. A new tube for single lung ventilation. Chest 1987; 92:761–763.
86. MacGillivray RG. Evaluation of a new tracheal tube with a movable bronchus blocker. Anaesthesia 1988; 43:687–689.
87. Benumof JL, Gaughan S, Ozaki GT. Operative lung constant positive airway pressure 1992; 74:406–410.
88. Burton NA, Watson DC, Brodsky JB, Mark JBD. Advantages of a new polyvinyl chloride double-lumen tube in thoracic surgery. Ann Thorac Surg 1983; 36:78–84.
89. Campos JH, Massa FC. Is there a better right-sided tube for one-lung ventilation? A comparison of the right-sided double-lumen tube with the single-lumen tube with right-sided enclosed bronchial blocker. Anesth Analg 1998; 86:696–700.
90. Slinger P. The Univent tube is the best technique for providing one-lung ventilation. Con: the Univent tube is not the best method of providing one-lung ventilation. J Cardiothor Vasc Anesth 1993; 7:108–112.

91. Temeck BK, Schafer PW, Park WY, Harmon JW. Epidural anesthesia in patients undergoing thoracic surgery. Arch Surg 1989; 124:415–418.
92. Tenling A, Joachimsson PO, Tyden H, Wegenius G, Hedenstierna G. Thoracic epdidural anesthesia as an adjunct to general anesthesia for cardiac surgery: effects on ventilation–perfusion relationships. J Cardiothorac Vasc Anesth 1999; 13:258–264.
93. Della Rocca G, Coccia C, Pompei L, Costa MG, Pierconti F, Di Marco P, Tommaselli E, Pietropaoli P. Post-thoracotomy analgesia: epidural vs intravenous morphine continuous infusion. Minerva Anestesiol 2002; 68:681–693.
94. Scheinin B, Scheinin R, Asantila R, Lindberg R, Viinamaki O. Sympatho-adrenal and pituitary hormone responses during and immediately after thoracic surgery—modulation by four different pain treatments. Acta Anaesthesiol Scand 1987; 31: 762–767.
95. Salomaki TE, Leppaluoto J, Laitinen JO, Vuolteenaho O, Nuutinen LS. Epidural versus intravenous fentanyl for reducing hormonal, metabolic, and physiologic responses after thoracotomy. Anesthesiology 1993; 79: 672–679.
96. Watanabe S, Noguchi E, Yamada S, Hamada N, Kano T. Sequential changes of arterial oxygen tension in the supine position during one-lung ventilation. Anesth Analg 2000; 90:28–34.
97. Kerr JH, Smith AC, Prys-Roberts C, Meloche R, Foex P. Observations during endobronchial anaesthesia. II. Oxygenation. Br J Anaesth 1974; 46:84–92.
98. Szegedi LL, Bardoczky GI, Engelman EE, d'Hollander AA. Airway pressure changes during one-lung ventilation. Anesthesiology 1997; 84:1034–1037.
99. Weiler N, Eberle B, Heinrichs W. Adaptive lung ventilation (ALV) during anaesthesia for pulmonary surgery: autonomic response to transitions to and from one-lung ventilation. J Clin Monit Comput 1998; 14:245–252.
100. Tugrul M, Camci E, Karadeniz H, Senturk M, Pembeci K, Akpir K. Comparison of volume controlled with pressure-controlled ventilation during one-lung anaesthesia. Br J Anaesth 1997; 79:306–310.
101. Kacmarek RM. Ventilator-associated lung injury. Int Anesthesiol Clin 1999; 37:47–64.
102. Slinger PD, Hickey DR. The interaction between applied PEEP and auto-PEEP during one-lung ventilation. J Cardiothorac Vasc Anesth 1998; 12:133–136.
103. Yokota K, Toriumi T, Sari A, Endou S, Mihira M. Auto-positive-end-expiratory pressure during one-lung ventilation using a double-lumen endobronchial tube. Anesth Analg 1996; 82:1007–1010.
104. Bardoczky GI, d'Hollander AA, Cappello M, Yernault JC. Interrupted expiratory flow on automatically constructed flow-volume curves may determine the presence of intrinsic positive end-expiratory pressure during one-lung ventilation. Anesth Analg 1998; 86:880–884.
105. Inomata S, Nishikawa T, Saito S, Kihara S. "Best" PEEP during one-lung ventilation. Br J Anaesth 1997; 78:754–756.
106. Katz JA, Laverne RG, Fairley HB, Thomas AN. Pulmonary oxygen exchange during endobronchial anesthesia: effects of tidal volume and PEEP. Anesthesiology 1982; 56:164–171.
107. Malmkvist G. Maintenance of oxygenation during one-lung ventilation. Effect of intermittent reinflation of the collapsed lung with oxygen. Anesth Analg 1989; 68:763–766.
108. Capan LM, Turndorf H, Chandrakant P, Ramanathan S, Acinapura A, Chalon J. Optimization of arterial oxygenation during one-lung anesthesia. Anesth Analg 1980; 59:847–851.
109. Hogue CW Jr. Effectiveness of low levels of nonventilated lung continuous positive airway pressure in improving arterial oxygenation during one-lung ventilation. Anesth Analg 1994; 79:364–367.
110. Cohen E, Eisenkraft JB. Positive end-expiratory pressure during one-lung ventilation improves oxygenation in patients with low arterial oxygen tensions. J Cardiothorac Vasc Anesth 1996; 10:578–582.
111. Scherer RW, Vigfusson G, Hultsch E, Van Aken H, Lawin P. Prostaglandin F_{2a} improves oxygen tension and reduces venous admixture during one-lung ventilation in anesthetized paralyzed dogs. Anesthesiology 1985; 62:23–28.
112. Chen TL, Lee YT, Wang MJ, Lee JM, Lee YC, Chu SH. Endothelin-1 concentrations and optimisation of arterial oxygenation and venous admixture by selective artery infusion of prostaglandin E1 during thoracotomy. Anaesthesia 1996; 51:422–426.
113. Steudel W, Hurford WE, Zapol WM. Inhaled nitric oxide: basic biology and clinical applications. Anesthesiology 1999; 91:1090–1121.
114. Rich GF, Lowson SM, Johns RA, Daugherty MO, Uncles DR. Inhaled nitric oxide selectively decreases pulmonary vascular resistance without impairing oxygenation during one-lung ventilation in patients undergoing cardiac surgery. Anesthesiology 1994; 80: 57–62.
115. Freden F, Wei SZ, Berglund JE, Frostell C, Hedenstierna G. Nitric oxide modulation of pulmonary blood flow distribution in lobar hypoxia. Anesthesiology 1995; 82:1216–1225.
116. Hambraeus-Jonzon K, Bindslev L, Frostell C, Hedenstierna G. Individual lung blood flow during unilateral hypoxia: effects of inhaled nitric oxide. Eur Respir J 1998; 11:565–570.
117. Freden F, Berglund JE, Hedenstierna G. Pulmonary blood flow distribution in lobar hypoxia: influence of cardiac output and nitric oxide inhalation. Scand Cardiovasc J 1999; 33:215–221.
118. Fradj K, Samain E, Delefosse D, Farah E, Marty J. Placebo-controlled study of inhaled nitric oxide to treat hypoxaemia during one-lung ventilation. Br J Anaesth 1999; 82:208–212.

119. Lester GD, DeMarco VG, Norman WM. Effect of inhaled nitric oxide on experimentally induced pulmonary hypertension in neonatal foals. Am J Vet Res 1999; 60:1207–1212.
120. Wilson WC, Kapelanski DP, Benumof JL, Newhart JW II, Johnson FW, Channick RN. Inhaled nitric oxide (40 ppm) during one-lung ventilation, in the lateral decubitus position, does not decrease pulmonary vascular resistance or improve oxygenation in normal patients. J Cardiothorac Vasc Anesth 1997; 11: 172–176.
121. Rocca GD, Passariello M, Coccia C, Costa MG, Di Marco P, Venuta F, Rendina EA, Pietropaoli P. Inhaled nitric oxide administration during one-lung ventilation in patients undergoing thoracic surgery. J Cardiothorac Vasc Anesth 2001; 15:218–223.
122. Doering EB, Hanson CW III, Reily DJ, Marshall C, Marshall BE. Improvement in oxygenation by phenylephrine and nitric oxide in patients with adult respiratory distress syndrome. Anesthesiology 1997; 87:18–25.
123. Dembinski R, Max M, Lopez F, Kuhlen R, Sunner M, Rossaint R. Effect of inhaled nitric oxide in combination with almitrine on ventilation–perfusion distributions in experimental lung injury. Intensive Care Med 2000; 26:221–228.
124. Papazian L, Bregeon F, Gaillat F, Thirion X, Roch A, Cortes E, Fulachier V, Saux P, Jammes Y, Auffray JP. Inhaled NO and almitrine bismesylate in patients with acute respiratory distress syndrome: effect of noradrenalin. Eur Respir J 1999; 14:1283–1289.
125. Lu Q, Mourgeon E, Law-Koune JD, Roche S, Vezinet C, Abdennour L, Vicaut E, Puybasset L, Diaby M, Coriat P. Dose–response curves of inhaled nitric oxide with and without intravenous almitrine in nitric oxide-responding patients with acute respiratory distress syndrome. Anesthesiology 1995; 83:929–943.
126. Moutafis M, Liu N, Dalibon N, Kuhlman G, Ducros L, Castelain MH, Fischler M. The effects of inhaled nitric oxide and its combination with intravenous almitrine on Pao2 during one-lung ventilation in patients undergoing thoracoscopic procedures. Anesth Analg 1997; 85:1130–1135.
127. Moutafis M, Dalibon N, Colchen A, Fischler M. Improving oxygenation during bronchopulmonary lavage using nitric oxide inhalation and almitrine infusion. Anesth Analg 1999; 89:302–304.
128. Moutafis M, Dalibon N, Liu N, Kuhlman G, Fischler M. The effects of intravenous almitrine on oxygenation and hemodynamics during one-lung ventilation. Anesth Analg 2002; 94:830–834.
129. Zeldin RA, Normadin D, Landtwing BS, Peters RM. Postpneumonectomy pulmonary edema. J Thorac Cardiovasc Surg 1984; 87:359–365.
130. Algar FJ, Alvarez A, Salvatierra A, Baamonde C, Aranda JL, Lopez-Pujol FJ. Predicting pulmonary complications after pneumonectomy for lung cancer. Eur J Cardiothorac Surg 2003; 23:201–208.
131. Turnage WS, Lunn JJ. Postpneumonectomy pulmonary edema. A retrospective analysis of associated variables. Chest 1993; 103:1646–1650.
132. Shapira OM, Shahian DM. Postpneumonectomy pulmonary edema. Ann Thorac Surg 1993; 56:190–195.
133. Waller DA, Gebitekin C, Saunders NR, Walker DR. Noncardiogenic pulmonary edema complicating lung resection. Ann Thorac Surg 1993; 55:140–143.
134. Caras WE. Postpneumonectomy pulmonary edema: can it be predicted preoperatively? Chest 1998; 114: 928–931.
135. Verheijen-Breemhaar L, Bogaard JM, van den Berg B, Hilvering C. Postpneumonectomy pulmonary oedema. Thorax 1988; 43:323–326.
136. Mathru M, Blakeman BP. Don't drown the "down lung". Chest 1993; 103:1644–1645.
137. Swartz DE, Lachapelle K, Sampalis J, Mulder DS, Chiu RC, Wilson J. Perioperative mortality after pneumonectomy: analysis of risk factors and review of the literature. Can J Surg 1997; 40:437–444.
138. Bleehen NM. Radiotherapy for small cell lung cancer. Chest 1986; 89:268S–276S.
139. Kaminski JM, Langer CJ, Movsas B. The role of radiation therapy and chemotherapy in the management of airway tumors other than small-cell carcinoma and non-small-cell carcinoma. Chest Surg Clin N Am 2003; 13:149–167.
140. Toy E, Macbeth F, Coles B, Melville A, Eastwood A. Palliative thoracic radiotherapy for non-small-cell lung cancer: a systematic review. Am J Clin Oncol 2003; 26:112–120.
141. Yang GY, Matthews RH. Prophylactic cranial irradiation in small-cell lung cancer. Oncologist 2000; 5: 293–298.
142. Pottgen C, Stuschke M. The role of prophylactic cranial irradiation in the treatment of lung cancer. Lung Cancer 2001; 33:S153–S158.
143. Tada T, Minakuchi K, Matsui K, Kawase I, Fukuda H, Nakajima T. Radiation pneumonitis following multi-field radiation therapy. Radiat Med 2000; 18: 59–61.
144. Kvale PA, Simoff M, Prakash UB. Lung cancer. Palliative care. Chest 2003; 123:284S–311S.
145. Barlow CS, Rudd RM. Chemotherapy and radiotherapy of bronchial carcinoma. Hosp Med 2003; 64: 144–149.
146. Donat SM, Levy DA. Bleomycin associated pulmonary toxicity: is perioperative oxygen restriction necessary? J Urol 1998; 160:1347–1352.
147. Curran WJ. New chemotherapeutic agents: update of major chemoradiation trials in solid tumors. Oncology 2002; 63:29–38.
148. Mauer AM, Ansari RH, Hoffman PC, Krauss SA, Taber D, Tembe SA, Gabrys GT, Cotter T, Schumm LP, Szeto L, Vokes EE. Phase I/II investigation of paclitaxel, ifosfamide and carboplatin for advanced non-small-cell lung cancer. Ann Oncol 2003; 14: 722–728.

149. Masters GA, Declerck L, Blanke C, Sandler A, DeVore R, Miller K, Johnson D. Phase II Trial of gemcitabine in refractory or relapsed small-cell lung cancer: eastern cooperative oncology group trial 1597. J Clin Oncol 2003; 21:1550–1555.
150. Hoang T, Traynor AM, Schiller JH. Novel therapies for lung cancer. Surg Oncol 2002; 11:229–241.
151. Wong AS, Hon Yoon K. Paraneoplastic Raynaud phenomenon and idiopathic thrombocytopenic purpura in non-small-cell lung cancer. Am J Clin Oncol 2003; 26:26–29.
152. Diacon AH, Schuurmans MM, Colesky FJ, Bolliger CT. Paraneoplastic bilateral proptosis in a case of non-small cell lung cancer. Chest 2003; 123:627–629.
153. Beckles MA, Spiro SG, Colice GL, Rudd RM. Initial evaluation of the patient with lung cancer: symptoms, signs, laboratory tests, and paraneoplastic syndromes. Chest 2003; 123:97S–104S.
154. Richardson GE, Johnson BE. Paraneoplastic syndromes in thoracic malignancies. Curr Opin Oncol 1991; 3:320–327.
155. Seneviratne U, de Silva R. Lambert–Eaton myasthenic syndrome. Postgrad Med J 1999; 75:516–520.
156. Nair SG, Kumar BS, Rajan B. Poorly differentiated carcinoma of the lung presenting with Lambert–Eaton myasthenic syndrome. Am J Clin Oncol 2000; 23: 58–59.
157. Sakura S, Saito Y, Maeda M, Kosaka Y. Epidural analgesia in Eaton–Lambert myasthenic syndrome. Effects on respiratory function. Anaesthesia 1991; 46:560–562.
158. Itoh H, Shibata K, Nitta S. Neuromuscular monitoring in myasthenic syndrome. Anaesthesia 2001; 56: 562–567.
159. Wudel LJ Jr, Nesbitt JC. Superior vena cava syndrome. Curr Treat Options Oncol 2001; 2:77–91.
160. Baker GL, Barnes HJ. Superior vena cava syndrome: etiology, diagnosis, and treatment. Am J Crit Care 1992; 1:54–64
161. Urban T, Lebeau B, Chastang C, Leclerc P, Botto MJ, Sauvaget J. Superior vena cava syndrome in small-cell lung cancer. Arch Intern Med 1993; 153:384–387.
162. Porte H, Metois D, Finzi L, Lebuffe G, Guidat A, Conti M, Wurtz A. Superior vena cava syndrome of malignant origin. Which surgical procedure for which diagnosis? Eur J Cardiothorac Surg 2000; 17:384–388.
163. Shah R, Sabanathan S, Lowe RA, Mearns AJ. Stenting in malignant obstruction of superior vena cava. J Thorac Cardiovasc Surg 1996; 112:335–340.
164. Courtheoux P, Alkofer B, Al Refai M, Gervais R, Le Rochais JP, Icard P. Stent placement in superior vena cava syndrome. Ann Thorac Surg 2003; 75:158–161.
165. Shaw RR. Pancoast's tumor. Ann Thorac Surg 1984; 37:343–345.
166. Kichari JR, Hussain SM, Den Hollander JC, Krestin GP. MR imaging of the brachial plexus: current imaging sequences, normal findings, and findings in a spectrum of focal lesions with MR-pathologic correlation. Curr Probl Diagn Radiol 2003; 32:88–101.
167. Remmen HJ, Lacquet LK, Van Son JA, Morshuis WJ, Cox AL. Surgical treatment of Pancoast tumor. J Cardiovasc Surg (Torino) 1993; 34:157–161.
168. Orringer MB, Marshall B, Iannettoni MD. Transhiatal esophagectomy for treatment of benign and malignant esophageal disease. World J Surg 2001; 25: 196–203.
169. Collard JM. High-grade dysplasia in Barrett's esophagus. The case for esophagectomy. Chest Surg Clin N Am 2002; 12:77–92.
170. Kim LS, Koch J. Do we practice what we preach? clinical decision making and utilization of endoscopic ultrasound for staging esophageal cancer. Am J Gastroenterol 1999; 94:1847–1852.
171. Butsch J, Christein JD, Millikan K. Prognostic factors relating to esophageal cancer. Minerva Chir 2002; 57:789–794.
172. Kato H, Kuwano H, Nakajima M, Miyazaki T, Yoshikawa M, Ojima H, Tsukada K, Oriuchi N, Inoue T, Endo K. Comparison between positron emission tomography and computed tomography in the use of the assessment of esophageal carcinoma. Cancer 2002; 94: 921–928.
173. Cooper DK. The incidence of postoperative infection and the role of antibiotic prophylaxis in pulmonary surgery. A review of 221 consecutive patients undergoing thoracotomy. Br J Dis Chest 1981; 75:154–160.
174. Pieper R, Book K, Nord CE. Microbial flora associated with pulmonary neoplasms. Scand J Thorac Cardiovasc Surg 1984; 18:259–261.
175. Bryant LR, Dillon ML, Mobin-Uddin K. Prophylactic antibiotics in noncardiac thoracic operations. Ann Thorac Surg 1975; 19:670–676.
176. Ziomek S, Read RC, Tobler HG, Harrell JE Jr, Gocio JC, Fink LM, Ranval TJ, Ferris EJ, Harshfield DL, McFarland DR, et al. Thromboembolism in patients undergoing thoracotomy. Ann Thorac Surg 1993; 56: 223–226.
177. Massard G, Moog R, Wihlm JM, Kessler R, Dabbagh A, Lesage A, Roeslin N, Morand G. Bronchogenic cancer in the elderly: operative risk and long-term prognosis. Thorac Cardiovasc Surg 1996; 44:40–45.
178. Dartevelle PG, Chapelier AR, Macchiarini P, Lenot B, Cerrina J, Ladurie FL, Parquin FJ, Lafont D. Anterior transcervical-thoracic approach for radical resection of lung tumors invading the thoracic inlet. J Thorac Cardiovasc Surg 1993; 105:1025–1034.
179. Korst RJ, Burt ME. Cervicothoracic tumors: results of resection by the "hemi-clamshell" approach. J Thorac Cardiovasc Surg 1998; 115:286–294.
180. Dartevelle P, Macchiarini P. Surgical management of superior sulcus tumors. Oncologist 1999; 4:398–407.
181. Ducic Y, Crepeau A, Ducic L, Lamothe A, Corsten M. A logical approach to the thoracic inlet: the Dartevelle approach revisited. Head Neck 1999; 21:767–771.

182. Vanakesa T, Goldstraw P. Antero-superior approaches in the practice of thoracic surgery. Eur J Cardiothorac Surg 1999; 15:774–780.
183. Fadel E, Missenard G, Chapelier A, Mussot S, Leroy-Ladurie F, Cerrina J, Dartevelle P. En bloc resection of non-small cell lung cancer invading the thoracic inlet and intervertebral foramina. J Thorac Cardiovasc Surg 2002; 123:676–685.
184. Bilaceroglu S, Cagiotariotaciota U, Gunel O, Bayol U, Perim K. Comparison of rigid and flexible transbronchial needle aspiration in the staging of bronchogenic carcinoma. Respiration 1998; 65:441–449.
185. Cappellari JO, Haponik EF. Bronchoscopic needle aspiration biopsy. Am J Clin Pathol 2000; 113: S97–S108.
186. Salathe M, Soler M, Bolliger CT, Dalquen P, Perruchoud AP. Transbronchial needle aspiration in routine fiberoptic bronchoscopy. Respiration 1992; 59: 5–8.
187. Kandasamy R, Sivalingam P. Use of sevoflurane in difficult airways. Acta Anaesthesiol Scand 2000; 44: 627–629.
188. Davies L, Mister R, Spence DP, Calverley PM, Earis JE, Pearson MG. Cardiovascular consequences of fibreoptic bronchoscopy. Eur Respir J 1997; 10: 695–698.
189. Gronnebech H, Johansson G, Smedebol M, Valentin N. Glycopyrrolate vs. atropine during anaesthesia for laryngoscopy and bronchoscopy. Acta Anaesthesiol Scand 1993; 37:454–457.
190. Williams T, Brooks T, Ward C. The role of atropine premedication in fiberoptic bronchoscopy using intravenous midazolam sedation. Chest 1998; 113: 1394–1398.
191. Cowl CT, Prakash UB, Kruger BR. The role of anticholinergics in bronchoscopy. A randomized clinical trial. Chest 2000; 118:188–1892.
192. Peacock AJ, Benson-Mitchell R, Godfrey R. Effect of fiberoptic bronchoscopy on pulmonary function. Thorax 1990; 45:38–41.
193. Suratt PM, Smiddy JF, Gruber B. Deaths and complications associated with fiberoptic bronchoscopy. Chest 1976; 69:747–751.
194. Lukomsky GI, Ovchinnikov AA, Bilal A. Complications of bronchoscopy: comparison of rigid bronchoscopy under general anesthesia and flexible fiberoptic bronchoscopy under topical anesthesia. Chest 1981; 79:316–321.
195. Plummer S, Hartley M, Vaughan. Anaesthesia for telescopic procedures in the thorax. Br J Anaesthesia 1998; 80:223–234.
196. Hautmann H, Gamarra F, Henke M, Diehm S, Huber RM. High frequency jet ventilation in interventional fiberoptic bronchoscopy. Anesth Analg 2000; 90: 1436–1440.
197. Kestin IG, Chapman JM, Coates MB. Alfentanil used to supplement propofol infusions for oesophagoscopy and bronchoscopy. Anaesthesia 1989; 44:994–996.
198. Smith CO, Shroff PF, Steele JD. General anesthesia for bronchoscopy. The use of the Sanders bronchoscopic attachment. Ann Thorac Surg 1969; 8:348–354.
199. Carden E, Burns WW, McDevitt NB, Carson T. A comparison of Venturi and side-arm ventilation in anesthesia for bronchoscopy. Can Anaesth Soc J 1973; 20:569–574.
200. Toloza EM, Harpole L, Detterbeck F, McCrory DC. Invasive staging of non-small cell lung cancer: a review of the current evidence. Chest 2003; 123:157S–166S.
201. Grondin SC, Liptay MJ. Current concepts in the staging of non-small cell lung cancer. Surg Oncol 2002; 11:181–190.
202. McNeill TM, Chamberlain JM. Diagnostic anterior mediastinotomy. Ann Thorac Surg 1966; 2:532–529.
203. Bowen TE, Zajtchuk R, Green DC, Brott WH. Value of anterior mediastinotomy in bronchogenic carcinoma of the left upper lobe. J Thorac Cardiovasc Surg 1978; 76:269–271.
204. Selby JH Jr, Leach CL, Heath BJ, Neely WA. Local anesthesia for mediastinoscopy: experience with 450 consecutive cases. Am Surg 1978; 44:679–682.
205. Rendina EA, Venuta F, De Giacomo T, Ciccone AM, Moretti MS, Ibrahim M, Coloni GF. Biopsy of anterior mediastinal masses under local anesthesia. Ann Thorac Surg 2002; 74:1720–1722.
206. Vaughan RS. Anaesthesia for mediastinoscopy. Anaesthesia 1978; 33:195–198.
207. Lee J, Salvatore A. Innominate artery compression simulating cardiac arrest during mediastinoscopy: a case report. Anesth Analg 1976; 55:748–749.
208. Petty C. Right radial artery pressure during mediastinoscopy. Anesth Analg 1979; 58:428–430.
209. Garry BP, Bivens HE. Blood pressure monitoring during mediastinoscopy. Can J Anaesth 1989; 36:365.
210. Goh MH, Liu XY, Goh YS. Anterior mediastinal masses: an anaesthetic challenge. Anaesthesia 1999; 54:670–674.
211. Furgang FA, Saidman LJ. Bilateral tension pneumothorax associated with mediastinoscopy. J Thorac Cardiovasc Surg 1972; 63:329–333.
212. Vueghs PJ, Schurink GA, Vaes L, Langemeyer JJ. Anesthesia in repeat mediastinoscopy: a retrospective study of 101 patients. J Cardiothorac Vasc Anesth 1992; 6:193–195.
213. Olak J. Parasternal mediastinotomy (Chamberlain procedure). Chest Surg Clin N Am 1996; 6:31–40.
214. Mason AC, Krasna MJ, White CS. The role of radiologic imaging in diagnosis complications of video-assisted thoracoscopic surgery. Chest 1998; 113:820–825.
215. Yim AP, Izzat MB, Lee TW, Wan S. Video-assisted thoracic surgery: a renaissance in surgical therapy. Respirology 1999; 4:1–8.
216. McKenna RJ Jr. The current status of video-assisted thoracic surgery lobectomy. Chest Surg Clin N Am 1998; 8:775–785.
217. Demmy TL, Krasna MJ, Detterbeck FC, Kilne GG, Kohman LJ, DeCamp MM Jr, Wain JC. Multicenter

VATS experience with mediastinal tumors. Ann Thorac Surg 1998; 66:187–192.
218. Kawahara K, Maekawa T, Okabayashi K, Hideshima T, Shiraishi T, Yoshinaga Y, Shirakusa T. Video-assisted thoracoscopic esophagectomy for esophageal cancer. Surg Endosc 1999; 13:218–223.
219. Moffatt SD, Mitchell JD, Whyte RI. Role of video-assisted thoracoscopic surgery and classic thoracotomy in lung cancer management. Curr Opin Pulm Med 2002; 8:281–286.
220. Landreneau RJ, Wiechmann RJ, Hazelrigg SR, Mack MJ, Keenan RJ, Ferson PF. Effect of minimally invasive thoracic surgical approaches on acute and chronic postoperative pain. Chest Surg Clin N Am 1998; 8: 891–906.
221. Yim AP. VATS major pulmonary resection revisited—controversies, techniques, and results. Ann Thorac Surg 2002; 74:615–623.
222. Baraka A. Hazards of carbon dioxide insufflation during thoracoscopy. Br J Anaesth 1998; 81:100.
223. Mehta MP. The contemporary role of radiation therapy in the management of lung cancer. The contemporary role of radiation therapy in the management of lung cancer. Surg Oncol Clin N Am 2000; 9: 539–561.
224. Simon GR, Wagner H. Small cell lung cancer. Chest 2003; 123:259S–271S.
225. Jett JR, Scott WJ, Rivera MP, Sause WT. Guidelines on treatment of stage IIIB non-small cell lung cancer. Chest 2003; 123:221S–225S.
226. Bethencourt DM, Holmes EC. Muscle-sparing posterolateral thoracotomy. Ann Thorac Surg 1988; 45: 337–339.
227. Ashour M. Modified muscle sparing posterolateral thoracotomy. Thorax 1990; 45:935–938.
228. Nomori H, Horio H, Fuyuno G, Kobayashi R. Non-serratus-sparing antero-axillary thoracotomy with disconnection of anterior rib cartilage. Improvement in postoperative pulmonary function and pain in comparison to posterolateral thoracotomy. Chest 1997; 111:572–576.
229. Daniels LJ, Balderson SS, Onaitis MW, D'Amico TA. Thoracoscopic lobectomy: a safe and effective strategy for patients with stage I lung cancer. Ann Thorac Surg 2002; 74:860–864.
230. McKenna RJ Jr, Wolf RK, Brenner M, Fischel RJ, Wurnig P. Is lobectomy by video-assisted thoracic surgery an adequate cancer operation? Ann Thorac Surg 1998; 66:1903–1908.
231. Solaini L, Bagioni P, Prusciano F, Di Francesco F, Poddie DB. Video-assisted thoracic surgery (VATS) lobectomy for typical bronchopulmonary carcinoid tumors. Surg Endosc 2000; 14:1142–1145.
232. McKenna RJ Jr. Lobectomy by video-assisted thoracic surgery with mediastinal node sampling for lung cancer. J Thorac Cardiovasc Surg 1994; 107:879–881.
233. Hoier-Madsen K, Schulze S, Moller Pedersen V, Halkier E. Management of bronchopleural fistula following pneumonectomy. Scand J Thorac Cardiovasc Surg 1984; 18:263–266.
234. Yokomise H, Takahashi Y, Inui K, Yagi K, Mizuno H, Aoki M, Wada H, Hitomi S. Omentoplasty for postpneumonectomy bronchopleural fistulas. Eur J Cardiothorac Surg 1994; 8:122–124.
235. al-Kattan K, Cattelani L, Goldstraw P. Bronchopleural fistula after pneumonectomy for lung cancer. Eur J Cardiothorac Surg 1995; 9:479–482.
236. Chan EC, Lee TW, Ng CS, Wan IY, Sihoe AD, Yim AP. Closure of postpneumonectomy bronchopleural fistula by means of single, perforator-based, latissimus dorsi muscle flap. J Thorac Cardiovasc Surg 2002; 124:1235–1236.
237. Refaely Y, Paley M, Simansky DA, Rozenman Y, Yellin A. Transsternal transpericardial closure of a postlobectomy bronchopleural fistula. Ann Thorac Surg 2002; 73:635–636.
238. Pinsonneault C, Fortier J, Donati F. Tracheal resection and reconstruction. Can J Anaesth 1999; 46:439–455.
239. Grillo HC, Mathisen DJ. Primary tracheal tumors: treatment and results. Ann Thorac Surg 1990; 49: 69–77.
240. D'Cunha J, Maddaus MA. Surgical treatment of tracheal and carinal tumors. Chest Surg Clin N Am 2003; 13:95–110.
241. Bricker DL, Parker TM, Dalton ML Jr. Cardiopulmonary bypass in anesthetic management of resection. Its use for severe tracheal stenosis. Arch Surg 1979; 114:847–849.
242. Konstantinov IE, Peterffy A. Cardiopulmonary bypass for tracheal tumor resection: revival of an old technique? Ann Thorac Surg 1998; 66:1865–1866.
243. Grillo HC. Surgery of the trachea. In: Keen G, ed. Operative Surgery and Management. 2nd ed. Bristol: Wright, 1987:776–784.
244. Briccoli A, Manfrini M, Rocca M, Lari S, Giacomini S, Mercuri M. Sternal reconstruction with synthetic mesh and metallic plates for high grade tumours of the chest wall. Eur J Surg 2002; 168:494–499.
245. Mansour KA, Thourani VH, Losken A, Reeves JG, Miller JI Jr, Carlson GW, Jones GE. Chest wall resections and reconstruction: a 25-year experience. Ann Thorac Surg 2002; 73:1720–1725.
246. Walsh GL, Davis BM, Swisher SG, Vaporciyan AA, Smythe WR, Willis-Merriman K, Roth JA, Putnam JB Jr. A single-institutional, multidisciplinary approach to primary sarcomas involving the chest wall requiring full-thickness resections. Thorac Cardiovasc Surg 2001; 121:48–60.
247. Abramson AL, Ladner W. The anesthetic management of the patient with an anterior mediastinal mass. Anesthesiology 1984; 60:144–147.
248. Prakash UB, Abel MD, Hubmayr RD. Mediastinal mass and tracheal obstruction during general anesthesia. Mayo Clin Proc 1988; 63:1004–1011.
249. Graeber GM, Shriver CD, Albus RA, Burton NA, Collins GJ, Lough FC, Zajtchuk R. The use of computer

tomography in the evaluation of mediastinal masses. J Thorac Cardiovasc Surg 1986; 91:662–666.
250. Miller RD, Hyatt RE. Obstructing lesions of the larynx and trachea: clinical and physiologic characteristics. Mayo Clin Proc 1969; 44:145–161.
251. Acres JC, Kryger MH. Clinical significance of pulmonary function tests: upper airway obstruction. Chest 1981; 80:207–211.
252. Pullerits J, Holzman R. Anaesthesia for patients with mediastinal masses. Can J Anaesth 1989; 36:681–688.
253. Narang S, Harte BH, Body SC. Anesthesia for patients with a mediastinal mass. Anesthesiol Clin North Am 2001; 19:559–579.
254. Stephens KE Jr, Wood DE. Bronchoscopic management of central airway obstruction. J Thorac Cardiovasc Surg 2000; 119:289–296.
255. Lee P, Kupeli E, Mehta AC. Therapeutic bronchoscopy in lung cancer. Laser therapy, electrocautery, brachytherapy, stents, and photodynamic therapy. Clin Chest Med 2002; 23:241–256.
256. Simoff MJ. Endobronchial management of advanced lung cancer. Cancer Control 2001; 8:337–343.
257. Edell ES, Cortese DA, McDougall JC. Ancillary therapies in the management of lung cancer: photodynamic therapy, laser therapy, and endobronchial prosthetic devices. Mayo Clin Proc 1993; 68:685–690.
258. Conacher ID, Paes LL, McMahon CC, Morritt GN. Anesthetic management of laser surgery for central airway obstruction: a 12-year case series. J Cardiothorac Vasc Anesth 1998; 12:153–156.
259. Tsang V, Goldstraw P. Endobronchial stenting for anastomotic stenosis after sleeve resection. Ann Thorac Surg 1989; 48:568–571.
260. Wilson GE, Walshaw MJ, Hind CR. Treatment of large airway obstruction in lung cancer using expandable metal stents inserted under direct vision via the fiberoptic bronchoscope. Thorax 1996; 51:248–252.
261. Wood DE. Airway stenting. Chest Surg Clin N Am 2001; 11:841–860.
262. Gelb AF, Zamel N, Colchen A, Tashkin DP, Maurer JR, Patterson GA, Epstein JD. Physiologic studies of tracheobronchial stents in airway obstruction. Am Rev Respir Dis 1992; 146:1088–1090.
263. Eisner MD, Gordon RL, Webb WR, Gold WM, Hilal SE, Edinburgh K, Golden JA. Pulmonary function improves after expandable metal stent placement for benign airway disease. Chest 1999; 115:1006–1011.
264. Zannini P, Melloni G, Chiesa G, Carretta A. Self-expanding stents in the treatment of tracheobronchial obstruction. Chest 1994; 106:86–90.
265. Shafer JP, Allen JN. The use of expandable metal stents to facilitate extubation in patients with large airway obstruction. Chest 1998; 114:1378–1382.
266. Scheinhorn DJ, Chao DC, Stearn-Hassenpflug M. Approach to patients with long-term weaning failure. Respir Care Clin N Am 2000; 6:437–461.
267. Kumar P, Roy A, Penny DJ, Ladas G, Goldstraw P. Airway obstruction and ventilator dependency in young children with congenital cardiac defects: a role for self-expanding metal stents. Intensive Care Med 2002; 28:190–195.
268. Cavaliere S, Venuta F, Foccoli P, Toninelli C, La Face B. Endoscopic treatment of malignant airway obstructions in 2,008 patients. Chest 1996; 110:1536–1542.
269. Taber SW, Buschemeyer WC III, Fingar VH, Wieman TH. The treatment of malignant endobronchial obstruction with laser ablation. Surgery 1999; 126: 730–733.
270. Miller JI, Phillip TW. Neodymim:YAG laser and brachytherapy in the management of inoperable bronchogenic carcinoma. Ann Thorac Surg 1990; 50: 190–196.
271. Suh JH, Dass KK, Pagliaccio L, Taylor ME, Saxton JP, Tan M, Mehta AC. Endobronchial radiation therapy with or without neodymium yttrium aluminum garnet laser resection for managing malignant airway obstruction. Cancer 1994; 73:2583–2588.
272. Vourc'h G, Fischler M, Personne C, Colchen A, Toty L. Anesthetic management during Nd-YAG laser resection for major tracheobronchial obstructing tumors. Anesthesiology 1984; 61:636–637.
273. Warner ME, Warner MA, Leonard P. Anesthesia for neodymium-YAG (Nd-YAG) laser resection of major airway obstructing tumors. Anesthesiology 1984; 60:230–232.
274. Duckett JE, McDonnel TJ, Unger M, Parr GVS. General anaesthesia for Nd:YAG laser resection of obstructing endobronchial tumours using the rigid bronchoscope. Can Anaesth Soc J 1985; 32:67–72.
275. Hanowell LH, Martin WR, Savelle JE, Foppiano LE. Complications of general anesthesia for Nd:YAG laser resection of endobronchial tumors. Chest 1991; 99: 72–76.
276. Blomquist S, Algotsson L, Karlsson SE. Anaesthesia for resection of tumours in the trachea and central bronchi using the Nd-Yag-laser technique. Acta Anaesthesiol Scand 1990; 34:506–510.
277. Jackson KA, Morland MH. Anaesthesia for resection of lesions of the trachea and main bronchi using the neodymium yttrium aluminum garnet (Nd YAG) laser. A report of 75 treatments in 52 patients. Anaesth Intensive Care 1990; 18:583–585.
278. McCaughan JS Jr, Barabash RD, Penn GM, Glavan BJ. Nd:YAG laser and photodynamic therapy for esophageal and endobronchial tumors under general and local anesthesia. Effects on arterial blood gas levels. Chest 1990; 98:1374–1378.
279. Sutedja G, Koppenol W, Stam J. Nd-YAG laser under local anaesthesia in obstructive endobronchial tumours. Respiration 1991; 58:238–240.
280. George PJ, Garrett CP, Nixon C, Hetzel MR, Nanson EM, Millard FJ. Laser treatment for tracheobronchial tumours: local or general anaesthesia? Thorax 1987; 42:656–660.
281. Stanopoulos IT, Beamis JF Jr, Martinez FJ, Vergos K, Shapshay SM. Laser bronchoscopy in respiratory

failure from malignant airway obstruction. Crit Care Med 1993; 21:386–391.
282. Dumon J, Shapshay S, Bourcereau J, Cavaliere S, Meric B, Garbi N, Beamis J. Principles for safety in application of neodymium-YAG laser in bronchoscopy. Chest 1984; 86:163–168.
283. Vanderschueren RG, Westermann CJ. Complications of endobronchial neodymium-Yag (Nd:Yag) laser application. Lung 1990; 168(suppl):1089–1094.
284. Rooney S, Goldiner PL, Bains MS, Hilaris B, Jain S. Anesthesia for the application of endotracheal and endbronchial radiation therapy. J Thorac Cardiovasc Surg 1984; 87:693–697.
285. Gaspar LE. Brachytherapy in lung cancer. J Surg Oncol 1998; 67:60–70.
286. Seagren SL, Harrell JH, Horn RA. High dose rate intraluminal irradiation in recurrent endobronchial carcinoma. Chest 1985; 86:810–814.
287. Lo Cicero J, Metzdorff M, Almgren C. Photodynamic therapy in the palliation of late stage obstructing non-small cell lung cancer. Chest 1990; 98:97–100.
288. Lam S. Photodynamic therapy of lung cancer. Semin Oncol 1994; 21:15–19.
289. Sutedja TG, Postmus PE. Photodynamic therapy in lung cancer. A review. J Photochem Photobiol B 1996; 36:199–204.
290. Metz JM, Friedberg JS. Endobronchial photodynamic therapy for the treatment of lung cancer. Chest Surg Clin N Am 2001; 11:829–839.
291. Banerjee A, George J. Bronchoscopic photodynamic diagnosis and therapy for lung cancer. Curr Opin Pulm Med 2000; 6:378–383.
292. Carlin BW, Harrell JH II, Moser KM. The treatment of endobronchial stenosis using balloon catheter dilatation. Chest 1988; 93:1148–1151.
293. Homasson JP, Renault P, Angebault M, Bonniot JP, Bell NJ. Bronchoscopic cryotherapy for airway structures caused by tumors. Chest 1986; 90:159–161.
294. Vergnon JM, Schmitt T, Alamartine E, Barthelemy JC, Fournel P, Emonot A. Initial combined cryotherapy and irradiation for unresectable non-small cell lung cancer. Preliminary results. Chest 1992; 102: 1436–1440.
295. Maiwand MO, Homasson JP. Cryotherapy for tracheobroncial disorders. Clin Chest Med 1995; 16: 427–443.
296. Mathur PN, Wolf KM, Busk MF, Briete WM, Datzman M. Fiberoptic bronchoscopic cryotherapy in the management of tracheobronchial obstruction. Chest 1996; 110:718–723.
297. Petrou M, Kaplan D, Goldstraw P. Bronchoscopic diathermy resection and stent insertion: a cost effective treatment of tracheobronchial obstruction. Thorax 1993; 48:1156–1159.
298. Boxem T, Muller M, Venmans B, Postmus P, Sutedja T. Nd-YAG laser vs bronchoscopic electrocautery for palliation of symptomatic airway obstruction: a cost-effective study. Chest 1999; 116:1108–1112.
299. Coulter TD, Mehta AC. The heat is on: impact of endobronchial electrosurgery on the need for Nd-YAG laser photoresection. Chest 2000; 118:516–521.
300. van Boxem AJ, Westerga J, Venmans BJ, Postmus PE, Sutedja G. Photodynamic therapy, Nd-YAG laser and electrocautery for treating early-stage intraluminal cancer: which to choose?. Lung Cancer 2001; 31: 31–36.
301. Urba S. Combined modality therapy of esophageal cancer—standard of care? Surg Oncol Clin N Am 2002; 11:377–386.
302. Doty JR, Salazar JD, Forastiere AA, Heath EI, Kleinberg L, Heitmiller RF. Postesophagectomy morbidity, mortality, and length of hospital stay after preoperative chemoradiation therapy. Ann Thorac Surg 2002; 74:227–231.
303. Mathisen DJ, Grillo HC, Wilkins EW Jr, Moncure AC, Hilgenberg AD. Transthoracic esophagectomy: a safe approach to carcinoma of the esophagus. Ann Thorac Surg 1988; 45:137–143.
304. Christein JD, Hollinger EF, Millikan KW. Prognostic factors associated with resectable carcinoma of the esophagus. Am Surg 2002; 68:258–262.
305. Swanson SJ, Linden P. Esophagectomy for esophageal cancer. Minerva Chir 2002; 57:795–810.
306. Davis PA, Law S, Wong J. Colonic interposition after esophagectomy for cancer. Arch Surg 2003; 138: 303–308.
307. Ikeguchi M, Maeta M, Kaibara N. Respiratory function after esophagectomy for patients with esophageal cancer. Hepatogastroenterology 2002; 49:1284–1286.
308. Daly JM, Fry WA, Little AG, Winchester DP, McKee RF, Stewart AK, Fremgen AM. Esophageal cancer: results of an American College of Surgeons patient care evaluation study. J Am Coll Surg 2000; 190: 562–572.
309. Tandon S, Batchelor A, Bullock R, Gascoigne A, Griffin M, Hayes N, Hing J, Shaw I, Warnell I, Baudouin SV. Peri-operative risk factors for acute lung injury after elective oesophagectomy. Br J Anaesth 2001; 86:633–638.
310. Bailey SH, Bull DA, Harpole DH, Rentz JJ, Neumayer LA, Pappas TN, Daley J, Henderson WG, Krasnicka B, Khuri SF. Outcomes after esophagectomy: a ten-year prospective cohort. Ann Thorac Surg 2003; 75:217–222.
311. Smyrnios NA, Connolly A, Wilson MM, Curley FJ, French CT, Heard SO, Irwin RS. Effects of a multifaceted, multidisciplinary, hospital-wide quality improvement program on weaning from mechanical ventilation. Crit Care Med 2002; 30:1224–1230.
312. Kaye J, Ashline V, Erickson D, Zeiler K, Gavigan D, Gannon L, Wynne P, Cooper J, Kittle W, Sharma K, Morton J. Critical care bug team: a multidisciplinary team approach to reducing ventilator-associated pneumonia. Am J Infect Control 2000; 28:197–201.
313. Critical care services and personnel: recommendations based on a system of categorization into two levels of

care. American College of Critical Care Medicine of the Society of Critical Care Medicine. Crit Care Med 1999; 27:422–426.
314. Kindgen-Milles D, Buhl R, Loer SA, Muller E. Nasal CPAP therapy: effects of different CPAP levels on pressure transmission into the trachea and pulmonary oxygen transfer. Acta Anaesthesiol Scand 2002; 46:860–865.
315. Auriant I, Jallot A, Herve P, Cerrina J, Le Roy Ladurie F, Fournier JL, Lescot B, Parquin F. Noninvasive ventilation reduces mortality in acute respiratory failure following lung resection. Am J Respir Crit Care Med 2001; 164:1231–1235.
316. Thys F, Roeseler J, Reynaert M, Liistro G, Rodenstein DO. Noninvasive ventilation for acute respiratory failure: a prospective randomised placebo-controlled trial. Eur Respir J 2002; 20:545–555.
317. D'Arsigny C, Goldberg P. Mechanical ventilation for respiratory failure postthoracotomy. Chest Surg Clin N Am 1998; 8:585–610.
318. Fialkow L, Vieira SR, Fernandes AK, Silva DR, Bozzetti MC. Acute respiratory distress syndrome research group.Acute lung injury and acute respiratory distress syndrome at the intensive care unit of a general university hospital in Brazil. An epidemiological study using the American–European consensus criteria. Intensive Care Med 2002; 28:1644–1648.
319. Slinger PD. Perioperative fluid management for thoracic surgery: the puzzle of postpneumonectomy pulmonary edema. J Cardiothorac Vasc Anesth 1995; 9:442–451.
320. Takagi K, Yamamori H, Morishima Y, Toyoda Y, Nakajima N, Tashiro T. Preoperative immunosuppression: its relationship with high morbidity and mortality in patients receiving thoracic esophagectomy. Nutrition 2001; 17:13–17.
321. Daly JM, Redmond HP, Gallagher H. Perioperative nutrition in cancer patients. J Parenter Enteral Nutr 1992; 16(6 suppl):100S–105S.
322. Aiko S, Yoshizumi Y, Sugiura Y, Matsuyama T, Naito Y, Matsuzaki J, Maehara T. Beneficial effects of immediate enteral nutrition after esophageal cancer surgery. Surg Today 2001; 31:971–978.
323. Bengmark S, Gianotti L. Nutritional support to prevent and treat multiple organ failure. World J Surg 1996; 20:474–481.
324. Kemper M, Weissman C, Hyman AI. Caloric requirements and supply in critically ill surgical patients. Crit Care Med 1992; 20:344–348.
325. Hazelrigg SR, Cetindag IB, Fullerton J. Acute and chronic pain syndromes after thoracic surgery. Surg Clin North Am 2002; 82:849–865.
326. Shulman M, Sandler AN, Bradley JW, Young PS, Brebner J. Postthoracotomy pain and pulmonary function following epidural and systemic morphine. Anesthesiology 1984; 61:569–575.
327. Furrer M, Rechsteiner R, Eigenmann V, Signer C, Althaus U, Ris HB. Thoracotomy and thoracoscopy: postoperative pulmonary function, pain and chest wall complaints. Eur J Cardiothorac Surg 1997; 12:82–87.
328. Kavanagh BP, Katz J, Sandler AN. Pain control after thoracotomy: a review of current techniques. Anesthesiology 1994; 81:737–759.
329. Boulanger A, Choiniere M, Roy D, Boure B, Chartrand D, Choquette R, Rousseau P. Comparison between patient-controlled analgesia and intramuscular meperidine after thoracotomy. Can J Anaesth 1993; 40:409–415.
330. Grant RP, Dolman JF, Harper JA, White SA, Parsons DG, Evans KG, Merrick CP. Patient-controlled lumbar epidural fentanyl compared with patient-controlled intravenous fentanyl for post-thoracotomy pain. Can J Anaesth 1992; 39:214–219.
331. Slinger P, Shennib H, Wilson S. Postthoracotomy pulmonary function: a comparison of epidural versus intravenous meperidine infusions. J Cardiothorac Vasc Anesth 1995; 9:128–134.
332. Etches RC, Gammer TL, Cornish R. Patient-controlled epidural analgesia after thoracotomy: a comparison of meperidine with and without bupivacaine. Anesth Analg 1996; 83:81–86.
333. Rawal N. Treating postoperative pain improves outcome. Minerva Anestesiol 2001; 67(S1):200–205.
334. Senturk M, Ozcan PE, Talu GK, Kiyan E, Camci E, Ozyalcin S, Dilege S, Pembeci K. The effects of three different analgesia techniques on long-term postthoracotomy pain. Anesth Analg 2002; 94:11–15.
335. Sandler AN. Post-thoracotomy analgesia and perioperative outcome. Minerva Anestesiol 1999; 65: 267–274.
336. Gray JR, Fromme GA, Nauss LA, Wang JK, Ilstrup DM. Intrathecal morphine for post-thoracotomy pain. Anesth Analg 1986; 65:873–876.
337. Lubenow TR, Faber LP, McCarthy RJ, Hopkins EM, Warren WH, Ivankovich AD. Postthoracotomy pain management using continuous epidural analgesia in 1,324 patients. Ann Thor Surg 1994; 58:924–929.
338. Brodsky JB, Chaplan SR, Brose WG, Mark JBD. Continuous epidural hydromorphone for postthoracotomy pain relief. Ann Thorac Surg 1990; 50:888–893.
339. Whiting WC, Sandler AN, Lau LC, Chovaz PM, Slavchenko P, Daley D, Koren G. Analgesic and respiratory effects of epidural sufentanil in patients following thoracotomy. Anesthesiology 1988; 69:36–43.
340. George KA, Wright PMC, Chisakuta A. Continuous thoracic epidural fentanyl for post-thoracotomy pain relief: with or without bupivacaine? Anaesthesia 1991; 46:732–736.
341. Guinard J-P, Mavrocordatos P, Chiolero R, Carpenter RL. A randomized comparison of intravenous versus lumbar and thoracic epidural fentanyl for analgesia after thoracotomy. Anesthesiology 1992; 77: 1108–115.
342. Rosseel PMJ, van den Broek WGM, Boer EC, Prakash O. Epidural sufentanil for intra- and postoperative analgesia in thoracic surgery: a comparative

study with intravenous sufentanil. Acta Anaesthesiol Scand 1988; 32:193–198.
343. Hansdottir V, Bake B, Nordberg G. The analgesic efficacy and adverse effects of continuous epidural sufentanil and bupivacaine infusion after thoracotomy. Anesth Analg 1996; 83:394–400.
344. Brose WG, Tanelian DL, Brodsky JB, Mark JBD. CSF and blood pharmacokinetics of hydromorphone and morphine following lumbar epidural administration. Pain 1991; 45:11–15.
345. Roxburgh JC, Markland CG, Ross BA, Kerr WF. Role of cryoanalgesia in the control of pain after thoracotomy. Thorax 1987; 42:292–295.
346. Gough JD, Williams AB, Vaughan RS, Khalil JF. The control of post-thoracotomy pain. A comparative evaluation of thoracic epidural fentanyl infusions and cryo-analgesia. Anaesthesia 1988; 43:780–783.
347. Benedetti F, Amanzio M, Casadio C, Cavallo A, Cianci R, Giobbe R, Mancuso M, Ruffini E, Maggi G. Control of postoperative pain by transcutaneous electrical nerve stimulation after thoracic operations. Ann Thorac Surg 1997; 63:773–776.
348. Sabanathan S, Smith PJB, Pradhan GN, Hashimi H, Eng J, Mearns AJ. Continuous intercostal nerve block for pain relief after thoracotomy. Ann Thorac Surg 1988; 46:425–426.
349. Kaiser AM, Zollinger A, De Lorenzi D, Largiader F, Weder W. Prospective, randomized comparison of extrapleural versus epidural analgesia for posthoracotomy pain. Ann Thorac Surg 1998; 66:367–372.
350. Mann LJ, Young GR, Williams JK, Dent OF, McCaughan BC. Intrapleural bupivacaine in the control of postthoracotomy pain. Ann Thorac Surg 1992; 53:449–454.
351. Ferrante FM, Chan VWS, Arthur GR, Rocco AG. Intrapleural analgesia after thoracotomy. Anesth Analg 1991; 72:105–109.
352. Schneider RF, Villamena PC, Harvey J, Surick BG, Surick IW, Beattie EJ. Lack of efficacy of intrapleural bupivacaine for postoperative analgesia following thoracotomy. Chest 1993; 103:414–416.
353. Gaeta RR, Macario A, Brodsky JB, Brock-Utne JG, Mark JBD. Pain outcomes after thoracotomy: lumbar epidural hydromorphone versus intrapleural bupivacaine. J Cardiothorac Vasc Anesth 1995; 9: 534–537.
354. Richardson J, Sabanathan S, Shah RD, Clarke BJ, Cheema S, Mearns AJ. Pleural bupivacaine placement for optimal postthoracotomy pulmonary function: a prospective, randomized study. J Cardiothorac Vasc Anesth 1998; 12:166–169.
355. Perttunen K, Kalso E, Heinonen J, Salo J. I.V. diclofenac in post-thoracotomy pain. Br J Anaesth 1992; 68:474–480.
356. Rhodes M, Conacher I, Morritt G, Hilton C. Nonsteroidal antiinflammatory drugs for postthoracotomy pain. A prospective controlled trial after lateral thoracotomy. J Thorac Cardiovasc Surg 1992; 103:17–20.
357. Singh H, Bossard RF, White PF, Yeatts RW. Effects of ketorolac versus bupivacaine coadministration during patient-controlled hydromorphone epidural analgesia after thoracotomy procedures. Anesth Analg 1997; 84:564–569.
358. Perttunen K, Nilsson E, Kalso E. I.v. diclofenac and ketorolac for pain after thoracoscopic surgery. Br J Anaesth 1999; 82:221–227.
359. Alexander R, El-Moalem HE, Gan TJ. Comparison of the morphine-sparing effects of diclofenac sodium and ketorolac tromethamine after major orthopedic surgery. J Clin Anesth 2002; 14:187–192.
360. Burgess FW, Anderson M, Colonna D, Sborov MJ, Cavanaugh DG. Ipsilateral shoulder pain following thoracic surgery. Anesthesiology 1993; 78:365–368.
361. Kenny GN. Potential renal, haematological and allergic adverse effects associated with nonsteroidal anti-inflammatory drugs. Drugs 1992; 44(5 suppl):31–36.
362. Deviere J. Do selective cyclo-oxygenase inhibitors eliminate the adverse events associated with nonsteroidal anti-inflammatory drug therapy? Eur J Gastroenterol Hepatol 2002; 14(1 suppl):S29–S33.
363. Thomsen AB, Becker N, Eriksen J. Opioid rotation in chronic non-malignant pain patients. A retrospective study. Acta Anaesthesiol Scand 1999; 43:918–923.
364. McGraw T, Stacey BR. Gabapentin for treatment of neuropathic pain in a 12-year-old girl. Clin J Pain 1998; 14:354–356.
365. Rose MA, Kam PC. Gabapentin: pharmacology and its use in pain management. Anaesthesia 2002; 57: 451–462.
366. Savage C, McQuitty C, Wang D, Zwischenberger JB. Postthoracotomy pain management. Chest Surg Clin N Am 2002; 12:251–263.
367. Venn RM, Grounds RM. Comparison between dexmedetomidine and propofol for sedation in the intensive care unit: patient and clinician perceptions. Br J Anaesth 2001; 87:684–690.
368. Weinbroum AA, Ben-Abraham R. Dextromethorphan and dexmedetomidine: new agents for the control of perioperative pain. Eur J Surg 2001; 167:563–569.
369. Cerfolio RJ, Bass C, Katholi CR. Prospective randomized trial compares suction versus water seal for air leaks. Ann Thorac Surg 2001; 71:1613–1617.
370. Cerfolio RJ, Bass CS, Pask AH, Katholi CR. Predictors and treatment of persistent air leaks. Ann Thorac Surg 2002; 73:1727–1730.
371. Rice TW, Okereke IC, Blackstone EH. Persistent air-leak following pulmonary resection. Chest Surg Clin N Am 2002; 12:529–539.
372. Deiraniya AK. Cardiac herniation following intrapericardial pneumonectomy. Thorax 1974; 29:545–552.
373. Gonzalez RP, Holevar MR. Role of prophylactic antibiotics for tube thoracostomy in chest trauma. Am Surg 1998; 64:617–620.
374. Bardell T, Petsikas D. What keeps postpulmonary resection patients in hospital?. Can Respir J 2003; 10: 86–89.

375. Hull RD, Pineo GF. Prophylaxis of deep venous thrombosis and pulmonary embolism. Current recommendations. Med Clin North Am 1998; 82:477–493.
376. Fennerty MB. Pathophysiology of the upper gastrointestinal tract in the critically ill patient: rationale for the therapeutic benefits of acid suppression. Crit Care Med 2002; 30(6 suppl):S351–S355.
377. MacLaren R, Jarvis CL, Fish DN. Use of enteral nutrition for stress ulcer prophylaxis. Ann Pharmacother 2001; 35:1614–1623.
378. Tryba M, Cook D. Current guidelines on stress ulcer prophylaxis. Drugs 1997; 54:581–596.
379. Hiramoto JS, Terdiman JP, Norton JA. Evidence-based analysis: postoperative gastric bleeding: etiology and prevention. Surg Oncol 2003; 12:9–19.
380. Steinberg KP. Stress-related mucosal disease in the critically ill patient: risk factors and strategies to prevent stress-related bleeding in the intensive care unit. Crit Care Med 2002; 30(suppl):S362–S364.
381. Groeben H. Effects of high thoracic epidural anesthesia and local anesthetics on bronchial hyperreactivity. J Clin Monit Comput 2000; 16:457–463.
382. Brown RH, Greenberg RS, Wagner EM. Efficacy of propofol to prevent bronchoconstriction: effects of preservative. Anesthesiology 2001; 94:851–855.
383. Kaliner M. Mechanisms of glucocorticosteroid action in bronchial asthma. J Allergy Clin Immunol 1985; 76:321–329.
384. Ho AM, Lee A, Karmakar MK, Dion PW, Chung DC, Contardi LH. Heliox vs air–oxygen mixtures for the treatment of patients with acute asthma: a systematic overview. Chest 2003; 123:882–890.
385. Kim EA, Lee KS, Shim YM, Kim J, Kim K, Kim TS, Yang PS. Radiographic and CT findings in complications following pulmonary resection. Radiographics 2002; 22:67–86.
386. Warner DO. Preventing postoperative pulmonary complications: the role of the anesthesiologist. Anesthesiology 2000; 92:1467–1472.
387. Poole PJ, Black PN. Mucolytic agents for chronic bronchitis or chronic obstructive pulmonary disease. Cochrane Database Syst Rev 2000; 2:CD001287.
388. Niederman MS. Appropriate use of antimicrobial agents: challenges and strategies for improvement. Crit Care Med 2003; 31:608–616.
389. Rello J, Catalan M, Diaz E, Bodi M, Alvarez B. Associations between empirical antimicrobial therapy at the hospital and mortality in patients with severe community-acquired pneumonia. Intensive Care Med 2002; 28:1030–1035.
390. Neuhaus T, Ewig S. Defining severe community-acquired pneumonia. Med Clin North Am 2001; 85: 1413–1425.
391. Marik PE. The clinical features of severe community-acquired pneumonia presenting as septic shock. Norasept II Study Investigators. J Crit Care 2000; 15:85–90.
392. Avendano CE, Flume PA, Silvestri GA, King LB, Reed CE. Pulmonary complications after esophagectomy. Ann Thorac Surg 2002; 73:922–926.
393. Stephan F, Boucheseiche S, Hollande J, Flahault A, Cheffi A, Bazelly B, Bonnet F. Pulmonary complications following lung resection: a comprehensive analysis of incidence and possible risk factors. Chest 2000; 118:1263–1270.
394. Ferguson MK, Durkin AE. Preoperative prediction of the risk of pulmonary complications after esophagectomy for cancer. J Thorac Cardiovasc Surg 2002; 123:661–669.
395. Schweizer A, de Perrot M, Hohn L, Spiliopoulos A, Licker M. Massive contralateral pneumonia following thoracotomy for lung resection. J Clin Anesth 1998; 10:678–680.
396. Bhattacharyya N, Kotz T, Shapiro J. Dysphagia and aspiration with unilateral vocal cord immobility: incidence, characterization, and response to surgical treatment. Ann Otol Rhinol Laryngol 2002; 111:672–679.
397. DeLegge MH. Aspiration pneumonia: incidence, mortality, and at-risk populations. J Parenter Enteral Nutr 2002; 26(6 suppl):S19–S24.
398. Heitmiller RF, Jones B. Transient diminished airway protection after transhiatal esophagectomy. Am J Surg 1991; 162:442–446.
399. Marik PE. Aspiration pneumonitis and aspiration pneumonia. N Engl J Med 2001; 344:665–671.
400. Lowrey LD, Anderson M, Calhoun J, Edmonds H, Flint LM. Failure of corticosteroid therapy for experimental acid aspiration. J Surg Res 1982; 32:168–172.
401. Wynne JW, DeMarco FJ, Hood CI. Physiological effects of corticosteroids in foodstuff aspiration. Arch Surg 1981; 116:46–49.
402. Drakulovic MB, Bauer TT, Torres A, et al. Supine body position as a risk factor for nosocomial pneumonia in mechanically ventilated patients: a randomised trial. Lancet 1999; 354:1851–1858.
403. Halm EA, Teirstein AS. Management of community acquired pneumonia. N Engl J Med 2002; 347: 2039–2045.
404. Craven DE, De Rosa FG, Thornton D. Nosocomial pneumonia: emerging concepts in diagnosis, management, and prophylaxis. Curr Opin Crit Care 2002; 8: 421–429.
405. Arozullah AM, Khuri SF, Henderson WG, Daley J. Participants in the National Veterans Affairs Surgical Quality Improvement Program. Development and validation of a multifactorial risk index for predicting postoperative pneumonia after major noncardiac surgery. Ann Intern Med 2001; 135:847–857.
406. Stoutenbeek CP, van Saene HK. Nonantibiotic measures in the prevention of ventilator-associated pneumonia. Semin Respir Infect 1997; 12:294–299.
407. Hoffken G, Niederman MS. Nosocomial pneumonia: the importance of a de-escalating strategy for antibiotic

treatment of pneumonia in the ICU. Chest 2002; 122:2183–2196.
408. Kollef MH. The prevention of ventilator-associated pneumonia. N Engl J Med 1999; 340:627–634.
409. Collard HR, Saint S, Matthay MA. Prevention of ventilator-associated pneumonia: an evidence-based systematic review. Ann Intern Med 2003; 138:494–501.
410. Strange C, Sahn SA. The definitions and epidemiology of pleural space infection. Semin Respir Infect 1999; 14:3–8.
411. Vallieres E. Management of empyema after lung resections (pneumonectomy/lobectomy). Chest Surg Clin N Am 2002; 12:571–585.
412. Schneiter D, Kestenholz P, Dutly A, Korom S, Giger U, Lardinois D, Weder W. Prevention of recurrent empyema after pneumonectomy for chronic infection. Eur J Cardiothorac Surg 2002; 21:644–648.
413. Abbas Ael-S, Deschamps C. Postpneumonectomy empyema. Curr Opin Pulm Med 2002; 8:327–333.
414. Vikram HR, Quagliarello VJ. Diagnosis and management of empyema. Curr Clin Top Infect Dis 2002; 22:196–213.
415. Smolle-Juttner F, Beuster W, Pinter H, Pierer G, Pongratz M, Friehs G. Open-window thoracostomy in pleural empyema. Eur J Cardiothorac Surg 1992; 6: 635–638.
416. Hollaus PH, Wilfing G, Wurnig PN, Pridun NS. Risk factors for the development of postoperative complications after bronchial sleeve resection for malignancy: a univariate and multivariate analysis. Ann Thorac Surg 2003; 75:966–972.
417. Light RW, Rodriguez RM. Management of parapneumonic effusions. Clin Chest Med 1998; 19:373–382.
418. Poe RH, Marin MG, Israel RH, Kallay MC. Utility of pleural fluid analysis in predicting tube thoracostomy/decortication in parapneumonic effusions. Chest 1991; 100:963–967.
419. Cassina PC, Hauser M, Hillejan L, Greschuchna D, Stamatis G. Video-assisted thoracoscopy in the treatment of pleural empyema: stage-based management and outcome. J Thorac Cardiovasc Surg 1999; 117: 234–238.
420. Hamm H, Light RW. Parapneumonic effusion and empyema. Eur Respir J 1997; 10:1150–1156.
421. Balci AE, Eren S, Ulku R, Eren MN. Management of multiloculated empyema thoracis in children: thoracotomy versus fibrinolytic treatment. Eur J Cardiothorac Surg 2002; 22:595–598.
422. Renner H, Gabor S, Pinter H, Maier A, Friehs G, Smolle-Juettner FM. Is aggressive surgery in pleural empyema justified? Eur J Cardiothorac Surg 1998; 14:117–122.
423. Landreneau RJ, Keenan RJ, Hazelrigg SR, Mack MJ, Naunheim KS. Thoracoscopy for empyema and hemothorax. Chest 1996; 109:18–24.
424. Angelillo-Mackinlay T, Lyons GA, Piedras MB, Angelillo-Mackinlay D. Surgical treatment of postpneumonic empyema. World J Surg 1999; 23:1110–1113.
425. Coote N. Surgical versus non-surgical management of pleural empyema. Cochrane Database Syst Rev 2002; (2):CD001956.
426. Deepika K, Kenaan CA, Barrocas AM, Fonseca JJ, Bikazi GB. Negative pressure pulmonary edema after acute upper airway obstruction. J Clin Anesth 1997; 9:403–408.
427. Lathan SR, Silverman ME, Thomas BL, Waters WC IV. Postoperative pulmonary edema. South Med J 1999; 92:313–315.
428. Fitzmaurice BG, Brodsky JB. Airway rupture from double-lumen tubes. J Cardiothorac Vasc Anesth 1999; 13:322–329.
429. Hofmann HS, Rettig G, Radke J, Neef H, Silber RE. Iatrogenic ruptures of the tracheobronchial tree. Eur J Cardiothorac Surg 2002; 21:649–652.
430. Kaloud H, Smolle-Juettner FM, Prause G, List WF. Iatrogenic ruptures of the tracheobronchial tree. Chest 1997; 112:774–778.
431. Chow JL, Coady MA, Varner J, Cannon W, Spain D, Brock-Utne JG. Management of acute complete tracheal transection caused by non-penetrating trauma—report of a case and review of the literature. J Cardiothorac Vasc Anesth. 2004; 18:475–478.
432. Jougon J, Ballester M, Choukroun E, Dubrez J, Reboul G, Velly JF. Conservative treatment for post-intubation tracheobronchial rupture. Ann Thorac Surg 2000; 69:216–220.
433. Gabor S, Renner H, Pinter H, Sankin O, Maier A, Tomaselli F, Smolle Juttner FM. Indications for surgery in tracheobronchial ruptures. Eur J Cardiothorac Surg 2001; 20:399–404.
434. Tcherveniakov A, Tchalakov P, Tcherveniakov P. Traumatic and iatrogenic lesions of the trachea and bronchi. Eur J Cardiothorac Surg 2001; 19:19–24.
435. Meyer M. Iatrogenic tracheobronchial lesions—a report on 13 cases. Thorac Cardiovasc Surg 2001; 49:115–119.
436. Sirbu H, Busch T, Aleksic I, Schreiner W, Oster O, Dalichau H. Bronchopleural fistula in the surgery of non-small cell lung cancer: incidence, risk factors, and management. Ann Thorac Cardiovasc Surg 2001; 7:330–336.
437. Wain JC. Management of late postpneumonectomy empyema and bronchopleural fistula. Chest Surg Clin N Am 1996; 6:529–541.
438. Deschamps C, Bernard A, Nichols FC III, Allen MS, Miller DL, Trastek VF, Jenkins GD, Pairolero PC. Empyema and bronchopleural fistula after pneumonectomy: factors affecting incidence. Ann Thorac Surg 2001; 72:243–247.
439. Cerfolio RJ. The incidence, etiology, and prevention of postresectional bronchopleural fistula. Semin Thorac Cardiovasc Surg 2001; 13:3–7.
440. Puskas JD, Mathisen DJ, Grillo HC, Wain JC, Wright CD, Moncure AC. Treatment strategies for bronchopleural fistula. J Thorac Cardiovasc Surg 1995; 109: 989–995.

441. Hubaut JJ, Baron O, Al Habash O, Despins P, Duveau D, Michaud JL. Closure of the bronchial stump by manual suture and incidence of bronchopleural fistula in a series of 209 pneumonectomies for lung cancer. Eur J Cardiothorac Surg 1999; 16:418–423.
442. Tsai FC, Chen HC, Chen SH, Coessens B, Liu HP, Wu YC, Lin PC. Free deepithelialized anterolateral thigh myocutaneous flaps for chronic intractable empyema with bronchopleural fistula. Ann Thorac Surg 2002; 74:1038–1042.
443. Watanabe S, Watanabe T, Urayama H. Endobronchial occlusion method of bronchopleural fistula with metallic coils and glue. Thorac Cardiovasc Surg 2003; 51:106–108.
444. Muskett A, Burton NA, Karwande SV, Collins MP. Management of refractory empyema with early decortication. Am J Surg 1988; 156:529–532.
445. Deslauriers J, Jacques LF, Gregoire J. Role of Eloesser flap and thoracoplasty in the third millennium. Chest Surg Clin N Am 2002; 12:605–623.
446. Benjaminsson E, Klain M. Intraoperative dual-mode independent lung ventilation of a patient with bronchopleural fistula. Anesth Analg 1981; 60:118–119.
447. Chow JL, Alfille PH. Postpneumonectomy pulmonary edema. In: Bailin MT, ed. The Harvard Department of Anaesthesia Electronic Anesthesia Library (HEAL) on CD-ROM. Philadelphia: Lippincott-Raven, 2001.
448. Ruffini E, Parola A, Papalia E, Filosso PL, Mancuso M, Oliaro A, Actis-Dato G, Maggi G. Frequency and mortality of acute lung injury and acute respiratory distress syndrome after pulmonary resection for bronchogenic carcinoma. Eur J Cardiothorac Surg 2001; 20:30–36.
449. Ware LB, Matthay MA. The acute respiratory distress syndrome. N Engl J Med 2000; 342:1334–1349.
450. Deslauriers J, Aucoin A, Gregoire J. Postpneumonectomy pulmonary edema. Chest Surg Clin N Am 1998; 8:611–631.
451. van der Werff YD, van der Houwen HK, Heijmans PJ, Duurkens VA, Leusink HA, van Heesewijk HP, de Boer A. Postpneumonectomy pulmonary edema. A retrospective analysis of incidence and possible risk factors. Chest 1997; 111:1278–1284.
452. Parquin F, Marchal M, Mehiri S, Herve P, Lescot B. Post-pneumonectomy pulmonary edema: analysis and risk factors. Eur J Cardiothorac Surg 1996; 10: 929–932.
453. Jordan S, Mitchell JA, Quinlan GJ, Goldstraw P, Evans TW. The pathogenesis of lung injury following pulmonary resection. Eur Respir J 2000; 15:790–799.
454. Martin TR, Nakamura M, Matute-Bello G. The role of apoptosis in acute lung injury. Crit Care Med 2003; 31:S185–S188.
455. The Acute Respiratory Distress Syndrome Network. Ventilation with lower tidal volumes as compared with traditional tidal volumes for acute lung injury and the acute respiratory distress syndrome. N Engl J Med 2000; 342:1301–1308.
456. Mathisen DJ, Kuo EY, Hahn C, Moncure AC, Wain JC, Grillo HC, Hurford WE, Wright CD. Inhaled nitric oxide for adult respiratory distress syndrome after pulmonary resection. Ann Thorac Surg 1998; 66:1894–1902.
457. Brambrink AM, Brachlow J, Weiler N, Eberle B, Elich D, Joost T, Koller M, Huth R, Heinrichs W. Successful treatment of a patient with ARDS after pneumonectomy using high-frequency oscillatory ventilation. Intensive Care Med 1999; 25:1173–1176.
458. Meduri GU, Chinn AJ, Leeper KV, et al. Corticosteroid rescue treatment of progressive fibroproliferation in late ARDS: patterns of response and predictors of outcome. Chest 1994; 105:1516–1527.
459. Thompson BT. Glucocorticoids and acute lung injury. Crit Care Med 2003; 31:S253–S257.
460. Symbas PN. Chest drainage tubes. Surg Clin North Am 1989; 69:41–46.
461. Loran DB, Woodside KJ, Cerfolio RJ, Zwischenberger JB. Predictors of alveolar air leaks. Chest Surg Clin N Am 2002; 12:477–488.
462. Toloza EM, Harpole DH Jr. Intraoperative techniques to prevent air leaks. Chest Surg Clin N Am 2002; 12:489–505.
463. Yu PY, Lee LW. Pulmonary artery pressures with tension pneumothorax. Can J Anaesth 1990; 37:584–586.
464. Brandenhoff P, Hoier-Madsen K, Struve-Christensen E. Pneumopericardium after pneumonectomy and lobectomy. Thorax 1986; 41:55–57.
465. Barton ED. Tension pneumothorax. Curr Opin Pulm Med 1999; 5:269–274.
466. Beards SC, Lipman J. Decreased cardiac index as an indicator of tension pneumothorax in the ventilated patient. Anaesthesia 1994; 49:137–1341.
467. Watts BL, Howell MA. Tension pneumothorax: a difficult diagnosis. Emerg Med J 2001; 18:319–320.
468. Debaene B, Plaud B, Dilly MP, Donati F. Residual paralysis in the PACU after a single intubating In: dose of nondepolarizing muscle relaxant with an intermediate duration of action. Anesthesiology 2003; 98: 1042–1048.
469. Kim KS, Lew SH, Cho HY, Cheong MA. Residual paralysis induced by either vecuronium or rocuronium after reversal with pyridostigmine. Anesth Analg 2002; 95:1656–1660.
470. Bevan DR. Neuromuscular blockade. Inadvertent extubation of the partially paralyzed patient. Anesthesiol Clin N Am 2001; 19:913–922.
471. Murray MJ, Cowen J, DeBlock H, Erstad B, Gray AW Jr, Tescher AN, McGee WT, Prielipp RC, Susla G, Jacobi J, Nasraway SA Jr, Lumb PD. Clinical practice guidelines for sustained neuromuscular blockade in the adult critically ill patient. Crit Care Med 2002; 30:142–156.
472. Zwienenberg M, Muizelaar JP. Acute quadriplegia myopathy in the intensive care unit: time to look at a mechanistic approach. Crit Care Med 2000; 28: 260–261.

473. Larsson L, Li X, Edstrom L, Eriksson LI, Zackrisson H, Argentini C, Schiaffino S. Acute quadriplegia and loss of muscle myosin in patients treated with nondepolarizing neuromuscular blocking agents and corticosteroids: mechanisms at the cellular and molecular levels. Crit Care Med 2000; 28:34–45.
474. Hund E. Myopathy in critically ill patients. Crit Care Med 1999; 27:2544–2547.
475. Rena O, Papalia E, Oliaro A, Casadio C, Ruffini E, Filosso PL, Sacerdote C, Maggi G. Supraventricular arrhythmias after resection surgery of the lung. Eur J Cardiothorac Surg 2001; 20:688–693.
476. Rho RW, Bridges CR, Kocovic D. Management of postoperative arrhythmias. Semin Thorac Cardiovasc Surg 2000; 12:349–361.
477. Christians KK, Wu B, Quebbeman EJ, Brasel KJ. Postoperative atrial fibrillation in noncardiothoracic surgical patients. Am J Surg 2001; 182:713–715.
478. Hollenberg SM, Dellinger RP. Noncardiac surgery: postoperative arrhythmias. Crit Care Med 2000; 28(10 suppl):145–150.
479. Chung MK. Cardiac surgery: postoperative arrhythmias. Crit Care Med 2000; 28(suppl):136–144.
480. Amar D, Zhang H, Leung DH, Roistacher N, Kadish AH. Older age is the strongest predictor of postoperative atrial fibrillation. Anesthesiology 2002; 96: 352–356.
481. Solomon AJ. Treatment of postoperative atrial fibrillation: a nonsurgical perspective. Semin Thorac Cardiovasc Surg 1999; 11:320–324.
482. Ferguson JD, DiMarco JP. Contemporary management of paroxysmal supraventricular tachycardia. Circulation 2003; 107:1096–1099.
483. Basta M, Klein GJ, Yee R, Krahn A, Lee J. Current role of pharmacologic therapy for patients with paroxysmal supraventricular tachycardia. Cardiol Clin 1997; 15:587–597.
484. Backlund M, Laasonen L, Lepantalo M, Metsarinne K, Tikkanen I, Lindgren L. Effect of oxygen on pulmonary hemodynamics and incidence of atrial fibrillation after noncardiac thoracotomy. J Cardiothorac Vasc Anesth 1998; 12:422–428.
485. Kannel WB, Wolf PA, Benjamin EJ, Levy D. Prevalence, incidence, prognosis, and predisposing conditions for atrial fibrillation: population-based estimates. Am J Cardiol 1998; 82(8A):2N–9N.
486. Maisel WH, Rawn JD, Stevenson WG. Atrial fibrillation after cardiac surgery. Ann Intern Med 2001; 135:1061–1073.
487. Crystal E, Connolly SJ, Sleik K, Ginger TJ, Yusuf S. Interventions on prevention of postoperative atrial fibrillation in patients undergoing heart surgery: a meta-analysis. Circulation 2002; 106:75–80.
488. Lanza LA, Visbal AI, DeValeria PA, Zinsmeister AR, Diehl NN, Trastek VF. Low-dose oral amiodarone prophylaxis reduces atrial fibrillation after pulmonary resection. Ann Thorac Surg 2003; 75:223–230.
489. Jakobsen CJ, Bille S, Ahlburg P, Rybro L, Hjortholm K, Andresen EB. Perioperative metoprolol reduces the frequency of atrial fibrillation after thoracotomy for lung resection. J Cardiothorac Vasc Anesth 1997; 11:746–751.
490. Oka T, Ozawa Y, Ohkubo Y. Thoracic epidural bupivacaine attenuates supraventricular tachyarrhythmias after pulmonary resection. Anesth Analg 2001; 93: 253–259.
491. Jideus L, Joachimsson PO, Stridsberg M, Ericson M, Tyden H, Nilsson L, Blomstrom P, Blomstrom-Lundqvist C. Thoracic epidural anesthesia does not influence the occurrence of postoperative sustained atrial fibrillation. Ann Thorac Surg 2001; 72:65–71.
492. Dell'Orfano JT, Naccarelli GV. Update on external cardioversion and defibrillation. Curr Opin Cardiol 2001; 16:54–57.
493. Fishman AP. Clinical classification of pulmonary hypertension. Clin Chest Med 2001; 22:385–391.
494. Riedel B. The pathophysiology and management of perioperative pulmonary hypertension with specific emphasis on the period following cardiac surgery. Int Anesthesiol Clin 1999; 37:55–79.
495. Meyrick B, Reid L. Pulmonary hypertension. Anatomic and physiologic correlates. Clin Chest Med 1983; 4:199–217.
496. Gomez A, Bialostozky D, Zajarias A, Santos E, Palomar A, Martinez ML, Sandoval J. Right ventricular ischemia in patients with primary pulmonary hypertension. J Am Coll Cardiol 2001; 38:1137–1142.
497. Gavazzi A, Ghio S, Scelsi L, Campana C, Klersy C, Serio A, Raineri C, Tavazzi L. Response of the right ventricle to acute pulmonary vasodilation predicts the outcome in patients with advanced heart failure and pulmonary hypertension. Am Heart J 2003; 145: 310–316.
498. Reed CE, Spinale FG, Crawford FA Jr. Effect of pulmonary resection on right ventricular function. Ann Thorac Surg 1992; 53:578–582.
499. Raymond RJ, Hinderliter AL, Willis PW, Ralph D, Caldwell EJ, Williams W, Ettinger NA, Hill NS, Summer WR, de Boisblanc B, Schwartz T, Koch G, Clayton LM, Jobsis MM, Crow JW, Long W. Echocardiographic predictors of adverse outcomes in primary pulmonary hypertension. J Am Coll Cardiol 2002; 39:1214–1219.
500. Zales VR, Pahl E, Backer CL, Crawford S, Mavroudis C, Benson DW Jr. Pharmacologic reduction of pretransplantation pulmonary vascular resistance predicts outcome after pediatric heart transplantation. J Heart Lung Transplant 1993; 12:965–972.
501. Runo JR, Loyd JE. Primary pulmonary hypertension. Lancet 2003; 361:1533–1544.
502. Givertz MM, Hare JM, Loh E, Gauthier DF, Colucci WS. Effect of bolus milrinone on hemodynamic variables and pulmonary vascular resistance in patients with severe left ventricular dysfunction: a rapid test

for reversibility of pulmonary hypertension. J Am Coll Cardiol 1996; 28:1775–1780.
503. Maxey TS, Smith CD, Kern JA, Tribble CG, Jones DR, Kron IL, Crosby IK. Beneficial effects of inhaled nitric oxide in adult cardiac surgical patients. Ann Thorac Surg 2002; 73:529–532.
504. Lowson SM, Doctor A, Walsh BK, Doorley PA. Inhaled prostacyclin for the treatment of pulmonary hypertension after cardiac surgery. Crit Care Med 2002; 30:2762–2764.
505. Hache M, Denault AY, Belisle S, Couture P, Babin D, Tetrault F, Guimond JG. Inhaled prostacyclin (PGI2) is an effective addition to the treatment of pulmonary hypertension and hypoxia in the operating room and intensive care unit. Can J Anaesth 2001; 48:924–929.
506. Atz AM, Adatia I, Wessel DL. Rebound pulmonary hypertension after inhalation of nitric oxide. Ann Thorac Surg 1996; 62:1759–1764.
507. Pearl JM, Nelson DP, Raake JL, Manning PB, Schwartz SM, Koons L, Shanley TP, Wong HR, Duffy JY. Inhaled nitric oxide increases endothelin-1 levels: a potential cause of rebound pulmonary hypertension. Crit Care Med 2002; 30:89–93.
508. Lepore JJ, Maroo A, Pereira NL, Ginns LC, Dec GW, Zapol WM, Bloch KD, Semigran MJ. Effect of sildenafil on the acute pulmonary vasodilator response to inhaled nitric oxide in adults with primary pulmonary hypertension. Am J Cardiol 2002; 90:677–680.
509. Stiebellehner L, Petkov V, Vonbank K, Funk G, Schenk P, Ziesche R, Block LH. Long-term treatment with oral sildenafil in addition to continuous IV epoprostenol in patients with pulmonary arterial hypertension. Chest 2003; 123:1293–1295.
510. Asamura H. Early complications. Cardiac complications. Chest Surg Clin N Am 1999; 9:527–541.
511. Foroulis C, Kotoulas C, Konstantinou M, Lioulias A. The use of pedicled pleural flaps for the repair of pericardial defects, resulting after intrapericardial pneumonectomy. Eur J Cardiothorac Surg 2002; 21:92–93.
512. Collet e Silva FS, Jose Neto F, Figueredo AM, Fontes B, Poggetti RS, Birolini D. Cardiac herniation mimics cardiac tamponade in blunt trauma. Must early resuscitative thoracotomy be done?. Int Surg 2001; 86:72–75.
513. Carrillo EH, Heniford BT, Dykes JR, McKenzie ED, Polk HC Jr, Richardson JD. Cardiac herniation producing tamponade: the critical role of early diagnosis. J Trauma 1997; 43:19–23.
514. Baaijens PF, Hasenbos MA, Lacquet LK, Dekhuijzen PN. Cardiac herniation after pneumonectomy. Acta Anaesthesiol Scand 1992; 36:842–845.
515. Tsang TS, Freeman WK, Miller FA Jr, Seward JB. Teardrop sign: echocardiographic features in cardiac herniation. J Am Soc Echocardiogr 1998; 11:74–76.
516. Self RJ, Vaughan RS. Acute cardiac herniation after radical pleuropneumonectomy. Anaesthesia 1999; 54: 564–566.
517. Schamaun M. Postoperative pulmonary torsion: report of a case and survey of the literature including spontaneous and posttraumatic torsion. Thorac Cardiovasc Surg 1994; 42:116–121.
518. Cable DG, Deschamps C, Allen MS, Miller DL, Nichols FC, Trastek VF, Pairolero PC. Lobar torsion after pulmonary resection: presentation and outcome. J Thorac Cardiovasc Surg 2001; 122:1091–1093.
519. Nonami Y, Ishikawa T, Ogoshi S. Lobar torsion following pulmonary lobectomy. A case report. J Cardiovasc Surg (Torino) 1998; 39:691–693.
520. Wong PS, Goldstraw P. Pulmonary torsion: a questionnaire survey and a survey of the literature. Ann Thorac Surg 1992; 54:286–288.
521. Garzon AA, Gourin A. Surgical management of massive hemoptysis. A ten-year experience. Ann Surg 1978; 187:267–271.
522. Ong TH, Eng P. Massive hemoptysis requiring intensive care. Intensive Care Med 2003; 29:317–320.
523. Garzon AA, Cerruti MM, Golding ME. Exsanguinating hemoptysis. J Thorac Cardiovasc Surg 1982; 84: 829–833.
524. Jougon J, Ballester M, Delcambre F, Mac Bride T, Valat P, Gomez F, Laurent F, Velly JF. Massive hemoptysis: what place for medical and surgical treatment?. Eur J Cardiothorac Surg 2002; 22:345–351.
525. Lee TW, Wan S, Choy DK, Chan M, Arifi A, Yim AP. Management of massive hemoptysis: a single institution experience. Ann Thorac Cardiovasc Surg 2000; 6:232–235.
526. Robinson CL. The management of chylothorax. Ann Thorac Surg 1985; 39:90–95.
527. Johnstone DW. Postoperative chylothorax. Chest Surg Clin N Am 2002; 12:597–603.
528. Markham KM, Glover JL, Welsh RJ, Lucas RJ, Bendick PJ. Octreotide in the treatment of thoracic duct injuries. Am Surg 2000; 66:1165–1167.
529. Demos NJ, Kozel J, Scerbo JE. Somatostatin in the treatment of chylothorax. Chest 2001; 119:964–966.
530. Wemyss-Holden SA, Launois B, Maddern GJ. Management of thoracic duct injuries after oesophagectomy. Br J Surg 2001; 88:1442–1448.
531. Shimizu K, Yoshida J, Nishimura M, Takamochi K, Nakahara R, Nagai K. Treatment strategy for chylothorax after pulmonary resection and lymph node dissection for lung cancer. J Thorac Cardiovasc Surg 2002; 124:499–502.
532. Le Pimpec-Barthes F, D'Attellis N, Dujon A, Legman P, Riquet M. Chylothorax complicating pulmonary resection. Ann Thorac Surg 2002; 73:1714–1729.
533. Wurnig PN, Hollaus PH, Ohtsuka T, Flege JB, Wolf RK. Thoracoscopic direct clipping of the thoracic duct for chylopericardium and chylothorax. Ann Thorac Surg 2000; 70:1662–1665.
534. Bonavina L, Saino G, Bona D, Abraham M, Peracchia A. Thoracoscopic management of chylothorax complicating

esophagectomy. J Laparoendosc Adv Surg Tech A 2001; 11:367–369.

535. Sieczka EM, Harvey JC. Early thoracic duct ligation for postoperative chylothorax. J Surg Oncol 1996; 61:56–60.
536. Swanson SJ, Batirel HF, Bueno R, Jaklitsch MT, Lukanich JM, Allred E, Mentzer SJ, Sugarbaker DJ. Transthoracic esophagectomy with radical mediastinal and abdominal lymph node dissection and cervical esophagogastrostomy for esophageal carcinoma. Ann Thorac Surg 2001; 72:1918–1924.
537. Hemmerling TM, Schmidt J, Jacobi KE, Klein P. Intraoperative monitoring of the recurrent laryngeal nerve during single-lung ventilation in esophagectomy. Anesth Analg 2001; 92:662–664.
538. de Leeuw M, Williams JM, Freedom RM, Williams WG, Shemie SD, McCrindle BW. Impact of diaphragmatic paralysis after cardiothoracic surgery in children. J Thorac Cardiovasc Surg 1999; 118:510–517.
539. Commare MC, Kurstjens SP, Barois A. Diaphragmatic paralysis in children: a review of 11 cases. Pediatr Pulmonol 1994; 18:187–193.
540. Guy TS, Montany PF. Thoracoscopic diaphragmatic plication. Surg Laparosc Endosc 1998; 8:319–321.
541. Chervin RD, Guilleminault C. Diaphragm pacing for respiratory insufficiency. J Clin Neurophysiol 1997; 14:369–377.
542. Lai DT, Paterson HS. Mini-thoracotomy for diaphragmatic plication with thoracoscopic assistance. Ann Thorac Surg 1999; 68:2364–2365.
543. Bhuiyan MS, Mallick A, Parsloe M. Post-thoracotomy paraplegia coincident with epidural anaesthesia. Anaesthesia 1998; 53:583–586.
544. Chan LL, Kumar AJ, Leeds NE, Forman AD. Post-epidural analgesia spinal cord infarction: MRI correlation. Acta Neurol Scand 2002; 105:344–348.
545. Gravereaux EC, Faries PL, Burks JA, Latessa V, Spielvogel D, Hollier LH, Marin ML. Risk of spinal cord ischemia after endograft repair of thoracic aortic aneurysms. J Vasc Surg 2001; 34:997–1003.
546. Griepp RB, Ergin MA, Galla JD, Lansman S, Khan N, Quintana C, McCollough J, Bodian C. Looking for the artery of Adamkiewicz: a quest to minimize paraplegia after operations for aneurysms of the descending thoracic and thoracoabdominal aorta. J Thorac Cardiovasc Surg 1996; 112: 1202–1213.
547. Medalion B, Bder O, Cohen AJ, Hauptman E, Schachner A. Delayed postoperative paraplegia complicating repair of type A dissection. Ann Thorac Surg 2001; 72:1389–1391.
548. Vander Salm TJ, Cereda JM, Cutler BS. Brachial plexus injury following median sternotomy. J Thorac Cardiovasc Surg 1980; 80:447–452.
549. Morin JE, Long R, Elleker MG, Eisen AA, Wynands E, Ralphs-Thibodeau S. Upper extremity neuropathies following median sternotomy. Ann Thorac Surg 1982; 34:181–185.
550. Stoelting RK. Brachial plexus injury after median sternotomy: an unexpected liability for anesthesiologists. J Cardiothorac Vasc Anesth 1994; 8:2–4.
551. Muller JM, Erasmi H, Stelzner M, Zieren U, Pichlmaier H. Surgical therapy of oesophageal carcinoma. Br J Surg 1990; 77:845–857.
552. Urschel JD. Esophagogastrostomy anastomotic leaks complicating esophagectomy: a review. Am J Surg 1995; 169:634–640.
553. Dewar L, Gelfand G, Finley RJ, Evans K, Inculet R, Nelems B. Factors affecting cervical anastomotic leak and stricture formation following esophagogastrectomy and gastric tube interposition. Am J Surg 1992; 163:484–489.
554. Giuli R, Gignoux M. Treatment of carcinoma of the esophagus: retrospective study of 2,400 patients. Ann Surg 1980; 192:44–52.

22

Anesthetic Management of Cardiac Tumors

DILIP THAKAR

Division of Anesthesia and Critical Care, The University of Texas M.D. Anderson Cancer Center, Houston, Texas, U.S.A.

ASHISH SINHA

Department of Anesthesiology, Louisiana State University Health Science Center, New Orleans, Louisiana, U.S.A.

Tumors of the heart are rare and primary tumors of the heart are far less common than metastatic tumors of the heart. The diagnosis of intracardiac tumors is a challenge and this is especially difficult in the case of myxoma, which causes a variety of nonspecific signs and symptoms. It is important for the anesthesiologist to understand the pathophysiology of cardiac tumor because many are resectable and some require diagnostic procedures that rely on anesthetic support. Diagnostic modalities such as magnetic resonance imaging (MRI), computed tomography (CT), two-dimensional echocardiography, transesophageal echocardiography (TEE), and three-dimensional echocardiography promote early and accurate diagnoses and help to define the anatomical relationship between the tumor and intracardiac structures. Nevertheless, a high index of suspicion remains the most important instrument in the diagnosis of cardiac tumors (1–3).

Primary cardiac tumors can arise from any cardiac structure. Although rare, myxoma is one of the most common benign tumors. Other rare benign tumors; include; lipoma, papillary fibroelastoma, rhabdomyoma, fibroma, hemangioma, teratoma, mesothelioma of the atrioventricular (AV) node, granular cell tumor, neurofibroma, lymphangioma, and hamartoma. The common malignant tumors of the heart include angiosarcoma of the atrial wall, rhabdomyosarcoma, and mesothelioma involving the AV node. Most metastatic tumors in the heart arise from lung cancer, breast cancer, lymphoma, and melanoma (4,5). Extension of a tumor via the inferior vena cava, superior vena cava, and pulmonary veins into the cardiac chambers is not unusual. Renal cell carcinoma, Wilms' tumor, hepatoblastoma, and uterine leiomyomatosis can extend to the right side of the heart via the inferior vena cava (6). Melanoma has a tendency to metastasize to the pericardium and heart.

I. CLINICAL PRESENTATION

Cardiac tumors can produce a variety of signs and symptoms depending upon the tumor type, location and size, and the release of chemical substances by the tumor (Table 1). Cardiac tumors in asymptomatic patients may be diagnosed by CT, MRI, or echocardiography as part of a routine examination. Other patients may present with signs and symptoms of cardiac or extracardiac tumor manifestation. Occasionally,

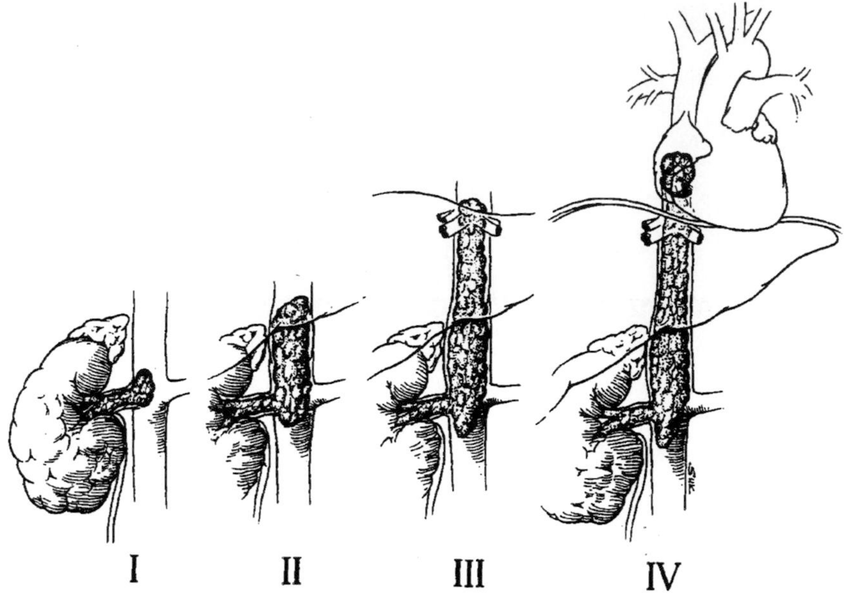

Figure 1 Classification system depicting the level of inferior vena cava involvement by a tumor thrombus. *Source*: From Ref. 32

cardiac tumors, especially angiosarcomas, can produce hemorrhagic pericardial effusion or tamponade. The mechanical effect of a tumor on the intracardiac blood flow varies with changes in body position, particularly if the tumor is mobile and pedunculated.

Myocardial tumors can cause conduction disturbances, arrhythmias, congestive heart failure, or myocardial rupture. A left atrial tumor may mimic the manifestations of mitral valve stenosis, mitral regurgitation, or systemic embolization. Right atrial tumors frequently produce the signs and symptoms of right heart failure, pulmonary embolism, and right-to-left shunting due to pulmonary hypertension. Occasionally, a large right-heart tumor can cause mechanical dysfunction of the tricuspid or pulmonic valve (Figs. 1 and 4). Patients with tumors of the left ventricle, which are predominantly intracavitary in location, may present with symptoms due to the obstruction of the left ventriclar outflow tract.

II. SPECIFIC CARDIAC TUMORS

A. Myxomas

Myxomas are the most common benign primary tumors of the heart. Microscopically, myxomas resemble an organized mural thrombus, and their origin is suspected to be subendocardial in nature. Most sporadic myxomas are single tumors that originate in the left atrium (Fig. 2), in the region of the fossa ovalis, and project into the left atrium. Familial myxomas may produce multiple tumors that can arise from different sites in the cardiac chambers. The gelatinous consistency of these tumors makes fragmentation and embolization common. A familial type, frequently called "Carneys syndrome," consists of myxoma of the skin and breast, spotty pigmentation of the skin, and endocrine over activity i.e., (pituitary adenoma, adrenocortical disease, and/or testicular tumors). Occasionally, patients present with peripheral nerve tumors (schwannomas) (9–12).

Familial myxoma appears to have autosomal dominant transmission. The etiology of myxoma appears to be excessive proliferation of certain mesenchymal cells and excessive glucosaminoglycan production. Routine

Table 1 Clinical Signs and Symptoms of Cardiac Tumors

Symptoms	Signs
Dyspnea	Systolic murmur
Paroxysmal dyspnea	Diastolic murmur
Fever	Pulmonary hypertension
Weight loss	Right-heart failure
Dizziness	Left-heart failure
Syncope	Anemia
Sudden death	Tumor plop (third heart sound)
Chest pain	Arrhythmia
Cachexia	Clubbing
Malaise	Raynaud's sign
Arthralgia	Systemic embolic necrosis
Rash	Pulmonary emboli
Hemoptysis	Stroke

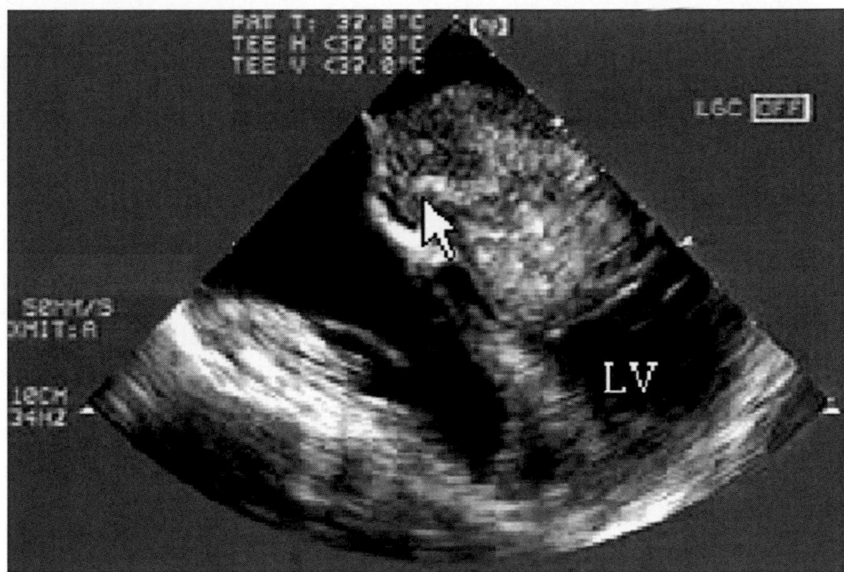

Figure 2 TEE (midesophageal four chamber view) image of an atrial myxoma originating from the left side of the interatrial septum (apex of arrow). The myxoma prolapses into the left ventricle (LV) during systole to produce inflow obstruction. The base of the arrow is located on the anterior leaflet of the mitral valve. *Abbreviations*: LV, left ventricle.

screening of first-degree relatives of such patients may improve the early diagnosis of this tumor, particularly if the patient is young and presents with multiple tumors, except those which are located in the left atrium.

The clinical presentation of cardiac myxoma varies from patient to patient and depends on the tumor size, location, consistency, and familial nature. Patients may present with the signs and symptoms of pulmonary or systemic embolization or mechanical effects on the cardiac chambers and valves. Endocrine manifestations may cause hypertension and acromegaly, skin involvement could result in pigmentation, and nerve compression may lead to sciatica.

Anesthetic considerations in the treatment of patient with myxoma depend on the tumor's intracardiac location and on the presence or absence of pulmonary hypertension, intracardiac shunting, and any mechanical effect of the tumor on the intracardiac blood flow caused by a change in position and preload. A pedunculated left atrial tumor can obstruct blood flow through the mitral valve when there is a sudden decrease in preload caused by a change in body position. Preoperative assessment should include a determination of the presence or absence of the systemic manifestations of adrenal hyperplasia, pituitary adenoma, and nerve compression. Patients with acromegaly may have soft-tissue overgrowth in the airway, which may lead to obstructive sleep apnea, difficult intubation, myopathy, hyperlipidemia, cardiomyopathies, and glucose intolerance. Excessive cortisol secretion (Cushing's syndrome) may cause systemic hypertension, hyperglycemia, skeletal muscle weakness, obesity, and an increased risk of infections.

B. Less Common Benign Tumors

Papillary fibroelastoma is a villous tumor composed of nonencapsulated connective tissue covered by a single layer of endothelium. These lesions are 3–4 cm in diameter with a frond-like appearance that resembles a sea anemone. They are most commonly located on the ventricular surface of the aortic valve and the atrial surface of the mitral valve. Most of the patients are clinically asymptomatic, but rarely, papillary fibroelastoma can cause embolization, mechanical valvular dysfunction, and obstruction of coronary blood flow, if it arises from the aortic valve. Papillary fibroelastoma should be differentiated from Lambl's excrescences and nodules of Arantius. See Table 2 for a summary of normal cardiac structures that can mimic cardiac tumors on diagnostic imaging.

Rhabdomyomas, which occur in infants and children, are multiple tumors that involve the myocardium. The common clinical presentation is right or left ventricular failure and intracavitary obstruction. Approximately 80% of patients may have associated tuberous sclerosis, which is characterized by adenoma sebaceum, mental retardation, hamartomas, and epilepsy (13–15).

Table 2 Normal Cardiac Structures that Mimic Cardiac Tumors on Diagnostic Imaging

(1) Epicardial adipose tissue
(2) Left atrial appendage
(3) Cumedin ridge
(4) Nodules of Arantius
(5) Lambl's excrescences
(6) Mitral valve myxomatous degeneration
(7) Chordal redundancy
(8) Hypertrophic papillary muscle
(9) Moderator band
(10) Central venous catheter
(11) Trabeculation
(12) Lipomatous hypertrophy of interatrial septum
(13) Crista terminalis
(14) Atrial septal aneurysm
(15) Coronary sinus dilatation

Fibromas are nonencapsulated connective tissue tumors that occur predominantly in children younger than 10 years and these range in size from 3 to 10 cm. Occasionally, calcifications and islands of bone formation may be seen on chest radiographs of patients with fibromas. Clinical manifestations may include right or left ventricular failure, conduction abnormalities, and mechanical obstruction of intracardiac flow.

Lipoma and lipomatous hypertrophy occur at any age. Lipomas are usually well encapsulated, 1–15 cm in diameter and can be sessile or polypoid. They are usually located in subendocardial, subpericardial, and intramuscular tissues. The clinical manifestation may vary depending on the location of the tumor. In contrast to lipomas, lipomatous hypertrophy is nonencapsulated, involves the interatrial septum, is 1–7 cm in diameter, and is more common in morbidily obese, elderly female patients. In most cases, the lipomatous hypertrophy protrudes toward the right atrium (14).

Mesothelioma is a rare and cystic, cardiac tumor. It usually involves the AV node and causes complete heart blockade, cardiac tamponade, and ventricular fibrillation.

C. Malignant Cardiac Tumors

Angiosarcoma is one of the most common malignant primary cardiac tumors. Other, more rare, forms are rhabdomyosarcoma, fibrosarcoma, malignant fibrohistiocytoma, and lymphoma. Angiosarcomas are rapidly growing tumors that typically arise from the right atrium and may be sessile or polypoid. Patients may present with a bloody pericardial effusion or a tamponade. Many patients present with progressive chest pain, right-heart failure, conduction abnormalities, arrhythmias, obstruction of the superior and inferior vena cava, swelling of the face and extremities, and sudden death. Preoperative chemotherapy and radiation therapy can reduce the size and the mechanical effects of the tumor (15–18).

Primary sarcoma of the pulmonary artery (Fig. 3) is an extremely rare tumor with multiple origins: angiosarcomas derived from the endothelium, leiomyosarcomas derived from arterial smoot muscle, and undifferentiated or "myointimal sarcomas" derived from myointimal cells. The prognosis for patients with pulmonary artery sarcoma is poor despite attempted multimodal therapy. This is largely related to delay and difficulty in diagnosis that results from the paucity of symptoms and physical findings. Symptoms are typically nonspecific (commonly dyspnea, tachypnea, chest pain, cough, and hemoptysis) and typically originate from tumor embolism to the lungs or from obstruction of the right ventricular outflow tract. In fact, the vast majority of patients are admitted to the hospital or undergo surgery for presumed thromboembolism.

Favorable outcome is dependent upon early diagnosis and aggressive management. This factor belies the importance of considering pulmonary artery sarcoma in the differential diagnosis for a patient presenting with a pulmonary arterial mass or pulmonary hypertension. Suspicion should be especially heightened in patients who present with atypical features of pulmonary embolism, such as the lack of predisposing factors for thromboembolism, persistence or recurrence of symptoms despite adequate anticoagulant or thrombolytic therapy, and atypical radiological features (e.g. unilateral hilar enlargement or unilateral pulmonary perfusion).

III. EXTRACARDIAC TUMORS WITH CARDIAC INVOLVEMENT

A. Renal Cell Carcinoma

It is estimated that 3–10% of renal cell carcinomas involve the inferior vena cava. Other tumors that extend to the right side of the heart via the inferior vena cava are hepatocellular carcinoma, Wilms' tumor, and uterine leiomyomatosis. The 5-year survival rate after complete resection for patients with renal cell tumors ranges from 30% to 60%. The most common clinical presentation is painless hematuria, an abdominal mass, and swelling of the lower extremities with prominent collateral veins. The levels of tumor thrombus are defined by four categories, based on the extent of surgical dissection required to remove the thrombus and these categories are similar to those described in Figure 1.

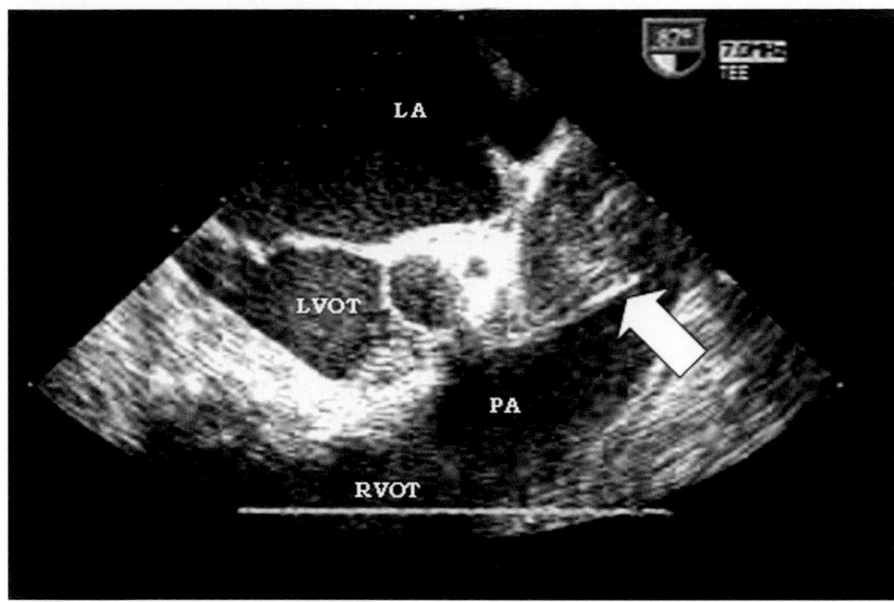

Figure 3 TEE (midesophageal RVOT long axis plane) revealed near occlusion of the pulmonary artery by an echogenic mass within the proximal pulmonary trunk, but did not involve the pulmonary value or RV outflow tract. The white arrow points to a pedunculated portion, with increased echogenicity, of the mass that was mobile with cardiac contraction. *Abbreviations*: LA, left atrium; LVOT, left ventricular outflow tract; RVOT, right ventricular outflow tract; PA, pulmonary artery.

B. Carcinoid Tumors

Metastatic carcinoid tumor of the heart is very rare because of the early diagnosis and treatment of the primary gastrointestinal tumor. The tumor secrets serotonin, kallidin (bradykinin), histamine, and tachykinins (neuropeptide K, neurokinin A, and substance P). The metabolism of these chemicals occurs in the liver.

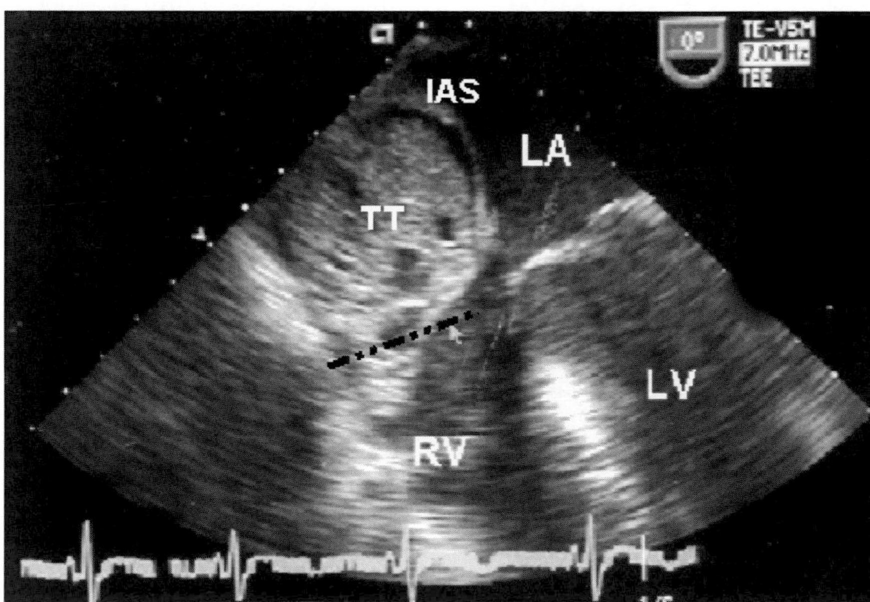

Figure 4 Transesophageal image (mid-esophageal; four chamber view) showing a large renal cell tumor thrombus extending through the right atrium and tricuspid valve into the right ventricle. The level of the tricuspid value is depicted by a broken line. *Abbreviations*: LA, left atrium; IAS, inter-atrial septum; LV, left ventricle; RV, right ventricle.

Table 3 Differentiation Among Tumor, Thrombus, and Vegetation by Echocardiography

Characteristics	Tumors	Vegetation	Thrombus
Location	Any site	Usually valve CVC line	Left atrial appendage Left ventricular apex
Echo appearence	Variable	Variable Found on the upstream side of valve Moves independent of valve	Laminated, if organized
Other associated abnormality	Myxoma syndrome Carcinoid syndrome	Fever Positive blood culture Evidence of endocarditis	Abnormal rhythm Mitral stenosis Ventricular wall motion abnormality

Once the tumor has metastasized to the liver, portal circulation is bypassed and the symptoms of carcinoid syndrome can occur. Tricuspid regurgitation and pulmonary stenosis are the most common symptoms of valvular lesions. Involvement of the mitral or aortic valve is rare but can occur with a right-to-left shunt or in the presence of a bronchial carcinoid tumor. The infiltrative fibrotic changes in the valves are probably the result of a chemical released by the tumor (Table 3).

Endocardial and myocardial involvement can cause a decrease in right-ventricular compliance and elevated right-sided pressure. The treatment of tricuspid valvular involvement is surgical replacement of the valve, and valvectomy or valvotomy for the pulmonary valve.

IV. DIAGNOSTIC METHODS

A clinical history and physical examination are as important as echocardiography, CT, MRI, and angiography in the diagnosis of cardiac tumors. Systolic and diastolic murmurs, neck vein distention, and edema of the extremities may or may not be present. Chest radiography may show areas of calcification and cardiomegaly, and electrocardiography may show conduction abnormalities or ischemic changes. Transesophageal echocardiography is more sensitive and specific than transthoracic echocardiography (TTE) and provides better visualization of cardiac chambers and a better understanding of the tumor location, size, and attachment and the dynamic changes occurring in the tumor with each cardiac cycle. CT and MRI of the heart help to discriminate tumor from normal tissue and determine the extent of the tumor. Computed tomography also helps to determine the degree of myocardial invasion and the involvement of pericardial and extracardiac structures. MRI may be considered when it is necessary to know the size, shape, and surface characteristics of the tumor. MRI examination can also provide additional information regarding tissue composition (22–27).

Table 4 Common Tumors of the Heart in Adults

Benign	Maligant	Metastatic
Myxoma	Angiosarcoma	Lung, liver, lymphoma, leukemia
Lipoma	Rhabdomyosarcoma	Breast
Fibroelastoma	Mesothelioma	Melanoma
Hemangioma	Lymphoma	Stomach and colon

V. ANESTHETIC MANAGEMENT OF CARDIAC TUMORS

Surgical resection is the treatment of choice for most benign cardiac tumors, whereas lymphosarcomas of the heart frequently respond to chemotherapy and radiation therapy. Orthotopic heart transplants have been performed in patients with primary cardiac tumors. Removal of most intramural and intracavitary tumors requires a cardiopulmonary bypass machine. Venous cannulation is usually performed via the femoral or azygous vein or the superior and inferior vena cava to avoid manipulation of a right atrial tumor (Table 4). Central venous access for fluid resuscitation is selected very carefully. Anesthesiologists should be familiar with the anatomic location of the tumor and the risk of tumor dislodgement during central venous access. Changes in preload, afterload, contractility, mechanical ventilation, and patient position can precipitate intracardiac shunting and mechanical obstruction of intracardiac blood flow. Pulmonary embolism and systemic embolism have been attributed to tumor manipulation. Patients with carcinoid tumors of the heart may be treated with preoperative octreotide, cyproheptadine, corticosteroid, and aprotinin. Drugs that release histamine and catacholamines should be avoided in patients with carcinoid tumors. A pulmonary artery catheter can be placed after the tumor is removed. Intraoperative use of TEE is very helpful to identify the extent of tumor spread, and for venous cannulation, hemodynamic monitoring, and recognition of any intracardiac shunting. Very little information exists in support of an anesthetic agent of choice in cardiac tumors. Intravenous and inhalation agents are equally safe, if used carefully (28–31).

REFERENCES

1. Reynan K. Frequency of primary tumors of the heart. Am J Cardiol 1996; 77:107.
2. Lam KYL, Dickens P, Chan ACL. Tumors of the heart. Arch Pathol Lab Med 1993; 117:1027.
3. Tazela ar HD, Locke TJ, McGregir CGA. Pathology or surgically excised primary cardiac tumors. Mayo Clin Proc 1992; 67:957.
4. Salcedo EE, Cohen GI, White RD, Davison MB. Cardiac tumors: diagnosis and treatment. Curr Probl Cardiol 1992; 17:73.
5. Hanson EC. Cardiac tumors: a current perspective. NY State J Med 1992; 92:41.
6. Godwin JF. Symposium on cardiac tumors. The spectrum of cardiac tumors. Am J Cardiol 1968; 21:307.
7. Carney JA, Hruska LS, Beauchamp GD, Gordon H. Dominant inheritance of the complex of myxomas, spotty pigmentation and endocrine overactivity. Mayo Clin Proc 1986; 61:165.
8. Van Gelder HM, O'Brien DJ, Staples ED, Alexander JA. Familial cardiac myxoma. Ann Thorac Surg 1992; 53:419.
9. Kopman RJ, Happle R. Autosomal dominat transmission of the Name syndrome (nevi, atrial myxoma, mucinosis of the skin and endocrine overactivity). Hum Genet 1991; 86:300.
10. Carney JA, Gordon J, Carpenter PC, et al. The complex of myxomas, spotty pigmentation and endocrine overactivity. Medicine 1985; 64:270.
11. Vidaillet HJ Jr, Seward JB, Fyke FE, et al. "Syndrome myxoma": a subset of patients with cardiac myxoma associated with pigmented skin lesions and peripheral and endocrine neoplasm. Br Heart J 1987; 57:247.
12. Bennet WS, Skelton TN, Lehan PH. The complex of myxomas, pigmentation and endocrine overactivity. Am J Cardiol 1990; 65:399.
13. Shahian DW, Labib SB, Chang G. Cardiac papillary fibroelastoma. Ann Thorac Surg 1995; 59:538.
14. LiMandri G, Homma S, Di Tullio MR, et al. Detection of multiple papillary fibroelastomas of the tricuspid valve by transesophageal echocardiography. J Am Soc Echo 1994; 7:315.
15. Pomerance A. Papillary "tumors" of the heart valves. J Pathol Bacteriol 1981; 87:135.
16. Putnam JB, Sweenay MS, Colon R, et al. Primary cardiac sarcomas. Ann Thorac Surg 1991; 51:906.
17. Burke AP, Cowan D, Virmani R. Primary sarcoma of the heart. Cancer 1992; 69:387.
18. Thomas CR, Johnson GW, Stoard MF, Clifford S. Primary malignant cardiac tumors: update 1992. Med Pediatr Oncol 1992; 20:519.
19. Charuzi Y, Bolger A, Beeder C, Lew AS. A new echocardiographic classification of left atrial myxoma. Am J Cardiol 1985; 55:614.
20. Dennis MA, Appareti K, Manco-Johnson ML, et al. The echocardiographic diagnosis of multiple fetal cardiac tumors. Ultrasound Med 1985; 4:327.
21. Panidis LP, Mimtz GS, McAllisterm M. Hemodynamic consequences of the left atrial myxomas as assessed by Doppler ultrasound. Am Heart J 1986; 111:927.
22. Edwards LC III, Louie EK. Transthoracic and transesophageal echocardiography for the evaluation of cardiac tumors, thrombi, and valvular vegetations. Am J Card Imag 1994; 8:45.
23. Shyu K-G, Chen J-J, et al. Comparison of transthoracic and transesophageal echocardiography in the diagnosis of intracardiac tumors in adults. J Clin Ultrasound 1994; 22:381.
24. Azuma T, Ohira A, Akagi H, et al. Transvenous biopsy of a right atrial tumor under transesophageal echocardiography guidance. Am Heart J 1996; 131:402.
25. Bough E, Bodem W, Gandsman E, et al. Radionuclide diagnosis of left atrial myxoma with computer-generated functional images. Am J Cardiol 1986; 52: 1365.
26. Bleiweis MS, Georgiou D, Brundage BH. Detection of intracardiac masses by ultrafast computed tomography. Am J Card Imag 1994; 8:63.
27. Fujita N, Caputo GR, Higgins CB. Diagnosis and characterization of intracardiac masses by magnetic resonance imaging. Am J Card Imag 1994; 8:69.
28. Crespo MG, Pulpon LA, Pradas G, et al. Heart transplantation for cardiac angiosarcoma: should its indication be questioned? J Heart Lung Transplant 1993; 12:527.
29. Welch M, Bazaral MG, Schmidt R, et al. Anesthetic management for surgical removal of renal carcinoma with caval or atrial tumor thrombus using dêp hypothermic circulatory arrest. J Cardiothorac Anes 1989; 3: 580–586.
30. Burt JD, Bowsher WG, Joyce G, et al. The management of renal cell carcinoma with inferior vena-caval involvement. Aut NZ J Surg 1993; 63:25–290.
31. Hasnain JU, Watson RJ. Transesophageal echocardiography during resection of renal cell carcinoma involving the inferior vana cava. South Med J 1994; 87: 273–275.
32. Nesbitt JC, Soltero ER, Dinney CP, Walsh GL, Schrump DS, Swanson DA, Pisters LL, Willis KD, Putnam JB, Jr. Surgical management of renal cell carcinoma with inferior vena cava tumor thrombus. Ann Thorac Surg 1997; 63:1592–1600.

23

Perioperative Care of Patients with Liver Neoplasms

JAMES F. ARENS and DEBRA L. KENNAMER

Department of Anesthesiology, The University of Texas M.D. Anderson Cancer Center, Houston Texas, U.S.A.

At the University of Texas M.D. Anderson Cancer Center, more than 250 patients a year undergo surgery for primary or metastatic liver neoplasms. Hepatocellular carcinoma is the most common primary hepatic tumor, with an annual incidence approaching 1 million new patients (1). Most patients presenting with liver neoplasms, however, have metastatic disease. The liver is second only to lymph nodes as a common site for solid tumor metastatic disease. Therefore, it is not uncommon for the liver to be the only site of metastatic disease in patients with colorectal adenocarcinoma disease (Table 1).

Patients with metastatic liver tumors seldom survive more than 1 year without treatment. Systemic or regional chemotherapeutic treatment rarely improves long-term survival for patients with primary or metastatic hepatic malignancies and, furthermore, the toxicities of these treatments adversely affect the patient's quality of life. In contrast, surgical resection has produced 5-year survival rates of 25–40% for patients with metastatic colorectal cancer (2). Additionally, surgical palliation can ameliorate symptoms related to excess hormone production in patients with symptomatic neuroendocrine tumors.

Increasing long-term survival is therefore a surgical challenge for patients with primary and some metastatic liver cancers. Hepatic resection may be indicated for a number of conditions including the treatment of primary benign or malignant tumors of the liver or biliary tract and for metastatic lesions. Unfortunately, <20% of patients with disease confined to the liver are eligible for curative resection (3). Patients may be ineligible for resection because of tumor size, multifocal disease with more than four or five lesions, multiple metastatic tumors involving both lobes of the liver, proximity of tumor to key vascular or biliary structures that precludes margin-negative resection, or inadequate hepatic function related to coexistent liver disease, e.g., cirrhosis.

Modern diagnostic imaging modalities have greatly improved preoperative staging of liver tumors. Specifically, high-speed helical computed tomography (CT) and organ-specific scanning protocols have improved preoperative staging of colorectal liver metastases. Magnetic resonance imaging (MRI), especially used in conjunction with liver-specific contrast agents, is more sensitive for the detection of early hepatocellular carcinoma (HCC). Additionally, improved anatomic scans of extrahepatic sites have reduced the number of patients who undergo unnecessary laparotomies. Despite these technologic advancements, 15–20% of patients whose tumors are determined to be resectable preoperatively have conflicting findings with intraperitoneal ultrasound performed at surgery.

Table 1 Etiology of Primary and Metastatic Liver Tumors in 242 Patients Who Presented (05/2001–04/2003) with Surgically Resectable Lesions to the University of Texas M.D. Anderson Cancer Center

Primary and metastatic liver tumors	N	Primary and metastatic liver tumors	N
Colon cancer	128	Pancreas carcinoma	4
Hepatocellular carcinoma	29	Renal cell carcinoma	4
Breast cancer	13	Melanoma	3
Primary biliary carcinoma	11	Sarcoma	3
Leiomyosarcoma	11	Benign diagnosis	2
Carcinoid	10	Ovarian carcinoma	2
Other	8	Adrenal carcinoma	1
Cholangiocarcinoma	6	Ocular	1
Neuroendocrine tumors	5	*Total number of patients*	*242*

The primary adverse effects of liver resection include biliary leakage, bleeding, and postoperative liver dysfunction or failure. Biliary leakage is a potential complication especially when the biliary system requires reconstruction, e.g., following resection of a cholangiocarcinoma. Massive intraoperative hemorrhage has been reported with elective liver resections (4). Bleeding usually occurs from the inferior vena cava and hepatic veins during parenchymal transection. High and posterior placed tumors especially being difficult to isolate and therefore at increased risk of hemorrhage. Furthermore, HCC frequently associated with cirrhotic livers can create difficult resection because of decreased functional parenchymal reserve, anatomical distortion, coexisting portal hypertension, and fragile collateral vasculature.

Substantial blood loss increases morbidity, including hepatic insufficiency, and mortality (5). In fact, patients who receive multiple transfusions have been shown to have shorter cancer-free survival compared with patients who do not require transfusion (6). Maneuvers employed to minimize intraoperative blood loss include anatomical resection of the liver segments (Fig. 1), resection under vascular exclusion of the liver, and resection at a low central venous pressure (CVP). Using these techniques, the average reported blood loss for a group of 212 patients who had major hepatic resections at our institution was 426 ml. In patients, who did not require transfusion, a 74% reduction in perioperative complications was observed.

Preventing postoperative hepatic insufficiency and failure is a major challenge to the surgical team. Postoperative liver failure and associated mortality are related to the amount of functional parenchyma resected and stage of preoperative liver disease. Additional predictors of postresection liver failure and increased mortality include increased intraoperative blood loss, postoperative increase in serum bilirubin, and postoperative abdominal sepsis.

Major liver resection is associated with a substantial loss of liver tissue (Fig. 2). The average percentages of the liver resected are as follows: right trisegmentectomy, 85%; right lobectomy, 65%; left lobectomy, 35%; and segmental or wedge resection, 3–15% (1). The total liver volume (TLV) and hepatic segment volumes as measured by CT are shown in Table 2 (7). Not surprisingly, larger hepatic resections are associated with increased incidence of postresection morbidity and mortality (8). Surgical resection of $< 50\%$ of functional hepatic parenchyma is associated with a negligible risk of clinically significant hepatic insufficiency. Patients with otherwise normal hepatic parenchyma and normal serum hepatic function tests can survive resection of up to 80% of their liver volume, as the remaining 20% of normal liver remnant may regenerate and provide adequate hepatic function. Patients with abnormal liver function related to fatty infiltration or cirrhosis (associated with ethanol

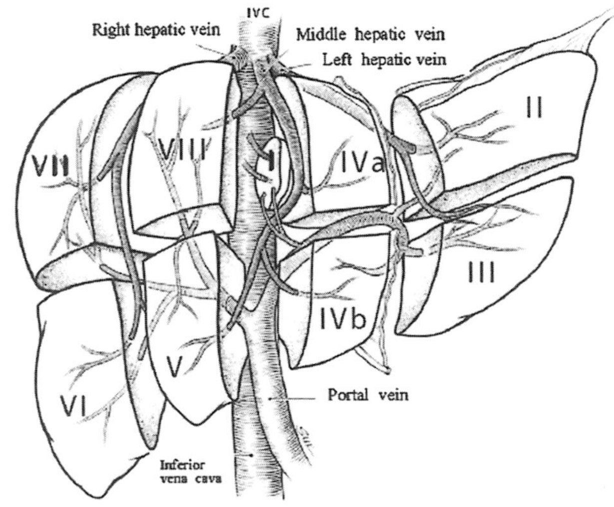

Figure 1 Anatomical diagram illustrating the segmental anatomy of the liver.

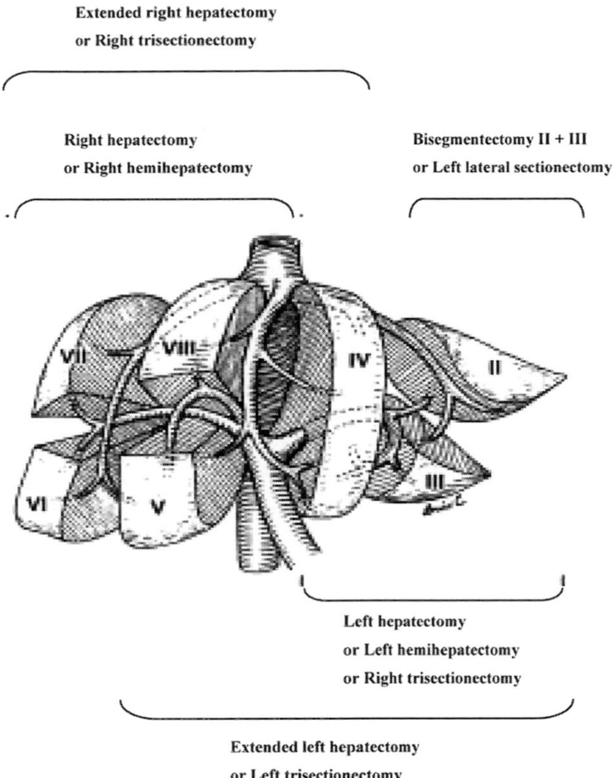

Figure 2 The Brisbane 2000 terminology of liver resections. *Source*: From Ref. 38.

ingestion or chronic viral infection), however, cannot tolerate resection of a large volume of liver and usually require >40% liver remnant.

Preoperative assessment of functional hepatic reserve is therefore recommended in patients with coexisting liver disease, e.g., patients with cirrhosis who have HCC. Hepatic synthetic function may be better evaluated by albumin, prothrombin time, or pseudocholinesterase determinations, whereas the bilirubin level can evaluate hepatic excretory function. Conventional biochemical markers of hepatobiliary disease, however, correlate poorly with the degree of hepatic dysfunction because of the lack of specificity (exception is prothrombin time) of individual tests. Nevertheless, these markers are helpful in combination for monitoring hepatic abnormalities.

Tests of global liver function such as the indocyanine green test, galactose elimination capacity, and aminopyrine breath test may have a role in predicting the outcome of surgery. These functional liver studies use compounds that are naturally synthesized and metabolized by hepatocytes. In cirrhotic or otherwise diseased livers, the rates of metabolism or clearance of these compounds are decreased. Some compounds used in these functional studies have a clearance rate that reflects changes in hepatic microcirculation and the decreased blood flow associated with cirrhosis (1). Indocyanine green, an anionic dye that is bound by lipoproteins, cleared by the liver, and excreted unconjugated in bile, is used to assess functional hepatic reserve. The disadvantage of indocyanine green clearance is that it is dependent on liver blood flow and does not truly assess hepatocyte function. Tests that are independent on liver blood flow include the aminopyrine and phenylalanine breath tests. In these tests, the patient ingests radiolabeled ^{14}C aminopyrine or phenylalanine, and expired $^{14}CO_2$ is measured to determine the amount of hepatic demethylation or oxidation. A less expensive test involves intravenous administration of lidocaine to determine the rate of microsomal metabolism of lidocaine to monoethylgylinexylidide. Although these tests may only quantitate specific enzymatic pathways, they may be helpful in identifying patients who are at low risk for postoperative liver failure in the presence of pre-existing liver disease.

The most commonly used approach for the prediction of perioperative risk is based on the system developed by Child and Turcotte (9) to predict mortality after portocaval shunt surgery. However, this system has never been prospectively validated in patients undergoing other types of surgery. Furthermore, it involved subjective assessments of nutrition and encephalopathy and thus could not be reliably used for retrospective studies. A modification proposed by Pugh et al. (10) replaced nutritional status with the prothrombin time (an independent predictor of mortality) in the assessment of patients undergoing esophageal transection. The Child–Pugh scoring system (Table 3) allows for simple, reliable, and reproducible prediction of a patient's risk for liver failure and has been shown to correlate with perioperative mortality in patients undergoing nonshunt surgery and cirrhotic patients undergoing abdominal procedures. Patients with a Child–Pugh score of <7 are considered candidates for liver resection. In contrast, patients with

Table 2 Modified Child–Pugh Score

Segment(s)	Volume (cm^3)		TLV (%)	
Total liver	1518 ± 353	(911–2729)	100	
Right liver	997 ± 279	(467–1881)	65 ± 7	(49–82)
Left liver	493 ± 127	(205–827)	33 ± 7	(17–49)
Segment IV	251 ± 70	(101–429)	17 ± 4	(10–29)
Bisegment II + III	242 ± 79	(101–490)	16 ± 4	(5–27)
Segment I	28 ± 9	(8–60)	2 ± 0	(1–3)

Values expressed as mean ± standard deviation; range is shown in parentheses.

Table 3 Perioperative Coagulation Status at Specific Time Intervals Associated with Epidural Instrumentation for Analgesia Following Hepatic Resection

	Points[a]		
Presentation	1	2	3
Albumin (g/dL)	> 3.5	2.8–3.5	< 2.8
Prothrombin time			
Seconds prolonged	< 4	4–6	> 6
INR	< 1.7	1.7–2.3	> 2.3
Bilirubin (mg/dL)[b]	< 2	2–3	> 3
Ascites	Absent	Slight–moderate	Tense
Encephalopathy	None	Grade I–II	Grade III–IV

[a] Class A = 5–6, B = 7–9 points, and C = 10–15 points.
[b] For cholestatic diseases (e.g., primary biliary cirrhosis), the bilirubin level is disproportionate to the impairment of hepatic function, and an allowance should be made. For these conditions, assign one point for bilirubin level < 4 mg/dL, two points for bilirubin 4–10 mg/dL, and three points for bilirubin >10 mg/dL.
Source: Adapted from Patel: Mayo Clin Proc 1999; 74(6):593–599.

serum bilirubin concentrations greater than twice the normal value or patients with radiologically detectable ascites should not undergo liver resection. Additionally, patients with signs of active hepatitis are at increased risk of postoperative ascites, renal failure, gastrointestinal bleeding, and death (8).

I. PORTAL VENOUS EMBOLIZATION

To increase the number of patients who may undergo potentially curable surgical resection, selective portal venous embolization (PVE) can be used to selectively induce hypertrophy in the nondiseased portion of the liver of patients in whom the liver remnant remaining after resection would be too small to provide adequate function (11). Preoperative interruption of the portal flow in the liver territories planned to be removed, induces their atrophy and the compensatory hypertrophy of the segments spared by the resection. This interruption can be induced by the surgical ligation of the portal branches or more commonly by percutaneous intraportal injection of polyvinyl alcohol particles and microcoils prior to the surgical resection. Preoperative portal vein embolization is usually indicated when the remnant liver is expected to account for < 25–40% of the TLV. Feasibility is close to 100% and the risk comparable to that of a percutaneous liver biopsy.

The regeneration process usually peaks within the 2 weeks of PVE. Liver regeneration is, however, slower in patients with cirrhosis or diabetes mellitus. Two to four weeks after PVE, a repeat CT is done to determine the level of regeneration or disease spread. If liver hypertrophy has occurred and there is no spread of disease, resection is then performed. Embolization results in ~12% increase of the predicted liver remnant, thus ensuring safe and potentially curative extensive hepatectomies in a group of patients preoperatively determined to be only marginally eligible for resection.

II. ANESTHETIC MANAGEMENT

A. Preoperative Evaluation

Patients scheduled for liver resection should receive a thorough preoperative anesthetic assessment that includes neurological, cardiovascular, pulmonary, hepatic, and renal evaluations. Patients with cirrhosis should be tested for present or past hepatitis B or C infections, alcoholic cirrhosis, and liver function assessed according to the Child–Pugh criteria (Table 3). It is not uncommon for patients who present with colorectal metastatic liver tumors to have been previously treated with systemic chemotherapeutic agents and radiation therapy to the pelvis and therefore any organ dysfunction resulting from these therapies should also be assessed.

B. Anesthesia for Hepatic Resection

Prior to induction of general anesthesia, and unless the epidural route is contraindicated, an epidural catheter is placed for postoperative analgesia. The epidural catheter is usually sited at the mid-to-low thoracic level. A balanced endotracheal general anesthetic consisting of a volatile agent, narcotic and muscle relaxant is used for the surgical procedure. Continuous monitoring of the patient's arterial and central venous pressure (CVP) is routinely performed. Although hemorrhage is a rare occurrence at our institution, it is important to have sufficient venous access in the event of massive blood loss. We routinely use an 8F central venous catheter and at least one large bore peripheral intravenous catheter. Furthermore, it is important to maintain a low central venous pressure (CVP 0–5 mmHg) to facilitate minimal intraoperative blood loss. This is achieved primarily by fluid restriction. Rarely, intravenous nitroglycerine infusion has been used when fluid restriction alone does not sufficiently lower the CVP. If there is massive blood loss in the fluid restricted patient, it is extremely important to have adequate venous access and the proper equipment available to perform a rapid, massive transfusion. Blood should be immediately available.

Because liver resections require a large abdominal incision, it is important to monitor the patient's body temperature. Forced air-warming devices can be routinely used on both the upper and lower extremities to maintain normal body temperature.

C. Intraoperative Anesthetic Management

Fluid management is critical in patients undergoing liver resection and may be considered in two phases. The first phase starts with the placement of the preinduction intravenous catheter and ends with completion of the hepatic parenchymal resection and hemostasis. The second phase begins after removal of the specimen and completion of hemostasis.

During the first phase, fluid is restricted in an effort to minimize CVP and, therefore, minimize blood loss. Blood loss may occur during vascular control of the porta hepatis. However, injury to the hepatic veins during parenchymal dissection or at their junction with the inferior vena cava is the most common cause of hemorrhage (12). The blood loss from vascular injury is directly proportional to the pressure gradient across the vessel wall and the fourth power of the radius of the injury. Lowering the CVP decreases both the pressure component and minimizes the radial component by decreasing vessel distention.

The maintenance of low CVP precludes vena cava distention and facilitates mobilization of the liver. It also facilitates the dissection of the major hepatic and retrohepatic veins. More importantly, it minimizes blood loss during parenchymal transection. Additionally, low CVP facilitates control of inadvertent venous injury.

Although minimizing fluids to maintain low CVP may seem simple, it can be challenging. Factors contributing to this challenge include the fact that patients present for surgery in a relatively dehydrated state because of their preoperative bowel preparation. Maintenance of an adequate level of anesthesia and acceptable perfusion pressure may be tricky. In addition, the patient may be placed in a reverse Trendelenberg position during the resection which may decrease perfusion pressure. Because fluid restriction is critical to the hepatic resection, short-term blood pressure support with vasoconstrictive agents, such is ephedrine or low-dose phenylephrine, may be necessary.

During dissection, mobilization of the liver, and isolation of the vessels, it is not unusual for the surgeon to temporarily compress the vena cava resulting in a sudden decrease in arterial pressure. Communication between the surgeon and anesthesiologist is therefore essential.

Urine output during the resection is often minimal, and in patients with normal renal function, 0.5 mL/kg/hr is considered acceptable. Small crystalloid fluid boluses may, however, be necessary to maintain this minimal acceptable urine output. Fortunately, this portion of the surgery is not prolonged and is usually limited to 1–3 hr in duration.

Admittedly, this degree of fluid restriction is not appropriate for all patients and open dialogue between the surgeon and anesthesiologist regarding the intraoperative fluid management of patients with significant cardiac, renal, or other comorbid conditions is essential. Clearly, there are patients who have pre-existing conditions in which even short-term severe fluid restriction is relatively contraindicated.

The second phase of fluid management begins when the specimen has been removed and hemostasis has been achieved. The goal of this phase is to render the patient normovolemic and hemodynamically stable. Hydration may be achieved with crystalloid and/or colloid solutions in a short period of time. If significant blood loss occurred, then transfusion of packed red blood cells is done to achieve a final hemoglobin concentration of 8–10 g/dL.

One could argue that loss of sympathetic tone could further decrease the CVP and help decrease the blood loss during the resection. But the potential for hemorrhage during liver resection is very real. Rendering the patient relatively hypovolemic makes most anesthesiologists uncomfortable at best. Therefore, it is recommended that the epidural is activated only during this second phase, after hemostasis and rehydration has been achieved. Prior to the second phase of fluid management, fluids are restricted to maintain a low CVP. Activation of the epidural with local anesthetic results in blocking the patient's sympathetic tone to some degree. Because these patients are dehydrated from preoperative fasting and the presurgical bowel preparation, loss of sympathetic tone may result in an unacceptable degree of hypotension. Additionally, if there is major blood loss during the resection, loss of sympathetic tone may adversely contribute to the hemodynamic changes that occur with rapid, massive blood loss.

The choice of drugs used in the epidural is basically one of personal preference. Epidural narcotics may have a profound respiratory depressant effect on patients who are particularly sensitive because they have had a large percentage of their liver removed. Occasionally, the degree of respiratory depression is difficult to predict. The use of even low concentrations of local anesthetics (0.125% bupivacaine) can be associated with profound hypotension in the hypovolemic patient. It is therefore important to render patients normovolemic prior to administering local anesthetics.

The vast majority of patients having liver resections are extubated in the operating room. In patients who have a large hepatic resection or lesser hepatic resection accompanied by radiofrequency ablation of several lesions, the metabolism of narcotics and muscle relaxants is dramatically slowed. If prolonged arousal and muscle relaxation are to be avoided, the anesthetic plan needs to be altered so that the dose of both narcotics and muscle relaxants can be significantly reduced.

Patients are monitored in postanesthesia care unit or the surgical intensive care unit overnight. Most patients receive the remainder of their care on a post-surgical floor where nursing staff are familiar with the care for these types of patients. The average hospital stay after liver resection is 5 days.

D. Postoperative Pain Management

Unless there is an absolute contraindication to epidural analgesia, the patient is offered patient controlled epidural analgesia. Admittedly, epidural analgesia in patients whose coagulation may be compromised after liver resection may be controversial. We feel that the benefits of epidural analgesia significantly outweigh the risks. These patients have large upper-abdominal incisions, which cause pulmonary compromise, including reduced vital capacity, tidal volume, functional residual capacity, and forced expiratory volume at one second, which increases the patient's risk for hypoxemia, atelectasis, and pneumonia. Additionally, some of these patients require chest tubes postoperatively. The excellent analgesia afforded with epidural pain control helps prevent pulmonary complications and allows patients to ambulate comfortably by the first postoperative day.

The combinations of low-dose anesthetics and narcotics and the advantages of each are well described. Most commonly, we use an infusion of bupivacaine 0.075% and fentanyl 5–10 mcg/mL. However, it is recommended that the epidural infusion be tailored to the individual patient. Several important points should be remembered when managing pain in these patients. These patients usually have greater analgesia requirements immediately after surgery. However, their ability to metabolize narcotic and local anesthetic agents is altered and therefore it is not unusual for a patient's analgesic requirements to change dramatically during the postoperative period. In younger patients who are otherwise healthy, an infusion of bupivacaine 0.075% with 10 mcg/mL of fentanyl may be appropriate for the first 12 hours of the postoperative period. Thereafter, depending on the amount of liver removed and degree of somnolence, the fentanyl concentration is decreased to 5 mcg/mL. In elderly, or debilitated patients, the initial epidural infusion is usually bupivacaine 0.075% with fentanyl 5 mcg/mL and it may be necessary to decrease the fentanyl concentration to 2.5 mcg/mL in some patients.

Additionally, coagulation may be altered after liver resection, resulting in increased risk of epidural hematoma. Prothrombin time (PT) usually increases after liver resection and peaks on the first or second postoperative day (Fig. 3) and correlates with the extent of hepatic resection (13). Additionally, in patients undergoing major liver resections (three segments or more), the platelet count decreases and reaches a nadir on the third postoperative day. Coagulation abnormalities are treated with appropriate blood products, such as plasma and/or platelets. The prothrombin time usually normalizes within 5–7 days postoperatively. The epidural catheter, however, is usually removed after the third postoperative day after documenting that the INR is <1.5 (correlating with clotting factor activity greater than 40%) (14). Coagulation status at the time of epidural catheter removal is deranged in approximately 10% of patients (Table 4) (13). Therefore, continuous neurologic function monitoring is extremely important in the postoperative period, with sensory and motor function being evaluated every 4 hr postoperatively. It is also important

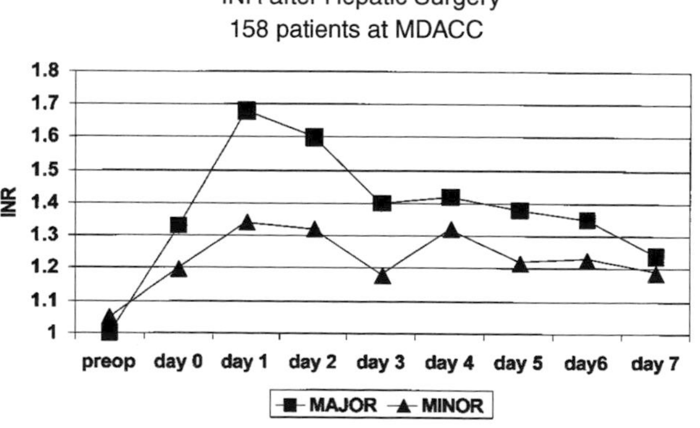

Figure 3 Changes in INR in the perioperative course following major and minor hepatic resection.

Table 4 Perioperative Coagulation Status at Time Intervals Related to Epidural Instrumentation

Epidural status	At insertion	In situ	At removal
INR	1.02 ± 0.11	–	1.28 ± 0.20
Abnormal INR (percent of patients)	1.9	67.7	8.9
PTT (sec)	29.8 ± 3.4	–	27.9 ± 3.2
Abnormal PTT (percent of patients)	1.3	1.9	1.3
Platelets (K/UL)	239 ± 74	–	155 ± 55
Platelets <100 K/UL (percent of patients)	0.64	19	12

to stress to the patients that they should report any motor or sensory deficits immediately. Patients with an INR >1.5 should additionally receive neurologic assessment for at least 24 hours after epidural catheter removal.

Patients often complain of right shoulder pain after surgery. This may be referred diaphragmatic pain caused by the surgical retractors or from air under the diaphragm. This shoulder pain is not usually relieved by the epidural but responds well with one or two small doses of a systemic narcotic. Systemic narcotic infusions are also used in patients who are not candidates for epidural analgesia. It is important to remember that the metabolism of these patients is altered and accumulation of narcotics can occur in the postoperative period.

E. Perioperative Antibiotic Treatment and Postoperative Nutrition

Perioperative antibiotics are routinely administered prior to the beginning of the surgical procedure and continued for the first five postoperative days.

Oral nutrition should be started as early as possible after liver resection. Fluid and sodium restriction with a low-sodium diet is advisable in order to prevent the formation of ascites (15). Postoperative ascites is treated with furosemide and low-sodium albumin. When massive ascites accumulates, paracentesis is indicated to avoid disruption of the surgical incision, leakage of ascitic fluid, and infection.

III. SURGICAL MANAGEMENT

A. Resection Procedure

For this procedure, the patient is positioned supine with arms extended laterally on padded arm boards. Draping extends from the nipple line to below the umbilicus and from midaxillary line to midaxillary line. Electrocardiogram leads should be positioned lateral to this area. The type of incision made depends on the type of resection that is to be performed. A bilateral subcostal incision is usually sufficient.

Once the abdomen is opened, the peritoneal cavity is explored for metastatic disease and the liver explored for masses. The surgeon then mobilizes the right and left sides of the liver, taking care not to injure the spleen during mobilization of the left side of the liver. At this time, intraoperative ultrasound (IOUS) is then used to define the number, location, and anatomic relationship of the hepatic lesions. Intraoperative ultrasound is important in hepatic resection as it allows the precise location and extent of the tumor(s) to be defined. These details are essential for the selection, planning, and performance of the surgical procedure. Intraoperative ultrasound is more sensitive in detecting hepatic lesions than CT or MRI and therefore plays an essential role in detecting smaller previously undiscovered metastatic lesions. It is not unusual that IOUS will determine that a tumor previously thought to be resectable by CT or MRI is, in fact, not resectable.

B. Vascular Control

The liver, a highly vascularized structure, has a dual blood supply with 75% of the blood derived from the portal vein and 25% from the hepatic artery. Hepatic blood flow is about 1500 mL/min. Importantly, although the hepatic artery supplies only 25% of the blood flow, it supplies 50% of the liver's oxygen supply. Hepatic resections require control of the vessels supplying blood to the portion of the liver to be resected. In addition, blood supply to and venous drainage from the liver remnant must be maintained.

Various surgical techniques have been developed to achieve vascular exclusion and are central to allowing an aggressive surgical approach to hepatic tumors. The type of vascular occlusion is selected according to the tumor site, underlying liver disease, the patient's cardiovascular status, and surgeon's expertise. Communication between the anesthesiologist and surgeon regarding monitoring and prevention of complications is essential. The following is a brief description of the techniques commonly used and their hemodynamic effects.

C. Hepatic Vascular Inflow Occlusion (Pringle Maneuver)

Vascular isolation of the liver is most commonly achieved through the Pringle maneuver. This maneuver allows control of vascular inflow by clamping the hepatic artery and portal vein (the hepatic pedicle). It should be remembered that occlusion of the inflow has no effect on the back flow of blood and bleeding from the hepatic veins. Hepatic pedicle may be applied continuously or intermittently. Under normothermic conditions, continuous clamping occlusion to a normal liver is safe for up to 60 minutes; however, more than 30 minutes invariably causes ischemic damage to the liver, with an incidence of complications that is proportional to the length of clamping. However, at our institution inflow occlusion rarely exceeds 20 minutes.

Intermittent clamping can extend warm ischemia time up to 120 minutes. Intermittent clamping usually consists of 15–20 minutes of clamping followed by 5 min of reperfusion until the hepatic transection is completed (16). When the hepatic pedicle is released, the transected plane bleeds and significant blood loss is possible during the reperfusion period. Although intermittent clamping is associated with more blood loss than continuous clamping, postoperative liver function is better preserved, especially in patients with abnormal liver function. Furthermore, intermittent inflow occlusion allows surgical resection of difficult hepatectomies that would otherwise be considered impossible in patients with abnormal liver parenchyma (17).

The hemodynamic response to inflow occlusion includes 5% decrease in pulmonary artery pressure, 10% decrease in mean arterial pressure, 40% increase in systemic vascular resistance, and 10% decrease in cardiac output (18). The decrease in venous return is secondary to the compression of splanchnic and hepatic contributions to venous return (19). This results in a decreased right atrial pressure and decrease in blood loss from the hepatic veins. Although there is a described increase in systemic vascular resistance, and only a slight decrease in cardiac output, it is the authors' experience that significant hypotension can occasionally be observed during hepatic resection. Inflow occlusion plus the surgical manipulation of the liver and compression of the inferior vena cava during this time can cause severe hypotension. When this occurs, the surgeon is notified, the pressure is allowed to normalize, and surgery resumed. Occasionally, pharmacologic intervention is required to allow the surgeon to proceed with the resection. The hypotension is usually short lived and probably exaggerated by the attempt to keep the patient's CVP low until the resection is complete.

D. Hemihepatic Vascular Clamping

Hemihepatic vascular clamping interrupts the arterial and venous inflow to the right or left side of the liver. Advantages of this clamping technique include the absence of ischemic injury to the liver remnant, absence of splanchnic congestion, minimal hemodynamic consequences, and clear demarcation of the limits of the resection. The disadvantage of this technique is that significant blood loss may occur at the resection plane.

E. Hepatic Vascular Exclusion

Hepatic vascular exclusion (HVE) includes total occlusion of vascular inflow and outflow to and from the liver, thereby completely isolating the liver from the circulation. Clamps are applied to the hepatic artery, portal vein, and both the infrahepatic and suprahepatic inferior vena cava. Hepatic vascular exclusion produces profound hemodynamic changes, including 25% decrease in pulmonary artery pressure, 10% decrease in systemic blood pressure, 80% increase in systemic vascular resistance, 40% decrease in cardiac output, and 50% increase in heart rate. The venous return from the inferior vena cava is interrupted, thus decreasing the cardiac output by 40–60% (20). It is clear that HVE requires arterial, pulmonary artery catheter, and/or, TEE monitoring. TEE is helpful in determining whether vasopressor support or volume expansion is required.

The hemodynamic consequences of HVE are difficult to predict preoperatively and depend upon the anesthetic technique as well as the individual patient's ability to tolerate these cardiovascular challenges. Complications seen after HVE include pulmonary dysfunction, spontaneous splenic rupture, and injury to the caudate lobe. The pulmonary dysfunction is secondary to large volume resuscitations and phrenic nerve injury, resulting in atelectasis, pleural effusion, and abdominal collections (21). There is also a moderate and transient increase in serum creatinine.

Fortunately, HVE has few indications. These include resections of lesions involving the cavo-hepatic junction or when backflow bleeding occurs due to an inability to control the CVP. Hepatic vascular exclusion is rarely if ever used at The University of Texas M.D. Anderson Cancer Center and in fact not been used for the past 3 years.

F. Inflow Occlusion with Extrahepatic Control of Major Hepatic Veins

The goal of this procedure is to achieve HVE without interruption of the inferior vena cava. This technique is technically more demanding than HVE with interruption of the inferior vena cava. Extrahepatic control of the main hepatic veins, however, is associated with risks of massive blood loss or air embolism loss should a vein tear. Inflow occlusion is achieved by clamping the hepatic pedicle and outflow occlusion achieved by clamping the hepatic veins. Advantages to this technique include hemodynamic stability, the possibility of intermittent inflow occlusion, and possibility of partial hepatic exclusion thereby preventing backflow bleeding and also air embolism.

Transection of the liver parenchyma is usually performed with the Cavetron Ultrasonic Surgical Aspirator (CUSA), an ultrasonic dissector. An anatomical approach to surgical dissection and the use of the ultrasonic dissector are key to reducing surgical blood loss, with control of residual bleeding by Argon beam coagulation. More recently, vascular staplers have been used to achieve inflow control and control the hepatic veins. When used in combination with maintenance of low CVP, these devices are associated with decreased warm ischemic time, decreased blood loss, and decreased total surgical time. These techniques should be used judiciously and are not appropriate for tumors located near the vascular pedicle.

An incidental cholecystectomy is usually performed with any hepatic resection. If a right hepatic lobectomy is to be done, the gallbladder is removed because of technical concerns and if a left hepatic lobectomy is performed, the gallbladder is removed because of the danger of bile sludging. In either scenario, should acute cholecycystitis occur following a hepatic resection, a cholecystectomy would technically be very difficult to perform because of adhesions.

In some cases, the liver mass may be attached directly to the diaphragm and a hole may be made through the diaphragm during dissection. When this occurs, a chest tube may need to be placed prior to closure, or the air is evacuated during a Valsalva maneuver provided by the anesthesiologist as the diaphragm is closed.

IV. OUTCOME AFTER LIVER RESECTION

Despite the advances made in surgical technique and patient selection perioperative morbidity and mortality still occurs in about 40% and 7%, respectively, for patients with liver cirrhosis. The main cause of death includes liver failure, ascites, and infection. The 5-year survival rate after resection for HCC in patients with cirrhosis is 45% (range: 8–79%), with disease free survival of around 30% (22).

According to The University of Texas M.D. Anderson Cancer Center's surgical database of 358 patients treated from 1992 to 2002, the 4-year survival rate for patients with colorectal liver metastases after sugical resection, resection and RFA, and RFA only were 65%, 36%, and 22%, respectively (39).

V. LAPAROSCOPIC LIVER RESECTION

Laparoscopy is commonly used in oncologic surgery to stage gastrointestinal malignancies. However, laparoscopic liver resection has not advanced as far as other abdominal procedures, such as splenectomy or adrenalectomy. Reasons include the size of the liver, its attachment to the retroperitoneum and diaphragm, the risk of major hemorrhage, the ability to achieve margin-negative resection of tumors, and the risk of CO_2 embolism. Other technical hurdles include the necessity for ultrasound identification of the tumors since manual palpation is not feasible, localization of the vasculature requiring division, adequate exposure and retraction, and parenchymal transection. Additionally, hemorrhage is much more difficult to control with a laparoscopic approach. Laparoscopic liver resection is, however, performed in cases that involve small, peripheral tumors requiring limited excision.

VI. RADIOFREQUENCY TISSUE ABLATION

Only 5–15% of patients with either newly diagnosed HCC or metastatic colorectal cancers are candidates for curative liver resection. Multifocal disease, proximity to key vascular or biliary structures, or inadequate functional hepatic reserve associated with cirrhosis renders some patients ineligible for curative liver resections. Other treatment modalities have been developed to control and potentially cure liver disease. One such modality is radiofrequency ablation (RFA), a new, innovative technology used to treat patients with unresectable primary and metastatic hepatic cancers (22). An RFA electrode may be advanced into a tumor percutaneously, laparoscopically, or during laparotomy.

Radiofrequency ablation operates on the premise that tumor cells are more sensitive to hyperthermic damage than normal cells and can thus be destroyed by local application of thermal energy. Radiofrequency ablation uses high frequency, alternating current (200–1200 MHz) and emits an energy source from the tip of the electrode into the surrounding tissue. This causes ionic movement that results in frictional heating within the tissue. The zone of thermal injury is precisely controlled because agitation of the ions within the tissue occurs only around the electrode. The final size of the region of heat-ablated tissue is proportional to the square of the RF current. The RF power delivered by a monopolar electrode decreases in proportion to the square of the distance from the electrode. Tissue temperature decreases with increasing distance from the electrode with a zone of coagulative necrosis extending about 0.5–1.0 cm away from the RF needle electrode. RFA treatment typically results in local tissue temperatures exceeding 100°C with subsequent denaturation of intracellular proteins, breakage of DNA strands resulting in clumping of chromatin, and destruction of cell membranes (23). Tissue microvasculature is also destroyed and thrombosis occurs in all vascular branches <3 mm in diameter (24).

The RFA electrodes are 20 cm long and 15–18 gauge diameter with the active tip being arranged in different lengths or configurations (single probe, cluster probe). Electrodes are internally cooled, have an insulated shaft and a noninsulated distal tip. It is sometimes necessary to use the single probe several times for a large lesion rather than one application of the cluster probe. An RFA treatment usually lasts 8–12 minutes. As RF energy is applied to the treatment probe a hyperechoic focus, which is attributed to tissue vaporization, and cavitation develops around the electrode. Hyperechoic microbubbles can escape into the hepatic veins as the proteins in the tumor break down and release nitrogen.

Because RFA results in increased temperatures, it is common to observe a marked increase in the patient's temperature. Active warming should be suspended and the patient's temperature allowed to return to normal. Active cooling is generally not necessary.

Indications for surgical RFA at The University of Texas M.D. Anderson Cancer Center include patients who have no preoperative or intraoperative evidence of extrahepatic disease. Radiofrequency ablation is usually limited to patients having tumor types with probability of liver-only metastases. Additionally, patients with neuroendocrine liver metastases who have functional endocrine syndromes may have ablation of multiple tumors to palliate symptoms. Patients with solitary liver tumors in a nonresectable location can be treated with RFA as well. Radiofrequency ablation and liver resection may be combined in patients with bilobar liver tumors. It is not uncommon for the surgeon to resect the portion of the liver with the large tumors and use RFA to obliterate the smaller lesions in the opposite lobe.

Radiofrequency ablation has some limitations based on the size of the tumor. Larger tumors have a high recurrence rate secondary to incomplete coagulative necrosis of the malignant cells (25–27). The RFA technology is being developed to treat larger tumors.

VII. PERCUTANEOUS RFA

Interventional radiologists can perform percutaneous RFA of liver lesions under ultrasound, CT, or MRI guidance. For lesions involving the right lobe, an intercostal approach with the patient in the left lateral decubitus position is preferred. For left-lobe lesions, a subcostal approach is used (28).

Percutaneous RFA is painful as heat is applied to superficial lesions near the liver capsule or in the parahilar region. Anesthesia for percutaneous RFA ranges from monitored anesthesia care (conscious sedation) with the administration of analgesics and anxiolytics to general anesthesia. When RFA involves larger or multiple lesions, general anesthesia is usually best. General anesthesia is preferable, in our opinion, because patients have unpredictable pain thresholds and anxiety levels. Additionally, general anesthesia allows ventilation to be controlled with temporary suspension of respiration to facilitate probe placement.

Preoperative evaluation for percutaneous RFA of liver requires routine screening for comorbid conditions, including evaluation of coagulation (prothrombin time, partial thromboplastin time, and platelet count). A prolonged PT or PTT <40% of control, an INR <1.8, and a platelet count greater than 40 K /UL are recommended as minimum acceptable values.

The anesthesia approach used to manage patients who undergo percutaneous RFA of liver lesions should be tailored to the patient's comorbid condition(s). The greatest anesthetic challenge may be the location in which these procedures are performed, which is outside of the operating room in the radiology suite. Although new interventional radiology suites are designed with anesthesia delivery in mind, technologic advancements have rendered some anesthetizing locations somewhat obsolete. It is important to have access to necessary supplies and equipment that one may need when positioning patients in the lateral decubitus position, including padding and extremity support. Grounding the patient undergoing RFA is an extremely important and specific procedure since inadequate grounding can result in severe second- and third-degree burns to the patient (29). Grounding pads, each with a surface area of 400 cm^2, should be placed symmetrically on the patient's thighs (two pads per thigh) or back (two pads).

VIII. COMPLICATIONS OF PERCUTANEOUS RFA

In a large, multicenter study of more than 3500 percutaneous RF-ablated liver lesions the reported morbidity and mortality rates were 2.2% and 0.3%, respectively (29). Causes of mortality included peritonitis resulting in multiorgan failure, tumor rupture with associated massive hemorrhage, and bile duct stenosis resulting in liver failure. Complications of special interest to the anesthesiologist in the perioperative period include peritoneal bleeding, visceral organ injury (e.g., perforation of the colon), hemothorax, diaphragmatic paresis, pulmonary embolism, pneumothorax, and cardiac arrest. Minor complications or side effects occurred in <5% of the patients and included pain, elevated temperature, and pleural effusion. Temperatures of 40°C have been noted in patients undergoing prolonged RFAs. It is important to note that second- and third-degree grounding pad burns occurred in patients before multiple grounding pads were used, but none have been reported since multiple grounding pads have become routine.

IX. LAPAROSCOPIC RFA

Laparoscopic RFA offers the advantage of being able to use laparoscopic ultrasound, which provides better resolution than transcutaneous ultrasound. Using laparoscopic ultrasound guidance, the RFA electrode is advanced percutaneously into the tumor for treatment and allows precise positioning of the multiple array RFA needle. This is particularly important when the tumor is located near blood vessels. Additionally, the presence of extrahepatic disease can be assessed during laparoscopy.

Radiofrequency ablation during open laparotomy is preferred in patients with large (>4 cm in diameter) tumors, multiple tumors, if the tumor is adjacent to a major intrahepatic blood vessel, or if the patient has a history of extensive intra-abdominal surgery. Open RFA procedures have the advantage of allowing temporary occlusion of hepatic inflow to be performed thereby facilitating RFA of large tumors, hypervascular tumors, or tumors near major vessels. Furthermore, because RFA utilizes heat generation to destroy tumor cells, the temperature response to a given amount of heat is critical. The amount of blood flow to a tumor is a determinant of this temperature response (30,31). Temperature and blood flow are inversely related. By occluding blood flow to a given area, the cooling effect of blood flow on perivascular tumor cells is therefore minimized (32). As previously mentioned, open RFA is often combined with surgical resection of tumors that are too large to ablate in one lobe, and ablation of smaller tumors in the opposite lobe. Radiofrequency ablation of hepatic tumors is often accompanied by a transient 2- to 3-fold elevation above baseline in serum liver function tests. These values return to normal within 1 month of the procedure.

The anesthetic management for laparoscopic RFA is essentially routine anesthetic management for laparoscopy. Laparoscopy and pneumoperitoneum induce a number of pathophysiologic changes that have been described in detail elsewhere. Emphasis on the placement of the grounding pads is important to prevent thermal injury to the patient. Our practice is to place four pads in symmetric positions on the patient's thighs.

X. ETHANOL INJECTION THERAPY

Injection of pure ethanol (absolute alcohol) into a tumor causes cell dehydration, protein denaturation, coagulative necrosis, and small vessel occlusion. An injection of 0.5 mL of absolute ethanol results in a 1 cm area of necrosis (33). The advantages of ethanol injection include safety, simplicity, repeatability, and minimal expense. Additionally, it causes minimal damage to the surrounding uninvolved liver parenchyma. Ethanol injection can be used for vascular tumors of the liver.

In patients with HCC, ethanol injection resulted in 1-, 3-, and 5-year survival rates of 94–97%, 47–68%, 26–40%, respectively (34). Ethanol injection is particularly effective in focal HCC because the tumor is soft and vascular. The soft consistency of the tumor promotes distribution of the ethanol and vascular necrosis. Additionally, HCC is very vascular so that ethanol not only causes dehydration and necrosis of the tumor cells, but also tumor ischemia as ethanol enters the arterial circulation resulting in small vessel thrombosis.

Ethanol injection can also be performed percutaneously under ultrasound guidance. The amount of ethanol to be injected is calculated based on the size of the tumor. However, because of pain, the patient may not tolerate injection of the total calculated amount. The patient may have to undergo several injections before the entire volume is injected. Additionally, ethanol may also be injected during laparotomy. The systemic absorption of ethanol is variable, thus, ethanol injection may affect the patient's mental status in the postoperative period. Platelet counts should be followed after ethanol injection, as the platelet count tends to drop after ethanol injection.

XI. HEPATIC ARTERY INFUSION

Hepatic artery infusion (HAI) of chemotherapeutic agents is sometimes used to treat nonresectable liver tumors, or as an adjuvant therapy after liver resection. Intrahepatic delivery of chemotherapeutic drugs has several advantages in that liver metastases are perfused primarily by the hepatic artery (whereas the normal liver parenchyma is perfused by both the hepatic artery and portal vein) (35), and high local drug concentrations can be achieved delivering drug directly to the liver via the hepatic artery with minimal systemic toxicity. This may prevent the stepwise progression of metastases confined to the liver from spreading to the lungs and other organs, thus prolonging patient survival. Intrahepatic drug delivery is especially useful in drugs with a steep dose–response curve and those with a high total body clearance.

The side effects of systemic chemotherapeutic agents are infrequent with HAI delivery. The most common problems associated with HAI are hepatic toxicity and ulcer disease (36,37).

Preoperative preparation of patients for HAI pump insertion includes staging of their disease to rule out extrahepatic disease, arteriogram, preoperative bowel preparation, and intravenous antibiotics. A small midline incision is made to expose the vessels. The arterial catheter is usually placed in the gastroduodenal artery as opposed to the hepatic artery since direct placement of the catheter into the hepatic artery risks thrombosis of the vessel.

Anesthetic management for placement of the HAI pump is the same as for any routine intra-abdominal surgery. The anesthetic should be tailored to the patient's pre-existing condition(s). Complications associated with HAI pump placement are the same as those associated with laparotomy and include atelectasis, pneumonia, urinary tract infection, and wound infection.

ACKNOWLEDGMENTS

The authors would like to recognize the superb surgical expertise of the two liver surgeons with whom they worked primarily, Drs. Steven Curley and Jean-Nicholas Vauthey. They also recognize the professionalism and expertise of the surgical nursing team who facilitate the entire intraoperative course of events.

REFERENCES

1. Curley SA, Cusack JC Jr, Tanabe KK, et al. Advances in the treatment of liver tumors. Curr Probl Surg 2002; 39:449–571.
2. Shumate CR. Hepatic resection for colorectal cancer metastases. In: Curley SA, ed. Liver Cancer. New York, NY: Springer-Verlag, 1998:136–149.
3. Tuttle TM. Hepatectomy for noncolorectal metastases. In: Curley SA, ed. Liver Cancer. New York, NY: Springer-Verlag, 1998:201–211.
4. Farid H, O'Connell T. Hepatic resections: changing mortality and morbidity. Am Surg 1994; 60:748–752.
5. Gozzetti G, Mazziotti A, Grazi GL, et al. Liver resection without blood transfusion. Br J Surg 1995; 82: 1105–1110.
6. Matsumata T, Ikeda Y, Hayashi H, et al. The association between transfusion and cancer-free survival after curative resection for hepatocellular carcinoma. Cancer 1993; 72:1866–1871.
7. Abdalla EK, Denys A, Chevalier P, et al. Total and segmental liver volume variations: implications for liver surgery. Surgery 2004; 135:404–410.
8. Ko S, Nakajima Y, Kanehiro H, et al. Significant influence of accompanying chronic hepatitis status on recurrence of hepatocellular carcinoma after hepatectomy. Result of multivariate analysis. Ann Surg 1996; 224:591–595.
9. Child CG, Turcotte JG. Surgery and portal hypertension. Major Probl Clin Surg 1964; 1:1–85.
10. Pugh RN, Murray-Lyon IM, Dawson JL, et al. Transection of the oesophagus for bleeding oesophageal varices. Br J Surg 1973; 60:646–649.
11. Abdalla EK, Hicks ME, Vauthey JN. Portal vein embolization: rationale, technique and future prospects. Br J Surg 2001; 88:165–175.
12. Edwards WH Jr, Blumgart LH. Liver resection in malignant disease. Semin Surg Oncol 1987; 3:1–11.
13. Norman PH, Daley MD, Hogervorst S, et al. Epidural analgesia for hepatic surgery. Anesthesiology 2003; 99: A1295.
14. Horlocker TT, Wedel DJ, Benzon H, et al. Regional anesthesia in the anticoagulated patient: defining the risks (the second ASRA Consensus Conference on Neuraxial Anesthesia and Anticoagulation). Reg Anesth Pain Med 2003; 28:172–197.
15. Sakamoto Y, Inoue K, Takayama T, Makuuchi M. Perioperative management for patients with chronic liver injury and the strategy for preventing postoperative liver failure. Nippon Geka Gakkai Zasshi 1997; 98:663–666.
16. Man K, Fan ST, Ng IO, et al. Prospective evaluation of Pringle maneuver in hepatectomy for liver tumors by a randomized study. Ann Surg 1997; 226:704–711. Discussion 11–13.
17. Wu CC, Hwang CR, Liu TJ, P'Eng FK. Effects and limitations of prolonged intermittent ischaemia for hepatic resection of the cirrhotic liver. Br J Surg 1996; 83:121–124.
18. Belghiti J, Noun R, Zante E, et al. Portal triad clamping or hepatic vascular exclusion for major liver resection. A controlled study. Ann Surg 1996; 224: 155–161.

19. Guyton AC, Lindsey AW, Abernathy B, Richardson T. Venous return at various right atrial pressures and the normal venous return curve. Am J Physiol 1957; 189: 609–615.
20. Huguet C, Gavelli A, Chieco PA, et al. Liver ischemia for hepatic resection: where is the limit? Surgery 1992; 111:251–259.
21. Roy A, Lapointe R, Dagenais M, et al. [Right diaphragmatic paralysis after liver transplantation]. Ann Chir 1993; 47:810–815.
22. Curley SA. Radiofrequency ablation of malignant liver tumors. Oncologist 2001; 6:14–23.
23. McGahan JP, Brock JM, Tesluk H, et al. Hepatic ablation with use of radio-frequency electrocautery in the animal model. J Vasc Interv Radiol 1992; 3: 291–297.
24. Izzo F, Barnett CC Jr, Curley SA. Radiofrequency ablation of primary and metastatic malignant liver tumors. Adv Surg 2001; 35:225–250.
25. Curley SA, Izzo F, Delrio P, et al. Radiofrequency ablation of unresectable primary and metastatic hepatic malignancies: results in 123 patients. Ann Surg 1999; 230:1–8.
26. Curley SA, Izzo F, Ellis LM, et al. Radiofrequency ablation of malignant liver tumors in 304 patients. Proc ASCO 2000; 248A.
27. Curley SA, Izzo F, Ellis LM, et al. Radiofrequency ablation of hepatocellular cancer in 110 patients with cirrhosis. Ann Surg 2000; 232:381–391.
28. Livraghi T, Goldberg SN, Lazzaroni S, et al. Hepatocellular carcinoma: radio-frequency ablation of medium and large lesions. Radiology 2000; 214:761–768.
29. Livraghi T, Solbiati L, Meloni MF, et al. Treatment of focal liver tumors with percutaneous radio-frequency ablation: complications encountered in a multicenter study. Radiology 2003; 226:441–451.
30. Patterson J, Strang R. The role of blood flow in hyperthermia. Int J Radiat Oncol Biol Phys 1979; 5: 235–241.
31. Kolios MC, Sherar MD, Hunt JW. Large blood vessel cooling in heated tissues: a numerical study. Phys Med Biol 1995; 40:477–494.
32. Sturesson C, Liu DL, Stenram U, Andersson-Engels S. Hepatic inflow occlusion increases the efficacy of interstitial laser-induced thermotherapy in rat. J Surg Res 1997; 71:67–72.
33. Sugiura N, Takara K, Ohto M. [Percutaneous intratumoral injection of ethanol under ultrasound imaging for treatment of small hepatocellular carcinoma]. Acta Hepatologica Japonica 1983; 24:920.
34. Livraghi T, Giorgio A, Marin G, et al. Hepatocellular carcinoma and cirrhosis in 746 patients: long-term results of percutaneous ethanol injection. Radiology 1995; 197:101–108.
35. Breedis C, Young G. The blood supply of neoplasms in the liver. Am J Pathol 1954; 30:969–977.
36. Kemeny N, Daly J, Oderman P, et al. Hepatic artery pump infusion: toxicity and results in patients with metastatic colorectal carcinoma. J Clin Oncol 1984; 2:595–600.
37. Hohn DC, Stagg RJ, Price DC, Lewis BJ. Avoidance of gastroduodenal toxicity in patients receiving hepatic arterial 5-fluoro-2-deoxyuridine. J Clin Oncol 1985; 3:1257–1260.
38. Strasberg SM, Survey ftIH-P-BATC. The Brisbane 2000 Terminology of Liver Anatomy and Resections. HPB 2000; 2:333–339.
39. Abdalla EK, Vauthey JN, Ellis LM, et al. Recurrence and outcomes following hepatic resection, radiofrequency ablation, and combined resection/ablation for colorectal liver metastases. Ann Surg 2004; 239: 818–825.

24

Perioperative Care for Major Abdominal Surgery: Stomach, Pancreas, Small Intestine, Colon, Rectum, Anus

KAREN CHEN
Department of Critical Care, The University of Texas M.D. Anderson Cancer Center, Houston, Texas, U.S.A.

PETER HSU
Department of Anesthesiology, The University of Texas M.D. Anderson Cancer Center, Houston, Texas, U.S.A.

I. INTRODUCTION

Malignancies of the intra-abdominal alimentary tract include cancers of the stomach, pancreas, small intestine, colon, rectum, and anus. The patterns of these tumors are varied, and the treatment for each is unique.

Marked progress has been made in perioperative management. Anesthetic and operative mortalities have been reduced, and extensive resections may now be performed with relative safety. As a result, a substantial increase in the cure rate of gastrointestinal cancers has been achieved (1).

Advances in surgical technique, anesthesia, and supportive services (blood products, antibiotics, fluid and electrolyte management, and post-operative support services) have allowed for increasingly radical and extensive surgeries. The caveat being that these complex procedures should only be undertaken in medical centers that have the multi-disciplinary expertise to support these patients.

In general, cancer patients have the highest incidence of protein-calorie malnutrition seen in hospitalized patients, with significant malnutrition occurring in more than 30% of cancer patients undergoing major upper gastrointestinal procedures. Clinically significant malnutrition occurs as a result of diminished nutritional intake, increased nutrient losses, and tumor-induced derangements in host metabolism. In those patients with malignant obstruction of the gastrointestinal tract, the tumor itself may induce diminished nutrient intake. Current treatment modalities including gastrointestinal resection, chemotherapy, and radiotherapy typically exacerbate these metabolic derangements, further increasing the risk of post-operative morbidity and death. The presence of malnutrition in cancer patients has prognostic importance. In a review of more than 3000 cancer patients, DeWys et al. (2) identified significantly improved survival in those patients who maintained their weight compared to those that had lost 6% of their body weight. Nutrition support is therefore vital to improving nutritional status and thereby reducing the risks of post-operative complications (3).

II. ANESTHESIOLOGIST'S CONCERNS

As with all major operations, good preoperative assessment must be practiced. General considerations should take into account the patient's age, comorbid conditions, exertion tolerance, performance status such as exemplified by the Karnofsky score and risks of the particular procedure. This starts with a thorough history and physical.

Due to the varied nature of the multiple operations, each entails slightly different concerns.

A. Cancers of the Stomach

Adenocarcinoma of the stomach (ACS) is the second most common cancer worldwide. There are two distinct biologic and etiologic subtypes of ACS, the epidemic-intestinal type, and the endemic diffuse-infiltrative type. The epidemic form causes high mortality around the world from Central and South American countries such as Brazil, Chile, Colombia, Costa Rica, and Venezuela to Asian nations such as Korea, Japan, and southern China. Additionally, the prevalence is high in European countries such as Germany, Italy, Iceland, Portugal, and Romania. The highest incidence worldwide is in the nation of Japan and thought to be associated with dietary factors such as food preservation techniques. In the United States, ACS is the 10th most common type of fatal cancer.

The incidence doubles with each decade of life with the male:female ratio being 2:1 in high-risk and 3:2 in low-risk populations.

Environment and diet are major risk factors for ACS, associated with chronic atrophic gastritis and intestinal metaplasia of the gastric mucosa. The ACS is postulated to be a multi-hit mechanism (4).

Heavy smoking in combination with drinking of alcoholic beverages have been associated with the development of ACS, especially in those older than 60 (5). Caffeine intake along with smoking has also been noted to increase the incidence of ACS (6). Interestingly, alcohol alone has not proven to be a carcinogen in the development of ACS.

Symptoms include early satiety, anorexia, and dysphagia. The most common presentation is weight loss followed by epigastric pain followed by nausea and vomiting. These symptoms may have a significant impact on the induction of anesthesia, possibly necessitating a rapid sequence induction or an awake intubation.

Although older patients have an increased risk of gastric carcinoma, they are at much higher risk of complications during surgical intervention. As exemplified by a study by Nagy et al. (7) in older patients (>55 years of age), the duration of post-operative artificial ventilation was significantly longer and the prevalence of septic complication was higher than in younger patients. All post-operative deaths recorded in this series occurred in the group of elderly patients.

In contrast, a study of 792 gastric cancer patients by Dumanski et al. (8) states that the increased risk is not due to the age but rather due to the severity of the primary disease, other coexisiting diseases, and the duration and extensiveness of the operation. They conclude that upon perfection of the surgical and anesthetic techniques, radical surgical intervention is acceptable for all patients to better treat patients with more advanced cancers.

Late complications from ACS include malignant peritoneal and pleural effusions, which may significantly impair the respiratory status of the patient. Other manifestations are obstruction of the gastric outlet; gastroesophagael junction or small bowel; bleeding in the stomach or from esophageal varices; jaundice; distant metastasis; malnutrition and cachexia from tumor load; and thromboembolic events from vascular catheters placed for nutritional supplementation.

Operations longer than 6 hr were associated with significantly longer post-operative ventilation period, need for longer intensive care unit stay and longer post-operative stay. The prevalence of pulmonary complications was proportional to the duration of the operation. An analysis of post-operative data demonstrates that post-operative pain control with a continuous epidural is superior to other methods because it shortens the length of stay in the intensive care unit and the post-operative hospitalization. Nutritional support is essential after esophageal anastomosis till oral feeding can start. One can conclude for that in the treatment of ACS careful selection of patients, appropriate intra- and post-operative management, with adequate post-operative pain control can reduce post-operative morbidity and length of inpatient stay (7).

B. Cancers of the Pancreas

Annually, approximately 150,000 deaths worldwide are attributed to pancreatic cancer, making it one of the five leading causes of cancer-related mortality and one of the most aggressive human tumors. Despite advances in chemotherapy, resection is still the only option that offers a chance of cure for pancreatic cancer patients (9).

Pancreatic cancer is the fifth leading cause of cancer related death for both men and women and is responsible for 5% of all cancer deaths (10). Because of the infrequency of diagnosing localized pancreatic tumors while they are still surgically resectable as well as lack of effective systemic therapies, incidence rates are virtually equal to mortality rates. These tumors have early vascular dissemination, often with subclinical liver metastases not noted on imaging studies.

Patient survival depends on the extent of disease and performance status at diagnosis (11). The extent of disease is best categorized as resectable, locally advanced or metastatic. Survival duration is superior in patients who receive preoperative or post-operative chemoradiation. However, disease recurrence following a potentially curative surgical resection remains relatively common; up to 86% have local recurrence, 25% have peritoneal recurrence and liver metastases occur in 50% (12–14). When surgery and chemoradiation are used to maximize regional tumor control, liver metastases become the dominant form of tumor recurrence and occur in 25–53% of patients (11). As expected, median survival for localized disease is much better than that for metastatic disease with survival ranging from 3 to 6 months.

An increased risk for pancreatic cancer exists in patients of advanced age, male gender, black race and Jewish religion. Most patients that develop pancreatic cancer range between ages 60 and 80 at diagnosis (15). There is a male preponderance in this disease, but the incidence in women is increasing, possibly due to tobacco smoking (10). Overall, pancreatic cancer incidence and mortality statistics are similar throughout the world.

An association between diabetes mellitus and pancreatic cancer has long been postulated, but the exact mechanism has not been elucidated and not all studies support this relationship (16). Some authors postulate that diabetes is an early manifestation of pancreatic cancer (17,18) and others that it is a predisposing factor (19,20). The underlying mechanisms of the association between diabetes mellitus and pancreatic carcinoma remain obscure.

The association between pancreatitis and an increased incidence of pancreatic cancer has been suspected; however, the magnitude of the risk remains uncertain. Chronic pancreatitis patients have a 13- to 18-fold increase in the incidence of pancreatic cancer (21). Somewhat in contrast, Karlson et al. (22) found that after 10 years or more, the excess risk of pancreatic cancer in patients with pancreatitis declined and was of borderline significance. There may be an increased incidence of carcinoma in patients with hereditary pancreatitis (23).

Patients who have undergone surgery for peptic ulcer disease appear to be at an increased risk for pancreatic cancer (24,25). An association may also exist between *Helicobacter pylori* and pancreatic cancer (26).

The management of individuals who are at increased risk of pancreatic cancer remains controversial; the options range from close observation to aggressive surgical intervention (27,28).

The most firmly established risk factor associated with pancreatic cancer is cigarette smoking (29–32). Approximately 30% of pancreatic cancers can be attributed to smoking (33). The risk of pancreatic cancer increases as the amount and duration of smoking increases and long-term (>10 years) smoking cessation reduces risk by 30% compared to current smokers (29,33,34).

Various dietary factors have been implicated in the development of pancreatic carcinoma. In general, high intakes of saturated fats or meats increase risk, whereas high intakes of fruits and vegetables reduce it (35–37). The data on coffee consumption and excessive alcohol intake are conflicting. Some studies have suggested an increased risk (38–41), though most recent literature has failed to prove such an association (19,34,38,42).

Most patients with pancreatic neoplasms present with jaundice due to extrahepatic biliary obstruction. Small tumors in the pancreatic head located near the intrapancreatic bile duct may obstruct and cause the patient to seek medical attention while the tumor is still localized. Unfortunately, most tumors are found after they have become locally advanced or metastatic due to late or no signs of biliary obstruction.

When jaundice is not present, patients complain of nonspecific symptoms. Pain is a frequent complaint: especially dull, constant pain localized to the middle or upper back or vague, intermittent epigastric pain. Other associated symptoms include anorexia, weight loss, fatigue, malabsorption, and steatorrhea. Rarely is diarrhea a major complaint. Patients often present with simultaneous glucose intolerance (43–45). On physical examination, important staging information must be obtained, including performance status, cardiopulmonary function, and the presence or absence of left supraclavicular adenopathy and ascites.

In the preoperative evaluation of these patients, the coexistent disease processes and malnutrition are important. The surgical resection of pancreatic masses is a long, complex procedure; therefore, patients should be optimized from nutritional as well as cardiopulmonary states in order to assure optimal recovery.

C. Cancers of the Small Intestine

The small intestine accounts for nearly 90% of the alimentary tract's mucosal surface area, but it is the site of a small percentage of intestinal neoplasms, and only rarely is a malignancy found (46). The reasons for this may include the rapid transit of contents through the small bowel, local protective mechanisms, or lack of carcinogens in contact with the mucosal surface (47,48). Statistics show that less than 3% of alimentary tract tumors and less than 1% of all malignancies arise from the small bowel (49). In comparison with colorectal cancers, small bowel tumors are 30 times less frequent in incidence; and when comparing mortality rates, colorectal carcinoma accounts for 50 times more loss of life than small bowel tumors.

Most small bowel tumors are benign. These include leiomyoma, adenoma, and lipoma with rare incidences of fibromas, fibromyxomas, neurofibromas, ganglioneuromas, hemangiomas, and lymphangiomas. The malignant tumors include adenocarcinoma, carcinoids, lymphomas, sarcomas, and its subtypes including Kaposi's sarcomas as seen in end-stage human immunodeficiency virus infections.

Many small bowel tumors are asymptomatic until late in the course due to slow growth and the ease with which the contents of the small bowel can pass even with a partially obstructing lesion. Half are incidental findings on autopsy; the remainder present with symptoms of partial obstruction: nausea and vomiting, crampy abdominal pain or nonspecific weight loss. Occult blood loss and microcytic anemia are common presenting signs. Studies reveal that a significant period of time may pass between the onset of symptoms and the definitive diagnosis of small bowel tumors (50,51). Many patients eventually diagnosed with small intestinal tumors present emergently with symptoms of bowel obstruction or perforation. Therefore, a rapid sequence induction or awake intubation often may be needed in these patients. Unfortunately, many of these patients may be malnourished or dehydrated with multiple electrolyte abnormalities, but due to the emergent nature of the operation optimization may not be possible. Therefore, understanding of the disease process is essential in the care of these fragile patients.

The diagnosis of these tumors is usually made with the aid of imaging studies. Contrast or barium studies or computed tomography scans are usually the best in diagnosing these lesions (52,53).

The treatment of small bowel tumors is usually surgical, with simple resection for benign lesions and more aggressive surgery for malignant lesions. Overall, the survival for adenocarcinomas, carcinoids, lymphomas and sarcomas was better in 328 cases from a population based registry than for all other organs, only surpassed by cancers of the prostate, breast, and colorectum (54).

Endocrine tumors of the gut, also known as carcinoid tumors, may present with a different set of symptoms, including flushing, diarrhea, cyanosis and intermittent respiratory distress. Fortunately, only a small percentage of patients have these symptoms with the remainder either asymptomatic or have symptoms of obstruction.

In those with the carcinoid syndrome, pretreatment with the synthetic somatostatin analog octreotide has proven beneficial in preventing the symptoms of a carcinoid crisis (55).

D. Cancers of the Colon and Rectum

Cancers of the colon and rectum are now the second most common causes of death from cancer in the United States (56). A decline in both incidence and mortality is in progress (57). Advances in colonoscopy, multi-modality adjuvant primary treatment of colon cancer, and curative resections with supplementary therapy all have played a role in bringing the decline in mortality. Application of large bowel screening using both tests for fecal occult blood and periodic endoscopy in known genetic and age-defined high-risk groups have allowed for surgical interruption of the carcinogenic process (58). Genetic and marker studies seek to define a higher risk population to undergo regular colorectal mucosal surveillance to diagnose and remove polyps before they undergo carcinogenic transformation. Screening with or without genetic guidance has proven cost effective.

The estimated number of new cases of colorectal cancer in the United States for 2000 was 130,200. Cancer of the colon will account for 27,800 male and 28,500 female deaths (56). Colorectal cancer survival falls as tumor grade and age increase. Males do slightly worse so there may be some protective benefits of female hormones (59). Hypotheses postulating the association of high dietary fat intake in the etiology of colon cancer and the protective role of dietary fiber continue to be supported (60,61). Dietary calcium may have a protective role in the development of colorectal cancer, at least partly because of the conversion of fecal bile acids to insoluble salts (62). Other theories including a high potassium to sodium intake ratio may be beneficial in the prevention of colorectal cancer (63). Other environmental factors linked to colorectal cancer include alcohol usage, tobacco exposure, and certain occupational exposures such as those to glass and brewery workers.

The estimated proportion of colorectal cancers that is attributable to hereditary causes varies between 5% and 20% (64). Some inherited familial polyposes include Gardner's syndrome, Peutz-Jeghers syndrome, Turcot's syndrome and juvenile polyposis.

Chemopreventive agents seek to block the action of carcinogens during the latent period before the appearance of cancer (65). Antioxidants are considered to be agents suitable for chemoprevention trials because they block oxidative damage to DNA resulting from free radical formation (65). Unfortunately, two large clinical trials did not show a statistically significant advantage in susceptible populations (66,67).

On the other hand, both aspirin and NSAID's have been linked to a 50% reduction in the incidence of colon cancer, but none of these trials were randomized-control trials (68). Most cancers in the large bowel are adenocarcinomas with two-thirds of these cancers located in the rectum, rectosigmoid or sigmoid colon. The remaining third is found in the remainder of the colon (69). Many of these cancers begin as adenomatous polyps. Recently, there has been a proximal migration in the occurrence of colon cancers. This statistical change is due to the decline in the incidence of rectal cancers for unknown reasons. Incidentally, squamous carcinoma and adenosquamous carcinomas have also been reported but these are rare (70).

Due to the location of the tumor, patients' presentations differ. Often these symptoms reveal large tumors, which have grown undetected because of avoided, or omitted rectal examinations, fecal occult blood tests, sigmoidoscopies or colonoscopies. Thus, patients who present with anemia of unknown origin should have an examination of both the upper and lower gastrointestinal tract, preferably by endoscopy. During active bleeding, the sequence of evaluation should be based on the patient's symptoms, the rapidity and acuity of bleeding and which other studies have already been performed. In general, colonoscopy is preferred over radiographic examinations and a full colonoscopy is preferable to a sigmoidoscopy. Hemorrhoids and constipation are common ailments. A bleeding hemorrhoid may obfuscate a more proximal bleeding source.

Anemia is the most common indication of cecal and right colon cancers and may be the only clue leading to early diagnosis. While some patients may present with abdominal pain or have a palpable mass on physical examination, others may present with fever of unknown origin, a sign of an abscess resulting from a perforated, ascending colonic tumor. In young familial cancers, metastatic disease may be the first sign.

In contrast, the most common symptom in descending or sigmoid colon and middle to upper rectum circumferential adenocarcinoma is an alteration in bowel habit. New bouts of constipation or diarrhea or alternating periods of both is usually the first sign. This may be accompanied by abdominal cramping, which may be mild, severe, or chronic. Occasionally, patients present with the classic "pencil" or "ribbon" stool, due to an almost totally constricting adenocarcinoma. This presentation is more common in the younger patient. Younger individuals with colorectal cancer have been reported to have worse prognosis stage for stage, usually due to a more aggressive tumor (71).

On the other hand, patients with distal rectal carcinomas may present with spotting of blood in their stool, especially during the early stages of development. Numerous benign and inflammatory lesions may also present with similar symptoms. Physical examination should include a digital examination and endoscopy of the anus, rectum, and sigmoid. More advanced symptoms may include tenesmus, the feeling of having to defecate without stool in the anal canal, or pain on defecation. These symptoms often reflect an ulcerated tumor and often invasion of the superficial sphincter muscle by the cancer. An abdominoperineal resection with colostomy is the primary treatment once diagnosis has been established.

Once surgical intervention is contemplated, initial work-up should include a good history and physical examination, including a pertinent family history. Establishment of a risk factor should increase the suspicion of the examiner. Digital and when appropriate, endoscopic examination should be part of every work-up. Endoscopic screening of the large bowel and rectum should be performed in every patient presenting with symptoms (72,73). The major advantage of endoscopy is increased specificity and sensitivity, with the additional advantage of obtaining a biopsy if a lesion is seen and possibly even one-step definitive treatment.

In the preoperative work-up, other tests may be needed. These include but are not limited to CEA, liver function tests, CT or MRI scan or even a PET scan. Pathologic examination is the major source of prognostic parameters, which includes tumor depth, invasion, and the presence or absence of lymph node involvement. Other important tests include those aimed to delineate the extent of coexistent diseases. Diagnostic and therapeutic maneuvers to improve cardiopulmonary function should be executed. Colorectal surgery, with the exception of complete obstruction, is not an emergency. Diagnostic tests that starve the patient and contribute to weight loss should be avoided, since low residue dietary supplements are available.

Overall evaluation of the patient prior to surgery is the key to success. Therapeutic plans should be established before surgery is commenced. Considerations should include the patient's age, comorbid conditions, and risk of a given surgical procedure.

E. Cancers of the Anus

Cancer in the anal area is rare, with only 2–3% of large bowel tumors arising in this area (56), though recent data suggest the incidence is increasing (74).

In the majority of patients, no etiologic factor has been identified. Though such factors as anal intercourse and the human papilloma virus may be associated with anal carcinoma (75–77).

Immunosuppresion clearly increases the risk of developing anal carcinomas (78). In patients who have anal carcinomas, a higher association with smoking has been noted (75,79). Others have postulated an antiestrogenic mechanism of smoking in anal carcinogenesis (80).

III. SURGICAL CONCERNS

A. Cancers of the Stomach

Gastric carcinomas are classified according to the long axis of the stomach. Approximately 42% (30–65%) of cancers arise in the lower part, 39% in the middle part (half body and half fundus), 16% in the upper part, and approximately 10% (10–20%) in the entire organ. Based on the short axis, 39% involve the lesser curvature, 17% the posterior wall, 12% the anteroinferior wall, 11% the greater curvature, and 10–20% the entire organ. The upper third, the gastroesophagael junction lesions, can be further divided into three subgroups: (i) distal esophageal, (ii) cardiac (true junction), and (iii) subcardial-fundus (81,82).

Cancers found in the upper and middle stomach are usually more advanced, as the more invasive endemic variant is located here. Both the pattern and frequency of spread of adenocarcinomas of the stomach are highly predictable. Therefore, the design of surgery and regional chemoradiation is based on this. Local contiguous extension is common with invasion through the wall and to adjacent organs (spleen, pancreas, bile duct, liver, transverse colon). Direct extension into the duodenum accompanies 25% of distal tumors (83). Local and regional relapse may occur in 70% of patients with initial invasion of surrounding organs. The risk of local failure is an important consideration and constitutes an indication for extensive resection of esophagus or duodenum when affected.

Lymph node metastases occur when a tumor invades lymphatics within the gastric wall and enters the lymph nodes. These lymph node metastases are critical in staging, prognostication, and surgery. It is imperative that the surgeon obtains adequate introperative biopsies of lymph nodes because of the possibility of declaring inoperability in a patient with enlarged reactive lymph nodes without metastases.

Peritoneal carcinomatosis is the most common form of distant metastasis for adenocarcinoma of the stomach. More than 50% have initial or clinically significant failure in the peritoneum. Debulking, when it does not increase the risk of surgery, is recommended because survival based on observation alone is not promising.

Gastric cancers metastasize to the liver via the portal vein (40%) and are carried to other organs such as lung and bone. Large metastases tend to form in the liver and diffuse small metastases in the lungs.

There is a large difference in the surgical technique for gastric cancer between Western and Asian populations. The survival in the Japanese is far greater than that noted in the Western world. There are few centers in the United States that have developed expertise in the treatment of gastric cancer. Therefore, outcome may be significantly improved by a surgeon who performs the procedure frequently.

Gastric cancers are extremely varied, and surgical techniques vary depending on the tumor, location, invasiveness, and patient's medical condition. In Japan, surgeons advocate extensive surgical resection. Often guided by computer-derived algorithms based on tumor location, histology, and differentiation, they are performing more extensive surgery with decreasing mortality (83).

Some patients with gastric cancer may benefit from staging laparoscopy with a placement of a feeding jejunostomy tube if the patient is not undergoing immediate resection (84). During staging laparoscopy, a significant portion of patients (up to 23%) may have peritoneal disease that were originally deemed resectable by imaging studies.

A potentially curative operation (resection stage 0, R_0) is defined as complete removal of all gross disease with a negative margin of resection. An R_1 resection is one performed with residual microscopic disease. An R_2 resection is one in which gross residual disease is left behind such as liver metastases. Patients with localized disease are most likely to benefit from surgery, and conversely the patients most likely to be long-term survivors are those that undergo resection.

The various types of gastrectomy include: (1) subtotal gastrectomy (used in tumors of the antrum or distal body), (2) total gastrectomy, and (3) proximal subtotal gastrectomy or esophago-gastrectomy either via transperitoneal or transthoracic approach.

In most circumstances, survival for those who have a total gastrectomy is better, but nutritionally those who undergo a subtotal gastrectomy fare better. The goals of gastric cancer surgery are to obtain negative margins and preserve as much function as possible. In contrast, a study by Gouzi in France failed to show any benefit in survival of total gastrectomy over subtotal gastrectomy in patients with distal stomach lesions. Therefore, subtotal gastrectomy is the procedure of choice if the distal gastric tumor can be removed with negative margins since these patients have better nutritional outcome.

The macroscopic and histologic boundaries of cancer are different. For example, 2 cm beyond the macroscopic margin of a superficial tumor, 3 cm beyond that of a localized cancer and 5 cm beyond that of an infiltrating tumor are considered acceptable. In tumors of the lower stomach, it is necessary to resect the pyloric ring and at least 2 cm of the duodenum.

Lesions of the gastroesophagael junction are divided into three groups for surgical considerations: (a) Barrett's (esophageal dysplasia), (b) the cardia, and (c) the fundal primary (81). The major concern of a proximal gastrectomy over a esophagogastrectomy is the lack of a complete nodal dissection of the lesser curvature. Thus, unless too much esophagus must be resected and the distal stomach is used as the conduit, a total gastrectomy is preferable.

Operations of the proximal stomach and cardia tumors are considered palliative. There may be a role for surgery in less advanced, proximal lesions particularly when combined with preoperative chemoradiotherapy. More investigation is needed to determine the extent of resection and adjuvant therapy required. In Japan, extensive lymph node dissections are considered standard. In Germany and the United States, most surgeons prefer more conservative procedures, but they still recommend different procedures for each part of the stomach (81,85,86). Most expert Western surgeons still favor radical subtotal gastrectomy, thus preserving the spleen, but do undertake en bloc resections for patients when this is the only way to remove all recognizable tumor (85). For noninvasive gastric cancer, surgery alone is sufficient with a 96% survival rate.

Gastric cancers can directly extend into adjacent organs. These patients require a combined resection for cure; this may include partial hepatectomy, and resections of the pancreatic head, duodenum, or transverse colon. More aggressively, in Japan, pancreatic tail resections and splenectomy are planned procedures for advanced cancers of the proximal stomach (85). Resection of two or more adjacent organs in advanced gastric adenocarcinoma is associated with a greater risk of developing a complication. Achieving an R_0 resection should still be considered the goal, even in locally advanced gastric cancer, but resection of additional organs should be performed judiciously (87).

Techniques for anastomosis after total gastrectomy include esophagojejunostomy, Roux-en-Y, as well as various loop procedures and various jejunal interpositions. Some people advocate the jejunal interposition technique for those with an excellent prognosis due to the improved nutritional status of these patients. There is no significant difference in leakage rates between sewn vs. stapled anastomosis; acceptable complication rates range from 4% to 8%. Therefore, anastomotic technique should be left to the surgeon's preference. In the western hemisphere, only 50% of patients present with resectable tumors, 33% undergo open-and-close laparotomy, and 15–20% have some palliative procedure (81,83).

Palliative procedures are undertaken to increase the patient's comfort and not with the intent of cure. Attempts at curative surgery are inappropriate for patients with metastases to remote distant lymph nodes, peritoneal carcinomatosis, unresectable hepatic metastases, pulmonary metastases, or direct extension into organs that cannot be completely resected. Palliative surgery includes wide local excision, partial gastrectomy, total gastrectomy, gastrointestinal anastomosis, and bypass. These procedures are undertaken with the goals of oral intake of food, alleviation of pain, and removal of the primary tumor as much as possible. Resection of the primary cancer is performed for emergency treatment for hemorrhage, chronic blood loss, stenosis, or perforation and rarely, for pain. Unfortunately, criteria for selecting the specific palliative procedure are not well definied. The patient's performance status, general health, extent of disease, likelihood to respond to adjuvant therapy should all factor into the clinical decision-making process for palliative surgery (83).

Palliative surgery may produce more morbidity than primary surgery; therefore, strict criteria for eligibility should be identified. Unexplained poor performance, deteriorating vital organ function, or rapidly increasing ascites do not respond well to palliative surgery. As a general rule, if no significant symptoms exist, palliative surgery should not be pursued. Well-selected palliative surgery is cost effective. It does not increase total cost of care compared with no surgery if the patient is relatively young, has tumor of the body or antrum, and is node negative (88). Although the median survival is only 10 months, failure to perform this procedure decreases the median survival time by two-thirds.

B. Cancers of the Pancreas

Almost all malignant neoplasms of pancreatic origin (95%) arise from the exocrine pancreas and have features consistent with adenocarcinoma (89). Infiltration of perineural spaces is characteristic of pancreatic adenocarcinoma (90,91). Once the tumor involves the superior mesenteric artery, infiltration of this neural plexus is characteristic. Extended pancreatic resection that requires arterial resection fails to achieve a negative margin and has not improved survival duration (92).

The use of laparoscopy remains controversial. With high-quality CT imaging, only 4–15% of patients are found to have CT occult extrapancreatic disease (93–95). Therefore, the routine use of laparoscopy would not be beneficial in most patients.

Diagnostic and therapeutic endoscopic biliary decompression is performed in the majority of pancreatic cancer patients prior to definitive treatment planning. In patients who are brought to the operating room for a planned pancreaticoduodenectomy, who are found to have locally advanced or metastatic disease, an operative biliary bypass may be done. At our institution, the preferred choice is a Roux-en-Y choledochojejunostomy. For patients who have locally advanced or metastatic disease based on imaging techniques, debate remains over the benefits of surgical bypass vs. endoscopic stenting (96–98). Thereby, a selective approach to biliary decompression should be based on tumor burden and patient's performance status (99). A multidisciplinary approach to the management of these patients is essential; it is imperative to keep an open dialogue between the medical oncologist, gastroenterologist, interventional radiologist, and surgeon.

Accurate preoperative assessment of resectability is the most critical aspect of the diagnostic and treatment sequence for patients with pancreatic cancer. If the primary tumor cannot be resected completely, surgery provides no survival advantage. However, only 30–50% of patients who undergo the procedure with curative intent have their tumors successfully removed; most are found to have unsuspected liver or peritoneal metastases or local invasion of the mesenteric vessels (100–102). For those who undergo laparotomy and are found to have unresectable disease, this procedure results in a perioperative morbidity rate of 20–30%, a mean hospital stay between 1 and 2 weeks and a median survival after surgery of only 6 months (101,103,104). In contrast to the case for gastric or colorectal cancer, there is no benefit for palliative resection in pancreatic adenocarcinoma.

The standard surgical resection for malignant tumors of the pancreatic head and periampullary region is pancreaticoduodenectomy, which involves removal of the pancreatic head, duodenum, gallbladder, and bile duct with or without removal of the gastric antrum. The current technique has evolved from the procedure first described by Whipple et al. (105) in 1935.

In our institution, a bilateral subcostal or midline incision is made by which the abdomen is carefully examined to exclude extrapancreatic disease. The need for frozen section lymph node biopsy analysis remains controversial. Positive lymph nodes are a prognostic factor predictive of decreased survival duration (106–108). However, 60–90% of specimens are found to have microscopic metastases on permanent frozen section specimens (109–111). Therefore, in a low-to-moderate risk patient with localized resectable disease, lymph node metastases are not an absolute contraindication to pancreaticoduodenectomy when used in a combined modality treatment plan. On the other hand, a high risk patient (due to other coexisting medical morbidities or oncologic concerns) with suspicious adenopathy, a positive regional lymph node may be viewed as a contraindication to surgery.

The technique of pancreaticoduodenectomy currently used in the United States incorporates selected aspects of the traditional Whipple procedure and emphasizes the importance of removing all soft tissue to the right side of the superior mesenteric artery (112). The high incidence of local recurrence after standard pancreaticoduodenectomy requires that close attention be paid to the retroperitoneal margin (also referred to as the mesenteric margin).

Despite the use of post-operative adjuvant external beam radiotherapy and 5-florouracil chemotherapy after pancreaticoduodenectomy for localized tumor, disease recurs in the tumor bed in up to 50% of patients (113). The available data regarding the efficacy of intraoperative radiotherapy (IORT) are derived from retrospective or prospective single center studies and one small randomized trial (114–117). The results of these studies indicate that IORT can be safely combined with pancreaticoduodenectomy and current chemoradiation regimens. Although local control may be improved with IORT, marked increases in survival have not been demonstrated.

After pancreaticoduodenectomy with or without IORT, gastrointestinal reconstruction is performed in a counterclockwise direction (112,118). Two recognized complications associated with gastrointestinal reconstruction after pancreaticoduodenectomy are leak at the pancreaticojejunostomy and delayed gastric emptying, which may be more common after pylorus preservation surgery (119). These patients with delayed gastric emptying complain of nausea, vomiting, and post-prandial fullness; which virtually resolves in 4–12 weeks in all patients. Therefore, routinely placing gastrostomy and jejunostomy tubes at the time of surgery avoids patient morbidity due to temporary gastric emptying dysfunction. In this way, patients can be discharged from the hospital while they are receiving enteral feeding and allowed to progress to oral diet at their own pace as tolerated.

Prognostic factors in patients with localized, potentially resectable disease are used to guide treatment recommendations especially in those patients with other comorbid conditions. However, it does not guide the usage of adjuvant therapy. Since up to 80% of patients develop recurrence after a curative pancreaticoduodenectomy, all patients with exocrine pancreatic cancer should receive adjuvant therapy regardless of pathologic findings (120). The prognostic factors include the radiographic appearance of local tumor extension as it predicts the eventual margin of resection status (107,110,121). The most important margin is the retroperitoneal or mesenteric margin along the right lateral border of the superior mesenteric artery. Other prognostic factors predictive of decreased survival rate include metastatic disease in regional lymph nodes, poorly differentiated histology and increased size of the primary tumor. Other factors that have been examined but in multi-variate analysis did not show any significance include the number of red cell transfusions and operative time (107,110). These probably reflect tumor characteristics, namely the larger tumors with less likelihood of a clear margin resection.

Adjuvant therapy may be initiated either preoperatively or post-operatively. The Gastrointestinal Tumor Study Group (GITSG) was the first to study the strategy of post-operative adjuvant chemoradiation to improve survival duration in pancreatic cancer patients. The data showed a survival advantage for those that received adjuvant therapy (122). Subsequently, other groups have reached similar results showing that adjuvant therapy improves survival duration (108,123–126).

Because of the risk that planned post-operative adjuvant therapy will be delayed or not delivered due to unforeseen medical or surgical complications (108,123,127), some institutions initiated studies of chemoradiation administered preoperatively (128,129). The results suggest that preoperative adjuvant therapy has some advantages (120): 1) because chemotherapy and radiation are given first, delayed surgical recovery has no impact on the delivery of multi-modality therapy (14,130); 2) due to the high frequency of retroperitoneal positive-margin resections, surgical excision is not adequate therapy for most patients (108,121); 3) patients found to have distant metastases on restaging imaging studies will not be subject to an unnecessary laparotomy (14). Utilizing a preoperative (neoadjuvant) approach, overall treatment time is reduced, a greater proportion of patients receive all components of therapy, and patients with rapidly progressive disease are spared the side effects of surgery as metastatic disease may be found at restaging following chemoradiation (prior to surgery) (131).

Despite its potential benefits, preoperative chemoradiation is associated with toxicities. In one study, up to one-third of the patients required a hospital admission for the gastrointestinal side effects of the chemotherapy (132). The Eastern Cooperative Oncology Group reported 51% of patients required a hospital admission during or within 4 weeks of the therapy (126). The small survival advantage seen with chemoradiation and surgery compared with surgery alone likely stems from the improved local and regional control of the tumor. Since pancreatic cancer responds poorly to 5-FU based chemotherapy, more promise is being shown by gemcitabine, a deoxycytidine capable of inhibiting DNA replication and repair. In patients with advanced pancreatic cancer, gemcitabine shows better results than 5-FU (133). In addition, this study showed better control of symptomatology (weight gain, pain control, performance status). Gemcitabine is also a potent radiation sensitizer of human pancreatic cancer cells. Gemcitabine has a prolonged inhibitory effect on DNA synthesis of tumors compared to normal tissues when combined with irradiation (134). The results of gemcitabine with locally advanced pancreatic cancer suggest that gemcitabine may be a useful adjunctive therapy.

In summary, pancreaticoduodenectomy should only be performed in patients whose tumors appear to be resectable on high quality CT imaging studies and who have a good Karnofsky performance score. In addition, adjuvant chemoradiation and combined multi-modality therapy should be used in addition to surgery, being preoperatively or post-operatively. Due to the lower mortality rates in centers with vast experiences with these procedures, patients with a potentially resectable disease should be referred to a center that performs at least five such procedures a year (135–137). Specialized centers have reported improved hospital morbidity, mortality and survival after pancreaticoduodenectomy; however, disease-specific survival after surgical resection remains dismal. An emphasis, therefore, has been placed upon the accurate preoperative staging of patients in order to identify those patients who would benefit from a complete surgical resection. Surgical staging that incorporates the use of laparoscopic techniques now complements nonsurgical methods of staging, including helical CT scans. While there is no defined preoperative staging approach, it is imperative that centers identify areas of expertise and experience with available modalities in any combination to effect accurate staging. Once patients have been accurately staged and deemed resectable, there exist various methods for resection of pancreas lesions, which include the standard "Whipple procedure," pylorus-preserving pancreaticoduodenectomy, regional pancreatectomy, total pancreatectomy, and en bloc vascular resection, where appropriate (138).

Due to recent advances in operative technique, anesthesia and critical care, the 30-day in-hospital mortality rate is less than 2% for pancreaticoduodenectomy when performed at major referral centers by experienced staff (107,139,140). In contrast, data from some university medical centers and the Department of Veterans Affairs report mortality rates ranging from 7.8% to more than 10% (141–143). Other studies have demonstrated that higher patient volume is associated with lower surgical mortality rates (135,144). Birkmeyer et al. (136,137) suggested a linear relationship between surgical volume and outcome, stating that the referral of pancreatic cancer patients to high-volume hospitals (defined as those hospitals performing more than five pancreaticoduodenectomies per year) could potentially prevent more than 100 deaths per year. Furthermore, in an analysis of survival duration, after adjustment for case mix and perioperative deaths, Birkmeyer et al. (137) found that those that underwent surgery at high-volume centers had a lower late mortality rate. In conclusion, the authors suggest that those patients considering a pancreaticoduodenectomy at low-volume hospitals be given the option for referral to high-volume centers.

Recent studies have highlighted the correlation between the number of pancreatic resections per year and post-operative mortality. Thus, large centers of pancreatic surgery have mortality rates below 5%, whereas centers with lower caseloads have mortality rates exceeding 10%. Standards have been established for the surgical treatment of pancreatic cancer; however, these are often not based on evidence derived from randomized, controlled studies. Resection for pancreatic cancer is carried out if there are no metastases present and if the tumor is locally resectable; i.e., if there is no complex vessel invasion. However, an isolated infiltration of the portal vein is not considered a contraindication for surgery (9).

As illustrated in a large-volume, single-institution review of 616 patients, examining factors influencing long-term survival, completeness of resection and tumor characteristics including tumor size and degree of differentiation are important independent prognostic indicators. Adjuvant chemoradiation is a strong predictor of outcome and likely decreases the independent significance of tumor location and nodal status (145).

Some patients with unresectable pancreatic carcinoma may present with gastric outlet obstruction. Currently, controversy exists regarding the necessity of gastric bypass either via laparotomy or laparoscopy vs. conservative management with observation after endoscopic biliary decompression (146–148). The primary goal for palliative interventions in patients with advanced pancreatic cancer should be to relieve symptoms such as pain, obstructive jaundice or the development of gastric outlet obstruction with minimal morbidity and to maintain or improve the quality of life for patients with an expected limited survival (149).

C. Cancers of the Small Intestine

In most instances, the surgical resection must include wide margins, resection of lymph nodes, and removal of the supporting mesentery. Lymphadenectomy is usually not necessary in leiomyosarcoma due to its lack of lymphatic metastases. Duodenal tumors may require pancreaticoduodenectomy if malignant, whereas tumors of the terminal ileum may require a right hemicolectomy to ensure resection and wide margins.

The most common benign tumor of the small bowel is the leimyoma. Accounting for 22% of all benign small bowel tumors in one series (150). These usually present with obstruction or with bleeding. Bleeding was seen in 40–67% and obstruction in 25–40% (151,152). Differentiation of the leiomyoma from that of leiomyosarcoma may be difficult therefore treatment should consist of surgical resection with wide margins, typically of 5 cm or more.

The second most common benign tumor of the small bowel is the lipoma, which accounts for about 20% of such tumors (152). Approximately 60% of the lipomas are found in the ileum, with the remainder equally divided between the duodenum and jejunum (153). Intussusception is the cause of surgical exploration in 50% of these cases. Treatment consists of local excision for small tumors and segmental resections for larger tumors.

Adenomas make up about 14% of small bowel benign tumors (152). Occasionally, adenomas cause symptoms by acting as the leading point for intussusception. These are most commonly located in the duodenum, usually picked up by endoscopy. Many consider these premalignant and almost all specimens greater than 5 cm contain malignant changes. Concurrent anemia, jaundice, and duodenal obstruction are predictive of malignancy (154).

Hemangiomas represent about 10% of benign small bowel tumors (152,155,156). Seventy percent of patients present with bleeding, but intussusception and obstruction can also occur (156,157). Treatment consists of resection of the lesion; though preoperative angiography may be helpful in localizing the precise site of bleeding.

Lymphangiomas, which are malformations of sequestered lymphatic tissue that fail to communicate with the normal lymphatic system, may be up to 4% of small bowel tumors (157–160). They most commonly present with obstruction, but occasionally with GI bleeding (161,162). Primary resection with adequate margins and primary anastomosis appears to be appropriate and adequate therapy.

Adenocarcinomas are the most common malignant tumors in the small bowel. They usually present late in life, around the seventh decade, and are found equally in the duodenum and jejunum (45%) each and least commonly in the ileum. The etiology of adenocarcinomas is unclear, although they have been associated with nontropical sprue (163,164) and regional enteritis (165,166). There is a slightly increased risk for tumors associated with Crohn's disease to occur in the terminal ileum, and they usually occur 10 years younger than the general population (167,168). Celiac sprue is known to predispose to intestinal lymphoma but it has also been associated with adenocarcinoma (164).

Symptoms of adenocarcinoma of the small bowel range from obstructive symptoms, such as vomiting and jaundice for those with duodenal tumors, to indistinct abdominal pain, weight loss, and anemia for more distal lesions. Pain is the most common complaint manifested in about 30–70% of patients. Weight loss is noted in about 50%. Obstruction is found in up to 70% and 71% had overt or clinical evidence of gastrointestinal tract bleeding (169).

Metastases occur via the lymphatics, hematogenously or by direct extension through the serosal surfaces into the peritoneal cavity. Adenocarcinomas tend to present late with either lymph node involvement or distant metastases (170).

The primary treatment of adenocarcinomas is surgical removal, including lymph nodes and vascular pedicle. A 5 cm margin of resection is considered acceptable. Depending on the location of the tumor, a hemicolectomy or even a pancreaticoduodenectomy may be deemed necessary. Even with such aggressive surgical resection, five-year survival in patients with node-positive disease is quite dismal at about 30% (171,172).

If the tumor is deemed inoperable, introperative radiotherapy may be beneficial in centers specialized for this (173). Other alternatives include external beam radiation or chemotherapy usually with 5-fluorouracil and nitrosoureas.

The carcinoid is an infrequently seen but well-studied tumor of the small bowel. They commonly occur in the small intestine as well as in the appendix, stomach, and rectum. Unlike adenocarcinomas, they usually arise in the distal small intestine rather than the more proximal segments with a slight male preponderance and usually in the sixth decade of life (174,175).

Most common presenting symptoms include intermittent abdominal pain, nausea, vomiting, bleeding and diarrhea (176). Around 30% of patients with carcinoid tumors will present with metastatic disease, with size as a good potential predictor of metastasis (176). Treatment consists of aggressive surgical resection. In this special subset of population, pretreatment with the synthetic somatostatin analog, octreotide, helps to prevent carcinoid crisis (55).

Gastrointestinal stromal tumors are a group of neoplasms derived from embryonic mesoderm. Malignant gatrointestinal stromal tumors, also known as sarcomas, constitute about 20% of malignant small bowel tumors (150). Most present either with symptoms of bowel obstruction or as GI bleeding. They usually present in patients older than 50 years, with no gender preference. Due to the rapid growth of these tumors, they often outgrow their blood supply, become necrotic and ulcerate, thereby explaining the chronic blood loss and microcytic anemia noted in these patients (177).

As with other tumors of the small bowel, the primary treatment of these tumors is surgical resection with wide margins. With sarcomas, lymph node dissection is not as critical, as lymphatic spread is rare. Other adjuvant treatment in patients with sarcoma includes radiation therapy, though lower doses are usually tolerated in the abdomen and chemotherapy with doxorubicin-based regimens (178).

Primary lymphomas of the GI tract only account for about 5% of all lymphomas, but 20–25% of all primary small bowel tumors found at laparotomy are lymphomas (179). Symptoms are similar to other tumors of the small bowel, including abdominal pain, nausea, vomiting and GI bleeding, occult, or frank. Presentation with an acute abdomen due to perforation may occur in some patients (177). Others may present with systemic signs of lymphoma, such as fever and lymphadenopathy. Diagnosis is aided with a CT scan with oral contrast. Treatment of these tumors should be surgical resection with adjuvant chemotherapy. In patients with unresectable lymphoma, radiation and chemotherapy are recommended (180).

Possible causes of small bowel lymphomas include celiac disease, though this disease association is uncommon (181). Lymphomas have developed following cyclosporine therapy for organ transplant. They usually present on average about 20 months after initiation of cyclosporine. Small bowel involvement was noted in 28% of these patients. All patients responded well to treatment, consisting of resection, conventional chemotherapy and radiation therapy, acyclovir and reduction of immunosuppresion (182). Small bowel lymphomas also occur in AIDS patients (183).

The most common tumor of the small bowel in children is non-Hodgkin's lymphoma, with the distal ileum the most common site. In a study, 36% of the high-grade gastrointestinal lymphomas had the small intestine as the primary site. Treatment was surgical resection and post-operative chemotherapy, since radiotherapy was of limited value in such rapidly growing tumors (184).

There is a particular subtype of small bowel lymphoma especially common in the Middle East, especially in southern Iran. In this part of the world, they are the most common neoplasm! This is found in children and young adults, usually from lower socioeconomic classes with a background of malnutrition (185,186). This lymphoma behaves more aggressively and appears to portend a poorer prognosis.

D. Cancers of the Colon and Rectum

Once a colorectal cancer develops, it is essential to establish the extent of disease. Whether the specimen is obtained endoscopically or surgically, similar principles apply: the entire cancer must be removed with a thorough pathologic analysis of depth and margins in particular. Once the tumor is beyond endoscopic removal, treatment of early stages is with surgery. If at the time of diagnosis, metastases are discovered, a combination of surgical and other therapeutic modalities is indicated. Occasionally, prolonged survival may be achieved with resection of isolated lung or liver metastases (187).

A biologic understanding of the disease is necessary to establish a therapeutic treatment plan. If the tumor arises spontaneously, a standard resection encompassing the lymphatic drainage is sufficient. If the cancers arise in a pedunculated polyp, endoscopic removal is adequate. A right hemicolectomy is appropriate for tumors arising from the cecum, ascending colon or hepatic flexure. Transverse colon cancers may be resected with a segmental and/or an extended right or left hemicolectomy. A tumor in the splenic flexure or descending colon requires a left hemicolectomy. Recently, multiple studies have shown that the choice of surgeon and the degree of monitoring and quality control applied appear to have a strong favorable impact on outcome, especially in rectal surgery (188,189).

The most important aspect of treatment for colorectal cancer is the adequacy of initial surgery and the appropriateness of multi-modality treatment for high risk patients. The major principles of surgical resection of colon and rectal cancer are: (1) removal of the entire cancer with enough bowel proximal and distal to the tumor mass to encompass the possibility that there has been submucosal lymphatic tumor spread; (2) removal of regional mesenteric draining lymphatics; (3) adequate visual, tactile, and now intraoperative ultrasound staging at the time of primary resection; and (4) minimization of psychological and functional consequences of surgery without sacrificing any of the first three precepts. Thus, the right hemicoloctomy, transverse colectomy, or left hemicolectomy are founded on *anatomic* structures, specifically the ileocolic, middle colic and left colic arteries, defining what is both a convenient anatomic boundary for standard colonic resection and also providing for adequate lymph node drainage.

The surgical convention for rectal cancer has been changing steadily. Older standards dictated that any distally located adenocarcinoma of the rectum that could be palpated digitally requires abdominoperineal resection, as first standardized by Miles. Standard techniques for low anterior resection and abdominoperineal resection have changed little over the years (190), with the exception of automatic stapling devices (191). Combined modality therapy reduces but does not eliminate the risks of local recurrence. The reduction is one-thirds to two-thirds but mostly for distant metastases. Unfortunately, improved local control does not correspond to improved overall survival. On extremely high-risk patients or selected superficial distal exophytic tumors, local treatment modalities including multiple coagulation sessions, local excision and endocavitary irradiation (192–194). The primary surgical approach must be the cornerstone of any appropriate therapy combination. Resection must be macroscopically complete and the microscopic tumor burden must be made as small as possible if adjuvant therapy is to achieve its maximum benefit.

Surgical cure of colorectal cancer is determined by the size, extent and stage of the tumor and its biologic behavior. For example, smaller superficial tumors without vascular or lymphatic invasion can be easily resected with a high chance of cure. In contrast, patients with deeper larger, ulcerated tumors invading into blood vessels and lymphatics are less likely to be cured by surgery alone, even if the margins are clear.

There are improving prospects and investigational options for advanced colorectal cancer. Surgery creates these opportunities for adjuvant therapy. These include radiation therapy, chemo and immunotherapy and even gene therapy, which is looming on the horizon. Systemic and adjuvant therapy can improve quality of life and duration of survival.

Finally, the most important aspect of treatment for colorectal cancer is the adequacy of initial surgery and the appropriateness of multi-modality treatment for patients who are identified as having a high risk of recurrence. Ideal surgery still provides the best chance for curing a patient with colon or rectum cancer, and the vigor of a follow-up plan and even salvage surgery and multi-modality therapy cannot make up for inadequate primary treatment.

E. Cancers of the Anus

The surgical approach for anal carcinomas has changed; there is no longer need for a colostomy. Successful multi-modality therapy has allowed sphincter preservation for even large primary tumors. In contrast, melanoma of anal canal still has a dismal prognosis.

Anal canal carcinomas are defined as tumors that are either wholly or partially situated across the dentate line (195). Tumors below are considered anal margin carcinomas. Anal margin and anal canal tumors have significant differences in treatment and survival.

Treatment is based on appropriate assessment of extent of disease. Physical exam should include a search for supraclavicular or inguinal adenopathy, hepatomegaly, abdominal masses or ascites or satellite lesions in the gluteal folds. The primary lesion should be evaluated by digital exam, anoscopy, and proctoscopy for size, location, invasion, depth, and extent of inguinal lymphadenopathy (196). Tumor grade has been reflective of prognosis (197).

Over the past 25 years, the preferred treatment has evolved from radical surgery to definitive chemoradiation, which has proven to be highly effective in achieving cures and preserving anal sphincter function with acceptable toxicity. Surgery has been limited to diagnostic biopsy of the tumor and suspicious lymph nodes and post-treatment biopsy as needed. Only very small superficial lesions of the anal canal are treated with local excision (198,199). Multiple regimens of chemoradiation including mitomycin and 5-florouracil and higher radiotherapy have shown efficacy (200–202).

Today the majority of patients are treated by combined multi-disciplinary therapy; therefore, adjacent organ resection (APR) and pelvic lymphadenectomy are reserved for those who fail first-line treatment (203).

Multi-modality therapy is definitely the treatment of choice for anal carcinoma with nodal involvement (204). Surgery should be used for diagnosis, for sampling the involved nodes or for salvage after an isolated node recurrence.

Anorectal melanoma is a rare disease, accounting for 1–2% of all anal cancer, with poor prognosis. Most patients present with bleeding, pain, or a detectable mass. No statistically significant survival difference was noted for those who underwent an APR as compared with those with a wide local excision (205). Distant and multiple sites of recurrence are common despite aggressive operative treatment by APR. There is no definitive way of treatment but some studies have shown increased survival when chemotherapy was added to local excision (206).

These patients should be treated as others with melanoma with adjuvant therapy, such as immunotherapy, chemotherapy or further investigational trials (207).

IV. COMPLICATIONS/PERIOPERATIVE CONCERNS

A. General

As with other cancer patients, common problems include venous thromboembolism, respiratory complications, infectious complications, and exacerbation of pre-existing comorbid conditions. Braga et al. (208) note that transfusion of more than 1000 mL of blood is an independent risk factor in the development of infection post-operatively in patients undergoing operations for gastrointestinal cancer.

The issue with nutrition is still unclear but definite benefit is seen with supplemental nutrition in the cachectic patient. Braga et al. (209) find that perioperative enteral nutrition significantly reduces post-operative infections and length of stay in patients undergoing surgery for cancer. Bozzetti et al. (210) conclude that if perioperative TPN is continued post-operatively, the complication rate reduces by about one-third and decreases mortality in severely malnourished gastric carcinoma patients.

B. Stomach

Early post-operative complications include anastomotic leakage, bleeding, ileus, chloecystitis, pancreatitis, respiratory infections, and thromboembolism. Reoperation may be required for anastomotic problems or medically unmanageable bleeding. Later complications include dumping syndrome, pernicious anemia, reflux esophagitis, and osteoporosis. Immunocompromise and deficiency of vitamins B1, B6, and B12 are not uncommon post-gastrectomy (211).

Post-gastrectomy management include education and diet modification which may need to be supplemented with vitamins and occasionally gastric motility agents.

Dhar et al. (212) report that patients transfused with only packed red blood cells vs. whole blood or other blood products had significantly higher rates of disease free survival in gastric resections.

C. Pancreas

Pancreatoduodenectomy may be followed by serious complications chiefly associated with exocrine pancreatic secretion. Somatostatin and its analogs are able to inhibit pancreatic secretion and thus have been advocated for the prevention of complications following pancreatic surgery (213).

Complications after pancreatic resections remain frequent despite a decreasing mortality. Pancreatic leakages represent a relevant part of those complications but data on risk factors for their occurrence are rare. Although easily managed in the majority of cases, pancreatic leakage still represents a relevant post-operative complication after pancreatic resection, especially in patients with malignant disease. Patients with impaired renal function are at increased risk of developing perioperative pancreatic leakage (214).

In one study by Carrabetta et al. (215), perioperative complications consist of gastroplegia (33%), pancreatic fistula (22%), biliary fistula (7.3%), abdominal abscess (5.5%), and hemoperitoneum (1.8%). Five patients died within 30 days after surgery (9%).

Although perioperative mortality following pancreaticoduodenectomy for cancer has a general reported incidence of 1–4% at high volume centers experienced with the operation, morbidity however still remains high with that of delayed gastric emptying, pancreatic anastomotic leak or fistula, intra-abdominal abscess, and hemorrhage as the leading reported complications (138). Researchers have investigated several agents and strategies to decrease or prevent the potential morbidity of these complications including the use of octreotide, drainage of the pancreatic bed, and institution of early enteral feeding (138).

D. Colorectal

The acute morbidity and mortality from surgery for colorectal carcinoma should be low. Significant, coexisting disease increases both mortality and morbidity. Typically in large studies, extremes of age have higher morbidity and mortality. In addition, male gender is another independent factor leading to worse outcomes.

Morbidity rates (mainly thromboembolic, infectious, and anastomotic problems) should be less than 10%. Operations for acute obstructions where adequate bowel preparation cannot occur, the decision to perform intraoperative bowel prep or a temporary colostomy may obviate the increased risk of a leak if primary anastomosis is performed. Addition of either oral preparative antibiotics or parenteral antibiotics perioperatively decreases the wound infection rate (216).

Blood transfusion is thought to affect adversely the rates of infection, complications, and actual survival, but not the actual rate of relapse (217).

Patients with locally advanced or metastatic disease may require preoperative or post-operative adjuvant radiation therapy. Preoperative adjuvant therapy has the advantages of decreased toxicity, increased biologic effectiveness, improved surgical resectability and increased chance of sphincter preservation. Radiation therapy given preoperatively may be more effective than an equivalent dose given post-operatively. Surgery may limit the oxygen supply to the tumor bed; therefore, limiting the effectiveness of the radiation therapy. Another advantage is sterilization of tumor cells in the perirectal tissues as well as allowing the patient to undergo a sphincter-sparing procedure once the tumor has been reduced in size by radiation. Potential disadvantages of preoperative radiation include delayed definitive excision of the tumor, potential for increased surgical complications, delayed wound healing, and lack of surgical pathologic staging.

V. CONCLUSIONS

In order to achieve optimal results in cancer surgery, including those of the major intrabdominal organs, a multi-disciplinary team approach must be utilized. One cannot overemphasize the importance of good preoperative preparation, anesthetic care, experienced surgeon and scrutinizing post-operative care in minimizing the morbidity and mortality of these procedures.

We conclude that careful selection of patients, appropriate intra- and post-operative management, with adequate post-operative pain control can reduce post-operative morbidity and length of inpatient stay.

Although multiple patient factors including demographics, coexisting diseases, ASA physical status, tumor characteristics, nutritional status all play an important role in risk stratification of patients, one variable that should not be overlooked is the experience of the multi-disciplinary team caring for the patients with such complex pathophysiological derangements undergoing major intrabdominal surgery. Only the experience acquired over time regarding the perioperative treatment of these complex patients seems to lower the rate of post-operative compications (218).

REFERENCES

1. Mayer RJ, O'Connell MJ, Tepper JE, Wolmark N. Status of adjuvant therapy for colorectal cancer. J Natl Cancer Inst 1989; 81:1359.
2. DeWys WD, Begg C, et al. Prognostic effect of weight loss prior to chemotherapy in cancer patients. Eastern Cooperative Oncology Group. Am J Med 1980; 69: 491–497.

3. Daly JM, Redmond HP, et al. Perioperative nutrition in cancer patients. JPEN J Parenter Enteral Nutr 1992; 16(suppl 6):100S–105S.
4. Correa P. Carcinoma of the stomach. Proc Nutr Soc 1985; 44:11.
5. Staszewski J. Smoking and cancer of the alimentary tract in Poland. Br J Cancer 1969; 22:247.
6. Kurita H. Clinico epidemiological study of stomach cancer and considering sex and age differences. Jpn J Cancer Clin 1974; 20:580.
7. Nagy K, Muranyi M, et al. Perioperative treatment after esophagogastric surgery. Magy Seb 2001; 3:138–143.
8. Dumanskii LU, Shtutin SA, et al. The complications in surgical treatment of gastric cancer in elderly and senile patients. Klin Khir 2001; 3:50–53.
9. Friess H, Kleeff J, Fischer L, et al. Surgical standard therapy for cancer of the pancreas. Chirurg 2003; 3:183–190.
10. Greenlee RT, Murray T, Bolden S, Wingo PA. Cancer statistics, 2000. Ca Cancer J Clin 2000; 50:13.
11. Evans DB, Pisters PWT, Lee JE, et al. Preoperative chemoradiation strategies for localized adenocarcinoma of the pancreas. J Hepatobiliary Pancreat Surg 1998; 5:242–250.
12. Foo ML, Gunderson LL, Nagorney DM, et al. Patterns of failure in grossly resected pancreatic ductal adenocarcinoma treated with adjuvant irradiation+ 5-florouracil. Int J Radiat Oncol Biol Phys 1993; 26:483.
13. Johnstone PA, Sindelar WF. Patterns of disease recurrence following definitive therapy of adenocarcinoma of the pancreas using surgery and adjuvant radiotherapy: correlations of a clinical trial. Int J Radiat Oncol Biol Phys 1993; 27:831.
14. Pisters PWT, Abbruzzese JL, Janjan NA, et al. Rapid-fractionation preoperative chemoradiation, pancreaticoduodenectomy, and intraoperative radiation therapy for resectable pancreatic adenocarcinoma. J Clin Oncol 1998; 16:3843–3850.
15. Gold EB, Gold SB. In epidemiology of and risk factors for pancreatic cancer. Surg Oncol Clin N Am 1998; 7:67.
16. Gullo L. Diabetes and the risk of pancreatic cancer. Ann Oncol 1999; 10(suppl 4):79.
17. Mack TM, Yu MC, Hanisch R, et al. Pancreas cancer and smoking, beverage consumption, and past medical history. J Natl Cancer Inst 1986;76:49.
18. Gullo L, Pezzilli R, Morselli-Labate AM. Diabetes and the risk of pancreatic cancer. N Engl J Med 1994; 331:81.
19. Shibata A, Mack TM, Paganini-Hill A, et al. A prospective study of pancreatic cancer in the elderly. Int J Cancer 1994; 58:46.
20. Silverman DT, Schiffman M, Everhart J, et al. Diabetes mellitus, other medical conditions and familial history of cancer as risk factors for pancreatic cancer. Br J Cancer 1999; 80:1830.
21. Talamini G, Falconi M, Bassi C, et al. Incidence of cancer in the course of chronic pancreatitis. Am J Gastroenterol 1999; 94:1253–1260.
22. Karlson BM, Ekbom A, Josefsson SD, et al. The risk of pancreatic cancer following pancreatitis; an association due to confounding factors? Gastroenterology 1997; 113:587–592.
23. Lowenfels AB, Maisonneuve P, Di Magno EP, et al. Hereditary pancreatitis and the risk of pancreatic cancer. International Hereditary Pancreatitis Study Group. J Natl Cancer Inst 1997; 89:442–446.
24. Warshaw AL, Fernandez-del Castillo C. Pancreatic carcinoma. New Engl J Med 1992; 326:455.
25. Offerhaus GJA, Tersmette AC, Tersmette KW, et al. Gastric, pancreatic and colorectal carcinogenesis following remote peptic ulcer surgery. Mod Pathol 1988; 1:352.
26. Raderer M, Wrba F, Kornek G, et al. Association between *Helicobacter pylori* infection and pancreatic cancer. Oncology 1998; 55:16.
27. Steinberg WM, Barkin J, Bradley EL III, et al. Workup of a patient with familial pancreatic cancer. Pancreas 1999; 18:219.
28. Brentnall TA, Bronner MP, Byrd DR, et al. Early diagnosis and treatment of pancreatic dysplasia in patients with a family history of pancreatic cancer. Ann Intern Med 1999; 131:247.
29. Talamini G, Bassi C, Falconi M, et al. Alcohol and smoking as risk factors in chronic pancreatitis and pancreatic cancer. Dig Dis Sci 1999; 44:1303.
30. Mulder I, van Genugten NL, Hoogenven RT, et al. The impact of smoking on future pancreatic cancer; a computer simulation. Ann Oncol 1999; 10(suppl 4):74.
31. Partanen TJ, Vainio HU Ojajarvi IA, et al. Pancreas cancer, tobacco smoking and consumption of alcoholic beverages: a case–control study. Cancer Lett 1997; 116:27.
32. Harnack LJ, Anderson KE, Zheng W, et al. Smoking, alcohol, coffee, and tea intake and incidence of cancer of the exocrine pancreas: the Iowa Women's Health Study. Cancer Epidemiol Biomarkers Prev 1997; 6:1081.
33. Silverman DT, Dunn JA, Hoover RN, et al. Cigarette smoking and pancreas cancer; a case–control study based on direct interviews. J Natl Cancer Inst 1994; 86:1510.
34. Zheng W, McLaughlin JK, Gridley G, et al. A cohort study of smoking, alcohol consumption and dietary factors for pancreatic cancer (United States). Cancer Causes Control 1993; 4:477.
35. Lyon JL, Slattery ML, Mahoney AW, et al. Dietary intake as a risk factor for cancer on the exocrine pancreas. Cancer Epidemiol Biomarkers Prev 1993; 2:513.
36. Woutersen RA, Appel MJ, van Garderen-Hoetmer A, et al. Dietary fat and carcinogenesis. Mutat Res 1999; 443:111.
37. Ohba S, Nishi M, Miyake H. Eating habits and pancreas cancer. Int J Pancreatol 1996; 20:37.
38. Olsen GW, Mandel JS, Gibson RW, et al. A case–control study of pancreatic cancer and cigarettes, alcohol, coffee, and diet. Am J Public Health 1989; 79:1016.

39. MacMahon B, Yen S, Trichopoulos D, et al. Coffee and cancer of the pancreas. N Engl J Med 1981; 304:630.
40. Lin RS, Kesssler IL. A multi-factorial model for pancreatic cancer in man. JAMA 1981; 245:147.
41. Hakulinen T, Lehtimaki L, Lehtonon M, et al. Cancer morbidity among two male cohorts with increased alcohol consumption in Finland. J Natl Cancer Inst 1974; 52:1711.
42. Friedman GD, van den Eeden SK. Risk factors for pancreatic cancer: an exploratory study. Int J Epidemiol 1993; 22:30.
43. Permert J, Ihse I, Jorfeldt L, et al. Pancreatic cancer is associated with impaired glucose metabolism. Eur J Surg 1993; 159:101.
44. Permert J, Larsson J, Fruin AB, et al. Islet hormone secretion in pancreatic cancer patients with diabetes. Pancreas 1997; 15:60–68.
45. Pour PM. The role of Langerhans islets in exocrine pancreatic cancer. Int J Pancreatol 1995; 17:217.
46. Rochlin DB, Lingmire WP. Primary tumors of the small intestine. Surgery 1961; 50:586.
47. Mittal VK, Bodzin JH. Primary malignant tumors of the small bowel. Am J Surg 1980; 140:396.
48. Williamson RC, Welch CE, Malt RA. Adenocarcinoma and lymphoma of the small intestine. Distribution and etiologic associations. Ann Surg 1983; 197:172.
49. Landis SH, Murray T, Bolden S, Wingo PA. Cancer statistics 1999. CA Cancer J Clin 1999; 49:8–31.
50. Parson J, Gray GF, Thorbjarnarson B. Pseudomyxoma peritonei Arch Surg 1970; 101:545.
51. Zollinger RM, Sternfeld WC, Schreiber H. Primary neoplasms of the small intestine. Am J Surg 1986; 151:654.
52. Silberman H, Crichlow RW, Caplan HS. Neoplasms of the small bowel. Ann Surg 1974; 180:157.
53. Dudiak KM, Johnson CD, Stephens DH. Primary tumors of the small intestine: CT evaluation. AJR AM J Roentgenol 1989; 152:995.
54. DiSario JA, Burt RW, Vargas H, McWhorter WP. Small bowel cancer: epidemiological and clinical characteristics from a population based registry. Am J Gastroenterol 1994; 89:699–701.
55. Ahlman H, Ahlund L, Dahlstrauom A. SMS 201–995 and provocation tests in preparation of patients with carcinoids for surgery or hepatic arterial embolization. Anesth Analg 1988; 67:1142.
56. Greenlee RT, Murray T, Bolden SA, et al. Cancer statistics. CA Cancer J Clin 1999; 50:7–33.
57. Wingo PA, Tong T, Bolden S. Cancer statistics 1995. CA Cancer J Clin 1995; 45:8–30.
58. Winawer SJ, Zauber AG, Ho MN. Prevention of colorectal cancer by colonoscopic polypectomy. The National Polyp Study Workgroup. N Engl J Med 1993; 329:1977–1981.
59. Potter JD. Hormones and colon cancer. J Natl Cancer Inst 1995; 87:1039–1040.
60. Wynder EL, Shigematsu T. Environmental factors of cancer of the colon and rectum. Cancer 1967; 20:1520.
61. Burkitt DP. Epidemiology of cancer of the colon and rectum. Cancer 1971; 28:3.
62. Thompson MH, Hill MJ. Etiology and mechanisms of carcinogenesis: diet, luminal factors and colorectal cancer. In: Faivre J, Hill MJ, eds. Causation and Prevention of Colorectal Cancer. Amsterdam: Excerpta Medica, 1987:99–120.
63. Kune GA, Kune S, Watson LF. Dietary sodium and potassium intake and colorectal cancer risk. Nutr Cancer 1989; 12:351.
64. Burt RW, Bishop DT, Lee RG, et al. Inheritance of colonic adenomatous polyps and colorectal cancer. Prog Clin Biol Res 1988; 279:189.
65. DeCosse JJ. Antioxidants. Prog Clin Biol Res 1988; 279:131.
66. De Cosse JJ, Miller HH, Lesser ML. Effect of wheat fiber and vitamins C and E on rectal polyps in patients with familial adenomatous polyps. J Natl Cancer Inst 1989; 81:1290.
67. McKeown-Eyssen G, Holloway C, Jazmaji V. A randomized trial of vitamins C and E in the prevention of recurrence of colorectal polyps. Cancer Res 1988; 48:4701.
68. Peleg II, Maibach HT, Brown SH, et al. Aspirin and non-steroidal anti-inflammatory drug use and the risk of subsequent colorectal cancer. Arch Intern Med 1994; 154:394–399.
69. Dayal Y, DeLellis RA. The gastrointestinal tract. In: Cotran RS, Kumar V, Robbins SL, eds. Pathologic Basis of Disease. 4th ed. Philadelphia: WB Saunders, 1989:882–902.
70. Michelassi F, Mishlove L, Stipa F, Block GF. Squamous cell carcinoma of the colon. Dis Colon Rectum 1988; 31:228.
71. Behbehani A, Sakwa M, Ehrlichman R. Colorectal cancer in patients under age 40. Ann Surg 1985; 202:620.
72. Lindsay DC, Freeman JGB, Cobden I, Record CO. Should colonoscopy be the first investigation for colonic disease? BMJ 1988; 296:167.
73. Ott DJ, Chen YM, Gelfand DW, et al. Single-contrast vs. double contrast barium enema in the detection of colonic polyps. AJR Am J Roentgenol 1986; 146:993.
74. Melbye M, Rabkin C, Frisch M, Biggar RJ. Changing patterns of anal cancer incidence in the United States, 1940–1989. Am J Epidemiol 1994; 139:772–780.
75. Daling JR, Weiss NS, Hislop G, et al. Sexual practices, sexually transmitted diseases, and the incidence of anal cancer. N Engl J Med 1987; 317:973–977.
76. Frisch M, Glimelius B, van den Brule AJ, et al. Sexually transmitted infection as a cause of anal cancer. N Engl J Med 1997; 337:1350–1358.
77. Zur Hausen H. Human papillomaviruses and their possible role in squamous cell carcinomas. Curr Top Microbiol Immunol 1977; 78:1–30.
78. Penn I. Cancers of the anogenital region in renal transplant recipients. Cancer 1986; 58:611–616.

79. Daniell HW. Re: causes of anal carcinoma. JAMA 1985; 254:358.
80. Frisch M, Glimelius B, Wohlfahrt J, et al. Tobacco smoking as a risk factor in anal carcinoma: an antiestrogenic mechanism? J Natl Cancer Inst 1999; 91:708–715.
81. AH Holscher, M Schuler, JR Siewert. Surgical treatment of gastric cancer: carcinomas of the gastroesophagael junction. In: Holtz J, Meyer HJ, Schmoll HJ, eds. Gastric Carcinoma. New York: Springer-Verlag, 1989:60.
82. Siewert JR, Holscher AH, Becker K, Gossner W. Cardia-cancer attempt at a therapeutically relevant classification. Chirugie 1987; 58:25.
83. Bruckner HW, Morris JC, Mansfield P. Neoplasms of the stomach. In: Holland JF, Frei E, eds. Cancer Medicine. 5th ed. Hamilton, Canada: BC Decker, 2000.
84. Fujimaki M Soga J, Wada K, et al. Total gastrectomy for gastric cancer. Clinical considerations on 431 cases. Cancer 1972; 30:660.
85. Adam YG, Effron G. Trends and controversies in the management of carcinoma of the stomach. Surg Gynecol Obstet 1989; 169:371.
86. Douglass HO, Nava HR. Gastric adenocarcinoma. Management of the primary disease. Semin Oncol 1985; 12:32.
87. Martin RC, Jaques DP, et al. Achieving RO resection for locally advanced gastric cancer: is it worth the risk of multi-organ resection? J Am Coll Surg 2002; 94:568–577.
88. Clark JL, Nava HR, Douglass HO Jr. Survival following potentially curative resection for stomach cancer. Proc Am Soc Clin Oncol 1988; 7:106.
89. Cunilla AL, Fitzgerald PJ. Tumors of the Exocrine Pancreas. Washington, DC: Armed Forces Institute of Pathology, 1984.
90. Kayahara M, Nagakawa T, Futagami F, et al. Lymphatic flow and neural plexus invasion associated with carcinoma of the body and tail of the pancreas. Cancer 1996; 78:2485–2491.
91. Nakai T, Koh K, Kawabe T, et al. Importance of microperineural invasion as a prognostic factor in ampulllary carcinoma. Br J Surg 1997; 84:1399–1401.
92. Evans DB, Lee JE, Leach SD, et al. Vascular resection and intraoperative radiation therapy during a pancreaticoduodenectomy: rationale and technique. Adv Surg 1995; 29:235.
93. Gloor B, Todd KE, Reber HA. Diagnostic workup of patients with suspected pancreatic carcinoma: the Univerity of California–Los Angeles approach. Cancer 1997; 79:1780–1786.
94. Friess H, Kleeff J, Silva JC, et al. The role of diagnostic laparoscopy in pancreatic and periampullary malignancies. J Am Coll Surg 1998; 186:675–682.
95. Rumstadt B, Schwab M, Schuster K, et al. The role of laparoscopy in the preoperative staging of pancreatic carcinoma. J Gastrointest Surg 1997; 1:245–250.
96. Andersen JR, Soren SM, Kruse A, et al. Randomized trial of endoscopic endoprosthesis versus operative bypass in malignant obstructive jaundice. Gut 1989; 30:1132.
97. Smith AC, Dowsett JF, Hatfield ARW, et al. Prospective randomized trial of bypass surgery versus endoscopic stenting in patients with malignant obstructive jaundice. Gut 1989; 30:A1513.
98. Shepherd HA, Royle G, Ross AP, et al. Endoscopic biliary endoprosthesis in the palliation of malignant obstruction of the distal common bile duct: a randomized trial. Br J Surg 1988; 75:1166.
99. Luque-deLeon E, Tsiotos GG, Balsiger B, et al. Staging laparoscopy for pancreatic cancer should be used to select the best means of palliation and not only to maximize the resectability rate. J Gastrointest Surg 1999; 3:111–118.
100. Geer RJ, Brennan MF. Prognostic indicators for survival after resection of pancreatic adenocarcinoma. Am J Surg 1993; 165:68.
101. Lillemoe KD, Sauter PK, Pitt HA, et al. Current status of surgical palliation of periampullary carcinoma. Surg Gyneco Obstet 1993; 176:1.
102. Kelsen DP, Portenoy R, Thaler H, et al. Pain as a predictor of outcome in patients with operable pancreatic carcinoma. Surgery 1997; 122:53–59.
103. de Rooij PD, Rogatako A, Brennan MF. Evaluation of palliative surgical procedures in unresectable pancreatic cancer. Br J Surg 1991; 78:1053.
104. DiFronzo LA, Egrari S, O'Connell TX. Choledochoduodenostomy for palliation in unresectable pancreatic cancer. Arch Surg 1988; 133:820–825.
105. Whipple AO, Parson WV, Mullin CR. Treatment of carcinoma of the ampulla of Vater. Ann Surg 1935; 102:763.
106. Cameron JL, Crist DW, Sitzmann JV, et al. Factors influencing survival after pancreaticoduodenectomy for pancreatic cancer. Am J Surg 1991; 161:120.
107. Yeo CJ, Cameron JL, Sohn TA, et al. Six hundred fifty consecutive pancreaticoduodenectomies in the 1990s. Ann Surg 1997; 226:248–260.
108. Yeo CJ, Abrams RA, Grochow LB, et al. Pancreaticoduodenectomy for pancreatic adenocarcinoma:postoperative adjuvant chemoradiation improves survival. Ann Surg 1997; 225:621–636.
109. Trede M, Chir B, Schwall G, Saeger H. Survival after pancreaticoduodenectomy:118 consecutive resections without an operative mortality. Ann Surg 1990; 211:447.
110. Yeo CJ, Cameron JL, Lillemoe KD, et al. Pancreaticoduodenectomy for cancer of the head of the pancreas: 201 patients. Ann Surg 1995; 221:721.
111. Tepper J, Nardi G, Suit H. Carcinoma of the pancreas: review of MGH experience from 1963–1973. Cancer 1976; 37:1519.
112. Evans DB, Lee JE, Pisters PWT. Pancreaticoduodenectomy (Whipple operation) and total pancreatectomy for cancer. In: Nyhus LM, Baker RJ, Fischer JF, eds. Mastery of Surgery. 3rd ed. Boston: Little, Brown, 1997:1233–1249.

113. Gunderson LL, Willett CG. Pancreas and hepatobiliary tract. In: Perez C, Brady L, eds. Principles and Practice of Radiation Oncology. 3rd ed. Philadelphia: Lippincott-Raven, 1997:1467–1488.
114. Hiraoka T, Watanabe E, Mochinaga M, et al. Intraoperative irradiation combined with radical resection for cancer of the head of the pancreas. World J Surg 1984; 8:766–769.
115. Hiraoka T. Extended radical resection of cancer of the pancreas with intraoperative radiotherapy. Ballieres Clin Gastroeneterol 1990; 4:985–993.
116. Coquard R, Ayzac L, Gilly N, et al. Intraoperative radiotherapy in resected pancreatic cancer feasibility and results. Radiother Oncol 1997; 44:271–275.
117. Sindelar WF, Kinsella TJ. Studies of intraoperative radiotherapy in carcinoma of the pancreas. Ann Oncol 1999; 10(suppl 4):S226–S230.
118. Evans DB, Roh M. Pancreaticoduodenectomy. In: Roh M, Ames RC, eds. Atlas of Advanced Surgical Oncology. London: Mosby-Year Book, 1994:42.
119. Warshaw AL, Torchiana DL. Delayed gastric emptying after pylorus-preserving pancreaticoduodenectomy. Surg Gynecol Obstet 1985; 160:1.
120. Evans DB, Pisters PWT, Lee JE, et al. Preoperative chemoradiation strategies for localized adenocarcinoma of the pancreas. J Hepatobiliary Pancreatic Surg 1998; 5:242–250.
121. Willett CG, Lewansrowski K, Warshaw AL, et al. Resection margins in carcinoma of the head of the pancreas: implications for radiation therapy. Ann Surg 1993; 217:144.
122. Gastrointestinal Study Tumor Group. Further evidence of effective adjuvant combined radiation and chemotherapy following curative resection of pancreatic cancer. Cancer 1987; 59:2006.
123. Klinkenbijl JH, Jeekel J, Sahmoud T, et al. Adjuvant radiotherapy and 5-florouracil after curative resection for the cancer of the pancreas and periampullary region, phase III trial of the EORTC gastrointestinal tract cancer cooperative group. Ann Surg 1999; 230: 776–784.
124. Demeure MJ, Doffek KM, Komorowski RA, et al. Molecular metastases in stage I pancreatic cancer: improved survival with adjuvant chemoradiation. Surgery 1998; 124:663–669.
125. Abrams RA, Grochow LB, Chakravarthy A, et al. Intensified adjuvant therapy for pancreatic and periampullary adenocarcinoma: survival results and observations regarding patterns of failure, radiotherapy dose and Ca 19-9 levels. Int J Radiat Oncol Biol Phys 1999; 44:1039–1046.
126. Hoffmann JP, Lipsitz S, Pisansky T, et al. Phase II trial of preoperative radiation therapy and chemotherapy for patients with localized, resectable adenocarcinoma of the pancreas: an Eastern Cooperative Oncology Group Study. J Clin Oncol 1998; 16: 317–323.
127. Crucitti F, Doglietto GB, Frontera D, et al. Integrated radiosurgical treatment of resectable pancreatic head carcinoma. Pancreas 1998; 16:31–39.
128. Evans DB, Rich TA, Byrd DR, et al. Preoperative chemoradiation and pancreaticoduodenectomy for adenocarcinoma of the pancreas. Arch Surg 1992; 127:1335–1339.
129. Hoffmann JP, Weese JL, Solin LJ. A single institutional experience with preoperative chemoradiation for stage I-III pancreatic adenocarcinoma. Am Surg 1993; 59:772.
130. Spitz FR, Abbruzzese JL, Lee JE, et al. Preoperative and post-operative chemoradiation strategies in patients treated with pancreaticoduodenectomy for adenocarcinoma of the pancreas. J Clin Oncol 1997; 226:248–260.
131. Wayne JD, Abdalla EK, et al. Localized adenocarcinoma of the pancreas: the rationale for preoperative chemoradiation. Oncologist 2002; 1:34–45.
132. Staley CA, Lee JE, Cleary KA, et al. Preopertaive chemoradiation, pancreaticoduodenectomy, and intraoperative radiation therapy for adenocarcinoma of the pancreatic head. Am J Surg 1996; 171:118–125.
133. Burris HA III, Moore MJ, Andersen J, et al. Improvements in survival and clinical benefit with gemcitabine as first-line therapy for patients with advanced pancreas cancer: a randomized trial. J Clin Oncol 1997; 15:2403–2413.
134. Lawrence TS, Chang EY, Hahn TM, et al. Radiosensitization of pancreatic cancer cells by 2,2-difluoro-2-deoycytidine. Int J Radiat Oncol Biol Phys 1996; 34:867–872.
135. Lieberman MD, Killburn H, Lindsey M, Brennan MF. Relation of perioperative deaths to hospital volume among patients undergoing pancreatic resection for malignancy. Ann Surg 1995; 222:638–645.
136. Birkmeyer JD, Finlayson SR, Tosteson AN, et al. Effect of hospital volume on in-hospital mortality with pancreaticoduodenectomy. Surgery 1999; 125: 250–256.
137. Birkmeyer JD, Warshaw AL, Finlayson SR, Grove MR, Tosteson AN. Relationship between hospital volume and late survival after pancreaticoduodenectomy. Surgery 1999; 126:178–183.
138. Spanknebel K, Conlon K. Advances in the surgical management of pancreatic cancer. Cancer J 2001; 4: 312–323.
139. Lowy AM, Lee JE, Pisters PWT, et al. Prospective randomized trial of octreotide to prevent pancreatic fistula after pancreaticoduodenectomy for malignant disease. Ann Surg 1997; 226:632–641.
140. Fernandez-del Castillo C, Rattner DW, Warshaw AL. Standards for pancreatic resection in the 1990s. Arch Surg 1995; 130:295.
141. Doerr RJ, Yildiz I, Flint LM. Pancreaticoduodenectomy: university experience and resident education. Arch Surg 1990; 125:463.

142. Edge SB, Schmieg RE, Rosenlof LK, et al. Pancreas cancer resection outcome in American university centers. Cancer 1993; 71:3502.
143. Wade TP, Radford DM, Virgo KS, et al. Complications and outcomes in the treatment of pancreatic adenocarcinoma in the United States veteran. J Am Coll Surg 1994; 179:38.
144. Sosa JA, Bowman HM, Tielsch JM, et al. Statewide regionalization of pancreaticoduodenectomy and its effect on in-hospital mortality. Ann Surg 1998; 228: 71–78.
145. Sohn TA, Yeo CJ, et al. Resected adenocarcinoma of the pancreas-616 patients: results, outcomes, and prognostic indicators. J Gastrointest Surg 2000; 6: 567–579.
146. Lillemoe KD, Cameron JL, Hardacre JM, et al. Is prophylactic gastrojejunostomy indicated for unresectable periampullary cancer? A prospective randomized trial. Ann Surg 1999; 230:322–328.
147. Espat NJ, Brennan MF, Conlon KC. Patients with laparoscopically staged unresectable carcinoma do not require subsequent surgical biliary or gastric bypass. J Am Coll Surg 1999; 188:649–657.
148. Raikar GV, Melin MM, Ress A, et al. Cost-effective analysis of surgical palliation vs. endoscopic stenting in the management of unresectable pancreatic cancer. Ann Surg Oncol 1996; 3:470–475.
149. Molinari M, Helton WS, et al. Palliative strategies for locally advanced unresectable and metastatic pancreatic cancer. Surg Clin North Am 2001; 3: 651–666.
150. Shandalakis JE, Gray SW, Shepard D, et al. Smooth Muscle Tumors of the Alimentary Tract. A Review of 2525 Cases. Springfield Il: Charles C Thomas, 1962:1–468.
151. River L, Silverstein J, Tope JW. Collective review: benign neoplasms of the small intestine. A critical comprehensive review with reports of 20 new cases. Inst Abstr Surg 1956; 102:1.
152. Wilson JM, Melvin DB, Gray G. Benign small bowel tumor. Ann Surg 1975; 181:247.
153. Smith FR, Mayo CW. Submucous lipomas of the small intestine. Am J Surg 1950; 80:922.
154. Bjork KJ, Davis CJ, Nagorney DM, Mucha P. Duodenal villous tumors. Arch Surg 1990; 125:961.
155. Good CA. Tumors of the small intestine. AJR Am J Roentgenol 1963; 89:685.
156. Boyle L, Lack EE. Solitary cavernous hemangioma of the small intestine. Arch Pathol Lab Med 1993; 117:939.
157. Warkel RL, Cooper PH, Helwig EB. Adenocarcinoid. A mucin producing tumor of the appendix. A study of 39 cases. Cancer 1978; 42:2781.
158. Darling RC, Welch CE. Tumors of the small intestine. N Engl J Med 1959; 260:397.
159. Gentry RW, Dockerty MS, Claggett OT. Vascular malformations and vascular tumors of the gastrointestinal tract. Int Abstr Surg 1949; 88:281.
160. Raiford TS. Tumors of the small intestine. Arch Surg 1932; 25:122.
161. Barquist E, Apple S, Jensen D, Ashley S. Jejunal lymphangioma: an unusual cause of gastrointestinal bleeding. Dig Dis Sci 1997; 42:1179.
162. Hanagiri T, Baba M, Shimabukuro T. Lymphangioma in the small intestine: report of a case and review of the Japanese literature. Surg Today 1992; 22:363.
163. Petreshock EJ, Pessah M, Menachemi E. Adenocarcinoma of the jejunum in association with celiac sprue. J Clin Gastroenterol 1989; 11:320.
164. Straker RJ, Gunasekaran S, Brady PG. Adenocarcinoma of the jejunum in association with celiac sprue. J Clin Gastroenterol 1989; 11:320.
165. Gonzalez-Moreno S, Shmookler BM, Sugarbaker PH. Appendiceal mucocele: contraindication to laparascopic appendectomy. Surg Endosc 1998; 12:1177.
166. Nesbit RR Jr, Elbadawi NA, Morton JH, Cooper RA Jr. Carcinoma of the small bowel. A complication of regional enteritis. Cancer 1976; 37:2948.
167. Frank JD, Shorey BA. Adenocarcinoma of the small bowel as a complication of Crohn's disease. Gut 1973; 14:120.
168. Goldman LI, Bralow SP, Cox W Peale AR. Adenocarcinoma of the small bowel complicating Crohn's disease. Cancer 1970; 26:1119.
169. Moertel CG. Small intestine. Holland JF, Frei E, eds. Cancer Medicine. 2nd ed. Philadelphia: Lea & Febiger, 1982:1808–1818.
170. Brophy C, Cahow CE. Primary small bowel malignant tumors. Am Surg 1989; 55:408.
171. Ouriel K, Adams JT. Adenocarcinomas of the small intestine. Am J Surg 1984; 147:66.
172. Hancock RJ. An 11-year review of primary tumors of the small bowel including the duodenum. Can Med J 1970; 103:1177.
173. Sindelar WF, Kinsella TJ. Intraoperative radiotherapy for locally advanced cancers. South Med J 1989; 82:358.
174. Moertel CG. An odyssey in the land of small tumors. J Clin Oncol 1987; 5:1503.
175. Sjoblom SM. Clinical presentation and prognosis of gastrointestinal carcinoid tumors. Scand J Gastroenterol 1988; 23:779.
176. Saha S, Hoda S, Godfrey R, et al. Carcinoid tumor of the gastrointestinal tract : a 44 year experience. South Med J 1989; 82:1501.
177. Herbsman H, Wetstein L, Rosen Y. Tumors of the small intestine. Curr Prob Surg 1980; 17:121.
178. Jacobs EM. Combination chemotherapy of metastatic testicular germinal cell tumors and soft part sarcomas. Cancer 1970; 25:324.
179. Moertel CG, Reitemeier RJ. Advanced Gastrointestinal Cancer. New York: Harper & Row, 1969.
180. Fu K, Stewart R. Radiotherapeutic management of small intestinal lymphoma with malabsorption. Cancer 1973; 31:286.

181. Harris OD, Cooke WT, Thompson H, et al. Malignancy in adult coeliac disease and idiopathic steatorrhoea. Am J Med 1967; 42:899.
182. Penn I. Cancers following cyclosporine therapy. Transplantation 1987; 43:32.
183. Collier PE. Small bowel lymphoma associated with AIDS. J Surg Oncol 1986; 32:131.
184. Takahashi H, Hansmann ML. Primary gastrointestinal lymphoma in childhood. Cancer Res Clin Oncol 1990; 116:190.
185. Al-Saleem T, Al-Bahrani Z. Malignant lymphoma of the small intestine in Iraq. Cancer 1973; 31:291.
186. Salem PA, Nassar VH, Shahid MJ. A Mediterranean abdominal lymphoma or immunoproliferative small intestinal disease. Part I: clinical aspects. Cancer 1977; 40:2991.
187. Steele G Jr, Ravikumar TS. Resection of hepatic metastases from colorectal cancer: biological perspectives. Ann Surg 1989; 188:210–217.
188. Enker WE. Total mesorectal excision—the new golden standard of surgery for rectal cancer. Ann Med 1997; 29:127–133.
189. Cunningham JD, Enker W, Cohen A. Salvage therapy for pelvic recurrence following curative rectal cancer resection. Dis Colon Rectum1997; 40:393–400.
190. Goligher JC. Surgery of the Anus, Rectum and Colon. London: Bailliere Tindall, 1975.
191. Beart RW Jr, Kelley KA. Randomized prospective evaluation of the EEA stapler for coloectal anastomoses. Am J Surg 1981; 141:143.
192. Madden JL, Kandalaft S. Electrocoagulation in the treatment of cancer of the rectum. Ann Surg 1971; 174:530.
193. Mason AY. Malignant tumors of the rectum: local excision. Clin Gastroenterol 1974; 4:582.
194. Papillon J. Rectal and Anal cancers: Conservative Treatment by Irradiation—an Alternative to Radical Surgery. Berlin: Springer-Verlag, 1982.
195. Morson BC. The pathology and results of treatment of squamous cell carcinoma of the anal canal and anal margin. Proc R Soc Med 1960; 53:414–420.
196. Enker WE, Heilweil M, Janov AJ, et al. Improved survival in epidermoid carcinoma of the anus in association with pre-operative multi-disciplinary therapy. Arch Surg 1986; 121:1386–1390.
197. Goldman S, Auer G, Erhardt K, et al. Prognostic significance of clinical stage, histologic grade, and nuclear DNA content in squamous-cell carcinoma of the anus. Dis Colon Rectum 1987; 30:444–448.
198. Greenall MJ, Quan SHQ, Stearns MW, et al. Epidermoid cancer of the anal margin. Am J Surg 1985; 149:95–101.
199. Kuehn PG, Eisenberg H, Reed JF. Epidermoid carcinoma of the perianal skin and anal canal. Cancer 1968; 22:932–938.
200. Flam M, John M, Pajak TF, et al. Role of mitomycin in combination with florouracil and radiotherapy, and of salvage chemoradiation in the definitive nonsurgical treatment of epidermoid carcinoma of the anal canal: results of a phase III randomized intergroup study. J Clin Oncol 1996; 14:2527–2539.
201. Flam M, John M, Pajak TF, et al. Role of mitomycin in combination with florouracil and radiotherapy, and of salvage chemoradiation in the definitive nonsurgical treatment of epidermoid carcinoma of the anal canal: results of a phase III randomized intergroup study—author update. In: Mayer RJ, ed. Classical Papers and Current Comments—Highlights of Clinical Gastrointestinal Cancer Research. Vol. 3. Philadelphia: Lippincott, Williams and Wilkens, 1999:539–552.
202. Grabenbauer GG, Matzel KE, Schneider IH, et al. Sphincter preservation with chemoradiation in anal canal carcinoma: abdominoperineal resection in selected cases? Dis Colon Rectum 1998; 41:441–450.
203. Stearns MW Jr, Urmacher C, Sternberg SS, et al. Cancer of the anal canal. Curr Probl Cancer 1980; 4: 1–44.
204. Peiffert D, Bey P, Pernot M, et al. Conservative treatment by irradiation of epidermoid cnacers of the anal canal: prognostic factors of tumoral control and complications. Int J Radiat Oncol Biol Phys 1997; 37: 313–324.
205. Brady MS, Kavolius JP, Quan SHQ. Anorectal melanoma: a 64-year experience at Memorial Sloan-Kettering cancer center. Dis Colon Rectum 1995; 38: 146–151.
206. Siegel B, Cohen D, Jacob ET. Surgical treatment of anorectal melanomas. Am J Surg 1983; 146:336–338.
207. Rosenberg SA, Speiss P, Lafreniere R. A new approach to the adoptive immunotherapy of cancer with tumor infiltrating lymphocytes. Science 1986; 233: 1318–1321.
208. Braga M, Vignali A, et al. Association between perioperative blood transfusion and post-operative infection in patients having elective operations for gastrointestinal cancer. Eur J Surg 1992; 10:531–536.
209. Braga M, Gianotti L et al. Perioperative immunonutrition in patients undergoing cancer surgery: results of a randomized double-blind phase 3 trial. Arch Surg 1999; 4:428–433.
210. Bozzetti, F, Gavazzi C, et al. Perioperative total parenteral nutrition in malnourished, gastrointestinal cancer patients: a randomized, clinical trial. JPEN J Parenter Enteral Nutr 2000; 1:7–14.
211. Kurashige S, Akuzawa Y, Fujii N, et al. Effect of vitamin B complex and the immunodeficiency produced by surgery of gastric cancer patients. Jpn J Exp Med 1988; 58:197.
212. Dhar DK, Kubota H, et al. A tailored perioperative blood transfusion might avoid undue recurrences in gastric carcinoma patients. Dig Dis Sci 2000; 9: 1737–1742.
213. Gouillat C. Somatostatin for the prevention of complications following pancreatoduodenectomy. Digestion 1999; (suppl 3):59–63.

214. Adam U, Makowiec F, et al. Pancreatic leakage after pancreas resection. An analysis of 345 operated patients. Chirurg 2002; 5:466–473.
215. Carrabetta S, De Cian F, et al. Pancreatic cancer. Analysis of 149 cases in our 17-year experience. G Chir 1998; 6–7:265–270.
216. Lau WY, Chu KW, Poon GP, Hok K. Prophylactic antibiotics in elective colorectal surgery. Br J Surg 1988; 75:782.
217. Donohue JH, Williams S, Cha S, et al. Perioperative blood transfusions do not affect disease recurrence of patients undergoing curative resection of colorectal carcinoma: a Mayo North central cancer treatment group study. J Clin Oncol 1995; 13:1671–1678.
218. Crucitti F, Doglietto GB, et al. Assessment of risk factors for pancreatic resection for cancer. World J Surg 1998; 3:241–247.

25

Perioperative Care of Patients with Endocrine Neoplasms

M. F. M. JAMES and D. M. DENT
Departments of Anaesthesia and Surgery, University of Cape Town, Cape Town, South Africa

The focus of this chapter is on neoplasms that secrete hormonally active substances, producing characteristic endocrine features that require specific management. Neoplasms arising in endocrine tissue, but without hormonal significance, will not be considered, as these are considered as simple anatomical lesions and not specifically as endocrine tumors.

I. PITUITARY TUMORS

Pituitary tumors can produce an array of hormones, with varying consequences. Approximately 25% of tumors are nonfunctional and present with the consequences of a space-occupying lesion at the base of the brain, including visual disturbances, headache, and rarely, panhypopituitarism. The management of these types of tumors is the neurosurgical management of a space-occupying lesion in the sella turcica, together with consideration of hormone replacement where appropriate.

A. Physiology

The pituitary gland consists of anterior and posterior parts that are histologically and embryologically distinct. The anterior lobe develops from the dorsal portion of Rathke's pouch and the posterior lobe as a downward protrusion from the floor of the third ventricle. The pituitary gland produces 14 or more hormonally active substances, of which those with recognized physiological effects are listed in Table 1. In addition, a variety of gastrointestinal and other polypeptides may be found within the lobes of the pituitary gland.

B. Pathophysiology

The majority of pituitary tumors are benign adenomas arising in the anterior part of the gland. Asymptomatic microadenomas of the pituitary reported incidentally at autopsy may occur as frequently as 11–25% (1,2) and these may present as "incidentalomas" during investigation of unrelated conditions. Such an incidental finding does not justify screening for hormone activity, but, as a quarter of these tumors may grow to a significant size, it may be appropriate to observe such patients carefully with repeated MR imaging scans (3). The prevalence of clinically relevant pituitary tumors is estimated to be ~0.02%. The frequency distribution of pituitary tumors presenting for surgery in a carefully documented series of 1043 patients is shown in Table 2. The predominant consequences of pituitary tumors are summarized in Table 3.

The majority of pituitary tumors are of little endocrine significance to the anesthetist. The commonest functioning pituitary tumors are prolactinomas. Most of these ($\pm 90\%$) are microadenomas and most commonly

Table 1 Pituitary Hormones

Anterior pituitary
Luteinizing hormone
Follicle-stimulating hormone
Growth hormone
Thyroid-stimulating hormone
Adrenocorticotrophic hormone
Prolactin
Melanocyte stimulating hormone
Posterior pituitary
Oxytocin
Vasopressin (antidiuretic hormone, ADH)

occur in women, when they typically present with galactorrhea and secondary amenorrhea, whereas those occurring in men result in impotence and infertility.

The glycopeptide-secreting tumors, which may produce thyroid-stimulating hormone (TSH), follicle-stimulating hormone (FSH), or luteinizing hormone (LH), are all uncommon and are usually inactive but may present with postmenopausal bleeding in women and rarely with premature puberty. Thyroid-stimulating hormone-secreting pituitary tumors are very rare but may be suspected in patients with hyperthyroidism associated with a normal or elevated TSH concentration. Apart from the appropriate management of the hyperthyroidism associated with excess TSH production, the management of these tumors presents no special anesthetic problems.

From an endocrine anesthesia viewpoint, the most important hormone-producing pituitary tumors are those secreting growth hormone (GH) and adrenocorticotrophic hormone (ACTH).

C. Acromegaly

Acromegaly is a chronic, debilitating condition characterized by progressive disfigurement and disability. Virtually, all cases (>99%) are caused by a GH-secreting pituitary adenoma. Very rarely, the syndrome may be the result of production of GH-releasing hormone by other tissues such as hypothalamic gangliocytoma, peripheral endocrine tumors arising from the pancreas and thymus, or midgut carcinoid. The incidence of the condition appears to be 3–4 per million of the population, and most patients present in the fourth to sixth decades (4). Growth hormone-hypersecretion before epiphyseal fusion results in pituitary gigantism, but this is uncommon. The physical changes resulting from acromegaly are slow to develop and insidious in onset; consequently, patients frequently do not notice the changes and the mean time to diagnosis from the onset of symptoms is in the region of 6 years.

Table 2 Frequency of Occurrence of Various Types of Pituitary Tumors

Prolactinomas	27.3%
Nonfunctioning tumors	25.2%
GH-secreting adenomas	14.0%
GH-prolactin secreting tumors	8.4%
Cushing's disease	8.0%
Gonadotrophin adenomas	6.4%
Silent ACTH-producing adenomas	6.0%
Plurihormonal adenomas	3.7%
TSH-secreting adenomas	1.0%

Source: From Ref. 138.

Table 3 Consequences of Pituitary Tumors

Hypersecretion with systemic hormonal effects
Prolactin LH and FSH excess with reproductive problems
TSH production with hyperthyroidism
ACTH production with Cushing's disease
GH excess with acromegaly
Mass effect
Visual changes
Raised ICP
Headache
Nonspecific
Infertility
Epilepsy
Pituitary hypofunction
Incidental

Excess GH produces a wide-ranging clinical syndrome that affects almost all organ systems in the body (Table 4). Although the clinical picture may make the diagnosis obvious, random measurement of GH may be misleading, as GH release is intermittent and the hormone has a short half-life (5). Insulin-like growth factor 1 (IGF-1), which regulates the release of GH, has a longer half-life, and a single elevated IGF-1 is a useful measure of sustained GH activity. The release of GH is normally inhibited by rising blood-glucose levels, and a failure of a 75 gm oral glucose load to suppress GH concentrations strongly supports the diagnosis.

Medical management of acromegaly is feasible, as GH release is well controlled with dopamine agonists and octreotide, although the need for parenteral administration and the increased incidence of gallstones with the latter agent limits its use (6). However, for most patients, trans-sphenoidal hypophysectomy will be the treatment of choice, with or without subsequent radiotherapy.

1. Anesthesia

The patient with acromegaly presents a considerable anesthetic challenge. Preoperative assessment must

Table 4 Consequences of Acromegaly

System	Process	Consequences
Integumentary	Thickening of skin and subcutaneous tissues	Coarsening of facial features; thickening of fingers; spade-shaped hands; carpal tunnel syndrome; skin tags
	Stimulation of cutaneous glands	Seborrheic skin; hypertrichosis; excessive sweating
Musculoskeletal	Bony overgrowth	Prognathism; jaw malocclusion; prominent supraorbital ridge; kyphoscoliosis and backache; osteoporosis; osteoarthrosis; joint pains
	Muscle overgrowth	Increased lean body mass; myopathy and weakness
Cardiovascular	Cardiac enlargement	Cardiomegaly; left ventricular hypertrophy; ECG abnormalities; myocardial interstitial fibrosis; cardiac failure; arrhythmia risk
	Unknown	Hypertension; accelerated atherosclerosis
Respiratory	Soft tissue overgrowth	Large tongue; enlargement of pharyngeal mucosa; thickening of vocal cords; narrowing of entire upper airway; upper airway obstruction, snoring, and sleep apnea; chronic obstructive lung disease
Gastrointestinal	Organomegaly	Enlarged liver and kidney (asymptomatic); increased hernia incidence; colonic polyps; increased risk of esophageal, gastric, and colonic cancer
Reproductive	Altered gonadotrphin production	Hypogonadism; galactorrhea; loss of libido; abnormal menstruation; infertility
Metabolic	Anti-insulin effect	Decreased glucose tolerance; diabetes mellitus
	Increased bone turnover	Raised urinary calcium; hyperphosphatemia; renal stones
Central nervous system	Mass effects	Headache; epilepsy; raised intracranial pressure; visual field defects

include a full cardiovascular evaluation, including echocardiography where it is appropriate to evaluate left ventricular function. It has been suggested that, where significant left ventricular dysfunction with cardiac failure is present, medical management with somatostatin should be used prior to surgery, until cardiac function has improved (7). Hypertension normally responds readily to standard antihypertensive medication and should be controlled preoperatively. Neurological evaluation should include visual field assessment and a search for the signs and symptoms of raised intracranial pressure. Glucose tolerance should be assessed, as it is advisable to maintain plasma glucose concentrations at <8 mmol/L in patients undergoing neurosurgical procedures. Blood glucose is generally higher in acromegalic patients than matched controls (8). Respiratory function (including blood-gas analysis) should be evaluated and a careful history taken looking for symptoms associated with sleep apnea such as daytime somnolence and snoring.

In planning the anesthesia, standard techniques for a neurosurgical procedure should be adopted, but, in addition, preparation must be made for managing possible airway problems. Acromegaly is associated with difficulties in airway management and intubation, and a careful preoperative airway evaluation should be performed, including indirect laryngoscopy, and, possibly, nasopharyngeal endoscopy. In a retrospective study of 28 patients undergoing pituitary tumor excision for acromegaly over a 10-year period, airway management was difficult in 11/28 and intubation was difficult in 12/28 of patients; for three patients, fiber-optic intubation was required (8). However, even fiber-optic airway management is no guarantee of success, as the hypertrophy of the soft tissues of the upper airway may make visualization of the vocal cords difficult using fiber-optic endoscopy (9). A prospective study of 128 patients found an incidence of difficult intubation (Cormack and Lehane Grade III) of 33%; Mallampati classes 3 and 4 were significantly associated with difficult intubation but did not predict all difficult intubations (10). The intubating laryngeal mask has been used successfully, but experience is limited (11). Laryngeal thickening also results in a narrowed glottic inlet, and a smaller diameter tube than anticipated from the patient's age and size may be needed. The airway involvement has been graded on a four-point scale, with grade 1 indicating no involvement, grade 2 reflecting nasal and laryngeal hypertrophy only, and grade 3 indicating glottic involvement; the presence of grade 2 and grade 3 involvement is categorized as grade 4 (12). It has been recommended that elective tracheostomy should be performed in the presence of the involvement of grade 3 or grade 4, but fiber-optic intubation has proved satisfactory in several other studies (5). It has also been recommended that awake, fiber-optic intubation should be performed, but most recent studies have reported the performance of laryngoscopy, with fiber-optic intubation where necessary, after the induction of anesthesia. In contrast to the statements in the older literature, recent reports have not suggested that maintenance of ventilation using a facemask is frequently difficult or impossible (5,8,9), provided that large-size facemasks and laryngoscope blades are used. Nevertheless, standard procedures for management of a difficult airway should be followed. Facilities for the emergency management of a failed intubation should be available where a difficult intubation is anticipated. Once the airway is secured, a pharyngeal pack should be inserted to prevent blood tracking down the esophagus, as blood in the stomach is a potent emetic in the postoperative period. The upper airway soft tissues may also be very friable, and bleeding may pose a problem. It is generally advised that a topical vasoconstrictor agent is applied to the nasopharyngeal mucosa, but cocaine is not recommended because it may induce unexpected adverse effects (13). A mixture of phenylephrine and lidocaine has proven to be efficacious (14).

The anesthetic technique should aim at hemodynamic stability and rapid recovery. For all pituitary surgery, 100 mg of hydrocortisone should be given at induction of anesthesia. In the presence of raised intracranial pressure, total intravenous anesthesia should be considered. Nitrous oxide should probably be avoided, not only because of its adverse effects on cerebral circulation and metabolism (15–17), but also because of the risk of air embolus and pneumocephalus, as the patient will be in a head-up position (18). Nasal vasoconstrictors will probably be required by the surgeon but, now as there are a number of good options, cocaine is probably best avoided in these patients who have an inherent risk of myocardial injury and arrhythmia (19,20). The trans-sphenoidal approach is intensely stimulating during access to the pituitary fossa, and this period may require deep anesthesia to control pain-induced increases in blood pressure. Remifentanil has recently been recommended for this type of procedure, not only for the good hemodynamic control, but also for the rapidity of recovery (21). However, a recent review of 28 cases suggested that hypertension was relatively mild and easily controlled (8). Hyperventilation to reduce brain volume is not recommended, as this may result in the tumor retreating into the cranium. Some surgeons use a lumbar CSF drain, so that the intracranial pressure can be more easily controlled injecting 0.9% saline into the CSF when an increase in pressure is required to deliver the tumor into the pituitary fossa, and draining CSF later if reduction in CSFP is needed, e.g., to control CSF leak from the operative site. Controlled hypercapnia has also been suggested to achieve similar purposes (22). Blood sugar should be controlled within a narrow range of 4.5–8 mmol/L throughout the procedure, using a continuous infusion of insulin if necessary. Intraoperative GH measurement to establish complete tumor excision improves the outcome in patients with noninvasive GH-secreting rnacroadenomas (23).

At the end of the procedure, smooth and rapid emergence from anesthesia is essential to allow early neurosurgical assessment and maintenance of respiratory and cardiovascular variables (5). The decision to extubate the patient should be based on the preoperative assessment of the airway, on any indication of preoperative sleep apnea, and on the state of consciousness of the patient. In their survey, Seidman et al. (8) found that 20 out of 28 patients could be extubated in the operating room. It should be remembered that airway difficulties may be increased by the presence of nasal packs and that there may be significant amounts of blood in the naso- and oropharynx. Careful oropharyngeal toilet should be performed before the removal of the endotracheal tube.

2. *Postoperative Care*

Postoperatively, patients should be managed in a neurosurgical intensive care or high dependency unit for at least 24 hr. Retropharyngeal bleeding, the presence of nasal packs, and the likelihood of upper airway obstruction and sleep apnea imply an increased risk of respiratory obstruction in the early recovery period. Obviously, nasal CPAP is not an option at this time, and careful airway monitoring for the first postoperative night is essential. Diabetes insipidus is always a risk with pituitary surgery and urine output, and specific gravity should be monitored routinely postoperatively, supported by regular plasma and urinary osmolality determinations if problems appear. Should polyuria develop, a diagnosis of diabetes insipidus should be confirmed clinically before treatment is instituted; the standard criteria include increased plasma osmolality (>295 mOsm/kg), hypotonic urine (<300 mOsm/kg), and a urine output > 2 ml/kg per hour. Patients are frequently able to compensate simply by increasing their oral intake, as the problem often resolves over a few days. Where treatment is required, the problem is easily managed with desmopressin acetate (DDAVP) (24) in a dose of 0.1 μg intravenous, although oral preparations and a nasal spray are also available for the conscious patient. All patients are likely to require cortisol replacement at least in the initial postoperative period. A standard regimen recommends hydrocortisone 50 mg BD on the first postoperative day, 25 mg BD on the second, reducing to 20 mg in the morning and 10 mg in the evening on the third day (25). By the time of hospital discharge, the dose could be reduced to 15 mg in the morning and 5 mg in the evening. The adrenal–cortical axis should be evaluated in the standard manner, once the patient has fully recovered from the surgery.

D. Cushing's Disease

Adrenocorticotrophic hormone-producing tumors of the pituitary occur with a similar frequency to those producing GH and lead to overstimulation of the adrenal glands and excess circulating cortisol. Most of these tumors are microadenomas and 80% occur in women. In paraneoplastic conditions, ectopic production of ACTH-like substances may occur, mainly from bronchial carcinoid or thymic tumors (26), and this source accounts for about 10% of all cases of endogenous Cushing's syndrome. The effects of overproduction of cortisol are mainly metabolic, with protein catabolism, excess gluconeogenesis, abnormalities of fat metabolism, abnormalities of reproductive function, and impaired stress–response and wound healing. The consequences are protean and, like excess GH, affect most systems in the body (Table 5).

As with other endocrine neoplasms, the diagnosis is frequently delayed, as the onset of symptoms may be subtle and gradual. In a recent European survey, the mean interval between onset and diagnosis was ~4 years (27). As various conditions may produce Cushing's syndrome and as the metabolic consequences of this condition may be the result, at least in part, of a number of other disease states, the diagnosis may be difficult and should be carried out in a specialist center. Primary screening is usually performed with the overnight dexamethasone suppression test. In this test, increased urinary cortisol should be markedly reduced in a morning collection of urine by a dose of 1–2 mg dexamethasone taken in the previous evening, and ACTH concentrations should fall to very low levels in the absence of an ACTH-producing tumor. Although this is a simple, outpatient procedure, a high level of patient compliance is required, so that this test is frequently not reliable. Stimulation with corticotrophin releasing hormone (CRH) should produce a marked increase in ACTH in pituitary disease, whereas this response is absent in patients with adrenal tumors or ectopic ACTH production. High-dose dexamethasone for 48 hr should suppresses cortisol production in pituitary-dependent Cushing's syndrome, and final confirmation of Cushing's disease is selective inferior petrosal sinus sampling before and after CRH stimulation.

The prognosis for Cushing's disease is reasonably good. Trans-sphenoidal hypophysectomy is the treatment of choice (28) resulting in a cure or prolonged remission in around 80% of sufferers, with a recurrence rate of around 10%. Rarely, where the primary tumor is not amenable to surgery or where hypophysectomy has been unsuccessful, bilateral adrenalectomy may be performed. However, more commonly, this procedure is performed for symptomatic relief in patients with ectopic ACTH production from a nonresectable tumor.

1. *Preoperative Preparation*

Hypertension is common (80% of cases) due to increased aldosterone production with increased renin–angiotensin production and may be difficult to control preoperatively, frequently requiring three or more antihypertensive agents (29). Control of hypertension and hyperglycemia should be optimized and the administration of H_2-receptor antagonists

Table 5 Consequences of Cortisol Excess

System	Consequences
Integumentary	Purple striae on abdomen, buttocks, and thighs; easy bruising; hirsutism; acne
Musculoskeletal	Proximal myopathy and weakness; osteoporosis; vertebral collapse
Cardiovascular	Left ventricular hypertrophy; ECG abnormalities; hypertension (85%)
Gastrointestinal	Esophageal reflux
Respiratory	Sleep apnea (32%)
Reproductive	Virilization in women due to hypersecretion of the adrenal androgens; oligomenorrhea; loss of libido; impotence in males
Metabolic	Decreased glucose tolerance; diabetes mellitus (60%)
	Altered fat metabolism: "moon" face, central obesity, "buffalo hump"
	Increased mineralocorticoid activity: hyponatremia, hypokalemia, metabolic alkalosis
Central nervous system	Psychiatric symptoms: depression, agitated psychosis (60–70% of patients)

considered in patients with reflux esophagitis. Control of excess cortisol production can be achieved preoperatively with the use of cortisol biosynthesis inhibitors such as metyrapone, etomidate, or ketoconazole (30), but this is not widely advocated except in severe cases. Octreotide has not been successful in controlling Cushing's disease (31).

2. *Anesthesia*

There is no evidence of an increase in airway problems in Cushing's disease, despite the increased incidence of sleep apnea. Extensive monitoring, including pulmonary artery catheter placement and invasive arterial pressure monitoring, has been advocated as fluid management, and cardiovascular instability may present particular problems. Peripheral vascular access may prove difficult, and the skin fragility means that care must be taken with adhesive strapping, as the skin is easily damaged. The use of sutures rather than strapping to secure vascular access catheters should be considered. Otherwise, the principles of anesthetic management are similar to those of other hypophyseal procedures, as outlined earlier for acromegaly. Care must be taken with patient positioning, as the osteoporosis renders the patient at risk from fractures, and scrupulous antiseptic procedures should be adopted, as the patients have diminished resistance to infection. Prophylactic antibiotics using a cephalosporin (e.g., cephuroxime 1.5 g) at induction and at 3 hr-intervals are currently recommended in the United Kingdom for these procedures (5).

3. *Postoperative*

Again, the principles of management are similar to those for acromegalic patients, although the airway problems are considerably less severe. Postoperative hormone replacement, as outlined earlier, is imperative for these patients, and patients are likely to require a longer period of steroid support than is the acromegalic patient.

II. PARATHYROID TUMORS

A. Parathyroid Function

The parathyroid glands are derived embryologically from endodermal tissue of the third and fourth pharyngeal pouches. The inferior parathyroid glands are associated developmentally with the thymus gland and, occasionally, may migrate with the thymus into the thorax. However, more usually, they are associated with the inferior thyroid poles, whereas the superior parathyroid glands are associated with the lateral lobes of the thyroid gland. This embryological origin makes the association of the parathyroid glands with the multiple endocrine neoplasia (MEN) syndromes difficult to explain, but it is suggested that elements of neuronal crest tissue are contained within the parathyroid glands.

Parathyroid hormone (PTH) has a half-life in the circulation of 2–3 min (32) and regulates extracellular ionized calcium ($[Ca^{2+}]_0$) and magnesium ($[Mg^{2+}]_0$) concentrations by direct effects on the bone and the kidney and indirect actions (via calcitriol production) on the gut. When the $[Ca^{2+}]_0$ concentration in the plasma falls, there is rapid increase in the concentration of PTH (33) that stimulates osteoblastic activity directly, with indirect stimulation of osteoclastic activity (32), resulting in an increase in bone turnover with release of calcium into the circulation.

In the kidney, PTH acts on the thick ascending limb of the loop of Henle and in the distal convoluted tubule to increase reabsorption of Ca^{2+}. In the proximal tubule, PTH inhibits the reabsorption of inorganic phosphate, thus increasing phosphate excretion. Parathyroid hormone also stimulates the conversion of vitamin D to the active 1,25-dihydroxy-cholecalciferol (calcitriol) in the kidney. Calcitriol stimulates intestinal uptake of calcium and may also have an effect on osteoclast activity.

The discovery of an extracellular, G-protein-coupled, calcium-sensing receptor (CaR) has helped to clarify some of the mechanisms by which calcium and its regulating factors interact (34). The CaR system regulates parathyroid secretion, with an increase in $[Ca^{2+}]_0$, inhibiting the release of PTH. The relationship between $[Ca^{2+}]_0$ and PTH release is a very tight one with a steep dose–response curve. Remarkably, small changes in the circulating concentration of either Ca^{2+} or Mg^{2+} are sensed by the CaR and produce corresponding changes in the secretion of PTH (35). In the kidney, stimulation of the CaR by excessive $[Ca^{2+}]_0$ or $[Mg^{2+}]_0$ leads to inability to concentrate the urine and the polyuria (36).

Parathyroid hormone-related protein is a 141-amino acid peptide, functionally similar to PTH, which is produced by certain malignant tumors, particularly squamous cell tumors of the head and neck and also tumors arising from kidney, breast, and lymphoid tissue.

B. Hyperparathyroidism

Among endocrine neoplasms, primary hyperparathyroidism is a relatively common disorder with an incidence of about 25 per 100,000 of the population. The majority of patients with primary hyperparathyroidism

Table 6 Features of Hyperparathyroidism

Organ system	Symptoms and signs
Renal	Polyuria,* polydipsia,* and diabetes insipidus;* nephrocalcinosis and renal stones; diminished bicarbonate absorption and renal tubular acidosis; phosphate and magnesium loss; glycosuria*
Cardiovascular	Hypertension, diminished circulating blood volume,* ECG changes: short QT interval, prolonged PR interval
Gastrointestinal	Abdominal pain, weight loss, vomiting;* peptic ulceration; pancreatitis
Skeletal	Osteitis fibrosa cystica; bone pain; demineralization; pathological fractures; joints: chondrocalcinosis, pseudogout, ligamentous calcification
Central nervous system	Depression; personality changes; memory loss; psychosis;* fatigue
Metabolic	Electrolyte abnormalities; muscle weakness

* denotes features usually found in acute disequilibrium states.

(>90%) have a single parathyroid adenoma, and the rest have multiple lesions that are usually part of MEN disorders. Less than 1% of all parathyroid tumors is malignant.

Chromosomal abnormalities of the PTH gene have been associated with some parathyroid adenomas and it has been suggested that loss of a tumor suppressor gene may also play a role, although such a gene has not been identified yet. However, although genetic mutations may explain the development of parathyroid adenomas, they do not explain the failure of response of the parathyroid cells to normal calcium regulation.

The presentation of primary hyperparathyroidism may be subtle and may remain clinically undetected as a number of patients are asymptomatic for many years. However, all patients with hyperparathyroidism have elevated plasma calcium concentrations, and the principle features of hypercalcemia due to hyperparathyroidism are summarized in Table 6. Untreated, these patients have a significantly higher mortality than the general population, and even after tumor excision, the risk of death is higher than the normal population (32).

1. *Management*

Mild hypercalcemia is seldom symptomatic, and many argue that it rarely warrants special treatment. An NIH Consensus statement suggested that modest calcium elevations in older patients without bone disease could be managed nonoperatively (37). On the other hand, others argue that as many as one-third of patients will develop complications within 10 years. Principal among these is progressive osteopenia, which would adversely affect middle-aged women (38). Further arguments relate to subtle psychological changes that may be difficult to detect but improve after parathyroidectomy (39).

Disequilibrium hypercalcemia refers to a progressive and rapid rise in calcium levels (usually >3 mmol/L and sometimes reaching 6 mmol/L), with the clinical features of disequilibrium (Table 6). This state constitutes a medical emergency and sometimes necessitates admission to an intensive-care ward. The most crucial factor is the re-establishment of cardiovascular homeostasis and adequate renal function, rather than the reduction of the plasma Ca^{2+} to any predetermined value. Hypercalcemia induces a diuresis due to the stimulation of the renal CaR (mentioned earlier) and, consequently, patients with disequilibrium hypercalcemia are usually severely fluid depleted. Fluid replacement should be with saline solutions using a central venous line. Saline diuresis may produce hypokalemia and hypomagnesemia with a resultant increase in risk of cardiac dysrhythmias, and potassium and magnesium supplementation should be considered. There is no literature to support any specific plasma calcium concentration as a cut-off value above which anesthesia becomes unacceptably hazardous. Once the plasma volume is re-expanded, the patient stabilized and the disease confirmed by emergency PTH measurement, an emergency parathyroidectomy should be performed. The operation leads to an almost immediate correction of the condition (39).

Various other approaches to hypercalcemia have been used but are of questionable value. The place of diuretics such as furosemide is controversial; the main therapeutic thrust being to establish normovolemia and a saline diuresis. Correction of hypophosphatemia will inhibit the absorption of calcium from the gut, increase bone uptake of calcium, and correct the cardiac and skeletal muscle weakness that accompanies phosphate deficits. However, the use of sodium phosphate to lower calcium concentrations can no longer be recommended due to the risk of calcium phosphate deposition in the tissues. Other agents that will lower the plasma Ca^{2+} include plicamycin (mithramycin), calcitonin, and glucocorticoids. Plicamycin, a cytotoxic, impedes osteoclastic bone resorption but may have renal, hepatic, and hematological toxic effects and must be used with caution. The diphosphonates (pamidronate, etidronate, clodronate) also inhibit osteoplastic activity. All these newer agents will take several days to be effective, and their use to lower $[Ca^{2+}]_0$ prior to parathyroidectomy is seldom necessary. Diphosphonates are usually prescribed for the hypercalcemia found in metastatic cancer.

Preoperative preparation for conventional parathyroidectomy should include a full cardiovascular workup, as these patients have an increased risk of hypertension and may have nonspecific ECG abnormalities, thrombo-embolic disease, and stroke. The main anesthetic considerations for a patient undergoing parathyroidectomy are fluid balance management, neuromuscular blockade, and the possibility of cardiac dysrhythmias. In a well-prepared patient, whose fluid balance and electrolyte status has been corrected preoperatively, invasive pressure (venous or arterial) monitoring should not be necessary. The response to muscle relaxants may be unpredictable, and neuromuscular transmission monitoring is essential if muscle relaxants are used (40), as abnormal responses may occur (41). There is no reason to avoid using a laryngeal mask airway, apart from the slight distortion of the neck it may produce, and this obviates the need for muscle relaxation. Increasingly, there is a trend towards regional anesthesia, particularly where improved tumor location techniques permit unilateral neck exploration. Superficial cervical plexus blockade with local anesthetic supplementation is a simple, safe technique for either unilateral or bilateral parathyroid exploration and may be performed on an outpatient basis on suitable patients (42–45). However, bilateral deep cervical plexus blockade should not be necessary (46) and carries the risk of bilateral phrenic nerve paralysis.

It is important to localize the adenoma preoperatively. The dictum "the best means of localization is with an experienced parathyroid surgeon" is outdated, as technetium-99m sestamibi scanning has a high degree of accuracy in localization and has superseded ultrasonography and CT scan. Further, accurate preoperative localization permits minimally invasive surgery; only one quadrant, instead of four, being explored (47,48). The adenoma may be localized preoperatively, and at surgery, a small cut made over the site and the lesion removed. Localization may be enhanced and facilitated by the use of an isotope probe (49).

In the immediate postoperative period, airway problems may occur due to recurrent laryngeal nerve injury. The "hungry bone syndrome" of rapid reuptake of calcium, phosphate, and magnesium into bone, following the removal of a parathyroid tumor and the consequent hypocalcemia, may precipitate cardiac arrhythmias, and very occasionally, life-threatening laryngeal spasm. The condition is usually found with secondary and tertiary (renal) hyperparathyroidism. In primary disease, it may only occur when severe osteopenia (as evidenced radiologically, by alkaline phosphatase elevation or by densitometry) is present. Such hypocalcemia may occur within hours of surgery where there is marked bone disease.

The patient experiences tingling of the lips, nose, and fingers. Treatment consists of intravenous calcium gluconate and oral calcium glubionate or carbonate.

III. GASTROENTEROPANCREATIC TUMORS

A. Carcinoid Tumors

The term carcinoid was originally introduced to describe intestinal tumors that resembled but were less aggressive than the more common intestinal adenocarcinomas. Carcinoid tumors represent about 2% of all malignant tumors of the gastrointestinal tract, with an overall incidence of tumors found at autopsy of 1–2 per 100,000 people (50), although the incidence of symptomatology is approximately one-quarter of that. The tumors are derived from enterochromaffin cells and may be found in any tissue derived from endoderm, although the gastrointestinal tract is the most common sight for their development. The cells giving rise to these tumors have the capacity for amine precursor uptake and decarboxylation. They may arise not only from the gut, but also from the lungs and bronchi. Carcinoid tumors contain and secrete a large number of amine and peptide hormones including serotonin, corticotrophin, histamine, dopamine, substance P, neurotensin, prostaglandins, and kallikrein (which stimulates the production of bradykinin and tachykinins). Despite this array of biologically active substances contained within these tumors, only a minority (5–8%) of patients with carcinoid tumors progress to develop carcinoid syndrome.

Traditionally, carcinoid tumors were classified according to their embryonic site of origin, arising from the foregut, midgut, and hindgut. Although it is now more customary to classify the tumors according to their functional status, this anatomical classification is still of some value, as the tumors arising from each of these anatomically distinct areas may behave quite

Table 7 Abbreviated Table of Sites, Secretions, Behavior, and Associations of Carcinoid Tumors

Site	Secretion	Behavior	Comment
Respiratory			
Typical carcinoid	Serotonin, corticotropin	Indolent	
Atypical carcinoid (139)	Serotonin, histamine	Malignant, metastasizing	
Gastric			
Type 1	Nil, hypergastrinemia from hypochlorhydria	Well differentiated, noninvasive	CAG-A, multiple, fundus, body
Type 2		Well differentiated, noninvasive	ZE syndrome, MEN 1
Type 3		Invasive	Sporadic, solitary
Small bowel	Serotonin, substance P	Indolent	Carcinoid syndrome
Appendix	Serotonin, substance P	Indolent	
Colon	Serotonin, substance P	Invasive	Right sided
Rectum	Nil	Well differentiated	

Note: CAG-A, chronic atrophic gastritis type A.
Source: Adapted from Ref. 53.

differently (Table 7). Tumors arising from embryological foregut may occur in the thymus, lung, stomach, pancreas, and proximal duodenum; of these, the lung and stomach are the commonest sites, with only occasional carcinoid tumors being reported from the other areas. Tumors arising from the lung and the thymus are particularly likely to contain histamine and may give rise to a very vivid red and patchy flushing. They may also secrete ACTH, resulting in Cushing's syndrome (26,51). Gastric carcinoids may take various forms. Benign tumors arise from mucosal cells and occur as multiple tumors in the fundus or body of the stomach and may be associated with atrophic gastritis and pernicious anemia. Tumors associated with the MEN type 1 (MEN-1) are more likely to be malignant and to metastasize (see in what follows).

Midgut structures giving rise to carcinoids include the distal duodenum, jejunum, appendix, and proximal colon, deriving their blood supply from the superior mesenteric artery and draining into the portal venous system. Small bowel carcinoid tumors are relatively slow growing but are much more likely to metastasize than tumors arising from other sites, with the exception of carcinoid of the appendix which has a low metastatic tendency, possibly because these tumors generally arise from a different cell type (52). However, the appendix is the commonest single site for the occurrence of carcinoid tumors, and these tumors generally present with symptoms related to anatomical distortion such as abdominal pain and intestinal obstruction, rather than hormone-related symptomatology. Midgut tumors are particularly likely to produce large quantities of serotonin. The primary midgut tumors are generally small (5–10 mm in diameter) and are multiple in up to one-third of patients; however, metastases arising from these sites may be large. Hindgut tumors of the distal colon and rectum generally secrete hormones (pancreatic polypeptide, peptide YY, human chorionic gonadotropin, and chromogranin A) that do not cause any specific clinical symptoms and most commonly present with problems related to the mass, including abdominal pain, intestinal obstruction, and bleeding. Other sites for the development of carcinoid tumors include the kidney, ovary, testes, and prostate. As it is almost exclusively the midgut carcinoids that produce the classical features of carcinoid disease, it has been suggested that the term "carcinoid tumor" should be assigned to midgut carcinoid, whereas carcinoid tumors arising from elsewhere are termed neuroendocrine tumors related to their anatomical site. Classification has now been extended to include histologic variations and behavior (53).

The majority of gastrointestinal carcinoid tumors do not present with the classical hormone-related constellation of symptoms. The reasons for this are not fully understood but may relate to the production of biologically inactive forms of the hormones, to the release of subphysiological concentrations of active peptides into the bloodstream, or, most probably, to the rapid degradation of the peptides and amines in the blood, the liver, and the lungs. These tumors may offer a more classical surgical presentation with abdominal pain, intermittent intestinal obstruction, and gastrointestinal bleeding. The symptoms are often vague and generalized, and this may result in a delay in diagnosis. Computerized tomography of the abdomen may demonstrate liver enlargement and metastatic deposits in lymph nodes associated with diffuse abdominal symptoms of discomfort, borborygmus, and diarrhea. As a result of the nonspecific symptomatology, patients may present for surgery without the diagnosis having been made and with the consequent risk of the development of carcinoid crisis during the surgical procedure. Some of the gastrointestinal symptoms experienced by patients with carcinoid tumors may be due to local secretion of some of the hormonally active substances produced by the tumor. Neuroendocrine cells contain high levels of Chromogranin A (CgA), an acid glycoprotein that appears to play a role in the formation of secretary granules. The detection of circulating CgA is a marker of a variety of neuroendocrine neoplasms and, in carcinoid tumors, is an independent marker of a poor prognosis.

Bronchial carcinoids are generally very slow growing and have a very low level of metastatic activity and may be detected on routine chest X-ray in an otherwise asymptomatic patient. However, these tumors may also present with bronchial obstruction, obstructive pneumonitis, pleuritic pain, atelectasis, and dyspnea (41%). The anesthetic management of these patients may represent a considerable clinical challenge (54), and carcinoid crisis has been reported following surgical intervention in bronchial carcinoid (55). The results of surgical excision are generally excellent with an 80% 10-year survival rate (51,56).

The management of carcinoid tumors is essentially surgical, and complete removal of the tumor will often result in a cure, unless there are widespread metastases. Carcinoid tumors are generally resistant to standard chemotherapy, although chemoembolization of hepatic metastases, together with standard chemotherapy, may reduce the size of the secondary tumors and control symptomatology reasonably well. Radiotherapy has generally been unsuccessful, although high dose radioactive octreotide has shown partial responses in the few patients treated so far (57). Interferon-α (IFNα) has been shown to produce antitumor effects in 50–80% of carcinoid tumor patients and has demonstrated antiproliferative effects in carcinoid tumor cells (58). The resection of isolated liver metastases may also be successful, but many midgut carcinoid tumors have multiple, widespread liver metastases that are not generally amenable to surgical cure. Liver transplantation has occasionally been performed in an attempt to remove multiple hepatic metastases, but the technique is too new to evaluate the benefits in terms of long-term outcome, although good short-term responses have so far been achieved (59). In a recent survey, the 5-year survival rate was 93% for patients with localized disease, 74% for those with regional spread, but only 19% for those with distant metastases.

1. *Carcinoid Syndrome*

The carcinoid syndrome occurs when various hormones produced by the tumor are released into the systemic circulation. It is generally assumed that carcinoid syndrome only becomes manifest, once metastatic disease is present, as the liver normally metabolizes the active peptides and amines before they reach the systemic circulation. However, in rare cases, notably but not exclusively, those where the tumors occur in regions not drained by the portal system (such as the lungs or ovaries), carcinoid syndrome may occur without hepatic metastases. Rectal carcinoid, despite having direct access to the systemic circulation, rarely causes carcinoid syndrome, as these tumors do not produce the classical array of active amines and peptides.

Diarrhea and flushing are the commonest symptoms of the carcinoid syndrome, although the relationship between the two symptoms is variable, the hormonal cause of each of these problems is different, and the hormones have different release patterns and duration of effect. The various causes of periodic flushing are summarized in Table 8. The flush reaction may have various manifestations from the typical varying, patchy red, plethoric appearance thought to be related to the production of tachykinins and to more serious generalized facial flushing with swelling and lachrymation. This latter presentation is thought to be associated with excess histamine release and is commoner with bronchial carcinoids; it may be associated with hypotension, exacerbation of diarrhea, and palpitations. This is the most severe type of flush reaction and is sometimes part of the carcinoid crisis. It is of relevance that upper airway edema and difficulties with intubation have not been reported as a feature of this type of facial flushing. The diarrhea is characterized by watery stools, colicky abdominal pain, and urgency of defecation. The gastro-intestinal symptomatology may respond to ondansetron (60). It may be associated with significant fluid and electrolyte abnormalities that should be looked for and corrected prior to anesthesia.

Bronchoconstriction and hypotension may be severe and resistant to conventional therapy, particularly in the perioperative period. The suggested relationship between the various secretary products of

Table 8 Causes of Episodic Flushing

Carcinoid syndrome
Medullary thyroid carcinoma
Pheochromocytoma
Diabetes, autonomic neuropathy
Menopause, hot flashes
Diencephalic seizures
Panic attacks
Mastocytosis

carcinoid tumors and the clinical symptoms is illustrated in Table 9.

Carcinoid heart disease occurs in the majority of patients with the carcinoid syndrome, with abnormal echocardiographic findings in up to 70% of patients (61). The characteristic lesions are plaque formation and the thickening of pulmonary and tricuspid valves leading to valvular insufficiency and occasionally stenosis. Tricuspid insufficiency is the most common finding in patients with carcinoid heart disease, but the pathophysiological mechanisms are not entirely understood. It is thought that serotonin and tachykinin damage the valvular endothelium resulting in platelet adhesion, valvulitis, and fibroblast proliferation, leading to the formation of carcinoid plaques (62). Tricuspid incompetence is the commonest finding in patients with carcinoid heart disease. Left-sided valvular lesions are uncommon (53), probably because the lung reduces the high concentrations of serotonin and tachykinins, to which the right heart is subjected. Valve surgery is the only definitive treatment. Although cardiac surgery carries a high perioperative mortality, marked symptomatic improvement occurs in survivors. Surgical intervention should, therefore, be considered when cardiac symptoms become severe (63). Myocardial metastatic carcinoid disease can also occur (64).

The diagnosis of carcinoid syndrome is based initially on the symptomatology and supported by biochemical tests. Urinary 5HIAA is the standard initial confirmatory test, although false positives may occur in patients taking chlorpromazine or who have recently ingested bananas, avocado, pineapple, walnuts, chocolate, or coffee. Plasma CgA is almost invariably elevated in metastatic carcinoid and is a useful marker of the success of treatment. Patients with foregut carcinoids should also undergo determination of ACTH or GH if they present with symptoms suggestive of Cushing's disease or acromegaly. Ultrasound and computerized tomography have been used for the detection of the metastases, with contrast-enhanced CT being superior to MRI scanning. Tumor localization with somatostatin scintigraphy is extremely useful in identifying multiple tumors but may be superseded by positron emission tomography in the future (65).

The cardiac status of patients with carcinoid syndrome should be evaluated by echocardiography preoperatively, given the high incidence of cardiac involvement. Carcinoid-associated cardiac disease and

Table 9 Clinical Effects, Mediators, and Treatment of Carcinoid Syndrome

Clinical effects	Proposed mediators	Treatment
Flushing	Tachykinins (neurokinin A, substance P, neuropeptide K)	Somatostatin analogues (others: IFNα, glucocorticoids, phenothiazine,α-adrenergic block; avoid alcohol) H_1- and H_2-receptor blocking drugs (chlorpheniramine, ranitidine, cimetidine)
	Histamine	
	Vasoactive peptides	Somatostatin analogues
Hypotension	Histamine	Check fluids; myocardial depressants, somatostatin analogues, angiotensin, vasopressin, methoxamine, (epinephrine–care!)
Diarrhea	Serotonin (5HT)	Somatostatin analogues [others: *para*-chlorophenylalanine, 5HT antagonists (cyproheptadine, methysergide ondansetron), loperamide, IFNα]
	Prostaglandins E and F	
	Bile acid loss	Cholestyramine
	Bacterial contamination	Doxycycline
Abdominal cramps	Small bowel obstruction	Surgical decompression
Dyspnea		
Wheezing (broncho constriction)	Serotonin	Somatostatin analogues, bronchodilators (care!) (β-adrenergic agonists, theophylline); chlorpheniramine, nebulized ipratropium bromide
	Substance P	
	Bradykinin	
Carcinoid heart disease	Growth factors, 5HT(?)	Valvular replacement (tricuspid, pulmonary) diuretics
Skin lesions	Niacin deficiency	Nicotinamide
Palpitations (tachycardia, hypertension)	Serotonin	Somatostatin analogues, ketanserin, (others: labetolol, esmolol, increased depth of anesthesia)

right-heart failure are significant predictors of postoperative morbidity and mortality (66). Careful fluid and electrolyte assessment and correction may be required, and the need for intraoperative measurements of electrolytes and glucose should be anticipated.

The major intraoperative concern is the occurrence of carcinoid crisis with severe hyper/hypotension and bronchospasm. As with most other endocrine tumors, the rarity of the condition has precluded prospective studies of preoperative preparation and anesthetic techniques in large number of patients. Prior to the advent of somatostatin, the generally recommended approach to patients with carcinoid syndrome was preoperative preparation with a variety of serotonin antagonists including ketanserin, methysergide, and cyproheptadine (67,68). However, introduction of somatostatin and its longer-acting analogue, octreotide, proved so immediately and obviously efficacious (69–71) as to reduce previous forms of perioperative management to the status of secondary level therapy. Five types of somatostatin receptors have been identified, and carcinoid tumors are particularly rich with type 2 (sst_2). Binding of somatostatin and its analogues to the sst_2 receptor mediates both antitumor effects and inhibition of hormone release. In addition, somatostatin has regulatory effects on GH and GH secretion and also regulates the release of gastrointestinal and pancreatic hormones. The half-life of somatostatin is 3 min, whereas that of its analogues, octreotide, lanreotide, and octastatin (all of which are octapeptides), is of the order of 100–120 min, making these agents easier to use in the treatment of patients with carcinoid syndrome. The efficacy of intraoperative administration of octreotide was confirmed recently in a retrospective study of 119 patients, but these authors were neither able to establish a reduction in intraoperative complication rate in patients receiving preoperative octreotide alone, nor could demonstrate a reduction in the rate of postoperative complications from the intraoperative use of octreotide (66). There is no single accepted guideline for the perioperative use of octreotide, and there are significant side effects including nausea, abdominal cramping, hypenglycemia, and (rarely) bradycardia and thrombocytopenia (72). The benefit of preoperative octreotide is not established, but some recommendations include the administration of 100 μg subcutaneously prior to surgery. It is generally recommended that 50–100 μg octreotide be given intravenously at induction. An intravenous infusion at a rate of 50–100 μ/hr can be used intraoperatively, with further bolus doses given intraoperatively as required for the control of symptoms. As intraoperative blood loss may be considerable, the presence of hypovolemia must always be considered should hypotension prove unresponsive octreotide. Hypotension refractory to octreotide may respond to the kallikrein inhibitor, aprotonin, and histamine antagonists, usually as a combination of H_1- and H_2-receptor blockers may be helpful, particularly in predominantly histamine-secreting tumors such as a gastric or bronchial carcinoid. Invasive monitoring should be used in most cases and may include central venous pressure monitoring, direct arterial pressure measurement, and possibly the use of pulmonary artery catheters. Whether or not it is advisable to place a pulmonary artery catheter in a patient with tricuspid and pulmonary valvular disease is unclear. Theoretically, transesophageal echocardiography should provide more useful information than pulmonary artery catheterization, as pulmonary artery dynamics may be significantly disrupted particularly during a carcinoid crisis. However, there is no firm scientific evidence on which to base recommendations.

There is also no scientific basis for recommending any one anesthetic technique in preference to any other. Histamine-releasing agents should, theoretically, be avoided, but most of the currently available anesthetic agents have been used in conjunction with carcinoid syndrome. Shorter acting agents may be preferred, as increased levels of serotonin may be associated with delayed emergence from anesthesia, and agents that release catecholamines should be avoided. Regional anesthesia is controversial, as the high-quality postoperative pain relief available from regional techniques is likely to be advantageous, but intraoperative management of hypotension associated with neuraxial blockade may be problematic. Although most texts recommend the avoidance of catecholamines, as all of the catecholamines have been reported to trigger carcinoid crises, there are also reports of good responses to epinephrine and phenylephrine in patients with otherwise unresponsive hypotension (73). Judicious use of small doses of direct-acting catecholamines, titrated against patient responsiveness, may be justified for both refractory bronchospasm and for cardiovascular support. Both phenylephrine and ephedrine have been extensively used during carcinoid resections (66). Bronchospasm should be managed in the first instance with deepening levels of volatile anesthesia and non-catecholamine bronchodilators such as ipratropium bromide. Antihistamines may be useful, but inhaled β-agonists should not be withheld if bronchospasm fails to respond to other measures.

IV. SURGICAL ASPECTS

The principles that underpin surgery for carcinoid tumors are similar to those for any epithelial tumor (e.g., ectodermal, neuroendocrine), with one important difference: palliative or "debulking" procedures are more readily undertaken where there is debilitating humoral secretion. Although excisional or debulking surgery is the most successful form of ablation, other modalities such as cryoablation, chemical ablation, or angioembolization may be used where surgery is not possible. Surgical resection is of benefit in patients with limited hepatic metastases (53) and may result in prolonged amelioration of symptoms and survival (74). Liver transplantation in highly selected cases may be successful, with up to 69% 5-year survival (75,76).

A. Pulmonary Carcinoids

Patients with pulmonary carcinoids may be asymptomatic, and the lesion found on routine chest roentgenogram is more usually with the symptoms of chest malignancy: cough, hemoptysis, recurrent infection, wheezing, and chest pain. Each of about 2% may present with the carcinoid or Cushing's syndromes. Preoperative biopsy is essential and is achieved by the bronchoscopic route for central tumors, and CT guided aspiration cytology for the more peripheral ones. Survival rates are 60–90%, depending on the degree of differentiation and stage of tumor.

The principles of surgery are complete removal of the primary tumor, with a draining lymphadenectomy. There are numerous surgical strategies, and these depend on the stage of the lesion. Wedge or segmental resections are usually undertaken. Endoscopic approaches are unlikely to achieve full tumor removal and should probably only be used palliatively. Imprint cytology or frozen section histology will help plan the extent of resection and lymphadenectomy. A multidisciplinary team approach offers potentially excellent results (54).

B. Gastric Carcinoids

There are three types of gastric carcinoids (Table 8) that differ in their pathogenesis and behavior. The majority of gastric carcinoids is type 1 and associated with chronic atrophic gastritis type A (CAG-A). The CAG-A induces hypergastrinemia, which is postulated, in turn, to cause enterochromaffin hyperplasia and carcinoid tumors. Most tumors are encountered in later life and have multiple lesions situated in the fundus or body of the stomach. Type 2 gastric carcinoids are also attributed to the hypergastrinemia found in the Zollinger Ellison syndrome. These are usually found in patients with MEN-1, and it is important that the other components of the syndrome (pituitary, pancreatic islet, parathyroid) be sought. Type 3 carcinoids are sporadic and malignant.

The surgical strategy chosen depends on the type, size, and number of the lesions. Because of the indolence of the first two types, small lesions (1 cm) are usually removed endoscopically and the biopsy site regularly monitored. Larger lesions may require segmental resection or gastrectomy. Multiple lesions may require a total gastrectomy. The inherent malignancy of the type 3 lesions mandates an approach similar to that for gastric carcinoma.

C. Carcinoids of Small Bowel

Carcinoid tumors of the small bowel are usually located in the distal ileum and are frequently multiple. Presenting in later life, they usually cause anemia and abdominal pain, and the diagnosis is made with difficulty; as a result, many present with nodal and liver metastases. The lesions may be accompanied by extensive mesenteric fibrosis.

The management is by surgical resection of both the affected bowel and mesentery, often in the presence of hepatic metastases (77).

D. Appendiceal Carcinoids

Over 90% of appendiceal carcinoids are asymptomatic, located at the tip of the appendix, and are <2 cm in diameter. More proximally located tumors may cause appendicitis and be a surprise finding at appendicectomy. The likelihood of nodal and hepatic metastases is size dependent and considerably more likely with tumors over 2 cm in size. The carcinoid syndrome usually occurs only when liver metastases are present.

Moertel's extensive review (78) provides guidance in management. Simple appendicectomy would suffice in tumors smaller than 2 cm. Moertel advises right hemicolectomy for larger lesions, but it is difficult to understand why a cecectomy would not be adequate.

E. Colonic and Rectal Carcinoids

Most tumors are found in the right side of the colon, usually the cecum. The symptoms are the same as those for colonic cancer and the carcinoid syndrome is found in <5% of them.

The surgical management strategies are the same as those for carcinoma of the colon; small rectal carcinoid is excised locally, with expectation of cure (79), but the larger ones are management using the surgical principles that govern rectal carcinoma.

Postoperatively, patients undergoing carcinoid tumor resection should be managed in a high care environment, as ongoing hemodynamic disturbances, metabolic disruptions, and release of mediators from residual tumor may pose significant problems. Good quality analgesia should improve the management of these patients, although there are no specific studies to support this proposition. As it is impossible to predict likelihood of continued mediated release, octreotide infusions should be continued postoperatively. Although it is generally recommended that histamine-releasing drugs should be avoided, there is no evidence that morphine, which releases histamine only at a cutaneous level, is contraindicated. Other short-acting, potent opioids such as fentanyl and sufentanil have been used successfully, and there would seem no reason to avoid nonsteroidal anti-inflammatory agents as part of a planned postoperative analgesic regime. Epidural analgesia is widely recommended. Antiemetic treatment is best provided with a serotonin antagonist such as ondansetron (80).

Kinney et al. (66) concluded that most people with metastatic carcinoid tumors could undergo intra-abdominal surgery safely. In their series, no intraoperative complications occurred in patients who received octreotide intraoperatively. Overall, perioperative complications and death were strongly associated with the presence of carcinoid heart disease and high elevated urinary 5HIAA output. A summary of the perioperative approach to carcinoid disease is presented in Table 10.

V. PHEOCHROMOCYTOMA

Pheochromocytomas are uncommon catecholamine-secreting tumors derived from neural crest tissues and may arise either from adrenal medulla or from other neural crest derivatives, mainly the sympathetic chain. True pheochromocytomas are those arising from the adrenal medulla, whereas those arising from the sympathetic chain are generally referred to as paraganglionomas or extra-adrenal pheochromocytomas. This latter group may arise from many locations from the base of the skull to the urinary bladder, with the commonest extra-adrenal site being the organ of Zuckerkandl in the para-aortic area. Catecholamine-producing tissues contain chromaffin cells so named as a result of the characteristic staining pattern seen when they are exposed to potassium dichromate. The cells are rich in chromogranin A, but CgA estimations in pheochromocytoma patients do not appear to have the same diagnostic and prognostic relevance they have in carcinoid disease (81). Less commonly, catecholamine-secreting tumors may arise from other tissues, including ganglioneuroblastoma, ganglioneuroma, and neuroblastoma. Familial pheochromocytoma is inherited as an autosomal dominant trait alone or as a component of the MEN type 2 syndromes (MEN-2A and MEN-2B), von Hippel-Lindau disease, or, in rare cases, neurofibromatosis type 1 (82,83). The remaining 90% of pheochromocytomas are classified as sporadic or nonsyndromic (84). However, recent evidence has suggested that there may be a genetic or familial basis for the development of pheochromocytoma of up to 25% of affected individuals (85). Malignant tumors are more likely to occur in association with the genetically determined forms of pheochromocytoma and are also commoner in association with extra-adrenal pheochromocytomas. Malignancy is difficult to diagnose, as there are no specific histological appearances. The diagnosis depends on the behavior of the tumor, particularly on the development of metastatic disease and tumor occurrence in sites not associated with neuroendocrine crest tissue.

A. Clinical Features

Although catecholamine excess is the hallmark of pheochromocytoma, an array of other neuropeptides may be found in association with these tumors,

Table 10 Evidence-Based Summary of Management Strategies for Carcinoid Disease

Condition	Management strategy	Level of evidence	Recommendation	References
Carcinoid syndrome				
Preoperative management	Somatostatin, octreotide	3, 4	B	59,70–72,140,141
Intraoperative control	Somatostatin, octreotide	3, 4	B	55,66,69,142
	Ketanserin, antihistamines, aprotonin	5	D	67,143,144
Carcinoid tumors				
Local lesion and mesenteric nodes	Local excision	3, 4	A	26,77,145–149
Liver metastases	Local excision with or without ablation of liver secondaries	5	D	74,146,150,151
	Orthotopic liver transplantation	5	D	75,76

including PTH, ACTH, tachykinins, and neuropeptide Y; the latter may contribute to hypertension, particularly during a crisis, which appears partially resistant to α-adrenergic blockade (86) but is not particularly useful in diagnosis (87).

The clinical features of pheochromocytoma are frequently diagnostic but may also present with a bewildering variety of symptoms. A triad of excessive sweating, headache, and palpitations occurs in over 90% of patients on careful inquiry but may not be the presenting symptoms. Patients may present with anxiety, tremor, nausea, vomiting and weight loss, chest and abdominal pain, peripheral vascular disease, cardiac failure, and cerebral vascular accident. Hypertension is classically episodic but may be sustained in up to 50% of patients (88). Heart rate may be either rapid or slow, and arrhythmias may or may not be present. Left ventricular failure and pulmonary edema may be present, particularly if the patient has developed a catecholamine-induced cardiomyopathy. An array of vascular pathology may be seen including peripheral vascular ischemia with tissue loss, myocardial infarction, cerebral vascular accident, and renal failure. Abdominal pain, presumably due to bowel ischemia, together with chronic constipation and pseudo-obstruction may lead to an erroneous diagnosis of an acute abdomen. Pheochromocytoma crisis may present with severe pounding headache, sweating, pallor, palpitations, and a feeling of impending doom. The onset may be sudden, but the duration is generally short. However, a minority of patients with pheochromocytoma will have experienced such a crisis. Metabolic problems, including weight loss and frank diabetes mellitus, may be presenting signs, and occasionally, patients may present in diabetic ketoacidosis (89). A significant proportion of pheochromocytomas are diagnosed at autopsy.

B. Diagnosis

Traditionally, diagnosis of pheochromocytoma relied on the measurement of catecholamines metabolites vanillylmandelic acid (VMA) and metanephrines in a 24-hr urine sample. However, VMA measurements have a sensitivity of only 60% but combined with metanephrine estimations on three separate occasions should give a sensitivity and specificity of around 90%. High performance liquid chromatography (HPLC) measurement of plasma and urine catecholamines provides greater specificity (95%) but without improvement in sensitivity, as sampling during periods of tumor quiescence may miss the diagnosis. Plasma epinephrine concentrations of >400 pg/mL and plasma norepinephrine concentrations exceeding 2000 pg/mL are generally diagnostic. In borderline cases, the clonidine suppression test, in which plasma catecholamines are estimated before and after an oral dose of 0.3 mg clonidine, may be a useful differentiating test (90). A fall in plasma norepinephrine of 30% or to <500 pg/mL implies that the elevated catecholamines are unlikely to be derived from a pheochromocytoma (91).

HPLC measurement of plasma free metanephrines produced 99% sensitivity, although the specificity was only 89% (92). This implies that a negative result on this estimation virtually excludes the diagnosis of pheochromocytoma. Once the diagnosis is suspected, CT scanning of both adrenals should be performed (93). It should be remembered that contrast media can precipitate pheochromocytoma crisis, and intravenous contrast should only be used if the patient has received appropriate adrenergic blockade. If this is negative or if malignancy or multiple tumors are suspected, radionuclide scanning with ^{123}I-MIBG should be performed. The tricyclic antidepressants, guanethidine and labetalol, may interfere with the test, but propranolol, α-blocking drugs, and calcium antagonists do not. Occasionally, octreotide scintigraphy has revealed small tumors not detected with MIBG (94,95). In cases where biochemistry suggests the presence of a pheochromocytoma, but other imaging tests have failed, positron emission tomographic scanning using the noradrenaline-receptor imaging agent 6-[18F]fluorodopamine offers a highly effective method for tumor localization (96,97).

C. Preoperative Assessment

Patient evaluation should include a detailed cardiovascular assessment, looking particularly for evidence of catecholamine-induced cardiomyopathy. A chest X-ray and 12-lead ECG should be performed and evidence of myocardial dysfunction evaluated. Left atrial enlargement secondary to left ventricular diastolic dysfunction is common but seldom poses a management problem. Left ventricular hypertrophy is frequently seen, as are ST and T-wave abnormalities, but there appears to be little point in attempting to correct these by medical management. These changes generally abate, once the excess catecholamine source is removed. Target organ damage from hypertension should be sought.

D. Preoperative Preparation

Medical management, predominantly with α-adrenergic blockade, prior to surgery is generally regarded as desirable (88,98–100) but is not universally accepted as essential. The rarity of these tumors means that large, randomized, prospective controlled trials on preoperative preparation are unlikely to be performed. Boutros et al. (101) reported a series of 63 patients of whom six patients received phenoxybenzamine, 28 patients received prazosin, and the remaining 29 patients received no preoperative α-blockade; there were no discernible differences between the groups in terms of outcome. However, Steinsapir et al. (102) reported markedly higher perioperative mortality (2/7) in patients who did not receive α-blockade when compared with those who were treated preoperatively (0/26). In another study, phenoxybenzamine appeared to provide better hemodynamic stability during the perioperative period than either prazosin or labetalol, but only 14 patients were studied in total (103). Phenoxybenzamine is a noncompetitive, nonselective α-adrenergic blocking agent that has the advantage that it forms an irreversible covalent bond with the α-adrenergic receptor, and thus the blockade cannot be overcome during a surge of release of catecholamines. It is generally the favored agent for this purpose. However, it produces significant postural hypotension, lethargy, and nasal congestion that patients find unpleasant and, in excessive doses, can result in postoperative hypotension (86). In one study, the mean dosage of phenoxybenzamine was 44 mg/day (range 10–240 mg/day) (100) and the average duration of treatment 10–14 days, although shorter periods have been advocated (103). Alternative approaches have been suggested, including the use of selective α_1-blocking drugs, including prazosin, and, more recently, the longer acting agent doxazosin (104,105). A recent comparative study of phenoxybenzamine, prazosin, and doxazosin failed to demonstrate any clinical differences in patients pretreated with one of the three agents (106). The place of β-adrenergic blockade is controversial, and it is the author's personal practice to avoid using these drugs if at all possible; it seems sensible to avoid β-adrenergic blockade at the time of tumor removal, and therefore, long-acting β-blockers should be withdrawn at least three half-lives prior to surgery. Where necessary, intraoperative β-blockade can be provided with the shorter acting agent, esmolol. Calcium channel blocking drugs have a theoretical appeal, in that they not only produce peripheral vasodilation, but may also inhibit calcium-mediated release of catecholamines and other neurotransmitter substances. They have been beneficial in the control of blood pressure in patients with moderate hypertension (86) and have been used intraoperatively with some success (107,108). However, failure of hemodynamic control with these drugs has also been reported, and, as the experience with them is less extensive than that with the α-adrenergic blocking agents, they cannot currently be regarded as first-line therapy.

There are no absolute guidelines as to the adequacy of preparation of a patient prior to surgery. Suggested guidelines have included the following:

- Supine arterial pressure not greater than 160/90 mmHg
- Orthostatic hypotension, with the arterial pressure not falling below 90/50 mmHg
- ECG free of ST segment and T-wave changes for at least 2 weeks
- Not more than one premature ventricular contraction every 5 min (109)

None of these criteria has been adequately validated, although they are largely sensible, and poor perioperative outcomes have occurred in patients who did not meet these criteria preoperatively (110). Paradoxically, failure to achieve adequate control by medical means may be an indication for relatively urgent surgery, which is the only mechanism for controlling the excess catecholamine production. However, there is little evidence to support the recommendation on ECG changes, as these seldom resolve within the relatively short-time frame that is now thought appropriate for preoperative preparation. It is probably more appropriate to proceed with anesthesia and surgery, unless the patient clearly has myocardial ischemia.

Satisfactory expansion of blood volume is difficult to estimate. There is little evidence that patients with relatively stable disease have significantly diminished blood volume, but patients who have recently suffered a hypertensive crisis may have significantly diminished blood volume. In these circumstances, regular monitoring of hematocrit may be helpful. There is no accepted rule regarding the duration of adequate preoperative preparation, although the study by Russell and colleagues (103) suggested that 5–7 days should generally be sufficient. The most practical guide is to increase α-blockade on a daily basis until adequate hemodynamic control is achieved and then to proceed to surgery.

E. Anesthetic Management

Various approaches to the management of anesthesia have been recommended. Most anesthetic agents have been used with relative safety, although it is generally recommended that agents releasing histamine should be avoided, as should agents that might induce tachycardia such as atropinics. Droperidol inhibits the reuptake of catecholamines (111) and is probably best avoided. Oral premedication with a benzodiazepine is generally all that is required. Where phenoxybenzamine has been used, it should be omitted on the morning of surgery, as it has a very long half-life. The β-blockade, where utilized, should also be withdrawn timeously, so that the patient is not under β-blockade at the time of tumor excision. Whether or not epidural anesthesia is performed as part of the anesthetic technique is largely a matter of choice, although the presence of additional sympathetic blockade will not enhance hemodynamic control due to catecholamine release and may make management of hypotension after tumor extirpation more difficult. Theoretically, desflurane, which may stimulate sympathetic discharge, and halothane, which may predispose to ventricular arrhythmia, should be avoided, but there is no scientific evidence to support either of these suggestions.

Prior to induction of anesthesia, good, high-capacity intravenous access should be obtained and direct arterial pressure monitoring established. Induction of anesthesia may be followed by either hypotension or hypertension, and a range of pharmacological agents to handle either of these eventualities should be immediately to hand. However, it is unwise to administer vasopressor agents at this time. Once the patient is stabilized, central venous access should be established for both monitoring and drug administration purposes. There is little evidence to support the use of pulmonary artery catheters in these patients, even where cardiomyopathy has been shown to be present preoperatively. However, transesophageal echocardiography can be extremely valuable, particularly in terms of assessing adequate ventricular filling and myocardial performance.

Intraoperative hemodynamic control has been performed with a variety of α-adrenergic blocking agents, β-adrenergic blocking agents, and direct acting vasodilators (Table 11). Sodium nitroprusside has been the most widely used vasodilator, although it may be difficult to titrate the infusion with sufficient accuracy to control the very rapid changes in blood pressure that frequently occur during tumor handling. Phentolamine has been used but has also proved difficult to control adequately. On the basis that calcium antagonism will oppose both the release of catecholamines and their peripheral effects, calcium channel blocking drugs have recently been used for intraoperative control with some success, particularly with nicardipine (108,112) at a rate of 2–6 μg/kg per min, often with accompanying β-adrenergic blockade. However, nicardipine has a long half-life of 4–6 hr. A similar rationale applies to the use of magnesium sulfate, given as an initial bolus of 2–4 gm with an infusion of 2 gm/hr and intermittent 2 gm boluses to a maximum of 26 gm. Good results have been achieved with this technique, often as a sole agent or in emergency situations (86,99,109,113–121). Magnesium has the additional advantages of excellent control of catecholamine-induced arrhythmia's (122) rapid onset and fast elimination through the kidneys. An immediate antagonist is available in the form of calcium chloride. Successful treatment of intraoperative hypertension and pulmonary edema with magnesium sulfate has been reported in a patient in whom maximum dosage of sodium nitroprusside had failed to control the hypertensive crisis (115). Once the tumor is removed, vasodilator therapy should be withdrawn and aggressive volume expansion undertaken. Care should be taken to ensure an adequate hematocrit, as this is a vital component of peripheral resistance in a maximally vasodilated patient. Brief periods of adrenergic support, particularly with phenylephrine, may be necessary immediately after tumor excision, but it should be possible to withdraw all adrenergic support by the end of the procedure. Persistent requirements for hemodynamic support should alert the attending clinicians to the possibility of occult hemorrhage. Blood sugar monitoring should be performed at hourly intervals throughout the procedure.

A range of surgical approaches is available, and the surgical technique should be determined by the size and location of the tumor, the possibility of multiple

Table 11 Evidence-Based Summary of Pheochromocytoma Management

Management strategy	Level of evidence	Recommendation	References
Preoperative management			
Phenoxybenzamine	3, 4	C	88,100,103,152,152–155
Prazosin	4	C	101,156–162
Doxazosin	3, 4	More studies needed	104,105,163–165
Calcium-channel blockers	4	D	166–168
β-Blockade	4	E	169,170
Intraoperative control			
Sodium nitroprusside	3, 4	C	
Phentolamine	4	D	171–176
Magnesium sulfate	4	D	86,99,109,113–121,177
Calcium channel blockers	4	D	108,112, 166–168,178–180

tumor sites, and the skill of the operator. Laparoscopic removal of small tumors has received considerable recent support (108,123–131), but the creation of a capnoperitoneum has been associated with increased hemodynamic instability (108,112,125), leading to the abandonment of the procedure due to the development of pulmonary edema in one report (132).

F. Postoperative Care

Postoperatively, patients should be admitted to high care facility for continuing monitoring. Ventilatory support should not be necessary, unless dictated by the nature of surgery and the site and size of the tumor. Provided that adequate hemodynamic control was established intraoperatively, postoperative hemodynamic instability should not occur, and if hypotension is problematic, the possibility of bleeding should be considered. Elevated blood pressures, together with persistently elevated plasma catecholamines, may be seen for several days following surgery, presumably because of uptake and storage of catecholamines in sympathetic nerve terminals, and does not necessarily imply incomplete tumor excision. Withdrawal of catecholamines may produce marked alterations in insulin sensitivity, and blood sugar monitoring should be performed on an hourly basis for 24 hr. Postoperative analgesia may be provided with any technique with which the practitioners are familiar.

The long-term prognosis is generally good, with 75% of patients returning to normal hemodynamic states. Catecholamine-induced cardiomyopathy has a surprisingly good prognosis, and normal myocardial performance and architecture can be re-established following complete tumor removal. Some patients will remain persistently hypertensive, but the hypertension is not paroxysmal and can be regarded as "essential" hypertension. Patients with paraganglionomas, multiple tumors, or MENs have an increased risk of tumor recurrence and should be monitored on an annual basis for at least 5 years following tumor excision. However, recurrence of tumors as late as 15 years after original excision has been reported.

VI. MULTIPLE ENDOCRINE NEOPLASIA

Multiple endocrine neoplasia is characterized by the occurrence of tumors involving two or more endocrine glands in a single patient (133). The diagnosis may, initially, be difficult to make, as the endocrinopathies may manifest themselves many years apart, and it is only recently that genetic screening has become available for these syndromes. There are two major forms—MEN-1 and MEN-2 (Table 12). In MEN-1, the typical combination of endocrine pathologies includes tumors of the pituitary, parathyroid, and pancreatic islet cells (Wermer's syndrome). MEN-2 comprises two major variants: MEN-2A characterized by medullary carcinoma of the thyroid linked with pheochromocytoma and inconsistently with parathyroid hyperplasia (Sipple's syndrome) and MEN-2B in which sufferers have, in addition, a marfanoid habitus (but without the ocular and vascular lesions) and mucosal neuromas, but without parathyroid involvement. Most of these syndromes are genetically linked and are usually inherited as an autosomal dominant, although occasional sporadic occurrences have been documented. It is possible that as genetic identification proceeds, more of the cases currently labeled as sporadic will be shown to have a genetic basis. The rarity of these syndromes and the complexity of their management mean that, wherever possible, these patients should be referred to specialist centers for their management.

A. Type 1 MEN Syndromes

In the MEN-1 (Wermer's) syndrome, over 95% of patients have primary hyperparathyroidism, and the most commonly associated pancreatic islet-cell tumor is gastrinoma (133). However, unlike the isolated form

Table 12 Patterns of MEN

MEN-1	
Parathyroid	95% of cases
Pancreatic islet cells	Frequency: 50–75%
	Gastrinoma
	PPoma
	Insulinoma
	Others
Anterior pituitary	Prolactin 60%
	GH 25%
	ACTH 3%
	Nonfunctional
Associated tumors	Carcinoid
	Adrenal cortex
	Lipomas
MEN-2A	
Medullary thyroid Ca	
Pheochromocytoma	
Parathyroid hyperplasia	
MEN-2B	
Medullary thyroid Ca	
Pheochromocytoma	
Associated conditions	Marfanoid habitus
	Mucosal neuromas
	Megacolon

of primary hyperparathyroidism, all four parathyroid glands are usually involved synchronously or metachronously, either with multiple adenomas or hyperplasia. Consequently, parathyroid surgery for MEN-1 has a markedly higher failure rate than that for isolated parathyroid adenoma. Both partial parathyroidectomy and total parathyroidectomy with autotransplantation of parathyroid tissue into the forearm have met with mixed results, with both hypo- and hypercalcemia resulting (134). Intraoperative measurement of PTH may be particularly valuable in ascertaining complete excision of multiple tumors (135). The associated gastrinomas are also frequently multiple, and again, surgery is less successful in MEN-1 patients than in patients with isolated tumors (136). Tumors secreting pancreatic polypeptide are also frequently found in association with MEN-1, but no pathological sequelae have been associated with these tumors. Insulinomas make up one-third of the pancreatic islet-cell tumors seen in MEN-1 syndromes. Anterior pituitary tumors occur with varying frequency in patients with MEN-1, but when they are present, 60% produce prolactin, 25% secrete GH, and 3% secrete ACTH. Treatment of the pituitary tumors is similar to that for patients without MEN-1 syndromes.

B. Type 2 MEN Syndromes

The defining tumor of this group is medullary thyroid carcinoma (MTC). The majority of MTC cases are probably spontaneous (75%), but the remainder occurs as an autosomal dominant condition, usually associated with other endocrine neoplasias. Three versions of MEN-2 are recognized: MTC, hyperparathyroidism and pheochromocytoma (MEN-2A, Sipple's syndrome, the commonest); MTC, pheochromocytoma, marfanoid habitus, and mucosal adenomas (MEN-2B, about 5% of MEN-2), and familial MTC. On the one hand, MEN-2A may run a relatively indolent course and up to one-third may never present with symptoms. On the other hand, MEN-2B has a more aggressive pattern of behavior with a younger onset of symptoms and impaired survival, perhaps accounting for its lower frequency (137). Medullary thyroid carcinoma disseminates by direct local and lymphatic spread within the neck and upper mediastinum, and by hematogenous spread to liver, bone, and lung. The presentation is usually as a result of the neck swelling from the MTC, but occasionally endocrine pathologies may occur from catecholamine secretion or because MTC can produce paraneoplastic syndromes with secretion of variety of polypeptide hormones. Management in the first instance is by total thyroidectomy and dissection of the regional lymph nodes. Prior to surgery, the patient should be fully investigated for other associated pathologies, particularly pheochromocytoma, although these tumors are seldom active at the time of presentation. However, bilateral pheochromocytomas frequently coexist and, during surgery, may behave in the same manner as overt catecholamine-secreting tumors. Whether or not prophylactic α-blockade should be instituted in these patients is not established, but it would seem reasonable not do so, unless the pheochromocytomas are to be excised. It is also not established whether or not simultaneous thyroidectomy and removal of the pheochromocytomas should be performed or whether they should be done as staged procedures, particularly in patients in whom the pheochromocytoma is asymptomatic. The management of patients with this type of MEN involves full genetic screening, genetic counseling of family members, and consideration of early management of genetic susceptible patients. In other respects, the perioperative care of these patients is related to the underlying pathology as detailed in previous sections of this chapter.

VII. CONCLUSIONS

Endocrine neoplasms present major clinical challenges in terms of diagnosis, preoperative preparation, anesthetic management, and surgical technique. These complex conditions are best managed by co-coordinated teams of physicians, surgeons, anesthesiologists, and oncologists with skill and experience in the management of endocrine conditions.

REFERENCES

1. Burrow GN, Wortzman G, Rewcastle NB, Holgate RC, Kovacs K. Microadenomas of the pituitary and abnormal sellar tomograms in an unselected autopsy series. N Engl J Med 1981; 304:156–158.
2. Molitch ME, Russell EJ. The pituitary "incidentaloma". Ann Int Med 1990; 112:925–931.
3. Molitch ME. Pituitary incidentalomas. Endocrinol Metab Clin North Am 1997; 26:725–740.
4. Melmed S. Acromegaly. N Engl J Med 1990; 322: 966–977.
5. Smith M, Hirsch NP. Pituitary disease and anaesthesia. Br J Anaesth 2000; 85:3–14.
6. Lamberts SW, Hofland LJ, de Herder WW, Kwekkeboom DJ, Reubi JC, Krenning EP. Octreotide and related somatostatin analogs in the diagnosis and treatment of pituitary disease and somatostatin receptor scintigraphy. Front Neuroendocrinol 1993; 14: 27–55.
7. Hashimoto K, Yamanaka M, Uchida H, Saito Y, Kosaka Y. [A patient with acromegalic heart disease—a case report]. Masui 1997; 46:951–954.

8. Seidman PA, Kofke WA, Policare R, Young M. Anaesthetic complications of acromegaly. Br J Anaesth 2000; 84:179–182.
9. Hakala P, Randell T, Valli H. Laryngoscopy and fibreoptic intubation in acromegalic patients. Br J Anaesth 1998; 80:345–347.
10. Schmitt H, Buchfelder M, Radespiel-Troger M, Fahlbusch R. Difficult intubation in acromegalic patients: incidence and predictability. Anesthesiology 2000; 93:110–114.
11. Shung J, Avidan MS, Ing R, Klein DC, Pott L. Awake intubation of the difficult airway with the intubating laryngeal mask airway. Anaesthesia 1998; 53:645–649.
12. Southwick JP, Katz J. Unusual airway difficulty in the acromegalic patient—indications for tracheostomy. Anesthesiology 1979; 51:72–73.
13. Latorre F, Klimek L. Does cocaine still have a role in nasal surgery? Drug Saf 1999; 20:9–13.
14. Latorre F, Otter W, Kleemann PP, Dick W, Jage J. Cocaine or phenylephrine/lignocaine for nasal fibreoptic intubation? Eur J Anaesthesiol 1996; 13: 577–581.
15. Girling KJ, Cavill G, Mahajan RP. The effects of nitrous oxide and oxygen on transient hyperemic response in human volunteers. Anesth Analg 1999; 89:175–180.
16. Matta BF, Lam AM. Nitrous oxide increases cerebral blood flow velocity during pharmacologically induced EEG silence in humans. J Neurosurg Anesthesiol 1995; 7:89–93.
17. Strebel S, Kaufmann M, Anselmi L, Schaefer HG. Nitrous oxide is a potent cerebrovasodilator in humans when added to isoflurane. A transcranial Doppler study. Acta Anaesthesiol Scand 1995; 39: 653–658.
18. Satapathy GC, Dash HH. Tension pneumocephalus after neurosurgery in the supine position. Br J Anaesth 2000; 84:115–117.
19. Meyer DR. Comparison of oxymetazoline and lidocaine versus cocaine for outpatient dacryocystorhinostomy. Ophthal Plast Reconstr Surg 2000; 16: 201–205.
20. Smith GA, Strausbaugh SD, Harbeck-Weber C, Cohen DM, Shields BJ, Powers JD, Barrett T. Prilocaine-phenylephrine and bupivacaine-phenylephrine topical anesthetics compared with tetracaine-adrenaline-cocaine during repair of lacerations. Am J Emerg Med 1998; 16:121–124.
21. Gemma M, Tommasino C, Cozzi S, Narcisi S, Mortini P, Losa M, Soldarini A. Remifentanil provides hemodynamic stability and faster awakening time in transsphenoidal surgery. Anesth Analg 2002; 94:163–168.
22. Korula G, George SP, Rajshekhar V, Haran RP, Jeyaseelan L. Effect of controlled hypercapnia on cerebrospinal fluid pressure and operating conditions during transsphenoidal operations for pituitary macroadenoma. J Neurosurg Anesthesiol 2001; 13: 255–259.
23. Abe T, Ludecke DK. Recent primary transnasal surgical outcomes associated with intraoperative growth hormone measurement in acromegaly. Clin Endocrinol (Oxf) 1999; 50:27–35.
24. Cusick JF, Hagen TC, Findling JW. Inappropriate secretion of antidiuretic hormone after transsphenoidal surgery for pituitary tumors. N Engl J Med 1984; 311:36–38.
25. Powell M, Lightman SL. Postoperative management. In: Powell M, Lightman SL, eds. Management of Pituitary Tumors: A Handbook. London: Churchill-Livingstone, 1996:145–158.
26. de Perrot M, Spiliopoulos A, Fischer S, Totsch M, Keshavjee S. Neuroendocrine carcinoma (carcinoid) of the thymus associated with Cushing's syndrome. Ann Thorac Surg 2002; 73:675–681.
27. Bochicchio D, Losa M, Buchfelder M. Factors influencing the immediate and late outcome of Cushing's disease treated by transsphenoidal surgery: a retrospective study by the European Cushing's Disease Survey Group. J Clin Endocrinol Metab 1995; 80: 3114–3120.
28. Lamberts SW, van der Lely AJ, de Herder WW. Transsphenoidal selective adenomectomy is the treatment of choice in patients with Cushing's disease. Considerations concerning preoperative medical treatment and the long-term follow-up. J Clin Endocrinol Metab 1995; 80:3111–3113.
29. Torpy DJ, Mullen N, Ilias I, Nieman LK. Association of hypertension and hypokalaemia with Cushing's syndrome caused by ectopic ACTH secretion. A series of 58 cases. Ann NY Acad Sci 2002; 970:134–144.
30. Morris D, Grossman A. The medical management of Cushing's syndrome. Ann NY Acad Sci 2002; 970: 119–133.
31. Lamberts SW, Uitterlinden P, Klijn JM. The effect of the long-acting somatostatin analogue SMS 201–995 on ACTH secretion in Nelson's syndrome and Cushing's disease. Acta Endocrinol (Copenh) 1989; 120:760–766.
32. Mihai R, Farndon JR. Parathyroid diseases and calcium metabolism. Br J Anaesth 2000; 85:29–43.
33. Marks KH, Kilav R, Naveh-Many T, Silver J. Calcium, phosphate, vitamin D, and the parathyroid. Pediatr Nephrol 1996; 10:364–367.
34. Hebert SC. Extracellular calcium-sensing receptor: implications for calcium amd magnesium handling in the kidney. Kidney Int 1996; 50:2129–2139.
35. Wada M, Nagano N, Nemeth EF. The calcium receptor and calcimimetics. Curr Opin Nephrol Hypertens 1999; 8:429–433.
36. Brown EM, Pollak M, Hebert SC. The extracellular calcium-sensing receptor: its role in health and disease. Ann Rev Med 1998; 49:15–29.
37. NIH conference. Diagnosis and management of asymptomatic primary hyperparathyroidism: consensus development conference statement. Ann Intern Med 1991; 114:593–597.

38. Silverberg SJ, Bone HG III, Marriott TB, Locker FG, Thys-Jacobs S, Dziem G, Kaatz S, Sanguinetti EL, Bilezikian JP. Short-term inhibition of parathyroid hormone secretion by a calcium-receptor agonist in patients with primary hyperparathyroidism. N Engl J Med 1997; 337:1506–1510.
39. Chan AK, Duh QY, Kate MH, Siperstein AE, Clark OH. Clinical manifestations of primary hyperparathyroidism before and after parathyroidectomy. A case–control study. Ann Surg 1995; 222:402–412.
40. Dougherty TB, Cronau LH Jr. Anesthetic implications for surgical patients with endocrine tumors. Int Anesthesiol Clin 1998; 30:31–44.
41. Al Mohaya S, Naguib M, Abdelatif M, Farag H. Abnormal responses to muscle relaxants in a patient with primary hyperparathyroidism. Anesthesiology 1986; 65:554–556.
42. Chen H, Sokoll LJ, Udelsman R. Outpatient minimally invasive parathyroidectomy: a combination of sestamibi-SPECT localization, cervical block anesthesia, and intraoperative parathyroid hormone assay. Surgery 1999; 126:1016–1021.
43. Ditkoff BA, Chabot J, Feind C, Lo GP. Parathyroid surgery using monitored anesthesia care as an alternative to general anesthesia. Am J Surg 1996; 172: 698–700.
44. Lo GP. Bilateral neck exploration for parathyroidectomy under local anesthesia: a viable technique for patients with coexisting thyroid disease with or without sestamibi scanning. Surgery 1999; 126: 1011–1014.
45. Norman J, Denham D. Minimally invasive radioguided parathyroidectomy in the reoperative neck. Surgery 1998; 124:1088–1092.
46. Saxe AW, Brown E, Hamburger SW. Thyroid and parathyroid surgery performed with patient under regional anesthesia. Surgery 1988; 103:415–420.
47. Wei JP, Burke GJ. Cost utility of routine imaging with Tc-99m-sestamibi in primary hyperparathyroidism before initial surgery. Am Surg 1997; 63:1097–1100.
48. Norman J, Chheda H, Farrell C. Minimally invasive parathyroidectomy for primary hyperparathyroidism: decreasing operative time and potential complications while improving cosmetic results. Am Surg 1998; 64:391–395.
49. Goldstein RE, Billheimer D, Martin WH, Richards K. Sestamibi scanning and minimally invasive radioguided parathyroidectomy without intraoperative parathyroid hormone measurement. Ann Surg 2003; 237:722–730.
50. Modlin IM, Sandor A. An analysis of 8305 cases of carcinoid tumors. Cancer 1997; 79:813–829.
51. Fink G, Krelbaum T, Yellin A, Bendayan D, Saute M, Glazar M, Kramer MR. Pulmonary carinoid: presentation, diagnosis, and outcome in 142 cases in Israel and review of 640 cases from the literature. Chest 2001; 119:1647–1651.
52. Wilander E, Lundqvist M, Oberg K. Gastrointestinal carcinoid tumors. Histogenetic, histochemical, immunohistochemical, clinical and therapeutic aspects. Prog Histochem Cytochem 1989; 19:1–88.
53. Kulke MH, Mayer RJ. Carcinoid tumors. N Engl J Med 1999; 340:858–868.
54. Fischer S, Kruger M, Mcrae K, Merchant N, Tsao MS, Keshavjee S. Giant-bronchial carcinoid tumors: a multidisciplinary approach. Ann Thorac Surg 2001; 71:386–393.
55. Karmyjones R, Vallieres E. Carcinoid crisis after biopsy of a bronchial carcinoid. Ann Thorac Surg 1993; 56:1403–1405.
56. Filosso PL, Rena O, Donati G, Casadio C, Ruffini E, Papalia E, Oliaro A, Maggi G. Bronchial carcinoid tumors: surgical management and long-term outcome. J Thorac Cardiovasc Surg 2002; 123:303–309.
57. Öberg K. Carcinoid syndrome. In: Grossman A, ed. Clinical Endocrinology. 2nd ed. Oxford: Blackwell Science Ltd, 1998:607–620.
58. Zhou Y, Wang S, Yue BG, Gobl A, Oberg K. Effects of interferon alpha on the expression of p21cip1/waf1 and cell cycle distribution in carcinoid tumors. Cancer Invest 2002; 20:348–356.
59. Claure RE, Drover DD, Haddow GR, Esquivel CO, Angst MS. Orthotopic liver transplantation for carcinoid tumor metastatic to the liver: anesthetic management. Can J Anaesth 2000; 47:334–337.
60. Wilde MI, Markham A. Ondansetron. A review of its pharmacology and preliminary clinical findings in novel applications. Drugs 1996; 52:773–794.
61. Lundin L, Norheim I, Landelius J, Oberg K, Theodorsson-Norheim E. Carcinoid heart disease: relationship of circulating vasoactive substances to ultrasound-detectable cardiac abnormalities. Circulation 1988; 77:264–269.
62. Westberg G, Wangberg B, Ahiman H, Bergh CH, Beckman-Suurkula M, Caidahl K. Prediction of prognosis by echocardiography in patients with midgut carcinoid syndrome. Br J Surg 2001; 88: 865–872.
63. Connolly HM, Nishimura RA, Smith HC, Pellikka PA, Mullany CJ, Kvols LK. Outcome of cardiac surgery for carcinoid heart disease. J Am Coll Cardiol 1995; 25:410–416.
64. Ksai VS, Ahsanuddin AN, Gilbert C, Orr L, Moran J, Sorrell VL, Ahsanudin AN. Isolated metastatic myocardial carcinoid tumor in a 48-year-old man. Mayo Clin Proc 2002; 77:591–594.
65. Oberg K. Carcinoid tumors: molecular genetics, tumor biology, and update of diagnosis and treatment. Curr Opin Oncol 2002; 14:38–45.
66. Kinney MA, Warner ME, Negorney DM, Rubin J, Schroeder DR, Maxson PM, Warner MA. Perianaesthetic risks and outcomes of abdominal surgery for metastatic carcinoid tumors. Br J Anaesth 2001; 87: 447–452.

67. Padfield NL. Carcinoid syndrome: comparison of pretreatment regimes in the same patient. Ann R Coll Surg Engl 1987; 69:16–17.
68. Patel KD, Dalal FY. Anaesthetic management of a patient with carcinoid tumor undergoing myocardial revascularization. Can Anaesth Soc J 1980; 27:260–263.
69. Marsh HM, Martin JK Jr, Kvols LK, Gracey DR, Warner MA, Warner ME, Moertel CG. Carcinoid crisis during anesthesia: successful treatment with a somatostatin analogue. Anesthesiology 1987; 66:89–91.
70. Roy RC, Carter RF, Wright PD. Somatostatin, anaesthesia, and the carcinoid syndrome. Peri-operative administration of a somatostatin analogue to suppress carcinoid tumor activity. Anaesthesia 1987; 42:627–632.
71. Parris WC, Oates JA, Kambam J, Shmerling R, Sawyers JF. Pretreatment with somatostatin in the anaesthetic management of a patient with carcinoid syndrome. Can J Anaesth 1988; 35:413–416.
72. Dierdorf SF. Carcinoid tumor and carcinoid syndrome. Curr Opin Anaesthesiol 2003; 16:343–347.
73. Hamid SK, Harris DN. Hypotension following valve replacement surgery in carcinoid heart disease. Anaesthesia 1992; 47:490–492.
74. Nave H, Mossinger E, Feist H, Lang H, Raab H. Surgery as primary treatment in patients with liver metastases from carcinoid tumors: a retrospective, unicentric study over 13 years. Surgery 2001; 129:170–175.
75. Lang H, Oldhafer KJ, Weimann A, Schlitt HJ, Scheumann GF, Flemming P, Ringe B, Pichlmayr R. Liver transplantation for metastatic neuroendocrine tumors. Ann Surg 1997; 225:347–354.
76. Le Treut YP, Delpero JR, Dousset B, Cherqui D, Segol P, Mantion G, Hannoun L, Benhamou G, Launois B, Boillot O, Domergue J, Bismuth H. Results of liver transplantation in the treatment of metastatic neuroendocrine tumors. A 31-case French multicentric report. Ann Surg 1997; 225:355–364.
77. Moertel CG. Karnofsky memorial lecture. An odyssey in the land of small tumors. J Clin Oncol 1987; 5: 1502–1522.
78. Moertel CG, Weiland LH, Nagorney DM, Dockerty MB. Carcinoid tumor of the appendix: treatment and prognosis. N Engl J Med 1987; 317:1699–1701.
79. Mani S, Modlin IM, Ballantyne G, Ahlman H, West B. Carcinoids of the rectum. J Am Coll Surg 1994; 179:231–248.
80. Graham GW, Unger BP, Coursin DB. Perioperative management of selected endocrine disorders. Int Anesthesiol Clin 2000; 38:31–67.
81. Taupenot L, Harper KL, O'Conner DT. The chromogranin–secretogranin family. N Engl J Med 2003; 348: 134–149.
82. Drolet P, Girard M. [The use of magnesium sulfate during surgery of pheochromocytoma: apropos of 2 cases] L'utilisation du sulfate de magnesium pendant la chirurgie du pehochromocytome: a propos de deux cas. Can J Anaesth 1993; 40:521–525.
83. Eng C, Crossey PA, Milligan LM. Mutations in the RET protooncogene and the von Hippel-Lindau disease tumor suppressor gene in sporadic and syndromic phaeochromocytomas. J Med Genet 1995; 32:934–937.
84. Dluhy RG. Pheochromocytoma–death of the axiom. N Engl J Med 2002; 346:1486–1488.
85. Neumann HP, Bausch B, McWhinney SR, Bender BU, Gimm O, Franke G, Schipper J, Klisch J, Altehoefer C, Zerres K, Januszewicz A, Eng C, Smith WM, Munk R, Manz T, Glaeskar S, Apel TW, Treier M, Reineke M, Walz MK, Hoang-Vu C, Brauckhoff M, Klein-Franke A, Klose P, Schmidt H, Maier-Woelfle M, Peczkowska M, Szmigielski C, Eng C. Germ-line mutations in nonsyndromic pheochromocytoma. N Engl J Med 2002; 346:1459–1466.
86. Bravo EL. Pheochromocytoma. An approach to anithypertensive management. Ann NY Acad Sci 2002; 970:1–10.
87. Grouzmann E, Fathi M, Gillet M, de Torrente A, Cavadas C, Brunner H, Buclin T. Disappearance rate of catecholamines, total metanephrines, and neuropeptide Y from the plasma of patients after resection of pheochromocytoma. Clin Chem 2001; 47:1075–1082.
88. Hull CJ. Phaeochromocytoma. Diagnosis, preoperative preparation and anaesthetic management. Br J Anaesth 1986; 58:1453–1468.
89. Ishii C, Inoue K, Negishi K, Tane N, Awata T, Katayama S. Diabetic ketoacidosis in a case of pheochromocytoma. Diabetes Res Clin Pract 2001; 54: 137–142.
90. Bravo EL, Terazi RC, Fouad FM, Vidt DG, Gifford RWJ. Clonidine-suppression test: a useful aid in the diagnosis of pheochromocytoma. N Engl J Med 1981; 305:623–626.
91. Lenz T, Rosa A, Schumm-Draeger P, Schulte KL, Geiger H. Clonidine suppression test revisited. Blood Press 1998; 7:153–158.
92. Lenders JW, Pacak K, Eisenhofer G. New advances in the biochemical diagnosis of pheochromocytoma: moving beyond catecholamines. Ann NY Acad Sci 2002; 970:29–40.
93. Mayo-Smith WW, Boland GW, Noto RB, Lee MJ. State-of-the-art adrenal imaging. Radiographics 2001; 21:995–1012.
94. Meunier JP, Tatou E, Bernard A, Brenot R, David M. Cardiac pheochromocytoma. Ann Thorac Surg 2001; 71:712–713.
95. van der HE, de Herder WW, Bruining HA, Bonjer HJ, de Krijger RR, Lamberts SW, van de Meiracker AH, Boomsma F, Stijnen T, Krenning EP, Bosman FT, Kwekkeboorn DJ. [(123)In]metaiodobenzylguanidine and [(111)In]octreotide uptake in begnign and malignant pheochromocytomas. J Clin Endocrinol Metab 2001; 86:685–693.
96. Pacak K, Goldstein DS, Doppman JL, Shulkin BL, Udelsman R, Eisenhofer G. A "pheo" lurks: novel approaches for locating occult pheochromocytoma. J Clin Endocrinol Metab 2001; 86:3641–3646.

97. Hoegerlc S, Nitzsche E, Altehoefer C, Ghanem N, Manz T, Brink I, Reincke M, Moser E, Neumann HP. Pheochromocytomas: detection with 18F DOPA whole body PET—initial results. Radiology 2002; 222:507–512.
98. Bravo EL, Gifford RWJ. Current concepts. Pheochromocytoma: diagnosis, localization and management. N Engl J Med 1984; 311:1298–1303.
99. O'Riordan JA. Pheochromocytomas and anesthesia. Int Anesthesiol Clin 1997; 35:99–127.
100. Kinney MA, Warner ME, vanHeerden JA, Horlocker TT, Young WF Jr, Schroeder DR, Maxson PM, Warner MA. Perianesthetic risks and outcomes of pheochromocytoma and paraganglioma resection. Anesth Analg 2000; 91:1118–1123.
101. Boutros AR, Bravo EL, Zanettin G, Straffon RA. Perioperative management of 63 patients with pheochrocytoma. Cleve Clin J Med 1990; 57:613–617.
102. Steinsapir J, Carr AA, Prisant M, Bransome ED. Metyrosine and pheochromocytoma. Arch Intern Med 1997; 157:901–906.
103. Russell WJ, Metcalfe IR, Tonkin AL, Frewin DB. The preoperative management of phaeochromocytoma. Anaesth Intensive Care 1998; 26:196–200.
104. Prys-Roberts C. Phaeochromocytoma—recent progress in its management. Br J Anaesth 2000; 85:44–57.
105. Prys-Roberts C, Farndon JR. Efficacy and safety of doxazosin for perioperative management of patients with pheochromocytoma. World J Surg 2002; 26:1037–1042.
106. Kocak S, Aydintug S, Canakci N. Alpha blockade in preoperative preparation of patients with pheochromocytomas. Int Surg 2002; 87:191–194.
107. Combemale F, Carnaille B, Tavernier B, Hautier B, Thevenot A, Scherpereel P, Proye C. Exclusive use of calcium channel blockers and cardioselective betablockers in the pre- and per-operative management of pheochromocytomas. 70 cases. Ann chir 1998; 52:341–345.
108. Atallah F, Bastide-Heulin T, Soulie M, Crouzil F, Galiana A, Samii K, Virenque C. Haemodynamic changes during retroperitoneoscopic adrenalectomy for phaeochromocytoma. Br J Anaesth 2001; 86:731–733.
109. Desmonts JM, Merty J. An anaesthetic management of patients with pheochromocytoma. Br J Anaesth 1984; 56:781–789.
110. Shupak RC. Difficult anesthetic management during pheochromocytoma surgery. J Clin Anesth 1999; 11:247–250.
111. Oh TE, Turner CW, Ilett KF, Waterson JG, Paterson JW. Mechanism of the hypertensive effect of droperidol in pheochromocytoma. Anaesth Intensive Care 1978; 6:322–327.
112. Joris JL, Hamoir EE, Harstein GM, Meurisse MR, Hubert BM, Charlier CJ, Lamy ML. Hemodynamic changes and catecholamine release during laparoscopic adrenalectomy for pheochromocytoma. Anesth Analg 1999; 88:16–21.
113. Beeton AG, Shipton EA, Katz BJ. Unexplained hypertension during induction of a patient with phaeochromocytoma. S Afr J Surg 1992; 30:165–167.
114. Bullough A, Karadia S, Watters M. Phaeochromocytoma: an unusual cause of hypertension in pregnancy. Anaesthesia 2001; 56:43–46.
115. Niruthisard S, Chatrkaw P, Laornual S, Sunthornyothin S, Prasertsri S. Anesthesia for one-stage bilateral pheochromocytoma resection in a patient with MEN type IIa: attenuation of hypertensive crisis by magnesium sulfate. J Med Assoc Thai 2002; 85:125–130.
116. Pitt-Miller P, Primus E. Use of magnesium sulphate as adjunctive therapy for resection of phaeochromocytoma. West Indian Med J 2000; 49:73–75.
117. Pivalizza EG. Magnesium sulfate and epidural anesthesia in pheochromocytoma and severe coronary artery disease. Anesth Analg 1995; 81:414–416.
118. Poopalalingam R, Chin EY. Rapid preparation of a patient with pheochromocytoma with labetolol and magnesium sulfate. Can J Anaesth 2001; 48:876–880.
119. Huddle KR, Mannell A, James MF, Plant ME. Phaeochromocytoma. A report of 10 patients. [Review] [18 refs]. S Afr Med J 1991; 79:217–220.
120. James MF. The use of magnesium sulfate in the anesthetic management of pheochromocytoma. Anesthesiology 1985; 62:188–190.
121. James MF. Use of magnesium sulphate in the anaesthetic management of phaeochromocytoma: a review of 17 anaesthetics. Br J Anaesth 1989; 62:616–623.
122. Mayer DB, Miletich DJ, Feld JM, Albrecht RF. The effects of magnesium salts on the duration of epinephrine-induced ventricular tachyarrhythmias in anesthetized rats. Anesthesiology 1989; 71:923–928.
123. Brunt LM, Moley JF, Doherty GM, Lairmore TC, DeBenedetti MK, Quasebarth MA. Outcomes analysis in patients undergoing laparoscopic adrenalectomy for hormonally active adrenal tumors. Surgery 2001; 130:629–634.
124. Chiu M, Crosby ET, Yelle JD. Anesthesia for laparoscopic adrenalectomy (pheochromocytoma) in an anemic adult Jehovah's witness. Can J Anaesth 2000; 47:566–571.
125. Darvas K, Pinkola K, Borsodi M, Tarjanyi M, Winternitz T, Horanyi J. General anaesthesia for laparoscopic adrenalectomy. Med Sci Monit 2000; 6: 560–563.
126. Gill IS. The case for laparoscopic adrenalectomy. J Urol 2001; 166:429–436.
127. Guazzoni G, Cestari A, Montorsi F, Lanzi R, Nava L, Centemero A, Rigatti P. Eight-year experience with transperitoneal laparoscopic adrenal surgery. J Urol 2001; 166:820–824.
128. Janetschek G, Neumann HP. Laparoscopic surgery for pheochromocytoma. Urol Clin North Am 2001; 28:97–105.

129. Kazaryan AM, Mala T, Edwin B. Does tumor size influence the outcome of laparoscopic adrenalectomy? J Laparoendosc Adv Surg Tech A 2001; 11:1–4.
130. Salomon L, Rabii R, Soulie M, Mouly P, Hoznek A, Cicco A, Saint F, Alame W, Antiphon P, Chopin D, Plante P, Abbou CC. Experience with retroperitoneal laparoscopic adrenalectomy for pheochromocytoma. J Urol 2001; 165:1871–1874.
131. Toniato A, Piotto A, Pagetta C, Bernante P, Pelizzo MR. Technique and results of laparoscopic adrenalectomy. Langenbecks Arch Surg 2001; 386:200–203.
132. Tauzin-Fin P, Hilbert G, Krol-Houdek M, Gosse P, Maurette P. Mydriasis and acute pulmonary oedema complicating laparoscopic removal of phaechromocytoma. Anaesth Insentive Care 1999; 27:646–649.
133. Thakker RV. Multiple endocrine neoplasia type 1. In: Grossman AB, ed. Clinical Endocrinology. 2nd ed. Oxford: Blackwell Science Ltd, 1998:621–634.
134. Mallette LE, Blevins T, Jordan PH, Noon GP. Autogenous parathyroid grafts for generalised primary hyperplasia: contrasting outcome in sporadic versus multiple neoplasia type 1. Surgery 1987; 101:738–745.
135. Tonelli F, Spini S, Tommasi M, Gabbrielli G, Amorosi A, Brocchi A, Brandi. Intraoperative parathormone measurement in patients with multiple endocrine neoplasia type 1 syndrome and hyperparathyroidism. World J Surg 2000; 24:556–562.
136. Sheppard BC, Norton JA, Doppman JL, Maton PL, Gardner JD, Jensen RT. Management of islet cell tumors in patients with multiple endocrine neoplasia. Surgery 1989; 106:1081–1086.
137. Eng C, Ponder BAJ. Multiple endocrine neoplasia type 2 and medullary thyroid carcinoma. In: Grossman A, ed. Clinical Endocrinology 2nd ed. Oxford: Blackwell Science Ltd, 1998:635–650.
138. Kovacs K, Horvath E. Pathology of pituitary tumors. Endocrinol Metab Clin North Am 1987; 16:529–551.
139. Arrigoni MG, Woolner LB, Bernatz PE. Atypical carcinoid tumors of the lung. J Thorac Cardiovasc Surg 1972; 64:413–421.
140. Kaltsas G, Korbonits M, Heintz E, Mukherjee JJ, Jenkins PJ, Chew SL, Reznek R, Monson JP, Besser GM, Foley R, Britton KE, Grossman AB. Comparison of somatostatin analog and meta-iodobenzylguanidine radionuclides in the diagnosis and localization of advanced neuroendocrine tumors. J Clin Endocrinol Metab 2001; 86:895–902.
141. Watson JT, Badner NH, Ali MJ. The prophylactic use of octreotide in a patient with ovarian carcinoid and valvular heart disease. Can J Anaesth 1990; 37:798–800.
142. Warner RRP, Mani S, Profeta J, Grunstein E. Octreotide treatment of carcinoid hypertensive crisis. Mt Sinai J Med 1994; 61:349–355.
143. Hughes EW, Hodkinson BP. Carcinoid syndrome: the combined use of ketanserin and octreotide in the management of an acute crisis during anaesthesia. Anaesth Intensive Care 1989; 17:367–370.
144. Propst JW, Siegel LC, Stover EP. Anesthetic considerations for valve replacement surgery in a patient with carcinoid syndrome. J Cardiothorac Vasc Anesth 1994; 8:209–212.
145. Asbun HJ, Calabria RP, Calmes S, Lang AG, Bloch JH. Thymic carcinoid. Am Surg 1991; 57:442–445.
146. Hellman P, Lundstrom T, Ohrvall U, Eriksson B, Skogseid B, Oberg K, Tiensuu JE, Akerstrom G. Effect of surgery on the outcome of midgut carcinoid disease with lymph node and liver metastases. World J Surg 2002; 26:991–997.
147. Newton JR Jr, Grillo HC, Mathisen DJ. Main bronchial sleeve resection with pulmonary conservation. Ann Thorac Surg 1991; 52:1272–1280.
148. Peterffy A, Konstantinov IE. Resection of distal tracheal and carinal tumors with the aid of cardiopulmonary bypass. Scand Cardiovasc J 1998; 32:109–112.
149. Rau BK, Harikrishnan KM, Krishna S. Endoscopic laser ablation of duodenal carcinoids: a new treatment modality. J Clin Laser Med Surg 1995; 13:37–38.
150. Munke H, Schworer H, Stockmann F, Ramadori G. Treatment of hepatic metastasized carcinoids with percutaneous ethanol injection. Follow up of five cases. Tumordiagnostik Therapie 1997; 18:133–137.
151. de Vries H, Verschueren RC, Willemse PH, Kema IP, de Vries EG. Diagnostic, surgical and medical aspect of the midgut carcinoids. Cancer Treat Rev 2002; 28:11–25.
152. Emerson CE, Rainbird A. Use of a 'hospital-at-home' service for patient optimization before resection of phaeochromocytoma. Br J Anaesth 2003; 90:380–382.
153. Hack HA, Brown TC. Preoperative management of phaeochromocytoma—a paedatric perspective. Anaesth Intensive Care 1999; 27:112–113.
154. Hermayer KL, Szpiech M. Diagnosis and management of pheochromocytoma during pregnancy: a case report. Am J Med Sci 1999; 318:186–189.
155. Kopf D, Goretzki PE, Lehnert H. Clinical management of malignant adrenal tumors. J Cancer Res Clin Oncol 2001; 127:143–155.
156. Yuasa S, Bandai H, Yura T, Sumikura T, Takahashi N, Uchida K, Yamamoto N, Tanaka H, Aono M, Fujioka H. Successful resection of pheochromocytoma in a hemodialysis patient. Am J Nephrol 1992; 12:111–115.
157. Katoh K. [A study on blood pressure variation—the clinical validation of continuous direct blood pressure recording in patients with pheochromocytoma]. Hokkaido Igaku Zasshi 1991; 66:769–779.
158. Rechavia E, Mager A, Sagie A, Strasberg B, Sclarovsky S. Prazosin's effect in high renin hypertension complicating pheochromocytoma. Clin Cardiol 1991; 14:533–535.
159. Chojnowski K, Feltynowski T, Wocial B, Chodakowska J, Filipecki S, Januszewicz W. [Prazosin in the preoperative management of patients with phaeochromocytoma]. Pol Tyg Lek 1989; 44:280–284.

160. Havlik RJ, Cahow CE, Kinder BK. Advances in the diagnosis and treatment of pheochromocytoma. Arch Surg 1988; 123:626–630.
161. Sasaki M, Takenawa J, Kanamaru H, Komatz Y. [Preoperative management of pheochromocytoma with prazosin: report of three cases]. Hinyokika Kiyo 1986; 32:61–66.
162. Pinaud M, Souron R, Le Neel JC, Lopes P, Murat A, L'hoste F. Bilateral phaeochromocytomas in pregnancy: anaesthetic management of combined caesarean section and tumor removal. Eur J Anaesthesiol 1985; 2:395–399.
163. Miura Y, Yoshinaga K. Doxazosin: a newly developed, selective alpha 1-inhibitor in the management of patients with pheochromocytoma. Am Heart J 1988; 116:1785–1789.
164. Sendo D, Katsuura M, Akiba K, Yokoyama S, Tanabe S, Wakabayashi T, Sato S, Otaki S, Obata K, Yamagiwa I, Hayasaka K. Severe hypertension and cardiac failure associated with neuroblastoma: a case report. J Pediatr Surg 1996; 31:1688–1690.
165. Taylor SH. Efficacy of doxazosin in specific hypertensive patient groups. Am Heart J 1991; 121: 286–292.
166. Combemale F, Carnaille B, Tavernier B, Hautier MB, Thevenot A, Scherpereel P, Proye C. [Exclusive use of calcium channel blockers and cardioselective beta-blockers in the pre- and per-operative management of pheochromocytomas. 70 cases]. Ann Chir J 1998; 52:341–345.
167. Proye C, Thevenin D, Cecat P, Petillot P, Carnaille B, Verin P, Sautier M, Racadot N. Exclusive use of calcium channel blockers in preoperative and intraoperative control of pheochromocytomas: hemodynamics and free catecholamine assays in ten consecutive patients. Surgery 1989; 106:1149–1154.
168. Takahashi S, Nakai T, Fujiwara R, Kutsumi Y, Tamai T, Miyabo S. Effectiveness of long-acting nifedipine in pheochromocytoma. Jpn Heart J 1989; 30:751–757.
169. Sheaves R, Chew SL, Grossman AB. The dangers of unopposed beta-adrenergic blockade in phaeochromocytoma. Postgrad Med J 1995; 71:58–59.
170. Shapiro B, Fig LM. Management of pheochromocytoma. Endocrinol Metab Clin North Am 1989; 18:443–481.
171. Adams HA, Hempelmann G. [Anesthesia for patients with pheochromocytoma. Our own results and a review]. Anasthesiol lntensived Notfallmed Schmerzther 1993; 28:500–509.
172. Anton AH, Sherman BW, Lina AA, Acheson LS. An atrial pheochromocytoma-induced hypertensive crisis resistant to nitroprusside. Ind J Clin Pharmacol Ther Toxicol 1993; 31:89–92.
173. Sugiyama Y, Inagaki Y, Hagihira T, Kamibayashi T, Sumikawa K, Yoshiya I. [A hypertensive crisis during surgery in a patient with neuroblastoma.] Masui 1992; 41:677–681.
174. Newell K, Prinz RA, Braithwaite S, Brooks M. Pheochromocytoma crisis. Am J Hypertens 1988; 1: 189S–191S.
175. Stenstrom G, Haijamae H, Tisell LE. Influence of preoperative treatment with phenoxybenzamine on the incidence of adverse cardiovascular reactions during anaesthesia and surgery for phaeochromocytoma. Acta Anaesthesiol Scand 1985; 29:797–803.
176. Nicholson JP Jr, Vaughn ED Jr, Pickering TG, Resnick LM, Artusio J, Kleinert HD, Lopez-Overjero JA, Laragh JH. Pheochromocytoma and prazosin. Ann Intern Med 1983; 99:477–479.
177. Minami T, Adachi T, Fukuda K. An effective use of magnesium sulfate for intraoperative management of laparoscopic adrenalectomy for pheochromocytoma in a pediatric patient. Anesth Analg 2002; 95:1243–1244.
178. Colson P, Ribstein J. [Simplified strategy for anesthesia of pheochromocytoma.] Ann. Fr Anesth Reanim 1991; 10:456–462.
179. Colson P, Ryckwaert F, Ribstein J, Mann C, Dareau S. Haemodynamic heterogeneity and treatment with the calcium channel blocker nicardipine during phaeochromocytoma surgery. Acta Anaesthesiol Scand 1998; 42:1114–1119.
180. Fujiwara M, Zaha M, Odashiro M, Kawamura J, Hayashi I, Mizoguchi H. [Use of diltiazem in the anesthetic management of epinephrine predominant pheochromocytoma.] Masui 1992; 41:1175–1179.

26

Perioperative Care for Breast and Gynecological Neoplasms

TROY S. BROWNE
Intensive Care and High Dependency Unit, Tauranga, New Zealand

ANEES CHAGPAR and KELLY K. HUNT
Department of Surgical Oncology, The University of Texas M.D. Anderson Cancer Center, Houston, Texas, U.S.A.

PEDRO RAMIREZ
The University of Texas M.D. Anderson Cancer Center, Houston, Texas, U.S.A.

I. PERIOPERATIVE CARE OF BREAST CANCER

A. Introduction

Breast cancer is the most common malignancy of women today, with more than 210,000 cases diagnosed in the United States in 2003 alone (1). This disease affects a heterogeneous population from otherwise healthy young women to elderly patients with a myriad of comorbid conditions. The perioperative management of patients with breast cancer must therefore be individualized and must take into account not only the physiologic well being of the patient, but also her psychological and emotional needs. The approach to such patients requires a multidisciplinary team including surgical oncologists, anesthesiologists, medical oncologists, radiation oncologists, plastic surgeons, social workers, genetic counselors, nurses, and others.

*Drs. Chagpar and Hunt authored the breast cancer portion and Dr. Ramirez authored the gynecologic portion of this chapter.

B. Preoperative Management

A detailed history and physical examination are of paramount importance. The history is directed not only at determining oncologic risk factors and progression of disease, but also at assessing the patient's physiologic state.

It is important to determine whether there is a palpable abnormality and, if so, how long it has been present. Has it been increasing in size? Is it associated with any other symptoms—pain, nipple discharge, nipple retraction, lymphadenopathy, or systemic findings? Correlation with mammographic and sonographic findings is also critical. Family history of cancer is useful in gaining insight into potential underlying genetic abnormalities. A complete gynecological history may also shed some light on the patient's risk factors. Determination of the patient's past medical and surgical history, medication use and allergies, and any problems with anesthesia or bleeding is crucial. A social history for alcohol use, drug use, and smoking is equally important.

The physical examination must be thorough and include examination of not only the breasts and nodal basins, but also the cardiopulmonary system, abdomen musculoskeletal system, and neurological systems. It is important to note whether the patient has difficulty in lying flat or abducting the arm, as this may affect positioning in the operating room and postoperative recovery after lymph node surgery.

Pathologic evaluation of radiologically suspicious areas or palpable masses is critical in the determination of malignancy. Core needle biopsy (CNB) is generally the technique of choice in obtaining tissue preoperatively to aid in surgical planning, as this technique can distinguish invasive from noninvasive disease and has been shown to have a high concordance with subsequent surgical findings (2). Core needle biopsy can be performed under stereotactic or ultrasound guidance and has been shown to decrease the time from identification of the radiologic abnormality to pathologic diagnosis and reduce the cost compared to needle localization with excision biopsy (3). There are some patients in whom CNB is not indicated because of any of a variety of patient and tumor factors (e.g., small breast size, architectural distortion, vague mass, faint calcifications). In these patients, needle localization biopsy is indicated (4).

Once the diagnosis of invasive malignancy is established, an appropriate staging workup should be performed. This includes diagnostic bilateral mammography to document any other lesions in the breast and sonography as necessary (for distinguishing solid vs. cystic mass lesions). Sonography of the nodal basins is also useful in patients with palpable nodal disease and those with larger tumors (in whom there is a greater likelihood of nodal disease). If the sonographic appearance is worrisome, fine-needle aspiration biopsy of the lymph node is recommended. Further staging includes chest radiography and, in patients with larger tumors or symptoms suggestive of potential distant metastases, bone scan, computed tomography (CT) of the abdomen and pelvis, and potentially CT or magnetic resonance imaging of the brain. The common sites of metastasis are highlighted by the current method of breast cancer staging described in Table 1 (5). From this Tumor-Node-Metastasis (TNM) staging method, breast cancers can be grouped into grades as in Table 2 (5).

If there is no evidence of distant metastatic disease, an open discussion then ensues with the patient as to her options. In the case of locally advanced disease or inflammatory breast carcinoma, or if there is evidence of a large tumor or nodal disease, it may be advisable to consider neoadjuvant chemotherapy (NACT) prior to surgery. In such instances, consultation with other members of the multidisciplinary team, including medical oncologists, radiation oncologists, and plastic surgeons, may be beneficial in planning appropriate therapeutic interventions.

Surgery for breast cancer involves two components:

1. Treatment of the lesion in the breast.
2. Evaluation of nodal status.

In terms of treating the breast, The National Surgical Adjuvant Breast and Bowel Project B-06 demonstrated the equivalence of mastectomy and breast-conserving surgery (BCS) (lumpectomy) regarding the patient's survival (6). However, the rate of local recurrence is reported to be higher with BCS than with mastectomy. This rate can be effectively reduced with the addition of postoperative radiation therapy (6). Table 3 summarizes recommendations for breast radiotherapy after BCS (7).

The alternative to breast conservation is mastectomy. This can be performed either with or without reconstruction. Skin-sparing mastectomy with reconstruction offers patients a better cosmetic outcome and has been shown to be oncologically safe (8). If this option is chosen, preoperative consultation with the plastic surgery team is important in allowing patients to understand the reconstructive options available, the timing of the reconstruction, and the risks associated with the procedure. Table 4 offers guidelines to assist in the choice between lumpectomy and mastectomy (9).

For patients who have clinically negative lymph node basins at presentation, nodal evaluation begins with sentinel lymph node biopsy. If findings on pathologic examination of the sentinel node are positive, a complete axillary node dissection is performed. This is done for staging and prognosis, as nodal status has been shown to be the most important predictor of survival (10). Preoperative lymphoscintigraphy, though not always needed for sentinel node identification, does provide a useful road map (11). The practice at the M.D. Anderson Cancer Center is to perform lymphoscintigraphy with 2.5 mCi of filtered technetium Tc 99 sulfur colloid the day prior to the planned surgery. Lymphoscintigraphy can be performed on the same day of surgery with a lower dose of radiocolloid (0.5 mCi). There is currently much debate surrounding the management of patients with drainage to the internal mammary nodes seen on lymphoscintigraphy (12). In general, in patients with dual drainage (to both the axilla and the internal mammary nodes), it is good practice to remove the axillary sentinel node alone. However, if drainage is noted only to the internal mammary nodes, it could be argued on the basis of the revised American Joint Committee on Cancer (AJCC) staging system (13) that removal of the internal mammary sentinel node is warranted.

Table 1 TNM Staging System for Breast Cancer

Primary tumor (T)	
TX	Primary tumor cannot be assessed
T0	No evidence of primary tumor
Tis	Carcinoma in situ
Tis (DCIS)	Ductal carcinoma in situ
Tis (LC1S)	Lobular carcinoma in situ
Tis (Paget)	Paget's disease[a] of the nipple with no tumor
T1	Tumor $\leq$2 cm in greatest dimension
T1mic	Microinvasion $\leq$0.1 cm in greatest dimension
T1a	Tumor $>$0.1 cm but not $>$0.5 cm in greatest dimension
T1b	Tumor $>$0.5 cm but not $>$1 cm in greatest dimension
T1c	Tumor $>$1 cm but not $>$2 cm in greatest dimension
T2	Tumor $>$2 cm but not $>$5 cm in greatest dimension
T3	Tumor $>$5 cm in greatest dimension
T4	Tumor of any size with direct extension to (a) chest wall or (b) skin, only as described below
T4a	Extension to chest wall, not including pectoralis muscle
T4b	Edema (including peau d'orange) or ulceration of the skin of the breast, or satellite skin nodules confined to the same breast
T4c	Both T4a and T4b
T4d	Inflammatory carcinoma
Regional lymph nodes (N)	
NX	Regional lymph nodes cannot be assessed (e.g., previously removed)
N0	No regional lymph node metastasis
Nl	Metastasis in movable ipsilateral axillary lymph node(s)
N2	Metastases in ipsilateral axillary lymph nodes fixed or matted, or in clinically apparent[b] ipsilateral internal mammary nodes in the absence of clinically evident axillary lymph node metastasis
N2a	Metastasis in ipsilaterol axillary lymph nodes fixed to one another (matted) or to other structures
N2b	Metastasis only in clinically apparent[b] ipsilateral internal mammary nodes and in the absence of clinically evident axillary lymph node metastasis
N3	Metastasis in ipsilateral infraclavicular lymph node(s), or in clinically apparent[b] ipsilateral internal mammary lymph node(s) and in the presence of clinically evident axillary lymph node metastasis; or metastasis in ipsilateral supraclavicular lymph node(s) with or without axillary or internal mammary lymph node involvement
N3a	Metastasis in ipsilateral infraclavicular lymph node(s) and axillary lymph node(s)
N3b	Metastasis in ipsilateral internal mammary lymph node(s) and axillary lymph node(s)
N3c	Metastasis in ipsilateral supraclavicular lymph node(s)
Regional lymph nodes (pN)[c]	
pNX	Regional lymph nodes cannot be assessed (e.g., previously removed or not removed for pathologic study)
pN0	No regional lymph node metastasis histologically, no additional examination for isolated tumor cells[d]
pN0(i−)	No regional lymph node metastasis histologically, negative for isolated tumor cells
pN0(i+)	No regional lymph node metastasis histologically, positive isolated tumor cells not $>$0.2 mm
pN0(mol−)	No regional lymph node metastasis histologically, negative molecular findings (RT–PCR)
pN0(mol+)	No regional lymph node metastasis histologically, positive molecular findings (RT–PCR)
pNlmi	Micrometastasis ($>$0.2 mm, none $>$2.0 mm)
pNl	Metastasis in one to three axillary lymph nodes and/or in internal mammary nodes with microscopic disease detected by sentinel lymph node dissection but-not clinically apparent[e]
pNla	Metastasis in one to three axillary lymph nodes
pNlb	Metastasis in internal mammary nodes with microscopic disease detected by sentinel

(*Continued*)

Table 1 TNM Staging System for Breast Cancer (*Continued*)

	lymph node dissection but not clinically apparent[e]
pNlc	Metastasis in one to three axillary lymph nodes and in internal mammary lymph nodes with microscopic disease detected by sentinel lymph node dissection but not clinically apparent[e,f]
pN2	Metastasis in four to nine axillary lymph nodes or in clinically apparent[b] internal mammary lymph nodes in the absence of axillary lymph node metastasis
pN2a	Metastasis in four to nine axillary lymph nodes (at least one tumor deposit >2.0 mm)
pN2b	Metastasis in clinically apparent[b] internal mammary lymph nodes in the absence of axillary lymph node metastasis
pN3	Metastasis in 10 or more axillary lymph nodes, or in infraclavicular lymph nodes, or in clinically apparent[b] ipsilateral internal mammary lymph nodes in the presence of one or more positive axillary lymph nodes; or in more than three axillary lymph nodes with clinically negative microscopic metastasis in internal mammary lymph nodes; or in ipsilateral supraclavicular lymph nodes
pN3a	Metastasis in 10 or more axillary lymph nodes (at least one tumor deposit >2.0 mm) or metastasis to the infraclavicular lymph nodes
pN3b	Metastasis in clinically apparent[b] ipsilateral internal mammary lymph nodes in the presence of one or more positive axillary lymph nodes; or in more than three axillary lymph nodes and in internal mammary lymph nodes with microscopic disease detected by sentinel lymph node dissection but not clinically apparent[e]
pN3c	Metastasis in ipsilateral supraclavicular lymph nodes
Distant metastasis (M)	
MX	Distant metastasis cannot be assessed
M0	No distant metastasis
Ml	Distant metastasis

Note: IHC, immunohistochemistry; RT–PCR, reverse transcriptase–polymerase chain reaction.

[a] Paget's disease associated with a tumor is classified according to the size of the tumor.

[b] Clinically apparent is defined as detected by imaging studies (excluding lymphoscintigraphy) or by clinical examination.

[c] Classification is based on axillary lymph node dissection with or without sentinel lymph node dissection. Classification based solely on sentinel lymph node dissection without subsequent axillary lymph node dissection is designated (sn) for "sentinel node" [e.g., pN0(i+)(sn)].

[d] Isolated lumor cells are defined as single tumor cells or small cell clusters not greater than 0.2 mm, usually detected only by immunohistochemical or molecular methods but which may be verified on hematoxylin and eosin stains. Isolated tumor cells do not usually show evidence of metastatic activity (e.g, proliferation or stromal reaction).

[e] Not clinically apparent is defined as not detected by imaging studies (excluding lymphoscintigraphy) or by clinical examination.

[f] If associated with more than three positive axillary lymph nodes, the internal mammary nodes are classified as pN3b to reflect increased tumor burden.

Source: Adapted with permission from the American Joint Committee on Caner (AJCC), Chicago, IL. The original source for this material is the AJCC Cancer Staging Manual, 6th ed (2002) published by Springer-Verlag, New York (www.springer-ny.com).

1. Chemotherapy in the Management of Breast Cancer

Chemotherapy in breast cancer is an area of considerable on-going research. Health Canada convened a Steering Committee to produce clinical practice guidelines for the treatment of breast cancer.

Table 5 lists the updated recommendations for adjuvant systemic therapy for women with node-negative breast cancer (14).

Table 6 lists the updated recommendations for adjuvant systemic therapy for women with node-positive cancer (15).

To assist patients in making an informed decision regarding choice of treatment (e.g., BCS with chemotherapy vs. mastectomy), they need to be educated about the common side effects of chemotherapy and antiestrogen therapy (tamoxifen).

2. Side Effects of Chemotherapy (16)

Commonly used chemotherapy regimens are anthracycline/cyclophosphamide (AC) combinations and cyclophosphamide/methotrexate/5-fluorouracil (CMF) combinations. Currently available data with adjuvant paclitaxel/anthracycline combinations in node positive breast cancer do not permit definitive recommendations of the use of taxanes in the adjuvant setting (17). Frequent side effects of chemotherapy are:

- Nausea and vomiting (more severe but briefer with AC combination)

Table 2 TNM Stage Grouping for Breast Cancer

Stage grouping			
0	Tis	N0	M0
I	T1[a]	N0	M0
IIA	T0	N1	M0
	T1[a]	N1	M0
	T2	N0	M0
IIB	T2	N1	M0
	T3	N0	M0
IIIA	T0	N2	M0
	T1[a]	N2	M0
	T2	N2	M0
	T3	N1	M0
	T3	N2	M0
IIIB	T4	N0	M0
	T4	N1	M0
	T4	N2	M0
IIIC	Any T	N3	M0
IV	Any T	Any N	M1

[a]T1 includes T1mic.
Source: Adapted with permission from the American Joint Committee on Cancer (AJCC), Chicago, IL. The original source for this material is the AJCC Cancer Staging Manual, 6th ed (2002) published by Springer-Verlag, New York (www.springer-ny.com).

- Fatigue
- Weight gain (14% of patients)
- Temporary hair loss, complete hair loss with AC, and with CMF, only 40% of patients have severe hair loss (30% have no hair loss at all)
- Mild irritation of the eyes, mucous membranes, and bladder
- Temporary cessation of menstruation (may be permanent in older women)
- Immunosuppression leading to increased risk of infection, and about 2% of patients suffer fevers requiring hospitalization
- Severe side effects are rare (<1%); however, there is a small risk of heart damage with AC and a small risk of leukemia later in life (1 per 1000 to 1 per 10,000), and chemotherapy can also be fatal

3. *Side Effects of Tamoxifen (16)*

Tamoxifen is an antiestrogen drug, useful in estrogen receptor (ER)-positive breast cancer treatment (improvement in survival of 9%). Common side effects of treatment are

Table 3 Recommendations for Breast Radiotherapy after BCS

Women who undergo BCS should be advised to have postoperative breast irradiation. Omission of radiation therapy after BCS increases the risk of local recurrence.

Contraindications to breast irradiation include pregnancy, previous breast irradiation (including mantle irradiation for Hodgkin's disease), and inability to lie flat or to abduct the arm. Scleroderma and systemic lupus erythematosus are relative contraindications.

A number of different fractionation schedules for breast irradiation have been used. Although the most common fractionation schedule in Canada to date has been 50 Gy in 25 fractions, recent data from a Canadian trial demonstrate that 42.5 Gy in 16 fractions is as good as this more traditional schedule.

Irradiation to the whole breast rather than partial breast irradiation is recommended.

There is insufficient evidence to recommend breast irradiation with brachytherapy implants or intraoperative radiation therapy. Further evaluation of these treatments in randomized trials is required.

Additional irradiation to the lumpectomy site (boost irradiation) reduces local recurrence but can be associated with worse cosmesis compared with no boost. A boost following breast irradiation may be considered in women at high risk of local recurrence.

Physicians should adhere to standard treatment regimens to minimize the adverse effects of breast irradiation.

When choices are being made between different treatment options, patients must be made aware of the acute and late complications that can result from radiation therapy.

Breast irradiation should be started as soon as possible after surgery and not later than 12 weeks after, except for patients in whom radiation therapy is preceded by chemotherapy. However, the optimal interval between BCS and the start of irradiation has not been defined.

The optimal sequencing of chemotherapy and breast irradiation is not clearly defined for patients who are also candidates for chemotherapy. Most centers favor the administration of chemotherapy before radiation therapy. Selected chemotherapy regimens are sometimes used concurrently with radiation therapy. There is no evidence that concurrent treatment results in a better outcome, and there is an increased chance of toxic effects, especially with anthracycline-containing regimens.

Patients should be offered the opportunity to participate in clinical trials whenever possible.

Source: Reproduced with permission from Whelan T, Olivotto I, Levine M, for the Steering Committee on Clinical Practice Guidelines for the Care and Treatment of Breast Cancer. Clinical practice guidelines for the care and treatment of breast cancer: breast radiotherapy after breast-conserving surgery (summary of the 2003 update). CMAJ 2003; 168:437–439.

Table 4 Guidelines to Assist in the Choice Between Lumpectomy and Mastectomy

For patients with stage I or II breast cancer, BCS followed by radiotherapy is generally recommended. In the absence of special reasons for selecting mastectomy, the choice between BCS and mastectomy can be made according to the patient's circumstances and personal preferences.

Mastectomy should be considered in the presence of any of the following:

- Factors that increase the risk of local recurrence such as extensive malignant-type calcifications visible on the mammogram, multiple primary tumors or failure to obtain tumor-free margins
- Physical disabilities that preclude lying flat or abducting the arm, thus preventing the use of radiotherapy
- Absolute contraindications for radiotherapy such as pregnancy in the first or second trimester or previous irradiation of the breast, or relative contraindications such as systemic lupus erythematosus or scleroderma
- Large tumor size in proportion to breast size
- The patient's clear preference for mastectomy.

The factors that are not contraindications for BCS are the presence of a centrally located tumor mass, axillary lymph node involvement, or the presence of breast implants.

In some cases, preoperative chemotherapy can shrink a large primary tumor and allow for BCS.

Before deciding between BCS and mastectomy, the physician must make a full and balanced presentation to the patient concerning the pros and cons of these procedures.

Whenever an open biopsy is performed on the basis of even modest suspicion of carcinoma, the procedure should be, in effect, a lumpectomy using wide local excision of the intact tumor surrounded by a cuff of tumor-free tissue (determined by palpation and visual inspection).

The following recommendations should be observed to provide optimum clinical and cosmetic results:

- Tumor-involved margins should be revised
- Separate incisions should be used for removal of the primary tumor and for the axillary dissection except when these coincide anatomically
- Curvilinear incisions, concentric with the areolar margin, or transverse incisions are recommended over radial incisions
- Drains and approximation sutures should not be used in the breast parenchyma.

Source: Reproduced with permission from Scarth H, Cantin J, Levine M, Steering Committee on Clinical Practice Guidelines for the Care and Treatment of Breast Cancer. Clinical practice guidelines for the care and treatment of breast cancer: mastectomy or lumpectomy? The choice of operation for clinical stages I and II breast cancer (summary of the 2002 update). CMAJ 2002; 167:154–155.

- Hot flashes in 20% of patients
- Deep vein thrombosis risk (1%), with a small attendant risk of pulmonary embolism (potentially fatal)
- Increased risk of endometrial cancer (1:500) and, therefore, all women taking tamoxifen should report all vaginal bleeding (even spotting)
- Cataracts (very rarely)
- Two positive side effects are reduction of the chance of cancer in the opposite breast and decrease in osteoporosis

Patients must be educated in the preoperative setting about their disease, their treatment options, and the associated risks, so that they may make informed decisions regarding their surgical management. The risks discussed must include those risks germane to any surgical procedure, such as the risks associated with anesthesia, bleeding, and infection, as well as the risks pertinent to the specific procedure being performed. In particular, patients should be informed of the risks of sentinel lymph node biopsy—the potential for blue staining of the skin and anaphylaxis if lymphazurin (blue dye) is used (18), and the potential that an intraoperatively negative sentinel node may be found to harbor malignancy on the final pathology review (19), necessitating a second procedure for axillary clearance. Complete axillary lymph node dissection has been found to be associated with numbness in the upper inner aspect of the arm in 78% of patients as a result of sacrifice of the intercostobrachial nerves (20), with decreased range of motion about the shoulder in 9% of patients (20), and with lymphedema resulting in an increase of >2 cm in arm circumference in 16% of patients (20). In terms of surgery on the breast itself, patients should be informed of the possibility of numbness and bruising and should be informed that the final pathology review may reveal involved or close margins that may necessitate further surgery. Skin-sparing mastectomies with immediate reconstruction are associated with risks specific to the type of reconstruction being considered, and the patient should discuss these risks with the plastic surgeon, as well as the surgical oncologist. For example, a bilateral mastectomy with TRAM flap carries with it increased surgical and anesthetic risk. Being able to access a resource center and talk to breast cancer survivors is often helpful to patients and their families in

Table 5 Updated Recommendations for Adjuvant Systemic Therapy for Women with Node-Negative Breast Cancer

Before deciding whether to use adjuvant systemic therapy, the prognosis without adjuvant therapy should be estimated.
A patient's risk for recurrence can be categorized as low, intermediate, or high on the basis of tumor size, histologic or nuclear grade, ER status, and lymphatic and vascular invasion.
For each individual, the choice of adjuvant therapy must take into account the potential benefits and possible side effects. These must be fully explained to each patient.
Pre- and postmenopausal women who are at *low risk* of recurrence can be advised not to have adjuvant systemic treatment. Women who are at low risk, if seeking treatment, may consider tamoxifen.
Women at *high risk* should be advised to have adjuvant systemic therapy. Chemotherapy should be recommended for all premenopausal women (<50 years of age) and for postmenopausal women (≥ 50 years of age) with ER-negative tumors. Tamoxifen should be recommended as first choice for postmenopausal women with ER-positive tumors. For this last group of patients, further benefit is obtained from the addition of chemotherapy to tamoxifen, but the expected incremental toxicity must also be considered. Whether tamoxifen following chemotherapy should be routinely recommended for premenopausal women with ER-positive tumors is unclear.
For women at *intermediate risk* with ER-positive tumors, tamoxifen should normally be the first choice. For those who decline tamoxifen, chemotherapy may be considered.
For most patients over 70 years of age who are at high risk, tamoxifen is recommended for ER-positive tumors. For those with ER-negative disease who are in robust good health, chemotherapy is a valid option.
There are two recommended chemotherapy regimens: six cycles of CMF; four cycles of AC. More intensive combinations such as CEF (cyclophosphamide, epirubicin, and 5-fluorouracil) and AC-Taxol have not yet been evaluated in node-negative disease.
Tamoxifen should normally be administered at a dose of 20 mg daily for 5 years.
Patients should be encouraged to participate in therapeutic trials whenever possible.

Source: Reproduced from Levine M. Clinical practice guidelines for the care and treatment of breast cancer: adjuvant systemic therapy for node-negative breast cancer (summary of the 2001 update). CMAJ 2001; 164:213.

surgical decision-making. At the M.D. Anderson Cancer Center, patients are given an educational package in the preoperative setting that reviews not only their planned surgical procedure and the associated risks, but also what to expect postoperatively and the community resources available to patients.

In the preoperative setting, an anesthesiologist sees the patients, so that they may be adequately evaluated in terms of their suitability for general anesthesia and that their questions regarding types of anesthesia and the associated risks may be answered. This preoperative consultation is scheduled as soon as the physician and the patient have decided on the surgical procedure that will be performed and whether the assistance of additional surgical teams (e.g. plastic surgery) is required.

Laboratory values are checked to ensure an adequate hemoglobin level, white blood cell count (especially in patients who recently completed NACT), platelet count, and coagulation profile. Patients' medications are reviewed, and patients are informed which medications they are to take in the morning of surgery. Patients are advised not to eat or drink after midnight of the day before surgery. Sometimes, further consultations are required to complete a patient's preoperative workup. These might include cardiology consultation in patients with pacemakers or a significant history of cardiac or pulmonary disease.

C. Intraoperative Management

In the intraoperative setting, the focus is not only on the technical performance of the surgery, but also on the thoughtful prevention of potential risks. The correct side of surgery is reconfirmed verbally with the patient and by checking her films and chart. The correct breast and/or nodal basin should be marked by the surgical team at the preoperative visit and reconfirmed on the morning of surgery.

Patients are brought into the operating theater, where they are positioned supine with the arm of the affected side abducted on an arm board. If axillary surgery (either in the form of a sentinel lymph node biopsy or complete axillary dissection) is planned, a rolled towel or sheet is placed vertically under the back and under the shoulder of the patient on the correct surgical side. The arm is then cushioned on stacked sheets, so that there is no stress at the shoulder joint and care is taken to support the wrist.

It is well known that patients undergoing surgery are at increased risk of deep venous thrombosis (DVT) and subsequent pulmonary embolus (PE) (21). Malignancy is an added risk factor for DVT (22), as are chemotherapy (23) and tamoxifen (24). It is, therefore, standard practice that intermittent pneumatic compression devices be used for DVT prophylaxis (25). The use of prophylactic anticoagulation has been

Table 6 Updated Recommendations for Adjuvant Systemic Therapy for Women with Node-Positive Cancer

Premenopausal women

- Chemotherapy should be offered to all premenopausal women with stage II breast cancer.
- Acceptable treatment regimens are those using CMF, or doxorubicin (Adriamycin) and cyclophosphamide (AC), or CEF. In terms of breast cancer outcomes, CMF and AC are equivalent, and CEF is superior to CMF. Cyclophosphamide, epirubicin, and 5-fluorouracil is associated with more side effects than CMF. Personal preference and quality of life influence the choice of chemotherapy regimen. The addition of taxanes to anthracycline-containing regimens remains under active investigation. Currently available data concerning line addition of taxanes to anthracycline-containing regimens are inconclusive, although highly informed and motivated patients may choose this treatment. Participation in approved clinical trials should be strongly encouraged.
- Potential toxic effects of chemotherapy should be fully discussed with patients.
- Systemic adjuvant chemotherapy should begin as soon as possible after the surgical incision has healed.
- The recommended duration of therapy is at least six cycles (6 months) for CMF or CEF and at least four cycles (2–3 months) for AC.
- The recommended CMF regimen consists of 14 days of oral cyclo-phosphamide with intravenous methotrexate and 5-fluorouracil on days 1 and 8. This is repeated every 28 days for six cycles.
- When possible, patients should receive the full standard dosage. High-dose chemotherapy with stem-cell support is not recommended.
- Ovarian ablation is effective in premenopausal women with ER-positives tumors.However, chemotherapy has been better studied and is considered the intervention of choice. Ovarian ablation should be recommended to women who decline chemotherapy and have ER-positive tumors.
- In the future, a small benefit may be shown for the combination of ovarian ablation and chemotherapy in women with node-positive, ER-positive tumors. At present, there is insufficient evidence for this to be recommended.
- Tamoxifen can be recommended in premenopausal women with ER-positive tumors, who refuse chemotherapy or ovarian ablation.
- Whether tamoxifen should routinely be recommended after chemotherapy in premenopausal women is unclear.
- Before recommending hormonal therapy in premenopausal women, both the long-term side effects and its effects on recurrence must be considered.

Postmenopausal women

- Postmenopausal women with stage II, ER-positive cancer should be offered adjuvant tamoxifen.
- The recommended duration of tamoxifen therapy is 5 years.
- No other hormonal intervention apart from tamoxifen can be recommended for postmenopausal patients.
- Women with ER-negative tumors who are fit to receive chemotherapy (generally younger than 70 years) should be offered CMF or AC. Personal preference and quality of life influence the choice of chemotherapy regimen.
- Women with ER-positive tumors gain an additional benefit from taking chemotherapy in addition to tamoxifen. This is an option for a motivated, well-informed patient.

All ages

- The routine use of bisphosphonates as adjuvant therapy is not recommended.
- Patients should be offered the opportunity to participate in clinical trials whenever possible.

Source: Reproduced from Levine M. Clinical practice guidelines for the care and treatment of breast cancer: adjuvant systemic therapy for node-positive breast cancer (summary of the 2001 update). CMAJ 2001; 164:644–646.

debated in the literature, but, in general, this practice is thought to have the same effect as mechanical prophylaxis (25), with the added risk of bleeding complications (26).

The use of prophylactic antibiotics in breast surgery remains a source of debate in the literature. Although it is clear that prophylactic antibiotics are generally not needed in class I cases (such as most breast cancer operations) (27), the use of antibiotics may be warranted in some patients. These include patients who are having implants placed and patients who have comorbid conditions such as diabetes or cachexia. At the M.D. Anderson Cancer Center, the practice is to use one intravenous (IV) dose of a first generation cephalosporin prior to the skin incision.

In patients undergoing sentinel lymph node biopsy, lymphazurin is generally injected into the breast parenchyma around the primary tumor to aid the surgeon in identifying the sentinel node. Another technique that aids the surgeon in identification of the sentinel node is use of a handheld gamma probe (Neoprobe Corp, Dublin, OH, U.S.A.), which detects radioactivity from the previously injected radiocolloid. Lymphazurin has been associated with a 1.1% incidence of anaphylactic reactions (18). At the M.D. Anderson Cancer Center, the practice is to give prophylaxis in the form of a cocktail of 100 mg of hydrocortisone, 50 mg of diphenhydramine, and 20 mg of famotidine IV prior to the induction of anesthesia for all patients in whom lymphazurin will be used. However, the anesthesiologist and surgeon must still be aware of the potential for allergic reactions and must be prepared to treat them appropriately, should they occur. Although many of the reactions that have been reported include skin reactions with urticaria, blue hives, and a generalized rash or pruritis (28), cardiovascular collapse has also been reported (18). After prompt recognition of cardiovascular collapse, all anesthetic agents should be stopped, 100% oxygen should be administered, and IV fluids should be given rapidly. Vasopressors may be used to restore blood pressure (e.g., epinephrine 0.1–0.3 mg boluses IV), along with diphenhydramine 50 mg IV and methylprednisolone 125 mg IV. Patients with allergic reactions should be monitored closely in the hospital postoperatively for at least 24 hr. Anesthesiologists should also be aware of the potential cyanotic discoloration of the patient, as the blue dye circulates through the venous system (29). This can be accompanied by a transient decrease in pulse oxygen saturation seen after the injection of the lymphazurin, mimicking a hypoxic event. Communication between the surgeon and the anesthesiologist is therefore important.

When an axillary lymph node dissection is planned, communication between the surgeon and the anesthesiologist is critical. Many surgeons prefer in this situation not to have the patient paralyzed in order to evaluate intraoperatively the function of the long thoracic and thoracodorsal nerves. If paralytics are needed for anesthesia, this information should be communicated to the surgeon.

At the M.D. Anderson Cancer Center, there is also close collaboration between radiologists, pathologists, and surgeons in the intraoperative evaluation of specimens. In the setting of BCS, the specimen is oriented by the surgeon and hand-delivered to the pathologist, who then inks the specimen. A whole specimen radiograph is obtained when there is a nonpalpable abnormality; the specimen is then sectioned by the pathologist and again inspected grossly, followed by an additional radiograph of the sectioned specimen. The radiologist reviews both the whole specimen and sliced specimen radiographs and confers with the pathologist. Then, they advise the surgeon about whether further excision of individual margins is needed. This approach of collaborative intraoperative assessment of margin status significantly decreases the need for further surgery for margin control (30).

At the M.D. Anderson Cancer Center, the sentinel lymph node is processed intraoperatively using touch-preparation techniques, and the intraoperative findings dictate the need for further axillary dissection. The sensitivity of assessment of touch preparations in the identification of sentinel node metastases has been found to be as low as 53% (31), and therefore, in some cases such as T1 tumors, the intraoperative evaluation may be deferred to final pathology. The sensitivity of assessment of touch preparations is similar to the sensitivity of intraoperative assessment using frozen sections (31), but the touch preparation technique allows assessment of the intact lymph node without microsectioning and avoids any difficulty in interpretation due to freezing artifact.

D. Postoperative Care

In most cases, BCS and sentinel lymph node biopsy are performed on an outpatient basis. Patients are discharged on the same day, as surgery with oral analgesics provided for pain control. Most patients do not require antiemetics beyond the immediate postoperative setting, but these are provided if continued nausea is encountered. Patients who undergo a mastectomy or axillary node dissection, in whom drains are left in place, may be admitted for 23-hr observation and discharged on the following morning. These patients and their designated caregivers are instructed in drain care and wound care preoperatively by nurse educators and video presentations. Patients are taught how to care for their drains and are asked to record their temperature once a day and the amount of drainage twice daily. Patients are asked to return for drain removal when the output is < 30 mL per day or no later than 3 weeks after surgery. They are informed of the warning signs of infection, including erythema, discharge, and fever and chill, and are told to return if they have any of these symptoms. In addition, patients are given written instructions in arm exercises to prevent shoulder stiffness and decreased range of motion. These are modified for patients with drains.

At the M.D. Anderson Cancer Center, patients are seen about 1–2 weeks following surgery to review the final pathology report with the patient and assess the incision sites. Following this, consultations are scheduled for the patient as appropriate with medical and radiation oncologists. Patients continue to have surveillance with physical examinations and mammograms and have follow-up visits on a regular basis determined by the stage of disease and use of adjuvant therapies.

E. Conclusions

The cornerstone of the perioperative management of breast cancer patients is the multidisciplinary team approach individualized to the patient. From multidisciplinary collaboration in the preoperative setting to plan optimal therapy, to the collaboration of specialists in the patient's intraoperative and postoperative course, co-operation among the various specialties is critical. This forms the foundation of quality cancer care.

Acknowledgments

The authors are grateful to Mary Elliott for assistance in manuscript preparation and to Stephanie Deming for her critical reading of the manuscript.

II. PERIOPERATIVE CARE OF GYNECOLOGIC CANCER

A. Introduction

Patients with gynecologic cancers typically suffer from a number of medical problems in addition to the cancer. The most common of which are obesity, old age, malnutrition, cardiac, pulmonary, and renal insufficiency. Therefore, it is imperative that patients with gynecologic malignancies undergo a multidisciplinary evaluation prior to surgery. Ultimately, the goals of the surgical team should be to minimize the perioperative complications and optimize the care of the patient. Attention to details of history and presentation in the perioperative period are crucial to prevent or minimize morbidity for all patients undergoing gynecologic surgery. This chapter will review the recommended preoperative evaluations and common comorbid conditions in patients with ovarian epithelial, uterine, and cervical cancer and will then offer suggestions for minimizing the risk of or the severity of intraoperative and postoperative complications in these patients.

B. Epithelial Ovarian Cancer

Elderly women represent the fastest-growing segment of the U.S. population. In 1994, 33 million Americans (12.6%) were ≥65 years of age. The proportion of the population ≥65 years of age will increase to 20% in 2030. In 2050, 5% of the total population will be ≥80 years of age (32). The largest number of patients with ovarian cancer is found in the 60–64-year age group. Advancing age is a significant risk factor for developing ovarian cancer; however, there is also a genetic predisposition with a strong link to the *BRCA1* and *BRCA2* genes (at least 5–10% of cases) (33). Other risk factors are early menarche, late menopause, and null parity. The oral contraceptive reduces the risk of ovarian cancer by 30–60% (33). Seventy five to eighty percent of elderly women with ovarian cancer present with advanced (stage III or IV) disease (34). In addition to the significant decrease in physiologic reserve that is typical in elderly patients, a number of other medical comorbid conditions are commonly seen in patients diagnosed with an ovarian malignancy. These include hypertension, cardiac disease, and pulmonary disease (35). Malignant pleural effusions and intraparenchymal disease may further compromise respiratory function when patients with ovarian cancer undergo extensive tumor-reductive surgery. An equally important preoperative factor that contributes to a poor outcome in patients with ovarian cancer is the significant proportion of women with gynecologic malignancies, who have associated nutritional compromise. Although less common, other complicating medical factors in patients with ovarian cancer include renal and liver disease, anemia, and endocrine disorders such as obesity.

In patients with ovarian cancer, the routine preoperative evaluation includes complete history and physical examination (including pelvis), complete blood cell count, measurement of serum electrolyte levels, baseline liver function tests, measurement of the serum CA-125 level and imaging studies, including routine chest radiography, and computerized tomography of the abdomen and pelvis. A preoperative IV pyelogram and barium enema may be useful to evaluate the urinary tract and bowel.

1. *The Role of Ovarian Cancer-Associated Antigen (CA 125) Levels*

Ovarian cancer generally presents late with advanced disease (36). The serum CA 125 antigen level remains the "gold standard" for ovarian cancer tumor markers. A high CA 125 level (>35 U/mL) indicates an 85% chance of epithelial ovarian cancer (33); however, normal levels do not exclude residual disease (37). Current screening techniques for early detection involve a combination of CA 125 levels and transvaginal ultrasound (36). Other benign gynecological problems (e.g., endometriosis) and other malignancies have also been associated with elevated CA 125 levels (38,39). The further usefulness of CA 125 levels for the early detection of ovarian cancer is limited by the fact that elevated levels are found in only < 50% of patients with disease confined to one ovary (i.e., it does not detect early disease very well) (36). Microarray technology (using DNA techniques) and proteomics (the study of the protein environment or proteome of a population of cells) are the promising new techniques in the early detection of ovarian cancer (36). CA 125 levels remain useful in the follow up and restaging of patients who had elevated CA 125 levels at the time of diagnosis (40,41).

2. *Staging Ovarian Cancer*

Ovarian cancer is a surgically staged disease. The AJCC and the International Federation of Gynecology and Obstetrics (FIGO) both offer similar staging systems. Table 7 shows both these systems of staging ovarian cancer (42).

The initial treatment of ovarian cancer is usually surgery. The surgical intention is to confirm the diagnosis, stage the patient with apparent early disease, and perform tumor debulking (cytoreduction) in patients with advanced disease (33). There is strong evidence to suggest that survival and response to treatment are much improved in the setting of microscopic disease or minimal (<2 cm in largest diameter) residual disease (43). The Gynecologic Oncology Group has established a 1-cm residual tumor criterion for their trials (44). A structured surgical approach to ovarian cancer is given in Fig. 1 (45).

3. *Chemotherapy for Epithelial Ovarian Cancer*

Epithelial ovarian cancer is chemosensitive. Chemotherapy should always be administered following recommendations from an oncologist, as there are several regimens available and much current research in progress. Typically, chemotherapy is considered to be adjuvant (given postsurgically) or neoadjuvant (given presurgically to reduce tumor bulk). Correct surgical staging is critical to determine which patients can forego adjuvant chemotherapy. The regimen of cisplatin (75 mg/m^2) and paclitaxel (135 mg/m^2) given over 24 hr every 3 weeks for a total of six cycles should be considered first line treatment following surgery (33). Carboplatin (another platinum-based alkylating compound) is often substituted for cisplatin, as it has less neurotoxicity and nephrotoxicity and can be administered on an outpatient basis (33). Other common side effects of platinum compounds are electrolyte disturbances, peripheral neuropathy, metallic taste changes, nausea and vomiting, teratogenicity, bone marrow suppression, and alopecia. Paclitaxel is a plant taxoid from the Pacific yew tree bark and interferes with mitosis. Common side effects include anemia, immunosuppression, alopecia, nausea and vomiting, joint and muscle pains, nerve pain, and peripheral neuropathy. Figure 2 shows an approach to planning adjuvant chemotherapy (46).

Follow-up recommendations include physical examinations every 3–6 months with measurement of CA 125 levels. A persistently elevated CA 125 level can

Table 7 Staging Systems of Ovarian Carcinoma: AJCC and FIGO

TNM	FIGO	
T1	*Stage I*	Tumor limited to the ovaries (one or both)
T1a	Stage IA	Tumor limited to one ovary; capsule intact; no tumor on ovarian surface; no malignant cells in ascites or peritoneal washings[a]
T1b	Stage IB	Tumor limited to both ovaries; capsules intact; no tumor on the ovarian surface; no malignant cells in ascites or peritoneal washings[a]
T1c	Stage IC	Tumor limited to one or both ovaries with any of the following: capsule ruptured, tumor on ovarian surface, malignant cells in ascites or peritoneal washings
T2	*Stage II*	Tumor involves one or both ovaries with pelvic extension
T2a	Stage IIA	Extension and/or implants on uterus and/or tube(s); no malignant cells in ascites or peritoneal washings
T2b	Stage IIB	Extension to other pelvic tissues; no malignant cells in ascites or peritoneal washings
T2c	Stage IIC	Pelvic extension (2a or 2b) with malignant cells in ascites or peritoneal washings
T3 and/or N1	*Stage III*	Tumor involves one or both ovaries with microscopically confirmed peritoneal metastasis outside the pelvis and/or regional lymph node metastasis
T3a	Stage IIIA	Microscopic peritoneal metastasis beyond pelvis
T3b	Stage IIIB	Macroscopic peritoneal metastasis beyond pelvis $\leq$2 cm in greatest dimension
T3c and/or N1	Stage IIIC	Peritoneal metastasis beyond pelvis >2 cm in greatest dimension and/or regional lymph node metastasis
M1	*Stage IV*	Distant metastasis (excludes peritoneal metastasis)

Note: Staging of ovarian carcinoma is based on findings at clinical examination and by surgical exploration. The histologic findings are to be considered in the staging, as are the cytologic findings of any effusions. Biopsy should be obtained from suspicious areas outside of the pelvis. Liver capsule metastases are T3/stage III; liver parenchymal metastasis, M1/stage IV. Pleural effusion must have positive cytology results for M1/stage IV.

[a] The presence of nonmalignant ascites is not classified. The presence of ascites does not affect staging unless malignant cells are present.

Source: Reproduced with permission from Ref. 33.

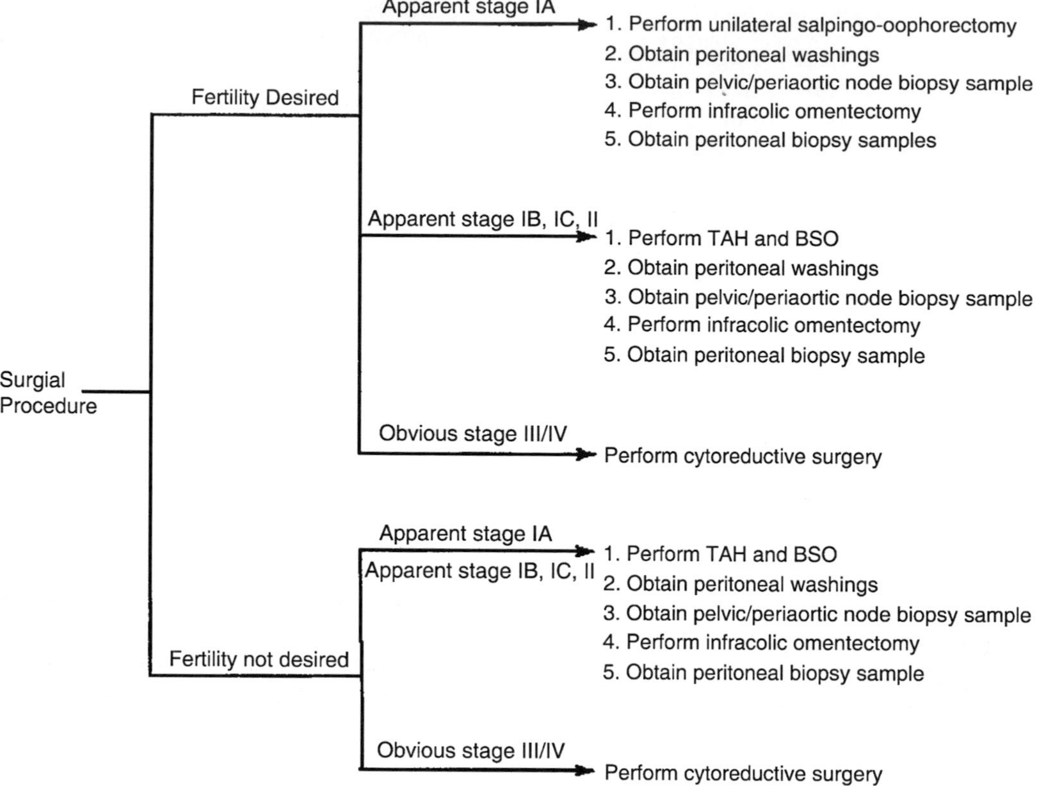

Figure 1 Selection of surgical procedure for ovarian cancer.

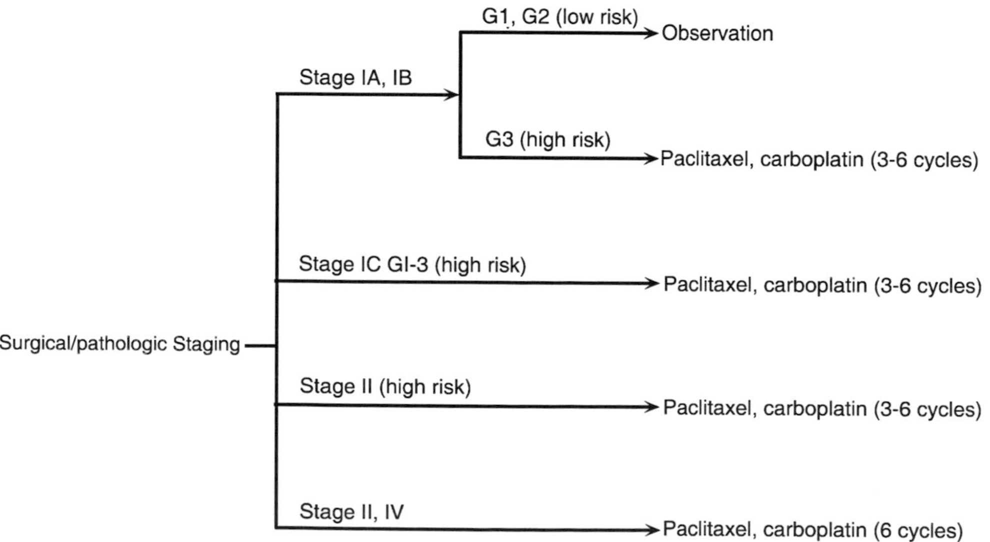

Figure 2 Postsurgical treatment. *Source*: From Ref. 46.

be used to predict persistent disease if the level was elevated prior to treatment. However, disease may still be present in up to 44% of patients with a CA 125 level <35 U/mL (33).

The concept governing NACT is to shrink advanced tumors prior to surgery, hopefully allowing for a more effective resection. The ovarian cancer is diagnosed by fine-needle biopsy or aspiration of malignant ascites. Neoadjuvant chemotherapy is indicated if there is evidence of disease in the thorax or unresectable disease in the abdominal and pelvic cavity. Ovarian cancer is deemed unresectable if the CT scan shows attachment of the omentum to the spleen or disease >2 cm on the diaphragm, liver surface, parenchyma, pleura, mesentery, gallbladder fossa, or suprarenal nodes (47). After three courses of NACT, the patient undergoes re-evaluation to determine whether surgery is an option.

Like NACT and second-look laparotomy, the role of radiation therapy in ovarian cancer should be regarded as experimental (33,48,49).

Unfortunately, in 10–15% of patients, achieving optimal cytoreduction requires one or multiple bowel resections, as well as splenectomy. These additional procedures increase surgical time and also increase blood loss, the need for IV fluid replenishment, and the exposure of the abdominal and pelvic cavity to a contaminated environment. All of these factors may have an adverse impact on the patient's postoperative course. The most common complications in patients undergoing tumor-reductive surgery are wound infections, cardiac complications, deep vein thrombosis, pulmonary embolism, genitourinary fistulae, reoperation because of bleeding, and small bowel obstruction.

C. Uterine (Endometrial) Cancer

The median age at diagnosis for patients with adenocarcinoma of the endometrium is 61 years. Obesity, nulliparity, late menopause, diabetes, and hypertension are common risk factors associated with this disease (50,51). In addition to age, this patient population is predisposed to cardiac, pulmonary, and wound complications after surgery.

In a patient diagnosed with an endometrial malignancy, the preoperative evaluation includes complete history and physical examination; baseline laboratory work, including a complete blood cell count, measurement of electrolyte levels, and liver function tests; and chest radiography, to rule out the possibility of pulmonary metastases or any other pulmonary abnormalities. Metastatic spread is usually the local invasion of vagina, bladder and bowel, lymph node, and peritoneal seeding. Spread distant from the abdomen is late (52). However, even cerebellar metastasis has been described (53).

American Joint Committee on Cancer stages uterine endometrial carcinoma, as shown in Table 8.

The surgical treatment of patients with endometrial cancer depends on the disease stage. Fortunately, this neoplasm presents with clinical symptoms early, (and therefore at a curable stage), as the neoplasm will still be confined to the uterus (54). Generally, for early disease (stage I or II), the routine recommendation is a total abdominal hysterectomy, bilateral salpingo-

Table 8 Staging Table for Endometrial Adenocarcinoma

TNM	FIGO	
T1	I	Tumor confined to corpus uteri
T1a	IA	Tumor limited to endometrium
T1b	IB	Tumor invades less than one-half of the myometrium
T1c	IC	Tumor invades one-half or more of the myometrium
T2	II	Tumor invades cervix but does not extend beyond uterus
T2a	IIA	Tumor limited to the glandular epithelium of the endocervix. There is no evidence of connective tissue stormal invasion
T2b	IIB	Invasion of the stromal connective tissue of the cervix
T3	III	Local and/or regional spread as defined below
T3a	IIIA	Tumor involves serosa and/or adnexa (direct extension or metastasis) and/or cancer cells in ascites or peritoneal washings
T3b	IIIB	Vaginal involvement (direct extension or metastasis)
N1	IIIC	Regional lymph node metastases to pelvic and/or para-aortic lymph nodes
T4	IVA	Tumor invades bladder mucosa and/or bowel mucosa (bullous edema is not sufficient evidence to classify a tumor as T4)
M1	IVB	Distant metastasis includes metastasis to intra-abdominal lymph nodes other than para-aortic, and/or inguinal lymph nodes; excludes metastasis to vagina pelvic serosa, or adnexa

oophorectomy. Pelvic and para-aortic lymph node sampling remains controversial (55). Since 1988, endometrial cancer has been staged surgically. Irradiation is now rarely administered preoperatively to this group of patients (56). Patients with node-positive disease or with incomplete surgical staging should receive postoperative radiation in the nodal distribution (56), with patients suffering para-aortic nodal involvement receiving an extended field. Whole abdomen radiation is controversial. Combination radiation and chemotherapy holds further promise (51,57).

Given that the majority of patients with endometrial cancer are obese, the issues that need to be dealt with in the operating room typically relate to poor exposure. Obese patients must be positioned carefully to avoid further compromising ventilation during general anesthesia. Gas exchange is impaired, because obesity reduces functional residual capacity. This effect can be reduced by the addition of positive end expiratory pressure (58). Thus, there are limitations on the positioning of these patients (minimal Trendelenberg position is ideal). In addition, when exposure is poor, the operating time is typically longer and blood loss is increased, along with the rate of blood transfusion. In the postoperative period, there are additional concerns (59). An epidural anesthetic for postoperative analgesia provides safer and more effective analgesia than opiate analgesia (58). Obesity predisposes to wound breakdown and separation (59). When this situation arises, the patient usually remains in bed for a prolonged period, and this can lead to further complications such as potentially fatal venous thromboembolic (VTE) events. The most important aspect of managing VTE is prevention (60). Common predisposing factors to VTE in this group of patients are increased age, obesity, abdominal surgery, cancer, cardiac and respiratory failure and postoperative immobility (61). Venous thromboembolism is a common but under-diagnosed condition in cancer patients (62). Clinical diagnosis is unreliable (63), and in contrast, venography remains the "gold standard"; magnetic resonance venography is a valid alternative when ultrasound is inconclusive (62,64). It has been shown that extension of the DVT up the inferior vena cava occurs frequently, but that this is not associated with an increased incidence of VTE disease (65). In theater, compression stockings or pneumatic calf compression devices should be used to minimize DVT. Postoperatively, all patients should receive at least subcutaneous prophylactic heparin (unless contraindicated) (60).

If an extensive node dissection is performed, the patient is at risk of developing chronic lymphedema, especially if the patient has received postoperative pelvic radiation.

D. Cervical Cancer

In the United States, cervical cancer is the third most common gynecologic malignancy. The disease is generally diagnosed in the fifth decade (which is earlier than the mean age for breast, lung, and ovarian cancer) (66). Risk factors for occurrence are exposure to human papilloma virus through early sexual exposure (<16 years), multiple (>4) partners, and genital warts. Other risk factors are exposure to cigarette smoke, immunosuppression, and HIV (66).

Once a tissue diagnosis of invasive carcinoma has been established, the disease is staged clinically—mainly on the basis of the size of the tumor and its extension into the pelvis (66). The FIGO system for staging cervical cancer is given in Table 9 (67).

Critical-care issues are frequently encountered in patients who undergo radical hysterectomies for early (stage IA2–IIA) disease or pelvic exenteration for a central recurrence. Common issues encountered in this group of patients in the perioperative period typically include thromboembolic prophylaxis (discussed in the previous section), management of intraoperative hemorrhage, transfusion requirements, and close monitoring and replacement of fluid and electrolytes, along with acid–base disturbances.

The recommended preoperative evaluation for patients with cervical cancer scheduled to undergo radical hysterectomy includes a complete history and physical examination; documentation of invasive disease by cervical biopsies or conization; laboratory studies, including a complete blood cell count, measurement of serum electrolyte levels, and baseline liver function tests; and routine chest radiography. For patients scheduled to undergo pelvic exenteration, CT or magnetic resonance imaging of the abdomen and pelvis is also performed. Intravenous pyelogram and barium enema may also be useful in planning surgery (66).

Table 10 describes a treatment algorithm for cervical cancer (68).

The objective of a radical hysterectomy is to remove the tissue adjacent to the cervix and vaginal fornices in addsition to the uterus, cervix, and upper-third of the vagina, preserving intact the urinary system and rectum. The parametria and paracolpos need to be removed because they are the first tissues involved by contiguous invasion and local lymphatic extension of cervical cancer. Generally, the cardinal ligaments and the uterosacral ligaments are resected. The most frequently reported intraoperative complication of radical hysterectomy is blood loss, with averages ranging from 800 mL to 1500 mL and approximately one-third to two-thirds of patients requiring a blood

Table 9 The FIGO System for Staging Cervical Cancer

Stage	Description
0	Carcinoma in situ, intraepithelial carcinoma
I	Invasive carcinoma strictly confined to cervix
IA	Invasive carcinoma identified microscopically (all gross lesions, even with superficial invasion, should be assigned to stage IB)
IA1	Measured invasion of stroma ≤3.0 mm in depth and no wider than 7.0 mm
IA2	Measured invasion of stroma >3.0 mm but no greater than 5.0 mm in depth and no wider than 7.0 mm
IB	Preclinical lesions greater than stage IA or clinical lesions confined to cervix
IB1	Clinical lesions of ≤4.0 cm in size
IB2	Clinical lesions >4.0 cm in size
II	Carcinoma extending beyond cervix but not to pelvic sidewall; carcinoma involves vagina but not its lower third
IIA	Involvement of upper two-thirds of vagina, no parametrial involvement
IIB	Obvious parametrial involvement
III	Carcinoma extending onto pelvic wall; on rectal examination, there is no cancer-free space between tumor and pelvic sidewall; the tumor involves lower third of the vagina and all patients with hydronephrosis or nonfunctioning kidney are included unless known to be the result of other causes
IIIA	Involvement of lower third of the vagina; no extension to pelvic sidewall
IIIB	Extension to pelvic sidewall and/or hydronephrosis or nonfunctioning kidney
IV	Carcinoma extends beyond true pelvis or clinically involves mucosa of bladder or rectum; bullous edema does not allow a case to be designated as stage IV
IVA	Spread of growth to adjacent organs
IVB	Spread to distant organs

Table 10 Treatment Algorithm for Cervical Cancer

Stage	Clinical features	Treatment
IA1	Invasion ≤3.0 mm	If patient desires fertility, conisation of cervix If the patient does not, simple hysterectomy (abdominal or vaginal)
	With lymphovascular space invasion	Hysterectomy with or without pelvic lymphadenectomy
IA2	3.0–5.0 mm invasion, <7.0 mm lateral spread	Radical hysterectomy with pelvic lymphadenectomy
		Radiotherapy
IB1	Tumor ≤4 cm	Radical hysterectomy with pelvic lymphadenectomy plus chemoradiotherapy for poor prognostic surgical–pathological factors[a]
		Radiotherapy
IB2	Tumor >4 cm	Radical hysterectomy with pelvic lymphadenectomy plus chemoradiotherapy for poor prognostic surgical and pathological factors[a]
		Chemoradiotherapy
		Chemoradiotherapy with adjuvant hysterectomy
IIA	Upper-two-thirds vaginal involvement	Radical hysterectomy with pelvic lymphadenectomy
		Chemoradiotherapy
IIB	With parametrial extension	Chemoradiotherapy
IIIA	Lower-third vaginal involvement	Chemoradiotherapy
IVA	Local extension within pelvis	Chemoradiotherapy Primary pelvic exenteration
IVB	Distant metastases	Palliative chemotherapy Chemoradiotherapy

[a] Pelvic lymph node metastases: large tumor; deep cervical stromal invasion; lymphovascular space invasion; positive vaginal or parametrial margins.

Source: Reprinted with permission from Ref. 66.

transfusion (69,70). Overall, 5–10% of patients may have significant intraoperative complications other than blood loss. These include injury to major blood vessels and injury to the bladder, ureter, obturator nerve, and rectum. The most common postoperative complications are wound complications and infectious processes. More serious complications may also arise, such as deep vein thrombosis, pulmonary embolism, ureteral stricture and fistula, bladder fistula, bladder dysfunction, and lymphocele formation (66).

Recurrent cervical cancer generally occurs in three sites. These are the pelvic sidewall (presumably in lymph node bearing areas), distal sites (para-aortic lymph nodes or other distal nodes), and bony metastasis (typically vertebral) (71). Owing to the limited radiation tolerance of pelvic organs such as small bowel, bladder, and rectum, reirradiation is generally not an option in patients with persistent or recurrent cervical cancer after maximal radiation (71). In patients with carcinoma of the cervix recurrent to the central pelvis after irradiation, total pelvic exenteration with removal of the pelvic organs, including the bladder and rectosigmoid, remains the only treatment modality with curative potential (71). In some cases, the procedure can be limited to anterior exenteration with removal of the bladder and preservation of the rectosigmoid or posterior exenteration with removal of the rectosigmoid and preservation of the bladder. The most common complication of pelvic exenteration is blood loss (median of 3000 mL). Other serious complications that may arise are sepsis (occurs in 10% of patients), wound dehiscence (10%), urinary fistula or obstruction (6%), intestinal leak (8%), small bowel obstruction (5%), PE (1.5%), and postoperative hemorrhage (2.5%) (72).

1. Chemotherapy for Cervical Cancer

Gynecologic Oncology Group studies have evaluated chemotherapy for cervical cancer, and because of poor response rates, its use should be considered palliative (71,73). Cisplatin (platinum) -based chemotherapy has shown reasonable activity (20–38%) in recurrent carcinomas of the cervix, but median survival was short at 6 months (71). Although response rates of up to 50% have been shown with combination chemotherapy, no significant increase in survival was noted, and toxicity is increased with combination chemotherapy (71,73). Neoadjuvant chemotherapy is being experimented in patients with advanced disease, and ~20% of patients do achieve a clinical response. However, there are too few randomized controlled studies to determine the effectiveness of NACT approaches over standard treatments (74).

Patients undergoing this extensive abdominal surgery will require general anesthesia. An epidural anesthetic may be performed prior to induction of general anesthesia as part of a combined technique. The epidural anesthetic can then be continued to provide postoperative analgesia. Whether this combined technique confers additional benefit to the patient over general anesthesia alone remains unanswered, as there are conflicting reports in the literature (75–79). In a large systematic review of 141 trials, Rodgers et al. (75) concluded that neuraxial blockade reduced postoperative mortality and complications due to reduction of deep vein thrombosis, pulmonary embolism, transfusion requirements, pneumonia, respiratory depression, myocardial infarction, and renal failure. Rodgers et al. comment that the size of some of these benefits remains uncertain and that further research should be conducted to understand how these effects occur. Grass (76) states that there is increasing evidence that epidural anesthesia and analgesia (EAA) can improve surgical outcome by reducing similar common postoperative complications that are listed earlier. Grass also adds that large multicenter prospective randomized studies are required to assess the definite impact of EAA on morbidity and mortality, ICU time, length of hospital stay, and cost of healthcare. The Multicenter Australian Study of Epidural Anesthesia (the MASTER Anesthesia Trial) (79), published in 2002, was a multicenter randomized controlled trial looking at outcome in 915 patients undergoing major abdominal surgery, who were deemed to be at high risk because of the presence of one or more important comorbidities. The conclusion was that apart from lower pain scores in the first three postoperative days and less respiratory failure in the epidural group, there was no reduction in adverse morbid outcomes between the two groups. There were also no major adverse effects of epidural catheter insertion (79). A year later, Peyton et al. (77) published a predetermined subgroup analysis of the same data aimed at identifying specific patients at risk of complications. There was no difference in outcome between the epidural and control groups in patients at increased risk of respiratory or cardiac complications, or undergoing aortic surgery, nor in the group with failed epidural block. There was a small reduction in the length of postoperative ventilation in the control group ($p = 0.048$), and there were no differences in the length of ICU or hospital stay (77). This paper was criticized in the accompanying editorial (78), where aspects of protocol design, evolution, and timeliness in research and statistical design of the study were analyzed. On the balance of the current evidence, it would appear that epidural analgesia confers at least equal postoperative benefit.

However, no individual case should be cancelled because of failure to establish an epidural anesthetic.

E. General Recommendations for Minimizing Risk of Complications

Fever is one of the most common postoperative problems. It is generally defined as a body temperature of at least 38°C on two occasions at least 4 hr apart, excluding the first 24 hr after surgery. In patients with gynecologic cancer who have fever after surgery, in addition to the routine evaluation, a pelvic examination must be performed to exclude the possibility of a vaginal cuff hematoma or abscess. After the first 48 hr after surgery, the most common sites of infection causing fever include the pulmonary system, wounds, and the urinary tract (80). Once infection is suspected, patients should have wound swabs and blood, urine, and sputum cultures taken before further antibiotic treatment is commenced. Once a specific site of infection is suspected, the exact choices of antibiotics (both prophylactic preoperatively and therapeutic postoperatively) are best determined by following the local hospital infectious disease guidelines. Peripheral venous cannulae are a source of infection, and therefore these should be changed every 72 hr (81). Central venous catheters should be replaced, once infection is suspected. There is no evidence that duration of catheterization is a specific risk factor for the development of sepsis (81).

F. Fluid and Electrolyte Imbalances

Fluid and electrolyte imbalances are influenced by several factors: the patient's comorbid conditions prior to the surgery, the extent of surgical resection, and the intraoperative complications. Patients undergoing radical tumor-reductive surgery for ovarian cancer, patients undergoing prolonged staging procedures for endometrial cancer, and patients undergoing radical hysterectomies or pelvic exenterations will require more fluid replenishment during the immediate postoperative period. Isotonic solutions (D5W in lactated Ringer's solution administered at a rate of 150 mL/hr) are ideal (82. Diuretic therapy to treat decreased urinary output should be avoided, because this may further deplete the intravascular volume. Patients with acute blood loss will need replacement with aggressive transfusions of isotonic fluid and/or blood component therapy. Plasma-volume expanders such as albumin, dextran, and hetastarch (all of which contain high-molecular-weight particles) can also be used. Transfusion of blood is not without complications. Vincent et al. (83) demonstrated in a large western European intensive care unit observational study that although mortality increased for all patients as organ failure increased, mortality was higher for transfused patients at all levels of organ dysfunction, with the exception of those with the most severe organ dysfunction. This effect was attributed to immunosuppression, as opposed to other complications of blood transfusion. Of note, patients transfused for acute bleeding had similar pretransfusion hemoglobin levels to those with other indications for transfusion, indicating that clinicians use hemoglobin level as a major determinant in the decision to transfuse patients. The overall mean pretransfusion hemoglobin was 8.4 g/dL. The need for blood transfusion should be seriously considered in postoperative cancer patients, as there is an increase in postoperative infectious complications (84) and morbidity from early recurrence of cancer (85).

G. Cardiac and Pulmonary Complications

It is estimated that 40% of all deaths after major gynecologic procedures are directly related to pulmonary embolism (86). Pulmonary embolism is the most frequent cause of death in the postoperative period in patients with uterine or cervical cancer (87,88). Preoperative risk factors for thromboembolic events in patients with gynecologic malignancies include older age, higher tumor stage, history of deep vein thrombosis, lower-extremity edema, and obesity, and history of radiation therapy (89). As most adverse events in patients with gynecologic cancer occur within the first 5 days after surgery, it is important for the patient to have external pneumatic compression stockings for that length of time. In a randomized prospective study, Maxwell et al. (90) compared the use of low-dose unfractionated heparin with the use of pneumatic calf compression stockings for the prevention of venous thrombosis in patients with gynecologic cancers. There were ~100 patients in each group, and no significant difference in the incidence of postoperative venous thrombosis was observed. However, 34 patients in the prophylactic heparin arm and only 17 patients using pneumatic compressing stockings required transfusions during their postoperative course.

Hypercoagulability should be assumed in cancer patients and may be caused by increased levels of clotting factors, cytokines, cancer procoagulant A, or increased release of tissue plasminogen activator (91). The American College of Obstetricians and Gynecologists have developed a practice bulletin on the prevention of DVT and pulmonary embolism. They class patients undergoing gynecologic surgery for malignancy as high risk for DVT and recommend the following alternatives (92):

1. Pneumatic compression should be placed intraoperatively and continued until the patient is fully ambulatory; or
2. Unfractionated heparin (5000 U) should be administered 8 hr before surgery and continued postoperatively until discharge; or
3. Dalteparin (5000 antifactor-Xa U) should be administered 12 hr before surgery and once a day thereafter; or
4. Enoxaparin (40 mg) should be administered 12 hr before surgery and once a day thereafter.

Given that most patients with gynecologic malignancies are elderly; cardiac and pulmonary problems are frequently encountered in this population. Coronary artery disease is responsible for most cardiac problems in patients undergoing major abdominal surgery. The majority of postoperative myocardial infarctions occur during the first 3 days after surgery; therefore, it is important to maintain very close monitoring of patients with previously diagnosed coronary artery disease during this period. Typically, pneumonia and pulmonary embolism are the most common causes of pulmonary complications in the postoperative period. Risk factors for such complications include upper abdominal surgery, a history of smoking, diabetes, older age, and obesity (93). Two common problems encountered with this group of patients are uncontrolled diabetes and uncontrolled hypertension. Unfortunately, patients with gynecologic malignancies cannot afford a delay in surgical intervention, and cardiac and pulmonary status must be optimized as rapidly as possible through a multidisciplinary approach utilizing the appropriate medical specialists. One role of the general internist often is to co-ordinate the patients' care (91).

The number of comorbid medical conditions and the number of postoperative complications can predict the length of hospitalization in patients undergoing surgery for gynecologic malignancies. In a recent study, Dean et al. (94) reviewed the medical records of 187 women who had surgery for known or suspected gynecologic cancers. The authors found that women with two or more comorbid medical conditions had significantly longer mean hospital stays (9 days) than those with none or just one comorbid medical condition (6 days). Women with two or more postoperative complications had significantly longer mean hospital stays (12 days) than those with none or just one complication (6 days). It is imperative that patients with multiple comorbid medical conditions are thoroughly evaluated, so that the potential for perioperative complications be minimized.

REFERENCES

1. American Cancer Society. Cancer Facts and Figures 2003; 9 (http://www.cancer.org/downloads/STT/CAFF2003PWSecured.pdf).
2. Parker SH, et al. Percutaneous large-core breast biopsy: a multi-institutional study. Radiology, 1994; 193(2): 359–364.
3. Lind DS, et al. Stereotactic core biopsy reduces the reexcision rate and the cost of mammographically detected cancer. J Surg Res 1998; 78(1):23–26.
4. Meric F, Hunt KK. Surgical options for breast cancer. In: Robb GL, Hunt KK, Strom EA, Ueno NT, eds. Breast Cancer. New York: Springer-Verlag, 2001:187–222.
5. Singletary SE, et al. Revision of the American Joint Committee on cancer staging system for breast cancer. J Clin Oncol 2002; 20(17):3630–3631.
6. Fisher B, et al. Twenty-year follow-up of a randomized trial comparing total mastectomy, lumpectomy, and lumpectomy plus irradiation for the treatment of invasive breast cancer. N Engl J Med 2002; 347(16): 1233–1241.
7. Whelan T, Olivotto I, Levine M. Clinical practice guidelines for the care and treatment of breast cancer: breast radiotherapy after breast-conserving surgery (summary of the 2003 update). CMAJ 2003; 168(4):437.
8. Kroll SS, et al. The oncologic risks of skin preservation at mastectomy when combined with immediate reconstruction of the breast. Surg Gynecol Obstet 1991; 172(1):17–20.
9. Scarth H, Cantin J, Levine M. Clinical practice guidelines for the care and treatment of breast cancer: mastectomy or lumpectomy? The choice of operation for clinical stages I and II breast cancer (summary of the 2002 update). CMAJ 2002; 167(2):155.
10. Donegan WL. Tumor-related prognostic factors for breast cancer. CA Cancer J Clin 1997; 47(1):28–51.
11. Upponi SS, et al. Sentinel lymph node biopsy in breast cancer—is lymphoscintigraphy really necessary? Eur J Surg Oncol 2002; 28(5):479–480.
12. Noguchi M. Relevance and practicability of internal mammary sentinel node biopsy for breast cancer. Breast Cancer 2002; 9:329–336.
13. Singletary SE, Alfred C, Ashley P, et al. Revision of the American Joint committee on cancer staging systems for breast cancer. J Clin Oncol 2002; 20:3628–3636.
14. Levine M. Steering Committee on Clinical Practice Guidelines for the Care and Treatment of Breast Cancer. Clinical practice guidelines for the care and treatment of breast cancer: adjuvant systemic therapy for node-negative breast cancer (summary of the 2001 update). Erratum. CMAJ 2001; 164(4):465.
15. Levine M. Clinical practice guidelines for the care and treatment of breast cancer: adjuvant systemic therapy for node-positive breast cancer (summary of the 2001 update). CMAJ 2001; 164(5):644.

16. The Steering Committee on Clinical Practice Guidelines for the Care and Treatment of Breast Cancer. CMAJ 1998; 158(suppl 3):S1–S82.
17. Aapro MS. Adjuvant therapy of primary breast cancer: a review of key findings from the 7th international conference, St. Gallen, February 2001. Oncologist 2001; 6(4):376–385.
18. Albo D, et al. Anaphylactic reactions to isosulfan blue dye during sentinel lymph node biopsy for breast cancer. Am J Surg 2001; 182(4):393–398.
19. Cserni G. The potential value of intraoperative imprint cytology of axillary sentinel lymph nodes in breast cancer patients. Am Surg 2001; 67:86–91.
20. Lin PP, et al. Impact of axillary lymph node dissection on the therapy of breast cancer patients. J Clin Oncol 1993; 11(8):1536–1544.
21. Kakkar VV and De Lorenzo F. Prevention of venous thromboembolism in general surgery. Baillieres Clin Haematol 1998; 11(3):605–619.
22. Heit JA, et al. Relative impact of risk factors for deep vein thrombosis and pulmonary embolism: a population-based study. Arch Intern Med 2002; 162(11): 1245–1248.
23. Otten HM, et al. Risk assessment and prophylaxis of venous thromboembolism in non-surgical patients: cancer as a risk factor. Haemostasis 2000; 30(suppl 2): 72–76; discussion 63.
24. Cushman M, et al. Effect of tamoxifen on venous thrombosis risk factors in women without cancer: the breast cancer prevention trial. Br J Haematol 2003; 120(1):109–116.
25. Marshall JC. Prophylaxis of deep venous thrombosis and pulmonary embolism. Can J Surg 1991; 34(6):551–554.
26. Bakker XR and Roumen RM. Bleeding after excision of breast lumps. Eur J Surg 2002; 168(7):401–403.
27. Gupta R, et al. Antibiotic prophylaxis for post-operative wound infection in clean elective breast surgery. Eur J Surg Oncol 2000; 26(4):363–366.
28. Montgomery LL, et al. Isosulfan blue dye reactions during sentinel lymph node mapping for breast cancer. Anesth Analg 2002; 95(2):385–388; table of contents.
29. Coleman RL, et al. Unexplained decrease in measured oxygen saturation by pulse oximetry following injection of lymphazurin 1% (isosulfan blue) during a lymphatic mapping procedure. J Surg Oncol 1999; 70(2):126–129.
30. Chagpar A, Yen T, Whitman G, et al. Intraoperative margin assessment reduces re-excision rates in breast conservation surgery for ductal carcinoma in situ. Am J Surg 2000; 186(4):371–377.
31. Creager AJ, et al. Intraoperative evaluation of sentinel lymph nodes for metastatic breast carcinoma by imprint cytology. Mod Pathol 2002; 15(11):1140–1147.
32. Cobbs EL, Ralapati AN. Health of older women. Med Clin North Am 1998; 82(1):127–144.
33. Partridge EE and Barnes MN. Epithelial ovarian cancer: prevention, diagnosis, and treatment. CA Cancer J Clin 1999; 49(5):297–320.
34. DiSaia PJ, Creasman WT. Epithelial ovarian cancer. eds. Clinical Gynecologic Oncology. Mosby, Inc., 2002: 289–350.
35. Mangano DT. Peri-operative cardiac mortality: epidemiology, cost and therapies. Annual Meeting of the Society of Gynecologic Oncology. San Francisco, CA, 1999.
36. Bandera CA, Ye B, Mok SC. New technologies for the identification of markers for early detection of ovarian cancer. Curr Opin Obstet Gynecol 2003; 15(1):51–55.
37. Makar AP, et al. CA 125 measured before second-look laparotomy is an independent prognostic factor for survival in patients with epithelial ovarian cancer. Gynecol Oncol 1992; 45(3):323–328.
38. Berek JS, et al. CA 125 serum levels correlated with second-look operations among ovarian cancer patients. Obstet Gynecol 1986; 67(5):685–689.
39. Atack DB, et al. CA 125 surveillance and second-look laparotomy in ovarian carcinoma. Am J Obstet Gynecol 1986; 154(2):287–289.
40. Hogberg T, Kagedal B. Long-term follow-up of ovarian cancer with monthly determinations of serum CA 125. Gynecol Oncol 1992; 46(2):191–198.
41. Mogensen O. Prognostic value of CA 125 in advanced ovarian cancer. Gynecol Oncol 1992; 44(3):207–212.
42. Partridge EE, Barnes MN. Epithelial ovarian cancer: prevention, diagnosis, and treatment. CA Cancer J Clin 1999; 49(5):304.
43. Hoskins WJ, et al. The effect of diameter of largest residual disease on survival after primary cytoreductive surgery in patients with suboptimal residual epithelial ovarian carcinoma. Am J Obstet Gynecol 1994; 170(4):974–979; discussion 979–980.
44. Berman ML. Future directions in the surgical management of ovarian cancer. Gynecol Oncol 2003; 90(2 Pt 2):S33–S39.
45. Partridge EE, Barnes MN. Epithelial ovarian cancer: prevention, diagnosis, and treatment. CA Cancer J Clin 1999; 49(5):306.
46. Partridge EE, Barnes MN. Epithelial ovarian cancer: prevention, diagnosis, and treatment. Cancer J Clin 1999; 49(5):312.
47. Nelson BE, Rosenfield AT, Schwartz PE. Preoperative abdominopelvic computed tomographic prediction of optimal cytoreduction in epithelial ovarian carcinoma. J Clin Oncol 1993; 11(1):166–172.
48. Gallo A, Frigerio L. Neoadjuvant chemotherapy and surgical considerations in ovarian cancer. Curr Opin Obstet Gynecol 2003; 15(1):25–31.
49. Ozols RF. Outcome issues in ovarian cancer. Oncology (Huntingt) 1995; 9(suppl 11):135–139.
50. Robertson G. Screening for endometrial cancer. Med J Aust 2003; 178(12):657–659.
51. Fiorica JV. Update on the treatment of cervical and uterine carcinoma: focus on topotecan. Oncologist 2002; 7(suppl 5):36–45.

52. AJCC. American Joint Committee on Cancer: AJCC Cancer Staging Manual. Vol. Corpus Uteri. 5th ed. Philadelphia: Lippincott–Raven, 1997.
53. Sewak S, Muggia FM, Zagzag D. Endometrial carcinoma with cerebellar metastasis: a case report and review of the literature. J Neurooncol 2002; 58(2):137–140.
54. Sonoda Y. Optimal therapy and management of endometrial cancer. Expert Rev Anticancer Ther 2003; 3(1): 37–47.
55. Huh WK, et al. Endometrial carcinoma. Curr Treat Options Oncol 2001; 2(2):129–135.
56. Grigsby PW. Update on radiation therapy for endometrial cancer. Oncology (Huntingt) 2002; 16(6):777–786, 790; discussion 791, 794–795.
57. McMeekin DS, Tillmanns T. Endometrial cancer: treatment of nodal metastases. Curr Treat Options Oncol 2003; 4(2):121–130.
58. Adams JP, Murphy PG. Obesity in anaesthesia and intensive care. Br J Anaesth, 2000; 85(1):91–108.
59. Byrne TK. Complications of surgery for obesity. Surg Clin North Am 2001; 81(5):1181–1193, vii–viii.
60. Williams MT, et al. Venous thromboembolism in the intensive care unit. Crit Care Clin 2003; 19(2):185–207.
61. Anderson FA Jr, Spencer FA. Risk factors for venous thromboembolism. Circulation 2003; 107(23 suppl 1): I9–I16.
62. Gomes MP, Deitcher SR. Diagnosis of venous thromboembolic disease in cancer patients. Oncology (Huntingt) 2003; 17(1):126–135, 139; discussion 139–144.
63. Tovey C, Wyatt S. Diagnosis, investigation, and management of deep vein thrombosis. BMJ 2003; 326(7400): 1180–1184.
64. Spritzer CE, Arata MA, Freed KS. Isolated pelvic deep venous thrombosis: relative frequency as detected with MR imaging. Radiology 2001; 219(2):521–525.
65. Borst-Krafek B, et al. Proximal extent of pelvic vein thrombosis and its association with pulmonary embolism. J Vasc Surg 2003; 37(3):518–522.
66. Waggoner SE. Cervical cancer. Lancet 2003; 361(9376): 2217–2225.
67. Waggoner SE. Cervical cancer. Lancet 2003; 361(9376): 2218.
68. Waggoner SE. Cervical cancer. Lancet 2003; 361(9376): 2220.
69. Levrant SG, Fruchter RG, Maiman M. Radical hysterectomy for cervical cancer: morbidity and survival in relation to weight and age. Gynecol Oncol 1992; 45(3):317–322.
70. Soisson AP, et al. Radical hysterectomy in obese women. Obstet Gynecol 1992; 80(6):940–943.
71. Selman AE, Copeland LJ. Surgical management of recurrent cervical cancer. Yonsei Med J 2002; 43(6): 754–762.
72. Morrow CP, Curtin JP, eds. Surgery for cervical neoplasia. In: Gynecologic Cancer Surgery. Churchill-Livingstone, 1996:451–568.
73. Berman ML. Advances in cervical cancer management from North American cooperative group clinical trials. Yonsei Med J 2002; 43(6):729–736.
74. Moore DH. Neoadjuvant chemotherapy for cervical cancer. Expert Opin Pharmacother 2003; 4(6):859–867.
75. Rodgers A, et al. Reduction of postoperative mortality and morbidity with epidural or spinal anaesthesia: results from overview of randomised trials. BMJ 2000; 321(7275):1493.
76. Grass JA. The role of epidural anesthesia and analgesia in postoperative outcome. Anesthesiol Clin North America 2000; 18(2):407–428, viii.
77. Peyton PJ, et al. Perioperative epidural analgesia and outcome after major abdominal surgery in high-risk patients. Anesth Analg 2003; 96(2):548–554, table of contents.
78. de Leon-Casasola OA. When it comes to outcome, we need to define what a perioperative epidural technique is. Anesth Analg 2003; 96(2):315–318.
79. Rigg JR, et al. Epidural anaesthesia and analgesia and outcome of major surgery: a randomised trial. Lancet 2002; 359(9314):1276–1282.
80. Harris WJ. Early complications of abdominal and vaginal hysterectomy. Obstet Gynecol Surv 1995; 50(11):795–805.
81. Centers for Disease Control and Prevention. Guidelines for the prevention of intravascular catheter-related infections. MMWR 2002; 51(no. RR-10):9–11.
82. Arieff AI, deFronzo RA. Fluid, Electrolyte and Acid–Base Disorders. New York: Churchill–Livingstone, 1985.
83. Vincent JL, et al. Anemia and blood transfusion in critically ill patients. JAMA 2002; 288(12):1499–1507.
84. Jensen LS, Hokland M, Nielsen HJ. A randomized controlled study of the effect of bedside leucocyte depletion on the immunosuppressive effect of whole blood transfusion in patients undergoing elective colorectal surgery. Br J Surg 1996; 83(7):973–977.
85. Blumberg N, et al. Association between transfusion of whole blood and recurrence of cancer. Br Med J (Clin Res Ed) 1986; 293(6546):530–533.
86. Jeffcoate TN, Tindall VR. Venous thrombosis and embolism in obstetrics and gynaecology. Aust N Z J Obstet Gynaecol 1965; 5(3):119–130.
87. Clarke-Pearson DL, Jelovsek FR, Creasman WT. Thromboembolism complicating surgery for cervical and uterine malignancy: incidence, risk factors, and prophylaxis. Obstet Gynecol 1983; 61(1):87–94.
88. Creasman WT, Weed JC Jr. Radical hysterectomy. In: Schaefer G, Graber EA, eds. Complications in Obstetrics and Gynecologic Surgery. Hagerstown, MD: Harper & Row, 1981:389–398.
89. Clarke-Pearson DL, et al. Variables associated with postoperative deep venous thrombosis: a prospective study of 411 gynecology patients and creation of a prognostic model. Obstet Gynecol 1987; 69(2):146–150.
90. Maxwell GL, et al. Pneumatic compression versus low molecular weight heparin in gynecologic oncology

surgery: a randomized trial. Obstet Gynecol 2001; 98(6):989–995.
91. Manzullo EF, Weed HG. Perioperative issues in patients with cancer. Med Clin North Am 2003; 87(1): 243–256.
92. Ressel GW. ACOG practice bulletin on preventing deep venous thrombosis and pulmonary embolism. American College of Obstetricians and Gynecologists. Am Fam Physician 2001; 63(11):2279–2280.
93. Ghosh K, Montz FJ. Postoperative care: major benign and radical surgery. In: Gershenson DM, DeCherney A, Curry SL, eds. Operative Gynecology. Philadelphia: WB Saunders, 2001:89–121.
94. Dean MM, Finan MA, Kline RC. Predictors of complications and hospital stay in gynecologic cancer surgery. Obstet Gynecol 2001; 97(5 Pt 1):721–724.

27

Postanesthesia Care for Reconstructive Microvascular Surgery

MICHAEL J. MILLER

Department of Plastic Surgery, The University of Texas M.D. Anderson Cancer Center, Houston, Texas, U.S.A.

Reconstructive microvascular surgery has become an integral part of surgical oncology, permitting treatment of some solid tumors previously considered inoperable or associated with unacceptable morbidity. Microvascular surgery is a method to replace impaired tissues by transferring healthy tissue from a distant site on the patient's body. It is useful not only to replace normal tissues that are excised during tumor ablation, but also it can be used to treat adverse effects of nonsurgical therapies. For example, radiotherapy can sometimes cause chronic wounds or functional tissue impairment. Some chemotherapy regimens can cause transient immunosuppression that can provide an opportunity for destructive soft tissue infections to occur. Excising the impaired tissues and using microvascular surgery to transfer well-vascularized tissue into the defect can successfully treat both examples.

Microvascular surgical procedures are technically complex and require careful preoperative planning and postoperative care. It is important to be able to detect and treat unique problems that can occur as well as understand what steps are necessary to prevent them in the immediate postoperative period. This leads to some special considerations in postanesthesia care after reconstructive microvascular surgery. In this chapter, we review principles of caring for cancer patients after this complicated surgery.

I. PRINCIPLES OF RECONSTRUCTIVE MICROVASCULAR SURGERY

The basic principles of reconstructive microvascular surgery can help establish a rationale for postanesthesia care. All such surgery involves transferring units of tissue as surgical flaps. The term flap refers to any tissue that is transferred with preservation of the blood supply. Originally, actual flaps of skin were elevated while still attached at the base and rotated into an adjacent area of tissue need. Over time, however, the definition has broadened. Throughout the body are units of muscle, skin, fat, bone, and visceral tissue that are supplied by a single vascular supply and can be isolated and moved to another location as a flap.

The vessels perfusing the flap are called the vascular pedicle (Fig. 1). If the distance from the original location of the flap to the area of reconstruction is less than the length of the pedicle, the tissue can be transferred as a rotational or pedicled flap without disrupting the pedicle's vessels. If the tissue must be moved a greater distance, then the vessels can be divided and reattached to other vessels lying close to the area of reconstruction. The blood vessels involved are typically less than 5 mm in diameter, hence the term microvascular surgery. This procedure is known as a free tissue transfer or a free flap because, during transfer, the tissues are completely detached from or free of the patient.

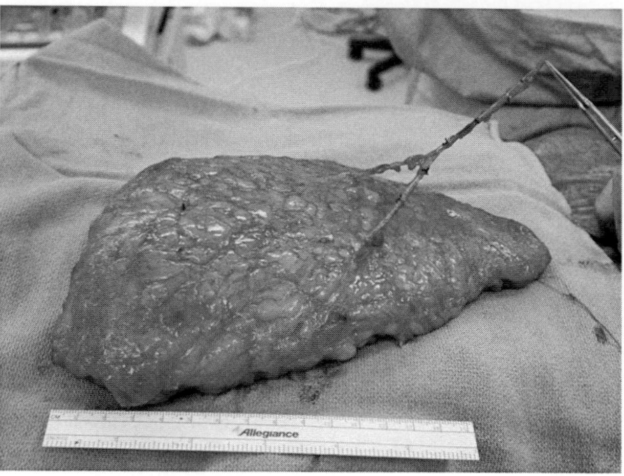

Figure 1 Example of a flap for microvascular transfer. It consists of skin and subcutaneous tissue harvested from the lower abdominal wall based on perforating vessels. These vessels will be anastomosed to others near to soft tissue defect.

During this time, there is an obligate period of total ischemia until the tissue is revascularized. Revascularization may require as long as 4 hr, depending on the nature of the tissue and location of the reconstruction. After the blood flow is re-established, tissue survival depends on continued patency at the microvascular anastomosis during the postoperative period.

Suturing the blood vessels creates an unavoidable injury to the vascular endothelium, which is thrombogenic. Platelet adherence is necessary for healing the endothelium, but excessive accumulation of platelets can occlude the pedicle vessel. A variety of factors contribute to unwanted platelet accumulation (Fig. 2). The principle factor that limits accumulation is the shearing force of blood flowing across the anastomosis. After 5–7 days, the endothelial surface is restored, and the risk of flap loss is substantially reduced. Maintain high flow across the microvascular anastomosis is therefore key to ensuring the success of reconstructive microvascular surgery. Any event that reduces flow during this critical period increases the risk of thrombosis, so avoiding decreased blood flow is essential in postoperative care of patients who have had this surgery.

Reconstructive microvascular surgery is often long and complicated. First, the procedure is usually combined with an ablative procedure, and both operations together can require many hours to complete. Moreover, microvascular surgery necessarily involves operating on at least two locations during the same operation: the area of the defect and the tissue donor site; additional flaps or tissue grafts (e.g., skin, cartilage, bone, vein, nerve) may be harvested from a third or fourth surgical site. All of these factors combined pose a considerable surgical trauma and physiological challenge to the patient. Also, in oncology, reconstructive microvascular surgery is often performed on patients of advanced age who may have comorbidities such as diabetes mellitus, high blood pressure, substance abuse, cardiopulmonary dysfunction, or vascular disease. Each coexisting disorder must be managed well to prevent it from threatening the overall recovery of the patient or the success of the free tissue transfer. Preoperative discussion between the anesthesiologist and the primary reconstructive surgeon should include positioning requirements, airway management, and which vascular sites should be selected for intravenous access and, if necessary, invasive hemodynamic monitoring.

II. POSTANESTHESIA CARE

The postanesthetic management of patients after free tissue transfer surgery requires a sound knowledge of circulatory physiology and attention detail. The principle that guides management is to support the patient with steps that maximize flow into the flap while ensuring a general safe recovery. Proper management minimizes the possibility of mechanical and physiological factors occurring that may result in decreased blood flow through the flap.

A. Emergence from Anesthesia

Gentle emergence of patients from anesthesia is vital after reconstructive microvascular surgery. Agitation, coughing, shivering, the Valsalva maneuver, or excessive movement can cause hemorrhage, formation of hematoma, or disruption of the microvascular anastomosis. The risk of these problems is particularly relevant for head and neck free flaps, which are prone to venous bleeding when the intrathoracic pressure suddenly increases and raises cervical venous pressure. Moreover, patients with head and neck cancer often have a history of alcohol abuse and can become agitated in the immediate postoperative period or later as symptoms of alcohol withdrawal appear. Extremity flaps can also be disrupted if there is excessive movement or thrashing during emergence. If any concern exists about how easily controlled a patient may be in the immediate postoperative period, the patient should remain intubated and sedated; neuromuscular paralysis may also be indicated for 12–24 hr after the procedure. After this time, the platelet coat on the microvascular anastomosis will be more mature and the tissues relatively less prone to disruption because

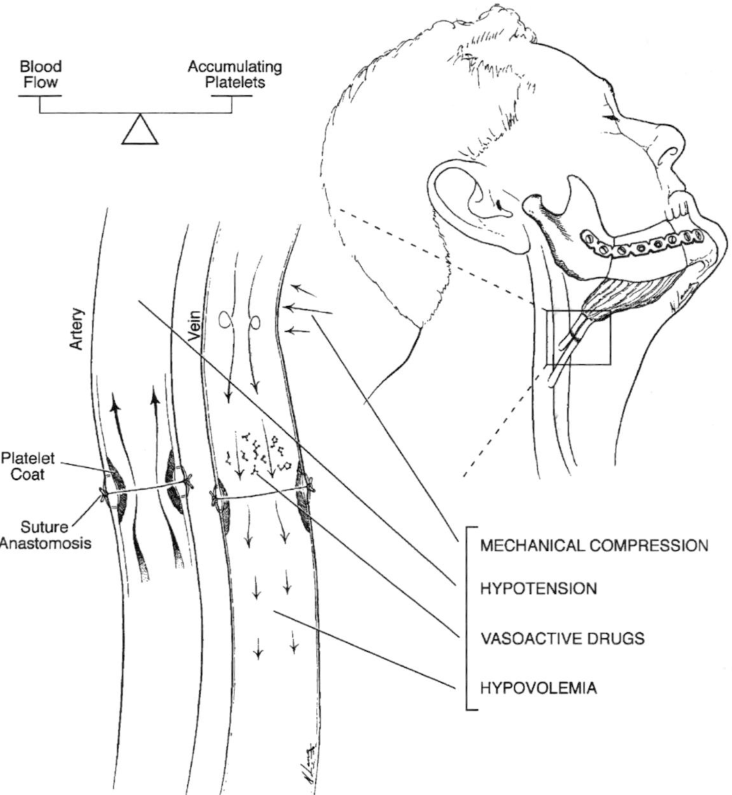

Figure 2 Successful microvascular surgery is related to the balance between blood flow and platelet accumulation at the site of the microanastomosis. There are four basic mechanisms that impair blood flow and promote thrombosis.

they have been stabilized internally by fibrin deposition. Alcohol withdrawal may be managed as with any other patient. No studies have been performed that specifically examine the effect of drugs like dexmedetomidine, clonidine, or benzodiazepines on microvascular patency, but no direct adverse effects would be expected unless dosages are sufficient to cause systemic hypotension. Nicotine patches should not be used because of evidence that acute nicotine exposure has an adverse effect on microvascular anastomotic patency (1), the cutaneous microvasculature (2), and free flap survival (3).

B. Patient Positioning

It is important to position the patient so that there is no compression on the area of the microvascular anastomosis or flap pedicle, especially if vein grafts have been used and the site of the microvascular anastomosis is a long distance from the location of the flap. For this reason, optimal positioning for the postoperative period should be discussed with the operating surgeon at the end of the surgery. Proper positioning can usually be determined with the area of the microvascular anastomosis still visible prior to closing the wounds.

Flaps placed on the head (e.g., oral cavity, midface, cranium) are often revascularized from the external carotid artery and internal jugular vein (Fig. 3). For this reason, relative movement between the head and neck can cause unfavorable changes in the geometry of the pedicle and lead to stretching, folding, or compression by adjacent soft tissues or subcutaneous drains. The head should be maintained in neutral position without excessive cervical rotation or flexion. A pillow is generally not used; with sedated patients it may be helpful to place sand bags on either side of the head. Special care must be taken to prevent patients from lying directly on flaps placed on the cranium. Similar concerns exist for tissues transferred to the torso. The most common torso flap is a transverse rectus abdominis musculocutaneous (TRAM) flap used for breast reconstruction. These flaps are often revascularized from vessels in the axilla, and it is important to keep the patient in a supine position with the arms slightly abducted to prevent compression of the pedicle. Positioning is also of particular importance in cases involving the extremities. The reconstructed extremity must be kept elevated

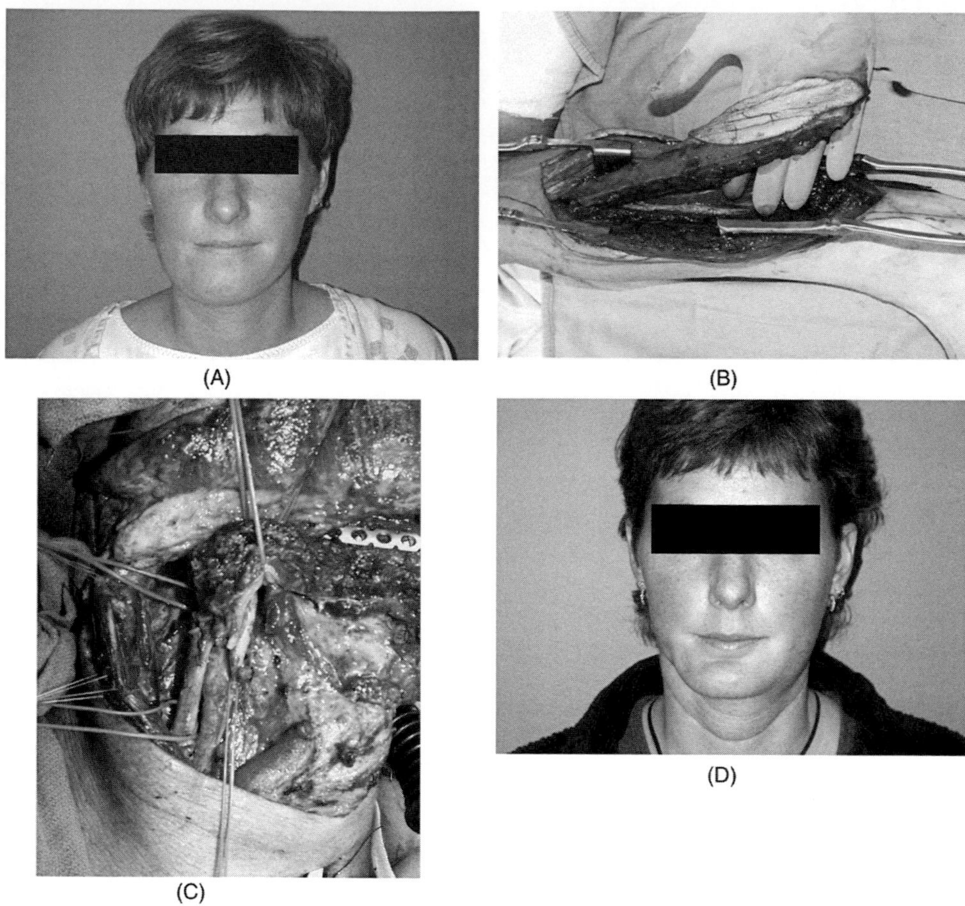

Figure 3 Example of microvascular reconstruction in the head and neck involving a left anterolateral mandible defect. (A) Preoperative appearance. (B) Fibula osteocutaneous flap prepared on the extremity. (C) Flap revascularization performed by microvascular anastomosis of the flap pedicle vessels (retracted by red latex vessel loop) to the external carotid artery and internal jugular vein. (D) Postoperative appearance.

to reduce soft tissue swelling and prevent elevated venous pressure that resists blood flow from the venous system of the flap. Circumferential dressings around the extremity at the level of the flap and pedicle must be avoided because of the risk of compression of the microvascular anastomosis.

C. Temperature Control

Patients who undergo reconstructive microvascular surgery are prone to a decrease in body temperature because of the length of the procedure and the need to operate simultaneously on different areas of the body. Large open wounds often exist for many hours, and there are few areas of the body to which blankets and other appliances intended to prevent heat loss can be applied. Systemic hypothermia can induce a coagulopathy (4) that potentially may lead to soft tissue bleeding, hematoma formation, and flap compromise. Although this degree of hypothermia is most often associated with major trauma, it remains a concern in these long and complicated microvascular surgeries.

More importantly, temperature directly affects the microcirculation in skin flaps. The skin is a thermoregulatory organ that responds locally to ambient temperature by adjusting the flow of blood through the cutaneous microcirculation through a direct local mechanism modulated by the autonomic nervous system. The autonomic nerves to the skin in surgical flaps are severed during harvest and the cutaneous microcirculation no longer has this systemic modulation. Skin flaps are therefore very sensitive to changes in air temperature and prone to vasoconstriction and decreased perfusion when exposed to a cool environment. In the postoperative period, continued systemic heat loss must be minimized and the transplanted flap kept warm. Postanesthesia body temperature should be monitored continuously. Keeping the ambient temperature warm in the postanesthesia care unit and covering the patient with warm blankets can effectively contribute to euthermia. Direct heating of the transferred tissue using a radiant source is not usually necessary and may be harmful because the flap tissue is insensate. The thermal threshold for tissue necrosis is 111.2°F (44°C), which can be exceeded if the heat source is positioned too closely to the surface of the flap (5). If warming lights are used, nursing guidelines must be in place and strictly followed.

D. Anesthesia-Care Devices

Devices used for postoperative care and monitoring must be carefully placed to prevent them from compressing the flap pedicle. For example, in cases of microvascular reconstructive surgery involving the head and neck, oxygen masks and tubing may cause compression and directly damage the flap or impair flow through the pedicle. Flaps used to restore defects around the nose, mouth, or chin are at risk for partial losses of tissue if there is direct pressure on some portion of the flap. Total loss of the flap can result if pedicle is lying in the subcutaneous tissues adjacent to the mouth and nose. Likewise, tracheostomy tubes should be sutured into place rather than being secured with collars passed circumferentially around the neck. Moreover, wire leads, arterial and venous lines, various catheters, wound drains, and other attachments must be placed so that they do not form a band across the patient's body surface and cause compression in the area of the flap or flap pedicle. Attention to these matters is most important when moving the patient from the operating room table to the transport stretcher or postanesthesia care bed.

E. Analgesia

Principles of immediate postoperative analgesia in cases of microvascular surgery are similar to those of any other major surgical procedure. The surgical stress response is well controlled intraoperatively by volatiles and potent analgesia, but as the patient enters the postoperative period, there is a surge in catecholamines that promote vasoconstriction and prothrombotic mediators (e.g., plasminogen-1 activator inhibitor (PAI-1), cortisol), each of which are unfavorable to flap perfusion. This stress response is controlled in the postoperative period by adequate analgesia.

Opioids are the mainstay of therapy, but, when used alone, generally do not provide sufficient pain control in many patients without also causing adverse effects, such as nausea, vomiting, and respiratory depression. Nausea and vomiting pose problems for a free flap in any location, but head and neck flaps are most at risk. Many head and neck flaps are set into the oral cavity or pharynx, and vomiting can disrupt the suture line causing complications even if the blood supply to the flap is not disturbed. The forceful Valsalva maneuver raises venous pressure in the head and neck, which might result in hematoma formation and compression of the flap pedicle.

Most investigators concur that multimodal analgesia (i.e., opioid analgesic agents combined with nonsteroidal anti-inflammatory drugs, regional blocks, local infiltration, etc.) results in lower pain scores and the need for fewer analgesics after surgery (6). These drugs and interventions themselves may not directly affect flap perfusion, but adverse effects, such as hypotension or hematoma formation, can impair the blood supply to the flap. Controversy exists about the safety of nonsteroidal anti-inflammatory drugs (e.g., ketorolac, diclofenac, ketoprofen) after major surgery because of concerns about the possibility of increased bleeding. One prospective, randomized multicenter European trial involving more than 11,000 patients demonstrated that ketorolac (Toradol; Roche Laboratories, Nutley, NJ) was an effective adjunct in postoperative pain control, associated with a 1.04% incidence of surgical site bleeding complications, and safe as diclofenac and ketoprofen for postoperative pain control (7). The risk of adverse effects can be reduced by minimizing the dosage, limiting the length of therapy to fewer than 5 days, and considering the use of other agents in vulnerable patients (e.g., elderly adults) (8). The benefits of using these agents in patients with postoperative pain that is difficult to control must be weighed against the risks of high-dosage narcotic drugs.

Finally, judicious use of regional analgesia should be considered in the postoperative period. Epidural blocks facilitate pain control and decrease catecholamine concentrations in plasma associated with the surgical stress response (9). One study suggested, however, that an epidural block might have a detrimental effect on microcirculation in flaps transferred to the lower extremity by decreasing mean arterial blood pressure and by diverting blood flow away from the flap to normal intact tissues. Despite these experimental findings, there have been no reports of increased flap complications in patients who have been given epidural analgesia.

F. Sedation and Neuromuscular Blockade

Movements of the patient can cause mechanical compression of the flap pedicle or disrupt the flap at the site of the reconstruction, especially in patients with head and neck free flaps. Flaps placed on the head are often revascularized from cervical vessels, thus introducing the potential for substantial changes with motion of the neck in the relationship between the flap and the site of the microvascular anastomosis. Neck flexion or rotation toward the side of the microvascular anastomosis can fold the pedicle and lead to decreased blood flow, whereas neck extension and rotation away from the side of the anastomosis can stretch the pedicle and possibly disrupt the anastomosis. Moreover, as mentioned previously, head and neck cancer patients often have a history of alcohol abuse and can become agitated in the immediate postoperative period or even later as symptoms of alcohol withdrawal emerge. Thus, maintaining heavy sedation or even neuromuscular blockade in these patients for at least the first 24 hr postoperatively is advisable so that fibrin deposition can seal and stabilize the tissues and undisturbed blood flow can occur through the site of the microvascular anastomosis. Neuromuscular blockade in patients with reconstructions outside of the head and neck is needed less frequently, but it should be considered in any patient for whom movement appears to have potential risk.

G. Hemodynamic Support and Fluid Management

Good overall hemodynamic support and maintenance of hydration are also essential to ensuring a successful outcome after reconstructive microvascular surgery (10,11). Measures instituted during surgery to produce optimal circulatory conditions must be maintained through the postoperative period. However, several aspects of reconstructive microvascular surgery can pose substantial challenges to fluid management. The combination of an ablative procedure with reconstruction can be associated with major blood loss, depending on the nature and location of the tumor. When assessing fluid balance, it is important to remember that insensible losses can be high, because the surgery is often long and involves large open wounds. Intraoperative records of fluid balance can be misleading and actual replacement needs underestimated (12).

The aim of fluid management is to maintain intravascular volume for optimal tissue perfusion and oxygen delivery, especially to the microsurgically transferred tissue. Laboratory studies suggest that tissue perfusion requirements in the flap after transfer are at least 30% greater than beforehand (13). Consequently, postoperative hypovolemia that appears to be well tolerated by the patient may actually pose a risk to the success of the surgery. Mild hypervolemia may even aid flap perfusion by increasing cardiac output with increased venous return and reflex peripheral vasodilatation (12). Therefore, adequate volume replacement with electrolyte solutions, plasma expanders, and blood products is indicated. The use of colloidal solutions may also be advantageous in order to reduce interstitial fluid formation in the flap. Surgical flaps are prone to swelling and accumulation of excess interstitial fluid because the lymphatic connections to the surrounding tissues have been severed. A hematocrit value of approximately 30–35% is suitable for oxygen transport and flap perfusion because the relationship between oxygen-carrying capacity and blood viscosity is ideal in this range (14).

Fluid management alone is sufficient to maintain optimal blood pressure and cardiac output in most microvascular surgery. At times, administration of vasoactive drugs is necessary, but such drugs must be used with caution because adverse effects on flap perfusion can occur independently of the systemic blood pressure. In one animal study (15), sodium nitroprusside in doses causing a 30% decrease in systemic vascular resistance and arterial pressure led to a severe reduction in free flap blood flow despite maintenance of cardiac output. Phenylephrine caused a significant decrease in flap blood flow when the drug entered the flap circulation, but it may not always cause problems in skin or muscle flaps if it is given systemically in doses that increase overall blood pressure. Finally, there was no evidence that dopamine administered in doses sufficient to promote renal perfusion or serve only as an inotrope is detrimental to flap perfusion.

Loop diuretics such as furosimide should be avoided in postoperative care of patients who have had reconstructive microvascular surgery, unless a patient needs prompt diuresis because of overwhelming volume overload with evidence of congestive heart failure. These drugs can cause transient intravascular volume depletion if the patient does not have true volume overload, and this depletion can have an adverse effect on blood flow through the venous microvascular anastomosis, particularly in the case of head and neck free flaps that have been revascularized from the internal jugular vein. The cervical veins collapse with volume depletion. When this happens, there is low blood flow in the recipient veins at the site of the microvascular anastomosis. This promotes platelet accumulation that can lead to thrombosis. This sequence of events can be severe enough to cause the recipient vessel, even the entire internal jugular vein, to obstruct and fill with thrombus beginning at the intimal injury caused by the microvascular anastomosis. Moreover, with volume depletion, there is a compensatory increase in the levels of circulating catecholamines (16). Although it has not been specifically studied in a clinical setting, a concern is that increased catecholamines may contribute to detrimental vasoconstriction within the flap microcirculation, analogous to directly perfusing the flap with vasopressors, thus decreasing blood flow and perfusion of the microcirculation. Therefore, if aggressive diuresis is indicated because of symptomatic and documented volume overload, it is best to be guided by direct monitoring of cardiac filling pressures using central venous or pulmonary artery wedge pressures.

H. Anticoagulation

The use of systemic anticoagulation in reconstructive microvascular surgery varies widely among surgeons (17), but most agree that routine anticoagulation is not indicated (18). When anticoagulation is chosen, the drugs of choice are aspirin, dextran 40, or heparin.

Aspirin impairs platelet function by acetylating platelet cyclo-oxygenase and thereby inhibiting production of thromboxane A_2, a prostaglandin that promotes platelet aggregation. A minimal dose of 100 mg is reported to completely suppress thromboxane A_2. Presumably, by this mechanism, aspirin is known to prevent graft occlusion in peripheral vascular surgery, coronary artery bypass, and digit replantation (19). Therefore, it is possible that there is some benefit to its use in routine free tissue transfer, but this has not been demonstrated.

Dextran 40 is the low-molecular weight (40,000) version of a polysaccharide that inhibits clotting by multiple mechanisms (20). In microvascular surgery, it may be administered as a continuous infusion (10%, 25 mL/hr). Dextran 40 is associated with some adverse effects in some patients. It has been observed to cause respiratory distress and anaphylaxis in reconstructive microvascular surgical patients (21). Therefore, an initial test dose is advisable prior to infusion.

Heparin is an antifibrin agent that prevents organized clot formation after platelets begin to accumulate. It is routinely used in macrovascular surgery to prevent thrombosis when major vessels are occluded to perform an anastomosis, but is associated with a high rate of hematoma formation in cases of reconstructive microvascular surgery (22). Results of animal studies have suggested that low-molecular weight heparin might confer benefit without increasing the occurrence of complications (23), but this has not been demonstrated clinically.

Finally, thrombolytics are indicated in free flap salvage surgery when actual thrombotic occlusion has occurred at the microvascular anastomosis (24). They are not relevant in the routine postoperative care of reconstructive microvascular surgery patients.

As suggested earlier, the role of routine systemic anticoagulation in reconstructive microvascular surgery is controversial. A retrospective review of practice using systemic anticoagulant in our early experience with reconstructive microvascular surgery at the University of Texas M.D. Anderson Cancer Center prior to 1994 (25) found that no anticoagulation was used in 44% of patients; low-dosage heparin (intraoperative intravenous bolus of 2000–3000 U followed by infusion of 100–400 U/hr) in 37% of patients; single intraoperative intravenous bolus of high-dosage heparin (5000 U) in 9% of patients; an infusion of high-dosage heparin (intraoperative intravenous bolus of 5000 U followed by infusion of 500–1200 U/hr) in 6% of patients; and an infusion of dextran 40 infusion (10% solution at 25 mL/hr) in 4% of patients. No significant differences in the rates of flap pedicle thrombosis were detected between these groups. Although the five groups in this study also had no detectable difference in intraoperative blood loss or incidence of hematoma formation, there remains a concern about increased incidence of bleeding complications with the use of systemic anticoagulation in cases of reconstructive microvascular surgery with no clearly documented benefit. We generally use systemic anticoagulation only when there is repeated microvascular anastomotic thrombosis without a cause that can be addressed by a technical or mechanical intervention (e.g., repeating the microvascular anastomosis, reposition the flap) during the operation.

I. Monitoring Flap Tissue Perfusion

Constant monitoring of tissue perfusion in the flap during the postoperative period is essential to maximize success in reconstructive microvascular surgery. The rate of success of free tissue transfer has steadily improved since it was first introduced as a clinical technique in the early 1970s (26). In a recently reported multicenter, multinational prospective study of free tissue transfer practice and outcomes, there was a 4.1% incidence of flap failure and 9.9% incidence of pedicle thrombosis requiring emergency reoperation (27). It was observed in this study that rates varied depending on the institution and experience of the microvascular surgeons. It was also noted that reconstruction in an irradiated field was associated with a fourfold increase in the risk of flap failure. Our experience at M.D. Anderson Cancer Center is consistent with these findings.

Frequent monitoring increases the success of free tissue transfer in the hours after completion of surgery (28,29). In a review of 1733 free tissue transfer operations performed at M.D. Anderson Cancer Center between 1990 and 1998, early detection of pedicle thrombosis was identified as the most important factor for successful salvage of flaps complicated by pedicle thrombosis (24). Consequently, flap perfusion must be monitored frequently in the postanesthesia care unit after surgery. Most flaps have an exposed portion visible for examination. The most important clinical signs to monitor are color, temperature, turgor, bleeding, and capillary refill time. The color of the visible flap skin should be compared with that of well-perfused skin in the surrounding area. With skin-grafted muscle flaps, the visible skin graft will have a poor color in the immediate postoperative period. If the graft is meshed, the underlying muscle may be visible and should appear red. If the color of the flap's skin is notably darker than surrounding tissues, then venous congestion might be present, and the surgeon should be notified. If the skin is paler, then arterial obstruction is possible. These color changes are visible in most patients except very dark-skinned people. When muscle flaps become venous congested, they appear dark blue or black, and there may be increased bleeding from the margins or exposed surfaces. The temperature of the flap should be warm, but this alone can be a misleading sign because even a poorly perfused flap can be warmed by heat transferred from surrounding tissues. The degree of turgor reflects the amount of fluid present in the flap tissues: a flap with arterial occlusion can seem flaccid and "deflated," whereas a flap with venous obstruction can feel tense and bulging. Bleeding from the flap edges can be another sign of increased pressure inside the flap due to venous obstruction. This is especially true if the bleeding appears to be new onset in the postoperative period. The most reliable clinical sign of adequate flap tissue perfusion is capillary refill time. This sign is elicited by gentle digital pressure enough to cause blanching on the surface of the flap. The pressure is released and the point of application observed for return of color. Normal capillary refill time is approximately 2 sec (i.e., the amount of time it takes to say, "capillary refill"). If the return is brisk (i.e., <2 sec), venous congestion and outflow compromise may be present. If it is prolonged (i.e., >2 sec), arterial occlusion might exist.

A familiarity with some of the devices available to assist evaluation of flap perfusion is necessary for optimal postanesthesia care of patients who have had reconstructive microvascular surgery. These devices are most useful for flaps that are difficult to assess by the clinical signs described above. Percutaneous Doppler ultrasound devices are the most commonly used aids because they can confirm the presence of blood flow if placed accurately over the flap pedicle. Other useful devices that have been used include continuous tissue oxygen monitors (30), photoplethysmography devices (31), laser Doppler flow meters (32), and implanted pulsed Doppler ultrasound probes (33,34). The most widely used of these specially designed devices is the implantable ultrasound probe. This device consists of a tiny (1 mm diameter) Doppler crystal that is implanted at the time of surgery immediately adjacent to the flap pedicle. It transmits a pulse of sound at frequency of 20 MHz and then receives the sound waves reflected from the formed elements circulating in the blood stream through the pedicle. With this or any other specialized device used for flap monitoring, it is important to communicate with the surgeon about to understand how to properly interpret information provided by the machine as well as how to troubleshoot possible problems to avoid false positive findings.

In summary, conclusions about the adequacy of flap tissue perfusion should not be based solely on any one clinical sign or device. Information from all sources must be considered together and followed over time. When a question arises about the adequacy of perfusion, the operating surgeon must be notified immediately and arrangements must be made to return the patient to the operating room as soon as possible. Depending on the types of tissue comprising the flap, it will usually be totally lost if perfusion is not re-established in less than 4 hr from the time of the occurrence of pedicle thrombosis and occlusion.

J. Preparations for Repeat Surgery

As previously stated, once a problem with perfusion of a microvascular flap has been identified, repeat surgery becomes imperative. Most often this reoperation will be a limited procedure compared with the initial reconstruction and will involve exploration of the microvascular anastomosis, identification of the cause of impaired perfusion, and steps to restore blood flow. This can range from simply repositioning of the flap pedicle to relieve a mechanical obstruction to a total revising the microvascular anastomosis that may even involve harvesting an interposition vein graft to allow revascularization of the flap from a different set of recipient vessels. In the most severe cases, a thrombectomy may be performed, a thrombolytic agent used to clear the pedicle and flap microcirculation of clot, and a new recipient vessel selected (35). The successful salvage of a failing free flap is directly related to the amount of time required to restore perfusion to the flap (28,36). Therefore, the standard postanesthesia care of every patient who has had reconstructive microvascular surgery must include preparedness on the part of the anesthesia and operating room staffs to accommodate such an emergency.

III. SUMMARY

Reconstructive microvascular surgery has become an integral part of surgical oncology. Microvascular surgery cases are technically complicated, usually lengthy, and are often performed in patients who may have significant comorbidities. Postanesthesia care requires an appreciation of the factors that affect the outcome in this specialized type of surgery and an attention to detail. The most important principle underlying the postanesthesia care of patients after this specialized surgery is to maintain maximum blood flow across the microvascular anastomosis to prevent excess platelet accumulation and flap pedicle thrombosis. Attention to detail is essential during emergence from anesthesia, positioning the patient, placement of anesthesia devices, and selection of medication for postoperative pain control and sedation. Sound knowledge of general circulatory physiology coupled with an appreciation for the unique physiology of tissue perfusion in surgical flaps is essential to proper hemodynamic support and fluid management in patients after microvascular surgery. Finally, postoperative monitoring of flap tissue perfusion is a team effort of everyone involved with postanesthesia care. Arrangements must be in place to facilitate prompt return of the patient to the operating room at the first sign of a problem. Close co-operation among operating room and postanesthesia care staffs provides the greatest chance of a successful outcome.

REFERENCES

1. Sachar K, Goel R, Weiss AP. Acute and chronic effects of nicotine on anastomotic patency following ischemia/reperfusion. J Reconstr Microsurg 1998; 14:179–184.
2. Black CE, Huang N, Neligan PC, Levine RH, Lipa JE, Lintlop S, Forrest CR, Pang CY. Effect of nicotine on vasoconstrictor and vasodilator responses in human skin vasculature. Am J Physiol Regul Integr Comp Physiol 2001; 281:R1097–R1104.
3. van Adrichem LN, Hoegen R, Hovius SE, Kort WJ, van Strik R, Vuzevski VD, van der Meulen JC. The effect of cigarette smoking on the survival of free vascularized and pedicled epigastric flaps in the rat. Plast Reconstr Surg 1996; 97:86–96.
4. Lynn M, Jeroukhimov I, Klein Y, Martinowitz U. Updates in the management of severe coagulopathy in trauma patients. Intensive Care Med 2002; 28:S241–S247.
5. Zukowski ML, Lord JL, Ash K. Precautions in warming light therapy as an adjuvant to postoperative flap care. Burns 1998; 24:374–377.
6. Jin F, Chung F. Multimodal analgesia for postoperative pain control. J Clin Anesth 2001; 13:524–539.
7. Forrest JB, Camu F, Greer IA, Kehlet H, Abdalla M, Bonnet F, Ebrahim S, Escolar G, Jage J, Pocock S, Velo G, Langman MJ. Ketorolac, diclofenac, and ketoprofen are equally safe for pain relief after major surgery. Br J Anaesth 2002; 88:227–233.
8. Reinhart DI. Minimising the adverse effects of ketorolac. Drug Saf 2000; 22:487–497.
9. Motamed S, Klubien K, Edwardes M, Mazza L, Carli F. Metabolic changes during recovery in normothermic versus hypothermic patients undergoing surgery and receiving general anesthesia and epidural local anesthetic agents. Anesthesiology 1998; 88:1211–1218.
10. Hynynen M, Eklund P, Rosenberg PH. Anaesthesia for patients undergoing prolonged reconstructive and microvascular plastic surgery. Scand J Plast Reconstr Surg 1982; 16:201–206.
11. Jakubowski M, Lamont A, Murray WB, de Wit SL. Anaesthesia for microsurgery. S Afr Med J 1985; 67: 581–584.
12. Sigurdsson GH. Perioperative fluid management in microvascular surgery. J Reconstr Microsurg 1995; 11: 57–65.
13. Hallock GG. Critical threshold for tissue viability as determined by laser Doppler flowmetry. Ann Plast Surg 1992; 28:554–558.
14. Macdonald DJ. Anaesthesia for microvascular surgery. A physiological approach. Br J Anaesth 1985; 57: 904–912.
15. Banic A, Krejci V, Erni D, Wheatley AM, Sigurdsson GH. Effects of sodium nitroprusside and phenylephrine on blood flow in free musculocutaneous flaps during general anesthesia. Anesthesiology 1999; 90:147–155.
16. Hasbak P, Petersen JS, Shalmi M, Lam HR, Christensen NJ, Christensen S. Role of the adrenal medulla in control of blood pressure and renal function during frusemide-induced volume depletion. J Hypertens 1995; 13:235–242.
17. Davies DM. A world survey of anticoagulation practice in clinical microvascular surgery. Br J Plast Surg 1982; 35:96–99.
18. Khouri RK. Avoiding free flap failure. Clin Plast Surg 1992; 19:773–781.
19. Collaboration AT. Collaborative overview of randomised trials of antiplatelet therapy—II: maintenance of vascular graft or arterial patency by antiplatelet therapy. Antiplatelet Trialists' Collaboration [comment]. Br Med J 1994; 308:159–168.
20. Johnson PC, Barker JH. Thrombosis and antithrombotic therapy in microvascular surgery. Clin Plast Surg 1992; 19:799–807.
21. Hein KD, Wechsler ME, Schwartzstein RM, Morris DJ. The adult respiratory distress syndrome after dextran infusion as an antithrombotic agent in free TRAM flap breast reconstruction. Plast Reconstr Surg 1999; 103: 1706–1708.
22. Pugh CM, Dennis RH II, Massac EA. Evaluation of intraoperative anticoagulants in microvascular free-flap surgery. J Natl Med Assoc 1996; 88:655–657.

23. Ritter EF, Cronan JC, Rudner AM, Serafin D, Klitzman B. Improved microsurgical anastomotic patency with low molecular weight heparin. J Reconstr Microsurg 1998; 14:331–336.
24. Yii NW, Evans GR, Miller MJ, Reece GP, Langstein H, Chang D, Kroll SS, Wang B, Robb GL. Thrombolytic therapy: what is its role in free flap salvage? Ann Plast Surg 2001; 46:601–604.
25. Kroll SS, Miller MJ, Reece GP, Baldwin BJ, Robb GL, Bengtson BP, Phillips MD, Kim D, Schusterman MA. Anticoagulants and hematomas in free flap surgery. Plast Reconstr Surg 1995; 96:643–647.
26. Khouri RK. Free flap surgery. The second decade. Clin Plast Surg 1992; 19:757–761.
27. Khouri RK, Cooley BC, Kunselman AR, Landis JR, Yeramian P, Ingram D, Natarajan N, Benes CO, Wallemark C. A prospective study of microvascular free-flap surgery and outcome [comment]. Plast Reconstr Surg 1998; 102:711–721.
28. Disa JJ, Cordeiro PG, Hidalgo DA. Efficacy of conventional monitoring techniques in free tissue transfer: an 11-year experience in 750 consecutive cases. Plast Reconstr Surg 1999; 104:97–101.
29. Hirigoyen MB, Urken ML, Weinberg H. Free flap monitoring: a review of current practice. Microsurgery 1995; 16:723–726; discussion 727.
30. Kamolz LP, Giovanoli P, Haslik W, Koller R, Frey M. Continuous free-flap monitoring with tissue-oxygen measurements: three-year experience. J Reconstr Microsurg 2002; 18:487–491; discussion 492–493.
31. Futran ND, Stack BC Jr, Hollenbeak C, Scharf JE. Green light photoplethysmography monitoring of free flaps. Arch Otolaryngol Head Neck Surg 2000; 126:659–662.
32. Jenkins S, Sepka R, Barwick WJ. Routine use of laser Doppler flowmetry for monitoring autologous tissue transplants. Ann Plast Surg 1988; 21:423–426.
33. Kind GM, Buntic RF, Buncke GM, Cooper TM, Siko PP, Buncke HJ Jr. The effect of an implantable Doppler probe on the salvage of microvascular tissue transplants. Plast Reconstr Surg 1998; 101:1268–1273; discussion 1274–1275.
34. Swartz WM, Izquierdo R, Miller MJ. Implantable venous Doppler microvascular monitoring: laboratory investigation and clinical results. Plast Reconstr Surg 1994; 93:152–163.
35. Wheatley MJ, Meltzer TR. The role of vascular pedicle thrombectomy in the management of compromised free tissue transfers. Ann Plast Surg 1996; 36:360–364.
36. Cho BC, Shin DP, Byun JS, Park JW, Baik BS. Monitoring flap for buried free tissue transfer: its importance and reliability. Plast Reconstr Surg 2002; 110:1249–1258.

28

Perioperative Care of Patients with Musculoskeletal Neoplasms

THAO P. BUI and ALAN W. YASKO

Department of Anesthesiology and Pain Management, The University of Texas M.D. Anderson Cancer Center, Houston, Texas, U.S.A.

I. INTRODUCTION

Musculoskeletal neoplasms are rare, heterogeneous tumors that arise from the connective tissues of the body including bone. These neoplasms exhibit diverse pathobiology ranging from latent to highly aggressive behavior. The malignant tumors, designated sarcomas, affect a broad spectrum of the population including young children through the elderly. In addition, bone is the third most common target for metastases from carcinomas and accounts for significant morbidity in patients with advanced cancer.

The management approach to these neoplasms is predicated on the type and aggressiveness of the disease entity. A multidisciplinary diagnostic approach for these rare neoplasms is preferable. A multidisciplinary approach to the treatment of the majority of malignant neoplasms is necessary to optimize patient outcome. Surgery is a key component of treatment of the musculoskeletal neoplasms. The surgical techniques applied to treat these tumors follow contemporary surgical oncologic principles.

The aim of this chapter is to familiarize the anesthesiologist with the management strategy for musculoskeletal neoplasms with an emphasis on surgical approaches to bone and soft tissue neoplasms and metastatic disease to bone. It is beyond the scope of this chapter to cover in detail all possible neoplasms and their disease- and site-specific management, however, a review of common surgical oncologic issues that impact anesthesia and the perioperative management of these patients will be presented.

II. GENERAL PRINCIPLES

Tumors that fall under the purview of orthopaedic oncologists include bone and soft tissue neoplasms of the extremities, spine, and pelvis. Other sites of tumor involvement including the chest wall, head, and neck region, abdomen, and retroperitoneum are addressed by other surgical oncologic specialists.

The diagnosis and treatment of bone and soft tissue neoplasms often requires a multidisciplinary team of experts in orthopaedic oncology, adult/pediatric oncology, musculoskeletal pathology, radiation oncology, diagnostic radiology, and anesthesiology to coordinate and optimize patient care. Benign and low-grade malignant neoplasms, in general, are treated with surgery and require less co-ordination of specialists. Aggressive benign and high-grade malignant neoplasms are treated with a multimodality approach of a combination of surgery and either radiation, chemotherapy or both.

The overwhelming majority of benign bone and soft tissue neoplasms is treated with local excision alone.

The adequacy of the surgical margin for these neoplasms depends, in large part, on the biological aggressiveness of the tumor. Benign tumors may be latent, active, or locally aggressive (1). The subset of bone and soft tissue neoplasms that are aggressive necessitate a more extensive surgical approach to achieve local tumor control. In general, complete excision is sufficient to treat benign neoplasms. En bloc resection with the intent to achieve wide surgical margins, similar to the treatment recommendation for sarcomas, is indicated rarely for benign neoplasms.

Current treatment strategies for musculoskeletal sarcomas have evolved over the past three decades with the emergence of effective chemotherapy, advances in diagnostic imaging modalities, and improvements in skeletal and soft tissue reconstructive techniques. A shift in the surgical management of extremity sarcomas from radical tumor extirpation procedures such as limb amputation toward limb-sparing approaches combining surgery with other therapies including chemotherapy and/or radiation has occurred. Technically demanding, yet more tissue-conserving surgical techniques have become predictably effective in preserving function without compromising local tumor control or overall patient survival in the majority of patients.

Bone and soft tissue sarcomas are excised surgically with a cuff of normal tissue attached to the tumor constituting a wide margin. For the majority of bone sarcomas, major skeletal reconstruction is necessary to maintain limb function. For many soft tissue sarcomas, complex soft tissue reconstruction is necessary to provide stable soft tissue coverage to maintain limb viability.

Multiagent chemotherapy regimens for bone and soft tissue sarcomas are harsh. The toxicities of these regimens impact the timing, nature, and ultimately the success of surgery. Current regimens active for the treatment of sarcomas include combinations of doxorubicin, ifosfamide, cisplatin, and methotrexate. All of these cytotoxic agents induce bone marrow suppression in addition to drug-specific toxicities including cardiotoxicity, nephrotoxity, neurotoxicity, and metabolic disturbances (2).

Radiation is used more frequently in the treatment of soft tissue sarcomas than bone sarcomas. Delivered locally to the site of a primary or metastatic tumor, radiation has consequences that are confined generally to the local tissues including skin, muscle, connective tissue, and bone. The addition of radiation as an adjunct therapy for the treatment of soft tissue sarcomas has reduced significantly the number of amputations performed to control the primary tumor. Although it may induce cytoreduction, the effect on the tissues surrounding the tumor within the radiation field can increase the complexity of the surgical procedure leading to a prolonged duration of surgery, increased intraoperative blood loss, and increased need for plastic surgery.

A. Bone Neoplasms

Benign bone tumors generally occur in patients of young and middle age. A wide spectrum of histologies is recognized that reflect the elements present within bone including bone marrow and osseous, cartilaginous and fibrous constituents. A detailed description of the demographic and site distribution, physical signs and symptoms, radiographic features and histopathology can be found in any of several bone pathology texts (3–5). Osteochondroma are the most common benign bone tumor. Rare benign tumors that occasionally become aggressive and undergo malignant transformation include giant cell tumors, chondroblastomas, osteoblastomas, and histiocytosis. Giant cell tumors are vascular, and resection may result in severe bleeding. Unlike other bone tumors, giant cell tumors are slightly more common in females. During pregnancy, they may grow inordinately rapidly. Resection is usually done after a fetus is believed to be viable. Both giant cell tumors and chondroblastomas are slow growing, but the treatment of choice is a complete resection of the lesion. Pulmonary metastasis rarely occurs (1–3%) with either giant cell tumors or chondroblastoma. When it does occur, it is usually found 3–20 years after resection. When histiocytosis includes systemic involvement, it is referred to as Hand–Schuller–Christian disease or Letterer–Siwe disease. Hand–Schuller–Christian disease is a clinical triad of skull lesions, exophthalmos, and diabetes insipidus. Letterer–Siwe disease affects patients less than 3 years old with fever, lymphadenopathy, hepatosplenomegaly, and multiple bone lesions. The presentation is similar to that of acute leukemia. Lung involvement is possible and can manifest as respiratory distress, tachypnea, retraction, and persistent cough. Patients may have chronic respiratory failure resulting from the development of multiple cysts or bullae, and pneumothorax may occur if the bullae rupture. These medical issues should be considered when indicated for the perioperative care of these patients (6–8).

Bone sarcomas generally affect children and young adults. Approximately 2400 new cases are identified annually in the United States (9). Osteosarcoma is the most common malignant primary bone tumor (excluding myeloma) comprising approximately 30% of all such malignancies. The annual incidence of osteosarcoma is approximately 800 cases per year in the United States. Hereditary retinoblastoma carries a risk of second cancers, 50% of which are osteosarcomas. Secondary osteosarcomas usually occur in older patients and at the site of another disease process. It is associated with previous radiation treatment of greater than 2500 cG and occurs 10–15 years after treatment. Paget's disease is also associated with osteosarcoma, and most commonly in the pelvis. Other bone conditions, such as fibrous dysplagia, bone infarct, osteochondroma, chronic osteomyelitis, chondrosarcoma, and osteogenesis imperfecta, have also been associated with secondary osteosarcomas. Osteosarcoma masses may be telangiectatic, fibrous, or cartilaginous. The telangiectatic variety contains aneurysmally dilated vascular spaces filled with blood that could pose a hemorrhagic risk during surgery. The majority of osteosarcomas is histologically high-grade and typically involves the ends of the long bones adjacent to major joints such as the knee (distal femur and proximal tibia), shoulder (proximal humerus), and hip (proximal femur). Pulmonary metastasis is common in 15% of patients but pulmonary wedge resection with good margins can be curative. Pulmonary metastasis and rapid relapse after treatment are poor prognostic factors. A combined chemotherapy and surgery approach to osteosarcoma is the current treatment standard.

Chondrosarcoma is the second most common malignant primary tumor of bone. Its annual incidence is approximately half that of osteosarcoma. Chondrosarcoma generally occurs in adults of middle age. The most common locations are the pelvis, ribs, proximal femur, and proximal humerus. Chondrosarcomas are resistant to chemotherapy and radiation. Surgical resection is the mainstay of treatment.

Ewing's sarcoma represents approximately 6% of all primary malignant bone tumors with an annual incidence of 200 cases. Ewing's sarcoma is the most common primary bone sarcoma in patients younger than 10 years of age. Ewing's sarcoma is usually found at the metaphysis (near the end) and diaphysis (shaft) of long bones and innominate bones of the pelvic girdle. Multiagent chemotherapy is the principal treatment for Ewing's sarcoma. Surgery, with or without local radiation, is used to optimize local tumor control.

The contemporary treatment paradigm for osteo sarcoma, Ewing's sarcoma, and other high-grade sarcomas such as malignant fibrous histiocytoma includes induction chemotherapy (approximately 12 week duration), surgery, and adjuvant chemotherapy for a duration predicated on the response to the preoperative chemotherapy. Current chemotherapy regimens for these sarcomas include combinations of doxorubicin, ifosfamide, cisplatin, high-dose methotrexate with leucovorin rescue, VP-16, etoposide, and vincristine.

Low-grade neoplasms of bone such as adamantinoma, chordoma, and low-grade variants of osteosarcoma are less frequently encountered and are treated by surgery alone. Of these, chordoma is of particular significance because the majority (50%) occurs in the sacrum. Chordoma is the most common primary bone malignancy found in the sacrum. Also after multiple myeloma, and excluding metastases, it is the second most common primary bone malignancy in the spine.

Multiple myeloma is the most common primary tumor of bone, accounting for 43% of primary malignancies of the bone. Multiple myeloma and metastatic cancer should be high on the differential diagnosis list for any patient over age 40 presenting with a new bone tumor. Diagnosis is by serum immunoelectrophoresis confirming monoclonal gammopathy. Approximately 20% of patients have no symptoms and are diagnosed by chance laboratory screening showing increased serum protein. Systemic therapy is the mainstay of treatment. Local radiation therapy is particularly effective for solitary lesions (plasmacytoma) and to palliate localized pain associated with symptomatic bone metastasis. Prognosis in general is poor, with a life expectancy of only 3 years after diagnosis. Both the axial (spine, pelvis, and ribs) and long bones are affected by multiple myeloma. A common presentation for multiple myeloma is a painful pathologic fracture, such as a vertebral collapse. The role of surgery in multiple myeloma is similar to that for bone metastases. Surgical intervention is required only for impending or established pathological fractures of the long bones, spine, and occasionally the pelvis. Systemic manifestations of the disease not associated with other bone tumors include anemia, thrombocytopenia, neutropenia, hypercalcemia, renal failure, and peripheral neuropathy. Hypercalcemia is from excessive bone destruction and renal insufficiency is from the deposition of large amount of protein into the renal tubules. Anemia, thrombocytopenia, neutropenia, and recurrent bacterial infections reflect bone marrow invasion by tumor cells.

Metastatic carcinoma is the most common neoplastic condition affecting bone. Most common metastatic tumors requiring orthopedic intervention arise from breast cancers, which accounts for more than 50% of all cases, followed by cancers of lungs, kidneys, prostate, gastrointestinal tract, thyroid, and other sites (10). Breast and prostate cancer tend to metastasize to the bone late in the course of the disease and thus make bones uncommon sites of primary disease. A late disease course means a likelihood of metastatic disease in other organs, leading to more cancer treatments and adverse effects. Other organ system abnormalities should be investigated and medically optimized preoperatively. Lung and kidney cancer tend to metastasize to the bones early and therefore are common sources of bone metastasis of unknown origin.

The axial skeleton and lower extremities, in particular, the hip region, are more commonly affected by metastatic bone disease. In general, many patients with bone metastasis will develop one or more pathologic fractures. Most pathologic fractures occur in the proximal femur, followed by the hip and humerus. Pathologic fractures are associated with an increased incidence of subsequent pulmonary metastases, which may be reduced by prophylactic fixation (11). The primary treatment of any patient with skeletal metastases is disease-specific systemic chemotherapy, hormonal therapy, and/or immunotherapy. Treatment of symptomatic bone lesions includes local radiation. Recent efforts to reduce skeletal events, such as a fracture with bisphosphonates and radiotherapeutics, have been promising (12–16); however, bone destruction secondary to metastatic disease continues to be a devastating consequence of advanced disease in patients. The majority of impending and established pathologic fractures can result in significant pain and limitation of limb function. Surgery can address the pain associated with tumor-induced bone destruction and provide durable stability for the diseased bone. Pain palliation and limb function restoration are achieved predictably.

B. Soft Tissue Neoplasms

Benign soft tissue tumors usually are of insignificant clinical consequence. A general reference of benign tumors is available to review the various histopathologic entities (17). Surgery is the primary treatment for these neoplasms.

Soft tissue sarcomas are a group of rare histologically diverse neoplasms that arise from mesenchymal tissues that are ubiquitous throughout the body. In the United States, approximately 8700 new cases of soft tissue sarcoma are identified annually. These sarcomas account for about 1% of all new cancers and 3700 patient deaths each year (9). There are nearly three dozen recognized histopathologic entities that represent the spectrum of disease of low-, intermediate- and high-grade soft tissue sarcoma.

Approximately half of the patients with soft tissue sarcomas are older than 60 years of age at diagnosis. Although they may arise in any site of the body, over 60% arise in an extremity or trunk. The remainder develops in the retroperitoneum (15%), viscera (15%), and head and neck region (10%). The majority of sarcomas is deep to the investing fascia and commonly juxtaposed to major neurovascular structures. They uncommonly involve regional lymph nodes and rarely invade bone or joints.

Although extremely heterogeneous in histopathology, soft tissue sarcomas generally are treated in a similar fashion and commonly are lumped together in treatment outcome analyses. Malignant fibrous histiocytoma, liposarcoma, and synovial sarcoma are the most common soft tissue sarcomas in adults. Rhabdomyosarcoma is the most common soft tissue sarcoma in children (18).

The mainstay of treatment of localized disease is surgical resection. Limb-sparing surgery combined with local radiation is the standard approach for large (>5 cm), intermediate- and low-grade extremity soft tissue sarcomas. Fewer than 10% of extremity tumors are treated with amputation. Patients for amputation often present with locally advanced disease or multifocal recurrent disease within the radiation field. The role of chemotherapy is less well defined in comparison to the treatment of bone sarcomas (19). Most current chemotherapy regimens include combinations of doxorubicin and ifosfamide.

III. ANESTHESIA PERSPECTIVES

A. Preoperative Evaluation

As with any surgical patient, a careful preoperative assessment of the cancer patient is critical to detect concurrent conditions that can complicate surgery. A patient's general health should be evaluated and correctable abnormalities should be treated. The evaluation also should include a detailed history of cancer therapies. Notable abnormalities may be a result of the cancer, cancer therapy, or medical comorbidities.

Common to musculoskeletal cancer patients is cyclical chemotherapy-induced bone marrow suppression resulting in anemia, neutropenia, and thrombocytopenia. Surgery usually is scheduled 2–3 weeks after the administration of the last dose of chemotherapy of the cycle to allow recovery of the blood counts. This immunosuppressed patient population has an increased likelihood of postoperative infections due to therapy-induced neutropenia. White blood cell counts of less than 3000/UL or absolute neutrophil counts of less than 1000/UL should be considered as a reason to delay surgery. Anemia and thrombocytopenia in these patients is common at the time of surgery, however, rarely do patients have complex acquired coagulopathy. A platelet count of at least 70,000/UL is considered adequate to proceed with surgery. An anemia characterized by hemoglobin of 8–10 g/dL is not uncommon.

Metabolic disturbances commonly result from the chemotherapy agents administered before surgery. Nausea and vomiting are common side effects of chemotherapy, and to some extent, radiation therapy. Treatment with metoclopramide and serotonin antagonist drugs may be helpful preoperatively. Malnutrition, dehydration, and electrolyte abnormalities all worsen with nausea and vomiting.

The patient's nutritional status should also be assessed. The albumin level is a good indication of the nutrition level, which is important for wound healing. Although postoperative hyperalimentation or tube feedings may be necessary in severely debilitated patients, healing is not commonly compromised in this patient population.

B. Disease and Disease-Specific Therapy Issues

Benign musculoskeletal neoplasms usually develop in young, healthy patients. It is rare for these patients to receive systemic cytotoxic therapy; therefore, the perioperative care routinely is less complicated. In general, most high-grade bone sarcomas that require multiagent systemic chemotherapy also arise in young patients. It is unusual for these patients to have nontherapy-related comorbidities that may effect anesthesia or surgical outcome. Sarcomas of bone and soft tissue present in patients over a wide range of ages, therefore it is difficult to generalize regarding the disease-specific fitness of a patient for surgery. Older patients with soft tissue and bone sarcomas receive similar agents, but often at reduced doses based on their lower tolerance, general health status, and medical comorbidities.

Chemotherapy-related toxicities can adversely impact anesthesia and surgery. An assessment of the severity of chemotherapy-induced efforts should always be performed during preoperative care. Patients who receive chemotherapy should have a comprehensive evaluation of pulmonary, cardiac, liver, and kidney function.

Cardiac function tests with electrocardiography and echocardiography are helpful to screen for abnormalities and assess ventricular function. Even though patients often are young, they may have decreased cardiac function and poor cardiac reserve. The most telling sign of possible undiagnosed cardiac dysfunction is resting tachycardia as shown by EKG. This should warrant further investigation with a clinical assessment of exercise function and, if indicated, more tests to determine left ventricular function.

Doxorubicin is cardiotoxic (20). Doxorubicin-induced cardiomyopathy is usually dose dependent. A cumulative dose of 400–500 mg/m^2 is associated with a 10% incidence of congestive heart failure and a 50% incidence of a subclinical decrease in left ventricular ejection fraction. A cumulative dose less than 350 mg/m^2 results in a much lower incidence of cardiomyopathy.

Methotrexate, cisplatin, and ifosfamide are nephrotoxic. Methotrexate at a high dose may precipitate in renal tubules and produce transient renal damage shown by elevated serum creatinine. Hydration and alkalanization help prevent renal damage. Ifosfamide is usually given with sodium mercaptoethylsulfonate (MESNA) to protect the bladder by neutralizing active ifosfamide metabolite in the urine. Potassium and bicarbonate wasting, known as Fanconi's renal tubular acidosis, are a major toxicity of ifosfamide/MESNA and should be treated accordingly (21). Liver function abnormalities also should be investigated because hepatic disease can affect coagulation and anesthetic metabolism may be altered. The chemotherapy regimens used for sarcomas are not hepatotoxic.

Radiation therapy is of concern in anesthetic management if there is a history of irradiation to the head and neck, because airway tissue may change and undergo fibrosis, rendering mask ventilation and laryngoscopy difficult. Head positioning with the procedure may also be difficult, because fibrosis of the tissue will make head movement difficult. Furthermore, irradiated bone tends to have a higher risk of bleeding, so proper preparations should be made.

Anesthesia for patients with advanced cancer carries inherent risks that are uncommon in the majority of patients with sarcomas. Although the perioperative mortality incidence is low, a generally higher risk of perioperative morbidity mandates an accurate evaluation of the patient's condition and careful management of vital organ function. Retrospective analyses of records of patients undergoing palliative operations for metastatic bone lesions have revealed perioperative lethal events that are varied and often unexpected. Examples from one study showed mortality from hepatic failure, unexpected cerebral tumor embolism, intraoperative cardiac arrest secondary to pulmonary embolism during intramedullary nailing, development of disseminated intravascular coagulation, acute renal failure, and superior vena cava syndrome causing life-threatening airway obstruction during general anesthesia with endotracheal intubation (22). Renal cell carcinoma, thyroid carcinoma, metastatic to bone, and multiple myeloma, consistently are associated with increased blood loss due to their high tumor vascularity. Renal cell cancers are hypervascular and the risk of hemorrhage is compounded because as many as 40% of patients have anemia as a result of chronic disease. This is a normochromic, normocytic anemia believe to be due to inability to use stored iron (23). However, 5% of patients may have erythrocytosis with hemoglobin >15 g/dL secondary to production of an erythropoietin-like substance. A small percentage of patients may have problems of amyloidosis, causing renal failure, polyneuromyopathy, and reversible hepatic dysfunction that usually resolves after a nephrectomy (24). These patients usually have undergone nephrectomy, so protecting any remaining renal function is important. Osseous metastases with hypercalcemia can be a concern in these patients. In the event of renal cell cancer, the anesthesia care team should be prepared for management of massive hemorrhage while preserving renal function.

In light of the palliative nature of the orthopedic procedure in metastatic bone disease, perioperative involvement of the anesthesia care team in the management of these patients is crucial to delineate and minimize medical risk. Indications for orthopedic surgical intervention in terminal cancer patients remain in debate, making proper surgical care challenging because the survival time is unpredictable. Surgery is delayed typically until the patient's medical condition is optimized.

C. Anatomic Site-Specific Issues

Knowledge of the nature and extent of the planned surgery is invaluable in optimizing the medical care unique to these patients. Both the tumor type and anatomic site involved are key determinants of the nature and extent of surgery and its attendant risks.

Bone neoplasms arise in the appendicular (extremities) and axial (spine, sacrum, and pelvis) skeleton. Soft tissue neoplasms occur wherever there is connective tissue. Surgery for musculoskeletal neoplasms, therefore, has variable attendant intra- and perioperative morbidity, in part, based on the complexity of the local anatomy. Surgery in the trunk and retroperitoneum is complicated by the complex anatomy in these regions, the locally advanced nature of many of the tumors in these areas, and the potential for massive hemorrhage.

Surgery in the extremities generally poses less inherent risk for the most serious complication of massive hemorrhage since access to large vessels is more easily gained and a pneumatic tourniquet can usually be applied to maintain hemostasis. Adjacent central vascular structures, the components of the brachial plexus and the lumbosacral plexus, and viscera pose greater risk of injury and operative morbidity. Moreover, the duration of surgery in the extremities generally is less than in the axial skeleton and trunk.

IV. SURGICAL MANAGEMENT

A. Bone Neoplasms

Benign tumors usually are amenable to intralesional excision by curettage with reconstruction using bone cement or bone graft (autogenic or allogeneic). A bolus of bone cement (polymethylmethacrylate) is used frequently to fill cavitary bone defects after tumor excision. This surgery is associated infrequently with significant blood loss intraoperatively. Occasionally, a benign tumor can cause significant bone destruction that precludes an intralesional approach. Giant cell tumors of bone and aneurysmal bone cysts are two benign neoplasms that can locally be destructive and achieve massive size with significant risk of intraoperative blood loss due to their high vascularity. En bloc excision with skeletal reconstruction similar to sarcomas is performed infrequently, but when local bone destruction in expendable bones such as the clavicle, proximal end of the fibula, and nonweight bearing portions of the pelvis, and scapula occurs it is appropriate.

For primary, high-grade bone sarcomas (osteosarcoma, Ewing's sarcoma, and malignant fibrous histiocytoma), surgery follows multiple cycles of induction chemotherapy. For others, surgery alone is the only treatment. Wide resection with en bloc removal of the tumor-bearing portion of the affected bone is performed either by limb-sparing resection or amputation. This approach is applicable to all bone sarcomas.

Bone resections fall into one of three types based on the anatomic site and extent of the involved bone to be excised. Because most bone sarcomas arise at the ends of a long bone near the joint, the majority of surgical excisions involve both the segment of tumor-bearing bone and adjacent joint (osteoarticular resection). Less frequently encountered is the clinical situation in which a malignant tumor arises within the shaft of the long bone far from the adjacent joint. The tumor-bearing segment of bone alone is resected (intercalary resection) to control the local tumor without sacrificing the adjacent joint. Less frequently, there may be extensive involvement along the length of the bone that precludes adequate resection and reconstruction without sacrificing the entire bone (femur and humerus). In this situation, a whole bone resection involving the proximal and distal joints is required.

Pelvic resections represent a unique challenge. A tumor arising in the pelvis can involve a segment of nonarticular bone (e.g., the iliac wing, pubis, or ischium) the acetabulum or both. The extent of the skeletal resection determines the functional deficits and influences the decision regarding the type of skeletal reconstruction, if any, to be offered to the patient to optimize function.

Operative risks are high with surgery of the bony pelvis and spine. Primary tumors arising within the sacrum and vertebrae are rare. Because of the unique anatomic considerations in these regions, tumors are seldom amenable to wide local excision. Metastatic disease to spine/sacrum, however, is very common (25).

B. Bone Metastases

Surgery is recommended for bone metastases of the long bones associated with an impending fracture, established fracture, and for symptomatic lesions that have failed to respond to nonsurgical therapy. In the spine, neural compression, loss of spinal stability, and intractable pain despite radiation are indications for surgery. The principal goal of surgery is to achieve stability of the affected bone to relieve mechanical pain and restore function. A secondary objective is to control local tumor to reduce tumor-associated pain, slow local progression of disease, and maintain the integrity of the construct used to stabilize the bone so function can be maintained. The surgical approach depends on the location and nature of the lesion, extent of local bone destruction, presence of a fracture, presence of multifocal involvement within a given bone, quality of the uninvolved bone, risk and potential complications attendant with a given surgical procedure, and general condition of the patient (12).

Most metastatic tumors requiring orthopedic intervention are lytic, destructive lesions arising from primary cancers of the breast, lung, and kidney. Although prostate cancer frequently metastasizes to bone, surgery is less frequently necessary because of the blastic (bone-forming) nature of the metastatic deposits. The axial skeleton and lower extremities, in particular the hip region, are most commonly regions affected by metastatic bone disease for which surgery is performed (26). The upper extremities are involved less frequently. In general, metastases distal to the knee and elbow are infrequent. Pathologic fracture is common. Most pathologic fractures occur about the hip joint (proximal femur and acetabulum).

The majority of most metastatic deposits are excised by curettage during surgical fixation of a fracture or stabilization of a bone with an impending fracture. Intramedullary nail fixation or joint arthroplasty are the two most commonly applied orthopaedic techniques to stabilize diseased bone. Plate fixation is used less frequently, but is effective in areas where a nail or arthroplasty is inappropriate. Bone cement is used to fill the bone defect or to augment stability at the site of pathologic fracture when a nail or plate fixation is used. En bloc resection of a metastases is uncommon, but can be appropriate for patients with a solitary bone lesion, extensive bone destruction, or failure of prior stabilization efforts due to local tumor progression.

As mentioned previously, metastases from renal cell carcinoma, thyroid carcinoma, and multiple myeloma present a unique challenge to the orthopaedic surgeon. All can be extremely vascular. Manipulation of the tumor during curettage or bone stabilization can result in massive hemorrhage. Selective transcatheter arterial embolization preoperatively is performed routinely to decrease tumor vascular and decrease intraoperative blood loss (27). For patients with vascular bone metastases, adequate intravenous access should be established and appropriate warming devices for multiple blood transfusions should be available. Central venous and direct arterial access should be performed to directly monitor volume status, perfusion pressure, and monitor blood values. Blood and blood products should be available, and strategies to ensure renal protection should be considered. Fenoldepam may be considered, because studies have shown improved outcome using dopamine 1-agonist receptors for renal protection to be effective (28).

C. Soft Tissue Neoplasms

Benign soft tissue tumors, like benign bone tumors, are amenable to local surgical excision. Intraoperative risks generally are low. Large intramuscular masses such as lipomas can be technically more challenging to excise, but rarely cause significant concerns from an anesthesia perspective. Soft tissue sarcomas are treated with wide local excision alone or in combination with radiation, chemotherapy, or both for large intermediate- and high-grade tumors. The tissue planes of dissection to extirpate large sarcomas often involve the adjacent neurovascular bundles. The risk for injury to major blood vessels can be higher. The potential for vascular resection and reconstruction or extensive blood loss can complicate surgery.

Adequate soft tissue reconstruction is central to the success of contemporary limb preservation for bone and soft tissue sarcomas. The treatment of local muscle flaps, free-tissue flaps transferring well-vascularized nonirradiated soft tissues provides durable protection for exposed bone, joint, blood vessels, and nerves expanding the number of patients who are eligible for limb preserving surgery. Preoperative wound-related complications are reduced significantly with a libel use of these soft tissue reconstruction techniques. Frequently, bone is involved by direct extension of a soft tissue sarcoma, composite soft tissue–bone resection may be performed to acquire both soft tissue and skeletal reconstructive efforts (29).

V. ANESTHESIA MANAGEMENT

A. Anesthetic Considerations in Specific Oncologic Orthopedic Procedures

Familiarity of specific oncologic orthopedic procedures is invaluable in the anesthetic care of these patients. Communication and discussion with the surgeon before the procedure is paramount. Procedure with possibility of massive hemorrhage requires appropriate anesthetic preparation. Prior knowledge of the patient's position during surgery is helpful. Proximal upper extremity procedure position is sloppy lateral or in beach chair and shifted to the edge of the table. The patient is placed in a slight reverse Trendelenburg sometimes flexed at the hip and knee. The patient's head, neck, and hip should be well secured. Stretch brachial plexus injury may result if head is severely rotated. Attention to pressure on the eyes and ears and securing of the airway are important because access after draping is limited. Procedure in the lateral or prone position also necessitate attention to the head and neck to be neutral position and securely padded in position to avoid misalignment with the spine. Use of bean bag may limits access to the patient. All invasive procedures for accessing and monitoring patient should be completed before positioning. Direct arterial blood pressure monitoring and following of hemoglobin levels are advisable if tourniquet cannot be used and significant blood loss may occur.

Orthopedic surgical procedures in the pelvis are more challenging and often accompanied by more hemorrhage. Pelvic tumors tend to grow relatively large before becoming symptomatic and often involve major vasculature or nerve roots. Preoperative assessment of tumor size, extension, invasion of pelvic veins, pelvic venous thrombosis, and expected blood loss is important for successful management. Magnetic resonance imaging, computed tomography, venography, and arteriography are helpful in this evaluation. Venography may reveal pre-existing thrombosis, and the insertion of temporary vena cava filter may prevent a fatal intraoperative pulmonary embolism resulting from surgical manipulation (11). Blood loss depends on the extent of the resection, type of tumor, and involvement of the acetabulum, sacrum, or blood vessels. If the procedure involves resection of the acetabulum or sacrum, then more blood loss should be expected. Acetabular resection is commonly done in patients with chondrosarcoma and may leave these patients bedridden for 2–3 weeks after surgery. Acetabular and sacral resection can require more than 40 units of packed red blood cells. Internal hemipelvectomy will result in more blood loss than external hemipelvectomy because of more extensive resection. Extraosseous involvement, such as invasion of the bladder, also results in higher blood loss. Hip disarticulation also carries a risk of large blood loss, though less than hemipelvectomy. Physiological derangement associated with large blood loss, such as hypothermia, large fluid shift, metabolic disturbances, and dilutional coagulopathy, should also be anticipated and early treatment should be planned. Communication with the surgeon before posting the procedure with the blood bank for ability to provide support for massive intraoperative hemorrhage is mandatory. Laboratory testing should be followed as discussed in the section on Blood loss management.

Hemipelvectomy, also known as hindquarter amputation, is most frequently indicated for neoplasms of the upper thigh, hip, or pelvis. On the other hand, internal hemipelvectomy is a limb-salvaging procedure used to preserve the ipsilateral extremity and neurovascular bundle to allow partial weigh bearing. The positioning of the patient during surgery is variable. Hemipelvectomy with a posterior or anterior flap usually requires the patient to be in a lateral, modified Trendelenburg, or semilateral 45° position with the table flex for anterior and posterior exposure. An internal hemipelvectomy patient is placed in a supine position with the proximal buttock padded and elevated, and the extremity prepped and draped freely for manipulation during surgery. Cystoscopy with placement of ureteral stents at the beginning is commonly performed as part of the surgical procedure. Hemipelvectomy is associated with considerable blood loss because of the possible involvement of iliofemoral vessels and the sacroiliac joint. The neurosurgery team may also be involved with the sacroiliac joint and neurovascular bundle lesions. Internal hemipelvectomy is associated with more excessive blood loss, because the entire innominate bone of the hemipelvis is resected (30). Blood loss ranges from less than 1 L to more than 20 L thus, adequate preparation is mandatory. In surgery of such long duration, attention to antibiotic readministration frequency to decrease postoperative wound infection is important. Plastic reconstruction with tissue flap is often necessary and maintenance of perfusion pressure is critical.

Intraoperatively, complications of thrombosis from tumor and blood vessel manipulation may manifest as hemodynamic instability, desaturation, secondary compartment syndrome, and renal insufficiency. Common postoperative complications of hemipelvectomy include flap necrosis, wound infection, poor wound healing, compartment syndrome, and renal insufficiency.

Sacral resection usually involves primary bone tumor chordoma, giant cell tumor, or recurrent rectal cancer. It is a complex surgery involving sacral nerve roots, bowels, and bones, thus requiring several surgical teams, including a general surgeon, a neurosurgeon, and an orthopedic surgeon. Patients often have had preoperative bowel preparation along with antibiotics. The patient's hydration status should be optimized before and after anesthetic induction for a smooth anesthetic course. The patient may assume several positions during the surgical procedure, including supine, lithotomy, or lateral positions for anterior exposure and prone for posterior exposure. Preparations should be made for extensive blood loss and its management.

Upper extremities resection of any structure of the shoulder girdle is challenging and complex. Forequarter amputation is a rare surgical option that is commonly performed only in special tertiary cancer centers. It is indicated in tumors of the shoulder girdle involving the axillary vessel and brachial plexus. This procedure is most commonly performed curatively in patients with high-grade soft tissue osteosarcoma or palliatively for pain in patients with metastatic cancer. Patients with soft tissue sarcoma, such as osteosarcoma, have often received adriamycin, and cardiac toxicity should be considered. This is a psychologically traumatic procedure and the major postoperative problem can be phantom limb pain. Adjuvant regional administration of epineural anesthesia has been found to be helpful. Forequarter amputation is less of a surgical challenge than hemipelvectomy. The patient's position is usually lateral. The surgical approach may be anterior or posterior depending on the tumor location. The risk of hemorrhage during dissection is from incursion into the subclavian or axillary artery or vein. The anterior approach carries more risk of uncontrolled hemorrhage. Tumors involving encasement of the neurovascular bundle also carry a higher risk of hemorrhage. A preoperative neurological examination may give as much information about this risk as radiological studies. Once vascular trunk exposure is complete and ligated, then the risk of uncontrolled hemorrhage is reduced.

Surgery to the spine for neoplasms is more a neurosurgical than orthopedic procedure. Anesthetic concerns include the risk of hemorrhage and issues related to the prone position. Risk for hemorrhage with spinal surgery is associated with areas involving large feeding veins, operative locations preclude the use of a tourniquet, or sometimes incorrect prone position. The establishment of appropriate monitoring and venous access before incision, correct positioning of the head, avoidance of injury to the eye globe, and chest and iliac crest support to decrease abdominal pressure and improve ventilation should be thought out.

B. Setup

For a given site, the duration of orthopaedic oncologic surgery is much greater than for standard orthopaedic procedures. The positioning of the patient during oncologic surgery is variable. All monitor placements and invasive procedures should be completed before positioning and surgical draping. This includes a standard ASA monitor, a Foley catheter for urine output, a large central access line for monitoring and fluid administration (12 gauge triple lumen), two large bore peripheral intravenous catheters (14–16 gauge), a direct arterial blood pressure monitor, and cardiac monitor if necessary. A long duration of surgery should be anticipated. The patient should be well secured to the operating table, and all pressure points should be checked and padded. The duration of surgery can be excessive with multiple adjustments and maneuvers of the operating table, and the patient may unnoticeably shift under the surgical drapes. Large surface areas of bone and soft tissue are exposed as a result of extensile approaches resulting in a loss of core body temperature. Warming of the operating room, warming of fluid, and the use of forced-air warming blankets will be helpful to maintain body temperature in a safe range.

Most surgery is performed with the patient in the supine position. Access to the anterior aspect of the lower extremities, knee joint, leg, and foot is achieved easily. The prone position limits an extensile approach for most parts of the body except for the back, buttocks, posterior thigh, and calf. Surgical approaches to the dorsal spine and are necessarily performed in this position. An incorrect prone position can put pressure on the abdomen and diaphragm and cause vena cava obstruction. This may result in more blood loss from increased distension and flow in the epidural venous plexus from vena cava obstruction. The prone position may place the operative site higher than the heart risking venous air emboli (VAE) (31,32). The causes of hemodynamic instability in spinal surgery are not always apparent. In the case of no obvious blood loss, unexplained hypotension during spinal surgery may be a result of a rare complication such as VAE or injury to major blood vessels.

The lateral position facilitates exposure to the pelvis, hip, lateral thigh, flank, and scapula. The beach-chair position is favored for anterior approaches to the cervical spine and shoulder. Irrespective of the patient's position, all pressure points should be well padded. In general, anesthetic considerations are usually more demanding and warrant more attention in procedures involving the shoulder girdle and hip, pelvis, and spine.

C. Fluid Management

Patients who have undergone preoperative chemotherapy frequently are dehydrated at the time of surgery. Hydration to maintain perfusion pressure to all organ systems is critical. Since anemia is common in these surgical patients, re-evaluation of the hemoglobin levels after hydration is important to establish an accurate baseline for before surgery commences. Patients with pelvic tumors often have a bowel preparation preoperatively. The patient's hydration status should be optimized before and after anesthetic induction for a stable anesthetic course.

Perfusion pressure is important also to reduce hemodynamic events that could compromise the viability of tissue transfers used to provide stable soft tissue coverage of acquired defects or over exposed bone or prosthetic implants. Judicious management of fluids, blood loss, and avoidance of the use of vasopressors is critical for myocutaneous flap viability. The use of vasodilators and a sympathetic blockade and avoidance of hypothermia all contribute to maintaining adequate perfusion pressure. Inhalation anesthetics are potent vasodilators and can increase tissue blood flow. The topical local anesthetic papaverine can prevent vasospasm and therefore can increase tissue blood flow (33). Direct vasodilators, such as nitroprusside, trimethaphan, and hydralazine, have no effect on vasospasm and may even decrease perfusion pressure if hypotension results (34). Phenylephrine should be avoided, because it decreases flap flow. Dopamine and dobutamine increase cardiac output but do not proportionally increase flap flow and should still be used with caution (35). Studies have shown a decrease in microcirculatory blood flow in free tissue flaps with the use of an epidural anesthesia, so caution is recommended (36,37). Maintenance of core body temperature improves coagulation and tissue blood flow by decreasing vasoconstriction (38,39).

D. Blood Loss Management

Bleeding tends to be of greater concern in this patient population because of both local and systemic factors. Local factors include the inherent vascularity of the tumor, site of the disease (proximal to a site where a pneumatic tourniquet can be applied), relation of the tumor to adjacent blood vessels, preoperative irradiation of the tumor, and large surface area of muscle through which the planes of dissection commonly are performed. Systemic factors include the preoperative anemia, lowered core body temperature, and intraoperative coagulopathy. Blood loss from transected bone and muscle and manipulation of major blood vessels is more difficult to control surgically. The extent of blood loss is often underestimated, because collection by surgical sponges in addition to suction collection often is not accounted for.

Induced hypotension has been shown to reduce intraoperative blood loss (40). Reducing systolic pressure to 20 mmHg from baseline or lowering of MAP to 55–65 mmHg has been shown to decrease blood loss and transfusion up to 50% and reduce operating time (41,42). Hypotension can be induced with a combination of general anesthesia and sympathetic blockade with neural-axial anesthesia or with intravenous hypotensive agents such as nitroglycerin, nitroprusside, volatile anesthetic, trimethaphan, calcium channel blockers, and alpha and beta antagonists. Risks associated with induced hypotension should be considered. Cord ischemia, neurological deficits, and blindness have been reported in the literature (43,44). Patients such as the elderly or those with preoperative hypertension and vascular disease should be carefully chosen for this technique. Hypotensive anesthesia is probably a relative contraindication in such patients but studies with this large patient population have shown this is a safe anesthesia technique with a low complication rate (45).

Transfused blood and blood products have been associated with immunomodulation and increased postoperative infection, transmission of infectious disease, acute lung injury, and increased cost.

Therefore, preparedness for massive transfusions with a fluid warmer and rapid fluid infuser should be set up. Physiological derangement associated with large blood loss, such as hypothermia, large fluid shift, metabolic disturbances, and dilutional coagulopathy should also be anticipated and early treatment should be planned. Communication with the surgeon before posting the procedure with the blood bank for ability to provide support for massive intraoperative hemorrhage is mandatory. Laboratory testing to follow the red cell count, coagulation cascade including prothrombin time, prolong activated thrombin time, platelet count, fibrinogen level, arterial blood gas analysis, and ionized calcium level should be promptly available and performed regularly (1–2 hr). At our institution, instant assessment of the hemoglobin level is available in the operating room through the use of Hemocues.

Platelets, fresh frozen plasma, and cryoprecipitate should be available to replace clotting factors to maintain hemostasis. Thrombelastographic monitoring is also useful in assessing clotting factor activity, platelet function, and fibrinolytic processes. Before surgery, the patient can donate autologous blood for use during surgery if blood loss estimates can be determined with relative certainty not to exceed more than three or four units. The theory is that the patient's own blood is safer than banked blood. Autologous blood may minimize the risk of exposure to infection seen with homologous blood transfusion, but it does not decrease the risk of a reaction due to type crossing, because that risk is often related to human error from the wrong blood units being given. In addition, as in hemodilution, factors of preoperative anemia and predictable massive intraoperative blood loss also limit the use autologous blood donation. Autologous blood recovered from the tumor bed with a cell saver during resection surgery is not an option in the cancer patient. This method of blood salvage is contraindicated because of the risk of tumor cell dissemination.

One mechanism that contributes to increased blood loss in major orthopedic operations involves an imbalance of the coagulation and fibrinolytic systems in response to major bleeding, vascular, endothelial and bone trauma, and absorption of bone cement. This has been observed in patients undergoing total hip surgery, in which sequential intrapulmonary and systemic activation of coagulation and fibrinolysis contributed to perioperative blood loss (46).

Aprotinin, epsilon amino-caproic acid (EACA), and transexaminic acid have been shown to reduce intraoperative bleeding and transfusion requirements in many surgeries including orthopedic surgery. The mechanism of aprotinin's blood sparing effect is probably through a protective effect on platelet membrane binding function and inhibition of intraoperative fibrinolysis by inhibition of plasmin, the kinin–kallikrein system, and intrinsic coagulation pathway (47–50). EACA is also a competitive inhibitor of plasmin by blocking lysine sites on fibrinogen, fibrin, and platelet receptors. EACA has benefits similar to those of aprotinin in reducing blood loss and transfusion requirements but at a lower cost and less risk of anaphylaxis. Transexaminic acid works in a similar manner. Studies of transexaminic acid use in orthopedic surgery have shown no noticeable benefit (51,52). To date, the data on the ability of aprotinin and EACA to reduce perioperative blood loss and transfusion requirements in major orthopedic oncology procedures remain questionable and conflicting (53,54). Some studies showed a dramatic reduction in bleeding and blood transfusion in major orthopedic procedures (55–57). Moderate hypotension with systolic blood pressure in the range of 80–90 mmHg and large aprotinin loading dose (1–2 million KIU) and maintenance infusion (500,000 KIU/Hr) was associated with 58% reduction in homologous blood transfusion (54). Other study showed the use of aprotinin and EACA did not reduce perioperative blood loss or transfusion requirements in patients with malignancies undergoing major orthopedic surgery (53). The benefit of in reducing perioperative transfusion requirements is probably dose related. Therefore, despite multiple studies proving the benefits of antifibrinolytic agents in major orthopedic surgery, the routine prophylactic use of these expensive drugs in orthopedic oncology cases remains questionable, and the risk of side effects remains unclear. Though aprotinin has anticoagulant properties, its inhibition of plasmin and protein C may be of theoretical concern, because those effects could produce a hypercoagulable state. Studies have not shown an increase in the deep vein thrombosis (DVT) rate but rather a trend toward a lower incidence of DVT in patients treated with aprotinin (54–56).

Desmopressin can decrease blood loss by increasing the von Willebrand factor to promote platelet adhesiveness to the vascular endothelium and therefore hemostasis. An intravenous dose of 0.3 μg/kg is used, and the hemostatic effect is almost immediate. Desmopressin reduces blood loss in congenital or acquired platelet disorder in patients with certain types of hemophilia, uremia, or chronic liver disease (58,59). However, it does not reduce blood loss in healthy patients with no coagulopathy (60,61).

Erythropoietin therapy has been used to increase perioperative hemoglobin level. Recombinant human erythropoietin (rHuEPO) has been used to stimulate erythropoesis to permit increase preoperative autologous blood collection and reduce allogeneic transfusion risk. Worldwide clinical trial on perisurgical use of rHuEPO showed a strong correlation between increase hemoglobin and reduction of allogeneic transfusion. An average increase in hemoglobin of 2 g/dL with rHuEPO therapy can reduce allogeneic exposure from a baseline of 40% of all patients in orthopedic surgery down to 10% (62–64). Patient undergoing elective orthopedic surgery with hemoglobin levels between 10 and 13 g/dL can be candidate for erythropoietin therapy. Appropriate dosages range from 300 to 600 U/kg weekly 2–3 week prior to surgery. The erythropoesis-stimulating protein, known as darbepoetin-alfa, has shown more promise than rHuEPO for convenience and practicality for preoperative preparation of anemic patient. Darbepoetin-alfa has faster onset, dose–response relationship, and longer half-life so one shot may be sufficient. This drug is currently in phase III study (65,66).

In conclusion, there are many strategies available to minimize perioperative blood loss and the need for transfusion in major orthopedic oncologic procedures. No one technique is superior in all cases. Studies have not shown that using a combination of these techniques to varying degrees seems to be the best course to minimize blood loss and transfusion risk (67–70).

E. Metabolic Disturbances

Therapy-related electrolyte imbalances such as hypokalemia, hypomagnesemia, and hypophosphatemia are common. Hypercalcemia in patients with metastatic bone disease warrants special attention. Hypercalcemia can be a life-threatening complication of bone destruction from bone metastases. It occurs in 10–20% of patients and tends to occur late in the clinical course of the disease. Clinical symptoms of hypercalcemia include weakness, nausea, vomiting, dehydration, polyuria, anorexia, lethargy, confusion, stupor, and coma. Multiple myeloma and breast carcinoma are more commonly associated with hypercalcemia due to localized bone disease by mediating local osteolytic factors causing bone resorption and destruction. Tumors such as renal, ovarian, lung cancer, and squamous cell carcinoma can systemically activate skeletal osteoclasts and cause hypercalcemia by secreting parathyroid hormone-related protein. Hypercalcemia may develop in patients with lymphoma due to lymphoid cells producing bone-resorbing lymphokines or lymphoid cells increasing the production of dihydroxyvitamin D causing an increase in intestinal absorption of calcium.

Treatment of hypercalcemia in conjunction with a malignancy starts with restoring intravascular blood volume with intravenous fluids to increase the urinary excretion of calcium. After restoration of blood volume, intravenous biphosphonates (e.g., clodronate, pamidronate, and zoledronate) are administered to inhibit osteoclastic bone activation, and reduce serum calcium levels. Normocalcemia is usually achieved in 3–5 days in most patients. In an emergency, calcitonin is an option to inhibit osteoclast-mediated bone resorption and enhance urinary calcium excretion. Another option for the treatment of hypercalcemia is gallium nitrate. Gallium nitrate is also an osteoclast inhibitor, and its administration schedule involves a 5-day continuous IV infusion. Long-term efficacy in reducing pathological fractures, spinal cord compression, and hypercalcemia is well documented, and its administration is safe and well tolerated with minimal side effects (71). New, promising options for treatment of bone metastases include the development of recombinant osteoprotegerin and an antiparathyroid-hormone-related monoclonal antibody (72).

F. Methylmethacrylate and Hemodynamic Instability

It is common to observe hemodynamic changes resulting from the insertion of bone cement (polymethylmethacrylate) into the medullary cavity of long bones for fixation of prosthetic devices. Hemodynamic changes can occur during cementation due to unreacted monomer, which can be a potent, direct vasodilator and can stimulate mast cell degranulation, release of histamine, and can cause myocardial depression. Insertion of the prosthesis into the cement increases intramedullary pressures and may result in forcing marrow content and air into the bloodstream. The piston–cylinder effect in the femur can produce intraluminal pressures that can exceed one atmosphere. Normal marrow pressure is 30–50 mmHg but can increase up to 600 mmHg during intramedullary reaming (73). Embolization of fat, bone marrow, cement, and bone fragments may occur during the insertion of the prosthesis but procedure in long bones such as the femur carry an even higher risk.

Emboli can result in systemic hypotension, pulmonary hypertension, or hypoxemia. Monitoring pulse oximetry for desaturation and end-tidal CO_2 to detect embolization may be helpful during reaming and cementing. Care should be taken to ensure that the patient is adequately hydrated before and during the procedure. Vasopressors can be used as necessary to maintain stable blood pressure. Maximizing inspired oxygen concentration will help offset hypoxemia, and discontinuing the use of nitrous oxide several minutes before this point in surgery will decrease the risk of air being entrained and therefore air emboli. Transesophageal monitoring may aid in differentiating between hypovolemia and deteriorating right heart function from an embolism (74).

G. Thromboembolism

Venous thromboembolism is a major cause of morbidity in orthopedic surgery. Risk factors include a hypercoagulable state associated with cancer, major surgery, advanced age, prolonged immobility, and a previous history of thromboembolism. Intraoperative use of a tourniquet or positioning of a limb causing a kinking of a blood vessel can decrease blood flow, thereby increasing the risk of thromboembolism. Patients with a history of DVT, pulmonary embolism, or severe cardiac and pulmonary disease may benefit from preoperative insertion of a temporary vena cava filter.

Without pharmacologic prophylaxis, the incidence of DVT has been reported to be as high as 40–80%, and the incidence of pulmonary embolism as shown by clinical and laboratory data is 1–24%. The incidence of fatal pulmonary embolism is 0.2–13%. Pharmacologic prophylaxis, however, is not used routinely for patients following major musculoskeletal tumor resection procedures. Transection through muscle planes and bone commonly result in large surface areas of potentially bleeding tissues. Large hematomas can develop in the dead space resulting from resection of a large soft tissue tumors or segments of unreconstructed bone. Patients who undergo bone stabilization procedures or joint arthroplasty that do not result from large tissue dissection to remove tumor, however, routinely are treated pharmacologically for DVT prophylaxis. Accepted regimens include subcutaneous heparin, low molecular-weight heparins and heparinoid, and warfarin. Low molecular-weight heparin (LMWH) can be effective and produces less platelet inhibition and therefore less bleeding (75).

Other prevention measures include pneumatic compression, regional anesthesia, and early postoperative mobilization. Routine use of elastic stockings and pneumatic compression devices should be instituted before, during, and after surgery. Hypotension associated with anesthesia induction can cause venous stasis, and the placement of a lower extremity compression device before hypotension episode is more effective.

Regional anesthesia with a neural-axial blockade may decrease perioperative DVT and intraoperative blood loss (76–79). Regional anesthetics decrease the rate of DVT through several mechanisms: a sympathetic blockade and epinephrine use improve blood flow and reduce venous stasis; a hypercoagulable response to the stress of surgery decreases with a central neural blockade; and local anesthetics may have a direct effect on platelet aggregation. Postoperatively, regional anesthetics promote early ambulation. The regional technique cannot be recommended in all patients for DVT prophylaxis, because there is no indication that the rate can be reduced to zero or that decreasing the rate of DVT will decrease the death rate. The risks and benefits of regional anesthesia must be weighed in partially anticoagulated patients.

The actual incidence of neural-axial blockade and neurological dysfunction due to spinal hematoma is unknown. Estimates in the literature are 1 in 150,000 for epidural and 1 in 220,000 for spinal anesthetic (80,81). Perioperative anticoagulation increases the frequency of spinal hematoma. This includes the concomitant use of antiplatelet drugs, standard heparin, and dextran. The incidence of spinal hematoma with LMWH anticoagulation is 1 in 40,800 with spinal and 1 in 3100 with continuous epidural anesthetic. These risks can be minimized if the LMWH dose is maintained for 24 hr after catheter placement. The LMWH dose should be not given for 10–12 hr before catheter removal and should not be restarted until 2 hr after catheter removal. Institution of LMWH in the presence of an indwelling catheter is risky. There is no laboratory test to follow the risk of bleeding. Antifactor Xa monitoring is not recommended, because its activity is not predictive of bleeding risk (81). The choice of treatment for spinal hematoma is decompression laminectomy. Recovery is not likely if postponed for more than 10–12 hr. One series reported less than 40% of patients had partial or good recovery of neurological function after spinal hematoma (82).

H. Fat Embolism

Clinically, evident fat embolism syndrome (FES) rarely manifests despite long bone medullary canal manipulation. Despite echocardiographic evidence of a high incidence of embolic phenomena (83), one study detected embolic showers in 97 out of 111 orthopedic procedures, with hypoxemia occurring during instrumentation in 59% of these procedures. These embolic showers may continue postoperatively, as shown by transesophageal echocardiography (84). Fat emboli have been found to occur regularly in dogs during femur prosthesis instrumentation (74,85). Thus, unrecognized fat embolism occurs regularly, but not all fat emboli develop in FES. Contributing factors, such as trauma, shock, hypovolemia, sepsis, or DIC, may trigger fat emboli to cause FES. The clinical incidence of FES varies from $<1\%$ to 19%, depending on the diagnostic clinical criteria (86). Mortality can be significant, ranging from 10% to 20%. Knowledge of and familiarity with the criteria for the diagnosis of fat emboli syndrome is important for early appropriate treatment. Diagnosis using Gurd's criteria requires the presence of at least one major and four minor factors. Major criteria are petechiae rash (usually on the axilla, neck, conjunctiva, and oral mucous membrane), PaO_2 <60 mmHg; FiO_2 <4, central venous system depression, pulmonary edema, and thrombocytopenia. Minor criteria are tachycardia >110 beats per minutes, hyperthermia >38.5°C, retinal fat emboli, urinary fat globules, sputum fat globules, increased sedimentation rate, and unexplained anemia. Treatments include the reversal of contributing factors and ventilatory support (87).

Pulmonary dysfunction is the most common manifestation of FES. The routine use of pulse oximetry allows early detection and treatment. An asymptomatic latent period of 12–48 hr may precede any clinical manifestation. Embolic showers continue postoperatively, and fragments can cause pulmonary embolization. Emboli may coalesce, forming thrombotic masses up to 8 cm in diameter post, yet a mortem examination may show evidence of fat macroemboli (86). Not all episodes of FES are obvious or fit the criteria for diagnosis. A fulminate episode can occur hours after surgery. Unexplained severe hypoxemia, respiratory failure, severe neurological impairment, or DIC should prompt the inclusion of FES as part of a differential diagnosis. Appropriate treatment includes hemodynamic resuscitation and aggressive therapy support. Corticosteroid therapy may be beneficial, with up to a 10-fold reduction of FES in one series (87). However, the optimum timing and dose in relation to outcome have yet to be elucidated. Pharmacological support, such as aspirin, heparin, and dextran has not been proven effective. Early administration of oxygen actually prevents the onset of FES possibly by preventing hypoxemia and, therefore, catecholamine response and fat mobilization (88). Approximately 10–44% of patients with pulmonary dysfunction from FES require mechanical ventilation, and, the condition usually resolves in 3–7 days (89–91).

I. Postoperative Pain Management

Bone pain associated with metastatic devices can be incapacitating, and the assessment of a patient's analgesic requirements is helpful in determining and planning the perioperative anesthetic. Pain evaluation includes an assessment of preoperative analgesic regimens including nonsteroidal anti-inflammatory agents, narcotics, and adjuvant tricyclic mood modulators. Patients may have baseline high narcotic tolerance before surgery and often require more analgesia intraoperatively and postoperatively. Tricyclic antidepressants have inherent analgesic effects and potentiate the analgesic effects of opioids. Many patients have and are treated for chronic pain, so communication and collaboration with the chronic or postoperative pain service should be sought to optimize the patient's perioperative pain management.

Nononcologic orthopedic surgical procedures lend themselves to the use of regional anesthesia, because it allows for both intraoperative surgical anesthesia and postoperative pain relief. Regional anesthesia offers the advantages of improved postoperative analgesia and less nausea, vomiting, respiratory depression, and cardiac depression. It also improved perfusion through the sympathetic blockade, thus decreasing blood loss and thromboembolic risk. However, these benefits must be weighed against certain risks in this patient population. In the setting of orthopedic neoplasms, several factors can make the choice of a strictly regional anesthetic technique not advisable. Surgical procedures involving the resection of tumors are often unpredictable. Extensive, complex, and wide resection are often required for a cancer-free margin, and thus long durations on the OR table are often uncomfortable and not well tolerated if the patient is only sedated and a regional block is used to provide anesthesia. Regional anesthesia is often not ideal if massive intraoperative blood loss is expected, because the consequent hemodynamic instability and coagulopathy can be of concern. In addition, tumors often involve neurological structures and the risk of injury with regional anesthesia is controversial. Regional anesthesia can also interfere with postoperative neurological assessments. The presence of epidural disease due to tumor spread often contraindicates the use of a regional epidural or spinal technique. Chemotherapy may cause neurotoxicity, so any preexisting neurological deficits should be elucidated and well documented before a regional anesthetic is used. Common chemotherapy agents associated with neurotoxicities include cisplatin and vincristine. Therefore, in cancer patient requiring orthopaedic procedures, regional anesthesia should be thoughtfully implemented to augment perioperative anesthetic care, but the issues unique to these patients should be considered.

Regional adjuvant anesthesia should be considered for patients undergoing amputation. The phantom limb pain incidence for cancer patients is unpredictable, but can be severe. Phantom pain is likely the result of differentiation from the loss of sensory input in a limb. Pre-existing pain prior to surgery is associated with a higher incidence of phantom limb pain, which can be as high as 80%. It has been proposed that pre-emptive analgesia with epidural administration of an analgesic may prevent long-term phantom pain, but published results have been contradictory and controversial (92). Analgesia via the placement of a catheter within the amputated nerve sheath has also been advocated and studied. The phantom pain incidence was found to decrease to 67% from the historic incidence of 80% in one retrospective study (93). Other studies showed no difference in the phantom pain incidence from that previously reported using either a nerve sheath catheter or an epidural catheter (94,95). Local anesthetic perineural catheter analgesia is just as effective as epidural analgesia yet more easily managed. In conclusion, randomized trials with epidurals, regional nerve blocks, and mechanical vibratory stimulation provide inconsistent results and little evidence to guide the clinician in the treatment of phantom pain.

Perioperative epidural and neural sheath catheter infusions provide effective postoperative analgesia and may decrease the severity of phantom limb pain, though not the incidence of its occurrence (92,96). Investigations have shown that oral dextomethorphan (DM) alleviates neuropathic pain in both animal and human models, and it has been used successfully to reduce postamputation phantom limb pain (97). This beneficial effect is through the interaction of DM with pain mediated centrally by *N*-methyl-D-aspartate receptors. DM is an NMDA receptor antagonist. Oral DM administration is also associated with reduced pain intensity, sedation, and analgesic requirements for patients undergoing surgery for bone and soft tissue malignancy (97,98). NMDA receptor antagonists are effective for both neuropathic phantom limb pain and postoperative surgical pain.

VI. INTENSIVE CARE AND POSTOPERATIVE PERSPECTIVES

Most patients require no more than routine postoperative recovery support after extubation. Postoperative management after orthopaedic oncologic surgery depends on the nature and extent of the surgical procedure and coexisting medical conditions. Most patients are able to recover in the postanesthesia care unit. Admission to the surgical intensive care unit is based on the duration and extent of the surgical procedure, pre-existing disease status, massive hemorrhage, and pain therapy. Most intensive care admission is for management of consequent of massive blood transfusion. Correction of fluid and electrolyte abnormalities, acquired coagulopathy, hypothermia, and acidosis may be required. Patients are at risk of respiratory complication of the shock lung. Patients require ventilatory support until the massive volume shift has equilibrated. Postoperative intensive care allows for adequate administration of fluid and transfusion requirements during rewarming and maximum therapy for pain relief.

Patients on ventilators need sedation for comfort, but any sedation given to spinal surgery patients should allow for evaluation of the neurological function of motor control of the extremities at all times. Placement of an epidural cathether, usually done under direct vision in surgery, is helpful for analgesic control. Limb-salvage procedures that involve manipulation or resection of large vessels or the application of free tissue transfers require monitoring of postoperative coagulation. Pulse oximetry in affected lower extremities helps to assess the adequacy of circulation. An arterial Doppler is used to assess the adequacy of flap perfusion if a tissue flap is used to cover a defect.

Extensive oncologic procedures involving bone call for continuous postoperative recording of vital signs, serial determination of hematocrit, careful observation of postoperative bleeding, and adequate hydration. Patients should be monitored carefully for hypoxia, tachycardia, and changes in mental status. Flap viability is also closely monitored postoperatively with Doppler flow. Current management to preserve blood flow in microvascular anastomoses includes antithrombotic (heparin), fibrinolytic (streptokinase, low molecular-weight dextran), and smooth muscle relaxant (papaverine, local anesthetic) agents. A desaturation episode due to postoperative fat embolism is possible. Fat emboli should always be suspected in unexplained hypoxemia accompanied by systemic inflammatory response syndrome with multiple organ failure. Early recognition is important, and treatment includes oxygen administration, fluid management, and judicious anticoagulation therapy. Verification of the circulatory and neurological integrity of affected limb is also an important issue. Treatment is nonspecific and supportive. The goal of treatment is early resuscitation and stabilization to minimize the stress response and hypovolemia (86).

VII. CONCLUSIONS

The anesthesia management of oncologic surgical patients with musculoskeletal neoplasms can be challenging. Preoperative assessment and medical optimization are critical. Knowledge of specific cancers and procedures is invaluable to the care of these patients. Both disease- and site-specific factors influence the nature and extent of surgery. The majority of patients are young without comorbidities. Chemotherapy-related adverse affects can be minimized with a thorough preoperative anesthesia evaluation and appropriate intraoperative maneuvers.

Postoperative pain management is an integral component to the perioperative management of these patients. Patients should be aggressively managed. Regional anesthesia with epidural catheter placement for postoperative analgesia can be extremely effective in controlling pain in the early postoperative period. Procedure-appropriate preparation with invasive lines for monitoring, blood and fluid resuscitation should be established prior to surgical incision. Strategies to minimize blood loss should be considered. In the future, erythropoietin therapy shows promise as the new arsenal to decrease allogeneic blood transfusion exposure. Knowledge of common cause of hemodynamic instability in orthopaedic oncology surgery should be reviewed for prompt diagnosis and treatment. In summary, management of the patient with a musculoskeletal neoplasm can be complex, but familiarity of common problems presented in these patients can greatly improve their perioperative outcome.

ACKNOWLEDGMENT

Acknowledgment to David Galloway from the Department of Scientific Publications for proofreading this manuscript.

REFERENCES

1. Simon MA, Springfield D. Natural history. In: Simon MA, Springfield D, eds. Surgery for Bone and Soft-tissue Tumors. Philadelphia, PA: Lippincott-Raven, 1998:3–7.
2. Holland JF, Frei EI. Cancer Medicine. Hamilton, ON: BC Decker, 2003.
3. Dorfman HD, Czerniak B. Bone Tumors. St. Louis, MO: Mosby Inc., 1998.
4. Huvos AG. Bone Tumors. Diagnosis, Treatment, and Prognosis. Philadelphia, PA: W.B. Saunders Company, 1991.
5. Unni KK. Dahlin's Bone Tumors. General Aspects and Data on 11,087 Cases. 5th ed. Philadelphia, PA: Lippincott-Raven, 1996.
6. Rosen GFC, Mankin H, Selch M. Neoplasm of the bone and soft tissue. In: Bast RKD, Pollock R, Weichselbam R, Holland J, Frie E, Gamser T, eds. Cancer Medicine. Hamilton: B.C. Decker, 2000, Section 35.121.
7. Heck R. Benign (occasionally aggressive) and Malignant tumors of bone. In: STC, ed. Campbell's Operative Orthopaedics. 10th ed. Philadelphia: Mosby, 2003:813–848.
8. Kelley K. Langerhans' cell histiocytosis. In: Bast RKD, Pollock R, Weichsebaum R, Holland J, Frei E, Gansler T, eds. Cancer Medicine. Hamilton: B.C. Decker, 2000, Section 39.138E.
9. Jemal A, Tiwari RC, Murray T, et al. Cancer statistics, 2004. CA Cancer J Clin 2004; 54:8–29.
10. Sabo D, Bernd L. [Surgical management of skeletal metastases of the extremities]. Orthopade 1998; 27:274–281.
11. Winkler M, Marker E, Hetz H. The peri-operative management of major orthopaedic procedures. Anaesthesia 1998; 53(suppl 2):37–41.
12. Heiner JP, Kinsella TJ, Zdeblick TA. Management of Metastatic Disease to the Musculoskeletal System. St. Louis, MO: Quality Medical Publishing Inc., 2002.
13. Frassica DA. General principles of external beam radiation therapy for skeletal metastases. Clin Orthop 2003; S158–S164.
14. Hortobagyi GN. Novel approaches to the management of bone metastases. Semin Oncol 2003; 30:161–166.
15. Ramaswamy B, Shapiro CL. Bisphosphonates in the prevention and treatment of bone metastases. Oncology (Hunting) 2003; 17:1261–1270; discussion 70–72, 77–78, 80.
16. Siegel HJ, Luck JV Jr, Siegel ME. Advances in radionuclide therapeutics in orthopaedics. J Am Acad Orthop Surg 2004; 12:55–64.
17. Weiss SW, Goldblum JR. Enzinger and Weiss's Soft Tissue Tumors. 4th ed. St. Louis, MO: Mosby, 2001.
18. Pollock RE, Morton DL. Principles of surgical oncology. In: Holland JF, Frei EI, ed. Cancer Medicine. 6th ed. Hamilton, ON: B.C. Decker, 2003:568–584.
19. Adjuvant chemotherapy for localised resectable soft-tissue sarcoma of adults: meta-analysis of individual data. Sarcoma Meta-analysis Collaboration. Lancet 1997; 350:1647–1654.
20. Singal PK, Iliskovic N. Doxorubicin-induced cardiomyopathy. N Engl J Med 1998; 339:900–905.
21. Logothetis CJ, Assikis V, Sarriera JE. Urologic complications. In: Kufe DW, Pollock RE, Weichselbaum RR, et al, eds. Cancer Medicine. Hamilton, ON: B.C. Decker, 2003:2517–2523.
22. Tsukeoka T, Kochi T, Koide K, et al. [The risk of palliative operation for bone metastasis]. Masui 1997; 46:1634–1638.
23. Ritchie JKP, Shapiro C. Renal cell carcinoma. In: Bast RKD, Pollock R, Weichselbaum R, Holland J, Frei E, Gansler T, eds. Cancer Medicine. Hamilton: B.C. Decker Inc., 2000, Section 30–105.
24. Loughlin KR, Gittes RF, Partridge D, Stelos P. The relationship of lactoferrin to the anemia of renal cell carcinoma. Cancer 1987; 59:566–517.
25. Bell RS. Treatment of axial skeleton bone metastases. Clin Orthop 2003; S198–S200.
26. Marco RA, Sheth DS, Boland PJ, et al. Functional and oncological outcome of acetabular reconstruction for the treatment of metastatic disease. J Bone Joint Surg Am 2000; 82:642–651.
27. Chatziioannou AN, Johnson ME, Pneumaticos SG, et al. Preoperative embolization of bone metastases from renal cell carcinoma. Eur Radiol 2000; 10: 593–596.
28. Sheinbaum R, Ignacio C, Safi HJ, Estrera A. Contemporary strategies to preserve renal function during cardiac and vascular surgery. Rev Cardiovasc Med 2003; 4(suppl 1):S21–S28.
29. Miller MJ, Yasko AW. Reconstruction options in sarcoma. In: Pollock RE, ed. Soft Tissue Sarcomas. Hamilton, ON: B.C. Decker, 2002:279–305.
30. Sugarbaker PKC, Malawer M. Summary of alternative approaches to hemipelvectomy. In: Sugarbaker PMM, ed. Musculoskeletal Surgery for Cancer. New York: Thieme, 1992, Chapter 13.

31. Albin MS, Ritter RR, Pruett CE, Kalff K. Venous air embolism during lumbar laminectomy in the prone position: report of three cases. Anesth Analg 1991; 73:346–349.
32. Artru AA. Venous air embolism in prone dogs positioned with the abdomen hanging freely: percentage of gas retrieved and success rate of resuscitation. Anesth Analg 1992; 75:715–719.
33. Geter RK, Winters RR, Puckett CL. Resolution of experimental microvascular spasm and improvement in anastomotic patency by direct topical agent application. Plast Reconstr Surg 1986; 77:105–115.
34. Banic A, Krejci V, Erni D, et al. Effects of sodium nitroprusside and phenylephrine on blood flow in free musculocutaneous flaps during general anesthesia. Anesthesiology 1999; 90:147–155.
35. Cordeiro PG, Santamaria E, Hu QY, Heerdt P. Effects of vasoactive medications on the blood flow of island musculocutaneous flaps in swine. Ann Plast Surg 1997; 39:524–531.
36. Lanz OI, Broadstone RV, Martin RA, Degner DA. Effects of epidural anesthesia on microcirculatory blood flow in free medial saphenous fasciocutaneous flaps in dogs. Vet Surg 2001; 30:374–379.
37. Erni D, Banic A, Signer C, Sigurdsson GH. Effects of epidural anaesthesia on microcirculatory blood flow in free flaps in patients under general anaesthesia. Eur J Anaesthesiol 1999; 16:692–698.
38. Macdonald DJ. Anaesthesia for microvascular surgery. A physiological approach. Br J Anaesth 1985; 57:904–912.
39. Bird TM, Strunin L. Anaesthetic considerations for microsurgical repair of limbs. Can Anaesth Soc J 1984; 31:51–60.
40. Rosberg B, Fredin H, Gustafson C. Anesthetic techniques and surgical blood loss in total hip arthroplasty. Acta Anaesthesiol Scand 1982; 26:189–193.
41. Patterson BM, Healey JH, Cornell CN, Sharrock NE. Cardiac arrest during hip arthroplasty with a cemented long-stem component. A report of seven cases. J Bone Joint Surg Am 1991; 73:271–277.
42. Mandel RJ, Brown MD, McCollough NC III, et al. Hypotensive anesthesia and autotransfusion in spinal surgery. Clin Orthop 1981; 27–33.
43. Dilger JA, Tetzlaff JE, Bell GR, et al. Ischaemic optic neuropathy after spinal fusion. Can J Anaesth 1998; 45: 63–66.
44. Grundy BL, Nash CL Jr, Brown RH. Deliberate hypotension for spinal fusion: prospective randomized study with evoked potential monitoring. Can Anaesth Soc J 1982; 29:452–462.
45. Sharrock NE, Mineo R, Urquhart B. Haemodynamic effects and outcome analysis of hypotensive extradural anaesthesia in controlled hypertensive patients undergoing total hip arthroplasty. Br J Anaesth 1991; 67:17–25.
46. Dahl OE, Pedersen T, Kierulf P, et al. Sequential intrapulmonary and systemic activation of coagulation and fibrinolysis during and after total hip replacement surgery. Thromb Res 1993; 70:451–458.
47. Lentschener C, Benhamou D. The blood sparing effect of aprotinin should be revisited. Anesthesiology 1998; 89:1598–1600.
48. Dietrich W, Spannagl M, Jochum M, et al. Influence of high-dose aprotinin treatment on blood loss and coagulation patterns in patients undergoing myocardial revascularization. Anesthesiology 1990; 73:1119–1126.
49. Royston D. High-dose aprotinin therapy: a review of the first five years' experience. J Cardiothorac Vasc Anesth 1992; 6:76–100.
50. Harke H, Gennrich M. [Aprotinin-ACD-blood: I. Experimental studies on the effect of aprotinin on the plasmatic and thrombocytic coagulation (author's translation)]. Anaesthesist 1980; 29:266–276.
51. Engel JM, Hohaus T, Ruwoldt R, et al. Regional hemostatic status and blood requirements after total knee arthroplasty with and without tranexamic acid or aprotinin. Anesth Analg 2001; 92:775–780.
52. Neilipovitz DT, Murto K, Hall L, et al. A randomized trial of tranexamic acid to reduce blood transfusion for scoliosis surgery. Anesth Analg 2001; 93:82–87.
53. Amar D, Grant FM, Zhang H, et al. Antifibrinolytic therapy and perioperative blood loss in cancer patients undergoing major orthopedic surgery. Anesthesiology 2003; 98:337–342.
54. Capdevila X, Calvet Y, Biboulet P, et al. Aprotinin decreases blood loss and homologous transfusions in patients undergoing major orthopedic surgery. Anesthesiology 1998; 88:50–57.
55. Lentschener C, Cottin P, Bouaziz H, et al. Reduction of blood loss and transfusion requirement by aprotinin in posterior lumbar spine fusion. Anesth Analg 1999; 89: 590–597.
56. Murkin JM, Shannon NA, Bourne RB, et al. Aprotinin decreases blood loss in patients undergoing revision or bilateral total hip arthroplasty. Anesth Analg 1995; 80: 343–348.
57. Janssens M, Joris J, David JL, et al. High-dose aprotinin reduces blood loss in patients undergoing total hip replacement surgery. Anesthesiology 1994; 80:23–29.
58. Keegan MT, Whatcott BD, Harrison BA. Osteogenesis imperfecta, perioperative bleeding, and desmopressin. Anesthesiology 2002; 97:1011–1013.
59. Sieber PR, Belis JA, Jarowenko MV, Rohner TJ Jr. Desmopressin control of surgical hemorrhage secondary to prolonged bleeding time. J Urol 1988; 139: 1066–1067.
60. Guay J, Reinberg C, Poitras B, et al. A trial of desmopressin to reduce blood loss in patients undergoing spinal fusion for idiopathic scoliosis. Anesth Analg 1992; 75:405–410.
61. Reynolds LM, Nicolson SC, Jobes DR, et al. Desmopressin does not decrease bleeding after cardiac operation in young children. J Thorac Cardiovasc Surg 1993; 106:954–958.

62. Faris P. Use of recombinant human erythropoietin in the perioperative period of orthopedic surgery. Am J Med 1996; 101:28S–32S.
63. Goldberg MA, McCutchen JW, Jove M, et al. A safety and efficacy comparison study of two dosing regimens of epoetin alfa in patients undergoing major orthopedic surgery. Am J Orthop 1996; 25:544–552.
64. de Andrade JR, Jove M, Landon G, et al. Baseline hemoglobin as a predictor of risk of transfusion and response to Epoetin alfa in orthopedic surgery patients. Am J Orthop 1996; 25:533–542.
65. Smith RE Jr, Jaiyesimi IA, Meza LA, et al. Novel erythropoiesis stimulating protein (NESP) for the treatment of anaemia of chronic disease associated with cancer. Br J Cancer 2001; 84(suppl 1):24–30.
66. Heatherington AC, Schuller J, Mercer AJ. Pharmacokinetics of novel erythropoiesis stimulating protein (NESP) in cancer patients: preliminary report. Br J Cancer 2001; 84(suppl 1):11–16.
67. Hur SR, Huizenga BA, Major M. Acute normovolemic hemodilution combined with hypotensive anesthesia and other techniques to avoid homologous transfusion in spinal fusion surgery. Spine 1992; 17:867–873.
68. Burbi L, Gregoretti C, Borghi B, Pignotti E. Effects of predeposit and intentional perioperative haemodilution on blood saving program in major orthopaedic surgery. Int J Artif Organs 1999; 22:635–639.
69. Dennis DA. Blood conservation in revision total hip arthroplasty. Semin Arthroplasty 1992; 3:246–256.
70. Mertes N, Booke M, Van Aken H. Strategies to reduce the need for peri-operative blood transfusion. Eur J Anaesthesiol Suppl 1997; 14:24–32; discussion 3–4.
71. Kenan S, Hortobagyi GN. Skeletal complications. In: Bast RCJ, Kufe DW, Pollock RE, et al., eds. Cancer Medicine. Hamilton, ON: B.C. Decker, 2000:2279–2290.
72. Hortobagyi GN. Novel approaches to the management of bone metastases in patients with breast cancer. Semin Oncol 2002; 29:134–144.
73. Wenda K, Runkel M, Degreif J, Ritter G. Pathogenesis and clinical relevance of bone marrow embolism in medullary nailing—demonstrated by intraoperative echocardiography. Injury 1993; 24(suppl 3):S73–S81.
74. Dambrosio M, Tullo L, Moretti B, et al. [Hemodynamic and respiratory changes during hip and knee arthroplasty. An echocardiographic study]. Minerva Anestesiol 2002; 68:537–547.
75. Hirsh J, Dalen J, Guyatt G. The sixth (2000) ACCP guidelines for antithrombotic therapy for prevention and treatment of thrombosis. American College of Chest Physicians. Chest 2001; 119:1S–2S.
76. Sharrock NE, Ranawat CS, Urquhart B, Peterson M. Factors influencing deep vein thrombosis following total hip arthroplasty under epidural anesthesia. Anesth Analg 1993; 76:765–771.
77. Davis FM, Laurenson VG, Gillespie WJ, et al. Leg blood flow during total hip replacement under spinal or general anaesthesia. Anaesth Intensive Care 1989; 17:136–143.
78. Modig J. Influence of regional anesthesia, local anesthetics, and sympathicomimetics on the pathophysiology of deep vein thrombosis. Acta Chir Scand Suppl 1989; 550:119–124. discussion 24–27.
79. Thorburn J, Louden JR, Vallance R. Spinal and general anaesthesia in total hip replacement: frequency of deep vein thrombosis. Br J Anaesth 1980; 52: 1117–1121.
80. Horlocker TT, Wedel DJ. Neurologic complications of spinal and epidural anesthesia. Reg Anesth Pain Med 2000; 25:83–98.
81. Horlocker TT, Wedel DJ, Benzon H, et al. Regional anesthesia in the anticoagulated patient: defining the risks (the second ASRA Consensus Conference on Neuraxial Anesthesia and Anticoagulation). Reg Anesth Pain Med 2003; 28:172–197.
82. Vandermeulen EP, Van Aken H, Vermylen J. Anticoagulants and spinal-epidural anesthesia. Anesth Analg 1994; 79:1165–1177.
83. Christie J, Robinson CM, Pell AC, et al. Transcardiac echocardiography during invasive intramedullary procedures. J Bone Joint Surg Br 1995; 77:450–455.
84. Pell AC, Christie J, Keating JF, Sutherland GR. The detection of fat embolism by transoesophageal echocardiography during reamed intramedullary nailing. A study of 24 patients with femoral and tibial fractures. J Bone Joint Surg Br 1993; 75: 921–925.
85. Kallos T, Enis JE, Gollan F, Davis JH. Intramedullary pressure and pulmonary embolism of femoral medullary contents in dogs during insertion of bone cement and a prosthesis. J Bone Joint Surg Am 1974; 56: 1363–1367.
86. Mellor A, Soni N. Fat embolism. Anaesthesia 2001; 56: 145–154.
87. Gurd AR, Wilson RI. The fat embolism syndrome. J Bone Joint Surg Br 1974; 56B:408–416.
88. Lindeque BG, Schoeman HS, Dommisse GF, et al. Fat embolism and the fat embolism syndrome. A double-blind therapeutic study. J Bone Joint Surg Br 1987; 69: 128–131.
89. Bulger EM, Smith DG, Maier RV, Jurkovich GJ. Fat embolism syndrome. A 10-year review. Arch Surg 1997; 132:435–439.
90. Arthurs MH, Morgan OS, Sivapragasam S. Fat embolism syndrome following long bone fractures. West Indian Med J 1993; 42:115–117.
91. ten Duis HJ. The fat embolism syndrome. Injury 1997; 28:77–85.
92. Halbert J, Crotty M, Cameron ID. Evidence for the optimal management of acute and chronic phantom pain: a systematic review. Clin J Pain 2002; 18:84–92.
93. Morey TE, Giannoni J, Duncan E, et al. Nerve sheath catheter analgesia after amputation. Clin Orthop 2002; 281–289.
94. Lambert A, Dashfield A, Cosgrove C, et al. Randomized prospective study comparing preoperative epidural and intraoperative perineural analgesia for

the prevention of postoperative stump and phantom limb pain following major amputation. Reg Anesth Pain Med 2001; 26:316–321.
95. Enneking FK, Scarborough MT, Radson EA. Local anesthetic infusion through nerve sheath catheters for analgesia following upper extremity amputation. Clinical report. Reg Anesth 1997; 22:351–356.
96. Gehling M, Tryba M. [Prophylaxis of phantom pain: is regional analgesia ineffective?]. Schmerz 2003; 17: 11–19.
97. Ben Abraham R, Marouani N, Weinbroum AA. Dextromethorphan mitigates phantom pain in cancer amputees. Ann Surg Oncol 2003; 10:268–274.
98. Weinbroum AA, Gorodetzky A, Nirkin A, et al. Dextromethorphan for the reduction of immediate and late postoperative pain and morphine consumption in orthopedic oncology patients: a randomized, placebo-controlled, double-blind study. Cancer 2002; 95:1164–1170.
99. Holmes FF, Fouts TL. Metastatic cancer of unknown primary site. Prog Clin Cancer 1973; 5:21–24.

29

Perioperative Care of Intraoperative Chemotherapy and Radiation: Limb and Peritoneal Perfusion Procedures

RICHARD E. ROYAL and PAUL F. MANSFIELD

Division of Surgical Oncology, The University of Texas M.D. Anderson Cancer Center, Houston, Texas, U.S.A.

I. INTRODUCTION

One limitation of systemic chemotherapy is that toxicity of a nontargeted organ restricts the amount of drug that can be administered to a patient, often to a dose lower than is necessary for killing the treated malignancy. This limitation may be overcome in diseases that are regionally confined by delivering the chemotherapy in an isolated perfusion system where systemic absorption and exposure of distant organs are minimized. These systems allow for high doses of chemotherapy to be delivered to an isolated region or organ within the patient. Not infrequently, such a high dose can be used in this fashion that it would be lethal if delivered systemically, but when sequestered in the region of the malignancy, may have a high enough dose to be tumoricidal and tolerable.

For example, a chemotherapeutic agent may cause bone marrow suppression, and thus has neutropenia as its dose-limiting toxicity. By perfusing an organ, body region or cavity using an isolated circuit, and delivering the agent for a short period of time, little systemic absorption occurs, and the bone marrow is spared exposure to the agent. Therefore, a higher dose of chemotherapy can be delivered through the isolated circuit, one that is more likely to be cytotoxic to the malignant cells, but with a low systemic concentration and therefore a low systemic toxicity.

This is the rationale for the delivery of chemotherapeutic agents using an isolated circuit: to maximize cytotoxicity while minimizing the dose-limiting toxicity seen by systemic administration of any given agent.

Hyperthermia is an additional modality frequently added to isolated perfusion. Tumor cells have been shown to be particularly sensitive to hyperthermia with cell death induced at a lower temperature than normal tissue (1,2). To take advantage of this unique property, the perfusate can be heated prior to perfusion of the organ or region. This in turn results in hyperthermia of the isolated treatment field.

There are several limitations to this hyperthermic isolated perfusion. By definition, this approach is only applicable to regionally isolated malignancies. Tumors with systemic spread will not be adequately treated with this approach. Only in rare circumstances should isolated perfusion be used in patients with disease outside the perfusion field (3). Also, because a region or body organ must be physically isolated, an operation is usually required for the delivery of the drug. The operation required is often quite extensive. This exposes the patient to the risks of the procedure in addition to any of those of the treatment and oftentimes restricts the treatment to a one-time application.

The initial applications of hyperthermic isolated perfusion were delivered through a vascular circuit to an extremity. After isolating the vascular system to an organ or region (such as an extremity), vascular cannulae, advanced into the artery and vein of the organ or region, are attached to a cardiopulmonary bypass circuit including a roller pump, oxygenator, and heater. With this circuit, a separate vascular circulation is established for the organ or region and chemotherapy can be delivered to this sequestered region.

This vascular model of regional treatment has also been applied using isolated lung perfusion (4,5), isolated liver perfusion (6,7), and as well as isolated limb perfusion. Isolated limb perfusion, in the upper or lower extremity, is the most widely applied scenario of vascular perfusions.

Isolated perfusion can also be applied using a nonvascular circuit. This is the method used when circulating chemotherapy through a body cavity. The afferent cannula is placed usually in the upper portion of the cavity and the efferent cannulae placed at the opposing end of the cavity. A high-dose chemotherapy solution is then circulated through the cavity attempting to obtain uniform distribution over all the surfaces of the cavity. This has been utilized for pelvic perfusion (8), pleural perfusion (9,10), but is most widely utilized for perfusion of the entire peritoneal cavity as first described by Spratt et al. (11) 1980 in.

We will focus on isolated limb perfusion and peritoneal perfusion in this chapter as prototypic examples of regional perfusions. Unique perioperative issues arise with each of these types of regional perfusion. These issues may be related to the procedure itself, to the chemotherapeutic agent or hyperthermia delivered, as well as to any systemic leak of the regional perfusate. In this type of dynamic system, it is often difficult to separate the contribution any one component may have to the pathophysiology of any given perioperative event. We will address indications, technique, and results of each of these procedures and then the major issues surrounding the perioperative care of these patients.

II. OPERATIVE PROCEDURES

A. Isolated Limb Perfusion

1. Indications

Isolated limb perfusion (ILP), while first described for melanoma, has emerged as a methodology also used in the management of other tumors such as soft-tissue sarcomas in an attempt to convert a situation where amputation is necessary to one where limb salvage may be achieved. Creech and the group at Tulane University first described the technique in 1958 (12). Following the successful development of animal models for limb, liver, and midgut perfusion, the technique was extended to a man with more than 80 intransit (regional) melanoma metastases in a lower extremity. He was perfused with melphalan using normothermia and achieved a durable complete response. He was disease free at his death 16 years following treatment (13).

The procedure has evolved as a standard approach for patients with stage IIIA and IIIAB melanoma by the old MD Anderson staging criteria (Table 1). These are patients who would be considered under the current American Joint Commission on Cancer/International Union Against Cancer (AJCC/UICC) staging system to have stage III disease under either the N2 or N3 category (14). Isolated limb perfusion has also been studied in stages I and II of disease, in an attempt to prevent the development of intransit disease. While there are significant problems with the design and targeted populations in these studies, it has offered no benefit as an adjuvant and is not recommended as a treatment for melanoma without intransit disease present (15). Isolated limb perfusion has also been used for soft-tissue sarcoma in an attempt to convert an otherwise unresectable tumor into one that can be excised with a limb sparing procedure (16). Isolated limb perfusion also has anecdotally been used for other histologies such as Merkle cell tumor.

2. Procedure

Following the establishment of general anesthesia, the vessels supplying the affected limb are isolated. In the arm, the axillary vessels, and for perfusions below the knee, the superficial femoral vessels are isolated. Most frequently, a full perfusion of the lower extremity is employed. Through a retroperitoneal approach, the deep inguinal lymph nodes are excised and the external iliac artery and vein of the involved leg isolated. Collaterals are controlled or ligated from the common iliac vessels to below the level of the inguinal ligament, to minimize leak into the systemic circulation.

Table 1 The M.D. Anderson Staging System

Stage	Definition
I	Primary disease
II	Local recurrences of satellites within 3 cm of the original tumor
IIIA	Intransit disease more than 3 cm from primary tumor
IIIB	Regional node involvement
IIIAB	Intransit disease and positive nodes
IV	Distant metastases (includes positive iliac or supraclavicular nodes)

Cannulae placed into the lumen of the iliac vessels are advanced to the level of the common femoral artery and vein and an isolated circulation established with a cardiopulmonary bypass circuit comprised of a reservoir, roller pump, heat exchanger, and membrane oxygenator. A tourniquet above the level of the tips of the cannulae prevents flow along small collaterals between the limb and the systemic circulation, and defines the proximal extent of perfusion. The actual proximal limit of the perfusion is usually several centimeters below the actual level of the tourniquet. The perfusion circuit is primed with banked blood (either allogeneic of autologous) and saline and the inflow heated to establish hyperthermia. The perfusate flows through the inflow cannulae into the limb's arterial system, circulates throughout the limb and flows from the vein into the outflow cannulae. The extremity is also wrapped in sterile warming blankets to maintain extremity temperature, which is monitored using four thermistor probes placed beneath the skin surface. Chemotherapy introduced into the reservoir can then be circulated in an isolated fashion to treat the limb.

At the conclusion of perfusion, the limb is flushed with low molecular weight dextran and the cannulae removed and systemic circulation re-established to the limb with vascular repair. The limb may be wrapped to minimize posttreatment edema. Fasciotomies may be necessary in some cases and rarely may need to be completed at the conclusion of perfusion in a limb with marked early edema.

3. *Response*

The response rates to ILP have been studied mainly in patients with melanoma. Primarily, melphalan has been the chemotherapeutic agent used in the perfusion circuit. The addition of tumor necrosis factor-alpha (TNF) has been advocated by some authors, but conclusive results regarding the effectiveness of this regimen are still pending. After the initial, very impressive results by the Dutch group reported in abstract form in the early 1990s, attempts to corroborate these results in the United States have been marked by various frustrations. In the late 1990s Lienard et al. presented the results of a randomized phase II study with similar excellent results, for both arms of this study where interferon-gamma was the variable. In this study, 64 patients with melanoma were treated by ILP with TNF, melphalan with or without interferon-gamma. Overall, a complete response was measured in 47 patients and a partial response in 14 patients with median overall survival just over 29 months and the interferon-gamma seemed to add little to the response rates (17). The biggest frustration has been the intermittent nature of the availability of TNF. Fraker et al. at the NCI with palliative ILP using melphalan or melphalan and TNF treated patients with systemic melanoma and bulky limb disease. The patients treated with melphalan alone showed a 17% complete response rate, while those treated with melphalan and TNF showed a complete response rate of 64%. Also, patients with stage III disease have been treated in a multicenter trial including the NCI and MD Anderson Cancer Center using TNF and melphalan vs. melphalan alone. Published results of this trial are still pending, but an interim analysis shows a complete response rate of melphalan plus TNF and melphalan alone of 80% and 61% respectively (18). The American College of Surgeons Oncology Group (ACOSOG) trial Z0020 is ongoing and compares these two regimens in the treatment of stage III melanoma, though this trial as well has been closed on at least two occasions due to lack of the availability of TNF.

Noncomparative trials have shown a therapeutic effect of ILP applied to patients with melanoma. Fraker et al. (19) at the NCI found, in 38 patients with melanoma treated by ILP utilizing interferon-gamma, melphalan, and escalating doses of TNF, a complete response in 23 patients and a partial response in 11 patients. Interestingly, patients who are perfused with TNF will have visible treatment effects against the tumor within 24 hr indicating an alternative method of action from the melphalan alone.

B. Continuous Hyperthermic Peritoneal Perfusion

1. *Indications*

Continuous hyperthermic peritoneal perfusion (CHPP) is designed to treat regional malignancy that has metastasized to the peritoneal cavity and peritoneal surfaces. Weisberger et al. (20) are credited with the first intraperitoneal delivery of chemotherapeutic agents in 1955. Spratt et al. (11) are credited with performing the first hyperthermic peritoneal perfusion in a person in 1980. Speyer et al. (21) further explored intraperitoneal therapy (without hyperthermia) by carefully analyzing chemotherapeutic concentration and absorption in human subjects. CHPP evolved from this early work through extensive application as a treatment modality in Japan for gastric cancer but has come full circle and is now used primarily for appendiceal tumors in this country.

This treatment strategy is based on the redistribution phenomenon of peritoneal carcinomatosis that has been described by Sugarbaker (22) for pseudomyxoma peritoneii. In this model of tumor spread, tumor cells are released within the peritoneal cavity and circulate with the peritoneal fluid. Tumor cells that lack adhesion properties deposit on peritoneal surfaces by gravity, or at sites of peritoneal fluid reabsorption. These deposited cells are immobilized by extruded mucin, proliferate, and establish neovascularity becoming established metastatic implants. Disease is thus limited to the peritoneal cavity, not disseminating through the lymphatic or vascular systems. There has been a recent report with intriguing potential ramifications from a randomized trial in the Netherlands where perfusion was found to be highly beneficial for patients with carcinomatosis from colon cancer (23). There are currently discussions underway in this country to conduct a similar type study. In the absence of a clinical trial, we currently employ this approach for patients with tumors of the appendix (with some histologic restrictions) that have spread to the peritoneal cavity.

2. *Procedure*

Treatment is delivered to patients under general anesthesia. Optimal intraoperative monitoring includes the use of a transduced arterial catheter and pulmonary artery catheter for hemodynamic monitoring. Core temperature must be monitored continuously. An esophageal temperature probe is adequate for this and the patient is initially passively cooled to below 35°C (with some using temperatures below 34°C). This is accomplished by not heating the infused intravenous fluids or inspired gases, keeping the room cool with a cooling blanket and in some circumstances packing the patient in ice.

A critical part of an effective CHPP is the resection and debridement of all visible tumor, minimizing implants to less than 2 mm thickness to optimize drug penetration of any remaining disease, as drug may adequately penetrate only about 5 mm. This is accomplished both by resection of encased organs, and debridement of isolated implants or plaques of implanted tumor. Heated chemotherapy can then be delivered to bathe the remaining surfaces and any microscopic residual disease.

Organs most frequently resected for debulking include the greater and lesser omentum, right colon, gallbladder, spleen, sigmoid colon, uterus with salpinx, and ovaries. Less commonly, the pancreatic tail, stomach, or total abdominal colon are removed. The excision of the right hemicolon can eliminate encasing disease; it is also indicated regardless of tumor bulk when treating patients with appendiceal cancer to effect a nodal dissection of the primary nodal basin and has been shown in one study to advance median survival (24). Remaining implants may then be excised from peritoneal surfaces. Resection of implants on the parietal peritoneum is predictably easier than debridement of those on visceral peritoneum. Additional length of colon or small bowel may be resected for regions of visceral peritoneal plaques of tumor covering these organs.

Peritoneal stripping has been advocated by Sugarbaker (25). This includes stripping of the peritoneum superiorly covering the posterior surface of the rectus sheaths in continuity with the peritoneum covering each hemi-diaphragm exposing both the muscular and tendonous portions of the diaphragm. This is a region frequently involved with plaques of tumor. Glisson's capsule over the surface of the liver may occasionally need to be partially stripped with cautery ablation of remaining discontinuous islands of tumor on the liver surface. Argon beam coagulation can aid in maintaining hemostasis when stripping Glisson's capsule. The colon is mobilized bilaterally and peritoneum stripped at the lateral gutters when involved with tumor. The pelvic peritoneum is stripped anteriorly off the inferior portion of the rectus and the bladder; laterally, peritoneum is stripped off the iliac vessels and ureters to the level of the vagina in women or seminal vesicles in men when tumor deposits are in these areas. The uterus or rectosigmoid colon may then be resected if necessary to remove pelvic disease en-bloc with involved peritoneum and organs.

Some argue against extensive peritoneal striping noting that exposure of subperitoneal tissue may increase the absorption of perfusate and systemic toxicities from the chemotherapeutic agent as well as increase surgical morbidity (26). We typically will use peritonectomy if necessary to remove bulk disease particularly from the diaphragm. Following complete debulking of intraperitoneal disease, all remaining adhesions are lysed to expose all peritoneal surfaces.

Efferent and afferent cannulae are then placed within the peritoneal cavity. Several methods have been described but can generally be broken down into open and closed techniques. At the MD Anderson Cancer Center (MDACC), we use a closed technique by placing a catheter superiorly with a "Y" connector to establish inflow into each subdiaphragmatic space and a custom made collector is placed in the pelvis with an outflow channel exiting through the lower portion of the midline wound and the skin temporarily is closed around them as well as multiple temperature probes. The outflow catheters are passed through this outflow channel into the reservoir. This prevents obstruction of the outflow tract by intraperitoneal structures. Temperature probes placed in six different locations under the peritoneum as well as two needle probes into the substance of the liver in a standardized fashion allow for continuous thermal monitoring. We close the midline wound at the level of the skin. This allows for perfusion of the wall of the midline wound and preserves the integrity of the fascia for ultimate closure. Some authors advocate an open coliseum technique in which the wound edge is tethered and suspended to an oval self-retaining retractor fixed around the wound.

The circulation is established with a reservoir, roller pump, heat exchanger, inflow cannulae, and outflow cannulae in the circuit. Heated chemotherapy solution is then circulated for a period of 60–120 min. An assistant agitates the abdomen throughout the perfusion period to avoid streaming of the perfusate and maximally expose all surfaces. In an open technique, the operator manipulates the intra-abdominal contents to expose all surfaces.

The most common drugs used include mitomycin C and cisplatin. Dosing of these agents as well as the degree of hyperthermia, flow rates, volume of perfusate, and duration of perfusion vary from center to center and specific technique used. We typically will run the flow rate at 3.0–3.5 L/min. We most commonly use single agent mitomycin C at total doses between 37.5 and 65 mg in volumes between 5.0 and 6.5 L, based on patient size and previous chemotherapy exposure.

At the conclusion of the perfusion, and removal of the catheters, any necessary anastomoses are completed. Theoretically, this minimizes the risk of tumor deposits becoming lodged within the suture line, sequestered from the perfusate.

3. *Response*

CHPP has been applied to patients with various histologies; all of which develop a pattern of peritoneal spread including carcinomatosis from high-grade and low-grade malignancies of stomach, small bowel, appendix, and colon, as well as sarcomatosis and peritoneal mesothelioma. The most frequent application in this country is in patients with what is commonly called pseudomyxoma peritoneii. This is in fact a spectrum of diseases with various degrees of aggressiveness which is most commonly divided into two basic groups, disseminated peritoneal adenomucinosis (DPAM) or peritoneal mucinous adenocarcinomatosis (PMCA), both or which most commonly originate in the appendix. In Japan, the most frequent application is in patients with gastric adenocarcinoma where 5-year survivors have been reported, though these are relatively few and concerns over selection bias exist and acceptance has not been widespread (27). CHPP is very effective for the management of ascites with over 80% of patients experiencing relief of their ascites after perfusion.

Most studies of the use of CHPP in gastric cancer have been conducted in Asia and have been retrospective or prospective but only rarely, randomized trials. In a nonrandomized trial, Fujimoto et al. (28) demonstrated in a trial of 112 patients with advanced gastric cancer, those treated by gastrectomy with CHPP had 3- and 5-year survival rates superior to that of patients receiving gastrectomy with no peritoneal treatment (81% vs. 49% and 45% vs. 16%, respectively). Patients in each group had T3 or T4 tumors, some with peritoneal spread and were randomly assigned to one of the treatment arms. More recently, the same group has shown improvement in peritoneal recurrence and overall survival when CHPP is used as an adjuvant treatment in early stage gastric cancer (29). Also, in gastric cancer, Fujimura et al. (30) reported a 3-arm study of 58 patients randomized to hyperthermic perfusion, normothermic perfusion, and resection alone. In this study, patients undergoing hyperthermic perfusion had a better survival and lower peritoneal recurrence rates than for patients undergoing surgery alone. In an extension of this study, Yonemura et al. (31) from the same group reported a larger randomized group with similar results and a benefit of hyperthermic over normothermic perfusion.

For patients with appendiceal malignancies, Sugarbaker and Chang (32) the Washington Hospital Center in a nonrandomized study reported on 385 patients treated with CHPP, and found that complete tumor resection and low-grade histology can result in prolonged survival following CHPP compared to those without complete resection or with high-grade tumors. Loggie et al. (26) at Wake forest University in a phase II study demonstrated a 52% 3-year survival in patients treated for appendiceal cancer. This group also found that survival was related to ability to obtain at least an R1 resection. In their study of patients with various GI malignancies, 3-year survival in an R0/R1 resection was 62% in contrast to an R2 resection with survival of 22%. Additionally patients with ascites had a significantly lower median survival than those patients treated without ascites at the start of treatment. The Sugarbaker and Loggie series are each completed without a control study cohort, and are not directly comparable due to differences in debulking, perfusion technique, differences in histologies treated, and differences in chemotherapies utilized. At MDACC, our first 24 patients treated with CHPP for DPAM or PMCA experienced a >75% 5-year actuarial survival (33).

III. INTRAOPERATIVE ISSUES

These issues will be looked at from the perspectives of both CHPP and ILP. While they share some similarities, there are profound differences in the impact each of these may have on the patient.

A. Hemodynamics

Intraoperative hemodynamic monitoring is an important element in the efficient care of the perfusion patient. Intraoperative monitoring with a radial arterial line and pulmonary artery catheter as has been mentioned previously, is utilized in most situations. Both ILP and CHPP may be associated with significant fluid shifts and while significant blood loss is more common with CHPP, it can also occur with ILP, particularly in the reoperative setting. With CHPP using the closed technique where the patient is shaken to enhance distribution, the EKG monitor frequently will have extensive motion artifact. The arterial waveform, however, should be maintained. Close attention to the maintenance of urine output is essential during any perfusion.

Insensible and third space losses can be significant with both procedures, but may be profound during CHPP. The procedure has a prolonged course through a large abdominal wound, and a large volume of ascites is not infrequently drained during the course of debulking. Insensible losses can be increased by hyperthermia in both CHPP and ILP.

Additionally, during the course of the actual perfusion, a depression in systemic vascular resistance (SVR) is characteristically measured. Tachycardia and increased cardiac output accompany this (34,35).

Also, in CHPP, the administration of intravenous cimetidine used by some surgeons to minimize the inflammatory response to thermal injury is accompanied by a depression of the patient's systemic blood pressure (36). This effect is strongly affected by the rate of infusion.

All of these effects can be minimized with the early hydration of the patient. Pulmonary capillary wedge pressure and urine output can be a guide to maximally hydrating the patient early in the operative course. During the actual perfusion, an intravenous fluid rate of 1500 cc/hr may be required and forced diuresis may occasionally be necessary to keep the urine output greater than 100 cc/hr. More often, however, these patients will have a significant diuresis, particularly postoperatively, which must be monitored carefully as it may continue despite a low central venous pressure (CVP). The precise cause of this diuresis is unknown. We find it good practice in the first 24 hr to give fluids sufficient to maintain the CVP within a target range of 6–12 mmHg depending upon the patient. Careful attention to this detail is important in all perfusions, but especially in perfusions with cisplatin, where a higher urinary output is required. In these cases, one may also consider use of fenoldopam in the early posttreatment course for renal protection. As these cases are frequently long with significant fluid shifts, the patients usually spend a day or two in the intensive care unit (ICU), and usually not extubated until the first postoperative day.

B. Hyperthermia

During CHPP, the treated region is typically heated to a temperature greater than 40°C, while for ILP this is usually in the 39–40°C range. This is accomplished primarily through the heating of in-flow perfusate. The circulating perfusate whether through the vascular circulation in a limb perfusion, or through flow over exposed surfaces in peritoneal perfusion then heats the treated region to a hyperthermic range. This exposes residual malignancy in the treatment field to thermal levels that may be lethal to malignant cells but tolerated by normal tissue. Hyperthermia appears to alter the absorption of chemotherapeutic agents when concurrently administered. Increased temperature is associated in vitro with increased intracellular drug absorption and a steepening of the log cell death curves (2).

During ILP, heating of the perfusate alone is usually insufficient to keep up with insensible heat loss from the extremity; therefore, the limb is wrapped in heating blankets to maintain temperature. Heating must be monitored to avoid direct thermal injury to the skin when using this method. Central core heating is not a concern during ILP.

Systemic temperature rises almost immediately with the establishment of hyperthermia in the treatment field during CHPP. To avoid toxic systemic hyperthermia, the patient is usually cooled to <35.0°C prior to perfusion. This can be accomplished through passive measures, by initiating the procedure in a cool room, without heating the infused intravenous fluids or inspired gases. During perfusion, the systemic temperature rise may be delayed by the use of a cooling blanket underneath or overlying the patient. A Baer type of cooling blanket set to ambient temperature is usually sufficient. Other cooling methods used have included packing the patient's body and head in ice. Depending on the inlet temperature used, we do not find this to be necessary, though it may help minimize hair loss in patients who absorb a significant amount of the drug.

In CHPP, hyperthermia in the treatment field has been implicated in causing a "scald injury" to the peritoneal surface which results in increased microvascular permeability, peritoneal edema, increased third space losses, and hypoalbuminemia. Cimetidine may protect the peritoneal surface from this injury. Boykin et al.'s early work exposed anesthetized animals to cutaneous scalding. The administration of cimetidine blocked ultrastructural changes of the microvasculature associated with cutaneous scald injury (37). Also, fluid requirements for resuscitation in these animals were decreased (38). Extending this premise, Fujimoto et al. (39) have advocated the use of intravenous cimetidine initiated prior to perfusion as an adjunct to prevent scald injury to the peritoneum and pathophysiologic changes that precipitate capillary leak into the peritoneal cavity. His groups studied 24 patients, half of whom received cimetidine immediately before hyperthermic perfusion for gastric cancer. The patients who received cimetidine exhibited hypotension and lower measured levels of catecholamines, felt to be secondary to elevated levels of histamine following H2 receptor blockade. Unfortunately, the level of injury to the peritoneum could not be measured. In a previous study from this same group, a decrease in the loss of protein was also associated with the use of cimetidine (36).

Shido et al. (40) dispute hyperthermia as the cause of peritoneal injury, noting that in seven patients treated with normothermic perfusion peritoneal protein levels during perfusion and in the immediate postoperative period were not different than patients treated with hyperthermia. They suggest these findings support the contention that cimetidine infusion does not prevent peritoneal injury.

We do administer a large dose of cimetidine (40 mg/kg up to a total dose of 3.2 g) given as a slow IV infusion prior to beginning the perfusion. Hypotension is characteristically noted at the initiation of cimetidine administration, which is controlled, with the infusion of fluid and but more easily by adjusting the flow rate of the drug.

The liver is fairly sensitive to hyperthermia and temperatures above 42°C are lethal to the liver. We therefore try to keep the systemic temperature below 39.5°C. As a side note because of the sensitivity of the liver to hyperthermia, we are extremely reluctant to perfuse patients who have even the earliest findings of cirrhosis. We believe that early cirrhosis was a mitigating factor in one of the three patients who have suffered postoperative mortality after CHPP at the MD Anderson.

C. Perfusate Leak

1. ILP

This issue is of far greater concern for ILP than for CHPP. Isolation of the treatment field should establish a complete separation of the perfused circuit from the systemic circuit. Leak can occur either from the perfused to systemic or systemic to perfused circuits. The former is the potentially more dangerous and great efforts have been made to minimize leak from the perfused circuit into the systemic system, particularly with the advent of the use of some of the biologic agents, namely TNF. Frequently, this separation was not complete and leak rates of 10% or more were experienced. Grossly, a change in reservoir volume during a stable period of perfusion can indicate a leak into or out of the perfusion circuit.

A perfusion to systemic leak increases the toxicity of the chemotherapeutic agent to the patient. Tolerated levels of leak differ between chemotherapeutic agents. In most agents, if a large enough leak exists, it can result in a lethal toxicity. For some agents, this may be as little as 5–10%, so close monitoring of leak into the systemic circulation is imperative. The most important factor for minimizing leak is complete and full dissection of all of the collateral vessels.

Monitoring of leak from vascular isolated perfusion circuits can be accomplished by several methods. The standard adopted by most centers is by continuous intraoperative radioisotope monitoring, although other methods have been described.

Radioisotope monitoring is established by the introduction of radiolabeled erythrocytes or albumin into the perfusion circuit typically with I^{131} or Tc^{99}. A scintillation counter is placed in a precordial position and calibrated. A high dose of the radioisotope should circulate only through the perfusion circuit and treated field. An increase in counts of the circulation flowing through the heart can be used to calculate the percent leakage accurately for a perfusion to systemic leak (41). Also the monitoring system can be set to account for isotope decay. The use of this method is limited in lung and liver perfusion where precordial counts are obscured by the close proximity of perfused organs.

In an alternate method, fluorescence can be injected into the perfusion circuit. A Wood's lamp can then be used to inspect the perfused limb demarcating at the proximal extent of perfusion. Fluorescence of the skin outside of the limb or in the urine indicates a leak. The major limitation of this method is that this is a one-time test with an all or none result. When needed, fluorescein injection can be used as needed as a single test in a patient being continuously monitored by another method. We will typically use this as an initial test to detect any major leak prior to using the radioisotope.

Of historical note, systemic leak can also be measured using intermittent aliquots of systemic blood drawn from the patient during ILP. Hafstrom et al. (42) describe the measurement of melphalan in blood drawn intermittently from patient systemic circulation during ILP with melphalan. This measures the leak directly by quantifying the toxic agent but is limited by the delay in obtaining actual drug levels.

In a variation of this, Cattel et al. (43) describe the analysis of drawn blood for radioactivity in patients with radiolabeled albumin in the perfusion circuit. This method allows rapid analysis, and eliminates the need for the precordial gamma counter, but is not continuous.

Stanley et al. (44) from Boston University recently reported an innovative method of monitoring for systemic leak. In a single patient undergoing ILP, the anesthetic gas desflurane introduced into the isolated limb circuit could be measured in expired gases when a leak was artificially induced. The level of desflurane in expired gases rapidly returned to insensible when the artificial leak was reversed. This method has not been validated in a clinical study. Ideally, a prospective cohort of patients would be monitored by this method and simultaneously by continuous radio-isotope analysis to validate the accuracy of desflurane monitoring before widespread acceptance could occur. Desflurane can easily be introduced into the perfusion circuit, and monitoring of expired gas measured through commonly available equipment is nearly routine. However, this method does require that the patient not be anesthetized with inhalation agents during perfusion.

Most minor leaks can be minimized by control of the patient's systemic pressure and perfusion circuit pressure. Maintaining a gradient of systemic to limb mean arterial pressure and central venous to limb venous pressure can promote a slight systemic to limb leak. This direction of leak should be minimized though; a systemic to limb leak can dilute the drug delivered to the treatment field, decreasing the effectiveness of the delivered agent.

2. *CHPP*

A modest loss of perfusate or absorption of drug occurs in all patients undergoing CHPP. In our experience, by the end of 2 hr approximately half of the mitomycin C has been absorbed systemically and about 75% of the perfusate is recovered at the end of the procedure. A dramatic loss of perfusate from the circuit in patients treated with CHPP may indicate an injury to the diaphragm with loss of perfusate across the diaphragm into the pleural space. Patients who have had peritoneal stripping of the diaphragm can sustain a small injury allowing this type of leak. We typically maintain a small level of positive end expiratory pressure (10–15 mm Hg) during the perfusion to minimize any leak. When this has been suspected, we obtain an on table chest x-ray to determine if there is a leak and if so on which side if clinical findings are equivocal. If there is a leak, it can be handled in one of two ways: (1) the perfusion could be halted, pleural space evacuated and diaphragm repaired prior to resuming perfusion, or (2) a chest tube can be placed with connective tubing to return the fluid to the circuit. The first method may be preferable if the leak is obvious early in the perfusion.

IV. POSTOPERATIVE ISSUES

A. Complications of ILP

The immediate postoperative period of ILP is characteristically marked by both initial hypothermia and/or hyperthermia, and elevated fluid requirements. These effects are usually self-limited and resolve within 24 hr of the procedure.

Postoperative complications are not uncommon and vigilant attention for their onset can result in early intervention and relief of symptoms, and possible prevention of a catastrophic outcome. The most serious potential complication is compartment syndrome, which, while rare, can result in loss of limb. The extremity must be monitored frequently and a low threshold be maintained for considering fasciotomies. Almost all patients will develop what appears to be a blistering sunburn in the treated extremity; it is most severely seen on the sole of the foot.

Several groups have measured morbidity in the postoperative period. Systemic complications are sporadic, but regional toxicity is common. Morbidity recorded in two European multicenter trials utilizing TNF and melphalan in the perfusate is shown (Table 2).

Fraker et al. (19) at the National Cancer Institute (NCI) developed an objective scale to carefully analyze

Table 2 Regional Complications from Isolated Limb Perfusion

	European Multicenter Trial[a]	Netherlands Cancer Insititute[b]
Year	1998	1999
N	832	64
Wound infection	56 (13.3)	8 (12.5)
Deep venous thrombosis	10 (2.7)	2 (3.1)
Neuralgia	17 (4.0)	4 (6.3)
Pain	175 (42.7)	37 (57.8)

[a] Koops.
[b] Lienard.

the toxicity in five tissue groups. In a series of 38 patients treated with ILP utilizing escalating TNF, melphalan, and interferon-gamma, all patients developed some degree of skin toxicity characterized by erythema to desquamation and necrosis, 19 had toxicity greater than grade 1. Thirty-five patients developed subcutaneous edema, 21 with greater than grade 1 toxicity. Muscle morbidity including myalgias and atrophy was noted in 22 patients, 5 with greater than grade 1 toxicity. Peripheral nerve morbidity ranging from paresthesias to neuropathy was noted in 18 patients, none with toxicity greater than grade 1. Vascular toxicity was seen in a single patient, and resulted in the amputation of the treated extremity.

Tissue injury in the early postoperative period may result in long-term disability. Olieman et al. (45) with the University of Groningen found long-term morbidity to be minimal following ILP with melphalan. Ninety-seven patients from the institution were entered into an EORTC trial randomizing patients treated with wide local excision to additional adjuvant ILP compared with no perfusion. Eighty-three patients were evaluable at 12 months. Comparing the two groups, the patients in the ILP group were more likely to complain of subjective events, such as a prickling sensation when the weather changes, but no skin muscle, or mobility morbidity could be found by objective measures. Conversely, Vrouenaets et al. (46) with the Netherlands Cancer Institute evaluated the patients from their institution who were enrolled in the same multicenter trial. Of 109 patients enrolled, 65 were evaluable when examined at >15 months following treatment. Forty percent of the patients treated with lower extremity ILP exhibited limited extension at the ankle, 24% of patients in this group had atrophy of the treated limb. The mean degree of abduction at the shoulder was restricted in those patients treated with ILP of the upper extremity. This reflects our own experience at the MD. Anderson; long-term limb disability is often mild, but may be seen in patients following limb perfusion manifested most frequently as limited mobility across a joint and atrophy.

B. Complications of CHPP

As with ILP, patients after CHPP will experience significant fluctuations of body core temperature. There is also frequently a diuresis, which often begins during CHPP and continues for 24 hr postoperatively. This can actually lead to hypovolemia if it is not recognized and treated. We typically will give postoperative fluids at a rate of 125–150 cc/hr with additional boluses as needed to maintain a CVP within a range of 6–12 mmHg or pulmonary capillary wedge pressure of 12–15 mmHg.

Ileus is also a frequent complication in patients treated with CHPP. Delayed bowel function could be predicted due to bowel manipulation, bowel resection, peritonectomy, extensive lysis of adhesions, and intestinal edema following the CHPP. Esquivel et al. (47) with the Washington Hospital Center found in 45 consecutive perfusions a median postoperative ileus of 21 days. Bartlett et al. (48) at the NCI found a shorter duration of ileus with median time to regular diet of 8 days. Glehan et al. (49) with the University of Lyon, although not reporting overall return of bowel function, noted that 2 of their 56 patients had a delay of bowel function to 11 and 14 days. Differences in ileus severity may be due to the chemotherapeutic agent, treatment temperature, and duration of treatment used, with patients receiving mitomycin C having the greatest incidence of ileus (50). In about half of our patients, a gastric ileus occurs, which can last for up to 6 weeks. Because of this, we routinely place a gastrostomy-tube at the completion of the procedure. The added benefit of this is that the stomach is then permanently fixed to the anterior abdominal wall and should the patient have disease recurrence and develop a bowel obstruction, a palliative gastrostomy tube can easily be placed. Curiously, the small bowel works and we will use a feeding jejunostomy-tube placed at time of surgery and thus have a median hospitalization of 17 days.

The next most frequent intra-abdominal complications of CHPP are noted in Table 3 and include anastomotic/enteric leak and abscess formation. Intra-abdominal complications are likely related to the tumor debulking procedures including resection and peritonectomy, although it is difficult to separate the effects of hyperthermia and chemotherapy in these procedures. We believe that the perfusion roughly doubles the risk of a leak from a bowel anastamosis to about 5%.

Postoperative pulmonary complications ranging from atelectasis to adult respiratory distress syndrome (ARDS) have been described in patients following peritoneal perfusion. Intraoperatively during closed CHPP, abdominal distension and decreased diaphragmatic excursion likely result from the circulation of the large volume of perfusate through the peritoneal cavity. Predictably, slightly higher airway pressures are required to maintain ventilation during the actual perfusion.

Chen et al. (51) at Wake Forest University described postoperative pulmonary complications seen in 48 patients treated with CHPP using a closed technique. They found 76% developed atelectasis, 64% developed effusions, and 24% pulmonary edema. Pneumonia and

Table 3 Intra-abdominal Complications Following CHPP

	Washington Hospital Center	National Cancer Institute	Netherlands Cancer Institute	Lyon-Sud University
Year	1999	1998	2001	2003
N	200	27	46	56
Pancreatitis	12 (6.0)	NA	1 (2.1)	NA
Fistula	9 (4.5)	1 (3.7)	6 (13)	7 (12.5)
Anastamotic leak /bowel perforation	6 (3.0)	0 (0.0)	10 (21.7)	1 (1.8)
Abcess	5 (2.5)[a]	1 (3.7)	4 (8.6)	1 (1.8)
Bile leak	4 (2.0)	NA	NA	NA
Severe ascites	NA	2 (7.4)	NA	NA

[a] Sterile abcesses in this series, Percent in parenthesis.
Abbreviations: NA, not applicable.

pneumothorax were less frequent developing in 5% of patients for each. This group did not note any patients developing ARDS. Stephens et al. (52) at the Washington Hospital Center has reported that in 200 patients treated with CHPP, 6 patients had effusions which required drainage, 5 patients experienced pneumothorax and 1 patient suffered a pulmonary embolus. In a separate report, two patients with SIRS were described by Alonso et al. (53), each requiring prolonged intubation without identification of an infectious agent.

Loggie et al. (26) note that while atelectasis and pleural effusions are common following treatment, the majority do not call for medical intervention This has been our experience also, effusions occur in almost all patients, however, only a handful of patients have ever required intervention for this. If dyspnea limits recovery, a single thoracentesis is usually sufficient for treatment. Atelectasis is self-limiting, and with adequate pain control (we routinely employ an epidural catheter), normal postoperative pulmonary toilet is usually all that is required.

McQuelloan et al. (54) with Wake Forest University evaluated the functional status and quality of life in 64 patients the treated with CHPP by the closed technique. Multiple validated scales were used for analysis. Functional status in the majority of patients returned to baseline or improved above baseline levels by three months following surgery. Quality of life decreased postoperatively and returned to baseline by three months. In the subset of patients with ascites, improved quality of life occurred earlier in their postoperative course and rebounded to a level higher than their preoperative quality of life.

For several weeks after perfusion, patients can develop unexplained fevers, which eventually resolve without any source ever being found despite exhaustive attempts to locate one. Nevertheless fever in the postoperative patient must be taken seriously and investigated fully.

V. CHEMOTHERAPY SPECIFIC COMPLICATIONS

Chemotherapy can induce unique complications when the agent is delivered by isolated perfusion; the morbidity is specific for the agent utilized. Two common agents used for ILP are melphalan and TNF alpha, and two agents commonly used for CHPP are cisplatin and mitomycin C. We will discuss concerns specific to each of these agents. The degree of systemic toxicity, particularly in CHPP, is a function of dose of drug utilized, duration of perfusion and the extent of dissection.

A. Melphalan

Although melphalan contributes to local toxicity in ILP, its effects are augmented by the addition of hyperthermia and other therapeutic agents such as TNF (55). To minimize local edema in the perfused limb, we routinely elevate the patients treated limb above the level of the patient's heart for the first 48 hr postoperatively. Lower extremities are elevated on pillows in such a fashion that pressure to the heel is minimized to avoid pressure necrosis and/or the foot of the bed is raised. Close monitoring for edema and muscle compromise should include frequent extremity exam, pain level assessment, and vascular checks in the first 48 hr postoperatively.

Systemic effects of melphalan are minimal, but are evident when patients develop a significant perfusion circuit to systemic leak. In patients who experience a leak >10%, routine evaluation with complete blood count, differential and platelet count should be performed as profound bone marrow suppression can occur. Neutropenia is treated with Filgrastim.

B. Tumor Necrosis Factor Alpha

TNF is a constitutive immunomodulator of normal physiology, but even modest doses present in the systemic circulation can exhibit lethal effects through profound shock. In ILP, regional toxicity is exacerbated by the addition of TNF and leak must be strictly controlled due to the severe hypotension exhibited in patients with >5% leak (56,57).

Following the cessation of ILP, and the re-establishment of systemic circulation to the isolated limb, patients treated with TNF exhibit a more profound shock-like picture than those not treated with TNF. Christoforidis et al. (58) at Lausanne carefully measured hemodynamics in 69 patients treated with ILP using melphalan alone or combined with TNF. The patients treated with TNF exhibited a more profound depression in SVR, increase in cardiac index and tachycardia. The TNF group required more fluid for resuscitation and more pressor administration to maintain systolic pressures. TNF, when used in liver perfusion, resulted in elevated levels of inflammatory cytokines IL-6 and IL-8 and hypotension in patients for the first 48 hr postoperatively (6). Secondary inflammatory mediators or washout of TNF itself may contribute to the loss of vascular tone and high output shock in the early postoperative period.

As our understanding of the effects of TNF increases, interventions to control the hemodynamic effects of the drug should evolve further. Hohenberger and the group at Humboldt University demonstrated that limb perfusion patients treated with systemic pentoxifylline during TNF limb perfusion had lower levels of systemic IL-6 and LPS binding protein, and required less pressors postoperatively (59). Nevertheless, sound surgical technique and keeping any leak to a minimum is essential to minimizing toxicity from this agent.

C. Cisplatin

Nephrotoxicity can be seen following CHPP using cisplatin due to systemic absorption. Adequate hydration can help minimize the nephrotoxicity of cisplatin. Prior to perfusion, CVP should be greater than 12, or if a PA catheter is available, pulmonary capillary wedge pressure should exceed 15. During perfusion, aggressive hydration, mannitol, and forced diuresis should be used to maintain a urine output greater than 200 cc/hr. Hydration must continue during the first 24 postoperative hours to maintain a urine output greater than 200 cc/hr for the first 12 hr and 100 cc/hr the second 12 hr.

The intravenous administration of sodium thiosulfate is an important intervention during cisplatin-based CHPP to minimize nephrotoxicity. This drug remains within the vascular system, and binds cisplatinum effectively eliminating some of the cisplatin that has migrated into the systemic circulation.

In a dose escalation phase 1 study, Bartlett et al. (48) at the National Cancer Institute treated patients with tumor debulking and CHPP. Cisplatin was administered through a dose escalation scheme, and patients developed high-grade nephrotoxicity at a dose of 350 mg/m^2. Kunisaki et al. (60) at Yokohama City University treated 45 patients with adjuvant cisplatin, mitomycin C, and etopiside by CHPP after gastrectomy for gastric adenocarcinoma. Sodium thiosulfate was not used and 7% of the patients developed renal failure defined as a serum creatinine greater than 3.0. With the use of multiple agents, the contribution of cisplatin to this toxicity is not completely clear.

Cisplatin has been used in ILP, and in dose escalation studies, Fletcher et al. (61) at Oregon Health Sciences University found that local toxicities, such as rhabdomyolysis, myoglobinuria, and neuropathy limited cisplatin dose rather than nephrotoxicity.

D. Mitomycin C

The primary morbidity of mitomycin C (MMC) relates to its systemic effect of bone marrow suppression and resultant neutropenia and thrombocytopenia. Witcamp et al. (50) at the Netherlands Cancer Institute noted in 46 patients treated with CHPP using MMC that 22 patients developed neutropenia, 4 patients developed thrombocytopenia. The neutropenia led to the postoperative death of one patient in this series. Loggie et al. (26) at Wake Forest University found in 84 patients treated with MMC-based CHPP that 32 patients developed neutropenia and 44 patients developed thrombocytopenia. The suppression in this series tended to be grade 1 or 2 toxicity. In these series, neutropenia occurred within 10 days of CHPP and were of short duration.

This mirrors our own experience at the MD Anderson with MMC-based CHPP. Thrombocytopenia is infrequently seen, and is characteristically self-limiting and rarely requires intervention. Close attention to the patient's absolute neutrophil count particularly starting about postoperative day 6 reveals 30–50% of patients will develop some degree of neutropenia and in about 20–30% of patients will require the use of Filgrastim. As mentioned earlier this neutropenia is seen prior to postoperative day 10, in contrast to the neutropenia at 4–6 weeks seen with intravenous MMC. We routinely administer Filgrastim when the ANC drops below 1000 or if the drop is very precipitous sometimes before this occurs. Neutropenic fevers are not infrequent during this period. While renal failure is a known complication of mitomycin C, we have not seen this effect in our patients, perhaps because the total systemic dose the kidneys are exposed to is relatively low.

VI. SUMMARY

Isolated perfusion provides a means of delivering high levels of chemotherapy to malignancies while sparing the potentially lethal systemic side effects of these agents. The delivery requires an extensive operation, and is usually combined with regional hyperthermia to augment antitumor effect. This combination results in unique physiologic responses and a morbidity pattern, which can be complex. Intraoperative monitoring and intervention can ameliorate some side effects of the treatment. Additionally close monitoring for postoperative complications can facilitate early intervention and potentially avoid serious morbidity. Perhaps more than any other operations, these procedures truly require a team approach.

REFERENCES

1. Oleson JR, Calderwood SK, Coughlin CT, et al. Biological and clinical aspects of hyperthermia in cancer therapy. Am J Clin Oncol 1988; 11:368–380.
2. Barlogie B, Corry PM, Drewinko B. In vitro thermochemotherapy of human colon cancer cells with cis-dichlorodiammineplatinum(II) and mitomycin C. Cancer Res 1980; 40:1165–1168.
3. Fraker DL, Alexander HR, Andrich M, et al. Palliation of regional symptoms of advanced extremity melanoma by isolated limb perfusion with melphalan and high-dose tumor necrosis factor. Cancer J Sci Am 1995; 1:122.
4. Pass HI, Mew DJ, Kranda KC, et al. Isolated lung perfusion with tumor necrosis factor for pulmonary metastases. Ann Thorac Surg 1996; 61:1609–1617.
5. Schrump DS, Zhai S, Nguyen DM, et al. Pharmacokinetics of paclitaxel administered by hyperthermic retrograde isolated lung perfusion techniques. J Thorac Cardiovasc Surg 2002; 123:686–694.
6. Lans TE, Bartlett DL, Libutti SK, et al. Role of tumor necrosis factor on toxicity and cytokine production after isolated hepatic perfusion. Clin Cancer Res 2001; 7:784–790.
7. Lindner P, Fjalling M, Hafstrom L, et al. Isolated hepatic perfusion with extracorporeal oxygenation using hyperthermia, tumour necrosis factor alpha and melphalan. Eur J Surg Oncol 1999; 25:179–185.
8. DeCian F, Bachi V, Mondini G, et al. Pelvic perfusion in the adjuvant therapy of locally advanced rectal cancer. Feasibility trial and initial clinical experience. Dis Colon Rectum 1994; 37:S106–S114.
9. Matsuzaki Y, Shibata K, Yoshioka M, et al. Intrapleural perfusion hyperthermo-chemotherapy for malignant pleural dissemination and effusion. Ann Thorac Surg 1995; 59:127–131.
10. Refaely Y, Simansky DA, Paley M, et al. Resection and perfusion thermochemotherapy: a new approach for the treatment of thymic malignancies with pleural spread. Ann Thorac Surg 2001; 72:366–370.
11. Spratt JS, Adcock RA, Muskovin M, et al. Clinical delivery system for intraperitoneal hyperthermic chemotherapy. Cancer Res 1980; 40:256–260.
12. Creech O Jr, Krementz ET, Ryan RF, et al. Chemotherapy of cancer: regional perfusion utilizing an extracorporeal circuit. Ann Surg 1958; 148:616–632.
13. Krementz ET, Sutherland CM, Muchmore JH: Isolated hyperthermia chemotherapy perfusion for limb melanoma. Surg Clin North Am 1996; 76:1313–1330
14. Greene FL, Page DL, Fleming ID, et al. Melanoma of the skin. In: Greene FL, ed. AJCC Cancer Staging Manual. 6th ed. Philadelphia, PA: Lippincott Raven Publishers, March 2002: 209–220.
15. Molife R, Hancock BW. Adjuvant therapy of malignant melanoma. Crit Rev Oncol Hematol 2002; 44: 81–102.
16. Feig BW. Isolated limb perfusion for extremity sarcoma. Curr Oncol Rep 2000; 2:491–494.
17. Lienard D, Eggermont AM, Koops HS, et al. Isolated limb perfusion with tumour necrosis factor-alpha and melphalan with or without interferon-gamma for the treatment of in-transit melanoma metastases: a multicentre randomized phase II study. Melanoma Res 1999; 9:491–502.
18. Alexander HR Jr, Fraker DL, Bartlett DL. Isolated limb perfusion for malignant melanoma. Semin Surg Oncol 1996; 12:416–428.
19. Fraker DL, Alexander HR, Andrich M, et al. Treatment of patients with melanoma of the extremity using hyperthermic isolated limb perfusion with melphalan, tumor necrosis factor, and interferon-gamma: results of a tumor necrosis factor dose-escalation study. J Clin Oncol 1996; 14:479–489.
20. Weisberger AS, Levine B, Storaasli JP. Use of nitrogen mustard in treatment of serous effusions of neoplastic origin. J Am Med Assoc 1955; 159:1704–1707.
21. Speyer JL, Collins JM, Dedrick RL, et al. Phase I and pharmacological studies of 5-fluorouracil administered intraperitoneally. Cancer Res 1980; 40:567–572.
22. Sugarbaker PH: Pseudomyxoma peritonei. A cancer whose biology is characterized by a redistribution phenomenon. Ann Surg 1994; 219:109–111.
23. Verwaal VJ, van Ruth S, de Bree E, et al. Randomized trial of cytoreduction and hyperthermic intraperitoneal

chemotherapy versus systemic chemotherapy and palliative surgery in patients with peritoneal carcinomatosis of colorectal cancer. J Clin Oncol 2003; 21: 3737–3743.
24. Nitecki SS, Wolff BG, Schlinkert R, et al. The natural history of surgically treated primary adenocarcinoma of the appendix. Ann Surg 1994; 219:51–57.
25. Sugarbaker PH. Peritonectomy procedures. Cancer Treat Res 1996; 82:235–253.
26. Loggie BW, Fleming RA, McQuellon RP, et al. Cytoreductive surgery with intraperitoneal hyperthermic chemotherapy for disseminated peritoneal cancer of gastrointestinal origin. Am Surg 2000; 66:561–568.
27. Yonemura Y, Bandou E, Kinoshita K, et al. Effective therapy for peritoneal dissemination in gastric cancer. Surg Oncol Clin N Am 2003; 12:635–648.
28. Fujimoto S, Takahashi M, Mutou T, et al. Survival time and prevention of side effects of intraperitoneal hyperthermic perfusion with mitomycin C combined with surgery for patients with advanced gastric cancer. Cancer Treat Res 1996; 81:169–176.
29. Fujimoto S, Takahashi M, Mutou T, et al. Successful intraperitoneal hyperthermic chemoperfusion for the prevention of postoperative peritoneal recurrence in patients with advanced gastric carcinoma. Cancer 1999; 85:529–534.
30. Fujimura T, Yonemura Y, Muraoka K, et al. Continuous hyperthermic peritoneal perfusion for the prevention of peritoneal recurrence of gastric cancer: randomized controlled study. World J Surg 1994; 18:150–155.
31. Yonemura Y, de Aretxabala X, Fujimura T, et al. Intraoperative chemohyperthermic peritoneal perfusion as an adjuvant to gastric cancer: final results of a randomized controlled study. Hepatogastroenterology 2001; 48:1776–1782.
32. Sugarbaker PH, Chang D. Results of treatment of 385 patients with peritoneal surface spread of appendiceal malignancy. Ann Surg Oncol 1999; 6:727–731.
33. Mansfield PF. Appendiceal malignancy: where do we stand? Ann Surg Oncol 1999; 6:715–716.
34. Esquivel J, Angulo F, Bland RK, et al. Hemodynamic and cardiac function parameters during heated intraoperative intraperitoneal chemotherapy using the open "coliseum technique". Ann Surg Oncol 2000; 7: 296–300.
35. Shime N, Lee M, Hatanaka T. Cardiovascular changes during continuous hyperthermic peritoneal perfusion. Anesth Analg 1994; 78:938–942.
36. Fujimoto S, Kokubun M, Shrestha RD, et al. Prevention of scald injury on the peritoneo-serosal surface in advanced gastric cancer patients treated with intraperitoneal hyperthermic perfusion. Int J Hyperthermia 1991; 7:543–550.
37. Boykin JV Jr, Eriksson E, Sholley MM, et al. Histamine-mediated delayed permeability response after scald burn inhibited by cimetidine or cold-water treatment. Science 1980; 209:815–817.
38. Boykin JV Jr, Crute SL, Haynes BW Jr. Cimetidine therapy for burn shock: a quantitative assessment. J Trauma 1985; 25:864–870.
39. Fujimoto S, Takahashi M, Kobayashi K, et al. Metabolic changes in cimetidine treatment for scald injury on the peritoneo-serosal surface in far-advanced gastric cancer patients treated by intraperitoneal hyperthermic perfusion. Surg Today 1993; 23:396–401.
40. Shido A, Ohmura S, Yamamoto K, et al. Does hyperthermia induce peritoneal damage in continuous hyperthermic peritoneal perfusion? World J Surg 2000; 24:507–511.
41. Daryanani D, Komdeur R, Ter Veen J, et al. Continuous leakage measurement during hyperthermic isolated limb perfusion. Ann Surg Oncol 2001; 8:566–572.
42. Hafstrom L, Hugander A, Jonsson PE, et al. Blood leakage and melphalan leakage from the perfusion circuit during regional hyperthermic perfusion for malignant melanoma. Cancer Treat Rep 1984; 68:867–872.
43. Cattel L, Buffa E, De Simone M, et al. Melphalan monitoring during hyperthermic perfusion of isolated limb for melanoma: pharmacokinetic study and 99mTc-albumin microcolloid technique. Anticancer Res 2001; 21:2243–2248.
44. Stanley G, Sundarakumaran R, Crowley R, et al. Desflurane as a marker of limb-to-systemic leak during hyperthermic isolated limb perfusion. Anesthesiology 2000; 93:574–576.
45. Olieman AF, Schraffordt Koops H, Geertzen JH, et al. Functional morbidity of hyperthermic isolated regional perfusion of the extremities. Ann Surg Oncol 1994; 1:382–388.
46. Vrouenraets BC, in't Veld GJ, Nieweg OE, et al. Long-term functional morbidity after mild hyperthermic isolated limb perfusion with melphalan. Eur J Surg Oncol 1999; 25:503–508.
47. Esquivel J, Vidal-Jove J, Steves MA, et al. Morbidity and mortality of cytoreductive surgery and intraperitoneal chemotherapy. Surgery 1993; 113:631–636.
48. Bartlett DL, Buell JF, Libutti SK, et al. A phase I trial of continuous hyperthermic peritoneal perfusion with tumor necrosis factor and cisplatin in the treatment of peritoneal carcinomatosis. Cancer 1998; 83:1251–1261.
49. Glehen O, Mithieux F, Osinsky D, et al. Surgery combined with peritonectomy procedures and intraperitoneal chemohyperthermia in abdominal cancers with peritoneal carcinomatosis: a phase II study. J Clin Oncol 2003; 21:799–806.
50. Witkamp AJ, de Bree E, Kaag MM, et al. Extensive surgical cytoreduction and intraoperative hyperthermic intraperitoneal chemotherapy in patients with pseudomyxoma peritonei. Br J Surg 2001; 88:458–463.
51. Chen MY, Chiles C, Loggie BW, et al. Thoracic complications in patients undergoing intraperitoneal heated chemotherapy with mitomycin following cytoreductive surgery. J Surg Oncol 1997; 66:19–23.
52. Stephens AD, Alderman R, Chang D, et al. Morbidity and mortality analysis of 200 treatments with cytoreductive surgery and hyperthermic intraoperative

intraperitoneal chemotherapy using the coliseum technique. Ann Surg Oncol 1999; 6:790–796.

53. Alonso O, Sugarbaker PH. Adult respiratory distress syndrome occurring in two patients undergoing cytoreductive surgery plus perioperative intraperitoneal chemotherapy: case reports and a review of the literature. Am Surg 2000; 66:1032–1036.
54. McQuellon RP, Loggie BW, Fleming RA, et al. Quality of life after intraperitoneal hyperthermic chemotherapy (IPHC) for peritoneal carcinomatosis. Eur J Surg Oncol 2001; 27:65–73.
55. Vrouenraets BC, Eggermont AM, Hart AA, et al. Regional toxicity after isolated limb perfusion with melphalan and tumour necrosis factor-alpha versus toxicity after melphalan alone. Eur J Surg Oncol 2001; 27:390–395.
56. Vrouenraets BC, Klaase JM, Nieweg OE, et al. Toxicity and morbidity of isolated limb perfusion. Semin Surg Oncol 1998; 14:224–231.
57. Fraker DL, Alexander HR. Isolated limb perfusion with high-dose tumor necrosis factor for extremity melanoma and sarcoma. Important Adv Oncol 1994; 179–192.
58. Christoforidis D, Chassot PG, Mosimann F, et al. Isolated limb perfusion: distinct tourniquet and tumor necrosis factor effects on the early hemodynamic response. Arch Surg 2003; 138:17–25.
59. Hohenberger P, Latz E, Kettelhack C, et al. Pentoxifyllin attenuates the systemic inflammatory response induced during isolated limb perfusion with recombinant human tumor necrosis factor-alpha and melphalan. Ann Surg Oncol 2003; 10:562–568.
60. Kunisaki C, Shimada H, Nomura M, et al. Lack of efficacy of prophylactic continuous hyperthermic peritoneal perfusion on subsequent peritoneal recurrence and survival in patients with advanced gastric cancer. Surgery 2002; 131:521–528.
61. Fletcher WS, Pommier RF, Woltering EA, et al. Pharmacokinetics and results of dose escalation in cis-platin hyperthermic isolation limb perfusion. Ann Surg Oncol 1994; 1:236–243.

30

Anesthesia for the Patient in Remote Diagnostic and Therapeutic Locations

JOHN C. FRENZEL

Department of Anesthesiology and Pain Medicine, The University of Texas M.D. Anderson Cancer Center, Houston, Texas, U.S.A.

I. INTRODUCTION

Over the past decade, the demand for anesthesia services outside the operating room (OR) has increased dramatically because of technologic, scientific, and economic forces. As a result, anesthesia providers are spending more of their time away from the OR, providing anesthetic care to patients undergoing procedures in remote locations. Patients with cancer present a mix of challenges to the anesthesiologist. These patients are commonly much more educated about their disease and treatment options than are patients with other diseases. They have often undergone more therapies and diagnostic interventions than have other patients and as a result refuse to accept the repetitive discomfort accompanying these tests and procedures. Also, patients with chronic pain can have a striking tolerance to opioids and benzodiazepines, making careful patient monitoring and dose titration essential to conducting a safe and effective anesthetic. These patients are often physically debilitated by the disease process itself or the side effects of chemotherapy or radiation treatments. A successful anesthesia service that cares for patients with cancer in areas of the hospital outside the OR requires a careful blend of equipment, personnel, and administration.

II. MANAGING CLINICAL STRUCTURE

Hospital-based anesthesia practices have traditionally been centered in the OR. Hospitals attempt to maximize the productivity of staff and equipment while caring for each patient using strict booking, scheduling, and staffing rules and guidelines. As the practices of surgery and anesthesia have evolved, the ORs have become a limited and, hence, tightly controlled resource. Anesthesiologists and surgeons are keenly aware of the need to move patients efficiently through the process and cooperate to facilitate patient flow.

However, when implemented in other areas of the hospital the systems, procedures and processes that work well within the OR are ineffective and cumbersome. Gastroenterologists, radiologists, and radiation therapy personnel, for example, arrange the flow of patients through their care areas in a manner optimized for their style of practice. Effective integration of anesthesia services into these clinical practices requires changes not only in patient flow in the care area, but also changes in scheduling, staffing, and provider expectations in the hospital's anesthesia service.

In institutions with higher patient volumes and many remote patient care areas, it may be advantageous to create an administrative manager position, a person whose responsibility it would be to coordinate remote anesthesia services. This individual would be the central contact for all issues concerning remote cases, including scheduling patient flow and staffing. They would be the "facilitator," eliminating bottlenecks, and solving problems while having a broad overview of the remote service as a whole and functioning as the central liaison between the anesthesiology OR scheduler, providers in the remote locations, and patients throughout the system. An effective coordinator also would gather data on patient flow, satisfaction and help engineer process improvement.

The creation of an effective remote anesthesia service requires managing different expectations of provider availability, patient flow, and scheduling. Formal communication paths would need to be established to facilitate the effective integration of the OR with the remote locations. Mechanisms would need to be put in place to measure and integrate quality assurance and patient satisfaction data, which would be used to improve patient and provider satisfaction, and patient outcomes.

III. SITE ASSESSMENT

As anesthesia services begin serving remote sites, consideration must be given to the basic infrastructure required for patient safety. Given the urgent and critical nature of caring for anesthetized patients, all of the necessary equipment, pharmaceuticals, and support staff are focused on and organized around the main hospital ORs. This model does not exist in remote locations and cannot be duplicated there in a cost-effective manner.

The American Society of Anesthesiologists (ASA) has issued several statements addressing the standards of care required for patients sedated or anesthetized outside the OR, the most recent of which was approved in October 1994 (1). The standards address patient support (oxygen, suction, emergency equipment, and electricity), provider safety (scavenging of waste gases, and electrical grounding) and usability issues (adequate space, communications, and lighting). These standards are addressed in the very early planning stages of traditional operating facilities, and are part of the modern OR environment. In remote locations, however, these standards are never formally addressed. When providing remote services, it is incumbent upon the hospital administration and the anesthesia team to correct any deficiencies to meet the minimum requirements.

Providing effective and efficient remote anesthesia services requires the development of individualized models of patient flow tailored to the specific environment. This process begins with a thorough survey to assess the adequacy of the existing infrastructure, preoperative and postoperative patient care facilities, and provider support services (pharmacy, disposable supply stock, and anesthesia tech support), and identify what will be necessary to create an environment able to support a high-quality anesthetic service.

IV. EQUIPMENT

The mobility, size, weight, and cost of the anesthetic equipment and supplies needed to support the specific mission are constraining factors. Standard anesthesia machines, monitors, and OR drug carts are simply too cumbersome and delicate to transport, and they are not necessarily appropriate for the clinical situation at the remote location. The anesthetic requirements of patients at remote locations are often limited in scope because the location usually provides only one circumscribed service. As such, much of the equipment commonly found in the OR is unnecessary in the remote location. Only after the proposed site has been surveyed and the mission has been delineated, can equipment choices be made.

V. MOBILE CARTS

The ASA published standards for basic anesthetic monitoring in October 1998. These standards apply to all anesthesia care, both in and out of the OR. The ASA requires that the patient's oxygenation, ventilation, circulation, and temperature all be continually evaluated during the course of the anesthetic. With current levels of electronic integration, deploying an anesthetic cart with seven channels of monitoring (electrocardiography, pulse oximetry, capnography, noninvasive blood pressure, arterial line, temperature, and inspired O_2 concentration), disposable supplies, oxygen, suction, and pharmaceuticals is possible. This type of equipment not only exceeds the minimum ASA standards, but also gives a provider flexibility in providing quality care to compromised patients in a broad range of situations (2).

Many suppliers offer mobile carts with modular components, which allow anesthesia departments to tailor the cart to the specific requirements of a remote service. The low cost and small footprint of these carts make it cost effective to create task and service specific platforms. The resulting package can easily be transported by one person and provides a level of monitoring that enables the anesthesiologist to care for debilitated patients in locations far removed from the OR.

VI. PHYSICALLY REMOTE SITUATIONS

In the magnetic resonance imaging (MRI) and radiation therapy suites, where the physical environment surrounding the patient is harmful, the provider must monitor the patient from outside the room for extended periods. These situations require specialized equipment. In radiation therapy, for example, the anesthesia provider can use a standard set of monitors but must be in a position to view their output via either a slave display or closed-circuit television. High-radiation environments are particularly damaging to semiconductors; therefore, a dedicated set of equipment should be used in the radiation therapy suite. Accelerated device failure is not uncommon, and the intense radiation in this area routinely subjects equipment to ionizing radiation levels far in excess of manufacturer tolerances. Dedicating individual units to these areas helps to speed failure analysis and repair at biomedical equipment shops. Because damage from radiation tends to manifest itself as failure of integrated circuits, these defects are more likely to result in the effective destruction of the device and catastrophic failure of the equipment.

Magnetic resonance imaging also presents a unique set of monitoring challenges. The environment demands specially designed equipment that can absorb intense radiofrequency energy and tolerate strong magnetic fields. Commonly found in larger institutions, MRI-certified anesthesia machines enable a provider to administer general anesthesia in the MRI suite without damage to the image quality or monitoring equipment. Some specialized supplies, such as nonferrous laryngoscopes, are also needed (3). Other equipment, such as infusion pumps, contains high amounts of ferric materials and must be kept away from the magnet.

VII. COMMUNICATION

In the hospital's ORs, voice communication is usually not a problem. The fixed location and long life of an operating suite enables the allocation of resources necessary to provide excellent voice and data communication services. These services are extremely important in facilitating high-quality care with minimum waste of critical resources such as time or personnel. Until anesthesia services began to be delivered in remote sites throughout the hospital, this infrastructure was taken for granted. In remote locations, however, providers are much more dependent on existing infrastructure found at a particular site.

Telephones are a necessary item, and must be accessible to the anesthesiologist at all times. In urgent or emergent situations, the phone is a lifeline that can quickly bring assistance, supplies, or advice. As institutions grow, communication problems become increasingly manifest. The challenges of patient and provider management multiply. Those in charge of the OR schedule begin to lose situational awareness, and inefficiencies develop. In larger facilities, wireless communication can play an important role. Cellular phones with full voice, paging, and text messaging can be ideal, although many institutions have banned their use, and spotty coverage within buildings can make them unreliable. Cellular providers can improve internal building coverage by installing special base stations and using other techniques. This solution is expensive, however, and is usually undertaken as part of a hospital-wide infrastructure initiative. Several companies have created special microcellular phone systems and wireless voice over internet protocol (WiFi-VoIP) equipment designed for hospital use. These systems are excellent substitutes for cellular phones, but they are expensive. Two-way paging systems are another option for contacting providers in remote locations if the voice component can be based on landlines. These devices enable users to send and receive text messages. They are easy to use, light, rugged, dependable, and inexpensive and are useful for routine, non-time-critical messaging.

VIII. DOCUMENTATION STANDARDS

Anesthesia record keeping in the OR has moved increasingly toward computer-based and automated formats, but record keeping in remote locations has continued to lag behind technologically for many reasons. Remote locations have different record keeping needs that fit poorly into preexisting charting templates. Often remote site cases are shorter, making automation not worth the time and effort. Short turnover times between cases limit the amount of time available to initialize the system. Finally, automated recorders are not compact enough to be portable and offer a comfortable user interface. As technology evolves and systems improve, these shortcomings will eventually be addressed.

In institutions with a higher volume of cases, custom records or documentation sets may need to be created. These customized sets yield several benefits. First, they can reduce provider cognitive workload because the record matches the case at hand and anticipates common user needs. A well-designed charting document allows the anesthesiologist to focus on the case, not the record. Secondly, the custom record can be tailored to capture charges accurately and completely, increasing revenue and billing compliance. This alone can have an enormous effect on the revenue realized from remote services.

IX. PREOPERATIVE AND POSTOPERATIVE EVALUATIONS

Over the past decade, the preoperative assessment process has undergone a dramatic shift as the number of outpatient and same-day surgical procedures performed has increased. Anesthesiologists have adapted to these changes by providing preoperative evaluation clinics in which patients can be assessed days or weeks prior to surgery. The purpose of the preoperative visit, however, remains unchanged. It is time to establish a relationship with the patient, review the medical record, discuss the medical history, assess the physical condition, perform any necessary tests, and determine the appropriate preoperative medications (4).

Many patients are unable to be evaluated before the day of the procedure. For most healthy patients (ASA classifications 1 and 2), this makes little difference. As long as the patients have fasted adequately to minimize stomach volume, they are at low risk for complications. Patients with cancer, however, tend to be more debilitated and have higher ASA classifications. As such, preoperative screening becomes more important. Patients undergoing lengthy or extensive procedures would also benefit from preoperative evaluations. As discussed in the section on managing clinical structure, adapting patient flow at remote sites to patient flow models in the OR benefits patients as well as providers, and the same can be said for preoperative evaluation. The benefits of this coordination are manifest in fewer case cancellations and more optimally prepared patients.

Preoperative evaluations work well if the schedule and evaluation are coordinated. However, difficulties arise when the patients require further evaluation that results in a delay of their procedure. Clear lines of communication must be established so that the patient, anesthesiologist, and procedurist understand why the delay is necessary and what additional information or therapy is required.

Postanesthetic recovery requires specialized nurses and the infrastructure needed to support them. In smaller institutions, remote recovery units are not cost effective because of the smaller patient loads; so patient recovery is completed either by the anesthesia provider, or the patient is transferred to the OR postanesthesia recovery unit. Larger institutions can provide remote recovery areas because of higher patient volumes. Postoperative care, in these remote areas, has to conform to hospital standards of nurse training, equipment, and physician supervision.

In October 1994, the ASA House of Delegates adopted a set of standards for postanesthesia care (5). These standards apply to postanesthesia care in all locations. The document covers transport, supervision, and discharge of the patient, but the guidelines focus primarily on care of the typical OR patient. When assessing a remote location, these criteria need to be referenced when creating patient flow models and recovery care plans. These guidelines must be followed and yet remain within the budgeted limits of staffing, and remote facilities available. Accommodating these various constraints must involve the hospital's Department of Anesthesia.

X. ANESTHETIC MANAGEMENT

Anesthetic procedures performed outside the OR range from light sedation to general anesthesia. Providers of remote services must be prepared and able to safely administer this range of care using mobile equipment in unfamiliar surroundings. These cases are commonly outpatient services, and share many of their characteristics and qualities. Postoperative pain is minimal, and the procedures result in little blood loss or fluid shifts. The focus is on rapid-onset, short-lived anesthetic agents with minimal adverse side effects, or residual action. Providers have many compounds from which to choose that have been specifically developed and tailored to fulfill these requirements. The technique ultimately chosen depends on the situation, the patient, and the provider.

A clear and common taxonomy must be used when describing sedation and anesthesia. The ASA guidelines contain a very useful standard for classifying anesthetic depth. They describe the range of anesthesia from sedation to general anesthesia using objective terminology. This chapter adheres to this taxonomy as summarized in Table 1.

XI. SEDATION

Sedation is a state of anesthesia in which the patient has anxiolysis and mild analgesia but is still able to respond purposefully to verbal or tactile stimulation. Respiratory and cardiovascular functions are unimpaired and the patient is able to support his or her own airway. Drugs such as propofol, midazolam, and fentanyl and newer agents such as dexmedetomidine are used to induce sedation. Older inhalational agents, such as nitrous oxide, can be used but they require effective scavenging systems for waste gas removal.

Sedation for procedures performed outside the OR is commonly provided without any sort of anesthesia

Table 1 Continuum of Depth of Sedation

	Minimal sedation ("anxiolysis")	Moderate sedation/analgesia ("conscious sedation")	Deep sedation/analgesia	General anesthesia
Responsiveness	Normal response to verbal stimulation	Purposeful response to verbal or tactile stimulation	Purposeful response following repeated or painful stimulation	Unarousable, even with painful stimulus
Airway	Unaffected	No intervention required	Intervention may be required	Intervention often required
Spontaneous ventilation	Unaffected	Adequate	May be inadequate	Frequently inadequate
Cardiovascular function	Unaffected	Usually maintained	Usually maintained	May be impaired

Source: From Ref. 13.

provider in attendance. In many institutions, a nursing-based sedation service is the norm. These services commonly have long histories of good outcomes and provide adequate care to the general patient population (6). Providers of these services operate within a strict set of guidelines, oftentimes using weight-based "recipes" for sedation. Therein lies the problem. Cancer patients present a unique challenge. They usually have higher tolerances to narcotics and are often more debilitated by complex drug regimens and coexisting disease processes. They need much more individualized treatment and care tailored to their specific physical state. Sedation protocols become less useful when drug therapies need to be specifically tailored to the patient. Therefore, in cases where patients are more debilitated and procedures more invasive, hospitals must establish strict guidelines that delineate clinical privileges and minimal levels of training for individuals administering and monitoring sedation.

Anesthesiologists are pivotal in the creation, implementation, monitoring, and quality assurance of these hospital guidelines (7). In many institutions, increased involvement by anesthesiologists in sedation procedures outside the OR is a direct result from misadventures involving sedation provided by nonanesthesia personnel (8). At a minimum, policy defining levels of sedation, training, required patient evaluations, drugs used, and monitoring equipment is needed. The ASA addresses many of these issues in its practice guideline, "Guidelines for Sedation and Analgesia by Non-Anesthesiologists" (9).

XII. DEEP SEDATION

The term deep sedation refers to a level of anesthesia in which purposeful movement can be elicited with painful stimuli. At this level of sedation, patients may not be able to support his or her own airway, or maintain adequate ventilation. Drugs commonly used are propofol, fentanyl, and midazolam. Older drugs such as ketamine, diazepam, and barbiturates can be useful, but they have pharmacokinetic profiles and adverse effects that limit their use (10).

Providers administering deep sedation must be skilled in airway management, as the level of anesthesia may change from deep sedation to spontaneous breathing general anesthesia. Deep sedation is commonly required for bone marrow biopsies and other diagnostic tests. Constant vigilance of anesthetic depth and ventilation is necessary, and equipment to assist patient ventilation and maintain airway patency must be readily at hand. Capnography is a critical monitor in these cases, allowing the anesthesiologist to directly assess the frequency and pattern of respiration. This device can provide early warning of apnea, leading a fall in the reading of the pulse oxymeter by a large margin.

XIII. GENERAL ANESTHESIA

General anesthesia is a state in which the patient is unarousable even with extremely painful stimuli. Respiration is often impaired, and circulation may be affected. Management of the airway is often necessary, ranging from intubation to the use of a laryngeal mask airway. Depending on the length of the procedure and the depth of anesthesia required, an inhalational technique with a relatively insoluble agent like desflurane or sevoflurane delivered via an anesthesia machine may be indicated. In locations where an anesthesia machine cannot be accommodated, total intravenous anesthesia using propofol is an option.

Endoscopic retrograde cholangiopancreatography (ERCP), which is commonly performed in remote locations, is a procedure in which general anesthesia is often indicated. In these cases, a spontaneously breathing general anesthetic without an endotracheal tube may be necessary so that the endoscopist can manipulate the scope freely. Because access to the airway is shared with a gastroenterologist, total intravenous technique is often used (11). The patient is often positioned prone during the procedure, increasing the difficulty of airway access and management (12).

Particularly painful procedures in invasive radiology such as computed tomography guided needle biopsies or radiofrequency ablation of liver metastases also require the depth and stability of general anesthesia. Controlling the airway and respiration is necessary, as the patient is not easily accessible to the anesthesia provider, and must remain motionless for extended periods. Children oftentimes require a general anesthetic in which adults in similar situations can tolerate deep sedation.

XIV. FUTURE DIRECTIONS AND TRENDS

Over the past two decades, the number of cost-effective outpatient diagnostic and therapeutic services has increased dramatically. This trend should accelerate as more imaging and treatment modalities are developed. Anesthesiologists must keep pace with the trend by offering sedation and anesthesia services outside the OR for procedures on debilitated patients. The increasing cost of healthcare has led providers to focus more on minimally invasive and outpatient surgical procedures, and this same economic force will shape diagnostic testing. The future will find anesthesiologists practicing further away from the OR and on patients with advanced disease states and more impaired physical status. Delivering high-quality, cost-effective care in remote sites will be an ongoing challenge. All patient care departments must be prepared to offer outpatient services and learn to provide high-quality care efficiently and with high patient satisfaction.

XV. CONCLUSIONS

The demand for anesthesia services in remote locations will continue to increase as minimally invasive testing, diagnostic, and treatment procedures multiply in number and scope. The question is not if remote practice will grow, because it will. Rather, the question is how we can efficiently integrate this growing facet of the practice so that patients in remote locations will receive the same quality of care and the providers can perform as efficiently as their colleges in the traditional OR setting.

REFERENCES

1. Guidelines for Nonoperating Room Anesthetizing Locations. The American Society of Anesthesiologists, Approved by the House of Delegates, Oct 19, 1994.
2. Gagne DJ, Malay MB, Hogle NJ, Fowler DL. Bedside diagnostic minilaparoscopy in the intensive care patient. Surgery 2002; 131(5):491–496.
3. Karlik SJ, Heatherley T, Pavan F, Stein J, Lebron F, Rutt B, Carey L, Wexler R, Gelb A. Patient anesthesia and monitoring at a 1.5-T MRI installation. Magn Reson Med 1988; 7(2):210–221.
4. Basic Standards for Preanesthetic Care. The American Society of Anesthesiologists, Approved by the House of Delegates, Oct 14, 1987.
5. Standards for Postanesthesia Care. The American Society of Anesthesiologists, Approved by the House of Delegates, Oct 12, 1988, last amended Oct 19, 1994.
6. Beebe DS, Tran P, Bragg M, Stillman A, Truwitt C, Belani KG. Trained nurses can provide safe and effective sedation for MRI in pediatric patients. Can J Anesth 2000; 47(3):205–210.
7. Patterson CH. Sedation, anesthesia update—Standards Interpretation Group at the Joint Commission. Nurse Manage 2002; 33(1):22.
8. Malviya S, Voepel-Lewis T, Eldevik OP, Rockwell DT, Wong JH, Tait AR. Sedation and general anesthesia in children undergoing MRI and CT: adverse events and outcomes. Br J Anesth 2000; 84(6):743–748.
9. Practice Guidelines for Sedation and Analgesia by Non-Anesthesiologists. The American Society of Anesthesiologists, Approved by the House of Delegates, Oct 25, 1995, last amended Oct 17, 2001.
10. Green SM, Denmark TK, Cline J, Roghair C, Abd Allah S, Rothrock SG. Ketamine sedation for pediatric critical care procedures. Pediatr Emergency Care 2001; 17(4):244–248.
11. Osborn I, Cohen J, Soper R, Roth L. Laryngeal mask airway—a novel method of airway protection during ERCP: comparison with endotracheal intubation. Poster Presentation at the American Society for Gastrointestinal Endoscopy. Vol. 53. May 20–23, 2001:AB80.
12. Koshy G, Nair S, Norkus EP, Hertan HI, Pitchumoni CS. Propofol versus midazolam and meperidine for conscious sedation in GI endoscopy. Am J Gastroenterol 2000; 95(6):1476–1479.
13. Practice Guidelines for Sedation and Analgesia by Non-Anesthesiologists, Definition of General Anesthesia and Levels of Sedation/Analgesia. Approved by ASA House of Delegates, Oct 13, 1999.

31

Oncologic Emergencies: Pulmonary Embolus, Superior Vena Cava Syndrome, Cardiac Tamponade, and Respiratory Emergencies

NICOLE D. SWITZER

Department of General Internal Medicine, The University of Texas M.D. Anderson Cancer Center, Houston, Texas, U.S.A.

ARUN RAJAGOPAL

Section of Cancer Pain Management, Department of Anesthesiology, The University of Texas M.D. Anderson Cancer Center, Houston, Texas, U.S.A.

I. INTRODUCTION

Oncologic emergencies are any acute, cancer-related events that require immediate medical attention without which the patient may experience severe or life-threatening consequences. Initial symptoms may be mild, such as a low-grade fever that may rapidly progress to sepsis in an immunocompromised patient. Or, symptoms may be severe, such as a sudden loss of neuromuscular function suggesting a spinal cord compression. In this chapter, the emphasis will be on oncologic emergencies that have in common the symptom of "respiratory distress." Medical and perioperative management of pulmonary embolus, pericardial tamponade, pleural effusion, superior vena cava syndrome, hemothorax, and airway obstruction will be discussed.

II. PULMONARY EMBOLUS

A. Overview

Cancer patients are particularly prone to develop pulmonary emboli for a variety of reasons. Thromboembolic phenomena are most common in adenocarcinomas of the breast, colon, and lung, reflecting their prevalence among the different types of cancer. Adjusted for their relative prevalence, carcinomas of the pancreas, ovary, and brain tend to cause the most thromboembolic phenomena (1). There may be increased emboli related to the tumor, increased risk of hypercoagulability related to the underlying malignancy or chemotherapy, increased rates of venous stasis, or platelet abnormalities. More than 90% of pulmonary emboli originate from thrombi in the deep venous circulation in the calves. About 80% will spontaneously resolve without embolization. The remaining 20% will extend proximally into the ileo-femoral veins and it is the fracture and migration of these propagating thrombi that result in clinically significant pulmonary emboli (2).

The hemodynamic consequences of pulmonary embolisms are related both to the actual mechanical obstruction of the pulmonary vascular bed and neurohumoral reflexes, which cause vasoconstriction of the pulmonary vascular bed. Pulmonary vascular resistance increases and in severe cases, may result in pulmonary hypertension and right ventricular failure.

B. Signs and Symptoms

Signs and symptoms of pulmonary emboli depend on the size and/or number of the emboli themselves as well as the patient's preexisting cardiopulmonary status. In patients with preexisting lung disease, a relatively small embolus may cause acute right ventricular failure and systemic hypotension. There is no single symptom or sign or combination of clinical findings that is pathognomonic of a pulmonary embolism. However, since they are considerably more common in cancer patients, the clinician should maintain a high index of suspicion for their occurrence.

Symptoms of pulmonary emboli include pleuritic chest pain, dyspnea, cough, hemoptysis, and diapheresis. Patients may also report a vague sense of apprehension and anxiety, possibly related to underlying dyspnea. Much less commonly and usually in larger pulmonary emboli, a pulmonary embolus may also present a syncopal episode.

The signs of pulmonary embolism include tachycardia, tachypnea, crackles, and the attenuation of the pulmonic component of the second heart sound. A low-grade fever is present in about 40% of the cases; cyanosis, wheezing, and cardiac arrhythmias are seen in a less than a quarter of the cases. Shock is unusual and is generally associated with massive pulmonary emboli. Pulmonary emboli may mimic other clinical entities such as pneumonia, pericarditis, myocardial infarction, pneumothorax, and rib fractures.

C. Diagnostic Studies

About 90% of patients who have pulmonary emboli have PaO_2 under 80 mmHg but only about 30% have a PaO_2 below 60 mmHg. Nearly all patients with pulmonary emboli have an abnormal EKG, but the most common abnormality is simple tachycardia. Tachycardia is seen in about 44% of the patients with pulmonary emboli and ST-T wave changes are seen in about 35–49% of the cases. Acute right heart strain on an EKG is characteristic but uncommon. Since a D-dimer level >500 mg/mL is highly sensitive but not specific for the presence of thrombus, this test is most useful when it is negative (3). D-dimer levels are elevated in a variety of clinical settings such as malignancies, recent surgery, pneumonia, myocardial infarction, trauma, or sepsis. D-dimer levels of <500 mg/mL have been associated with a negative predictive value of about 94% regardless of the pretest probabilities for emboli (4).

Imaging studies used to work up pulmonary emboli include the plain chest radiograph, a ventilation/perfusion (VQ) scan, ultrasonography for venous thrombosis, pulmonary angiography, and CT/MRI scans (5). Chest radiographs are frequently abnormal although this is often related to coexisting pulmonary or cardiac disease. Pulmonary infiltrates are the most common finding. Rarely, the transient clearing (avascularity) of the normal radiographic appearance of pulmonary tissue is seen distal to an embolus (Westermark's sign). Ventilation/perfusion scans are interpreted as low, indeterminate, or high probability for pulmonary emboli. The diagnostic value of V/Q scans is enhanced by noting some basic principles. A significantly abnormal chest radiograph makes interpretation of V/Q scans difficult and a completely normal ventilation/perfusion scan rules out clinically significant pulmonary emboli. Although Doppler ultrasonography of the lower extremities does not specifically diagnose a pulmonary embolus, it should be noted that about 40% of patients with deep venous thromboses (DVT) and no symptoms of pulmonary emboli will have radiographic evidence of pulmonary emboli.

Pulmonary angiography remains the "gold standard" test for the diagnosis of pulmonary embolism because of its very high sensitivity and specificity. The finding of an intraluminal defect or an arterial cut-off on the pulmonary angiogram is diagnostic of pulmonary emboli. However, it is an invasive and expensive test and it can be difficult to interpret. In experienced hands and in conjunction with a reasonable degree of suspicion and V/Q lung scanning, pulmonary angiography may be a cost-effective tool in diagnosing pulmonary embolism. Relative contraindications to pulmonary angiography include severe pulmonary hypertension, ventricular arrhythmias, left bundle branch block, and renal insufficiency or failure.

The advances in CT and MRI scanning may supplant pulmonary angiography as the "gold standard" because of their noninvasiveness, sensitivity, and usefulness in the setting of a baseline significantly abnormal plain chest radiograph. Helical or spiral CT scanning and magnetic resonance angiography (MRA) are also used now in the diagnosis of pulmonary embolism. Spiral CT has a reported sensitivity for the diagnosis of between 63% and 98%. This test is more sensitive for the detection of emboli in the proximal pulmonary arteries and less so in the segmental arteries; specificity is about 80–95%. MRA is available at fewer centers but reports similar specificity and sensitivity.

D. Treatment

Once the diagnosis is established, it is imperative to insure that no further embolization occur if possible. If a patient is hemodynamically stable and there are no contraindications to anticoagulation, the patient should be placed on either heparin or low-molecular weight heparin immediately. A recent study demonstrated a lower risk of recurrent thromboemboli on low-molecular weight heparin vs. oral anticoagulation (6). If a recurrent embolism occurs in the setting of adequate anticoagulation, the patient should have an inferior vena cava (IVC) filter placed (7). If anticoagulation is contraindicated (e.g., a recent hemorrhage, recent surgery, high vascularity of tumor with risk of bleeding), an IVC filter should be placed immediately. A hemodynamically stable patient with a large pulmonary embolus should be followed in the ICU with the aim toward obtaining right atrial pressures of 15–20 mmHg.

For patients who are hemodynamically unstable, the treatment algorithm is considerably more complicated. The patient's cardiovascular hemodynamics may need to be stabilized with intravenous fluid resuscitation and possible inotropic support. The patient must then be anticoagulated to help prevent further clot formation and migration. Although fluid resuscitation augments preload as well as improving hypotension, caution is indicated as excessive increases in preload may further distend the right ventricle and precipitate right ventricular ischemia.

Unless there are contraindications to anticoagulation, even with only a high clinical suspicion of pulmonary embolus, anticoagulation should be started before all diagnostic studies are completed. Anticoagulation with unfractionated heparin is initiated with a dose of 5–10,000 units, depending on patient size, followed by a continuous infusion of 18 units/kg/hr. Most people rapidly become therapeutically anticoagulated with this regimen and the goal is a partial thromboplastin time (PTT) of 60–80 or $1\frac{1}{2}$ times the reference control. In stable patients, an alternative regimen is to use low-molecular weight heparin. Its advantages include efficacy, safety, and ease of administration. Warfarin is started after therapeutic levels of PTT are achieved and is usually started at about 5 mg/day. Heparin should be continued until adequate anticoagulation is (INR 2-3) achieved with oral warfarin, usually for at least 5 days. Anticoagulation therapy is continued for 3–6 months after a single event but may be continued indefinitely in patients with active cancer (8).

Thrombolytic agents may result in substantial improvements in right ventricular hemodynamics although there have been no clinical trials to date, which have been large enough to conclusively demonstrate a survival advantage. Thrombolytics are considered for unstable patients with major pulmonary emboli (9). The NIH consensus conference on major pulmonary embolism recommended thrombolytics for all patients in whom more than 40% of the pulmonary artery is obstructed by clot (10). Other indications for thrombolytics include evidence of right ventricular dysfunction or severe hypoxemia. Currently, there are three thrombolytic agents approved for use in major pulmonary emboli: urokinase, streptokinase, and tissue plasminogen activator (TPA). TPA can be infused more rapidly and thus may result in quicker thrombolysis. As mentioned above for the heparins, any anticoagulant is contraindicated in patients who have had recent intracranial surgery, trauma within the prior 2 months, currently have an intracranial neoplasm, hemorrhagic CVA, or has had internal hemorrhage within the prior 6 months.

Indications for a surgical embolectomy include refractory systemic hypotension, right atrial thrombus as seen by echocardiography, pulmonary artery pressures > 35 mmHg, and failed prior anticoagulation therapy, if indicated. Survival after an emergency embrectomy can exceed 80% as long as a patient has not had a cardiac arrest. Survival rates from an emergency embolectory after cardiac arrests are dismal. Another option is the use of transvenous catheters for removal of pulmonary emboli. Recently, self-expanding stents and catheters with rotating heads have been developed and are increasingly being used with success in setting of major pulmonary emboli.

E. Anesthetic Considerations

The majority of clinically significant pulmonary emboli are treated nonsurgically with the exception of the hemodynamically unstable patient. Even in these patients, the nonsurgical treatment options outlined above are considered the first-line options and very few patients require surgical embolectomies. Thus, patients presenting to the operating room for pulmonary embolectomies are generally in much poorer health. Due to the relatively small number of pulmonary emboli needing surgical intervention, very few prior well-established guidelines exist. However, pulmonary emboli can occur in the context of other operative procedures (e.g., some orthopedic procedures, cesarean sections) and may need to be addressed urgently (11). There are several short case series describing surgical embolectomies and the overall consensus seems to involve at least partial cardiopulmonary bypass (12–14). In one case series, in which two out of five patients died, the authors note that of the two who died, one was during induction of anesthesia and the other was during pulmonary angiography (15). The authors submit that for pulmonary embolectomies, it may be clinically advantageous to implement partial cardiopulmonary bypass *before* anesthetic induction.

A complete discussion of cardiopulmonary bypass is beyond the scope of this chapter and is discussed elsewhere. For general guidelines in providing anesthetic care for pulmonary embolectomies, the following are suggested:

1. Patients presenting for surgical relief of a pulmonary embolus are critically ill and the time between progression of the embolus and death may be brief. Thus, the anesthesiologist should be prepared for all cardiovascular contingencies.
2. Depending on the patient's clinical condition, it may be advantageous to implement femoral artery–femoral vein partial bypass prior to induction of anesthesia.
3. Maintain appropriate anticoagulation throughout the perioperative period and reverse as indicated.
4. Adequate large-bore intravenous access should be established since significant amounts of blood loss may occur quickly.
5. The anesthesiologist should have inotropic support readily available. Dobutamine has a favorable profile on both right ventricular contractility and cardiac output and is a vasodilator in both systemic and pulmonary vascular beds. Norepinephrine, in combination with dobutamine, is helpful as an inotropic combination in shock related to pulmonary embolism. Dopamine is generally less useful because of tachycardia. Isoproterenol is not indicated as it may reduce preload and in the setting of shock, may have adverse consequences.
6. Maintain the patient's acid–base and electrolyte status as close to baseline as possible. Hematocrit will fall during bypass and is considered acceptable. Slight hypothermia is maintained at about 28°C.
7. Supplemental doses of opioids, benzodiazepines, and neuromuscular blocking agents may be needed during bypass.

III. SUPERIOR VENA CAVA (SVC) SYNDROME

A. Overview

The superior vena cava (SVC) is the main avenue for venous return from the part of the body above the heart, which includes the upper extremities, head and neck, and upper thorax. Anatomically, the SVC is surrounded by the trachea, ascending aorta, right mainstem bronchus, right pulmonary artery, thoracic vertebrae, and an assortment of lymph nodes. Enlargement of any of these structures may compress the SVC and impede venous return to the heart, a condition termed "SVC syndrome." In the cancer patient, the majority of patients with SVC syndrome have lung cancer (65–85%) or lymphoma (±8%). Nonmalignant causes of SVC syndrome are less than 10%.

B. Signs and Symptoms

Facial edema is the most common symptom associated with SVC syndrome although dyspnea is the most commonly reported symptom. Since the differential diagnosis of dyspnea is considerably broader than facial edema, patients with dyspnea and SVC syndrome are usually initially worked up for other causes. Other symptoms include cough, swelling of the upper extremity, chest pain, headache, and dysphagia. Common signs include distension of the veins of the neck or chest wall, general edema of the upper extremities or face, cyanosis, or mental status changes.

C. Diagnostic Studies

Although a chest radiograph may identify a mediastinal mass, a thoracic CT or MRI remains an essential and important part of the workup. A CT or MRI can help delineate the exact anatomy and location of the tumor. In addition, if the patient needs a general anesthetic, a CT or MRI may help determine if the patient can maintain airway patency during induction. Finally, treatment for SVC syndrome is dependent on a histological diagnosis and CT or MRI may help in obtaining a tissue sample.

In addition to the imaging studies above, it is essential to obtain a proper tissue diagnosis to guide therapy. If extramediastinal sites show the presence of tumor, consideration should be given for a fine-needle aspiration or excision biopsy of these. If this is nondiagnostic, the patient may need to undergo a bronchoscopy, mediastinoscopy, or thoracotomy to obtain tissue.

D. Treatment

Treatment of SVC syndrome is dependent on histologic diagnosis (e.g., small-cell vs. non-small-cell lung cancer vs. lymphoma). For most patients, symptomatic relief can be attained with a combination of radiotherapy, chemotherapy, and/or stent placement (16). Recently, it has been suggested that stenting should be considered as a first-line treatment for symptomatic relief since it does not bias the administration of subsequent chemotherapy or radiation (17). The treatment algorithm for SVC syndrome is summarized in Fig. 1. A recent meta-analysis of the efficacy of steroids vs. radiotherapy vs. chemotherapy for treatment of SVC syndrome caused by carcinoma of the bronchus found that, in general, synchronous chemotherapy and/or radiotherapy relieved symptoms in a majority of

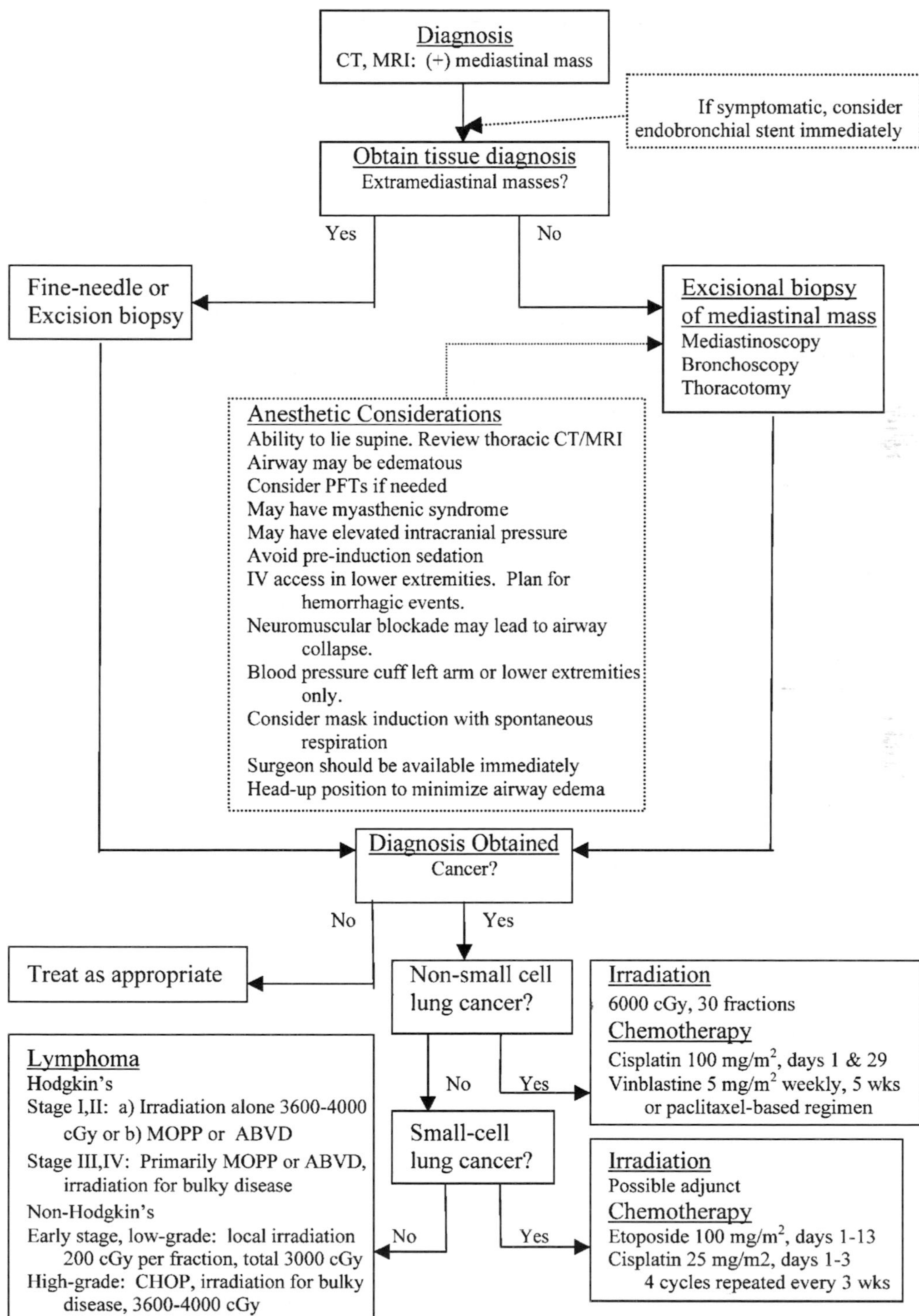

Figure 1 Diagnosis and treatment algorithm for SVC syndrome. *Abbreviations*: MOPP: mustard, oncovin, procarbazine, prednisone; ABVD: adriamycin, bleomycine, vincristine, dacarbazine; CHOP: cyclophosphamide, adriamycin, oncovin, prednisone.

patients with small-cell and non-small-cell lung cancer (18). Recurrence rates were between 17% and 20%. Insertion of a stent relieved symptoms in >95% of patients although optimal timing of stent insertion was not known; morbidity was also higher with concurrent administration of thrombolytics. Finally, this study concluded that the role of steroids remains uncertain.

E. Anesthetic Considerations

Although symptomatic relief may be achieved with the above modalities, definitive treatment necessitates a histologic diagnosis. Thus, most patients with severe SVC syndrome are likely to undergo general anesthesia to obtain a tissue diagnosis. Patients with SVC syndrome present a unique set of challenges to the anesthesiologist since the risk of total airway collapse is quite high during induction (19). The following general guidelines may be helpful in preparing to anesthetize patients with SVC syndrome:

1. Assessment of the patient's ability to tolerate the induction is critical in anesthetizing a patient with SVC syndrome. The patient should be questioned about the ability to lie supine and the development of cough or dyspnea should be noted. CT or MRI studies should be reviewed to determine the exact location of the mass.
2. On examination, check for differences in wheezing, stridor, or cyanosis between the supine and upright positions. The anesthesiologist should be aware that SVC syndrome may lead to airway edema and adjust tube size accordingly.
3. If airway compression is noted, consider obtaining a set of pulmonary function tests (PFT) with flow-volume loops in upright and supine positions. These may help determine whether an obstruction is intra- or extrathoracic.
4. Note that some patients with lung cancer may have myasthenic syndrome (Eaton–Lambert syndrome) and may be unusually sensitive to the effects of nondepolarizing neuromuscular blockade.
5. Note that some patients with SVC syndrome may also have elevated intracranial pressure and adjust anesthetics accordingly.
6. Minimize or avoid preinduction sedation.
7. Have adequate intravenous access available and plan for hemorrhagic events. Intravenous access should be established in the femoral vein since the SVC is partially compressed.
8. Note that mediastinoscopy may compress the innominate artery and lead to erroneous blood pressure measurements on the right upper extremity. Thus, the blood pressure cuff should be on the left arm or lower extremities.
9. During induction, if possible, avoid neuromuscular blockade altogether. The possibility that loss of neuromuscular tone may lead to complete airway collapse is high. A mask induction with sevoflurane/oxygen in a spontaneously breathing patient is preferred. A surgeon familiar with rigid bronchoscopy should be immediately available to stent the airway if collapse occurs.
10. The patient should be positioned in the slightly head-up position to minimize venous engorgement in the upper half of the body and minimize airway edema. However, note that this position increases the risk of cerebral embolism.
11. Note that other complications may include airway rupture or hemorrhagic events with the mediastinoscope and preparations for emergent thoracotomy should be ready.

IV. CARDIAC TAMPONADE

A. Overview

Pericardial effusions may develop secondary to neoplastic involvement of the pericardium, radiation to the thoracic area, infectious processes, uremia in end-stage renal disease patients, or some connective tissue diseases (e.g., lupus, rheumatoid arthritis) (20,21). In cancer patients, accumulation of fluid in the pericardium can occur by alteration of vascular permeability, obstruction of lymphatic efferents, and hemorrhagic events in tumors. Neoplastic pericarditis may be seen in patients with lung cancer, metastatic breast cancer, renal cell, certain lymphomas, leukemia, and primary melanoma. Most tumors involving the heart are of metastatic origin and metastatic pericardial effusions are the most common cause of cardiac tamponade. Radiation pericarditis usually follows treatments of >4000 cGy delivered to ports including more than 30% of the heart. Pericardial effusions are an ominous, late finding in metastatic cancer with only a minority of patients surviving a year beyond diagnosis. Two-thirds of malignant pericardial effusions are asymptomatic and are incidental findings on routine cardiac echocardiograms, chest CT scans, or postmortem examination.

Rapidly accumulating pericardial effusions are more likely to cause hemodynamic effects because the pericardium cannot gradually stretch to accommodate the increasing volume. Intrapericardial pressure is dependent on four factors: (1) the total amount of fluid in the pericardial space, (2) rate of accumulation of fluid, (3) intravascular volume, and (4) the distensibility of the pericardial sac. The intrapericardial pressure at which venous filling of the ventricle is impaired, 15 mm of mercury, is characterized as cardiac tamponade. In acute tamponade, the hemodynamic result of impaired ventricular filling can result in reduced stroke volume, compensatory rise in heart rate, rise in venous pressure, and possible shock and death.

B. Signs and Symptoms

Signs and symptoms of pericardial effusion and/or cardiac tamponade are shortness of breath, pleuritic chest pain, orthopnea, and weakness. Pain may be present if there is an underlying inflammatory process, such as infectious pericarditis. Painless pericardial effusions may be due to uremia or neoplastic involvement. The patient may have tachycardia, a friction rub, hypotension, jugular venous distension, organomegaly, and/or lower extremity edema although a normal examination does not rule out the diagnosis. In cardiac tamponade, the patient may develop tachycardia, tachypnea, a narrow pulse pressure, and relatively preserved systolic pressure. Pulsus paradoxus may be present but is not diagnostic and can also be seen in other processes. Beck's triad (distended neck veins, muffled heart sounds, and decreased blood pressure) may be present in only 30% of patients with cardiac tamponade.

C. Diagnostic Studies

Central venous pressure is increased and the patient may have peripheral edema and ascites. Additional testing that may be beneficial include a chest x-ray and EKG. On a chest x-ray, an enlarged cardiac silhouette may indicate a pericardial effusion although this could occur with cardiomegaly as well. An EKG may show low voltage in both the frontal and precordial leads and electrical alternans may be seen although the absence of these on the EKG does not preclude the diagnosis. Although pericardial effusions may be seen on CT or MRI, these tools do not quantitate the amount of fluid. The most useful test for this a 2D echocardiogram.

D. Treatment

Treatment of pericardial tamponade depends on many factors, whether the tamponade is acute vs. chronic, malignant vs. nonmalignant, and whether the patient can tolerate a general anesthetic vs. a bedside procedure (22) (see Fig. 2). In patients who are hemodynamically compromised, an echocardiography-guided pericardiocentesis with placement of a drainage catheter is the treatment of choice. This procedure can be performed at bedside. Using a bedside echocardiogram is generally quite safe. Complications include pericardial hemorrhage from inadvertent damage to a coronary artery or pneumothorax, which is more commonly seen in patients with coexisting emphysema. The catheter is then left in place with daily drainage until the output is <50 mL in 24 hr. Reaccumulation of fluid in malignant pericardial effusions is relatively common.

If reaccumulation is a problem, the placement of a pericardial window may be indicated. This procedure is usually done in the operating room although it could be done under local anesthesia at bedside in the intensive care unit. For some patients, malignant pericardial effusions may be treated with systemic chemotherapy or even thoracic radiation. Occasionally, local chemotherapy or sclerosing agents are injected into the pericardium although these are associated with a fair degree of comorbidity and may be painful (23).

E. Anesthetic Considerations

Although some treatment may be initiated at bedside or under local anesthesia, placement of a pericardial window is best done in the operating room in anticipation of other contingencies (e.g., hemorrhagic event, hemodynamic compromise, etc.). In the oncologic patient, the anesthesiologist should be aware of the anesthetic implications of prior chemotherapy, prior surgery or radiation, and patient's prior consumption of chronic pain medication. These are discussed elsewhere in this book.

The anesthesiologist should prepare for possible sternotomy or thoracotomy and the patient is positioned and prepared as such. In addition to standard anesthetic equipment and monitoring, the anesthesiologist should have a rapid infusion device and patient warming system. Massive blood loss should be expected and both large-bore peripheral intravenous catheters and central venous catheterization is recommended. Adequate availability of blood should be determined. Depending on the degree of blood loss, the anesthesiologist should monitor the patient's coagulation status. The patient may need to be monitored in the ICU postoperatively.

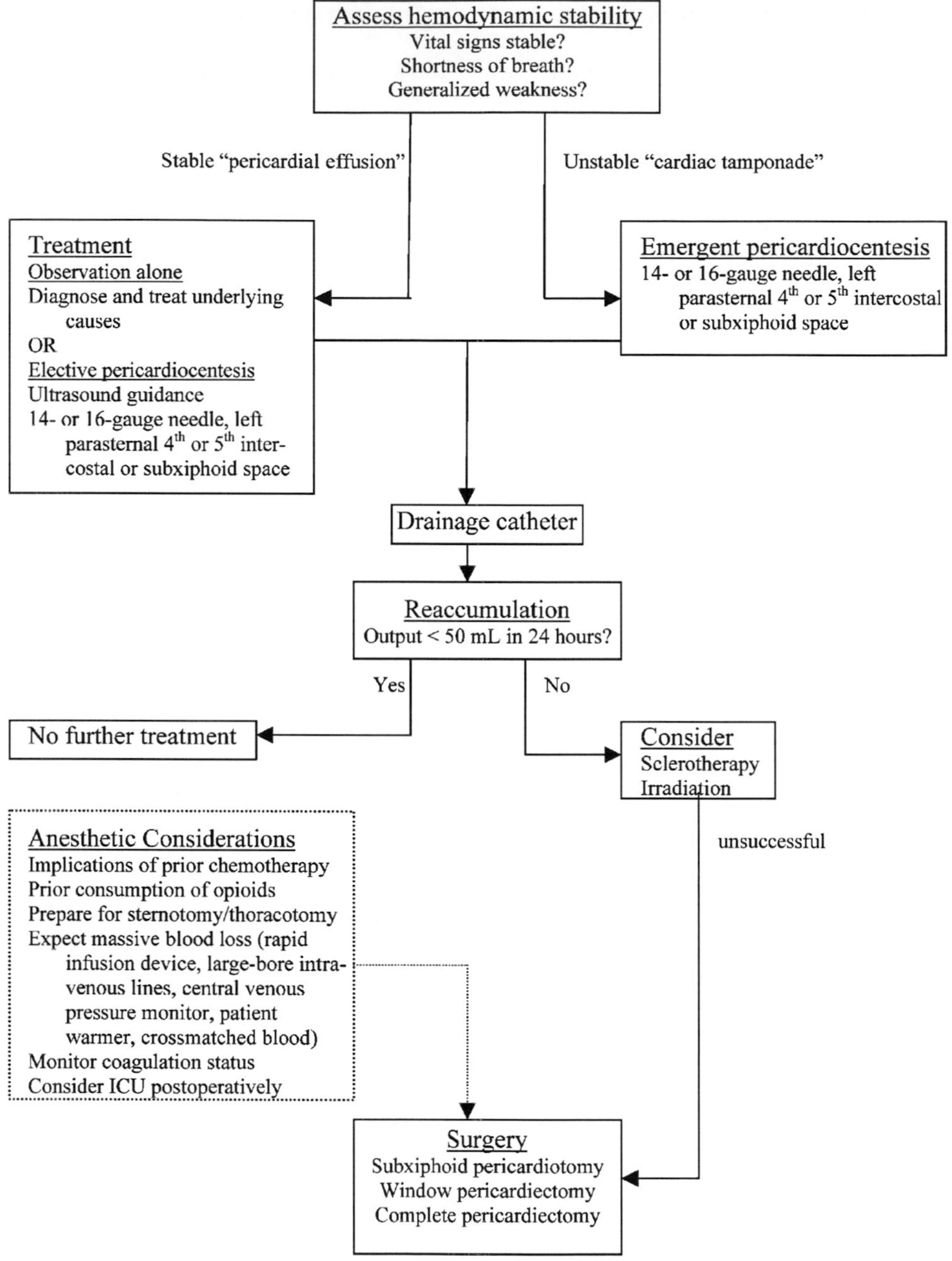

Figure 2 Treatment algorithm for cardiac tamponade.

V. RESPIRATORY EMERGENCIES

A. Pleural Effusion and Hemothorax

The most common causes of exudative pleural effusions are cancer and pneumonia. The major causes of malignant pleural effusions are primary lung, breast, ovarian, lymphoma, and gastric carcinomas. Hemothorax may develop from spontaneous hemorrhage within a tumor, invasion of tumor into blood vessels, or postoperative complications.

Typical symptoms are dyspnea, cough, and occasional pleuritic chest pain. Physical findings may include decreased breath sounds over the area of the effusion, dullness to percussion, and vocal fremitus. Rarely, the patient may develop bulging of intercostal spaces and tracheal deviation. Diagnosis is generally made by plain chest radiograph which, when combined with decubitus views, can detect effusions as little as 100 mL. CT scans are sensitive for even smaller effusions. Arterial blood gas measurements may show decreased pO_2 and increased pCO_2.

Initial treatment of pleural effusions is by noninvasive or minimally invasive procedures (see Fig. 3). These may be by thoracentesis, tube thoracostomy, and instillation of sclerosing agents (tetracycline, doxycycline, talc) or antineoplastic agents (24–26). Surgical procedures that may be beneficial include video-assisted thoracoscopic surgery (VATS) (27) and implanted pleuro-peritoneal pump reservoir. This latter device allows the flow of pleural fluid into the peritoneal cavity either when a preset pressure is reached or by manual decompression. An obvious disadvantage of an implanted device is the risk of obstruction or infection.

Other procedures that may be helpful in chronic effusions or empyemas are construction of an Eloesser

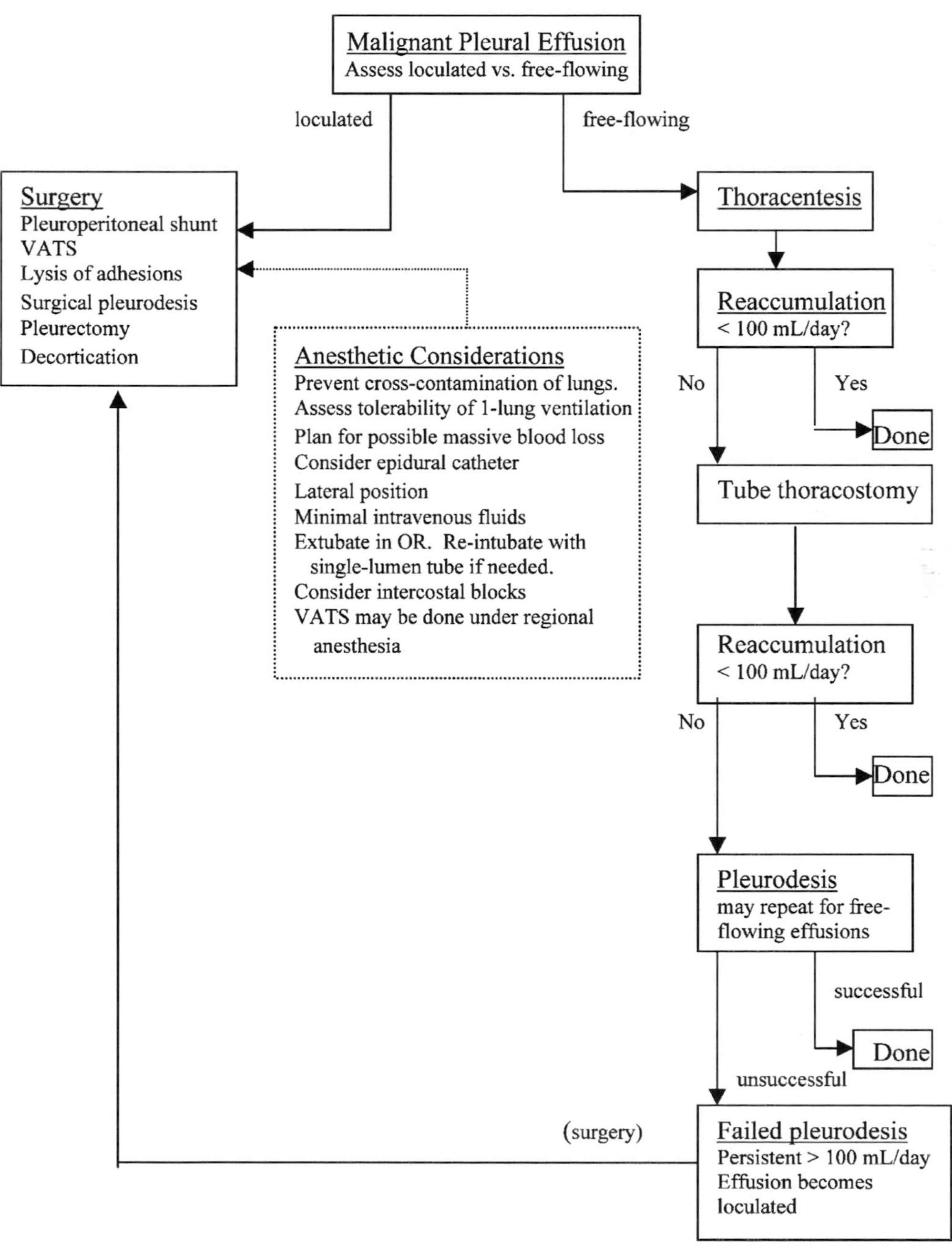

Figure 3 Treatment algorithm for malignant pleural effusion.

(28) flap or a variant called the Clagett procedure (29). In these procedures, an epithelial-lined permanent opening is made in the chest wall for chronic drainage. These are usually done after a pneumonectomy and are generally well tolerated physiologically.

For hemothoraces, the initial treatment is placement of a thoracostomy tube. If the patient's recent history or hemodynamic status indicate continued hemorrhage, the patient should be taken to the operating room for definitive treatment.

B. Anesthetic Considerations

In general, initial treatment is performed at bedside under local anesthesia. For more involved procedures and implantation of pleuro-peritoneal drains, general anesthesia may be needed in the operating room.

For all surgical procedures except VATS, the following general guidelines are suggested:

1. Strict precautions should be observed to protect the nonaffected lung from being contaminated by the affected lung.
2. Preoperative assessment should include an evaluation of the patient's ability to tolerate one-lung ventilation.
3. Consideration should be given for a thoracic epidural catheter unless the patient has symptoms of systemic bacteremia.
4. Large-bore intravenous access should be established in the unlikely event of significant hemorrhagic events. This is more likely for treatment of a hemothorax.
5. Consideration should be given for an awake intubation with a spontaneously breathing patient.
6. Intubate the patient with a double-lumen tube to allow isolation of lungs.
7. Patient position is usually lateral.
8. Avoid the use of nitrous oxide since hypoxemia during single-lung ventilation is unpredictable.
9. Intravenous fluids should be kept to a minimum because of the increased risk of right-heart failure in an overhydrated patient.
10. Extubate, if possible, in the OR. If reintubation is required, a single-lumen tube should suffice.

For the VATS procedure, the above guidelines are appropriate and may be used safely although there are some minor differences that may be helpful:

1. This procedure may be done with sedation and local anesthesia although the patient should be warned beforehand of the slight dyspnea that may develop from pneumothorax during initial entry into the pleural cavity.
2. For regional anesthesia, intercostal blocks may also be used in addition to a thoracic epidural catheter.
3. The patient may not necessarily need an awake intubation. This depends on the clinical situation.

C. Airway Obstruction

An airway obstruction is an acute emergency and must be treated promptly. Airway obstructions can be classified into upper and lower airway obstruction. In the cancer setting, these types of obstruction are common in head and neck cancers such as primary carcinomas of the trachea, tongue base, lung, thyroid, hypopharynx, and larynx. Primary bronchogenic carcinomas and some carcinoid tumors may also cause airway obstruction. They may also be the result of metastatic spread of breast, sarcoma, melanoma, esophagus, renal, and colon malignancies. Rarely, lymphomas may cause airway compromise with associated edema. Finally, certain chemotherapeutic regimens may cause drug reactions that involve increased airway edema and obstruction.

Symptoms of upper airway obstruction include restlessness, tachypnea, stridor (present with >80% cross-sectional airway obstruction), and hoarseness. If these symptoms are accompanied by nasal flaring, puffing of the cheeks, intercostal retraction, or paradoxical breathing, the patient may need urgent intervention for relief of the obstruction. Cyanosis is a very late sign of airway obstruction. Note that aspiration can also cause airway obstruction. Aspiration may be seen in certain cancers that cause vocal cord paralysis, either by direct invasion of the recurrent laryngeal nerves or by affecting cranial nerve function.

Symptoms of lower airway obstruction include gradual increase in shortness of breath, cough, and focal wheezing. Occasionally, if a large lesion in a mainstem bronchus causes sudden airway collapse, the patient may develop acute dyspnea.

Treatment of an acute upper airway obstruction is shown in Fig. 4. For a lower airway obstruction, if the patient is stable, the following procedures may be beneficial:

a. Flexible or rigid bronchoscopy for balloon bronchoplasty followed by placement of an endobronchial stent or endobronchial laser to enlarge the obstructed region. Complications include pneumothorax, bronchospasm, pneumomediastinum, or airway perforation.

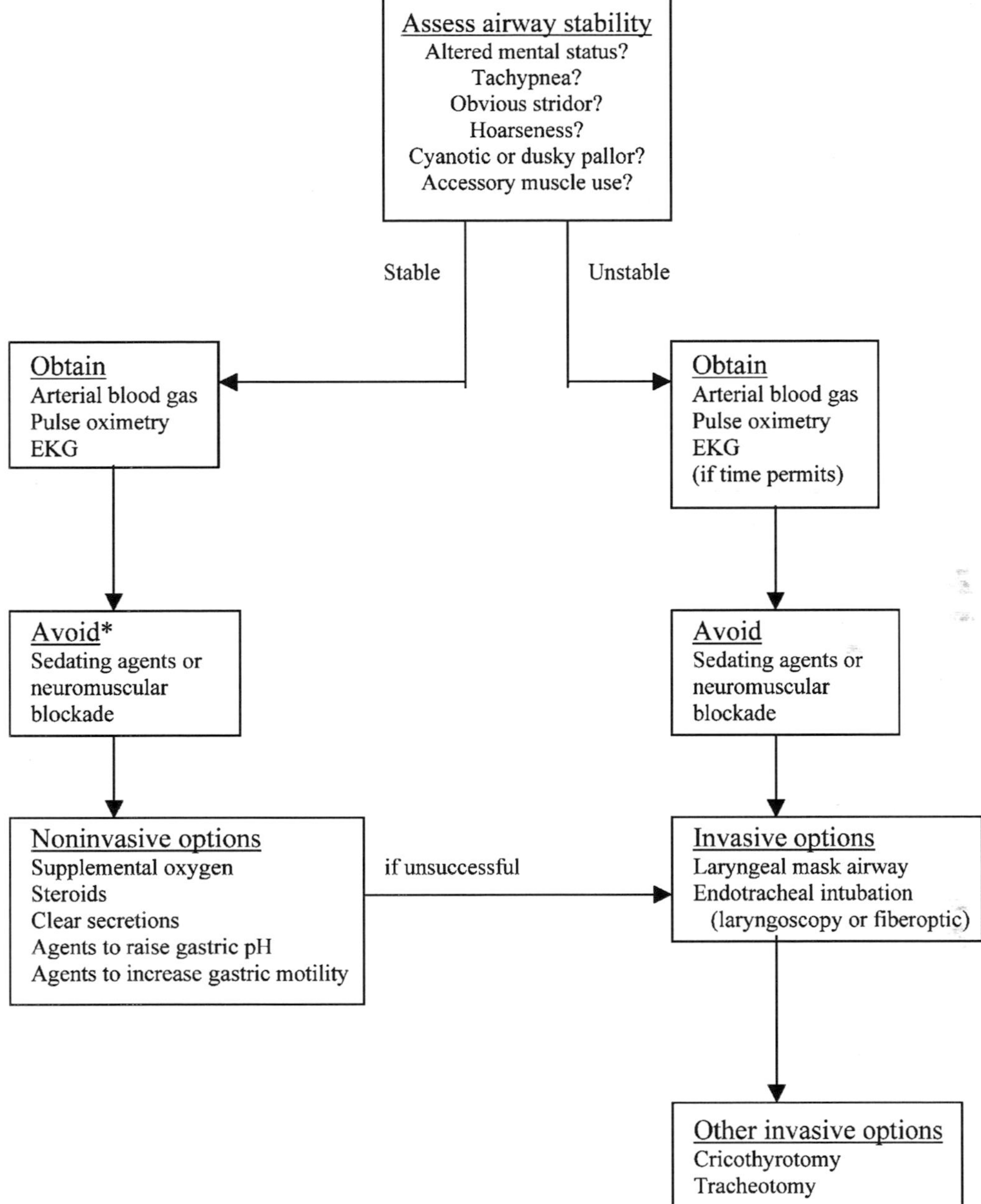

*In some settings, intravenous morphine has been shown to relieve distress associated with dyspnea.

Figure 4 Treatment algorithm for the compromised airway.

b. Tracheobronchial stent placement.
c. Cryosurgery: generally considered safer than laser surgery and may be used for more distal obstruction. Cryotherapy may act synergistically with certain types of radiation therapy or chemotherapy.
d. Brachytherapy: bronchoscopic placement of catheters next to an obstructing lesion followed by implantation of radioactive pellets into the catheters. This is a useful procedure for patients where surgery is not feasible. Since postradiation edema may transiently worsen airway obstruction, this procedure should not be attempted with high-grade obstructions unless a stent or laser ablation is first performed.

D. Anesthetic Considerations

The hallmark of treating an acute airway obstruction is to secure the airway while the patient maintains spontaneous ventilation. In the cancer setting, the most common cause of upper airway obstruction is from an enlarging mass (tumor or hematoma) or radiation induced changes. As the degree of obstruction progresses, the airway may be held patent by neuromuscular tone. If this is abolished by neuromuscular blockade, complete collapse and obstruction of the airway may result and attempts to secure the airway may be unsuccessful.

The airway is best secured by the patient breathing spontaneously. A small dose of an anticholinergic agent (e.g., atropine 0.02 mg/kg) may be given to minimize vagal reflexes. It is strongly advised to have an experienced anesthesiologist and ENT surgeon immediately available. Inhalation induction is achieved with a combination of oxygen and sevoflurane. Caution should be exercised in selection of the ET tube. A smaller size may be needed. Intravenous access is usually established after the patient is induced. Once the airway is secured, intravenous adjuvant agents (e.g., opioids) may be titrated for comfort.

If an operative procedure is indicated for relief of the airway obstruction, the surgeon may proceed after the airway is secured. In the postoperative period, the patient's airway is kept intubated until it is ascertained that the airway will remain patent upon endotracheal tube removal. This may be achieved by a "leak test," in which deflation of the cuff accompanied by a positive pressure breath should allow air to "leak" around the endotracheal tube.

Possible postoperative complications include pulmonary edema and accidental extubation. Pulmonary edema can occur after relief of an airway obstruction and is treatable with intermittent positive pressure ventilation.

REFERENCES

1. Lee AY, Levine MN. Venous thromboembolism and cancer: risks and outcomes. Circulation 2003; 107(23 suppl 1):I17–I21.
2. Kearon C. Natural history of venous thromboembolism. Circulation 2003; 107(23 suppl 1):I22–I30.
3. Palareti G, Legnani C, Cosmi B, Guazzaloca G, Pancani C, Coccheri S. Risk of venous thromboembolism recurrence: high negative predictive value of D-dimer performed after oral anticoagulation is stopped. Thromb Haemost 2002; 87:7–12.
4. Bounameaux H, DeMoerloose P, Perriera A, Miron M. D-dimer testing in suspected venous thromboembolism: an updata. QJM 1997; 90:437–442.
5. Weg JG. Current diagnostic techniques for pulmonary embolism. Semin Vasc Surg 2000; 13:182–188.
6. Lee AY, Levine MN, Baker RI, Bowden C, Kakkar AK, Prins M, Rickles FR, Julian JA, Haley S, Kovacs MJ, Gent M. Low-molecular-weight heparin versus a coumarin for the prevention of recurrent venous thromboembolism in patients with cancer. N Engl J Med 2003; 349:146–153.
7. Schleich JM, Morla O, Laurent M, Langella B, Chaperon J, Almange C. Long-term follow-up of percutaneous vena cava filters: a prospective study in 100 consecutive patients. Eur J Vasc Endovasc Surg 2001; 21:450–457.
8. Couturaud F, Grand'Maison A, Kearon C. Optimal duration of anticoagulant treatment of venous thromboembolism. Presse Med 2000; 29:1379–1385.
9. Goldhaber SZ. Modern treatment of pulmonary embolism. Eur Respir J Suppl 2002; 35:22s–27s.
10. NIH Consensus Development Conference: thrombolytic therapy in thrombosis. Ann Intern Med 1980; 93:141.
11. Oda K, Sato N, Ishii H, Agatsuma T, Hashimoto K, Sato S. Acute massive pulmonary embolism occurring during orthopedic surgery. Kyobu Geka 2003; 56(5): 356–359.
12. Pargger H, Stulz P, Friedli D, Gachter A, Gradel E, Skarvan K. Massive intraoperative pulmonary embolism. Diagnosis and control following embolectomy with transesophageal echocardiography. Anaesthesist 1994; 43:398–402.
13. Goldberg ME, Moore JH, Jarrell BE, Seltzer JL. Anaesthetic technique for transvenous pulmonary embolectomy. Can Anaesth Soc J 1986; 33:79–83.
14. Haiderer O, Lexer G, Gulle HD, Weiss H. Massive pulmonary embolism: case report of successful embolectomy with transatrial vena cava blockade. Wien Med Wochenschr 1983; 133:549–552.
15. Ruberti U, Odero A, Giordanengo F, Miani S. Surgical treatment of massive pulmonary embolism. Personal cases. Minerva Chir 1979; 34:525–536.
16. Wudel LJ, Nesbitt JC. Superior vena cava syndrome. Curr Treat Options Oncol 2001; 2:77–91.
17. Lanciego C, Chacon JL, Julian A, Andrade J, Lopez L, Martinez B, Cruz M, Garcia-Garcia L. Stenting as first option for endovascular treatment of malignant superior vena cava syndrome. AJR Am J Roentgenol 2001; 177:585–593.
18. Rowell NP, Gleeson FV. Steroids, radiotherapy, chemotherapy and stents for superior vena caval obstruction in carcinoma of the bronchus: a systematic review. Clin Oncol (R Coll Radiol) 2002; 14:338–351.
19. Narang S, Harte BH, Body SC. Anesthesia for patients with a mediastinal mass. Anesthesiol Clin North America 2001; 19:559–579.
20. Palacios IF. Pericardial effusion and tamponade. Curr Treat Options Cardiovasc Med 1999; 1:79–89.

21. Keefe DL. Cardiovascular emergencies in the cancer patient. Semin Oncol 2000; 27:244–255.
22. Campione A, Cacchiarelli M, Ghiribelli C, Caloni V, D'Agata A, Gotti G. Which treatment in pericardial effusion? J Cardiovasc Surg (Torino) 2002; 43:735–739.
23. Martinoni A, Cipolla CM, Civelli M, Cardinale D, Lamantia G, Colleoni M, DeBraud F, Susini G, Martinelli G, Goldhirsh A, Fiorentini C. Intrapericardial treatment of neoplastic pericardial effusions. Herz 2000; 25:787–793.
24. Bertolaccini L, Zamprogna C, D'Urso A, Massaglia F. The treatment of malignant pleural effusions: the experience of a multidisciplinary thoracic endoscopy group. Tumori 2003; 89:233–236.
25. Antunes G, Neville E, Duffy J, Ali N. BTS guidelines for the management of malignant pleural effusions. Thorax 2003; 58:29–38.
26. Love D, White D, Kiroff G. Thoracoscopic talc pleurodesis for malignant pleural effusion. ANZ J Surg 2003; 73:19–22.
27. Allen MS, Deschamps C, Jones DM, Trastek VF, Pairolero PC. Video-assisted thoracic surgical procedures: the Mayo experience. Mayo Clin Proc 1996; 71: 351–359.
28. Thourani VH, Lancaster RT, Mansour KA, Miller JI Jr. Twenty-six years of experience with the modified Eloesser flap. Ann Thorac Surg 2003; 76:401–405; discussion 405–406.
29. Gharagozloo F, Trachiotis G, Wolfe A, DuBree KJ, Cox JL. Pleural space irrigation and modified Clagett procedure for the treatment of early postpneumonectomy empyema. J Thorac Cardiovasc Surg 1998; 116:943–948.

SUGGESTED READINGS

Jaffe RA, Samuels SI, eds. Anesthesiologist's Manual of Surgical Procedures. 2nd ed. Philadelphia: Lippincott Williams & Wilkins, 1999.

Practice Guidelines for Management of the Difficult Anesthesiology. American Society of Anesthesiologists Task Force on Management of the Difficult Airway. Anesthesiology 2003; 98:1269–1277.

Putnam JB Jr. Malignant pleural effusions. Surg Clin North Am 2002; 82(4):867–883.

Saclarides TJ, Millikan DW, Godellas CV, eds. Surgical Oncology: An Algorithmic Approach. New York: Springer-Verlag Publishers, 2003.

Yeung SJ, Escalante CP. Holland Frei Oncologic Emergencies. Hamilton, Ontario: BC Decker, Inc., 2002.

32

Transfusion Therapy and the Cancer Patient

LAWRENCE T. GOODNOUGH

Departments of Pathology and Medicine, Stanford University School of Medicine, Stanford, California, U.S.A.

GEORGE DESPOTIS

Departments of Pathology and Immunology and Anesthesiology, Washington University School of Medicine, St. Louis, Missouri, U.S.A.

I. CURRENT BLOOD RISKS

Rates of disease transmission could previously be measured by simply following transfusion recipients over time (1). Current viral disease transmission rates are now too low to measure, so that mathematical models (2,3) are needed to estimate blood risks. The models are based on the fact that disease transmission is thought to occur primarily in the window period (the time after a blood donor is infectious but before any donor screening tests are positive). These models also disregard the fact that due to underlying disease, patients who receive transfusions have 1-year and 10-year mortality rates of about 24% and 52%, respectively, and may not live long enough to develop transfusion-transmitted disease (4). Estimated risks of transfusion-transmitted diseases (5) are lower than ever before (6,7). These risks have declined substantially by the implementation of nucleic acid testing (NAT) that has shortened infectious window periods and has substantially reduced the estimated risks of post-transfusion hepatitis C and Human immunodeficiency virus (HIV) (Table 1).

A. Viral Transmission

The first descriptions of transfusion associated-HIV infection occurred in late 1982 and early 1983 (8). Blood banks began direct questioning for specific high risk behaviors (9) and gave donors the opportunity to selfexclude their blood after donation (10). Even prior to antibody screening for HIV, these measures resulted in an impressive decrease in transfusion-associated HIV (11), illustrated in Fig. 1 (12). After implementation of HIV antibody testing in March 1985, only five cases of transfusion-associated HIV infection were reported over the subsequent 5 years, compared to 714 cases reported in the year prior to HIV testing (13).

Additional testing for a related HIV-2 virus has had only a small impact in the United Sates, as only three positive donors out of 74 million donations have been found (14). To further decrease the risk of transfusion-transmitted HIV disease, in late 1995, blood banks began to test donors for p24 antigen (15). In a little more than a year of screening, only two blood donors (p24 antigen positive/anti-HIV antibody negative)

Table 1 Some Estimated Risks of Blood Transfusion

	Estimated frequency of occurence per million units (per actual unit)
Infectious	
Virus	
Hepatitis B	139 (1/60,000–1/200,000)
Hepatitis C	29 (1/800,000–1/1.7 × 10^6)
Human immunodeficiency	12 (1/1.4–2.4 × 10^6)
Bacteria	
Red Cells	2 (1/500,000)
Platelets	2,000 (1/2,000)
Acute hemolytic transfusion reactions	1–4 (1/250,000–1,000,000)
Delayed hemolytic transfusion reactions	1,000 (1/1,000)

Source: From Ref. 5.

were identified that were otherwise acceptable, out of ~6 million donations.

The labeling of blood from paid donors in 1972 and the implementation of third generation hepatitis B surface antigen screening tests led to a marked reduction in transfusion-transmitted hepatitis B (Fig. 1), so that it now comprises only about 10% of all cases of post-transfusion hepatitis (16). Although about 35% of hepatitis B cases will develop acute disease, only 1–10% of patients develop chronic infection (17). A reduction in non-A, non-B post-transfusion hepatitis occurred when potential HIV-positive donors were excluded (18) and again when donors were tested for the surrogate markers aminolevulenic transferase as a marker for acute liver inflammation and anti-HBc (antibody to hepatitis B core antigen as evidence of previous hepatitis B infection) (12). The risk of transmission of non-A, non-B hepatitis was greatly reduced after implementation of a test for hepatitis C virus (HCV) antibody (19). The probable risk of transfusion-transmitted HCV is now estimated to be 1:800,000–1:1.7×10^6 transfusions with NAT testing in place (5). Although blood transfusion accounted for a substantial proportion of HCV infections acquired more than 10 years ago, it now rarely accounts for HCV infection (20). For post-transfusion HCV infection, 85% of infections become chronic, 20% of infections lead to cirrhosis, and 1–5% of infections lead to hepatocellular carcinoma; the combined mortality

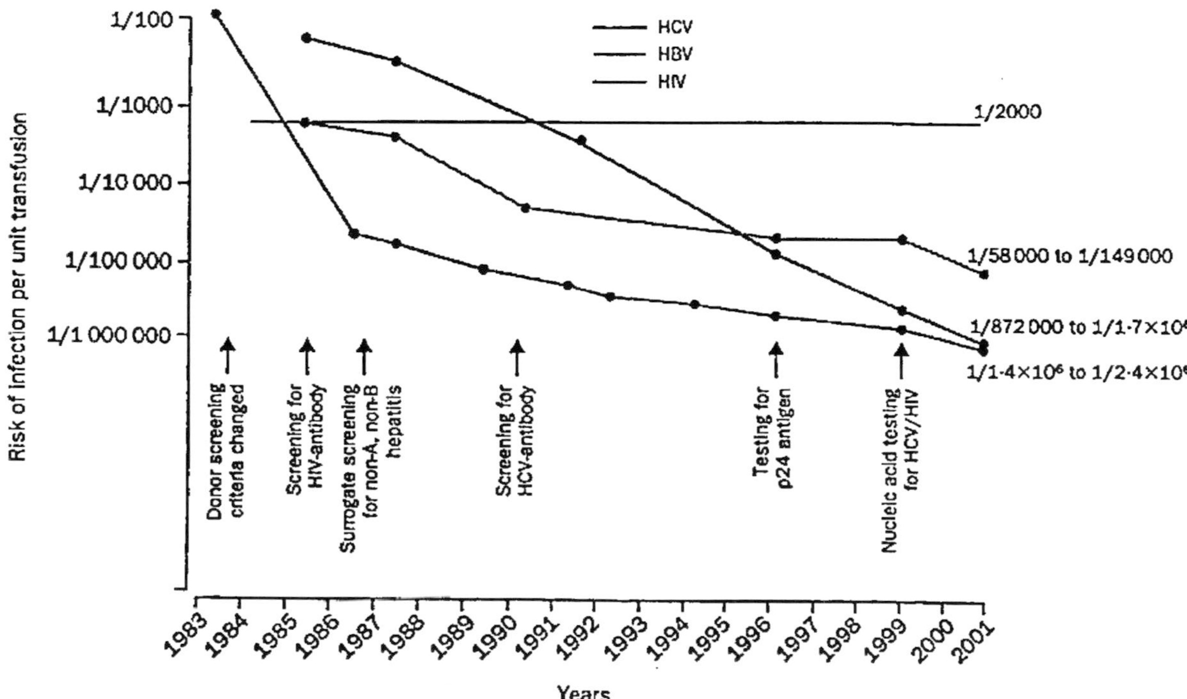

Figure 1 The risks of transfusion-related transmission of human immunodeficiency virus (HIV) hepatitis B virus (HBV), and hepatitis C virus (HCV) in the United States. Each unit represents exposure to one donor. The risk of each of these infections has declined dramatically since 1983, the year the criteria for donor screening were changed. Further declines have resulted from the implementation of testing of donor blood for antibodies to HIV beginning in 1985; surrogate testing for non-A, non-B hepatitis beginning in 1986–1987; testing for antibodies to HCV beginning in 1990; testing for HIV p24 antigen beginning in late 1995; and nucleic acid testing in 1999. *Source*: From Refs. 7 and 12.

from transfusion-transmitted HCV liver disease is 14.5% over 20.6 years to 28.3 years from cirrhosis and hepatocellular carcinoma, respectively (21,22).

Hepatitis A transmission by blood transfusion has been estimated to occur in one in 1,000,000 U (17). The lack of a chronic carrier state for hepatitis A and the presence of symptoms that would exclude blood donation during the brief viremic phase of the illness explain why hepatitis A is so uncommonly associated with blood transfusion.

In recent years, blood centers have implemented NAT of minipools (16–24 donation samples/pool) from blood donations to reduce HIV and HCV transmissions occurring during the infectious window period (before serologic conversion). Current estimates of the risk per unit of blood in the post-NAT era are illustrated in Fig. 1 (6,7,12). To date, three cases of HIV transmission by units from two donors who were negative by both minipool NAT and HIV serology (anti-HIV antibody and HIV p24 antigen) have occurred (23,24), and one documented case of apparent HCV transmission by a unit negative by both minipool NAT and HCV serology has been reported from Germany (25). In contrast to the successes at risk reduction for HIV and HCV, the risk of hepatitis B virus (HBV) transmission remains approximately 1:50,000 in western countries; the window period would be shortened only modestly with minipool testing due to the slow replication rate of HBV, but greater risk reduction may be achieved with single donor testing by NAT.

B. Blood Bacterial Contamination

1. *Red Cells*

The most commonly implicated organism in bacterial contamination of red cells is *Yersinia enterocolitica*. In the United States, a contamination rate of less than one per million red cell units has been described (26). Onset of clinical symptoms typically occurs acutely during transfusion, with a mortality rate of 60% and median time to death of only 25 hr (27).

2. *Platelets*

Currently, the greatest risk of transfusion-transmitted disease is bacterial contamination of platelets. Unlike viruses, bacteria have the potential to proliferate from low levels (<1 CFU/mL) at the time of collection to very high levels ($>1 \times 10^8$ CFU/mL) during the liquid storage period of blood components. As platelets are stored for up to 5 days at 20–24°C, they constitute an excellent growth medium for bacteria. Culture surveillance suggests that bacterial contamination of platelet concentrates and apheresis platelets occurs in approximately 1:1000–1:2000 U (28,29). Although the true prevalence of severe episodes of transfusion-associated bacterial sepsis is not known, it is estimated to occur with one-fourth to one-sixth of contaminated transfusions (30–32). With 4 million (1 million apheresis platelets and 3 million platelet concentrates) platelet units transfused yearly in the United States alone, it would be expected that 2000–4000 bacterially contaminated units would be transfused and be associated with 333–1000 cases of severe and possibly fatal sepsis. Pooled platelet concentrates have a higher risk than apheresis platelets (a function of the number of units pooled, reflecting the increased donor exposure and number of phlebotomies required to obtain the products) (33).

Recent reports from Europe and North America have advocated the use of automated liquid media culture systems for the testing of platelets in order to reduce the risk of bacterial contamination (34–38). Culturing of platelets is currently mandatory in Belgium (Flemish speaking part) and in the Netherlands. Although not mandatory, culturing of platelets is also performed by the majority of blood centers in Sweden, Norway, and Denmark and in selected sites in the United Kingdom, Yugoslavia, Germany, Canada, and the United States. Culturing is typically performed after some storage time has elapsed (e.g., 1–2 days) to allow for bacterial growth to optimize detection. Bacterial detection processes are mandated to be in place for the United States in 2003. The use of bacterial culturing is used as a rationale to propose that the shelf life of platelets be extended to 7 days (34–40).

Another promising approach is pathogen inactivation (e.g., psoralens with ultraviolet (UV) irradiation), with the potential to eliminate both viral and bacterial contaminants in platelets (41). However, these techniques have difficulty in inactivating spore-forming bacteria (e.g., *Bacillus* sp.) (42). Another concern is that such processing leads to decreased platelet recovery and in vivo survival (thereby leading to the need for increased platelet transfusions) (43). This phenomenon was observed in the U.S. clinical trial utilizing apheresis platelets, with lower post-transfusion corrected count increments (CCI) and increased platelet transfusion requirements for maintenance of hemostasis, when compared with untreated platelets (44). Additionally, potential concerns regarding costs and limited availability (e.g., the pivotal U.S. phase III trial for platelet products was conducted with products derived from apheresis technology from one vendor) leave the eventual role of this technology uncertain.

C. Cytomegalovirus Infection

Cytomegalovirus (CMV) infection has been a substantial cause of morbidity and mortality in oncology patients who are immunocompromised. Patients predominately at risk are those who receive allogeneic bone marrow/stem cell transplantation due to a combination of preparative regimens and immunosuppressive regimens or complications [cyclosporin and steroid therapy and/or graft-vs.-host disease (GVHD)] (45,46). These patients have a prevalence of CMV infection of up to 60%, with up to half of these developing CMV disease (47). Transfusion of cellular blood components from CMV-seropositive donors is a major cause of seroconversion in CMV-negative recipients. This problem is markedly reduced (but not entirely eliminated) when CMV-seronegative products are used for transfusing CMV-seronegative donor-recipient transplant patients. Cytomegalovirus seroconversion has been reported in 1–4% of patients (47); a recent analysis of our own program identified CMV viremia in only one (2.5%) of 39 CMV-negative donor-recipient pairs undergoing allogeneic peripheral stem cell transplantation (48). Of note, an analysis of 59 patients receiving allogeneic peripheral blood stem cell (PBSC) transplant, who received two prophylactic granulocyte infusions from their same stem cell donor, found that stem cell infusion and two subsequent granulocyte infusions from CMV-positive donors did not alter the risk of viremia when compared with stem cells and granulocytes from CMV-negative donors (34.5% vs. 26.6% incidence of CMV viremia).

Cytomegalovirus infection and CMV disease are much less common in patients undergoing autologous bone marrow/stem cell transplantation, despite evidence that seroconversion or CMV urinary excretion occurs at equivalent prevalence rates as in allogeneic transplant recipients (49). Cytomegalovirus disease has been described in autologous transplant patients (50) but is not currently recognized to be a significant clinical problem (51). Nevertheless, some guidelines recommend that CMV-negative blood products be used in seronegative patients undergoing autologous bone marrow/stem cell transplantation (52). One report compared patients undergoing autogolous transplant with CD34-selected PBMCs with patients undergoing transplant with unselected peripheral stem cells (53). Overall, seven (25%) of the 31 CD34-selected patients developed CMV disease within 100 days of transplant and four (13%) died as a result of their infection. Of the 237 unselected PBMC, 10 (4%) developed CMV disease and five (2%) died. Of note, 35% and 31% of these autogolous transplant patients, received methylprednisone steroid therapy (1–2 mg/kg per day); the use of steroid therapy post-transplant was highly significant for the development of CMV infection.

Cytomegalovirus-negative blood products have traditionally been provided from community donors who are seronegative by either an enzyme-linked immunoassay or a latex agglutination testing. Cytomegalovirus-seronegative individuals comprise 10–50% of the blood-donor population, so that red blood cell inventory considerations are important for some communities, and platelet inventory considerations affect virtually all transplant programs. Considerable investigation into leukodepletion technology has been invested in order to determine whether these products can be considered to be as "CMV-safe" as blood products that are seronegative.

One randomized, controlled clinical trial (54) of bone marrow transplant patients compared the value of CMV-seronegative blood products with CMV-unscreened blood products that were subjected to bedside leukofiltration. Four (1.3%) of 252 patients in the CMV-seronegative cohort developed CMV infection, with no CMV disease or fatalities; six (2.4%) of 250 patients in the leukodepleted cohort developed CMV disease, of whom five patients died. The filtered cohort had an increased probability of developing CMV disease by day 100 (2.4% vs. 0%, $p = 0.03$). Even when the investigators eliminated CMV infections that occurred within 21 days of transplant, two cases of fatal CMV disease occurred in the filtered arm compared with none in the leukodepletion arm. These "treatment failures" may be ascribed to receiving unfiltered blood in error (54) or to the "failure rate" of bedside leukoreduction filters (55), but the conclusion by the authors of this study that leukodepleted blood products are "CMV safe" remains controversial (56). Endogenous viral (such as CMV) activation ascribed to transfusion is a potential consideration (57); however, a report of the Viral Activation Transfusion Study indicated that the use of leukodepleted blood components had no value in prevention of HIV or CMV viral activation in patients with HIV infection (58).

Guidelines by the American Association of Blood Banks (AABB) have suggested that CMV-seronegative or leukoreduced blood products be used for all CMV-negative transplant recipients, both autologous and allogeneic, as well as patients receiving chemotherapy likely to induce severe neutropenia (52). However, in a consensus conference developed by the Canadian Blood Services, seven of 10 panelists concluded that patients considered at risk for CMV disease should receive CMV-negative blood products, even when blood components are leukoreduced (59,60).

Institutional policies for our leukemia/stem cell transplant program at Washington university in St. Louis are in what follows. Any patient undergoing allogeneic or autologous transplant, solid organ or bone marrow/stem cells, if CMV serology is negative or unknown, is to receive CMV-seronegative blood products. If CMV-negative platelet products are not available, a bedside leukoreduction filter is offered. Patients who are known to be CMV-positive may receive CMV-unscreened products. Patients who are considered to be candidates for allogeneic stem cell transplant whose CMV status is negative or unknown also receive negative CMV blood products. These include patients diagnosed with AML, ALL, CML, CLL, aplastic anemia, and myelodysplastic syndromes.

D. Other Infectious Agents

The risk of B19 parvovirus transmission depends on both the incidence in blood donors, which is highly variable from year to year, and the patient setting. Infection is generally not clinically significant except in certain clinical settings such as in pregnant women (where hydrops fetalis may develop), in patients with hemolytic anemia (where aplastic crises may develop), or in immunodeficiency states (where chronic aplastic anemia may develop) (61).

In recipients of blood infected by HTLV-I/II, 20–60% will develop infection. Blood stored more than 14 days and noncellular blood products such as cryoprecipitate and fresh frozen plasma do not appear to be infectious. Myelopathy can occur in individuals infected with HTLV-I or HTLV-II due to blood transmission (62). One case of adult T-cell leukemia has also been reported following a blood transfusion (63). In 1988, a first generation HTLV test was licensed for use in blood donor screening in the United States. Because these tests were able to detect only from 46% to 91% of HTLV-II infections, screening was implemented for HTLV-II and HTLV-I. Other infectious agents such as Epstein-Barr virus, leishmaniasis, lyme disease, brucelosis, malaria, babesiosis, toxoplasmosis, Chagas' disease, and most recently West Nile virus are rarely transmitted via transfusion.

Advances in blood safety from viral disease transmission now mean that the current mortality from blood transfusion arises as much from other risks, particularly administrative error leading to ABO-related hemolysis, or bacterial contamination. These other estimated risks of transfusion (5) are summarized in Table 1.

Several cases of malaria transmitted by blood transfusion are identified yearly. The Food and Drug Administration (FDA) revised deferral criteria for malaria risk in 1994 (64), but another revision is being considered; 103 cases of transfusion-transmitted disease were reported to the Centers for Disease Control (CDC) from 1958 to 1998, with an estimated occurrence rate of 0.25 per million units transfused (65). Two-thirds of these occurred in donors who should have been excluded under current screening criteria, but the remaining one-third were from donors whose last travel exceeded the time limits (a minimum of 3 years for immigrants or residents from endemic areas) in the FDA guidelines (66). Transfusion-transmitted malaria is similarly a potential infectious threat in Europe.

Chagas' disease (*Trypanosoma cruzi*) is endemic in many parts of central and South America. Transfusion-transmitted Chagas' disease is a major concern because *T. cruzi* establishes a chronic, asymptomatic carrier, state in most infected persons (Table 1) (67,68). Donor history screening for risk factors associated with *T. cruzi* infection have poor specificity; in one study, 39.5% of donors at a Los Angeles hospital were judged to be at risk for *T. cruzi* infection, and of these one in 500 was confirmed antibody positive (69). To date, seven cases of transfusion-transmitted and three cases of transplant-associated Chagas' disease (from one organ donor) in the United States and Canada have been reported (70,71). Although donor screening or *T. cruzi* antibody is important in endemic conditions in Latin and South America (Table 1), there is no direct evidence currently to suggest that the introduction of routine donor screening for antibodies to *T. cruzi* in all donors would measurably improve the safety of the U.S. blood supply. A pilot program to screen and test blood donors for *T. cruzi* infection is currently underway in Canada.

Transfusion-associated babesioses is another example of a transmissible zoonotic disease. Red cells and platelets prepared from asymptomatic donors have been implicated in more than 30 transfusion-transmitted cases. Asplenic, elderly, or severely immunocompromised patients are at the greatest risk of developing hemolytic anemia, coagulopathy, and renal failure. No test is currently available for mass screening to detect asymptomatic carriers of *Babesia* species (72).

Donor referral criteria to deal with the potential problems of Creutzfeldt-Jakob disease (CJD) and variant CJD (vCJD) have been implemented beginning in 1987. Although CJD has been transmitted from human to human by transplantation of dura matter or cornea, injection of pituitary growth hormone, or reuse of EEG electrodes (73), there are no reported cases of transmission by blood transfusion. Newer epidemiological studies confirm earlier studies that failed to show a link between transfusion and transmission of CJD (74).

Concerns regarding the potential transmission of circulating prions, were verified in a report of CJD possibly transmitted by blood transfusion (74A); strategies that have been implemented, such as donor deferral schemes, universal leukoreduction, etc., are therefore considered precautionary. Deferral of donors who have spent more than 6 months in the United Kingdom from 1980 through 1996 was implemented in the United States in April 2000, in a preemptive effort to minimize a potential risk of vCJD while avoiding disruption of the blood supply. As of April 2002, more than 100 patients, mostly in the United Kingdom, as well as five patients in France, have been diagnosed with vCJD. As a further measure to reduce the potential risk of vCJD by transfusion, new donor deferrals were implemented in the United States in October 2002: cumulative time spent from 1980 to present were more than 3 months in the United Kingdom, more than 5 years in Europe, or more than 6 months on a U.S. military base in Europe. These criteria have been estimated to reduce by 90% the total donor person-days of exposure to the putative agent of vCJD, with an estimated loss of ~5% of the U.S. donor pool (75). The impact of these enhanced donor-screening measures has been most severe in the metropolitan New York City region, which in the past derived ~25% of its blood inventory via importation from the European Union.

E. Leukoreduction of Blood Components

Leukocytes are known to have a number of biologic effects associated with allogeneic blood transfusion (Table 2). The potential clinical importance of these effects, which are the focus of the current debate over the merits of "universal" leukoreduction (cellular components with $<5 \times 10^6$ leukocytes) includes febrile-associated transfusion reactions (FATR), transfusion-related alloimmunization to platelets (TRAP), and transfusion-related immunomodulation (TRIM). Several recent reviews (76,77) of this topic, along with commentaries (78–81) regarding the use of leukodepleted blood components, have been published. The Blood Products Advisory Committee (BPAC) to the Food and Drug Administration (FDA) voted 13–0 on 18th September 1998 in favor of universal leukoreduction of blood components (82), but the minutes stated that many committee members agreed there were insufficient good studies, and everyone wanted more data (ABC newsletter, 9/25/98). To date, both leukoreduced and nonleukoreduced blood components remain FDA approved.

Table 2 Potential Adverse Effects of Leukocytes in Blood Components

Immunologic effects
Alloimmunization (HLA and leukocyte antigens)
Febrile reactions
Refractoriness to platelet transfusion
Transplant rejection
Transfusion-induced acute lung injury
Graft-vs.-host disease
Immunomodulation (possibly)
Infectious disease[a]
Cytomegalovirus infection
HTLV-I infection
Epstein-Barr virus infection

Note: HLA, human leukocyte antigen; HTLV-1, human T-cell lymphotrophic virus-I.
[a] Caused exclusively by leukocytes in blood components.
Source: From Ref. 79.

Febrile-associated transfusion reactions occur in only 0.5% of red cell transfusions (83); of these, 18% and 8% of patients experience a second or third FATR. Approximately 18% of platelet transfusions are associated with FATR (84); although the prevalence of platelet-associated FATR can be as high as 30% in frequently transfused populations such as oncology patients, reactions characterized as severe occur in only 2% of platelet transfusions (84–86). These reactions are caused mostly by plasma supernatants (87), and platelets leukoreduced by bedside filtration have not been found to reduce the overall prevalence of FATR (84–86). Bedside leukoreduction filters are now recognized to cause significant hypotensive events by activation of the bradykinin/kininogen systems, particularly in patients taking angiotensin-converting enzyme inhibitors (88). There is general agreement that bedside leukoreduction filters are not an appropriate technology to address FATR; the Canadian Blood Service implemented prestorage universal leukoreduction in order to address the problem of FATR (89). However, two retrospective studies (90,91) indicated that leukoreduction did not affect the incidence of transfusion reactions or other indices of morbidity, and a prospective study found no benefit from leukoreduction when patients were evaluated for in-hospital mortality, length of stay, and hospital costs (92).

The issue of alloimmunization to platelet transfusions (TRAP) was studied in an NHLBI-sponsored multicenter trial of newly diagnosed patients with leukemia (85). The study found that clinical platelet refractoriness associated with HLA antibody seropositivity was reduced from 18% of patients transfused with unprocessed platelet concentrates compared with 8% of patients receiving leukoreduced apheresis platelets, leukoreduced platelet concentrates, or psoralen/UV-B treated platelets. Although this difference achieved statistical significance, no important clinical differences were found among the patient cohorts, including prevalence of transfusion reactions, hemorrhagic events, mortality, length of stay, number of platelet transfusions, or number of red cell transfusions. A possible clinical benefit has been proposed for these patients during later hospitalizations for therapy, such as bone marrow/stem cell transplantation. However, a subsequent study indicates that clinical platelet refractoriness in this setting is multifactorial and dependent on patient and treatment variables, rather than the presence of HLA antibodies (93). Furthermore, an audit of transplant programs found that two-thirds of hemorrhagic events occurred in patients whose morning platelet count exceeded $20,000/mm^3$; clinical bleeding episodes were frequently related to disease or anatomic pathophysiology (ulcers, infections, GVHD) rather than to the degree of thrombocytopenia (94). The debate regarding "low dose" vs. "high dose" platelet transfusions is in part related to some of these issues (95).

Transfusion-related immunomodulation (TRIM) has been previously cited to be clinically important in two clinical settings, namely, patients undergoing renal transplantation (96) and women with multiple miscarriages (97). One commentary supporting universal leukoreduction concluded that allogeneic leukocytes were shown to be beneficial and widely accepted to be clinically effective in the treatment of recurrent spontaneous abortions (98); however, a multicenter, controlled study published shortly thereafter found no evidence of such an effect, and the authors recommended against allogeneic mononuclear infusions as a treatment for unexplained, recurrent miscarriage (99). Similarly, patients transfused before renal transplantation have been identified to have superior 1-year renal allograft survival compared with untransfused patients (96). Nevertheless, when patients who are untransfused prior to surgery are subsequently analyzed for blood transfused at the time of transplantation surgery, no effect is found for 1-year renal allograft survival (96).

Whether allogeneic blood exposure causes clinically significant immune suppression in any other settings remains a subject of debate. A number of observational, retrospective reports have described an association between exposure to allogeneic blood, with earlier recurrences of malignancy or increased rates of postoperative infection (76). Only a few prospective studies of this issue have been performed in order to clarify the potential immunomodulatory effects of allogeneic transfusion (100). A study of 120 patients undergoing curative resection of colorectal carcinoma failed to demonstrate a difference in relapse free survival time or a difference in the prevalence of serious postoperative infection between patients randomized to allogeneic or autologous transfusion (101). In another study of 423 patients, there was no difference in relapse-free survival time or in infectious complications when comparing allogeneic vs. autologous red-cell transfusions (102). Houbiers et al. (103) compared transfusion of leukocyte-depleted (a three $\log_{10}$ reduction) components with buffy coat-depleted components (a one $\log_{10}$ reduction) and found no difference in cancer recurrence risk after colorectal surgery (103). van de Watering et al. (104) found no effect of leukoreduction on postoperative infection rates in cardiac surgery patients, which was the primary study outcome; they also concluded that the use of leukoreduced units was associated with half (3.4%) of the 7.8% 60-day mortality rate observed in the control group. However, mortality in this study was a secondary outcome, with no stratification at randomization for patients who presented with preoperative risk factors known to be predictive for postoperative morbidity and mortality (105).

Although the data available at present raise questions about the potential immunosuppressive effect of allogeneic blood transfusion, they do not allow formulation of a definitive statement about its clinical importance and, consequently, whether universal leukoreduction is appropriate (106). Similarly, although some guidelines suggest that leukoreduced products are "CMV safe" (80), data to support this conclusion are scant (54–56). Table 3 lists the indications and nonindications for leukoreduction published in a review in 1992 (79); these continue to be applicable, pending future additional data that cause re-evaluation.

II. BLOOD TRANSFUSION

The therapeutic goal of a blood transfusion is to improve oxygen delivery and consumption according to the physiologic need of the recipient. The usual response to an acute reduction in [Hgb] in the normovolemic state is to increase cardiac output to maintain adequate oxygen delivery (Ref. 107, Fig. 2). The heart is therefore the principal organ at risk in acute anemia. Myocardial anaerobic metabolism, indicating inadequate O_2 delivery, occurs when lactate metabolism in the heart converts from lactate uptake to lactate production. The normal whole-body oxygen-extraction ratio (the ratio of oxygen consumption to oxygen delivery) is 20–25%. The oxygen-extraction ratio approaches 50% when myocardial lactate production occurs, indicating anaerobic metabolism. In a normal heart, this lactate production and an oxygen-extraction ratio of 50% occur at a [Hgb] of approximately

Table 3 Indications and Nonindications for Leukocyte Reduced Blood Components

Established indications
Prevention of recurrent nonhemolytic febrile transfusion reactions to red blood cell transfusions
Prevention or delay of alloimmunization to leukocyte antigens in selected patients who are candidates for transplantation transfusion on a long-term basis (see text)
Possible indications (under review)
Prevention of the platelet-refractory state caused by alloimmunization
Prevention of recurrent febrile reactions during platelet transfusions
Prevention of cytomegalovirus transmission by cellular blood components
Nonindications
Prevention of transfusion-associated GVHD
Prevention of transfusion-related acute lung injury due to the passive administration of antileukocyte antibody
Patients who are expected to have only limited transfusion exposure
Acellular blood components (e.g., fresh frozen plasma, cryoprecipitate)

Source: From Ref. 79.

3.5–4 g/dL (108). In a model of coronary stenosis, the anaerobic state occurs at a [Hgb] of approximately 6–7 g/dL. (109). No single number, either extraction ratio or [Hgb], can serve as an absolute indicator of transfusion need. However, the use of such a physiologic value in conjunction with clinical assessment of the patient status permits a rational decision regarding the appropriateness of transfusion prior to the onset of hypoxia or ischemia (110).

A. Mortality

If a transfusion is appropriate, then a benefit should occur. In a literature assessment of the benefit of transfusion, data on mortality are the clearest. In a review

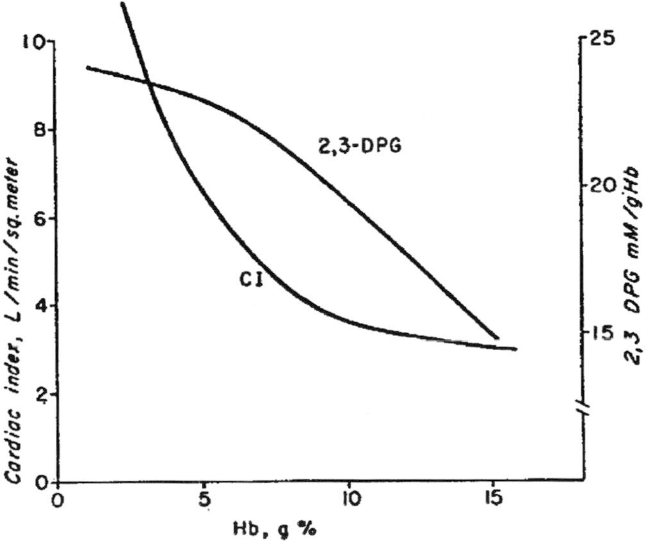

Figure 2 Effect of anemia on cardiac index and diphosphoglycerate. *Source*: From Ref. 107.

of 16 reports of the surgical outcomes in Jehovah's witnesses who underwent major surgery without blood transfusion, mortality associated with anemia occurred in 1.4% of the 1404 operations (111). In one large study, the risk of death was found to be higher in patients with cardiovascular disease than in those without (112). A follow-up analysis (113) of a subset of these patients reported that the odds of death in patients with a postoperative Hgb level of <8 g/dL increased 2.5 times for each gram decrease in Hgb level, whereas no deaths occurred in 98 patients with postoperative levels of 7.1–8.0 g/dL, 34.4% of 32 patients with postoperative levels of 4.1–5.0 g/dL died. These data suggest that in surgery-induced anemia, survival in patients at risk is improved if blood transfusion is administered to maintain Hgb >7 g/dL. In a large, retrospective study of elderly patients who underwent surgical repair of hip fracture, the use of perioperative transfusion in patients with hemoglobin levels as low as 8.0 g/dL did not appear to influence 30-day or 90-day mortality (114).

In a multi-institutional study (115), 418 critical-care patients received red-cell transfusions when the [Hgb] dropped below 7.0 g/dL, with [Hgb] maintenance in the range of 7.0–9.0 g/dL, and 420 patients received transfusions when the [Hgb] declined below 10.0 g/dL, with [Hgb] levels maintained in the range of 10.0–12.0 g/dL. The 30-day mortality rates were not different in the two groups (18.7% vs. 23.3%, $p=0.11$), indicating that a transfusion threshold as low as 7.0 g/dL is as safe as a higher transfusion threshold of 10.0 g/dL in critical-care patients. A follow-up analysis found that the more restrictive strategy of red blood cell transfusion appeared to be safe in most patients with cardiovascular disease; but among a subgroup of 257 patients with ischemic heart disease, there was an insignificant ($p>0.30$) decrease in overall survival among the patients treated according to the restrictive transfusion strategy (116). Clearly, more data are needed to determine when transfusion in this setting is beneficial, particularly in patients known to have risk factors for ischemic heart or cerebral disease.

A study by Wu et al. (117) analyzed the relationships among anemia, blood transfusion, and mortality in a retrospective analysis of nearly 80,000 elderly (>65 years) patients hospitalized for acute myocardial infarction. In this study, lower hematocrit values on admission were associated with higher 30-day mortality rates. Secondly, anemia (defined as hematocrit <39%) was present on hospital admission in nearly half (43.7%) of patients and was clinically significant (i.e., ≤33%) in 10.4% of patients. Finally, transfusion in patients with hematocrit levels <33% at admission was associated with significantly lower 30-day mortality.

B. Morbidity

Data on the relationship between transfusion and morbidity are less clear. A reduction in morbidity may be possible with transfusion in critically ill patients, especially those with hypoxia or sepsis, by optimizing oxygen delivery and minimizing the frequency of potential complications. In one study (118), hemodynamic and oxygen transport measurements were examined in five severely burned male patients who did not receive blood transfusions for 36–48 hr after the operative incision. The [Hgb] level was then raised 3 g/dL with multiple transfusions. Although transfusion raised the red cell mass significantly and increased oxygen delivery, the physiologic benefit seemed marginal. The O_2 extraction ratio, in particular, was not markedly deranged before the transfusion, which indicates that the compensation for the anemia was quite adequate. In addition, there was no change in oxygen consumption, which suggests that blood transfusion may not benefit critically ill patients without known risk factors.

In a report by Babineau et al. (119), the benefit of transfusion was examined in 30 surgical intensive care unit patients who were normovolemic and hemodynamically stable. Once again, transfusion increased the [Hgb] level and total oxygen delivery but had a negligible effect on oxygen consumption. There were no important hemodynamic benefits in this group of patients. One can conclude from these data that the assumed benefit of an increase in the red cell mass does not always translate into a true benefit in terms of oxygen transport in critically ill patients.

Silent perioperative myocardial ischemia has been observed in patients undergoing noncardiac (120), as well as cardiac (121), surgery. A study of elderly patients who were undergoing elective, noncardiac surgery found that intraoperative or postoperative myocardial ischemia was more likely to occur in patients with hematocrits below 28%, particularly in the presence of tachycardia (122). Hemoglobin levels ranging from 6.0 to 10.0 g/dL—a range in which indicators other than [Hgb] may identify patients who may benefit from blood—therefore need to be the most closely scrutinized (110,123). In the absence of a physiologic need or known risk factors in a stable, nonbleeding patient, a decline in [Hgb] level alone is not a good reason to give a transfusion (124).

C. Guidelines for Transfusion

Guidelines for blood transfusion have been issued by several organizations including the National Institutes of Health consensus conference on perioperative transfusion of red cells (125), the American College of Physicians (126), the American Society of Anesthesiologists (123), and the Canadian Medical Association (127). These guidelines recommend that blood not be transfused prophylactically and suggest that in patients without risk factors, the threshold for transfusion should be a hemoglobin level of 6.0–8.0 g/dL. A [Hgb] of 8.0 g/dL seems an appropriate threshold for transfusion in surgical patients with no risk factors for ischemia, whereas a threshold of 10–11 g/dL can be justified for patients who are considered at risk. A recent mathematical analysis suggested that surgical blood losses that exceed 70–120% (e.g., 3500–6000 mL in a 70-kg patient with a 5 L blood volume) of patients' baseline estimated blood volumes are necessary before any blood transfusion (128), but this model assumes a perisurgical red cell transfusion trigger of between 18% and 21% HCT. The study by Hebert et al. (115) concluded that critically ill patients could tolerate Hgb levels as low as 70 g/L, but that no conclusions could be made for patients with risk factors for cardiac or cerebral ischemia. Evidence is accumulating that patients with known risk factors may benefit from higher hemoglobin transfusion thresholds (116,117). With substantial improvements in blood safety (7), concern has been expressed that patients are now at risk for undertransfusion (129). The study by Wu et al. (117) provides evidence for the first time that patients with a specific clinical presentation are affected adversely by the underuse of transfusion. On the basis of this study, hematocrit levels have been recommended to be maintained above 33% in patients who present with acute myocardial infarction (130).

Table 4 Transfusion of Platelets[a] in the United States

	1989	1992	1994	1997	1999	2001
Concentrates	5,146	4,688	3,582	3,396	3,036	2,614
Apheresis	352 (26%)	607 (44%)	714 (54%)	940 (62%)	1,003 (60%)	1,264 (74%)
Total transfusions	6,958	8,330	7,866	9,037	9,054	10,196

[a] Thousands of units. One apheresis unit = six concentrates.
Source: From Refs. 131–133.

III. PLATELET TRANSFUSIONS

Use of intensive chemotherapy regiments in oncology and in bone marrow/stem cell transplantation programs has increased the demand for platelet products, particularly in patients with severe thrombocytopenia or bleeding complications. Use of apheresis platelet transfusions has also increased substantially from 365,000 U in 1989 to 1,003,000 U in 1999 (Table 4) (131–133); this increase is being driven partly by the need for alternative platelet inventories to support cardiac surgery, oncology, and PBSC transplantation programs but partly by use of leukoreduced platlet products (134). Emerging issues in platelet transfusion therapy include (1) re-evaluation of the platelet threshold for prophylactic transfusion and (2) modification of platelet transfusion dose.

A. Threshold for Transfusion

Several studies have evaluated prophylactic platelet transfusion thresholds for patients with thrombocytopenia because of myelosuppressive therapy. Bernstein et al. (135) found that most patients undergoing stem cell transplantation received prophylactic platelet transfusions when their platelet counts were 10,000–20,000 cells/μL, indicating that a threshold of 20,000 cells/μL was most common (Fig. 3). Only 9% of hemorrhagic events reported in this study occurred when platelet counts were < 10,000 cells/μL.

Two prospective, randomized studies evaluated the relative merits of platelet transfusion thresholds of 10,000–20,000 cells/μL for leukemia patients undergoing chemotherapy (136,137). Rebulla et al. (136) found that the lower transfusion threshold was associated with 22% fewer platelet transfusions. In an analysis of hemorrhagic complications, number of red cell transfusions, duration of hospital stay, and mortality, no differences were seen between the two thresholds. In a second study, Wandt et al. (137) showed that a platelet threshold of 10,000 cells/μL was safe and effective aganist the 20,000 cells/μL threshold. Of 105 patients in this study, two (1.9%) died of hemorrhagic complications, each with a platelet count >30,000 cells/μL at the time of death.

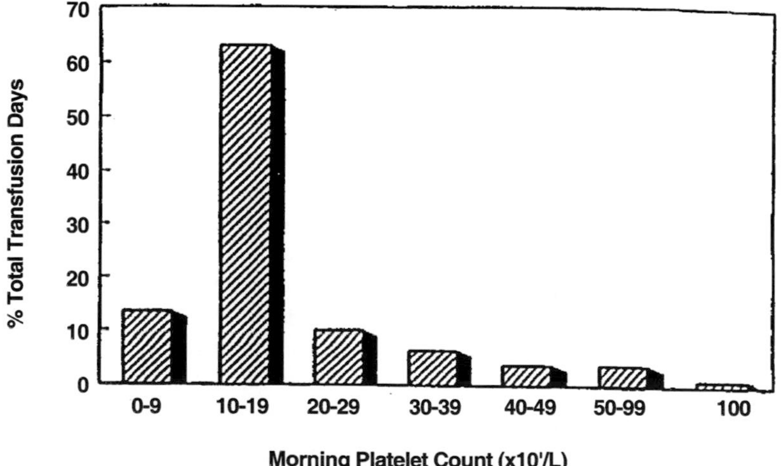

Figure 3 Percentage of patient days in which platelet transfusions were administered to patients with a range of morning platelet counts. In a multicenter study of patients undergoing autologous (n = 456) or allogeneic (n = 335) hematopoietic stem cell transplantation, nearly two-thirds of patients received prophylactic platelet transfusion when platelet counts were between 10,000 and 20,000/mm^3. *Source*: From Ref. 135.

Table 5 Platelet Doses Used in Several Recent Studies[a]

T-1 Study	T-1 Platelet dose ($\times 10^{11}/mm^3$)
TRAP study (85)	
Six unmodified pooled platelet concentrates	4.5 ± 1.2[a]
Six F-PC filtered units[b]	3.7 ± 1.1[a]
One F-AP filtered unit[c]	3.7 ± 1.3[a]
Goodnough et al. (139)	
One apheresis unit	4.2 ± 1.1[a]
Rubella et al. (136)	
Apheresis	2.8 (1.1 to 5.9)[d]
Pooled concentrates	2.2 (1.4 to 5.0)[d]

[a] Median ± SD.
[b] F-PC filtered, pooled platelet concentrates from random donors.
[c] F-AP filtered platelets obtained by apheresis from single random donors.
[d] Median (range).

B. Dose

Standards of the AABB require that 75% of apheresis products contain $>3 \times 10^{11}$ platelets, and that 75% of platelet concentrates contain $>5.5 \times 10^{10}$ platelets (138); however, no consensus exists for a standardized platelet dose. Table 5 presents the platelet doses used in several recent studies and shows the broad range of platelet doses used. In an evaluation of our own hospital-based apheresis program, 32% of products contained between 3 and 4×10^{11} platelets and 32% of products contained $4–5 \times 10^{11}$ platelets (139). Leukoreduction of apheresis platelets or platelet concentrates results in ~20% loss of platelets (85).

Mathematical modeling has suggested that low-dose platelet therapy would be more beneficial in thrombocytopenic patients who are receiving prophylactic platelet transfusions (140). The relationship between patient platelet count and in vivo platelet survival is illustrated in Fig. 4 (141). A fixed platelet requirement for hemostasis is estimated to be 7100/mm^3 per day, and platelet consumption above this threshold is mainly a result of platelet senescence. For patients who become thrombocytopenic due to myeloablative therapy, platelet survival decreases with increasing severity of thrombocytopenia. Thus, platelet survival is 5–7 days in patients with platelet counts in the normal range but only 1–2 days in patients with platelet counts of 10,000–20,000 cells/μL—levels at which most thrombocytopenic patients are maintained to prevent hemorrhage. One mathematical model predicted that low-dose platelet therapy provides a 22% decrease in donor exposures (and total number of platelets) while maintaining patients at a platelet threshold $>10{,}000$ cells/μL (140), even with a shorter transfusion-free interval and a greater daily relative risk of receiving additional transfusions (142).

A randomized clinical trial was conducted to address the issue of high-dose platelet therapy (143). Standard, high, and very high platelet doses (4.6×10^{11}, 6.5×10^{11}, and 8.9×10^{11} platelets, respectively) were administered to patients receiving prophylactic platelet transfusions. The high and very high dose cohorts had greater incremental increases in platelet count and prolonged time to next transfusion than the standard dose cohort. Interestingly, the platelet half-life estimate (i.e.,

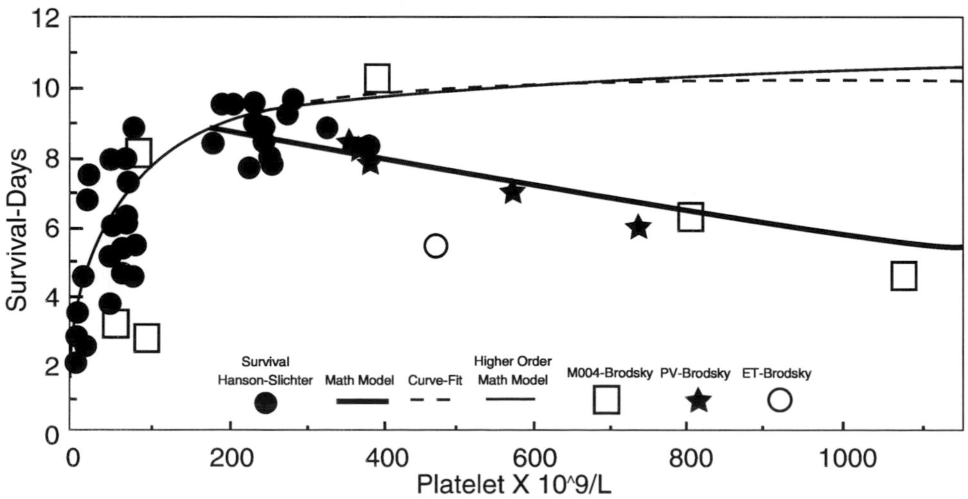

Figure 4 The relationship between patient platelet count and in vivo platelet survival. Survival data are points obtained from normal individuals and patients with hypoplastic or aplastic marrows (141) and patients with myeloproliferative disease. *Source*: From Ref. 140.

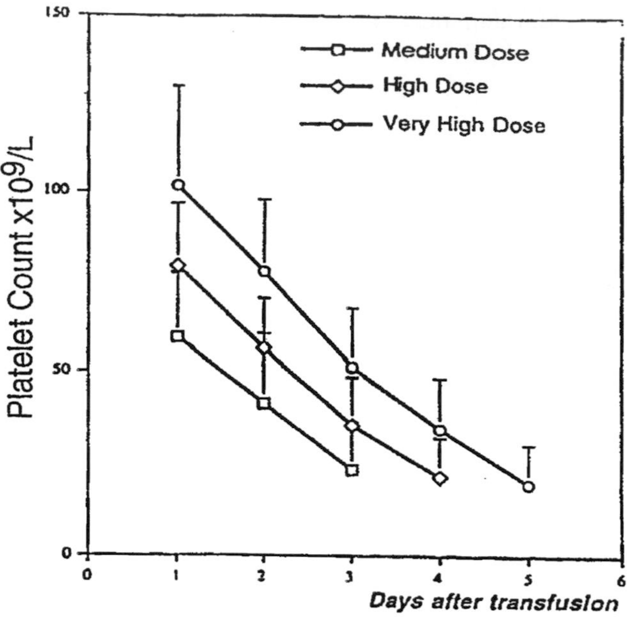

Figure 5 Platelet count and platelet decline after transfusion. The half-disappearance of platelets (i.e., slope) after transfusion of standard, high, and very high platelet doses is not different among the three cohorts over a five-day post-transfusion interval. *Source*: From Ref. 143.

slopes) for the patient cohorts was not different for post-transfusion platelet counts ranging from ~50,000 to 110,000 cells/μL (Fig. 5). These data suggest that the in vivo platelet lifespan of transfused platelets cannot be normalized in this setting, even at higher platelet counts. Further studies of platelet transfusion dosage strategies are needed.

C. Patient Response

Patient response to platelet transfusion varies. When thrombocytopenic patients undergoing hematopoietic stem cell transplantation were analyzed for platelet CCI after transfusion, a bell-shaped or polynomial distribution was found (Fig. 6), and patient-specific factors accounted for this distribution (42). Factors usually associated with response to platelets (e.g., history of previous transfusion, pregnancy, presence of HLA or platelet-specific antibodies) did not significantly correlate with CCI. These findings suggest that administration of leukoreduced platelets is not clinically important in prevention of platelet refractoriness in patients undergoing stem cell transplantation (140).

In summary, platelet transfusion dose is variable and patient's response to transfusion varies. Furthermore, thrombocytopenic patients can be maintained safely at prophylactic transfusion thresholds of 10,000 cells/μL. Finally, the likelihood of hemorrhagic complications correlates poorly with degree of thrombocytopenia in patients undergoing myeloablative chemotherapy. These findings, the results of the TRAP study (86) and our own observations, indicate that the use of specialized products (apheresis platelets and leukoreduced platelets) needs to be reassessed in the context of emerging technologies.

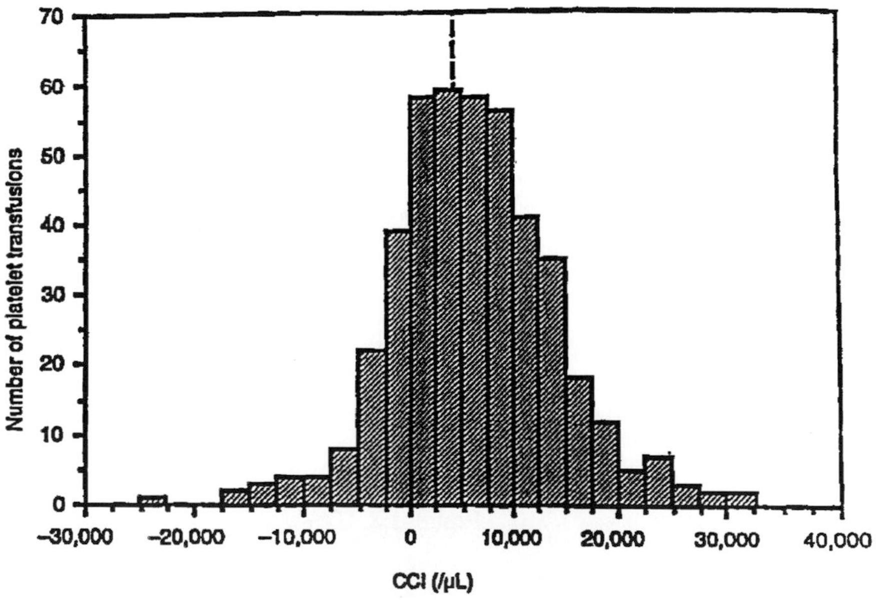

Figure 6 Distribution of 16-hr CCI for 439 platelet transfusions in 42 stem cell transplantation recipients. *Source*: From Ref. 144.

IV. CONCLUSION

Thrombocytopenia remains a significant clinical problem for patients with cancer. Management approaches include watchful waiting, platelet transfusions, and use of pharmacologic agents. Although platelet transfusions remain the gold standard for prophylaxis and treatment of thrombocytopenia, transfusion-transmitted diseases, infection, and platelet refractoriness are associated with their use. Because of these complications and the expense of platelet therapy, studies have examined the clinical evidence behind the widely used platelet transfusion trigger of 20,000 cells/μL and found that values of 5,000–10,000 cells/μL are safe for selected patients. Finally, the likelihood of hemorrhagic complications correlates poorly with degree of thrombocytopenia in patients undergoing myeloablative chemotherapy. These findings, the results of the TRAP study and our own observations, indicate that the use of specialized products (apheresis platelets and leukoreduced platelets) needs to be reassessed.

REFERENCES

1. Aach RD, Szmuness W, Mosley JW, Hollinger FB, Kahn RA, Stevens CE, Edwards VM, Werth J. Serum alanine aminotransferase of donors in relation to the risk of non-A, non-B hepatitis in recipients: the transfusion-transmitted viruses study. N Engl J Med 1981; 304:989–994.
2. Schreiber GB, Busch MP, Kleinman SH, Korelitz JJ. The risk of transfusion-transmitted viral infections. N Engl J Med 1996; 334:1685–1690.
3. Lackritz EM, Satten GA, Aberle-Grasse J, Dodd RY, Raimondi VP, Janssen RS, Lewis F, Notari EP, Petersen LR. Estimated risk of transmission of the human immunodeficiency virus by screened blood in the United States. N Engl J Med 1995; 333:1721–1725.
4. Vamvakas EC, Taswell HF. Long-term survival after blood transfusion. Transfusion 1994; 34:471–477.
5. Goodnough LT, Brecher ME, Kanter MH, Aubuchon JP. Transfusion medicine, part I. Blood transfusion. N Engl J Med 1999; 340:438–447.
6. Dodd RY, Notari EP, Stramer SL. Current prevalence and incidence of infectious disease markers and estimated window-period risk in the American red cross blood donor population. Transfusion 2002; 42: 975–979.
7. Goodnough LT, Shander A, Brecher ME. Transfusion medicine: looking to the future. Lancet 2003; 361: 161–169.
8. Joint statement on acquired immune deficiency syndrome (AIDS) related to transfusion. Transfusion 1983; 23:87–88.
9. Silvergleid AJ, Leparc GF, Schmidt PJ. Impact of explicit questions about high-risk activities on donor attitudes and donor referral patterns. Results in two community blood centers. Transfusion 1989; 29: 362–364.
10. Petersen LR, Lackritz E, Lewis W, Smith DS, Herrera G, Raimondi V, Aberle-Grasse J, Dodd RY. The effectiveness of the confidential unit exclusion option. Transfusion 1994; 34:865–869.
11. Busch MP, Young MJ, Samson SM, Mosley JW, Ward JW, Perkins HA, and the Transfusion Safety Study Group. Risk of human immunodeficiency virus (HIV) transmission by blood transfusions before the implementation of HIV-1 antibody screening. Transfusion 1991; 31:4–11.
12. AuBuchon JP, Birkmeyer JD, Busch MP. Safety of the blood supply in the United States: opportunities and controversies. Ann Int Med 1997; 127:904–909.
13. Selik RM, Ward JW, Buehler JW. Trends in transfusion-associated acquired immune deficiency syndrome in the United States, 1982–1991. Transfusion 1993; 33:890–893.
14. MMWR Update: HIV-2 infection among blood and plasma donors—United States, June 1992–June 1995. MMWR 1995; 44:603–606.
15. Stramer SL, Grasse JA, Brodsky JP, Busch MP, Lackritz EM. US blood donor screening with p24 antigen (Ag): one year experience. Transfusion 1997; 37(suppl):1S.
16. Domen RE. Paid-versus-volunteer blood donation in the United States: a historical review. Transfusion Med Reviews 1995; 9:53–59.
17. Dodd RY. Adverse consequences of blood transfusion: quantitative risk estimates. In: Nance ST, ed. Blood Supply: Risks Perceptions, and Prospects for the Future. Bethesda, MD: American Association of Blood Banks, 1994:1–24.
18. Stevens CE, Aach RD, Hollinger FB, Mosley JW, Szmuness W, Kahn R, Werch J, Edwards V. Hepatitis B virus antibody in blood donors and the occurrence of non-A, non-B hepatitis in transfusion recipients: an analysis of the transfusion-transmitted viruses study. Ann Intern Med 1984; 101:733–738.
19. Alter HJ, Purcell RH, Shih JN, Melpolder JC, Houghton M, Choo QL, Kuo G. Detection of antibody to hepatitis C virus in prospectively followed transfusion recipients with acute and chronic non-A and non-B hepatitis. N Eng J Med 1989; 321: 1494–1500.
20. MMWR. Recommendations for prevention and control of hepatitis C virus (HCV) infection and HCV-related chronic disease. USHHS. Oct 16, 1998.
21. Conry-Cantilena C, van Raden M, Gibble J, Melpolder J, Shakil AO, Viladomiu L, Cheung L, DiBisceglie A, Hoofnagle J, Shih JW, Kaslow R, Ness P, Alter HJ. Routes of infection, viremia, and liver disease in blood donors found to have hepatitis C virus infection. N Engl J Med 1996; 334:1691–1696.

22. Tong MJ, El-Farra NS, Reikes AR, Ruth L. Clinical outcomes after transfusion-associated hepatitis C. N Engl J Med 1995; 332:1463–1466.
23. Delwart E, Kalmin N, Jones S, Ladd D, Tobler L, Tsui R, Busch M. First Case of HIV transmission by an RNA-screened blood donation. 9th Conference on Retroviruses and Opportunistic Infections, Feb 24–28, 2002 Washington State Convention and Trade Center, Seattle, WA (http://www.retroconference.org/2002/Posters/13519.pdf).
24. HIV-tainted blood infects two in Florida (http://www.cbsnews.com/stories/2002/07/19/health/main515694.shtml).
25. da Silva, Cardoso M, Koerner K, Kubanek B. The first case of HCV seroconversion after 3 years of HCV NAT screening in Baden-Wurttemberg. Transfusion 2000; 40(11):1422–1423.
26. Red blood cell transfusions contaminated with *Yersinia enterocolitica*—United States, 1991–1996, and initiation of a national study to detect bacteria-associated transfusion reactions. MMWR 1997; 46: 553–555.
27. Cookson ST, Arduino MJ, Aguero SM, Jarvis WR, and the Yersinia Study Group. *Yersinia entercolitica*-contaminated red blood cells—an emerging threat to blood safety. 1996 Interscience Conference on Antimicrobial Agents and Chemotherapy, ABS New Orieans 1996; 2352.
28. Yomtovian R, Lazarus HM, Goodnough LT, Hirschler NV, Morrissey AM, Jacobs MR. A prospective microbiologic surveillance program to detect and prevent the transfusion of bacterially contaminated platelets. Transfusion 1993; 33:902–909.
29. Leiby DA, Kerr KL, Campos JM, Dodd RY. A retrospective analysis of microbial contaminants in outdated random-donor platelets from multiple sites. Transfusion 1997; 37(3):259–263.
30. Goldman M, Blajchman MA. Blood product-associated bacterial sepsis. Transfus Med Reviews 1991; 5:73–83.
31. AABB. Association Bulletin #96–6. Bacterial contamination of blood components. AABB Faxnet, No 294, August 1996. American Association of Blood Banks.
32. Jacobs MR, Palavecino E, Yomtovian R. Don't bug me: the problem of bacterial contamination of blood components—challenges and solutions. Transfusion 2001; 41:1331–1334.
33. Ness PM, Braine HG, King K, Barrasso C, Kickler T, Fuller A, Blades N. Single-donor platelets reduce the risk of septic platelet transfusion reactions. Transfusion 2001; 41:857–861.
34. Ollgaard M, Albjerg I, Georgen J. Monitoring of bacterial growth in platelet concentrates—one year's experience with the BactAlert™ System. Vox Sanguinis 1998; 74(suppl 1):1126.
35. Laan E, Tros C. Improved safety and extended shelf-life of leuco-depleted platelet concentrates by automated bacterial screening. Transfusion 1999; 39:5S.
36. Vucetic D, Taseski J, Balint B, Mirovic V. The use of BacTAlert system for bacterial screening in platelet concentrates. Vox Sanguinis 2000; 78(suppl 1):P371.
37. McDonald CP, Roy A, Lowe P, Rogers A, Green G, Vegoda J, Earley J, Barbara JAJ. The first experience in the United Kingdom of the bacteriological screening of platelets to increase shelf life to 7 days. Vox Sanguinis 2000; 78(suppl 1):P375.
38. Brecher ME, Means N, Jere CS, Heath D, Rothenberg S, Stutzman LC. Evaluation of an automated culture system for detecting bacterial contamination of platelets: an analysis of 15 contaminating organisms. Transfusion 2001; 41:477–482.
39. AuBuchon JP, Cooper LK, Leach MF, Herschel LH, Roger JC. Bacterial culture of platelet units and extension of storage to 7 days. Transfusion 2001; 41S:1S.
40. Brecher ME, Holland PV, Pineda AA, Tegtmeier GE, Yomtovian R. Growth of bacteria in inoculated platelets: implications for bacteria detection and the extension of platelet storage. Transfusion 2000; 40: 1308–1312.
41. Lin L, Cook DN, Wiesehahn GP, Alfonso R, Behrman B, Cimino GD, Corten L, Damonte PB, Dikeman R, Dupuis K, Fang YM, Hanson CV, Hearst JE, Lin CY, Londe HF, Metchette K, Nerio AT, Pu JT, Reames AA, Rheinschmidt M, Tessman J, Isaacs ST, Wollowitz S, Corash L. Photochemical inactivation of viruses and bacteria in platelet concentrates by use of a novel psoralen and long-wavelength ultraviolet light. Transfusion 1997; 37:423–435.
42. Knutson F, Alfonso R, Dupuis K, Mayaudon V, Lin L, Corash L, Hogman CF. Photochemical inactivation of bacteria and HIV in buffy-coat-derived platelet concentrates under conditions that preserve in vitro platelet function. Vox Sanguinis 2000; 78(4):209–216.
43. Corash L, Behrman B, Rheinschmidt M, Wages D, Snyder E, Raife T, Kagen L, Baril L, Davis K, Metzel P, Walsh J, Smith D, Shafer S, Cimino G, Hei D, Tessman J, Lin L, Buchholz DH. Post-transfusion viability and tolerability of photochemically treated platelet concentrates. Blood 1997; 90:267a.
44. McCullough J, Vesole D, Benjamin RJ, Slichter S, Pineda A, Snyder E. Pathogen-inactivated platelets using Helinx™ technology are hemostatically effective in the thrombocytopenia patient. Blood 2001; 98:45a.
45. Sayers MH, Anderson KC, Goodnough LT, Kurtz SF, Lane TA, Pisciotto P, Silberstein LE. Reducing the risk for transfusion-transmitted cytomegalovirus infection. Ann Intern Med 1992; 116:55–62.
46. Rubie H, Attal M, Campardou AM, Gayet-Mengelle C, Payen C, Sanguignol F, Catol JP, Charlet JP, Robert A, Huguet F, Puel J, Pris J, Laurent G. Risk factors for cytomegalovirus in BMT recipients transfused exclusively with seronegative blood products. Bone Marrow Transplant 1993; 11:209–214.

47. Bowden RA, Sayers M, Fluornoy N, Newton B, Banaji M, Thomas ED, Meyers JD. Cytomegalovirus immune globulin and seronegative blood products to prevent primary cytomegalovirus infection after marrow transplantation. N Engl J Med 1986; 314: 1006–1010.
48. Vij R, DiPersio JF, Venkatraman P, Trinkaus K, Goodnough LT, Brown R, Khoury HJ, Devine SM, Oza A, Shenoy S, Blum W, Adkins D. Donor CMV serostatus has no impact on CMV viremia or disease when prophylactic granulocyte transfusions are given following allogeneic peripheral blood stem cell transplantation. Blood 2003; 101:2067–2069.
49. Wingard JR, Chen DYH, Burns WH, Fuller DJ, Braine HG, Yeager AM, Kaiser H, Burke PJ, Graham ML, Santos GW, Saral R. Cytomegalovirus infection after autologous bone marrow transplantation with comparison to infection after allogeneic bone marrow transplantation. Blood 1988; 71:1432–1437.
50. Verdonck LF, van der Linden JA, Bast BJEG, Meling FGJG, de Gast GC. Influence of cytomegalovirus-infections on the recovery of humoral immunity after autologous bone marrow transplant. Exp Hematol 1987; 15:864–868.
51. Wingard JR, Sostrin MB, Vriessendorp HM, Mellits ED, Santos GW, Fuller DJ, Braine HG, Yeager AM, Burns WH, Saral R. Interstitial pneumonitis following autologous bone marrow transplantation. Transplantation 1988; 46:61–65.
52. American Association of Blood Banks. Leukocyte reduction for the prevention of transfusion-transmitted cytomegalovirus (TT-CMV). AABB Bulletin 1997; 17:391.
53. Holmberg LA, Boeckh M, Hooper H, Leisenring W, Rowley S, Heimfeld S, Press O, Maloney DG, McSweeney P, Corey L, Maziarz RT, Appelbaum FR, Bensinger W. Increased incidence of cytomegalovirus disease after autologous CD34-selected peripheral blood stem cell transplantation. Blood 1999; 94: 4029–4035.
54. Bowden RA, Slichter SJ, Sayers M, Weidorf D, Cays M, Schoch G, Banaji M, Haake R, Welk K, Fisher L, McCullough J, Miller W. A comparison of filtered leukocyte reduced and cytomegalovirus (CMV)-seronegative blood products for the prevention of transfusion-associated CMV infection after marrow transplant. Blood 1985; 86:3598–3603.
55. Ledent E, Berlin G. Inadequate white cell reduction from red cell concentrates by filtration. Transfusion 1994; 34:765–768.
56. Landaw EM, Kanter M, Petz LD. Safety of filtered leukocyte-reduced blood products for the prevention of transfusion-associated cytomegalovirus infection. Blood 1996; 87:4910–4911.
57. Adler SP, Baggett J, McVoy M. Transfusion-associated cytomegalovirus infections in seropositive cardiac patients. Lancet 1985; 1:743–746.
58. AABB. VATS study shows no benefit of leukocyte reduction for HIV-Infected patients. AABB Weekly Report 1999; 5:1–2.
59. Lepaucis A, Brown J, Costello B, Delage G, Freedman J, Hume H, King S, Kleinman S, Mazzulli T, Wells G. Prevention of posttransfusion CMV in the era of universal WBC reduction: a consensus statement. Transfusion 2001; 41:560–569.
60. Blajchman MA, Goldman M, Freedman JJ, Sher GD. Proceedings of a consensus conference: prevention of post-transfusion CMV in the era of universal leukoreduction. Transfusion Med Reviews 2001; 15:1–20.
61. Luban NLC. Human parvoviruses; implications for transfusion medicine. Transfusion 1994; 34:821–827.
62. Gout O, Baulac M, Gessain A, Semah F, Saal F, Peries J, Cabrol C, Fougault-Fretz C, Laplane D, Sigaux F, de The G. Rapid development of myelopathy after HTLV-I infection acquired by transfusion during cardiac transplantation. N Engl J Med 1990; 322:383–388.
63. Kanno M, Nakamura S, Matsuda T. Adult T-cell leukemia with HTLV-I associated myelopathy after complete remission of acute myelogenous leukemia. N Eng J Med 1998; 338:333.
64. Nahlen BL, Lobel HO, Cannon SE, Campbell CC. Reassessment of blood donor selection criteria for United States travelers to malarious areas. Transfusion 1991; 31:786–788.
65. Guerrero IC, Weneger BG, Schultz MG. Transfusion malaria in the United States, 1972–1981. Ann Int Med 1983; 99:221–226.
66. Mungai M, Tegtmeier G, Chamberland M, Parise M. Transfusion-transmitted malaria in the United States from 1963 through 1999. N Engl J Med 2001; 344:1973–1978.
67. Schmunis GA. Trypanosomo Cruzi, the etiologic agent of Chagas' disease: status in the blood supply in endemic and non-endemic countries. Transfusion 1991; 31:547–557.
68. Schmunis GA, Zueker F, Cruz JR, Cuchi P. Safety of blood supply for infectious disease in Latin American countries. Am J Trop Med Hug 2001; 65:924–930.
69. Shulman IA, Appelman S, Saxena S, Hiti AL, Kirchhoff LV. Specific antibodies to *Trupansoma cruzi* among blood donors in Los Angeles, California. Transfusion 1997; 37:727–731.
70. Cimo PL, Luper WE, Scouroso MA. Transfusion-associated Chagas' disease in Texas: report of a case. Tex Med J 1993; 89:48–50.
71. CDC. Chagas disease after organ transplantation. United States, 2001 (http://www.coc.gov/mmwr/preview/mmwrhtm/mm511093.htm).
72. McQuiston JH, Childs JE, Chamberland ME, Tabor E. Transmission of tick-borne agents of disease by blood transfusion: a review of known and potential risks in the United States. Transfusion 2000; 40: 274–284.

73. Brown P, Preece MA, Will RG. Friendly fire in medicine: hormones, homografts, and Creutzfeldt–Jacob disease. Lancet 1992; 340:24–27.
74. Dodd RY, Sullivan MT. Creutzfeldt–Jacob disease and transfusion safety: tilting at icebergs? (editorial). Transfusion 1998; 38:221–223.
74a. Llewelyn CA, Hewill PE, Knight RW, et al. Possible Transmission of variant creutzfeldt disease by blood transfusion. Lancet 2004; 356:417–419.
75. Revised preventative measures to reduce the possible risk of transmission of CJD and vCJD by blood and blood products (http://www.fda.gov/cber/gdlins/cjdvcjd.htm).
76. Bordin JO, Heddle NM, Blajchman MA. Biologic effects of leukocytes present in transfused cellular blood products. Blood 1994; 84:1703–1721.
77. Landers DF, Hill GE, Wong KC, Fox IJ. Blood transfusion-induced immunomodulation. Anesth Analg 1996; 82:187–204.
78. Vamvakas EC, Dzik WH, Blajchman MA. Deleterious effects of transfusion-associated immunomodulation: appraisal of the evidence and recommendations for prevention. In: Vamvakas, ed. Immunomodulatory Effects of Blood Transfusion. Bethesda, MD: AABB Press, 1999:253–285.
79. Lane TA, Anderson KC, Goodnough LT, Kurtz S, Moroff G, Pisciotto PT, Sayers M, Silberstein LE. Leukocyte reduction in blood component therapy. Ann Int Med 1992; 117:151–162.
80. British Committee for Standards in Haematology, Blood Transfusion Task Force. Guidelines on the clinical use of leukocyte-depleted blood components. Transfusion Med 1998; 8:59–71.
81. Brown P, Cervenakova L, McShane LM, Barber P, Rubenstein R, Drohan WN. Further studies of blood infectivity in an experimental model of transmissible sponge for encephalopathy, with an explanation of why blood components do not transmit Creutzfeldt–Jacob disease in humans. Transfusion 1999; 39: 1169–1178.
82. AABB. PAC recommends universal leukoreduction. AABB Newsbriefs 1998; 20:16.
83. Menitove JE, McElligott MC, Aster RH. Febrile transfusion reaction: what blood component should be given next? Vox Sang 1982; 42:318–321.
84. Chambers LA, Kruskall MS, Pacini DG, Donovan LM. Febrile reactions after platelet transfusion: the effect of single vs. multiple donors. Transfusion 1990; 30:219–221.
85. TRAP Study Group. Leukocyte reduction and ultraviolet B irradiation of platelets to prevent alloimmunization and refractoriness to platelet transfusions. N Engl J Med 1997; 337:1861–1869.
86. Goodnough LT, Riddell J, Lazarus H, Chafel TL, Prince G, Hendrix D, Yomtovian R. Prevalence of platelet transfusion reactions before and after implementation of leukocyte-depleted platelet concentrates by filtration. Vox Sang 1993; 65:103–107.
87. Heddle NM, Klama L, Singer J, Richards C, Fedak F, Walker I, Kelton JG. The role of plasma in transfusion reactions. N Engl J Med 1994; 331:625–628.
88. Shiba M, Tadokoro K, Sawanobori M, Nakajima K, Suzuki K, Juji T. Activation of the contact system by filtration of platelet concentrates with a negatively charged white cell removal filter and measurement of venous blood bradykinin level in patients who received filtered platelets. Transfusion 1997; 37:457–462.
89. Leukoreduction: The techniques used, their effectiveness and costs. Canadian coordinating office for health technology assessment (ECOHTA), 1998 (http://www.ccohta.ca).
90. Uhlmann EJ, Isriggs E, Walher M, Fechtel M, Goodnough LT. Pre-storage universal leukoreduction of RBC does not affect the incidence of transfusion reactions. Transfusion 2001; 41:997–1000.
91. Hebert PC, Fergusson D, Blajchman MA, Wells GA, Kmetic A, Coyle D, Heddle N, Germain M, Goldman M, Toye B, Schweitzer I, van Walraven C, Devine D, Sher GD. Clinical outcomes following institution of the Canadian universal leukoreduction program for red blood cell transfusions. JAMA 2003; 289:1941–1949.
92. Dzik WH, Anderson SK, O'Neill EM, Assmann SF, Kalish LA, Stowell CP. A prospective, randomized clinical trial of universal WBC reduction. Transfusion 2002; 42:1114–1122.
93. Ishida A, Handa M, Wakui M, Okamoto S, Kamakura M, Ikeda Y. Clinical factors influencing posttransfusion platelet increment in patients undergoing hematopoietic progenitor cell transplantation—a prospective analysis. Transfusion 1998; 38: 839–847.
94. Bernstein SH, Nademanee AP, Vose JM, Tricot G, Fay JW, Negrin RS, DiPersio J, Rondon G, Champlin R, Barnett MJ, Cornetta K, Herzig GP, Vaughan W, Geils G Jr, Keating A, Messner H, Wolff SN, Miller KB, Linker C, Cairo M, Hellmann S, Ashby M, Stryker S, Nash RA. A multicenter study of platelet recovery and utilization in patients after myeloblative therapy and hematopoietic stem cell transplantation. Blood 1998; 91:3509–3517.
95. Goodnough LT, Kuter D, McCullough J, Brecher ME. Apheresis platelets: emerging issues related to donor platelet count, apheresis platelet yield, and platelet transfusion dose. J Clin Apher 1998; 13:114–119.
96. Opelz G, Terasaki PI. Improvement of kidney-graft survival with increased numbers of blood transfusions. N Engl J Med 1978; 299:799–803.
97. Mowbray JF, Gibbings C, Liddell H, Reginald PW, Underwood JL, Beard RW. Controlled trial of treatment of recurrent spontaneous abortion by immunization with paternal cells. Lancet 1985; 1:941–943.

98. Blajchman MA. Transfusion-associated immunomodulation and universal white cell reduction: are we putting the cart before the horse? Transfusion 1999; 37:667–670.
99. Ober C, Karrison T, Odem RR, Barnes RB, Branch DW, Stephenson MD, Baron B, Walker MA, Scott JR, Schreiber JR. Mononuclear cell immunization in prevention of recurrent miscarriages: a randomized trial. Lancet 1999; 354:365–369.
100. Vamvakas EC. Transfusion-associated cancer recurrence and postoperative infection: meta-analysis of randomized, controlled clinical trials. Transfusion 1996; 36:175–186.
101. Heiss MM, Mempel W, Delanoff C, Jauch KW, Gabka C, Mempel M, Dieterich HJ, Eissner HJ, Schildberg FW. Blood transfusion-modulated tumor recurrence: first results of a randomized study of autologous versus allogeneic blood transfusion in colorectal cancer surgery. J Clin Oncol 1994; 12: 1859–1867.
102. Busch OR, Hop WC, van Papendrecht H, Marquet RL, Jeekel J. Blood transfusions and prognosis in colorectal cancer. N Engl J Med 1993; 328:1372–1376.
103. Houbiers JG, van de Watering LM, Hermans J, Verwey PJM, Bijnen AB, Pahlplatz P, Schattenkerk ME, Wobbes T, de Vries JE, Klementschlitsch P, van de Maas AHM, van de Velde CJH. Randomized controlled trial comparing transfusion of leukocyte-depleted or buffy-coat-depleted blood in surgery for colorectal cancer. Lancet 1994; 344:573–578.
104. van de Watering LMG, Hermans J, Houbiers JGA, van den Broek PJ, Bouter H, Boer F, Harvey MS, Huysmans HA, Brand A. Beneficial effects of leukocyte depletion of transfused blood on postoperative complications in patients undergoing cardiac surgery. A randomized clinical trial. Circulation 1998; 97: 562–568.
105. Hattler BG, Madia C, Johnson C, Armitage JM, Hardesty RL, Kormos RL, Pham SM, Payne DN, Griffith BP. Risk stratification using the Society of Thoracic Surgeons program. Ann Thor Surg 1994; 58:1348–1352.
106. Corwin HL, Aubuchon JP. Is leukoreduction of blood components for everyone? JAMA 2003; 289: 1993–1995.
107. Finch CA, Lenfant C. Oxygen transport in man. N Engl J Med 1972; 286:407–415.
108. Levy PS, Chavez RP, Crystal GJ, Kim SJ, Eckel PK, Sehgal LR, Sehgal HL, Salem MR, Gould SA. Oxygen extraction ratio: a valid indicator of transfusion need in limited coronary reserve?. J Trauma 1992; 32: 769–774.
109. Levy PS, Kim SJ, Eckel PK, Chavez R, Ismail EF, Gould SA, Ramez Salem M, Crystal GJ. Limit to cardiac compensation during acute isovolemic hemodilution: influence of coronary stenosis. Am J Physiol 1993; 265:H340–H349.
110. Goodnough LT, Despotis GJ, Hogue CW. On the need for improved transfusion indicators in cardiac surgery. Ann Thor Surg 1995; 60:473–480.
111. Kitchens CS. Are transfusions overrated? Surgical outcome of Jehovah's Witnesses [Editorial]. Am J Med 1993; 94:117–119.
112. Carson JL, Duff A, Poses RM, Berlin JA, Spence RK, Trout R, Novecek H, Strom BL. Effect of anaemia and cardiovascular disease on surgical mortality and morbidity. Lancet 1996; 348:1055–1060.
113. Carson JL, Novock H, Berlin JA, Gould SA. Mortality and morbidity in patients with very low postoperative Hgb levels who decline blood transfusion. Transfusion 2002; 42:812–818.
114. Carson JL, Duff A, Berlin JA, Lawrence VA, Poses RM, Huber EC, O'Hara DA, Noveck H, Strom BL. Perioperative blood transfusion and postoperative mortality. JAMA 1998; 279:199–205.
115. Hebert PC, Wells G, Blajchman MA, Marshall J, Martin C, Pagliarello G, Tweeddale M, Schweitzer I, Yetisir E, and the Transfusion Requirements in Critical Care Investigators for the Canadian Critical Care Trials Group. A multicenter, randomized, controlled clinical trial of transfusion requirements in critical care. N Engl J Med 1999; 340:409–417.
116. Hebert PC, Yetisir E, Martin C, Blajchman MA, Wells G, Marshall J, Tweeddale M, Pagliarello G, Schweitzer I. Is a low transfusion threshold safe in critically ill patients with cardiovascular disease? Crit Care Med 2001; 29:227–234.
117. Wu WC, Rathore SS, Wang Y, Radford MJ, Krumholtz KM. Blood transfusion in elderly patients with acute myocardial infarction. N Engl J Med 2001; 345:1230–1236.
118. Gore DC, DeMaria EJ, Reines HD. Elevations in red blood cell mass reduce cardiac index without altering the oxygen consumption in severely burned patients. Surg Forum 1992; 43:721–723.
119. Babineau TJ, Dzik WH, Borlase BC, Baxter JK, Bistrian BR, Benotti PN. Reevaluation of current transfusion practices in patients in surgical intensive care units. Am J Surg 1992; 164:22–25.
120. Mangano DT, Browner WS, Hollenberg M, London MJ, Tubau JF, Tateo IM. Association of perioperative myocardial ischemia with cardiac morbidity and mortality in men undergoing noncardiac surgery. N Engl J Med 1990; 323:1781–1788.
121. Rao TLK, Montoya A. Cardiovascular, electrocardiographic and respiratory changes following acute anemia with volume replacement in patients with coronary artery disease. Anesth Dev 1985; 12:49–54.
122. Hogue CW Jr, Goodnough LT, Monk TG. Perioperative myocardial ischemic episodes are related to hematocrit level in patients undergoing radical prostatectomy. Transfusion 1998; 38:924–931.
123. ASA Task Force. Practice guidelines for blood component therapy: a report by the American Society of

Anesthesiologists Task Force on blood component therapy. Anesthesiology 1996; 84:732–747.
124. Welch HG, Mehan KR, Goodnough LT. Prudent strategies for elective red blood cell transfusion. Ann Int Med 1992; 116:393–440.
125. NIH. Consensus Conference: perioperative red cell transfusion. JAMA 1988; 260:2700–2703.
126. American College of Physicians. Practice strategies for elective red blood cell transfusion. Ann Int Med 1992; 116:403–406.
127. Expert Working Group. Guidelines for red blood cell and plasma transfusions for adults and children. Can Med Assoc J 1997; 156(suppl 11):S1–S24.
128. Weiskopf RB. Efficacy of acute normovolemic hemodilution assessed as a function of fraction of blood volume lost. Anesthesia 2001; 94:439–446.
129. Lenfant C. Transfusion practices should be audited for both undertransfusion and overtransfusion (Letter). Transfusion 1992; 32:873–874.
130. Goodnough LT, Bach RG. Anemia, transfusion, and mortality. N Engl J Med 2001; 345:1272–1274.
131. Wallace EL, Churchill WH, Surgenor DM, An J, Cho G, McGurk S, Murphy L. Collection and transfusion of blood and blood components in the United States, 1992. Transfusion 1995; 35:802–812.
132. Wallace EL, Churchill WH, Surgenor, Cho GS, McGurk S. Collection and transfusion of blood and blood components in the United States, 1994. Transfusion 1998; 38:625–636.
133. National Blood Data Resource Center. Comprehensive Report on Blood Collection and Transfusion in the United States in 2001. Bethesda Maryland, National Blood Data Resource Center 2003.
134. Pall Corp. Demand leukocyte-depleted blood for more complete patient protection. Ann Thor Surg 1997; 60:A20-A21.
135. Bernstein SH, Nademanee AP, Vose JM, Tricot G, Fay JW, Negrin RS, DiPersion J, Rondon G, Champlin R, Barnett MJ, Cornetta K, Herzig GP, Vaughan W, Geils G, Keating A, Messner H, Wolff SN, Miller KB, Linker C, Cairo M, Hellmann S, Ashby M, Stryker S, Nash RA. A multicenter study of platelet recovery and utilization in patients after myeloablative therapy and hematopoietic stem cell transplantation. Blood 1998; 91:3509–3517.
136. Rebulla P, Finazzi G, Marangoni F, Avvisati G, Gugliotta L, Tognoni G, Barbue T, Mancelli F, Sirchia G. The threshold for prophylactic platelet transfusions in adults with acute myeloid leukemia. N Engl J Med 1997; 337:1870–1875.
137. Wandt H, Frank M, Ehninger G, Schneider C, Brack N, Daoud A, Fackler-Schwalbe I, Fischer J, Gackle R, Geer T, Harms P, Loffler B, Ohl S, Otremba B, Raab M, Schonrock-Nabulsi P, Strobel G, Winter R, Link H. Safety and cost effectiveness of a $10 \times 10^9/L$ trigger for prophylactic platelet transfusions compared with the traditional $20 \times 10^9/L$ trigger: a prospective comparative trial in 105 patients with acute myeloid leukemia. Blood 1998; 91:3601–3606.
138. American Association of Blood Banks. In: Menitove JE, eds. Standards for Blood Banks and Transfusion Services. Bethesda, MD: American Association of Blood Banks, 2002.
139. Goodnough LT, Ali S, Despotis GJ, Dynis M, Dipersio JF. Economic impact of donor platelet count and platelet yield in apheresis products: relevance for emerging issues in platelet transfusion therapy. Vox Sang 1999; 76:43–49.
140. Hersh JK, Hom EG, Brecher ME. Mathematical modeling of platelet survival with implications for optimal transfusion practice in the chronic platelet transfusion dependent patient. Transfusion 1998; 38: 637–644.
141. Hanson SR, Slichter SJ. Platelet kinetics in patients with bone marrow hypoplasia: evidence for fixed platelet requirements. Blood 1985; 66:1105–1109.
142. Klumpp TR, Herman JH, Gaughan JP, Russo RR, Christman RA, Goldberg SL, Ackerman SJ, Bleeker GC, Mangan KF. Clinical consequences of alterations in platelet transfusion dose: a prospective, randomized double-blind trial. Transfusion 1999; 39:674–681.
143. Norol F, Bierling P, Roudot-Throvac F, Le Coeur FF, Rieux C, Lavaux A, Kuentz M, Deudari N. Platelet transfusion: a dose–response study. Blood 1998; 92:1448–1453.
144. Ishida A, Handa M, Wakui M, Okamoto S, Kamakura M, Ikeda Y. Clinical factors influencing post-transfusion platelet increment in patients undergoing hematopoietic pregenitor cell transplantation — a prospective analysis. Transfusion 1998; 38:839–847.

33

Principles of Medical ICU Oncology

SPENCER S. KEE

Department of Anesthesiology and Pain Medicine, The University of Texas M.D. Anderson Cancer Center, Houston, Texas, U.S.A.

I. INTRODUCTION

An estimated 556,500 patients in the United States died of cancer in 2003, making cancer responsible for one in every four deaths in the United States. When adjusted for normal life expectancy, the 5-yr relative survival rate for all cancers combined is 62% (1). The emergency center at M.D. Anderson Cancer Center registered approximately 14,000 patient visits in the year 2000 and approximately 40% of these visits resulted in admission to the hospital. Of the hospital admissions, 94% were admitted to a floor bed and 6% were admitted to the intensive care unit (ICU) (2).

The MICU at M.D. Anderson admitted 844 patients during the years 2002–2003. Of these patients admitted, 277 received mechanical ventilation, which represents more than 32% of admitted patients.

Our admissions come from the in-patient floor units, the emergency center, and as transfers from other hospitals elsewhere. Broadly, the indications for admission to the MICU can be divided into three categories:

1. Complications from the cancer from the primary site or from metastasis causing compression, organ invasion, bleeding, effusions, hormonal and antibody dysfunction, electrolyte disturbance, or infection.
2. Complications of treatment of the cancer e.g., tumor lysis syndrome, neutropenic fever, bleeding diathesis, renal failure, altered mental status, cardiac failure, arrhythmia, radiation recall, bronchiolitis obliterans, graft-versus-host disease, and hypersensitivity reactions.
3. Incidental serious illness such as acute coronary syndrome, severe diarrhea, acute upper intestinal bleed, cerebrovascular accidents, pulmonary embolus, Stevens–Johnson syndrome.

Prior to admission, it is vital to ascertain the patient's wishes about resuscitation and treatment goals. It is not uncommon for further courses of chemotherapy or radiation to be planned and given during the course of the ICU admission. It is helpful at this stage to inform the patient and relatives of the invasive environment of the ICU—noisy, lack of privacy, intrusive, disorienting, and isolating (3,4). A clear understanding of the aim or purpose of the ICU admission should be communicated to the patients and their significant others. This allows redirection of any misconceived expectations and re-establishes a realistic perspective for the patient and their significant others.

The issue of communication is paramount to achieving patient satisfaction and an acceptable outcome by the family or significant others. The need for critical care support should not be based on the type of cancer but on the functional status of the patient (5). If invasive procedures are imminent to stabilize or treat the patient, then consent should be sought from the patients if they are capable. This can be in the form of a universal consent form with eight common procedures included on the form and patient/empowered designate is asked to sign (6). We do not do this in our institute, preferring to obtain consent as needed. We feel this ensures proper communication with the patients or their representative.

This is also an opportune time to consider whether a "Do Not Resuscitate" order or treatment limitation option is appropriate. Our published figures demonstrate that the outcome is grim when we examine those patients who received CPR in the ICU with respect to hospital discharge (mortality of 98%). The exceptions to this, the surviving 2% discharged from hospital, were when the cause of the arrest was ventricular tachycardia or ventricular fibrillation, which was promptly treated (7). We also demonstrate a higher incidence of CPR in hematological malignancies and a higher mortality rate following CPR in hematological malignancies compared to solid malignancies (7).

Where further oncological treatment is planned off-site from the ICU (such as radiation, imaging, and surgery), it is imperative to be able to coordinate the care and transport of the patient particularly if the patient is receiving dialysis and mechanical ventilation. Communication between primary teams, critical care teams, and family/patient support structures underpin the daily treatment received in critical care units. New developments and findings and their relevance need to be communicated in a cohesive manner and concerns addressed promptly.

II. ANESTHESIA TEAM PERSPECTIVE

Assessment of the patient's airway, breathing, and circulation is part of the primary survey after reviewing the history and events leading to admission to the ICU. For patients in respiratory distress, estimation of respiratory reserve function is the pivotal factor in determining how emergently the mechanical ventilatory support is needed. The history will reveal how rapidly and progressively the respiratory function is being compromised. Examination of the airway and respiratory system may localize a functional lesion and a chest radiograph may be available for comment. The presence of tachypnea and the inability to speak in sentences are sensitive indicators of urgent mechanical support. The respiratory therapists will prepare mechanical ventilatory support if this is required.

Airway assessment will determine the safest method for securing the airway if mechanical ventilation is contemplated. The presence of stridor or wheeze may indicate airway obstruction. Comprehensive airway support with such elements, as double lumen endobronchial tubes, flexible fiberoptic laryngoscopes, emergent tracheotomy kits, intubating LMA, cook airway exchange catheters as well as nasal and oral airway devices, must be made available if difficulty is anticipated. In the ideal circumstance, surgical airways should be inserted in the operating room environment under controlled conditions and under local anesthesia.

The circulatory assessment will allow prediction of how the patient will respond to positive pressure ventilation and affect the choice of anesthesia induction agents as well as continued sedation after mechanical ventilation is initiated. The presence of an arterial line allows assessment of "swing" with the patient's respiration cycle and this will alert the practitioner to the possibility of undiagnosed hypovolemia, cardiac tamponade, tension pneumothorax, or low output cardiac states. Large bore peripheral or central venous access catheters should be placed prior to mechanical ventilation. This allows intravenous volume resuscitation to be initiated prior to the drop in cardiac output. This drop in cardiac output results from the loss of circulating catecholamines once the patient is sedated and loss of venous return in the presence of positive pressure ventilation.

Qualitative cardiac output assessment can be made by considering the hourly urine output, peripheral perfusion, level of consciousness, and the character of the patient's pulse. Quantitative cardiac output can be derived from the esophageal Doppler monitor, the Lidco/Pulseco arterial waveform analyzer device, transthoracic echocardiogram, transesophageal echocardiogram, and from the pulmonary artery floatation catheter.

The timing of resuscitation and mechanical ventilation can be difficult to achieve in a controlled manner, but generally where more data are available, there is less disruption to the cardiac output. Laboratory results and patient's condition will influence the choice of agents for hypnosis, paralysis, and analgesia for placement of the endotracheal tube. Awake fiberoptic placement of the endotracheal tube may be needed in cases of difficult airways such as occurring in head and neck tumors or infective masses in the airway. In patients with severe hypocoagulation disorders, the dysfunction should be corrected prior to intubation and central venous access.

Efficient floatation of the PAFC can be achieved with minimal arrhythmia by attention to detail. The patient is placed in semi-Fowler's position with a lateral tilt so that the patient's right side is lower. Premature ventricular contractions indicate that the balloon is in the ventricular outflow tract. The application of positive pressure inspiratory pause (Valsalva maneuver) at this time will encourage rapid passage of the balloon tip into the pulmonary artery. Once the catheter tip is in the pulmonary artery, then the Valsalva maneuver is discontinued . (8). Judicious use of intravenous fluids with vasoconstrictor/vasodilator/beta-blockade will preserve cardiac output during the transition from spontaneous breathing to controlled/assisted mechanical ventilation.

Important background information such as the presence of cardiac tamponade, airway obstruction from the tumor/infection, large anterior mediastinal masses, severe coronary artery disease, bronchospasm, and myopathy will all influence the conduct of endotracheal intubation and initial ventilation management.

III. ONCOLOGY TEAM PERSPECTIVE

The need for ICU admission is precipitated by either a new phenomenon or a progressive deterioration in known patient. A discussion of the goals and expectations of the ICU stay should be addressed prior to admission. The patient's wishes, functional status, and his oncological diagnosis must be evaluated to determine the likelihood of success of further intervention (9). This entails a detailed reassessment of the likelihood of achieving a cure, palliative relief of symptoms, or active management of end-of-life issues with the patient and the critical care team.

Factors that have an increased risk of death are those patients who require ventilation within 24 hr of admission to the ICU, have leukemia, have a progression or recurrence of their malignancy, have received an allogeneic bone transplant, developed cardiac arrhythmias, exhibit disseminated intravascular coagulopathy, or need vasopressor treatment (10). However, if surgery was performed with curative intent, then this factor was protective in terms of outcome.

Cancer patients who are admitted to the ICU during or immediately postcardiopulmonary compression and resuscitation fared much worse than other admissions unless the cause of the arrest was a ventricular arrhythmia that was resuscitated promptly (7). Communication with the critical care team and the patient and the family is vital for realistic goal directed treatment.

Side effects and complications of the oncological treatment may become worse or arise de novo and this often complicates the clinical course in the unit. They will depend on the type of cytotoxic agent, immunosuppression agent, site of radiation as well as the planned support devices such as plasmapharesis, leukopharesis, and plasma phototherapy. The cell line that is implicated will dictate treatment of bone marrow suppression. Absolute neutropenic patients will be isolated in a protective environment, given broad-spectrum antibiotics, antiviral, and antifungal cover usually on an empirical basis. It is worthy to note that neutropenia does not affect outcome in critically ill cancer patients (11). Colony stimulating factors such as granulocyte colony stimulating factor (GCSF) or granulocyte-macrophage colony stimulating factor (GMCSF) may be used to stimulate white cell line recovery (12). White cell transfusions may be used for short-term protection in high-risk patients (13). Anemia may be supported by red cell transfusions and erythropoietin analogues. Severe thrombocytopenia is treated with platelet transfusions.

Patients who are status-post bone marrow transplantation are already on antirejection therapy such as tacrolimus, prednisolone, cyclophoshamide, azothiaprine, mycophenolate, OKT3, or thymoglobulin. Evidence of graft-versus-host disease should be sought, followed and treatment tailored to circumstance (14,15). In patients who have received bone marrow transplants, we have shown that the survivability drops from 65.7% to 18.8% when these patients are intubated and ventilated (16). Furthermore, patients who had peripheral stem cell transplants fared better than those who received bone marrow transplants and patients with autologous transplants survived better than those with allogeneic transplants (16).

Acute tumor lysis syndrome results from the acute dissolution of bulky tumors sensitive to the chemotherapy or radiation and is commonly seen in leukemia and lymphoma. It can also be seen in solid tumors but it is less frequent. Recombinant urate oxidase has replaced allopurinol in dealing with the hyperuricemia having been shown to be superior and is available in intravenous formulation (17–19). Maintenance of adequate diuresis will control the hyperkalemia and hyperphosphatemia otherwise dialysis will need to be instituted.

Hypercalcemia has an incidence of 10–20% in patients with malignancy. The severity of the hypercalcemia is related to the clinical condition with altered mental status, dehydration, arrhythmia, and renal insufficiency determining if crisis is present. Treatment is centered on rehydration with saline, decreasing calcium removal from bone and increasing calcium excretion (20). Frusemide will increase calcium excretion once the patient is rehydrated. Biphosphonates prevent calcium mobilization from bone and may alleviate bone pain (21). Zoledronate has been shown to provide a faster return to normal levels in hypercalcemia of malignancy (22,23). Calcitonin has been shown to be a safe agent in malignancy-related hypercalcemia (24,25).

Lower airway obstruction with respiratory failure due to tumor growth/invasion of the major tracheobronchial tree can present as an emergency. These are usually inoperable primary tumors of the esophagus or lung and may be associated with hemoptosis and dyspnea. Temporary tracheal intubation and mechanical ventilation may be required to allow fiberoptic placement of tracheal or bronchial stent as a palliative measure to provide subjective relief for the patient (26). The tumor may be amenable to endobronchial argon plasma coagulation, which would also provide treatment for endoluminal hemoptosis (27).

Pericardial tamponade requires admission to the ICU. Malignancies of the lung, breast, and leukemia/lymphoma tissues account for three quarters of these cases (28). Once the patient has appropriate monitors and intravenous access attached, a percutaneous pericardial catheter is inserted with local anesthesia and under ultrasound guidance (29,30). The degree of pulses paradoxus can be evident on examination of the arterial transducer waveform. The catheter is left in place for several days to observe the rate of reaccumulation of the effusion. In the immunocompromised patient, aspergillus pericarditis should be considered if there is evidence of pulmonary aspergillosis and evidence of pericarditis (31). Percutaneous double balloon pericardiotomy has been shown to be safe and effective in relieving large malignant pericardial effusions that have a tendency to reaccumulate (32).

Enterocolitis and typhlitis occur in certain chemotherapeutic regimes that render the patient severely neutropenic. Typically, this is a patient with leukemia on induction chemotherapy. Diagnosis rests on neutropenic fever, abdominal pain, and tenderness (33). Abdominal CT scan will demonstrate cecal distention and circumferential thickening of the cecal wall, which may have low attenuation secondary to edema (34). Treatment consists of medical support with antibiotics, bowel rest, and supplemental nutrition (35).

IV. INTENSIVE CARE TEAM PERSPECTIVE

Stabilization of the patient's acute problem and improvement in functional status are the goals of treatment. Further monitoring parameters for the patient's condition are required and this usually involves placement of invasive lines such as central venous catheters, arterial lines, Foley catheters, and Dobhoff tubes, etc. Consent issues have been addressed earlier in this chapter. Frequently, patients may need their coagulation profile or platelet count corrected prior to invasive procedures.

Sepsis and the systemic inflammatory response syndrome (as generally defined (36)) are common disorders in the MICU and this should be treated by a combination approach similar to that seen in cancer treatment and HIV infection (37). A systemic inflammatory response in the presence of infection or malignancy reflects excessive stimulation of immune responses to cellular triggers such as cytokines (38). A logical approach to treatment is dependent on understanding the pathophysiologic basis of sepsis (39). A more detailed discussion is presented in another chapter within this book.

Tighter and more stringent hyperglycemic control (blood glucose <110 mg/dL) in critically ill patients has been shown to have a positive outcome benefit in mortality ($p<0.0001$), critical illness neuropathy ($p<0.0001$), bacteremia ($p<0.02$), and inflammation ($p<0.0006$) (40). This simple approach can have far reaching effects in patient outcome and its importance cannot be overstated.

Ventilator-associated pneumonia occurs between 7% and 41% of patients on mechanical ventilation (41). The onset, outcome, and financial burden have been elucidated (42,43). Strategies to prevent the incidence have been unremarkable (41,44) with the possible exception of chest physiotherapy in an Australian study (45). Lung protective strategies to reduce volutrauma have been shown to reduce cytokine release when compared to conventional ventilation (46), and this has deep implications in any ventilated patient with an inflammatory process. These cytokines were increased within 1 hr of starting conventional mechanical ventilation (tidal volumes = 12 mL/kg body weight) (46). At our institute, our ideal tidal volume is 7 mL/kg body weight.

Transfusion related acute lung injury (TRALI) is probably an under-reported complication of blood transfusion. It is clinically indistinguishable from adult respiratory distress syndrome (ARDS) or acute lung injury (ALI) when less severe. Two groups were at risk of developing TRALI: patients with hematologic malignancies ($p<0.0004$) and patients with cardiac disease ($p<0.0006$) (47). The TRALI appears to be precipitated by donor or recipient antibodies to the respective recipient or donor WBC antigens resulting in monocyte activation (48). The mechanism of pulmonary injury is as yet unknown.

Diffuse alveolar hemorrhage is usually a complication of vasculitis and connective tissue diseases (49,50). In the oncological patient, it is more commonly seen in status-post bone marrow transplant recipients. The cause is unknown, the mortality is high, and the treatment is largely empirical (51,52). Favorable prognostic factors are early (as opposed to late) development of alveolar hemorrhage and autologous (as opposed to homologous) marrow transplants (52), whereas the presence of active graft-versus-host disease is strong predictor of poor outcome (53). Bronchoscopy and bronchoalveolar lavage are important to confirm alveolar hemorrhage as well as to exclude other causes of pulmonary bleeding (54). This is crucial as high dose steroid regimen is the mainstay of treatment (55). Tuberculosis may mimic alveolar hemorrhage after bone marrow transplant (56). Treatment with steroids, DDAVP, aminocaproic acid, blood products, and recombinant factor VIIa have been used where the bleeding has been very aggressive (57).

Patients who have a prolonged stay in the ICU have a tendency to develop critical illness myopathy and critical illness polyneuropathy. Tight normoglycemic with intensive insulin regimes have been shown to decrease the incidence of critical illness polyneuropathy as well as affecting other markers such as renal failure and length of stay (58). The neuropathy is an acute axonal neuropathy that recovers once the underlying sepsis is controlled. The myopathy is associated with the presence of sepsis, steroid administration, and muscle relaxant use (59,60). Treatment is supportive and directed at the underlying cause. One paper suggests that the acute myopathy with thick filament (myosin) loss may be the common pathway in both the neuropathy and well as the myopathy (61).

Deep vein thrombosis (DVT) is more common in patients admitted to the ICU (62). Treatment with low dose heparin prophylaxis reduces the incidence dramatically (62). Patients with cancer are at higher risk of bleeding, thrombosis, and disseminated intravascular coagulation (63,64), and some of these mechanisms have been demonstrated (65). Mobilization, TED hose, sequential compression devices, and prophylactic heparin remain the mainstay of prevention. The effect of heparins on cancer progression and angiogenesis has been indeterminate (66). There is some evidence that patients with cancer are more likely to develop heparin-induced thrombocytopenia (67).

Gastrointestinal bleeding is a common complication of critically ill patients. Approximately 15% may be amenable to injection sclerotherapy or thermal coagulation via upper gastroendoscopy (68). The risk of rebleeding is 15–20% and proton pump inhibitors have demonstrated that they prevent rebleeding (69,70). It is important to stress that proton pump inhibitors have not been shown to prevent stress ulcers, only rebleeding from stress ulcers (71,72).

Pancreatitis is an occasional complication seen in the oncological ICU. The management in the acute phase is nonspecific and supportive (73,74). Clinical and radiographic prognostic indices were not helpful in predicting course or complication rate of the pancreatitis (75). Adjuvant therapy with octreotide showed initial success at a dose of 100 μg TID IV (76), and subsequent trials demonstrating some effect at higher doses when given subcutaneously (77). However, a larger multicenter trial has not confirmed these benefits (78).

Acute myocardial ischemia and heart failure and renal failure are dealt with in their relevant chapters.

V. CONCLUSIONS

Critically ill oncological patients have a reversible element in their functional state. This may be true despite their oncological disease state. Our challenge is to correct that element in an appropriate manner that is cognizant of the wishes of the patient and within the goals of the primary oncological team. Oncological critical care is a rapidly evolving field due to the constant innovation applied by highly motivated oncological teams in their search to eradicate cancer. However, the core principles of critical care medicine remain unchanged. Attention to detail and maintaining open communications between all care-givers and the patient will be more likely to generate a satisfactory ICU stay for all involved. This is especially true when the outcome is negative.

REFERENCES

1. Society AC. Cancer, Facts and Figures, 2003. New York: American Cancer Society, 2003:2.
2. Yeung SJ, Escalante CP. Holland Frei Oncologic Emergencies. Houston, Texas: BC Decker Inc, 2002.
3. Donchin Y, Seagull FJ. The hostile environment of the intensive care unit. Curr Opin Crit Care 2002; 8(4): 316–320.
4. Nelson JE, et al. Self-reported symptom experience of critically ill cancer patients receiving intensive care [comment]. Crit Care Med 2001; 29(2):277–282.
5. Azoulay E, et al. Predictors of short-term mortality in critically ill patients with solid malignancies. Intensive Care Med 2000; 26(12):1817–1823.
6. Nicole D, Brian G, Kress JP, McAtee J, Herlitz J, Hall J. Improving the process of informed consent in the critically ill. JAMA 2003; 289(15):1963–1968.
7. Wallace K, et al. Outcome and cost implications of cardiopulmonary resuscitation in the medical intensive care unit of a comprehensive cancer center. Supportive Care Cancer 2002; 10(5):425–429.
8. Szabo Z. A simple method to pass a pulmonary artery flotation catheter rapidly into the pulmonary artery in anaesthetized patients. Br J Anaesthesia 2003; 90(6):794–796.
9. Groeger JS, Aurora RN. Intensive care, mechanical ventilation, dialysis, and cardiopulmonary resuscitation. Implications for the patient with cancer. Crit Care Clin 2001; 17(3):791–803.

10. Groeger JS, et al. Outcome for cancer patients requiring mechanical ventilation. J Clin Oncol 1999; 17(3): 991–997.
11. Kress JP, et al. Outcomes of critically ill cancer patients in a university hospital setting. Amer J Respir Crit Care Med 1999; 160(6):1957–1961.
12. Ozer H, et al. 2000 update of recommendations for the use of hematopoietic colony-stimulating factors: evidence-based, clinical practice guidelines. American society of clinical oncology growth factors expert panel [comment]. J Clin Oncol 2000; 18(20):3558–3585.
13. Price TH. Granulocyte transfusion in the G-CSF era. Int J Hematol 2002; 76(suppl 2):77–80.
14. Vogelsang GB, Wagner JE. Graft-versus-host disease. Hematol Oncol Clin N Am 1990; 4(3):625–639.
15. Dey B, Sykes M, Spitzer TR. Outcomes of recipients of both bone marrow and solid organ transplants. A review. Medicine 1998; 77(5):355–369.
16. Price KJ, et al. Prognostic indicators for blood and marrow transplant patients admitted to an intensive care unit. Amer J Respir Crit Care Med 1998; 158(3):876–884.
17. Baeksgaard L, Sorensen JB. Acute tumor lysis syndrome in solid tumors—a case report and review of the literature. Cancer Chemother Pharmacol 2003; 51(3):187–192.
18. Pui CH, et al. Recombinant urate oxidase for the prophylaxis or treatment of hyperuricemia in patients with leukemia or lymphoma. J Clin Oncol 2001; 19(3): 697–704.
19. Goldman SC, et al. A randomized comparison between rasburicase and allopurinol in children with lymphoma or leukemia at high risk for tumor lysis. Blood 2001; 97(10):2998–3003.
20. Chisholm MA, Mulloy AL, Taylor AT. Acute management of cancer-related hypercalcemia. Ann Pharmacother 1996; 30(5):507–513.
21. Coleman RE. Management of bone metastases. Oncologist 2000; 5(6):463–470.
22. Major P. The use of zoledronic acid, a novel, highly potent bisphosphonate, for the treatment of hypercalcemia of malignancy. Oncologist 2002; 7(6):481–491.
23. Major P, et al. Zoledronic acid is superior to pamidronate in the treatment of hypercalcemia of malignancy: a pooled analysis of two randomized, controlled clinical trials. J Clin Oncol 2001; 19(2):558–567.
24. Ralston SH, et al. Treatment of cancer associated hypercalcaemia with combined aminohydroxypropylidene diphosphonate and calcitonin. Br Med J Clin Res Ed 1986; 292(6535):1549–1550.
25. Wisneski LA. Salmon calcitonin in the acute management of hypercalcemia. Calcified Tissue Int 1990; 46(suppl):S26–S30.
26. Vonk-Noordegraaf A, Postmus PE, Sutedja TG. Tracheobronchial stenting in the terminal care of cancer patients with central airways obstruction. Chest 2001; 120(6):1811–1814.
27. Morice RC, et al. Endobronchial argon plasma coagulation for treatment of hemoptysis and neoplastic airway obstruction. Chest 2001; 119(3):781–787.
28. Hancock EW. Neoplastic pericardial disease. Cardiol Clin 1990; 8(4):673–682.
29. Laham RJ, et al. Pericardial effusion in patients with cancer: outcome with contemporary management strategies. Heart 1996; 75(1):67–71.
30. Vaitkus PT, Herrmann HC, LeWinter MM. Treatment of malignant pericardial effusion. JAMA 1994; 272(1):59–64.
31. Walsh TJ, Bulkley BH. Aspergillus pericarditis: clinical and pathologic features in the immunocompromised patient. Cancer 1982; 49(1):48–54.
32. Wang HJ, et al. Technical and prognostic outcomes of double-balloon pericardiotomy for large malignancy-related pericardial effusions. Chest 2002; 122(3): 893–899.
33. Pastore D, et al. Typhlitis complicating induction therapy in adult acute myeloid leukemia. Leukemia Lymphoma 2002; 43(4):911–914.
34. Horton KM, Corl FM, Fishman EK. CT evaluation of the colon: inflammatory disease. Radiographics 2000; 20(2):399–418.
35. Schlatter M, Snyder K, Freyer D. Successful nonoperative management of typhlitis in pediatric oncology patients. J Pediatr Surgery 2002; 37(8):1151–1155.
36. Bone RC, et al. Definitions for sepsis and organ failure and guidelines for the use of innovative therapies in sepsis. The ACCP/SCCM consensus conference committee. American college of chest physicians/society of critical care medicine [comment]. Chest 1992; 101(6):1644–1655.
37. Cross AS, Opal SM. A new paradigm for the treatment of sepsis: is it time to consider combination therapy? Ann Intern Med 2003; 138(6):502–505.
38. Bone RC. Toward a theory regarding the pathogenesis of the systemic inflammatory response syndrome: what we do and do not know about cytokine regulation. Crit Care Med 1996; 24(1):163–172.
39. Glauser MP. Pathophysiologic basis of sepsis: considerations for future strategies of intervention. Crit Care Med 2000; 28(suppl 9):S4–S8.
40. Van den Berghe G, et al. Outcome benefit of intensive insulin therapy in the critically ill: insulin dose versus glycemic control [comment]. Crit Care Med 2003; 31(2):359–366.
41. Fagon JY. Prevention of ventilator-associated pneumonia. Intensive Care Med 2002; 28(7):822–823.
42. Rello J, et al. Epidemiology and outcomes of ventilator-associated pneumonia in a large US database [comment]. Chest 2002; 122(6):2115–2121.
43. Warren DK, et al. Outcome and attributable cost of ventilator-associated pneumonia among intensive care unit patients in a suburban medical center [comment]. Crit Care Med 2003; 31(5):1312–1317.
44. Collard HR, Saint S, Matthay MA. Prevention of ventilator-associated pneumonia: an evidence-based systematic review [comment]. Ann Intern Med 2003; 138(6):494–501.

45. Ntoumenopoulos G, et al. Chest physiotherapy for the prevention of ventilator-associated pneumonia. Intensive Care Med 2002; 28(7):850–856.
46. Stuber F, et al. Kinetic and reversibility of mechanical ventilation-associated pulmonary and systemic inflammatory response in patients with acute lung injury. Intensive Care Med 2002; 28(7):834–841.
47. Silliman CC, et al. Transfusion-related acute lung injury: epidemiology and a prospective analysis of etiologic factors. Blood 2003; 101(2):454–462.
48. Kopko PM, et al. TRALI: correlation of antigen–antibody and monocyte activation in donor–recipient pairs. Transfusion 2003; 43(2):177–184.
49. Green RJ, et al. Pulmonary capillaritis and alveolar hemorrhage. Update on diagnosis and management [erratum appears in Chest 1997; 112(1):300]. Chest 1996; 110(5):1305–1316.
50. Specks U. Diffuse alveolar hemorrhage syndromes. Curr Opin Rheumatol 2001; 13(1):12–17.
51. Lewis ID, DeFor T, Weisdorf DJ. Increasing incidence of diffuse alveolar hemorrhage following allogeneic bone marrow transplantation: cryptic etiology and uncertain therapy. Bone Marrow Transplant 2000; 26(5):539–543.
52. Afessa B, et al. Outcome of diffuse alveolar hemorrhage in hematopoietic stem cell transplant recipients. Amer J Respir Crit Care Med 2002; 166(10):1364–1368.
53. Huaringa AJ, et al. Outcome of bone marrow transplantation patients requiring mechanical ventilation [comment]. Crit Care Med 2000; 28(4):1014–1017.
54. Huaringa AJ, et al. Bronchoalveolar lavage in the diagnosis of pulmonary complications of bone marrow transplant patients. Bone Marrow Transplant 2000; 25(9):975–979.
55. Raptis A, et al. High-dose corticosteroid therapy for diffuse alveolar hemorrhage in allogeneic bone marrow stem cell transplant recipients. Bone Marrow Transplant 1999; 24(8):879–883.
56. Keung YK, et al. Mycobacterium tuberculosis infection masquerading as diffuse alveolar hemorrhage after autologous stem cell transplant. Bone Marrow Transplant 1999; 23(7):737–738.
57. Hicks K, Peng D, Gajewski JL. Treatment of diffuse alveolar hemorrhage after allogeneic bone marrow transplant with recombinant factor VIIa. Bone Marrow Transplant 2002; 30(12):975–978.
58. Mesotten D, Van den Berghe G. Clinical potential of insulin therapy in critically ill patients. Drugs 2003; 63(7):625–636.
59. Bird SJ, Rich MM. Critical illness myopathy and polyneuropathy. Curr Neurol Neurosci Rep 2002; 2(6):527–533.
60. Hund E. Neurological complications of sepsis: critical illness polyneuropathy and myopathy. J Neurol 2001; 248(11):929–934.
61. Sander HW, Golden M, Danon MJ. Quadriplegic areflexic ICU illness: selective thick filament loss and normal nerve histology. Muscle Nerve 2002; 26(4): 499–505.
62. Cade JF. High risk of the critically ill for venous thromboembolism. Crit Care Med 1982; 10(7):448–450.
63. Schwartzberg LS, Holbert JM. Hemorrhagic and thrombotic abnormalities of cancer. Crit Care Clin 1988; 4(1):107–128.
64. DeSancho MT, Rand JH. Bleeding and thrombotic complications in critically ill patients with cancer. Crit Care Clini 2001; 17(3):599–622.
65. Prandoni P, Piccioli A, Girolami A. Cancer and venous thromboembolism: an overview. Haematologica 1999; 84(5):437–445.
66. Smorenburg SM, Van Noorden CJ. The complex effects of heparins on cancer progression and metastasis in experimental studies. Pharmacol Rev 2001; 53(1):93–105.
67. Andreescu AC, et al. Evaluation of a pharmacy-based surveillance program for heparin-induced thrombocytopenia. Pharmacotherapy 2000; 20(8):974–980.
68. Lewis JD, Shin EJ, Metz DC. Characterization of gastrointestinal bleeding in severely ill hospitalized patients [comment]. Crit Care Med 2000; 28(1):46–50.
69. Lau JY, et al. Effect of intravenous omeprazole on recurrent bleeding after endoscopic treatment of bleeding peptic ulcers [comment]. N Engl J Med 2000; 343(5):310–316.
70. Conrad SA. Acute upper gastrointestinal bleeding in critically ill patients: causes and treatment modalities. Crit Care Med 2002; 30(suppl 6):S365–S368.
71. Jung R, MacLaren R. Proton-pump inhibitors for stress ulcer prophylaxis in critically ill patients. Ann Pharmacother 2002; 36(12):1929–1937.
72. Yang YX, Lewis JD. Prevention and treatment of stress ulcers in critically ill patients. Semin Gastrointestinal Dis 2003; 14(1):11–19.
73. Mitchell RM, Byrne MF, Baillie J. Pancreatitis. Lancet 2003; 361(9367):1447–1455.
74. Werner J, et al. Modern phase-specific management of acute pancreatitis. Digestive Dis 2003; 21(1):38–45.
75. Liu TH, et al. Acute pancreatitis in intensive care unit patients: value of clinical and radiologic prognosticators at predicting clinical course and outcome. Crit Care Med 2003; 31(4):1026–1030.
76. Fiedler F, et al. Octreotide treatment in patients with necrotizing pancreatitis and pulmonary failure. Intensive Care Med 1996; 22(9):909–915.
77. Nikou GC, et al. The significance of the dosage adjustment of octreotide in the treatment of acute pancreatitis of moderate severity. Hepato-Gastroenterol 2001; 48(42):1754–1757.
78. Uhl W, et al. A randomised, double blind, multicentre trial of octreotide in moderate to severe acute pancreatitis. Gut 1999; 45(1):97–104.

34

Delirium and Substance Withdrawal

ALAN D. VALENTINE and JACQUELINE BICKHAM

Department of Neuro-Oncology (Psychiatry Section), The University of Texas M.D. Anderson Cancer Center, Houston, Texas, U.S.A.

I. INTRODUCTION

Delirium is a common and serious complication of perioperative and intensive care of cancer patients (1,2). It is associated with increased morbidity and mortality, as well as increased length and cost of hospital stay (3–5). It is a variable with potential impact on long-term disposition of patients who survive hospitalization. The unexpected development of delirium is often very frightening for family members, even more so than the malignancy itself (6).

Several factors complicate assessment and management of delirium. The nomenclature is itself confusing and imprecise. Over 30 terms (e.g., acute confusional state, acute brain failure, encephalopathy) have been used in the literature to describe the same syndrome (7). Because it is so common in intensive care settings development of delirium unfortunately may be regarded almost as a natural consequence of critical care (the so-called "ICU psychosis") (8–10). The diagnosis of delirium is often not straightforward. Signs and symptoms of delirium are commonly seen with other behavioral disorders (e.g., agitation, anxiety, depression); the risk of misdiagnosis is significant (11).

A separate but often related issue, which this chapter will address, is that of withdrawal from licit and illicit substances, particularly alcohol. While alcohol withdrawal delirium (delirium tremens) is the classic model for agitated delirium (12), withdrawal syndromes associated with other substances (e.g., narcotics, nicotine) present in ways that if less dangerous, are still significant complications of acute care and sources of physical and emotional distress for patients.

Delirium, as defined by Lipowski, is a transient organic syndrome characterized by acute onset, global impairment of cognitive function, altered level of consciousness, inability to attend, psychomotor agitation or retardation, and disruption of sleep–wake cycle (12). This definition is somewhat more inclusive of behavioral phenomena than the criteria required for diagnosis in the Diagnostic and Statistical Manual (DSM IV) of the American Psychiatric Association (13) (Table 1). Several points are relevant to both definitions of delirium. First, delirium is not a disease state itself. It is a syndromal manifestation of one or more underlying pathophysiological processes. These processes are by definition "organic" in nature. Delirium is not caused by a preexisting psychological condition nor is it a "functional" reaction to stress. While altered reality testing is a hallmark of delirium, the other required symptoms distinguish delirium from psychosis as the latter term is used in the psychiatric literature. This is one of the reasons why the term "ICU psychosis" is inappropriate (14). Second, delirium is a dynamic syndrome. Levels

Table 1 DSM IV Criteria for Delirium

1. Disturbance of consciousness (i.e., reduced clarity of awareness of the environment) with reduced ability to focus, sustain, or shift attention.
2. Change in cognition (i.e., memory deficit, disorientation, language disturbance) or development of a perceptual disturbance that is not better accounted for by a preexisting or evolving dementia.
3. Development of the disturbance over a short period of time (usually hours–days) with fluctuating course during the day.
4. Evidence from the history, physical examination, or laboratory findings that the disturbance is caused by physiological consequences of a medical condition.

Source: From Ref. 13.

of arousal, degrees of cognitive impairment, and psychomotor behavior vary greatly between patients and may even fluctuate markedly in a given individual. Patients may experience "lucid intervals" in which their mental function appears to have normalized, only to lapse back into a state of confusion.

II. PREVALENCE

Delirium is one of the most common behavioral disorders experienced by hospitalized patients (15–17). The elderly are at particular risk for development of delirium during admission, with rates of over 60% reported in some series (18,19). Given current models of clinical practice and an aging population, the prevalence of delirium will increase with time.

In the oncology setting, cognitive disorders including delirium are the second most frequently encountered psychiatric disorders (20). Only mood disorders are seen more often. In end-stage disease as many as 85% of cancer patients may experience delirium (21,22).

Prevalence rates for delirium in perioperative and critical care settings vary greatly. Most of the surgical literature involves assessment of delirium after orthopedic and cardiac surgery. In postoperative populations, rates of 7–52% have been reported, with differences attributed to factors including study methodology, setting, disease site, and age of population (15,23). Delirium is one of the most common complications of surgery in the elderly. Fifteen to twenty percent of geriatric patients who come to surgery develop delirium as a postoperative complication (12,24,25). Rates of >40% have been detected in patients taken to surgery for hip fracture (26,27). While also highly variable, recent studies of delirium after heart surgery suggest that rates of delirium in this setting are somewhat lower (approximately 12–25%), with older age strongly associated with increased risk (23,28,29).

There is little data available specifically related to rates of postoperative delirium in cancer patients. In their study of altered mental status in cancer patients, Tuma and DeAngelis found that delirium occurred in the postoperative period in 32% of cancer patients with delirium, though the surgical experience was considered to be a contributing, not directly causal factor (1).

III. CLINICAL PRESENTATIONS OF DELIRIUM

Clinical manifestations of delirium can vary greatly from patient to patient. Subtypes of delirium including hyperactive, hypoactive, and mixed forms have been described (12,30).

The hyperactive form of delirium includes behaviors that are likely most consistent with what clinicians routinely associate with delirium. These include increased psychomotor activity to the point of agitation or combativeness, rapid or pressured speech that is often (not always) illogical, hyperalertness or hypervigilance, hallucinations and delusions, impulsive and/or disinhibited behavior, and fluctuations of mood and affect over a range of emotional states including irritability and hostility, paroxysmal sadness and euphoria. In the intensive care setting such presentations can constitute an active emergency, the patient being at risk to pull lines, desaturate or self-extubate, fall, or injure bystanders. It is also this form of delirium that is most frightening to family members, because it is unexpected and often so uncharacteristic of the patient's baseline personality.

The hypoactive form of delirium is often so subtle in its manifestations that it is not noticed or is attributed to another problem, usually depression. The patient demonstrates decreased motor activity, speech and thought processes that are slowed (to the point of being blocked) though often as illogical as in the hyperactive form, a decreased level of arousal and indifference or lack of attention to external stimuli, and a flat, unreactive affect. While patients in such a state are not obvious dangers to themselves or others, the potential consequences of an unrecognized and treated hypoactive delirium are as (or more) serious as those associated with hyperactive states.

A mixed form of delirium is characterized by features of both the hyperactive and hypoactive forms. The behaviors of a patient in a mixed-form delirium may vary from day-to-day or within a day, often without warning and without any predictability in the variability. Such variation only makes management more difficult.

Lucid intervals are characterized by periods in which the patient appears cognitively and behaviorally intact. It may appear that the delirium has resolved only to have the patient return to previous or new abnormal behaviors.

Delirium typically develops over a period of hours or a few days. In the perioperative setting, the patient might easily enter a delirious state coming out of anesthesia-induced sedation. Deliria due to infection, metabolic dyscrasias, or drug intoxications might develop more slowly at first, and then become more obvious as cognitive dysfunction becomes more pervasive. Prodromal states of irritability, anxiety, or illogical thinking might be observed before level of consciousness is affected, or before frankly altered mentation is observed.

Patients vulnerable for delirium will often experience symptoms at night or in the early morning. Such presentations are so common that the imprecise and nonspecific term "sundowning" has entered the informal medical lexicon (31). Nighttime agitation places the delirious patient at risk for gradual disruption of sleep–wake cycle, further exacerbating delirium (12,25). In intensive care settings where there may be considerable activity and sensory stimulation at all hours, a frank diurnal variation in onset or intensity of delirium may be less noticeable. In this setting, it may also be more difficult to approximate a normal sleep–wake cycle, and control of the variable may be more easily obtained if/when the patient is moved out of the ICU.

Autonomic dysfunction may be encountered. The delirious patient may experience changes of heart rate, blood pressure, temperature, and respiratory rate. While elevations in these parameters may simply be due to exertion in the agitated patient, autonomic instability can also be seen in patients with "quiet" delirium and may be due to a significant pathophysiological process that is driving the delirium.

IV. CAUSES OF DELIRIUM

Cancer patients in perioperative and intensive care settings are vulnerable to a wide variety of insults capable of causing delirium. In the perioperative/intensive care setting it is quite likely that more than one process will be involved, and the etiology of the altered mental status will be considered multifactorial. Very common causes of delirium, including effects of drugs (withdrawal, intoxication, side effects), metabolic abnormalities, and systemic infection should be considered in all cases of delirium.

A. Drugs

Medication effects may be the most common precipitants of delirium in hospitalized patients, and the list of drugs with any potential to cause altered mental status is extremely long (32,33) (Table 2). Altered mental status thought secondary to effects of anesthesia is common and some investigators choose not to include the initial 24 postoperative hours in studies of delirium (34,35). Route of delivery of anesthesia does not appear to influence development of delirium (36). Other medications that are routinely associated with altered mental status in this setting include opioid analgesics, benzodiazepine sedative-hypnotics, corticosteroids, antiarrhythmics, and sympathomimetics (37).

Table 2 Drugs Associated with Delirium (Partial List)

Anesthetics
General: halothane, enflurane
Anticholinergics
Atropine, scopalamine, benztropine
Anticonvulsants
Phenytoin, carbamazepine
Antiarrhythmics
Lidocaine, mexiletine procainamide, amiodarone, quinidine, digoxin
Antihypertensives
β-Blockers, clonidine, methyldopa
Antiviral agents
Acyclovir, gancyclovir, fuscarnet, interferon
Antifungal agents
Amphotericin
Antibiotics
Cephalosporins, chloramphenicol, tetracyclines, sulfonamides
Corticosteroids
Immunosuppressants
Cyclosporine, FK-506
H_1-receptor antagonists
Diphenhydramine
H_2-receptor antagonists
Cimetidine, ranitidine
Prokinetic drugs
Metoclopramide
Respiratory agents
Albuterol, theophylline
Narcotic analgesics
Nonsteroidal anti-inflammatory drugs
Sedative-hypnotic drugs
Barbiturates, benzodiazepines
Antineoplastic agents
Cytosine arabinoside, ifosphamide, methotrexate, interleukin

Source: From Refs. 12, 16, 17, 32, 33, 37, 41, 61.

Anticholinergic drugs have long been associated with a characteristic hyperactive delirium and anticholinergic processes are the best-studied causes of delirium (38–40).

Geriatric patients are at potentially higher risk for drug-induced delirium because of altered (slowed) drug metabolism and because of the higher rate of baseline cognitive impairment.

In the oncology setting, many antineoplastic therapies have been associated with delirium, but there are relatively few common offenders. These include methotrexate, cytosine arabinoside, ifosfamide, and cyclofosphamide (16). Biological response modifiers, especially interleukin-2 and interferon alpha are, especially if used in combination, associated with delirium and sometimes with a prolonged encephalopathic state (41).

B. Other Causes

Electrolyte and metabolic abnormalities are common causes of postoperative delirium, with hypoxia (often related to respiratory failure or anemia or both) the most frequent precipitant (12,25,42).

Altered mental status can be the first sign of evolving infection. Especially in setting where there might be associated respiratory or metabolic dysfunction (e.g., pneumonia, septic shock), consideration of possible infection in the assessment and management of the altered patient is indicated.

Delirium can also be caused by direct and indirect effects of primary brain tumors and cancer metastatic to the central nervous system.

V. ASSESSMENT OF DELIRIUM

Assessment for delirium in the postoperative and ICU settings is in some ways straightforward, but also associated with unique difficulties. The diagnosis of delirium is a clinical one and is based history and observation of the patient, physical examination and laboratory studies. As has been noted earlier, presentations of delirium can closely resemble other neuropsychiatric disorders and conditions in which there is not global impairment of central nervous system function (Tables 3 and 4).

Table 3 Evaluation of the Delirious Patient

History and chart review; attention to medications
Clinical interview and mental status examination
Physical examination; attention to neurologic status
Laboratory assessment: complete blood count with differential and platelets, electrolytes, creatinine, BUN, calcium, magnesium, albumin, liver function tests, thyroid, glucose, RPR function tests, O_2 saturation/arterial blood gases
Chest x-ray, EKG
Urine, blood cultures, cerebral spinal fluid studies, if indicated
Serum/urine drug and alcohol screens, serum drug levels
As indicated: B_{12} and folate levels, serum drug levels, EEG, brain CT/MRI

Table 4 Differential Diagnosis of Delirium

Dementia
Major depression
Substance intoxication, withdrawal
Schizophrenia/schizophreniform disorder
Bipolar mania
Brief psychotic disorder
Nonspecific agitation
Unrelieved pain
Hypoxia
Anxiety, fear
Akathisia

A. Screening Instruments

Several screening instruments are available to assist in the assessment of delirious patients. The mini-mental state examination (MMSE) may be the most frequently used screen of cognitive function and is often employed to assess delirious patients (43). However, the MMSE does not distinguish delirium from dementia and patients may score poorly on the test for a number of reasons not directly related to delirium (17,44).

The confusion assessment method (CAM) developed by Inouye et al. is frequently designed to allow nonpsychiatric clinicians to screen for presence of delirium (45). It has been modified and other rating instruments developed for use in ICU settings with patients who are intubated or otherwise unable to communicate (46,47). Even frequently used instruments such as the CAM have a significant associated error rate and patients who score above threshold levels on these scales should go on to careful clinical evaluation. Other instruments including the Delirium Rating Scale (DRS) and the Memorial Delirium Assessment Scale (MDAS) are used more to assess severity of delirium and can be used to follow patients over time and assess response to therapy, and also as research instruments (48,49).

B. Clinical Evaluation and Mental Status Examination

The clinical evaluation of a patient thought to be delirious will include elements of history, observation and interview of the patient, and mental status examination (12). The patient is likely to be an unreliable or unavailable (e.g., intubated) historian, so it is necessary to rely on family members, nursing staff, and others for information on the time course and characteristics (including diurnal variation with symptoms worse at night) of changes in behavior, arousal, and cognitive function. History of use of medications, use or discontinuation of alcohol and illicit drugs, baseline cognitive function, and other events (e.g., falls) is critical in consideration of possible evolving delirium. Observation and clinical interview of the patient includes assessment of level of arousal, psychomotor agitation or retardation, stability of affect, distractibility, and assessment for presence of illusions, hallucination, and delusions. It is important to keep in mind that the patient in the early or prodromal stages of a delirium may show little evidence of abnormality to observation.

Depending on the patient's status, it may or may not be possible to complete a detailed mental status examination. The mental status examination should test attention, orientation, memory, abstract thinking, and speed and dynamics of thought (12,25). Often the MMSE is used to provide a quantifiable assessment of cognitive function, though again it should be noted that this is not adequate by itself for evaluation.

C. Physical Examination

While the diagnosis of delirium can be made without ever touching the patient, careful physical examination provides information crucial to the search for precipitating and potentially dangerous causes of altered mental status, and will often influence the choice of diagnostic tests. Current and recent vital signs should be assessed. Cardiovascular and pulmonary examinations should be performed. The neurological examination should be emphasized, with assessment for lateralizing signs and increased intracranial pressure.

D. Laboratory Assessment and Other Tests

Most of the information desired from laboratory assessment of possible delirium is readily available in ICU/perioperative settings. This includes serum chemistries: electrolytes, creatinine, blood urea nitrogen, calcium, magnesium, liver function assays, thyroid functions, as well as urinalysis and complete blood count with differential and platelet count. Chest x-ray and EKG should be reviewed or obtained. Serum drug levels should be checked in patients on some medications including immunosuppressants (e.g., cyclosporine), anticonvulsants, cardiac drugs (e.g., digoxin), psychotropics (e.g., lithium, tricyclic antidepressants), and patients known or suspected of use of illicit drugs. Vitamin B12 and serum folate levels should be checked in patients known or suspected to be alcohol dependent.

Other tests should be considered in certain settings, but are probably not routinely necessary. Neuroimaging (CT, MRI) may be helpful if physical examination reveals focal neurologic signs, and in the absence of other obvious causes of delirium, or when delirium persists despite appropriate treatment. The electroencephalogram (EEG) will almost always reveal diffuse, nonspecific slowing in the delirious patient. While EEG evaluation is probably not routinely necessary, it should be obtained in cases of suspected seizures. It may also be useful in attempts to distinguish delirium from other causes of similar behavior (e.g., dementia, severe depression, "functional" psychiatric disorders) (50,51).

VI. MANAGEMENT

The potential consequences of delirium are such that it should be prevented or detected and treated as early as possible. Patients who might be expected to develop delirium (e.g., geriatrics, known cognitive impairment, alcohol dependence) should be monitored closely and evaluated frequently. Preoperative assessment that predicts and allows for early intervention has potential to significantly impact morbidity and costs associated with intensive treatment (52,53).

A. Behavioral and Environmental Management

The physical environment of the ICU is itself a potential impediment to the management of delirium. Especially in open ward type units, patients are vulnerable to excessive sensory stimulation including bright light and noise. Ideally, the ICU is constructed to support nonpharmacological treatment of delirium (Table 5). The patient should be treated in a room that is sheltered from other activity in the ICU. Attempts to minimize disruption of sleep–wake cycles should be made; lights should be on during the day and if possible long periods of daytime sleep should be avoided. The patient should be frequently reoriented and any sensory deficits should be addressed (i.e., glasses, hearing aids). At night low-level background light and noise (music or television) should be maintained. Often the presence of family members is comforting to a frightened, delirious patient. Whether in the ICU or in a regular hospital room, a patient in a hyperactive or mixed delirium must be closely

Table 5 Behavioral Aids to Management of Delirium

Maintain background light and sound
Music or television
Lights dimmed at night
Reorient patient frequently
Calendars, message boards
Minimize sensory deprivation
Replace glasses or hearing aides
Facilitate patient contact with family and other support systems
Maintain communication with family, caregivers
Use physical restraints only if absolutely necessary
Check patient and release restraints frequently
Consider one-on-one attendant as alternative

Table 6 Medications for Management of Delirium

Antipsychotics	
Haloperidol[a]	0.5–5 mg q 30 min–12 hr PO, IM, IV
Droperidol[a]	0.625–2.5 mg IV q 3–4 hr
Chlorpromazine[a]	25–100 mg q 4–12 hr PO, IM, IV
Risperidone	0.5–2 mg q 12 hr PO
Olanzapine	2.5–5 mg q 12–24 hr PO
Benzodiazepines	
Lorazepam[a]	0.5–2 mg q 1–4 hr PO, IM, IV
Midazolam[a]	0.03 mg/kg/hr titrate to effect IV
Anesthetics	
Propofol[a]	0.5 mg/kg/hr titrate to effect IV
Alpha agonists	
Dexmedtomidine[a]	1 mcg/kg over 10 min followed by continuous infusion 0.2–0.7 mcg/kg/hr

[a]May be administered by continuous infusion.

monitored to prevent accidental self-harm (i.e., falls, pulled IV lines, and catheters). If family cannot be present and nursing obligations preclude close observation, it is useful to arrange for a sitter to be in the room with the patient. This can minimize the need for physical restraints, which are sometimes necessary but should be avoided if possible. Because the behaviors associated with delirium are often unexpected and frightening for family members (and sometimes patients), it is important to keep them informed about the process taking place and efforts to control it (6).

B. Pharmacotherapy

A delirious patient in the ICU who is physically agitated or overtly psychotic will usually require pharmacologic stabilization while attempts are made to treat the underlying cause(s) of the delirium. Drugs from several different classes have been used to treat delirium in the ICU and postoperative setting, including neuroleptics, benzodiazepine sedative-hypnotics, and anesthetic agents (Table 6).

1. *Antipsychotics*

Usually the goal of treatment is to control the behaviors and cognitive dysfunction associated with delirium without causing excess sedation (54). Antipsychotics are very useful for this purpose and of the several available drugs in this class haloperidol is the drug of choice (16,54–56). Reasons for this include its potent activity as an antipsychotic drug. Its significant dopamine receptor blockade activity is desirable in treatment of a syndrome associated with excessive dopamine activity. Though not approved for intravenous administration, haloperidol is routinely and effectively given by this route, facilitating rapid delivery and usually with minimal anticholinergic toxicity, extrapyramidal effects, or effects on cardiac, respiratory, and hepatic function (57–60).

The initial and total haloperidol doses required to treat delirium vary greatly. Variations of the dosing protocol used at the Massachusetts General Hospital are frequently employed (61). Typically, mild agitation would be treated with 0.5–2.0 mg IV, moderate to severe agitation 5 mg, and very severe agitation 10 mg. Dosing is repeated q 30 min prn until control is achieved. The patient can then be put on scheduled doses of haloperidol q 4–6 hr (with prn doses available). Alternatively, haloperidol is given on a prn basis for 24 hr and the first day's total administered the second day in divided doses. If the patient does well, the haloperidol can then be tapered by 25% per day. If control of severe agitation is not achieved with 2–3 doses of haloperidol, it is often useful to add lorazepam 1–2 mg to the regimen. Delirious patients requiring frequent prn doses of haloperidol may benefit from a continuous infusion of the drug (62). It is rare for patients to require more than 100 mg of IV haloperidol per day but total administered doses of >1 g have been reported (63). On one occasion, we have administered IV haloperidol in continuous infusion at 11 mg/hr over 24 hr.

Though intravenous haloperidol is usually well tolerated, it has been associated with QTc interval prolongation and ventricular arrhythmia (torsades de pointes), usually in patients with histories of heart disease and/or receiving high (>50 mg/day) doses of the drug. Cardiac monitoring with measurement of QTc intervals is recommended, with reduction or discontinuation of haloperidol if QTc interval increase 25% over baseline (64,65). Compared to oral dosing, IV administration of haloperidol is much less likely to cause extrapyramidal side effects or akathisia (motor restlessness). A prudent precaution in intubated patients treated with high dose or continuously infused haloperidol is to give benzotropine against possible undetected laryngospasm. Akathisia should be suspected if motor agitation increases with escalation of haloperidol doses (54).

Alternative antipsychotic medications include droperidol and chlorpromazine. Both may be given IV and their sedating/calming effects are desirable in management of an acutely agitated patient (66,67). However, both drugs are potent alpha-adrenergic antagonists with significant hypotensive effects that can seriously complicate care of critically ill patients, and droperidol has been associated with QTc prolongation and cardiac dysrhythmias.

The atypical antipsychotics (e.g., risperdal, olanzapine, quetiapine, ziprasidone) have been used to treat delirium and are attractive because their side effect profiles are generally more benign than traditional antipsychotics, but the lack of available IV administration may limit their utility in ICU settings (68–70). Olanzapine in particular has been used in the management of delirious cancer patients and is available in a zydis formulation that quickly dissolves with oral administration, which may increase its potential utility (71,72).

2. *Benzodiazepines*

Benzodiazepines (BZPs) are the drugs of choice for treatment of alcohol withdrawal delirium (see below). In the ICU, parenterally administered benzodiazepines (e.g., midazolam, lorazepam) are also often used to treat delirium caused by other insults. The drugs are attractive because of ease of administration and desirable sedative-hypnotic effects. However, used alone BZPs will not improve cognitive dysfunction associated with delirium and, especially in patients with baseline cognitive impairment (e.g., dementia, some geriatrics), they are likely to exacerbate cognitive dysfunction and may increase psychomotor agitation (73). Dependence and tolerance are associated with long-term use of BZPs and if withdrawn abruptly the patient is vulnerable for withdrawal seizures.

Benzodiazepines are more effectively used in combination or alternating with neuroleptics, and may decrease the dose requirements for both drugs (57,60). Continuous infusions of midazolam or lorazepam may be desirable if intent is to sedate the patient and in palliative care settings (74).

3. *Propofol*

The anesthetic propofol is now in regular use in intensive care settings for sedation (see sedation chapter). Its rapid onset of action is a great advantage in management of an acutely agitated patient. Like benzodiazepines, propofol does not have antipsychotic properties and will not treat cognitive dysfunction associated with delirium. Its use may be indicated in management of refractory delirium and alcohol withdrawal delirium (75,76).

4. *Dexmedetomidine*

Dexmedtomidine is a potent, highly selective alpha (2)-adrenoceptor agonist. It has a number of advantages in the treatment of perioperative delirium. The drug has sedative-hypnotic effects as well as anesthetic-sparing and analgesic effects. The main advantage of its use is that it creates no significant respiratory depressant effects (77).

This drug is promising in the treatment of perioperative delirium even over some more traditionally selected drugs. In one study, four patients with delirium associated with agitation refractory to haloperidol were responsive to dexmedtomidine (78).

5. *Other Agents*

In cases of anticholinergic delirium, treatment with parenteral physostigmine can reverse symptoms. Patients must be monitored closely because of physostigmine's short duration of action and because of associated toxicity including hypotension and bradycardia (79,80). Analgesics should be maintained in patients known or suspected of being in pain. Though opioid and other analgesics may contribute to delirium, pain is also a risk factor and at the least complicates assessment of an agitated patient (81,82). Opioid rotation or dose reduction may improve mental status and decrease motor agitation, and may have particular utility in end-of-life care (83).

VII. SUBSTANCE WITHDRAWAL

Intoxication/withdrawal states, whether from licit or illicit substances, can result in serious behavioral syndromes and have the potential for significantly complicating patient care in the perioperative and critical care settings. Most recreational drugs (e.g., cocaine, phencyclidine, amphetamine) can induce agitation, and tend to do so in a dose-dependent fashion. When the intoxication is accompanied by attentional deficits and alterations of the sensorium, it may be clinically indistinguishable from other forms of delirium. In postoperative cancer patients, intoxication states arising from the use of licit drugs are more likely to be encountered. Relevant examples include intoxication induced by opiates, benzodiazepines, and anticholinergic medications. Removal of the offending agent and supportive care are generally the treatments of choice. In some cases, administration of a reversing agent (e.g., naxolone, flumazenil, physostigmine) may be indicated.

A substance withdrawal state arises following abrupt reduction or cessation of a substance that has been used regularly and heavily over a prolonged period of time. The resulting constellation of symptoms tends to be substance specific and may vary in intensity from mild discomfort to a full-blown, life-threatening abstinence syndrome (13). In general, nonspecific symptoms such as anxiety, restlessness, irritability, and dysphoria can be seen in patients withdrawing from most habituating substances (e.g., nicotine, opiates, stimulants, sedative-hypnotics). More specific signs (e.g., pupillary dilation, diaphoresis, tachycardia) tend to be opposite of those characteristically observed during the intoxication state of a particular substance (85). The resulting emotional distress can greatly impact the course of hospital care insofar as the patient's ability to comply with the treatment plan may be compromised. The changes in mood and behavior have the potential for alienating the patient from the treatment team and can adversely influence the patient's perception of the hospitalization. The mainstay of treatment in withdrawal syndromes is to provide supportive care and appropriate sedation (84). In some cases, reintroduction of the drug or an equivalent substitute for the drug followed by gradual tapering is an effective intervention. Amelioration of distressing physical symptoms with adjunct medications (e.g., loperamide for loose stooling, acetaminophen for headache, ondansetron for vomiting) often improves the patient's morale and overall sense of well-being.

Though clearly unpleasant, not all withdrawal states are associated with the same degree of risk in terms of morbidity and mortality. Opioid withdrawal, for example, may give rise to a multitude of somatic complaints (e.g., tremor, insomnia, headache, nausea, vomiting, diarrhea, abdominal cramps, musculoskeletal pain) but is rarely fatal (85). Serious neurological symptoms, such as convulsions or delirium, typically do not occur (86). Of the licit and illicit substances known to precipitate withdrawal syndromes, only withdrawal from the central nervous system depressants (e.g., alcohol, sedative-hypnotics) has been associated with the development of frank delirium.

Alcohol and sedative-hypnotics (e.g., barbiturates, benzodiazepines) exert inhibitory effects on the CNS by facilitating GABA-A receptor-mediated transmission and impeding glutaminergic receptor-mediated transmission. Chronic administration leads to upregulation of GABA receptors and downregulation of glutaminergic receptors. The result is an overall state of GABA deficiency. When the alcohol or sedative-hypnotic is suddenly withdrawn, a syndrome of CNS hyperexcitability ensues (14). Alpha-adrenergic and dopaminergic neurotransmitter systems also have a role in the pathogenesis of acute withdrawal from CNS depressants. Many of the specific withdrawal symptoms observed (e.g., elevated blood pressure, hallucinations) can be described in terms of dysregulation of these two systems (87).

The withdrawal syndromes associated with alcohol and sedative-hypnotics are clinically similar. In their most severe form, symptoms can include confusion, disorientation, autonomic hyperactivity, psychomotor agitation, tremulousness, and seizures. Delirium tremens, or alcohol withdrawal delirium, is the prototypic example of delirium induced by substance withdrawal.

A. Alcohol Withdrawal Delirium

Alcohol withdrawal delirium occurs in approximately 5% of patients withdrawing from alcohol (88). It is associated with a mortality rate of 1–15% (84). Given that as many as 15–20% of primary care and hospitalized patient have alcohol abuse issues, the number at risk for developing alcohol withdrawal delirium is significant (86). The manifestations of alcohol withdrawal emerge within 6–48 hr following the cessation of or significant reduction in the amount of alcohol usually consumed (88). Withdrawal symptoms can escalate to alcohol withdrawal delirium within 24–72 hr (84). Several risk factors for the development of alcohol withdrawal have been described in the literature. In his study of 334 alcohol-dependent patients, Palmistiera identified five risk factors for alcohol withdrawal delirium: (1) current infectious disease, (2) tachycardia (defined as a heart rate over 120 beats per minute at admission), (3) signs of alcohol withdrawal in the presence of an alcohol concentration of more than 1 g/L of body fluid, (4) a history of epileptic seizures, and (5) a history of delirium (89). In a case–control study done by Fiellin et al., elevated blood pressure, medical comorbidity, and prior history of complicated alcohol withdrawal increased the risk of developing alcohol withdrawal delirium (90).

Alcohol withdrawal delirium can be a significant source of complications in the medically ill. In a sample of 17 consecutive patients presenting for mandibular reconstruction, Gallivan et al. found that flap survival rate was only 25% for patients who experienced alcohol withdrawal delirium, and 85% in patients who did not (91). This is a strong argument for the early identification of the patient at risk for development of severe alcohol withdrawal and the preoperative treatment of alcohol dependence.

B. Management of Alcohol Withdrawal

There are several options available to the physician in the treatment of alcohol withdrawal. The lynchpins of withdrawal therapy are detoxification and supportive care, including adequate hydration, correction of electrolyte abnormalities, and replacement of nutritional deficiencies (e.g., thiamine, folate). Proper replacement of magnesium, pyridoxine, and niacin will reduce the risk of alcohol withdrawal seizures.

1. Benzodiazepines

The preferred pharmacologic treatment of alcohol withdrawal delirium is the use of benzodiazepines. Benzodiazepines have been shown to reduce withdrawal severity, reduce incidence of delirium and reduce the incidence of seizures (92). Alcohol, benzodiazepines, and barbiturates produce cross-tolerance. As such, they may effectively substitute for one another in the management of acute withdrawal (14). With regard to barbiturates, there are only a few controlled studies supporting their use in alcohol withdrawal delirium. This is in contrast to the numerous studies in the literature supporting the use of benzodiazepines (86). The use of barbiturates is further limited by the fact that barbiturates have a relatively narrow therapeutic index, and a high propensity to produce respiratory depression (84). Oral and IV ethanol are still used by some surgical services to prevent or to treat alcohol withdrawal delirium. In one study of 32 hospitals surveyed, 50% had alcohol available on the formulary (93). There are compelling arguments against the use of alcohol for the prevention or treatment of alcohol withdrawal delirium. Randomized, controlled studies are lacking (94). Ethanol is more toxic than benzodiazepines, more difficult to administer and requires monitoring of serum levels (93). Ethanol has a short pharmacologic half-life, numerous drug–drug interactions, and a narrow therapeutic index (94). The underlying message to the addicted patient is also potentially harmful. Administration of alcohol by a physician or under a physician's orders does not communicate that continued dependence on alcohol is dangerous and ill advised.

All benzodiazepines are equally efficacious in treating symptoms of alcohol withdrawal (92). Several factors, including patient age, severity of withdrawal symptoms, requirement for supportive care, liver status, history of seizures, and detoxification setting should be taken into account when selecting which benzodiazepine to use. In ambulatory patients, longer acting benzodiazepines (e.g., chlordiazepoxide, diazepam) confer several advantages: their elimination is gradual, they have less abuse potential than shorter acting benzodiazepines, and they are easier to taper (85). For patients admitted to the hospital, especially unstable patients requiring critical care, the short to intermediate-acting benzodiazepines are preferred. Lorazepam and midazolam for example, are more titratable, can be reliably given by most routes (PO, IM, IV), can be given by continuous infusion, and have a lower risk of accumulation and overdose (14,85). Lorazepam has the added advantage of not requiring an intact liver for its metabolism. Unlike most of the other benzodiazepines, lorazepam does not undergo hepatic oxidation–reduction reactions. Lorazepam is metabolized via glucuronide conjugation, which may occur in nonhepatic tissues. Lorazepam is thus especially favorable in patients with hepatic insufficiency (14,85).

Appropriate dosing of benzodiazepines in alcohol withdrawal depends on several factors, including patient age, weight, symptom severity, quantity of alcohol consumption, drug half-life, and route of administration. Patients may vary greatly in their requirement for benzodiazepines. Doses should be titrated as indicated to control withdrawal symptoms.

There are several different dosing strategies. More stable patients can be given a loading dose of a long-acting benzodiazepine, after which the medication is allowed to clear naturally without further dosing (85). This approach is not recommended for critical care patients. An alternate strategy is the symptom-triggered dosing strategy. Patients are administered a dose of medication only when their symptoms reach a certain threshold of severity as measured by a standardized rating scale. Patients who undergo detoxification by this method do so more rapidly, and require significantly less medication than with fixed-dose administration (95). This approach has been used mainly as a treatment for uncomplicated alcohol withdrawal. A third strategy involves the administration of fixed doses of benzodiazepines followed by a gradual taper over a series of days (86). General practice guidelines recommend decreasing the total daily dose by 10–20% per 24 hr.

The benzodiazepines used most frequently in the intensive care unit setting are lorazepam, midazolam, and diazepam (84). Of the three, both midazolam and diazepam have active metabolites and depend on the liver for their metabolism. Lorazepam has an intermediate duration of action, with a half-life of 10–20 hr. It has reliable absorption by both oral and intramuscular routes. It may be given intravenously through intermittent dosing or by continuous infusion. It has a somewhat slower onset of action than either midazolam or diazepam. Lorazepam is generally given in 0.5–2 mg doses by slow IV infusion. The dosing interval may vary from 30 min to 8 hr. Parameters that may be used to determine adequacy of dose or dosing interval include heart rate, blood pressure, degree of agitation, and level of sedation. If frequent dosing is required to control breakthrough agitation, the total dose required in 24 hr can be given in the form of a continuous infusion. Lorazepam can be unstable in solution however, and may precipitate in the IV tubing during prolonged infusion (84). Midazolam is a short-acting benzodiazepine with an onset of action of 1–5 min and an elimination half-life of 1.5–3.5 hr (14). It is reliably absorbed when administered by both oral and intramuscular routes. It undergoes rapid redistribution to the fatty tissues and thus is more effective as a sedative when given by continuous infusion. Midazolam is associated with dose-dependent respiratory depression; however, this effect is minimal when midazolam is administered by continuous infusion. Its use is recommended for no more than 48–72 hr (84). Diazepam is a highly lipophilic, long-acting benzodiazepine with a rapid onset of action. Sedation is accomplished in 2–3 min following IV administration. It is not reliably absorbed when administered intramuscularly. The half-life of the parent compound is approximately 20–50 hr. The active metabolites may persist for much longer. Diazepam thus has a potential for prolonged sedation following chronic administration. This makes it an undesirable agent for use in the postoperative or critical care patient (84).

Agitation and autonomic hyperactivity in rare circumstances may persist in spite of aggressive treatment with benzodiazepines and adjunct sedatives (e.g., haloperidol). If the patient's respiratory status or hemodynamic stability is compromised, the use of a rapidly titratable, short-acting sedative-anesthetic agent (e.g., propofol) may be indicated. Airway support in the form of endotracheal intubation and mechanical ventilation may be necessary.

2. *Other Agents*

There are several other agents that may serve as adjuvant treatments in alcohol withdrawal delirium. Adrenergic medications (e.g., beta-receptor antagonists, alpha-2-receptor agonists) are useful in managing the symptoms of autonomic hyperactivity. There is no evidence, however, that they prevent delirium or seizures (92). The anticonvulsants carbamazepine and valproic acid have been shown to be efficacious in attenuating withdrawal symptoms in patients withdrawing from alcohol (86). There is insufficient evidence available to determine whether or not these agents can prevent withdrawal seizures. Antipsychotic agents may be useful in the treatment of agitation and restlessness. The newer, atypical antipsychotics are associated with fewer side effects but are only available for oral use. Ziprasidone was recently formulated to include an injectable form; however, its use has only been recommended for the intramuscular route. There are no studies documenting the use of ziprasidone in the treatment of alcohol withdrawal delirium. Haloperidol has been shown to be efficacious in reducing agitation in patients withdrawing from alcohol. It is associated with fewer cardiovascular side effects than the phenothiazines, and is less sedating (14). When used by the intravenous route, the likelihood of extrapyramidal side effects is significantly reduced (96). It can be given in bolus doses or as a continuous infusion. A history of alcohol abuse, however, may be a risk factor for the development of torsades de pointes in patients receiving haloperidol for agitation (64). The anesthetic agent propofol may prove to be useful in the management of alcohol delirium. However, there is currently little data available to support its use in nonintubated patients (84).

The emergence of alcohol delirium in the postoperative patient is a serious concern. Identifying the at-risk patient and taking steps to prevent the onset of symptoms may reduce morbidity and improve overall outcome in this patient group.

REFERENCES

1. Tuma R, DeAngelis LM. Altered mental status in patients with cancer. Arch Neurol 2000; 57(12):1727–1731.
2. Tune L, Carr S, Cooper T, Klug B, Golinger RC. Association of anticholinergic activity of prescribed medications with postoperative delirium. J Neuropsychiatry Clin Neurosci 1993; 5(2):208–210.
3. Ely EW, Gautam S, Margolin R, Francis J, May L, Speroff T, et al. The impact of delirium in the intensive care unit on hospital length of stay. Intensive Care Med 2001; 27(12):1892–1900.
4. Caraceni A, Nanni O, Maltoni M, Piva L, Indelli M, Arnoldi E, et al. Impact of delirium on the short term prognosis of advanced cancer patients. Italian Multicenter Study Group on Palliative Care. Cancer 2000; 89(5):1145–1149.
5. Franco K, Litaker D, Locala J, Bronson D. The cost of delirium in the surgical patient. Psychosomatics 2001; 42(1):68–73.
6. Breitbart W, Gibson C, Tremblay A. The delirium experience: delirium recall and delirium-related distress in hospitalized patients with cancer, their spouses/caregivers, and their nurses. Psychosomatics 2002; 43(3):183–194.
7. Lipowski ZJ. Update on delirium. Psychiatr Clin North Am 1992; 15(2):335 346.
8. Curtis T. 'Climbing the walls' ICU psychosis: myth or reality? Nurs Crit Care 1999; 4(1):18–21
9. Fricchione G. What is an ICU psychosis? Harvard Ment Health Lett 1999; 16(6):7
10. McGuire BE, Basten CJ, Ryan CJ, Gallagher J. Intensive care unit syndrome: a dangerous misnomer. Arch Inter Med 2000; 160(7):906–909.

11. Grossman S, Labedzki D, Butcher R, Dellea L. Definition and management of anxiety, agitation, and confusion in ICUs. Nurs Connect 1996; 9(2):49–55.
12. Lipowski ZJ. Delirium: Acute Confusional States. New York: Oxford University Press, 1990.
13. Diagnostic and Statistical Manual of Mental Disorders. 4th ed. Washington, DC: American Psychiatric Association, 1994.
14. Crippen D. Life-threatening brain failure and agitation in the intensive care unit. Crit Care (Lond) 2000; 4(2):81–90.
15. Bucht G, Gustafson Y, Sandberg O. Epidemiology of delirium. Dement Geriatr Cogn Disord 1999; 10(5): 315–318.
16. Breitbart W, Cohen KR. Delirium. In: Holland JC, ed. Psycho-oncology. New York: Oxford University Press, 1998:564–573.
17. Liptzin B. Clinical diagnosis and management of delirium. In: Stoudemire A, Fogel BS, Greenberg DB, eds. Psychiatric Care of the Medical Patient. 2nd ed. New York: Oxford University Press, 2000:581–597.
18. Inouye SK. Delirium in hospitalized older patients. Clin Geriatr Med 1998; 14(4):745–764.
19. Inouye SK. Delirium in hospitalized older patients: recognition and risk factors. J Geriatr Psychiatr Neurol 1998; 11(3):118–125.
20. Derogatis LR, Morrow GR, Fetting J. The prevalence of psychiatric disorders among cancer patients. JAMA 2003; 249:751–757.
21. Massie MJ, Holland J, Glass E. Delirium in terminally ill cancer patients. Am J Psychiatry 1983; 140(8): 1048–1050.
22. Lawlor PG, Gagnon B, Mancini IL, Pereira JL, Hanson J, Suarez-Almazor ME, et al. Occurrence, causes, and outcome of delirium in patients with advanced cancer: a prospective study. Arch Intern Med 2000; 160(6): 786–794.
23. van der Mast RC. Postoperative delirium. Dement Geriatr Cogn Disord 1999; 10(5):401–405.
24. Beliveau MM, Multach M. Perioperative care for the elderly patient. Med Clin North Am 2003; 87(1): 273–289.
25. Lipowski ZJ. Delirium (acute confusional states). JAMA 1987; 258(13):1789–1792.
26. Holmes JD, House AO. Psychiatric illness in hip fracture. Age Ageing 2000; 29(6):537–546.
27. Galanakis P, Bickel H, Gradinger R, Von Gumppenberg S, Forstl H. Acute confusional state in the elderly following hip surgery: incidence, risk factors and complications. Int J Geriatr Psychiatry 2001; 16(4):349–355.
28. Eriksson M, Samuelsson E, Gustafson Y, Aberg T, Engstrom KG. Delirium after coronary bypass surgery evaluated by the organic brain syndrome protocol. Scand Cardiovasc J 2002; 36(4):250–255.
29. Gokgoz L, Gunaydin S, Sinci V, Unlu M, Boratav C, Babacan A, et al. Psychiatric complications of cardiac surgery postoperative delirium syndrome. Scand Cardiovasc J 1997; 31(4):217–222.
30. Liptzin B, Levkoff SE. An empirical study of delirium subtypes. Br J Psychiatry 1992; 161:843–845.
31. Burney-Puckett M. Sundown syndrome: etiology and management. J Psychosoc Nurs Ment Health Serv 1996; 34(5):40–43.
32. Brown TM, Stoudemire A. Psychiatric Side Effects of Prescription and Over-the-Counter Medications. Washington, DC: American Psychiatric Press Inc., 1998.
33. Brown TM. Drug-induced delirium. Semin Clin Neuropsychiatry 2000; 5(2):113–124.
34. Rasmussen LS, Moller JT. Central nervous system dysfunction after anesthesia in the geriatric patient. Anesthesiol Clin North Am 2000; 18(1):59–70.
35. Boucher BA, Witt WO, Foster TS. The postoperative adverse effects of inhalational anesthetics. Heart Lung J Acute Crit Care 1986; 15(1):63–69.
36. Parikh SS, Chung F. Postoperative delirium in the elderly. Anesth Analg 1995; 80(6):1223–1232.
37. Marcantonio ER, Juarez G, Goldman L, Mangione CM, Ludwig LE, Lind L, et al. The relationship of postoperative delirium with psychoactive medications. JAMA 1994; 272(19):1518–1522.
38. Tune LE, Damlouji NF, Holland A, Gardner TJ, Folstein MF, Coyle JT. Association of postoperative delirium with raised serum levels of anticholinergic drugs. Lancet 1981; 2(8248):651–653.
39. Tune LE. Post-operative delirium. Int Psychogeriatr 1991; 3:325–332.
40. Trzepacz PT. Delirium. Advances in diagnosis, pathophysiology, and treatment. Psychiatr Clin North Am 1996; 19(3):429–448.
41. Meyers CA, Valentine AD. Neurological and psychiatric adverse effects of immunological therapy. CNS Drugs 1995; 3:56–58.
42. Winawer N. Postoperative delirium. Med Clin North Am 2001; 85(5):1229–1239.
43. Folstein MF, Folstein SE, McHugh PR. "Mini-mental state." A practical method for grading the cognitive state of patients for the clinician. J Psychiatr Res 1975; 12(3):189–198.
44. Anthony JC, LeResche L, Niaz U, Von Korff MR, Folstein MF. Limits of the 'mini-mental state' as a screening test for dementia and delirium among hospital patients. Psychol Med 1982; 12(2):397–408.
45. Inouye SK, van Dyck CH, Alessi CA, Balkin S, Siegal AP, Horwitz RI. Clarifying confusion: the confusion assessment method. A new method for detection of delirium. Ann Intern Med 1990; 113(12):941–948.
46. Bergeron N, Dubois MJ, Dumont M, Dial S, Skrobik Y. Intensive care delirium screening check list: evaluation of a new screening tool. Intensive Care Med 2001; 27(5):859–864.
47. Bergeron N, Skrobik Y, Dubois MJ. Delirium in critically ill patients. Crit Care (Lond) 2002; 6(3):181–182.
48. Trzepacz PT, Baker RW, Greenhouse J. A symptom rating scale for delirium. Psychiatry Res 1988; 23(1): 89–97.

49. Breitbart W, Rosenfeld B, Roth A, Smith MJ, Cohen K, Passik S. The Memorial Delirium Assessment Scale [comment]. J Pain Symptom Manage 1997; 13(3): 128–137.
50. Jacobson SA, Leuchter AF, Walter DO. Conventional and quantitative EEG in the diagnosis of delirium among the elderly. J Neurol Neurosurg Psychiatry 1993; 56(2):153–158.
51. Rabins PV, Folstein MF. Delirium and dementia: diagnostic criteria and fatality rates. Br J Psychiatry 1982; 140:149–153.
52. Inouye SK. Prevention of delirium in hospitalized older patients: risk factors and targeted intervention strategies. Ann Med 2000; 32(4):257–263.
53. Marcantonio ER, Goldman L, Mangione CM, Ludwig LE, Muraca B, Haslauer CM, et al. A clinical prediction rule for delirium after elective noncardiac surgery. JAMA 1994; 271(2):134–139.
54. Hassan E, Fontaine DK, Nearman HS. Therapeutic considerations in the management of agitated or delirious critically ill patients. Pharmacotherapy 1998; 18(1): 113–129.
55. Boland RJ, Goldstein MG, Haltzman SD. Psychiatric management of behavioral syndromes in intensive care units. In: Stoudemire A, Fogel BS, Greenberg DB, eds. Psychiatric Care of the Medical Patient. New York: Oxford University Press, 2000:299–314.
56. Shapiro BA, Warren J, Egol AB, Greenbaum DM, Jacobi J, Nasraway SA, et al. Practice parameters for intravenous analgesia and sedation for adult patients in the intensive care unit: an executive summary. Society of Critical Care Medicine. Crit Care Med 1995; 23(9):1596–1600.
57. Adams F. Emergency intravenous sedation of the delirious, medically ill patient. J Clin Psychiatry 1988; 49(suppl):22–27.
58. Akechi T, Uchitomi Y, Okamura H, Fukue M, Kagaya A, Nishida A, et al. Usage of haloperidol for delirium in cancer patients. Support Care Cancer 1996; 4(5): 390–392.
59. Crippen DW. Pharmacologic treatment of brain failure and delirium. Crit Care Clin 1994; 10(4):733–766.
60. Fish DN. Treatment of delirium in the critically ill patient. Clin Pharm 1991; 10(6):456–466.
61. Cassem NH, Murray GB. Delirious patients. In: Cassem NH, Stern TA, Rosenbaum JF, Jellinek MS, eds. Massachusetts General Hospital Handbook of General Hospital Psychiatry. St. Louis, Missouri: Mosby Inc., 1997:101–122.
62. Fernandez F, Holmes VF, Adams F, Kavanaugh JJ. Treatment of severe, refractory agitation with a haloperidol drip. J Clin Psychiatry 1988; 49(6):239–241.
63. Sanders KM, Murray GB, Cassem NH. High-dose intravenous haloperidol for agitated delirium in a cardiac patient on intra-aortic balloon pump. J Clin Psychopharmacol 1991; 11(2):146–147.
64. Metzger E, Friedman R. Prolongation of the corrected QT and torsades de pointes cardiac arrhythmia associated with intravenous haloperidol in the medically ill. J Clin Psychopharmacol 1993; 13(2):128–132.
65. Lawrence KR, Nasraway SA. Conduction disturbances associated with administration of butyrophenone antipsychotics in the critically ill: a review of the literature. Pharmacotherapy 1997; 17(3):531–537.
66. Frye MA, Coudreaut MF, Hakeman SM, Shah BG, Strouse TB, Skotzko CE. Continuous droperidol infusion for management of agitated delirium in an intensive care unit. Psychosomatics 1995; 36(3):301–305.
67. Shale JH, Shale CM, Mastin WD. A review of the safety and efficacy of droperidol for the rapid sedation of severely agitated and violent patients. J Clin Psychiatry 2003; 64:500–505.
68. Sipahimalani A, Masand PS. Use of risperidone in delirium: case reports. Ann Clin Psychiatry 1997; 9(2): 105–107.
69. Schwartz TL, Masand PS. The role of atypical antipsychotics in the treatment of delirium. Psychosomatics 2002; 43(3):171–174.
70. Leso L, Schwartz TL. Ziprasidone treatment of delirium. Psychosomatics 2002; 43(1):61–62.
71. Passik SD, Cooper M. Complicated delirium in a cancer patient successfully treated with olanzapine. J Pain Symptom Manage 1999; 17(3):219–223.
72. Breitbart W, Tremblay A, Gibson C. An open trial of olanzapine for the treatment of delirium in hospitalized cancer patients. Psychosomatics 2002; 43(3):175–182.
73. Breitbart W, Marotta R, Platt MM, Weisman H, Derevenco M, Grau C, et al. A double-blind trial of haloperidol, chlorpromazine, and lorazepam in the treatment of delirium in hospitalized AIDS patients. Am J Psychiatry 1996; 153(2):231–237.
74. Stiefel F, Fainsinger R, Bruera E. Acute confusional states in patients with advanced cancer. J Pain Symptom Manage 1992; 7(2):94–98.
75. Coomes TR, Smith SW. Successful use of propofol in refractory delirium tremens. Ann Emerg Med 1997; 30(6):825–828.
76. McCowan C, Marik P. Refractory delirium tremens treated with propofol: a case series. Crit Care Med 2000; 28(6):1781–1784.
77. Mantz J. Dexmedtomidine. Drugs Today (BARC) 1999; 35(3):151–157.
78. Romero C, Bugedo G, Bruhn A, Mellado P, Hernandez G, Castillo L. Preliminary experience with dexmedtomidine treatment of confusional state and hyperadrenergic states at an intensive care unit. Rev Esp Anestesiol Reanim 2000 Oct; 49(8):403–406.
79. Heiser JF, Gillin JC. The reversal of anticholinergic drug-induced delirium and coma with physostigmine. Am J Psychiatry 1971; 127(8):1050–1054.
80. Stern TA. Continuous infusion of physostigmine in anticholinergic delirium: case report. J Clin Psychiatry 1983; 44(12):463–464.
81. Coyle N, Breitbart W, Weaver S, Portenoy R. Delirium as a contributing factor to "crescendo" pain: three case reports. J Pain Symptom Manage 1994; 9(1):44–47.

82. Lynch EP, Lazor MA, Gellis JE, Orav J, Goldman L, Marcantonio ER. The impact of postoperative pain on the development of postoperative delirium. Anesth Analg 1998; 86(4):781–785.
83. Bruera E, Franco JJ, Maltoni M, Watanabe S, Suarez-Almazor M. Changing pattern of agitated impaired mental status in patients with advanced cancer: association with cognitive monitoring, hydration, and opioid rotation. J Pain Symptom Manage 1995; 10(4):287–291.
84. Cohen IL, Gallagher TJ, Pohlman AS, Dasta JF, Abraham E, Papdokos PJ. Management of the agitated intensive care unit patient. Crit Care Med 2002; 30(1 suppl):S97–S123.
85. Mack AH, Franklin JE Jr, Frances RJ. Substance use disorders. In: Hales RE, Yudofsky SC, eds. The American Psychiatric Publishing Textbook of Clinical Psychiatry. Washington, DC: American Psychiatric Publishing Inc., 2000:309–377.
86. Kosten T, O'Connor PG. Management of drug and alcohol withdrawal. N Engl J Med 2003; 348(18): 1786–1795.
87. Stanley KM, Amabile CM, Simpson KN, Couillard D, Norcross ED, Worrall CL. Impact of an alcohol withdrawal syndrome practice guideline on surgical patient outcomes. Pharmacotherapy 2003; 23(7):843–854.
88. Myrick H, Anton RF. Treatment of alcohol withdrawal. Alcohol Health Res World 1998; 22(1):38–43.
89. Palmstierna T. A model for predicting alcohol withdrawal delirium. Psychiatr Serv 2001; 52(6):820–823.
90. Fiellin DA, O'Connor PG, Holmboes ES, Horowitz RI. Risk for delirium tremens in patients with alcohol withdrawal syndrome. Subst Abus 2002; 23(2):83–94.
91. Gallivan KH, Reiter D. Acute alcohol withdrawal in free flap mandibular reconstruction outcomes. Arch Facial Plastic Surg 2001; 3(4):264–266.
92. Mayo-Smith MF. Pharmacological management of alcohol withdrawal. A meta-analysis and evidence-based practice guideline. JAMA 1997; 278(2):144–151.
93. Rosenbaum M, McCarty T. Alcohol prescription by surgeons in the prevention and treatment of delirium tremens: historic and current practice. Gen Hosp Psychiatry 2002; 24:257–259.
94. DiPaula B, Tommasello A, Solounias B, McDuff D. An evaluation of intravenous ethanol in hospitalized patients. J Subst Abuse Treat 1998; 15(5):437–442.
95. Daeppen JB, Gache P, Landry U, Sekera E, Schweizer V, Gloor S, Yersin B. Symptom-triggered vs. fixed schedule doses of benzodiazepine for alcohol withdrawal: a randomized treatment trial. Arch Intern Med 2002; 162(10):1117–1121.
96. Sanders KM, Minnema AM, Murray GB. Low incidence of extrapyramidal symptoms in treatment of delirium with intravenous haloperidol and lorazepam in the intensive care unit. J Intensive Care Med 1989; 4:201–204.

35

Neutropenia and Sepsis in Cancer Patients

KENNETH V. I. ROLSTON

Department of Infectious Diseases, Infection Control and Employee Health, Section of Infectious Diseases, The University of Texas M.D. Anderson Cancer Center, Houston, Texas, U.S.A.

EDWARD B. RUBENSTEIN

Medical Supportive Care, The University of Texas M.D. Anderson Cancer Center, Houston, Texas, U.S.A.

I. INTRODUCTION

Infection continues to be the most common complication seen in cancer patients with neutropenia (1). Most of the attention has been focused on patients with hematologic malignancies and recipients of hematopoietic stem-cell transplantation (HSCT), since these patients have severe and prolonged neutropenia and a high risk of developing a serious infection (2). However, most infections in cancer patients occur in patients who are not neutropenic (3). Some of these, particularly in patients with solid tumors, occur in the perioperative period following surgical treatment for the underlying malignancy (4). Some infections require surgical intervention for appropriate management, creating special problems related to neutropenia and thrombocytopenia. Invasive diagnostic procedures are also impacted by the presence of severe neutropenia and thrombocytopenia, which generally go hand in hand. A substantial number of cancer patients require critical care in an intensive care unit for infection-related (septic shock, respiratory insufficiency, etc.) or other medical complications, raising issues related not only to the management of the infection itself, but also infection prevention and infection control, in this high-risk environment. The increasing use of vascular access catheters and other external medical devices has created a unique spectrum of infection, and challenging issues regarding the management of device-related infections (5). This chapter focuses on infections in neutropenic and non-neutropenic patients and discusses the growing problem of antimicrobial resistance and measures to combat it.

II. INFECTION IN NEUTROPENIC PATIENTS

A. Risk Factors

Patients with hematologic malignancies and recipients of HSCT are at particular risk of developing infectious complications since they often experience episodes of severe ($ANC \leq 100/mm^3$) and prolonged ($\geq$14 days) neutropenia (6). In addition, many of these patients have qualitative defects in neutrophil function and are at risk even when not neutropenic. In many patients, neutropenia is superimposed on other immunological defects (impaired cellular or humoral immunity) associated with underlying malignancy, which can have an impact on the spectrum of infection. The use of antibacterial and antifungal prophylaxis, and of external devices such as central venous catheters, also influences the nature and spectrum of infection in such patients.

B. Spectrum

In approximately 50% of febrile episodes in neutropenic patients, all microbiologic cultures are negative and no clinical sites of infection are identified (6). These are defined as episodes of "unexplained fever," and probably represent low-grade infections, since most of them respond to empiric antibiotic therapy. It is important to recognize that a substantial proportion of patients who are initially thought to have unexplained fever, subsequently develop a documented infection (7). Approximately 20–25% of febrile neutropenic patients will have a "clinically documented infection," i.e., negative cultures but a clinical site such as cellulitis, pneumonia, or enterocolitis (6). These infections can be associated with substantial morbidity, since most of them involve deep-tissue sites.

Patients who have positive microbiological cultures from normally sterile sites are categorized as having microbiologically documented infections. The most common sites of infection include the bloodstream, the urinary tract, and skin/skin structure infections. Bacterial infections predominate in the early phases of neutropenia. Prolonged neutropenia increases the risk of invasive fungal infections (candidiasis and aspergillosis). Viral infections (HSV, VZV, and CMV) are common in certain high-risk populations (HSCT recipients) (8–10). Community respiratory viruses have recently been shown to be a significant cause of morbidity and mortality, particularly in HSCT recipients and patients with hematologic malignancies (11–13). Table 1 lists the common pathogens from neutropenic patients and includes organisms from all sites of infection (not just bloodstream infections) and polymicrobial infections as well. It is important to recognize that institutional differences in the spectrum/epidemiology of infections do occur, and that the spectrum is also likely to change over time.

Table 1 Common Pathogens Isolated from Neutropenic Patients

Bacterial
Gram-positive:
Coagulase-negative staphylococci
Staphylococcus aureus (including MRSA)
Viridans streptococci (including penicillin-resistant isolates)
Enterococcus spp. (including VRE)
Corynebacterium spp.
Bacillus spp.
Beta-hemolytic streptococci (Groups A, B, C, G, F)
Gram-negative:
Escherichia coli
Pseudomonas aeruginosa
Klebsiella spp.
Enterobacter spp.
Citrobacter spp.
Stenotrophomonas maltophilia
Acinetobacter spp.
Fungal
Candida spp.
Aspergillus spp.
Fusarium spp.
Zygomycetes
Trichosporon beigelii
Viral
Herpes viruses (HSV, VZV, CMV, EBV, HHV-6)
Respiratory syncytial virus (RSV)
Influenza A and B viruses
Parainfluenza viruses
Adenovirus

C. Treatment

Standard treatment consists of the prompt administration of broad-spectrum, empiric antibiotic therapy. Febrile neutropenic patients can now be subdivided into "low-risk" and "non-low-risk" subsets based either on clinical criteria, or on statistically derived risk prediction rules (14,15). Low-risk patients (children and adults) can safely be managed without hospital admission using oral, sequential, or parenteral antibiotic regimens (2,16–19). All other patients receive hospital-based, parenteral antibiotic regimens—listed in Table 2. Empiric therapy produces response rates in approximately 60–80% of febrile neutropenic episodes (2). Most of these patients remain relatively stable and do not require critical care or surgical (diagnostic and/or therapeutic) intervention. In patients failing to respond to empiric therapy, alteration of the initial regimen and the administration of empiric antifungal (and in some cases antiviral) agents is the next therapeutic step (1,2). Some patients with significant cutaneous lesions, solitary or diffuse pulmonary lesions, hepatic lesions, cerebral lesions, or lesions at other deep-tissue sites might need an invasive procedure in order to make a specific diagnosis. With the possible exception of cutaneous biopsies, the limiting factor for such procedures is the presence of severe thrombocytopenia. If a specific diagnosis is made (e.g., aspergillosis, CMV, PCP, and mycobacterial infection), then specific therapy directed at the offending pathogen(s) is administered.

Table 2 Therapeutic Options in Febrile Neutropenic Patients

Out-patient regimens
Parenteral
Aztreonam + clindamycin
Ciprofloxacin + clindamycin
Ceftriaxone + amikacin
Ceftazidime or cefepime
Oral
Ciprofloxacin + amoxicillin/clavulanate
Ciprofloxacin + clindamycin
Hospital-based, broad-spectrum regimens
Combination therapy
Aminoglycoside + cefepime or ceftazidime
Aminoglycoside + piperacillin/tazobactam
Aminoglycoside + imipenem or meropenem
Vancomycin can replace the aminoglycoside in the combinations listed above
Monotherapy
Cefepime
Imipenem
Meropenem
Piperacillin/tazobactam

A small proportion of high-risk febrile neutropenic patients (generally with hematologic malignancies/HSCT and pre-existing medical morbidity) will develop complications that require critical care. These include severe SIRS/septic shock, progressive respiratory insufficiency, acute renal failure, DIC and other hematologic complications, neurological complications, and multiple organ system failure. Such patients are best managed in an intensive care unit by a critical care team skilled in providing overall supportive care, which can include intubation, mechanical ventilation, and other respiratory support; transfusions, pressors, and other measures for hemodynamic stability; dialysis and other measure for renal insufficiency; antimicrobial agents, hematopoietic growth factors, WBC transfusions, and activated protein C for infection management; and the ability to rapidly provide specialty medical or surgical consultations as the need arises.

III. INFECTIONS IN NON-NEUTROPENIC PATIENTS

A. Risk Factors

Although some patients with solid tumors receive chemotherapy that is myelosuppressive enough to cause significant neutropenia, over 90% of infections seen in solid tumor patients develop when they are not neutropenic (20). Factors predisposing these patients to the development of infections (many of which occur perioperatively) include lengthy and extensive surgical procedures, large tumor burden with lesions that produce significant obstruction, the use of vascular access catheters, stents, shunts, and prosthetic and other medical devices, and the need in some patients for care in an intensive care unit, which can increase the risk of infection with nosocomial, multidrug resistant organisms. The specific site(s) and nature of these infections will largely depend on the type of surgery, location of foreign medical devices, and location of the obstructing lesion(s). The most common sites of infection in such patients are listed in Table 3.

B. Spectrum

Most infections in patients with solid tumors are caused by the patients' resident microflora. Acquisition of nosocomial pathogens occurs after hospitalization, particularly, following prolonged or multiple antibiotic exposure. The distribution of causative pathogens generally mirrors the normal flora at a particular site of infection, or the nosocomial flora of a specific unit or institution (21). For example, surgical wound infections and catheter-related infections are caused most often by organisms colonizing the skin (coagulase-negative staphylococci, *Staphylococcus aureus*, *Streptococcus* species, *Bacillus* species, etc.), although opportunistic gram-negative organisms (*Acinetobacter* species, *Pseudomonas aeruginosa*, *Stenotrophomonas maltophilia*) and some moulds (*Aspergillus* species, the zygomycetes) are significant pathogens in the nosocomial setting. In contrast, most upper and lower respiratory infections are caused by the resident oropharyngeal microflora (*Streptococcus pneumoniae*, *Haemophilus influenzae*, mouth anaerobes) with *Staphylococcus* spp. and gram-negative bacilli gaining predominance in the hospital. Enteric gram-negative bacilli (*Escherichia coli*, *Enterobacter* species, *Pseudomonas* species, *Enterococcus* species) and intestinal anaerobes (*Bacteroides* and *Clostridium* species) dominate abdominal and pelvic sites of infection. Polymicrobial infections have been increasing in frequency particularly when there is tissue involvement (22,23). Examples include pneumonia, complicated or extensive wound infections with necrosis, neutropenic enterocolitis/typhlitis, perirectal infections, necrotizing fasciitis, and other skin and skin structure infections (20,24–26). Catheter-associated infections may also be polymicrobial in nature. Occasionally, bacterial, fungal, and/or viral infections coexist. *Candida* species frequently colonize debilitated hospitalized patients, particularly patients who have received multiple

Table 3 Common Sites of Infection in Patients with Solid Tumors

Tumor type	Infection sites
Central nervous system	Surgical wound infection; epidural or subdural abscess; brain abscess; shunt-related infection; meningitis/ventriculitis; aspiration pneumonia; urinary tract (catheter-related) infection
Head and neck	Surgical wound infection/facial cellulitis; sinusitis; mastoiditis; deep facial tissue infection; aspiration/postoperative pneumonia; cavernous (or other) sinus infection; meningitis; brain abscess; retropharyngeal/paravertebral abscess; craniofacial osteomyelitis
Breast	Surgical wound infection; mastitis; breast abscess; lymphangitis/cellulitis secondary to axillary node infection
Upper gastrointestinal	Surgical wound infection; gastric perforation and abscess; feeding tube related infections; aspiration pneumonia; mediastinitis; tracheoesophageal fistula with pneumonitis; empyema
Lower gastrointestinal and pelvic	Surgical wound infection; abdominal/pelvic abscess; peritonitis; typhlitis/enterocolitis; necrotizing fasciitis; perianal/perirectal infection; infected hemorrhoids; acute or chronic urinary tract infection; sacral-coccygeal osteomyelitis
Hepatobiliary and pancreatic	Surgical wound infection; ascending cholangitis with or without bacteremia; peritonitis; hepatic, pancreatic, or subdiaphragmatic abscess
Genitourinary and prostate	Acute and/or chronic pyelonephritis; prostatitis; cystitis; urethritis; catheter-related complication urinary tract infection, epididymitis; surgical wound infection; orchitis
Cutaneous	Cellulitis; subcutaneous tissue infection; myositis; fasciitis; lymphangitis and lymphadenitis
Lung and mediastinum	Surgical wound infection; pneumonia (postobstructive): empyema; tracheoesophageal fistula and associated infections; mediastinitis/mediastinal abscess
Bone, joints, cartilage	Surgical wound infection; skin and subcutaneous tissue infection, bursitis, synovitis; tendonitis; septic arthritis; osteomyelitis; infected prosthesis, myositis

courses of broad-spectrum antibacterial therapy. Candidemia and candiduria are not uncommon in this setting (*Candida* species are now recognized as the fourth most commonly isolated nosocomial pathogens) although disseminated candidiasis is uncommon in solid tumor patients (27–29). Colonization with *Candida* spp. is therefore not sufficient reason for antifungal therapy in such patients. Excessive use of prophylactic/empiric antifungal therapy particularly with azole antifungal agents has contributed to the emergence of resistant species such as *Candida krusei* and *Candida glabrata* (30,31). Invasive mould infections, viral infections (CMV, VZV, EBV, and community respiratory viruses), and parasitic infections are quite rare in solid tumor patients. A breakdown of the predominant pathogens according to the site(s) of infection is shown in Table 4.

C. Treatment

The general principles of managing infections in neutropenic patients with solid tumors are similar to those applied to neutropenic patients with hematologic malignancies. However, the frequency of documented infections in solid tumor patients who are not neutropenic is much greater than in patients who are neutropenic. Consequently, the need for empiric therapy is much less, and the opportunity to use specific or targeted therapy based on local epidemiological/susceptibility data is much greater.

Many solid tumors produce lesions that cause significant obstruction and lead to the development of acute or chronic postobstructive infections. Common situations include the following:

- Postobstructive pneumonitis in patients with lung cancer or metastatic pulmonary lesions.
- Ascending cholangitis and local abscesses in patients with hepatobiliary obstruction due to tumor masses.
- Tubo-ovarian and urinary tract infections due to local obstruction in patients with gynecological malignancies.

Additionally, the development of a sinus tract or fistula, and the perforation of a viscus, is not uncommon in patients with obstructive lesions, or those that have undergone certain surgical procedures. Surgical intervention is a critical component in these settings, and antimicrobial therapy is often a secondary modality.

IV. DEVICE-RELATED INFECTIONS

Vascular access devices (VADs) are indispensable tools in the management of patients with cancer. They provide many advantages, including easy vascular access and the ability to administer medications, blood products, parenteral nutrition, and large volumes of fluids, when indicated. Although the frequency of VAD-related infection is low, a large number of manifestations, including local site infection, catheter-related bloodstream infection, septic and nonseptic thrombophlebitis, endocarditis, osteomyelitis, and disseminated infections, can occur. Nearly all indwelling intravascular catheters develop a biofilm which provides a protective milieu for the existence of bacteria that are the source for such infections. Vascular access device-related infections are associated with substantial morbidity, some mortality, and significant increase

Table 4 Common Pathogens According to Site of Infection in Solid Tumor Patients

Site of infection	Predominant organism
Bloodstream	*Staphylococcus* species, *Streptococcus* spp., *Enterococcus* spp., *Enterobacteriaceae*, *Pseudomonas* spp., *Stenotrophomons maltophilia*, *Candida* species
Respiratory tract (including lung abscess and empyema)	*S. pneumoniae*, *H. influenzae*; *M. catarrhalis*; *Staphylococcus*, *Streptococcus* spp., *Enterobacteraceae*, nonfermentative gram-negative bacilli, *Legionella* spp., mouth anaerobes (*Peptococcus*, *Peptostreptococcus*, *Fusobacterium*) mycobacteria
Intraabdominal/pelvic	Enteric gram-negative bacilli, nonfermentative gram-negative bacilli, *Enterococcus* spp., intestinal anaerobes (*Bacteroides* + *Clostridium* spp.), *Candida* species
Skin/skin structure	*Staphylococcus* species, *Streptococcus* species, gram-negative bacilli, anaerobes
Central nervous system	*S. pneumonial*, *H. influenzae*, *Neisseria* spp., *Staphylococcus* spp., *Streptococcus* spp., mouth anaerobes, gram-negative bacilli, *Listeria monocytogenes*, *Cryptococcus neoformans*
Central venous catheter related	*Staphylococcus* species, *Streptococcus* species, gram-negative bacilli, *Candida* spp., rapidly growing mycobacteria
Biliary tract	Enteric gram-negative bacilli, *Enterococcus* spp., anaerobes, *Candida* spp., *Staphylococcus* spp.
Bone and joint	*Staphylococcus* spp., *Streptococcus* spp., gram-negative bacilli (anaerobes and fungi uncommon)

in healthcare expenditure (5,32). The organisms isolated most frequently include coagulase-negative staphylococci and *S. aureus* (including MRSA). However, gram-negatives such as *P. aeruginosa*, *S. maltophilia*, and *Acinetobacter* spp., the rapidly growing mycobacteria, and *Candida* spp. are not uncommon, particularly in cancer patients (32,33). A detailed discussion regarding diagnosis and management of catheter-related infections is beyond the scope of this chapter. National guidelines for the management of these infections have been published (5). They can be summarized as follows:

- Patients with short-term catheters and noncomplicated bloodstream infections can be treated with (and often respond to) a short course of parenteral antibiotic therapy with or without removal of the infected device.
- In patients with complicated extraluminal (tunnel or pocket site) infection, the catheter must be removed and antibiotic therapy given for 10–14 days.
- In patients with septic thrombophlebitis or distant foci such as endocarditis, management consists of prompt removal of the infected device and appropriate antimicrobial therapy for 4–6 weeks.

V. SPECIAL CONSIDERATIONS

Hematopoietic growth factors (G-CSF and GM-CSF) and granulocyte transfusions are not recommended for routine use. Situations in which they might be helpful include documented infections refractory to appropriate therapy, disseminated fungal infections, and deep-tissue infections such as pneumonia (34,35). Human activated protein C (Drotrecogin alfa) is indicated in patients with severe sepsis associated with acute, multiple organ dysfunction (36). It has, however, not been fully evaluated in neutropenic/thrombocytopenic patients. Since it can increase the risk of bleeding, such studies (which are ongoing) will help clarify its role in this high-risk population.

Routine antibacterial, antifungal, and antiviral prophylaxis for all neutropenic patients is not recommended (2). High-risk patients may benefit from antibacterial prophylaxis (usually a fluoroquinolone), antifungal prophylaxis (fluconazole or itraconazole), and antiviral prophylaxis (acyclovir). Pre-emptive therapy (rather than prophylaxis) is the current recommendation for suspected CMV disease. Prophylaxis with TMP/SMX (or an alternative agent in patients allergic to TMP/SMX) is recommended for all patients at risk for infection in *Pneumocystis jiroveci*. All prophylaxes should be given for the shortest duration possible (i.e., the period of maximum risk).

A. Antimicrobial Resistance

The frequent use of antimicrobial agents for prophylaxis, pre-emptive, or specific therapy in neutropenic and non-neutropenic cancer patients is unavoidable. This has led to tremendous selective pressure and the emergence of several gram-positive and gram-negative organisms that are multidrug resistant. These organisms are listed in Table 5, although a detailed discussion

Table 5 Resistant Organisms of Particular Concern in Cancer Patients

Organisms	Treatment choices
Gram-positive	
Methicillin-resistant staphylococci	Vancomycin, linezolid, daptomycin TMP/SMX[a], rifampin, minocycline
Vancomycin-resistant enterococci	Linezolid, quinupristin–dalfopristin, daptomycin, combination regimens
Penicillin-resistant streptococci (*S. pneumoniae* and viridans streptococci)	Vancomycin, gatifloxacin, moxifloxacin
Gram-negative	
Pseudomonas aeruginosa (multidrug resistant)	Piperacillin/tazobactam, combination regimens, colistin, polymyxin B
Stenotrophomonas maltophilia	TMP/SMX, newer quinolones, beta lactam + beta lactamase inhibitor, rifampin, combination regimens
ESBL[b] producing gram-negative bacilli	Carbapenems, quinolones, aminoglycosides, combination regimens
Fungi	
Candida species (*C. glabrata*, *C. krusei*)	Caspofungin, amphotericin B (including lipid formulations)
Fusarium spp.	Voriconzaole, combinations (?)
Zygomycetes	Posaconazole (?)

[a] Extended spectrum beta-lactamase.
[b] Trimethoprim/sulfamethoxazole.

is beyond the scope of this chapter. Among the gram-positive pathogens, methicillin-resistant staphylococci (*S. aureus* and coagulase-negative species), penicillin-resistant streptococci (pneumococci and viridans or α-hemolytic streptococci), and vancomycin-resistant enterococci are isolated most often and are generally resistant to most agents used in empiric regimens (6). Current therapeutic options are listed in Table 5. Among gram-negative bacilli, multidrug resistant *P. aeruginosa*, *S. maltophilia*, and ESBL producing organisms are of great concern, and often require treatment with combination regimens (Table 5). *Candida* species other than *C. albicans*, and certain moulds (*Fusarium* spp., the zygomycetes), are the fungi of greatest concern, often with limited therapeutic options. Infection prevention and strict adherence to infection-control practices are of utmost importance in the management of these infections.

Increasing antimicrobial resistance particularly in high-risk populations such as febrile neutropenic patients is of such concern that the Centers for Disease Control (CDC) has recently developed a 12-step plan to combat antimicrobial resistance in hospitalized patients (37). The four major components of this plan include strategies for:

- Infection prevention
- Appropriate therapy
- Control of antibiotic usage
- Infection control/prevention of transmission

These measures need to be implemented and strictly adhered to, in order to minimize the selection and spread of resistant organisms particularly in patients receiving critical care in intensive care units.

VI. SUMMARY

Infections are common in neutropenic and non-neutropenic cancer patients. The prompt administration of empiric antibiotic therapy in neutropenic patients is critical. Low-risk neutropenic patients can be treated with parenteral or oral regimens in the outpatient setting. Moderate-to-high-risk patients require hospital-based parenteral therapy. Some patients develop complications that require surgical intervention and/or critical care. Infections related to vascular access catheters, prosthetic devices, or other foreign bodies create special problems, and not infrequently, result in the removal of these devices, if long-term suppressive therapy is unsuccessful. The development of multidrug resistant organism is of great concern. Strategies to prevent the emergence and spread of such organisms have been developed and need to be implemented and adhered to, particularly in high-risk patients receiving critical care.

REFERENCES

1. Pizzo PA. Management of fever in patients with cancer and treatment induced neutropenia. N Engl J Med 1993; 328:1323–1332.
2. Hughes WT, Armstrong D, Bodey GP, Bow EJ, Brown AE, Calandra T, Feld R, Pizzo PA, Rolston KVI, Shenep JL, Young LS. Guidelines for the use of antimicrobial agents in neutropenic patients with cancer. Clin Infect Dis 2002; 34:730–751.
3. Yadegarynia D, Rolston KV, Tarrand J, Raad I. Current spectrum of bacterial infections in patient with hematological malignancies (HM) and solid tumors (st) [abstr no. 139]. 40th Annual Meeting of Infectious Diseases Society of America, Chicago, IL, Oct 24–27, 2002.
4. Rolston KVI. Infections in patients with solid tumors. In: Rolston KVI, Rubenstein EB, eds. Textbook of Febrile Neutropenia. United Kingdom: Martin Dunitz, 2001:91–109.
5. Mermel LA, Farr BM, Sheretz RJ, Raad II, O'Grady N, Harris JS, Craven DE. Infectious Diseases Society of America, American College of Critical Care Medicine, Society for Healthcare Epidemiology of America. Guidelines for the management of intravascular catheter-related infection. Clin Infect Dis 2001; 32: 1249–1272.
6. Rolston KVI, Bodey GP. Infections in patients with cancer. In: Holland JF, Frei E, eds. Cancer Medicine. 6th ed. Ontario: BC Decker, 2003:2633–2658.
7. Rubenstein EB, Kim YJ, Legha R, Rolston KVI on behalf of the MASCC Infectious Disease Study Section. Documented infections in febrile neutropenic patients (pts) presenting with apparent fever of undetermined origin (fuo): a wolf in sheep's clothing. [abstr no. 8]. 12th MASCC International Symposium, Washington, DC, Mar 23–25, 2000.
8. Maltezou HC, Kafetzis DA, Abi-said D, Mantzouranis EC, Chan KW, Rolston KVI. Viral infections in children undergoing hematopoietic stem cell transplants. Pediatr Infect Dis J 2000; 19:307–312.
9. Maltezou HC, Petropoulos D, Gardner M, Abi-Said D, Mantzouranis EC, Rolston KVI, Chan KW. Varicella-zoster virus infection in children with hematopoietic stem cell transplants. Int J Pediatr Hematol Oncol 1998; 5:345–351.
10. Nguyen Q, Champlin R, Giralt S, Rolston K, Raad I, Jacobson K, Ippoliti C, Hecht D, Tarrand J, Luna M, Whimbey E. Late cytomegalovirus pneumonia in adult allogeneic blood and marrow transplant recipients. Clin Infect Dis 1999; 28:618–623.
11. Yousuf HM, Englund J, Couch R, Rolston K, Luna M, Goodrich J, Lewis V, Mirza NQ, Andreeff M, Koller C, Elting L, Bodey GP, Whimbey E. Influenza among hospitalized adults with leukemia. Clin Infect Dis 1997; 24:1095–1099.

12. Lewis VA, Champlin R, Englund J, Couch R, Goodrich JM, Rolston K, Przepiorka D, Mirza NQ, Yousuf HM, Luna M, Bodey GP, Whimbey E. Respiratory disease due to parainfluenza virus in adult bone marrow transplant recipients. Clin Infect Dis 1996; 23:1033–1037.
13. Couch RB, Englund JA, Whimbey E. Respiratory viral infections in immunocompetent and immunocompromised persons. Am J Med 1997; 102:2–9.
14. Talcott JA, Seigel RD, Finberg R, Goldman L. Risk assessment in cancer patents with fever and neutropenia: a prospective, two-center validation of a prediction rule. J Clin Oncol 1992; 10:316–322.
15. Klastersky J, Paesmans M, Rubenstein E, Boyer M, Elting L, Feld R, Gallagher J, Herrstedt J, Rapaport B Rolston K, Talcott J. The MASCC Risk Index: a multinational scoring system to predict low-risk febrile neutropenic cancer patients. J Clin Oncol 2000; 18: 3038–3051.
16. Rubenstein EB, Rolston K, Benjamin RS, Loewy J, Escalante E, Manzullo E, Hughes P, Moreland B, Fender A, Kennedy K, Holmes F, Elting L, Bodey GP. Outpatient treatment of febrile episodes in low risk neutropenic cancer patients. Cancer 1993; 71:3640–3646.
17. Mullen CA, Petropoulos D, Roberts WM, Rytting M, Ziph T, Chan KW, Culbert SJ, Danielson M, Jeha S, Kuttesch JF, Rolston K. Outpatient treatment of febrile neutropenia in low risk pediatric cancer patients. Cancer 1999; 86:126–134.
18. Malik IA, Khan WA, Karim M, Aziz Z, Khan MA. Feasibility of outpatient management of fever in cancer patients with low-risk neutropenia: results of a prospective randomized trial. Am J Med 1995; 98:224–231.
19. Rolston K. New trends in patient management: risk-based therapy for febrile patients with neutropenia. Clin Infect Dis 1999; 29:515–521.
20. Yadegarynia D, Tarrand J, Raad I, Rolston K. Current spectrum of bacterial infections in cancer patients. Clin Infect Dis 2003; 37:1144–1145.
21. Wisplinghoff H, Seifert H, Wenzel RP, Edmond MB. Current trends in the epidemiology of nosocomial bloodstream infections in patients with hematological malignancies and solid neoplasms in hospitals in the United States. Clin Infect Dis 2003; 36:1103–1110.
22. Adachi JA, Yadegarynia D, Rolston K. Spectrum of polymicrobial bacterial infection in patients with cancer, 1975–2002 (abstr 4). American Society for Microbiology. Polymicrobial Diseases, Lake Tahoe, NV, Oct 19–23, 2003.
23. Pulimood S, Ganesan L, Alangaden G, Chandrasekar P. Polymicrobial candidemia. Diagn Microbiol Infect Dis 2002; 44:353–357.
24. Gomez L, Martino R, Rolston KV. Neutropenic enterocolitis: spectrum of the disease and comparison of definite and possible cases. Clin Infect Dis 1998; 27: 695–699.
25. Rolston KVI, Bodey GP. Diagnosis and management of perianal and perirectal infection in the granulocytopenic patient. In: Remington J, Swartz MN, eds. Current Clinical Topics in Infectious Diseases. Boston: Blackwell Scientific Publications, 1993:164–171.
26. Elting LS, Rubenstein EB, Rolston KVI, Bodey GP. Outcomes of bacteremia in patients with cancer and neutropenia; observations from two decades of epidemiological and clinical trials. Clin Infect Dis 1997; 25:247–259.
27. Rolston KVI. Infections in patients with solid tumors. In: Glauser MP, Pizzo PA, eds. Management of Infections in Immunocompromised Patients. London: W.B. Saunders Company Ltd., , 2000:117–140.
28. Phaller MA, Jones RN, Doern GV, Sader HS, Messer SA, Houston A, Coffman S, Hollis RJ. The Sentry Participant Group. Bloodstream infections due to *Candida* species: SENTRY Antimicrobial Surveillance Program in North America and Latin America, 1997–1998. Antimicrob Agents Chemother 2000; 44:747–751.
29. National Nosocomial Infectious Surveillance (NNIS) System Report, data summary from January 1990–May 1999, issued June 1999, 1999; 27:520–532.
30. Viscoli C, Girmenia C, Marinus A, Collette L, Martino P, Vandercam B, Doyen C, Lebeau B, Spence D, Krcmery V, De Pauw B, Meunier F. Candidemia in cancer patients: a prospective, multicenter surveillance study by the Invasive Fungal Infection Group (IFIG) of the European Organization for Research and Treatment of Cancer (EORTC). Clin Infect Dis 1999; 28:1071–1079.
31. Mullen CA, Abd El-Baki H, Samir H, Tarrand JJ, Rolston KV. Non-albicans *Candida* is the most common cause of candidemia in pediatric cancer patients. Support Care Cancer 2003; 11:321–325.
32. Raad II. Intravascular-catheter-related infections. Lancet 1998; 351:893–898.
33. Raad II, Hanna HA. Intravascular catheter-related infections. Arch Intern Med 2002; 162:871–878.
34. Update of recommendations for the use of hematopoietic colony-stimulating factors: evidence-based clinical practice guidelines. J Clin Oncol 1996; 14:1957–1960.
35. Hubel K, Dale DC, Engert A, Liles WC. Current status of granulocyte (neutrophil) transfusion therapy for infectious diseases. J Infect Dis 2001; 183:321–328.
36. Bernard GR, Vincent JL, Laterre PF, LaRosa SP, Dhainaut JF, Lopez-Rodriguez A, Steingrub JS, Garber GE, Helterbrand JD, Ely EW, Fisher CJ Jr. Recombinant human protein C Worldwide Evaluation in Severe Sepsis (PROWESS) Study Group. Efficacy and safety of recombinant human activated protein C for severe sepsis. N Engl J Med 2001; 344:699–709.
37. Centers for Disease Control (CDC). Twelve steps to prevent antimicrobial resistance among hospitalized adults. Available at http://www.cdc.gov/ drugresistance/healthcare/ha/12steps.HA.htm. Accessed August 12, 2003.

36

Acute Coronary Syndrome in Cancer Patients

S. WAMIQUE YUSUF and EDWARD T. H. YEH
Department of Cardiology, The University of Texas M.D. Anderson Cancer Center, Houston, Texas, U.S.A.

I. INTRODUCTION/BACKGROUND

About 150 years ago, Virchow postulated that three features predispose to thrombus formation, namely abnormalities in blood constituent, vessel wall, and blood flow. Although originally Virchow was referring to venous thrombosis, the concepts hold true to arterial thrombosis as well. A number of patients with cancer show abnormalities in each component of Virchow's triad leading to a prothrombotic or hypercoagulable state (1), with consequent vascular disorders ranging from venous and arterial thrombosis to myocardial infarction. The understanding of atherosclerosis and subsequent coronary ischemia has evolved over the years. Hyperlipidemia has traditionally been implicated in the pathogenesis of coronary atheroma, but cholesterol deposits in the arterial wall do not fully explain all the feature of proliferation of smooth muscle cells (2). Inflammation is a key factor in the development of cardiovascular disease (2), and atherogenesis is increasingly being recognized as an inflammatory disease (2,3). There is evidence that the entry of inflammatory cells such as monocytes into the arterial wall plays a pivotal role in this disease (3,4). Any inflammatory stimulus, such as oxidized LDL or infection, alters the endothelial lining of the artery to make it "sticky" through the expression of adhesion molecules (such as vascular cell adhesion molecule-1 and inter-cellular adhesion molecule-1) and the secretion of chemokines (such as monocyte chemo attractant protein-1) on the luminal surface. The sticky endothelium attracts or captures circulating monocytes or other inflammatory cells onto the arterial surface. Once monocytes are arrested on the surface of the endothelium, they travel across the junction between two endothelial cells and become tissue macrophages, which can ingest lipid deposits to form foam cells. With the continuous entry of monocots into the arterial wall, the lesion develops from the initial fatty streak to the more advanced fibrous plaque (2). Coronary artery disease (CAD) in patients with malignancy is multifactorial in nature. In addition to athersoclerosis, thrombosis, endothelial damage, and chemotherapy, it is known that in a number of patients without traditional risk factors for CAD, radiotherapy (XRT) contributes to the causation of CAD (5). The precise mechanism responsible for radiation-induced CAD is not clearly defined but is thought to relate to damage to the vascular endothelium leading to significant fibrosis (6,7). Radiation itself can cause medial degeneration in the coronary arteries, but cholesterol feeding of the animals markedly increased the degree of atherosclerosis in the rabbits (8). These findings suggest that the combined effect of irradiation and some other risk factors are necessary to produce significant radiation-induced atherosclerosis. Various chemotherapeutic agents, notably 5-flurouracil (and its analogue capecitabine), cisplastin, vinblastin, bleomycin, and cyclophosphamide, are associated with cardiotoxicity including coronary spasm, acute vascular toxicity, reversible cardiomyopathy, thromboembolism, prinzmetal angina, and myocardial infarction (MI) (9–14). The etiological mechanism behind these vascular events may be due to activation of clotting factors following disturbances of microcirculation caused by the release of toxic substance from necrotic tissue and or malignant cells (15). Patients with bone marrow transplant (BMT) are known to develop syndrome X with insulin resistance, hyperinsulinemia, and metabolic disturbance (16). This may predispose these patients to early coronary atherosclerosis. One report found gynecological cancer to be one of many coronary risk factors (17), and now there is increasing awareness that cancer cells are involved not only in activating the blood coagulation but also causing injury to endothelial lining of blood vessels and activation of platelets. Coronary atherosclerotic disease is the underlying substrate in nearly all patients with acute myocardial infarction (AMI). The initiating lesion is a fissure in the vessel wall, which results as a loss in the integrity of the plaque cap. The fissure or even frank plaque rupture leads to exposure of subendothelial matrix elements such as collagen, stimulating platelet activation, and thrombus formation. Tissue factor is released which directly activates the coagulation cascade and promotes the formation of fibrin. If an occlusive thrombus forms, patient may develop an acute ST segment elevation MI, unless the subtended myocardium is richly collateralized. On the other hand if the thrombus formation is not occlusive, the patient may develop unstable angina or nonspecific ST changes on the electrocardiogram (ECG) (ST depression or T wave changes). The most common cause of unstable angina and non-ST elevation myocardial infarction (NSTEM1) is due to coronary artery narrowing caused by a thrombus that develops on a disrupted atherosclerotic plaque and is usually non-occlusive (18). A less common cause is intense vasospasm of a coronary artery (prinzmetal angina). This intense vasospasm is caused by vascular smooth muscle or by endothelial dysfunction (18). Plaque that, rupture or fissure, tends to have a thin fibrous cap, a high lipid content, few smooth muscle cells, and a high proportion of macrophages and monocytes (4,19). All AMI is not necessarily due to plaque rupture or a fissure event. A myocardial supply and demand mismatch can be invoked as a cause of infarct in a small subset of patients, as may occur in the peri-operative setting. Arterial inflammation, caused by or related to infection, may cause plaque destabilization and rupture and precipitate acute coronary syndrome (ACS). Activated macrophages and T lymphocytes located at the shoulder of a plaque increase the expression of enzymes like metalloproteinases that may cause thinning and disruption of plaque leading to ACS (18). Other factors, which are extrinsic to coronary artery bed, may precipitate ACS. These include: (1) increased myocardial oxygen requirements such as fever, tachycardiar, and thyrotoxicosis; (2) reduce coronary blood flow e.g., hypotension; and (3) reduce myocardial oxygen delivery such as anemia or hypoxemia. One of the common and challenging clinical manifestations of cardiovascular disease in cancer patient is ACS.

II. ACUTE CORONARY SYNDROME

The ACS is an abbreviation that encompasses any clinical symptoms that are compatible with acute myocardial ischemia. It includes: acute myocardial infarction (ST elevation and Non-ST elevation) as well as unstable angina. The emphasis is for early diagnosis and management of these patients. Patients who are considered to have ACS should be placed in an environment with continuous ECG monitoring and defibrillation capability, where a 12 lead ECG can be taken expeditiously and definitely interpreted within 10 min (18). The most urgent priority for early evaluation is to identify patients with AMI who are candidates for reperfusion therapy and to recognize other potentially catastrophic causes of similar presentation like aortic dissection.

III. ETIOLOGY OF ACS IN CANCER PATIENTS

Coronary atherosclerotic disease is the underlying substrate in majority of the patients. In the remainder of patients, besides radiation-induced CAD, various chemotherapeutic agents (9,20,21), coronary embolization due to papillary fibroelastomas (22), and atrial myxomas (23–25) can present with ACS. Malignancy involving the heart can present with symptoms and ECG findings of AMI (26) and papillary fibroelastoma is known to cause sudden cardiac death (27). In patients with acute leukemia, occurrence of AMI and various ECG changes could be due to leukemic infiltration into the myocardium or pericardium, effects of antileukemic therapy such as chemotherapy or radiation therapy, occlusion of a major coronary artery by leukemic infiltrate, secondary disorders of coagulation caused by leukemic process, with embolization in a hypercoagulable state or hemorrhages in the myocardium or intima of a coronary artery in association with disseminated intravascular coagulation, thrombocytopenia, or hyperfibrinolysis. Platelets are integral part of thrombosis in ACS, but thrombocytopenia per se does not prevent from occurrence of ACS in patients who have thrombocytopenia (28–30). In patients with idiopathic thrombocytopenic purpura (ITP), infusion of intravenous immunoglobin has been reported to cause ACS (31). Thus most patients with malignancy have underlying atherosclerosis but some patients have unusual pathology for ACS and the presence of hematological abnormalities and metastasis creates a diagnostic and therapeutic dilemma (Table 1).

IV. PRESENTATION

Most patients present with chest pain, although women, diabetics, and elderly may present with atypical symptoms (18). Clinically patients with malignancy, most commonly present with angina or myocardial infarction, however there are reports of coronary spasm and sudden death in patients previously treated with radiotherapy (5). Sudden death in these patients is thought either due to diffuse fibrointimal hyperplasia of coronary vessels or left main stenosis and ostial lesions (5,7).

V. RISK STRATIFICATION

Patients can be risk stratified, based on symptoms, examination, ECG, and cardiac markers. Presence of any of these features, such as chest or left arm pain as chief symptom reproducing prior angina, known CAD, transient mitral regurgitation, hypotension, pulmonary edema, rales, ECG changes, and elevated cardiac markers puts the patient at high likelihood that symptoms and signs represent ACS (18). Similarly history, character of pain, clinical findings, ECG changes, and cardiac markers can identify a group of patients with unstable angina who are at high risk of death or nonfatal myocardial infarction (18).

Table 1 Etiology of CAD in Cancer Patients

1. Coronary atherosclerosis
2. Cardiac metastasis
   Coronary tumor embolization
   Coronary compression
   Coronary ostial lesion
3. Tumor-related coagulation disorder (especially in patients with leukemia)
   Coronary embolization from tumor or nonbacterial endocarditis
   Coronary thrombosis from dessiminated intravascular coagulation
4. Antitumor therapy
   Radiation
   Chemotherapy
5. Infection and inflammation

VI. EXAMINATION

The major objective in physical examination is to exclude other potentially catastrophic conditions with similar presentation like aortic dissection and to identify the precipitating cause of myocardial ischemia, like pneumonia, hypoxia, fever, anemia, tachycardia, uncontrolled hypertension or thyrotoxicosis, and other comorbid conditions such as pulmonary disease. Frequently, except for the presence of tachycardia and fourth heart sound, the examination in these patients may be unremarkable. Careful evaluation for acute mitral regurgitation, and LV dysfunction (rales, S3 gallop) should be done, for such patients are at a higher likelihood of severe underlying CAD and are at higher risk for poor outcome. Presence of bruits, pulse deficit that suggests extra cardiac vascular disease, identifies patients with higher likelihood of significant CAD. Physical examination is critical in making important alternative diagnosis in patients with chest pain. Aortic dissection is suggested by pain in the back, unequal pulses, or murmur of aortic regurgitation. Acute pericarditis is suggested by pericardial friction rub, and cardiac tamponade may be evidenced by pulsus paradox. Pneumothorax, if large, will lead to tracheal deviation, hyperesonnace, and decreased air entry.

VII. INVESTIGATIONS

A. Biochemical Cardiac Markers

1. Myoglobin

Myoglobin is a low molecular heme protein found in both cardiac and skeletal muscle and is not cardiac specific. It may be detected as early as 2 hr after the onset on AMI and remains elevated for less than 24 hr. It lacks cardiac specificity, but because of its high sensitivity, a negative test for myoglobin when blood is sampled within first 4–8 hr onset is useful in ruling out AMI (Table 2) (18).

2. CK-MB

The earliest marker of myocardial necrosis, myoglobin, is sensitive but lacks specificity. Later appearing markers like CK-MB isoform is useful for the extremely early diagnosis (less than 4 hr). However, its disadvantage is its loss of specificity in the setting of skeletal muscle disease or injury including surgery. It has also low sensitivity

Table 2 Serum Markers of Acute Myocardial Infarction

	Myoglobin	cTnI	cTnT	CK-MB	MB-isoforms
First detectable (hr)	1–2	2–4	2–4	3–4	2–4
Peak (hr)	4–8	10–24	10–24	10–24	6–12
Duration (days)	0.5–1.0	5–10	5–14	2–4	0.5–1.0

cTnI indicates troponin I; cTnT indicates troponin T.
Source: From Ref. 32.

during early (<6 after symptoms onset) or later after symptom onset (>36 hr and for minor damage) (18).

3. *Troponins*

Both TnT and TnI are more specific but have lower sensitivity for the very early detection of myocardial necrosis (e.g., <6 hr) after symptoms onset. If the early (less than 6 hr) troponin test is normal, then a measurement should be repeated after 8–12 hr after symptoms onset (18). It remains elevated in the serum up to 10–14 days after release. Thus, if a patient who had an AMI several days earlier presents with recurrent ischemic chest discomfort, a single, slightly elevated cardiac troponin level may represent either old or new myocardial damage. Serum myoglobin although less specific than the troponin may be helpful in this case. A negative myoglobin value suggests that the elevated troponin be related to recent (less than 10–14 days) but not AMI (18).

B. Treatment of Myocardial Infarction

In treating patients with AMI, a targeted clinical examination and a 12 lead ECG should be done within 10 min and in appropriate patients the door to needle time for thrombolysis should be <30 min (32). Once the diagnosis is established, patient should be managed upon ECG findings (Tables 3 and 4) with important difference between non-ST elevation and ST elevation MI being that the latter group should be considered for thrombolytic therapy, whereas in patients with non-ST-elevation, there is no role of thrombolytics and in some circumstance it may even be harmful (33). In patients with malignancy, other conditions with ECG changes that can be interpreted as ischemia should be excluded (Table 5).

1. *Thrombolytic Therapy*

All patients with ST elevation or presumably new LBBB who present within 12 hr of onset of symptoms in the absence of contraindications and intracranial metastasis (Table 6) should be considered for thrombolytics (32). Patients with ST segment depression should not be thrombolyzed, unless ST depression in lead V1–V4 is thought to be due to posterior myocardial infarction (32). In patients with metastasis and thrombocytopenia, the safety profile of thrombolytics is unknown and in view of the potential bleeding complication, in general, these patients should not receive thrombolytic therapy. Also, in patients with widespread metastasis and normal platelet count, the safety profile of thrombolytics is unknown, although at our institution thrombolytic therapy has been given to a similar patient without any bleeding complications.

2. *Oxygenation*

It is a routine clinical practice to administer oxygen to patients with ACS and ACLS guidelines (34)

Table 3 Treatment of ST Elevation Myocardial Infarction

General treatment measures
1. Aspirin 160–325 mg (chew and swallow)
2. Adequate analgesia: morphine 2–4 mg as needed
3. Oxygen

Specific treatment measures
1. Reperfusion therapy: goal door to needle time <30 min; door to balloon inflation 90 ± 30 min
2. Conjunctive antithrombotics: aspirin, plavix, heparin
3. Adjunctive therapies:
   Beta-blockers if eligible
   Intravenous nitroglycerin (for anti-ischemic and antihypertensive effect)
   Ace-inhibitors [especially if large or anterior MI, heart failure without hypotension (SBP > 100), previous MI]

Source: Modified from Ref. 32.

Table 4 Treatment of Non-ST Elevation Myocardial Infarction

General treatment measures
1. Bed rest and correct any underlying precipitating or contributing factors
2. Analgesia: morphine 2–4 mg IV q 1–3 hr prn (for pain and anxiety)
3. Oxygen supplement

Specific treatment measures
1. IV Nitroglycerin infusion (for anti-ischemic and antihypertensive effect)
2. Antiplatelets and antithrombin agents
   a. Aspirin 162–325 mg and/or plavix 75 mg/d (loading 300 mg) PO
   b. Lovenox (enoxaparin) 1 mg/kg subc q 12 hr for unstable angina and non-Q myocardial infarction patients
      Or
   c. IV Heparin 5,000 u bolus, followed by 800–1,000 u/h infusion
   d. Platelet glycoprotein IIb/IIIa receptor antagonists
      [a]Integrilin/eptifibatide for acute coronary syndrome (serum creatinine <2.0 mg/dL): 180 μg/kg IV bolus, then infusion of 2 μg/kg/min unto 72 hr, until discharge or CABG; for percutaneous coronary interventions: (serum creatinine <2.0 mg/dL) 180 μg/kg bolus followed by a continuous infusion of 2.0 μg/kg/min infusion unto 18–24 hr (minimum of 12 hr) and a second 180 μg/kg bolus 10 min after the first bolus. (for creatinine between 2.0–4.0 mg/dL: continuous infusion of 1.0 μg/kg/min)
      [a]Report/abciximab 0.25 μg/kg bolus, then 0.125 μg/kg/min infusion for 12 hr before and during percutaneous coronary interventions
      [a]Aggrastat/tirofiban 0.4 μg/kg/min bolus for 30 min, then 0.1 μg/kg/min infusion for unto 72 h for acute coronary synd
3. Beta-blockers: if no contraindication
      IV Atenolol (tenormin) 5 mg, repeated in 10 min prn and followed by PO 25–100 mg/day
      IV Metoprolol (lopressor) 2–5 mg q 5 min to total 15 mg total dose, and followed by PO 25–100 mg bid
      IV Esmolol, ultrashort acting, start 500 μg/kg bolus, followed by infusion of 50–200 μg/kg/min as needed
4. ACE-inhibitor (especially if large or anterior MI, heart failure without hypotension (SBP > 100), previous MI)
5. Intervention: angioplasty (PTCA) with or without stent, coronary bypass (CABG) as indicated

[a] Combination of aspirin and plavix may result in higher bleeding complications; hence, this combination should be used with caution in patients with malignancy.

recommending oxygen 4 L/min. Although experimental results indicate that breathing oxygen may limit ischemic myocardial injury (35,36), whether this therapy reduces mortality or morbidity in patients with AMI is unknown. In patients with severe congestive heart failure (CHF) and pulmonary edema, mechanical ventilation is needed and should not be delayed.

3. Antiplatelets

Aspirin in a dose of 160–325 mg should be given promptly and continued indefinitely on a daily basis thereafter (32). In patients unable to swallow or with nausea or known upper gastrointestinal disorders, aspirin suppositories (325 mg) can be used safely (32). The use of aspirin is contraindicated in active gastrointestinal ulceration, hypersensitivity to aspirin, and thrombocytopenia (37). Clopidogrel (plavix) should be given to patients who are allergic to aspirin (18). Plavix should be added to aspirin therapy in patients with unstable angina and non-ST elevation MI (18).

Table 5 Condition Associated with EGG Changes That Can Be Interpreted as Ischemia

Pericarditis
Early repolarization
Digitalis use
Intracranial pathology
Pneumothorax
Hypocalcemia
Tumor involvement of heart

4. Beta-Blockers and Ace-Inhibitors

Unless there are contraindications, most patients with AMI should receive these medications (32).

VIII. SPECIAL PROBLEMS IN CANCER PATIENTS

Management of AMI in patients with malignancy is similar to general population but with important differences. This is a group of patients, which has effectively been excluded from all trials of ACS or heart failure, making it impossible to develop an evidence-based approach to these patients. Thrombocytopenia and metastasis, which are common in patients with malignancy, prevent the use of aspirin, plavix, heparin,

Table 6 Contraindications and Cautions for Thrombolytic Therapy

Contraindications
Previous hemorrhagic stroke at any time: other strokes or cerebrovascular events within last 1 year
Known intracranial neoplasm
Active internal bleeding (does not include menses)
Suspected aortic dissection
Cautions/relative contraindications
Severe uncontrolled hypertension on presentation (BP >180/110)[a]
History of prior cerebrovascular accident or known intracerebral pathology not covered in contraindications
Current use of anticoagulants in therapeutic doses; known bleeding diathesis
Recent trauma (within 2–4 weeks), including head injury or traumatic or prolonged (>10 min) CPR or major surgery (<3 week)
Noncompressable vascular punctures
Recent (2–4 weeks) internal bleeding
For streptokinase/anistreplase:prior exposure (especially within 5 days–2 year) or prior allergic reaction
Pregnancy
Active peptic ulcer
History of chronic hypertension

[a] Severe uncontrolled hypertension: could be an absolute contraindication in low risk patients.
Source: Modified from Ref. 32.

glycoprotein 11b 111a inhibitors, and thrombolytics: a group of drugs, which form the cornerstone of management in these patients. Hence, these medications and even aspirin alone are denied to the majority of patients with thrombocytopenia who present with ACS. However, successful coronary intervention with the use of aspirin, plavix, and heparin (without any bleeding complication) has been reported in a patient with thrombocytopenia (28). Despite thrombocytopenia and treatment with both aspirin and plavix, thrombotic stent occlusion has been reported (28), suggesting that patients with malignancy, despite being thrombocytopenic, are predisposed to thrombotic vascular complications. In patients with ITP, successful percutaneous coronary intervention (29) and coronary artery bypass graft (CABG) with intra-aortic balloon pump (IABP) insertion and supportive platelet transfusion have been reported (31,38). In patients with thrombocytopenia and AMI, aspirin and plavix together (28) and aspirin alone (30) have been used without any bleeding complications. Despite thrombocytopenia, thrombus was noted on cardiac catheterization (30). For patients with XRT-induced atherosclerosis, both percutaneous intervention and CABG have been used (5). Theoretically, reocclusion could be a problem in these patients and reocclusion in both stent and bypass graft has been reported (28,39), although the exact incidence of this problem in cancer population is unknown. In these patients because of mediastinal fibrosis, surgical intervention and CABG may be associated with higher incidence of complications (5). Also XRT-induced involvement of mammary arteries may prevent usage of this for arterial conduits (40). Concomitant carotid atherosclerosis, which is known to be associated with XRT therapy (41), potentially puts these patients at higher risk for peri-operative complications.

IX. COMPLICATIONS OF MYOCARDIAL INFARCTION

A. Arrhythmias

1. *Atrial Fibrillation*

Atrial fibrillation (AF) associated with AMI often occurs within the first 24 hr and is usually transient. Reperfusion therapy has decreased the incidence of this arrhythmia, which carries an independent prognostic value (42). The occurrence of AF is associated with excess sympathetic activity, hypokalemia, hypomagnesaemia, and hypoxia, underlying chronic lung disease and ischemia of sinus node or left atrial circumflex arteries.

2. *Treatment*

When hemodynamic compromise occurs, immediate cardio version is indicated, beginning with 100 J, then 200, then 300 J, then 360 J, if lower energies fail (32,34). In the absence of CHF or severe pulmonary disease, one of the most effective means of slowing the ventricular rate in AF is the use of intravenous beta-adrenoceptor blocking agents such as atenolol (2.5–5.0 mg over 2 min to a total of 10 mg in 10–15 min) or metoprolol (2.5–5.0 mg every 2–5 min to a total of 15 mg over 10–15 min). Heart rate, blood pressure, and the ECG should be monitored, and treatment should be halted when therapeutic efficacy is achieved or if systolic blood pressure falls below 100 mmHg or heart rate below 50 bpm during treatment (32). Intravenous digoxin can also be used to slow the heart rate (32). Diltiazem and verapamil can also be used, but because of their negative inotropic effect and concerns regarding the use of calcium channel blockers in AMI, these agents are not recommended as first line drugs, despite their effectiveness in slowing the heart rate (32). Heparin therapy should be given to all patients with AF (32). Transient AF does not obligate the patient to receive long-term anticoagulation or antiarrhythmic agents, but if such treatment is elected, it is appropriate to limit their use to 6 weeks if sinus rhythm has been restored (32).

X. VENTRICULAR FIBRILLATION

Primary ventricular fibrillation (VF) remains an important contributor to risk of mortality during the first 24 hr after AMI. Primary VF should be distinguished from secondary VF, which occurs in the presence of severe CHF or cardiogenic shock. Late VF develops more than 48 hr after onset of infarction. The incidence of primary VF is highest (around 3–5%) in the first 4 hr after MI and declines markedly thereafter (43). Contrary to prior belief, primary VF appears to be associated with a significantly higher in-hospital mortality, but those persons who survive to hospital discharge have the same long-term prognosis as patients who do not experience primary VF (44).

XI. PROPHYLAXIS

With the exception of beta-blockers, no other medications are recommended or have proved useful in prevention of VF after AMI. Traditionally, lidocaine was used for prophylaxis of VF in patients with MI, but a meta-analysis of randomized trials of prophylaxis with lidocaine has shown a reduction in the incidence of primary VF by about 33%, but this was offset by a trend toward increased mortality, probably from fatal episodes of bradycardia and asystole (45). Routine administration of intravenous beta-adrenoceptor blockers to patients without hemodynamic or electrical (AV block) contraindications is associated with a reduction in incidence of early VF. Intravenous followed by oral beta-adrenoceptor blockers should be given in the absence of contraindications. Suitable regimens include intravenous metoprolol (5 mg every 2 min for 3 doses, if tolerated, followed by 50 mg orally twice a day for at least 24 hr and then increased to 100 mg twice a day). An alternative regimen is atenolol (5–10 mg intravenously followed by 100 mg orally on a daily basis). The association of VF and hypokalemia is neither sensitive nor specific, but in one study the risk of VF was 8% in patients with admission potassium of <3 mmol/L and 0.9% in patients with potassium of >4 mmol/L (46). Of the 25 patients with low potassium (<3 mmol/L), only two developed VF, the others had an uncomplicated course (46). Both hypokalemia and hypomagnesaemia may act as arrythmogenic risk factor, and although randomized clinical trial data do not exist to confirm the benefits of repletion of potassium and magnesium deficits in preventing VF, it is a sound clinical practice to maintain serum potassium levels at greater than 4.0 mEq/L and magnesium levels at greater than 2.0 mEq/L in patients with AMI.

XII. TREATMENT

The VF should be treated with an unsynchronized electric shock using an initial energy of 200 J. If this is unsuccessful, a second shock using 200–300 J and, if necessary, a third shock using 360 J are indicated (34). The VF that is not easily converted by defibrillation may be treated with additional adjunctive measures. Epinephrine 1 mg intravenously should be given and repeated every 3–5 min or vasopressin 40 units intravenous as a single dose should be given (34). For persistent and recurrent VF and ventricular tachycardia (VT), amiodarone in a dose of 300 mg intravenously can be given (34). If pulseless VT/VF recurs, then consider administration of a second dose of 150 mg intravenously (34). There are no firm data to help define an optimal management strategy for prevention of recurrent VF in patients who have sustained an initial episode of VF in the setting of AMI. It seems prudent to correct any electrolyte and acid–base disturbances and administer beta-adrenoceptor-blocking agents to inhibit increased sympathetic activity and prevent ischemia (34).

XIII. VENTRICULAR TACHYCARDIA

Several definitions have been used for VT in the setting of AMI. Nonsustained VT lasts less than 30 sec, whereas sustained VT lasts more than 30 sec and/or causes earlier hemodynamic compromise requiring immediate intervention. Based on electrocardiographic appearance, VT has also been categorized as monomorphic or polymorphic. While short bursts (fewer than 5 beats) of nonsustained VT of either monomorphic or polymorphic configuration may be seen frequently, contemporary epidemiological data do not suggest that they are associated with a sufficiently increased risk of sustained VT or VF to warrant a recommendation of prophylactic therapy (32). In patients with recent AMI and left ventricular dysfunction, the tendency to suppress PVCs with certain medications like encainide and flecainide may be associated with an increased mortality (47). The vast majority of post-MI VT and VF occur within the first 48 hr of MI. Sustained VT or VF occurring outside of this time frame deserves careful evaluation, including consideration of electrophysiology studies.

XIV. MANAGEMENT STRATEGIES FOR VENTRICULAR TACHYCARDIA

Rapid polymorphic-appearing VT should be considered similar to VF and managed with an unsynchronized discharge of 200 J, while monomorphic VT with rates greater than 150 bpm can usually be treated with a 100-J synchronized discharge (34). Episodes of sustained VT that are somewhat better tolerated hemodynamically may initially be treated with one of the following drug regimens: (1) amiodarone: 150 mg infused over 10 min followed by a constant infusion of 1.0 mg/min for 6 hr and then a maintenance infusion at 0.5 mg/min; (2) lidocaine: bolus 1.0–1.5 mg/kg. Supplemental boluses of 0.5–0.75 mg/kg every 5–10 min to a maximum of 3 mg/kg total loading dose may be given as needed. Loading is followed by infusion of 2–4 mg/min (30–50 µg/kg/min). In older patients and those with CHF or hepatic dysfunction, infusion rates should be reduced to avoid lidocaine toxicity; (3) procainamide: 20–30 mg/min loading infusion, up to 12–17 mg/kg. This may be followed by an infusion of 1–4 mg/min. Infusion rates should be lower in the presence of renal dysfunction. Rare episodes of drug-refractory-sustained polymorphic VT ("electrical storm") have been reported in cases of AMI. Anecdotal evidence suggests that these may be related to uncontrolled ischemia and increased sympathetic tone and are best treated by intravenous beta-adrenoceptor blockade (48), intravenous amiodarone (49), IABP, or emergency revascularization (32). Ventricular tachyarrhythmia is not an indication for emergency CABG, except in rare circumstances when refractory ventricular tachyarrhythmia is thought to be due to ischemia (32). The IABP support can be used for intractable ventricular arrythmia with hemodynmic instability (32).

XV. HEART FAILURE AND LOW-OUTPUT SYNDROMES

A. Left Ventricular Dysfunction

Pump failure due to AMI is manifested clinically by a weak pulse, poor peripheral perfusion with cool and cyanotic limbs, obtundation, and oliguria. Blood pressure is usually low, and there are variable degrees of pulmonary congestion. A third heart sound may be audible. The treatment of left ventricle (LV) dysfunction is determined by the specific hemodynamic derangements that are present, most importantly (1) pulmonary capillary wedge pressure (PAWP), (2) cardiac output (measured with a balloon flotation catheter), and (3) systemic arterial pressure (preferably measured with an intra-arterial cannula). Patients with adequate systolic blood pressure (SBP >100 mm Hg), modest elevation in PAWP (>18 mm Hg) and preserved cardiac output can be managed with (1) modest diuresis (best accomplished with intravenous frusemide) in combination with (2) after load and preload reduction, using nitroglycerin. Nitroglycerin offers a greater degree of venodilation than sodium nitroprusside and relieves ischemia by dilating epicardial coronary arteries. In the early hours of acute infarction, when ischemia often contributes substantially to LV dysfunction, nitroglycerin is the more appropriate agent. Its intravenous infusion should be initiated at 5 µg/min and increased gradually until mean systolic arterial pressure falls by 10–15% but not below 90 mm Hg. The institution of ACE-inhibitor therapy is also appropriate in this setting. The patient with more severe LV dysfunction has a depressed cardiac output, an abnormally high left-sided filling pressure, and systolic arterial pressure less than 90 mm Hg; this patient has, or is rapidly approaching, cardiogenic shock. If the patient is markedly hypotensive, intravenous norepinephrine should be administered until systolic arterial pressure rises to at least 80 mm Hg, at which time a change to dopamine may be attempted, beginning at 5–15 µg/kg/min. Once arterial pressure is brought to at least 90 mm Hg, intravenous dobutamine may be given simultaneously in an attempt to reduce the magnitude of the dopamine infusion. In addition, consideration should be given to initiating intra-aortic balloon counterpulsation. Mechanical reperfusion by PTCA or CABG of occluded coronary arteries may improve survival in patients with AMI and cardiogenic shock (50).

B. Right Ventricular Infarction and Dysfunction

Right ventricular (RV) infarction encompasses a spectrum of disease states ranging from asymptomatic mild RV dysfunction through cardiogenic shock.

1. Clinical Diagnosis

Evidence of RV ischemia should be sought in all patients with acute inferior MI. The clinical triad of hypotension, clear lung fields, and elevated jugular venous pressure in the setting of an inferior MI is characteristic of RV ischemia. Although specific, this triad has a sensitivity of less than 25% (51). Distended neck veins alone or the presence of Kussmaul's sign (distention of the jugular vein on inspiration) is both sensitive and specific for RV ischemia in patients with an inferior AMI (52). These findings may be masked in the setting of volume depletion and may only become evident after adequate volume loading. A right atrial pressure of 10 mmHg or greater and greater than 80% of pulmonary wedge pressure is a relatively sensitive and specific finding in patients with RV ischemia (53). Demonstration of 1 mm ST-segment elevation in the right precordial lead V_{4R} is the single most predictive electrocardiographic finding in patients with RV ischemia (54). Echocardiography can be helpful in patients with suspicious but nondiagnostic findings as it may show regional wall motion abnormalities and RV involment. The RV infarct besides causing RV dilation and asynergy can also lead to right-to-left shunting through a patent foramen ovale (55). This latter finding should be suspected when persistent hypoxia in this setting is not responsive to supplemental oxygen (55).

Table 7 Treatment of Right Ventricular Infarct

Maintenance of right ventricular preload
Volume loading (intravenous normal saline)
Avoidance of nitrates, diuretics, and morphine
Maintenance of AV synchrony
AV sequential pacing for complete heart block
Prompt cardioversion for atria fibrillation
Inotropic support
Dobutamine
Reduction of right ventricular afterload (in the presense of LV dysfunction)
IABP
Vasodilators (sodium nitroprusside)
Reperfusion
Thrombolytics
Direct angioplasty

Source: Modified from Ref. 32.

XVI. MANAGEMENT OF RIGHT VENTRICULAR ISCHEMIA/INFARCTION

Treatment of RV infarction (Table 7) includes early maintenance of RV preload, reduction of RV after load, inotropic support of the dysfunctional right ventricle, and early reperfusion. Because of their influence on preload, drugs routinely used in management of LV infarction, such as nitrates and diuretics, may reduce cardiac output and produce severe hypotension when the right ventricle is ischemic. Indeed, a common clinical presentation for RV infarction is profound hypotension following administration of sublingual nitroglycerin, with the degree of hypotension often out of proportion to the electrocardiographic severity of the infarct. Volume loading with normal saline alone often resolves accompanying hypotension and improves cardiac output (56). Although volume loading is a critical first step in the management of hypotension associated with RV ischemia, inotropic support (in particular, dobutamine) should be initiated promptly if cardiac output fails to improve after 0.5–1 L of fluid has been given. Another important factor for sustaining adequate RV preload is maintenance of atrioventricular (AV) synchrony. High-degree heart block is common, occurring in as many as half of these patients (57). The AV sequential pacing leads to a significant increase in cardiac output and reversal of shock, even when ventricular pacing alone has not been of benefit (58). The AF may occur in up to one-third of patients with RV ischemia (59) and has profound hemodynamic effects. Prompt cardioversion from AF should be considered at the earliest sign of hemodynamic compromise. When LV dysfunction accompanies RV ischemia, the right ventricle is further compromised because of increased RV afterload and reduction in stroke volume (60). In such circumstances, the use of afterload-reducing agents such as sodium nitroprusside or an intra-aortic counterpulsation device is often necessary to "unload" the left and subsequently the right ventricle. In patients with RV infarct, successful reperfusion leads to an improvement in RV ejection fraction and reduces the incidence of complete heart block (61,62). Prognosis RV involment in patients with acute inferior MI is an independent predictor of prognosis (63) with an in-hospital mortality of 31% compared only 6% with inferior infarct and no RV involvement (63).

XVII. MECHANICAL DEFECTS AFTER ACUTE MYOCARDIAL INFARCTION

Mechanical defects can occur after AMI and include acute mitral valve regurgitation, post infarction ventricular septal defect (VSD), LV free wall rupture, and LV aneurysm. Sudden and/or progressive hemodynamic deterioration with low cardiac output and/or pulmonary edema should lead to prompt consideration of these defects and rapid institution of diagnostic and therapeutic measures. These defects, when they occur, usually present within the first week after AMI. On physical examination, the presence of a new cardiac murmur indicates the possibility of either VSD, mitral regurgitation, or, occasionally, ventricular rupture. A precise diagnosis can usually be established with transthoracic or transesophageal echocardiography. Use of a balloon flotation catheter is helpful for both diagnosis and monitoring of therapy. With a VSD and left-to-right shunting, oxygen saturation will be higher in the pulmonary artery compared with the right atrium; in this instance, thermodilution cardiac output and pulmonary artery samples for mixed venous oxygen saturation will be falsely elevated. With acute mitral regurgitation, a large V wave may be evident on the pulmonary artery wedge pressure tracing. With ventricular rupture and pericardial tamponade, equalization of diastolic pressure may be seen. In general, prompt surgical repair is indicated. Although there is a need to minimize invasive angiographic procedures before early surgical correction of the ruptured septum, initial coronary arteriography to assess the coronary anatomy seems warranted in most cases. Insertion of an IABP can help stabilize the patient. Surgical consultation should be obtained when a mechanical defect is suspected for medical treatment alone is associated with extremely high mortality. Occassionally, incomplete rupture of heart may lead to a pseudoaneurysm formation, which should also be treated surgically.

REFERENCES

1. Lip GYH, Chin BSP, Blann AD. Cancer and prothrombotic state. Lancet Oncol 2002; 3:27–34.
2. Yeh ETH, Anderson HV, Pasceri V, Willerson JT. C-Reactive protein. Linking inflammation to cardiovascular complications. Circulation 2001; 104:974–975.
3. Ross R. Atherosclerosis: an inflammatory disease. N Engl J Med 1999; 340:115–126.
4. Libby P. Molecular bases of the acute coronary syndromes. Circulation 1995; 91:2844–2850.
5. Oran F, Brusca A, Conte MR, Presbitero P, Figliomeni MC. Severe coronary artery disease after radiation therapy of chest and mediastinum: clinical presentation and treatment. Br Heart J 1993; 69:496–500.
6. Om A, Ellahham S, Vetrovec GW. Radiation induced coronary artery disease. Am Heart J 1992; 124:1598–1602.
7. Brosius FC, Waller BF, Roberts WC. Radiation induced analysis of the 16 young (aged 15–33 years) necropsy patients who received over 3500 rads to the heart. Am J Med 1981; 70:519–530.
8. Amromin GD, Gilden horn HL, Solomon RD, Nadkarni BB, Jacobs ML. The synergism of x-irradiation and cholesterol fat feeding on the development of coronary artery lesions. J Atheroscler Res 1964; 4: 325–334.
9. Lestuzzi C, Viel E, Picano E, Meneguzzo N. Coronary vasospasm as a cause of effort related myocardial ischemia during low dose chronic continuous infusion of 5-Fluorouracil. Am J Med 2001; 111:316–318.
10. Schwarzer S, Eber B, Greinix H, Lind P. Non-Q-wave myocardial infarction associated with bleomycin and etoposide chemotherapy. Eur Heart J 1991; 12:748–750.
11. Stefenelli T, Kuzmuts R, Ulrich W, Glogar D. Acute toxicity after combination chemotherapy with cisplastin, vinblastine and bleomycin for testicular cancer. Eur Heart J 1988; 9:552–556.
12. Steffenelli T, Zielinski C, Mayr W, Scoheithauer W. Prinzmetal angina during cyclophosphamide therapy. Eur Heart J 1988; 9:1155–1157.
13. Cheriparambil KM, Vasireddy H, Kuruvilla A, Gambarin B, Makan M, Saul BI. Acute reversible cardiomyopthy and thromboembolism after cisplastin and 5-FU chemotherapy. Angiology 2000; 51:873–878.
14. Frickhofen N, Bck FJ, Jung B, Fuhr HG, Andrasch H, Sigmund M. Capecitabine can induce acute coronary syndrome similar to 5-Fluouracil. Ann Oncol 2002; 13:797–801.
15. Gordon SG, Franks JJ, Lewis FB. Cancer procoagulant A, a factor X activating procoagulant from malignant tissue. Thrombos Res 1975; 6:127–132.
16. Taskinen M, Saarinen-Pihkala UM, Hovi L, Lipsanen-Nyman M. Impaired glucose tolerance and dyslipidemia as late effects after bone marrow transplantation in childhood. Lancet 2000; 356:993–997.
17. Thompson SG, Greenberg G, Meade TW. Risk factors for stroke and myocardial infarction in women in the United Kingdom as assessed in general practice: a case control study. Br Heart J 1989; 61:403–409.
18. Braunwald E, Antman EM, Beasley JW, Califf RM, Chetlin MD, Hochman JS, Jones RH, Kereiakas D, Kupersmith J, Levin TN, Pepine CJ, Schaeffer JW, Smith EE III, Steward DE, Theroux P. ACC/AHA 2002 guideline update for the management of patients with unstable angina and non-ST segment elevation/ myocardial infarction. A report of the American College of Cardiology/American Heart Association task force on Practice guidelines (Committee on the management of patients with unstable angina). J Am Coll Cardiol 2002; Available at www.acc.org.
19. Moreno PR, Bernadi VH, Palacios IF, Newell JB, Fuster V, Fallon JT. Macrophage infiltration in acute coronary syndromes. Implications for plaque rupture. Circulation 1994; 90:775–778.
20. Schwarzer S, Eber B, Greinix H, Lind P. Non-Q-wave myocardial infarction associated with bleomycin and etoposide chemotherapy. Eur Heart J 1991; 12: 748–750.
21. Frickhofen N, Bck FJ, Jung B, Fuhr HG, Andrasch H, Sigmund M. Capecitabine can induce acute coronary syndrome similar to 5-Fluouracil. Ann Oncol 2002; 13:797–801.
22. Takada A, Saito K, Ro A, Tokudome S, Murai T. Papillary fibroelastoma of the aortic valve: a sudden

death case of coronary embolism with myocardial infarction. Forensic Sci Int 2000; 113:209–214.
23. Abascal V, Kasznica J, Aldea G, Davidoff R. Left atrial myxoma and acute myocardial infarction, a diagnosis duo in the thrombolytic therapy. Chest 1996; 109(4): 1106–1108.
24. Panos A, Kalangos A, Sztajzel J. Left atrial myxoma presenting with acute myocardial infarction. Case report and review of literature. Int J Cardiol 1997; 62:73–75.
25. Denniston AKO, Beattie JM. An unusual case of multiple infarcts. Postgrad Med J 2002; 78:431.
26. Daher IN, Luh JY, Duarte AG. Squamous cell lung cancer simulating an acute myocardial infarction. Chest 2003; 123:304–306.
27. Takada A, Saito K, Ro A, Tokudome S, Murai T. Papillary fibroelastoma of the aortic valve: a sudden death case of coronary embolism with myocardial infarction. Forensic Sci Int 2000; 113:209–214.
28. Jachmann-Jahn U, Cornel OA, Lauds U, Hop HW, Meuthen I, Krakau M, O'Brien B. Acute anterior myocardial infarction as first manifestation of acute myeloid leukemia. Ann Hematol 2001; 80:677–681.
29. Fuchi T, Kondo T, Sase K, Takahashi M. Primary percutaneous transluminal coronary angioplasty for acute myocardial infarction in a patient with idiopathic thrombocytopenic purpura. Jpn Circ J 1999; 63: 133–136.
30. Pervez H, Potti A, Mehdi SA. Simultaneous presentation of acute mylengenous leukemia and acute myocardial infarction. J Clin Oncol 2003; 21(7):1416–1421.
31. Crouch ED, Watson LE. Intravenous immunoglobulin related acute coronary syndrome and coronary angiography in idiopathic thrombocytopenic purpura. Angiology 2002; 53:113–117.
32. Ryan TG, Antman EM, Brooks NH, Califf RM, Hillis LD, Hiratzka LF, Rapaport E, Riegel B, Russell RO, Smith E III, Weaver WD. ACC/AHA guidelines for the management of acute myocardial infarction: 1999 update: a report of the American College of Cardiology/American Heart Association Task force on Practice guidelines (Committee on the Management of acute myocardial infarction). J Am Coll Cardiol 1999; Available at www.acc.org.
33. Fibrinloytic therapy trialists (FTT) collaborative group. Indications for thrombolytic therapy in acute myocardial infarction. Collaborative overview of early mortality and major morbidity result from all randomized trails of more than 1000 patients. Lancet 1994; 343: 311–322.
34. ACLS Provider Manual. American Heart Association, 2001.
35. Moroko PR, Radvany P, Braunwald E, Hale S. Reduction of infarct size by oxygen inhalation following acute coronary occlusion. Circulation 1975; 52:360–368.
36. Madias JE, Hood WB Jr. Reduction of precordial ST elevation in patients with anterior myocardial infarction by breathing oxygen. Circulation 1976; 53(suppl I): I198–I200.
37. Blann AD, Landray MJ, Lip GYH. ABC of antithrombotic therapy. An overview of antithrombotic therapy. BMJ 2002; 325:762–765.
38. Mathew TC, Vasudevan RV, Leb L, Pezzella SM, Pezzella AT. Coronary artery bypass graft in idiopathic thrombocytopenic purpura. Ann Thorac Surg 1997; 64:1059–1062.
39. Waard de DEP, Verhorst PMJ, Visser CA. Exercise induced syncope as late consequence of radiotherapy. Int J Cardiol 1996; 57:289–291.
40. Katz NM, Hall AW, Cerqueira MD. Radiation induced valvulitis with late leaflet rupture. Heart 2001; 86:e20.
41. Basavaraju SK. Pathophysiological effects of radiation on atherosclerosis development and progression and the incidence of cardiovascular complications. Am Assoc Phys Med 2002; 29(10):2391–2403.
42. Behar S, Zahavi Z, Goldbourt U, Reicher-Reiss H. Long-term prognosis of patients with paroxysmal atrial fibrillation complication acute myocardial infarction. SPRINT Study Group. Eur Heart J 1992; 13:45–50.
43. Campbell RW, Murray A, Julian DG. Ventricular arrhythmias in first 12 hours of acute myocardial infarction. Natural history study. Br Heart J 1981; 46:351–357.
44. Behar S, Goldbourt U, Reicher-Reiss H, Kaplinsky E. Prognosis of acute myocardial infarction complicated by primary ventricular fibrillation: principal investigators of the SPRINT study. Am J Cardiol 1990; 66: 1208–1211.
45. MacMahon S, Collins R, Peto R, Koster RW, Yusuf S. Effects of prophylactic lidocaine in suspected acute myocardial infarction: an overview of results from the randomized, controlled trials. JAMA 1988; 260: 1910–1916.
46. Campbell RWF, Higham D, Adams P, Murrary A. Pottasium—its relevance for arrhythmias complicating acute myocardial infarction. J Cardiovasc Pharm 1987; 10:S25–S27.
47. Echt DS, Liebson PR, Mitchell LB, Peters RW, Obias-Manno D, Barke AH, Aresberg D, Baker A, Friedman L, Greene HL, et al. Mortality in patients receiving encainide, flecainide or placebo. The cardiac arrhythmia suppression trial. N Engl J Med 1991; 324: 781–788.
48. Nademanee K, Taylor RD, Bailey WM. Management and long-term outcome of patients with electrical storm. J Am Coll Cardiol 1995; 25:187A. Abstract.
49. Scheinman MM, Levine JH, Cannom DS, Friehling T, Kopelman HA, Chilson D, Platia EV, Wilber DJ, Kowey PR; for the Intravenous Amiodarone Multicenter Investigators Group. Dose-ranging study of intravenous amiodarone in patients with life-threatening ventricular tachyarrhythmias. Circulation. 1995; 92: 3264–3272.
50. Hochman JS, Boland J, Sleeper LA, Porway M, Brinkler J, Col J, Jacobs A, Slater J, Miller D, Wasserman H, Menegus MA, Talley JD, McKinlay S, Sanborn T, LeJemtel T; and the SHOCK Registry Investigators. Current spectrum of cardiogenic shock

and effect of early revascularization on mortality. Results of an international registry. Circulation 1995; 91:873–881.
51. Dell'Italia LJ, Starling MR, O'Rourke RA. Physical examination for exclusion of hemodynamically important right ventricular infarction. Ann Intern Med 1983; 99:608–611.
52. Dell'Italia LJ, Starling MR, Crawford MH, Boros BL, Chaudhuri TK, O'Rourke RA. Right ventricular infarction: identification by hemodynamic measurements before and after volume loading and correlation with noninvasive techniques. J Am Coll Cardiol 1984; 4:931–939.
53. Cohn JN, Guiha NH, Broder MI, Limas CJ. Right ventricular infarction: clinical and hemodynamic features. Am J Cardiol 1974; 33:209–214.
54. Robalino BD, Whitlow PL, Underwood DA, Salcedo EE. Electrocardiographic manifestations of right ventricular infarction. Am Heart J 1989; 118:138–144.
55. Manno BV, Bemis CE, Carver J, Mintz GS. Right ventricular infarction complicated by right to left shunt. J Am Coll Cardiol 1983; 1:554–557.
56. Goldstein JA, Vlahakes GJ, Verrier ED, Dchiller NB, Botvinick E, Tyberg JV, Parmley WW, Chatterjee K. Volume loading improves low cardiac output in experimental right ventricular infarction. J Am Coll Cardiol 1983; 2:270–278.
57. Braat SH, De Zwaan C, Brugada P, Coenegracht JM, Wellens HJ. Right ventricular involvement with acute inferior wall myocardial infarction identifies high risk of developing atrioventricular nodal conduction disturbances. Am Heart J 1984; 107:1183–1187.
58. Love JC, Haffajee CI, Gore JM, Alpert JS. Reversibility of hypotension and shock by atrial or atrioventricular sequential pacing in patients with right ventricular infarction. Am Heart J 1984; 108:5–13.
59. Sugiura T, Iwasaka T, Takahashi N, Nakamura S, Taniguchi H, Nagahama Y, Matsutani M, Inada M. Atrial fibrillation in inferior wall Q-wave acute myocardial infarction. Am J Cardiol 1991; 67:1135–1136.
60. Fantidis P, Castejon R, Fernandez Ruiz A, Madero-Jarabo R, Cordovilla G, Sanz Galeote E. Does a critical hemodynamic situation develop from right ventriculotomy and free wall infarct or from small changes in dysfunctional right ventricle afterload? J Cardiovasc Surg (Torino) 1992; 33:229–234
61. Braat SH, Ramentol M, Halders S, Wellens HJ. Reperfusion with streptokinase of an occluded right coronary artery: effects on early and late right and left ventricular ejection fraction. Am Heart J 1987; 113:257–260.
62. Schuler G, Hofmann M, Schwarz F, Mehmel H, Manthey J, Tillmanna H, Hartmann S, Kubler W. Effect of successful thrombolytic therapy on right ventricular function in acute inferior wall myocardial infarction. Am J Cardiol 1984; 54:951–957.
63. Zehender M, Kasper W, Kauder E, Schonthaler M, Geibel A, Olschewski M, Just H. Right ventricular infarction as an independent predictor of prognosis after acute inferior myocardial infarction. N Engl J Med 1993; 328:981–988.

37

Critical Care of the Cancer Patient with Pulmonary Infiltrates

VICKIE R. SHANNON and BURTON F. DICKEY

Department of Pulmonary Medicine, The University of Texas M.D. Anderson Cancer Center, Houston, Texas, U.S.A.

I. INTRODUCTION

Evaluation of the cancer patient with new or worsening pulmonary infiltrates remains a complex and pervasive clinical challenge and a frequent dilemma for the intensivist. Despite tremendous technological advancements in imaging, hemodynamic assessment, and more sensitive culture techniques that facilitate the diagnosis of pulmonary disorders, mortality rates for the critically ill patient with cancer-related pulmonary infiltrates remain disturbingly high (1,2). These rates may exceed 90% among those patients with associated acute respiratory failure requiring mechanical ventilation (2–7). Life-threatening lung disease has become increasingly prevalent as more aggressive radiation and cancer protocols have been implemented. Cancer treatment protocols result in further suppression of an already impaired host defense system and render the cancer patient highly susceptible to both infectious and noninfectious pulmonary complications. Thus, the threat of lung disease among patients with cancer is pervasive and mortality rates among this group of patients remain high, despite novel and aggressive therapeutic interventions.

The etiologic spectrum of pulmonary infiltrates in the cancer patient is broad and includes those that occur as a consequence of the cancer itself or as a result of its treatment (Table 1). For instance, cancer has a unique propensity to invade and obstruct contiguous structures. This activity may lead to a variety of complications within the lung, including acute airway obstruction, superior caval syndrome, atelectasis, massive hemoptysis, pneumothorax, pneumonia, and pleural effusions. Pleural diseases, including pneumothorax, empyema, and hemothorax, may occur as a consequence of necrosis of tumor within the periphery of the lung. Prolonged bedrest, major surgery, and hypercoaguability are well-recognized substrates for pulmonary embolism. Analgesia, excessive sedation, and chemotherapy-related mucositis render the debilitated cancer patient at risk for aspiration. Adding to these is a spectrum of noninfectious pulmonary complications induced by cancer therapy, including pulmonary edema, alveolar hemorrhage, bronchospasm, interstitial pneumonitis, pulmonary veno-occlusive disease, and obliterative bronchiolitis with or without organizing pneumonia. Finally, the success of cancer treatment modalities of radiation, chemotherapy, and hematopoietic stem cell transplantation (HSCT) occurs at a cost—the exhaustion of immune resources. The depression of host immune defense mechanisms renders the cancer patient vulnerable to inexorable pulmonary infections triggered by opportunistic and nosocomial pathogens. Thus, pulmonary infiltrates among critically ill cancer patients may result from a variety of infectious and

Table 1 Major Etiologies of Pulmonary Infiltrates in Critically Ill Patients with Cancer

Conditions caused by cancer	Conditions caused by cancer or its R_X[a]	Conditions caused by cancer R_X
Lymphangitic carcinomatosis	Pneumonia	Interstitial pneumonitis
Pulmonary leukostasis with hyperleukocytosis	Atelectasis	Drug toxicity
Tumor embolism	Massive hemoptysis	Radiation toxicity
	Airway obstruction	TRALI
	Thromboembolic disease	Fat embolism syndrome
	Pulmonary edema	Venous air embolism
	Pulmonary hemorrhage syndromes	Idiopathic pneumonia syndrome
	Pulmonary veno-occlusive disease	
	BOOP (cryptogenic organizing pneumonitis)	

[a]R_x = treatment; TRALI = transfusion-related acute lung injury.

noninfectious etiologies. The devastating impact of pulmonary infiltrates on patient outcome underscores the urgent need for a concise approach to the diagnosis and treatment of patients in this setting. Accordingly, a pragmatic approach to the diagnosis and treatment of pulmonary infiltrates among critically ill cancer patients is the central focus of this chapter. The information provided is designed to highlight current insights and therapeutic advancements while underscoring diagnostic dilemmas and areas of uncertainty that warrant further study and investigation.

II. INFECTIOUS PULMONARY COMPLICATIONS AMONG CRITICALLY ILL PATIENTS WITH CANCER

A. Incidence

The prevalence of pneumonia is dependent upon the study population and the nature of the underlying neoplasm. Nearly 2/3 of patients with leukemia and 60% of recipients of hematopoietic stem cell transplants will develop pneumonia during the course of their illness. (8–12). Pneumonia decisively contributes to overall mortality among 40–60% of all stem cell transplant recipients, 60% of patients with leukemia, and 40% of patients with solid tumors (13–15). Rates of pneumonia, including fatal pneumonia, have escalated as more aggressive cancer treatment protocols have been implemented.

Although pneumonia is the overall leading infectious cause of death in critically ill patients with cancer (13,16,17), precise estimates of the incidence of pulmonary infections in this group of patients are incompletely understood, linked in part to several fundamental problems. The critically ill, debilitated cancer patient may be too clinically unstable to undergo definitive testing. Therefore, the diagnosis is often based on conjecture rather than specific imaging, microbiologic, or histologic data. Indistinct definitions of infection vs. colonization further contribute to imprecise estimates. Atypical presentations of lung infections are common in this setting. Conventional clinical symptoms of cough, fever, and sputum production may be absent despite overwhelming pneumonia. During the period of marrow recovery following chemotherapy or HSCT, the chest radiograph may be profoundly abnormal in the absence of detectable infection, while a normal chest radiograph in the setting of neutropenic fever may belie the presence of pneumonia. Successful identification of underlying infectious etiologies is further confounded by comorbid illnesses, such as acute respiratory distress syndrome (ARDS), pulmonary edema, alveolar hemorrhage, and atelectasis that closely mimic infectious diagnoses. The intensivist caring for the cancer patient with pulmonary infiltrates must have a fundamental understanding of the indistinct interface between infectious diagnoses and noninfectious comorbidities as well as other inherent diagnostic challenges that commonly confound the evaluation of these patients.

B. Host Defenses

The predilection for pulmonary infection and the susceptibility to particular opportunistic pathogens may be gleaned from knowledge of the patient's cancer diagnosis, antecedent treatment regimens, and the functional status of the immune system. A composite sketch of the prototype cancer patient admitted to the intensive care unit demonstrates numerous potential breaches in local host defenses as well as all three components of the immune system. This breakdown in host defense mechanisms may occur as a direct result of the cancer itself or its treatment. Thus, the predilection to infection in the cancer patient is best understood by examining the effects of cancer and its treatment on host defenses including local, innate, and adaptive immunity (Tables 2–4).

Table 2 Infectious Etiologies of Pulmonary Infiltrates Associated with Specific Immune Defects: Deficiencies of Local Defenses

	Type of microorganism		
Associated conditions	Bacterial	Fungal	Viral
Mucositis	*Streptoccoccus* spp.	Aspergillus	Herpes simplex
Altered glottic function	*Staphylococcus* spp.	Candida	Varicella-zoster
Indwelling catheters	*Pseudomonas* spp.	Mucoraceae	
Endotracheal tubes	Enterobacteriaceae	Fusaria	
Venipunctures	Corynebacterium		

1. Impairment of Physical Barriers to Infection

Breach of cutaneous and mucosal barriers as a consequence of chemotherapy or by local invasion of tumor may predispose the cancer patient to infection. Cancer patients are further burdened by iatrogenic alterations in mechanical barriers including percutaneous, foley, and nasogastric catheters, which facilitate the development of infection (18). The biofilm of nasogastric catheters and endotracheal tubes imposes a direct infection risk to the lungs by serving as a conduit for chronic colonization of pathogenic organisms (19,20). In addition, these catheters alter mucociliary activity and interfere with coordinated glottic function, thereby enhancing the risk for aspiration. The upper airways are a common site of colonization of potential nosocomial pathogens, many of which exhibit enhanced antibiotic resistance and virulence. Breaches in local defense barriers confer a significant infection risk only when other host defenses are overwhelmed, as by heavy innoculum, resistant or virulent organisms, or when other components of the immune system are compromised.

2. Impairment of Local Innate Lung Defense Mechanisms: Epithelial Cells, Mast Cells, and Macrophages

The first point of contact of microbial pathogens entering the lungs are the epithelial cells that line the airways and alveoli, and the lining fluid that bathes their apical surface. Lung epithelial cells constitutively

Table 3 Infectious Etiologies of Pulmonary Infiltrates Associated with Specific Immune Defects: Deficiencies in Innate Immunity

		Type of microorganism	
Defect	Associated conditions	Bacterial	Fungal
Neutrophil disorder			
Neutropenia	Mucositis	*Psuedomonas aerginosa*	Aspergillus
	Acute leukemia	*Staphylococcus aureus*	Candida
	Hodgkin's lymphoma	Coagulase negative staphylococci	Mucoraceae
	Tumor infiltration of BM	Viridans streptococci	Fusaria
	Infectious/infiltration of BM	*Enterobacteria*	Cryptococcus
	Chemotherapy	*Corynebacterium jeikeium*	*Pseudoallescheria* spp.
	Radiation therapy	Enterococci	*Histoplasma* spp.
		Bacteroides fragilis	*Coccidiodies* spp.
		Treponema pallidum	*Paracoccidioides* spp.
		Rickettsia	*Blastomyces* spp.
		Chlamydia	
Altered chemotaxis	Chemotherapy	*Staphylococcus aureus*	Aspergillus
Altered phagocytosis	Radiation therapy	*Escherichia coli*	Candida
	Hyperglycemia	Streptococci	Mucoraceae
	Acidosis		
	Corticosterooids		
	Uremia		
	Hodgkin's lymphoma		

Table 4 Infectious Etiologies of Pulmonary Infiltrates Associated with Specific Immune Defects: Deficiencies of Adaptive Immunity

Defect	Associated conditions	Type of microorganism			
		Bacterial	Fungal	Viral	Protozoal/parasitic
Humoral	Multiple myeloma CLL Waldenstrom's Chemotherapy Corticosteroids	*Streptococcus pneumoniae* *Haemophilus influenzae* GNRs (encapsulated) *Neisseria* spp. *Salmonella* *E. coli* *Pseudomonas* *Plasmodium* spp.		Influenza virus Arbovirus Echovirus	
CMI	Hodgkin's Non-Hodgkin's Hairy cell leukemia T-cell leukemia Lymphocytic leukemia Corticosteroids Chemotherapy	Mycobacteria Legionella Nocardia Rhodococcus Listeria Brucella Bartonella	Aspergillus Histoplasma Coccdioides Pneumocytsis Candida Cryptococcus Blastomycoses	Cytomegalovirus Herpes simplex Varicella-zosters Influenza RSV[a] Adenovirus Measle virus	Toxoplasma Ameba Strongyloides Giardia Cryptosporidium Isospora Microsporidium Salmonella

[a] RSV=Respiratory syncytial virus.

secrete a variety of antimicrobial macromolecules into the lining fluid that include lactoferrin, lysozyme, defensins, mucins, secretory IgA, and complement components, and upon stimulation they are able to augment this repertoire (21). They also release chemotactic signals that attract circulating leukocytes. Unlike epithelial cells of the gut, lung epithelial cells are relatively long lived and slowly dividing, making them less susceptible to the acute cytoxicity of chemotherapeutic agents. Nonetheless, it is likely that chemotherapy reduces their ability to express genes encoding microbial defensive polypeptides, though this is not well studied. Whereas antimetabolites, such as as cytarabine, show very little epithelial toxicity in comparison to the degree of myelosuppression, alkylating agents such as cyclophosphamide show substantial epithelial toxicity (22).

The principle resident immune cells of the skin and mucosal surfaces are mast cells and macrophages. The role of mast cells in the initiation of acute allergic reactions mediated through IgE receptors is well known, but their essential role in defense against severe bacterial infections has only recently been recognized (23,24). Mast cells act as sentinels of the immune system, residing within the surface epithelia and submucosa and continuously sampling the environment through innate immune receptors such as those for microbial products and complement components. Upon detection of microbial pathogens, they rapidly release eicosanoids and preformed inflammatory mediators, such as proteases, cytokines, and vasoactive signaling molecules that allow extravasation of protective plasma proteins and recruitment of immune effector cells. Similarly, macrophages are long-lived resident immune cells of the skin and mucosa that help form the first line of defense in their role as professional phagocytes, by signaling other leukocytes through the release of cytokines and chemokines, and by presenting antigens to immune cells (23,24). As long-lived, nondividing cells, mast cells and macrophages are relatively resistant to cancer chemotherapeutic agents compared to the rapidly dividing cells of the bone marrow. Nonetheless, their function may be altered, particularly by corticosteroids. Among patients undergoing HSCT, for example, cytoreductive therapy results in profound impairments in alveolar macrophage chemotaxis, phagocytosis, and killing during the first 4 months following transplantation. Full recovery of these mechanisms typically occurs at 6–12 months following HSCT (25).

3. *Impairment of Recruitable Innate Immune Cells: Alterations in Qualitative and Quantitative Neutrophil Function*

Neutrophils are critical effectors of innate immunity that represent an essential line of defense against pathogens at mucosal surfaces and other points of entry (24). These avidly phagocytic cells are the central cellular defense against infections caused by bacterial and fungal organisms (17,26,27). Neutropenia is defined as a neutrophil count of < 500/mL, or < 1000/mL with a predicted low nadir in the neutrophil count to < 500/mL within 2 days of the initial test. Both the number of circulating neutrophils and the duration of neutropenia are important determinants of infection. Patients with protracted neutropenia lasting more than 10 days and neutrophil counts of less than 100/mL are at greatest risk for infection. At least 50% of these patients who become febrile will have established or occult infection, with the lungs, alimentary tract, and skin being the major anatomic sites for infection (28,29). For example, profound neutropenia is extremely common among patients with acute myeloid leukemia and the incidence of pneumonia in this group of patients may exceed 80% (13,30,31). Neutropenia may be fostered by chemotherapy, radiation therapy, or infectious infiltration of the bone marrow. Chemotherapy may induce both absolute agranulocytosis by direct myelotoxicity and functional neutropenia by interfering with the phagocytic and chemotactic activity of neutrophils (32,33). Functional neutropenia is commonly seen in patients with refractory non-Hodgkin's lymphoma, or relapsed/untreated acute leukemia. A number of other factors may also contribute to functional neutropenia, especially in the critically ill patient with cancer. These include radiation therapy and administration of glucocorticosteroids. In addition, common cancer-related disorders such as hypovolemia, prolonged hypoxemia, acidosis, and poorly controlled hyperglycemia are common in the cancer setting and have been shown to cause dysfunctional neutrophils. Specific pathogens causing pneumonia that are commonly encountered in neutropenic patients are listed in Table 2.1. *Pseudomonas aeroginosa* remains the most common and the most life-threatening gram-negative pathogen among neutropenic patients. The incidence of pneumonias caused by gram-positive organisms including *Staphylococcus aureus*, *Streptococcus viridans*, and *Streptococcus pneumoniae* has increased by nearly 40% among neutropenic patients over the past decade (34), owing in part to the increased use of intravascular catheters and the expanded use of antimicrobial prophylaxis directed at aerobic gram-negative organisms. Neutropenia that persists for more than 7 days is significantly associated with increased rates of severe fungal pneumonias. Specific fungal infections may result from opportunistic nosocomial pathogens (*Aspergillus*, *Candida*, *Mucoraceae*, *Cryptococcus*) or reactivation of indolent endemic organisms (*Histoplasma capsulatum*, *Coccidiodes immitis*, *Paracoccidioides brasiliensis*, *Blastomyces dermatidides*).

4. *Impairment of Adaptive Immunity*

Altered Humoral Responses

B-cell dysfunction is a common sequela of lymphoreticular malignancies as well as aggressive cytoreductive chemotherapeutic protocols. Lymphoreticular malignancies including multiple myeloma, chronic lymphocytic leukemia, and Waldenstom's macroglobulinemia may directly cause immunoglobulin dyscrasias and associated hypogammaglobulinemia (35,36). Loss of proper B-cell function is tightly linked to profound impairments of humoral immunity, including impaired neutralization of toxins and disorders of immunoglobulin production, antibody-dependent cellular cytotoxicity, and complement activation. Defects in opsonization, owing to functional or anatomic asplenism, are a common problem among patients with lymphoreticular malignancies. Thus, qualitative as well as quantitative depression of the alternative complement pathway, which is housed in the spleen, may be seen. Bacterial organisms that require opsonization with complement (C_3, C_5) for elimination may proliferate in hypocomplementemic states. Thus, infection caused by *S. pneumonia* and other encapsulated organisms may cause fulminant and often lethal infections during this time period. Other bacterial pathogens (*Neisseria menigitidis*, *Pseudomonas aeruginosa*, *Haemophilus influenzae* and encapsulated strains of gram-negative bacilli) and viral organisms (influenza and enteroviruses) are noted with increased frequency. Adding to this, defects in antibody-dependent lymphocyte cytolytic activity lead to unchecked parasitic infections. Importantly, isolated defects in humoral defense do not confer an increased risk for fungal pathogens (Table 4).

Altered Cellular Immune Response

The cellular arm of adaptive immunity is dependent on intact macrophage and T-lymphocyte interactions. Consequently, disorders that affect T-lymphocyte and macrophage function, including prolonged administration of corticosteroids or other immunosuppressive agents, lymphoreticular malignancies of T-cell origin, and viral illnesses may severely depress the cellular arm of the immune system. Patients with certain cancers, including Hodgkin's disease, hairy cell leukemia, adult T-cell leukemia, and lymphocytic leukemia have markedly impaired T-lymphocyte function. In addition, multiple agents in the armamentarium of cancer therapy, antineoplastic agents, glucocorticosteroid therapy, and agents used for prophylaxis as well as treatment of established graft-versus-host disease may induce profound lymphopenia (Table 4). Defective cellular immunity gives rise to infections by unusual pathogens, including intracellular bacteria (mycobacterial species, *Legionella*, and *Listeria monocytogenes*), *Nocardia*, *Salmonella*, *Brucella*, *and Rhodococcus*. Viral infections among this group of patients may reflect primary infection or recrudescence of latent disease. The most frequently encountered viral pathogen in this setting is *Cytomegalovirus*. Other common viral infections include those caused by *Respiratory syncytial virus* (RSV), *Influenza virus* and *Adenovirus*. The virulence of these infections in the immunocompromised host is highlighted by mortality rates of 50–90% (37–42).

C. Altered Host Defense Following HSCT

1. *Deficiencies in Innate and Adaptive Immunity*

Over the past decade, hematopoietic stem cell transplants have emerged as standard therapy for a variety of malignant and nonmalignant diseases. Tremendous progress in our understanding of the human leukocyte antigen (HLA) system, advances in pretransplant preparative regimens and measures of intensive support following transplant have resulted in improved patient outcomes. Despite these advances, many of patients succumb to lethal complications, usually within the first 3 months following transplantation. Pulmonary disease occurs in 40–60% of transplant recipients and is the proximal cause of death in up to 80% of these patients. Susceptibility to lung injury following transplantation is tightly linked to the dynamically changing immunologic status of the patient and is roughly predictable based on the amount of time that has elapsed since transplantation. The intent of the pretransplant cytoablative regimen is to eradicate the underlying malignancy and mitigate the ability of the recipient to reject the allograft by inducing profound immune suppression. Risk factors, including the transplant allotype, underlying disease, intensity of chemoradiotherapy regimens prior to transplant, HLA compatibility between the donor and the recipient, rate of immune recovery, and T-cell depletion of the graft greatly influence the later development of infection. Accordingly, infection rates, including fatal pneumonias among recipients of allogeneic transplants are much higher than that seen among autologous transplant recipients because of more stringent preparative chemotherapeutic regimens, delayed recovery of T and B-cell functions, histoincompatible donor stem cells and the development of GVHD among this group of patients.

The posttransplant period may be divided to reflect three stages of major impairment of specific arms of the host defense system, which roughly correlate with the periods of highest vulnerability to infection. In the post-HSCT patient population, the differential diagnosis of unexplained pulmonary infiltrates may be narrowed, therefore, by knowledge of the timetable for immune reconstitution following the chemoablative regimens. The chronologic development of pulmonary complications following transplantation may vary significantly, however, depending on the rate of immune recovery and the presence of graft-versus-host disease (GVHD) (17,38,43). The approach to the patient with pulmonary infiltrates following HSCT requires an understanding of the evolution of immune defects that occur as a consequence of therapy and the associated unique susceptibility of these patients to the sequential pathogens that emerge during the evolution of immune reconstitution (Fig. 1). Exploitation of this knowledge may help to simplify the often daunting task of streamlining the differential diagnosis.

2. *Periods of Immune Recovery Following HSCT*

Preengraftment Period

The early or preengraftment period occurs within the first 3 weeks after transplantation and is heralded by profound neutropenia and lymphopenia (17,38,44) Predictably, bacterial infections, particularly those caused by gram-negative organisms (*Pseudomonas*, *Enter obacteriaceae*, and *Stenotrophomonas maltophilia Legionella*, *Escherichia coli*, *and Acinetobacter*) have been the major culprits of infection and may cause fatal pneumonias during this time period. Aggressive prophylactic strategies following HSCT using antimicrobial agents that target gram-negative organisms have resulted in the resurgence of gram-positive pathogens, including *Streptococcus pneumoniae* and *Staphylococcus aureus* (45). Simultaneous deficiencies in the humoral immune system during this time increase the propensity for infections caused by gram-negative rods, such as *Hemophilus influenzae*, *Neisseria meningitis*, and *Pseudomonas*, and to encapsulated organisms, *Streptococcus*. Early depression of humoral immunity also facilitates the emergence of viral infections, in particular those caused by HSV and respiratory viruses (*RSV, Parainfluenza virus, Rhinovirus, Influenza virus types A and B*). The respiratory viruses occur with seasonal fluctuations. Despite aggressive prophylactic and preemptive antifungal strategies, fungal infections during the early posttransplant period remain a persistent threat and a leading cause of mortality. Both the degree and duration of neutropenia influence the development of fungal pneumonias, with most occurring as the number of neutrophils falls below $100/mm^3$ and the period of neutropenia extends beyond 7 days. The dominant

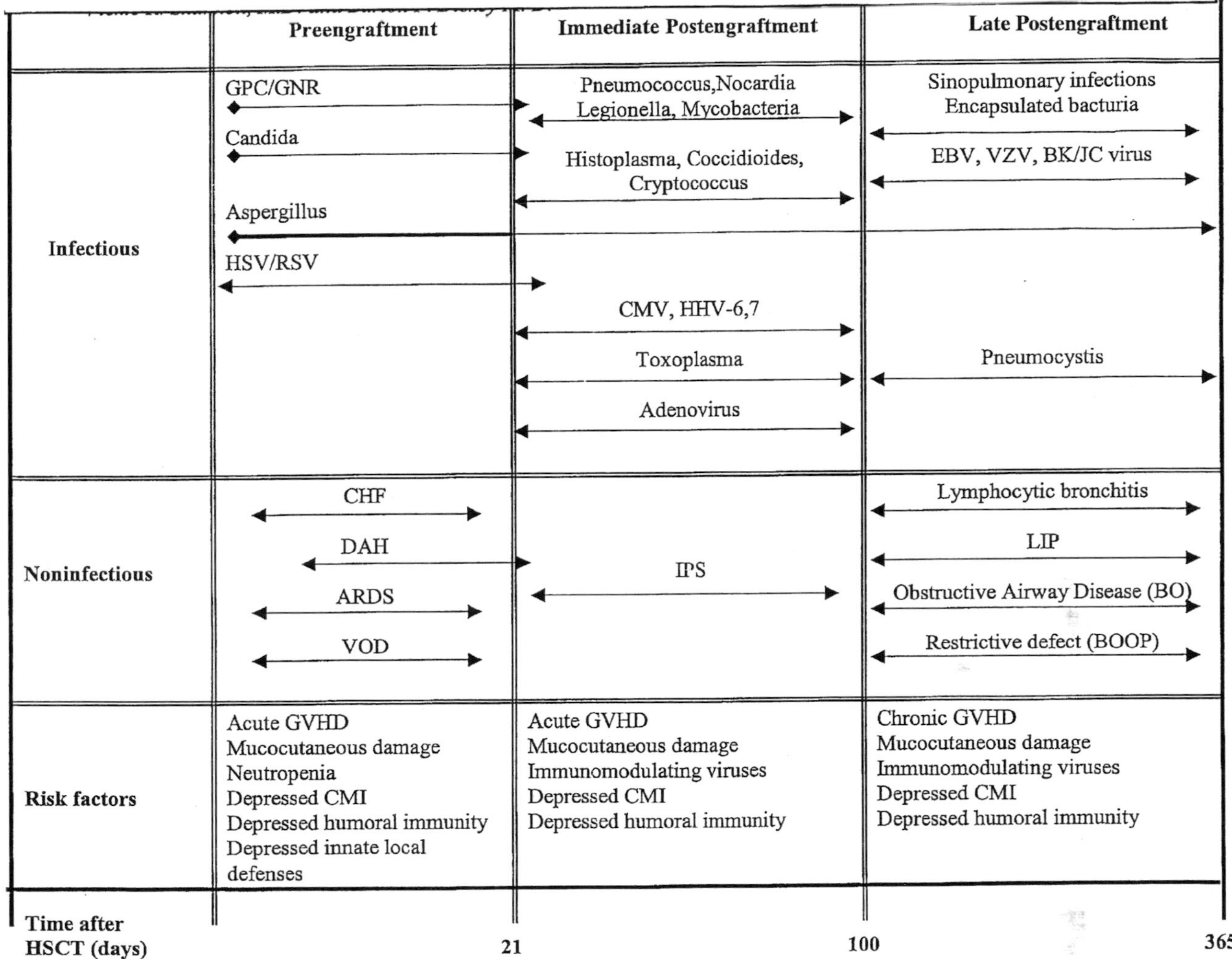

Figure 1 Temporal relationship between HSCT and the development of pulmonary complications. ARDS, acute respiratory distress syndrome; BO, obliterative bronchiolitis; BOOP, bronchiolitis obliterans with organizing pneumonia; CHF, congestive heart failure; CMV, cytomegalovirus; CMI, cell mediated immunity; DAH, diffuse alvelar hemorrhage; EMV, Epstein–bar virus GNR, gram-negative rods; GPC, gram-positive cocci; GVHD, graft-versus-host disease; HHV-6,7, human herpes virus 6,7; HSCT, hematopoietic stem cell transplant; HSV, herpes simplex virus; IPS, idiopathic pneumonia syndrome; LIP, lymphocytic interstitial pneumonitis; RSV, respiratory syncytial virus; VOD; veno-occlusive disease; VZV, varicella zoster virus.

fungal infections encountered during this time period include the filamentous fungal pathogens (*Aspergillus*, *Fusarium*, and *Mucormycosis*) and *Candida* species. Diligent prophylactic protocols with azol derivatives during the neutropenic period significantly reduce the risk of *Candida pneumonias*. Triazole-resistant strains of *Candida glabrata* and *Candida kruseii* have emerged at increased rates, however, presumably secondary to these aggressive prophylactic strategies (46,47). Neutrophil recovery typically occurs within 14–21 days following transplantation. Although tissue and blood lymphocytes may demonstrate partial reconstitution of cytotoxic and proliferative activity within the first 3 months following transplant, full recovery of lymphocyte function characteristically does not occur until 12 months or more following transplantation.

Intermediate Postengraftment Period

Engraftment marks the beginning of the intermediate or postengraftment stage. This period may last from 3 weeks to 3 months posttransplantation and is characterized by profound suppression of both the cellular and humoral arms of the host defense system. Persistent suppression of these two arms of the immune system drives the development of peculiar bacterial and nonbacterial pathogens, including *Legionella*, *Mycobacteria*, *Norcardia*, and *Salmonella* during this posttransplant phase. *Aspergillus*, *Pneumocystis carinii* and endemic fungi (*Histoplasmosis*, *Coccidioidomycosis*) also occur at increased rates. Other opportunistic mycoses caused by *Fusarium*, *Zygomycetes*, resistant Candida, and *Pseudallaesceria boydii* have been increasingly recognized during this period. Rare infections by typical and atypical mycobacteria may occur as a consequence of reactivation or de novo disease. Viral pneumonias caused by immunomodulating viruses (CMV, *HSV*) and those typically found in the community (*Adenovirus*, *Rhinovirus*, *RSV*) may be particularly troublesome during this time period. Pretransplant donor serology that is positive for CMV strongly influences the emergence of CMV infection in the seronegative transplant recipient. Reactivation of a dormant viral organism accounts for the preponderance of viral infections in the postengraftment period. Seasonal fluctuations of enteric viruses (Norwalk virus, coxsackie virus, echovirus, rotavirus) may also be seen.

Late Postengraftment Period

The late postengraftment period is marked by severe and unrelenting impairment of cellular and humoral immunity. These persistent immune derangements, coupled with mucocutaneous damage and hyposplenism, underlie the bulk of the infections that occur during this period. The late postengraftment period typically occurs 3 or more months following transplantation and is exquisitely linked to the appearance of chronic GVHD. Disseminated infections caused by VZV, EBV, and a resurgence of recalcitrant late bacterial infections caused by *Staphylococci*, *Streptococcus pneumoniae*, *Neisseria meningitides*, *Haemophilus influenza*, and gram-negative bacteria, including *Pseudomonas* species are common during this period. Increased rates of pneumonia caused by PCP are also seen during the late postengraftment stage as a consequence of relaxation of prophylactic strategies against this organism.

3. *Central Role of Graft-vs.-Host Disease Following HSCT*

The scourge of fatal pulmonary disease following allogeneic stem cell transplants is often propagated by the development of graft-vs.-host disease (GVHD). GVHD is an inherently immunosuppressive disorder that arises when immunocompetent donor T-lymphocytes are transfused into a HLA nonidentical recipient. This triggers a series of host responses resulting in injury to a variety of targeted tissues, including the skin, liver, and gastrointestinal tract. GVHD complicates 25–75% of all transplants and may be divided into acute (occurring within the first 100 days) and chronic (occurring at day 100 or greater) forms. Both acute and chronic GVHD are characterized by inherent deficiencies in humoral and cellular immune function (48). Patients frequently have significant disruptions of mucosal barriers of the gut and skin secondary to GVHD. Adding to this, protocols for prophylaxis and the treatment of established GVHD primarily involve the use of immunosuppressive agents. Thus, the susceptibility to infection is markedly amplified by the development of this disorder.

Signs and symptoms, including liver dysfunction, diarrhea, and an exfoliative skin rash, may signal the development acute GVHD, depending on the major organ system that is involved. Roughly 1/3 of patients that survive beyond the first 100 days following allogeneic transplantation will develop chronic GVHD. Functional asplenia, scleroderma-like changes and clinical features resembling a variety of other autoimmune multisystem diseases are prominent features of the chronic form of this disease. Chronic GVHD commonly targets the lungs and imposes increased vulnerability to infectious (sinopulmonary infections, *Pneumocystis carinii* pneumonia, *Aspergillus*, chronic aspiration, infections due to encapsulated bacteria) and noninfectious (lymphoid interstitial pneumonia, bronchitis, bronchiolitis obliterans, BOOP) diseases.

D. Evaluation of the Critically Ill Patient with Pulmonary Infiltrates

1. *History and Physical Examination*

Although the clinical assessment of the cancer patient with pulmonary infiltrates is often ambiguous, critical clues to the diagnosis may be found in the history, physical examination, and diagnostic work-up. For example, a history of recent travel to areas endemic for *Histoplasmosis* (Ohio-Mississippi river valley), *Coccidiodomycosis* (southwestern United States, Central and South America), multidrug-resistant mycobacterial disease (inner-city New York), or *Babesiosis* (northeastern United States) may have clinical relevance in this setting. Because many infections occur as a result of reactivated disease, a history of antecedent infection with *Aspergillus*, *Cytomegalovirus*, *Herpes simplex*, or *Varicella zoster virus* may also yield helpful clues to the diagnosis. Knowledge of prior antibiotic therapy is also helpful. For example, HSCT recipients are routinely prescribed preemptive antimicrobial therapy with gancyclovir and trimethoprim–sulfamethoxazole during the early and intermediate posttransplant period. These antibiotics substantially reduce the risk of HSV and PCP, respectively, but also occasionally promote a shift in the microbial spectrum to more virulent pathogens. Trimethoprim–sulfamethoxazole, as well as the flouroquinolones, demonstrates variable coverage against gram-positive organisms. Neutropenic patients who receive these antibiotics are, therefore, at increased risk for the development of *Streptoccocus viridans* pneumonia, an aggressive pneumonia associated with toxic shock syndrome and leading to ARDS and death. The predilection for CMV pneumonia among HSCT recipients with positive CMV serologies prior to transplantation is dramatically reduced with gancyclovir therapy (49,50). Thus, suspicion for CMV pneumonia in this group of patients with pulmonary infiltrates is diminished. Similarly, the risk of CMV infection among seronegative patients who receive HSCT cells from seropositive donors is markedly increased. Accordingly, the differential diagnosis of unexplained pulmonary infiltrates in this group of patients should include CMV pneumonia.

The clinical bedside assessment of patients with pulmonary infiltrates may be underwhelming; productive cough, fever, dyspnea, and chest pain are nonspecific findings that are variably present, depending on the underlying disorder and severity of the disease. The intensivist, therefore, is often required to make clinical and therapeutic decisions based on a paucity of clinical signs and symptoms. In the general population, temperature elevations are reported in up to 78% of patients with pneumonia (51). Chemotherapeutic agents and concomitant glucocorticosteroid therapy, however, may mask fever in the patient with cancer. In addition, fever may be the presenting symptom of many comorbid illnesses that mimic pneumonia in the cancer patient, including radiation pneumonitis, drug toxicity, pulmonary embolic disease, alveolar hemorrhage, and thermoregulatory problems associated with polypharmacy. Similarly, the presence of rigors coupled with cough and fever is highly predictive of pneumonia in the general population; in the cancer setting, these symptoms are frequently seen as a consequence of certain cancer chemotherapeutic regimens. Cough may be minimal in the debilitated cancer patient with severe pneumonia. Cough and dyspnea may be substantive in the absence of pneumonia, however, among those patients with distorted airway anatomy secondary to chemoradiotherapy or tumors involving the proximal airway. Rales and egophony, two physical findings suggestive of chest consolidation, may be absent. The interpretation of other auscultatory findings suggestive of pneumonia, including wheeze, rales, and dullness to percussion, is obscured by coexisting and confounding entities with similar clinical presentations. For example, centrally obstructing bronchial masses may cause focal wheeze as well as percussion dullness. Rales commonly occur with exacerbations of bronchitis or congestive heart failure, two entities that frequently coexist with or closely resemble pneumonia in the cancer patient. Despite these limitations, the physical examination is a key component of the overall evaluation. Clues to the diagnoses may be gleaned from extrathoracic manifestations of the lung infection. Nodular skin lesions, for example, may suggest the diagnosis of disseminated mycobacterial or fungal disease. Concomitant sinus disease offers support for *Mucormycosis* or *Legionella* species as potential etiologies of the pneumonia. In addition, the physical examination is the final arbiter in determining the severity of the pneumonia. In the pneumonia severity scores outlined by the British Thoracic Society and the Pneumonia Severity Index, substantial weight is placed on components of the physical examination (52,53).

2. *Diagnostic Imaging*

Chest radiography is a powerful tool that unquestionably influences clinical decision making in the evaluation of the cancer patient with pulmonary infiltrates. Knowledge of the classic radiographic patterns of infectious and noninfectious disorders is often very informative. Atypical radiographic presentations among this group of patients, however, are common and chest radiography alone usually cannot delineate with precision the underlying etiology. Adding to this, chest radiography in the debilitated and/or unstable cancer patient is often limited to a supine, anteroposterior portable chest film, precluding definitive confirmation of abnormalities that may be seen on the lateral radiograph. Infiltrate morphology and the anatomic localization of the radiographic abnormalities may have helpful diagnostic implications (Table 5). Radiographic changes may include focal (involving one lung) or diffuse (both lungs involved), reticular, or reticulonocular opacities with or without consolidation. Bacterial and fungal pneumonias typically cause focal radiographic changes although some infections, including those caused by viral pathogens and other organisms, such as *Puneumocystis carinii*, *Legionella*, *Mycoplasma*, disseminated *Histoplasma*, and *Strongyloides* may cause diffuse disease. Nodules (< 3 cm) or masses (> 3 cm) with or without cavitation occur frequently. An associated halo or crescent sign strongly suggests the diagnosis of fungal pneumonia. The presence of pleural effusion, and hilar or mediastinal adenopathy are distinctive attributes of some infectious diagnoses, although overlapping features between infectious and noninfectious categories of disease are common. The presence of a predominant alveolar or interstitial process may also streamline the diagnosis. Alveolar filling opacities appear as ground-glass attenuations on chest

Table 5 Differential Diagnosis of Pulmonary Infiltrates Based on Appearance and Rate of Progression of Chest Radiographic Abnormalities

	Rate of radiographic appearence/progression			Rate of radiographic resolution
Abnormality on chest radiograph	< 1 day	1–7 days	> 7 days	< 3 days
Infectious				
Focal consolidation	GPC; GNR	Legionella, CMV[a]; fungi; *Mycobacteria* spp.	Resistant GNR; Legionella; *Mycobacteria* spp.; Pneumocystis; fungi; Nocardia; viruses	
Diffuse infiltrates	GPC; GNR	GPC; GNR; viruses; fungi; *Mycobacteria* spp.	Pneumocystis; viruses; Mycobacteria; Nocardia; fungi;	
Nodular infiltrates	*Staphylococcus aureus*; GNR CMV; VZV; *Aspergillus* spp.	Legionella, *Aspergillus* spp.; other fungi; GNR; *Mycobacteria* spp.	Fungal; Nocardia; *Mycobacteria* spp.; pneumocystis	
Noninfectious				
Focal consolidation	Pulmonary hemorrhage; pulmonary edema[a]	Hyperacute radiation pneumonitis; drug toxicity; BOOP; IPS[a];	Radiation pneumonitis drug toxicity; primary or metastatic disease	Pulmonary hemorrhage; pulmonary edema
Diffuse infiltrates	Leukoagglutinin reaction	Hyperacute radiation BOOP; IPS; thromboembolic disease	Posttransplant lymphoproliferataive disorder; lymphangitic spread of tumor; radiation pneumonitis; thromboembolic disease	Pulmonary hemorrhage; pulmonary edema
Nodular infiltrates		Pulmonary infarction	Pulmonary infarction; lung cancer; metastatic disease	

[a] Indicates atypical radiographic manifestation.

radiographs or computed tomography (CT) and broadly reflect the presence of water (pulmonary edema), blood (alveolar hemorrhage) pus (infection), or protein (alveolar proteinosis) within the distal airspaces. The spectrum of diseases causing predominantly interstitial process is much broader and includes infectious and noninfectious etiologies. The diagnosis may also be suggested by the rapidity with which the radiographic changes evolve. For example, fleeting infiltrates that evolve over a 24–72 hr period are typically caused by edema or blood, whereas those with underlying inflammatory etiologies typically resolve over days to weeks. As a general rule, the doubling time for most neoplastic processes is greater than 3–4 weeks. Thus, focal infiltrates with more rapid doubling times are typically nonneoplastic in origin.

Conventional chest radiographs may fail to detect lung infiltrates during early stage disease or periods of severe neutropenia. Hence, normal chest radiographs in these settings should be interpreted with caution. Thoracic CT is an important tool in the early identification of lung disease among immunocompromised patients. Computed tomography scan examination of the chest offers several advantages over routine chest radiography. First, the use of cross-sectional images often makes it possible to distinguish between densities that would be superimposed on plain radiographs. Computed tomography is far superior to plain chest radiography in distinguishing subtle differences in density, thereby providing a more accurate distinction between adjacent structures. These features permit better recognition of hilar, mediastinal, and pleural disease. The addition of contrast material to the study allows differentiation of masses from adjacent vascular structures. Furthermore, cross-sectional imaging and the use of high resolution CT scan techniques may identify subtle parenchymal patterns that are nearly pathognomonic for certain types of diseases, lymphangitic spread, bronchiectasis, and diffuse parenchymal disease. In a recent study, the presence of a halo sign on CT and ground-glass attenuation surrounding segmental or nodular areas of consolidation in neutropenic patients accurately correlated with pulmonary invasive aspergillosis on surgical lung biopsy (54). These techniques may obviate the need for lung tissue sampling in the future.

3. *Culture Analysis of Respiratory Secretions*

Examination of expectorated sputum and endotracheal tube secretions is woefully problematic in the critical care setting. The retrieval of adequate sputum samples in the debilitated cancer patient with an ineffective cough is often difficult. Concerns regarding the contamination of sputum by potentially pathogenic bacteria that colonize the upper airway are a ubiquitous problem, especially in this patient setting. Contamination decreases the diagnostic specificity and sensitivity of sputum Gram's stain and culture from lower respiratory tract specimens. Recovery of certain pathogenic bacteria (*Legionella*, *Mycobacterium tuberculosis*, *Nocardia*) and endemic fungi (*Histoplasma*, *Coccidioidomycosis*, *Blastomycosis*) from the airway, however, are felt to be diagnostic of lower tract disease (55). Overall, the diagnostic utility of sputum Gram's stain and culture is felt to be low, and its impact on antimicrobial management is minimal (56). Furthermore, the yield of sputum analysis in the diagnosis of cancer-related noninfectious disorders, such as treatment-related lung injury and malignancies other than centrally obstructing tumors, is negligible (57).

4. *Novel Molecular Diagnostic Techniques*

Until recently, attempts to establish a definitive etiological diagnosis of pneumonia relied primarily on microbiologic testing. Even with the most rigorous testing, culture-based analyses of respiratory samples fail to detect responsible organisms causing pneumonia in greater than 50% of cases (58,59). Promising new advances in microbial detection have utilized molecular diagnostic techniques, such as polymerase chain reaction (PCR). These molecular tools employ antigen and nucleic acid detection assays to provide rapid etiological diagnoses of pneumonia. New antigen and nucleic acid detection assays for *Legionella pneumophilia*, *Streptococcus pneumonia*, *Pneumocystis carinii*, and certain types of viral pneumonias are currently being investigated. These tests will require further study before they are approved by the FDA for routine diagnoses of pneumonia. Key parameters such as sensitivity, specificity, reproducibility, and optimal sample types need to be determined before theses tests become commercially available (60). Recently an aspergillus-specific polymerase chain reaction and the detection of Aspergillus antigen (Galactomannan assay) using the sandwich enzyme-linked immunosorbent assay (ELISA) were successfully introduced into clinical practice for the early detection of invasive fungal infections (61,62). The sensitivity of these nonculture based detection methods has been high in some studies (61,63,64). Issues regarding variations in different PCR assays, reproducibility, false-positive results, and optimal sample source for detection of the fungal organism currently hinder the widespread utilization of these diagnostic tools. Similarly, extensive use of ELISA assays for the detection of galactomannan has been thwarted by a high frequency of false-positive results and, accordingly, a low positive predictive value (65,66).

5. *Invasive Procedures*

Fiberoptic bronchoscopy (FOB) with bronchoalveolar lavage (BAL) is increasingly used as the procedure of choice for the assessment of undiagnosed pulmonary infiltrates in cancer patients. Abundant studies have investigated the utility of BAL among immunocompromised hosts with pulmonary infiltrates and demonstrated diagnostic yields of 25–80% (67–72). Despite the inherent increased risks associated with invasive procedures in this group of patients, FOB is felt to be a safe procedure, even among mechanically ventilated patients and in the setting of thrombocytopenia and coagulopathy (70,73,74). The procedure may be used to identify a broad array of infectious and noninfectious diagnoses. In particular, the sensitivity of BAL in detecting organisms that have a high alveolar load (*Pneumocystis carinii, Mycobacteria, Histoplasma, CMV*, and other viruses) is quite high ($>80\%$) in published studies (75,76). Inconclusive results on analysis of BAL fluid, however, may not indicate absence of infection as prior antibiotic therapy may significantly diminish the sensitivity and specificity of bronchoscopically obtained quantitative cultures (77,78). An important exception to this concept is the absence of *Pneumocystis carinii* or mycobacteria on BAL fluid, in which case discontinuation of antimicrobial agents targeting these organisms may be warranted (75,76,79). Bronchoalveolar lavage with transbronchial biopsies is rarely performed in patients with hematologic malignancies, especially in the posttreatment setting for several reasons. Low platelet counts may be prohibitive for this procedure. Secondly, transbronchial biopsies have been found to be of only incremental value in the evaluation of these patients with suspected pneumonia over BAL alone (75,80–82). The utility of FOB with TBBx in the evaluation of suspected noninfectious pulmonary diagnoses is well established. Transbronchial biopsies may be helpful in the assessment of patients with suspected pulmonary diseases that require histologic confirmation, such as bronchiolitis obliterans with organizing pneumonia (BOOP), diffuse alveolar damage (DAD), or interstitial pneumonitis (IP). Thoracotomy with open-lung biopsy or thoracoscopic lung biopsy may be useful in some patients with hematologic malignancies and undiagnosed pulmonary infiltrates, especially those with focal abnormalities on chest radiographs. The yield of this procedure and impact on therapeutic decision making has been variable (32–82% and 28–69%, respectively) and appears to be lowest among mechanically ventilated patients with neutropenia, diffuse infiltrates, or recent pneumotoxic chemotherapy '(15,83). Etiologic diagnoses of focal lung lesions or pleural-based nodules or masses may also be amenable to percutaneous transthoracic needle aspiration or biopsy. Although the experience in this procedure among critically ill patients with hematologic malignancies is limited, its utility in the diagnosis of invasive fungal infections and malignancy is generally favorable (84).

E. Specific Pathogens

1. *Bacterial Infections*

Only those diverse causes of infectious and noninfectious pulmonary morbidity that frequently cause life-threatening disease will be considered in this section. Bacterial pneumonias caused by legionella, Nocardia, and mycobacterial organisms in the cancer setting frequently cause severe disease and are a common reason for ICU admission. These bacterial pneumonias, therefore, will be discussed separately.

Pneumonia is the most frequent source of infection encountered among patients with cancer. Although specific types of infection commonly reflect the ecology of the hospital, pneumonia caused by bacterial organisms remains the most common source of infection, especially during the early stages of immune exhaustion following chemotherapy. Bacterial pathogens account for the majority of all postobstructive pneumonias and up to half of all lung infections during the first 100 days posttransplantation (8,12,85,86). Fulminant pneumonias caused by gram-negative pathogens, including Pseudomonas and Enterobacteriaceae are common in this setting. Selection pressures induced by aggressive prophylactic strategies targeting gram-negative organisms during periods of severe neutropenia have resulted in a resurgence of *Streptococcus pneumonia*, *Staphylococcus* and a growing number of other gram-positive organisms as significant pulmonary pathogens (87). The widespread use of indwelling central venous catheters and mucosal excoriation associated with high-dose chemotherapy also contribute to the shift in the microbial spectrum of pulmonary pathogens in this setting (19,88,89). Sporadic emergence of multidrug resistant organisms, including methicillin-resistant *S. aureus* and pan-resistant *Stenotrophomonas maltophilia* species, have also been observed, owing in part to the use of broad-spectrum antibiotics in these patients. These infections are particularly recalcitrant to therapy and are associated with a poor outcome. Among those pneumonias caused by gram-negative bacteria, the source of infection is rarely identified. Infections cause by gram-positive organisms, however, as well as Enterobacter and Acinetobacter, can be frequently traced to an infectious nidus, such as an indwelling intravascular catheter. Removal of these catheters is critical to a successful outcome, especially in the setting of prolonged neutropenia or relapsed disease. Bacterial pneumonia caused by aspiration of gram-positive and anaerobic organisms is of particular concern in neutropenic patients requiring narcotic analgesics or those with oral mucositis. Mixed bacterial infections have also been increasingly isolated in the immunocompromised host. Neutropenic patients who receive prophylactic antibiotic coverage with trimethoprim/sufamethoxazole or fluoroquinolones are at higher risk for the development of streptococcal shock syndrome because of the less predictable coverage by these antibiotics against gram-positive organisms (90). Palmar desquamation, associated with a generalized rash, and rapidly progressive pneumonia are clues to the diagnosis of this frequently fatal disease (Fig. 2). Mortality rates for pneumonia caused by *S. viridans* in the neutropenic patient are, in fact, higher than any of the other gram-positive organisms. Both gram-positive and gram-negative pathogens may be realized as the dominant cause of late infections in HSCT patients with chronic GVHD.

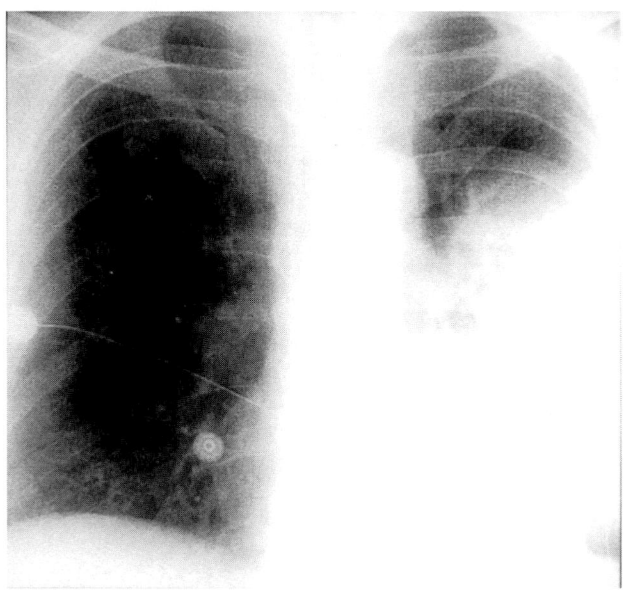

Figure 2 A 26-year-old woman with acute myelogenous leukemia and neutropenic fever who developed severe mucositis, dyspnea, and palmar desquamation following 3 weeks of quinolone prophylaxis after a hematopoietic stem cell transplantation. Cultures of BAL specimens grew *Streptococcus viridans*.

Pneumonia caused by bacteria in the setting of profound neutropenia defies all rules. Atypical presentations are common. The radiographic appearance of lobar consolidations typical of bacterial pneumonias is less common. Instead, bacterial pneumonias are often manifest by diffuse interstitial infiltrates or patchy areas of dense alveolar consolidation. Nodular lesions with or without cavitation have been described in infections caused by *Staphylococcus*, *Nocardia*, *Pseudomonas*, and fungal pathogens. Parapneumonic effusions are common. Fulminant infections occasionally present with negligible radiographic change in the setting of profound neutropenia. Minimal cough and low-grade fever may belie the seriousness of the disease. Furthermore, radiographic enhancement of pulmonary infiltrates despite appropriate therapy may occur coincident with neutrophil recovery.

Nocardia

Pulmonary nocardiosis is a clinically significant cause of infectious morbidity in the cancer patient. In a recent review, the incidence of pulmonary nocardiosis was 60 cases per 100,000 admissions to a major cancer center (91). The responsible organism, Nocardia, is a ubiquitous, slow growing actinomycetes fond in soil. Morphologic features include thin, branched filaments. Additional properties of partial acid-fast staining help to distinguish this opportunistic pathogen from other organisms (91,92). Patients with defects in cell-mediated immunity are at the highest risk for development of this disease. Hematopoietic stem cell and solid organ transplantation as well as a history of prolonged steroid administration and the use of other T-cell suppressive drugs, including tacrolimus, cyclosporin and fludarabine are recognized risk factors for the development of this disease. Comorbidities, including chronic lung disease, diabetes, splenectomy, alcoholism, end-stage renal disease, hypogammaglobulinemia, and GVHD add additional burdens of infection susceptibility. Whether GVHD facilitates the development of Nocardia directly or does so as a consequence of its attendant treatment with immunosuppressive therapy is unclear. Coinfections with *Aspergillus* species, *Pneumocystis carinii*, *CMV*, and other pathogens associated with impaired T-cell immunity are common (91,93,94). Neutropenia is not a common precursor and plays no significant role in the progression of this disease. While several species of Nocardia are capable of causing nocardiosis, *N. asteroides* is the most common and the most virulent pathogen. Nocardiosis primarily targets the lungs, although a variety of extrapulmonary manifestations of this disease are recognized. Extrapulmonary manifestations of nocardiosis, including cutaneous and soft tissue infections involving the pericardium, aorta, bones, kidneys and central nervous system may represent primary or disseminated disease. Nonproductive cough and fever are frequent symptoms of pulmonary disease, which typically develops over a 1–3 week period before diagnosis. Acute symptoms of pneumonia have also been reported among patients with severe immunosuppression. The classic radiographic pattern with nocardia pneumonia is a slowly progressive, nodular infiltrate, which may cavitate. Diffuse disease is associated with spread of infection to the central nervous system (CNS) and carries a poor prognosis. Diffuse multilobar infiltrates and slowly progressive nodular infiltrates are the major radiographic manifestations of the disease. Pulmonary abscess formation and pleural effusions have also been described. Nocardial empyema has been reported in up to 25% of patients (95). The clinical and radiographic manifestations of pulmonary nocardiosis may resemble *Mycobacterium tuberculosis*, however, fibrocavitary disease is less prominent in this disorder. The organism may be isolated in cultures of sputum, lung aspiration, or biopsy material. Colonies typically require 6–8 weeks for growth. Local spread from transcutaneous inoculation has been described as a complication of transtracheal aspiration. Isolation of *Nocardia* species from blood cultures is almost always associated with concomitant pulmonary disease or prosthetic valve endocarditis. Sulfonamides remain first-line therapy and may be given as single agents or in combination with beta-lactam or tetracycline antibiotics. Combination therapy with imipenem or amikacin plus a sulfa derivative provides bactericidal and bacteriostatic antimicrobial activity. Alternatively, treatment with amikacin, imipenem, cefuroxime, cefotaxime, or minocycline is a reasonable option for persons intolerant of sulfa drugs. Linezolid, a newer oxazoledinone, may also be used in combination with β-lactam antimicrobial agents with good response. Although the optimal duration of antimicrobial therapy has not been determined, prolonged antibiotic therapy (8–12 months) is favored in all patients to reduce the risk of disease relapse. Patients with severe immunosuppression or CNS disease may require more than 12 months of antibiotic therapy. The treatment of lung abscesses may be amenable to antibiotic therapy alone. A multimodality approach that utilizes surgical drainage and medical therapy, however, is occasionally indicated for the treatment of brain abscesses, soft tissue infections, and empyema. Mortality rates range from 5%–60% and vary with the degree of immune suppression, associated comorbidities, extent of disease, and timeliness of the diagnosis and therapy.

Legionella pneumophilia

Legionella species may cause life-threatening pneumonias, particularly in the immunocompromised host. The rapid development of ARDS leading to respiratory failure and death underscores the virulence of this pathogen (96–98). These fastidious, gram-negative organisms may be found in contaminated potable water systems, including water distribution systems and water-containing respiratory devices. Lower water temperatures (less than 60°C or 140°F), sediment accumulation, and the presence of commensal organisms play an important role in colonization of water distribution systems by *Legionella*. An increased predilection for *Legionella* pneumonia is associated with patients with chronic pulmonary disease, stem cell and organ transplantation, and patients with defects in cellular and humoral immunity. Certain types of cancers, such as hairy cell leukemia and head and neck malignancies, impose an increased infection risk for Legionella pneumonia. Patients with head and neck cancer have higher rates of cigarette smoking and an almost universal propensity for aspiration. A major mode of transmission is aspiration of contaminated water into the lower respiratory tract. Thus, patients with an increased propensity for aspiration, including head and neck cancer patients and patients with altered mental status have a higher risk for developing this disease.

L. pneumophilia is the *Legionella* species implicated in the overwhelming majority of pulmonary infections and is the responsible organism underlying both Pontiac fever and Legionnaire's disease. Unlike the self-limited flu-like symptoms that characterize Pontiac fever, Legionnaire's disease typically presents as a multisystem disorder with pneumonia as the predominant feature. Initial symptoms of Legionnaire's disease are indolent and nonspecific. Patients typically present with fever, malaise, lethargy, and generalized weakness after a 2–10 day incubation period.

High fever that is out of proportion to pulse rate has been reported in the literature, but the true incidence of this dissociation in unknown. The cough is initially dry but may become purulent or bloody as the disease progresses. Extrapulmonary symptoms, including nausea, vomiting, diarrhea, abdominal pain, headache, change in mental status, and pleuritic chest pain are frequent complaints and offer clues to the diagnosis. Bacteremic spread of disease may lead to pericarditis, endocarditis, sinusitis, pancreatitis, and cellulitis. Hyponatremia (serum sodium less than 130 mEq/L) occurs more frequently in Legionnaire's disease than in other types of pneumonia and connotes a poor prognosis. Severe disease is also associated with a constellation of other nonspecific findings, such as rash, rhabdomyolysis, disseminated intravascular coagulation, and peripheral neuropathy. The chest radiograph is heterogeneous and typically abnormal at the time of presentation (Fig. 3). Unilateral segmental or lobar alveolar opacities may give way to multilobar bilateral areas of consolidation as the disease progresses. Rapidly enlarging pulmonary nodules that progress to cavitation have also been described. Cavitation may occur in the setting of appropriate antibiotic therapy. Pleural effusions are common and may precede the development of parenchymal infiltrates. Abscess formation and pleural-based densities resembling pulmonary infarction are also common presentations.

The diagnosis of legionella is complicated by the overgrowth of commensal flora, which interferes with respiratory cultures. Culture of Legionella from enhanced culture media (buffered charcoal-yeast extract agar) may facilitate isolation of the organism and clinch the diagnosis. Legionella isolates have been detected in sputum, BAL fluid, blood, and soft tissues. Growth in culture may not become manifest for 3–5 days and culture-based delays in diagnosis and treatment are associated with sharp escalations in morbidity and mortality. Early detection may be provided by direct fluorescent antibody (DFA) staining of clinical specimens, indirect staining using enzyme-linked immunosorbent assays (ELISA) of serologic specimens, radioimmunoassay (RIA) of urine samples for soluble *L. pneumophilia* antigen, and radiolabeled DNA probes.

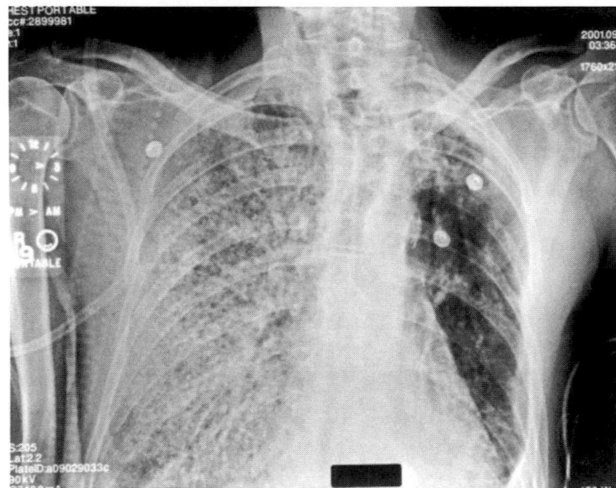

Figure 3 A 56-year-old man with laryngeal carcinoma who has been treated with prolonged systemic corticosteroids for severe COPD. The patient presented to the emergency room with fever, dry cough, and generalized weakness. DFA staining of BAL specimens was positive for *Legionella pneumophilia*.

Of these, DFA and RIA detection of urinary antigen are most widely used. *L. pneumophilia*, serogroup 1 is the pathogenic subtype that is responsible for more than 80% of Legionella infections. Antigen detection using DFA assay techniques reliably identifies this organism with sensitivities and specificities of 99% and 80%, respectively.

Monotherapy using quinolones (gemifloxacin, ofloxacin, levofloxacin, gatifloxacin, moxifloxacin, ciprofloxacin) or the newer macrolides (clarithromycin, azithromycin) remains the mainstay of therapy. The addition of rifampin to macrolide therapy may enhance the clinical efficacy of these drugs. Because of the potential for incomplete gastrointestinal absorption, initial drug therapy via the intravenous route is recommended. Three weeks of therapy are advocated, especially for severely immunosupressed patients. Delays in diagnosis and severe immunosuppression are two factors that adversely impact outcome, with mortality rates among this group of patients approaching 50%.

Mycobacterial Tuberculosis Pneumonia

Pneumonia caused by mycobacteria is increased in the cancer patient and the enriched predilection for disseminated disease among this group portends a poor prognosis. Increased rates of tuberculous (TB) and nontuberculous (NTB) mycobacterial pneumonia have been reported among patients with cancer (99–101). In particular, patients with head and neck cancers, lymphoproliferative disease, hairy cell leukemia, or chronic T-cell suppression related to cancer therapy are at highest risk for the development of active mycobacterial disease. Patients typically present with a subacute course, although disseminated disease may occur and tends to be rapidly fatal. Clinical and radiographic findings of protracted fever and cough, unexplained weight loss, and chest radiographs demonstrating upper lobe predominant disease or diffuse micronodular disease suggest the diagnosis (Fig. 4a–b). A nonproductive cough is characteristic, although blood-streaked hemoptysis is not unusual. Indirect evidence of mycobacterial infection may be derived from the PPD evaluation, which may be positive despite immunosuppression in 65% of patients (102). Definitive diagnosis can be derived from cultures and histology of BAL, protected brush specimens, transbronchial biopsies, or open-lung biopsy. Assays of respiratory tissue or secretions using polymerase chain reaction (PCR) techniques may expedite mycobacterial detection and advance early therapeutic strategies. Long-term, multidrug therapy is indicated. Depending on the characteristic mycobacterial sensitivities of the region in which

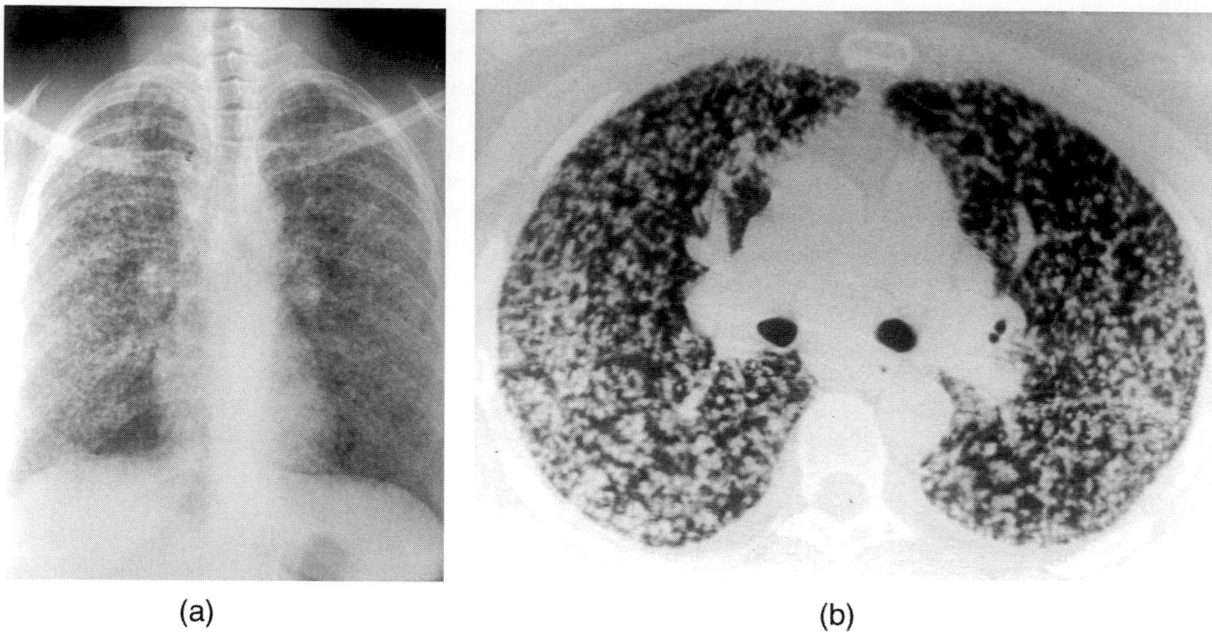

Figure 4 A 45-year-old Asian woman with progressive symptoms of dry cough, weight loss, low-grade fevers, and lethargy following an allogeneic hematopoietic stem cell transplantation for acute myelogenous leukemia. A chest radiograph (a) and CT scan (b) demonstrated extensive tiny nodular infiltrates. Postmortem analysis of lung and brain tissue was positive for *Mycobacteria tuberculosis.*

the patient lives, the patient may require quadruple antibiotic coverage to achieve adequate control of the disease. Unchecked infection owing to delays in diagnosis not only contributes substantially to fatal outcomes, but imparts significant infection risk to other patients and hospital personnel.

Nontuberculosis Mycobacterial Pneumonia

Among the NTB pneumonias, the most frequently encountered pathogens include *M. avium*–intracellulare complex (MAI), *M. cheloni*, and *M. kansasii*. Risk factors and clinical manifestations of NTB mimic those of TB. An insidious onset of low-grade fever, dry cough, and weight loss is typical. The spectrum of chest radiograph is abnormalities that range from normal studies to diffuse pulmonary involvement with cavitation. Bronchoscopy or open-lung biopsy is required for diagnosis. Like TB, a definitive diagnosis of NTB requires culture and histologic analysis of BAL or tissuesamples. Prolonged multiagent therapy is advocated for both MAI and *M. kansaii* pneumonias. Strategies to improve outcome among patients with MAI pneumonia include early diagnosis and multidrug therapy with a macrolide (clarithromycin or azithromycin), fluroquinolone (ciprofloxacin or ofloxacin), rifamycin (rifampin or rifabutin), plus clofazamine or ethambutol. The approach to *M. kansasii* is similar to M. TB. Successful treatment of either infection usually requires greater than 18 months of therapy.

2. Fungal Pneumonias

Of all of the types of infections caused by fungal pathogens, pneumonia is most common and the most virulent. The past decade has witnessed a resurgence of pathogenic fungal organisms causing intractable and often fatal pneumonias. This observation may relate, at least in part, to the parallel development of standard cancer treatment protocols that prolong the duration of neutropenia and the widespread use of aggressive antibiotic therapy for prophylaxis and established infections. Additional factors, including patient age, history of prior lung infection, presence of GVHD, and corticosteroid administration following marrow engraftment enhance the infection risk of fungal infection. Furthermore, successful efforts to reduce the toxicity of chemotherapy protocols place more patients at risk for the development of fungal infections who would have otherwise succumbed to the lethal complication of the drugs. Enhanced susceptibility to certain fungal pathogens in the setting of prolonged neutropenia is associated with the development of opportunistic fungal pneumonias caused by *Aspergillus, Candida, Mucoraceae* (*Mucormycosis, Rhizopus, Absidia*), *Fusaria and Cryptococcus.*

Prolonged neutropenia plays a critical pathogenic role in the development of invasive fungal infections. Reactivation of infections caused by *Histoplasma capsulatum*, *Coccidioides immitis*, *Paracoccidioides brasiliensis*, and *Blastomycoces dermatitidis* may occur especially among patients with cellular immunity. Both Candida and Aspergillus may colonize the proximal airway. Differentiation of colonization from infection by Aspergillus is based on the isolation of filamentous fungi in sputum or BAL fluid coupled with the clinical findings of neutropenic fever and lung infiltrates. This clinical scenario strongly supports the diagnosis of Aspergillus pneumonia and represents sufficient evidence to initiate treatment in most patients.

Candida Pneumonia

Candidal infections contribute substantially to the morbidity of recipients of certain types of chemotherapy and following stem cell transplantation. Current prophylaxis protocols, however, have diminished the incidence of *Candida* pneumonia and render fatal infections caused by this pathogen a relatively rare event (103,104). *Candida albicans* is the most common pathogenic Candidal species causing lung infection, although resistant *C. glabrata, C. tropicalis*, and *C. krusei* have been noted recently with increasing frequency (105). Both aspiration of upper airway contents and hematogenous dissemination from concomitant sources, such as the gastrointestinal or genitourinary tract, are common causes of Candidal pneumonia. Pure pneumonias caused by *Candida* are so rare that information regarding clinical and radiographic findings is culled from individual case reports and small retrospective studies (106,107). Micronodular lesions without an associated halo sign have been reported on chest radiographs. The diagnosis of *Candida* pneumonia should be considered among patients with progressive infiltrates unresponsive to antibiotic therapy and concomitant evidence of local invasion of the retina or mucosal surfaces of the gastrointestinal or genitourinary tracts. Frequent upper airway contamination by *Candida* confounds the diagnosis, which usually requires histopathologic evidence of tissue invasion for confirmation. In contrast to aspergillosis, skin and sinus involvement by *Candida* is unusual. The response to antifungal therapy with amphotericin B, lipid-complexed amphotericin B, and the triazole compounds has been variable.

Aspergillus Pneumonia

The most life-threatening fungal pneumonias in the cancer setting are those caused by invasive molds. Among these pathogens, *Aspergillus* is the most common and the most life threatening. Although more than 300 different species of *Aspergillus* have been described, the predominant species causing infection in humans include *A. niger*, *A. fumigatus*, *A. nidulans*, and *A. clavatus*. Recently, *A. versicolor* has been recognized as an emergent pathogen causing skin and lung lesions among patients with hematologic malignancies (108). A major risk factor cited in the development of *Aspergillus* pneumonia is prolonged neutropenia. Granulocyte counts of $<1 \times 10^9/L$ and lasting more than 7 days are associated with an increased risk. Higher granulocyte counts are not completely protective, especially in the setting of prolonged immunosuppression associated with corticosteroid administration, HSCT, and GVHD. Increased vulnerability is also seen among recipients of T-cell depleted marrow, presumably on the basis of associated delays in engraftment. The degree of immune suppression is a tenacious substrate for the development of Aspergillus infection. Thus, recipients of allogeneic stem cell transplants are at highest risk for the development this disease. Coinfection of *Aspergillus* with CMV disease has also been reported and may be explained in part by virus-induced granulocytopenia (109). Nosocomial dissemination via airborne contamination in buildings undergoing renovation or in contaminated air conditioning units represents major sources of *Aspergillus* infection and may cause outbreaks of this disease at single centers (110).

Patients typically present with nonspecific symptoms of fever, dry cough, and dyspnea. These symptoms, together with focal wheezing, hemoptysis, pleuritic chest pain, and a pleural friction rub are highly suggestive, although this constellation of symptoms is seen in only 30% of patients (16,43). A rapidly progressive hemorrhagic pneumonia with infarction and hemoptysis due to invasion of large blood vessels by *Aspergillus* may occur in some patients with fatal consequences. Blood-stream infection is also seen and heralds a poor prognosis. Extrathoracic sites of *Aspergillus* infection include the sinuses, skin, frontal cortex, or periorbital areas. These areas may occasionally represent sites of primary infection with secondary spread to the lungs. Skin lesions are characterized by concentrically enlarging nodules with central necrosis. Histologic assessment of biopsied skin lesions may yield the diagnosis. The spectrum of radiographic findings range from focal or diffuse infiltrates and nodules with or without cavitation to normal chest radiographs. The latter may be seen in the setting of severe neutropenia. Wedge-shaped pleural-based infiltrates consistent with the radiographic appearance of pulmonary infarction may also be seen. CT evidence of an air-crescent or halo sign is helpful in discriminating aspergillosis from other types of pneumonia (Fig. 5a). Bronchoscopic findings include pseudomembranes lining the bronchial mucosa and necrotic endobronchial disease (Fig. 5b–c). Pathologic changes include a necrotizing bronchopneumonia, tracheobronchitis, and sinopulmonary disease.

Histologic assessment of endobronchial and transbronchial biopsies may not be feasible because of prohibitive thrombocytopenia and the associated risk of bleeding and the vasotropic predilection of Aspergillus. Cytologic and microbiologic evaluation of BAL fluid is an effective diagnostic modality in patients with diffuse disease (111). False-negative results for Aspergillus on BAL fluid are seen in up to 30% of patients, however, presumably because the organism has invaded the interstitium. Although isolation of Aspergillus from sputum or BAL usually signals contamination in the normal host, detection of this organism in oral or airway secretions among severely immunosuppressed patients is usually sufficient to prove causation.

Early and aggressive therapy is indicated. Standard therapy includes intravenous amphotericin B or one of its liposomal derivatives. Liposomal preparations of amphotericin are less nephrotoxic and permit the use of larger doses of the drug (112,113). Caspofungin acetate (cancidas), a cell wall active echinocandin, was recently approved for the treatment of severe

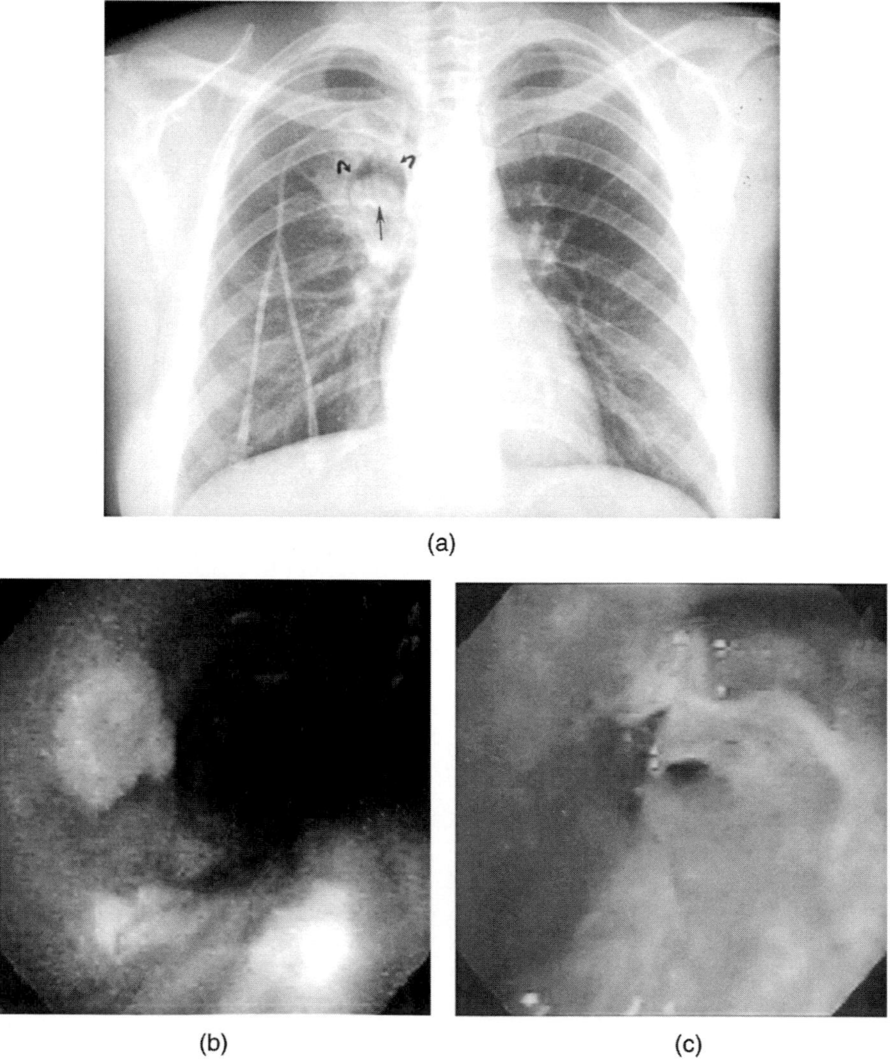

Figure 5 Prolonged neutropenia, dyspnea, and hemoptysis developed in a 29-year-old man following an allogeneic hematopoietic stem cell transplant. A chest radiograph (a) showed upper lobe cavitary lesion with a fungus ball (straight arrow) and an air crescent sign (curved arrows). Ulcerations (b) and pseudomembranes (c) were seen along the bronchial mucosa on bronchoscopic examination. Silver stains of BAL specimens were positive for *Aspergillus fumigatus*.

Aspergillus infections. The efficacy of azole compounds, such as itraconazole in the treatment of invasive aspergillosis, is currently being studied. The use of these agents in HSCT patients is limited due to unreliable enteral absorption (114). Voriconazole and posaconazole are two newer triazole antifungal agents that offer broad-spectrum activity against *Aspergillus* and other mold and yeast infections. Posaconazole has been held promise in the treatment of invasive fungal infections that are refractory to standard antifungal therapy. Despite aggressive therapy, the outcome of patients with established disease remains disappointing. The role of prevention in mitigating disease should not be overlooked. Preventive measures, such as the use of laminar airflow and HEPA filtration in patient rooms, have been shown to be highly protective in lowering the incidence of invasive aspergillus in the HSCT population. The benefit of prophylactic and preemptive strategies against *Aspergillus* using lipid complex Amphothericin B, itraconazole, the newer azoles and echinocandins in reducing mortality remains undefined. The utility of granulocyte transfusion in the treatment of neutropenia-related *Aspergillus* infection and other fungal diseases has not been definitively proven (115–117).

Other Invasive Mycoses

Other invasive mycoses, including *Fusaria* and *Mucormycoses*, *Pseudoallescheria boydii*, *Penicillium*, *Cladosporium, and Tricosporum* may cause recalcitrant and frequently fatal pneumonias. Patients at risk for the development of pneumonia caused by one of these organisms include those with leukemia, lymphoma, severe neutropenia, and patients with a history of prolonged corticosteroid therapy. The clinical and radiographic appearance of fusaria pneumonia may mimic aspergillosis. Concomitant involvement of the sinuses and skin and a predilection for vascular infarction and dissemination is common. Radiographic changes are nonspecific and identification of filamentous fungi in blood cultures or observation of subcutaneous nodules on physical examination suggests the diagnosis. The prognosis is dismal despite aggressive antifungal therapy. *Mucormycoses*, a zygomycetes, is a ubiquitous, broad-based fungus found in soil. Of the three clinical syndromes associated with mucormycoses (rhinocerebral, pulmonary, and gastrointestinal mucormycosis), pulmonary manifestations of this disease are the most life threatening. Pulmonary mucormycosis is transmitted by inhalation of spores by a susceptible host. Patients at highest risk for this form of the disease include those with leukemia, lymphoma, and those posttransplantation. The risk and severity of invasive mucormycosis is enhanced by prior deferoxamine therapy (118). The clinical presentation resembles invasive aspergillosis and includes fever and hemoptysis. Diffuse pneumonia with infarction and necrosis may rapidly progress to ARDS and death. Extrapulmonary disease may be caused by local spread of infection to contiguous structures, such as the heart and mediastinum as well as hematogenous spread to the brain. Surgical resection of early pulmonary infection may be curative, but is usually not a therapeutic option as most patients present with advanced multilobar disease. Medical therapy includes amphotericin B or its liposomal derivatives. The prognosis is poor. Mortality rates of 80% are unchanged over the years despite aggressive therapy.

Pneumocytis carinii Pneumonia

The institution of aggressive prophylactic protocols against pneumocytis carinii pneumonia (PCP) as standard therapy among cancer and HSCT patients has resulted in a dramatic decline in the incidence of PCP in this patient population. Susceptibility profiles for this disease include patients with lymphoproliferative disorders, HSCT recipients, and those receiving prolonged courses of high-dose corticosteroids. *Pneumocytis carinii* pneumonia among patients with solid tumors in the absence of other risk factors is unusual. The incidence of PCP is reported in less than 10% of patients following HSCT (43,119). Patients who are noncompliant with prophylactic therapy or those with allergies to sulfa drugs are at the highest risk for the development of this disease, which typically occurs more than 2 months after HSCT.

Patients characteristically present with an insidious onset of fever, nonproductive cough, dyspnea, and cyanosis. Occasionally, an acute fulminant course is seen in the posttransplant patient and among patients with a concomitant diagnosis of AIDS. Laboratory evidence of elevated lactate dehydrogenase, angiotensin-converting enzyme levels, fibrinogen levels, and erythrocyte sedimentation rate are nonspecific but supportive findings. Normal chest radiographs in the face of profound hypoxia are not uncommon. Alternatively, patients may present with minimal symptoms and grossly abnormal chest radiographs. A broad array of radiographic changes have been reported, including perihilar infiltrates, nodular densities, cavitation, lobar distribution, abscess formation, and spontaneous pneumothorax (Fig. 6a).

Unilateral predominance of disease and diffuse alveolar consolidation has also been described. Predominantly upper-lobe infiltrates mimicking tuberculosis are common in patients receiving aerosolized pentamidine prophylaxis. Air bronchograms may be seen in

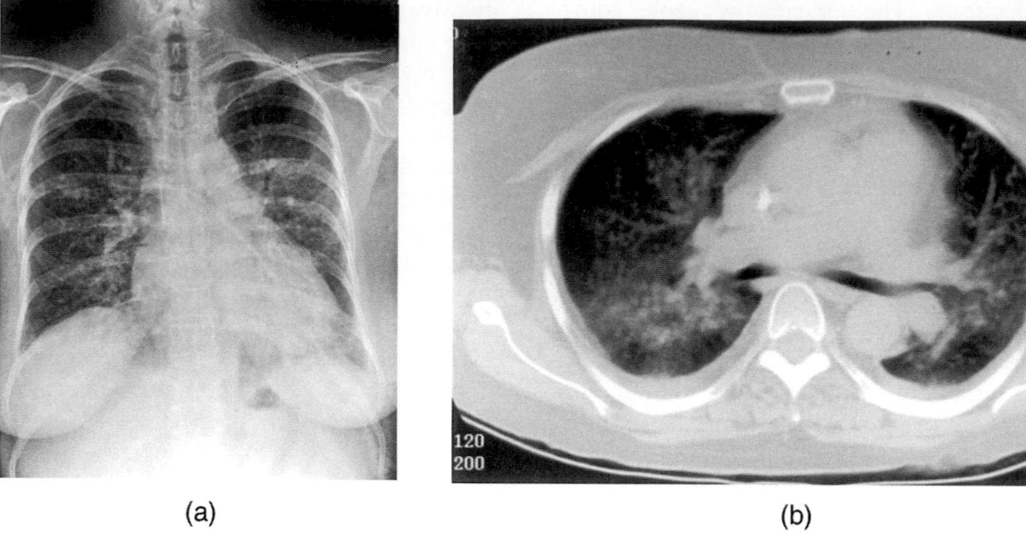

(a) (b)

Figure 6 Progressive dyspnea and dry cough developed 6 months following an allogeneic stem cell transplant from a matched unrelated donor. Bilateral diffuse infiltrates were noted on chest radiograph (a). Patchy areas of consolidation and ground-glass opacification with bilateral small effusions were seen on chest CT (b) Cytologic examination of BAL fluid revealed clusters of trophozoites and cysts, consistent with *Pneumocystis carinii* pneumonia.

more than half of the patients (43,119). Diffuse ground-glass attenuations on CT examination should heighten suspicion for PCP in the appropriate clinical setting (Fig. 6b). Cytologic or histologic analysis of respiratory secretions or biopsy tissue demonstrating evidence of intracytoplasmic cysts and trophozoites establishes the diagnosis. In patients with PCP and AIDS-related malignancies, the burden of infection is usually so large that BAL analysis is virtually always positive. In this subgroup of patients, examination of expectorated sputum induced with hypertonic saline is frequently diagnostic (120,121).

TMP-SMX dosed at 20 mg/kg/day of the TMP component is the mainstay of therapy. Intravenous pentamidine is appropriate therapy for patients with histories of allergy to sulfa-containing medications. Adjuvant corticosteroid therapy has proven efficacy in reducing inflammation and improving hypoxemia, azotemia, hypoglycemia, abnormalities of liver function, and rash. Severe bronchospasm has been reported with aerosolized pentamidine therapy. Other treatment options for mild-to-moderate disease include atovaquone, trimetrexate, or combined therapy with dapsone-TMP or clindamycin-primaquine. A high level of suspicion and early institution of therapy are pivotal to a successful outcome. Delayed therapy and untreated disease are almost uniformly fatal among immunocompromised patients. Because of the added infectious burden associated with *Pneumocystis carinii* and prolonged steroid therapy, PCP prophylaxis is recommended for this group of patients (122).

3. Viral Pneumonias

Viral infections caused by members of the Herpesviridae family (*HSV, CMV, EBV, VZV, human herpesvirus-6*), Measles virus, *Influenza* virus, respiratory syncytial virus, and adenovirus may cause disabling and rapidly fatal infections among patients with malignancy and among HSCT recipients (123,124). Suppressed immunity associated with HSCT, GVHD, and administration of T-cell suppressive therapies are well-defined risk factors. Viral infections threaten the success of 35–50% of HSCT recipients, usually within the first year of the transplant and the emergence of particular viral pathogens follows a fairly predictable timetable that closely correlates with the evolution of immune recovery following the transplant. Viral infections in cancer patients overwhelmingly reflect reactivation of latent disease. Seasonal variations of community acquired viral pneumonias caused by RSV and *Influenza* are seen in temperate regions. Common presentations of most viruses include symptoms suggestive of upper respiratory infection coupled with progressive, bilateral interstitial infiltrates on chest radiographs. Approximately 10% of affected patients develop disseminated disease with the gastrointestinal tract, lungs, brain, and liver being most frequently involved. Viral organisms have an early predilection for the distal airways, which correlates radiographically with patchy areas of centrilobular nodules, ground-glass attenuation and air-space consolidation on CT scan examinations. Bronchiolitis may also complicate the disease. Pathologic and radiographic correlates of this complication include epithelial necrosis and hyperinflation, respectively (125,126). The diagnosis of viral pneumonia often rests on the results of viral cultures. The adequacy of clinical airway samples as well as delay in transport may facilitate the overgrowth of competing bacterial and fungal organisms that frequently coexist in the lower airway, and impede the growth of viruses in culture. Thus, the incidence of viral pneumonia may be underestimated. Newer diagnostic techniques, such as immunohistochemistry, polymerase chain reaction, and in situ hybridization, have recently emerged as diagnostic tools of value in the early detection of viral infections.

Cytomegaloviral Pneumonia

Cytomegalovirus, a member of the herpes family of viruses, is an important cause of intractable pneumonitis in immunocompromised patients (127,128). Disordered immune response not only underlies the development of CMV pneumonia, but strong inferential evidence suggests that the immune response to CMV is pivotal in limiting dissemination of the virus following reactivation (129). Thus, recipients of stem cell and solid organ transplants are at the highest risk of developing a variety of infectious and noninfectious complications of CMV infection. Increased rates of CMV pneumonitis correlate with the intensity of the preconditioning regimen and the use of cytotoxic and T-cell immunosuppressive agents (methotrexate, OKT3, antithymocyte globulin, cyclosporin, tacrolimus) (130,131). Pretransplant conditioning regimens that include high-dose radiation, and pretransplant seropositivity for CMV also strongly influence the emergence of CMV pneumonitis (43,127,132). The presence of GVHD also contributes to CMV-related lung injury among HSCT recipients. Interestingly, CMV pneumonitis is rarely seen among patients with AIDS, suggesting that factors in addition to immunosuppression contribute to its occurrence in the posttransplant population. Anecdotal evidence, citing the capacity of CMV to modulate the expression of MHC molecules, cytokines, and natural killer (NK) cells, suggests that CMV infection is inherently immunosuppressive (133,134). A causal relationship between CMV and immunosuppression, however, has not been definitively proven because of the frequent coexistence of multiple variables acting simultaneously with CMV, such as preexisting immunosuppression owing to immunosuppressive drugs or other diseases (cancer, GVHD). Reactivation of latent disease represents the predominant source of CMV infection, although nosocomial acquisition through the use of infected blood or blood products or the transplanted organ occasionally occurs (135–140). This property of latency and reactivation is seen among all the herpesviruses and the balance of evidence suggests that CMV is carried in myeloid lineage progenitor cells of the bone marrow where latency and reactivation are felt to occur (141). It is worth pointing out that the virus is excreted in saliva, breast milk, urine, semen, and cervical secretions, suggesting that CMV persists in epithelial cells. Whether epithelial cells are a site of virus latency, however, has not been clearly established. Primary disease may rarely occur among seronegative patients and, in general, causes more severe disease (142).

CMV-related pneumonitis is the most frequent and the most serious manifestation of CMV disease in the posttransplant population. Although the virus may target a variety of organ systems, the apparent tropism of CMV for the lung may explain the higher rates of CMV pneumonitis in this group of patients vs. other clinical manifestations of the disease. Approximately one-third of patients with serologic evidence of CMV infection develop clinical syndromes of CMV disease. Clinical syndromes attributable to CMV include fever, hypoxia, pneumonitis, gastrointestinal ulcerations, leukopenia, atypical lymphocytosis, hepatitis, and arthritis. CMV pneumonitis may have an insidious or explosive onset that typically includes fever, malaise, hypoxia, dyspnea, and dry cough. Effective prophylaxis and preemptive treatment have resulted in a marked reduction in the rates of CMV pneumonitis. Currently, CMV pneumonitis complicates 12–20% of HSCT (49,143). The period of highest susceptibility is usually 6–12 weeks following transplantation. Radiographic changes are nonspecific and include diffuse interstitial infiltrates (Fig. 7). CT findings typically include mixed alveolar-interstitial infiltrates, such as ground-glass attenuation, consolidation, thickened interlobular septa, and bronchial dilation. Ground-glass attenuation typically results from hemorrhage, neutrophilic and fibrinous exudates, or hyaline membrane formation. Nodule formation, corresponding histopathologically to areas of inflammation or hemorrhage, has also been reported. The diagnosis is suggested by isolation of CMV from cultures of peripheral blood buffy coat. Findings of intranuclear inclusion bodies or cytomegalic cells within areas of inflammation and alveolar damage on sputum or BAL cytopathology or lung biopsy specimens are pathognomonic for CMV infection. The clinical utility of novel diagnostic strategies including the use of nucleic acid probes and amplification methods, such as PCR, is currently under investigation.

Early and aggressive therapy is critical to a successful outcome. Standard therapy for established disease

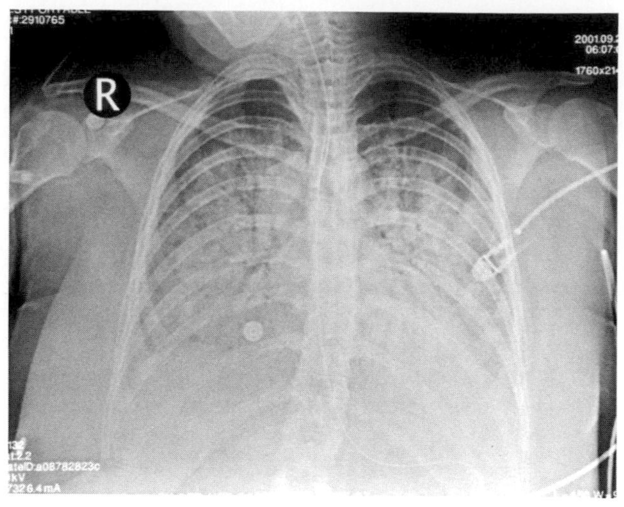

Figure 7 A 22-year-old woman who underwent an allogeneic hematopoietic stem cell transplantation, complicated by acute graft-versus-host disease and respiratory failure 2 months following transplantation. A chest radiograph demonstrated dense bilateral alveolar consolidation. *Cytomegalovirus* was confirmed on shell vial assay of BAL fluid.

includes combined treatment with intravenous gancyclovir together with immune globulin. Foscarnet, an inorganic pyrophosphate, has clinical efficacy against CMV disease that is equivalent to gancyclovir and represents a reasonable alternative in some patients. The extent of lung injury parallels CMV viral load in the blood and also dictates the length of therapy. Three to six-week therapy is usually indicated for treatment of established disease. Approximately 4–20% of HSCT recipients develop severe necrotizing pneumonitis leading to respiratory failure despite preemptive therapy. Antiviral therapy is woefully inadequate once respiratory failure occurs, and mortality rates are as high as 80–90% among this group of patients (127,144–146). The efficacy of risk-reduction strategies aimed at lowering the morbidity and mortality of CMV disease in the posttransplant period is well established (136,147). These strategies include adherence to stringent donor selection criteria, GVHD management, antiviral prophylaxis, and the use of CMV negative or irradiated blood products. A consensus on the optimal preventive antiviral regimen has not been unequivocally established. Questions regarding patient selection for CMV prophylaxis and duration of therapy remain. Nevertheless, gancyclovir is most frequently given as preventive therapy, usually during the first 1–3 months following transplantation and has resulted in significant reduction in the development of this disease. The success of these therapies is limited in part by drug toxicity. Drug-induced marrow suppression prompts discontinuation of gancyclovir in up to 40% of patients, often as early as 2 weeks into therapy. Emerging reports of resistant organisms following prolonged therapy with gancyclovir are also a concern (137,148). Foscarnet is also associated with significant side effects, including CNS disease, metabolic abnormalities, and dose-limiting nephropathy which limit the use of this drug. Foscarnet is currently available only as an intravenous formulation, which also hampers widespread use of this drug.

Herpes Simplex Virus (HSV) Pneumonia

Herpes simplex virus causes a variety of infections that typically target mucocutaneous surfaces and the central nervous system. Visceral involvement, including the lungs, occasionally occurs. HSV-related pulmonary injury typically occurs in the setting of severe immunosuppression or proximal airway trauma caused by intubation or smoke inhalation from burns or chronic cigarette smoke. These factors may facilitate lower respiratory tract infection with HSV by promoting squamous metaplasia. Recipients of HSCT are at increased risk for the development of HSV-related infections. Pneumonia in this group of patients tends to occur early (7–21 days following transplantation) and coincides with the period of posttransplant neutropenia. HSV-related gingivostomatitis is common among HSCT recipients. Associated pneumonias, however, are rare and cultures of HSV from the oropharynx do not automatically denote causality. The pathogenesis of HSV pneumonia is unclear. Reactivation of latent virus, possibly from the sensory ganglia most likely, plays a major role. The virus may be shed into the oropharynx and subsequently aspirated into the lower respiratory tract. Hematogenous spread of HSV infection among patients with sepsis has also been proposed (41,149,150). Polymicrobial infections are frequent with HSV pneumonias. Patients are typically coinfected with bacterial organisms. At bronchoscopy, the tracheobronchial epithelium may be lined with focal or diffuse ulcerations. The histopathologic correlates of these lesions include epithelial and alveolar necrosis and ulcerations with a variable polymorphonuclear inflammatory response (151). Until recently, definitive diagnosis required identification of HSV in BAL fluid by culture or positive hematoxylin and eosin (H&E) stains for viral inclusion bodies on BAL or lung tissue. PCR for HSV DNA and immunostaining of nuclear and cytoplasmic inclusion bodies have recently emerged as valuable diagnostic tools. These important diagnostic advances permit earlier detection of HSV with high sensitivity and specificity and offer the possibility of earlier treatment

(152,153). Presently issues regarding approval by the Food and Drug Administration for the routine use of PCR in the diagnosis of pneumonia hamper its widespread use. Other factors, such as the specificity, reproducibility, and optimal sample types for PCR, also require further investigation before this tool becomes part of the standard diagnostic armamentarium in the evaluation of pneumonia. Chest radiographs are almost always abnormal. A positive BAL for HSV in the setting of a normal chest radiograph most likely represents oropharyngeal contamination of the BAL sample rather than true disease. Common radiographic findings include bilateral opacities with an airspace or mixed airspace and diffuse interstitial pattern (Fig. 8) (142,150,154,155). Characteristic changes on CT include multifocal segmental or subsegmental areas of ground-glass attenuation. Associated pleural effusions are common. ARDS frequently occurs in the setting of HSV pneumonia (92,155). The radiographic appearance of ARDS mimics that of HSV pneumonia and confounds the diagnosis. Furthermore, the appearance of ARDS is a strong predictor of poor outcome. Mortality rates are high among patients with full-blown disease and patients with associated ARDS. Intravenous acyclovir remains the antiviral treatment of choice for established disease. The use of acyclovir as standard HSV prophylaxis during the neutropenic phase of HSCT has greatly reduced the incidence of disease following transplantation (156–158).

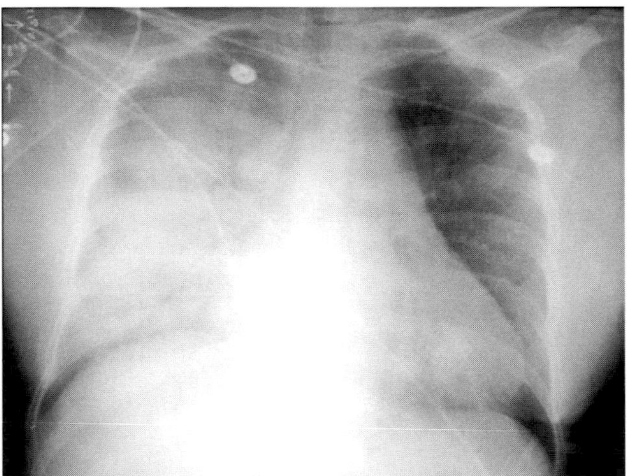

Figure 8 A 32-year-old male who presented with dry cough and severe dyspnea 3 weeks following an allogeneic transplant for treatment of acute leukemia. Postmortem examination of lung tissue revealed intranuclear inclusion bodies, consistent with *Herpes simplex* pneumonia.

Varicella Zoster (VZV) Pneumonia

Varicella zoster viral infection, a typically benign self-limiting disease in children, may cause fatal pneumonia in susceptible adults. Susceptibility profiles for VZV pneumonia include patients with lymphoproliferative disease and patients with altered cell-mediated immunity. These two risk factors are seen among 90% of patients with VZV pneumonia (159,160). Unlike HSV-1 pneumonia, pneumonia caused by VZV typically occurs as a late infection among allogenic transplant recipients, usually between 3 months and 1 year after transplantation and correlates with the period of most severe cellular immune deficiency. VZV in the transplant recipient may present as primary infection, or more commonly, as reactivation of latent disease. Disease reactivation typically is manifested clinically as localized shingles. Visceral involvement of disseminated disease to the skin, lungs, brain, and liver are poor prognosticators. Disease dissemination typically occurs during or 2–3 days after the appearance of a vesicular rash (161). Nonspecific symptoms of high fever, dry cough, dyspnea, pleuritic chest pain, and occasionally hemoptysis signal lung involvement by VZV. Pulmonary lesions appear coincident with the period of cutaneous dissemination and the characteristic rash of VZV is helpful in establishing the diagnosis. Furthermore, scrapings of the cutaneous lesions offer an opportunity for rapid diagnostic confirmation. Chest radiographic findings consist of extensive tiny (5–10 mm) nodular and interstitial infiltrates in a peribronchial distribution. Resolution of the nodules within a week following the disappearance of the skin lesions is typical, although in widespread disease they may persist for months. Persistent lesions typically calcify and may appear as numerous, well-circumscribed, tiny calcified nodules on subsequent films. Coalescence of nodules and ground-glass opacity may be seen on CT scan examinations of the chest. Pleural effusions and hilar adenopathy are rare. The appearance of GVHD confers an increased risk of VZV infection and facilitates the development of disseminated disease (160). Prophylactic antiviral therapy with acyclovir or gancyclovir reduces the risk of VZV reactivation, but only during the period of administration. Extending the period of prophylaxis until effective cellular immunity is established may abrogate excess susceptibility to VZV reactivation and reduce the sequelae of this disease. Intravenous acyclovir is frequently used for treatment of established VZV pneumonia, although no prospective clinical trials documenting the efficacy of this drug in this setting are available. Mortality remains high among HSCT recipients despite aggressive therapy.

Human Herpesvirus-6 (HHV-6)

Primary HHV-6 infection causes exanthem subitum, a self-limited febrile illness of infancy. Reactivated disease, however, is inherently immunosuppressive and is associated with a spectrum of clinical, biological, and molecular activities that mimic CMV. Human herpesvirus-6 is a DNA virus that is seen primarily among hematopoietic and solid tumor transplant recipients, and among patients with AIDS and lymphoproliferative disorders. Two distinct variants (variants A and B) exist. Variant B is responsible for most of the HHV-related disease that occurs in humans (162). The clinical sequelae of HHV-6 include interstitial pneumonitis, encelphalitis, and a skin rash resembling GVHD. Pneumonitis secondary to HHV-6 among HSCT recipients typically occurs within the first 2–3 weeks following transplantation. Patients typically present with dry cough, dyspnea, and interstitial infiltrates on chest radiographs. The pathogenic role of this virus in the development of pulmonary disease is not well understood. The presence of GVHD appears to be a significant risk factor for the development of HHV-6-related disease. Clinical manifestations of fever, encephalitis, and rash may suggest the diagnosis. Adequate therapy for HHV-6 is not available. Acyclovir and other thymidine kinase-dependent drugs demonstrate only marginal efficacy against HHV-6 in in vitro studies. Limited experience with ribavirin and foscarnet suggest that these agents may have some therapeutic efficacy against this infection (163).

Respiratory Syncytial Virus (RSV)

T-cell deficiency confers an increased risk for the development of RSV pneumonia. Hence, RSV pneumonia is seen with increased frequency among recipients of hematopoietic and solid organ transplants, as well as patients on chronic steroid and other T-cell suppressive therapy. The immediate postengraftment phase is the period of highest vulnerability following HSCT. Epidemic peaks of RSV infection typically occur between October and March in the United States. Transmission of infection is typically by direct contact of infected nasopharyngeal or ocular mucous membranes. Person to person spread by aerosolized droplets has been occasionally documented. Childhood infection with RSV is nearly universal; however, this does not protect adult patients from reinfection. Symptoms of upper respiratory infection—coryza, sinusitis, fever, cough—predominate during the early phase of the disease. The development of lower respiratory tract infection is heralded by the development of severe dyspnea associated with signs and symptoms suggestive of bronchiolitis or pneumonia. Chest radiographic findings commonly reveal bilateral interstitial infiltrates, indistinguishable from pneumonitis secondary to other causes. Symptoms may rapidly deteriorate to respiratory failure in the HSCT patient and mortality rates among this group of patients are high. The clinical presentation of *Influenza* as well as *Parainfluenza* viral pneumonia resembles that of RSV. The year-round appearance of *Parainfluenza* viral pneumonia may help to distinguish this infection from RSV-related pneumonia. Diagnostic strategies include viral cultures, immunofluorescent staining, antigen testing, or direct tissue examination. Standard treatment with aerosolized ribavirin and intravenous immune globulin (IVIG) may improve outcome if administered early, before the onset of respiratory failure (164,165).

Adenovirus

Adenovirus, a common cause of self-limited upper respiratory tract symptoms in children, may cause fulminant pneumonia in immunocompromised adults. Pneumonia owing to adenovirus is well described among HSCT recipients. Although reactivation of latent adenovirus and asymptomatic viral shedding into the stool or urine is almost universal following HSCT, active adenoviral disease among this group of patients has only been documented in 0.9–6.5% of patients (166,167). Recipients of T-cell-depleted bone marrow grafts have a higher risk of developing adenoviral infections. Adenoviral pneumonitis typically complicates HSCT during the immediate postengraftment period. Graft-versus-host disease represents a dominant risk factor for the development of adenoviral disease. The clinical spectrum of adenoviral disease is broad and varies from hepatitis, hemorrhagic cystitis, meningoencephalitis, myocarditis, tubulointerstitial nephritis, hemorrhagic colitis, and disseminated intravascular coagulation. Mortality rates of disseminated adenoviral infection exceed 50%. Viral inclusions, including "Cowdry A" or smudge cells, are two types of intranuclear adenoviral inclusions that are seen on cytologic analysis. These nuclear changes must be distinguished from those of HSV and CMV and from the cytopathic changes that occur secondary to reparative epithelial atypia, which often mimics adenoviral inclusions. Optimal therapy for this disease is not well defined. Various antiviral regimens have been tried with variable results.

Other Viral Pneumonias

Acute respiratory illnesses caused by Influenza A or B has been documented worldwide. Outbreaks of influenza are predominantly seen in the winter months and are characterized by malaise, fever, headache, and myalgia coupled with signs and symptoms of upper and lower respiratory tract infections. Pneumonia is the most frequent complication of influenza. Influenza type A most commonly underlies influenza pneumonia, although occasionally type B organisms are detected as the responsible culprit. Immunocompromised and elderly persons are at highest risk for the development of influenza pneumonia, which is often rapidly fatal among this group of patients. Among HSCT recipients, the incidence of influenza viral pneumonia is highest during the immediate postengraftment period. Nonspecific parenchymal opacities, interstitial infiltrates, and ground-glass attenuation may be observed on chest radiographs. Pleural effusions and hilar adenopathy are unusual findings. Parainfluenza virus is an RNA virus belonging to the genus paramyxovirus. These viruses occasionally cause fatal pneumonia in the immunocompromised host. Like Influenza- and CMV-related pneumonias, pneumonias caused by *Parainfluenza* virus also target the elderly and the immunocompromised host. Prodromal symptoms of fever, malaise, and upper respiratory tract illness caused by *Parainfluenza* virus are similar to those of other viral illnesses, including *Influenza, Adenovirus*, and RSV. Furthermore, similarities in clinical and radiographic features and patient susceptibility profiles among these viruses further confound the diagnosis of parainfluenza pneumonia. In contrast to the seasonal fluctuation in infections caused by RSV and *Influenza* virus, infections caused by *Parainfluenza* virus, may occur at any time during the year. The prognosis of fulminant pneumonia attributable to *Influenza* or *Parainfluenza* is poor. Antiviral interventions, including the use of aerosolized ribavirin and the newer neuraminidase inhibitors, are advocated in the treatment of *Parainflueza* pneumonia; however, their clinical benefit has not been clearly established.

F. Management of Neutropenia in the High-Risk Patient with Unexplained Fever

Untreated, infections in the setting of neutropenia may be rapidly fatal. Thus, all neutropenic patients with fever or clinical findings suggestive of infection should be promptly started on empiric antimicrobial therapy. Practice guidelines for the empiric treatment of the neutropenic cancer patient with unexplained fever have been established by the Infectious Disease Society of America (IDSA) in collaboration with the Neutropenia Guidelines Panel (168). These documents are updated regularly and provide evidence-based recommendations that are primarily derived from the treatment of patients with hematopoietic and lymphoproliferative malignancies, but may be applied to neutropenic febrile states associated with other neoplastic diseases as well. The IDSA guidelines are general recommendations that only provide an antibiotic template in the management of neutropenic fever. Factors such as the predominant nosocomial organism and resistance patterns of a particular hospital, underlying cause of neutropenia, anticipated time of hematopoietic recovery, previous microbial isolates from infected sites and any prior antibiotic regimen that the patient may have recently received should be considered in making antibiotic selections. Clinical risk-index scores may be used to stratify patients according to low, intermediate, and high-risk categories for severe infections. Clinical features, such as mucositis, protracted neutropenia, comorbid illnesses, and unstable signs and symptoms define the high-risk patient (169,170) (Table 6).

Antibiotic recommendations for the high-risk patient subgroup are shown in Fig. 9 and are based on the perceived need for vancomycin (Table 7). These schemes include monotherapy, two-drug therapy without a glycopeptide (vancomycin) and one- or two-drug therapy with a glycopeptide (vancomycin). If vancomycin is indicated, it should be given in combination with a carbapenam (imipenam-cilastin, merapenam) or a third or fourth generation cephalosporin (cefipime, ceftazidine), with or without an aminoglycoside. The need for continued vancomycin therapy should be assessed following 24–48 hr of therapy and discontinued if no vancomycin susceptible organism

Table 6 Risk Stratification for Severe Infection Among Neutropenic Patients

Low risk
Duration of neutropenia < 5 days
Absence of any high-risk factors
Intermediate risk
Duration of neutropenia 5–9 days
High risk
Duration of neutropenia > 10 days
Medical conditions associated with high risk for severe infection
1. Hypotension (systolic blood pressure < 90 mmHg or need for vasopressor support)
2. Respiratory failure
3. Need for ICU care
4. Disseminated intravascular coagulation
5. Severe bleeding requiring blood product support
6. Multiorgan system dysfunction including
Neurologic (confusion, altered mental status)
Renal (need for dialysis or other intervention)
Cardiac (arrhythmias or other EKG changes requiring treatment, congestive heart failure)

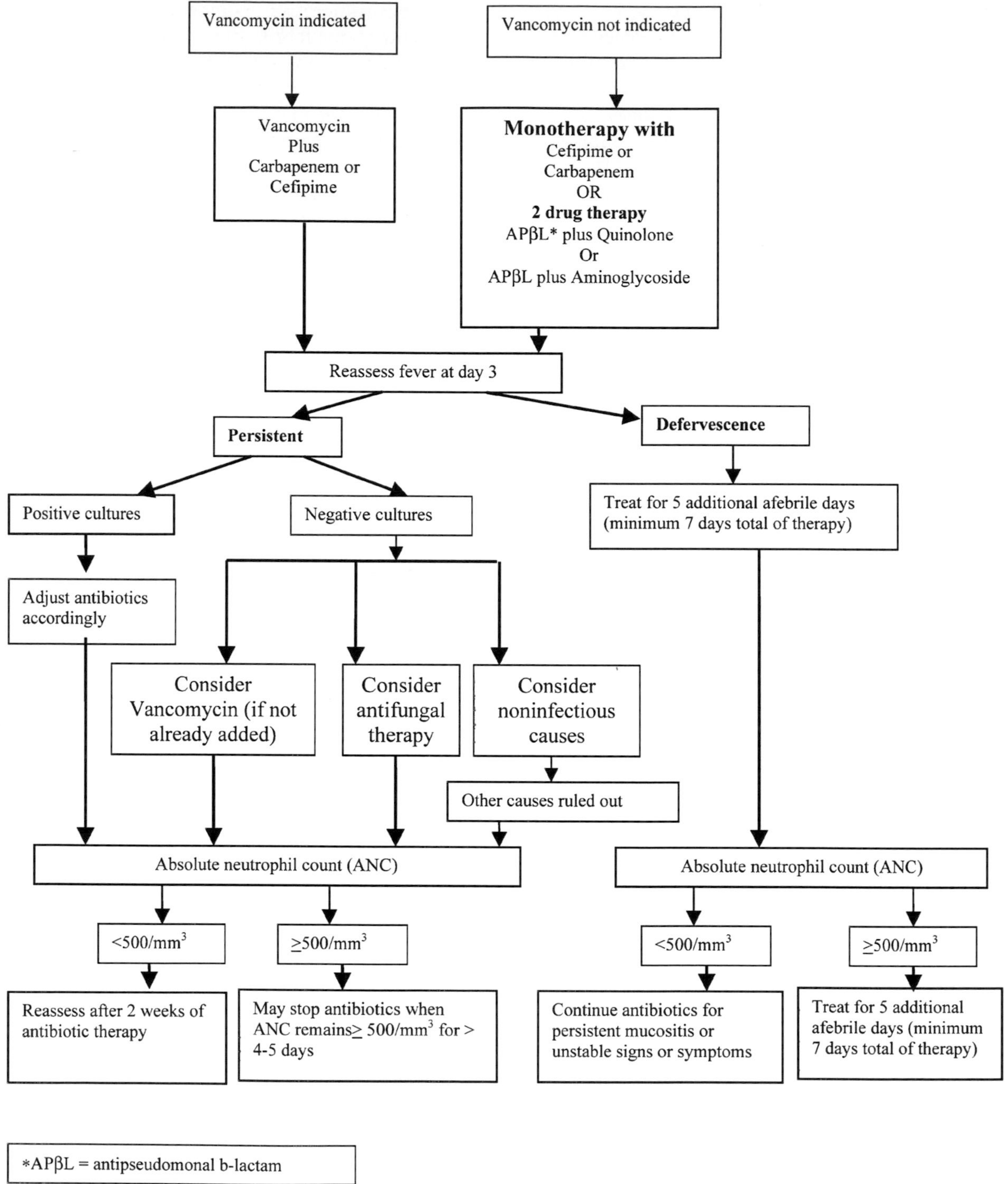

Figure 9 Guidelines for the treatment of febrile neutropenic fever in high risk patients.

is identified. Linezolid, the first Food and Drug administration (FDA)-approved oxazoledinone, and synercid are reasonable alternatives for the treatment of some gram-positive bacterial infections, including vancomycin-resistant enterococci.

Monotherapy or two-drug therapy without a glycopetide is recommended in the absence of a perceived need for vancomycin. Several studies have shown equivalent efficacy in the use of monotherapy vs. multiagent combinations for the management of the

Table 7 Indications for Vancomycin in the Treatment of High-Risk Patients with Neutropenic Fever

1. Known colonization with penicillin- or cephalosporin-resistant pneumococci or methicillin resistant *S. aureus*
2. Suspected serious catheter-related infection
3. Positive blood cultures for gram-positive bacteria before identification and susceptibility testing
4. Hemodynamic instability
5. Prior prophylaxis with quinolones

uncomplicated high-risk patient with neutropenic fever (168,171–174). Recommended antibiotic selections for monotherapy include a third or forth generation cephalosporin (cefipime, ceftazidine) or a cabapenam (imipenam-cilastin or meropenam). Ceftazidine as monotherapy provides inadequate coverage against gram-positive organisms, such as *Pneumococci* and *Viridans streptococci*. In addition, the extended-spectrum β-lactamases and type 1 β-lactamases show resistance to ceftazidine, limiting its utility as monotherapy. Other antimicrobial agents, including the quinolones and piperacillin-tazobactam, have been evaluated for use as monotherapy. Although the results have been generally favorable, the data are currently insufficient to establish a practice standard. Furthermore, the quinolones are widely used as prophylaxis among afebrile neutropenic patients, which limit their use as monotherapy for neutropenic fever.

Two-drug combinations may be applied for the management of complicated cases or if antimicrobial resistance is a problem. An aminoglycoside plus (1) an antipseudomonal uredopenicillin or carboxypenicillin (ticarcillin-clavulinate, piperacillin-tazobactam), (2) an antipseudomonas cephalosporin (cefipime, ceftazidine) or (3) a carbapenam (imipenam-cilastin, merapenam) are recommended in this setting. These regimens may offer synergistic activity against some gram-negative bacilli and mitigate the emergence of drug resistance during therapy. These potential advantages need to be weighed against the increased rates of nephrotoxicity, ototoxicity, and electrolyte disturbances associated with some of these drug combinations. If the offending pathogen is identified, the antibiotic regimen should be modified, if necessary, to reflect the culture and sensitivity of the identified organism. Antibiotic selections for definitive therapy should be chosen based on their maximal curative effect, minimal adverse effect, and cost-effectiveness. If the patient defervesces after 3–5 days of empiric or definitive antibiotic therapy, coverage should be continued for at least 7 days, or until cultures are sterile and the patient has clinically recovered. Preferably, the neutrophil count should be above 500 cells/mm^3 before treatment is stopped; however, exceptions to this recommendation are reasonable if the aforementioned responses have been achieved and prolonged neutropenia is anticipated. Discontinuation of antibiotics in the afebrile neutropenic patient should only be considered among those patients that have no evidence of catheter site infections, whose skin and mucous membranes are intact and who are not anticipating further ablative chemotherapy or invasive procedures.

High-risk patients with negative cultures and persistent fevers beyond 3–5 days of empiric antimicrobial therapy should be reassessed for modifications in the antibiotic regimen, including the addition of vancomycin (if indicated) or antifungal therapy. Systemic fungal infections, typically of *Candida* or *Aspergillus* origin, account for approximately one-third of febrile neutropenic episodes that persist beyond 1 week despite broad-spectrum antibiotic coverage. The addition of antifungal therapy with amphotericin B is therefore warranted, especially in the setting of profound and protracted neutropenia (ANC $<$ 500 cells/mm^3 for more than 7 days). Lipid formulations of amphotericin B are also available. These agents provide relatively equivalent antimycotic coverage with less drug-related toxicity (175–177). Voriconizole and caspofungin have recently met FDA approval for the treatment of refractory aspergillosis infections. Data regarding these relatively new agents are limited.

Antiviral therapy should be instituted in the febrile neutropenic patient if the clinical or laboratory assessment suggests evidence of viral disease. Local skin and mucous membrane infections that suggest the presence of herpes simplex virus or varicella-zoster may breach the skin and mucous membranes, thereby providing portals for the entry of bacterial and fungal pneumonias. These lesions should, therefore, be treated with antiviral therapy in the setting of febrile neutropenia, even if they are not the cause of fever.

The addition of granulocyte transfusions represents nonstandard therapy in the treatment of severely neutropenic patients with life-threatening infections. Although there is no convincing evidence from any large prospective clinical trials to support this practice, published case reports and pilot studies suggest clinical efficacy in the treatment of opportunistic fungal infections among patients with severe neutropenia (178–181). Fever and chills occur commonly during granulocyte transfusions. More severe reactions, including hypotension and respiratory distress, are rarely noted. The later may occur in association with the concomitant administration of granulocytes with amphotericin B. Other complications include alloimmunization, transmission of cytomegalovirus and other infectious diseases, and graft-vs.-host reactions. These adverse reactions should weigh into the decisions to initiate granulocyte transfusion therapy. Lastly, the addition of colony-stimulating factors, such as granulocyte colony-stimulating factor (G-CSF) or granulocyte-macrophage colony-stimulating factor (GM-CSF), may be considered when prolonged neutropenia is anticipated in the setting of worsening infection. Adjunctive therapy with G-CSF is generally added around days 3–5 in patients with established soft tissue infections and persistent neutropenia. Although these agents may shorten the duration of neutropenia, the routine use of these drugs for the treatment of uncomplicated neutropenic fever is not advocated (168). Anitmicrobial therapy for catheter-related infections is predicated on the susceptibility of the cultured organism. Catheter removal is advocated for tunnel or pocket infections caused by long-term catheters and for infections caused by *S. aureus* and *Candida* infections (182). The use of antimicrobial-coated catheters has been shown to reduce the rates of catheter-associated infections in recent studies (183,184).

G. Lung Injury Caused by Aspiration

A number of factors, such as ineffective cough reflex, impaired respiratory mucociliary clearance, altered mental status, and abnormalities of the airway cellular and immune function, may all contribute to an increased propensity to aspirate oropharyngeal and gastric contents. Aspiration pneumonitis results from the regurgitation of usually sterile gastric contents into the airway. Aspiration pneumonia, on the other hand, occurs when colonized secretions from the oropharyngx are inhaled. The cancer patient is at risk for both. The increased predilection to aspirate among the debilitated cancer patient has multifactorial etiologies. Two important defenses against aspiration—preservation of swallowing function and cough reflex—are often breached in the cancer patient. Chemoradiotherapy regimens may induce severe mucositis with associated dysphagia, a major risk factor for aspiration. The frequent use of sedating medications, supine positioning, the need for mechanical ventilation and nasogastric tube feeding also contribute to increased rates of aspiration. Gastroparesis is common among cancer patients, owing to sepsis, shock, surgery, or the frequent use of opiods and other drugs that may slow gastric motility. These factors, together with impaired mechanical, humoral, and cellular defense mechanisms that are inherent to this group of patients, frequently result in the development of clinically significant pneumonia (Table 8). Both the volume of the aspirated inoculum as well as the content of the aspirate strongly influence the likelihood of developing clinically significant lung injury. The historical importance of acid, first pointed out by Mendelson, in the pathogenesis of aspiration pneumonitis has been supported by more recent investigators. It is generally agreed that aspiration of gastric aspirates with a pH of less than 2.5 and a volume of greater than 0.3 mL/kg of body weight is associated with a poor outcome (185–187).

The earliest clinical response to significant gastric aspiration is due to the direct caustic effect of the acidic aspirate on the cells lining the alveolar–capillary interface. Infiltration of neutrophils into the alveoli and interstitium heralds the development of the inflammatory response, which occurs 4–6 hr later. The acidic gastric content is a poor medium for bacterial overgrowth, thus bacterial infection does not play a dominant role during the early phases of aspiration pneumonitis. Medications that alter gastric pH, such as proton-pump inhibitors, histamine H_2-receptor antagonists, and antacids may facilitate colonization of gastric contents by pathogenic bacteria. Enteral feeding, gastroporesis, and small bowel obstruction may have a similar effect in promoting gastric colonization. Under these conditions, the early response to gastric aspiration may be due to inflammation with superimposed bacterial infection. These considerations are important in designing treatment strategies for lung injury secondary to gastric aspiration. Aspiration pneumonia, by definition, results from inhalation of sufficiently large, nonsterile oropharyngeal material, the consequence of which is roentgenographically apparent changes on chest imaging studies. Pathogens underlying nosocomial vs. community-acquired aspiration pneumonias differ. In nosocomial aspirations, enteric gram-negative bacilli, gram-positive organisms, and mixed aerobic–anaerobic infections predominate.

Among patients with aspiration pneumonitis, the onset of symptoms may be dramatic and the event precipitating lung injury is usually known. The spectrum of symptoms may range from minimal wheezing, cough, and dyspnea to cyanosis, pulmonary edema, hypotension, hypoxemia and severe respiratory distress. Bronchospasm contributes significantly to early hypoxemia. Initial improvements in hypoxemia with control of bronchospasm may be seen. Refractory hypoxemia may develop 36–48 hr after large-volume gastric aspiration, owing to the loss of surfactant and destruction of type II pneumocytes. Progression to ARDS, respiratory failure, and death rapidly follow. Pneumonia resulting from aspiration of oropharyngeal contents, by contrast, often occurs more insidiously, frequently with no recollection of the inciting event.

Table 8 Clinical Features of Aspiration Pneumonitis and Pneumonia

	Aspiration pneumonitis	Aspiration pneumonia
Cause	Aspiration of acidic and particulate gastric contents	Aspiration of colonized oropharyngeal material
Primary type of lung injury	Chemical burn	Infectious process
Major risk factors	• Depressed/altered mental status • Gastroparesis • Supine positioning	• Dysphagia • Poor oral hygiene • Impaired mucociliary clearance • Ineffective cough • Disruption of G–E junction • Anatomical abnormalities of upper aerodigestive tract
Pathophysiology	Sterile chemical burn initially; subsequent bacterial infection may occur in some patients	Acute inflammatory response to gram-positive, gram-negative and, rarely, anaerobic bacteria caused by aspiration of colonized airway secretions
Clinical presentation	Cough, wheeze, SOB, hypoxemia, cyanosis, pulmonary edema; hypotension, ARDS	Cough, tachypnea, radiographic signs suggesting pneumonia
Aspiration event	Commonly witnessed	Witnessed aspiration uncommon
Clinical clues to diagnosis	Patient with altered/depressed mental status and new/worsening pulmonary infiltrates with associated respiratory distress	Patient with dysphagia and respiratory signs/symptoms associated with new/worsening pulmonary infiltrates in the dependent portions of the lungs
Management	Supportive only. Antibiotic therapy may be appropriate for patients with signs/symptoms >48 hr, small bowel obstruction, or prior use of antacids/antisecretory agents	Immediate antibiotic therapy is indicated

This type of pneumonia is, therefore, frequently inferred based on a compatible patient risk profile and radiographic evidence of pneumonia. Areas of geographic abnormalities on chest radiographs correlate with the patient position at the time of aspiration. Aspiration that occurs while the patient is in the upright position typically involves the basilar segments of the lower lobes, whereas the superior segments of the lower lobes and posterior segments of the upper lobes are more frequently affected by aspiration occurring in the supine position.

Management strategies for patients with lung injury secondary to aspiration of gastric contents focus on several interventions. Upper airway suctioning and aggressive pulmonary toileting are mandatory for witnessed aspiration. Early intubation for airway protection should be considered for selected patients (patients with decreased level of consciousness). If mechanical ventilation is required, application of PEEP is recommended to minimize airway collapse. Continuous positive airway pressure (CPAP) may be administered to nonintubated patients with mild-to-moderate respiratory distress. Antimicrobial therapy should be withheld for the first 48 hr following gastric aspiration unless the patient has risk factors, such as small bowel obstruction, that predispose to colonization of gastric contents. Prophylactic use of antibiotics is discouraged as this may only serve to select out more resistant organisms. When antibiotics are initiated, those with broad-spectrum activity are recommended. Selection of antimicrobials that target anaerobes may be appropriate in some cases. Targeted therapy based on culture results of lower respiratory tract samples (BAL, protected brush specimens) is advocated. Although steroid therapy may effect a more rapid improvement in lung injury patterns seen radiographically, the impact of steroid administration on overall outcome has not been found to be superior to placebo (188). In fact, in a prospective study by Wolfe et al. (189), the incidence of gram-negative bacterial pneumonia was higher among steroid-treated than placebo-treated patients with aspiration pneumonitis. Thus, the routine use of corticosteroid therapy is not recommended in the management of aspiration pneumonitis.

The approach to the person with aspiration pneumonia, on the other hand, requires early and aggressive antimicrobial therapy as up-front management of these patients. Antibiotic selection should be based on the setting in which the aspiration occurred (community vs. nosocomial) as well as the underlying immune status of the patient. Requisite antimicrobial regimens should be broad in spectrum and target gram-negative organisms with or without anaerobic coverage. Anaerobic coverage is indicated in patients with periodontal disease, putrid sputum, or evidence of necrotizing pneumonia (190).

III. NONINFECTIOUS PULMONARY COMPLICATIONS AMONG CRITICALLY ILL PATIENTS WITH CANCER

A. Pulmonary Hemorrhage Syndromes

1. *Massive Hemoptysis*

Although a strict definition of massive hemoptysis has not been established, this condition is variably defined as the expectoration of 100 mL of blood in a single episode to more than 600 mL of blood within a 24-hr period (191,192). Both the volume of blood as well as the hemodynamic and pulmonary response to hemoptysis are important factors in the clinical presentation of this disorder. Smaller volume or submassive bleeding into the airway may cause life-threatening airway obstruction, hypotension, or aspiration in patients with prior hemodynamic or pulmonary instability with equally devastating consequences. Thus, precise definitions of massive hemoptysis are elusive. Whether massive or submassive, this sentinel event is important not only because of its potential life-threatening consequences, but also as a sign of underlying disease.

Because the volume of blood expectorated may not necessarily reflect the seriousness of underlying disease, all patients with unexplained hemoptysis should undergo a thorough initial evaluation, even when the amount of blood expectorated is small. Among patients with hemoptysis, approximately 5% develop massive hemoptysis and nearly 1/3 of these patients have fatal hemorrhage (193). The risk of death from massive hemoptysis correlates strongly with the amount of blood expectorated. Other factors, including the rate of hemoptysis, amount of blood retained in the lungs, and underlying pulmonary reserve, are associated with risk of death from massive hemoptysis, regardless of the cause of bleeding. The usual cause of pulmonary hemorrhage-related deaths is asphyxiation rather than exsanguination.

Bleeding into the lungs may be due to localized lesions or diffuse disease. Although the distinction between localized vs. diffuse source of bleeding is usually readily obvious clinically, the diagnosis is occasionally confounded by similarities in clinical and radiographic features. Massive bleeds from focal lesions, such as bronchiectasis, neoplasms, pulmonary infarction, or radiation-induced lung injury, may be associated with aspiration of blood and simulate diffuse bleeding radiographically. Pulmonary hemorrhage syndromes have diverse and occasionally overlapping etiologies (Table 9). The spectrum of attributable con-

Table 9 Major Conditions Associated with Pulmonary Hemorrhage Syndromes in Patients with Cancer

Malignancy
Primary bronchogenic carcinoma
Metastatic disease
Pulmonary
Bronchiectasis
Bronchopleural fistula
Bullous emphysema
Chronic bronchitis
Pulmonary embolism with infarction
Infection
Necrotizing pneumonia (*Staphylococcus, Legionella, Klebsiella*)
Fungal pneumonia (*Aspergillus, Mucor, Coccidioides, Histoplasma*)
Mycetoma
Parasitic (strongyloidiasis, amebiasis, ascariasis)
Viral (*Varicella, Influenza*)
Mycobacterial pneumonia (tuberculosis, atypical mycobacteria)
Septic pulmonary emboli
Lung abscess
Tricuspid endocarditis
Hematologic
Neutrophil recovery following severe neutropenia
Severe thrombocytopenia
Platelet dysfunction
Coagulopathy
Disseminated intravascular coagulation
Drugs/toxins
Anticoagulants
Thrombolytic agents
Radiation
Vascular
Pulmonary embolism with infarction
Pulmonary hypertension
Fat embolism syndrome
Vascular prosthesis
Iatrogenic
Bronchoscopy
Swan-Ganz catheterization
Transtracheal needle aspiration
Lung biopsy
Endobronchial therapy (laser, APC, cryotherapy brachtherapy)
Pulmonary artery rupture

ditions associated with pulmonary hemorrhage in the cancer patient includes infectious (viral, fungal, bacterial, parasitic) and noninfectious (drug and radiation effects, tumor infiltration, bronchiectasis, pulmonary infarction, trauma) etiologies. Derangements in both the fibrinolytic and coagulation pathways are common in the cancer patient, resulting in an increased risk of both hemorrhage and thrombosis. Adding to this, sepsis and circulating tumor procoagulants may cause activation of the clotting cascade and chronic consumption with disseminated intravascular coagulation (DIC). Hematologic derangements, including severe neutropenia and thrombocytopenia, may result from cancer infiltration of the bone marrow and liver or occur as a consequence of chemoradiation therapy. Both neutropenia and granulocyte recovery may potentiate alveolar hemorrhage. The period of neutropenia may be protracted following certain types of chemotherapy or HSCT. Prolonged neutropenia is strongly correlated with the development of angioinvasive fungal pneumonias, including those caused by aspergillosis and mucormycosis. These necrotizing fungal organisms may cause vascular necrosis, leading to pulmonary infarction and hemorrhage, which may be massive. Pulmonary infections, irradiation-induced lung injury, sepsis, and lung injury secondary to certain cytotoxic agents are frequent sequelae cancer therapy. Each of these conditions may provoke the development of diffuse alveolar damage (DAD). DAD in the setting of thrombocytopenia or coagulopathy may cause intractable and fatal hemoptysis. Specific infections and chemotherapeutic agents that are associated with pulmonary hemorrhage syndromes are discussed elsewhere in this chapter. The noninfectious etiologies will be discussed in this section.

Neoplasms with the highest propensity to cause hemoptysis typically are large, centrally located tumors. Not surprisingly, squamous cell and small cell carcinoma of the lung, bronchial carcinoid tumors, and tracheobronchial carcinomas comprise 83% of the tumors associated with hemoptysis (Table 10).

Table 10 Neoplasms with the Highest Propensity for Massive Hemoptysis

Primary bronchogenic carcinoma	Metastatic carcinomas	Other
Squamous cell	Breast	Esophageal
Bronchial carcinoid	Renal cell	Mediastinal lymphoma
	Colon	
	Melanoma	
	Sarcoma	

Approximately 20% of patients with primary bronchogenic carcinoma develop hemoptysis. Fatal hemoptysis among this group of patients is, fortunately, rare (3%) (194). Metastatic disease, particularly those with an increased predilection for endobronchial spread of disease (melanoma, primary tumors of the breast, kidney, larynx, and colon) also have excess rates of pulmonary hemorrhage. Esophageal carcinoma and other mediastinal tumors may cause massive hemoptysis by direct extension of tumor into the tracheobronchial tree. Bleeding from this source may be fatal. Traumatic causes of pulmonary hemorrhage are uncommon and the hemoptysis associated with these conditions is frequently massive and fatal.

Ineffective cough plays a critical role in the development of respiratory failure and death in the debilitated cancer patient with massive hemoptysis. Therefore, patients with rapid ongoing bleeds, hemodynamic instability, ventilation impairment, severe dyspnea, or hypoxemia should be considered for early intubation to protect the airway. Initial management of the unstable patient should include volume resuscitation, supplemental oxygen, correction of preexisting coagulopathy, and cough suppression. In addition, lateral decubitus positioning with the bleeding lung in dependent position is recommended to minimize aspiration of blood to the contralateral lung. Localization of the bleeding site may not always be readily obvious on clinical exam but is an important adjunct to therapy. Once the bleeding site is identified, isolation of the nonbleeding lung may be accomplished by selective occlusion of the right or left mainstem bronchus under bronchoscopic guidance. Alternatively, unilateral intubation of the nonbleeding lung may be used to prevent aspiration of blood from the contralateral lung and to preserve gas exchange. Unilateral intubation of the left mainstem bronchus in the case of a massive right-sided bleed is appropriate. This approach is not recommended, however, in the case of a massive left-sided bleed because of the risk of occluding the right upper lobe. Endobronchial tamponade of the left mainstem bronchus using a Fogarty (balloon) catheter in the case of a massive left-sided bleed in preferred. Bronchoscopy is used to facilitate catheter placement. Both single-lumen and double-lumen catheters are commercially available. The later has the advantage of an additional inner channel that can be used to administer vasoactive and hemostatic topical agents (195). Because of theoretical concerns regarding ischemia of the bronchial mucosa and postobstructive pneumonia caused by balloon tamponade, the period of balloon inflation should not exceed 48 hr. Balloon catheters may be passed through either the fiberoptic or the rigid bronchoscope. Advantages of the later scope include greater access for suctioning, better airway control, and more effective retrieval of large clots from the airway than the fiberoptic bronchoscopes. Visualization of the distal airway is limited to the mainstem bronchi with these scopes, however, because of their larger diameter. The choice of bronchoscopic technique is primarily dictated by the clinician's training and comfort in using these instruments. Concurrent use of both scopes has the added advantages of optimizing clot removal and suctioning capacity with distal airway visualization.

Intubation using a double lumen endotracheal tube may be used to selectively isolate the nonbleeding lung. The propensity for airway obstruction secondary to clot formation and the difficulty in passing a bronchoscope through these smaller-lumen tubes limit their efficacy. Furthermore, these tubes are oftentimes difficult to place and may become dislodged easily with movement. These confounding factors restrict the widespread use of the double lumen tube, which is typically reserved for the critically unstable patient with severe bleeding and associated refractory hypoxemia.

Endobronchial instillation of hemostatic agents is often used in the acute management of massive endobronchial bleeds. Pharmacologic agents, including topical epinephrine (1:20,000 dilution), thrombin, and fibrinogen–thrombin combinations have been employed with variable success. These agents may be instilled directly into the bleeding bronchus through the fiberoptic bronchoscope. The use of iced saline lavage has been supported in some of the older literature, although more recent proof of its efficacy is lacking. Anecdotal reports of successful treatment of massive bleeds with vasopressin, corticosteroids, and tranexamic acid given systemically are also documented in the literature (196–198). Vasopressin, a potent vasoconstrictor, should be used with caution in patients with coronary artery disease or hypertension because of the potential for precipitating coronary artery ischemia. Finally, local intracavitary instillation of antifungal agents represents a viable option for the treatment of mycetoma-related massive hemoptysis when surgical intervention is not feasible. Antifungal drugs, including sodium or potassium iodide and amphotericin B, may be administered percutaneously or transbronchially into the fungal cavity directly with excellent control of hemoptysis (199).

Other treatment modalities, such as laser photocoagulation, argon plasma coagulation (APC), and electrocautery have had mixed results in the treatment of patients with massive hemoptysis. Endobronchial bleeds caused by central, exophytic intraluminal tumors may be controlled with laser photocoagulation using neodymium-yttrium-garnet laser (Nd:YAG) phototherapy. The photocoagulative, photoresective, and vaporization properties of Nd:YAG lasers permit curative resection of some central tumors while simultaneously controlling bleeding (196). This procedure typically is done under general anesthesia using rigid bronchoscopy although successful reports of Nd:YAG laser therapy, using fiberoptic bronchoscopy with topical anesthesia and conscious sedation only has been reported (200). Catastrophic complications of Nd:YAG laser therapy, including airway combustion, bronchial rupture, tissue perforation, hemorrhage, and death have been reported. In addition, the potential for ocular damage from accidental laser scatter requires that both patient and medical team use protective eyewear. Argon plasma coagulation (APC), a form of noncontact electrocoagulation, represents an alternative modality for definitive and palliative treatment of proximal endobronchial lesions. Unlike Nd:YAG laser therapy, the need for endotracheal intubation or general anesthesia is generally not necessary with APC therapy, as this procedure is routinely performed through the flexible bronchoscope (201). In addition, the risk of airway perforation is less with APC therapy, owing to a more shallow depth of tissue penetration (3 mm vs. Nd:YAG laser therapy 5 mm). Minimizing supplemental oxygen therapy during Nd:YAG laser and APC (preferably below 40% inspired oxygen) is recommended to reduce the risk of collateral thermal tissue damage (200,201).

The lungs are subserved by bronchial and pulmonary vascular circuits, each with independent and specialized functions. The high-pressure bronchial circulation may bleed profusely in disease states and is the major source of massive endobronchial bleeds. On rare occasions, massive hemoptysis may occur as a result of rupture or puncture of the low-pressure pulmonary artery circuit (202). The most common setting for this adverse event is following placement or manipulation of a Swan Ganz catheter. A herald bleed commonly presages this frequently fatal event. Selective angiography of the bronchial circuit may be used to identify the bleeding source. Embolization of the source vessel using polyvinyl alcohol foam, Gianturco steel coils, isobutyl-2-cyanoacrylate, or absorbable gelatin pledgets may offer short-term control of bleeding. Recurrent bleeds following successful embolization occur in 23–46% of patients, usually within the year following therapy (203–205). Significant adverse events of bronchial vessel cannulation and embolization are rare. Vessel perforation, intimal tears, and inadvertent embolization of the spinal artery have occasionally been reported. Adding to this, the spinal artery may arise aberrantly from the bronchial circulation. Embolization of the bronchial circulation under these circumstances may lead to inadvertent occlusion of spinal vessels with associated sequelae of spinal infarction and paraparesis. This unfortunate complication is seen in less than 1% of patients undergoing embolotherapy. A role for radiation therapy in the management of massive hemoptysis following failed embolization is suggested by individual case reports in the literature. Radiotherapy has been used successfully in this setting to treat persistent bleeds caused by rupture of a mycetoma or radiosensitive vascular tumors (206).

Patients with hemoptysis that is refractory to other therapeutic measures may be candidates for surgical therapy. These patients may have life-threatening cardiovascular compromise related to persistent bleeding and the escalated operative risks in this setting must be carefully weighed against any potential surgical benefit. Mortality rates among patients with massive hemoptysis vary widely, ranging from 0.9% to 50% among surgically treated patients and 1.6% to 80% among patients treated medically (207,208). The benefits of the surgical vs. medical approach to patients with massive hemoptysis have not been studied in any randomized prospective trials. Clinicians considering patients for surgical candidacy must carefully weigh the additional operative risks in the setting of severely compromised cardiopulmonary reserve against the potential surgical benefits. The approach to the cancer patient with massive hemoptysis is summarized in Fig. 10.

2. *Diffuse Alveolar Hemorrhage*

Various cancer-related conditions, including HSCT, left-ventricular failure, infections, pulmonary veno-occlusive disease, and certain drugs (cytotoxic medications, anticoagulants, amiodarone) have been implicated as causing diffuse alveolar hemorrhage (DAH). Although pneumonia is a known cause of focal alveolar bleed, strict definitions of DAH exclude infectious etiologies (209). Clinicopathologic findings that support the diagnosis of DAH include: (1) radiographic support for widespread alveolar injury, (2) progressively bloody BAL fluid taken from three different subsegmental bronchi, (3) cytologic analysis of BAL fluid demonstrating 20% or greater hemosiderin-laden macrophages, (4) abnormal

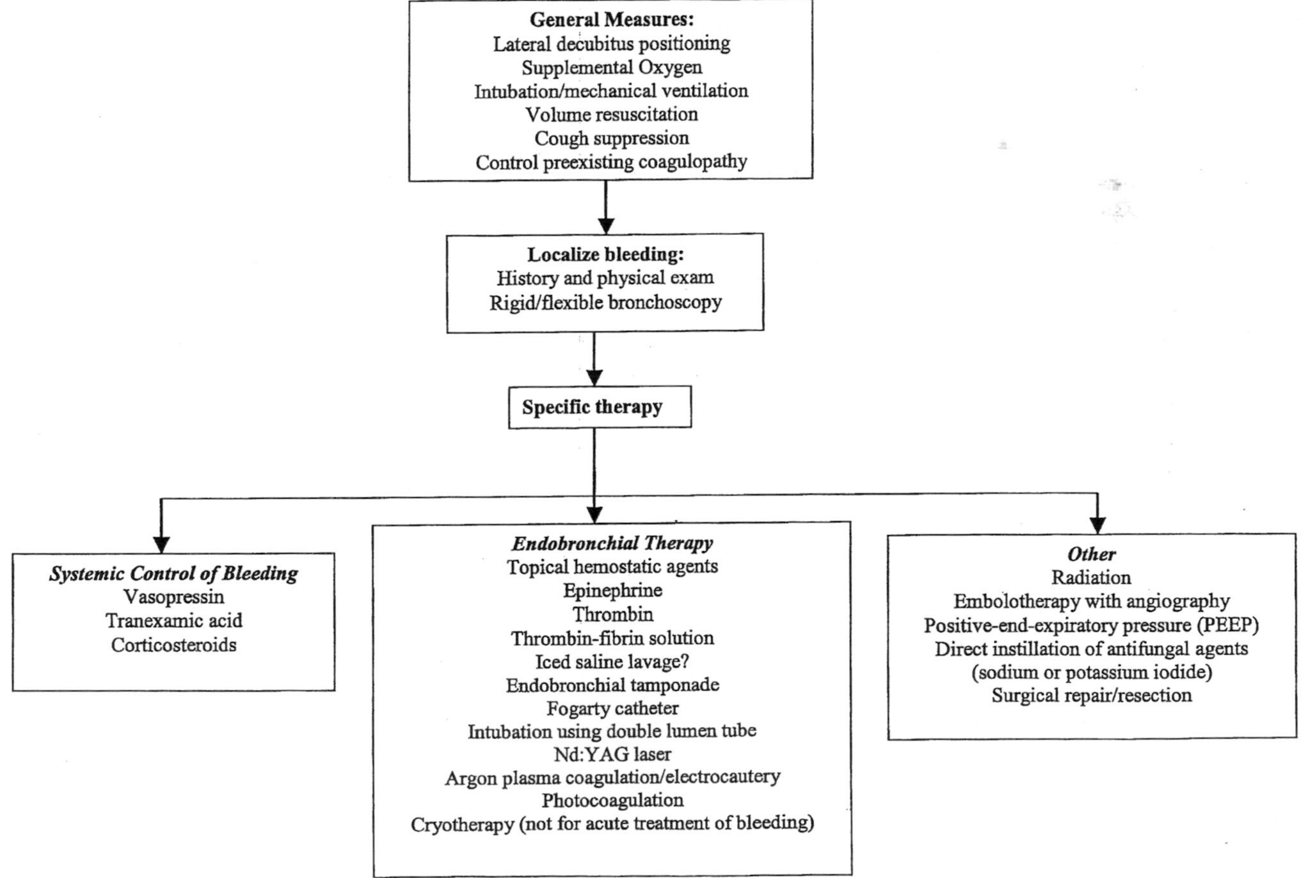

Figure 10 General principles in the management of patients with massive hemoptysis.

pulmonary physiology reflecting an increased alveolar–arterial gradient and a restrictive lung defect, (5) autopsy evidence of alveolar surfaces with greater than 30% blood and (6) the absence of a discernable infectious etiology. The incidence of DAH among autologous transplant recipients is 1–5%. Among allogeneic transplant recipients, the incidence is a bit higher (2–7%), perhaps reflecting the increased prevalence of immune suppression and GVHD among this group of patients. Although various reports site aggressive preconditioning chemotherapeutic regimens, pretransplant radiation regimen, older age, renal insufficiency, and the development of GVHD as prominent risk factors for the development of DAH, these factors were not consistently predictive of DAH in more contemporary reports (210–212). Interestingly, coagulopathy and thrombocytopenia are not recognized risk factors for the development of DAH. Thrombocytopenia and disordered coagulation frequently accompany DAH and are thought to aggravate the underlying condition. Hence, platelet and other blood product transfusions are frequently given as part of the treatment regimen for DAH, although the utility of blood products in mitigating this disorder has not been proven (211).

Diffuse alveolar hemorrhage typically occurs early following HSCT and accompanies neutrophil engraftment. Late-onset DAH has been increasingly reported and confers a less favorable outcome. The development of GVHD may be a risk factor for the development of late alveolar hemorrhage, which carries a worse prognosis (209,212). Leukocyte infiltration into the lungs is coincident with marrow recovery following HSCT and may amplify the lung injury through the release of inflammatory cytokines. These inflammatory mediators, including interleukin-12 and tumor necrosis factor-α have been implicated in the development of DAH (213). A role for inflammation in the development of DAH is supported by studies that show increased rates of DAH among patients with more than 20% neutrophils or any eosinophils on pretransplant bronchoscopy (214). Similarly, evidence of excess bronchial inflammation or airway erythema confers an increased risk of HSCT-related DAH. Recent evidence suggests that antecedent lung injury caused by infection, radiation, or drugs may facilitate the development of DAH by inducing endothelial damage and disrupting alveolar–capillary basement membranes.

The clinical presentation of DAH following HSCT is variable. Dyspnea, low-grade fever, dry cough, and an abnormal chest radiograph demonstrating diffuse, predominantly central alveolar infiltrates. Hemoptysis is unusual, occurring in only 0–25% of patients (128,211,212). Fine reticular opacities occur early and appear primarily over the middle and low lung zones (Fig. 11). CT findings characteristically include bilateral areas of ground-glass attenuation or consolidation. Although BAL returns yielding progressively bloody samples and the presence of $>20\%$ hemosiderin-laden macrophages are highly suggestive of DAH, neither of these findings are pathognomonic for the disease. Blood in the distal airways from any source may yield progressively bloody returns on BAL. Furthermore, cigarette smoking may cause an increase in hemosiderin-laden macrophages in the otherwise normal host. The delayed appearance of hemosiderin-laden macrophages into the airway (48–72 hr) and slow clearance of these cells from the airway following an alveolar bleed further confounds the diagnosis. A repeat bronchoscopy at 2–5 days following the initial bronchoscopic study may help to establish the diagnosis.

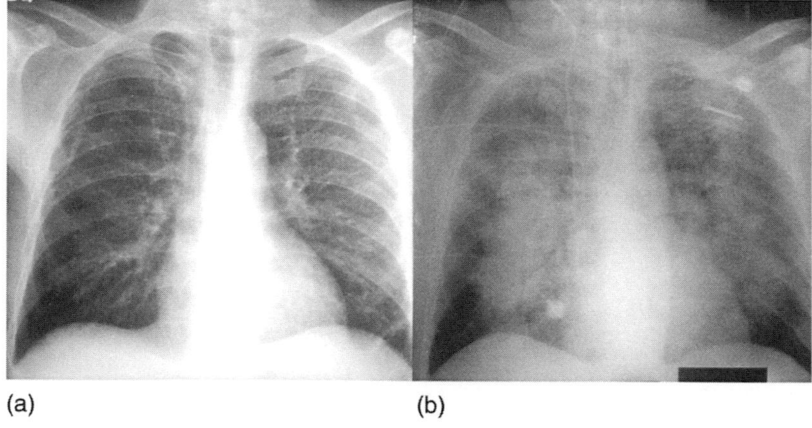

(a) (b)

Figure 11 A 22-year-old female with low-grade fever and cough productive of blood-tinged sputum 2 weeks following an allogeneic stem cell transplantation for acute leukemia. The admitting chest radiograph (a) was normal. A chest radiograph taken 24 hr following admission (b) revealed dense bilateral alveolar opacifications. BAL fluid analysis was consistent with the diagnosis of diffuse alveolar hemorrhage.

The recognition of inflammatory responses in the pathogenesis of DAH has prompted the use of steroids in the treatment of this disease. Multiple studies describe improved respiratory status with high-dose systemic corticosteroids, although a favorable impact on overall outcome has not been definitively shown (210,212). The optimal dose and duration of steroid therapy is not well defined. Steroid dosages have ranged from 0.25 to 2 g of methylprednisolone per day in divided doses for 4–5 days then tapered over 2–4 weeks (198,212,215). Individual case reports suggest a role for recombinant coagulation factor VIIa in the treatment of hemorrhage in HSCT recipients (216,217). This prothrombotic agent is currently being studied in a prospective placebo-controlled trial. The results of other treatment modalities, including plasma exchange, immunosuppressive therapy, and plasmapheresis in the treatment of alveolar hemorrhage have been disappointing. Despite aggressive therapy, respiratory failure occurs in 77–85% of patients with fulminant DAH. Associated mortality rates of 32–100% have been reported in these patients (209,210,212,218).

B. Idiopathic Pneumonia Syndrome

In 1993, the NIH adopted the term idiopathic pneumonia syndrome (IPS) to describe diffuse lung injury following HSCT without a discernable infectious etiology (219). The histopathologic correlates of IPS include interstitial pneumonitis and diffuse alveolar damage. Approximately 30–50% of patients with interstitial pneumonitis or diffuse alveolar damage meet the criterion for IPS. Less frequently bronchiolitis obliterans with or without organizing pneumonia are identified among patients with IPS. Transplant allotypes also influence the development of IPS. Earlier reports documented IPS among 30–50% of allogeneic and 20% of autologous transplant recipients. More recent investigations, however, suggest that the incidence of this disease is much lower than previously described (220). Several lines of indirect evidence implicate cytokines, including interleukin-1, interleukin-2, interleukin-6, and tumor necrosis factor in the pathogenesis of this disorder (219). In addition, the cumulative effects of radiation and chemotherapy (in particular methotrexate-based pretransplant regimens) on the lungs may play a role in the development of IPS. Other independent risk factors include older age, a low pretransplant Kanrnosky score, vascular injury caused by endotoxemia, and immunologically mediated lung damage associated with severe GVHD.

Idiopathic pneumonia syndrome is an inherently heterogeneous disorder with variable clinical expression and severity. Affected patients classically present 42–79 days following grafting with fever, dry cough, and dyspnea and radiographic evidence of diffuse, nonlobar interstitial infiltrates. The absence of infection on BAL with a second negative confirmatory test for infection performed 2–14 day following the initial examination supports the diagnosis (219,221). Systemic corticosteroid therapy may have a salutary effect in improving symptoms, although a proven benefit on overall outcome has not been established in any prospective trials. Immunomodulating regimens that include cyclosporin and IVIG for GVHD prophylaxis are associated with less severe disease and portend a better prognosis. The overall prognosis is poor. More than 70% of patients with IPS succumb to respiratory failure caused by the disease itself or superimposed respiratory infection (219,220).

C. Chemotherapy-Induced Lung Injury

Historically, conventional cancer interventions have exploited the disproportionate rate at which malignant cells divide relative to normal cells. The cytotoxic activities of ionizing radiation and many of the chemotherapeutic agents are based on this principle. Both ionizing radiation and cytotoxic agents, such as busulfan and bleomycin, for example, cause breaks in cellular DNA, rendering rapidly dividing cancer cells susceptible to errors in transcription and early cell death. Newer antineoplastic agents, such as the taxanes, inhibit mitotic activity by blocking microtubule formation, resulting in reduced cell survival. These conventional antitumor strategies have resulted in dramatic survival benefits among patients with certain types of cancers. The success of these strategies has resulted in an exponential growth in both the number and complexity of chemotherapy and radiation treatment regimens. Unfortunately, coincident with advances in treatment has been a parallel expansion in the incidence and spectrum of treatment-related toxicities, of which the lungs appear particularly susceptible. The damaging effects of radiation and the older cytotoxic agents, such as bleomycin and busulfan on the lungs, are well recognized. In addition, our emerging understanding of cancer biology has paved the way for new classes of drugs, including the taxanes, immunomodulating agents, and biologic response modifiers, which are also implicated in the development of lung toxicity. Lung injury owing to radiation and cytotoxic drugs substantially reduces the quality of life in cancer patients and may be life threatening. Moreover, treatment-related lung disease represents a major limitation to dose-intensification strategies, which ultimately impact antitumor activities.

The radiosensitizing and radio-recall effects of drugs, such as bleomycin, may potentiate the adverse effects of radiation on the lungs (222,223). Furthermore, synergistic interactions between high inspired oxygen therapy and radiation or bleomycin may enhance lung toxicity and result in life-threatening lung disease. In addition to the influence of oxygen and radiation therapy in the promoting drug-induced lung damage, patient age, cumulative dose of the drug, and the use of multidrug regimens contribute to excess lung injury. These risk factors also influence the dose of drug in which lung injury is manifested.

The adverse consequences of chemotherapy- and radiation-induced lung damage are associated with stereotyped clinical syndromes and histopathologic correlates. Damage to vascular endothelial cells type II and alveolar lining cells leading to edema of the alveolar interstitium are early pathologic findings. Fibroblast proliferation and hyaline membrane formation occur later and signal the onset of pulmonary fibrosis. Reactive infiltration of lymphocytes and macrophages are also frequent findings. Common histopathologic changes include diffuse alveolar damage (DAD), nonspecific interstitial pneumonitis (NSIP), noncardiogenic pulmonary edema (NCPE), bronchiolitis obliterans with (BOOP) or without (BO) organizing pneumonia, and hypersensitivity pneumonitis (HP). Pleural diseases (pneumothorax, pleural thickening, pleural effusions) and vascular diseases (veno-occlusive disease, thromboembolism) have also been described following chemoradiation therapy. Rarely, eosinophilic pneumonia is also seen. Knowledge of cancer therapies and their major patterns of lung injury are critical in the management of the cancer patient with undiagnosed pleuropulmonary disease.

A causal relationship between specific drugs and lung toxicity is often inferred from individual case reports. The diagnosis and precise estimates of the incidence of adverse lung, reactions resulting from individual anticancer drugs are confounded by several factors including: (1) infections that may coexist and/or closely mimic the radiographic and clinical presentation of lung toxicity, (2) inherent difficulties in identifying the individual culprit drug in a multidrug or multimodality regimen, and (3) the absence of clinical and biologic markers that distinguish drug-induced lung damage from infection or other causes. The diagnosis of lung disease owing to radiation or anticancer therapy thus relies on histologic confirmation of lung damage and the exclusion of alternative causes. Recognition of signs, symptoms, and risk factors are often critical to a good outcome. Premonitory symptoms of nonproductive cough, fever, dyspnea, malaise, and anorexia are common. These symptoms are usually indolent, progressing over several weeks. Exercise-induced hypoxemia is also an early finding (128,224). Occasionally patients may present with acute respiratory failure in the absence of prodromal symptoms. Clinical manifestations of toxicity usually occur during the course of chemotherapy, although lung injury due to agents, such as bleomycin, busulfan, and carmustine (BCNU), may occur weeks to years following completion of therapy (225–229). Pulmonary function testing is an imperfect test in this setting and the predictive potential for the detection of early toxicity has been variable. Nonetheless, these tests remain the diagnostic tool most frequently used in assessing lung reactions to cytotoxin and radiation-related lung injury. The diffusing capacity (DLco) is generally accepted as the most sensitive parameter within the battery of pulmonary function tests. Characteristic changes on pulmonary function tests include a restrictive ventilatory defect with an associated reduction in DLco. Obstructive ventilatory defects may also occur as a result of drug-induced bronchospasm or the development of obliterative bronchiolitis.

The exponential growth in the numbers of chemotherapeutic agents over the past decade has resulted in a staggering list of drugs that may cause lung injury. Table 11 chronicles those chemotherapeutic agents and their associated major patterns of lung injury. This section will review radiation-induced lung toxicity and several of the more prominent chemotherapeutic agents that cause clinically relevant pulmonary disease will be discussed.

1. *Alkylating Agents*

Busulfan

The earliest descriptions of cytotoxin-induced lung injury documented pulmonary fibrosis in two patients treated with the alkylating agent, busulfan (230). Since that time, the literature has been replete with reports of lung injury caused by busulfan and other alkylating agents, such as cyclophosphamide, melphalan, and chlorambucil. Among these, toxicity caused by busulfan and cyclophosphamide is the most common and the most well characterized. In contrast to other alkylating agents, lung injury caused by busulfan commonly results following single agent therapy (231,232). Lung toxicity typically follows a latency period of 3 or more years after completion of treatment. Shorter periods of only 6 weeks have also been reported (233,234). The major lung injury patterns associated with busulfan lung are interstitial pneumonitis and pulmonary fibrosis which occurs in 4–10% of busulfan-treated patients (Fig. 12). The chest radiograph typically discloses bibasilar reticular infiltrates—findings

Table 11 Major Patterns of Chemotherapy- and Radiation-Induced Lung Injury

Agent	HP	IP	PIE	Fibrosis	ARDS/ NCPE	Lung nodules	DAH	BOOP/ BO	Pleural effusion	Bronchospasm	VTE	PTX	Other
Alkylating agents													
Busulfan		+		+				+					PAP; PVOD: BAC
Cyclophosphamide		+		+	+			+		+			
Antimetabolites													
Cytosine arabinoside					+		+						Opportunistic infections
Fludarabine	+	+	+		+		+						Opportunistic infections
Methotrexate	+	+	+	+	+	+			+	+			NC granulomas; hilar LNs
Azathioprine		+					+			+			Airway edema; UAO
Cemcitabine		+		+	+					+			
Cytotoxic antibiotics													
Bleomycin		+	+	+		+		+				+	PVOD; acute chest pain
Mitomycin C		+		+			+			+[a]			TTP-HUS; hilar LNs
Nitroureas													
Carmustine		+		+	+							+	PVOD; NC granulomas
Lomustine		+		+	+							+	PVOD; NC granulomas
Taxanes													
Paclitaxel		+	+	+	+				+	+			
Docetaxel		+	+	+	+					+			
Immunotoxins/BRMs													
IL-2			+		+				+				Pulmonary hypertension
Tumor necrosis factor					+								
G-CSF/GM-CSF		+	+	+	+				+		+		Fat embolism
Trastuzumaab													
Rituximab										+			Angioedema
Infliximab			+										
Interferon-γ		+		+	+			+	+				Pulmonary hypertension sarcoidosis
Herceptin													Cardiogenic pulmonary edema
Gemtuzumab													Opportunistic infections
Gefitinib				+					+				
Imatinib	+		+						+				Opportunistic infections
Other													
Procarbazine	+	+	+	+					+				
Tamoxifen citrate											+		
L-Asperaginase										+	+		
Retinoic acid					+		+						
Thalidomide											+		
Etoptoside/teniposide										+			

[a] In association with vinca alkaloids.

HP, hypersensitivity pneumonitis; IP, interstitial pneumonitis; PIE, pulmonary infiltrates with eosinophils; NCPE, noncardiogenic pulmonary edema; DAH, diffuse alveolar hemorrhage; BOOP/BO, bronchiolitis obliterans with organizing pneumonia/obliterative bronchiolitis; VTE, venous thromboembolism; PTX, pneumothorax; HUS-TTP, hemolytic uremic syndrome-thrombotic thrombocytopenic purpura; hilar LNs = hilar lymphadenopathy; BAC, bronchoalveolar cell carcinoma; PAP, pulmonary alveolar proteinosis; PVOD, pulmonary veno-occlusive disease; NC granulomas, noncaseating granulomas.

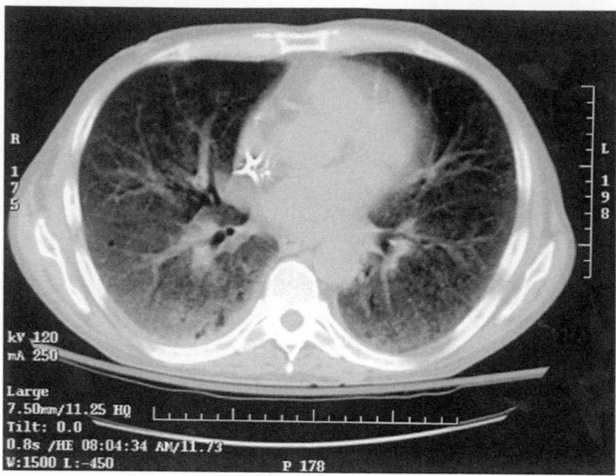

Figure 12 A 35-year-old man who developed progressive shortness of breath and dry cough 3 years after treatment with busulfan-based chemotherapy for acute myelogenous leukemia. CT scan of the chest demonstrated primarily bibasilar interstitial infiltrates. Gram stain and cultures of BAL specimens were negative. Fibroblast proliferation and dysplastic pneumocytes were seen on analysis of lung tissue, consistent with drug-induced lung disease.

that are typical of lung injury caused by other cytotoxic drugs. Intrathoracic lymphadenopathy, and pleural effusions are unusual findings. Pulmonary alveolar proteinosis and bronchoalveolar cell carcinoma have been anecdotally reported following busulfan therapy. Whether these citings reflect a causal or coincidental association between busulfan and these types of lung disease is unclear. The duration of therapy and total dose of the drug influence the development of pulmonary complications. Ginsberg and Comis (235) reported an increased incidence of pulmonary toxicity among patients whose total dose of busulfan exceeded 500 mg of the drug. Concomitant administration of other cytotoxic agents, including melphalan and uracil mustard may cause synergistic damage to the lung at lower total doses of busulfan. Busulfan-based chemotherapy is typically given over longer periods of time and the longer duration of therapy with this drug also appears to be associated with a higher incidence of lung toxicity. Busulfan-related lung disease carries a poor prognosis and mortality rates as high as 90% in fully developed cases have been reported (236,237). Treatment strategies include drug withdrawal and supportive therapy. Anecdotal reports describe salutary effects of corticosteroid administration in controlling symptoms; however, an effect on mortality has not been systematically proven (238).

Cyclophosphamide

This drug has broad application in the treatment of neoplastic and nonneoplastic diseases. Given its frequent administration, the overall prevalence of lung injury secondary to this drug is low. Accumulated reports suggest a 2% incidence of associated lung disease. Rates may be much higher, however, in the setting of high-dose cyclophosphamide administration or multiagent therapy. Cyclophosphamide given concomitantly with chemotherapeutic regimens that contains bleomycin, carmustine, etoposide, vincristine, or mitoxanthrone confers an increased risk. The major histopathologic change associated with cyclophosphamide-induced lung injury is interstitial pneumonitis with or without pulmonary fibrosis. Noncardiogenic (increased permeability) pulmonary edema following cyclophosphamide chemotherapy has also been reported (239). This may occur with or without diffuse alveolar damage. Interstitial pneumonitis is the most frequent pattern of cyclophosphamide-related lung toxicity. Clinical symptoms of interstitial pneumonitis typically occur early, within the first 2 weeks after the initiation of therapy. Early-onset symptoms tend to be reversible and respond nicely to drug withdrawal and corticosteroid administration. A late-onset pneumonitis with associated pulmonary fibrosis and bilateral pleural thickening is also seen. Late-onset pneumonitis carries a poor prognosis with associated mortality rates of 40% (240,241). Although corticosteroid therapy is frequently tried, the value of any specific therapy has not been established for late disease.

2. *Cytotoxic Antibiotics*

Bleomycin

Lung toxicity is the most serious and the most frequent side effect of bleomycin toxicity. The major patterns of bleomycin-induced lung injury are interstitial pneumonitis and pulmonary fibrosis. Up to 40% of recipients of the drug develop lung toxicity of varying severity. Toxicity is dose dependent and precipitous escalations in the incidence of lung injury are seen with cumulative doses above 450 units of the drug (242,243). Fatal pulmonary fibrosis has been documented, however, following doses as low as 50 units. The radiosensitizing and radiorecall properties of bleomycin potentiate the toxic effects of radiation on the lung, resulting in generalized pulmonary fibrosis that may extend well beyond the margins of the radiation field (222,223,228,244,245). The sequence of combined therapy with bleomycin and radiation therapy does not appear to influence the subsequent development of lung damage. In addition, the optimal interval between sequential therapy has not been established. Therefore, the minimal effective dosage of radiation and bleomycin is recommended when multimodality therapy is anticipated. Other factors that confer an increased susceptibility to bleomycin-induced lung disease include age >70, oxygen administration, route of administration, and multimodality therapy (223,246–248). Bleomycin given by continuous intravenous infusion as opposed to bolus injections has been associated with reduced rates of pulmonary toxicity (223,249,250). Several studies have suggested that renal failure may promote excess rates of bleomycin pulmonary toxicity (251–254). Enhanced rates of lung damage have been shown with bleomycin-containing chemotherapy regimens even at low dosages of the medication. Thus, recipients of multiagent regimens, including ABVD (doxarubicin, bleomycin, vinblastine, and dacarbazine), BACOP (bleomycin, adriamycin, cyclophosphamide, oncovin, and prednisone) and M-BACOD (methotrexate, bleomycin, adriamycin, cyclophosphamide, oncovin, and dexamethasone) should be closely monitored for signs of lung toxicity (14,255). A synergistic relationship between high inspired oxygen and bleomycin administration in the development of lung injury has been suggested (256,257), although the validity of this relationship has been challenged in the more recent literature (258). The threshold dose and duration of oxygen therapy that confers an increased risk of lung toxicity in bleomycin-treated patients has not been well established. Lung injury associated with fractions of inspired oxygen (FIO_2) as low as 30% has been documented in some studies (256,259). Clinical symptoms of pneumonitis and respiratory failure precipitated by ARDS may occur as early as 18 hr after oxygen exposure in bleomycin–treated patients. Several key issues regarding bleomycin-oxygen interactions remain unresolved. In particular questions regarding the threshold dose of supplemental oxygen associated with increased toxicity and the interval between oxygen and bleomycin therapy that mitigates the risk of lung injury remain unanswered. Restriction of supplemental oxygen levels to <25% FIO_2 and sequential oxygen–bleomycin treatment intervals of >3 months greatly decreased postoperative morbidity and mortality in one study (257). These unresolved issues resonate with the intensivist caring for the bleomycin-treated patient on mechanical ventilation and pose particular problems for bleomycin-treated patients undergoing surgical procedures with general anesthesia. In these settings, continuous monitoring of mixed venous oxygen levels may be helpful, especially when higher levels of oxygen supplementation are required.

Several patterns of bleomycin-related lung injury have been described, including: (1) interstitial pneumonitis progressing to chronic fibrosis, (2) hypersensitivity pneumonitis with associated peripheral eosinophilia resembling eosinophilic pneumonia, (3) bronchiolitis obliterans with organizing pneumonia, and (4) acute chest pain syndrome (128), (241,243,224,246,260). The syndrome of interstitial pneumonitis with fibrosis represents the most common pattern of bleomycin-related lung injury. With the exception of acute chest pain syndrome, the chest radiograph is typically abnormal at clinical presentation. The clinical presentation and radiographic findings of parenchymal pneumonitis/fibrosis is slowly progressive, evolving over 4–10 weeks after bleomycin therapy (Fig. 13a–b). A spectrum of abnormalities is seen on chest radiographs. Most commonly bibasilar reticular and fine nodular infiltrates initially involving the costophrenic angles are seen. Lobar infiltrates and pulmonary nodules mimicking metastatic disease have been reported. Although pleural thickening is a common finding, pleural effusions are uncommon and their presence should prompt evaluations for an alternative diagnosis. Other radiographic manifestations, including pneumomediastinum and pneumothorax, are rare findings (75,261,262). Histologic and radiographic evidence of bleomycin-induced pneumonitis is noted among 20% of patients in the absence of symptoms (122). Early diagnosis of bleomycin lung disease relies on the results of pulmonary function and radiographic testing, both of which are of poor predictive value in the early diagnosis of this disease. Open-lung biopsy may be necessary in some cases, although the exclusion of other processes by bronchoalveolar lavage and transbronchial biopsy may be sufficient for diagnosis when the index of suspicion for drug-induced lung injury is high. The risk of surgery must also be weighed against any potential benefit of establishing a definitive diagnosis.

Mortality rates associated with bleomycin-induced lung disease range from 13% to 83% (242,244,249, 255). The efficacy of corticosteroid therapy in the treatment of bleomycin-induced hypersensitivity pneumonitis is well documented. Prompt response to drug withdrawal and steroid therapy is expected among this group of patients. However, among patients with bleomycin-related pneumonitis/fibrosis, the response to steroid therapy is quite variable. Steroid treatment dosages have varied from 60 to 100 mg given over 1–3 months in most studies (263,264). Guidelines regarding the dosage and duration of steroid therapy among this group of patients are poorly defined.

Mitomycin

Mitomycin is extensively used in the treatment of cancers of gastrointestinal, gynecologic, breast, prostatic, and bronchogenic origin. The lung toxic effects of this cytotoxic antibiotic are primarily seen as a result of synergistic interactions with other cytotoxic agents, including the vinka alkyloids, cyclophosphamide

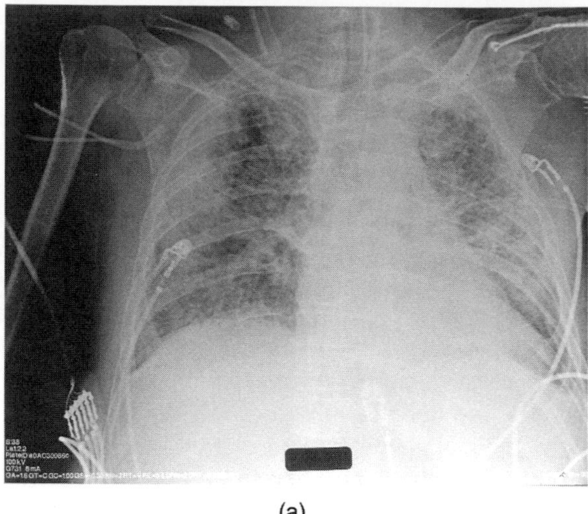

(a)

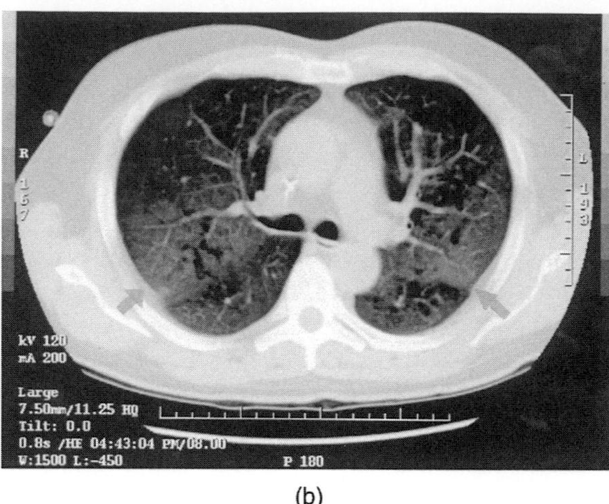

(b)

Figure 13 A 32-year-old male treated with bleomycin-based chemotherapy for germ cell tumor who developed respiratory failure following general anesthesia for surgical reduction of the tumor. A chest radiograph (a) and CT scan of the chest (b) showed diffuse alveolar infiltrates with areas of consolidation. Bilateral pleural thickening (arrows) was also noted. Cultures of BAL fluid were negative. Interstitial edema and an inflammatory infiltrate were reported on analysis of transbronchial biopsies. The findings were consistent with drug-induced lung disease.

and 5-fluorouricil. Lung injury may occur as a result of concomitant or sequential dosing schedules that include mitomycin with these agents. Interstitial pneumonitis, the most prominent pattern of mitomycin-associated lung disease, typically occurs 2–4 months following initiation of mitomycin therapy. Pulmonary fibrosis may occur as a late finding and carries a poor prognosis. Pulmonary veno-occlusive disease following mitomycin therapy has also been reported. Acute bronchospasm with or without associated pulmonary infiltrates is a well-recognized complication of mitomycin/vinca alkyloid regimens and occurs in 5% of patients. This complication has been reported with concomitant and sequential administration of these two drugs. The recommended interval of delay between administration of these agents that would limit the occurrence of this complication is not well defined. Signs and symptoms of airway obstruction in these patients may be prominent and severe. This complication of mitomycin therapy is usually steroid-responsive, and resolution of symptoms typically occurs within 24 hr of steroid therapy. Derangements on pulmonary function testing indicating airway obstruction and reductions in DLco may be severe and persist beyond resolution of clinical symptoms. Although a decline in DLco of greater than 20% portends a poor prognosis, serial pulmonary function testing has not been reliably shown to be predictive of pulmonary toxicity (265). Patients with gastrointestinal malignancies who receive treatment with mitomycin/vinca alkyloid combinations also have an increased predilection for noncardiogenic pulmonary edema. This life-threatening complication occurs as a component of a hemolytic uremic-like syndrome (266–268). Patients may present with pulmonary edema associated with microangiopathic hemolytic uremia, thrombocytopenia, and renal insufficiency in varying degrees of severity. Mitomycin-induced bronchospasm and interstitial pneumonitis are associated with an overall favorable prognosis. Withdrawal of the drug and corticosteroid therapy is associated with rapid clinical improvement (269). The hemolytic-uremic syndrome carries a poor prognosis. Mortality rates as high as 95% have been reported among patients with fulminant disease (267,270,271). The efficacy of various treatment strategies, such as the use of corticosteroids, plasmapheresis, and fresh frozen plasma in improving symptoms or altering the outcome has not been poven.

3. *Antimetabolites*

Methotrexate

The spectrum of lung injury patterns attributable to methotrexate is broad, and the incidence of lung toxicity due to this drug is probably underestimated, as toxic reactions are frequently attributed to the underlying disease process. Methotrexate-related lung toxicity and associated mortality rates are reported as 7% and 11%, respectively, among cancer recipients of high-dose therapy (272,273). The clinical patterns associated with methotrexate-induced lung injury may be sorted into acute and chronic forms of the disease. Noncardiogenic (increased permeability) pulmonary edema is the hallmark of acute lung injury caused by methotrexate therapy. This unpredictable sequela of methotrexate may quickly progress to respiratory failure and death. Chest pain accompanying an acute pleuritis occurs rarely, usually in association with pleural effusions. More commonly, patients present a hypersensitivity type of lung injury. This pattern of toxicity is characterized clinically by a constellation of symptoms, including nonproductive cough, low-grade fever, dyspnea, headache, malaise, fatigue, and an erythematous skin rash that may wax and wane without adjustments in therapy. Unilateral or bilateral effusions, and intrathoracic lymphadenopathy may occur in conjunction with diffuse bibasilar reticulonodular infiltrates (273). Noncaseating granulomas, interstitial eosinophilia, and a prominent cellular interstitial infiltrate consisting primarily of mononuclear cells seen on histologic sections of lung tissue are unique features of methotrexate-induced lung injury and help to distinguish toxicity due to this drug from other etiologies.

A relationship between serum corticosteroid levels and the development of methotrexate-related lung disease is suggested by studies that show increased rates of lung injury associated with rapid withdrawal of corticosteroids or prior adrenalectomy (243,274). Factors such as age, sex, total or cumulative dose, underlying lung disease, prior thoracic irradiation, or supplemental oxygen therapy do not appear to potentiate the development of lung injury in methotrexate-treated patients. The pathogenesis of methotrexate-induced lung injury has not been clearly elucidated. A hypersensitivity reaction has been postulated, based on the presence of peripheral blood eosinophilia and on histopathologic evidence of helper T-lymphocyte alvelolitis and granuloma formation on BAL fluid and lung biopsy specimens (272,275). A hypersensitivity response does not reliably recur with rechallenge of the drug, however, and thus may not represent the sole mechanism of injury. Methotrexate is available in oral, intravenous, intrathecal, or intramuscular formulations. The predominant site of methotrexate accumulation and toxicity is the lungs regardless of the method of delivery. Thus, a direct toxic effect on the lungs as the mechanism of lung injury has been postulated (276).

Spontaneous remission has been reported with methotrexate-induced pneumonitis and clinical remissions despite continuation of the drug have been reported with this form of lung injury. Thus, this form of lung toxicity usually confers a favorable prognosis and questions regarding the utility of steroid therapy in the treatment of this disease are unsettled. Steroid therapy is routinely used in the treatment of acute fulminant disease, although no associated improvement in outcome has been systematically documented in the literature.

Cytosine Arabinoside

The purine analog, cytosine Arabinoside (cytarbine, Ara-C) is a critical component of the treatment regimen for acute leukemias. Although severe myelosuppression, gastrointestinal toxicity, and cerebellar/cerebral toxicity are reported as the major impediments with high-dose ($3\,g/m^2$ for 8–12 consecutive doses) therapy, Ara-C may also trigger formidable reactions in the lungs. Noncardiogenic pulmonary edema (NCPE) is the most frequent and the most life-threatening adverse pulmonary event. High-dose therapy may trigger the development of ARDS. In addition, Ara-C given in combination with fludarabine triggers a precipitous and durable reduction of the CD_4 subset of T-lymphocytes, resulting in an increased risk of opportunistic infection by *Pneumocystis carinii*, *Cytomegalovirus*, and *Aspergillus* species (277). The pathogenic mechanism of NCPE in Ara-C-treated patients has not been fully elucidated, although increased capillary permeability involving the lung parenchymal, pleural, pericardial, and peritoneal surfaces is thought to underlie the development of this disorder. Postmortem examinations demonstrate a paucity of inflammatory cells in the setting of diffuse alveolar damage and massive pulmonary edema. Estimates of lung toxicity vary with the dose and schedule of the drug and ranges from 5% to 32%. An abrupt development of respiratory distress frequently hallmarks the onset of disease, which typically occurs 2–21 days into therapy (278,279). Drug withdrawal at the earliest signs of lung toxicity is critical to a successful outcome. Despite florid symptoms of toxicity, patients with NCPE typically do well and recovery is complete generally within 10 days of disease onset. A 10% mortality rate has been reported among those patients who develop NCPE, but may be much higher among the subgroup of patients who develop ARDS. Anecdotal reports support the use of high-dose corticosteroids in the treatment of Ara-C-related NCPE and ARDS.

Fludarabine

Fludarabine is a potent analog of Ara-A. This agent is widely used in the treatment of hematopoietic malignancies, including chronic lymphocytic leukemia, promyelocytic leukemia, non-Hodgkin's lymphoma, and Waldenstom's magroglobulinemia. Fludarabine is a principle component of the FLAG (Fludarabine, Ara-C, G-CSF) regimen, which has shown enhanced efficacy in the treatment of acute leukemias

(280,281). The incidence of fludarabine-related lung toxicity ranges form 14% to 69% of treated patients. Interstitial pneumonitis, pleural effusions, and an increased propensity for pneumonia represent the principal adverse pulmonary reactions to this agent. Interstitial pneumonitis tends to occur 3–28 days following the third or later course of therapy (282–284). Withdrawal of the agent coupled with corticosteroid therapy is generally associated with a favorable outcome (285). Spontaneous remission following drug withdrawal alone has also been reported. Like ARA-C, fludarabine may promote profound T-cell suppression, resulting in increased rates of pneumonia caused by opportunistic pathogens.

Azathioprine/6-Mercaptopurine

Azathioprine is the major metabolite of the purine analog, 6-mercaptopurine. These agents are widely used in the treatment of malignant diseases and as immunosuppressive therapy in the setting of organ transplantation and primary autoimmune disorders. A steroid-responsive interstitial pneumonitis has been reported following administration of either drug (8,286). In addition, both drugs may rarely incite hypersensitivity reactions, characterized by fever, bronchospasm, and dyspnea(287,288). Several reports of diffuse alveolar hemorrhage following azathiaprine therapy are also documented in the literature (289,290). Severe acute upper airway obstruction after azathioprine exposure has also been reported (291). Symptoms typically develop one week to several months following therapy. Drug withdrawal constitutes standard therapy. The indications for corticosteroids in the treatment of azathioprine- or 6-mercaptopurine-induced lung disease have not been well defined.

Gemcitabine

Gemcitabine is a nucleoside analog with therapeutic efficacy against a growing variety of solid tumors. In particular, this agent has shown clinical benefit in the treatment nonsmall cell lung cancer, and carcinomas of the pancreas, breast, and bladder. Early reports following the inception of gemcitabine touted a broad safety profile with side effects primarily limited to mild alopecia, nausea, malaise, and dose-limiting myelosupression. Pulmonary toxicity is increasingly cited in more recent reports of gemcitabine-related adverse events, and appears more common than initially anticipated (292–294). Prior or concurrent radiation therapy and combined therapy with taxane-, cyclophosphamide-, and cisplatin-based chemotherapy regimens appears to augment the risk of gemcitabine-induced lung toxicity(295,296). Transient mild bronchospasm and associated dyspnea during drug infusion may occur in 3–5% of patients and is likely related to an allergic phenomenon. The more serious patterns of gemcitabine-related lung injury include interstitial pneumonitis, pulmonary fibrosis, noncardiogenic pulmonary edema, and ARDS (Fig. 14a–b). These pulmonary events may be life threatening and characteristically occur 1 week to several months after multiple courses of therapy. Recognition of gemcitabine as the

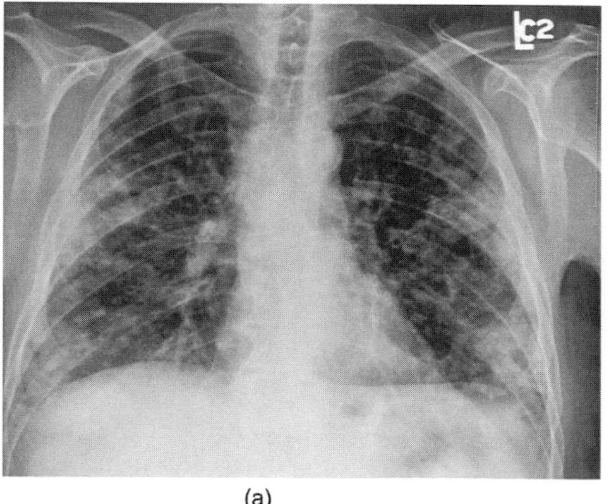

(a)

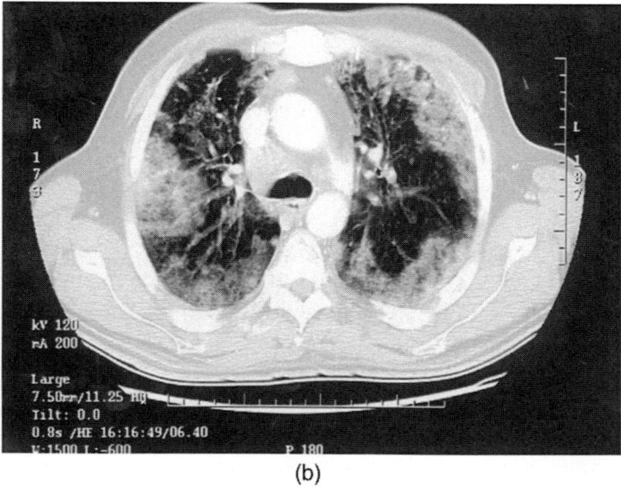

(b)

Figure 14 A 54-year-old man developed symptoms of severe shortness of breath 3 weeks following gemcitabine chemotherapy for treatment of primary bladder carcinoma. Chest radiograph (a) and CT scan of the chest (b) demonstrated marked areas of peripheral ground-glass opacity with areas of consolidation, which were new when compared to studies done 4 weeks prior. Postmortem analysis of lung tissue was consistent with a drug-induced lung disease.

offending agent and discontinuation of this drug is critical to a successful outcome. High-dose corticosteroid therapy is recommended, although the response to this treatment has been variable (296). Rechallenge of this agent following successful treatment of gemcitabine-related pulmonary edema is not recommended.

4. *Nitrosureas*

BCNU/CCNU

Among the various nitrosureas that are currently commercially available, only carmustine (BCNU), lomustine (CCNU), and semustine (methyl-CCNU) have been associated with clinically relevant pulmonary toxicity. Carmustine is the most frequently sited nitrosurea associated with lung toxicity. This agent is frequently prescribed as single agent therapy in the treatment of central nervous system tumors, which permits better definitions of the incidence and relevance of this drug in the development of lung disease. The prevalence of lung toxicity following BCNU therapy varies with drug dosage and the presence of preexisting lung disease but is generally reported to be within the range of 20–30%. In patients with preexisting underlying lung diseases, such as bronchiectasis, chronic obstructive pulmonary disease (COPD), recurrent pneumonia, or asthma, the propensity for BCNU lung injury is amplified. Cumulative dosages of BCNU that exceed $1500\,mg/m^2$ are associated with a 10-fold increase in BCNU toxicity (297). Synergistic lung damage between BCNU and prior radiation therapy or hyperoxia has not been firmly established. The clinical, radiographic, and histologic features of BCNU-related lung disease are similar to those caused by other cytotoxins. Clinical signs and symptoms tend to occur during administration of the drug, although reports of disease development years following completion of therapy occasionally appear in the literature. The major histopathologic derangement associated with BCNU lung toxicity is pneumonitis and associated clinical symptoms of dry cough, fever, and dyspnea typically evolve insidiously over weeks to months. Acute respiratory decompensation leading to ARDS and death has also been reported, predominantly among recipients of higher cumulative doses of the drug. A paucity of inflammatory infiltrate associated with areas of pulmonary fibrosis on histologic sections is commonly seen in advanced disease. Granuloma formation similar to Wegener's granulomatosis has also been described (298). A reduction in DLco typically marks the earliest physiologic alteration, which may precede the onset of clinical symptoms and radiographic changes by several weeks. Abnormalities on chest radiographs characteristically appear late in the course of disease. Adding to the usual reticular nodular infiltrates that are typically seen with cytotoxin-related lung injury, apical acinar shadows and spontaneous pneumothorax are seen and are unique features of this disease. Pneumothoraces may occur as unilateral or bilateral disease. Lung disease owing to BCNU may be recalcitrant and unremitting even with discontinuation of the drug. Full-blown toxicity results in fatal disease in 30–40% of affected patients. The impact of steroids in the management of BCNU-related lung disease is confounded by the fact that corticosteroid therapy is frequently added to the BCNU-based chemotherapy for treatment of central nervous system malignancies. Thus, the utility of corticosteroids in ameliorating symptoms and improving patient outcome is uncertain.

5. *Taxanes*

Paclitaxel/Docetaxel

Major advances in the understanding of the biology and mechanisms of cancer over the past two decades have occurred in tandem with seminal discoveries of new classes of chemotherapeutic agents. These newer classes of agents include the taxanes and targeted therapeutic agents, such as the immunotoxins and antineoplastic monoclonal antibiotics. The two commercially available taxanes, docetaxel (taxotere) and paclicaxel (taxol), are widely used in the treatment of a variety of malignancies, including lung, breast, and ovarian carcinomas. These mitochondrial-stabilizing agents exert their antineoplastic effects in part through mitotic arrest caused by inhibition of mitochondrial spindle activities. Early clinical trials described myelosuppression as a major complication of taxane use. Concomitant use of growth factors has largely eliminated this problem and has permitted the use of dose escalation strategies. Unfortunately, the emergence of new toxicities including lung toxicity has been associated with these more aggressive protocols.

The major taxane-induced lung toxicities include hypersensitivity reactions, pneumonitis, fluid retention, and pulmonary fibrosis (299–301). With the exception of fluid retention, which is largely seen following taxotere administration, the adverse effects of the different taxanes on the lung are similar. Hypersensitivity reactions have been reported following both taxol and taxotere administration, which may arise as a result of the drug or its diluent. Taxol is formulated in a highly allergenic polyoxyethyated castor oil (Cremophor EL) solvent. This solvent may educe mast cell activation and histamine release, triggering type 1 hypersensitivity reactions. Flushing, bronchospasm, urticaria, angioedema, puritis, and anaphylaxis plagued early reports of taxol-related toxicity in 25–30% of patients. These reactions typically occur within the first hour following drug administration and after the first or second dose of the drug. The incidence of these life-threatening symptoms has waned significantly with the routine use of prophylactic corticosteroids and histamine receptor antagonists. Although these prophylactic measures are not fully protective, severe reactions now occur in only 1–3% of patients (301,302). Mild hypersensitivity reactions including flushing and puritis are noted in as many as 40% of patients. These minor reactions do not predict the development of major ones. Standard prophylaxis varies with the taxane agent. Corticosteroid prophylaxis given as a single dose simultaneously with the histamine-blocking drugs may be protective in preventing paclitaxol-induced hypersensitivity reactions. Effective prophylaxis against docetaxol hypersensitivity reactions requires multiple doses of dexamethasone, given 12 hr prior to therapy and continued for 3–5 days following docetaxol administration (301,303). These measures may also mitigate the recurrence of hypersensitivity responses upon rechallenge with the drug, although recrudescence of symptoms may occur with redosing. Successful drug rechallenge following augmented antiallergic strategies has been reported among patients with an antecedent history of severe hypersensitivity reactions, although this approach has not been universally accepted (301,304).

Interstitial pneumonitis occurs among 3% of taxane-treated patients. This incidence may rise to 16% among patients receiving concurrent or sequential radiation therapy (305–307). Combined therapy with radiation or other chemotherapeutic agents, such as cisplatin, cyclophosphamide, or gemcitabine not only enhances the risk of lung toxicity, but also the severity of the disease (308,309). The etiology of taxol-induced interstitial lung disease is unknown although a cell-mediated hypersensitivity response to the drug has been postulated (306). Unlike the taxane-induced hypersensitivity reactions associated with airway disease and anaphylaxis, the risk of taxane-induced interstitial pneumonitis is not mitigated by premedication with steroids and antihistamine stabilizing agents. Bronchospasm and hypotension are not prominent components of taxane-induced interstitial lung disease. Patients typically present with dyspnea, hypoxia, dry cough, and diffuse infiltrates within 8–14 days of receiving the second or third course of taxane therapy. Respiratory symptoms tend to evolve acutely, over a 1–2 day period. Although most patients with taxane-related interstitial pneumonitis have a favorable prognosis, respiratory failure and death associated with ARDS and pulmonary fibrosis have been described (310). For most patients, complete resolution of symptoms following drug withdrawal and corticosteroid therapy is expected. A 2–3 week course of prednisolone at 30–60 mg per day is generally recommended. A higher dose of prenisolone (60–240 mg per day) with a more protracted taper may be necessary for patients with more severe conditions, such as acute respiratory failure.

Taxotere has been associated with the development of a dose-dependent syndrome of generalized fluid retention. This syndrome has been attributed to capillary leak and results in ascites, peripheral edema, and pleural effusions. Interestingly, pulmonary edema has not been described with this syndrome. Fluid retention typically occurs following several cycles of drug administration. Pretreatment with oral dexamethasone given 24 hr before and continuing for 3–5 days after taxotere administration successfully reduces the incidence as well as delays the development of this problem.

6. *Miscellaneous Cytotoxins*

L-*Asparaginase*

L-Asparaginase has by far the highest prevalence of hypersensitivity reactions of all of the antineoplastic agents. The enzyme is derived from *Escherichia coli* and primarily used in the treatment of T-cell lymphomas and acute lymphocytic leukemias. Hypersensitivity reactions have been reported in as many as 43% of patients, typically within one hour of administration of the drug. Intravenous injections, high-dose therapy, and repeated dosing of the drug confer an increased risk. Patients may present with a constellation of symptoms, including fever, dyspnea, bronchospasm, urticaria, laryngospasm, angioedema, rash, and abdominal pain after 2 weeks of injections given on a daily or thrice weekly schedule. More severe reactions, including anaphylaxis and death, occur in less than 10% of patients (311). Skin testing with L-asparaginase is recommended for all patients at the initiation of therapy and following the first week of drug administration. Patients with a positive skin test, defined as the formation of a wheal within the subsequent hour of testing, should undergo desensitization prior to administration of the drug. Skin test negativity does not fully predict drug safety. Thus, all patients should undergo treatment in facilities that are capable of treating anaphylaxis, regardless of prior skin test reactions. The utility of prophylactic steroid and antihistamines has not been established. An alternative form of the drug derived from the parasitic bacteria, *Erwinia*, is available for patients with a history of allergies to *E. coli.* Cross-reactivity to Erwinia-derived

L-asparaginase may develop over time. Rechallenge with the native drug is associated with an increased risk of adverse reactions, which may be severe. Pegaspara-gase, a less immunogenic analog of L-asparaginase, may represent a reasonable substitute for those patients with severe hypersensitivity reactions to the native drug. L-Asparaginase-induced reductions in antithrombin III, leading to increased rates of thromboembolic disease, have also been reported (312).

Procarbazine

Procarbazine, a cogener of the monoamine oxidase inhibitor 1-methyl-1–2-benzyl hydrazine, is typically used in combination with other chemotherapeutic agents in the treatment of lymphoma. Lung toxicity, manifested as a hypersensitivity pneumonitis, rarely complicates procarbazine chemotherapy. Several reports have documented the development of a severe interstitial pneumonitis following the administration of combination chemotherapy with mechlorethamine, vincristine, procarbazine, and prednisone (MOPP) for the treatment of Hodgkin's lymphoma (313). Symptoms of cough, fever dyspnea, hypoxemia, and dense interstitial opacities on chest radiographs may occur after the second or third cycle of the drug. Pleural effusions may accompany the interstitial infiltrates. Lung biopsies typically show evidence of mononuclear cell alveolitis and interstitial fibrosis. A peripheral blood and tissue eosinophilia and noncaseating granulomas are also frequent pathologic findings. Steroid therapy may hasten recovery, which tends to evolve slowly over a period of weeks to months. Airway disease, owing to procarbazine-induced hypersensitivity reactions, has also been reported. These self-limiting reactions also tend to occur with repeated courses of the drug. Re-exposure to procarbazine following successful treatment of lung toxicity is associated with a recrudescence of symptoms.

Tamoxifen Citrate

Tamoxifen citrate is an estrogen receptor antagonist with proven efficacy in the treatment of breast carcinoma. Patients taking tamoxifen have a 3-fold increased rate of thromboembolic events (Fig. 15) (314–316). The prothrombotic effect of tamoxifen may be exacerbated when given in combination with other chemotherapeutic agents, such as cyclophosphamide, methotrexate, and 5-flurouracil (CMF-tamoxifen) (314,316) .The pathophysiologic basis for the thrombogenicity of tamoxifen is not completely understood, although tamoxifen is known to cause decrements in protein C and antithrombin III levels (317,318).

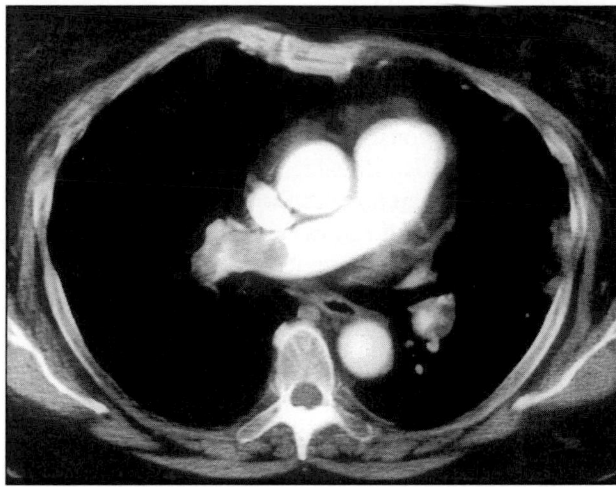

Figure 15 A 48-year-old woman with a history of breast carcinoma who had been maintained on tamoxifen chemotherapy who presented to the emergency room with an acute onset of dyspnea and right-sided pleuritic chest pain. A CT angiogram showed filling defects consistent with clot involving the bilateral main pulmonary arteries and their associated branches.

All-Trans Retinoic Acid (ATRA)

ATRA is a noncytotoxic chemotherapeutic agent that is commonly used to induce remissions in patients with acute promyelocytic leukemia. Lung toxicity hampers ATRA therapy in up to 26% of patients (319,320). Distinct pulmonary syndromes include noncardiogenic pulmonary edema, diffuse alveolar hemorrhage, and ARDS. A rise in the periperal blood white count commonly heralds the development of fever, dyspnea, weight gain, diffuse pulmonary infiltrates, pleural and pericardial effusions, generalized edema, and hypotension. Standard prophylaxis with high-dose corticosteroids has dramatically decreased the incidence of pulmonary toxicity. Dexamethasone, dosed at 10 mg every 12 hr, may rapidly reverse the pulmonary infiltrative process and improve patient outcome (320,321).

Thalidomide

Thalidomide, a sedating agent known for its devastating teratogenic effects in the 1960s, has reemerged with the discovery of its putative antiangiogenic properties and its ability to modulate proinflammatory cytokines, such as TNF and IL-2. The drug is currently approved only for the treatment of erythema nodosum leprosum (ENL) in the United States (322), but has been studied in a variety of malignant diseases and treatment-related disorders, including multiple myeloma (323,324), myelodysplastic syndromes (325,326), acute myeloid leukemias (327), renal cell carcinoma (328), and GVHD (329,330). Adverse events asso ciated with thalidomide therapy include peripheral neuropathy, constipation, somnolence, rash, and thromboembolic disease. Thromboembolic events, including pulmonary embolism, deep venous thrombosis, and clotting of central venous catheters, have been reported with thalidomide administration (331–333). Patients who receive thalidomide as a component of combination chemotherapy appear to be at particularly high risk, with thromboembolic events as high as 28% among this group of patients. Rates of thromboembolism appear highest among recipients of combined thalidomide and doxorubicin- and BCNU-based chemotherapy (334,335).

Etoposide/Teniposide

The podophyllotoxin derivatives, etoposide (VP16) and teniposide (VM26), are antitumor agents with activity against a variety of malignancies, including lymphomas, germ-cell tumors, and lung cancer. Hypersensitivity reactions represent the principal form of lung toxicity among these agents. Teniposide is formulated in a Cremaphor EL solvent similar to taxol, which may contribute to the increased rates of hypersensitivity reactions with this agent (336,337). Patients may present with flushing, bronchospasm, dyspnea, abdominal pain, and hypotension coincident with the first or second dose of the drug. Antihistamines, steroids, and epinephrine are standard therapy. The response is generally favorable. Prophylaxis with steroids and antihistamines frequently permits successful rechallenge of these drugs (338).

7. *Biologic Response Modifiers/Immunotoxins*

Advances in molecular biologic techniques have permitted the rapid isolation and analysis of DNA, RNA, and protein and identified pathways that are unique to cancer cell growth, survival, and metastasis. The exploitation of these pathways as specific tumor targets has provided novel strategies for the development of a new class of targeted anticancer therapeutics. This class of agents, collectively known as the biologic response modifiers, includes an expanding list of cytokines (interleukin-2, interferons, tumor necrosis factor), growth factors (granulocyte-stimulating growth factor, granulocyte colony-stimulating growth factor), and synthetic immunotoxin monoclonal antibodies (imitimab, transtuzumab, rituximab)). Early descriptions of the efficacy of each of these agents have been generally encouraging, although individual toxicity profiles, including pulmonary toxicity, have been substantive and treatment-limiting for some drugs.

Interleukin-2 (IL-2)

Interleukin-2 (IL-2) has become standard therapy in the treatment of cancers, such as renal cell carcinoma that are refractory to conventional therapy. Clinical toxicities associated with the use of this drug are extensive and occasionally life threatening. Dermatologic (erythema, mucositis, reactivation of psoriasis,) endocrine (hypothyroidism), cardiac (arrhythmias, myocarditis, myocardial depression), neurologic (altered mental status) musculoskeletal and flu-like symptoms top the list of potential adverse reactions. In addition, hematologic derangements, including eosinophilia, anemia, and thrombocytopenia may be seen (339,340). Pulmonary toxicity represents the most feared consequence of treatment. The major patterns of pulmonary toxicity include bronchospasm, pleural effusions, pulmonary infiltrates with eosinophilia, and cardiovascular collapse associated with noncardiogenic pulmonary edema. Acute permeability pulmonary edema is thought to represent a vascular leak syndrome. Pulmonary edema, hypotension, impaired renal function, and generalized edema with concomitant weight gain are prominent features of this disorder. The hemodynamic derangements include hypotension, increased cardiac output, and decreased peripheral vascular resistance, which closely mimic septic shock. The clinical consequences and physiologic derangements of IL-2-induced lung disease are not trivial—the need for mechanical ventilation and hemodynamic support is indicated in 15% of patients and 2–3% of patients die from refractory cardiopulmonary failure (341,342). Disease severity varies with the total dose and route of IL-2 administration. Continuous infusion of IL-2 is associated with decreased rates of clinical toxicity. Pulmonary infiltrates and associated symptoms of dyspnea tend to occur late in the course of treatment and are coincident with the development of eosinophilia. Tissue and peripheral eosinophilia associated with IL-2 therapy are mediated by interlcukin-5, a lymphocyte-derived cytokine that promotes eosinophil differentiation, activation, and proliferation (343). The associated release of major basic protein, a known endothelial toxin in vitro, by eosinophils may play a critical role in the development of capillary leak syndrome (344,345). Although the pathogenesis of capillary leak syndrome remains speculative, these observations support a role for eosinophils and toxic eosinophil products in the development of this disease. Cessation of IL-2 therapy, the judicious use of corticosteroid therapy and initiation of mechanical ventilation and hemodynamic supportive measures when indicated, frequently result in a favorable outcome.

Tumor Necrosis Factor Therapy

Tumor necrosis factor (TNF), a pleiomorphic cytokine, is broadly implicated in a variety of cellular activities, including growth promotion and inhibition, cytotoxicity, apoptosis, immunomodulation, inflammation, and angiogenesis. In addition, this cytokine induces a variety of cell surface molecules (IL-2, intercellular adhesion molecule-1, major histocompatibility complex class I and II) and cellular proteins (granulocyte-macrophage colony-stimulating factor, interferon, IL-1, IL-6, IL-8) that are involved in immune activation and inflammatory processes (346,347). The therapeutic efficacy of recombinant TNF (rTNF) as well as antibodies to this cytokine has been studied. Although early reports of rTNF in the treatment of advanced solid tumors were disappointing, more recent studies with locoregional administration of this agent through isolated limb infusions appear more encouraging (348–351). Furthermore, TNF has been found to enhance the efficacy of other antitumor drugs, such as melphalan and doxorubicin (351). Administration of rTNF may result in a profound capillary leak syndrome that closely mimics septic shock (352,353). Pulmonary hemorrhage following rTNF-a infusion has also been described (354). Antibodies to rTNF have only recently been developed and the potential role and toxicity profile of these agents in the management of disease are only beginning to emerge.

Infliximab, a chimeric IgG_1 monoclonal antibody that targets TNF, has recently gained FDA approval in the treatment of inflammatory bowel disease and rheumatoid arthritis (355,356). The utility of this agent in the treatment of graft-versus-host disease and in the management of certain tumors, such as multiple myeloma and lymphomas, has not been definitively established, although early reports appear encouraging (357). Enhanced rates of opportunistic infections, in particular pneumonias caused by tuberculosis aspergillus, nocardia, and Pneumocystis, have been reported following the use of this drug (358–360). Infections tend to develop within the first three to four doses of therapy. The reported frequency of tuberculosis appears much higher than other opportunistic infections and may be associated with the development of disseminated disease (358,359). Pulmonary infiltrates with eosinophilia (PIE syndrome) and eosinophilic pleural effusions have also been reported following the use of this drug.

Interferon

The interferons (IFN) represent a family of cytokines with diverse immunomodulatory effects. Emerging data suggest a role for these mediators in the treatment of a variety of malignant and nonmalignant diseases, including viral and antitumor activities. The oncologic indications for IFN include renal cell carcinoma, melanoma, HIV-associated Kaposi's sarcoma and a variety of lymphoproliferative malignancies. IFN administration induces an array of adverse reactions such as flu-like symptoms and disturbances of cardiovascular, hepatic and central nervous system function. Pulmonary complications subsequent to IFN therapy are unusual and potentially life threatening. Individual case reports have cited an association between IFN therapy and the development of interstitial pneumonitis, bronchiolitis obliterans with organizing pneumonia and pulmonary hypertension (361–363). There have been rare reports of sarcoidosis and thromboembolic events associated with the application of this drug (364–366).

Tyrosine Kinase Inhibitors

Gefitinib (Iressa), an oral selective inhibitor of the epidermal growth factor tyrosine kinase, is used in the treatment of patients with advanced nonsmall cell lung cancer. Acute interstitial pneumonitis has been reported among 2–3% of recipients of this drug and may be severe (367,368). This complication of therapy may occur 1–2 months following gefitinib therapy. The utility of corticosteroids in treating this disorder has not been established. Finally, imatinib (Gleevac) an inhibitor of c-kit and Bcr-Abl tyrosine kinase has shown efficacy in the treatment of chronic myeloid leukemia. Pulmonary edema occurs as a rare manifestation of the fluid retention syndrome associated with gleevec therapy. Gleevec-related lung toxicity, manifested as hypersensitivity pneumonitis, has been documented in case reports (369,370).

Granulocyte Colony-Stimulating Factor (G-CSF)

G-CSF is widely used to accelerate the recovery of myelopoiesis following myelosuppressive chemotherapy, stem cell transplantation, and radiation therapy. The spectrum of lung toxicity associated with G-CSF therapy includes acute permeability edema with or without ARDS, interstitial pneumonitis with eosinophilia and venous thrombosis. Drug withdrawal is usually sufficient to ameliorate clinical symptoms although fatal toxicity associated with G-CSF-related pneumonitis and ARDS has been reported (371–375).

Immunotoxin Therapy

Immunotoxin chemotherapy using monoclonal antibodies represents a robust and rapidly expanding class of antitumor agents directed against specific tumor antigens. The full spectrum of clinical toxicities associated with this relatively new class of anticancer agents continues to be defined. Rituximab, an anti-CD_{20} monoclonal antibody, is widely used in the treatment of non-Hodgkin's lymphoma. This agent may also be used as an "in vivo purging agent" prior to stem cell transplantation to remove residual $CD20^+$ lymphoma cells (376). Although the drug is fairly well tolerated, fever, chills, bronchospasm, hypotension, angioedema, and interstitial pneumonitis have been associated with infusion of this agent (377). Rituximab activity is known to release TNF and induce other biologic activities, including B-lymphocyte cytolysis, and compliment activation, which may underlie the development of interstitial pneumonitis. Infectious deaths in rituximab-treated patients owing to delayed recovery of neutrophils and lymphocytes following stem cell transplantation have also been reported (378–380). Transtuzumab (Herceptin), used either as single agent therapy or in combination with anthracyclines or paclitaxel, shows promising efficacy in the treatment of advanced breast cancers that demonstrate overexpression of the HER-2/neu protein. This monoclonal antibody targets the human epidermal growth factor (HER-2) receptor. Reports of major pulmonary events have been limited primarily to cardiogenic pulmonary edema, which tends to occur in patients with underlying significant cardiac disease or prior anthracycline therapy (381). Gemtuzumab ozogamicin (Mylotarg) targets the CD33 antigen found on the surface of AML leukemic blasts. An infusion-related symptom complex similar to that seen with the administration of other monoclonal antibodies frequently occurs with gemtuzumab therapy. Fever, dyspnea, and chills are prominent symptoms with initial infusion of the drug in 1/3 of patients and usually abate with subsequent therapy. An increased predilection for pneumonia has also been noted following administration of this drug.

D. Radiation-Induced Lung Injury

Clinically significant lung injury is a well-known sequela of thoracic radiation, occurring in approximately 5–15% of treated patients. Despite numerous studies and animal models of radiation-induced lung injury, the precise incidence and clinical diagnosis of this disorder are elusive and the complex pathogenic events leading to lung damage remain incompletely described. Although pneumonitis is a prominent feature of both radiation- and chemotherapy-induced lung disease, no unifying concept highlighting common mechanisms between these two disorders exists. The major clinical manifestations of radiation-related lung damage include a dose-dependent classical pneumonitis and pulmonary fibrosis. Recently, sporadic pneumonitis has been recognized as an acute form of radiation pneumonitis with features distinct from its classical counterpart. The type II pneumocytes and alveolar endothelial cells are most vulnerable to radiation. Radiation injury to these cells results in release of surfactant and inflammatory exudates into the interstitium and hyperplasia of type II pneumocytes. In addition, damage to the capillary endothelium leads to increased vascular permeability and congestion. Over the ensuing 2–3 months following thoracic radiation, oxidative lung injury caused by the release of reactive free radicals may give rise to clinically evident symptoms of pneumonitis. An exuberant inflammatory response triggered by locally released growth factors and cytokines, including transforming growth factor-β (TGF-β), interleukin-l(IL-l), tumor necrosis factor (TNF) and intercellular adhesion molecule-1 (ICAM-1) also contributes to the development of pneumonitis.

Classic pneumonitis marks the early phase of radiation-induced lung injury, which usually appears clinically at 2–3 months after the completion of radiotherapy. Patients typically present with gradually progressive symptoms of fever, exertional dyspnea, and nonproductive cough which peak at 3–4 months after radiotherapy. The radiographic changes of classic pneumonitis may range from subtle abnormalities, such as indistinct vascular margins to frank consolidations with or without air-bronchograms and are predominantly restricted to areas of previously irradiated lung. The development of pleural effusions coincident with the onset of pneumonitis has also been described. The absence of malignant cells on pleural fluid cytology and the propensity to spontaneously remit help to distinguish these effusions from those directly related to malignancy.

Pulmonary fibrosis is the histologic hallmark of the late phase of radiation damage to the lungs. Radiographic and histologic evidence of radiation-induced pulmonary fibrosis occurs regardless of prior overt clinical manifestations of pneumonitis. Pulmonary fibrosis may be clinically silent or associated with varying degrees of dyspnea. The physiologic consequences of radiation fibrosis include respiratory failure, pulmonary hypertension, and cor pulmonale, especially when large areas of the lungs are involved. The fibrotic changes occur insidiously over 6 months to a year after thoracic irradiation as a consequence of repair initiated by radiation tissue injury. Pulmonary hypertension may also occur as a result of radiation-induced pulmonary veno-occlusive disease (382). Characteristic radiographic findings that suggest pulmonary fibrosis include ipsilateral pleural thickening, volume loss, bronchiectasis, retraction of the lung parenchyma, tenting and elevation of the hemidiaphragm, and linear densities. As the disease progresses pneumothorax and hyperlucency of the ipsilateral lung may be seen. The radiographic appearance of fibrosis typically stabilizes over the ensuing 1–2 years following completion of radiation and persists unchanged thereafter.

Sporadic pneumonitis is thought to represent an acute hypersensitivity pneumonitis following thoracic irradiation. A pathologic hallmark of this lung reaction is a diffuse lymphocyte-predominant alveolitis on recovered BAL fluid and generalized bilateral uptake on gallium scan. The etiology of sporadic pneumonitis is unclear, although it is thought to be immunologically mediated. Minimal infiltrate corresponding to the radiation port is occasionally seen on chest radiographs although frequently these films are deceptively clear. Gallium scans and CT scans of the chest are more sensitive tools in detecting this disease. Patients frequently present with progressive dyspnea that is out of proportion to radiographic findings or the volume of lung irradiated. These symptoms typically begin 2–3 months following the completion of radiation and resolve within 6–8 weeks of onset without sequelae. Steroids are occasionally required to ameliorate symptoms.

Another manifestation of radiation-related lung injury is bronchiolitis obliterans with organizing pneumonia (BOOP) (383). Unlike radiation-induced pneumonitis, which typically presents with dyspnea, the salient clinical features of this lung reaction are dry cough and fever. This entity has been most frequently described among irradiated patients with breast cancer. Although radiation-related BOOP characteristically begins within the radiation portal, it may spread to the nonirradiated lung in up to 40% of patients. The prognosis is generally favorable. Steroid therapy may result in dramatic clinical improvement. Relapses with steroid withdrawal are common.

Both the onset and severity of radiation toxicity are influenced by risk factors, including dose of radiation, dose fractionation, volume of lung irradiated, geographic location of tumor within the lung, concomitant chemotherapy, prior radiotherapy, and underlying pulmonary reserve (384). Radiation pneumonitis rarely occurs with irradiated lung volumes of less than 10% or with fractionated total doses of radiation of less than 2000 cGy (384). The radiographic manifestations of toxicity typically appear at doses of 4000 cGy or above, are nearly universal with doses above 6000 cGy, and may be attenuated by administering the total dose of radiation in multiple small fractions (385,386). Rapid steroid withdrawal may also facilitate the development of radiation-induced toxicity by unmasking subclinical findings of pneumonitis. Synergistic effects causing severe lung toxicity have been reported with sequential or concurrent use of radiation with adriamycin, vincristine, bleomycin, cyclophosphamide, mitomycin C, and actinomycin D. These drugs not only potentiate the lung toxic effects of radiation, but also shorten the latency period after radiation exposure. Lung damage following combined chemoradiation therapy is typically not limited to the radiation site and may extend well outside the radiation field. Concomitant chemoradiation therapy regimens may also heighten the risk of radiation injury through the process of radiation recall. This phenomenon occurs when certain chemotherapeutic regimens are given after radiation therapy, resulting in the unmasking of subclinical damage within the treated radiation field. In radiation-recall, an exuberant inflammatory response develops within hours to days after the completion of chemotherapy. Unlike the diffuse lung injury seen with the synergistic interactions between radiation and certain chemotherapeutic agents, lung damage associated with radiation recall is typically limited to the previously irradiated site. The radiation-recall response may occur days to years after radiation therapy. Among the various antineoplastic agents that have been implicated in the radiation-recall response are the taxanes (paclitaxel), anthracyclines (adriamycin), alkylating agents (cyclophosphamide), cytotoxic antibiotics (actinomycin D), vinca alkyloids (vinblastine), antimetabolites (methotrexate, 5-flourouracil), hormonal agents (tamoxifen), and gemcitabine (305,387,388). Measurements of lung function including lung volumes and the transfer factor (DLco) prior to radiation do not reliably predict the later development of radiation-induced lung toxicity (389). Moreover, these parameters have not been shown to detect early radiation-induced lung damage with any degree of certainty. Nevertheless, these tests provide an objective assessment of the functional late affects of radiation lung injury. Serial measurements of these two parameters are frequently used to guide therapy.

The overall prognosis for radiation-induced lung disease is good for patients with mild-to-moderate disease. Mortality rates among patients with severe pneumonitis, however, are poor. In one recent study of lung cancer patients, the diagnosis of severe pneumonitis was associated with a 0% 3-year survival as compared to a 38.2% and 33.4% 3-year survival among patients with mild and moderate pneumonitis, respectively (389). The survival rates at 8 months among lung cancer patients with severe radiation pneumonitis reported by Graham et al. (384) were equally as bleak (0% at 8 months). Steroids are indicated for moderate-to-severe pneumonitis. Therapy is generally initiated at 0.5–1.0 mg/kg/day of prednisone or its equivalent at the time of diagnosis and tapered once a complete response is noted.

E. Pulmonary Embolic Disease

1. *Venous Thromboembolism*

Venous thromboembolism (VTE) represents a spectrum of disorders that range from localized deep venous thrombosis (DVT) to life-threatening massive pulmonary embolism (PE). Shock complicating massive pulmonary embolism occurs in 10% of patients with PE and is associated with a 30% mortality. VTE frequently complicates the management of critically ill cancer patients. The overall prevalence of DVT among critically ill medical and surgical patients in the absence of prophylaxis ranges from 22% to 80%, and varies with the underlying medical/surgical condition. Critically ill cancer patients are particularly vulnerable to VTE events. Cancer alone confers a 4-fold increased risk of thrombosis; associated threatment with certain chemotherapeutic agents raises the risk 6-fold (390,391). The need for prompt diagnosis and intervention is underscored by the 2- to 3-fold increased mortality rate in this already debilitated patient population.

The association between malignancy, the hypercoaguable state, and thromboembolic events was first described by Trousseau more than a century ago, and has since been confirmed by abundant clinical and pathologic observations (392–405). A classic example of cancer-related thromboembolic disease is the "Trousseau" syndrome, a recurrent, migratory thrombophlebitis that is most frequently associated with gastrointestinal malignancies. The "Budd–Chiari" syndrome, most notably associated with myeloproliferative disorders, and portal vein thrombosis, associated with hepatomas and carcinomas of the kidneys and adrenals in addition to myeloproliferative disorders provide other salient examples. The highest rates of cancer-related thromboembolic events have been reported among patients with mucin-producing adenocarcinomas of the gastrointestinal tract, pancreas, lung, kidneys, prostate, and ovaries (396,398,400, 401,403–408). Acute promyelocytic leukemias, myeloproliferative disorders, and primary carcinomas of the brain are also associated with an increased incidence of thromboembolic disease (394,409–411). Cancer-associated thromboembolic disease may occur at any time during the course of established malignancy or as the sentinel event among patients who subsequently are diagnosed with cancer. The incidence of subsequent malignant neoplasm in patients with no obvious risk factors for thrombosis is 2–25% (394,403, 412,413).

Thrombosis as the initial manifestation of cancer portends a worse prognosis, perhaps because VTE acts as a surrogate marker for a more aggressive cancer (406,411). Alternatively, VTE may appear as a more recalcitrant disease in patients with cancer. This would explain the higher incidence of recurrent PE and fatal PE among patients with malignancy.

Although the majority of thrombi originate in the large capacitance vessels of the pelvis and lower extremities, upper extremity thrombosis has been increasingly recognized and may be the presenting event among patients with occult or undiagnosed cancer (414–416). The near universal use of central venous catheters in the cancer patient profoundly contributes to increased rates of catheter-related clot formation. Right ventricular (RV) thrombi have been reported in patients with cor pulmonale and indwelling right atrial catheters (417). Factors such as catheter material (polyvinyl, noncoated polyurethane), non-heparin-bonded catheters, femoral and internal jugular sites of catheter placement and duration of cannulation of greater than 6 days confer an increased risk of central venous catheter-related thrombosis.

Each of the components of Virchow's triad—intimal injury, venous stasis, and altered coagulation—may contribute to the excess rates of thromboembolism in cancer (Table 12). Comorbid conditions such as prolonged bed rest, major surgery, and the use of central venous catheters are ubiquitous in the cancer setting and enhance the risk of venous thrombosis. In addition, hematopoietic colony-stimulating factors, hormonal therapy, and other antineoplastic agents augment this risk by interfering with normal hemostasis. These predisposing risk factors for the development of thromboembolic disease exert their effects cumulatively, resulting in a 3-fold increased risk of recurrent embolic events and a 2- to 3-fold increased risk of fatal thromboembolism. The hypercoaguable state of cancer is conditioned by interactions between tumor cells and the fibrinolytic and/or coagulation systems. Tumor cells are capable of expressing tissue factors and other cancer procoagulants that interfere with normal clotting-fibrinolytic pathways. The most common laboratory manifestations of these interactions include elevations in fibrinogen, fibrinogen degradation products, platelet counts, anticardiolipin antibodies and in clotting factors V, VIII, IX, and XI. In addition,

Table 12 Pathogenesis of Thromboembolism in Cancer Patients

Condition	Pathogenesis
Venous stasis	• Venous obstruction by tumor • Decreased mobility/prolonged bed rest • Increased blood viscosity • Increased venous pressure from tumoral compression of vessel
Vessel wall injury	• Direct tumor injury to endothelium • Chemotherapy-induced (BCNU, bleomycin, vincristine, adriamycin, taxanes)
Hypercoaguability	• Direct and indirect tumor-cell activation of clotting factors • Overexpression of tissue factor and other procoagulants • Chemotherapy-induced reductions in protein C and protein S (cyclophosphamide, methotrexate, tamoxifen) • Reductions in antithrombin III caused by surgery, chemotherapeutic agents (L-asparaginase, tamoxifen) and heparin
Platelet abnormalities	• Spontaneous platelet aggregation • Increased thrombopoietin • Reactive thrombocytosis (carcinomas of the breast, lung, stomach, ovary, colon)

reductions in plasma levels of inhibitors of coagulation, such as antithrombin III, and protein C and S, have also been reported (418). These derangements may directly contribute to the hypercoaguable state and the excess rates of thromboembolism among patients with cancer. Unfortunately, none of these abnormalities are specific for cancer. Nor can they be used to reliably predict the occurrence of thromboembolism in the cancer setting.

Under normal circumstances, the pulmonary circulation is very forgiving. Up to 50% of the normal pulmonary circulation may be obliterated without significant changes in pulmonary hemodynamics, right heart performance or ventilation/perfusion match. This is because much of the lung's tremendous redundant vascular bed is nonperfused at rest and is selectively recruited with rising cardiac outputs. This unique physiologic phenomenon permits optimization of the ventilation/perfusion balance during all phases of exercise. Thus, the abundant pulmonary vasculature underlies the lung's capacity to tolerate clots that truncate significant portions of the pulmonary circulation with little change in pulmonary hemodynamics, ventilation–perfusion (V/Q) match, or right heart performance. The large clot burden posed by massive pulmonary embolism or smaller clots in the setting of compromised cardiopulmonary reserve may overwhelm these compensatory mechanisms, resulting in acute elevations in pulmonary vascular resistance, altered RV performance, severe hypoxemia, and sudden death. Pulmonary embolism may cause acute elevations in RV afterload and parallel increases in RV wall tension. The compensatory response of the RV to increase its stroke volume against acute escalations in RV afterload is very limited. Thus, abrupt elevations in RV wall tensions above 40–50 mmHg cause the RV to progressively dilate and ultimately fail. Associated hemodynamic conditions, such as RV ischemia and dysfunction, and tricuspid regugitation further impair forward flow and contribute to hemodynamic collapse. Right-to-left intracardiac shunt secondary to the opening of a patent foramen ovale may occur in the setting of severe right atrial pressure elevations. The release of serotonin by platelets and bradykinin by the thrombus further aggravate RV failure by increasing pulmonary vascular resistance. These pathologic conditions further contribute to severely impaired ventilation/perfusion balance and lead to intractable hypoxemia.

The diagnosis of thromboembolism in the setting of cancer is often difficult, confounded by competing disorders with similar clinical findings. Clinical symptoms of pulmonary embolism, such as acute pleuritic chest pain associated with unexplained hypoxemia, tachycardia, and hemodynamic instability are highly suggestive of pulmonary embolism. These symptoms, however, may represent clinical manifestations of a preexisting compromised cardiopulmonary reserve and therefore mask any superimposed symptoms of PE. In addition, the clinical manifestations of thromboembolic events are notoriously imprecise and cannot be relied on to establish or exclude the diagnosis. Documented deep venous thrombosis predicts the presence of pulmonary embolism in only 50% of patients. Symptomatic pulmonary embolism may be associated with clinically silent thrombus involving the proximal vessels of the lower extremities. Dyspnea, the most common presenting symptom of PE, occurs in 70–90% of patients, but is a nonspecific complaint. The triad of dyspnea, pleuritic chest pain, and/or tachypnea was noted among 97% of patients with angiographically proven PE in one study (419). Angina secondary to RV ischemia has also been reported (419). In addition to respiratory symptoms and signs, patients with PE related to an upper extremity source may present with arm face and neck swelling and pain. Tumor infiltration or extrinsic compression of the axillary or subclavian veins may mimic these findings, making the diagnosis of PE related to an upper extremity clot even more of a clinical challenge.

Hemoptysis may occur 12–36 hr following the embolic event. This rare event more often complicates PE among patients with a significant prior history of cardiac or pulmonary dysfunction and indicates pulmonary infarction when it occurs. Pulmonary infarction may occur in up to 20% of patients with prior compromised cardiopulmonary reserve. On physical examination, unexplained tachypnea and tachycardia may offer clues to the diagnosis. Sinus tachycardia is the most common associated arrhythmia. Acute atrial arrhythmias, right axis deviation, (p-pulmonale) and T-wave inversion are other electrocardiographic (EKG) findings that typically occur with large clot burdens. The $S_1Q_3T_3$ pattern may occasionally occur and is more suggestive of PE. Evidence of T-wave inversion closely paralleled PE severity and was the most common EKG finding in one study (420). Derangements in blood gas measurements, including arterial oxygen partial pressure (PaO_2) and alveolar arterial PO_2 difference (PO_2) (421) do not reliably predict the presence or absence of PE. In the PIOPED study both of these parameters were normal in 38% of patients with normal prior cardiopulmonary reserve and in 14% of patients with antecedent cardiopulmonary disease (422). Moreover, although respiratory acidosis is the most common acid–base abnormality seen among patients wit acute PE, respiratory alkalosis has also been reported in the setting of massive PE and preexisting severe cardiopulmonary disease. An acute and unexplained drop in the systolic blood pressure of $\geq$40 mmHg, or a sustained drop in the systolic blood pressure to $\leq$90 mmHg, accompanied by tachycardia or an acute decline in FIO_2 should raise the suspicion for massive pulmonary embolism. In most patients, the constellation of signs and symptoms at presentation is sufficiently vague to warrant further invasive evaluations. An algorithm for the evaluation of the patient with suspected PE is shown in Fig. 16. The standard diagnostic evaluation may not be feasible in the critically ill patient with suspected PE because of hemodynamic instability. First-line diagnostic strategies in these patients frequently rely on pretest-probability of PE coupled with and emergent bedside transthoracic echocardiography. In the general population, patients may be started on empiric anticoagulant therapy until the definitive evaluation for PE can be done. In the cancer patient, however, hematologic failure may preclude the safe use of empiric anticoagulation and the risk of precipitating bleeding must be carefully weighed against any potential therapeutic benefits.

Although the findings on chest radiographs are nonspecific, chest radiography is essential to rule out competing pathology. Findings range from a normal chest radiograph to focal infiltrates, atelectasis, elevation of the ipsilateral hemidiaphragm, and hypoperfusion of the involved lung with associated enlargement of the pulmonary artery (Westermark's sign). The finding of Hamptom's hump, a pleural-based opacity in the setting of PE, suggests pulmonary infarction. This opacity is typically wedge shaped but may be of any configuration. Transthoracic or transesophageal echocardiography may yield valuable circumstantial evidence of pulmonary embolism and permits rapid bedside evaluation of the unstable patient. Evidence of right ventricular strain is seen in more than 40% of patients with documented PE and augurs a poor outcome (423). Findings such as cor pulmonale, dilatation of the pulmonary artery, and a dilated right ventricle may offer indirect evidence PE. Occasionally, retained right-sided mobile thrombi may appear as echodense material within the right atrium or ventricle (Fig. 17). Assays for D-dimer, the cross-linked degradation product of fibrin, have been extensively studied as potential markers with predictive value for the diagnosis of thromboembolism. Levels of D-dimer elevation may vary depending on the type of assay and the population studied. Acute thrombosis is virtually always associated with D-dimer levels of >500 ng/mL. Other nonthrombotic conditions such as malignancy, pneumonia, myocardial infarction, sepsis, surgery, hemorrhage, advancing age, pregnancy, and trauma may also cause acute elevations in D-dimer levels to this extent or greater. Moreover, in patients with cancer, the D-dimer assay has a significantly lower negative predictive value as compared with patients without cancer and thus cannot be used to reliably exclude thrombus formation in this group of patients (424). In a recent study by De Monye et al. (425), the sensitivity of D-dimer varied with the location of the embolus. The authors concluded that the sensitivity of the D-dimer assay was higher with pulmonary emboli involving segmental or larger arteries (94%) and could not be relied upon in excluding small subsegmental pulmonary emboli (50% sensitivity). Thus, D-dimer assays are of only incremental value in the diagnostic evaluation of the elderly patient with comorbid illnesses and/or subsegmental pulmonary emboli. The diagnosis of PE may be inferred in patients with acute respiratory symptoms and evidence of clot on lower extremity imaging studies, such as Doppler venous untrasonography, impedence plethysmography (IPG), contrast venography, or radioisotopic examinations.

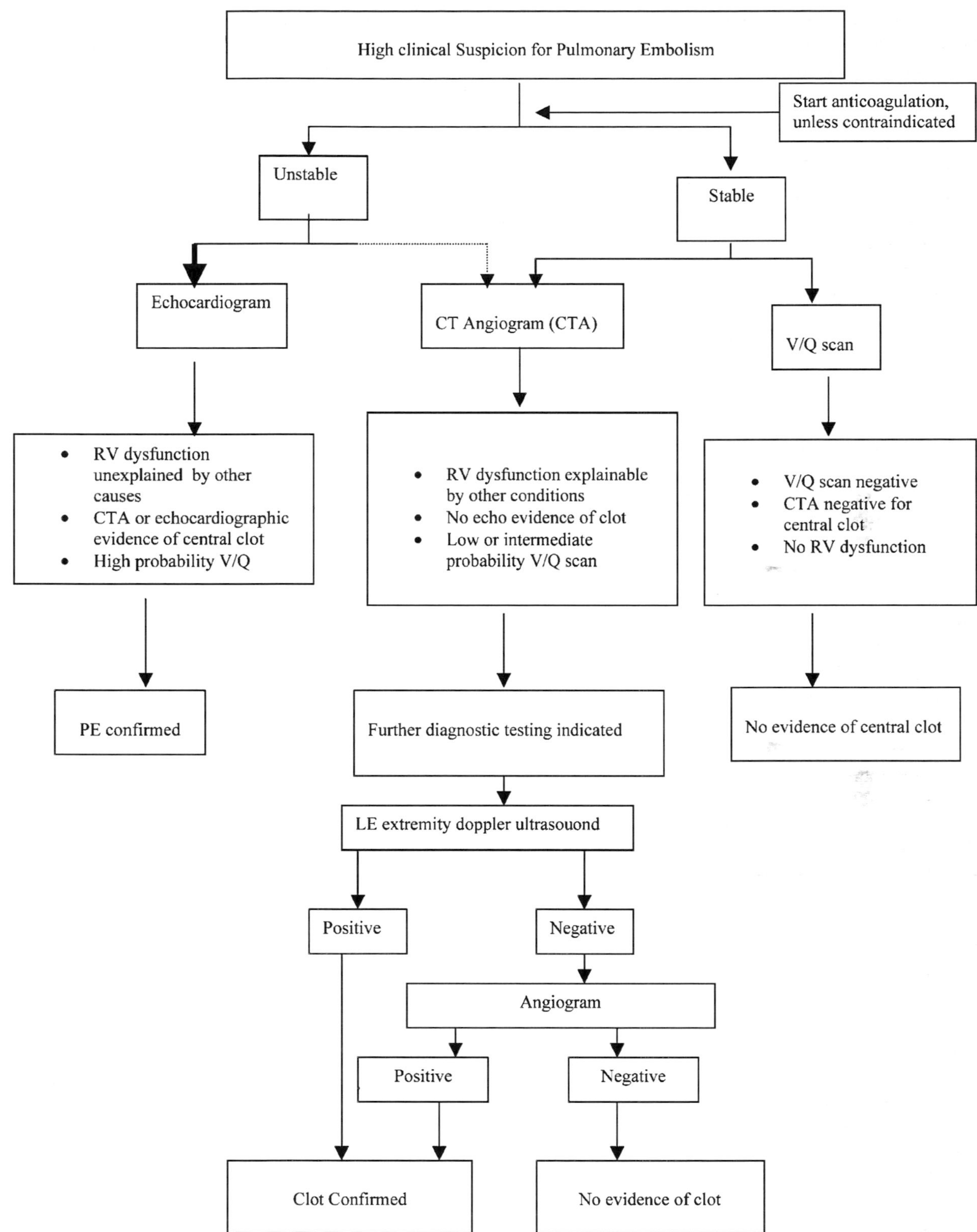

Figure 16 Algorithm for evaluation of pulmonary embolism.

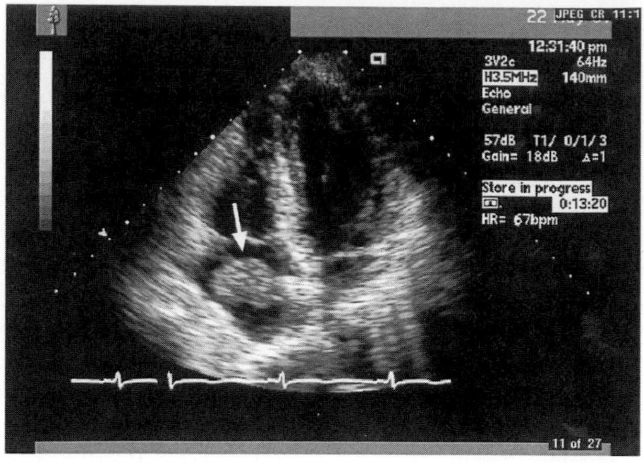

Figure 17 A patient with mucinous adenocarcinoma of the breast and acute symptoms of shortness of breath and severe hypoxemia. An echocardiogram showed a large clot occupying the right atrium (*arrow*).

The findings on physical examination, chest radiograph, echocardiogram, lower extremity imaging, and laboratory assays may create footprints of PE but cannot definitively establish the diagnosis. The definitive diagnostic evaluation relies on specific tests, including ventilation/perfusion (V/Q) scintigraphy, spiral CT, magnetic resonance imaging, and pulmonary angiography. For more than three decades, the V/Q scan has represented a critical component of the diagnostic armamentarium for PE. A normal V/Q scan effectively excludes the diagnosis of PE. A high probability scan is defined as 2 or more moderate to large perfusion defects (occupying >25% of the lung segment) with intact ventilation in radiographically normal areas of the lung. These studies are regarded as highly predictive of the presence of PE. More than 60% of patients, however, with suspected PE who undergo V/Q scanning have nondefinitive or intermediate probability studies (426). The approach to this group of patients is based on the initial clinical suspicion for PE and the underlying cardiopulmonary reserve. Spiral CT angiography has emerged over the past decade as an important tool in the evaluation of PE. This instrument reliably detects clots in the central (second- to fourth-order) bronchi with sensitivities and specificities of 90% (for both measures). In addition, the lung windows obtained with spiral CT imaging permit visualization of the lung parenchyma and offers additional information regarding competing diagnoses. CT evidence of acute PE is similar to the angiographic signs of PE and includes partial or complete filling defects and the "railway track" signs. Several shortcomings of CT angiography are recognized: accurate interpretation of the spiral CT images is heavily operator dependent; psuedo-filling defects caused by severe tachypnea may lead to interpretive errors and emboli within the distal (subsegmental) pulmonary vasculature cannot be reliably detected with this technique. Isolated thromboembolism at the subsegmental level occurs in 5–36% of patients (427). The significance of these smaller emboli is a matter of much debate. Treatment is generally advocated, however, especially in the setting of poor cardiopulmonary reserve. Thus, the CT angiogram is an excellent tool for detecting central clot. Because of the decreased sensitivity and specificity for distal thrombi, a negative CT angiogram does not rule out pulmonary embolism with the same degree of certainty as a normal V/Q scan. Patients with high clinical suspicion for PE and a negative CT angiogram or an intermediate probability V/Q scan may ultimately require pulmonary angiography for diagnosis. Conventional pulmonary angiography remains the gold standard for the diagnosis of PE. Although angiography is often touted as a high-risk procedure, the incidence of procedure-related deaths and morbidity were low (0.5% and 0.8%, respectively) in the PIOPED study (426). Partial studies that limit the injection of contrast to abnormal areas seen on V/Q or CT angiographic studies represent reasonable strategies designed to mitigate the patient's risk.

The goals of therapy in the management of the unstable patient with pulmonary embolism include stabilization of cardiovascular hemodynamics, and prevention of further clot formation and migration while allowing the endogenous fibrinolytic system to dissolve the existing thrombi. Other therapeutic options, including thrombolytic therapy and surgical or transvenous catheter embolectomy, are aimed at reducing the embolic burden and may be appropriate in select patients with life-threatening acute PE. These therapeutic options should be considered as up-front therapy in the hemodynamically unstable patient with massive pulmonary embolism (see below). Hemodynamic stabilization is paramount and independent of clot dynamics and thrombolysis. Volume resuscitation, aimed at improving hypotension and augmenting RV preload, should be administered judiciously. Overzealous fluid replacement may further distend the RV, aggravate RV ischemia, and precipitate further deterioration in RV function. Typically, right atrial pressures of 15–20 mmHg by central venous monitoring are sufficient to maintain adequate RV preload. If hypotension persists after 500–1000 cc of fluid resuscitation or despite RA pressures of 15–20 mmHg, the institution of vasoactive medications should be considered. Vasoactive agents, including dobutamine and norepinephrine, have been used to augment RV contractility in the treatment of shock-related PE;

however, the efficacy of these and other agents have not been validated in any large, randomized studies. Dobutamine, a potent vasodilator of the systemic and pulmonary vascular beds, may improve forward flow and cardiac output by reducing RV afterload. The α and β adrenoreceptor agonist activity of norepinephrine may enhance cardiac contractility and coronary blood flow and is preferred in the management of severe reductions in cardiac outputs and associated hypotension.

Strategies to prevent further clot formation typically involve the use of unfractionated heparin or low-molecular weight heparin (LMWH) preparations. Abundant studies have documented favorable bioavailability, equivalent efficacy, convenient dosing, an apparent lower incidence of heparin-induced thrombocytopenia, and recurrent VTE with LMWHs. The LMWHs have thus been increasingly used instead of unfractionated heparin (UFH) for VTE prophylaxis as well as in the treatment of stable patients with established thromboembolic disease. This switch has been supported by the American College of Chest Physicians (ACCP) in the 2001 consensus statement (428). Other advantages of LMWHs include the lack of a need for monitoring of coagulation profiles (except in special circumstances), and a possible survival benefit among patients with cancer (404,428). Several recent studies have suggested that long-term LMWH therapy may improve survival in patients with cancer, putatively due to the antiangiogenic effect of these drugs (139,404,429,430). Reduced rates of recurrent thromboembolism among patients treated with fractionated heparin vs. oral anticoagulant therapy have also been documented (429,431). For the treatment of the unstable ICU patient, UFH is still favored because of the shorter half-life and easy reversibility of this drug. Anticoagulation should be initiated immediately to patients with high clinical suspicion of PE, even before the diagnosis is firmly established, unless contraindicated. Weight-based normograms for heparin are recommended with the intent to achieve therapeutic levels of partial thromboplastin time (PTT) within 24 hr of initiation of therapy. Anticoagulation is adequate when a PTT of 1.5–2.0 times the control value is achieved. Delays in achieving full anticoagulation within the 24-hr time frame are associated with increased rates of recurrent thrombosis (432). Warfarin sodium (coumadin) may be added 2–3 days following the establishment of therapeutic levels of PTT. Depletion of factor VII and thrombin is required to achieve full anticoagulation. Because thrombin has a half-life of 5 days, overlap of warfarin sodium with heparin (either UF or LMWH) therapy is important. The therapeutic goal of warfarin sodium is reached when an international normalized ratio (INR) of 2–3 is achieved. Heparin reduces the INR by approximately 0.5. Thus, an optimal initial targeted INR of 2.0 on combined heparin and warfarin sodium therapy yields an effective INR of 1.5 with warfarin alone. The usual challenges of warfarin interactions with diet and concomitant drugs, its long half-life, and the narrow therapeutic window of this agent may frequently produce wide fluctuations in the INR and lead to excessive bleeding or recurrent thrombosis. In the cancer patient, drug-induced and cancer-related disturbances in gastrointestinal absorption and hepatic function and the frequent need to discontinue oral anticoagulants for invasive procedures make the use of these agents particularly problematic. LMWHs are increasingly used as an alternative to oral anticoagulation for the long-term treatment of VTE in the cancer patient. Their rapid onset of action and predictable clearance facilitate the ease of interrupting anticoagulation coverage for invasive procedures. Furthermore, the putative antineoplastic effects of these drugs, including antiangiogenesis activity, induction of tumor cell apoptosis, and inhibition of coagulation proteases make LMWH use particularly attractive in the cancer setting (433,434). Several meta-analyses comparing LMWH with UFH in the treatment of DVT among cancer patients demonstrated a survival advantage among those patients treated with LMWH (435–437). Other advantages of LMWHs over UFH include lower rates of heparin-induced thrombocytopenia (HIT) and a greater degree of thrombus regression and restoration of venous patency (438,439). The duration of anticoagulant therapy should be customized to the individual patient. In patients with recurrent PE, active cancer, or persistent risk factors for PE, life-long therapy may be appropriate. Among those patients with a single, uncomplicated PE event or with transient underlying risk factors, 3–6 months of therapy are generally recommended (440).

Strategies to reduce clot burden include the use of thrombolytic agents and surgical rheolytic embolectomy techniques. In general, each of these options is reserved for those patients with massive PE associated with hemodynamic instability. Echocardiographic evidence of severe RV dysfunction or documentation on imaging studies of greater than 40% occlusion of the pulmonary vascular bed by clot are also included as indications for one of these more aggressive therapies by some experts (441–444). No clinical trials to date have been sufficiently large to adequately assess a differential mortality benefit among patients with massive PE complicated by shock who received thrombolytics vs. those who received conventional therapy alone. Results of smaller studies, however, have consistently

Table 13 Indications and Contraindications to Thrombolytic Therapy

Indications
Pulmonary embolism with shock physiology
Pulmonary embolism with moderate-to-severe RV dysfunction?
Failure of conventional anticoagulation?
Clot obstructing more than 40% of pulmonary vasculature?
Contraindications
Absolute
Major intracranial surgery or trauma within the prior 2 months
Cerebrovascular hemorrhage within the prior 3–6 months
Active intracranial neoplasm
Major internal hemorrhage within the prior 6 months
Severe bleeding diatheses, including those associated with severe liver or renal disease
Relative
Prolonged cardiopulmonary resuscitation
Pregnancy or postpartum period within the prior 10 days
Nonhemorrhagic stroke within the prior 2 months
Major trauma or surgery (excluding CNS) within the prior 10 days
Thrombocytopenia (platelet count $<100{,}000/mm^3$)
Hemorrhagic retinopathy
Allergies to thrombolytic agents
Minor surgery to noncompressible vessels within the prior 10 days
Tissue biopsy within the prior 10 days
Peptic ulceration within the prior 3 months
Infective endocarditis/pericarditis
Uncontrolled hypertension (systolic BP $\geq$200 or diastolic BP $\geq$110 mmHg)
Aortic aneurysm

demonstrated a survival benefit among patients with PE-related shock who were treated with thrombolytic therapy (445–447). Consensus regarding the indications for thrmbolysis among hemodynamically stable patients with moderate-to-severe RV dysfunction remains unsettled (Table 13). In a recent study by Konstantinides (441), there was no difference in the mortality among patients with PE and echocardiographic evidence of RV dysfunction who were randomized to receive heparin with or without alteplase. Patients treated with heparin alone, however, were more likely to develop clinical deterioration and the associated need for escalation of treatment than patients treated with heparin plus thrombolytic therapy. Thus, properly selected, hemodynamically stable patients with echocardiographic evidence of moderate-to-severe RV dysfunction may benefit from thrombolytic therapy.

Several agents for thrombolysis are commercially available. These agents include tissue plasminogen activator (t-PA), streptokinase, and urokinase. Although the clinical efficacy of each of these agents is relatively similar, t-PA is most widely used because of its more rapid onset of action and minimal antigenic activity. Each of the thrombolytic agents facilitates accelerated clot lysis, resulting in substantial earlier improvements in RV hemodynamic parameters and radiographic derangements than the use of heparin alone. Successful thrombolysis is typically followed by long-term treatment with anticoagulation. Although the immediate impact of thrombolytic therapy on RV hemodynamics is significant, these findings have not correlated with improvements in outcome in any large prospective clinical trials. The potential benefit of thrombolytic therapy must be weighed against major hemorrhage, its primary complication. The incidence of major bleeding and fatal hemorrhage ranges from 8.4% to 21.9% and 2.2% to 7.8%, respectively (441,448,449). Intracranial hemorrhage, the most feared site of bleeding, occurs in up to 3.0% of thrombolysis-treated patients, a rate that is 10-fold higher than that seen in patients treated with heparin alone (447,448,450). Moreover, intracranial hemorrhage associated with thrombolytic therapy is associated with a 75% mortality rate compared to a 5% mortality rate among patients who develop intracranial hemorrhage while on heparin (450,451). Major bleeding may occur during thrombolytic therapy despite modifications in dose, rate of drug delivery, type of agent, or avoidance of vascular punctures prior to administration. The lytic agents may be given systemically or via selective catheterization of the pulmonary vessels with local delivery of the agents. The theoretic advantage of the later is decreased risk of major hemorrhagic complications. In addition, advancement of the catheter tip directly into the clot may be used to mechanically disrupt the thrombus. Local instillation of thrombolytics into central venous catheters is also advocated for the treatment of PE caused by catheter-related clot formation. The need for catheter replacement once patency of the line has been restored is unclear.

Reperfusion of the pulmonary artery may also be effected by surgical embolectomy. This approach predates the advent of catheter embolectomy and thrombolysis and no formal clinical trials comparing thrombolysis with embolectomy are available. In general, surgical embolectomy is reserved for patients with PE and refractory shock, echocardiographic evidence of RV thrombi, a mean pulmonary artery pressure of >35 mmHg, or contraindicated or failed thrombolytic therapy (452). Both surgical and catheter embolectomy are reserved for the extraction of large, centrally located clots. Perioperative cardiac arrest confers a dismal outcome. Mortality rates following surgical embolectomy are otherwise as high as 80% in some studies.

2. *Tumor Embolism*

The pulmonary vascular bed acts as a very efficient filter that traps any materials larger than 10 μm that gain access to the systemic circulation. Thus hematogenous seeding of a variety of substances, including thrombus, tumor cell aggregates, fat, and air may eventually become lodged within the pulmonary circulation. Tumor involvement of the pulmonary vascular bed may manifest as large proximal tumor emboli resembling acute pulmonary embolism, smaller microvascular tumor cell aggregates that occlude small airways, generalized microvascular disease with associated lymphangitic spread or a combination of these. Estimates of a 3–26% incidence of pulmonary tumor embolism among patients with cancer are primarily derived from autopsy series (453,454). Antemortem diagnosis is difficult, occurring in only 6% of patients with cancer. Clinically apparent tumor emboli typically occur in patients with known malignancy although it may occasionally appear as the sentinel event among patients with occult malignancy. Patients commonly present with subacute symptoms of dyspnea, cough, and echocardiographic evidence of pulmonary hypertension as the presenting manifestation of occult malignancy. Mucinous tumors originating in the breast, lung, stomach, and colon appear to confer the highest risk of tumor embolization. Tumor emboli also frequently complicate carcinomas of the kidneys, liver, prostate, and choriocarcinomas. Patients in blast crisis associated with acute myleloid and lymphocytic leukemias may develop leukemic sequestration and thrombi within the pulmonary vasculature that appears physiologically and clinically similar to tumor emboli associated with solid malignancies (455). Myeloid leukemias associated with elevated white blood counts of greater than 50,000/dL may also develop leukemic infiltration of the lung with pulmonary hypertension caused by leukemic sequestration and thrombi within the pulmonary vasculature.

Clinically apparent tumor embolism tends to occur in patients with established neoplastic disease, although occasionally it may be the sentinel event among patients with occult malignancy. Patients with large proximal tumor emboli may present with signs and symptoms indistinguishable from massive pulmonary embolism. More often subacute symptoms of cor pulmonale secondary to microvascular pulmonary arterial embolization occur and follow a more deliberate and progressive course. Symptoms of dyspnea, dry cough, chest, and abdominal pain occur insidiously over weeks to months. The physical examination may reveal tachypnea, tachycardia, an augmented second heart sound, ascites, and peripheral edema. Hypoxemia, respiratory acidosis, clear lungs, and echocardiographic evidence of right heart strain are other findings. Mean pulmonary artery pressures of greater than 50 mmHg are typical and suggest chronicity. The utility of echocardiography, therefore, is in discriminating acute vs. chronic disease, establishing the severity of pulmonary hypertension, and documenting the degree of RV dysfunction. The presence of pulmonary parenchymal or lymphatic disease on radiographic studies coupled with hypoxemia with pulmonary hypertension may be helpful in the diagnosis of lymphangitic carcinomatosis.

Except for the notable absence of plexiform lesions, pulmonary hypertension secondary to tumor embolism appears pathologically indistinguishable from pulmonary arterial hypertension secondary to other causes. Lung scintigraphy may demonstrate mottled subsegmental mismatched perfusion defects with normal ventilation. Although pulmonary angiography is the gold standard for the diagnosis of pulmonary thromboembolic disease, this diagnostic tool has poor sensitivity and specificity in the detection of tumor emboli. The diagnosis of tumor emboli is confirmed by the finding of malignant cells on cytologic analysis of aspirated blood from a wedged pulmonary artery catheter. The major utility to the antemortem diagnosis of tumor embolism is to identify potentially treatable disease in patients with chemosensitive tumors and to avoid the morbidity of long-term anticoagulation and/or inferior vena cava filter placement. Chemotherapy, embolectomy, and surgical resection of primary tumor may be reasonable therapeutic options in some patients.

3. *Venous Air Embolism*

Cancer patients routinely undergo a variety of procedures that place them at risk for venous air embolism. Central venous catheterization is nearly universal among cancer patients. In addition, gynecologic and surgical procedures and positive pressure ventilation add to the risk of venous air embolism. Each of these procedures may cause inadvertent communication between the atmosphere and the venous system, permitting ingress of atmospheric air into the venous circulation. Intravenous pressure may fall below atmospheric during periods of deep inspiration, hypovolemia, or upright positioning, favoring the ingress of gas along a negative pressure gradient. Reported rates of catheter-related VAE are 1 in 47 to 1 in 3000 catheter insertions. Several factors may influence the severity of VAE: the rate of air sufflation, the posture of the individual at the time gas enters the venous system, and the volume of air insufflated. Upright positioning at the time of air insufflation may produce catastrophic consequences. The pressure within the venous system and the cardiovascular status prior to the event also influence the outcome of gas embolism. Air emboli may impede pulmonary blood flow by acutely obstructing the apical part of the RV. An associated rise in pulmonary artery and right ventricular pressures follows. Cardiovascular collapse and death may quickly ensue. A high index of suspicion is required for diagnosis as few signs and symptoms are pathognomonic for this disease. Premonitory symptoms of chest pain, dyspnea, and lightheadedness may frequently occur. Livido reticularis, myocardial ischemia, and cerebral infarction are nonspecific findings. Auscultory findings of a "mill wheel" murmur and an air-fluid level in the pulmonary artery on chest radiograph are rare but specific findings. Intracardiac air is also an infrequent finding on contrast echocardiography. Capnography may demonstrate an abrupt fall in $ETCO_2$ and is advocated during surgical procedures. Intracavitary air is quickly absorbed and attempts to document this finding with radiographic studies may inappropriately delay therapy. The strong suspicion of gas embolism should prompt immediate action in an effort to restore blood flow and facilitate resorption of intravascular air. The patient should be placed in left lateral decubitus position at the first sign of VAE. This positioning may encourage migration of intravascular air into the RV and thereby improve blood flow. Central venous or pulmonary artery catheters may be utilized to aspirate intravascular air from the right atrium, ventricle, or pulmonary artery. Closed chest cardiac massage and 100% oxygen therapy are additional measures that may offer some therapeutic benefit. Hyperbaric oxygen (HBO) therapy may reduce the volume of intravascular gas but frequently requires transfer to a hyperbaric facility. Although early aggressive therapy is critical to a good outcome, the benefits of HBO therapy may be appreciated even when this treatment is delayed by 30–40 hr (456,457). Mortality rates in excess of 90% have been reported among patients with massive untreated VAE. Aggressive supportive care and HBO therapy can reduce these harrowing statistics to 30% and 10%, respectively.

4. *Fat Embolism Syndrome*

Fat embolism syndrome (FES) is characterized by a triad of global neurologic impairment, acute respiratory insufficiency, and petechial rash. Precise estimates of the incidence of FES are obscured by its varied clinical presentation. FES typically occurs following trauma to long bones. In the cancer setting, FES has been reported after bone marrow transplantation, in bone tumor lysis following nontraumatic orthopedic procedures, following administration of GM-CSF and with administration of the sedating medication, propofol (458–461). The clinical features of massive FES may resemble an acute thromboembolic event and may occur with as little as 20 cm^3 of bone marrow fat embolization (462). Dramatic increases in pulmonary pressures, acute corpulmonale, and sudden death may acutely occur as a consequence of acute obstruction by massive fat emboli. A number of other conditions, such as dermatologic and neurologic derangements, may occur as a result of increased pulmonary pressures and intrapulmonary shunt formation. Neurologic symptoms of confusion, seizures, and coma may be the presenting features of this disease. The findings of a petechial rash distributed over the axilla, anterior chest, and head and neck are nearly pathognomonic of FES. These dermatologic alterations are frequently late findings that occur in only 20–50% of patients and thus may not help in establishing the diagnosis. Lung parenchymal injury is usually fatty acid-mediated and occurs 24–72 hr after the initiating event. Clinical suspicion is heightened by findings of stainable fat in serum, urine, or BAL, although these results are neither sensitive nor specific for the diagnosis (463–465). Ventilation–perfusion studies demonstrate mottled perfusion defects with normal ventilation similar to that seen with tumor embolism. Overall, clinical outcome is quite good and permanent sequelae of FES are rare. The utility of corticosteroid therapy in as prophylaxis or in the treatment of established disease is not well defined (466,467). Current recommendations include supportive measures only.

F. Transfusion-Related Lung Injury

Patients with cancer, in particular those with hematologic malignancies, have a frequent and nearly universal requirement for transfusion of blood products. The transfusion of red blood cell platelets and fresh frozen platelets (FFP) predisposes these patients to the syndrome of transfusion-related lung injury (TRALI). A cardinal feature of this syndrome is noncardiogenic pulmonary edema. Patients frequently present with fever, hypotension, severe hypoxemia, and bilateral lung infiltrates during or immediately following blood or blood product transfusion. The pathogenesis of TRALI is unclear but putatively involves the passive transfer of granulocyte- or HLA-specific complement-activating antibodies from the donor to the recipient. Treatment of TRALI is generally supportive. Clinical symptoms and radiographic changes typically resolve in a 2–3 day period without permanent pulmonary sequelae (468,469). In approximately 20% of patients, symptoms and radiographic changes may persist for a week.

G. Pulmonary Veno-Occlusive Disease

Pulmonary veno-occlusive disease (PVOD) is a rare disorder that has been reported as a complication of hematopoietic stem cell transplantation and following administration of certain cancer chemotherapeutic agents, including BCNU and bleomycin. This frequently lethal condition targets the small pulmonary veins and is characterized pathologically by widespread narrowing and/or occlusion of small pulmonary veins and venules by organized thrombi. The resulting increase in pulmonary resistance is associated with increased hydrostatic pressure and pulmonary edema. Although the pathologic findings of PVOD appear strikingly similar to veno-occlusive disease of the liver, the pathogenesis of this disease remains uncertain. Pulmonary hypertension is a cardinal feature of this disorder and is typically associated with rapidly progressive dyspnea, hypoxia, respiratory failure, and cor pulmonale. The pulmonary capillary wedge pressure is normal to low, owing to the patency of the large pulmonary veins. Normal caliber large pulmonary veins associated with enlarged central pulmonary arteries on chest radiographs suggest the diagnosis. Radiographic findings of pulmonary edema, including multifocal areas of ground-glass attenuation, peribronchial cuffing, and diffuse interstitial edema with associated Kerley B lines, are common. Treatment involves discontinuation of the offending agent along with supportive care.

H. Pulmonary Edema and Acute Lung Injury in the Cancer Patient

Pulmonary edema occurs when the transudation of fluid from the pulmonary vessels exceeds the resorptive capacity of the pulmonary lymphatics and vasculature, resulting in the abnormal accumulation of extravascular fluid and solute in the lung. The predilection for pulmonary edema in the setting of cancer is legion. Older classification schemes for pulmonary edema sorted the diverse causes of this disorder into two major categories: hydrostatic or cardiogenic pulmonary edema and noncardiogenic pulmonary edema. This simple approach has been revised more recently based on recent advances in our understanding of the pathophysiology of this disorder. Pulmonary edema is now sorted into three major categories that reflect the underlying permeability characteristics of the microcirculation and the presence or absence of diffuse alveolar damage (DAD) (Table 14).

Normal permeability pulmonary edema is characterized by an imbalance of Starling forces and associated increased hydrostatic pressures within the lung microvasculature, leading to fluid filtration into the lungs. Pulmonary edema of cardiogenic and neurogenic etiologies and lung edema caused by pulmonary veno-occlusive disease are salient examples of normal permeability hydrostatic pulmonary edema. In addition, pulmonary edema caused by lung re-expansion, lymphatic obstruction and relief of upper airway obstruction are typically associated with normal microvascular permeability.

Increased permeability pulmonary edema is commonly referred to as primary or noncardiogenic pulmonary edema. Increased permeability pulmonary edema may be caused by a diverse array of insults to the lung that violate the integrity of the alveolar and microvascular surfaces, resulting in the accumulation of proteinaceous fluid within the interstitium. These permeability changes may occur with or without DAD. Acute lung injury (ALI) and adult respiratory distress syndrome (ARDS) are the sine qua non of pulmonary edema with DAD. Increased permeability pulmonary edema without DAD (capillary leak syndrome) is more often seen as a complication of heroin overdose, but has been reported following cocaine/crack cocaine use and is described in high-altitude pulmonary edema. In the cancer setting, this type of pulmonary edema frequently complicates cytokine administration. Two agents in particular, IL2 and TNF, may disrupt capillary endothelial cell integrity, leading to increased permeability edema without associated DAD. Both these drugs may also cause direct toxicity to the myocardium, leading to concurrent modest increases in pulmonary capillary wedge pressures and reductions in left ventricular ejection fractions. Although normal and increased permeability pulmonary edema represents distinct pathophysiologic mechanisms, there is considerable overlap. *Mixed* or overlap edema caused by both hydrostatic and increased permeability etiologies is seen following administration of certain cytokines as mentioned above and with neurogenic and re-expansion pulmonary edema. A brief discussion of these categories of pulmonary edema and their prominent precipitating factors is given below. Cytokined-related increased permeability pulmonary edema without DAD is discussed in the section under chemotherapy-induced lung injury.

Table 14 Cancer-Related Causes of Pulmonary Edema

I. Normal permeability
A. Increased intravascular hydrostatic pressure
  Increased left ventricular end-diastolic pressure
    Systolic dysfunction
      Arrhythmias
      Coronary artery disease
      Cardiomyopathy (congestive, restrictive, hypertrophic)
      High output states (severe anemia)
      Constrictive pericarditis
    Diastolic dysfunction
      Left ventricular hypertrophy
      Ischemia
      Pericardial effusion
    Volume overload/renal failure
    Constrictive pericarditis
    Mechanical ventilation (elevated intrathoracic pressure)
  Increased left atrial pressure
    Left atrial myxoma
    Mitral/aortic valve disease
  Increased pulmonary venous pressure
    Pulmonary veno-occlusive disease
    Fibrosing mediastinitis
  Neurogenic edema
    Seizures
    Hemorrhagic/embolic strokes
B. Decreased iterstitial hydrostatic pressure
  Mechanical ventilation/PEEP
  Re-expansion edema
  Surfactant depletion
II. Increased permeability
ALI/ARDS
  Infection/inflammation
    Sepsis syndrome
    Pneumonia
    Aspiration of gastric contents
    Pancreatitis
    Shock
  Disseminated intravascular coagulation
  Transfusion-related
    Massive blood transfusion
    Leukoagglutination reaction
  Drugs
    Chemotherapy (IL-2, bleomycin, mitomycin, Ara-C)
    Narcotics (oral and intravenous)
    Radiologic contrast media
    Aspirin
    Tricyclic antidepressants
  Embolic phenomenon
    Thromboembolism
    Fat embolism
    Air embolism
III. Mixed edema
Neurogenic
Postrelief of upper airway obstruction
Re-expansion
Postthoracotomy

1. Normal Permeability (Hydrostatic) Pulmonary Edema

Cardiogenic Pulmonary Edema

Cardiogenic pulmonary edema associated with systolic or diastolic dysfunction may occur as a result of cancer and its therapy. This form of pulmonary edema represents one of the major causes of normal permeability pulmonary edema in the cancer patient. Atrial myxoma, the most common primary cardiac tumor, typically arises from the left atrium and may cause dramatic elevations in left atrial pressures and associated normal permeability pulmonary. Other neoplastic diseases such as pheochromocytoma and carcinoid tumors may secrete mediators that precipitate cardiogenic shock and related pulmonary edema (470,471). Infections, caused by bacterial, viral, and fungal pathogens may cause severe myopericarditis and/or valvular disease that often lead to fatal myocardial failure and pulmonary edema. The cardiotoxic effects of the anthracyclines are well established. These agents may cause life-threatening cardiomyopathy with associated congestive heart failure and hydrostatic (cardiogenic) pulmonary edema. At standard doses, the effects of the alkylating agents, cyclophosphamide and ifosfamide, are associated with minimal adverse cardiac effects. These drugs are often used at high doses in an effort to effect marrow ablation. Severe cardiac injury manifested as myocarditis, pericarditis, malignant arrhythmias, myocardial depression, and congestive heart failure may develop in this setting with associated cardiogenic pulmonary edema. Signs and symptoms of cardiac toxicity and pulmonary edema are heralded by nonspecific ST-segment or T-wave changes and/or loss of QRS voltage, typically within 2 weeks of receiving either of these drugs. Cardiogenic pulmonary edema has also been reported during mitoxanthrone therapy and following the administration of the newer recombinant monoclonal antibody, herceptin (transtuzumab), especially in the setting of prior antracyclin therapy or antecedent cardiac disease (472). These agents impair left ventricular function leading to increased left ventricular end-diastolic pressure (LVEDP). 5-Fluorouracil may rarely precipitate acute coronary artery spasm, leading to myocardial ischemia, infarction, and cardiogenic pulmonary edema. Thoracic radiation therapy may precipitate myocardial dysfunction and cardiogenic pulmonary edema by direct toxicity to the pericardium and myocardium, leading to pericardial effusions and constriction and ultimately myocardial fibrosis. Catastrophic valvular disease and conduction abnormalities have also been reported following thoracic radiation. In addition, myocardial dysfunction attributed to radiation-induced accelerated coronary artery disease is well documented (473,474). Fibrosing mediastinitis, a rare consequence of mediastinal radiation, may also cause elevated pulmonary venous pressures and hydrostatic pulmonary edema. The risk of radiation-related cardiac disease is life long and may, in fact, be progressive over time, occurring years after completion of therapy (475). Mediastinal radiation and radiation doses of 3000 cGy or greater confer the greatest risk. Diastolic dysfunction occurs as a consequence of altered diastolic pressure–volume relationships that result in decreased end-diastolic volume for a given diastolic filling pressure. Disturbances in diastolic function may also lead to cardiogenic pulmonary edema. Several cancer-related conditions may result in diastolic dysfunction, including septic shock, large pericardial effusions, and elevated intrathoracic pressures associated with mechanical ventilation. Obliteration of upstream vasculature and subsequent elevation of pulmonary venous pressures occur with pulmonary veno-occlusive disease. This disorder is a rare complication of radiation and certain chemotherapeutic drugs and may also result in normal permeability pulmonary edema.

Radiographic changes owing to (cardiogenic) normal permeability pulmonary edema include increased cardiac silhouette, prominent central interstitial markings, perivascular cuffing, cephalization of pulmonary vessels, and the appearance of Kerley B lines. Pleural effusions are late findings that occur as the edema progresses. The radiographic findings of central distribution of pulmonary edema fluid, cephalization of pulmonary vessels, increased cardiac size are often used to distinguish cardiogenic from other causes of pulmonary edema. These radiographic findings are nonspecific, however, and cannot be relied on solely to determine the cause of edema formation (476,477). Nonetheless, familiarity with the predominant radiographic changes that are associated with pulmonary edema from various causes may help to narrow the differential diagnosis. Hemodynamic data derived from pulmonary artery catheterization are regarded as a definitive diagnostic tool in differentiating cardiogenic (hydrostatic) and increased permeability pulmonary edema. Cardiogenic pulmonary edema typically is manifest as high pulmonary capillary wedge pressures on invasive monitoring. Invasive monitoring is not an exact technique, however, and overlap of underlying causes may confound the diagnosis. For example, very low oncotic pressures may falsely lower the pulmonary artery wedge pressure in the setting of cardiogenic pulmonary edema. Conversely, the normal to low pulmonary capillary wedge pressure that is typically seen with conditions associated with increased permeability pulmonary edema may be elevated when any of these conditions is complicated by volume overload. Thus, hemodynamic monitoring should only be used as an adjunctive tool in the evaluation of selected patients and may be beneficial in the clinical management of selected patients with pulmonary edema. Furthermore, survival benefit in pulmonary artery-guided management of critically ill patients has not been demonstrated in any prospective study. Distinctions between cardiogenic and increased permeability pulmonary edema may also be gleaned from studies of the alveolar protein concentration in bronchoalveolar lavage fluid. An alveolar protein to plasma protein ratio of 0.6 or greater suggests increased permeability pulmonary edema (478,479).

Patients with cardiogenic pulmonary edema may present with pernicious symptoms of cough, dyspnea, and chest pain. Syncopal episodes and sudden death may be the sentinel events signaling cardiogenic edema in some cases. Early clinical signs include tachypnea and wheezing that may progress to diaphoresis, peripheral cyanosis, and frothy sputum production as edema progresses. Cardiogenic pulmonary edema owing to valvular disease may present abruptly and catastrophically. A new or changing murmur on cardiac examination is an important clue in making the diagnosis. A definitive diagnosis relies the constellation of findings gathered from the physical examination, chest radiographs, and echocardiographic data and pulmonary artery catheterization. Initial treatment strategies for cardiogenic pulmonary edema associated with circulatory collapse are targeted at patient stabilization. These supportive measures may include diuresis, inotropic support, after-load reduction, supplemental oxygenation, vasodilators, and morphine administration. These measures may help to mitigate further edema formation by reduce cardiac work and improve cardiac efficiency. Ventilatory support with CPAP, BiPAP, or intubation with mechanical ventilation may be indicated. Sedating medications are routinely used to facilitate intubation and optimization of mechanical ventilation strategies. Sedating medications should be selected carefully, as many of the standard sedating agents may aggravate hypotension by decreasing venous return. Preload reduction and increased venous capacitance may be achieved with sublingual or intravenous nitroglycerin. The use of this drug may be limited by the development of hypotension. Angiotensin-converting enzyme inhibitors (ACEI) or an ACE receptor blocker is frequently used for afterload reduction. Dopamine at low doses may increase cardiac contractility and renal blood flow, reduce systemic vascular resistance, and improve cardiac output without attendant increases in myocardial oxygen consumption or heart rate. This drug is thus advocated in the treatment of pulmonary edema complicated by hypotension. Sodium nitroprusside, a potent vasodilator, may be beneficial in the hypertensive patient with severe pulmonary edema.

Postobstructive Pulmonary Edema

Postobstructive, or negative pressure pulmonary edema, is a form of hydrostatic pulmonary edema that may occur as a consequence of large negative intrathoracic pressure swings that are created while attempting to forcefully inhale against an obstructed upper airway. The sudden marked drop in intrathoracic pressure is associated with an increase in venous return and a parallel decrease in intrapleural pressures. These physiologic alterations result in a high hydrostatic pressure gradient between the intravascular and extravascular compartments which promotes fluid filtration into the interstitial space and alveoli. Loss of intrinsic PEEP following relief of the obstruction also appears to play a role. Hence, conditions such as severe laryngospasm, choking, strangulation, endotracheal tube obstruction, bronchospasm, vocal cord paralysis, premature extubation, and neoplastic obstruction of the upper airway are identified risk factors for the development of this disorder (480–482). Patients may present with upper airway stridor or severe bronchospasm. Signs and symptoms typically develop within the first hour of the acute obstructing event. Radiographic patterns of postobstructive pulmonary edema are similar to those seen with cardiogenic pulmonary edema and include septal lines, peribronchial cuffing, and, in more severe cases, central alveolar edema. Unlike cardiogenic pulmonary edema, the cardiac silhouette is usually normal. Fatal outcomes are associated with delayed treatment. Thus, early recognition and treatment are imperative. Prompt resolution of the clinical symptoms and radiographic signs of edema typically occurs within 2–3 days with appropriate therapy. Diuretics, supplemental oxygen, and supportive therapy with PEEP delivered via continuous positive airway pressure (CPAP), bilevel positive airway pressure (BIPAP), or other modes of artificial ventilation are recommended.

Pulmonary Edema Secondary to Lymphatic Obstruction

Decreased lymphatic clearance with associated normal permeability pulmonary edema are frequent complications of a variety of neoplastic and nonneoplastic disorders. Both lymphatic obstruction by tumor and lymphangitic spread of disease may markedly interfere with lymph flow and are the most common causes of diminished lymphatic clearance in the cancer setting. Although lymphangitic tumor involvement of the lung may complicate any cancer, adenocarcinomas of the breast, stomach, pancreas, and prostate are most frequently associated with the development of this disorder. Pulmonary edema owing to lymphangitic spread of tumor may be clinically and radiographically indistinguishable from the underlying malignancy. Patients typically present with the insidious onset of dyspnea, nonproductive cough, and hypoxemia. Disabling dyspnea and cor pulmonale rapidly follow as fluid accumulation, neoplastic infiltration of interlobular septa and lymphatics, and superimposed tumor microemboli continue. Open-lung or transbronchial biopsies are required for definitive diagnosis, although rarely, examination of pulmonary microvascular cytology obtained from a wedged pulmonary artery catheter may establish the diagnosis. Despite treatment with chemotherapy or hormonal agents, the prognosis for patients with interstitial edema secondary to lymphangitic carcinomatosis is poor. The mean survival after diagnosis is only 3 months.

2. Increased Permeability Pulmonary Edema

Acute Respiratory Distress Syndrome and Acute Lung Injury

DEFINITIONS: Increased permeability pulmonary edema arises from a broad spectrum of insults to the pulmonary endothelial and epithelial surfaces. Historically, this form of pulmonary edema has been described as primary or noncardiogenic pulmonary edema and its associated major clinical syndromes are referred to as acute respiratory distress syndrome (ARDS) and acute lung injury (ALI). Not all permeability pulmonary edema results in ARDS. In 1994, the American-European Consensus conference published criteria for ARDS and ALI. These definitions characterize ARDS as an extreme manifestation of a spectrum of precipitating events resulting in severe lung injury and hypoxemia, and ALI as the less severe pulmonary disorder. Although these definitions of ARDS/ALI have been widely accepted, they are regarded as only an interim solution. Diagnostic criteria that more accurately reflect the underlying cause and other organ system involvement are not addressed in the current criteria and may be important. For example, ARDS attributable to direct pulmonary insults, such as pneumonia, may be clinically, radiographically and prognostically distinct from that due to indirect causes, such as sepsis or trauma. Furthermore, the concept that ALI is a "lesser- or pre-ARDS" condition has not been confirmed.

CANCER-RELATED RISK FACTORS AND INCIDENCE OF ARDS/ALI: The precipitating conditions that result in ARDS/ALI may be divided into those associated with direct lung injury and those that provoke indirect injury to the lungs in the setting of a systemic process (Table 14). Common causes of direct lung injury include pneumonia and aspiration of gastric contents. Sepsis and shock associated with trauma and multiple blood transfusions comprise the dominant causes of indirect lung injury. While this etiological dichotomy of ARDS/ALI provides a simplistic approach to this disorder, it is confounded by the fact that the inciting event(s) are often multifactorial or unknown. Furthermore, synergistic interactions between direct and indirect categories of lung injury significantly augment the risk of ARDS/ALI. Precise estimates of ARDS are unknown. An annual incidence of 22 per 100,000 population has been reported by the NIH Acute Respiratory Distress Syndrome Network (483). The incidence and prognosis of ARDS/ALI varies broadly, however, with the predisposed group and the precipitating conditions. For example, ARDS following cardiopulmonary bypass surgery occurs in 1–5% of patients. Ten to 38% of patients with sepsis develop ARDS (484–487). An additional 35% of patients with sepsis will develop some degree of ALI during the course of their illness. Thus, the incidence of some degree of lung injury in patients with sepsis syndrome is not trivial. Multiple studies identify sepsis, pneumonia, including aspiration pneumonia, and multiple blood transfusions as the most common risk factors for the development of ARDS (484,488–490). Synergistic interactions between these conditions further increase the susceptibility for ARDS/ALI. Each of the precipitating events for ARDS/ALI is over-represented among patients with cancer and thus the predilection for ARDS/ALI in the setting of malignancy is high. In addition, radiation and chemotherapy are prominent causes of lung injury that add to the burden of ARDS/ALI among this group of patients. Coexisting and competing diagnoses that may mimic ARDS/ALI in the cancer patient render precise estimates among this group of patients very difficult to define. Recent reports of improvements in outcome associated with ARDS in the general population have failed to show similar trends among certain subgroups of patients with malignancy and ARDS. In particular, mortality rates exceeding 80–90% have been consistently reported over the past decade among those patients with hematologic malignancies who develop respiratory failure and ARDS following marrow transplantation (3,491–494). Sepsis poses a substantial burden on the patient with cancer and represents one of the major risk factors for poor outcome among patients with ARDS. Recent studics have demonstrated that the incidence of sepsis and sepsis-related deaths are rising (171). Cancer-related sepsis syndromes have been predominantly attributed to bacterial and viral pathogens, although fungal infections associated with sepsis and ARDS have been increasingly recognized.

PATHOPHYSIOLOGY OF ARDS: ARDS is characterized by stereotyped, sequential pathologic changes within the lungs that occur regardless of the underlying cause. An early or exudative phase, resulting from severe injury to the alveolocapillary unit, typically occupies the first week following the precipitating event and is characterized by the extravasation of inflammatory fluid into the interstitial space. As the process unfolds, sloughing of the endothelial and alveolar lining cells permits free escape of proteinaceous fluid into the alveoli. The progression from interstitial to alveolar edema corresponds radiographically to areas of widespread but patchy consolidation. The type 1 epithelial cells are exquisitely susceptible to lung damage and suffer the bulk of injury to the epithelium. These cells undergo extensive necrosis and sloughing along the alveolar surface, leaving behind a denuded basement membrane. Injury to the type II pneumocyte also occurs, resulting in reduced surfactant turnover and disruption of normal epithelial ion transport activity. Impaired epithelial ion transport impedes the resorption of edema fluid from the airway. Hyaline membrane formation similar to that seen in infantile respiratory distress syndrome is a prominent feature that occurs early in the disease process. These changes are referred to as diffuse alveolar damage (DAD), the histopathologic hallmark of this disease. These morphologic alterations promote the development of microatelectasis and shunt formation and lead to severely impaired gas exchange and associated hypoxemia. The fibroproliferative phase of ARDS typically evolves over the ensuing 1–3 weeks following lung injury. There is considerable overlap, however, and proliferation of type II cells and the appearance of fibrosis are occasionally observed as early as 3 and 10 days, respectively, following lung injury (495,496). Fibroblast and type II pneumocyte proliferation and hyperplasia mark the onset of the fibroproliferative phase of this disease. Collagen deposition and the regeneration of type II pneumocytes are prominent features of this stage of ARDS, which occur as the lung attempts to repair itself. These reparative mechanisms occasionally result in the restoration of normal parenchymal architecture. Resolution of lung injury may occur after the exudative or fibroproliferative stage or progress. Alternatively, the exuberant deposition of

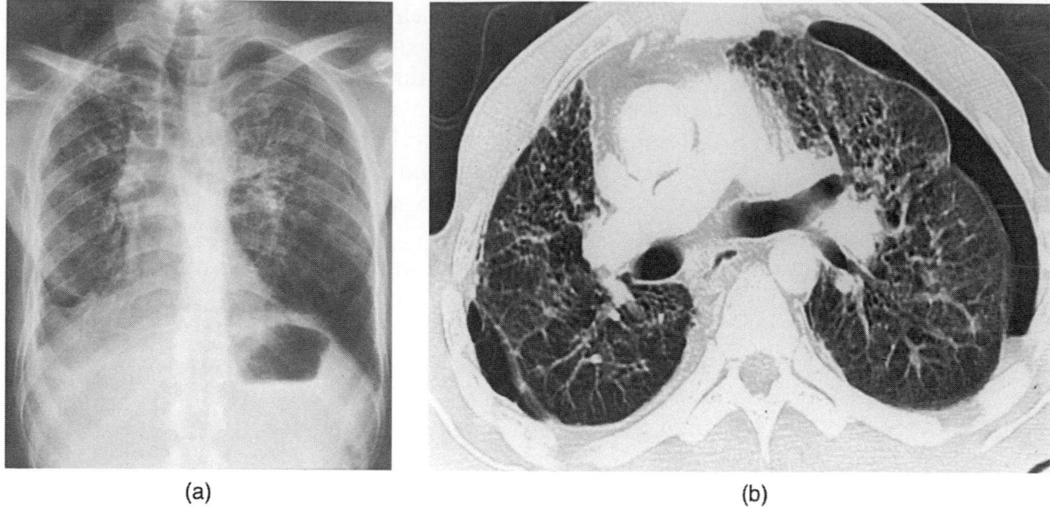

Figure 18 A 32-year-old male with Hodgkin's disease who developed pneumonia and ARDS following chemotherapy. A chest radiograph (a) and chest CT examination (b) demonstrated bilateral cystic airspace disease with extensive parenchymal fibrosis and associated pneumothorax. Postmortem examination confirmed the development of ARDS.

collagen results in widespread fibrosing alveolitis and a dense, noncompliant lung. Disease progression is primarily dictated by the efficacy of the therapeutic interventions and the severity and chronicity of lung injury, rather than the etiology of the underlying cause. During the final (fibrotic) stage of ARDS, the lung is completely remodeled by sparsely cellular fibrous tissue. Extensive intra-alveolar and interstitial fibrosis obliterates the airspace and further promotes deadspace ventilation and hypoxemia. Subpleural and intraparenchymal cyst formation during this stage may give rise to recurrent pneumothoraces (Fig. 18a–b). These changes are typically observed among ventilated patients who survive beyond 3–4 weeks from the onset of ARDS. Pulmonary vascular injury is also a prominent component of ARDS. Pulmonary vasoconstriction, thromboembolism, and interstitial edema may contribute to increased pulmonary vascular resistance and pulmonary hypertension during the early (exudative) phase of ARDS. Hemorrhagic infarcts are frequent pathologic findings that may appear as classic wedge-shaped or subpleural band-like lesions on chest radiographs. These early vascular derangements are potentially reversible. Pulmonary vascular remodeling occurs as a late, irreversible finding (495).

Inflammation and inflammatory cytokines are felt to play an important role in the pathogenesis of ARDS. Although neutrophilic inflammation has been implicated in the pathogenesis of this disease, the development of ARDS in the setting of profound neutropenia is well documented (497,498). Furthermore, the incidence and severity of lung injury does not appear to be increased following neutrophil stimulation with granulocyte-colony stimulating factor (498,499). Thus, other inflammatory mediators are likely to be important and the appearance of the neutrophil as the cause vs. the result of lung injury has not been fully clarified. Although no one cytokine has been shown to predict the development of ARDS, the proinflammatory cytokines, including tumor necrosis factor, interleukin (IL)-1, 6, and 8 have received the most attention. These agents may modulate ARDS by either initiating or amplifying the inflammatory response. The anti-inflammatory activities of tumor necrosis factor receptor (TNFr), interleukin-1 receptor antagonist, and interleukin-10 and 11 may also have a modulating effect on the development of acute lung injury (500,501). Activated protein C (APC) is a circulating plasma anticoagulant with antithrombotic and anti-inflammatory and profibrinolytic properties. This plasma protien is markedly reduced in ALI/ARDS, while circulating thrombomodulin is increased (502). These biological markers may play a central role in the pathogenesis ARDS/ALI. Reductions in APC during sepsis-related ARDS have been correlated with poor clinical outcomes (503). High-mobility group B1 protein (HMGB1) has recently been shown to play a central role in the development of sepsis and sepsis-related ARDS (299,504). The role of this nuclear binding protein in transcriptional regulation is well established (505). In addition, HMGB1 is a potent regulator of monocyte proinflammatory cytokines, including TNF-α, IL-1β, IL-1α, IL-6 (506). HMGB1-mediated cytokine release results in an inflammatory response in the lungs that is manifested as neutrophil accumulation, interstital edema, and the accumulation of proinflammatory cytokines. Anti-inflammatory cytokines, such as IL-10 and TGF-β, may counterreguate these proinflammatory mediators and downregulate the inflammatory response (507,508). The progression and severity of lung injury is defined by the balance of pro- and anti-inflammatory cytokine mediators. The relative contribution of each of these mediators in the development of lung injury is currently being investigated.

CLINICAL MANIFESTATIONS OF ARDS: Manifestations of ARDS/ALI are clinically apparent within 2–24 hr of the inciting event in 76% of patients and within 72 hr in 93% of patients. Acute respiratory failure and associated hypoxemia reflecting severe pulmonary injury may occur early, usually within 24–48 hr of the predisposing event. Superimposed multiorgan system failure is also seen and the associated clinical manifestations may vary widely, depending on the number and type of extrapulmonary organ systems in addition to the lungs that are involved. Fever and leukocytosis, owing to the inflammatory response associated with lung injury or the precipitating event, can be prominent. Changes on chest radiographs are not distinctive for ARDS. Focal symmetrical or asymmetrical infiltrates seen early on may quickly progress over several hours to diffuse areas of consolidation. The chest radiograph nonetheless has an important, albeit limited, role in ruling out associated complications, such as pneumothorax and infections. Radiologic signs that are seen in cardiogenic pulmonary edema, including Kerley B lines, cardiomegaly, and apical vascular redistribution are typically absent. Ground-glass opacification occurs early and gives way to frank consolidation on the chest radiograph as the alveolar inflammatory exudates progresses. CT scan examinations frequently reveal nonhomogeneous areas of opacification representing alveolar filling, consolidation, and atelectasis that typically occur in dependent lung zones. Despite CT evidence of patchy lung involvement, bronchoalveolar lavage studies indicate substantial inflammation, even in areas of radiographic sparing. Bronchoscopic examination with bronchoalveolar lavage is of proven utility in excluding competing diagnoses. For example, lymphocyte rich BAL fluid may indicate sarcoidosis, brochiolitis obliterans with organizing pneumonia (cryptogenic organizing pneumonia) or hypersensitivity pneumonitis. Elevated eosinophil counts (>15–20% of the total cell count) on BAL fluid suggest acute eosinoophilic pneumonia. Increased hemosiderin laden macrophages are consistent with diffuse alveolar hemorrhage. BAL fluid should also be submitted for cytologic analysis for viral inclusions, malignant cells, *Pneumocystis carinii*, and also for culture. Transbronchial biopsies are generally avoided because of the added risks associated with biopsies in mechanically ventilated patients. Prohibitive thrombocytopenia, a common problem in these patients, adds to the diagnostic conundrum. Open-lung biopsy is frequently nondiagnostic and may not justify the added risk of this procedure. Respiratory acidosis gives way to respiratory alkalosis as deadspace ventilation and the work of breathing increases. Because sepsis or the systemic inflammatory response syndrome (SIRS) often underlies ARDS, associated hematologic derangements, including anemia, thrombocytopenia, leukopenia, and leukocytosis are common findings. Acute renal insufficiency may add to the laboratory conundrums of ARDS, especially in the setting of sepsis or SIRS.

DIFFERENTIAL DIAGNOSIS OF ARDS: The differential diagnosis of ARDS is broad and many of the causes of diffuse lung disease may also cause ARDS (Table 15). In the cancer patient, common alternative diagnoses, such as congestive heart failure, sepsis, pneumonia, interstitial pneumonitis, diffuse alveolar hemorrhage, cryptogenic organizing pneumonia (BOOP) lymphanigitic carcinomatosis, and leukemic infiltration are important differential considerations.

ARDS OUTCOME AND TREATMENT: Treatment of ARDS/ALI involves aggressive supportive care coupled with strategies that attenuate the early inflammatory response and hasten the resolution of the syndrome. Advances in supportive care over the past decade have contributed to recent improvements in ARDS-related survival rates (509). Supportive measures, such as early identification and aggressive management of the precipitating condition(s), may strongly influence the duration of intensive care as well as the outcome of ARDS. Persistent sepsis that is refractory to therapy confers the highest rates of multiorgan system failure and death. Therefore, an aggressive search for sepsis or other underlying infections should be vigorously sought and treated. Prophylactic antibiotic therapy is of no proven benefit in the management of ARDS. β_2-Adrenergic stimulation may reduce alveolar edema by increasing alveolar sodium and fluid clearance. Data from several animal models of lung injury have shown that the judicious use of aerosolized β-agonists results in marked increases in alveolar fluid clearance (510). Intravenous administration of the β-2 vasoactive agonists, dobutamine, and dopamine, demonstrates similar effects on alveolar fluid clearance in animal models (511,512)Several small studies of the efficacy of β_2-agonist therapy in patients with ARDS/ALI have shown promising results with a trend towards improved oxygenation and decreased peak and plateau pressures (513).

Guidelines for nutritional support among patients in the ICU were summarized in a recent statement by a consensus group of the American College of Chest Physicians (514). The provision of nutrition among critically ill patients with ARDS/ALI is recommended, although controlled clinical trials are lacking. The goal of nutritional supplementation is to achieve a level of nutritional support that is commensurate with the patient's level of metabolism. Enteral feeding is associated with lower rates of infectious complications than parenteral support. Enteral feeding in the intubated patient with ARDS/ALI is preferred route of administration of nutritional support.

Fluid loading may improve oxygen consumption and tissue oxygen delivery. Careful attention to fluid homeostais is imperative, however, as a persistent positive fluid balance has been associated with a poor outcome (515–517). One approach to fluid management advocates preserving the lowest pulmonary capillary occlusion pressure (PCWP) with vasopressor support as needed to maintain an adequate cardiac index and blood pressure. No compelling data are currently available that support the use of any particular vasopressor or vasopressor combination. Dopamine or norepinephrine is frequently used to achieve a mean arterial pressure of 55–65 mmHg. Dobutamine, a positive inotropic agent that reduces systemic vascular resistance in some patients, is also frequently utilized. Avoidance of tissue hypoperfusion may be a difficult challenge with this strategy, confounded by the fact that no marker of tissue dysoxia is sensitive or specific enough to reliably guide fluid management. Tissue hypoperfusion to vital organs, such as the kidneys, may precipitate a spiraling downhill clinical course. Clinical indices, including urine output, blood pH, and base deficit, are frequently applied as surrogate markers of organ perfusion and should be used to guide therapy. Hemodynamic monitoring may provide additional information regarding the cardiac index and pulmonary arterial wedge pressure and may be especially useful in the setting of pulmonary hypertension and left ventricular dysfunction. An NIH-funded study designed to compare clinical outcomes of ARDS patients treated with fluid-conservative and fluid-liberal management schemes is currently in progress. Until prospective data from randomized trials are available, current recommendations support prudent restriction of intravenous fluids as long as systemic tissue perfusion is maintained by objective assessments. Vasopressors should be added as needed optimize end-organ tissue perfusion and normalize oxygen delivery (518).

Aggressive fluid resuscitation and inotropic therapy have also been used to achieve supraphysiologic levels of oxygen delivery in patients with acute lung injury. No studies have consistently shown any beneficial effects with this strategy, which, in fact, may adversely influence overall mortality among patients with ARDS/ALI (518). Nitric oxide (NO) is a potent endogenous pulmonary arterial vasodilator which enhances perfusion to aerated lung units and diverts blood flow from poorly ventilated or shunt regions. These ideal physiologic properties fueled earlier studies of gaseous nitric oxide in the treatment of ARDS/ALI-related pulmonary hypertension and hypoxemia. Initial enthusiasm in the use of NO in the treatment of ARDS is derived from the known effects of this agent as a selective vasodilator of the pulmonary vasculature. The results of several large, randomized double-blind controlled trials, however, have shown only modest and transient improvements in hypoxemia (432,519–521). The effect of NO on mortality and the duration of mechanical ventilation have been equally as disappointing (432,522). Attempts to lower pulmonary arterial pressures with other pulmonary vasodilators, including hydralazine and prostaglandin E2, have not been studied in any randomized, prospective trials. The use of intravenous prostacyclin has shown promising results as a pulmonary vasodilator, however its prohibitive effects on the systemic hemodynamics have limited its use (523). The results of aerosolized prostacyclin in animal models of ARDS in attenuating edema formation and improving ventilation-perfusion matching (524). The recognition of the role of inflammation in promoting ARDS/ALI prompted investigations of the utility of agents, such as high-dose glucocorticoids, anti-TNF-α, and anti-interleukin-1 in attenuating lung injury by modulating the inflammatory response. These trials have not convincingly shown any clinical benefit among ARDS/ALI patients that were treated with these agents. Salutory effects of HMGB1 antagonists have been demonstrated in animal models of sepsis-related ARDS (525), although data on higher species are currently unavailable. Two other anti-inflammatory agents, ibuprofen and ketoconazole, have been studied and their effect on ARDS/ALI mortality has been equally disappointing (526–528). In several recent small studies, patients randomized to receive high-dose steroids administered during late-phase (fibroproliferative phase) of ARDS/ALI demonstrated improved clinical outcomes (529,530). Larger studies are needed, however, to validate this therapeutic benefit. Activated protein C, a novel anti-inflammatory and anticoagulant agent, has been associated with reduced mortality among patients with sepsis-related ARDS/ALI (528,531). This novel therapy may become standard for selected patients with severe sepsis and associated end organ toxicity. Exogenous surfactant replacement therapy has also been proposed for treatment of adult patients with ARDS, based on its ability to mitigate surface tension at the air-fluid interface of small airways and alveoli. Although the beneficial effects surfactant-treated pediatric patients with neonatal respiratory distress syndrome is well documented, the results of this treatment modality in adults have been disappointing. Newer preparations of surfactant and methods of delivery are currently being evaluated (532,533).

Virtually all (90%) patients with full-blown ARDS require mechanical ventilation, usually within the first 72 hours of the onset of the disease. This life-saving therapy may facilitate adequate gas exchange and provide time for the lungs to heal. Mechanical ventilation may also be life threatening. Inspiratory airway pressures may be markedly elevated in mechanically ventilated patients with ARDS/ALI. Several factors, including poor lung compliance, elevated alveolar pressures at end-expiration owing to auto-PEEP or applied PEEP, and large tidal volume breaths on traditional modes of mechanical ventilation may contribute to increased inspiratory airway pressures. The associated excessive end-inspiratory volumes have been convincingly shown in numerous studies to produce a specific pattern of ventilator-induced lung injury (VILI) that is histologically similar to ARDS (534–538). This pattern of lung injury, referred to as volutrauma, is manifested as increased alveolar–capillary permeability, edema, decreased lung compliance, and atelectasis due to overdistention or stretch of the aerated lung (539–543). In addition, the repetitive collapse and reopening of injured lung units associated with mechanical ventilation may cause shearing of epithelial and endothelial cell layers and adds to the lung injury. This additional stress on the lungs promotes the release of mediators that enter the circulation and may cause distal organ dysfunction. Ventilator-induced lung injury is typically seen with conventional modes of ventilation. Interestingly, deaths related to ARDS are typically caused by multiorgan system disease rather than respiratory failure (544). The release of mediators into the circulation associated with VILI is one putative mechanism for the high rates of MOSF-related deaths among this group of patients. Adequate gas exchange may become exceedingly difficult to achieve as ARDS progresses and the lungs become less compliant. Various combinations of tidal volumes, positive end-expiratory pressure (PEEP), and FIO_2 are frequently used to optimize arterial oxygenation and gas exchange. Upward adjustments in these ventilator parameters not only add to the risk of VILI, but also increase the propensity for oxygen toxicity and barotrauma. Toxicity from high-inspired FIO_2 may act synergistically with VILI to exacerbate or perpetuate lung injury in patients with ARDS/ALI. The application of PEEP has been shown to reduce intrapulmonary shunt formation by recruiting small atelectatic and fluid-filled bronchioles and alveoli and preventing their closure during expiration. As a result, adequate arterial oxygenation may be achieved at a lower FIO_2. The salutary effects of PEEP may be offset by PEEP-induced increases inspiratory pressures, which add to the risk of volutrauma, barotrauma, and PEEP-associated circulatory depression. Pneumothorax, mediastinal emphysema, interstitial emphysema, and pneumatoceles may appear as clinical consequences of barotrauma, and the results of any one of these complications in the mechanically ventilated patient may be devastating. Excessive PEEP may precipitate circulatory collapse by decreasing cardiac output. Therefore, monitoring of oxygen transport and cardiac parameters may be warranted in some patients.

Overdistention of the lungs at end-inspiration and repetitive collapse of the lungs at end-exhalation are identified as two major contributors to VILI. Not surprisingly, these observations prompted a flury of investigations that were designed to address the optimal lung protective strategies for mechanically ventilated patients with ARDS/ALI. In a recent landmark paper by the Acute Respiratory Distress Syndrome Network (ARDSnet), lung ventilation strategies that restricted tidal volumes and inspiratory plateau pressures were associated with a 22% decrease in ARDS-related mortality (545). In addition, tidal volume reduction strategies were associated with longer ventilator-free days and fewer episodes of multisystem organ failure in this study. Based on compelling data from this study, lower tidal volume strategies that limit tidal volumes to $\leq 6\,\text{mL/kg}$ predicted body weight and plateau pressures to $\leq 30\,\text{cm}\ H_2O$ are recommended as standard therapy for most patients with ARDS/ALI who require mechanical ventilation. Smaller tidal volumes are often achieved at the expense of respiratory acidosis. Bicarbonate infusions and adjustments in respiratory rates may be required to maintain the arterial pH above 7.2. A $PaCO_2$ of 50–77 and pH of 7.20–7.30 appear to be well tolerated in most patients, although the levels of hypercapnia and acidosis that are truly benign are not well defined. Patients with conditions that may be worsened by permissive hypercapnea, such as sickle cell anemia and increased intracranial pressure, may not be candidates for this ventilator strategy.

Lung protective strategies may be accomplished using either volume-cycled or pressure-controlled modes of ventilation. For a given tidal volume, no studies have shown one mode of ventilation to be superior to the other with regard to rates of barotrauma or stretch-induced lung injury. The most appropriate method of mechanical ventilation in patients with ARDS, nonetheless, is a matter of intense and ongoing controversy. A combined lung protective approach with higher levels of PEEP has been recently proposed as a method of mitigating VILI while optimizing arterial oxygenation. In this strategy, the recruitment of atelectatic lung was augmented by raising the level of PEEP above the level at which alveoli collapse, defined as the lower inflection point on a pressure–volume curve (546). Levels of PEEP in this approach may be substantially higher than those typically used to support arterial oxygenation. The level of PEEP in which the adverse effects of PEEP outweigh the incremental benefit of lung recruitment is unknown. Larger prospective trials are needed to confirm the efficacy of this approach. Inverse ratio ventilation (IRV) recruits and stabilizes atelectatic alveoli by extending the duration of the inspiratory phase and shortening the expiratory phase of respiration. This theoretically results in shunt reduction and improvements in arterial oxygenation without associated increases in inspiratory airway pressures or tidal volume. Volume-cycled or pressure-controlled ventilation may be used to achieve IRV. Improved oxygenation with IRV ventilator strategies was initially felt to be on the basis of IRV-induced increases in mean arterial pressures (MAP). More recent studies, however, strongly suggest that the shortened exhalation times facilitates the development of auto-PEEP and improved gas exchange is likely on the basis of this mechanism (547,548). Significant levels of auto-PEEP may be associated with the development of barotrauma and hemodynamic compromise. Lung protection may therefore be difficult to achieve with IRV. Furthermore, this mode of ventilation is very uncomfortable for the patient and typically requires heavy sedation and neuromuscular blockade to optimize patient–ventilator interactions. With the growing awareness of potential complications associated with paralytic agents among critically ill patients coupled with the absence of data showing a survival benefit among patients who received IRV, this mode of ventilation has become less popular over the past few years. Other modes of ventilation, including airway pressure-release ventilation (APRV) and intermittent mandatory pressure-release ventilation (IMPRV), are similar to IRV but permit spontaneous breaths during the periods of prolonged airway pressure elevations. The need for heavy sedation and neuromuscular blockade is reduced with these modes of ventilation.

Furthermore, these ventilator strategies may reduce the work and oxygen cost of breathing while augmenting arterial oxygenation. Like IRV, lung protection is mitigated as enhanced oxygenation likely occurs as a result of air trapping and increased auto-PEEP.

High-frequency oscillatory ventilation (HFOV) has also been proposed as a ventilatory strategy in patients with respiratory insufficiency secondary to ARDS. The use of HFOV in this setting is attractive because the inherently low tidal volumes and small pressure swings delivered by this mode of ventilation putatively accomplish both goals of protective ventilation—avoidance of overdistention during inspiration and reduction in atelectasis at end-expiration (549). Although the use of HFOV in pediatric patients with acute respiratory distress is substantial, the application of this mode of ventilation in the treatment of adult patients with ARDS is only starting to emerge. The results of several small studies are encouraging. The merits of this instrument over conventional modes of ventilation among adult patients with ARDS, and the optimum strategy for the application of HFOV, however, remain undefined (550,551).

Patients with hypercapneic respiratory failure and limited acute hypoxemic failure may be candidates for noninvasive modes of ventilation. Noninvasive positive pressure ventilation (NPPV) may be appropriate in some patients with milder levels of respiratory distress. In the general population, this mode of ventilation is associated with fewer episodes of nosocomial pneumonia, briefer requirements for ventilator assistance, and reduced numbers of ICU days than conventional mechanical ventilation (552–554). Recent studies have demonstrated similar benefits following lung resection among patients with cancer and among other groups of immunocompromised patients with acute respiratory failure (555,556). The findings from these studies offer convincing evidence for the early use of noninvasive ventilatory strategies in selected immunocompromised patients with respiratory failure. Noninvasive positive pressure ventilation should be avoided in patients with hemodynamic instability, obtundation, delirium, high-risk of aspiration, difficulty clearing secretions, significant gastrointestinal bleeding, uncontrolled arrhythmias, or poor compliance. The inability of some patients to tolerate the tight-fitting mask further limits this form of ventilation.

Intriguing alternative paradigms, including extracorporeal membrane oxygenation (ECMO) and partial liquid ventilation (PLV), have been proposed for the treatment of patients with refractory hypoxemia secondary to severe ARDS. ECMO has been refined in newborns with severe respiratory failure and its efficacy validated in this patient population in numerous clinical trials. The benefits of ECMO among adult patients with refractory hypoxemia and pulmonary failure are currently undergoing investigation in a prospective, randomized trial.

Reduced surfactant function and increased surface tension contribute substantially to alveolar collapse in ARDS. This problem is exacerbated by the repetitive opening and closing of surfactant-deficient alveolar units during mechanical ventilation. Reductions in surface tension may be achieved using an "open-lung" approach to ventilation, a concept whereby the alveoli remain open at end-expiration in as much of the lung as possible. Extrinsic PEEP has been used to achieve this goal but the rise in inspiratory pressure, volume, and stretch with incremental increases in PEEP may perpetuate lung injury. Interest in PLV using perflourocarbons as a "liquid PEEP" to maintain open alveoli has emerged as a promising new treatment modality for ARDS. The physical properties of perflourocarbons—low surface tension, ability to dissolve oxygen at rates that are 17 times faster than water and the ability to spread quickly over the respiratory epithelium—render theses compounds ideally suited for liquid ventilation. Partial liquid ventilation has been safely performed in both children and adults in several small, uncontrolled trials (557,558). Reports of improved oxygenation decreased lung compliance, and reduced rates of nosocomial pneumonia using PLV have been documented in small studies; however, these observations require larger, controlled investigations for confirmation (559). Further work in this area is needed to determine whether the application of PLV confers a greater survival benefit over conventional ventilatory strategies. Issues regarding long-term toxicity, optimum dose, and ventilator strategies for PLV also need to be defined in clinical trials.

An extensive body of literature documents dramatic improvements in arterial oxygenation when patients with ARDS/ALI are turned from supine to prone position (560–564). The degree of improvement in oxygenation is quite variable but is frequently of sufficient magnitude to permit reductions in PEEP and FIO_2. This approach is based on the knowledge that lung distention is more uniform in the prone position and compressive forces, which facilitate airspace collapse, are mitigated with prone ventilation. Prone positioning may encourage dorsal lung recruitment, which results clinically in a dramatic and usually rapid improvement in gas exchange. Improvements in oxygenation are generally immediate and may be sustained with return of the patient to the supine position. Nonresponders to initial attempts at prone ventilation do not always constitute failures, as some patients may demonstrate improvement on subsequent attempts. Ostensibly, prone position has the potential to reduce VILI and oxygen toxicity in mechanically ventilated patients with ARDS. Despite these encouraging observations, no prospective randomized trials have shown that these changes translate to improved clinical outcome. In a recent study, the clinical outcome of ARDS patients treated with prone positioning for 6 hr per day was no different from those ventilated in the supine position (565,566). Longer periods of prone ventilation may be necessary to affect outcome. Guidelines regarding the optimal timing of prone positioning during the course of ARDS/ALI and duration of prone ventilation have not been established. Prone positioning requires the commitment of multiple ICU personnel. Dislodgement of intravenous catheters and endotracheal tubes and worsening oxygenation may occur during the process of repositioning the patient. Routine assessments of IV catheters and suctioning through the endotracheal tube are more problematic in the prone position. Thus, the role of nursing education in the management of prone positioning is pivotal to the success of this therapeutic intervention (567,568).

Neurogenic Pulmonary Edema

Neurogenic pulmonary edema (NPE) may arise as a direct result of acute severe brain insults caused by trauma, subarachnoid hemorrhage, seizures, or venous air embolism, cerebrovascular accidents and intracranial surgery. Many of these insults occur as a direct or indirect complication of primary central nervous system (CNS) malignancy, or metastatic CNS disease (569–571). NPE is seen in 50% of patients with severe brain injury. Areas of the brain that are most frequently cited as the origin of the pathophysiologic process leading to NPE include the medulla oblongata and the hypothalamus. Damage to these areas may lead to abrupt increases in intracranial pressures and subsequent pulmonary edema. The pathogenesis of neurogenic pulmonary edema remains controversial, although hydrostatic mechanisms and changes in vascular permeability have been implicated. Dyspnea, tachypnea, and cyanosis are prominent symptoms of NPE, which usually occur immediately following the brain insult. Copious respiratory secretions and a frequently ineffective cough in these patients with deteriorating CNS function are commonly associated with a "death rattle." Patients with NPE are often obtunded and the associated predilection for aspiration in these patients confounds the diagnosis and complicates therapy. Chest radiographic findings range from predominantly apical, homogeneous airspace consolidations to diffuse inhomogeneous areas of pulmonary edema. These changes are transient, typically resolving within 1–2 days of appearance. The treatment of NPE is primarily palliative. Airway management with intubation and endotracheal suction, and the institution of corticosteroids, loop diuretics, and morphine are appropriate palliative measures in some patients. Phenoxybenzamine, verapamil, propranolol, and antioxidants may offer protection against NPE in high-risk patients. Mortality rates associated with neurogenic pulmonary edema are high, conditioned primarily by the underlying CNS disease.

Re-expansion Pulmonary Edema

Cancer patients are susceptible to a variety of pleural diseases, including pneumothorax, hydrothorax, and hemothorax that may result in lung collapse. Evacuation of the pleural disease may cause re-expansion pulmonary edema, a rare and potentially fatal complication following rapid reinflation of a collapsed lung. Typically, more than 50% of the lung is involved in this process and the associated lung collapse is present for several days prior to therapy. Edema formation is commonly limited to the involved lung but may rarely progress to the contralateral side. The onset of pulmonary edema may be signaled by pernicious coughing and chest tightness during or immediately following thoracentesis or chest tube thoracostomy. These symptoms frequently escalate over the ensuing 24–48 hr and slowly resolve within 5–7 days of onset. In approximately 20% of patients, severe hypoxemia, respiratory failure leading to cardiovascular collapse, and death may occur (572,573). Lung injury is usually manifested as unilateral pulmonary edema in the re-expanded lung. The mechanism of re-expansion pulmonary edema is unclear, although increased microvascular permeability, reductions in perimicrovascular hydrostatic pressures and lung ischemia–reperfusion injury have been implicated.

Treatment primarily involves supportive care with hemodynamic support, supplemental oxygen, and intubation with mechanical ventilation, when necessary. Diuretic therapy should be administered cautiously, as aggressive diuresis may result in further decreases in intravascular volume and tissue perfusion. The use of underwater seal drainage during the initial 24–48 hr following chest tube thoracostomy may afford some protection against the development of re-expansion pulmonary edema. Negative pressure may then be applied to the chest tube if lung re-expansion has not been accomplished with simple underwater seal drainage. Pleural pressure monitoring during fluid evacuation may be appropriate in some patients with chronic, large-volume pleural effusions. Thoracentesis may safely continue as long as pleural pressures do not fall below −20 cm H_2O. These are general guidelines, however, and the occurrence of re-expansion pulmonary edema may not necessarily correlate with the absolute level of negative pleural pressure. Earlier studies advocated limiting the total amount of pleural fluid evacuation per thoracentesis in the absence of pleural pressure monitoring to 1.0 L (574). Although these guidelines have not been challenged in any recent prospective studies, several observations may permit safe removal of larger volumes of fluid. Patients with radiographic evidence of large pleural effusions causing contralateral shift of the mediastinum may tolerate removal of several liters of fluid as long as cough, dyspnea, or chest tightness do not occur. Ipsilateral mediastinal shift or the absence of contralateral shift of the mediastinum in the setting of a massive pleural effusion may be associated with a trapped lung or bronchial obstruction. Large-volume pleural fluid evacuation in this setting may be associated with a precipitous drop in pleural fluid pressures and an increased risk of re-expansion pulmonary edema. In the absence of pleural fluid monitoring in this group of patients, only small volumes of fluid (< 300 mL) should be removed at one sitting.

Postthoracotomy Pulmonary Edema

Diffuse lung injury following thoracotomy for lung or esophageal resection occurs in 5–10% of patients may threaten the success of an otherwise uneventful surgery (575,576). Respiratory failure in this setting is most frequently ascribed to pneumonia; however, in many cases a microbiological pathogen is never identified. An emerging body of evidence suggests that lung injury following thoracotomy is pathophysiologically similar to that of classic ARDS. Increased capillary hydrostatic pressure, alveolar inflammation, and increased permeability pulmonary edema are cardinal features of this disorder. The pathophysiologic mechanisms that underlie the development of postthorachotomy pulmonary edema are uncertain but may be related to single lung ventilation that occurs during the surgery. Several mechanisms have been postulated. During single lung ventilation most of the pulmonary blood flow passes through the ventilated lung. This may result in increased pulmonary capillary transmural pressures, damage to the pulmonary capillary endothelium, and edema formation. Intraoperative ventilation is usually accomplished using high FIO_2 values. In addition, normal or near-normal tidal volumes are generally maintained during ventilation of the single lung. Both of these measures cause damage to the single ventilated lung. Microatelectasis, which is nearly universal following general anesthesia, may represent a form of subclinical lung injury. Finally, reduced blood flow to the collapsed lung during surgery may lead to lung ischemia–reperfusion injury. Several important risk factors in the development of postthoracotomy pulmonary edema include perioperative mechanical ventilation with high pressures, low serum colloidal osmotic pressures, and transfusion of fresh frozen plasma. The administration of high ventilatory pressures intraoperatively is one of the putative mechanisms of acute lung injury. Additionally, the need for incremental increases in ventilatory pressures intraoperatively suggests poor lung compliance and may represent an early marker for postthoracotomy pulmonary edema. Interestingly right-sided pneumonectomy confers a higher risk for postpneumonectomy pulmonary edema than left-sided pneumonectomy. This observation is probably due to the smaller volume of the remaining (left) lung. The contribution of excessive intraoperative fluid administration and marked postsurgical diuresis (which reflects volume overload) in the development of postthoracotomy pulmonary edema has recently been in question (577–579). Severe dyspnea heralds the development of postthoracotomy pulmonary edema, which typically occurs within 48–72 hr of the surgery. Respiratory failure may quickly ensue. Radiographic evidence of pulmonary edema, including bilateral interstitial infiltrates, Kerley B lines, and peribronchial cuffing are important early clinical parameters that accompany

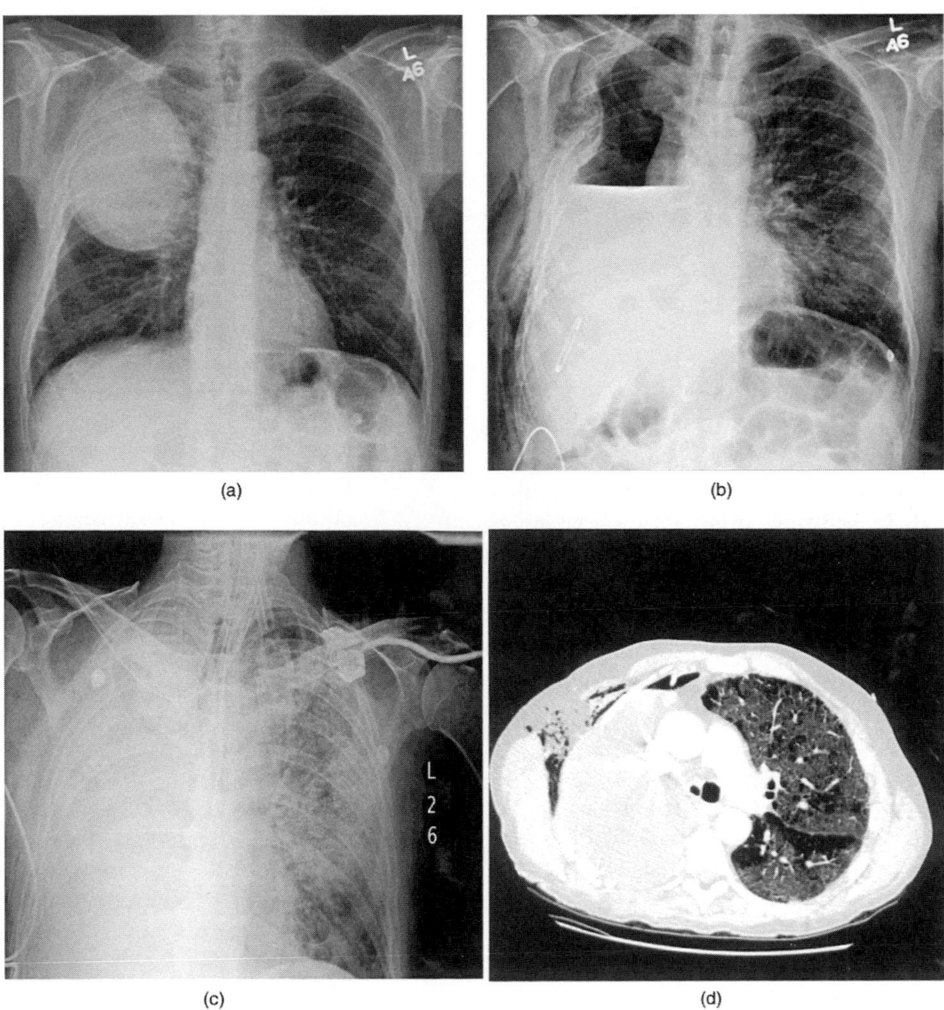

Figure 19 A 57-year-old man who developed acute respiratory failure several days after an uneventful open thoracotomy and pneumonectomy for a large bronchogenic tumor involving the right upper lobe. Radiographic evidence of pulmonary edema rapidly progressed to ARDS in the remaining lung. Chest radiograph prior to (a) and 3 days following (b) surgery. Chest radiograph and CT of the chest taken at day 10 (c–d) following surgery.

the development of this syndrome (Fig. 19a–e). Treatment is primarily supportive and includes reintubation, mechanical ventilation, and forced diuresis. Mortality rates associated with postthoracotomy pulmonary edema exceed 50% despite aggressive supportive measures (577). The role of intraoperative ventilatory strategies in the development of postthoracotomy pulmonary edema warrants further investigation.

IV. SUMMARY

A potent admixture of barrier breakdown and immune exhaustion associated with malignancy and its therapy render cancer patients exquisitely vulnerable to a wide variety infectious and noninfectious disorders. These disorders take an inexhorable toll on the lungs. The ubiquitous potential for lung damage with cancer treatment not only dictates the limits of therapy, but may also trump otherwise successful cancer treatment strategies. Significant advances in antineoplastic therapy, including more aggressive cytoreductive and multimodality protocols, challenge the limits of tolerance and offer the prospect of longer-term disease-free survival. In addition, targeted therapy using immunonodulators and hematopoietic cytokines have bolstered survival in certain groups of patients. New definitions of the suitable donor and recipient of stem cell transplantation have resulted in marked expansion of this therapeutic procedure to patients who were previously considered ineligible for this type of therapy. Surgical approaches to patients with resectable intrathoracic tumors are frequently used in combination with aggressive chemoradation regimens in an effort to improve survival. In addition, interventional bronchoscopy has emerged as standard therapy for some patients and offers pallation as well as definitive therapy for some patients with advanced intrathoracic tumors. In the wake of these significant achievements is an evolving list of pulmonary sequelae, which have become more numerous and complex as new cancer treatment strategies have emerged.

The intensivist is charged with the monumental task of integrating diverse sources of information in order to focus the differential diagnosis of pulmonary infiltrates in this inherently complex group of patients. Recognition of the indistinct interface between infection and comorbid conditions that often mimic infection is only one of many challenges that face the intensivist in caring for these patients. Balancing aggressive treatment protocols with strategies that limit further lung injury in the intensive care unit represents another. Advances in the treatment of critically ill patients with pulmonary infiltrates will occur as new strategies for earlier and more precise recognition of the underlying pulmonary diseases are established.

REFERENCES

1. Perlin E, Bang KM, Shah A, et al. The impact of pulmonary infections on the survival of lung cancer patients. Cancer 1990; 66:593–596.
2. Schapira DV, Studnicki J, Bradham DD, et al. Intensive care, survival, and expense of treating critically ill cancer patients. JAMA 1993; 269:783–786.
3. Groeger JS, Glassman J, Nierman DM, et al. Probability of mortality of critically ill cancer patients at 72 h of intensive care unit (ICU) management. Support Care Cancer 2003; 11:686–695. Epub 2003 Aug 2005.
4. Groeger JS, White P Jr, Nierman DM, et al. Outcome for cancer patients requiring mechanical ventilation. J Clin Oncol 1999; 17:991–997.
5. Jackson SR, Tweeddale MG, Barnett MJ, et al. Admission of bone marrow transplant recipients to the intensive care unit: outcome, survival and prognostic factors. Bone Marrow Transplant 1998; 21: 697–704.
6. Huaringa AJ, Leyva F, Giralt S. Outcome of bone marrow transplantation patients requiring mechanical ventilation. Crit Care Med 2000; 28:10, 14–17.
7. Maschmeyer G, Bertschat FL, Moesta KT, et al. Outcome analysis of 189 consecutive cancer patients referred to the intensive care unit as emergencies during a 2-year period. Eur J Cancer 2003; 39:783–792.
8. Krowka MJ, Rosenow EC, Hoagland HC. Pulmonary complications of bone marrow transplantation. Chest 1985; 87:237–246.
9. Kolbe K, Domkin D, Derigs H, et al. Infectious complications during neutropenia subsequent to peripheral blood cell transplantation. Bone Marrow Transplant 1997; 19:143–147.
10. Mossad S, Longworth D, Goormastic, et al. Early infectious complications in autologous bone marrow transplantation. A review of 219 patients. Bone Marrow Transplant 1996; 18:265–271.
11. Gonzales-Barca E, Fernandez-Sevillaa A, Carratala J, et al. Prospective study of 288 episodes of bacteremia in neutropenic cancer patients in a single institution. Eur J Clin Microbiol Infect Dis 1996; 15:291–296.
12. Raad I, Whimbey E, Rolston K, et al. A comparison of aztreonam plus vancomycin and imipenem plus vancomycin as initial therapy for febrile neutropenic cancer patients. Cancer 1996; 77:1386–1394.
13. Hildebrand F, Rosenow EI, Haberman T. Pulmonary complications of leukemia. Chest 1998; 80:1233–1239.
14. Hirsch A, Vander Els N, Straus DJ, et al. Effect of ABVD chemotherapy with and without mantle or mediastinal irradiation on pulmonary function and symptoms in early-stage Hodgkin's disease. J Clin Oncol 1996; 14:1297–1305.

15. Crawford S, Schwartz D, Petersen F, et al. Mechanical ventilation after marrow transplantation: risk factors and clinical outcome. Am Rev Respir Dis 1988; 137:682.
16. Aronchick J. Pulmonary infections in cancer and bone marrow transplant patients. Semin Roentgenol 2000; 35:140–151.
17. Collin BA, Ramphal R. Lower respiratory tract infections. Infect Dis Clin N Am 1998; 12:781–805.
18. Mermel LA. Prevention of intravascular catheter-related infections. Ann Intern Med 2000; 132:391–402.
19. Adair CG, Gorman SP, Feron BM, et al. Implications of endotracheal tube biofilm for ventilator-associated pneumonia. Intensive Care Med 1999; 25: 1072–1076.
20. Ibrahim EH, Tracy L, Hill C, et al. The occurrence of ventilator-associated pneumonia in a community hospital: risk factors and clinical outcomes. Chest 2001; 120:555–561.
21. Ganz T. Epithelia: not just physical barriers. PNAS 2002; 99:3357–3358.
22. Goodman L, Gilman A. Antineoplastic Agents. 10th ed. New York, NY: McGraw Hill, 2001.
23. Nathan C. Points of control in inflammation. Nature 2002; 420:846–852.
24. Cohen J. The immunopathogenesis of sepsis. Nature 2002; 420:885–891.
25. Winston D, Territo M, Ho W, et al. Alveolar macrophage dysfunction in human bone marrow transplant recipients. Am J Med 1982; 73:859–866.
26. Lehrer R, Cline M. Leukocyte candidacidal activity and resistance to systemic candidiasis in patients with cancer. Cancer 1971; 27:1211–1217.
27. Stossel T. Phagocytosis. N Engl J Med 1974; 290: 717–723.
28. Hughes WT, Armstrong D, Bodey GP, et al. 1997 guidelines for the use of antimicrobial agents in neutropenic patients with unexplained fever. Infectious Diseases Society of America. Clin Infect Dis 1997; 25: 551–573.
29. Schimpff SC. Empiric antibiotic therapy for granulocytopenic cancer patients. Am J Med 1986; 80:13–20.
30. Tenholder M, Hooper R. Pulmonary hemorrhage in the immunocompromised host—an elusive reality. Am Rev Respir Dis 1980; 121:A198.
31. Balducci L, Halbrook JC, Chapman SW, et al. Acute leukemia and infections: perspectives from a general hospital. Am J Hematol 1983; 15:57–63.
32. Hubel K, Hegener K, Schnell R, et al. Suppressed neutrophil function as a risk factor for severe infection after cytotoxic chemotherapy in patients with acute nonlymphocytic leukemia. Ann Hematol 1999; 78: 73–77.
33. Pickering LK, Ericsson CD, Kohl S. Effect of chemotherapeutic agents on metabolic and bactericidal activity of polymorphonuclear leukocytes. Cancer 1978; 42:1741–1746.
34. Marschmeyer G, Link H, Hiddemann W, et al. Pulmonary infiltrations in febrile patients with neutropenia. Cancer 1994; 73:2296–2304.
35. Fanger MW, Erbe DV. Fc gamma receptors in cancer and infectious disease. Immunol Res 1992; 11:203–216.
36. Hussein M. Multiple myeloma: an overview of diagnosis and management. Cleve Clin J Med 1994; 61: 285–298.
37. Englund J, Sullivan C, Jordan C, et al. Respiratory syncytial virus infection in immunocompromised adults. Ann Intern Med 1988; 109:203–208.
38. Reed E, Bowden R, Dandliker P, et al. Treatment of cytomegalovirus pneumonia with ganciclovir and intravenous cytomegalovirus immunoglobulin in patients with bone marrow transplants. Ann Intern Med 1988; 109:783–788.
39. Ringden O, Lonnqvist B, Paulin T, et al. Pharmacokinetics, safety and preliminary clinical experiences using foscarnet in the treatment of cytomegalovirus infections in bone marrow and renal transplant recipient. J Antimicrob Chemother 1986; 1986:373–387.
40. Emanuel D, Cunningham L, Jules-Elysee K, et al. Cytomegalovirus pneumonia after bone marrow transplantation successfully treated with the combination of ganciclovir and high dose intravenous immune globulin. Ann Intern Med 1988; 109:777–782.
41. Ramsey P, Fife K, Hackman R, et al. Herpes simplex virus pneumonia. Ann Intern Med 1982; 97:813–820.
42. Wendt C, Hertz M. Respiratory syncytial virus and parainfluenza virus infections in the immunocompromised host. Semin Respir Infect 1995; 10:224–231.
43. Soubani A, Miller K, Hassoun P. Pulmonary complications of bone marrow transplantation. Chest 1996; 109(4):1066–1077.
44. Clark J. The challenge of bone marrow transplantation (editorial). Mayo Clin Proc 1990; 65:111–114.
45. Spanik S, Kukuckova E, Pichna P, et al. Analysis of 553 episodes of monomicrobial bacteraemia in cancer patients: any association between risk factors and outcome to particular pathogen? Support Care Cancer 1997; 5:330–333.
46. Slavin S, Naparstek E, Nagler A, et al. Allogeneic cell therapy for relapsed leukemia after bone marrow transplantation with donor peripheral blood lymphocytes. Exp Hematol 1995; 23:1553–1562.
47. Goodman JL, Winston DJ, Greenfield RA, et al. A controlled trial of fluconazole to prevent fungal infections in patients undergoing bone marrow transplantation. N Engl J Med 1992; 326:845–851.
48. Seddik M, Seemayer TA, Lapp WS. The graft-versus-host reaction and immune function. III. Functional pre-T cells in the bone marrow of graft-versus-host-reactive mice displaying T cell immunodeficiency. Transplantation 1986; 41:238–242.
49. Goodrich JM, Bowden RA, Fisher L, et al. Ganciclovir prophylaxis to prevent cytomegalovirus disease after allogeneic marrow transplant. Ann Intern Med 1993; 118:173–178.

50. Winston DJ, Ho WG, Bartoni K, et al. Intravenous immunoglobulin and CMV-seronegative blood products for prevention of CMV infection and disease in bone marrow transplant recipients. Bone Marrow Transplant 1993; 12:283–288.
51. Marrie TJ, Durant H, Yates L. Community-acquired pneumonia requiring hospitalization: 5-year prospective study. Rev Infect Dis 1989; 11:586–599.
52. Neill AM, Martin IR, Weir R, et al. Community acquired pneumonia: aetiology and usefulness of severity criteria on admission. Thorax 1996; 51:1010–1016.
53. Fine MJ, Auble TE, Yealy DM, et al. A prediction rule to identify low-risk patients with community-acquired pneumonia. N Engl J Med 1997; 336:243–250.
54. Won HJ, Lee KS, Cheon JE, et al. Invasive pulmonary aspergillosis: prediction at thin-section CT in patients with neutropenia—a prospective study. Radiology 1998; 208:777–782.
55. Yellin A, Rosen A, Reichert N, et al. Superior vena cava syndrome. The myth—the facts. Am Rev Respir Dis 1990; 141(5p + 1):1114–1118.
56. Ewig S, Schlochtermeier M, Goke N, et al. Applying sputum as a diagnostic tool in pneumonia: limited yield, minimal impact on treatment decisions. Chest 2002; 121:1486–1492.
57. Crawford SW. Noninfectious lung disease in the immunocompromised host. Respiration 1999; 66: 385–395.
58. Reamer RH, Dey BP, White CA, et al. Comparison of monolayer and bilayer plates used in antibiotic assay. J AOAC Int 1998; 81:398–402.
59. Ewig S. Diagnosis of ventilator-associated pneumonia: nonroutine tools for routine practice. Eur Respir J 1996; 9:1339–1341.
60. Murdoch DR. Nucleic acid amplification tests for the diagnosis of pneumonia. Clin Infect Dis 2003; 36: 1162–1170. Epub 2003 Apr 1122.
61. Hebart H, Loffler J, Meisner C, et al. Early detection of aspergillus infection after allogeneic stem cell transplantation by polymerase chain reaction screening. J Infect Dis 2000; 181:1713–1719.
62. Erjavec Z, Verweij PE. Recent progress in the diagnosis of fungal infections in the immunocompromised host. Drug Resist Updat 2002; 5:3–10.
63. Maertens J, Verhaegen J, Lagrou K, et al. Screening for circulating galactomannan as a noninvasive diagnostic tool for invasive aspergillosis in prolonged neutropenic patients and stem cell transplantation recipients: a prospective validation. Blood 2001; 97: 1604–1610.
64. Sulahian A, Boutboul F, Ribaud P, et al. Value of antigen detection using an enzyme immunoassay in the diagnosis and prediction of invasive aspergillosis in two adult and pediatric hematology units during a 4-year prospective study. Cancer 2001; 91:311–318.
65. Verweij PE, Stynen D, Rijs AJ, et al. Sandwich enzyme-linked immunosorbent assay compared with Pastorex latex agglutination test for diagnosing invasive aspergillosis in immunocompromised patients. J Clin Microbiol 1995; 33:1912–1914.
66. Verweij PE, Meis JF. Microbiological diagnosis of invasive fungal infections in transplant recipients. Transplant Infect Dis 2000; 2:80–87.
67. Reichenberger F, Habicht J, Matt P, et al. Diagnostic yield of bronchoscopy in histologically proven invasive pulmonary aspergillosis. Bone Marrow Transplant 1999; 24:1195–1199.
68. Pizzo PA. Fever in immunocompromised patients. N Engl J Med 1999; 341:893–900.
69. Matthew P, Bozeman P, Krance RA. Bronchiolitis obliterans organizing pneumonia (boop) in children after allogeneic bone marrow transplantation. Bone Marrow Transplantation 1994; 13:221–223.
70. Dunagan DP, Baker AM, Hurd DD. Bronchoscopic evaluation of pulmonary infiltrates following bone marrow transplantation. Chest 1997; 111:135–141.
71. White P Jr, Bonacum J, Miller C. Utility of fiberoptic bronchoscopy in bone marrow transplant patients. Bone Marrow Transplantion 1997; 20:681–687.
72. Glazer M, Breuer R, Berkman N, et al. Use of fiberoptic bronchoscopy in bone marrow transplant recipients. Acta Haematol 1998; 99:22–26.
73. Weiss RB. Complications of fiberoptic bronchoscopy in thrombocytopenic patients. Chest 1993; 104: 1025–1028.
74. Casetta M, Blot F, Antoun S, et al. Diagnosis of nosocomial pneumonia in cancer patients undergoing mechanical ventilation. Chest 1999; 115:1641–1645.
75. White D, Rankin J, Stover D. Severe bleomycin-induced pneumonitis: clinical features and response to corticosteroids. Chest 1984; 86:723–728.
76. Pisani RJ, Wright AJ. Clinical utility of bronchoalveolar lavage in immunocompromised hosts. Mayo Clin Proc 1992; 67:221–227.
77. Torres A, el-Ebiary M, Padro L, et al. Validation of different techniques for the diagnosis of ventilator-associated pneumonia. Comparison with immediate postmortem pulmonary biopsy. Am J Respir Crit Care Med 1994; 149:324–331.
78. Rouby JJ, Martin De Lassale E, Poete P, et al. Nosocomial bronchopneumonia in the critically ill. Histologic and bacteriologic aspects. Am Rev Respir Dis 1992; 146:1059–1066.
79. Feller-Kopman D, Ernst A. The role of bronchoalveolar lavage in the immunocompromised host. Semin Respir Infect 2003; 18:87–94.
80. Dalhoff K, Braun J, Hollandt H, et al. Diagnostic value of bronchoalveolar lavage in patients with opportunistic and nonopportunistic bacterial pneumonia. Infection 1993; 21:291–296.
81. Rano A, Agusti C, Jimenez P, et al. Pulmonary infiltrates in non-HIV immunocompromised patients: a

diagnostic approach using non-invasive and bronchoscopic procedures. Thorax 2001; 56:379–387.
82. Hohenadel IA, Kiworr M, Genitsariotis R, et al. Role of bronchoalveolar lavage in immunocompromised patients with pneumonia treated with a broad spectrum antibiotic and antifungal regimen. Thorax 2001; 56:115–120.
83. White DA, Wong PW, Downey R. The utility of open-lung biopsy in patients with hematologic malignancies. Am J Respir Crit Care Med 2000; 161:723–729.
84. Egermayer P, Peacock AJ. Is pulmonary embolism a common cause of chronic pulmonary hypertension? Limitations of the embolic hypothesis. Eur Respir J 2000; 15:440–448.
85. Lossos I, Breuer R, Or R, et al. Bacterial pneumonia in recipients of bone marrow transplantation: a five year prospective study. Transplantation 1995; 60: 672–678.
86. Cordonnier C, Bernaudin J, Bierling P, et al. Pulmonary complications occurring after allogeneic bone marrow transplantation. Cancer 1986; 58:1047–1054.
87. Carratala J, Marron A, Fernandez-Sevilla A. Treatment of penicillin-resistant pneumococcal bacteremia in neutropenic patients with cancer. Clin Infect Dis 1997; 24:148–152.
88. Escande MC, Herbrecht R. Prospective study of bacteraemia in cancer patients. Results of a French multicentre study. Support Care Cancer 1998; 6:273–280.
89. Jones RN. Contemporary antimicrobial susceptibility patterns of bacterial pathogens commonly associated with febrile patients with neutropenia. Clin Infect Dis 1999; 29:495–502.
90. Bochud P, Calandra T, Francioli P. Bacteremia due to viridans streptococci in neutropenic patients. A review. Am J Med 1997; 3:256–264.
91. Danes C, Gonzalez-Martin J, Pumarola T, et al. Pulmonary infiltrates in immunosuppressed patients: analysis of a diagnostic protocol. J Clin Microbiol 2002; 40:2134–2140.
92. Baracco GJ, Dickinson GM. Pulmonary nocardiosis. Curr Infect Dis Rep 2001; 3:286–292.
93. Simpson GL, Stinson EB, Egger MJ, et al. Nocardial infections in the immunocompromised host: a detailed study in a defined population. Rev Infect Dis 1981; 3:492–507.
94. Rano A, Agussti C, Natividad B, et al. Prognostic factors of non-HIV immunocompromised patients with pulmonary infiltrates. Chest 2002; 122:253–261.
95. Lerner PI. Nocardiosis. Clin Infect Dis 1996; 22: 891–903; Quiz 904–895.
96. Schlossberg D, Bonoan J. Legionella and immunosuppression. Semin Respir Infect 1998; 13:128–131.
97. Sabria M, Campins M. Legionnaires' disease: update on epidemiology and management options. Am J Respir Med 2003; 2:235–243.
98. Valles J, Mesalles E, Mariscal D, et al. A 7-year study of severe hospital-acquired pneumonia requiring ICU admission. Intensive Care Med 2003; 29:1981–1988. Epub 2003 Sep 1910.
99. Tsiodras S, Samonis G, Keating MJ, et al. Infection and immunity in chronic lymphocytic leukemia. Mayo Clin Proc 2000; 75:1039–1054.
100. Jacobson K, Garcia R, Libshitz H, et al. Clinical and radiological features of pulmonary disease caused by rapidly growing mycobacteria in cancer patients. Eur J Clin Microbiol Infect Dis 1998; 17:615–621.
101. Levendoglu-Tugal O, Munoz J, Brudnicki A, et al. Infections due to nontuberculous mycobacteria in children with leukemia. Clin Infect Dis 1998; 27:1227–1230.
102. Fled R, Bodey G, Groschel D. Mycobacteriosis in patients with malignant disease. Arch Intern Med 1976; 136:67.
103. Saubolle MA. Fungal pneumonias. Semin Respir Infect 2000; 15:162–177.
104. Goodman ER, Hardy MA. Transplantation 1992: the year in review. Clin Transplant 1992; 285–297.
105. Wingard JR, Merz WG, Rinaldi MG, et al. Increase in Candida krusei infection among patients with bone marrow transplantation and neutropenia treated prophylactically with fluconazole. N Engl J Med 1991; 325: 1274–1277.
106. Engelhard D. Bacterial and fungal infections in children undergoing bone marrow transplantation. Bone Marrow Transplant 1998; 21:S78–S80.
107. Petrocheilou-Paschou V, Georgilis K, Kontoyannis D, et al. Pneumonia due to Candida krusei. Clin Microbiol Infect 2002; 8:806–809.
108. Reijula K, Tuomi T. Mycotoxins of aspergilli: exposure and health effects. Front Biosci 2003; 8:s232–s235.
109. Wingard JR, Beals SU, Santos GW, et al. Aspergillus infections in bone marrow transplant recipients. Bone Marrow Transplant 1987; 2:175–181.
110. Anaissie EJ, Stratton SL, Dignani MC, et al. Pathogenic molds (including Aspergillus species) in hospital water distribution systems: a 3-year prospective study and clinical implications for patients with hematologic malignancies. Blood 2003; 101:2542–2546. Epub 2002 Dec 2545.
111. McWhinney PH, Kibbler CC, Hamon MD, et al. Progress in the diagnosis and management of aspergillosis in bone marrow transplantation: 13 years' experience. Clin Infect Dis 1993; 17:397–404.
112. Ringden O, Andstrom EE, Remberger M, et al. Prophylaxis and therapy using liposomal amphotericin B (AmBisome) for invasive fungal infections in children undergoing organ or allogeneic bone-marrow transplantation. Pediatr Transplant 1997; 1:124–129.
113. Chopra R, Blair S, Strang J, et al. Liposomal amphotericin B (AmBisome) in the treatment of fungal infections in neutropenic patients. J Antimicrob Chemother 1991; 28:93–104.
114. Jeu L, Piacenti FJ, Lyakhovetskiy AG, et al. Voriconazole. Clin Ther 2003; 25:1321–1381.

115. Bhatia S, McCullough J, Perry EH, et al. Granulocyte transfusions: efficacy in treating fungal infections in neutropenic patients following bone marrow transplantation. Transfusion 1994; 34:226–232.
116. Price TH, Bowden RA, Boeckh M, et al. Phase I/II trial of neutrophil transfusions from donors stimulated with G-CSF and dexamethasone for treatment of patients with infections in hematopoietic stem cell transplantation. Blood 2000; 95:3302–3309.
117. Briones MA, Josephson CD, Hillyer CD. Granulocyte transfusion: revisited. Curr Hematol Rep 2003; 2: 522–527.
118. Boelaert JR, De Baere YA, Geernaert MA, et al. The use of nasal mupirocin ointment to prevent *Staphylococcus aureus* bacteraemias in haemodialysis patients: an analysis of cost-effectiveness. J Hosp Infect 1991; 19:41–46.
119. McCloud T, Naidich D. Thoracic disease in the immunocompromised patient. Radiol Clin North Am 1992; 30:525–554.
120. Bigby TD, Margolskee D, Curtis JL, et al. The usefulness of induced sputum in the diagnosis of *Pneumocystis carinii* pneumonia in patients with the acquired immunodeficiency syndrome. Am Rev Respir Dis 1986; 133:515–518.
121. Pitchenik AE, Ganjei P, Torres A, et al. Sputum examination for the diagnosis of *Pneumocystis carinii* pneumonia in the acquired immunodeficiency syndrome. Am Rev Respir Dis 1986; 133:226–229.
122. Stover DE, Kaner RJ. Pulmonary complications in cancer patients. CA Cancer J Clin 1996; 46:303–320.
123. Hale GA, Heslop HE, Krance RA, et al. Adenovirus infection after pediatric bone marrow transplantation. Bone Marrow Transplant 1999; 23:277–282.
124. Whimbey E, Ghosh S. Respiratory syncytial virus infections in immunocompromised adults. Curr Clin Top Infect Dis 2000; 20:232–255.
125. Yeldandi AV, Colby TV. Pathologic features of lung biopsy specimens from influenza pneumonia cases. Hum Pathol 1994; 25:47–53.
126. Palmer SM, Robinson LJ, Wang A, et al. Massive pulmonary edema and death after prostacyclin infusion in a patient with pulmonary veno-occlusive disease. Chest 1998; 113:237–240.
127. Winston D, Ho W, Champlin R. Cytomegalovirus infections after allogenic bone marrow transplantation. Rev Infect Dis 1990; 12:S776.
128. Jules-Elysee K, Stover D, Yahalom J, et al. Pulmonary complications in lymphoma patients treated with high-dose therapy and autologous bone marrow transplantation. Am Rev Respir Dis 1992; 146:485.
129. Reddehase MJ. The immunogenicity of human and murine cytomegaloviruses. Curr Opin Immunol 2000; 12:390–396.
130. Maltezou H, Whimbey E, Abi-Said D, et al. Cytomegalovirus disease in adult marrow transplant recipients receiving ganciclovir prophylaxis: a retrospective study. Bone Marrow Transplant 1999; 24:665–669.
131. Hadley S, Samore MH, Lewis WD, et al. Major infectious complications after orthotopic liver transplantation and comparison of outcomes in patients receiving cyclosporine or FK506 as primary immunosuppression. Transplantation 1995; 59:851–859.
132. de Maar EF, Verschuuren EA, Harmsen MC, et al. Pulmonary involvement during cytomegalovirus infection in immunosuppressed patients. Transpl Infect Dis 2003; 5:112–120.
133. Hengel H, Esslinger C, Pool J, et al. Cytokines restore MHC class I complex formation and control antigen presentation in human cytomegalovirus-infected cells. J Gen Virol 1995; 76:2987–2997.
134. Raftery MJ, Schwab M, Eibert SM, et al. Targeting the function of mature dendritic cells by human cytomegalovirus: a multilayered viral defense strategy. Immunity 2001; 15:997–1009.
135. Boeckh M, Leisenring W, Riddell SR, et al. Late cytomegalovirus disease and mortality in recipients of allogeneic hematopoietic stem cell transplants: importance of viral load and T-cell immunity. Blood 2003; 101: 407–414. Epub 2002 Sep 2012.
136. Boeckh MJ, Nichols WG. The impact of cytomegalovirus serostatus of donor and recipient before hematopoietic stem cell transplantation in the era of antiviral prophylaxis and preemptive therapy. Blood 2003; 26: 203–208.
137. Limaye AP, Corey L, Koelle DM, et al. Emergence of ganciclovir-resistant cytomegalovirus disease among recipients of solid-organ transplants. Lancet 2000; 356: 645–649.
138. Boeckh M, Nichols WG, Papanicolaou G, et al. Cytomegalovirus in hematopoietic stem cell transplant recipients: current status, known challenges, and future strategies. Biol Blood Marrow Transplant 2003; 9: 543–558.
139. Kakkar AK, Levine M, Pinedo HM, et al. Venous thrombosis in cancer patients: insights from the FRONTLINE survey. Oncologist 2003; 8:381–388.
140. Wingard JR. Viral infections in leukemia and bone marrow transplant patients. Leuk Lymphoma 1993; 11:115–125.
141. Sinclair J, Sissons P. Latent and persistent infections of monocytes and macrophages. Intervirology 1996; 39:293–301.
142. Ettinger N, Trulock E. Pulmonary considerations of organ transplantation. Am Rev Respir Dis 1991; 144:433–451.
143. Nguyen Q, Champlin R, Giralt S, et al. Late cytomegalovirus pneumonia in adult allogeneic blood and marrow transplant recipients. Clin Infect Dis 1999; 28:618–623.
144. Konoplev S, Champlin RE, Giralt S, et al. Cytomegalovirus pneumonia in adult autologous blood and marrow transplant recipients. Bone Marrow Transplant 2001; 27:877–881.

145. Ljungman P. Cytomegalovirus pneumonia: presentation, diagnosis, and treatment. Semin Respir Infect 1995; 10:209–215.
146. Manna A, Cordani S, Canessa P, et al. CMV infection and pneumonia in hematological malignancies. J Infect Chemother 2003; 9:265–267.
147. Ippoliti C, Morgan A, Warkentin D, et al. Foscarnet for prevention of cytomegalovirus infection in allogeneic marrow transplant recipients unable to receive ganciclovir. Bone Marrow Transplant 1997; 20: 491–495.
148. Drew WL, Stempien MJ, Andrews J, et al. Cytomegalovirus (CMV) resistance in patients with CMV retinitis and AIDS treated with oral or intravenous ganciclovir. J Infect Dis 1999; 179:1352–1355.
149. Graham BS, Snell JD Jr. Herpes simplex virus infection of the adult lower respiratory tract. Medicine (Baltimore) 1983; 62:384–393.
150. Ramsey PG, Fife KH, Hackman RC, et al. Herpes simplex virus pneumonia: clinical, virologic, and pathologic features in 20 patients. Ann Intern Med 1982; 97:813–820.
151. Nash G, Ross JS. Herpetic esophagitis. A common cause of esophageal ulceration. Hum Pathol 1974; 5:339–345.
152. Schmutzhard J, Merete Riedel H, Zweygberg Wirgart B, et al. Detection of herpes simplex virus type 1, herpes simplex virus type 2 and varicella-zoster virus in skin lesions. Comparison of real-time PCR, nested PCR and virus isolation. J Clin Virol 2004; 29: 120–126.
153. Akhtar N, Ni J, Stromberg D, et al. Tracheal aspirate as a substrate for polymerase chain reaction detection of viral genome in childhood pneumonia and myocarditis. Circulation 1999; 99:2011–2018.
154. Schuller D, Spessert C, Fraser VJ, et al. Herpes simplex virus from respiratory tract secretions: epidemiology, clinical characteristics, and outcome in immunocompromised and nonimmunocompromised hosts. Am J Med 1993; 94:29–33.
155. Aquino SL, Dunagan DP, Chiles C, et al. Herpes simplex virus 1 pneumonia: patterns on CT scans and conventional chest radiographs. J Comput Assist Tomogr 1998; 22:795–800.
156. Crumpacker CS. Use of antiviral drugs to prevent herpesvirus transmission. N Engl J Med 2004; 350:67–68.
157. Eisen D, Essell J, Broun ER, et al. Clinical utility of oral valacyclovir compared with oral acyclovir for the prevention of herpes simplex virus mucositis following autologous bone marrow transplantation or stem cell rescue therapy. Bone Marrow Transplant 2003; 31:51–55.
158. Trifilio S, Verma A, Mehta J. Antimicrobial prophylaxis in hematopoietic stem cell transplant recipients: heterogeneity of current clinical practice. Bone Marrow Transplant 2004; 2:735–739.
159. Taplitz RA, Jordan MC. Pneumonia caused by herpesviruses in recipients of hematopoietic cell transplants. Semin Respir Infect 2002; 17:121–129.
160. Steer CB, Szer J, Sasadeusz J, et al. Varicella-zoster infection after allogeneic bone marrow transplantation: incidence, risk factors and prevention with low-dose aciclovir and ganciclovir. Bone Marrow Transplant 2000; 25:657–664.
161. Rowland P, Wald ER, Mirro JR Jr, et al. Progressive varicella presenting with pain and minimal skin involvement in children with acute lymphoblastic leukemia. J Clin Oncol 1995; 13:1697–1703.
162. Yoshikawa T, Asano Y, Ihira M, et al. Human herpesvirus 6 viremia in bone marrow transplant recipients: clinical features and risk factors. J Infect Dis 2002; 185:847–853. Epub 2002 Mar 2019.
163. Kadakia MP. Human herpesvirus 6 infection and associated pathogenesis following bone marrow transplantation. Leuk Lymphoma 1998; 31:251–266.
164. Anaissie EJ, Mahfouz TH, Aslan T, et al. The natural history of respiratory syncytial virus infection in cancer and transplant patients: implications for management. Blood 2004; 103:1611–1617. Epub 2003 Oct 1612.
165. Broughton S, Greenough A. Effectiveness of drug therapies to treat or prevent respiratory syncytial virus infection-related morbidity. Expert Opin Pharmacother 2003; 4:1801–1808.
166. Flomenberg P, Babbitt J, Drobyski WR, et al. Increasing incidence of adenovirus disease in bone marrow transplant recipients. J Infect Dis 1994; 169:775–781.
167. Bruno B, Gooley T, Hackman RC, et al. Adenovirus infection in hematopoietic stem cell transplantation: effect of ganciclovir and impact on survival. Biol Blood Marrow Transplant 2003; 9:341–352.
168. Hughes WT, Armstrong D, Bodey GP, et al. 2002 guidelines for the use of antimicrobial agents in neutropenic patients with cancer. Clin Infect Dis 2002; 34:730–751.
169. Klastersky J. Empirical treatment of sepsis in neutropenic patients. Int J Antimicrob Agents 2000; 16: 131–133.
170. Talcott JA, Siegel RD, Finberg R, et al. Risk assessment in cancer patients with fever and neutropenia: a prospective, two-center validation of a prediction rule. J Clin Oncol 1992; 10:316–322.
171. Einsele H, Bertz H, Beyer J, et al. Infectious complications after allogeneic stem cell transplantation: epidemiology and interventional therapy strategies—guidelines of the Infectious Diseases Working Party (AGIHO) of the German Society of Hematology and Oncology (DGHO). Ann Hematol 2003; 82:S175–S185.
172. Link H, Bohme A, Cornely OA, et al. Antimicrobial therapy of unexplained fever in neutropenic patients—guidelines of the Infectious Diseases Working Party (AGIHO) of the German Society of Hematology and Oncology (DGHO), Study Group

Interventional Therapy of Unexplained Fever, Arbeitsgemeinschaft Supportivmassnahmen in der Onkologie (ASO) of the Deutsche Krebsgesellschaft (DKG-German Cancer Society). Ann Hematol 2003; 82: S105–S117.
173. Engervall P, Kalin M, Dornbusch K, et al. Cefepime as empirical monotherapy in febrile patients with hematological malignancies and neutropenia: a randomized, single-center phase II trial. J Chemother 1999; 11:278–286.
174. Behre G, Link H, Maschmeyer G, et al. Meropenem monotherapy versus combination therapy with ceftazidime and amikacin for empirical treatment of febrile neutropenic patients. Ann Hematol 1998; 76: 73–80.
175. Walsh T, Gonzalez C, Lyman C, et al. Invasive fungal infections in children: recent advances in diagnosis and treatment. Adv Pediatr Infect Dis 1995; 11:187–290.
176. Wingard JR. Approach to invasive fungal infection after blood or marrow transplantation. Transplant Proc 2000; 32:1543–1544.
177. Fleming RV, Walsh TJ, Anaissie EJ. Emerging and less common fungal pathogens. Infect Dis Clin North Am 2002; 16:915–933, vi–vii.
178. Hubel K, Engert A. Clinical applications of granulocyte colony-stimulating factor: an update and summary. Ann Hematol 2003; 82:207–213.
179. Hubel K, Engert A. Granulocyte transfusion therapy for treatment of infections after cytotoxic chemotherapy. Onkologie 2003; 26:73–79.
180. Strauss RG. Neutrophil (granulocyte) transfusions in the new millennium. Transfusion 1998; 38:710–712.
181. Di Mario A, Sica S, Salutari P, et al. Granulocyte colony-stimulating factor-primed leukocyte transfusions in candida tropicalis fungemia in neutropenic patients. Haematologica 1997; 82:362–363.
182. Fatkenheuer G, Buchheidt D, Cornely OA, et al. Central venous catheter (CVC)-related infections in neutropenic patients—guidelines of the Infectious Diseases 181 Working Party (AGIHO) of the German Society of Hematology and Oncology (DGHO). Ann Hematol 2003; 82:S149–S157. Epub 2003 Sep 2009.
183. Hanna HA, Raad II, Hackett B, et al. Antibiotic-impregnated catheters associated with significant decrease in nosocomial and multidrug-resistant bacteremias in critically ill patients. Chest 2003; 124:1030–1038.
184. Marciante KD, Veenstra DL, Lipsky BA, et al. Which antimicrobial impregnated central venous catheter should we use? Modeling the costs and outcomes of antimicrobial catheter use. Am J Infect Control 2003; 31:1–8.
185. Scott DB. Mendelson's syndrome. Br J Anaesth 1978; 50:977–978.
186. Schwartz DJ, Wynne JW, Gibbs CP, et al. The pulmonary consequences of aspiration of gastric contents at pH values greater than 2.5. Am Rev Respir Dis 1980; 121:119–126.
187. Knight PR, Rutter T, Tait AR, et al. Pathogenesis of gastric particulate lung injury: a comparison and interaction with acidic pneumonitis. Anesth Analg 1993; 77:754–760.
188. Sukumaran M, Granada MJ, Berger HW, et al. Evaluation of corticosteroid treatment in aspiration of gastric contents: a controlled clinical trial. Mt Sinai J Med 1980; 47:335–340.
189. Wolfe JE, Bone RC, Ruth WE. Effects of corticosteroids in the treatment of patients with gastric aspiration. Am J Med 1977; 63:719–722.
190. Marik PE. Aspiration pneumonitis and aspiration pneumonia. N Engl J Med 2001; 344:665–671.
191. Cahill BC, Ingbar DH. Massive hemoptysis. Assessment and management. Clin Chest Med 1994; 15: 147–167.
192. Lordan JL, Gascoigne A, Corris PA. The pulmonary physician in critical care* Illustrative case 7: assessment and management of massive haemoptysis. Thorax 2003; 58:814–819.
193. Cahill BC, Ingbar DH. Massive hemoptysis. Clin Chest Med 1994; 15:147–168.
194. Miller R, McGregor D. Hemorrhage from carcinoma of the lung. Cancer 1980; 46:200–205.
195. Freitag L. Development of a new balloon catheter for management of hemoptysis with bronchofiberscopes. Chest 1993; 103:593.
196. Dweik R, Mehta A. Bronchoscopic, management of malignant airway disease. Clin Pul Med 1996; 3:43–51.
197. Wong LT, Lillquist YP, Culham G, et al. Treatment of recurrent hemoptysis in a child with cystic fibrosis by repeated bronchial artery embolizations and long-term tranexamic acid. Pediatr Pulmonol 1996; 22:275–279.
198. Haselton DJ, Klekamp J, Christman B. Use of high-dose corticosteroids and high-frequency oscillatory ventilation for treatment of a child with diffuse alveolar hemorrhage after bone marrow transplantation: case report of the literature. Crit Care Med 2000; 28:245–248.
199. Rumbak M, Kohler G, Eastrige C. Topical treatment of life threatening haemoptysis from aspergillomas. Thorax 1996; 51(3):253–255.
200. Colt H. Laser bronchoscopy. Chest Surg Clin N Am 1996; 6:277–291.
201. Morice R, Ece T, Ece F, et al. Endobronichial argon plasma coagulation for treatment of hemoptysis and neoplastic airway obstruction. Chest 2001; 119:781–787.
202. Stoller J. Diagnosis and management of massive hemoptysis: A review. Respir Care 1992; 37:564–581.
203. Tanaka N, Yamakado K, Murashima S, et al. Superselective bronchial artery embolization for hemoptysis with a coaxial microcatheter system. J Vasc Interv Radiol 1997; 8:65–70.
204. Brinson G, Noone P, Mauro M, et al. Bronchial artery embolization for the treatment of hemoptysis in patients with cystic fibrosis. Am J Respir Crit Care Med 1998; 157:1951–1958.

205. Osaki S, Nakanishi Y, Wataya H, et al. Prognosis of bronchial artery embolization in the management of hemoptysis. Respiration 2000; 67:412–416.
206. Shneerson JM, Emerson PA, Phillips RH. Radiotherapy for massive haemoptysis from an aspergilloma. Thorax 1980; 35:953–954.
207. Kay PH. Surgical management of pulmonary aspergilloma. Thorax 1997; 52:753–754.
208. Knott-Craig CJ, Oostuizen JG, Rossouw G, et al. Management and prognosis of massive hemoptysis. Recent experience with 120 patients. J Thorac Cardiovasc Surg 1993; 105:394–397.
209. Afessa B, Tefferi A, Litzow MR, et al. Outcome of diffuse alveolar hemorrhage in hematopoietic stem cell transplant recipients. Am J Respir Crit Care Med 2002; 166:1364–1368.
210. Lewis ID, DeFor T, Weisdorf DJ. Increasing incidence of diffuse alveolar hemorrhage following allogeneic bone marrow transplantation: cryptic etiology and uncertain therapy. Bone Marrow Transplant 2000; 26:539–543.
211. Robbins RA, Linder J, Stahl MG, et al. Diffuse alveolar hemorrhage in autologous bone marrow transplant recipients. Am J Med 1989; 87:511–518.
212. Afessa B, Tefferi A, Litzow MR, et al. Diffuse alveolar hemorrhage in hematopoietic stem cell transplant recipients. Am J Respir Crit Care Med 2002; 166: 641–645.
213. Cooke KR, Kobzik L, Martin TR, et al. An experimental model of idiopathic pneumonia syndrome after bone marrow transplantation: I. The roles of minor H antigens and endotoxin. Blood 1996; 88:3230–3239.
214. Sisson J, Thompson A, Anderson J. Airway inflammation predicts diffuse alveolar hemorrhage during bone marrow transplantation in patients with Hodgkin disease. Am Rev Respir Dis 1992; 146:439–443.
215. Metcalf J, Rennard S, Reed E, et al. Corticosteroids as adjunctive therapy for diffuse alveolar hemorrhage associated with bone marrow transplatnation: University of Nebraska Medical Center Bone Marrow Transplant Group. Am J Med 1994; 96:327–334.
216. Hicks K, Peng D, Gajewski JL. Treatment of diffuse alveolar hemorrhage after allogeneic bone marrow transplant with recombinant factor VIIa. Bone Marrow Transplant 2002; 30:975–978.
217. Pastores SM, Papadopoulos E, Voigt L, et al. Diffuse alveolar hemorrhage after allogenieic stem-cell transplantation: treatment with recombinant factor VIIa. Chest 2003; 124:2400–2403.
218. Ben-Abraham R, Paret G, Cohen R, et al. Diffuse alveolar hemorrhage following allogeneic bone marrow transplantation in children. Chest 2003; 124: 660–664.
219. Clark JG, Hansen JA, Hertz MI. Idiopathic pneumonia syndrome after bone marrow transplantation. Am Rev Respir Dis 1993; 147:1601–1601.
220. Shankar G, Cohen DA. Idiopathic pneumonia syndrome after bone marrow transplantation: the role of pre-transplant radiation conditioning and local cytokine dysregulation in promoting lung inflammation and fibrosis. Int J Exp Pathol 2001; 82:101–113.
221. Clark J, Madtes D, Martin T. Idiopathic pneumonia after bone marrow transplantation: cytokine activation and lipopolysaccharide amplification in the bronchoalveolar compartment. Crit Care Med 1999; 27: 1800–1806.
222. Catane R, Schwade J, Turrisi A. Pulmonary toxicity after radiation and bleomycin: A review. Int J Radiat Oncol Biol Phys 1979; 5:1513–1528.
223. Samuels M, Johnson D, Holoye P. Large-dose bleomycin therapy and pulmonary toxicity: A possible role of prior radiotherapy. JAMA 1976; 235:1117–1120.
224. White D. New chemotherapy-induced pulmonary syndromes. Pulm Perspect 1995; 12:4–5.
225. Parish JM, Muhm JR, Leslie KO. Upper lobe pulmonary fibrosis associated with high-dose chemotherapy containing BCNU for bone marrow transplantation. Mayo Clin Proc 2003; 78:630–634.
226. Willenbacher W, Mumm A, Bartsch HH. Late pulmonary toxicity of bleomycin. J Clin Oncol 1998; 16:3205.
227. Hasleton PS, O'Driscoll BR, Lynch P, et al. Late BCNU lung: a light and ultrastructural study on the delayed effect of BCNU on the lung parenchyma. J Pathol 1991; 164:31–36.
228. Kreisman H, Wolkove N. Pulmonary toxicity of antineoplastic therapy. Semin Oncol 1992; 19:508–520.
229. Rubio C, Hill M, O'Brien M, et al. Idiopathic pneumonia syndrome after high-dose chemotherapy for relapsed Hodgkin's disease. Br J Cancer 1997.
230. Oliner H, Schwartz R, Rubio F. Interstitial pulmonary fibrosis following busulfan therapy. Am J Med 1961; 31:134–139.
231. Carr M. Chlorambucil induced pulmonary fibrosis: report of a case and review. Va Med Q 1986; 113: 667–680.
232. Goucher G, Rowland V, Hawkins J. Melphalan-induced pulmonary interstitial fibrosis. Chest 1980; 77:805–806.
233. Sostman H, Matthay R, Putnam C. Cytotoxic drug-induced lung disease. Am J Med 1977; 62:371–388.
234. Massin F. Busulfan-induced pneumopathy. Rev Mal Respir 1987; 3:3–10.
235. Ginsberg S, Comis R. The pulmonary toxicity of antineoplastic agents. Semin Oncol 1982; 9:34–51.
236. Brockstein BE, Smiley C, Al-Sadir J, et al. Cardiac and pulmonary toxicity in patients undergoing high-dose chemotherapy for lymphoma and breast cancer: prognostic factors. Bone Marrow Transplant 2000; 25:885–894.
237. Massin F, Fur A, Reybet-Degat O, et al. [Busulfan-induced pneumopathy]. Rev Mal Respir 1987; 4:3–10.
238. Burns W, McFarland W, Matthews M. Busulfan-induced pulmonary disease: Report of a case and review of the literature. Am Rev Respir Dis 1970; 101:408–413.

239. Maxwell I. Letter: Reversible pulmonary edema following cyclophosphamide treatment. JAMA 1974; 229:137–138.
240. Cooper JA Jr, Matthay RA. Drug-induced pulmonary disease. Dis Mon 1987; 33:61–120.
241. Cooper JA, White D, Matthay R. Drug-induced pulmonary disease. Part 1 Cytotoxic drugs. Adv Intern Med 1986; 42:231–268.
242. Blum R, Carter S, Agre K. A clinical review of bleomycin: a new antineoplastic agent. Cancer 1973:904–913.
243. Cooper J, White D, Matthay R. State of the art: Drug-induced pulmonary disease. Am Rev Respir Dis 1986; 133:321–340.
244. Einhorn L, Krause M, Hornback N, et al. Enhanced pulmonary toxicity with bleomycin and radiotherapy in oat cell lung cancer. Cancer 1976; 37:2414–2416.
245. Nygaard K, Smith-Erichsen N, Hatlevoll R, et al. Pulmonary complications after bleomycin, irradiation and surgery for esophageal cancer. Cancer 1978; 41:17–22.
246. Sleijfer S. Bleomycin-induced pneumonitis. Chest 2001; 120:617–624.
247. Comis RL. Bleomycin pulmonary toxicity: current status and future directions. Semin Oncol 1992; 19: 64–70.
248. Parvinen L, Kilkku P, Makinen E. Factors affecting the pulmonary toxicity of bleomycin. Acta Radiol 1983; 22:417–421.
249. Simpson AB, Paul J, Graham J, et al. Fatal bleomycin pulmonary toxicity in the west of Scotland 1991–95: a review of patients with germ cell tumours. Br J Cancer 1998; 78:1061–1066.
250. Chisholm RA, Dixon AK, Williams MV, et al. Bleomycin lung: the effect of different chemotherapeutic regimens. Cancer Chemother Pharmacol 1992; 30:158–160.
251. O'Sullivan JM, Huddart RA, Norman AR, et al. Predicting the risk of bleomycin lung toxicity in patients with germ-cell tumours. Ann Oncol 2003; 14:91–96.
252. Perry DJ, Weiss RB, Taylor HG. Enhanced bleomycin toxicity during acute renal failure. Cancer Treat Rep 1982; 66:592–593.
253. McLeod BF, Lawrence HJ, Smith DW, et al. Fatal bleomycin toxicity from a low cumulative dose in a patient with renal insufficiency. Cancer 1987; 60: 2617–2620.
254. Bennett WM, Pastore L, Houghton DC. Fatal pulmonary bleomycin toxicity in cisplatin-induced acute renal failure. Cancer Treat Rep 1980; 64:921–924.
255. Bauer K, Skarin A, Balikian J. Pulmonary complications associated with combination chemotherapy programs containing bleomycin. Am J Med 1983; 74: 557–563.
256. Goldiner P, Rooney S. In defense of restricting oxygen in bleomycin-treated surgical patients. Anesthesiolgy 1984; 61:225–227.
257. Mathes DD. Bleomycin and Hyperoxia Exposure in the Operating room. Anesthesia Analgesia 1995; 8: 624–629.
258. Donat SM, Levy DA. Bleomycin associated pulmonary toxicity: is perioperative oxygen restriction necessary? J Urol 1998; 160:1347–1352.
259. Goldiner PL, Schweizer O. The hazards of anesthesia and surgery in bleomycin-treated patients. Semin Oncol 1979; 6:121–124.
260. Zitnick R. Drug-induced lung disease: cancer chemotherapy agents. Respir Dis 1995; 16:855–865.
261. Leeser J, Carr D. Fatal pneumothorax following bleomycin and other cytotoxic drugs. Cancer Treat Rep 1985; 69:344–345.
262. Doll D. Fatal pneumothorax associated with bleomycin-induced pulmonary fibrosis. Cancer Chemother Pharmacol 1986; 17:294–295.
263. Maher J, Daly PA. Severe bleomycin lung toxicity: reversal with high dose corticosteroids. Thorax 1993; 48:92–94.
264. Jensen JL, Goel R, Venner PM. The effect of corticosteroid administration on bleomycin lung toxicity. Cancer 1990; 65:1291–1297.
265. Castro M, Krowka M, Schroeder D. Frequency and clinical implications of increased pulmonarty artery pressures in liver transplant patients. Mayo Clin Proc 1996; 71:543–551.
266. Gundappa RK, Sud K, Kohli HS, et al. Mitomycin-C induced hemolytic uremic syndrome: a case report. Ren Fail 2002; 24:373–377.
267. Medina PJ, Sipols JM, George JN. Drug-associated thrombotic thrombocytopenic purpura-hemolytic uremic syndrome. Curr Opin Hematol 2001; 8:286–293.
268. Pisoni R, Ruggenenti P, Remuzzi G. Drug-induced thrombotic microangiopathy: incidence, prevention and management. Drug Saf 2001; 24:491–501.
269. Luedke D, McLaughlin T, Daughaday c. Mitomycin c and vindesine associated pulmonary toxicity with variable clinical expression. Cancer 1984; 55:542–545.
270. Cantrell J, Phillips T, Schein P. Carcinoma-associated hemolytic uremic syndrome: A complication of mitomycin C chemotherapy. J Clin Oncol 1985; 3:723–734.
271. Schiebe ME, Hoffmann W, Belka C, et al. Mitomycin C-related hemolytic uremic syndrome in cancer patients. Anticancer Drugs 1998; 9:433–435.
272. Sostman H, Matthay R, Putnam C. Methotrexate-induced pneumonitis. Medicine 1976; 55:371–388.
273. Imokawa S, Colby TV, Leslie KO, et al. Methotrexate pneumonitis: review of the literature and histopathological findings in nine patients. Eur Respir J 2000; 15: 373–381.
274. Wall M, Wohl M, Jaffe N. Lung function in adolescents receiving high dose methotrexate. Pediatrics 1979; 63:741–746.
275. White R, McCurdy S, von Marensdorff H. Home prothrombin time monitoring after the initiation of warfarin therapy: a randomized, prospective study. Ann Intern Med 1989; 111:730–737.
276. Anderson L, Collins G, Ojima Y. A study of the distribution of methotrexate in human tissues and

tumours. Pulm Complications Cancer Therapy 1970; May 30(5):1344–1348.
277. Anaissie E, Kontoyionnis D, OBrien S. Infections in patients with chronic lymphocytic leukemia treated with fludarabine. Ann Inter Med 1998; 129:559–566.
278. Andersson B, Cogan B, Keating M. Subacute pulmonary failure complicating therapy with high-dose ara-C in acute leukemia. Cancer 1985; 56:2181–2184.
279. Jehn U, Goldel N, Rienmuller R. Non-cardiogenic pulmonary edema complicating intermediate and high-dose Ara C treatment for relapsed acute leukemia. Med Oncol Tumor Pharmacother 1988; 5:41–47.
280. McCarthy A, Pincher L, Hann I. FLAG (Fludarabine, high-dose cytarabine, and G- CSF) for refractory and high-risk relapsed acute leukemia in children. Med Ped Oncol 1995; 32:411–415.
281. Montillo M, Mirto S, Petti M. Fludarabine, cytarabine, and G-CSF (FLAG) for the treatment of poor risk acute myeloid leukemia. Am J Hematol 1998; 58:105–109.
282. Helman DL Jr, Byrd JC, Ales NC, et al. Fludarabine-related pulmonary toxicity: a distinct clinical entity in chronic lymphoproliferative syndromes. Chest 2002; 122:785–790.
283. Salvucci M, Zanchini R, Molinari A, et al. Lung toxicity following fludarabine, cytosine arabinoside and mitoxantrone (flan) treatment for acute leukemia. Haematologica 2000; 85:769–770.
284. Hurst PG, Habib MP, Garewal H, et al. Pulmonary toxicity associated with fludarabine monophosphate. Invest New Drugs 1987; 5:207–210.
285. Stoica GS, Greenberg HE, Rossoff LJ. Corticosteroid responsive fludarabine pulmonary toxicity. Am J Clin Oncol 2002; 25:340–341.
286. Bedrossian CW, Sussman J, Conklin RH, et al. Azathioprine-associated interstitial pneumonitis. Am J Clin Pathol 1984; 82:148–154.
287. Sinico RA, Sabadini E, Borlandelli S, et al. Azathioprine hypersensitivity: report of two cases and review of the literature. J Nephrol 2003; 16:272–276.
288. Fields CL, Robinson JW, Roy TM, et al. Hypersensitivity reaction to azathioprine. South Med J 1998; 91: 471–474.
289. Stetter M, Schmidl M, Krapf R. Azathioprine hypersensitivity mimicking Goodpasture's syndrome. Am J Kidney Dis 1994; 23:874–877.
290. Refabert L, Sinnassamy P, Leroy B, et al. Azathioprine-induced pulmonary haemorrhage in a child after renal transplantation. Pediatr Nephrol 1995; 9: 470–473.
291. Jungling A, Shangraw R. Massive airway edema after azathioprine. Anesthesiology 2000; 92:888–890.
292. Barlesi F, Villani P, Doddoli C, et al. Gemcitabine-induced severe pulmonary toxicity. Fundam Clin Pharmacol 2004; 18:85–91.
293. Le Chevalier T, Gottfreid M, Gatzmeier U, et al. A phase II multicenter study of gemcitabine in non-small cell lung cancers. Bull Cancer 1997; 84:282–288.
294. Crino L, Mosconi A, Scagliotti G, et al. Gemcitabine as second-line treatment for relapsing or refractory advanced non-small cell lung cancer: a phase II trial. Semin Oncol 1998; 25:23–26.
295. Maas KW, van der Lee I, Bolt K, et al. Lung function changes and pulmonary complications in patients with stage III non-small cell lung cancer treated with gemcitabine/cisplatin as part of combined modality treatment. Lung Cancer 2003; 41:345–351.
296. Sauer-Heilborn A, Kath R, Schneider CP, et al. Severe non-haematological toxicity after treatment with gemcitabine. J Cancer Res Clin Oncol 1999; 125:637–640.
297. Durant J, Norgard M, Murad TM, et al. Pulmonary toxicity associated with bischoloroethylnitrosourea (BCNU). Ann Intern Med 1979; 90:191–194.
298. Aronin PA, Mahaley MS Jr, Rudnick SA, et al. Prediction of BCNU pulmonary toxicity in patients with malignant gliomas: an assessment of risk factors. N Engl J Med 1980; 303:183–188.
299. Wang H, Yang H, Czura CJ, et al. HMGB1 as a late mediator of lethal systemic inflammation. Am J Respir Crit Care Med 2001; 164:1768–1773.
300. Merad M, Le Cesne A, Baldeyrou P, et al. Docetaxel and interstitial pulmonary injury. Ann Oncol 1997; 8: 191–194.
301. Markman M. Management of toxicities associated with the administration of taxanes. Expert Opin Drug Saf 2003; 2:141–146.
302. Rowinsky E, Donehower R. The clinical pharmacology of paclitaxel. Semin Oncol 1993; 3:16–25.
303. Micha JP, Rettenmaier MA, Dillman R, et al. Single-dose dexamethasone paclitaxel premedication. Gynecol Oncol 1998; 69:122–124.
304. Peereboom DM, Donehower RC, Eisenhauer EA, et al. Successful re-treatment with taxol after major hypersensitivity reactions. J Clin Oncol 1993; 11:885–890.
305. Schweitzer VG, Juillard GJ, Bajada CL, et al. Radiation recall dermatitis and pneumonitis in a patient treated with paclitaxel. Cancer 1995; 76:1069–1072.
306. Fujimori K, Yokoyama A, Kurita Y, et al. Paclitaxel-induced cell-mediated hypersensitivity pneumonitis. Diagnosis using leukocyte migration test, bronchoalveolar lavage and transbronchial lung biopsy. Oncology 1998; 55:340–344.
307. Taghian AG, Assaad SI, Niemierko A, et al. Risk of pneumonitis in breast cancer patients treated with radiation therapy and combination chemotherapy with paclitaxel. J Natl Cancer Inst 2001; 93:1806–1811.
308. Dunsford ML, Mead GM, Bateman AC, et al. Severe pulmonary toxicity in patients treated with a combination of docetaxel and gemcitabine for metastatic transitional cell carcinoma. Ann Oncol 1999; 10: 943–947.
309. Mileshkin L, Prince HM, Rischin D, et al. Severe interstitial pneumonitis following high-dose cyclophosphamide, thiotepa and docetaxel: two case reports and a review of the literature. Bone Marrow Transplant 2001; 27:559–563.

310. Wang GS, Yang KY, Perng RP. Life-threatening hypersensitivity pneumonitis induced by docetaxel (taxotere). Br J Cancer 2001; 85:1247–1250.
311. Muller HJ, Beier R, Loning L, et al. Pharmacokinetics of native *Escherichia coli* asparaginase (Asparaginase medac) and hypersensitivity reactions in ALL-BFM 95 reinduction treatment. Br J Haematol 2001; 114: 794–799.
312. Pitney W, Phadke K, Dean S. Antithrombin III deficiency during asparaginase therapy. Lancet 1980; 1: 493–494.
313. Mahmood T, Mudad R. Pulmonary toxicity secondary to procarbazine. Am J Clin Oncol 2002; 25:187–188.
314. Cuzic J, Forbes J, Edwards R. Firt results from the International Brezast Cancer Intervention Study (IBIS): a randomized prevention trial. Lancet 2002; 360:817–824.
315. Meier C, Jick H. Tamoxifen and risk of idiopathic venous thromboembolism. Br J Clin Pharmacol 1998; 45:608–612.
316. Pritchard J, Paterson A, Paul N. Increased thromboembolic complications with concurrent tamoxifen and themotherapy in a randomized trial of adjuvant therapy for women with breast cancer. National Cancer Institute of Canada Clinical Trials Group Breast Cancer Site Group. J Clin Oncol 1996; 14: 2731–2737.
317. Rogers JI, Murgo A, Fontana J, et al. Chemotherapy for breast cancer decreased plasma protein C and protein S. J Clin Oncol 1988; 6:276–281.
318. Lipton A, Harvey H, Hamilton R. Venous thrombosis as a side effect of tamoxifen treatment. Cancer Treat Rep 1984:887–889.
319. Frankel S, Eardley A, Lauwers G. The "retinoic acid syndrome" in acute promyelocytic leukemia. Ann Intern Med 1992; 117:292–296.
320. Tallman M, Andersoen J, Schiffer C. Clinical description of 44 patients with acute promyelocytic leukemia who developed the retinoic acid syndrome. Blood 2000; 95:90.
321. Wiley J, Firkin F. Reduction of pulmonary toxicity by prednisone prophylaxis during all-trans-retinoic acid treatment of acute promyelocytic leukemia. Leukemia 1995; 9:774–778.
322. Hastings RC, Trautman JR, Enna CD, et al. Thalidomide in the treatment of erythema nodosum leprosum. With a note on selected laboratory abnormalities in erythema nodosum leprosum. Clin Pharmacol Ther 1970; 11:481–487.
323. Alexanian R, Weber D. Recent advances in treatment of multiple myeloma and Waldenstrom's macroglobulinemia. Biomed Pharmacother 2001; 55:550–552.
324. Blade J, Rosinol L, Esteve J, et al. Thalidomide: a step forward in the treatment of malignant monoclonal gammopathies. Clin Lymphoma 2003; 3:247–248.
325. Zorat F, Shetty V, Dutt D, et al. The clinical and biological effects of thalidomide in patients with myelodysplastic syndromes. Br J Haematol 2001; 115: 881–894.
326. Barosi G, Grossi A, Comotti B, et al. Safety and efficacy of thalidomide in patients with myelofibrosis with myeloid metaplasia. Br J Haematol 2001; 114:78–83.
327. Steins MB, Padro T, Bieker R, et al. Efficacy and safety of thalidomide in patients with acute myeloid leukemia. Blood 2002; 99:834–839.
328. Motzer RJ, Berg W, Ginsberg M, et al. Phase II trial of thalidomide for patients with advanced renal cell carcinoma. J Clin Oncol 2002; 20:302–306.
329. Arora M, Wagner JE, Davies SM, et al. Randomized clinical trial of thalidomide, cyclosporine, and prednisone versus cyclosporine and prednisone as initial therapy for chronic graft-versus-host disease. Biol Blood Marrow Transplant 2001; 7:265–273.
330. Vogelsang GB. Acute and chronic graft-versus-host disease. Curr Opin Oncol 1993; 5:276–281.
331. Zangari M, Anaissie E, Barlogie B, et al. Increased risk of deep-vein thrombosis in patients with multiple myeloma receiving thalidomide and chemotherapy. Blood 2001; 98:1614–1615.
332. Camba L, Peccatori J, Pescarollo A, et al. Thalidomide and thrombosis in patients with multiple myeloma. Haematologica 2001; 86:1108–1109.
333. Osman K, Comenzo R, Rajkumar SV. Deep venous thrombosis and thalidomide therapy for multiple myeloma. N Engl J Med 2001; 344:1951–1952.
334. Fine HA, Wen PY, Maher EA, et al. Phase II trial of thalidomide and carmustine for patients with recurrent high-grade gliomas. J Clin Oncol 2003; 21:2299–2304.
335. Zangari M, Siegel E, Barlogie B, et al. Thrombogenic activity of doxorubicin in myeloma patients receiving thalidomide: implications for therapy. Blood 2002; 100:1168–1171.
336. Hudson MM, Weinstein HJ, Donaldson SS, et al. Acute hypersensitivity reactions to etoposide in a VEPA regimen for Hodgkin's disease. J Clin Oncol 1993; 11:1080–1084.
337. Szebeni J, Alving CR, Savay S, et al. Complement activation-related pseudoallergy caused by liposomes, micellar carriers of intravenous drugs, and radiocontrast agents. Crit Rev Ther Drug Carrier Syst 2001; 18:567–606.
338. Kellie S, Crist W, Pui C, et al. Cancer 1991:1070–1075.
339. Loetze M, Matory Y, Raynor A, et al. Clinical effects and toxicity of interleukin-2 in patients with cancer. Cancer 1986; 58:2764–2772.
340. Margolin KA. Interleukin-2 in the treatment of renal cancer. Semin Oncol 2000; 27:194–203.
341. Lee R, Lotze M, Skibber E, et al. Interleukin-2 administration causes reversible hemodynamic changes and left ventricular dysfunction similar to those seen in septic shock. Chest 1989; 94:750–754.
342. Lee RE, Lotze MT, Skibber JM, et al. Cardiorespiratory effects of immunotherapy with interleukin-2. J Clin Oncol 1989; 7:7–20.

343. Macdonald D, Gordon AA, Kajitani H, et al. Interleukin-2 treatment-associated eosinophilia is mediated by interleukin-5 production. Br J Haematol 1990; 76: 168–173.
344. Ayars G, Altman L, Gleich G, et al. Eosinophil and eosinophil granule-mediated pneumocyte injury. J Allergy Clin Immunol 1985; 76:595–604.
345. O'Hearn DJ, Leiferman KM, Askin F, et al. Pulmonary infiltrates after cytokine therapy for stem cell transplantation. Massive deposition of eosinophil major basic protein detected by immunohistochemistry. Am J Respir Crit Care Med 1999; 160:1361–1365.
346. Aderka D. The potential biological and clinical significance of the soluble tumor necrosis factor receptors. Cytokine Growth Factor Rev 1996; 7:231–240.
347. Beutler B, Cerami A. The common mediator of shock, cachexia, and tumor necrosis. Adv Immunol 1988; 42:213–231.
348. Lejeune FJ. Clinical use of TNF revisited: improving penetration of anti-cancer agents by increasing vascular permeability. J Clin Invest 2002; 110:433–435.
349. Lejeune FJ, Ruegg C, Lienard D. Clinical applications of TNF-alpha in cancer. Curr Opin Immunol 1998; 10:573–580.
350. Feldman ER, Creagan ET, Schaid DJ, et al. Phase II trial of recombinant tumor necrosis factor in disseminated malignant melanoma. Am J Clin Oncol 1992; 15:256–259.
351. Curnis F, Sacchi A, Corti A. Improving chemotherapeutic drug penetration in tumors by vascular targeting and barrier alteration. J Clin Invest 2002; 110: 475–482.
352. Tracey KJ, Cerami A. Tumor necrosis factor: a pleiotropic cytokine and therapeutic target. Annu Rev Med 1994; 45:491–503.
353. Villani F, Galimberti M, Mazzola G, et al. Pulmonary toxicity of alpha tumor necrosis factor in patients treated by isolation perfusion. J Chemother 1995; 7: 452–454.
354. Schilling PJ, Murray JL, Markowitz AB. Novel tumor necrosis factor toxic effects. Pulmonary hemorrhage and severe hepatic dysfunction. Cancer 1992; 69: 256–260.
355. Markham A, Lamb HM. Infliximab: a review of its use in the management of rheumatoid arthritis. Drugs 2000; 59:1341–1359.
356. Lang KA, Peppercorn MA. Promising new agents for the treatment of inflammatory bowel disorders. Drugs R D 1999; 1:237–244.
357. Couriel D, Hicks K, Ippoliti C. Infliximab for the treatment of graft-versus host disease in allogeneic transplant recipients. Proc Am Soc Clin Oncol 2000; 19:52a.
358. Keane J, Gershon S, Wise RP, et al. Tuberculosis associated with infliximab, a tumor necrosis factor alpha-neutralizing agent. N Engl J Med 2001; 345: 1098–1104.
359. Lim WS, Powell RJ, Johnston ID. Tubcrculosis and treatment with infliximab. N Engl J Med 2002; 346: 623–626.
360. Warris A, Bjorneklett A, Gaustad P. Invasive pulmonary aspergillosis associated with infliximab therapy. N Engl J Med 2001; 344:1099–1100.
361. Ogata K, Koga T, Yagawa K. Interferon-related bronchiolitis obliterans organizing pneumonia. Chest 1994; 106:612–613.
362. Kamisako T, Adachi Y, Chihara J, et al. Interstitial pneumonitis and interferon-alfa. Br Med J 1993; 306:896.
363. Fruehauf S, Steiger S, Topaly J, et al. Pulmonary artery hypertension during interferon-alpha therapy for chronic myelogenous leukemia. Ann Hematol 2001; 80:308–310.
364. Antoniou KM, Ferdoutsis E, Bouros D. Interferons and their application in the diseases of the lung. Chest 2003; 123:209–216.
365. Ravenel JG, McAdams HP, Plankeel JF, et al. Sarcoidosis induced by interferon therapy. AJR Am J Roentgenol 2001; 177:199–201.
366. Pietropaoli A, Modrak J, Utell M. Interferon-alpha therapy associated with the development of sarcoidosis. Chest 1999; 116:569–572.
367. Inoue A, Saijo Y, Maemondo M, et al. Severe acute interstitial pneumonia and gefitinib. Lancet 2003; 361:137–139.
368. Kris MG, Natale RB, Herbst RS, et al. Efficacy of gefitinib, an inhibitor of the epidermal growth factor receptor tyrosine kinase, in symptomatic patients with non-small cell lung cancer: a randomized trial. Jama 2003; 290:2149–2158.
369. Bergeron A, Bergot E, Vilela G, et al. Hypersensitivity pneumonitis related to imatinib mesylate. J Clin Oncol 2002; 20:4271–4272.
370. Druker BJ, Sawyers CL, Capdeville R, et al. Chronic myelogenous leukemia. Hematology (Am Soc Hematol Educ Program) 2001:87–112.
371. Gertz MA, Lacy MQ, Bjornsson J, et al. Fatal pulmonary toxicity related to the administration of granulocyte colony-stimulating factor in amyloidosis: a report and review of growth factor-induced pulmonary toxicity. J Hematother Stem Cell Res 2000; 9:635–643.
372. Couderc LJ, Stelianides S, Frachon I, et al. Pulmonary toxicity of chemotherapy and G/GM-CSF: a report of five cases. Respir Med 1999; 93:65–68.
373. Nakamura M, Sakemi T, Fujisaki T, et al. Sudden death or refractory pleural effusion following treatment with granulocyte colony-stimulating factor in two hemodialysis patients. Nephron 1999; 83: 178–179.
374. Goodman ER, Stricker P, Velavicius M, et al. Role of granulocyte-macrophage colony-stimulating factor and its receptor in the genesis of acute respiratory distress syndrome through an effect on neutrophil apoptosis. Arch Surg 1999; 134:1049–1054.

375. Ruiz-Arguelles GJ, Arizpe-Bravo D, Sanchez-Sosa S, et al. Fatal G-CSF-induced pulmonary toxicity. Am J Hematol 1999; 60:82–83.
376. Blum K, Bartlett N. Antibodies for the treatment of diffuse large cell lymphoma. Semin Oncol 2003; 30: 448–456.
377. Burton C, Kaczmarski R, Jan-Mohamed R. Interstitial pneumonitis related to rituximab therapy. N Engl J Med 2003; 348:2690–2691; discussion 2690–2691.
378. Tarella C, Ladetto M, Magni M. Rituximab-supplemented high dose chemotherapy with autografting in high risk B-diffuse large cell lymphoma: a multicenter, prospective study lof GITIL (Gruppo Italiano Terapie Inovative nei Linformi). Blood 2002; 100(suppl 2541): 2546.
379. Horwitz S, Negrin R, Stockerl-Goldstein K. Phase II trial of rituximab as adjuvant therapy to high dose chemotherapy and peripheral blood stem cell transplantation for relapsed and refractory aggressive non-Hodgkin's lymphoma. Blood 2001; 98(suppl 3671):3678.
380. Benelki M, Shafi F, Qureshi A. The effect of rituximab on peripheral blood stem cell mobilization in non-Hodgkin's lymphoma. Proc Am Soc Clin Oncol 2002; 21:1666.
381. Baselga J. Multinational studies of Herceptin (humanized anti-HER2 antibody) in HER2+ metastiatic breast cancer: phase III of Herceptin plus chemotherapy (CRx) vs. CRx alone in first-time and large phase II of Herceptin alone in advanced disease. Ann Ocol 1998; 9:47.
382. Kramer M, Estenne M, Berkman N, et al. Radiation-induced pulmonary veno-occlusive disease. Chest 1993; 104(4):1282–1284.
383. Arbetter KR, Prakash UB, Tazelaar HD, et al. Radiation-induced pneumonitis in the "nonirradiated" lung. Mayo Clin Proc 1999; 74:27–36.
384. Graham MV, Purdy JA, Emami B, et al. Clinical dose-volume histogram analysis for pneumonitis after 3D treatment for non-small cell lung cancer (NSCLC). Int J Radiat Oncol Biol Phys 1999; 45:323–329.
385. Abid SH, Malhotra V, Perry MC. Radiation-induced and chemotherapy-induced pulmonary injury. Curr Opin Oncol 2001; 13:242–248.
386. Libshitz HI. Radiation changes in the lung. Semin Roentgenol 1993; 28:303–320.
387. Jeter MD, Janne PA, Brooks S, et al. Gemcitabine-induced radiation recall. Int J Radiat Oncol Biol Phys 2002; 53:394–400.
388. D'Angio GJ, Farber S, Maddock CL. Potentiation of x-ray effects by actinomycin D. Radiology 1959; 73: 175–177.
389. Inoue A, Kunitoh H, Sekine I, et al. Radiation pneumonitis in lung cancer patients: a retrospective study of risk factors and the long-term prognosis. Int J Radiat Oncol Biol Phys 2001; 49:649–655.
390. Heit JA, Silverstein MD, Mohr DN, et al. Risk factors for deep vein thrombosis and pulmonary embolism: a population-based case–control study. Arch Intern Med 2000; 160:809–815.
391. Silverstein MD, Heit JA, Mohr DN, et al. Trends in the incidence of deep vein thrombosis and pulmonary embolism: a 25-year population-based study. Arch Intern Med 1998; 158:585–593.
392. Baron JA, Gridley G, Weiderpass E, et al. Venous thromboembolism and cancer. Lancet 1998; 351: 1077–1080.
393. Loreto MF, De Martinis M, Corsi MP, et al. Coagulation and cancer: implications for diagnosis and management. Pathol Oncol Res 2000; 6:301–312.
394. Rickles FR, Levine MN. Epidemiology of thrombosis in cancer. Acta Haematol 2001; 106:6–12.
395. Prandoni P, Lensing A, Buller H. Deep-vein thrombosis and the incidence of subsequent symptomatic cancer. N Engl J Med 1992; 327:1128–1133.
396. Prandoni P, Piccioli A, Pagnan A. Recurrent thromboembolism in cancer patients: incidence and risk factors. Semin Thromb Hemost 2003; 29:3–8.
397. Rocha AT, Tapson VF. Venous thromboembolism in intensive care patients. Clin Chest Med 2003; 24: 103–122.
398. Mandala M, Ferretti G, Cremonesi M, et al. Venous thromboembolism and cancer: new issues for an old topic. Crit Rev Oncol Hematol 2003; 48:65–80.
399. Schafer AI, Levine MN, Konkle BA, et al. Thrombotic disorders: diagnosis and treatment. Hematology (Am Soc Hematol Educ Program) 2003:520–539.
400. Han D, Lee KS, Franquet T, et al. Thrombotic and nonthrombotic pulmonary arterial embolism: spectrum of imaging findings. Radiographics 2003; 23: 1521–1539.
401. Zangari M, Barlogie B, Thertulien R, et al. Thalidomide and deep vein thrombosis in multiple myeloma: risk factors and effect on survival. Clin Lymphoma 2003; 4:32–35.
402. Lee AY. The role of low-molecular-weight heparins in the prevention and treatment of venous thromboembolism in cancer patients. Curr Opin Pulm Med 2003; 9:351–355.
403. Lee AY, Levine MN. Venous thromboembolism and cancer: risks and outcomes. Circulation 2003; 107: I17–I21.
404. Levine MN, Lee AY, Kakkar AK. From Trousseau to targeted therapy: new insights and innovations in thrombosis and cancer. J Thromb Haemost 2003; 1: 1456–1463.
405. Lee AY. Epidemiology and management of venous thromboembolism in patients with cancer. Thromb Res 2003; 110:167–172.
406. Sorensen HT, Mellemkjaer L, Olsen JH, et al. Prognosis of cancers associated with venous thromboembolism. N Engl J Med 2000; 343:1846–1850.

407. Levine MN. Management of thromboembolic disease in cancer patients. Haemostasis 2001; 31:68–69.
408. Thodiyil PA, Kakkar AK. Variation in relative risk of venous thromboembolism in different cancers. Thromb Haemost 2002; 87:1076–1077.
409. Bick RL. Alterations of hemostasis associated with malignancy: etiology, pathophysiology, diagnosis and management. Semin Thromb Hemost 1978; 5:1–26.
410. Levine M, Gent M, Hirsh J, et al. A comparison of low-molecular-weight heparin administered primarily at home with unfractionated heparin administered in the hospital for proximal deep-vein thrombosis. N Engl J Med 1996; 334:677–681.
411. Levitan N, Dowlati A, Remick SC, et al. Rates of initial and recurrent thromboembolic disease among patients with malignancy versus those without malignancy. Risk analysis using Medicare claims data. Medicine (Baltimore) 1999; 78:285–291.
412. Griffin MR, Stanson AW, Brown ML, et al. Deep venous thrombosis and pulmonary embolism. Risk of subsequent malignant neoplasms. Arch Intern Med 1987; 147:1907–1911.
413. Green KB, Silverstein RL. Hypercoagulability in cancer. Hematol Oncol Clin North Am 1996; 10: 499–530.
414. Shah MK, Burke DT, Shah SH. Upper-extremity deep vein thrombosis. South Med J 2003; 96:669–672.
415. Bona RD. Thrombotic complications of central venous catheters in cancer patients. Semin Thromb Hemost 1999; 25:147–155.
416. Girolami A, Prandoni P, Zanon E, et al. Venous thromboses of upper limbs are more frequently associated with occult cancer as compared with those of lower limbs. Blood Coagul Fibrinolysis 1999; 10:455–457.
417. Wanscher B, Frifelt J, Silverstein-Smith C. Thrombosis caused by polyurethane double-lumen subclavian superior vena cava catheter and hemodialysis. Crit Care Med 1988; 16:624.
418. Rickles FR, Levine M, Edwards RL. Hemostatic alterations in cancer patients. Cancer Metastasis Rev 1992; 11:237–248.
419. Stein P, Saltzman H, Weg J. Clinical characteristics of patients with acute pulmonary embolism. Am J Cardiol 1991; 68:1723–1724.
420. Ferrari E, Imbert A, Chevalier T. The EKG in pulmonary embolism. Chest 1997; 111:537.
421. Stein P, Goldhaber S, Henry J. Alveolar-arterial oxygen gradient in the assessment of acute pulmonary embolism. Chest 1995; 107:139–143.
422. Investigators CSbtP. Value of the ventilation/perfuperfusion scan in acute pulmonary embolism—results of the prospective investigation of pulmonary embolism diagnosis. JAMA 1990; 263:2753–2759.
423. Kasper W, Konstantinides S, Geibel A. Prognostic significance of right ventricular afterload stress detected by echocardiography in patients with clinically suspected pulmonary embolism. Heart 1997; 77: 346–349.
424. Putnam J Jr, Light R, Rodriguez R, et al. A randomized comparison of indwelling pleural catheter and doxycycline pleurodesis in the management of malignant pleural effusions. Cancer 1999; 10;86:1992–1999.
425. De Monye W, Sanson BJ, Mac Gillavry MR, et al. Embolus location affects the sensitivity of a rapid quantitative D-dimer assay in the diagnosis of pulmonary embolism. Am J Respir Crit Care Med 2002; 165:345–348.
426. Stein PD, Terrin ML, Hales CA, et al. Clinical, laboratory, roentgenographic, and electrocardiographic findings in patients with acute pulmonary embolism and no pre-existing cardiac or pulmonary disease. Chest 1991; 100:598–603.
427. Remy-Jardin M, Remy J, Deschildre F, et al. Diagnosis of pulmonary embolism with spiral CT: comparison with pulmonary angiography and scintigraphy. Radiology 1996; 200:699–706.
428. Haas S. Prevention of venous thromboembolism: recommendations based on the International Consensus and the American College of Chest Physicians Sixth Consensus Conference on Antithrombotic Therapy. Clin Appl Thromb Hemost 2001; 7:171–177.
429. Blot E, Gutman F, Thannberger A. Dalteparin compared with an oral anticoagulant for thromboprophylaxis in patients with cancer. N Engl J Med 2003; 349:1385–1387. Author reply 1385–1387.
430. Thodiyil P, Kakkar AK. Can low-molecular-weight heparins improve outcome in patients with cancer? Cancer Treat Rev 2002; 28:151–155.
431. Lee AY, Levine MN, Baker RI, et al. Low-molecular-weight heparin versus a coumarin for the prevention of recurrent venous thromboembolism in patients with cancer. N Engl J Med 2003; 349:146–153.
432. Dellinger R, Zimmerman J, Taylor R, et al. Effects of inhaled nitric oxide in patients with acute respiratory distress syndrome: results of a randomized phase II trial. Inhaled Nitric Oxide in ARDS Study Group. Crit Care Med 1998; 26:15–23.
433. Li HL, Ye KH, Zhang HW, et al. Effect of heparin on apoptosis in human nasopharyngeal carcinoma CNE2 cells. Cell Res 2001; 11:311–315.
434. Norrby K. Heparin and angiogenesis: a low-molecular-weight fraction inhibits and a high-molecular-weight fraction stimulates angiogenesis systemically. Haemostasis 1993; 23:141–149.
435. Siragusa S, Cosmi B, Piovella F, et al. Low-molecular-weight heparins and unfractionated heparin in the treatment of patients with acute venous thromboembolism: results of a meta-analysis. Am J Med 1996; 100:269–277.
436. Gould MK, Dembitzer AD, Doyle RL, et al. Low-molecular-weight heparins compared with unfractionated heparin for treatment of acute deep venous thrombosis. A meta-analysis of randomized, controlled trials. Ann Intern Med 1999; 130:800–809.
437. Dolovich LR, Ginsberg JS, Douketis JD, et al. A meta-analysis comparing low-molecular-weight heparins

with unfractionated heparin in the treatment of venous thromboembolism: examining some unanswered questions regarding location of treatment, product type, and dosing frequency. Arch Intern Med 2000; 160: 181–188.
438. Breddin HK, Hach-Wunderle V, Nakov R, et al. Effects of a low-molecular-weight heparin on thrombus regression and recurrent thromboembolism in patients with deep-vein thrombosis. N Engl J Med 2001; 344:626–631.
439. Warkentin TE, Levine MN, Hirsh J, et al. Heparin-induced thrombocytopenia in patients treated with low-molecular-weight heparin or unfractionated heparin. N Engl J Med 1995; 332:1330–1335.
440. Schulman S, Staffan G, MD, Margareta G. The duration of oral anticoagulant therapy after a second episode of venous thromboembolism. N Engl J Med 1997; 336:393–398.
441. Konstantinides S. Thrombolysis in submassive pulmonary embolism? Yes. J Thromb Haemost 2003; 1: 1127–1129.
442. Konstantinides S, Geibel A, Heusel G, et al. Heparin plus alteplase compared with heparin alone in patients with submassive pulmonary embolism. N Engl J Med 2002; 347:1143–1150.
443. Liu P, Meneveau N, Schiele F, et al. Predictors of long-term clinical outcome of patients with acute massive pulmonary embolism after thrombolytic therapy. Chin Med J (Engl) 2003; 116:503–509.
444. Goldhaber S, Haire W, Feldstein M. Alteplase versus heparin in acute pulmonary embolism: randomized trial assessing right-ventricular function and pulmonary perfusion. Lancet 1993; 341:507–511.
445. Agnelli G, Becattini C, Kirschstein T. Thrombolysis vs heparin in the treatment of pulmonary embolism: a clinical outcome-based meta-analysis. Arch Intern Med 2002; 162:2537–2541.
446. Jerjes-Sanchez C. Streptokinase and heparin versus heparin alone in massive pulmonary embolism: a randomized controlled trial. J Thromb Thrombolysis 1995; 2:227–229.
447. Goldhaber S. Contemporary pulmonary embolism thrombolysis. Chest 1995; 107:51s.
448. Goldhaber SZ. Thrombolysis for pulmonary embolism. N Engl J Med 2002; 347:1131–1132.
449. Levine GN, Hochman JS. Thrombolysis in Acute Myocardial Infarction Complicated by Cardiogenic Shock. J Thromb Thrombolysis 1995; 2:11–20.
450. Dalen J, Joseph A, Hirsh J. Thrombolytic therapy for pulmonary embolism: Is it effective? Is it safe? When is it indicated? Arch Intern Med 1997; 157: 2550–2556.
451. Levine M. Thrombolytic therapy for venous thromboembolism. Clin Chest Med 1995; 16:321–328.
452. Savelyev V. Massive pulmonary embolism: embolectomy or thrombolysis. Int Angiol 1985; 4:137–140.
453. Goldhaber SZ, Dricker E, Buring JE, et al. Clinical suspicion of autopsy-proven thrombotic and tumor pulmonary embolism in cancer patients. Am Heart J 1987; 114:1432–1435.
454. Veinot JP, Ford SE, Price RG. Subacute cor pulmonale due to tumor embolization. Arch Pathol Lab Med 1992; 116:131–134.
455. Lester T, Johnson J, Cuttner J. Pulmonary leukostasis as the single worst prognostic factor in patients with acute myelocytic leukemia and hyerleukocytosis. Am J Med 1985; 79:43.
456. Wherrett CG, Mehran RJ, Beaulieu MA. Cerebral arterial gas embolism following diagnostic bronchoscopy: delayed treatment with hyperbaric oxygen. Can J Anaesth 2002; 49:96–99.
457. Bitterman H, Melamed Y. Delayed hyperbaric treatment of cerebral air embolism. Isr J Med Sci 1993; 29:22–26.
458. Lipton JH, Russell JA, Burgess KR, et al. Fat embolization and pulmonary infiltrates after bone marrow transplantation. Med Pediatr Oncol 1987; 15:24–27.
459. Hagley SR, Lee FC, Blumbergs PC. Fat embolism syndrome with total hip replacement. Med J Aust 1986; 145:541–543.
460. Bilgrami S, Hasson J, Tutschka PJ. Case 23–1998: fat embolism. N Engl J Med 1999; 340:393–394.
461. Bairaktari A, Raitsiou B, Kokolaki M, et al. Respiratory failure after pneumonectomy in a patient with unknown hyperlipidemia. Anesth Analg 2001; 93: 292–293, 292nd contents page.
462. Nijsten MW, Hamer JP, ten Duis HJ, et al. Fat embolism and patent foramen ovale. Lancet 1989; 1:1271.
463. Vedrinne JM, Guillaume C, Gagnieu MC, et al. Bronchoalveolar lavage in trauma patients for diagnosis of fat embolism syndrome. Chest 1992; 102: 1323–1327.
464. Chastre J, Fagon JY, Soler P, et al. Bronchoalveolar lavage for rapid diagnosis of the fat embolism syndrome in trauma patients. Ann Intern Med 1990; 113: 583–588.
465. Huaman A, Nice W, Young I. Fat embolism syndrome. Premortem diagnosis by cryostat frozen sections. J Kans Med Soc 1969; 70:487–488.
466. Zhou DS, Wang F, Wang BM, et al. The diagnosis and treatment of severe cerebral fat embolism. Chin J Traumatol 2003; 6:375–378.
467. Kubota T, Ebina T, Tonosaki M, et al. Rapid improvement of respiratory symptoms associated with fat embolism by high-dose methylpredonisolone: a case report. J Anesth 2003; 17:186–189.
468. Goodnough LT, Brecher ME, Kanter MH, et al. Transfusion medicine. Second of two parts—blood conservation. N Engl J Med 1999; 340:525–533.
469. Kopko PM, Marshall CS, MacKenzie MR, et al. Transfusion-related acute lung injury: report of a

clinical look-back investigation. JAMA 2002; 287: 1968–1971.

470. Kaye J, Edlin S, Thompson I, et al. Pheochromocytoma presenting as life-threatening pulmonary edema. Endocrine 2001; 15:203–204.

471. Keefe DL. Cardiovascular emergencies in the cancer patient. Semin Oncol 2000; 27:244–255.

472. Keefe DL. Trastuzumab-associated cardiotoxicity. Cancer 2002; 95:1592–1600.

473. Veinot JP, Edwards WD. Pathology of radiation-induced heart disease: a surgical and autopsy study of 27 cases. Hum Pathol 1996; 27:766–773.

474. Hull MC, Morris CG, Pepine CJ, et al. Valvular dysfunction and carotid, subclavian, and coronary artery disease in survivors of hodgkin lymphoma treated with radiation therapy. JAMA 2003; 290:2831–2837.

475. Adams MJ, Hardenbergh PH, Constine LS, et al. Radiation-associated cardiovascular disease. Crit Rev Oncol Hematol 2003; 45:55–75.

476. Aberle DR, Wiener-Kronish JP, Webb WR, et al. Hydrostatic versus increased permeability pulmonary edema: diagnosis based on radiographic criteria in critically ill patients. Radiology 1988; 168:73–79.

477. Milne EN. What is "congested" in cardiac failure? A newer approach to plain film interpretation of cardiac failure. Rays 1997; 22:94–106.

478. Suzuki S, Tanita T, Koike K, et al. Evidence of acute inflammatory response in reexpansion pulmonary edema. Chest 1992; 101:275–276.

479. Fein A, Grossman RF, Jones JG, et al. The value of edema fluid protein measurement in patients with pulmonary edema. Am J Med 1979; 67:32–38.

480. Tarrac SE. Negative pressure pulmonary edema—a postanesthesia emergency. J Perianesth Nurs 2003; 18: 317–323.

481. Gropper MA, Wiener-Kronish JP, Hashimoto S. Acute cardiogenic pulmonary edema. Clin Chest Med 1994; 15:501–515.

482. Stalcup S, Mellins R. Mechanical forces producing pulmonary edema in acute asthma. N Engl J Med 1977; 297:592.

483. Goss CH, Brower RG, Hudson LD, et al. Incidence of acute lung injury in the United States. Crit Care Med 2003; 31:1607–1611.

484. Estenssoro E, Dubin A, Laffaire E, et al. Incidence, clinical course, and outcome in 217 patients with acute respiratory distress syndrome. Crit Care Med 2002; 30:2450–2456.

485. Sloane PJ, Gee MH, Gottlieb JE, et al. A multicenter registry of patients with acute respiratory distress syndrome. Physiology and outcome. Am Rev Respir Dis 1992; 146:419–426.

486. Messent M, Sullivan K, Keogh BF, et al. Adult respiratory distress syndrome following cardiopulmonary bypass: incidence and prediction. Anaesthesia 1992; 47:267–268.

487. Seidenfeld JJ, Pohl DF, Bell RC, et al. Incidence, site, and outcome of infections in patients with the adult respiratory distress syndrome. Am Rev Respir Dis 1986; 134:12–16.

488. Morrison RJ, Bidani A. Acute respiratory distress syndrome epidemiology and pathophysiology. Chest Surg Clin N Am 2002; 12:301–323.

489. Win N, Ranasinghe E, Lucas G. Transfusion-related acute lung injury: a 5-year look-back study. Transfus Med 2002; 12:387–389.

490. TenHoor T, Mannino DM, Moss M. Risk factors for ARDS in the United States: analysis of the 1993 National Mortality Followback Study. Chest 2001; 119:1179–1184.

491. Price K, Thall P, Kish S. Prognostic indicators for blood and marrow transplant patients admitted to an intensive care unit. Am J Respir Crit Care Med 1998; 158:876–884.

492. Veys P, Owens C. Respiratory infections following haemopoietic stem cell transplantation in children. Br Med Bull 2002; 61:151–174.

493. Barnes RA, Stallard N. Severe infections after bone marrow transplantation. Curr Opin Crit Care 2001; 7:362–366.

494. Bojko T, Notterman DA. Reversal of fortune? Respiratory failure after bone marrow transplantation. Crit Care Med 1999; 27:1061–1062.

495. Tomashefski JF Jr. Pulmonary pathology of acute respiratory distress syndrome. Clin Chest Med 2000; 21:435–466.

496. Katzenstein AL, Myers JL, Mazur MT. Acute interstitial pneumonia. A clinicopathologic, ultrastructural, and cell kinetic study. Am J Surg Pathol 1986; 10:256–267.

497. Ware LB, Matthay MA. The acute respiratory distress syndrome. N Engl J Med 2000; 342:1334–1349.

498. Laufe MD, Simon RH, Flint A, et al. Adult respiratory distress syndrome in neutropenic patients. Am J Med 1986; 80:1022–1026.

499. Nelson S. Novel nonantibiotic therapies for pneumonia: cytokines and host defense. Chest 2001; 119: 419S–425S.

500. Hamacher J, Lucas R, Lijnen HR, et al. Tumor necrosis factor-alpha and angiostatin are mediators of endothelial cytotoxicity in bronchoalveolar lavages of patients with acute respiratory distress syndrome. Am J Respir Crit Care Med 2002; 166:651–656.

501. Pittet JF, Mackersie RC, Martin TR, et al. Biological markers of acute lung injury: prognostic and pathogenetic significance. Am J Respir Crit Care Med 1997; 155:1187–1205.

502. Ware LB, Fang X, Matthay MA. Protein C and thrombomodulin in human acute lung injury. Am J Physiol Lung Cell Mol Physiol 2003; 285:L514–L521. Epub 2003 May 2016.

503. Yan SB, Helterbrand JD, Hartman DL, et al. Low levels of protein C are associated with poor outcome in severe sepsis. Chest 2001; 120:915–922.
504. Abraham E, Arcaroli J, Carmody A, et al. HMG-1 as a mediator of acute lung inflammation. J Immunol 2000; 165:2950–2954.
505. Bustin M. Regulation of DNA-dependent activities by the functional motifs of the high-mobility-group chromosomal proteins. Mol Cell Biol 1999; 19: 5237–5246.
506. Andersson U, Wang H, Palmblad K, et al. High mobility group 1 protein (HMG-1) stimulates proinflammatory cytokine synthesis in human monocytes. J Exp Med 2000; 192:565–570.
507. Tsunawaki S, Sporn M, Ding A, et al. Deactivation of macrophages by transforming growth factor-beta. Nature 1988; 334:260–262.
508. Oswald IP, Wynn TA, Sher A, et al. Interleukin 10 inhibits macrophage microbicidal activity by blocking the endogenous production of tumor necrosis factor alpha required as a costimulatory factor for interferon gamma-induced activation. Proc Natl Acad Sci USA 1992; 89:8676–8680.
509. Suchyta MR, Orme JF Jr, Morris AH. The changing face of organ failure in ARDS. Chest 2003; 124:1871–1879.
510. Saldias FJ, Comellas A, Ridge KM, et al. Isoproterenol improves ability of lung to clear edema in rats exposed to hyperoxia. J Appl Physiol 1999; 87: 30–35.
511. Tibayan FA, Chesnutt AN, Folkesson HG, et al. Dobutamine increases alveolar liquid clearance in ventilated rats by beta-2 receptor stimulation. Am J Respir Crit Care Med 1997; 156:438–444.
512. Barnard ML, Olivera WG, Rutschman DM, et al. Dopamine stimulates sodium transport and liquid clearance in rat lung epithelium. Am J Respir Crit Care Med 1997; 156:709–714.
513. Wright PE, Carmichael LC, Bernard GR. Effect of bronchodilators on lung mechanics in the acute respiratory distress syndrome (ARDS). Chest 1994; 106:1517–1523.
514. Cerra FB, Benitez MR, Blackburn GL, et al. Applied nutrition in ICU patients. A consensus statement of the American College of Chest Physicians. Chest 1997; 111:769–778.
515. Schuster DP. Fluid management in ARDS: "keep them dry" or does it matter? Intensive Care Med 1995; 21:101–103.
516. Mitchell JP, Schuller D, Calandrino FS, et al. Improved outcome based on fluid management in critically ill patients requiring pulmonary artery catheterization. Am Rev Respir Dis 1992; 145:990–998.
517. Schuller D, Mitchell JP, Calandrino FS, et al. Fluid balance during pulmonary edema. Is fluid gain a marker or a cause of poor outcome? Chest 1991; 100: 1068–1075.
518. Matthay A, Broaddus V. Fluid and hemodynamic management in acute lung injury. Semin Respir Crit Care Med 1994; 1994:271–288.
519. Gerlach H, Keh D, Semmerow A, et al. Dose–response characteristics during long-term inhalation of nitric oxide in patients with severe acute respiratory distress syndrome: a prospective, randomized, controlled study. Am J Respir Crit Care Med 2003; 167:1008–1015.
520. Rossaint R, Gerlach H, Schmidt-Ruhnke H, et al. Efficacy of inhaled nitric oxide in patients with severe ARDS. Chest 1995; 107:1107–1115.
521. Dellinger RP. Inhaled nitric oxide versus prone positioning in acute respiratory distress syndrome. Crit Care Med 2000; 28:572–574.
522. Pay en DM. Inhaled nitric oxide and acute lung injury. Clin Chest Med 2000; 21:519–529, ix.
523. Bone RC, Slotman G, Maunder R, et al. Randomized double-blind, multicenter study of prostaglandin E1 in patients with the adult respiratory distress syndrome. Prostaglandin E1 Study Group. Chest 1989; 96: 114–119.
524. Schermuly RT, Leuchte H, Ghofrani HA, et al. Zardaverine and aerosolised iloprost in a model of acute respiratory failure. Eur Respir J 2003; 22:342–347.
525. Ulloa L, Ochani M, Yang H, et al. Ethyl pyruvate prevents lethality in mice with established lethal sepsis and systemic inflammation. Proc Natl Acad Sci USA 2002; 99:12351–12356. Epub 12002 Sep 12353.
526. Bernard GR, Wheeler AP, Russell JA, et al. The effects of ibuprofen on the physiology and survival of patients with sepsis. The Ibuprofen in Sepsis Study Group. N Engl J Med 1997; 336:912–918.
527. listed" Na. Ketoconazole for early treatment of acute lung injury and acute respiratory distress syndrome: a randomized controlled trial. The ARDS Network. JAMA 2000; 283:1995–2002.
528. Matthay MA. Severe sepsis—a new treatment with both anticoagulant and antiinflammatory properties. N Engl J Med 2001; 344:759–762.
529. Meduri GU, Headley AS, Golden E, et al. Effect of prolonged methylprednisolone therapy in unresolving acute respiratory distress syndrome: a randomized controlled trial. JAMA 1998; 280:159–165.
530. Brun-Buisson C, Brochard L. Corticosteroid therapy in acute respiratory distress syndrome: better late than never? JAMA 1998; 280:182–183.
531. Bernard GR, Vincent JL, Laterre PF, et al. Efficacy and safety of recombinant human activated protein C for severe sepsis. N Engl J Med 2001; 344:699–709.
532. Poynter SE, LeVine AM. Surfactant biology and clinical application. Crit Care Clin 2003; 19:459–472.
533. Lewis JF, Brackenbury A. Role of exogenous surfactant in acute lung injury. Crit Care Med 2003; 31: S324–S328.
534. Gattinoni L, Carlesso E, Cadringher P, et al. Physical and biological triggers of ventilator-induced lung

injury and its prevention. Eur Respir J Suppl 2003; 47:15s–25s.

535. Adams AB, Simonson DA, Dries DJ. Ventilator-induced lung injury. Respir Care Clin N Am 2003; 9: 343–362.

536. Ricard JD, Dreyfuss D, Saumon G. Ventilator-induced lung injury. Eur Respir J Suppl 2003; 42:2s–9s.

537. Slutsky AS, Imai Y. Ventilator-induced lung injury, cytokines, PEEP, and mortality: implications for practice and for clinical trials. Intensive Care Med 2003; 29:1218–1221.

538. Michaud G, Cardinal P. Mechanisms of ventilator-induced lung injury: the clinician's perspective. Crit Care 2003; 7:209–210. Epub 2003 Jan 2024.

539. Dreyfuss D, Saumon G. From ventilator-induced lung injury to multiple organ dysfunction? Intensive Care Med 1998; 24:102–104.

540. Dreyfuss D, Saumon G. Ventilator-induced lung injury: lessons from experimental studies. Am J Respir Crit Care Med 1998; 157:294–323.

541. Parker JC, Hernandez LA, Longenecker GL, et al. Lung edema caused by high peak inspiratory pressures in dogs. Role of increased microvascular filtration pressure and permeability. Am Rev Respir Dis 1990; 142:321–328.

542. Tsuno K, Miura K, Takeya M, et al. Histopathologic pulmonary changes from mechanical ventilation at high peak airway pressures. Am Rev Respir Dis 1991; 143:1115–1120.

543. Parker J, Hernandez L, Peevy K. Mechanisms of ventilator-induced lung injury. Crit Care Med 1993; 21:131–143.

544. Montgomery A, Stager M, Coalson J, et al. Causes of mortality in patients with the adult respiratory distress syndrome. Am Rev Respir Dis 1985; 132:485–489.

545. Pinsky MR. Toward a better ventilation strategy for patients with acute lung injury. Crit Care 2000; 4:205–206. Epub 2000 Jul 2003.

546. Amato M, Barbas C, Medeiros D, et al. Effect of a protective-ventilation strategy on mortality in the acute respiratory distress syndrome. N Engl J Med 1998; 338:347–354.

547. Pesenti A, Marcolin R, Prato P, et al. Mean airway pressure vs. positive end-expiratory pressure during mechanical ventilation. Crit Care Med 1985; 13:34–37.

548. Mercat A, Titiriga M, Anguel N, et al. Inverse ratio ventilation (I/E = 2/1) in acute respiratory distress syndrome: a six-hour controlled study. Am J Respir Crit Care Med 1997; 155:1637–1642.

549. Husain S, Singh N. Bronchiolitis obliterans and lung transplantation: evidence for an infectious etiology. Semin Respir Infect 2002; 17:310–314.

550. Ritacca FV, Stewart TE. Clinical review: high-frequency oscillatory ventilation in adults—a review of the literature and practical applications. Crit Care 2003; 7:385–390. Epub 2003 Apr 2017.

551. Singh JM, Stewart TE. High-frequency mechanical ventilation principles and practices in the era of lung-protective ventilation strategies. Respir Care Clin N Am 2002; 8:247–260.

552. Ambrosino N. Noninvasive mechanical ventilation in acute on chronic respiratory failure: determinants of success and failure. Monaldi Arch Chest Dis 1997; 52:73–75.

553. Antonelli M, Conti G, Moro ML, et al. Predictors of failure of noninvasive positive pressure ventilation in patients with acute hypoxemic respiratory failure: a multicenter study. Intensive Care Med 2001; 27: 1718–1728. Epub 2001 Oct 1716.

554. Martin TJ, Hovis JD, Costantino JP, et al. A randomized, prospective evaluation of noninvasive ventilation for acute respiratory failure. Am J Respir Crit Care Med 2000; 161:807–813.

555. Auriant I, Jallot A, Herve P, et al. Noninvasive ventilation reduces mortality in acute respiratory failure following lung resection. Am J Respir Crit Care Med 2001; 164:1231–1235.

556. Hilbert G, Gruson D, Vargas F, et al. Noninvasive ventilation in immunosuppressed patients with pulmonary infiltrates, fever, and acute respiratory failure. N Engl J Med 2001; 344:481–487.

557. Hirschl RB, Pranikoff T, Wise C, et al. Initial experience with partial liquid ventilation in adult patients with the acute respiratory distress syndrome. JAMA 1996; 275:383–389.

558. Gauger PG, Pranikoff T, Schreiner RJ, et al. Initial experience with partial liquid ventilation in pediatric patients with the acute respiratory distress syndrome. Crit Care Med 1996; 24:16–22.

559. Sajan I, Scannapieco FA, Fuhrman BP, et al. The risk of nosocomial pneumonia is not increased during partial liquid ventilation. Crit Care Med 1999; 27: 2741–2747.

560. Chatte G, Sab JM, Dubois JM, et al. Prone position in mechanically ventilated patients with severe acute respiratory failure. Am J Respir Crit Care Med 1997; 155:473–478.

561. Blanch L, Mancebo J, Perez M, et al. Short-term effects of prone position in critically ill patients with acute respiratory distress syndrome. Intensive Care Med 1997; 23:1033–1039.

562. Stocker R, Neff T, Stein S, et al. Prone positioning and low-volume pressure-limited ventilation improve survival in patients with severe ARDS. Chest 1997; 111: 1008–1017.

563. Piedalue F, Albert RK. Prone positioning in acute respiratory distress syndrome. Respir Care Clin N Am 2003; 9:495–509.

564. Meade M. Prone positioning for acute respiratory failure improved short-term oxygenation but not survival. ACP J Club 2002; 136:55.

565. Gattinoni L, Tognoni G, Brazzi L, et al. Ventilation in the prone position. The Prone-Supine Study Collaborative Group. Lancet 1997; 350:815.

566. Gattinoni L, Tognoni G, Pesenti A, et al. Effect of prone positioning on the survival of patients with

acute respiratory failure. N Engl J Med 2001; 345: 568–573.

567. Marion BS. A turn for the better: "prone positioning" of patients with ards: a guide to the physiology and management of this effective, underused intervention. Am J Nursing 2001; 101:26–34.
568. Blanch L, Mancebo J, Perez M, et al. Short-term effects of prone position in critically ill patients with acute respiratory distress syndrome. Intensive Care Med 1997; 23:1033–1039.
569. Friedman JA, Pichelmann MA, Piepgras DG, et al. Pulmonary complications of aneurysmal subarachnoid hemorrhage. Neurosurgery 2003; 52:1025–1031; discussion 1031–1022.
570. Brambrink AM, Tzanova I. Neurogenic pulmonary oedema after generalized epileptic seizure. Eur J Emerg Med 1998; 5:59–66.
571. Keegan MT, Lanier WL. Pulmonary edema after resection of a fourth ventricle tumor: possible evidence for a medulla-mediated mechanism. Mayo Clin Proc 1999; 74:264–268.
572. Tarver RD, Broderick LS, Conces DJ Jr. Reexpansion pulmonary edema. J Thorac Imaging 1996; 11:198–209.
573. Sherman SC. Reexpansion pulmonary edema: a case report and review of the current literature. J Emerg Med 2003; 24:23–27.
574. Light R, Girard W, Jenkinson S, et al. Parapneumonic diseases. Am J Med 1980; 69:507–512.
575. Ruffini E, Parola A, Papalia E, et al. Frequency and mortality of acute lung injury and acute respiratory distress syndrome after pulmonary resection for bronchogenic carcinoma. Eur J Cardiothorac Surg 2001; 20:30–36; discussion 36–37.
576. Tandon S, Batchelor A, Bullock R, et al. Perioperative risk factors for acute lung injury after elective oesophagectomy. Br J Anaesth 2001; 86: 633–638.
577. Baudouin SV. Lung injury after thoracotomy. Br J Anaesth 2003; 91:132–142.
578. Jordan S, Mitchell JA, Quinlan GJ, et al. The pathogenesis of lung injury following pulmonary resection. Eur Respir J 2000; 15:790–799.
579. Williams E, Goldstraw P, Evans TW. The complications of lung resection in adults: acute respiratory distress syndrome (ARDS). Monaldi Arch Chest Dis 1996; 51:310–315.

38

Acute Renal Failure

JOHN R. FORINGER

Division of Renal Diseases and Hypertension, Houston Medical School and Section of Nephrology, The University of Texas M.D. Anderson Cancer Center, Houston, Texas, U.S.A.

ANDREW D. SHAW

Department of Critical Care Medicine, The University of Texas M.D. Anderson Cancer Center, Houston, Texas, U.S.A.

KEVIN W. FINKEL

Division of Renal Diseases and Hypertension, Houston Medical School and Section of Nephrology, The University of Texas M.D. Anderson Cancer Center, Houston, Texas, U.S.A.

Acute renal failure (ARF) is characterized by an abrupt decrease in glomerular filtration rate (GFR) over hours to days. It occurs in approximately 5% of all hospitalized patients and 30% of those in the intensive care unit (ICU) (1). The morbidity and mortality associated with ARF are well described. In ICU patients with ARF mortality rates approach 60–80% (2–4). Over the last 30 years there has been little change in mortality associated with hospital-acquired ARF. In 1979, the incidence of ARF was reported as 4.9% with an overall mortality of 29%. If the rise in creatinine was >3 mg/dL, then mortality increased to 64% (1). A more recent report in 1996 also looked at incidence and outcomes of ARF. Using the same definition for ARF as the previous study, the incidence of ARF was 7.4% (5). The overall mortality rate was 19.4%, while the mortality in patients with sepsis and ARF was 76% (5). Acute renal failure significantly increases hospital length of stay and cost of care (6,7). Additional morbidity and cost result from chronic dialysis therapy needed by 5–30% of surviving patients (8).

Numerous scoring systems relying on various clinical and laboratory data are used to predict mortality in ICU patients, such as APACHE II and III. Although all have reasonable utility, they perform poorly in patients with ARF (9,10). Newer prediction models such as the Cleveland Clinic Severity of Illness Score and the Liano Score have better accuracy in predicting mortality in ARF patients (10,11). However, the reliability of the scores appears to be institution specific. When applied to ICU patients in different hospitals, the predictive value falls (10). Therefore, to accurately define the prognosis of ICU patients with ARF, it may be necessary for individual institutions to develop site-specific scoring systems. Unfortunately, the absence of a centralized registry and widely accepted definition of ARF hinders the accurate recording of the incidence, etiology, and outcomes of ARF.

I. DEFINING ACUTE RENAL FAILURE

To date there is no standard definition for ARF. Acute renal failure is detected by a change in the serum creatinine concentration that serves as a surrogate for a change in GFR. However, no consensus exists on what degree of change in the creatinine level constitutes ARF.

This variability in the definition makes it difficult to compare individual treatment or intervention trials. It also delays the recognition of ARF in the clinical setting. Typically, ARF is defined as a 50% increase in serum creatinine if the baseline is $\leq$1.5 mg/dL, or a doubling of the value if the baseline is >1.5 mg/dL. The increase in serum creatinine is an insensitive measure of decreased GFR. Creatinine excretion occurs through both glomerular filtration and proximal tubular secretion. As filtration of creatinine declines tubular secretion will increase, thus no measurable change in the serum creatinine develops until there is a profound decrease in the GFR. In addition, the nonsteady state of creatinine levels in ARF makes it impossible to accurately determine GFR with the use of 24-hr urine collections or the Cockcroft-Gault formula. The Cockcroft-Gault formula is accepted as a standard method for estimating GFR only when the serum creatinine level is stable (12,13).

$$\mathrm{GFR} = \frac{140 - \mathrm{age}}{\mathrm{SCr}72} \times \text{Pt weight (0.85 for a woman)}$$

Pt weight = Patient's weight in kg; SCr = serum creatinine

The insensitivity in serum creatinine change as a marker for declines in GFR makes it difficult to identify early ARF and initiate timely intervention. This lack of sensitivity for identifying small declines in the GFR have led to attempts to develop biomarkers of tubular injury that are both sensitive and specific for early ARF. Recently described, kidney injury molecule-1 (KIM-1) is a novel protein that is expressed during tubular injury and acute tubular necrosis (ATN) (14). Urinary KIM-1 is being evaluated as a possible biomarker for the early diagnosis of ATN. Thus far, other urinary markers for the early detec tion of ATN have not been proven useful for clinical use.

II. EVALUATION OF ACUTE RENAL FAILURE

In the evaluation of ARF, the most useful clinical indices include the history, physical examination, and urinary output. Useful laboratory data are urinalysis, urinary specific gravity, examination of urinary sediment, and measurement of urine electrolytes. Under certain circumstances, evaluation of urine osmolality and staining for urine eosinophils are helpful. On the other hand, a 24-hr urine collection for creatinine clearance is of no value in differentiating the cause of ARF or in assessing the GFR when the creatinine level is increasing. Measurements of the serum blood urea nitrogen (BUN) and creatinine are routine for following the progression of ARF. When assessing the hemodynamic changes in critically ill patients and evaluating the adequacy of renal perfusion, central hemodynamic monitoring is often required.

The first indication of renal hypoperfusion or tubular injury may be changes in urine output. Prerenal azotemia with intact tubular function results in increased tubular sodium reabsorption and decreased water excretion. The glomerular hypoperfusion that occurs often results in a drop in the urine output to less than 0.5 mL/kg of body weight per hour. Oliguria, defined as a urine output < 400 mL/day, may ensue. Oliguria is present in approximately 50% of ARF cases regardless of cause. In the evaluation of suspected prerenal azotemia, urine indices are predictable based on the effect of norepinephrine, angiotensin II, aldosterone, and antidiuretic hormone (ADH) on renal blood flow and sodium and water reabsorption. Typical urine indices are illustrated in Table 1. During low urine flow states, tubular reabsorption of BUN increases and the serum BUN to creatinine ratio is often elevated to > 20:1. An increased BUN/creatinine ratio also develops with gastrointestinal bleeding, obstructive uropathy, and hypercatabolic states common in critically ill patients. With the increased avidity of the proximal and distal tubule for sodium, the urine sodium typically is <20 mEq/L. An alternative measure to evaluate the kidneys' ability to conserve sodium during oliguric ARF is the fractional excretion of sodium (FENa). The FENa has been adopted to distinguish intact tubular function (prerenal) from compromised

Table 1 Urinary Indices in the Differential of ARF

Index	Normal value	Prerenal azotemia	Acute tubular necrosis	Obstruction
Urinary volume	$\geq$0.5 mL/kg/hr	$\leq$0.5 mL/kg/hr	Variable	Variable
Urine specific gravity	1.003–1.025	$\geq$1.020	1.010	Variable
Urinary sodium	Variable	<20 mEq/L	>40 mEq/L	<40 mEq/L early >40 mEq/L late
FENa	<1%	<1%	> 3%	<1% early >3% late
BUN/creatinine ratio	10:1	>20:1	Variable	Variable

tubular function (ATN) in the *oliguric* patient. With simultaneous measurements of the plasma sodium (PNa) and creatinine (PCr) and the urine sodium (UNa) and creatinine (UCr), the FENa is calculated as follows:

$$\text{FENa}\ (\%) = \frac{\text{UNa} \times \text{PCr}}{\text{PNa} \times \text{UCr}} \times 100$$

The FENa is <1% (Table 1) in healthy people, demonstrating that <1% of the daily sodium load filtered by the kidneys is normally excreted in the urine. In the face of suppressed atrial natriuretic peptide release and high serum levels of aldosterone during prerenal azotemia, the FENa is also < 1% indicating intact tubular function. In contrast, in ATN the FENa is usually > 1% (15,16). Although the FENa can be a useful tool in differentiating prerenal azotemia from ATN, there are many pitfalls to its use when confounding factors are present. In chronic renal disease, impaired sodium and water reabsorption can increase the FENa despite the presence of prerenal azotemia. Similarly, administration of diuretics, bicarbonate, and saline can also raise the urine sodium content. In contrast, there are numerous reports of patients with ATN from radiocontrast, rhabdomyolysis, sepsis, transplant rejection, urinary obstruction, acute glomerulonephritis, and hepatorenal syndrome in which the FENa is < 1% (17). Therefore, the utility of calculating the FENa to differentiate prerenal azotemia from ATN is dependent on the patient's clinical disease and the use of ancillary urine and serum tests.

Urinalysis and examination of the urinary sediment can help differentiate the underlying etiology of ARF. Prerenal azotemia is typically associated with bland urinalysis or occasional fine granular and hyaline casts. In ATN, tubular epithelial cells, epithelial cell casts, and coarse granular casts are seen. Pyuria and white blood cell casts are indicative of glomerulonephritis, infection, or acute tubulointerstitial nephritis (TIN). Staining for the presence of urine eosinophils can help identify TIN, although, their detection is not a finding exclusive to TIN. Eosinophils have been seen in patients with rapidly progressive glomerulonephritis, bacterial prostatitis, acute cystitis, and postinfectious glomerulonephritis (18). Red blood cell casts indicate acute or rapidly progressive glomerulonephritis. Nephrotic range proteinuria suggests intrinsic glomerular disease. In hemoglobinuria and myoglobinuria, the urine dipstick is positive for large blood in the absence of red blood cells on microscopic analysis. The common causes of ARF and the typical urine findings are listed in Table 2.

III. CLASSIFICATION OF ACUTE RENAL FAILURE

The etiology of ARF is divided into prerenal, intrinsic renal, and postrenal causes according to the nature of the insult to the kidneys. The diagnostic and therapeutic approach to ARF depends on this classification scheme. Intrinsic renal failure can result from ischemic or nephrotoxic ATN, acute TIN, glomerulonephritis, or vascular syndromes such as atheroembolic disease. The majority of hospital-acquired ARF is secondary to prerenal azotemia and ATN.

A. Prerenal Azotemia

Prerenal azotemia accounts for approximately 70% of hospital-acquired ARF (1,19). Prerenal azotemia is a normal physiologic response to decreased renal perfusion pressure resulting in a hemodynamically mediated reduction in the GFR. No immediate injury occurs to the renal parenchyma and the GFR rapidly returns to normal with reversal of the hemodynamic insult. Overt pathologic changes can occur if the renal hypoperfusion is sustained. The decrease in glomerular ultrafiltration pressure can be secondary to a true decrease in the arterial blood volume or a decrease in the effective arterial blood volume as in congestive heart failure, cirrhosis, capillary leak syndromes, and sepsis. When the mean arterial pressure falls below 80–90 mmHg, there is a reduction in renal blood flow. Progression of the prerenal state can lead to ATN. Prerenal azotemia and ischemic ATN are manifestations of renal hypoperfusion. The severity and duration of the insult will dictate the likelihood of progression from prerenal azotemia to ischemic tubular damage.

Common causes of prerenal azotemia are listed in Table 3. In renal hypoperfusion states, GFR is maintained by the interplay of several neuro-humeral systems. The renin-angiotensin axis increases the vasomotor tone of the efferent arteriole while afferent arteriolar vasomotor tone decreases under the influence of nitric oxide, vasodilatory prostaglandins, and the kallikrein–kinin system. The sympathetic nervous system reacts to hypoperfusion with release of norepinephrine and ADH. With sustained reductions in renal blood flow, the ability of the kidney to maintain glomerular perfusion pressure is overwhelmed and the GFR declines resulting in azotemia and cellular hypoxia with ischemic tubular damage.

Table 2 Urinary Findings and Confirmatory Test in the Common Causes of ARF

	Prerenal azotemia	
Suggestive clinical findings	*Typical urine analysis*	*Confirmation*
Volume depletion Decreased EABV NSAID ACE-I or ARB	FENa $< 1\%$ UNa < 20 SG > 1.020	Rapid resolution of ARF with correction of renal hypoperfusion Invasive monitoring—CVP or PCWP
	Postrenal azotemia	
Abdominal or flank pain Palpable bladder Enlarged prostate Nephrolithiasis Urinary frequency, oliguria, or anuria	Hematuria without dysmorphic red blood cells, casts, or proteinuria Variable FENa and UNa	Abdominal X-ray Renal ultrasound IVP Retrograde pyelography
	Intrinsic renal azotemia	
Cause of ARF	*Typical urine analysis*	*Confirmation*
Acute tubulointerstitial nephritis	Positive urine WBC Urine eosinophils White cell cast Red blood cells Rarely red blood cell casts	Systemic eosinophilia Renal biopsy Biopsy of skin rash
Hemolysis	Urine supernatant is pink and heme + Hemoglobinuria	Elevated K^+, PO_4, and uric acid, LDH Hypocalcemia Peripheral smear with fragmented red blood cells
Hemolyic uremic syndrome and Thrombotic thrombocytopenic purpura	Urine red blood cells Heme +	Renal biopsy Peripheral smear with schistocytes and fragmented red cells Thrombocytopenia
Glomerulonephritis	Proteinuria Red blood cell casts White blood cell casts	Renal biopsy Serum antibody test
Radiocontrast	Early FENa $< 1\%$, UNa < 20 Progression to FENa $> 1\%$ and UNa > 20	Temporal relationship to the contrast infusion
Rhabdomyolysis	Urine supernatant heme + without red blood cells Myoglobinuria	Elevated creatinine kinase, PO_4, uric acid, K^+ Hypocalcemia Elevated serum myoglobin
Tumor lysis syndrome	Urate crystals	Elevated K^+, PO_4, uric acid Decreased Ca^{2+}
Ischemia	FENa $> 1\%$, UNa > 20 SG $= 1.010$ Muddy brown granular or tubule epithelial cell cast	Clinical assessment and urine findings usually sufficient

EABV = effective arterial blood volume; NSAID = nonsteroidal anti-inflammatory drugs; ACE-I = angiotensin converting enzyme inhibitor; ARB = angiotensin receptor blocker; FENa = fractional excretion of sodium; UNa = urine sodium concentration; SG = urine specific gravity; K^+ = serum potassium; PO_4 = serum phosphorous; Ca^{2+} = serum calcium.

Table 3 Causes of Prerenal Azotemia

Intravascular volume depletion
Cutaneous losses
Burns
Hyperthermia
Cutaneous graft vs. host disease
Cutaneous T-cell lymphoma
Gastrointestinal fluid loss
Vomiting
Diarrhea
Enterocutaneous fistula
Nasogastric suction
Renal losses
Drug-induced or osmotic diuresis
Diabetes insipidus
Adrenal insufficiency
"Third-space" losses
Capillary leak syndrome (graft vs. host disease, >interferon therapy, SIRS)
Pancreatitis
Hypoalbuminemia
Decreased effective arterial blood volume
Decreased cardiac output
Myocardial, valvular, pericardial disease
Pulmonary embolism
Pulmonary hypertension
Positive pressure ventilation
Cirrhosis
Nephrotic syndrome
Sepsis
Anesthesia
Impaired renal vascular autoregulation
Angiotensin-converting enzyme inhibitors
Angiotensin-receptor blockers
Nonsteroidal anti-inflammatory drugs
Cyclooxygenase 2 inhibitors
Cyclosporine A
Tacrolimus
Hypercalcemia
Hepatorenal syndrome

B. Specific Causes of Prerenal Azotemia

1. *Nonsteroidal Anti-inflammatory Drugs (NSAID)*

Nonsteroidal anti-inflammatory drugs can be divided into nonselective inhibitors of both cyclooxygenase-1 (COX-1) and cyclooxygenase-2 (COX-2) or selective inhibitors of COX-2. Patients at greatest risk for NSAID induced ARF include the elderly, and patients with congestive heart failure, advanced liver disease, atherosclerotic vascular disease, or chronic kidney disease (20,21). Special attention should be given to elderly patients treated with NSAIDs of any type. In a population-based study, the risk of ARF in the elderly increased by 58% with prescription NSAID use (22). The nonselective NSAIDs are inhibitors of the prostaglandins responsible for vasodilatation in the kidney and can promote prerenal azotemia in susceptible patients. The selective COX-2 inhibitors also cause a similar renal vasoconstriction. The renal safety profile of celecoxib (COX-2) is similar to ibuprofen. One selective COX-2 inhibitor, rofecoxib, was found to have a higher incidence of renal toxicity than the nonselective inhibitors or celecoxib (23). The renal toxicity of NSAIDs is increased when they are used in combination with other medications with the potential to alter the kidneys' ability to autoregulate glomerular filtration pressure such as angiotensin-converting enzyme (ACE) inhibitors and angiotensin receptor blockers (ARBs). The renal vascular changes associated with NSAID use are typically reversible although prolonged use can lead to permanent renal injury. Nonsteroidal anti-inflammatory drugs are also known to cause acute TIN in which case there is often a sudden change in GFR that may persist for days to weeks.

2. *Angiotensin-Converting Enzyme Inhibitors and Angiotensin Receptor Blockers*

The renin–angiotensin system contributes to the autoregulation of glomerular perfusion pressure and inhibition of this system has the potential to induce prerenal azotemia. Angiotensin-converting enzyme inhibitors reduce blood pressure by inhibiting the proteolytic cleavage of angiotensin I to angiotensin II. Angiotensin receptor blockers occupy the angiotensin receptor. Much like the prostaglandin inhibitors, ACE-inhibitors and ARBs increase the risk of ARF in patients on diuretic therapy, with volume depletion, congestive heart failure, or diabetes, and in the elderly (24,25). Their use in conjunction with NSAIDs, cyclosporine, and tacrolimus put patients at an even greater risk for ARF (24,26). The incidence of ARF is also higher in patients with chronic kidney disease of any etiology. Patients with chronic kidney disease usually depend on local angiotensin II production to maintain GFR in the face of decreased functional renal mass. Therefore, a decline in GFR when these patients receive ACE-inhibitors is not unexpected. The rise in serum creatinine is typically $<30\%$ and does not constitute ARF. More dramatic increases in serum creatinine suggest the presence of underlying renal vascular disease.

3. *Calcineurin-Inhibitors*

The calcineurin-inhibitors cyclosporine A (CSA) and tacrolimus are widely used as immunosuppressants in solid organ and bone marrow transplantation (BMT). CSA and tacrolimus cause both ARF and chronic renal failure. The nephrotoxicity seen in the critically ill patient is the result of direct afferent arteriolar vasoconstriction leading to a decrease in the glomerular filtration pressure and GFR. The vascular effect associated with CSA and tacrolimus is reversible with discontinuation of the drug. A dose reduction is sometimes enough to reverse the prerenal affect. Chronic nephrotoxicity is a potential complication with more prolonged use of the calcineurin-inhibitors. Proteinuria, tubular dysfunction, arterial hypertension, and rising creatinine are clinical findings consistent with chronic CSA or tacrolimus nephrotoxicity. It typically takes more than 6 months of therapy for the chronic changes to occur. Arteriolar damage, interstitial fibrosis, tubular atrophy, and glomerulosclerosis are found on renal biopsy specimens. The pathologic changes of the chronic nephrotoxicity are irreversible (27–29). A rare complication of CSA and tacrolimus therapy is hemolytic uremic syndrome (HUS). The mechanism of CSA or tacrolimus-induced HUS is direct damage to the vascular endothelium in a dose-dependent fashion. With discontinuation of the drug, patients may have partial recovery (30–32). Calcineurin-inhibitors have also been associated with hyperkalemia, thought to be secondary to tubular resistance to aldosterone (33).

4. *Hepatorenal Syndrome*

Hepatorenal syndrome (HRS) is a unique cause of renal vasoconstriction with a decline in GFR in the face of normal renal histology that occurs in the setting of liver failure. The clinical picture associated with HRS is that of a prerenal azotemia. In true HRS without confounding renal injuries, the renal failure will resolve with liver transplantation. The pathogenesis of HRS is not completely understood. Systemic and splanchnic vascular resistance is decreased leading to a decrease in the effective arterial volume and hypoperfusion of the renal vasculature. The compensatory response is an increase in the mediators of renal vasoconstriction including increased renin–angiotensin–aldosterone activity, ADH levels, sympathetic tone, and endothelin levels. The renal response is an increase in salt and water avidity leading to worsening ascites and edema (34,35). Clinically, HRS is characterized by oliguric ARF with very low urine sodium and bland urine sediment. The diagnosis of HRS is a diagnosis of exclusion. Other causes for the ARF should be ruled out including causes of prerenal azotemia, intrinsic renal disease, and obstructive nephropathy. Major and minor criteria have been established for the diagnosis of HRS (Table 4). Liver transplant is the definitive therapy for HRS. However, patients who develop HRS prior to transplant have worse graft and patient survival (36). Newer pharmacologic therapy with vasopressin analogs (e.g., ornipresson and terlipressin), which are splanchnic vasoconstrictors, has shown some benefit. However, the major complication associated with these medications is mesenteric ischemia (37–39). Oral midodrine (a selective α_1-adrenergic agonist) in combination with octreotide showed benefit in renal function in a small series of patients (40). *N*-acetylcysteine was shown to increase renal blood flow without changing the hemodynamic derangements associated with HRS (41). Several small studies have shown that transjugular intrahepatic portosystemic shunting (TIPS) has prolonged survival and improved renal function in patients with HRS (42,43). Given the poor prognosis of HRS, in a patient with rapid onset of renal failure, dialysis is usually not instituted unless the patient is a candidate for liver transplant or has a chance of hepatic recovery (34,35,44).

IV. OBSTRUCTIVE (POSTRENAL) NEPHROPATHY

Urinary tract obstruction is a relatively common cause of renal failure in patients with malignancy. Regardless of cause, obstruction of urinary flow leads to renal impairment, which early in the course of the condition is reversible if the obstruction is alleviated. Tubular function is initially affected; however, prolonged

Table 4 Diagnostic Criteria for Hepatorenal Syndrome

Major criteria
Acute or chronic liver disease with advanced hepatic failure and portal hypertension
Depressed GFR with a serum creatinine > 1.5 mg/dL or a creatinine clearance < 40 mL/min
Absence of shock, ongoing bacterial infection, fluid loss, and treatment with nephrotoxic medications
No sustained improvement in renal function after withdrawal of diuretics and fluid resuscitation with 1.5 L of isotonic saline
Proteinuria <500 mg/day and no evidence of obstructive nephropathy on ultrasound
Minor criteria
Oliguria
Urine sodium < 10 mEq/L
Urine osmolality > plasma osmolality
Urine red blood cells < 50 per high-power field
Serum sodium concentration < 130 mEq/L

Source: From Ref. 44.

obstruction leads to tubular damage and parenchymal atrophy. Commonly encountered causes of urinary tract obstruction in cancer patients are listed in Table 5.

Clinical manifestations of urinary tract obstruction vary depending on the location, duration, and degree of obstruction. In patients with complete bilateral obstruction or with an obstructed solitary kidney, anuria (<50 mL urine output in 24 hr) can be the presenting feature, whereas in patients with partial obstruction, the urinary output can vary from oliguria to polyuria. Although pain is more likely to be associated with acute blockage, obstruction may be totally asymptomatic and occur without overt clinical manifestations or suggestive laboratory findings (45). Therefore, obstructive nephropathy should always be considered as a cause of renal failure when an obvious prerenal or intrinsic renal cause is not identified.

Diagnosis of urinary tract obstruction can be difficult. Anuria, flank pain with a palpable mass, or a palpable bladder are obvious clues. The laboratory evaluation can be helpful. Hyperkalemia with a nonanion gap metabolic acidosis is suggestive of a renal tubular acidosis (RTA) associated with obstruction (46). The urinary sediment may be bland or demonstrate crystals or hematuria depending on the etiology of the obstruction. Patients may have very dilute urine due to the presence of an acquired form of nephrogenic diabetes insipidus (Table 6) (47).

Table 5 Causes of Obstruction in Cancer Patients

Intratubular
Uric acid crystals from tumor lysis syndrome
Methotrexate
Light chains from multiple myeloma
Acyclovir crystals
Ureteric obstruction
Stones
Blood clot
Sloughed renal papillae
Uric acid
Iatrogenic ligation
Extrinsic compression
Abscess
Hemorrhage
Tumor (lymphoma)
Radiation induced strictures
Transitional cell cancer
Bladder neck obstruction
Stones
Hemorrhagic cystitis (cyclophosphamide, holmium)
Prostatic hypertrophy
Bladder carcinoma
Neurogenic bladder (spinal cord compression)
Urethral obstruction
Stricture
Tumor

Table 6 Common Cause of Nephrogenic Diabetes Insipidus in Cancer Patients

Medications
Aminoglycosides
Amphotericin B
Cisplatin
Ifosfomide
Hypercalcemia
Metastatic bone disease
Multiple myeloma
Paraneoplastic syndromes
Renal cell carcinoma
Obstructive nephropathy
Recovery phase of acute tubular necrosis

Ultrasonography is the most useful test to evaluate for the presence of obstruction. Although hydronephrosis is usually demonstrated, there are circumstances when hydronephrosis is not seen despite urinary tract obstruction: (a) early in the course of obstruction (12–24 hr) when the collecting system is relatively noncompliant; (b) in the face of severe volume depletion when glomerular filtration is severely depressed; and (c) when the collecting system is encased by retroperitoneal lymphadenopathy or fibrosis. Conversely, the finding of hydronephrosis on ultrasound does not prove the presence of obstruction since it is also seen in high urinary flow states such as diuretic use and diabetes insipidus, pregnancy, previous obstruction, and congenital megaureter. The lack of functional obstruction can be verified in these cases by a normal renal scan with furosemide washout. In this test, an intravenously injected radioisotope will collect in the dilated collecting system but be promptly excreted by the increased urinary flow induced by the diuretic.

Once obstruction is identified, it should be corrected with either percutaneous nephrostomy tubes or ureteral stenting depending on local expertise and availability. The duration and severity of obstruction are the major determinants for the recovery of renal function after its correction. The longer the duration of obstruction, the less likely are the chances for complete renal recovery.

A. Postobstructive Diuresis

Postobstructive diuresis occurs when there is correction of complete bilateral obstruction or complete obstruction of a solitary kidney. It involves the production of a large volume of urine that results from a defect in urinary concentrating ability, impaired reabsorption of urinary sodium, and solute diuresis from retained urea and intravenous administration of sodium-containing solutions. Patients with relief of complete obstruction who are at risk for developing postobstructive diuresis should be carefully monitored. It has been recommended that for patients without pulmonary edema, congestive heart failure, or altered consciousness from uremia, urine losses be replaced by oral intake (48). Replacement fluids are given only if the patients develop orthostatic hypotension, tachycardia, hyponatremia, or a urine output more than 200 mL/ hr. On the other hand, in high-risk patients with altered sensorium, congestive heart failure, or pulmonary edema, replacement of half the hourly urine output with half-normal saline has been recommended. If the patient is hyponatremic, normal saline should be used instead (48).

V. INTRINSIC ACUTE RENAL FAILURE

Intrinsic ARF (Table 7) is associated with renal parenchymal injury. The most common cause of intrinsic renal failure is ATN. It accounts for approximately 85% of intrinsic ARF episodes in hospitalized patients (49). The etiology of the tubular injury may be nephrotoxic (35%) or ischemic (50%) in origin. However, ATN is often a multifactorial process, developing in the setting of a critical illness with nephrotoxic medications, renal hypoperfusion, and sepsis all playing a role. With prolonged episodes of renal hypoperfusion, cortical necrosis can occur and lead to irreversible renal failure. The pathophysiologic abnormalities that result in a fall in GFR include intrarenal vasoconstriction, decreased glomerular filtration pressure, intratubular obstruction, transtubular back-leak of filtrate, and interstitial inflammation. The clinical course of ATN is divided into three components: initiation, maintenance, and recovery. The period in which a patient first experiences a renal injury is the initiation phase of the ATN. The renal injury is potentially reversible if the precipitating insult is alleviated. With progression of the injury, parenchymal damage ensues and abrupt changes in the GFR occur. The maintenance phase can last several days to weeks during which the GFR remains depressed and the patient can have variable urine output. In the recovery phase, the GFR returns to normal as cellular regeneration and tubular repair occurs.

A. Specific Causes of Intrinsic Renal Failure

1. Radiocontrast Nephropathy (RCN)

Ten percent of hospital-acquired ARF is the result of contrast-induced nephrotoxicity making it one of the most common causes of ATN (5). Patients at particular risk for RCN are the elderly, diabetics, and patients with chronic kidney disease, congestive heart failure, or volume depletion. Patients receiving NSAIDs, ACE-inhibitors, ARBs, CSA, or tacrolimus are also

Table 7 Causes of Intrinsic Renal Azotemia in Cancer Patients

Acute tubular necrosis
Ischemic
Hypotension
Sepsis
Cardiopulmonary arrest
Exogenous nephrotoxins
Acyclovir
Aminoglycosides
Amphotericin B
Cisplatin
Cyclosporine
Foscarnet
Ifosfomide
Pentamidine
Radiocontrast
Intrinsic nephrotoxins
Myoglobinuria
Hemoglobinuria
Hyperuricosuria
Acute glomerulonephritis
Postinfectious
Endocarditis associated
Systemic vasculitis
HUS/TTP
Vascular syndromes
Renal artery thromboembolism
Renal vein thrombosis
Atheroembolic disease
Acute tubulointerstitial nephritis
Drug-induced
Penicillins
Cephalosporins
Bactrim
Fluoroquinolones
NSAID
Furosemide
Thiazides
Interferon-alfa
Infectious causes
Bacterial
Viral
Cytomegalovirus
Fungal
Tuberculosis
Malignancy
Lymphoma
Leukemia
Myeloma

at increased risk for RCN. Contrast nephropathy causes ARF by renal vasoconstriction and direct tubular injury (50,51). The vasoconstriction associated with RCN has been linked to vasoactive mediators such as calcium, endothelin, adenosine, and inhibition of the vasodilator nitric oxide. Oxidant injury through free radical oxygen species has also been implicated and has been a target of preventative measures (52). Clinically, patients usually have an elevation in the serum creatinine 24–48 hr after the exposure to the contrast. The creatinine typically peaks at 3–5 days and returns to baseline in 7–10 days. The diagnosis of RCN is often based on the temporal relationship. It is common to see an FENa $< 1\%$ with RCN secondary to the renal vasoconstriction and a prerenal-like picture. Although RCN is typically a transient event, it is associated with a hospital mortality rate five times greater than in matched controls who receive radiocontrast but do not develop ARF (53).

2. *Aminoglycosides*

Aminoglycosides cause ARF in approximately 10% of patients who are treated with them for more than 2–3 days. The serum creatinine typically rises 7–10 days after the drug is initiated. Aminoglycosides concentrate in the proximal tubular cells causing cellular damage. Once overt nephropathy develops, the urinalysis shows tubular epithelial cells and tubular cell casts. Proximal tubular injury is evident by wasting of electrolytes such as potassium, magnesium, and calcium in the urine (54). The FENa is typically $> 2\%$. Aminoglycosides can also cause nephrogenic diabetes insipidus because the tubulointerstitial injury inhibits adenylate cyclase activity leading to ADH resistance (55). Risk factors for aminoglycoside-induced ARF are advanced age, chronic kidney disease, volume depletion, liver disease, and prolonged use of the drug. Monitoring of aminoglycoside blood levels is important in preventing renal toxicity. Studies suggest that once daily dosing of aminoglycosides decreases the risk of ARF without altering the antimicrobial efficacy (56,57).

3. *Amphotericin B*

Amphotericin B and its liposomal derivatives are a common cause of ARF in the ICU, particularly in patients who have undergone bone marrow transplant. Eighty percent of patients who receive amphotericin B will develop some degree of renal impairment. The initial nephrotoxic injury from amphotericin B results from renal vasoconstriction of the preglomerular arterioles and predisposes the patient to an ischemic insult (58,59). Direct tubular toxicity follows. As with many tubular toxins, amphotericin B results in tubular wasting of potassium and magnesium. A hyperchloremic metabolic acidosis as well as a nephrogenic diabetes insipidus from ADH resistance are common findings (25,59,60). The newer liposomal forms of amphotericin B lack the solubilizing agent deoxycholate that contributes to tubular toxicity. Although the renal failure associated with amphotericin B is usually temporary and improves with discontinuation of the drug, reinstitution often results in recurrence of the ARF (61). In the prevention of amphotericin B-induced ARF, clinical studies have shown that hydration with normal saline prior to the amphotericin infusion provides some protection (62,63).

4. *Cisplatin*

Nephrotoxicity is the most common dose-limiting side effect of cisplatin administration. The primary site for clearance of cisplatin is the kidney. Cisplatin asserts its toxicity on the tubules resulting in a tubular wasting syndrome that is often severe. The proximal tubule is most affected but the distal nephron is also vulnerable. Electrolytes such as potassium, magnesium, calcium, and bicarbonate can be excreted in the urine in large amounts necessitating prolonged intravenous supplementation. The direct tubular toxicity associated with cisplatin is exacerbated in a low-chloride environment. In the intracellular compartment, chloride molecules are replaced with water molecules in the cis position of cisplatin, forming hydroxyl radicals that injure the neutrophilic binding sites on DNA (64,65). The decline in GFR associated with cisplatin toxicity usually occurs 7–14 days after the exposure. Doses of cisplatin $>50\ mg/m^2$ are sufficient to cause renal insufficiency. The renal injury is typically reversible but repeated doses of cisplatin in excess of $100\, mg/m^2$ may cause irreversible renal damage (65). Hydration and avoidance of concomitant nephrotoxins is the most effective way to prevent cisplatin-induced nephrotoxicity. Amifostine has been shown to reduce cisplatin nephrotoxicity (66).

5. *Ifosfamide*

Ifosfamide is an alkylating drug that causes renal toxicity either directly or through a metabolite. The metabolite of ifosfamide, chloracetaldehyde, causes direct tubular epithelial cell damage (67). The renal injury occurs throughout the kidney including the glomerulus, proximal and distal tubule, and interstitium. The proximal tubule is most seriously affected causing wasting of electrolytes similar to cisplatin. The degree of hypokalemia, hypophosphatemia, hypomagnesaemia, and hyperchloremic acidosis experienced with ifosfamide toxicity can be severe. Patients can develop Fanconi's syndrome with hypophosphatemic rickets and osteomalacia, as well as nephrogenic diabetes insipidus (68). A potential marker for ifosfamide nephrotoxicity is increased urinary beta 2-microglobulin excretion (69). Risk factors for ifosfamide nephrotoxicity include previous exposure to cisplatin, chronic kidney disease, and a cumulative dose >84 g/m^2 (70,71). Recent data suggest that amifostine may have a protective role against ifosfamide and cisplatin nephrotoxicity (72).

6. *Myoglobin*

The principal cause of the pigmented nephropathies is rhabdomyolysis. The majority of rhabdomyolysis cases are subclinical with mild elevations in the creatine kinase, lactic dehydrogenase, or aspartate aminotransferase. In severe cases, ARF may ensue from myoglobinuria. Rhabdomyolysis has been thought to cause ARF through three mechanisms: renal vasoconstriction, intratubular cast formation, and heme-mediated proximal tubular injury. It is also known that oxidant stress is increased with the release of heme proteins. Free heme proteins are suspected to reduce the formation of nitric oxide and increase endothelin levels leading to vasoconstriction and the decline in GFR. Intratubular obstruction occurs with the interaction of myoglobin and Tamm–Horsfall protein in an aciduric environment (73). The diagnosis of myoglobin-induced nephrotoxicity is suspected on history. The urine dipstick is commonly positive for blood with no red blood cells on microscopic examination. The FENa may be $< 1\%$ despite tubular injury. Evaluation of the urine sediment typically reveals heme-pigmented casts. Serum electrolyte derangements are common including, hyperkalemia, hyperphosphatemia, hyperuricemia, and hypocalcemia. In the recovery phase of rhabdomyolysis, hypercalcemia develops in 30% of patients secondary to increased levels of vitamin D and parathyroid hormone. Replacement of serum calcium should be withheld in asymptomatic patients to prevent severe hypercalcemia after recovery. To prevent and treat the ARF of rhabdomyolysis, aggressive hydration is effective. Alkalinization of the urine has also been advocated to increase the solubility of the heme proteins in the urine. Alkalinization may also reduce the production of reactive oxygen species thus reducing the oxidant stress (74).

7. *Multiple Myeloma*

Fifty percent of patients with multiple myeloma (MM) will develop some degree of renal functional impairment and 10% will require dialysis. The pathogenesis of MM-induced renal failure includes myeloma kidney, renal tubular dysfunction, light-chain deposition disease, amyloidosis, and plasma cell infiltration. Hypercalcemia can also complicate MM and induce renal failure. Patients with MM are at increased risk for other causes of renal failure, in particular contrast nephropathy. The overproduction of monoclonal immunoglobulin light chains is the primary factor associated with the renal disease of MM. The recommended diagnostic tool for identifying the presence of urinary light chains is urine protein electrophoresis with immunofixation. Light chains can combine with Tamm–Horsfall proteins to form casts that cause intratubular obstruction. Factors that influence tubular cast formation include low tubular flow rate, acidity of the urine, radiocontrast infusion, and distal nephron sodium, chloride, and calcium concentration. The therapy of MM-induced renal disease is limited to treating the MM. In patients with high tumor burdens, acute renal failure may ensue. Partial recovery of the GFR may occur in up to 50% of patients who undergo treatment of the MM (75). Small case series suggest that plasmapheresis improves renal survival in patients who require dialysis for ARF from myeloma kidney (76,77). However, renal biopsy may be necessary to identify those patients likely to respond to pheresis therapy. Given the limited clinical experience and need for biopsy, plasmapheresis for myeloma kidney has not gained wide acceptance.

Patients with MM are at increased risk for developing ARF from nephrotoxic injury, particularly radiocontrast. The incidence of contrast nephropathy in MM patients is 0.6–1.25% (78). It is postulated that iodinated contrast enhances the precipitation of intratubular proteins leading to obstruction. Adequate hydration and avoiding low urine flow states are the best protection against ARF in MM patients.

B. Hypercalcemia Associated with Multiple Myeloma

Hypercalcemia complicates MM in 15% of patients at presentation. Hypercalcemia induces prerenal azotemia by causing nephrogenic diabetes insipidus, renal vasoconstriction, and intratubular calcium deposition (79). When the serum calcium level is >13 mg/dL, most patients will have some degree of volume depletion. Volume repletion and a saline diuresis are essential to the therapy. Isotonic saline should be infused intravenously in large volumes to increase calcium excretion. Furosemide may be used to increase the calciuresis once volume depletion is corrected. Thiazide diuretics should be avoided because they decrease urinary calcium excretion. Bisphosphonates, pyrophosphate analogs with a high affinity for hydroxyapatite, may be necessary to control the serum calcium in severe cases (80,81). Pamidronate and clodronate, two second generation bisphosphonates, are commonly used preparations. Both drugs are potent inhibitors of osteoclast bone resorption without significant bone demineralization (82). Pamidronate can be given as a single intravenous dose of 30–90 mg and may normalize the calcium for several weeks (81). Calcitonin, derived from the thyroid C-cell, inhibits osteoclast activity. The onset of calcitonin is rapid but with a short half-life and is usually not given as a sole therapy (83). Plicamycin (mithramycin) is an inhibitor of RNA synthesis and impairs osteoclast activity. It is an effective means to acutely lower serum calcium. However, the multiple toxicities associates with plicamycin have made its use uncommon. Glucocorticoids are also effective in the therapy of hypercalcemia in patients with hematologic malignancies. Hemodialysis with a low calcium bath is the preferred method of reducing serum calcium levels in patients with a severely depressed GFR.

1. *Methotrexate*

Methotrexate (MTX) induced ARF is caused by the precipitation of the drug and its metabolites in the tubular lumen (65,84). High doses of MTX ($>1\,g/m^2$) increase the risk of ARF. Once ARF develops, the excretion of MTX is reduced and the systemic toxicity of MTX is increased. Hydration and high urine output is essential to preventing MTX renal toxicity. Isotonic saline infusion and furosemide may be necessary to keep the urine output >100 mL/hr. Alkalinization of the urine to a pH >7.0 is also recommended. Once ARF has developed, it may be necessary to remove the drug with dialysis. Hemodialysis, using high blood flow rates with a high-flux dialyzer is an effective method of removing methotrexate (85). High-dose leucovorin therapy can reduce the systemic toxicity associated with MTX and ARF (86,87).

2. *Tumor Lysis Syndrome*

Tumor lysis syndrome is often a dramatic presentation of ARF in patients with malignancy. It is characterized by the development of hyperphosphatemia, hypocalcemia, hyperuricemia, and hyperkalemia. Tumor lysis syndrome can occur spontaneously during the rapid growth phase of malignancies such as bulky lymphoblastomas and Burkitt and non-Burkitt lymphomas that have extremely rapid cell turnover rates (88). More commonly it is seen when cytotoxic chemotherapy induces lysis of malignant cells in patients with large tumor burdens. Tumor lysis syndrome has developed in patients with non-Hodgkin lymphoma, acute lymphoblastic leukemia, chronic myelogenous leukemia in blast crises, small cell lung cancer, and metastatic breast cancer (89). In most patients, the ARF is reversible after aggressive supportive therapy including dialysis.

The pathophysiology of ARF associated with tumor lysis syndrome is related to two main factors, preexisting volume depletion prior to the onset of renal failure, and the precipitation of uric acid and calcium phosphate complexes in the renal tubules and tissue (90). Patients may be volume depleted from anorexia or nausea and vomiting associated with the malignancy, or from increased insensible losses from fever or tachypnea. Therefore, it is important to establish brisk flow of hypotonic urine to prevent or ameliorate ARF associated with tumor lysis syndrome.

Hyperuricemia is either present before treatment with chemotherapy or develops after therapy despite prophylaxis with allopurinol (91). Uric acid is nearly completely ionized at physiologic pH, but becomes progressively insoluble in the acidic environment of the renal tubules. Precipitation of uric acid causes intratubular obstruction leading to increased renal vascular resistance and decreased GFR (92). Moreover, a granulomatous reaction to intraluminal uric acid crystals and necrosis of tubular epithelium can be found on biopsy specimens.

Hyperphosphatemia and hypocalcemia also occur in tumor lysis syndrome. In patients who do not develop hyperuricemia in tumor lysis syndrome, ARF has been attributed to metastatic intrarenal calcification or acute nephrocalcinosis (93). Tumor lysis with release of inorganic phosphate results in acute hypocalcemia and metastatic calcification resulting in ARF.

Therefore, ARF associated with tumor lysis syndrome is the result of the combination of volume depletion in the face of urinary precipitation of uric acid in the renal tubules and parenchyma, and acute nephrocalcinosis from severe hyperphosphatemia. Since patients at risk for tumor lysis often have intra-abdominal lymphoma, urinary tract obstruction can be a contributing factor in the development of ARF.

Given the aforementioned pathogenetic factors for ARF, patients who are undergoing treatment with malignancies likely to experience rapid cell lysis should receive vigorous intravenous hydration to maintain good urinary flow and urinary dilution. In addition, because uric acid is very soluble at physiologic pH, sodium bicarbonate should be added to the intravenous fluid to achieve a pH >6.5 in the urine. Alkalinization can be achieved by the administration of 100 mEq/L of sodium bicarbonate in 1 L of D_5W at a rate of 200 mL/hr. Since metabolic alkalosis can aggravate hypocalcemia, caution should be exercised when using alkali in patients with low serum calcium levels. It is advisable to stop the infusion if the serum bicarbonate level is >30 mEq/L. Allopurinol is administered to inhibit uric acid formation. Through its metabolite oxypurinol, allopurinol inhibits xanthine oxidase and thereby blocks the conversion of hypoxanthine and xanthine to uric acid. During massive tumor lysis, uric acid excretion can still increase despite the administration of allopurinol so that intravenous hydration is still necessary to prevent ARF. Since allopurinol and its metabolites are excreted in the urine, the dose should be reduced in the face of impaired renal function. Uricase has been recently approved for use in the United States. It converts uric acid to water-soluble allantoin, thereby decreasing serum uric acid levels and urinary uric acid excretion (94). The use of uricase may obviate the need for urinary alkalinization, but good urine flow with hydration should be maintained given the probability of pre-existing volume depletion.

Dialysis for ARF associated with tumor lysis syndrome may be required for the traditional indications of fluid overload, hyperkalemia, hyperphosphatemia, or hyperuricemia unresponsive to medical management. There is some interest in using dialysis in patients at high risk of tumor lysis syndrome to prevent the development of renal failure. In a small trial in five children, continuous hemofiltration was started prior to administration of chemotherapy and appeared to prevent renal failure in 80% of the patients (95). However, given that continuous dialysis is complicated, expensive, and not without risk, its routine use as prophylaxis cannot be recommended.

3. *Thrombotic Microangiopathy*

Thrombotic microangiopathy (TMA) in the form of hemolytic uremic syndrome and thrombocytopenic purpura (TTP) is a disease of multiple etiologies manifesting as nonimmune hemolytic anemia, thrombocytopenia, varying degrees of encephalopathy, and renal failure due to platelet thrombi in the microcirculation of the kidneys. Laboratory findings include elevated indirect bilirubin and LDH levels, and depressed serum haptoglobin values. The characteristic renal lesion consists of vessel wall thickening in capillaries and arterioles, with swelling and detachment of endothelial cells from the basement membranes and accumulation of subendothelial fluffy material (96). These vascular lesions are indistinguishable from those seen in malignant hypertension or scleroderma renal crisis.

Typically, HUS develops in children with hemorrhagic colitis from verotoxin-producing *E. coli* infection associated with ingestion of undercooked meat (97). Renal failure is pronounced and altered sensorium is not consistently present. In contrast, idiopathic TTP is usually seen in adult women where encephalopathy is the predominant clinical feature whereas renal involvement is less severe. However, because of similar laboratory findings and the great overlap in clinical features, these syndromes likely share the same pathogenesis, endothelial cell dysfunction (98).

In cancer patients, malignancy, chemotherapy, radiation, immunosuppressive agents, and BMT can induce endothelial dysfunction leading to TMA and renal failure (Table 8).

Treatment of renal failure and TMA in cancer patients is mainly supportive with initiation of dialysis as necessary. Stopping any causative medications is advised. However, the role of plasmapheresis remains controversial. Although all forms of TMA share the same underlying pathogenesis of endothelial cell injury and dysfunction, the actual inciting event may be different in each case and not amenable to plasmapheresis. As an example, plasmapheresis has not been found to be an effective therapy for HUS in children despite its clear benefit in the treatment of idiopathic TTP (99). In TTP, an autoantibody to the von Willebrand factor-cleaving protease has been described (100). Inhibition of the cleaving enzyme leads to unusually large von Willebrand multimers that may agglutinate circulating platelets at sites with high levels of intravascular shear stress and trigger TMA. Plasma infusion may provide an exogenous source of cleaving protease to compete with the autoantibody while plasmapheresis will remove the pathogenic antibody. In HUS, no autoantibody has been found and may explain the ineffectiveness of plasmapheresis in this disorder (101). Reports on the use of plasmapheresis in cancer

Table 8 Thrombotic Microangiopathy in Cancer Patients

Chemotherapy
Mitomycin C
Platinum
Bleomycin
Holmium
Immunosuppressive agents
Cyclosporine
Tacrolimus
Malignancy
Gastric carcinoma
Bone marrow transplantation
BMT nephropathy
Radiation
Acute radiation nephritis
Malignant hypertension

patients are confined to those with BMT nephropathy. Most studies are small case series that are unable to clearly demonstrate true benefit. Nevertheless, when faced with a patient with the clinical characteristics of severe TTP after BMT, a trial of plasmapheresis is probably warranted.

4. *Bone Marrow Transplantation*

Acute renal failure, defined as doubling of the baseline serum creatinine level, may occur in up to 50% of patients who undergo bone marrow transplantation, of which half will undergo hemodialysis (102). Initially, it was assumed that the cause of ARF was multifactorial in nature given the severity of illness and the amount of nephrotoxin exposure. Instead, three distinctive renal syndromes associated with BMT were described and are categorized according to the time of onset (103). Renal complications are more prevalent in patients that undergo allogeneic transplants. When autologous stem cell transplants became the predominant method of BMT, the incidence of these disorders decreased (104).

Within the first few days of transplantation, ARF may develop from hemoglobinuria caused by infusion of hemolyzed red blood cells (105). Preservation of bone marrow with dimethyl sulfoxide (DMSO) will cause hemolysis of red blood cells present in the stored specimen, and subsequent infusion will result in hemoglobinuria. Three mechanisms are involved in the pathogenesis of hemoglobinuric ARF: renal vasoconstriction, direct cytotoxicity of hemoglobin, and intratubular cast formation. By scavenging nitric oxide and stimulating the release of endothelin and thromboxane, hemoglobin causes renal vasoconstriction. Hemoglobin is also toxic to renal tubular epithelial cells either directly or through release of iron, and by generation of reactive oxygen species (106). Intratubular cast formation occludes urinary flow thereby decreasing GFR, and prolongs cellular exposure to the harmful effects of hemoglobin.

Another renal syndrome usually occurs between 10 and 21 days after transplantation and is associated with the development of veno-occlusive disease (VOD) of the liver (103). VOD of the liver is characterized by tender hepatomegaly, fluid retention with ascites formation, and jaundice. It is the result of fibrous narrowing of small hepatic venules and sinusoids triggered by the pretransplant cytoreductive regimen, and is more common after allogeneic than autologous BMT. The ARF is similar in appearance to hepatorenal syndrome. Patients have hyperdynamic vital signs along with hyponatremia, oliguria, and low urinary sodium concentration. The urinalysis shows minimal proteinuria and muddy brown granular casts as a result of bile salts and bilirubin in the urine.The patients are usually resistant to diuretics andspontaneous recovery is rare. Risk factors for the development of ARF include weight gain, hyperbilirubinemia, use of amphotericin B, and a baseline serum creatinine level >0.7 mg/dL. The development of ARF adversely affects survival. In patients who require dialysis, the mortality rate approaches 80%. Although VOD can be diagnosed by either direct measurement of sinusoidal pressures or liver biopsy, these procedures are difficult or hazardous in BMT patients. Therefore, the diagnosis of VOD is usually made on clinical criteria. However, studies have shown that clinical criteria alone may not be sufficient to recognize or exclude a diagnosis of VOD (107). Small trials using infusions of prostaglandin E, pentoxifylline, or low-dose heparin to prevent the development of VOD have been promising (108–110). However, their use is not commonplace because of the associated risks of bleeding.

A late stage renal manifestation of transplantation referred to as "BMT nephropathy" usually occurs more than 6 months after the procedure. It ischaracterized by the development of ARF with microangiopathic hemolytic anemia, worsening thrombocytopenia, hypertension, and fluid retention. Hence, BMT nephropathy is a form of HUS (111). Patients may also have varying degrees of encephalopathy resembling TTP. It occurs in patients who receive cyclosporine for prevention of graft-vs.-host disease as well as those who do not. Radiation may play a role since its incidence appears higher after allogeneic compared with autologous BMT (104). Although plasmapheresis therapy is often successful in treating idiopathic TTP, the results in BMT nephropathy have been disappointing (112). Prognosis of BMT nephropathy is variable. Those patients who present with a modest rise in creatinine concentration and normal level of consciousness may have either spontaneous resolution or slow progression to chronic hemodialysis. Those patients who present with a fulminant course of TTP uniformly do poorly despite aggressive dialysis and plasmapheresis and often succumb to the disease.

VI. TUBULOINTERSTITIAL NEPHRITIS

Acute tubulointerstitial nephritis is a common cause of ARF accounting for 10% of cases in hospitalized patients (113). On renal biopsy, an interstitial cellular infiltrate is the hallmark of TIN. The infiltrate is predominantly mononuclear with T- and B-lymphocytes, macrophages, and natural killer cells (114). Scattered neutrophils, eosinophils, basophils, and plasma cells are also present. The infiltrate results in interstitial edema, disruption of tubular basement membrane, and destruction of the interstitial architecture.

Similar to glomerulonephritis, most forms of acute TIN are immune mediated (115). Although earlier investigations concentrated on humeral mechanisms with deposition of antibody or antigen–antibody immune complexes in the tubular basement membrane, there is abundant evidence now to suggest that cell-mediated immune responses account for most cases of acute TIN (116–119). Experimental studies demonstrate that renal tubular epithelial cells can process and present target antigens to T-cells, as well as strongly express Class II MHC determinants when stimulated by proinflammatory cytokines such as interferon-γ and tumor necrosis factor-α.

The clinical features of TIN are variable and in part depend on the inciting process (120). In general, besides renal failure, disruption of the normal tubulointerstitial compartment will produce findings consistent with renal tubular dysfunction including urinary concentrating defect, hyperchloremic metabolic acidosis, hypo- or hyperkalemia, and hypomagnesaemia. Modest proteinuria can be present, but nephrotic range proteinuria is distinctly unusual and associated with use of only a few medications: NSAIDs, interferon-α, and methacillin.

A. Drug-Induced Acute Tubulointerstitial Nephritis

Drug reactions are a major cause of acute TIN in patients with cancer because they are exposed to a large number of medications of different classes. The most commonly implicated agents are the penicillins, cephalosporins, and NSAIDs. It can be difficult to establish a direct link between a particular drug and ARF because patients typically receive a variety of potentially nephrotoxic medications making it uncertain which is the responsible agent. Also, comorbid conditions are usually present that could cause renal dysfunction. Since renal biopsy to determine the etiology of ARF is not routine, the diagnosis of acute TIN is presumptive. Acute TIN occurs within days to a few weeks of exposure to a drug, and there is no relationship between its development and the cumulative dose. Most patients present with symptoms of edema, hypertension, diminished urine output, and renal failure. The classical manifestations of allergic phenomena such as skin rash, arthralgias, fever, and eosinophilia are present in only a minority of patients (121). Occasionally, flank pain is prominent feature of the presentation. The presence of urinary eosinophils is of limited utility in the evaluation of ARF (122). The finding of eosinophils in the urine has a positive predictive value (PPV) for diagnosing acute TIN of only 40%. Absence of urinary eosinophils is more helpful in excluding the diagnosis although the negative predictive value (NPV) is still only 70%. Hansel rather than Wright staining is the preferred method of detecting eosinophiluria (18). Therefore, the diagnosis of acute TIN requires a high index of suspicion and knowledge of the potential causes. Clues to the presence of acute TIN are listed in Table 9.

Treatment of drug-induced acute TIN is cessation of the causative agent. Small case series have reported significant clinical response to corticosteroid administration (120,123,124). There are no large randomized placebo-controlled trials to guide treatment. Given the potential side effects of corticosteroids, their use should be restricted to patients with progressive renal failure despite stopping the offending drug. Consideration of renal biopsy in these cases is strongly recommended since the clinical diagnosis of TIN is presumptive and the risks of corticosteroid use in critically ill patients are high. Drug-induced acute TIN has been associated with a wide spectrum of medications as listed in Table 10.

1. *Fluoroquinolones*

All members of this class have been reported to cause acute TIN (121). There is typically fever, rash, and eosinophilia, but no other systemic features of an allergic reaction. Granulomatous TIN as well as necrotizing vasculitis has been reported on kidney biopsy (125).

Table 9 Clinical Features of Acute Tubulointerstitial Nephritis

Absence of other major causes to explain renal failure
Prior implication of drug as a cause of acute TIN
Nonoliguric acute renal failure
Microscopic or gross hematuria
Pyuria
White blood cell casts
Eosinophilia
Eosinophiluria
Fever
Skin rash
Arthralgias
Hyperchloremic metabolic acidosis (RTA)
Urinary concentrating defect
Hypo- or hyperkalemia
Hypomagnesemia

Table 10 Medications Causing Acute Tubulointerstitial Nephritis

Antibiotics
Cephalosporins
Fluoroquinolones
Penicillins
Rifampin
Sulfonamides
Vancomycin
Biological agents
Interleukin 2
α-Interferon
Anti-inflammatory agents
NSAIDs
COX-2 inhibitors
Diuretics
Furosemide
Thiazide diuretics
Immunosuppressive agents
Azathioprine
OKT3
Miscellaneous
Allopurinol
Cimetidine/ranitidine/famotidine
Omeprazole
Pamidronate

2. *Sulfonamides*

Sulfonamides are a relatively uncommon cause of acute TIN considering their widespread use. Oliguric ARF from acute TIN has been reported with sulfadiazine and cotrimoxazole. There may or may not be features of systemic hypersensitivity. Renal biopsy reveals interstitial infiltrates with eosinophils and occasional granulomas (126).

3. *Penicillins*

Acute tubulointerstitial nephritis has been reported with all the penicillins (121). Renal manifestations include hematuria, proteinuria, and oliguric ARF. Fever, rash, arthralgias, eosinophilia, pyuria, and eosinophiluria may also be present, particularly associated with the use of methacillin.

4. *Cephalosporins*

All generations of cephalosporins produce nephrotoxicity. Most cases involve direct toxicity to the renal tubular cells, resulting in ATN. In addition, cephalosporins can produce hypersensitivity reactions with skin rash, fever, eosinophilia, hematuria, and TIN (120,121). In some reports, renal failure was the only finding. Cephalosporins are structurally similar to the penicillins and cross-reactivity has been reported in 1–20% of patients.

5. *Biological Agents*

A high incidence of ARF associated with the administration of interleukin-2 and α-interferon has been reported (127,128). Most cases are attributed to a systemic capillary leak syndrome resulting in volume depletion, hypotension, prerenal azotemia, and ARF. However, there are several cases of acute TIN in patients treated with interleukin-2 and α-interferon. Nephrotic syndrome or nephrotic range proteinuria can develop with TIN caused by α-interferon. Renal biopsy demonstrates tubulointerstitial inflammation and glomerular abnormalities of minimal change disease.

6. *Nonsteroidal Anti-inflammatory Drugs*

The incidence of acute TIN due to NSAIDs is unknown, but the condition must be considered in the differential diagnosis of ARF given the widespread availability of these over-the-counter agents (129,130). Nephrotic range proteinuria is present in 10% of cases. Acute renal failure is usually nonoliguric and hematuria may be present. Typical features of hypersensitivity including urinary eosinophilia are rare. Women are affected much more frequently than men, and onset may be weeks to months after the start of NSAID use. Although recovery usually occurs within days to weeks of cessation of the drug, up to 20% progress to chronic renal failure.

B. Infective Tubulointerstitial Nephritis

1. *Bacterial Infection*

Bacterial pyelonephritis may result in ARF (131). This occurs most commonly in the setting of an ascending urinary tract infection superimposed on obstructive nephropathy. In patients with urinary tract infection or pyelonephritis who develop ARF, urgent imaging of the kidneys and urinary tract is necessary to exclude the presence obstruction. Acute renal failure as a result of pyelonephritis can also occur in the absence of urinary tract obstruction. Occasionally, renal involvement results from hematogenous spread. In such cases, blood cultures are frequently positive and there may be evidence of overt sepsis. Clinical distinction from ATN secondary to septicemia and septic shock may therefore be difficult. Renal histopathologic findings reveal an acute polymorphonuclear infiltrate in the interstitium with microabscess formation.

The prognosis in acute bacterial TIN is significantly worse than for ATN. Whereas patients with ATN are expected to make full recovery, bacterial TIN often progresses to severe interstitial scarring and progressive chronic renal failure. Patients require prolonged antibiotic treatment to eradicate the infection and close monitoring to minimize chronic progressive renal damage.

2. *Renal Candidiasis*

Mucosal ulceration and long-dwelling intravascular catheters are major risk factors for invasion of the blood stream by candida species. Other important risk factors include prolonged hospitalization, prior exposure to antimicrobial agents, corticosteroid therapy, the postoperative state, surgical wounds, chronic indwelling urinary catheters, and underlying malignancy. The kidneys are particularly vulnerable to candidal invasion. Therefore, a positive culture of candida from urine in the septicemic patient is considered as proof of renal candidiasis (132). The candida organisms progressively penetrate the renal parenchyma, forming hyphae and microabcesses especially in the cortical regions. Involvement of renal vasculature may result in renal infarction and papillary necrosis. Penetration of the organisms into the renal tubules may result in multiple sites of tubular obstruction, or the formation of large aggregates of fungi within the collecting system in the form of fungal balls or bezoars (133). This complication should be suspected in the presence of flank pain and microscopic hematuria. Candida species differ in virulence capacity to involve the kidneys. *Candida albicans* and *C. tropicalis* have the greatest propensity to cause widespread metastatic disease and renal invasion.

The patient with renal candidiasis usually presents with fever, candiduria, and unexplained progressive renal failure (134). There usually are no symptoms referable to the kidneys, while there may be symptoms arising from involvement of other organs including skin, mucosa, muscle, and eyes. Contrary to the case with bacterial urinary tract infections, there is no consensus as to the critical concentrations of candiduria required for a diagnosis of renal candidiasis. High colony counts may be a reflection of colonization rather than infection in patients with indwelling bladder catheters or nephrostomy tubes. The presence of hyphae in the urine does not have diagnostic significance, while the absence of pyuria does not rule out a diagnosis of renal candidiasis especially in the severely neutropenic patient. Diagnosis is further complicated by the lack of any tests to localize infection to the kidneys. Candida casts are highly suggestive of renal infection but are an unusual finding. The presence of fungal bezoars in the upper urinary tract can be excluded with renal ultrasonography or other suitable imaging procedure. A useful diagnostic test in the catheterized patient with candiduria, bladder washings with amphotericin B will clear the urine of colonization but not renal candidosis (135).

3. *Zygomatosis*

Invasive zygomatosis (mucormycosis) occurs predominantly in immunocompromised patients. Patients present with bilateral flank pain, fever, hematuria, pyuria, and renal failure, with radiographic evidence of enlarged nonfunctioning kidneys (136). Mortality is high and nephrectomy is usually required along with systemic antifungal therapy.

4. *Adenovirus infections*

Opportunistic infections secondary to systemic adenovirus infection occur in immunocompromised patients. Adenovirus type II appears to have a predilection for urothelial membrane surfaces and infections of the urothelium are frequent. As a result, adenovirus type II has been associated with urinary tract obstruction and hemorrhagic cystitis in this patient population. There are several reports of acute TIN with oliguric ARF in the setting of a severe pneumonitis, hepatitis, meningoencephalitis, myocarditis, and hemorrhagic cystitis (137,138).

5. *Polyomavirus (BK-Type) Infection*

Polyomaviruses are ubiquitous, usually acquired in childhood, and have a predilection for the urothelial surfaces. They have been associated with renal dysfunction and urinary tract obstruction from ureteral ulcerations and strictures. An acute TIN (BK nephropathy) has been reported in patients who have received renal or bone marrow transplants (139). The diagnosis of BK nephropathy is suggested by the presence of inclusion-bearing cells in the urine ("decoy" cells) and the detection by polymerase chain reaction of BK-virus DNA in the serum.

6. *Epstein–Barr Virus Infection*

Epstein–Barr virus (EBV) is associated with acute TIN and renal failure in both immunocompetent and immunocompromised patients (140). Other renal lesions associated with EBV and infectious mononucleosis includes acute glomerulonephritis, HUS, and rhabdomyolysis-induced ARF (141).

7. *Disseminated Histoplasmosis*

Immunocompromised patients can develop multiple organ failure from disseminated histoplasmosis. The disease usually follows a rapidly progressive course with a high mortality rate. Although uncommon, ARF does occur (142,143). Biopsy specimens show aggregates of phagocytosed macrophages in the glomerular capillaries and the tubular interstitium.

VII. ACUTE RENAL FAILURE ASSOCIATED WITH LYMPHOMA AND LEUKEMIA

A. Lymphoma

Infiltration of the kidneys by lymphoma cells may be detected in up to 90% of cases at autopsy. However, clinical renal disease as a result of infiltration is rare, most commonly seen in highly malignant and disseminated disease (144–147). The diagnosis of renal failure resulting from lymphomatous infiltration is necessarily one of exclusion because more common explanations for renal failure usually exist. The diagnosis may be suspected from clinical features and imaging studies. Patients may present with flank pain and hematuria. Renal ultrasonography reveals diffusely enlarged kidneys sometimes with multiple focal lesions. Although definitive diagnosis depends on renal biopsy, this procedure often is impossible because of the presence of contraindications. In such cases, the following criteria support the diagnosis of renal failure as a result of lymphomatous infiltration: (1) renal enlargement without obstruction; (2) absence of other causes of renal failure; and (3) rapid improvement of renal failure after radiotherapy or systemic chemotherapy.

B. Cytotoxic Nephropathy/ Hemophagocytic Syndrome

Hemophagocytic syndrome (HPS) is a reactive disorder that results from intense macrophage activation and cytokine release (148). It has developed in patients with malignant lymphoma, severe bacterial and viral infections, and in patients receiving prolonged parenteral nutrition with soluble lipids. Patients present with fever, rash, respiratory failure, lymphadenopathy, and hepatosplenomegaly. There have been recent reports of HPS in association with occult peripheral T-cell lymphomas causing severe ARF (149). Renal biopsy specimens are characterized by an unusually severe degree of interstitial edema with limited interstitial cellular infiltrate. A number of cytokines, including interferon-γ, TNF-α, interleukin-6, macrophage colony-stimulating factor, and CD-8 are upregulated in HPS and may explain the marked macrophage activation and cytokine release. In patients with lymphadenopathy who develop unexplained multiple organ dysfunction, markedly elevated cytokine levels support the diagnosis.

C. Leukemia

Leukemic infiltration of the kidneys is present in 60–90% of patients with chronic lymphocytic leukemia (CLL). Although uncommon, many cases of renal failure attributable to leukemic infiltration are known (150–152). Ultrasound usually reveals bilateral renal enlargement. Chemotherapy often produces a dramatic improvement in renal function.

There are reports of patients with CLL who develop ARF from leukemic infiltration and are infected with polyomavirus (153). Urine from patients demonstrates viral inclusions in tubular cells ("decoy" cells) and blood is positive for BK virus DNA. Therefore, in leukemia patients with ARF considered due to leukemic infiltration, evidence for coexisting BK virus infection should be sought.

Patients with significantly elevated white cell counts can develop ARF from leukostasis. Leukemic cells occlude the peritubular and glomerular capillaries thereby decreasing GFR. Patients may be oliguric but their renal function often improves with therapeutic leukopheresis or chemotherapy. Leukostasis has been described in both acute and chronic leukemia.

VIII. RADIATION NEPHRITIS

Renal failure and hypertension develop when the kidneys are exposed to >2300 rad of radiation in fractionated doses over a period of 3–5 weeks (154). A characteristic of radiation injury is the long latent period between radiation and overt nephrotoxicity. The effects of DNA damage from radiation are not evident until cell division occurs. The latency period depends on the proliferation rate of a particular tissue. The recognition of radiation injury has led to treatment protocols that have significantly minimized exposure and the incidence of radiation nephropathy. In the past, abdominal radiation and total body irradiation for BMT were leading causes of radiation nephritis. Today, sequential radiosensitizing chemotherapy with radiation is a more prevalent mode (155).

Five clinical syndromes of radiation injury to the kidney are described: (1) acute radiation nephropathy; (2) chronic radiation nephropathy; (3) asymptomatic proteinuria; (4) benign hypertension; and (5) malignant hypertension.

A. Acute Radiation Nephropathy

Acute radiation nephropathy usually occurs after a latent period of 6–12 months (156,157). Patients present with ARF accompanied by microangiopathic hemolytic anemia with schistocytes, thrombocytopenia, hypertension, and fluid overload with edema. Renal biopsy findings are not specific to radiation injury and are typical of HUS. The onset of ARF can be abrupt and the degree of anemia and hypertension is severe. Although progression to chronic renal failure is the rule, there are reports of response to ACE-inhibitor therapy in stabilizing the renal function (158). The development of end stage renal disease (ESRD) is a poor prognostic event in these patients as survival on chronic dialysis is poor compared to that of age-matched nondiabetic and diabetic patients.

Malignant hypertension as a complication of radiation to the kidney has been reported as a feature of acute radiation nephropathy, but also occasionally as an isolated late manifestation presenting 18 months to 11 years after irradiation. The incidence of this complication is much less with the availability of the new classes of antihypertensive agents, in particular, the ACE-inhibitors.

IX. PREVENTION OF ACUTE TUBULAR NECROSIS

There currently exist no known therapeutic options to ameliorate ARF or hasten its recovery. Dialysis remains only a supportive measure to treat or prevent the metabolic and hypervolemic complications of renal failure. Therefore, prevention of ARF remains a keystone in the treatment of the critically ill patient.

A. General Measures

Most cases of ARF in the intensive care unit are the result of multiple factors including exposure to nephrotoxic agents and relative or frank renal hypoperfusion. Avoidance of potential nephrotoxins such as intravenous radiocontrast, aminoglycoside antibiotics, and antifungal agents, when possible, is prudent. Although NSAIDs generally have a low nephrotoxic risk, the potential renal vasoconstrictive effect of these agents should be remembered in selected patients, such as those with sepsis, heart failure, cirrhosis, nephrotic syndrome, volume depletion, and hypoalbuminemia. Single daily dosing of aminoglycoside antibiotics is associated with a lower risk of nephrotoxicity with equivalent antimicrobial efficacy compared to multiple dosing strategies (159). Drug modifications such as nonionic radiocontrast and lipid-emulsified amphotericin B may also reduce the incidence of ARF (160,161). Aggressive diuresis, particularly in conjunction with the use of ACE-inhibitors or ARBs must be avoided. Monitoring the serum levels of potential nephrotoxic drugs such as aminoglycosides, CSA, tacrolimus, and vancomycin is recommended.

Maintenance of adequate intravascular volume to preserve renal perfusion pressure is essential. Many critically ill patients have capillary leak associated with the systemic inflammatory response syndrome (SIRS) resulting in severe interstitial edema and renal hypoperfusion. Often these patients also are receiving intravenous vasopressor agents and positive pressure ventilation that further impair renal blood flow. How exactly to maintain effective arterial blood volume in such circumstances remains a contentious issue. Aggressive hydration with crystalloid solutions such as 0.9% sodium chloride can worsen interstitial edema and pulmonary function. Colloidal solutions such as various starches and human albumin might appear to be attractive alternatives, but there is little solid evidence that establishes their superiority in clinical trials (45,162,163). Systematic reviews of randomized controlled trials comparing crystalloids with colloids have yielded conflicting results. Some trials have found an increased mortality rate associated with the administration of human albumin and hydroxyethylstarch while others have not (164,165). So despite the importance of fluid therapy in the prevention of ARF, the nature of the optimum fluid resuscitation regimen remains a disputed topic. For the time being it appears that treatment of the underlying diagnosis, usually sepsis, and general supportive efforts, including ultrafiltration if necessary, are the mainstays of therapy.

In the critically ill patient, it is often difficult to predict when a potential insult to the kidneys will occur, making true prophylaxis difficult. However, the administration of intravenous radiocontrast is one exception. In this case, the administration of intravenous fluid, in the form of 0.45% sodium chloride, significantly decreased the incidence of ARF when compared to the administration of intravenous fluid with either mannitol or furosemide (166). Although radiocontrast is a renal tubular toxin, it also causes intense renal vasoconstriction, in part due to the release of endothelin, which may explain the salutatory effects of fluid administration. Another study suggests that a solution containing 0.9% sodium chloride is more efficacious than one containing 0.45% sodium chloride in preventing ARF (167).

B. Specific Measures

1. *Mucomyst® (n-Acetyl-Cysteine)*

Mucomyst is an antioxidant and causes renal vasodilatation by generating increased levels of nitric oxide (NO). Based on these effects, Mucomyst was used in several small human trials for the prevention of ARF from radiocontrast agents in high-risk individuals. The trials have shown that its administration results in a significantly smaller change in baseline serum creatinine values compared to changes in the placebo group (168,169). However, whether or not Mucomyst prevents severe ARF and the need for dialysis has not been determined. At this point, it is probably reasonable to provide Mucomyst prior to radiocontrast administration in patients at risk for the development of ARF. However, there exist no convincing data to support the routine administration of Mucomyst in other clinical circumstances to prevent the development of ARF.

2. *Low-Dose Dopamine*

Low-dose dopamine administration (1–3 μg/kg/min) to normal individuals causes renal vasodilatation and increased GRF, and acts as a proximal tubule diuretic. Due to these effects, numerous studies have used low-dose dopamine to either prevent or treat ARF in a variety of clinical settings. It has been given as prophylaxis for ARF associated with radiocontrast administration, repair of aortic aneurysms, orthotopic liver transplantation, unilateral nephrectomy, renal transplantation, and chemotherapy with interferon (170,171). Yet despite more than 20 years of clinical experience, prevention trials with low-dose dopamine all have been small, inadequately randomized, of limited statistical power, and with end-points of questionable clinical significance. Furthermore, there is concern for the potential harmful effects of dopamine, even at low doses. It can trigger tachyarrhythmias and myocardial ischemia, decrease intestinal blood flow, and suppress T-cell function (170–172). It has also been shown to increase the risk of RCN when given as prophylaxis to patients with diabetic nephropathy (173). Therefore, the use of low-dose dopamine for renal protection should be abandoned.

3. *Low-Dose Fenoldopam*

Fenoldopam is a pure dopamine type-1 receptor agonist that has similar hemodynamic effects to dopamine in the kidney without α- and β-adrenergic stimulation. Limited trials suggest administration of fenoldopam reduces the occurrence of ARF from radiocontrast agents and following repair of aortic aneurysms (174,175). However, as in the case of low-dose dopamine, there exists no randomized controlled trials to support its indiscriminate use and should be restricted to well-designed clinical studies.

4. *Diuretics*

Furosemide is a loop diuretic and vasodilator that may decrease oxygen consumption in the loop of Henle by inhibiting sodium transport, thus lessening ischemic injury. By increasing urinary flow, it may also reduce intratubular obstruction and back-leak of filtrate. Based on these properties, furosemide might be expected to prevent ARF. However, there is little data to support its use. Furosemide was found to be ineffective when used to prevent ARF after cardiac surgery, and to increase the risk of ARF when given to prevent contrast nephropathy (166,176).

Mannitol is an osmotic diuretic that can also scavenge free radicals. It may be beneficial when added to organ preservation solutions during renal transplantation and protect against ARF caused by rhabdomyolysis if given extremely early (177,178). Otherwise, mannitol has not been shown to be useful in the prevention of ARF. In fact, mannitol may aggravate ARF from radiocontrast agents (173).

5. *Atrial Natriuretic Peptide*

Atrial natriuretic peptide (ANP) causes vasodilatation of the afferent arteriole and constriction of the efferent arteriole resulting in an increased GFR. It also inhibits renal tubular sodium reabsorption. Most studies with ANP concern the treatment of established ARF. However, in two studies that administered ANP in renal transplant recipients to prevent primary renal dysfunction, no benefit was found (179,180). As with low-dose dopamine and mannitol, one study suggested that ANP prophylaxis might worsen renal function in diabetic patients receiving radiocontrast material (173).

6. *Insulin-Like Growth Factor-1*

Insulin-like growth factor-1 (IGF-1) increases renal blood flow and induces cell proliferation and differentiation. In addition, it reverses apoptosis. In animal models, it ameliorates renal injury associated with ischemia and may prevent injury following renal transplantation (181,182). IGF-1 has been given to a small group of patients in a single trial for prophylaxis of ARF following aortic aneurysm repair (183). IGF-1 was started postoperatively in a randomized placebo-controlled fashion. It was well tolerated, and produced a modest increase in the creatinine clearance in the treated group compared to the placebo group. However, no patients developed ARF necessitating dialysis. Hence, the role, if any, for IGF-1 in the prevention of ARF remains unknown.

X. TREATMENT OF ACUTE TUBULAR NECROSIS

Effective treatment of ARF in critically ill patients is lacking despite substantial advances in the understanding of its pathogenesis at a cellular and molecular level. This lack of efficacy results from numerous factors: the multifactorial nature of ARF in the intensive care unit, reliance on changes in serum creatinine levels to detect changes in GFR, varying definitions of ARF, the high mortality rate of ICU patients in general, and the lack of consensus on the timing and appropriate form of acute dialysis. Although a wide variety of agents including loop diuretics, low-dose dopamine, ANP, thyroid hormone, and IGF-1 are effective in animal models, they have not been effective in the treatment of ARF in the clinical setting (49,184).

The reasons that these therapies have been highly effective only in animals remain speculative. Most human trials involve moderately or severely ill patients in the ICU with multiple organ failure, whereas animal models of ARF rely on a single mechanism of injury in otherwise healthy animals (185). In addition, the time of the renal insult is known precisely in the models allowing for early administration of the intervention. In clinical trials, on the other hand, therapy is delayed because of reliance on a change of the serum creatinine level to indicate ARF. By the time the serum creatinine concentration has increased, there has been a significant decline in the GFR and the renal injury has been present for a prolonged period. Timing of the intervention may be critical to its success. Very early in ARF hemodynamic factors and oxidant injury may predominate while later inflammation may play a more prominent role. Unfortunately, there still exists no easily available reliable marker of early ARF. Therefore, therapy of ARF remains primarily supportive.

A. Low-Dose Dopamine

Numerous trials using low-dose dopamine to treat ARF have been reported in the last several years that suggest its use is beneficial (170,171,186). However, most studies were either uncontrolled case series or small randomized trials with limited statistical power. More recently, a large randomized placebo-controlled trial in 328 critically ill patients with early ARF sufficiently powered to detect a small benefit was reported (187). There was no effect of low-dose dopamine on renal function, need for dialysis, ICU or hospital length of stay, or mortality. These findings combined with the aforementioned potential deleterious effects of low-dose dopamine are strong arguments for abandoning its use entirely in ARF.

B. Diuretics

In patients with ARF, several studies have found no benefit of loop diuretics (188–192). Their use did not accelerate renal recovery, decrease the need for dialysis, or reduce mortality. It was shown that the mortality rate of oliguric patients who responded to furosemide with a diuresis was lower than those who did not (19,192). However, the clinical characteristics, severity of renal failure, and mortality rates were similar in patients with either spontaneous nonoliguric ARF or patients who became nonoliguric after furosemide. This implies that those patients able to respond to furosemide are less sick and have intrinsically less severe renal damage than nonresponders, rather than there existing any true therapeutic benefit to furosemide administration. Although administration of furosemide might improve fluid management if it induces a diuresis, a retrospective review of a recent trial in critically ill patients with ARF found diuretic use to be associated with an increased risk of death and nonrecovery of renal function (193). Most of the increased risk, however, was seen in those patients unresponsive to high doses of diuretics implying they had more severe disease. Therefore, diuretics should be used with caution in critically ill patients. Diuretics should be withdrawn if there is no response. In patients who experience an increase in urine output, volume status must be closely monitored since the injured kidneys are susceptible to further damage from mild changes in perfusion pressure. To maintain the diuresis, a continuous infusion of drug is probably preferable to intermittent bolus administration (194). Although there are no large randomized controlled trials, the overall evidence suggests that continuous infusion of diuretics as opposed to bolus administration is more effective and associated with less toxicity and delayed development of diuretic resistance.

C. Atrial Natriuretic Peptide

Atrial natriuretic peptide (ANP) improved renal blood flow and GRF in an uncontrolled trial of 11 patients who developed ARF after cardiac surgery (195). In an open-labeled trial, infusion of ANP to patients with ARF increased GFR and decreased the need for dialysis by nearly 50% (196). Based on these results, a randomized placebo-controlled trial of 504 critically ill patients with ARF was conducted (197). Despite the large size of the trial, ANP administration had no effect on 21-day dialysis-free survival, mortality, or change in plasma creatinine concentration. Although a subgroup analysis of the study suggested that ANP might be beneficial in those patients with oliguric renal failure, a subsequent similar trial in patients with oliguric renal failure failed to demonstrate any benefit of ANP (198). Hence, there is no convincing evidence to support the use of ANP in the treatment of ARF.

D. Insulin-like Growth Factor-1

Based on the positive effects of insulin-like growth factor-1 (IGF-1) in animal models of ARF, a randomized placebo-controlled trial was conducted in 72 critically ill patients with ARF (199). The results showed there was no difference in the two groups in post-treatment GFR, need for dialysis, or mortality. In anuric patients, IGF-1 administration was associated with a slower rate of improvement in urine output and GFR. So despite the ample evidence that IGF-1 accelerates renal recovery in animal models of ARF, there is no support for its use in humans.

E. Thyroxine

The administration of thyroid hormone following the initiation of ARF in a variety of ischemic and nephrotoxic animal models was found to be effective in promoting recovery of renal function (200–203). Based on these results, thyroxine was administered to 59 patients with ARF in a randomized placebo-controlled trial (204). Patients were well matched in baseline characteristics. Administration of thyroxine had no effect on any renal parameter. However, the trial was terminated early because of a significantly higher mortality rate in the patients who received thyroxine.

XI. RENAL REPLACEMENT THERAPY

Dialysis initially entered clinical practice more than 50 years ago, yet there is no consensus on the appropriate timing for initiation of dialysis, the dose or intensity of dialysis, or the mode of dialysis (intermittent vs. continuous) in patients with ARF. By tradition, clinical parameters such as severe electrolyte imbalance, pulmonary edema, intractable metabolic acidosis, azotemia (BUN>100 mg/dL), and uremia are used as indications for starting dialysis, but these parameters may be inappropriate in the critically ill patient. No studies have clearly defined the optimal time to initiate dialysis. Retrospective trials done more than 30 years ago suggested that maintaining a BUN level below 150 mg/dL conferred a survival benefit (205,206). In a later prospective trial, more intensive dialysis (maintaining the BUN level below 60 mg/dL compared to 100 mg/dL) did not improve mortality (207). Part of the problem is that the dialysis procedure itself may be harmful. Bleeding and infection from vascular access, and hypotension and arrhythmias from changes in volume may complicate dialysis. Studies also show that the dialysis procedure may prolong the course of ARF (208). Delayed recovery may result from hypotension or activation of an inflammatory cascade by the interaction of blood components with the dialyzer membrane (209).

A. Intensity of Dialysis

Once dialysis has been initiated, it has not been established how often and how long it should be prescribed. In other words, what is the optimal intensity of dialysis that provides the patient the benefits of the procedure without exposure to undue risk? Equally germane to the issue is identifying appropriate end-points to define "adequate" dialysis in an ICU patient. Survival rate appears most relevant. However, given the severity of the patients' comorbid diseases, it may be unrealistic to expect that various intensities of dialysis will impact mortality, or at the very least, to expect clinical trials to be powered sufficiently to prove any effect. Currently, there is interest in applying some form of measuring urea removal in patients with ARF to define dialysis adequacy analogous to the circumstance in chronic outpatient dialysis. The National Cooperative Dialysis Study demonstrated that morbidity and hospitalization rates were inversely related to the amount of urea removal per treatment in chronic stable hemodialysis patients (210). Whether such a relationship exists in acutely ill patients with higher urea generation rates because of hypercatabolism is unknown. Recent trials have begun to address this issue. A study from the Cleveland Clinic showed a link between dialysis intensity and outcome in ICU patients when underling comorbidity was accounted for using the Cleveland Clinic Severity of Illness Score (211). Dialysis had no effect on the outcome of patients with low or high severity scores, but a beneficial effect in those with intermittent scores. Higher delivery of dialysis as measured by the reduction of urea concentration was associated with a significant decrease in morbidity when compared to low-dose delivery in patients with an intermediate severity score. A more recent study in 72 critically ill patients with ARF randomized to daily or alternate day dialysis reported improved survival with the more intense regimen (212). However, in this study, the dose of dialysis per session was significantly lower than what would be considered adequate for a stable patient on chronic hemodialysis. It thereby proves that underdosing dialysis in a critically ill patient is detrimental but failed to define what should be considered adequate for such patients. Although one could take the position that more dialysis is better, given the aforementioned risks associated with dialysis, that attitude may be cavalier. In fact, in a trial recently reported in chronic renal failure patients, increasing the dose of dialysis beyond what is currently considered adequate conferred no additional benefit to patients (213). Therefore, "excessive" dialysis in critically ill patients may only increase the exposure to risk without imparting any additional benefit. Until these issues are resolved by ongoing clinical trials, it seems prudent to rely on clinical parameters such as electrolyte and acid–base balance, control of volume overload, and avoidance of azotemia (maintaining the BUN below 60 mg/dL) to guide dialytic therapy.

B. Mode of Dialysis

In the past, intermittent hemodialysis (IHD) was the treatment of choice for ARF. However, as a result of the rapid solute removal and large volume shifts associated with its use, patients with hemodynamic instability poorly tolerate it. Because of the risk of hypotension and the possibility of prolonging ARF, newer modes of dialysis to minimize hypotension have been devised. Continuous renal replacement therapy (CRRT) removes solute and fluid at a much slower rate than IHD thus minimizing hypotension (214,215). Use of CRRT was originally reserved for patients with hemodynamic instability or massive fluid overload who could not otherwise tolerate IHD. Although dialysis was usually successful in such patients, the mortality rate remained high due to the underlying severity of illness. Given the better hemodynamic profile of CRRT, as well as potentially better solute clearance and removal of inflammatory cytokines, it was thought that CRRT would lead to better outcomes in critically ill patients who could otherwise tolerate IHD.

CRRT and IHD have been compared in a number of nonrandomized or retrospective trials that have championed CRRT as the modality of choice in critically ill patients. However, prospective or randomized trials comparing IHD and CRRT have not found CRRT to confer a better outcome (216,217). This somewhat surprising finding may be the result of studying critically ill patients where multiple factors play a role in the ultimate outcome. For now, it appears that IHD and CRRT are equivalent methods of treatment for ARF in the ICU.

There is also interest in using CRRT for nonrenal indications including sepsis and acute respiratory distress syndrome (ARDS) (218). It is based on the assumption that dialytic removal of inflammatory cytokines such as TNF-α and interleukins improves survival (219). Small trials suggesting CRRT is beneficial all have serious methodological flaws. In addition, although cytokines can be removed by filtration and/or absorption to the filter, the actual quantity is low compared to endogenous clearance (220). Clearance is also indiscriminant and can remove cytokines that may be beneficial in the face of critical illness. Until adequate clinical trials are completed, the use of CRRT for nonrenal indications cannot be recommended.

REFERENCES

1. Hou SH, et al. Hospital-acquired renal insufficiency: a prospective study. Am J Med 1983; 74(2):243–248.
2. Albright RC Jr. Acute renal failure: a practical update. Mayo Clin Proc 2001; 76(1):67–74.
3. Brivet FG, et al. Acute renal failure in intensive care units—causes, outcome, and prognostic factors of hospital mortality; a prospective, multicenter study. French Study Group on Acute Renal Failure. Crit Care Med 1996; 24(2):192–198.
4. van Bommel EF, Leunissen KM, Weimar W. Continuous renal replacement therapy for critically ill patients: an update. J Intensive Care Med 1994; 9(6): 265–280.
5. Nash K, Hafeez A, Hou S. Hospital-acquired renal insufficiency. Am J Kidney Dis 2002; 39(5):930–936.
6. Huynh TT, et al. Determinants of hospital length of stay after thoracoabdominal aortic aneurysm repair. J Vasc Surg 2002; 35(4):648–653.
7. Dimick JB, et al. Complications and costs after high-risk surgery: where should we focus quality improvement initiatives? J Am Coll Surg 2003; 196(5):671–678.
8. Silvester W. Outcome studies of continuous renal replacement therapy in the intensive care unit. Kidney Int Suppl 1998; 66:S138–S141.
9. Douma CE, et al. Predicting mortality in intensive care patients with acute renal failure treated with dialysis. J Am Soc Nephrol 1997; 8(1):111–117.
10. Halstenberg WK, Goormastic M, Paganini EP. Validity of four models for predicting outcome in critically ill acute renal failure patients. Clin Nephrol 1997; 47(2):81–86.
11. Liano F, et al. Prognosis of acute tubular necrosis: an extended prospectively contrasted study. Nephron 1993; 63(1):21–31.
12. Robertshaw M, Lai KN, Swaminathan R. Prediction of creatinine clearance from plasma creatinine: comparison of five formulae. Br J Clin Pharmacol 1989; 28(3):275–280.
13. Vervoort G, Willems HL, Wetzels JF. Assessment of glomerular filtration rate in healthy subjects and normoalbuminuric diabetic patients: validity of a new (MDRD) prediction equation. Nephrol Dial Transplant 2002; 17(11):1909–1913.
14. Han WK, et al. Kidney injury molecule-1 (KIM-1): a novel biomarker for human renal proximal tubule injury. Kidney Int 2002; 62(1):237–244.
15. Espinel CH, Gregory AW. Differential diagnosis of acute renal failure. Clin Nephrol 1980; 13(2):73–77.

16. Miller TR, et al. Urinary diagnostic indices in acute renal failure: a prospective study. Ann Intern Med 1978; 89(1):47–50.
17. Zarich S, Fang LS, Diamond JR. Fractional excretion of sodium. Exceptions to its diagnostic value. Arch Intern Med 1985; 145(1):108–112.
18. Nolan CR III, Anger MS, Kelleher SP. Eosinophiluria—a new method of detection and definition of the clinical spectrum. N Engl J Med 1986; 315(24): 1516–1519.
19. Anderson RJ, et al. Nonoliguric acute renal failure. N Engl J Med 1977; 296(20):1134–1138.
20. Whelton A. Nephrotoxicity of nonsteroidal anti-inflammatory drugs: physiologic foundations and clinical implications. Am J Med 1999; 106(5B):13S–24S.
21. Bennett WM, Henrich WL, Stoff JS. The renal effects of nonsteroidal anti-inflammatory drugs: summary and recommendations. Am J Kidney Dis 1996; 28(1 suppl 1):S56–S62.
22. Griffin MR, Yared A, Ray WA. Nonsteroidal antiinflammatory drugs and acute renal failure in elderly persons. Am J Epidemiol 2000; 151(5):488–496.
23. Zhao SZ, et al. A comparison of renal-related adverse drug reactions between rofecoxib and celecoxib, based on the World Health Organization/Uppsala Monitoring Centre safety database. Clin Ther 2001; 23(9): 1478–1491.
24. Knight EL, et al. Predictors of decreased renal function in patients with heart failure during angiotensin-converting enzyme inhibitor therapy: results from the studies of left ventricular dysfunction (SOLVD). Am Heart J 1999; 138(5 Pt 1):849–855.
25. Schoolwerth AC, et al. Renal considerations in angiotensin converting enzyme inhibitor therapy: a statement for healthcare professionals from the Council on the Kidney in Cardiovascular Disease and the Council for High Blood Pressure Research of the American Heart Association. Circulation 2001; 104(16):1985–1991.
26. Adhiyaman V, et al. Nephrotoxicity in the elderly due to co-prescription of angiotensin converting enzyme inhibitors and nonsteroidal anti-inflammatory drugs. J R Soc Med 2001; 94(10):512–514.
27. Myers BD, Newton L. Cyclosporine-induced chronic nephropathy: an obliterative microvascular renal injury. J Am Soc Nephrol 1991; 2(2 suppl 1):S45–S52.
28. Myers BD, et al. The long-term course of cyclosporine-associated chronic nephropathy. Kidney Int 1988; 33(2):590–600.
29. Lopau K, et al. Tacrolimus in acute renal failure: does L-arginine-infusion prevent changes in renal hemodynamics? Transpl Int 2000; 13(6):436–442.
30. Medina PJ, Sipols JM, George JN. Drug-associated thrombotic thrombocytopenic purpura-hemolytic uremic syndrome. Curr Opin Hematol 2001; 8(5): 286–293.
31. Busca A, Uderzo C. BMT: bone marrow transplant associated thrombotic microangiopathy. Hematology 2000; 5(1):53–67.
32. Gharpure VS, et al. Thrombotic thrombocytopenic purpura associated with FK506 following bone marrow transplantation. Bone Marrow Transplant 1995; 16(5):715–716.
33. Kamel KS, et al. Studies to determine the basis for hyperkalemia in recipients of a renal transplant who are treated with cyclosporine. J Am Soc Nephrol 1992; 2(8):1279–1284.
34. Kramer L, Horl WH. Hepatorenal syndrome. Semin Nephrol 2002; 22(4):290–301.
35. Gines P, Arroyo V. Hepatorenal syndrome. J Am Soc Nephrol 1999; 10(8):1833–1839.
36. Gonwa TA, et al. Impact of pretransplant renal function on survival after liver transplantation. Transplantation 1995; 59(3):361–365.
37. Guevara M, et al. Reversibility of hepatorenal syndrome by prolonged administration of ornipressin and plasma volume expansion. Hepatology 1998; 27(1):35–41.
38. Uriz J, et al. Terlipressin plus albumin infusion: an effective and safe therapy of hepatorenal syndrome. J Hepatol 2000; 33(1):43–48.
39. Mulkay JP, et al. Long-term terlipressin administration improves renal function in cirrhotic patients with type 1 hepatorenal syndrome: a pilot study. Acta Gastroenterol Belg 2001; 64(1):15–19.
40. Angeli P, et al. Reversal of type 1 hepatorenal syndrome with the administration of midodrine and octreotide. Hepatology 1999; 29(6): 1690–1697.
41. Holt S, et al. Improvement in renal function in hepatorenal syndrome with N-acetylcysteine. Lancet 1999; 353(9149):294–295.
42. Guevara M, et al. Transjugular intrahepatic portosystemic shunt in hepatorenal syndrome: effects on renal function and vasoactive systems. Hepatology 1998; 28(2):416–422.
43. Brensing KA, et al. Long term outcome after transjugular intrahepatic portosystemic stent-shunt in non-transplant cirrhotics with hepatorenal syndrome: a phase II study. Gut 2000; 47(2):288–295.
44. Arroyo V, et al. Definition and diagnostic criteria of refractory ascites and hepatorenal syndrome in cirrhosis. International Ascites Club. Hepatology 1996; 23(1):164–176.
45. Klahr S. Obstructive nephropathy. Kidney Int 1998; 54(1):286–300.
46. Batlle DC, Arruda JA, Kurtzman NA. Hyperkalemic distal renal tubular acidosis associated with obstructive uropathy. N Engl J Med 1981; 304(7):373–380.
47. Schlueter W, Batlle DC. Chronic obstructive nephropathy. Semin Nephrol 1988; 8(1):17–28.
48. Vaughan ED Jr, Gillenwater JY. Diagnosis, characterization and management of post-obstructive diuresis. J Urol 1973; 109(2):286–292.
49. Star RA. Treatment of acute renal failure. Kidney Int 1998; 54(6):1817–1831.
50. Murphy SW, Barrett BJ, Parfrey PS. Contrast nephropathy. J Am Soc Nephrol 2000; 11(1):177–182.

51. Solomon R. Contrast-medium-induced acute renal failure. Kidney Int 1998; 53(1):230–242.
52. Bakris GL, et al. Radiocontrast medium-induced declines in renal function: a role for oxygen free radicals. Am J Physiol 1990; 258(1 Pt 2):F115–F120.
53. Levy EM, Viscoli CM, Horwitz RI. The effect of acute renal failure on mortality. A cohort analysis. JAMA 1996; 275(19):1489–1494.
54. Swan SK. Aminoglycoside nephrotoxicity. Semin Nephrol 1997; 17(1):27–33.
55. Humes HD, Weinberg JM. The effect of gentamicin on antidiuretic hormone-stimulated osmotic water flow in the toad urinary bladder. J Lab Clin Med 1983; 101(3):472–478.
56. Barza M, et al. Single or multiple daily doses of aminoglycosides: a meta-analysis. Br Med J 1996; 312(7027):338–345.
57. Hatala R, Dinh TT, Cook DJ. Single daily dosing of aminoglycosides in immunocompromised adults: a systematic review. Clin Infect Dis 1997; 24(5):810–815.
58. Sawaya BP, et al. Direct vasoconstriction as a possible cause for amphotericin B-induced nephrotoxicity in rats. J Clin Invest 1991; 87(6):2097–2107.
59. Sawaya BP, Briggs JP, Schnermann J. Amphotericin B nephrotoxicity: the adverse consequences of altered membrane properties. J Am Soc Nephrol 1995; 6(2):154–164.
60. Barton CH, et al. Renal magnesium wasting associated with amphotericin B therapy. Am J Med 1984; 77(3):471–474.
61. Sacks P, Fellner SK. Recurrent reversible acute renal failure from amphotericin. Arch Intern Med 1987; 147(3):593–595.
62. Branch RA. Prevention of amphotericin B-induced renal impairment. A review on the use of sodium supplementation. Arch Intern Med 1988; 148(11):2389–2394.
63. Llanos A, et al. Effect of salt supplementation on amphotericin B nephrotoxicity. Kidney Int 1991; 40(2):302–308.
64. Leibbrandt ME, et al. Critical subcellular targets of cisplatin and related platinum analogs in rat renal proximal tubule cells. Kidney Int 1995; 48(3):761–770.
65. Ries F, Klastersky J. Nephrotoxicity induced by cancer chemotherapy with special emphasis on cisplatin toxicity. Am J Kidney Dis 1986; 8(5):368–379.
66. Hensley ML, et al. American Society of Clinical Oncology clinical practice guidelines for the use of chemotherapy and radiotherapy protectants. J Clin Oncol 1999; 17(10):3333–3355.
67. Skinner R. Strategies to prevent nephrotoxicity of anticancer drugs. Curr Opin Oncol 1995; 7(4):310–315.
68. Skinner R, et al. Nephrotoxicity after ifosfamide. Arch Dis Child 1990; 65(7):732–738.
69. Lee BS, et al. Ifosfamide nephrotoxicity in pediatric cancer patients. Pediatr Nephrol 2001; 16(10): 796–799.
70. Skinner R, Cotterill SJ, Stevens MC. Risk factors for nephrotoxicity after ifosfamide treatment in children: a UKCCSG Late Effects Group study. United Kingdom Children's Cancer Study Group. Br J Cancer 2000; 82(10):1636–1645.
71. Aleksa K, Woodland C, Koren G. Young age and the risk for ifosfamide-induced nephrotoxicity: a critical review of two opposing studies. Pediatr Nephrol 2001; 16(12):1153–1158.
72. Hartmann JT, et al. The use of reduced doses of amifostine to ameliorate nephrotoxicity of cisplatin/ ifosfamide-based chemotherapy in patients with solid tumors. Anticancer Drugs 2000; 11(1):1–6.
73. Holt SG, Moore KP. Pathogenesis and treatment of renal dysfunction in rhabdomyolysis. Intensive Care Med 2001; 27(5):803–811.
74. Moore KP, et al. A causative role for redox cycling of myoglobin and its inhibition by alkalinization in the pathogenesis and treatment of rhabdomyolysis-induced renal failure. J Biol Chem 1998; 273(48):31731–31737.
75. Winearls CG. Acute myeloma kidney. Kidney Int 1995; 48(4):1347–1361.
76. Zucchelli P, et al. Controlled plasma exchange trial in acute renal failure due to multiple myeloma. Kidney Int 1988; 33(6):1175–1180.
77. Johnson WJ, et al. Treatment of renal failure associated with multiple myeloma. Plasmapheresis, hemodialysis, and chemotherapy. Arch Intern Med 1990 150(4):863–869.
78. McCarthy CS, Becker JA. Multiple myeloma and contrast media. Radiology 1992; 183(2):519–521.
79. Smolens P, Barnes JL, Kreisberg R. Hypercalcemia can potentiate the nephrotoxicity of Bence Jones proteins. J Lab Clin Med 1987; 110(4):460–465.
80. Lin JH. Bisphosphonates: a review of their pharmacokinetic properties. Bone 1996; 18(2):75–85.
81. Fleisch H. Bisphosphonates. Pharmacology and use in the treatment of tumour-induced hypercalcaemic and metastatic bone disease. Drugs 1991; 42(6):919–944.
82. Singer FR, Minoofar PN. Bisphosphonates in the treatment of disorders of mineral metabolism. Adv Endocrinol Metab 1995; 6:259–288.
83. Hosking DJ, Gilson D. Comparison of the renal and skeletal actions of calcitonin in the treatment of severe hypercalcaemia of malignancy. QJM 1984; 53(211): 359–368.
84. Condit PT, Chanes RE, Joel W. Renal toxicity of methotrexate. Cancer 1969; 23(1):126–131.
85. Wall SM, et al. Effective clearance of methotrexate using high-flux hemodialysis membranes. Am J Kidney Dis 1996; 28(6):846–854.
86. Kepka L, et al. Successful rescue in a patient with high dose methotrexate-induced nephrotoxicity and acute renal failure. Leuk Lymphoma 1998; 29(1–2):205–209.
87. Ackland SP, Schilsky RL. High-dose methotrexate: a critical reappraisal. J Clin Oncol 1987; 5(12): 2017–2031.
88. Cohen L, Magrath I, Poplack D, Ziegler JAcute tumor lysis syndrome. A review of 37 patients with Burkitt lymphoma. Am J Med 1980; 68:486–491.

89. Silverman P, Distelhorst CW. Metabolic emergencies in clinical oncology. Semin Oncol 1989; 16(6):504–515.
90. Arrambide K, Toto RD. Tumor lysis syndrome. Semin Nephrol 1993; 13(3):273–280.
91. Kjellstrand CMCD, von Hartitzsch B, Buselmeier TJ. Hyperuricemic acute renal failure. Arch Intern Med 1974; 133:349–359.
92. Conger J. Acute uric acid nephropathy. Semin Nephrol 1981; 1(1):69–74.
93. Boles JM, et al. Acute renal failure caused by extreme hyperphosphatemia after chemotherapy of an acute lymphoblastic leukemia. Cancer 1984; 53(11): 2425–2429.
94. Masera G, et al. Urate-oxidase prophylaxis of uric acid-induced renal damage in childhood leukemia. J Pediatr 1982; 100(1):152–155.
95. Saccente SL, Kohaut EC, Berkow RL. Prevention of tumor lysis syndrome using continuous veno-venous hemofiltration. Pediatr Nephrol 1995; 9(5):569–573.
96. Symmers W. Thrombotic microangiopathic haemolytic anaemia (thrombotic microangiopathy). Br Med J 1952; 2:897–903.
97. Riley LW, et al. Hemorrhagic colitis associated with a rare *Escherichia coli* serotype. N Engl J Med 1983; 308(12):681–685.
98. Remuzzi G, Ruggenenti P. The hemolytic uremic syndrome. Kidney Int 1995; 48(1):2–19.
99. Rizzoni G, et al. Plasma infusion for hemolytic-uremic syndrome in children: results of a multicenter controlled trial. J Pediatr 1988; 112(2):284–290.
100. Tsai H, Lian EC. Antibodies to von Willebrand factor-cleaving protease in acute thrombotic thrombocytopenic purpura. N Engl J Med 1998; 339(22):1585–1594.
101. Furlan M, et al. von Willebrand factor-cleaving protease in thrombotic thrombocytopenic purpura and the hemolytic-uremic syndrome. N Engl J Med 1998; 339(22):1578–1584.
102. Zager RA, et al. Acute renal failure following bone marrow transplantation: a retrospective study of 272 patients. Am J Kidney Dis 1989; 13(3):210–216.
103. Zager RA. Acute renal failure in the setting of bone marrow transplantation. Kidney Int 1994; 46(5): 1443–1458.
104. Gruss E, et al. Acute renal failure in patients following bone marrow transplantation: prevalence, risk factors and outcome. Am J Nephrol 1995; 15(6):473–479.
105. Smith DM, et al. Acute renal failure associated with autologous bone marrow transplantation. Bone Marrow Transplant 1987; 2(2):195–201.
106. Zager RA. Rhabdomyolysis and myohemoglobinuric acute renal failure. Kidney Int 1996; 49(2):314–326.
107. Carreras E, et al. On the reliability of clinical criteria for the diagnosis of hepatic veno-occlusive disease. Ann Hematol 1993; 66(2):77–80.
108. Attal M, et al. Prevention of hepatic veno-occlusive disease after bone marrow transplantation by continuous infusion of low-dose heparin: a prospective, randomized trial. Blood 1992; 79(11):2834–2840.
109. Gluckman E, et al. Use of prostaglandin E1 for prevention of liver veno-occlusive disease in leukaemic patients treated by allogeneic bone marrow transplantation. Br J Haematol 1990; 74(3):277–281.
110. Bianco JA, et al. Phase I–II trial of pentoxifylline for the prevention of transplant-related toxicities following bone marrow transplantation. Blood 1991; 78(5): 1205–1211.
111. Loomis LJ, et al. Hemolytic uremic syndrome following bone marrow transplantation: a case report and review of the literature. Am J Kidney Dis 1989; 14(4):324–328.
112. Silva VA, et al. Plasma exchange and vincristine in the treatment of hemolytic uremic syndrome/thrombotic thrombocytopenic purpura associated with bone marrow transplantation. J Clin Apheresis 1991; 6(1): 16–20.
113. Michel DM, Kelly CJ. Acute interstitial nephritis. J Am Soc Nephrol 1998; 9(3):506–515.
114. Rastegar A, Kashgarian M. The clinical spectrum of tubulointerstitial nephritis. Kidney Int 1998; 54(2): 313–327.
115. Kelly CJ. T cell regulation of autoimmune interstitial nephritis. J Am Soc Nephrol 1990; 1(2):140–149.
116. Eddy AA, et al. A relationship between proteinuria and acute tubulointerstitial disease in rats with experimental nephrotic syndrome. Am J Pathol 1991; 138(5): 1111–1123.
117. Neilson EG. Pathogenesis and therapy of interstitial nephritis. Kidney Int 1989; 35(5):1257–1270.
118. Neilson EG, et al. Molecular characterization of a major nephritogenic domain in the autoantigen of anti-tubular basement membrane disease. Proc Natl Acad Sci USA 1991; 88(5):2006–2010.
119. Wilson CB. Nephritogenic tubulointerstitial antigens. Kidney Int 1991; 39(3):501–517.
120. Linton AL, et al. Acute interstitial nephritis due to drugs: review of the literature with a report of nine cases. Ann Intern Med 1980; 93(5):735–741.
121. Rossert J. Drug-induced acute interstitial nephritis. Kidney Int 2001; 60(2):804–817.
122. Ruffing KA, et al. Eosinophils in urine revisited. Clin Nephrol 1994; 41(3):163–166.
123. Galpin JE, et al. Acute interstitial nephritis due to methicillin. Am J Med 1978; 65(5):756–765.
124. Pusey CD, et al. Drug associated acute interstitial nephritis: clinical and pathological features and the response to high dose steroid therapy. QJM 1983; 52(206):194–211.
125. Lien YH, et al. Ciprofloxacin-induced granulomatous interstitial nephritis and localized elastolysis. Am J Kidney Dis 1993; 22(4):598–602.
126. Cryst C, Hammar SP. Acute granulomatous interstitial nephritis due to co-trimoxazole. Am J Nephrol 1988; 8(6):483–488.
127. Webb DE, et al. Metabolic and renal effects of interleukin-2 immunotherapy for metastatic cancer. Clin Nephrol 1988; 30(3):141–145.

128. Ault BH, et al. Acute renal failure during therapy with recombinant human gamma interferon. N Engl J Med 1988; 319(21):1397–1400.
129. Clive DM, Stoff JS. Renal syndromes associated with nonsteroidal antiinflammatory drugs. N Engl J Med 1984; 310(9):563–572.
130. Kleinknecht D. Interstitial nephritis, the nephrotic syndrome, and chronic renal failure secondary to nonsteroidal anti-inflammatory drugs. Semin Nephrol 1995; 15(3):228–235.
131. Huang JJ, et al. Acute bacterial nephritis: a clinicoradiologic correlation based on computed tomography. Am J Med 1992; 93(3):289–298.
132. Ramsay AG, Olesnicky L, Pirani CL. Acute tubulo-interstitial nephritis from *Candida albicans* with oliguric renal failure. Clin Nephrol 1985; 24(6): 310–314.
133. Bhattacharya S, Bryk D, Wise GJ. Clinicopathological conference: renal pelvic filling defect in a diabetic woman. J Urol 1982; 127(4):751–753.
134. Wise GJ, Silver DA. Fungal infections of the genitourinary system. J Urol 1993; 149(6):1377–1388.
135. Wise GJ, Kozinn PJ, Goldberg P. Amphotericin B as a urologic irrigant in the management of noninvasive candiduria. J Urol 1982; 128(1):82–84.
136. Levy E, Bia MJ. Isolated renal mucormycosis: case report and review. J Am Soc Nephrol 1995; 5(12): 2014–2019.
137. Myerowitz RL, et al. Fatal disseminated adenovirus infection in a renal transplant recipient. Am J Med 1975; 59(4):591–598.
138. Erdogan O, et al. Acute necrotizing tubulointerstitial nephritis due to systemic adenoviral infection. Pediatr Nephrol 2001; 16(3):265–268.
139. Rosen S, et al. Tubulo-interstitial nephritis associated with polyomavirus (BK type) infection. N Engl J Med 1983; 308(20):1192–1196.
140. Frazao JM, et al. Epstein–Barr-virus-induced interstitial nephritis in an HIV-positive patient with progressive renal failure. Nephrol Dial Transplant 1998; 13(7):1849–1852.
141. Mayer HB, et al. Epstein–Barr virus-induced infectious mononucleosis complicated by acute renal failure: case report and review. Clin Infect Dis 1996; 22(6):1009–1018.
142. Nasr SH, et al. Granulomatous interstitial nephritis. Am J Kidney Dis 2003; 41(3):714–719.
143. Walker JV, et al. Histoplasmosis with hypercalcemia, renal failure, and papillary necrosis. Confusion with sarcoidosis. JAMA 1977; 237(13):1350–1352.
144. Kanfer A, et al. Acute renal insufficiency due to lymphomatous infiltration of the kidneys: report of six cases. Cancer 1976; 38(6):2588–2592.
145. Koolen MI, et al. Non-Hodgkin lymphoma with unique localization in the kidneys presenting with acute renal failure. Clin Nephrol 1988; 29(1):41–46.
146. Malbrain ML, et al. Acute renal failure due to bilateral lymphomatous infiltrates. Primary extranodal non-Hodgkin's lymphoma (p-EN-NHL) of the kidneys: does it really exist? Clin Nephrol 1994; 42(3): 163–169.
147. Miyake JS, Fitterer S, Houghton DC. Diagnosis and characterization of non-Hodgkin's lymphoma in a patient with acute renal failure. Am J Kidney Dis 1990; 16(3):262–263.
148. Gauvin F, et al. Reactive hemophagocytic syndrome presenting as a component of multiple organ dysfunction syndrome. Crit Care Med 2000; 28(9):3341–3345.
149. Holt S, et al. Cytokine nephropathy and multi-organ dysfunction in lymphoma. Nephrol Dial Transplant 1998; 13(7):1853–1857.
150. Comerma-Coma MI, et al. Reversible renal failure due to specific infiltration of the kidney in chronic lymphocytic leukaemia. Nephrol Dial Transplant 1998; 13(6): 1550–1552.
151. Pagniez DC, et al. Reversible renal failure due to specific infiltration in chronic lymphocytic leukemia. Am J Med 1988; 85(4):579–580.
152. Phillips JK, et al. Renal failure caused by leukaemic infiltration in chronic lymphocytic leukaemia. J Clin Pathol 1993; 46(12):1131–1133.
153. Boudville N, et al. Renal failure in a patient with leukaemic infiltration of the kidney and polyomavirus infection. Nephrol Dial Transplant 2001; 16(5): 1059–1061.
154. Krochak RJ, Baker DG. Radiation nephritis. Clinical manifestations and pathophysiologic mechanisms. Urology 1986; 27(5):389–393.
155. Cassady JR. Clinical radiation nephropathy. Int J Radiat Oncol Biol Phys 1995; 31(5):1249–1256.
156. Cohen EP. Radiation nephropathy after bone marrow transplantation. Kidney Int 2000; 58(2):903–918.
157. Moulder JE, Fish BL, Abrams RA. Renal toxicity following total-body irradiation and syngeneic bone marrow transplantation. Transplantation 1987; 43(4): 589–592.
158. Cohen EP, et al. Captopril preserves function and ultrastructure in experimental radiation nephropathy. Lab Invest 1996; 75(3):349–360.
159. Hatala R, Dinh T, Cook DJ. Once-daily aminoglycoside dosing in immunocompetent adults: a meta-analysis. Ann Intern Med 1996; 124(8):717–725.
160. Barrett BJ, Carlisle EJ. Metaanalysis of the relative nephrotoxicity of high- and low-osmolality iodinated contrast media. Radiology 1993; 188(1):171–178.
161. Sorkine P, et al. Administration of amphotericin B in lipid emulsion decreases nephrotoxicity: results of a prospective, randomized, controlled study in critically ill patients. Crit Care Med 1996; 24(8): 1311–1315.
162. Schierhout G, Roberts I. Fluid resuscitation with colloid or crystalloid solutions in critically ill patients: a systematic review of randomised trials. Br Med J 1998; 316(7136):961–964.
163. Choi PT, et al. Crystalloids vs. colloids in fluid resuscitation: a systematic review. Crit Care Med 1999 27(1): 200–210.

164. Schortgen F, et al. Effects of hydroxyethylstarch and gelatin on renal function in severe sepsis: a multicentre randomised study. Lancet 2001; 357(9260):911–916.
165. Boldt J, et al. Volume therapy in the critically ill: is there a difference? Intensive Care Med 1998; 24(1): 28–36.
166. Solomon R, et al. Effects of saline, mannitol, and furosemide to prevent acute decreases in renal function induced by radiocontrast agents. N Engl J Med 1994; 331(21):1416–1420.
167. Mueller C, et al. Prevention of contrast media-associated nephropathy: randomized comparison of 2 hydration regimens in 1620 patients undergoing coronary angioplasty. Arch Intern Med 2002; 162(3):329–336.
168. Durham JD, et al. A randomized controlled trial of *N*-acetylcysteine to prevent contrast nephropathy in cardiac angiography. Kidney Int 2002; 62(6):2202–2207.
169. Kay J, et al. Acetylcysteine for prevention of acute deterioration of renal function following elective coronary angiography and intervention: a randomized controlled trial. JAMA 2003; 289(5):553–558.
170. Burton CJ, Tomson CR. Can the use of low-dose dopamine for treatment of acute renal failure be justified? Postgrad Med J 1999; 75(883):269–274.
171. Denton MD, Chertow GM, Brady HR. "Renal-dose" dopamine for the treatment of acute renal failure: scientific rationale, experimental studies and clinical trials. Kidney Int 1996; 50(1):4–14.
172. Segal JM, Phang PT, Walley KR. Low-dose dopamine hastens onset of gut ischemia in a porcine model of hemorrhagic shock. J Appl Physiol 1992; 73(3): 1159–1164.
173. Weisberg LS, Kurnik PB, Kurnik BR. Risk of radiocontrast nephropathy in patients with and without diabetes mellitus. Kidney Int 1994; 45(1):259–265.
174. Tumlin JA, et al. Fenoldopam mesylate blocks reductions in renal plasma flow after radiocontrast dye infusion: a pilot trial in the prevention of contrast nephropathy. Am Heart J 2002; 143(5):894–903.
175. Sheinbaum R, et al. Contemporary strategies to preserve renal function during cardiac and vascular surgery. Rev Cardiovasc Med 2003; 4(suppl 1): S21–S28.
176. Lassnigg A, et al. Lack of renoprotective effects of dopamine and furosemide during cardiac surgery. J Am Soc Nephrol 2000; 11(1):97–104.
177. Better OS, et al. Mannitol therapy revisited (1940–1997). Kidney Int 1997; 52(4):886–894.
178. Bonventre JV, Weinberg JM. Kidney preservation ex vivo for transplantation. Annu Rev Med 1992; 43:523–553.
179. Ratcliffe PJ, et al. Effect of intravenous infusion of atriopeptin 3 on immediate renal allograft function. Kidney Int 1991; 39(1):164–168.
180. Sands JM, et al. Atrial natriuretic factor does not improve the outcome of cadaveric renal transplantation. J Am Soc Nephrol 1991; 1(9):1081–1086.
181. Petrinec D, et al. Insulin-like growth factor-I attenuates delayed graft function in a canine renal autotransplantation model. Surgery 1996; 120(2):221–225; discussion 225–226.
182. Miller SB, et al. Insulin-like growth factor I accelerates recovery from ischemic acute tubular necrosis in the rat. Proc Natl Acad Sci USA 1992; 89(24): 11876–11880.
183. Franklin SC, et al. Insulin-like growth factor I preserves renal function postoperatively. Am J Physiol 1997; 272(2 Pt 2):F257–F259.
184. Thadhani R, Pascual M, Bonventre JV. Acute renal failure. N Engl J Med 1996; 334(22):1448–1460.
185. Miller SB, et al. Rat models for clinical use of insulin-like growth factor I in acute renal failure. Am J Physiol 1994; 266(6 Pt 2):F949–F956.
186. Graziani G, Casati S, Cantaluppi A. Dopamine–furosemide therapy in acute renal failure. Proc EDTA 1982; 19:319–324.
187. Bellomo R, et al. Low-dose dopamine in patients with early renal dysfunction: a placebo-controlled randomised trial. Australian and New Zealand Intensive Care Society (ANZICS) Clinical Trials Group. Lancet 2000; 356(9248):2139–2143.
188. Cantarovich F, et al. High dose frusemide in established acute renal failure. Br Med J 1973; 4(5890): 449–450.
189. Minuth AN, Terrell JB Jr, Suki WN. Acute renal failure: a study of the course and prognosis of 104 patients and of the role of furosemide. Am J Med Sci 1976; 271(3):317–324.
190. Kleinknecht D, et al. Furosemide in acute oliguric renal failure. A controlled trial. Nephron 1976; 17(1):51–58.
191. Brown CB, Ogg CS, Cameron JS. High dose frusemide in acute renal failure: a controlled trial. Clin Nephrol 1981; 15(2):90–96.
192. Shilliday IR, Quinn KJ, Allison ME. Loop diuretics in the management of acute renal failure: a prospective, double-blind, placebo-controlled, randomized study. Nephrol Dial Transplant 1997; 12(12):2592–2596.
193. Mehta RL, et al. Diuretics, mortality, and nonrecovery of renal function in acute renal failure. JAMA 2002; 288(20):2547–2553.
194. Martin SJ, Danziger LH. Continuous infusion of loop diuretics in the critically ill: a review of the literature. Crit Care Med 1994; 22(8):1323–1329.
195. Sward K, Valson F, Ricksten SE. Long-term infusion of atrial natriuretic peptide (ANP) improves renal blood flow and glomerular filtration rate in clinical acute renal failure. Acta Anaesthesiol Scand 2001; 45(5):536–542.
196. Rahman SN, et al. Effects of atrial natriuretic peptide in clinical acute renal failure. Kidney Int 1994; 45(6):1731–1738.
197. Allgren RL, et al. Anaritide in acute tubular necrosis. Auriculin Anaritide Acute Renal Failure Study Group. N Engl J Med 1997; 336(12):828–834.

198. Lewis J, et al. Atrial natriuretic factor in oliguric acute renal failure. Anaritide Acute Renal Failure Study Group. Am J Kidney Dis 2000; 36(4):767–774.
199. Hirschberg R, et al. Multicenter clinical trial of recombinant human insulin-like growth factor I in patients with acute renal failure. Kidney Int 1999; 55(6): 2423–2432.
200. Siegel NJ, et al. Beneficial effect of thyroxin on recovery from toxic acute renal failure. Kidney Int 1984; 25(6):906–911.
201. Cronin RE, Newman JA. Protective effect of thyroxine but not parathyroidectomy on gentamicin nephrotoxicity. Am J Physiol 1985; 248(3 Pt 2): F332–F339.
202. Cronin RE, Brown DM, Simonsen R. Protection by thyroxine in nephrotoxic acute renal failure. Am J Physiol 1986; 251(3 Pt 2):F408–F416.
203. Sutter PM, et al. Beneficial effect of thyroxin in the treatment of ischemic acute renal failure. Pediatr Nephrol 1988; 2(1):1–7.
204. Acker CG, et al. A trial of thyroxine in acute renal failure. Kidney Int 2000; 57(1):293–298.
205. Parsons FM, Hobson F, Blagg CR, McCracken BH. Optimal time for dialysis in acute reversible renal failure. Lancet 1961; 1:129–134.
206. Kleinknecht D, et al. Uremic and non-uremic complications in acute renal failure: evaluation of early and frequent dialysis on prognosis. Kidney Int 1972; 1(3):190–196.
207. Gillum DM, et al. The role of intensive dialysis in acute renal failure. Clin Nephrol 1986; 25(5):249–255.
208. Conger J. Dialysis and related therapies. Semin Nephrol 1998; 18(5):533–540.
209. Hakim RM, Wingard RL, Parker RA. Effect of the dialysis membrane in the treatment of patients with acute renal failure. N Engl J Med 1994; 331(20): 1338–1342.
210. Lowrie EG, et al. Effect of the hemodialysis prescription of patient morbidity: report from the National Cooperative Dialysis Study. N Engl J Med 1981; 305(20):1176–1181.
211. Paganini EP, Tapolyai M, Goormastic M, Halstenberg W, Kozlowski L, LeBlanc M, Lee JC, Moreno L, Sakai K. Establishing a dialysis therapy patient outcome link in intensive care unit acute dialysis for patient with acute renal failure. Am J Kidney Dis 1996; 28(suppl 3):S81–S89.
212. Schiffl H, Lang SM, Fischer R. Daily hemodialysis and the outcome of acute renal failure. N Engl J Med 2002; 346(5):305–310.
213. Eknoyan G, et al. Effect of dialysis dose and membrane flux in maintenance hemodialysis. N Engl J Med 2002; 347(25):2010–2019.
214. Ronco C. Continuous renal replacement therapies in the treatment of acute renal failure in intensive care patients. Part 1. Theoretical aspects and techniques. Nephrol Dial Transplant 1994; 9(suppl 4):191–200.
215. Ronco C. Continuous renal replacement therapies in the treatment of acute renal failure in intensive care patients. Part 2. Clinical indications and prescription. Nephrol Dial Transplant 1994; 9(suppl 4):201–209.
216. Rialp G, et al. Prognostic indexes and mortality in critically ill patients with acute renal failure treated with different dialytic techniques. Ren Fail 1996; 18(4): 667–675.
217. Mehta RL, et al. A randomized clinical trial of continuous versus intermittent dialysis for acute renal failure. Kidney Int 2001; 60(3):1154–1163.
218. van Bommel EF. Should continuous renal replacement therapy be used for 'non-renal' indications in critically ill patients with shock?. Resuscitation 1997; 33(3): 257–270.
219. Bellomo R, et al. Preliminary experience with high-volume hemofiltration in human septic shock. Kidney Int Suppl 1998; 66:S182–S185.
220. Schetz M, et al. Removal of pro-inflammatory cytokines with renal replacement therapy: sense or nonsense? Intensive Care Med 1995; 21(2):169–176.

39

Complications of Bone Marrow Transplantation and Immunosuppression

SHUBHRA GHOSH and DANIEL R. COURIEL

Department of Blood and Marrow Transplantation, The University of Texas M.D. Anderson Cancer Center, Houston, Texas, U.S.A.

During the last two decades, blood and marrow transplantation (BMT) is being increasingly offered as a treatment option for patients with various hematologic and solid organ malignancies. Every year more than 3000 allogeneic transplants are performed in the United States. However, wider use of BMT is limited by the serious and often life-threatening complications associated with transplants.

Among the various complications of allogeneic BMT, one of the most serious is the occurrence of graft-versus-host disease (GvHD). In addition, GvHD or its treatment makes the patient susceptible to other acute and chronic complications, often life threatening. Some of these include opportunistic infections, diffuse pulmonary hemorrhage (DAH), thrombotic thrombocytopenic purpura (TTP), posterior reversible leukoencephalopathy syndrome (PRES), chronic GvHD, and post-transplant lymphoproliferative disorders (PTLD) among others. These complications related to GvHD have significant ramifications in terms of additional health-care costs while at the same time restricting the use of allogeneic BMT for a broader range of diseases.

This section will focus on severe complications resulting from GvHD and its treatment. Other transplant related complications have been addressed in another chapter.

Graft-versus-host disease is the reaction of the transplanted donor cells against the recipient's tissues, which are unable to respond due to myeloablation rendered by the preparative regimen. Graft-versus-host disease can occur anytime after transplantation, even as early as within the first two weeks after infusion before the patient has engrafted the transplanted cells (1,2). When GvHD occurs within the first 100 days post-transplant, it is known as acute GvHD, and when the signs and symptoms of GvHD occur after the initial 100 days post-transplant, it is defined as chronic. However, there is an ongoing debate regarding the definition of GvHD based on time post-transplant and some hematologists believe that acute GvHD usually manifests itself within the first 30–40 days while chronic GvHD can occur as early as 50 days post-transplant (1). In essence, certain subsets of patients develop clinical manifestations of acute GvHD beyond 100 days (3,4). Therefore, the main difference between acute and chronic GvHD is the clinical spectrum of each disease rather than the time of onset.

I. ACUTE GvHD

Acute graft-versus-host disease can occur in 10–100% of allogeneic BMT recipients. It occurs when T cells in the infused graft recognize host alloantigens as "non-self" and generate an attack on the host tissues and organs. The production of various cytokines and interleukins has been demonstrated in the development of acute GvHD (1). An increased level of tumor necrosis factor alpha (TNF) in the host serum has been implicated in both, the development of acute GvHD as well as the morbidity and mortality associated with it. Granulocyte-macrophage colony-stimulating factor (GM-CSF) and interferon gamma (IFN) have also been implicated in the development of acute GvHD.

The three conditions necessary for development of acute GvHD are summarized in Billingham's laws, which state that (5):

1. The graft must contain immunologically competent cells.
2. The host must possess important tissue antigens that are lacking in the donor.
3. The recipient must be incapable of mounting an effective immunologic response against the graft cells.

The risk of developing acute GvHD in a patient is directly related to the degree of HLA-histoincompatibility between the donor and the recipient (the risk being 30–50% in matched related recipients, ~70% in one antigen mismatched recipients and almost 100% in those receiving two or more antigen mismatched transplants) (1). The risk is also increased in older patients, those receiving female to male transplants (especially if the donor has had two or more viable pregnancies), recipients of matched unrelated donor transplants (MUD) and in recipients of non-T-cell-depleted transplants.

A. Signs and Symptoms of Acute GvHD

The most common presentation of acute GvHD is a rash in the extremities, which may spread to other parts of the body. Besides skin, the other commonly affected sites are the mucosa of the gastrointestinal tract manifest as profuse diarrhea with or without abdominal cramping and severe nausea and vomiting in case of upper GI involvement, and liver leading to elevated levels of total bilirubin and, sometimes, alkaline phosphatase in the blood. Other organs like the eyes and lungs may also be involved.

The management and outcome of acute GvHD is determined by the stage of organ involvement and the overall grade based on the stages of various sites involved. The staging and grading of acute GvHD as per the consensus conference is shown in Table 1 (6). Since lower grades respond better to treatment, the overall grade of acute GvHD has been shown to be an indicator of disease-free survival as well as overall survival (OS) for recipients of allogeneic transplants. Five-year leukemia free survival according to grade of acute GvHD has been reported to be ~60% with grade 0–1, ~55% with grade 2, ~32% with grade 3 and ~8% with grade 4 (7). Five-year overall survival has been reported to be 62% in those with grade 0–1 acute GvHD vs. 24% in patients with grade 2–4 acute GvHD (8).

B. Acute GvHD of the Skin

Skin is frequently the first site to get involved in acute GvHD and is characterized by a red, maculopapular rash often first noticed in the palms and soles, gradually spreading to involve other parts of the body. The rash may be accompanied by itching, pain on pressure, and erythema. The maculopapular rash may become confluent and in advanced cases, there is desquamation of skin. The most severe form of acute GvHD of the skin is associated with bullous formation and resembles toxic epidermal necrolysis (TEN), which is often fatal (9).

Toxic epidermal necrolysis, a serious condition that shares clinical, histological, and immunological similarities with acute GvHD, is often associated with toxic reaction to drugs like sulfonamides and manifestation of toxic epidermal necrolysis has also been linked to hyperacute GvHD occurring before the patient has engrafted post-transplant. However, even after emergency intervention, in most cases, outcome with stage 4 acute GvHD of the skin is poor and often fatal (10–14).

Early diagnosis of acute GvHD can often be difficult due to effects of drug toxicities, reactions to radiation therapy and viral infections presenting with similar clinical and histological features (15,16). Histological examination is often useful in establishing the diagnosis of acute GvHD, although in most cases where the clinical suspicion of acute GvHD is strong, treatment is started while awaiting a histologic diagnosis. A variety of changes have been associated with the pathogenesis of acute GvHD including infiltration with CD4+ and CD8+ lymphocytes, increased levels of cyclin A in keratinocytes and accumulation of Ki67 antigen (17–19).

C. Acute GvHD of the Gastrointestinal Tract

The gastrointestinal tract is one of the most frequently involved organs in acute GvHD. It is characterized by profuse diarrhea, which may be associated with severe

Table 1 Grading of Acute GvHD

Clinical grading of individual organ system

Organ	Grade	Description
Skin	+1	Maculo-papular eruption <25% of body area
	+2	Maculo-papular eruption 25–50% of body area
	+3	Generalized erythroderma
	+4	Generalized erythroderma with bullous formation and often with desquamation
Liver	+1	Bilirubin 2.0–3.0 mg/dL
	+2	Bilirubin 3.1.0–6.0 mg/dL
	+3	Bilirubin 6.1–15.0 mg/dL
	+4	Bilirubin >15.0 mg/dL
Gut	+1	Diarrhea >30 mL/kg or >500 mL/day
	+2	Diarrhea >60 mL/kg or >1000 mL/day
	+3	Diarrhea >90 mL/kg or >1500 mL/day
	+4	Diarrhea >90 mL/kg or >2000 mL/day, or severe abdominal pain, ileus

Overall grade	Grade				
	Skin	Liver	Gut		ECOG performance status
I	+1 to +2	0		0	0
II	+1 to +3	+1	and/or	+1	0–1
III	+2 to +3	+2 to +4	and/or	+2 to +3	2–3
IV	+2 to +4	+2 to +4	and/or	+2 to +4	3–4

If no skin disease the overall grade is the higher single organ grade
The % of skin involvement is based on the "Rule of Nine" for burns.
Volume of diarrhea applies to adults. For pediatric patients, volume of diarrhea is based on body surface area.

abdominal cramps. In the case of involvement of the upper GI tract, the patient experiences severe nausea and vomiting leading to loss of appetite, which may necessitate the use of nasogastric tube (20).

The pathogenesis of acute GvHD of the GI tract involves local damage to the GI mucosa causing translocation of endotoxins, which leads to cytokine release and promotes further inflammation and additional gastrointestinal damage (21,22). In a prospective study conducted in Fred Hutchinson Cancer Center in Seattle, patients were followed for GI bleeding over a 10-year period. It was found that both the incidence and mortality of GI bleeding from multiple GI sites, viral and fungal ulcers and GvHD significantly declined during the decade. However, severe bleeding after transplant remained an indicator of poor prognosis (23).

In another study reported from Johns Hopkins Oncology Center, in a series of 463 allogeneic transplant recipients, bleeding occurred in 40% and GvHD in 27%. The incidence of bleeding was higher in patients with GvHD as compared with non-GvHD, and correlated with the severity of GvHD. The higher bleeding incidence in GvHD was due to gastrointestinal hemorrhage, hemorrhagic cystitis, and pulmonary hemorrhage. The authors concluded that bleeding in these patients was associated with acute GvHD and as such GvHD was a risk factor for bleeding in transplant recipients and since the occurrence of bleeding was associated with poor outcome, it may be used as an indicator for the assessment of severity of GvHD (24).

In a patient with severe nausea and vomiting not relieved by antiemetics, upper GI endoscopic examination is often performed and biopsies obtained for histological examination to rule out GvHD. The findings in the stomach and duodenum vary from subtle mucosal erythema and edema to frank ulceration and mucosal slough. The biopsy reveals crypt epithelial cell apoptosis and dropout, crypt destruction, and lymphocytic infiltration of the epithelium and lamina propria. Either diffuse or focal involvement may be seen (25). In patients with lower GI involvement, endoscopy reveals apoptosis of individual cells in the mucosa. Severe disease may lead to loss of crypts and eventual sloughing of the mucosa, hemorrhagic ulceration of the upper jejunum, terminal ileum, and colon (26,27). Similar histology may be seen in the presence of viral infections, especially CMV, and the use of cytoreductive agents.

Radiographically, acute gastrointestinal GvHD characteristically appears on CT scans as multiple, diffuse, fluid-filled bowel loops with a thin, enhancing layer of bowel wall mucosa. Bowel wall thickening often is absent (28).

D. Acute GvHD of the Liver

In acute GvHD, the small bile ducts in the liver are damaged as a result of the reaction of transplanted donor cells against the recipient's tissues. This compromises the flow of bile and the clearance of bilirubin from the circulation. As a result, the bilirubin level rises in the blood and the patient starts to appear jaundiced. Depending on the amount of injury, the bile duct damage can be mild, moderate, or severe.

Transjugular biopsy of the liver can be useful in confirming the diagnosis of acute GvHD of the liver. In a study from Spain, 76 BMT recipients underwent 82 transjugular liver biopsies (29). Characteristic findings in the biopsy were used to modify the diagnosis in 45%, with both the diagnosis and treatment being modified in 30% of patients. In 15/35 patients suspected to have acute GvHD of the liver, the diagnosis was confirmed with biopsies and in 4/24 (17%), it was not. Also, in 15/26 patients suspected to have veno-occlusive disease (VOD), the diagnosis was histologically confirmed and in 2/33 (6%), it was not. It was concluded that transjugular liver biopsy was an effective, safe, and useful technique for evaluating BMT related liver dysfunction.

In a series published in 1980, 62 allogeneic BMT recipients with apparent drug toxicity, GvHD, and disseminated cytomegalovirus (CMV) infection underwent autopsy examinations (30). Twenty patients had acute cutaneous GvHD with associated hepatic dysfunction. Eight of the 20 also had disseminated CMV infection. Among the 12 patients without concomitant CMV infection, 5 had an early onset of GvHD and had predominantly periportal and focal midzonal hepatocellular necrosis, and 7 had acute GvHD with later onset with predominantly bile duct injury.

In severe cases, acute GvHD of the liver can lead to liver failure and death. The other conditions in the differential diagnosis of acute GvHD of the liver include infectious hepatitis, drug toxicity from cyclosporine or tacrolimus and VOD.

1. Veno-Occlusive Disease

Another common liver disorder seen early in recipients of BMT is VOD. The high-dose chemotherapy and total body irradiation used in the preparative regimen (especially in patients with leukemia/lymphoma/solid organ malignancies) may damage the hepatic blood vessels resulting in swelling and obstruction. This condition is known as VOD. Besides the preparative regimen, other risk factors include the history of prior transplant, transplants from HLA mismatched or unrelated donors and infectious hepatitis at the time of the preparative regimen. Unlike liver GvHD where bile ducts are primarily damaged, VOD is caused by injury to the blood vessels taking blood back to the heart. Veno-occlusive disease usually develops within the first three months post-transplant and is usually reversible. The fluid leaks from the damaged vessels and collects in the abdominal cavity causing ascites. If it persists, the increased intra-abdominal pressure can lead to shortness of breath. Over a period of time other complications can also develop. If renal clearance is affected, there is retention of salt and water leading to generalized edema. The build up of toxins in the circulation can affect the brain function and present as confusion.

Veno-occlusive disease should be suspected when there is a sudden gain in weight, enlarged liver, and icterus in a patient 7–21 days post-transplant with high-dose chemotherapy or total body irradiation. Other signs and symptoms include abdominal tenderness, increased bilirubin level, and elevated liver function tests. The management of VOD includes the discontinuation or reduction in the dosing of any drugs that could burden or injure the liver until the resolution of VOD. Diuresis and, if necessary, dialysis are used to reduce fluid overload and the patient is monitored for daily input and output. In some cases, packed red cell transfusion may also be required. In the majority of the cases, VOD resolves completely with conservative management and mortality is high only in severe cases (31–33).

E. Acute GvHD of the Lungs

The recipients of BMT are at increased risk of developing respiratory problems. The use of drugs like busulphan and methotrexate before transplant significantly increases the risk of pulmonary complications post-transplant as do pulmonary infections and these along with other complications like pulmonary edema and diffuse alveolar hemorrhage have been discussed in a separate chapter. Acute injury of the lungs related to GvHD is poorly defined. In a study conducted at Dana-Farber Cancer Institute, 24% of allogeneic transplant recipients developed severe pulmonary complications seen within 100 days post-transplant including diffuse alveolar hemorrhage, need for mechanical ventilation, or death from respiratory failure (34). GvHD prophylaxis with cyclosporine/methotrexate was found to be the single most important factor affecting the incidence of severe pulmonary complications, and T-cell depletion was associated with a significantly lower risk.

F. Acute GvHD of the Eye

Frequently, GvHD of the eye occurs as a serious problem especially in the setting of GvHD involving other sites. Immunosuppression with various chemotherapeutic agents and total body irradiation leads to high incidence of ophthalmologic complications including dry eye syndrome, viral keratitis, sterile conjunctivitis and uveitis, trophic disturbances of the cornea and later to chronic problems of severe drying and conjunctival and corneal scarring (35,36).

In a series of 263 allogeneic transplant recipients reported from Johns Hopkins Oncology Center, GvHD involving the conjunctiva was diagnosed in 24 patients 79% of whom presented with pseudomembrane formation due to denudation of conjunctival epithelium (37). In this study, 19/24 patients had conjunctival involvement with acute GvHD with a mortality of almost 90% and the other five cases were associated with severe chronic GvHD with 80% mortality. The authors concluded that conjunctival involvement by GvHD represented a distinct clinical finding and was a marker for severe systemic involvement by GvHD.

Conjunctival biopsies can be useful in establishing the diagnosis in some cases with low-grade GvHD or GvHD limited to the eye. In a study conducted in Melbourne, Australia, 41/44 transplant recipients followed by the ophthalmology team were found to have abnormal findings on conjunctival biopsy examinations among whom 64% had clinical and laboratory proven evidence of GvHD and six patients with no systemic evidence of GvHD had conjunctival histology specific for GvHD (38).

II. PREVENTION OF ACUTE GvHD

Various centers use cyclosporine or tacrolimus for the prophylaxis of GvHD. Methotrexate is often used in combination with these agents (39,40). The effectiveness of GvHD prophylaxis is generally assessed by the rate of GvHD and survival at 100–180 days. Several groups have demonstrated that tacrolimus is a more potent prophylactic agent than cyclosporine after allogeneic matched related and unrelated marrow transplantation. Two randomized studies showed the combination of tacrolimus with methotrexate to be superior to cyclosporine and methotrexate for the prevention of GvHD. Nash et al. observed 74% of grade II–IV acute GvHD with the cyclosporine/methotrexate versus 56% using tacrolimus/methotrexate ($P=0.0002$) (41) while Hiraoka et al. reported incidences of 48% and 20.6% respectively ($P<0.0001$) (42). The MD Anderson Cancer Center experience has shown tacrolimus to be superior to cyclosporine as the toxicities are more predictable and nephrotoxicity is easily controlled with tacrolimus by rigorously following blood levels and maintaining adequate hydration (43,44).

At many centers standard GvHD prophylaxis is currently done with cyclosporine or tacrolimus plus methotrexate with regular monitoring to maintain prophylactic levels of cyclosporine and tacrolimus (39). Mycophenolate mofetil has been also been tested with good results and favorable toxicity profile in combination with cyclosporin for acute GvHD prophylaxis (45).

Antithymocyte globulin is another agent frequently used in the prophylaxis of GvHD in patients receiving unrelated donor transplants (46–52).

Better selection of patients for transplants with lesser risk factors can go a long way in preventing the occurrence of GvHD.

III. MANAGEMENT OF ACUTE GvHD

The management of acute GvHD involves the use of various immunosuppressive agents. Topical steroids are widely used for grade I skin GvHD; however, their usefulness is not well defined. High-dose steroids are used as the first-line treatment for grade II or higher GvHD and various doses have been successfully tried in different situations (40,53–55). However, long-term use of steroids is associated with its own complications including myopathy, early development of cataract, chronic pulmonary complications, opportunistic infections, and diabetes to name a few.

In about 50% cases, acute GvHD is refractory to steroid therapy and the management of such cases is difficult (56–59). Various other immunosuppressive agents including tacrolimus, antithymocyteglobulin (ATG), Mycophenolate mofetil (MMF), and sirolimus (Rapamycin) have been tried with varying degrees of response (39,59–67).

Monoclonal antibodies including daclizumab, infliximab, visilizumab, and basiliximab have shown activity in the management of steroid resistant acute GvHD (68–74). Investigators are also exploring agents targeting CD2 molecule, a glycoprotein expressed on thymocytes, mature T lymphocytes, and natural killer cells which act as a costimulatory molecule for antigen-specific lymphocyte activation in the development of acute GvHD (75,76). ABX-CBL which targets CD147 (neurothelin/EMMPRIN) and XomaZyme-CD5 plus, a CD5-specific immunotoxin have also been studied as potential agents for prevention and management of acute GvHD (77–79).

Pentostatin, a purine neucleoside analog, reduces the number and function of lymphocytes. These immunosuppressant properties have prompted its use for the treatment of acute GvHD (80). In an attempt to avoid the side-effects of systemic steroids, oral (topical) agents beclomethasone and budesonide have been evaluated in clinical trials for acute gastrointestinal GvHD with some success (81–83).

Extra-corporeal photopheresis (ECP), which has been used for a long time for the treatment of cutaneous T-cell lymphoma, some autoimmune diseases, and rejection after solid organ transplantation, is recently being investigated for its role in treatment of acute GvHD (84–86).

In some cases of severe grade IV acute GvHD of the liver, refractory to treatment with corticosteroids and other immunosuppressive agents like IL2-receptor antibodies, liver transplantation has been used with some success (87).

IV. CHRONIC GvHD

Chronic graft-versus-host disease is a major complication in long-term survivors of allogeneic BMT. The incidence of chronic GvHD has been reported to be 20–50% post-matched related donor transplant and 40–72% post-unrelated donor transplant (88–93). Although prolonged systemic immunosuppressive therapy is often required in chronic GvHD, the GvHD-specific survival at 5 years post-transplant has been reported to be as high as 74% (94).

The majority of the patients develop chronic GvHD with a prior history of acute GvHD. In 15–20% cases, chronic GvHD can occur de novo after more than three months post-transplant. Therefore, acute GvHD is the single most important risk factor for the development of chronic GvHD (95). Older age, higher degree of HLA mismatching, and possibly CMV seropositivity also increase the risk of developing chronic GvHD (1). Unlike acute GvHD where T cells have been shown to be specific for host alloantigens, the pathophysiology of chronic GvHD is considered to have an autoimmune component in which activated T cells perceive autoantigens as foreign antigens. The immunopathogenesis of chronic GvHD is, in part, Th-2 mediated, resulting in a syndrome of immunodeficiency and an autoimmune disorder (96–101).

The most commonly targeted organs include the skin, mucosa of the gastrointestinal tract, liver, lung, eye, and the immune system but almost any organ can be affected with chronic GvHD (102,103). When chronic GvHD affects the secretory glands, it can cause various symptoms due to dryness from lack of mucous/saliva/tears/other lubricants. Chronic GvHD is graded as "limited" or "extensive" (Table 2) (6).

A. Signs and Symptoms of Chronic GvHD

Skin rash with or without itching, dryness, and tightening is frequently seen. Discoloration and lichenoid thickening and scleroderma are also common. Abnormal liver function tests and jaundice develop in chronic GvHD of the liver. Involvement of oral mucosa leads to dry mouth with or without sores/lichenoid plaques, and burning sensation related to acidic foods. There may be weight loss resulting from failure to thrive, heart burn, abdominal pain, dysphagia, and impaired nutrient absorption. Ocular symptoms include dry eyes with burning sensation and vision impairment. Pulmonary involvement is often in the form of bronchiolitis obliterans causing shortness of breath and wheezing. There may also be premature graying and partial hair-loss and joint stiffness and contractures limiting the range of movement. These signs and symptoms may be complicated due to opportunistic infections which frequently occur in these severely immunosuppressed patients.

B. Chronic GvHD of the Skin

Chronic GvHD of the skin can have different manifestations. It is characterized by thickened, lichenoid skin changes with or without darkening (104). In some cases, it may manifest as scleroderma and there have even been reports of bullous scleroderma as a manifestation of chronic GvHD (103,105–112). Acral scleroderma can cause severe limitation of range of

Table 2 Chronic GvHD

Limited	Localized skin involvement and/or hepatic dysfunction
Extensive	Generalized skin involvement or limited skin involvement or hepatic involvement and any of the following: a) Liver histology showing chronic progressive hepatitis, bridging necrosis, or cirrhosis b) Eye involvement (Schirmer's test with less than 5 mm wetting) c) Involvement of minor salivary glands or oral mucosa d) Involvement of any other organ

movement (113,114,116,117). Cytokine production may propagate the cytotoxic cascade and perpetuate the tissue injury in chronic cutaneous GvHD (100).

C. Chronic GvHD of the Oral Mucosa and Gastrointestinal Tract

Chronic GvHD of the gastrointestinal tract can affect any part of the digestive tract. Lichenoid plaques and dry mouth are seen in oral involvement, while dysphagia, burning sensation on ingestion of acidic food, and retrosternal pain are features of esophageal involvement. In severe forms, desquamative esophagitis may lead to esophageal strictures and web formation. Intestinal and colonic involvement can lead to prolonged malabsorption and diarrhea. Wasting and weight loss follow persistent symptoms (20,115).

D. Chronic GvHD of the Liver

Typically chronic GvHD of the liver presents as an indolent cholestatic disease in patients with involvement of other organ sites mostly, skin, mouth, and eye and is characterized by elevated bilirubin and alkaline phosphatase levels along with other liver function abnormalities. But, it can, sometimes, mimic acute viral hepatitis in its presentation. In a study reported from Seattle, 14 allogeneic transplant recipients with marked elevations of serum aminotransferases and a clinical resemblance to acute viral hepatitis were followed (116). They were 294 days (range 74–747) post-transplant and around taper/cessation of immunosuppression at the onset of abnormal liver function tests. Liver biopsies were performed on all the patients and showed changes characteristic of GvHD including damaged and degenerative small bile ducts. In cases where high-dose immunosuppressive therapy was administered, there was prompt improvement with normalization of bilirubin and liver function tests while in those where therapy was delayed there was worsening of liver function supported by histologic evidence of loss of small bile ducts and portal fibrosis. The authors concluded that liver GvHD can present as acute hepatitis in a patient who is receiving minimal/no immunosuppression and that a liver biopsy is necessary in making the correct diagnosis.

Secondary biliary cirrhosis has also been reported as a progression of chronic GvHD of the liver (96,117).

E. Chronic GvHD of the Lung

After the initial 100 days, pulmonary complications are seen in upto 15–20% of transplant recipients. Among those who develop chronic GvHD approximately 10% patients present with bronchiolitis obliterans usually 6–12 months post-transplant. Radiographically, it is characterized by thickening of bronchovascular interstitium with ground-glass opacities in the periphery of the lung. There may be patchy sub-pleural consolidation along with 5–15 mm nodules with well-defined margins. Bronchiolitis obliterans with organizing pneumonia can lead to respiratory distress and respiratory failure. Pulmonary fibrosis and restrictive airway disease can also occur many months post-transplant, sometimes in conjunction with chronic GvHD of the skin. Infections can be serious in these patients (103,118,119).

F. Chronic GvHD of the Eye

Keratoconjunctivitis and sicca syndrome can develop as a manifestation of chronic GvHD and persist for many years. Dry eye can lead to corneal ulceration and even perforation. Treatment of corneal ulceration in a patient with dry eye due to chronic GvHD is as important as it is difficult. In noninfectious ulcers, daily application of collagen-shields and frequent use of artificial tears may prevent severe ocular complications like corneal perforation (120). In a case reported from Spain, multilayer amniotic membrane transplantation was successfully used for reconstructing the ocular surface in a patient with severe dry eyes and calcareous corneal degeneration, with perforation (121).

Cataracts occur more frequently in patients who have received total body irradiation. When these patients develop GvHD of the eye, cataract surgery proves to be a greater challenge. However with aggressive management of dry eyes and other ocular surface problems, cataract surgery had excellent outcomes in patients with GvHD.

Topical steroids and topical cyclosporine are commonly used as first-line treatment for ocular GvHD. In refractory cases, successful treatment of chronic GvHD of the eye has been shown with the use of systemic corticosteroids and FK506 (123,124). Artificial tears are useful in relief of symptoms and also in preventing scarring of the conjunctival and corneal tissue. Some investigators have successfully used antologous serum eye drops, sometimes along with punctual plugs, to treat severe dry eye resulting from chronic GvHD in cases refractory to treatment with artificial tears (125).

G. Chronic GvHD of Musculoskeletal System

Myositis and myopathy can occur after prolonged steroid use and/or as a manifestation of chronic GvHD (102,111). Joint contractures and fascitis limiting the range of movement can seriously compromise the quality of life (126–129).

H. Post-Transplant Lymphoproliferative Disorder

Prolonged immunosuppression in a BMT recipient can lead to uncontrolled proliferation of Ebstein–Barr virus infected B cells with a rapidly progressive and often fatal condition known as post-transplant lymphoproliferative disorder (PTLD). It can present as benignly as a tonsillitis or as a rapidly growing Kaposi's sarcoma requiring emergency intervention. Usually, PTLD develops within 1 year post-transplant.

In a multi-institutional study conducted by the National Cancer Institute, 1% of 18,014 allogeneic transplant recipients developed PTLD over a 10-year period (130). Most of the patients were between 1 and 5 months post-transplant. Among those who developed PTLD within 1 year of transplant, the association was strongly significant for recipients of unrelated/HLA mismatched related transplants, T-cell-depleted donor marrow transplants and recipients of antithymocyte globulin/anti-CD3 monoclonal antibody as GvHD prophylactic/therapeutic agents ($p < 0.0001$). The presence of acute GvHD grade II–IV and a preparative regimen including irradiation were also significant factors for development of PTLD ($p = 0.02$). In the same study, the only significant factor associated with late onset PTLD (after 1 year post-transplant) was found to be the presence of chronic GvHD ($p = 0.01$).

In another study conducted in Helsinki, Finland during a period of 5 years, autopsy proven PTLD was diagnosed in 19/257 (7%) recipients of consecutive allogeneic non-T-cell-depleted grafts from HLA-identical siblings or unrelated donors, and in none of the surviving patients (131). Among them, the diagnosis was made when the patient was alive in 7/19 cases based on the histology and positive EBV staining of lymph node and kidney biopsies (one patient) or liver biopsy (one patient), the presence of EBV positive and CD20 positive atypical lymphocytes in blood (two patients), or the presence of high copy numbers of EBV-DNA in plasma by PCR (three patients). All the 19 patients had received ATG either for the treatment of steroid-resistant acute GvHD or as part of the conditioning regimen. In transplantations from a HLA-identical donor with a non-T-cell-depleted graft, the risk of PTLD correlated strongly with the intensity of the immunosuppressive treatment.

Post-transplant lymphoproliferative disorder can also prove to be fatal when the symptoms are confused with those due to GvHD, for example, intestinal infiltration of lymphoid cells in PTLD can mimic diarrhea due to gastrointestinal GvHD and the patient may require critical intervention unless the pathologic diagnosis is made at the onset of symptoms (132).

Patients with PTLD usually have high-titers of EBV antibody in blood. PCR, in a suspicious case, can be used for early diagnosis of the disease. Initial symptoms may start with fever, tonsillitis, cervical adenopathy, and diarrhea. Radiographically, depending on the sites involved, there may be multiple well-circumscribed lung nodules and areas of alveolar infiltrates or intestinal infiltrates. The management of PTLD includes immune-based therapies such as monoclonal anti-B-cell antibodies, interferon-alpha, EBV-specific cytotoxic T cells, donor lymphocyte infusion, and discontinuation of immunosuppressive drugs but mortality continues to be high in BMT recipients (133,134).

V. MANAGEMENT OF CHRONIC GvHD

As in acute GvHD, the first line of treatment for chronic GvHD is with corticosteroids. Usually chronic GvHD of the skin is more responsive than other sites. In a large randomized double-blind, placebo-controlled trial conducted in Fred Hutchinson Cancer Center, 126 patients either received prednisone (1 mg/kg every other day) or prednisone and azathioprine (1.5 mg/kg/day) as early treatment of extensive chronic GvHD with standard risk (platelet count $\geq 100{,}000/\mu L$) (135). The group receiving prednisone alone had a lower rate of infection and longer 5-year survival as compared to the group that received the combination ($p = 0.03$). In a subgroup of patients with thrombocytopenia who were treated only with prednisone, the survival was much poorer (136). Subsequent trials by the same group of investigators showed that a combination of cyclosporine with prednisone had a better response in high-risk patients with chronic GvHD and that treatment failure was lower with this combination in both high-risk as well as standard-risk patients (137,138).

In patients failing to respond to the combination of cyclosporine and prednisone, response has been seen with the use of tacrolimus (139,140). Fewer side-effects associated with tacrolimus suggest the need to investigate its use as a first-line treatment for chronic GvHD.

Photochemotherapy (PUVA) using ultraviolet A irradiation has been used with some success in refractory chronic cutaneous lichenoid GvHD and chronic oral GvHD (141–146). The major limiting factor for its wider use is the risk of developing photo toxicity of the skin and even basal cell carcinoma in the long run. Extra-corporeal photopheresis (ECP) has also been shown to be useful in the management of chronic GvHD involving skin and liver (85,147–149). Steroid-sparing effects were seen with the use of ECP in 32 patients with extensive chronic GvHD at MD Anderson Cancer Center with 64% patients able to reduce the steroid dose by at least half (150).

In recent years, thalidomide, alone or in combination with cyclosporine or other agents, has been used in extensive chronic GvHD (151–153). Mycophenolate mofetil (MMF) has been tried in multiple small trials alone or in combination with other immunosuppressive agents for steroid-refractory extensive chronic GvHD of the skin, mouth, liver, or gastrointestinal tract with response rates ranging from 25% to 77% (154–156).

Recently, in a phase II trial sirolimus (rapamycin) as a second or third-line therapy was found to cause some improvement in chronic GvHD and allow tapering of the steroid/tacrolimus/cyclosporine (157). However, side-effects such as renal failure, hemolytic-uremic syndrome, thrombocytopenia, and infections are the major drawbacks with this drug. In a phase II trial at the MD Anderson Cancer Center, 29 patients with steroid-refractory chronic GVDH were treated with the combination of tacrolimus and sirolimus (158). Sixty-eight patients responded, mostly with skin involvement, including five complete remissions. Toxicities included hyperlipidemia, hypertension, and reversible cytopenias.

In refractory chronic GvHD of the liver, ursodeoxycholic acid has been shown to improve serum biochemical markers of cholestasis along with immunosuppressive therapy in a study conducted in Seattle (159). All 12 patients showed improvement after treatment for 6 weeks but relapsed on discontinuation of ursodeoxycholic acid.

REFERENCES

1. Chao NJ. Graft-versus-host disease. In: Burt RK, Dee HJ, Lothian ST, Santos GW, eds. Bone Marrow Transplantation. Austin, TX: Lands Biosciences, 1998:478–497.
2. Couriel DR, Saliba R, Ghosh S, et al. Early acute GvHD: syndrome and clinical implications [abstr]. 2003 American Society of Hematology 45th Annual Meeting, San Diego, CA.
3. Lee SJ, Vogelsang G, Gilman A, et al. A survey of diagnosis, management, and grading of chronic GvHD. Biol Blood Marrow Transplant 2002; 8(1): 32–39.
4. Mielcarek M, Martin PJ, Leisenring W, et al. Graft-versus-host disease after nonmyeloablative versus conventional hematopoietic stem cell transplantation. Blood 2003; 102(2):756–762.
5. Bellingham RE. The biology of graft-versus-host reactions. Harvey Lectures 1966–67; 62:21–78.
6. Przepiorka D, Weisdort D, Martin P, et al. Consensus conference on acute GvHD grading. Bone Marrow Transplant 1995; 15:825–828.
7. Ringden O, Hermans J, Labopin M, et al. The highest leukaemia-free survival after allogeneic bone marrow transplantation is seen in patients with grade I acute graft-versus-host disease. Acute and Chronic Leukaemia Working Parties of the European Group for Blood and Marrow Transplantation (EBMT). Leuk Lymphoma 1996; 24(1–2):71–79.
8. Hagglund H, Bostrom L, Remberger M, et al. Risk factors for acute graft-versus-host disease in 291 consecutive HLA-identical bone marrow transplantrecipients. Bone Marrow Transplant 1995; 16(6): 747–753.
9. Itin PH, Lautenschlager S, Orth B, et al. A skin manifestation of graft-versus-host reaction following bone marrow transplantation. Schweizerische Medizinische Wochenschrift. Journal Suisse de Medecine 1996; 126(9):339–347.
10. Villada G, Roujeau JC, Cordonnier C, et al. Toxic epidermal necrolysis after bone marrow transplantation: study of nine cases. J Am Acad Dermatol 1990; 23(5 Pt 1):870–875.
11. Correia O, Delgado L, Barbosa IL, et al. Increased interleukin 10, tumor necrosis factor alpha, and interleukin 6 levels in blister fluid of toxic epidermal necrolysis. J Am Acad Dermatol 2002; 47(1):58–62.
12. Correia O, Delgado L, Barbosa IL, et al. CD8+ lymphocytes in the blister fluid of severe acute cutaneous graft-versus-host disease: further similarities with toxic epidermal necrolysis. Dermatology 2001; 203(3):212–216.
13. Takeda H, Mitsuhashi Y, Kondo S, et al. Toxic epidermal necrolysis possibly linked to hyperacute graft-versus-host disease after allogeneic bone marrow transplantation. J Dermatol 1997; 24(10):635–641.
14. Hewitt J, Ormerod AD. Toxic epidermal necrolysis treated with cyclosporine. Clin Exp Dermatol 1992; 17(4):264–265.
15. Hani N, Casper C, Groth W, et al. Stevens-Johnson syndrome-like exanthema secondary to methotrexate histologically simulating acute graft-versus-host disease. Eur J Dermatol 2000; 10(7):548–550.
16. Kharfan Dabaja MA, Morgensztern D, Markoe AM, et al. Radiation recall dermatitis induced by methotrexate in a patient with Hodgkin's disease. Am J Clin Oncol 2001; 24(2):211–213.
17. Nikaein A, Poole T, Fishbeck R, et al. Characterization of skin-infiltrating cells during acute graft-versus-host disease following bone marrow transplantation using unrelated marrow donors. Hum Immunol 1994; 40(1): 68–76.
18. Klimczak A, Lange A. Apoptosis of keratinocytes is associated with infiltration of CD8+ lymphocytes

and accumulation of Ki67 antigen. Bone Marrow Transplant 2000; 26(10):1077–1082.
19. Jerome KR, Conyers SJ, Hansen DA, Zebala JA. Keratinocyte apoptosis following bone marrow transplantation: evidence for CTL-dependent and -independent pathways. Bone Marrow Transplant 1998; 22(4): 359–366.
20. Weisdorf DJ, Snover DC, Haake R, et al. Acute upper gastrointestinal graft-versus-host disease: clinical significance and response to immunosuppressive therapy. Blood 1990; 76:624–629.
21. Cooke KR, Olkiewicz K, Erickson N, Ferrara JL. The role of endotoxin and the innate immune response in the pathophysiology of acute graft versus host disease. J Endotoxin Res 2002; 8(6):441–448.
22. Takatsuka H, Iwasaki T, Okamoto T, Kakishita E. Intestinal graft-versus-host disease: mechanisms and management. Drugs 2003; 63(1):1–15.
23. Schwartz JM, Wolford JL, Thornquist MD, et al. Severe gastrointestinal bleeding after hematopoietic cell transplantation, 1987–1997: incidence, causes, and outcome. Am J Gastroenterol 2001; 96(2): 385–393.
24. Nevo S, Enger C, Swan V, et al. Acute bleeding after allogeneic bone marrow transplantation: association with graft versus host disease and effect on survival. Transplantation 1999; 67(5):681–689.
25. Ponec RJ, Hackman RC, McDonald GB. Endoscopic and histologic diagnosis of intestinal graft-versus-host disease after marrow transplantation. Gastrointest Endosc 1999; 49(5):612–621.
26. Snover DC. Graft-versus-host disease of the gastrointestinal tract. Am J Surg Pathol 1990; 14(suppl 1): 101–108.
27. Saito H, Oshimi K, Nagasako K, et al. Endoscopic appearance of the colon and small intestine of a patient with hemorrhagic enteric graft-vs-host disease. Dis Colon Rectum 1990; 33(8):695–697.
28. Donnelly LF, Morris CL. Acute graft-versus-host disease in children: abdominal CT findings. Radiology 1996; 199(1):265–268.
29. Carreras E, Granena A, Navasa M, et al. Transjugular liver biopsy in BMT. Bone Marrow Transplant 1993; 11(1):21–26.
30. Beschorner WE, Pino J, Boitnott JK, et al. Pathology of the liver with bone marrow transplantation. Effects of busulfan, carmustine, acute graft-versus-host disease, and cytomegalovirus infection. Am J Pathol 1980; 99(2):369–385.
31. Litzow MR, Repoussis PD, Schroeder G, et al. Veno-occlusive disease of the liver after blood and marrow transplantation: analysis of pre- and post-transplant risk factors associated with severity and results of therapy with tissue plasminogen activator. Leuk Lymphoma 2002; 43(11):2099–2107.
32. McCarville MB, Hoffer FA, Howard SC, et al. Hepatic veno-occlusive disease in children undergoing bone-marrow transplantation: usefulness of sonographic findings. Pediatr Radiol 2001; 31(2):102–105.
33. Carreras E. Veno-occlusive disease of the liver after hemopoietic cell transplantation. Eur J Haematol 2000; 64(5):281–291.
34. Ho VT, Weller E, Lee SJ, et al. Prognostic factors for early severe pulmonary complications after hematopoietic stem cell transplantation. Biol Blood Marrow Transplant 2001; 7(4):223–229.
35. Jack MK, Hicks JD. Ocular complications in high-dose chemoradiotherapy and marrow transplantation. Ann Ophthalmol 1981; 13(6):709–711.
36. Franklin RM, Kenyon KR, Tutschka PJ, et al. Ocular manifestations of graft-vs-host disease. Ophthalmology 1983; 90(1):4–13.
37. Jabs DA, Wingard J, Green WR, et al. The eye in bone marrow transplantation. III. Conjunctival graft-vs-host disease. Arch Ophthalmology 1989; 107(9):1343–1348.
38. West RH, Szer J, Pedersen JS. Ocular surface and lacrimal disturbances in chronic graft-versus-host disease: the role of conjunctival biopsy. Aust NZ J Ophthalmol 1991; 19(3):187–191.
39. Jacobson P, Uberti J, Davis W, Ratanatharathorn V. Tacrolimus: a new agent for the prevention of graft-versus-host disease in hematopoietic stem cell transplantation. Bone Marrow Transplant 1998; 22(3): 217–225.
40. Chao NJ, et al. Cyclosporine, methotrexate, and prednisone compared with cyclosporine and prednisone for prophylaxis of acute graft-versus-host disease. N Engl J Med 1993; 329(17):1225–1230.
41. Nash RA, Pineiro LA, Storb R, et al. FK506 in combination with methotrexate for the prevention of graft-versus-host disease after marrow transplantation from matched unrelated donors. Blood 1996; 88:3634–3641.
42. Hiraoka A, Ohashi Y, Okamoto S, et al. Phase III study comparing tacrolimus (FK 506) with cyclosporine for graft-versus-host disease prophylaxis after allogeneic bone marrow transplantation. Bone Marrow Transplant 2001; 28:181–185.
43. Przepiorka D, Devine SM, Fay JW, et al. Practical considerations in the use of tacrolimus for allogeneic marrow transplantation. Bone Marrow Transplant 1999; 24:1053–1056.
44. Przepiorka D, Khouri I, Ippoliti C, et al. Tacrolimus and minidose methotrexate for prevention of acute graft-versus-host disease after HLA-mismatched marrow or blood stem cell transplantation. Bone Marrow Transplant 1999; 24:763–768.
45. Bornhauser M, Schuler U, Porksen G, et al. Mycophenolate mofetil and cyclosporine as graft-versus-host disease prophylaxis after allogeneic blood stem cell transplantation. Transplantation 1999; 67(4):499–504.
46. Schleuning M, Günther W, Tischer J, et al. Dose-dependent effects of in vivo antithymocyte globulin during conditioning for allogeneic bone marrow transplantation from unrelated donors in patients with

chronic phase CML. Bone Marrow Transplant 2003; 32(3):243–250.
47. Kabisch H, Erttmann R, Zander AR, et al. Influence of anti-thymocyte globulin as part of the conditioning regimen on immune reconstitution following matched related bone marrow transplantation. J Hematother Stem Cell Res 2003; 12(2):237–242.
48. Ayas M, Al-Mahr M, Al-Jefri A, et al. Does adding ATG to the GvHD prophylaxis regimen help reduce its incidence? Bone Marrow Transplant 2003; 31(4):311.
49. Duggan P, Booth K, Chaudhry A, et al. Unrelated donor BMT recipients given pretransplant low-dose antithymocyte globulin have outcomes equivalent to matched sibling BMT a matched pair analysis. Bone Marrow Transplant 2002; 30(10):681–686.
50. Bertz H, Potthoff K, Finke J. Allogeneic stem-cell transplantation from related and unrelated donors in older patients with myeloid leukemia. J Clin Oncol 2003; 21(8):1480–1484.
51. Finke J, Schmoor C, Lang H, et al. Matched and mismatched allogeneic stem-cell transplantation from unrelated donors using combined graft-versus-host disease prophylaxis including rabbit anti-T lymphocyte globulin. J Clin Oncol 2003; 21(3):506–513.
52. Graf Finckenstein F, Zabelina T, Durken M, et al. Unrelated donor stem cell transplantation in children: low toxicity using a GvHD-prophylaxis regimen with CSA, MTX, metronidazole, iv-immunoglobulin and ATG. Klinische Padiatrie 2002; 214(4):206–211.
53. Ruutu T, Niederwieser D, Gratwohl A, Apperley JF. A survey of the prophylaxis and treatment of acute GvHD in Europe: a report of the European Group for Blood and Marrow, Transplantation (EBMT). Chronic Leukaemia Working Party of the EBMT. Bone Marrow Transplant 1997; 19(8):759–764.
54. Ruutu T, Hermans J, van Biezen A, et al. How should corticosteroids be used in the treatment of acute GvHD? EBMT Chronic Leukemia Working Party. European Group for Blood and Marrow Transplantation. Bone Marrow Transplant 1998; 22(6):614–615.
55. Hings IM, Filipovich AH, Miller WJ, et al. Prednisone therapy for acute graft-versus-host disease: short-versus long-term treatment. A prospective randomized trial. Transplantation 1993; 56(3):577–580.
56. Weisdorf D, Haake R, Blazar B, et al. Treatment of moderate/severe acute graft-versus-host disease after allogeneic bone marrow transplantation: an analysis of clinical risk features and outcome. Blood 1990; 75(4):1024–1030.
57. Martin PJ, Schoch G, Fisher L, et al. A retrospective analysis of therapy for acute graft-versus-host disease: initial treatment. Blood 1990; 76(8):1464–1472.
58. Roy J, et al. Acute graft-versus-host disease following unrelated donor marrow transplantation: failure of conventional therapy. Bone Marrow Transplant 1992; 10(1):77–82.
59. Martin PJ, Schoch G, Fisher L, et al. A retrospective analysis of therapy for acute graft-versus-host disease: secondary treatment. Blood 1991; 77(8): 1821–1828.
60. Bloom EA, Barnes J. Use of FK506 for graft-versus-host disease (GvHD) following bone marrow transplantation. J Cell Biochem 1994; (suppl 18B):90 [abstr G401].
61. Furlong T, Storb R, Anasetti C, et al. Clinical outcome after conversion to FK 506 (tacrolimus) therapy for acute graft-versus-host disease resistant to cyclosporine or for cyclosporine-associated toxicities. Bone Marrow Transplant 2000; 26(9):985–991.
62. Khoury H, Kashyap A, Adkins DR, et al. Treatment of steroid-resistant acute graft-versus-host disease with anti-thymocyte globulin. Bone Marrow Transplant 2001; 27(10):1059–1064.
63. McCaul KG, Nevill TJ, Barnett MJ, et al. Treatment of steroid-resistant acute graft-versus-host disease with rabbit antithymocyte globulin. J Hematother Stem Cell Res 2000; 9(3):367–374.
64. Basara N, Blau WI, Romer E, et al. Mycophenolate mofetil for the treatment of acute and chronic GvHD in bone marrow transplant patients. Bone Marrow Transplant 1998; 22(1):61–65.
65. Basara N, Blau WI, Kiehl MG, et al. Efficacy and safety of mycophenolate mofetil for the treatment of acute and chronic GvHD in bone marrow transplant recipient. Transplant Proc 1998; 30(8):4087–4089.
66. Basara N, Kiehl MG, Blau W, et al. Mycophenolate mofetil in the treatment of acute and chronic GvHD in hematopoietic stem cell transplant patients: four years of experience. Transplant Proc 2001; 33(3): 2121–2123.
67. Kahan BD. Rapamycin: personal algorithms for use based on 250 treated renal allograft recipients. Transplant Proc 1998; 30(5):2185–2188.
68. Przepiorka D, Kernan NA, Ippoliti C, et al. Daclizumab, a humanized anti-interleukin-2 receptor alpha chain antibody, for treatment of acute graft-versus-host disease. Blood 2000; 95(1):83–89.
69. Couriel D, Hicks K, Ipolitti C, et al. Infliximab for the treatment of graft-versus-host disease in allogeneic transplant recipients: an update. Blood 2000; 96:400a.
70. Redei IK, Tanner A. Salvage therapy with infliximab for patients with severe acute and chronic GvHD. Blood 2001; 98:399a.
71. Magalhaes-Silverman MC-K, Hohl R, et al. Treatment of severe steroid refractory acute graft versus host disease with infliximab. Blood 2001; 98 [abstract 5208].
72. Kobbe G, Schneider P, Rohr U, et al. Treatment of severe steroid refractory acute graft-versus-host disease with infliximab, a chimeric human/mouse anti-TNFalpha antibody. Bone Marrow Transplant 2001; 28(1):47–49.
73. Carpenter PA, Appelbaum FR, Corey L, et al. A humanized non-FcR-binding anti-CD3 antibody, visilizumab, for treatment of steroid-refractory acute graft-versus-host disease. Blood 2002; 99(8): 2712–2719.

74. Pasquini RM, Moreira VA, Medeiros CR, et al. Basiliximab (BaMab)—a selective interleukin-2 receptor (IL-2R) antagonist—as therapy for refractory acute graft versus host disease following bone marrow transplantation. Blood 2000; 96:177a.
75. Moingeon P, Chang HC, Sayre PH, et al. The structural biology of CD2. Immunol Rev 1989; 111: 111–144.
76. Timonen T, Gahmberg CG, Patarroyo M. Participation of CD11a–c/CD18, CD2 and RGD-binding receptors in endogenous and interleukin-2-stimulated NK activity of CD3-negative large granular lymphocytes. Int J Cancer 1990; 46(6):1035–1040.
77. Deeg HJ, Blazar BR, Bolwell BJ, et al. Treatment of steroid-refractory acute graft-versus-host disease with anti-CD147 monoclonal antibody ABX-CBL. Blood 2001; 98(7):2052–2058.
78. Koehler M, Hurwitz CA, Krance RA, et al. XomaZyme-CD5 immunotoxin in conjunction with partial T cell depletion for prevention of graft rejection and graft-versus-host disease after bone marrow transplantation from matched unrelated donors. Bone Marrow Transplant 1994; 13(5):571–575.
79. Weisdorf D, Filipovich A, McGlave P, et al. Combination graft-versus-host disease prophylaxis using immunotoxin (anti-CD5-RTA [Xomazyme-CD5]) plus methotrexate and cyclosporine or prednisone after unrelated donor marrow transplantation. Bone Marrow Transplant 1993; 12(5):531–536.
80. Margolis J, Vogelsang G. An old drug for a new disease: pentostatin (Nipent) in acute graft-versus-host disease. Semin Oncol 2000; 27(2 suppl 5):72–77.
81. McDonald GB, Bouvier M. Hockenbery DM, et al. Oral beclomethasone dipropionate for treatment of intestinal graft-versus-host disease: a randomized, controlled trial. Gastroenterology 1998; 115(1):28–35.
82. Baehr PH, Levine DS, Bouvier ME, et al. Oral beclomethasone dipropionate for treatment of human intestinal graft-versus-host disease. Transplantation 1995; 60(11):1231–1238.
83. Bertz H, Afting M, Kreisel W, et al. Feasibility and response to budesonide as topical corticosteroid therapy for acute intestinal GvHD. Bone Marrow Transplant 1999; 24(11):1185–1189.
84. Edelson R, Berger C, Gasparro F, et al. Treatment of cutaneous T-cell lymphoma by extracorporeal photochemotherapy. Preliminary results. N Engl J Med 1987; 316(6):297–303.
85. Greinix HT, Volc-Platzer B, Rabitsch W, et al. Successful use of extracorporeal photochemotherapy in the treatment of severe acute and chronic graft-versus-host disease. Blood 1998; 92(9):3098–3104.
86. Greinix HT, Volc-Platzer B, Knobler RM. Extracorporeal photochemotherapy in the treatment of severe graft-versus-host disease. Leuk Lymphoma 2000; 36(5–6):425–434.
87. Marks DI, Dousset B, Robson A, et al. Orthotopic liver transplantation for hepatic GvHD following allogeneic BMT for chronic myeloid leukaemia. Bone Marrow Transplant 1992; 10(5):463–466.
88. Sanders JE. Chronic graft-versus-host disease and late effects after hematopoietic stem cell transplantation. Int J Hematol 2002; 76(suppl 2):15–28.
89. Remberger M, Ringden O, Blau IW, et al. No difference in graft-versus-host disease, relapse, and survival comparing peripheral stem cells to bone marrow using unrelated donors. Blood 2001; 98(6):1739–1745.
90. Storek J, Gooley T, Siadak M, et al. Allogeneic peripheral blood stem cell transplantation may be associated with a high risk of chronic graft-versus-host disease. Blood 1997; 90(12):4705–4709.
91. Beatty PG, Hansen JA, Longton GM, et al. Marrow transplantation from HLA-matched unrelated donors for treatment of hematologic malignancies. Transplantation 1991; 51(2):443–447.
92. Gaziev D, Polchi P, Galimberti M, et al. Graft-versus-host disease after bone marrow transplantation for thalassemia: an analysis of incidence and risk factors. Transplantation 1997; 63(6):854–860.
93. Urbano-Ispizua A, Garcia-Conde J, Brunet S, et al. High incidence of chronic graft versus host disease after allogeneic peripheral blood progenitor cell transplantation. The Spanish Group of Allo-PBPCT. Haematologica 1997; 82(6):683–689.
94. Lee JH, Lee JH, Choi SJ, et al. Graft-versus-host disease (GvHD)-specific survival and duration of systemic immunosuppressive treatment in patients who developed chronic GvHD following allogeneic haematopoietic cell transplantation. Br J Haematol 2003; 122(4):637–644.
95. Wagner JL, Flowers ME, Longton G, et al. The development of chronic graft-versus-host disease: an analysis of screening studies and the impact of corticosteroid use at 100 days after transplantation. Bone Marrow Transplant 1998; 22(2):139–146.
96. Epstein O, Thomas HC, Sherlock S. Primary biliary cirrhosis is a dry gland syndrome with features of chronic graft-versus-host disease. Lancet 1980; 1(8179): 1166–1168.
97. Ratanatharathorn V, Ayash L, Lazarus HM, et al. Chronic graft-versus-host disease: clinical manifestation and therapy. Bone Marrow Transplant 2001; 28(2):121–129.
98. Sevilla J, Gonzalez-Vicent M, Madero L, Diaz MA. Acute autoimmune hemolytic anemia following unrelated cord blood transplantation as an early manifestation of chronic graft-versus-host disease. Bone Marrow Transplant 2001; 28(1):89–92.
99. Muro Y, Kamimoto T, Hagiwara M. Anti-mitosin antibodies in a patient with chronic graft-versus-host disease after allogeneic bone marrow transplantation. Bone Marrow Transplant 1997; 19(9): 951–953.
100. Ochs LA, Blazar BR, Roy J, et al. Cytokine expression in human cutaneous chronic graft-versus-host disease. Bone Marrow Transplant 1996; 17(6):1085–1092.

101. Siegert W, Stemerowicz R, Hopf U. Antimitochondrial antibodies in patients with chronic graft-versus-host disease. Bone Marrow Transplant 1992; 10(3): 221–227.
102. Oya Y, Kobayashi S, Nakamura K, et al. Skeletal muscle pathology of chronic graft versus host disease accompanied with myositis, affecting predominantly respiratory and distal muscles, and hemosiderosis. Rinsho Shinkeigaku Clin Neurol 2001; 41(9):612–616.
103. Serrano J, Prieto E, Mazarbeitia F, et al. Atypical chronic graft-versus-host disease following interferon therapy for chronic myeloid leukaemia relapsing after allogeneic BMT. Bone Marrow Transplant 2001; 27(1): 85–87.
104. Scanlan KA, Propeck PA. Chronic graft-versus-host disease causing skin thickening on mammograms. Am J Roentgenol 1995; 165(3):555–556.
105. Lawley TJ, Peck GL, Moutsopoulos HM, et al. Scleroderma, Sjogren-like syndrome, and chronic graft-versus-host disease. Ann Intern Med 1977; 87(6): 707–709.
106. Gratwhol AA, Moutsopoulos HM, Chused TM, et al. Sjogren-type syndrome after allogeneic bone-marrow transplantation. Ann Intern Med 1977; 87(6):703–706.
107. Moreno JC, Valverde F, Martinez F, et al. Bullous scleroderma-like changes in chronic graft-versus-host disease. J Eur Acad Dermatol Venereol 2003; 17(2): 200–203.
108. Eming SA, Peters T, Hartmann K, et al. Lichenoid chronic graft-versus-host disease-like acrodermatitis induced by hydroxyurea. J Am Acad Dermatol 2001; 45(2):321–323.
109. Grundmann-Kollmann M, Behrens S, Gruss C, et al. Chronic sclerodermic graft-versus-host disease refractory to immunosuppressive treatment responds to UVA1 phototherapy. J Am Acad Dermatol 2000; 42(1 Pt 1):134–136.
110. Itin PH, Lautenschlager S, Orth B, et al. Skin manifestations of graft-versus-host reaction following bone marrow transplantation. Schweizerische Medizinische Wochenschrift. Journal Suisse de Medecine 1996; 126(9):339–347.
111. Blanche P, Dreyfus F, Sicard D. Polymyositis and chronic graft-versus-host disease: efficacy of intravenous gammaglobulin and methotrexate. Clin Exp Rheumatol 1995; 13(3):377–379.
112. Chosidow O, Bagot M, Vernant JP, et al. Sclerodermatous chronic graft-versus-host disease. Analysis of seven cases. J Am Acad Dermatol 1992; 26(1):49–55.
113. Kossard S, Ma DD. Acral keratotic graft versus host disease simulating warts. Aust J Dermatol 1999; 40(3):161–163.
114. Dilek I, Demirer T, Ustun C, et al. Acquired ichthyosis associated with chronic graft-versus-host disease following allogeneic peripheral blood stem cell transplantation in a patient with chronic myelogenous leukemia. Bone Marrow Transplant 1998; 21(11): 1159–1161.
115. McDonald GB, Sullivan KM, Schuffler MD, et al. Esophageal abnormalities in chronic graft-versus-host disease in humans. Gastroenterology 1981; 80(5 pt 1): 914–921.
116. Strasser SI, Shulman HM, Flowers ME, et al. Chronic graft-versus-host disease of the liver presentation as an acute hepatitis. Hepatology 2000; 32(6): 1265–1271.
117. Stechschulte DJ Jr, Fishback JL, Emami A, Bhatia P. Secondary biliary cirrhosis as a consequence of graft-versus-host disease. Gastroenterology 1990; 98(1): 223–225.
118. Wolff D, Reichenberger F, Steiner B, et al. Progressive interstitial fibrosis of the lung in sclerodermoid chronic graft-versus-host disease. Bone Marrow Transplant 2002; 29(4):357–360.
119. Schulenburg A, Herold C, Eisenhuber E, et al. Pneumatosis cystoides intestinalis with pneumoperitoneum and pneumoretroperitoneum in a patient with extensive chronic graft-versus-host disease. Bone Marrow Transplant 1999; 24(3):331–333.
120. Spraul CW, Lang GE, Lang GK. Corneal ulcer in chronic graft-versus-host disease: treatment with collagen shields. Klinische Monatsblatter fur Augenheilkunde 1994; 205(3):161–166.
121. Peris-Martinez C, Menezo JL, Diaz-Llopis M, et al. Multilayer amniotic membrane transplantation in severe ocular graft versus host disease. Eur J Ophthalmol 2001; 11(2):183–186.
122. Penn EA, Soong HK. Cataract surgery in allogeneic bone marrow transplant recipients with graft-versus-host disease. J Cataract Refract Surg 2002; 28(3): 417–420.
123. Ahmad SM, Stegman Z, Fructhman S, Asbell PA. Successful treatment of acute ocular graft-versus-host disease with tacrolimus (FK506). Cornea 2002; 21(4): 432–433.
124. Ogawa Y, Okamoto S, Kuwana M, et al. Successful treatment of dry eye in two patients with chronic graft-versus-host disease with systemic administration of FK506 and corticosteroids. Cornea 2001; 20(4): 430–434.
125. Ogawa Y, Okamoto S, Mori T, et al. Autologous serum eye drops for the treatment of severe dry eye in patients with chronic graft-versus-host disease. Bone Marrow Transplant 2003; 31(7):579–583.
126. Janin A, Socie G, Devergie A, et al. Fasciitis in chronic graft-versus-host disease. A clinicopathologic study of 14 cases. Ann Intern Med 1994; 120(12): 993–998.
127. Markusse HM, Dijkmans BA, Fibbe WE. Eosinophilic fasciitis after allogeneic bone marrow transplantation. J Rheumatol 1990; 17(5):692–694.
128. van den Bergh V, Tricot G, Fonteyn G, et al. Diffuse fasciitis after bone marrow transplantation. Am J Med 1987; 83(1):139–143.
129. Couriel DR, Beguelin GZ, Giralt S, et al. Chronic graft-versus-host disease manifesting as polymyositis:

an uncommon presentation. Bone Marrow Transplant 2002; 30:543–546.

130. Curtis RE, Travis LB, Rowlings PA, et al. Risk of lymphoproliferative disorders after bone marrow transplantation: a multi-institutional study. Blood 1999; 94(7):2208–2216.

131. Juvonen E, Aalto SM, Tarkkanen J, et al. High incidence of PTLD after non-T-cell-depleted allogeneic haematopoietic stem cell transplantation as a consequence of intensive immunosuppressive treatment. Bone Marrow Transplant 2003; 32(1):97–102.

132. Claviez A, Tiemann M, Wagner HJ, et al. Epstein–Barr virus-associated post-transplant lymphoproliferative disease after bone marrow transplantation mimicking graft-versus-host disease. Pediatric Transplant 2000; 4(2):151–155.

133. Winer-Muram HT, Gurney JW, Bozeman PM, Krance RA. Pulmonary complications after bone marrow transplantation. Radiol Clin North Am 1996; 34(1):97–117.

134. Loren AW, Porter DL, Stadtmauer EA, Tsai DE. Post-transplant lymphoproliferative disorder:a review. Bone Marrow Transplant 2003; 31(3):145–155.

135. Sullivan KM, et al. Prednisone and azathioprine compared with prednisone and placebo for treatment of chronic graft-v-host disease: prognostic influence of prolonged thrombocytopenia after allogeneic marrow transplantation. Blood 1988; 72(2):546–554.

136. Sullivan KM, Witherspoon RP, Storb R, et al. Prednisone and azathioprine compared with prednisone and placebo for treatment of chronic graft-v-host disease prognostic influence of prolonged thrombocytopenia after allogeneic marrow transplantation. Blood 1988; 72(2):546–554.

137. Sullivan KM, Witherspoon RP, Storb R, et al. Alternating-day cyclosporine and prednisone for treatment of high-risk chronic graft-v-host disease. Blood 1988; 72(2):555–561.

138. Sullivan KM, Goley T, Nims J, et al. Comparison of ciclosporin, prednisone or alternating-day CSP/Pred in patients with standard and high-risk chronic graft-versus-host disease. Blood 1993; 82:215a.

139. Kanamaru A, Takemoto Y, Kakishita E, et al. FK506 treatment of graft-versus-host disease developing or exacerbating during prophylaxis and therapy with cyclosporine and/or other immunosuppressants. Japanese FK506 BMT Study Group. Bone Marrow Transplant 1995; 15(6):885–889.

140. Carnevale-Schianca F, Martin P, Sullivan K, et al. Changing from cyclosporine to tacrolimus as salvage therapy for chronic graft-versus-host disease. Biol Blood Marrow Transplant 2000; 6(6):613–620.

141. Nagler A, Menachem Y, Ilan Y. Amelioration of steroid-resistant chronic graft-versus-host-mediated liver disease via tacrolimus treatment. J Hematother Stem Cell Res 2001; 10(3):411–417.

142. Hymes SR, Morison WL, Farmer ER, et al. Methoxsalen and ultraviolet A radiation in treatment of chronic cutaneous graft-versus-host reaction. J Am Acad Dermatol 1985; 12(1 Pt 1):30–37.

143. Atkinson K, Weller P, Ryman W, Biggs J. PUVA therapy for drug-resistant graft-versus-host disease. Bone Marrow Transplant 1986; 1(2):227–236.

144. Jampel RM, Farmer ER, Vogelsang GB, et al. PUVA therapy for chronic cutaneous graft-vs-host disease. Arch Dermatol 1991; 127(11):1673–1678.

145. Vogelsang GB, Wolff D, Altomonte V, et al. Treatment of chronic graft-versus-host disease with ultraviolet irradiation and psoralen (PUVA). Bone Marrow Transplant 1996; 17(6):1061–1067.

146. Altman JS, Adler SS. Development of multiple cutaneous squamous cell carcinomas during PUVA treatment for chronic graft-versus-host disease. J Am Acad Dermatol 1994; 31(3 Pt 1):505–507.

147. Owsianowski M, Gollnick H, Siegert W, et al. Successful treatment of chronic graft-versus-host disease with extracorporeal photopheresis. Bone Marrow Transplant 1994; 14(5):845–848.

148. Rossetti F, Dall'Amico R, Crovetti G, et al. Extracorporeal photochemotherapy for the treatment of graft-versus-host disease. Bone Marrow Transplant 1996; 18(suppl 2):175–181.

149. Alcindor T, Gorgun G, Miller KB, et al. Immunomodulatory effects of extracorporeal photochemotherapy in patients with extensive chronic graft-versus-host disease. Blood 2001; 98(5):1622–1625.

150. Apisarnthanarax N, Donato M, Körbling M, et al. Extracorporeal photopheresis in the management of steroid-refractory or steroid-dependent extensive cutaneous chronic graft-versus-host disease after allogeneic stem cell transplantation: feasibility and results. Bone Marrow Transplant 2003; 31:459–465.

151. Vogelsang GB, Farmer ER, Hess AD, et al. Thalidomide for the treatment of chronic graft-versus-host disease. N Engl J Med 1992; 326(16):1055–1058.

152. Rovelli A, Arrigo C, Nesi F, et al. The role of thalidomide in the treatment of refractory chronic graft-versus-host disease following bone marrow transplantation in children. Bone Marrow Transplant 1998; 21(6): 577–581.

153. Arora M, Wagner JE, Davies SM, et al. Randomized clinical trial of thalidomide, cyclosporine, and prednisone versus cyclosporine and prednisone as initial therapy for chronic graft-versus-host disease. Biol Blood Marrow Transplant 2001; 7(5):265–273.

154. Abhyankar S, Godder K, Christiansen N, et al. Treatment of resistant acute and chronic graft versus host disease with mycophenolate mofetil. Blood 1998; 92:340b.

155. Roberts T, Koc Y, Sprague K, et al. Mycophenolate mofetil for the treatment of chronic graft versus host disease of the liver. Blood 1999; 94:159a.

156. Busca A, Saroglia EM, Lanino E, et al. Mycophenolate mofetil (MMF) as therapy for refractory chronic GvHD (cGvHD) in children receiving bone marrow transplantation. Bone Marrow Transplant 2000; 25 (10): 1067–1071.

157. Johnston LF, Shizuru FS, Stockerl-Goldstein KE, et al. Rapamycin for treatment of chronic graft versus host disease. Biol Blood Marrow Transplant 2002; 8:87.
158. Couriel DR, Hicks K, Saliba R, et al. Sirolimus (Rapamycin) for treatment of steroid-refractory chronic graft versus host disease. Biol Blood Marrow Transplant 2003; 9(2). Abstract.
159. Fried RH, Murakami CS, Fisher LD, et al. Ursodeoxycholic acid treatment of refractory chronic graft-versus-host disease of the liver. Ann Intern Med 1992; 116(8):624–629.

40

Sedation in the ICU

LISA E. CONNERY and DOUGLAS B. COURSIN

Department of Anesthesiology, University of Wisconsin Medical School, University of Wisconsin Hospital and Clinics, Madison, Wisconsin, U.S.A.

One of our primary goals as physician is to promote patient safety and comfort. With recent advancements in technology and modern intensive care, we are able to improve outcomes in critically ill patients who in the past had little hope of survival. Aggressive critical care often involves life support measures and invasive techniques that are frequently uncomfortable and/or frightening. Patients with normal mentation may be aware that their life is threatened and yet often have little ability or opportunity to communicate with others. The stress of systemic derangement and organ failure often results in mental status changes or encephalopathy. These factors in addition to unpleasant aspects of the intensive care unit (ICU) environment may contribute to disorientation, agitation, and delirium in many critically ill patients. The inability of such patients to comprehend or cope with their circumstances often results in unsafe conditions for both the patient and staff members should they become combative or severely agitated. Sedation helps to alleviate anxiety, facilitates mechanical ventilation, and helps to modulate excessive humoral and hemodynamic manifestations of the stress response (1–6). Inadequate pain control may also contribute to the patient's distress or agitation and must be routinely assessed and treated as needed.

Older modes of mechanical ventilation were especially uncomfortable for patients who often found it difficult to synchronize their respiratory patterns with that of the ventilator. In the early 1980s, most ICUs administered deep sedation and analgesia and often initiated neuromuscular blockade in patients who required mechanical ventilation (7,8). Newer ventilatory modes with more physiological respiratory patterns are better tolerated. This enabled the intensivist to decrease the degree of sedation administered to many patients, with the notable exception of those with severe cases of acute respiratory distress syndrome (ARDS), where modes of ventilation such as pressure control ventilation, inverse ratio ventilation, and prone ventilation are often used. However, many patients who require mechanical ventilation still require some degree of sedation and/or analgesia in order to tolerate the endotracheal tube, to minimize the discomfort from associated injuries, surgical incisions, and stress of critical illness. In fact, more than 90% of critically ill patients receive sedatives and analgesics during their stay in intensive care (9).

Ideally, the practitioner wishes to keep the patient comfortable, calm, and safe. Amnestic effects of sedatives are often desirable as well, but especially so under circumstances where the patient requires neuromuscular blockade as a state of awareness, while chemically paralyzed condition has been described by many patients as being a terrifying experience. Undersedation is undesirable, but oversedation has also been recognized as contributing to the patient's morbidity, and indirectly, to mortality. Not surprisingly, sedatives comprise a large proportion of most ICU pharmacy budgets. The cost of sedatives and analgesics for critically ill patients has been estimated to be more than a billion dollars annually (9). Yet our armentatarium of sedatives is still relatively limited. The ideal sedative has been "profiled," but unfortunately does not exist at this time.

Concerns about many of these issues, as well as the need for some standardization of sedation assessment and monitoring, have lead to the development of sedation protocols. It is hoped that these will improve the quality of the patient's ICU experience and have ancillary benefits of minimizing oversedation, which may help to reduce intensive care costs. The Joint Commission on Accreditation of Healthcare Organizations (JCAHO) has advised that the assessment of the degree of pain should be considered the "fifth vital sign" (9). Others have also suggested that the proper use of sedation should be used with other criteria as a quality index for ICUs and should be considered the "sixth vital sign" in this patient population (9,10).

I. PATIENTS WITH MALIGNANCY

Admission to the ICU is not necessarily a preterminal event for cancer patients (Table 1). In particular, many pediatric oncology patients may attain long-term disease-free survival.

A recent study surveyed outcomes of children with malignancy admitted to a pediatric ICU (PICU). It found an acute survival rate of 73% and a long-term survival rate of 50% for all pediatric oncology patients admitted to the PICU. However, as with adults, the outcomes for bone marrow transplant patients are worse. Initiating mechanical ventilation in pediatric bone marrow transplant patients has been associated with very poor outcomes, with only 18% surviving (11). Another series, with a greater proportion of autologous transplants revealed a 30% long-term survival for the 20 children requiring ventilatory support (12).

Sivan et al. (13) also assessed the outcome of pediatric oncology patients in the PICU. They also found an overall mortality rate of 50%; however, only 20% of the septic patients survived. Children have a better prognosis than adults with similar disease, but in the setting of life-threatening complications their prognosis is still poor.

Khassawneh et al. (14) at the University of Arkansas studied all autologous peripheral blood stem cell transplantation (PBSCT) patients who required mechanical ventilation for more than 24 hr and who had not previously undergone mechanical ventilation. They found that 26% of all patients survived to hospital discharge, of whom 67% went on to achieve more than 6 months survival. Patients with isolated organ failure, or who only required vasopressors (considered a single organ failure), fared better, with a 32% hospital survival rate. Patients with such single organ failures represented 75% of those who underwent mechanical ventilation. Those with hepatic and renal failure, and patients with lung injury and the use of vasopressors, had dismal outcomes, however, with 6% hospital survival, and 0% 6 month survival. Rates of hospital survival after mechanical ventilation for patients who have received nonautologous bone marrow transplants have been reported to be significantly lower, at 4–13%. The authors suspected that the improved survival in patients with autologous transplants was related to more rapid engraftment, less treatment-related toxicity, and the absence of graft vs. host disease. They concluded that patients with

Table 1 Oncology/ICU Outcome Studies from 1998 to 2000

Study	Year	*N*	ICU survival (%)	Comments
Conti et al. (2)	1998	16	65	All noninvasive ventilation
Hauringa et al. (9)	2000	60	18	All BMT, all ventilated
Krongsgaard and Meidell (10)	1998	115	46	All BMT, 18% survival if ventilated
Price et al. (11)	1998	119	71	Includes surgical cases, all ventilated
Staudinger et al. (12)	2000	414	53	
Kress et al. (13)	1999	348	59	
Hayes et al. (14)	1998	39	27	All BMT, pediatric population
Azoulay et al. (15)	1999	75	43	All myeloma, BMT in 37%

BMT, bone marrow transplantation; ICU, intensive care unit.
Source: From Ref. 11.

autologous PBSCT should undergo mechanical ventilation.

Dalrymple et al. (15) retrospectively studied the course of all patients at The University of Texas M.D. Anderson Cancer Center, who were admitted and died with gynecological malignancies from 1992 to 1997. Twelve percent of deaths occurred in the ICU. The average interval between the last cycle of chemotherapy and death was 77 days. Twenty-one percent of patients received chemotherapy during their last hospitalization. They found that discussions about DNR orders were occurring earlier in relation to terminal events in the latter half of the time interval studied. Seventy-two percent of all DNR orders were placed within two weeks before death and 35% were placed within 72 hr before death. The authors also pointed out a shortened interval between the last cycle of chemotherapy and death during the latter study period (1995–1997), and expressed the concern that this apparently futile care may belie a need for more effective and frank communication between the patients and their caregivers.

Over the past few decades, the attitudes of patients and their families have changed regarding their wishes for their physician to inform them of their diagnosis and prognosis, shifting from a preference for information to be with held to favoring full disclosure (15). This has implications regarding the need for comfort care, withdrawal of support, and terminal sedation in the ICU.

II. THE ICU EXPERIENCE FROM THE PERSPECTIVE OF THE CANCER PATIENT

Most studies regarding patients' perspectives on their ICU experience have been surveys performed sometimes weeks or months after a patient's discharge from the ICU and thus are limited to the views of survivors alone and are subject to errors in recall. Nelson et al. (16) did a real-time symptom assessment of adult patients admitted to the ICU with either a current or former diagnosis of cancer. "Active" cancer was present in approximately 75% of the patients. Thirty-two percent of the patients died in the ICU. Palliative care specialists routinely consulted on these patients, and the impression of the care team providers was that liberal sedation and analgesia was being administered, although there was not any use of sedation or analgesia protocols. Patients selfreported symptoms daily using the Edmonton Symptom Assessment Scale. Fifty percent of eligible patients were able to respond. Symptoms of moderate to severe pain, anxiety, hunger and thirst, were reported by 55–75% of patients. Approximately, 35% reported feeling moderate to severe depression or dyspnea (16).

III. TERMINAL SEDATION

Patients with advanced cancer suffer not only from pain and fatigue, but also from depression and anxiety. More than one-third of patients dying with cancer experience depression (17). Oncologists need to acquire skill in end-of-life care and have to be able to make the transition from attempts to aggressively treat disease to palliative care in preterminal patients. Oncologists and intensivists are generally considered to be the experts in managing end-of-life care. A survey of the American Society of Clinical Oncology (ASCO) members in 1998 showed that more than 90% of oncologists felt comfortable treating the physical symptoms of cancer such as pain, nausea, and vomiting. However, only 50% felt comfortable managing depression. Many also expressed uneasiness discussing psychiatric issues and the end of life with their patients. The ASCO also found that those with less training in communication of end-of-life issues were also more likely to treat terminally ill patients with chemotherapy and to forego hospice care (17). This discomfort with dealing with psychiatric issues is apparently not limited to practitioners from the United States. Morita et al. surveyed Japanese oncologists and palliative care physicians and found that up to 50% surveyed chose continuous deep sedation as a possibility or a strong possibility for managing cases of depression and delirium. They found that physicians who were unsure about proper care for psychological distress and those who scored highly for symptoms of burnout were significantly more likely to use continuous deep sedation. They surmised that many oncologists may benefit from further education to help them to decide when a patient might benefit from referral to a psychiatrist and how best to utilize palliative care services. Others have expressed that such education should be a formal part of fellowship training in oncology (17).

In Morita's survey, four different vignettes of patients with terminal cancer were described. Two of the four theoretical patients were competent, nondepressed patients requesting terminal sedation for refractory physical and psychological distress. The other two patients' vignettes were described as having associated delirium or depression, which were viewed by experienced psychiatrists as treatable. Five treatment options were offered to the practitioners: (1) psychiatric treatment without sedation, (2) treatment with psychotropics, (3) mild sedation, (4) terminal sedation, and (5) patient-assisted suicide.

The practice of terminal sedation was defined by Morita et al. (18) in his study as the continuous administration of sedatives or opioids to the point where the patient almost or completely loses consciousness, with the primary goal for the patient not to suffer. He found that those who chose terminal sedation in cases where there was a strong possibility of the presence of a treatable psychiatric disorder were less confident with psychiatric care, were more likely to prefer symptomatic treatment for themselves, and scored higher for burnout. Morita expressed the concern that depression and delirium were being underdiagnosed and undertreated.

Those who tended to choose psychiatric treatment in cases with symptoms of depression and delirium were significantly more involved in end-of-life care, tended to be younger, more religious, were more likely to be specialized in palliative medicine, and demonstrated greater degrees of personal accomplishment (18). Physicians who regarded euthanasia as a treatment option in any of the cases demonstrated higher levels of depersonalization and were less involved in end-of-life care.

There was a high incidence of palliative sedation being chosen for use at the end of life in this study, for both physical and psychiatric distress. Patient assisted suicide/euthanasia was chosen as an option much less frequently. A survey of palliative care specialists in the U.K. and North America found that the use of deep sedation prior to death is also prevalent. Morita proposed guidelines for the use of palliative sedation in the terminally ill. After clarification of the terminal state of disease with the patient and identification of the treatment goals, palliative sedation may be initiated in the face of severe refractory distress that is unresponsive to other measures. Team consent or second opinion and informed consent from the patient and their family should proceed. The above process should be explicitly documented (18). One might also be concerned that physician burnout is not being pre-empted in this high-risk specialty as well.

IV. SEDATION

A discussion of general concepts of sedation in the critically ill follows. Sedation is a physiological state comprising anxiolysis, hypnosis, and amnesia.

Anxiolysis is the reduction of the physiological response to a real or perceived danger.

Amnesia refers to the impairment or cessation of memory caused by drug-induced, reversible modulation of synaptic communication (19).

Hypnosis is defined as a state of decreased motor activity that appears physically similar to sleep (19).

Sedation thus does not necessarily entail any component of analgesia. This differs from general anesthesia, defined by Kissin (20) in 1993 as a state comprising analgesia, amnesia, anxiolysis, and the suppression of hormonal, cardiovascular, and motor responses to noxious stimuli/surgical stimulation.

V. ANXIETY

Anxiety is defined by the DSM-IV (Diagnostic and Statistical manual of Mental Disorders) as the "apprehensive anticipation of future danger or misfortune accompanied by a feeling of dysphoria or somatic symptoms of tension" (21). This state of apprehension and autonomic arousal may be in response to a real or perceived threat. Benzodiazepines (BZDs) are appropriate if therapy is required.

VI. AGITATION

Agitation and delirium may affect as many as 57–70% of critically ill patients at one point or another (9,22). Agitation is characterized by the presence of violent motion and/or strong and tumultuous emotion. It is considered to be further along on the spectrum of emotional turmoil than is anxiety (23,24). The patient generally will be tachycardic and hypertensive, is often unintelligible, may have an exaggerated sense of pain, and will not follow commands. Agitation may be a manifestation of physiological derangement or some other cause of discomfort. Thus, it is imperative that the patient be evaluated and treated for reversible causes such as hypoxemia, pain, a full bladder, hypoglycemia, residual neuromuscular blockade, cerebral events or central nervous system (CNS) infections, electrolyte imbalances, hypoglycemia, and sepsis prior to initiating sedation. Pain is a common cause of agitation in the critically ill. Pain should always be specifically addressed and adequate analgesia supplied (25). Drug withdrawal syndromes may also be responsible for agitation. Physical restraints, frustration, the inability to synchronize their respirations with the ventilator, and other environmental factors may also be contributory (7,9,19). Agitation may provoke myocardial ischemia in predisposed patients (9). It can also result in dangerous outcomes, with potential harm to the patient and/or caregivers. Patients may selfextubate or remove other invasive devices such as intravenous or arterial cannulae, pulmonary artery catheters, or ventriculostomies (9). This situation mandates expeditious evaluation and may necessitate applying physical restraints in addition to the administration of sedatives or psychotropics before the patient manages to harm himself or his caregivers.

VII. DELIRIUM

The delirious state is characterized by an acute, potentially reversible impairment of consciousness and mentation, which tends to follow a fluctuating course. Patients often behave inappropriately, are disinhibited, disoriented, and may experience hallucinations or paranoid ideation. There may or may not be altered psychomotor activity (26). The autonomic nervous system is often hyperactive. The electroencephalogram (EEG) may demonstrate diffuse slowing (25). Delirium differs from dementia, which usually is irreversible and chronic in nature (25). Various triggers of delirium include numerous drugs, sepsis, endocrine, hepatic, or uremic encephalopathies, encephalitis, subarachnoid hemorrhage, and other acute CNS insults (25).

Delirium occurs frequently in the ICU, with an incidence of 15–40% (23). It is especially common in patients with terminal cancer and end stage acquired immune deficiency syndrome (AIDS), with a prevalence of 25–85% (27). Some associations or risk factors for delirium have been identified, and include preexisting dementia, advanced age, fever or hypothermia, sicker patients, use of psychotropic drugs, and an elevated blood urea nitrogen (BUN) level. Patients with three or more of these risk factors had a 60% incidence of delirium (25).

Several subtypes of delirium exist, including hyperactive, hypoactive, and mixed forms. Patients with hypoactive delirium may appear to be somnolent. Patients with hyperactive delirium are more likely to be aggressive, paranoid, and hallucinating (28).

Plasma anticholinergic activity is higher in intensive care patients with signs of delirium than in patients who do not exhibit these signs (25). Elderly patients are especially prone to develop delirium in the postoperative period. Patients with agitation and delirium also appear to have a higher mortality rate than critically ill patients without these problems. The onset of delirium in an elderly patient while hospitalized has been correlated with a risk of death of from 25% to 75% (22,27). Administration of BZDs or opiates to the delirious patient may paradoxically exacerbate his symptoms, possibly because of the further alteration in sensory perception produced by these agents (26). Haloperidol is considered the drug of choice for delirium.

Delirium may be underrecognized, misdiagnosed, and undertreated in cancer patients. Changes in mental status are often not appreciated or difficult to document if a baseline, screening mental status evaluation—such as the MiniMental State Evaluation or the Confusion Assessment Method (CAM)—was not performed on or prior to admission. The CAM, which is an instrument used for the assessment of delirium, has been modified to a form more appropriate for use in the critically ill patient, the CAM-ICU. The modified form has been validated, and found to be useful for the assessment of patients who are mechanically ventilated (29). Agitation from delirium is often misinterpreted as being due to pain alone. Unfortunately, opioids used to help alleviate pain, such as morphine sulfate, fentanyl, and levorphanol can result in confusion or delirium (27). A number of different chemotherapeutic agents, in addition to glucocorticoids, have also been reported to cause a confusional state. These drugs include methotrexate, vincristine and vinblastine, bleomycin, fluorouracil, and cisplatin (27).

Delirium or "terminal restlessness" is extremely common in patients with advanced cancer. A study performed assessing the use of breakthrough analgesics in delirious vs. nondelirious patients indicated that most breakthrough analgesic doses were being administered to delirious patients at night, when agitation and confusion are often worse. Nondelirious patients received breakthrough analgesics predominantly during the day (28).

Delirium is very distressing to the patient, and probably even more so for visiting family members. As there is often an exaggerated sense of pain and agitation in this state, there is often a lot of pressure from family members to escalate opioid doses. This can result in opioid toxicity in a situation where looking for a reversible cause and treating more specifically for delirium might be more appropriate. In a preterminal state, delirium may be irreversible. If the delirious state remains refractory after reasonable attempts have been made to find and treat potentially reversible causes, team members should consult and come to a consensus. If they concur that the patient has been appropriately evaluated, and that environmental and pharmaceutical interventions have been optimized, consideration should be given to sedating the patient for refractory, or "terminal anguish." This should be discussed with the patient's family, or healthcare representative (28).

VIII. ENVIRONMENT

Over time, we have come to realize that certain aspects of the ICU environment itself can have a dramatic impact on our patients' mental status. Noise levels are high, and lights are on 24 hr a day. Patients are frequently awakened for examinations, assessments, vital signs, x-rays, or procedures, and are often sleep deprived. Sleep disturbances have been associated with delirium, especially in the elderly. Melatonin, which helps to regulate the sleep–wake cycle, has been found to be decreased in hospitalized and postoperative patients. A recent case study reported successful treatment of a case of refractory delirium with melatonin, and apparently successful prevention of delirium in a patient with a history of postoperative delirium (30).

A number of nonpharmacological methods to help minimize confusion, agitation, and delirium have been employed. The presence of windows in the ICU can decrease the likelihood of mental status alterations by almost 50% (9). Noise level reduction, reducing bright lights, (avoiding total darkness with night lights) minimizing sleep interruptions, frequent verbal reorientation and reassurance, family visits, and the presence of calendars and clocks can also have a positive effect (9). Alternative nonpharmaceutical techniques have not been routinely employed as adjuncts in the United States; however, Chinese ICUs have employed acupuncture and acupressure (23). A recent study by Kober et al. (31) in Austria found that ambulance patients who received acupressure at the auricular acupuncture site were significantly more relaxed and anticipated less pain as tested by the Visual Analog Scale than those that received acupressure at a sham site. Transcutaneous electrical stimulation of another auricular acupuncture site (the lateralization control point) 3 cm anterior to the tragus was found to reduce the concentration of volatile anesthetic required to prevent movement in response to a noxious electrical stimulus in a randomized, double-blind trial published by Greif et al. (32). Volatile anesthetic requirements were reduced by $11 \pm 7\%$.

IX. SEDATION AND THE STRESS RESPONSE

Stress and pain result in elevation of serum catecholamine levels and a host of other neuroendocrine changes. The increase in catecholamines results in an increase in heart rate, contractility, and myocardial oxygen consumption. It also inhibits insulin production in favor of glucagon production, resulting in hyperglycemia. Free fatty acids and triglycerides also increase. The catecholamines and released substrates fuel the "fight or flight" response. Growth hormone, vasopressin, renin–angiotensin, cortisol, aldosterone, and other hormones also increase. The presence of tissue inflammation results in the release from macrophages of a variety of cytokines, including tumor necrosis factor, and interleukins 1, 6, and 8 (1–5,19,33). The balance of salt and water is shifted towards conservation, in attempts to maintain intravascular volume to help compensate for blood loss (34).

These survival mechanisms evolved in order for our species to have a better chance of surmounting life-threatening circumstances. However, negative consequences of these physiological adaptations include immunosuppression, hypercoagulability, catabolism, poor wound healing, and myocardial ischemia.

Myles et al. (35) reported their double-blind, randomized controlled trial comparing the use of remifentanil infusions, low dose fentanyl, and moderate dose fentanyl in outcomes after coronary artery bypass surgery. Higher doses of fentanyl (28 μg/kg) and remifentanil (0.85 μg/kg/min) were shown to reduce the incidence of perioperative infarction after coronary artery bypass grafting. Remifentanil also reduced the cortisol response to surgery, compared to both fentanyl groups. Alpha-2 adrenergic agonists, such as clonidine, have also been shown to attenuate the sympathetic response to surgery. Although it may be intuitive that modulating the stress response may be beneficial in critically ill patients, it remains unclear whether the use of sedation confers any survival benefit or improvement in outcome (33).

X. THE IDEAL ICU SEDATIVE

Criteria for the ideal sedative in the ICU have been described (23,36). Unfortunately, this ideal drug does not exist yet. Potential characteristics of the ideal sedative are described in Table 2.

XI. GOALS OF SEDATION

The Society of Critical Care Medicine (SCCM) advises that the critically ill patient should be sedated only after provision of adequate analgesia and finding and treating reversible causes for agitation. Once this has been accomplished, the primary goals of sedation are anxiolysis, hypnosis, and amnesia (7). Both underseda-

Table 2 Characteristics of the Ideal Sedative

Minimal cardiovascular depression
Provides analgesia
Provides amnesia
Rapid onset and offset
Easy to titrate to desired effect
No development of tolerance
No withdrawal syndromes
Does not support bacterial growth
Inexpensive
No significant drug interactions
Does not suppress adrenocortical axis

tion and oversedation are undesirable. The intensivist must strike a delicate balance with the sedation regimen, in order to optimize patient comfort, minimize the stress response, and (hopefully) decrease the incidence of post-traumatic stress syndrome, while avoiding any adverse hemodynamic effects and oversedation.

Oversedation is potentially dangerous. Times to extubation are prolonged in oversedated patients. Prolongation of mechanical ventilation and ICU stays predisposes the patient to nosocomial complications, such as pneumonia, thromboses, myoneuropathy, and other adverse events related to invasive procedures or monitoring, such as line sepsis, urinary tract infections, and airway complications, which can increase the mortality rate. Oversedated patients in a pharmacologically induced coma are also more likely to undergo unnecessary testing for evaluation of mental status changes/unresponsiveness such as computed tomography (CT) scans and magnetic resonance imaging scans (MRIs), which adds further to the costs accruing from a prolonged length of stay (9,19,25).

XII. SEDATION MONITORING

Individual patients will have different needs for sedation, which will change over time. Ideally, team members should specify a sedation goal for the patient that is appropriate for their circumstances at that point in time.

The JCAHO has defined several levels of sedation (7,23):

1. Minimal (anxiolysis): drug-induced state where the patient responds normally to verbal commands, either alone or accompanied by light tactile stimulation. Cognitive function may be impaired, but there is no depression of respiratory or cardiovascular function.
2. Moderate (conscious sedation): drug-induced depression of consciousness where patients respond purposefully to verbal commands, either alone or accompanied by light tactile stimulation. There is no need to assist with airway maintenance, and spontaneous respirations are adequate.
3. Deep: drug-induced depression of consciousness during which patients cannot be easily aroused, but respond purposefully following repeated or noxious stimulation. They may need assistance to maintain a patent airway. Spontaneous ventilation may be inadequate. Cardiovascular function is usually maintained.
4. Anesthesia: a drug-induced loss of consciousness (LOC) where patients are not arousable, even by painful stimulation.

Most patients in the ICU do not require deep sedation or anesthetic doses of sedation, which often can compromise the cardiovascular system. However, there are circumstances where this may be necessary, e.g., patients with severe ARDS requiring inverse ratio ventilation and neuromuscular blockade, patients with severe head injuries in barbiturate coma, and trauma patients with an open abdominal wound who require neuromuscular blockade and sedation to prevent evisceration. These patients clearly have different sedation goals than the stable postoperative patient who is expected to reach extubation criteria shortly, or a patient intubated for an exacerbation of chronic obstructive pulmonary disease.

XIII. SEDATION SCALES

The use of sedation scales helps to standardize patient assessment and minimize interobserver differences in patient evaluation (9). A variety of different sedation scales have been described and are in use. Ideally, a sedation scale should be easy for practitioners to learn and use, and should be reproducible. The scale should be able to adequately assess the range of clinical conditions of the patient, and should enable the practitioner to choose a clear endpoint for sedation for the patient. Not all sedation scales have been validated in clinical practice, and most do not include pain assessment (7,37). Tables 3 and 4 display some of the more commonly used, validated sedation scales.

Many institutions have initiated the use of sedation protocols, where patients who have been receiving continuous intravenous sedation have it held on a periodic basis. Recent studies showed that the use of a sedation protocol or daily interruption of continuous intravenous sedation resulted in a decreased duration of mechanical ventilation and ICU stay, fewer diagnostic tests to assess mental status changes, and fewer tracheotomies. Use of a sedation protocol also resulted in significant cost savings (7,9,25,38).

A discussion of concepts of sedation, subjective and objective methods of assessment, and specific agents for sedation follows.

XIV. CLINICAL SEDATION MONITORING

Subjective scoring systems are based on observing a patient's motor behavior. Thus, patients who have been rendered pharmaceutically immobile with neuromuscular blockade will not be able to be accurately assessed with this type of scale. The same is true for patients with physiological disorders such as critical illness myoneuropathy. Hypertension and tachycardia have traditionally been used as surrogate means of

Table 3 Scales Available in Full-Text Form and Tested for Validity and Reliability

Ramsay Scale		
1	Anxious and agitated or restless or both	
2	Cooperative, oriented, and tranquil	
3	Responding to commands only	
4	Brisk response to light glabellar tap	
5	Sluggish response to light glabellar tap	
6	No response to light glabellar tap	
Sedation–Agitation Scale		
7	Dangerous agitation	Pulling at ET tube, trying to remove catheters, climbing over bed rail, striking at staff, thrashing side-to-side
6	Very agitated	Does not calm despite frequent verbal reminding of limits, requires physical restraints, biting ET tube
5	Agitated	Anxious or mildly agitated, attempting to sit up, calms down with verbal instructions
4	Calm and cooperative	Calm, awakens easily, follows commands
3	Sedated	Difficult to arouse, awakens to verbal stimuli or gentle shaking, but drifts off again, follows simple commands
2	Very sedated	Arouses to physical stimuli, but does not communicate or follow commands, may move spontaneously
1	Unarousable	Minimal or no response to noxious stimuli, does not communicate or follow commands
Motor Activity Assessment Scale		
0	Unresponsive	Does not move with noxious stimuli
1	Responsive only to noxious stimuli	Opens eyes OR raises eyebrows OR turns head toward stimulus OR moves limbs with noxious stimuli
2	Response to touch	Opens eyes OR raises eyebrows OR turns head toward stimulus or moves limbs when touched or name is loudly spoken
3	Calm and cooperative	No external stimulus is required to elicit movement AND patient is adjusting sheets or clothes purposefully and follows commands
4	Restless and cooperative	No external stimulus is required to elicit movement AND patient is picking at sheets or tubes OR uncovering self BUT follows commands
5	Agitated	No external stimulus is required to elicit movement AND attempting to sit up OR move limbs out of bed AND does not consistently follow commands (e.g., will lie down when asked but soon reverts to attempts to sit up or move limbs out of bed)
6	Dangerously agitated, uncooperative	No external stimulus is required to elicit movement AND patient is pulling at tubes or catheters OR thrashing side-to-side OR striking at staff OR trying to climb out of bed AND does not calm down when asked

ET, endotracheal tube; noxious stimuli, suctioning OR five seconds of vigorous orbital, sternal, or nail bed pressure.
Source: From Ref. 9.

alerting practitioners to the presence of anxiety or agitation in these patients, but are nonspecific. In he operating room setting, it has also been shown that patients may experiencc awareness under anesthesia in the absence of hypertension or tachycardia (39).

XV. SUBJECTIVE SEDATION SCALES

Ramsay Sedation Scale: This scale has been widely used for many years. The Ramsay Scale scores the patient at one of six levels—three asleep, three awake. It has been criticized, however for not clearly distinguishing degrees of severity of agitation that are considered clinically significant, grouping mildly agitated and severely agitated patients in the same rating (Table 3) (7,19,25,40).

Riker Sedation–Agitation Scale (*SAS*): This scale was developed to address some of the perceived failings of the Ramsay Scale. It has seven levels, three descriptive levels of degrees of agitation, and three degrees of oversedation, with zero being used to describe a calm and co-operative patient. The Riker Scale was the first sedation scale to be formally tested, and it has been validated as reliable in clinical practice in the ICU (Tables 3 and 5) (7,23,41).

Table 4 "Time" (The COMFORT© Scale)

	Time
Alertness	
Deeply asleep	1
Lightly asleep	2
Drowsy	3
Fully awake and alert	4
Hyperalert	5
Calmness/agitation	
Calm	1
Slightly anxious	2
Anxious	3
Very anxious	4
Panicky	5
Respiratory response	
No coughing and no spontaneous respiration	1
Spontaneous respiration with little or no response to ventilation	2
Occasional cough or resistance to ventilator	3
Actively breathes against ventilator or coughs regularly	4
Fights ventilator; coughing or choking	5
Physical movement	
No movement	1
Occasional, slight movement	2
Frequent, slight movement	3
Vigorous movement limited to extremities	4
Vigorous movements including torso and head	5
Blood pressure (map) baseline	
Blood pressure below baseline	1
Blood pressure consistently at baseline	2
Infrequent elevations of 15% or more (1–3)	3
Frequent elevations of 15% or more (more than 3)	4
Sustained elevation of ≥15%	5
Heart rate baseline	
Heart rate baseline	1
Heart rate consistently at baseline	2
Infrequent elevations or 15% or more above baseline (1–3) during observation period	3
Frequent elevations of 15% or more above baseline (more than 3)	4
Sustained elevation of ≥15%	5
Muscle tone	
Muscles totally relaxed; no muscle tone	1
Reduced muscle tone	2
Normal muscle tone	3
Increased muscle tone and flexion of fingers and toes	4
Extreme muscle rigidity and flexion of fingers and toes	5
Facial tension	
Facial muscles totally relaxed	1
Facial muscle tone normal; no facial muscle tension evident	2
Tension evident in some facial expressions	3
Tension evident throughout facial muscles	4
Facial muscles contorted and grimacing	5

Source: From Ref. 38.

The COMFORT Scale: This scale was developed and validated as a subjective measure of distress for use in the pediatric population, but subsequently has been validated in adults. The advantage of the COMFORT Scale over the Ramsay Scale is that it is not based on evaluating responsiveness in a way that disturbs the patient from rest (41). Marx et al. (41) described the use of the COMFORT Scale for assessing the level of sedation of 85 mechanically ventilated children (Table 4). The target range of optimal sedation had COMFORT scores of 17–26.

The Motor Activity Assessment Scale (MAAS): This scale, an adaptation of the SAS, was tested in surgical ICU patients. The MAAS had a good inter-rater reliability, and a high correlation with a visual analog scale. There was a significant correlation between the MAAS, and heart and respiratory rate variations, respiratory rate variations, as well as the number of agitation associated events reported in the 30 min time interval just prior to scoring (9) (Table 3).

Devlin et al. (9) evaluated 23 different sedation assessment scales. They found that few had undergonepsychometric testing to evaluate them for their validity (the degree to which a sedation scale truly measures how agitated a patient is at that point in time), and their reliability for discriminating between patients.

The Ramsay Scale has been validated against the modified Glasgow Coma Scale and more recently against the Sedation Agitation Scale. It must be remembered, however, that there is no existing gold standard for sedation scales, and the format and content of the scales are similar (9). Comparisons of some of the scales have been made with objective means of neurological assessment. Of the scales assessed, the Ramsay Scale showed the highest degree of correlation with changes in auditory evoked potential latency. The reliability of

Table 5 Riker Sedation–Agitation Scale

Score	Description	Example
+3	Immediate threat to safety	Pulling at endotracheal tube or catheters, trying to climb over bedrail, striking at staff
+2	Dangerously agitated	Requiring physical restraints and frequent verbal reminding of limits, biting ETT, thrashing-side-to-side
+1	Agitated	Physically agitated, attempting to sit up, calms down to verbal instructions
0	Calm and cooperative	Calm, arousable, follows commands
–1	Oversedated	Difficult to arouse or unable to attend to conversation or commands
–2	Very oversedated	Awakens to noxious stimuli only
–3	Unarousable	Does not awaken to any stimulus

the Ramsay Scale, the Sedation–Agitation Scale (aka the Riker Sedation–Agitation Scale), the Motor Activity Assessment Scale (MAAS), the Hahneman Sedation Assessment Scale (HSAS), the Vancouver Interaction and Calmness Scale (VICS), the Richmond Agitation Assessment Score (RASS), and the Agitation/ Scale were found to be high (9).

XVI. NEUROMUSCULAR BLOCKADE

As previously discussed, the use of sedation scales largely based on assessment of motor activity level has significant limitations in certain populations of patients. There is general consensus that all patients who undergo neuromuscular blockade should be pharmacologically sedated. In a survey of 185 anesthesiologist intensivists, neuromuscular blockade was reported to be used most commonly (89%) to facilitate mechanical ventilation (41).

Patients who require neuromuscular blockade are among the most critically ill and hemodynamically compromised patients. It is difficult to determine what the correct degree of sedation is under such circumstances. Autonomic signs of inadequate sedation such as hypertension, tachycardia, sweating, and lacrimation are often absent in patients who report recall (42). Conversely, such autonomic signs are nonspecific in critically ill patients. Concerns about the accuracy of such assessment and the wish to provide adequate and safe sedation for all patients has led many to consider alternative, objective techniques for monitoring the level of sedation or awareness in ICU patients.

XVII. OBJECTIVED SEDATION MONITORING

A. The Bispectral Index (BIS)

The BIS was derived from bifrontal EEG recordings obtained from anesthetized patients with the intent of finding an index that would correlate well with degrees of hypnosis and specifically absence of recall. Individual elements of the EEG recordings that change with levels of hypnosis were converted via multivariate analysis to a linear, numeric index, ranging from 0, representing an isoelectric EEG, to 100 (fully awake) (7,43) (Table 6).

Amnesia generally occurs at BIS levels less than 64–80, although some cases of awareness under general anesthesia have been reported in the presence of very low BIS numbers (44). The BIS index itself does not indicate whether the patient is arousable or not. Volunteers in natural sleep had BIS levels less than 30, and were arousable, whereas patients anesthetized with volatile anesthetics or propofol were not arousable at similar BIS indices (44).

B. BIS in the ICU

Intensivists gained interest in the prospects of using the BIS monitor to function as an objective measure of sedation in critically ill patients, especially for those receiving neuromuscular blockade. Up to 36% of patients have reported recall during neuromuscular blockade in the ICU (45). Ancillary motivations for the use of the BIS monitor are as a potential tool to help minimize excessive sedation and secondarily reduce pharmaceutical costs, although the monitor itself, of course would be more costly than the use of subjective assessment protocols.

Table 6 The Bispectral Index

90–100	Awake
80	Some sedation
60	Moderate hypnosis
$\leq$40	Unconscious, moderate to deep hypnosis
0	Isoelectric EEG

The presence or absence of awareness per se is not the chief concern when sedating most patients in the ICU. Usually, the goal is to avoid both excessive and inadequate sedation. Since the BIS was derived from patients undergoing general anesthesia, and not from critically ill patients, some have questioned its applicability in the ICU population, where patients are sedated for prolonged periods. The ICU itself is a less controlled environment, and has the potential for introducing more noise and artifact than the operating room environment. Electromyography (EMG) interference has been noted to be more of a significant problem in recording consistent BIS indices in critically ill patients since fewer patients are undergoing neuromuscular blockade in the ICU, and there is a greater likelihood of spontaneous movement. This tends to increase the BIS score greater than expected clinically. Even so, The BIS has been reported to correlate with subjective sedation assessment scales (9,24,46).

Some authors have attempted to correlate subjective assessment scales with BIS monitor readings in the ICU. Nasraway et al. (43) performed a prospective, comparative single-blind observer study attempting to establish the correlation between the subjective Sedation–Agitation Scale and the BIS. None of the patients in this study received neuromuscular blockade. Wide variability in BIS scores was noted for any given SAS score. Correlation between the BIS and the SAS was improved, but still not impressive, when BIS values obtained in the presence of excessive muscle activity were excluded. The correlation improved with subgroup analysis when BIS values associated with excessive muscle movement were excluded. The authors concluded that regular and routine use of the BIS cannot be recommended to monitor critically ill patients who are not receiving neuromuscular blockade. (A figure that represented only 1% of the surgical patients admitted to the ICU at that institution.) Others have noted a wide range of BIS indices for any given Ramsay Sedation Scale (RSS) level of sedation, and speculated that the comparisons may be confounded since performing subjective assessments usually involves stimulating the patient and subsequently tends to increase concurrent BIS values (44). Abnormal EEGs are often associated with CNS pathology such as traumatic brain injuries and encephalopathy. Since the BIS is derived from the EEG, BIS readings may also be lowered by these disorders. It is unclear what goal the BIS index would be appropriate in such patients. Central nervous system injuries or disturbances are common in the ICU setting, leading some to question whether studies attempting to validate the use of the BIS as a sedation tool are accurate under such circumstances (9,45).

The unobtrusive nature of obtaining a BIS reading, and its ability to give continuous data, is seen as an advantage by others. Berkenbosch et al. (24) studied the correlation of three different sedation scales with BIS monitor readings in PICU patients requiring sedation and mechanical ventilation. The authors found that the BIS correlated with subjective sedation scores and was able to effectively differentiate clinically adequate from inadequate sedation. They found that it seemed less accurate for predicting oversedation, when using a BIS value of <40 as a criterion number for a state of deep hypnosis. Raising the criterion number to a value of 50 was more accurate, but many patients with BIS levels less than that still had what was deemed to be appropriate levels of sedation. The authors suggested that maintaining a BIS range of 50–70 seemed to minimize the likelihood of oversedation while still maintaining adequate sedation for the majority of their PICU patients (24).

Newer versions of the BIS software (4.0) have been designed to help minimize the influence of EMG artifact of the BIS index readings. Further studies are still needed to validate this technique. It remains unknown whether the use of the BIS monitor will help to improve outcomes for the critically ill patient, or help to minimize the cost of pharmaceuticals (9,46). O'Connor et al. (47) performed a cost analysis of the use of the BIS monitor to prevent awareness under general anesthesia. Their analysis was based on a variant of a standard model of cost, encompassing the range of potential incidences of awareness and the efficacy of the monitor for detecting the presence of awareness. Using this model, cost = price/(efficiency × incidence), assuming an incidence of awareness of 1/20,000 and an efficiency of 90% for detecting the presence of awareness, the cost of preventing a single case of awareness would be approximately U.S.$400,000. Using an incidence of 1/100, and an efficiency of 50%, the cost would be U.S.$2000 per case prevented. However, the incidence of awareness during sedation and neuromuscular blockade in the ICU is not clearly known at this time, nor is the efficiency of the BIS monitor for preventing awareness.

XVIII. AUDITORY EVOKED POTENTIALS

Auditory evoked potentials apply an auditory stimulus to the patient as a means of performing functional assessment of the auditory pathway (ear, auditory nerve, and brainstem). This technique has been useful for assessing neurological function in comatose patients, and has been tested as a sedation instrument. It requires the presence of functioning auditory nerves.

With increasing levels of anesthesia, the amplitude of the early cortical response decreases, and there is a prolongation of the latency. An index, the Auditory Evoked Potential Index (AEPI) can then be calculated. Auditory evoked potentials have been found to be a reliable measure of depth of sedation in the ICU setting. In a study by Gajraj et al., the AEPI was most accurate at determining the transition from consciousness to unconsciousness when compared to the BIS monitor, spectral edge frequency (SEF), and median frequency (MF) in patients sedated with propofol administered by a target-controlled infusion device (9,48).

XIX. CHOICE OF SEDATIVE

When choosing a sedative and analgesic regimen for a particular patient, considerations include the expectations for the duration of mechanical support, the patient's hemodynamic status and age, cost-effectiveness, and the particular organ dysfunctions or injuries that might predispose to metabolite accumulation or intolerance of the regimen. Many cancer patients are on chronic opioids and have developed tolerance to this class of agents. In patients who are not intubated, one must be very cautious when combining sedative-hypnotics and opioids due to the potentiation of respiratory depressant effects.

The Society of Critical Care Medicine (SCCM) has published updated guidelines for sedation and analgesia in the ICU (49).

XX. SCCM GUIDELINES FOR SEDATIVES

The SCCM recommends using midazolam or diazepam for rapid sedation of acutely agitated patients.

Lorazepam was recommended as the preferred agent for most patients, either by continuous infusion or by intermittent intravenous dosing, as midazolam infusions may result in prolonged sedation when used for more than 48 hr. The use of sedation guidelines or protocols is recommended (26,36,49).

Propofol is the recommended agent when it is important for the patient to be able to awaken quickly (e.g., head injured patients requiring periodic neurological exams). The caloric input from the lipid vehicle of propofol needs to be accounted for in the patient's nutritional assessment and management. Triglycerides should be followed during the first 2 days of the infusion.

Midazolam or propofol are recommended when only short-term (< 24 hr) sedation is anticipated. The additional cost of propofol may be offset by patients' rapid emergence on this regimen when used short term.

Haloperidol is preferred for the treatment of delirium.

The SCCM cautioned against the use of etomidate as a sedative infusion. Experience in Europe revealed such a manner of administration to be associated with adrenocortical insufficiency and an increase in mortality (26).

They also advised that ketamine, commonly used in burn units as an analgesic for dressing changes, need not be used as an intravenous sedative due to its tendency to cause tachycardia, hypertension, and increased intracranial pressure.

The barbiturates, thiopental and pentobarbital, are useful for the treatment of refractory intracranial hypertension and status epilepticus. Their use as routine sedatives is not advised, however, due to their adverse hemodynamic effects and accumulation (26).

XXI. BENZODIAZEPINES

Benzodiazepines have been the mainstay of sedatives in the ICU for years. They produce anxiolysis, sedation and anterograde amnesia by binding in a stereospecific manner to a particular site (the BZD receptor) on CNS GABA-A receptors, a subtype of the GABA receptor (19,26).

The amnestic effects of BZDs appear to be due to binding to GABA receptors in the limbic cortex (23). Hypnotic effects may be mediated at another site. Binding of BZDs to the GABA-A receptor results in enhanced binding of GABA, an inhibitory neurotransmitter. Benzodiazepines also exhibit anticonvulsant and muscle relaxant effects (19,26). They have no inherent analgesic activity.

Three types of ligands for GABA receptors exist: agonists, antagonists, and inverse agonists.

Agonists: Binding of an agonist results in an increase in chloride conductance and hyperpolarization of the neuron and enhances the receptor complex affinity for GABA. The cell becomes less excitable (19).

Antagonists: Occupy the receptor without affecting GABA binding affinity, thereby blocking GABA action.

Inverse agonists: are experimental agents that decrease the ability of GABA to interact with the receptor, resulting in CNS stimulation (19).

The potency of the different members of the BZD class is determined by the degree of their affinity for the receptor. Lorazepam has the greatest affinity for the receptor, and thus the greatest potency. Midazolam is more potent than diazepam.

The binding of BZDs to the GABA-A receptor is saturable. Chronic use of BZDs results in tolerance, meaning an increased dose required to achieve a similar effect. This may be related to changes in the BZD receptor density, affinity, or occupancy, and possibly due to changes in the volume of distribution of the drug. Acute tolerance has been observed in ICU settings as well. This has been noted as early as 24 hr after initiation of the drug. Benzodiazepines do depress the cardiovascular system and can cause respiratory depression at higher doses (19).

Paradoxical reactions: Patients may experience a paradoxical reaction to BZDs, becoming more agitated or delirious with its administration rather than sedated. Elderly patients and those with pre-existing CNS disorders, psychiatric disease, or substance abuse are more likely to manifest this type of a reaction. Discontinuation of the drug is advised. Administration of haloperidol may be more likely to achieve the desired effect in these patients, and can help control the increased agitation associated with the paradoxical response (19).

Metabolism: Benzodiazepines are metabolized by the liver, either by oxidative reduction, glucuronide conjugation, or both. Drugs that are metabolized by oxidative reduction are more affected by hepatic dysfunction, and have the potential for more drug–drug interactions than those that undergo glucuronide conjugation (such as lorazepam).

The degree to which a sedative is lipophilic is clinically pertinent, since this characteristic affects the rapidity of onset of the agent, and the degree that it will accumulate in fat stores. Midazolam and diazepam are more lipophilic than lorazepam, and thus readily cross the blood–brain barrier, resulting in a more rapid onset of effect. However, as they will be more likely to accumulate in adipose tissue, continued mobilization of the drug from fat stores after the drug has been discontinued may prolong recovery from sedation. This effect is more pronounced in the obese patient.

Clearance of a drug refers to the quantity of blood or plasma from which a substance is removed per unit of time. Context-sensitive $t_{1/2}$s reflect the amount of time that it takes for the plasma concentration of a drug to decrease 50% after a continuous infusion is stopped. It is felt to be more useful than the $t_{1/2}$ beta for assessing the time that it takes for drug concentrations to fall in cases where a patient has been on a continuous infusion for more than a few hours. Computer programs have enabled the invention of target-controlled infusion devices that assess the expected context-sensitive $t_{1/2}$ of a particular agent in combination with the duration of the infusion to help the clinician more accurately deliver sedatives in a manner that one can anticipate expected emergence times. When administered continuously, propofol and midazolam have shorter context-sensitive $t_{1/2}$s than lorazepam (19) (Table 7).

Lorazepam, midazolam, diazepam, and chlordiazepoxide are marketed in parenteral formulations. Lorazepam and midazolam are more useful in the ICU than diazepam and chlordiazepoxide. Diazepam and chlordiazepoxide both have active metabolites and have long half-lives, which makes them inappropriate for use as continuous infusions.

When BZDs and opioids are coadministered, they act synergistically to produce respiratory depression.

Benzodiazepines decrease the cerebral metabolic rate for oxygen ($CMRO_2$) consumption, and decrease cerebral blood flow (CBF), maintaining a relatively normal ratio of CBF to $CMRO_2$.

XXII. MIDAZOLAM

Midazolam is a short-acting BZD, which has characteristics very similar to those of diazepam except for its having a short duration of action which favors its being administered by continuous infusion (26). Midazolam undergoes changes in its conformation based upon the pH of the solution in which it is dissolved. These conformational changes affect the degree of lipid solubility of the drug. In acidic solutions, as dispensed by the manufacturer, midazolam exists in an open-ring form. This open-ring form is water-soluble and thus facilitates administration due to its compatibility with crystalloids. Upon exposure to blood, however, the pH of the solution rises more than the p*Ka* of midazolam (6.1), resulting in closure of the diazepine ring. Midazolam thus morphs into a lipid-soluble agent in the blood. This enables it to rapidly cross the blood–brain barrier, and thus considerably speeds the onset of its effects, estimated at one to two circulation times (19,50).

Midazolam is 95% protein-bound, has a volume of distribution of 1.1–1.7 L/kg, and has a clearance of 6.4–11.1 mL/kg/min. The $t_{1/2}$ alpha is 6–15 min, and $t_{1/2}$ beta is 1.7–2.6 hr (23). Its brief duration (approximately, 15 min after bolus administration) is due to rapid redistribution. Duration prolongs to 1–2 hr after short-term infusions. Wake-up times may be unpredictable after midazolam has been infused for more than 48–72 hr, where effects may last for more than 3–15 hr after discontinuing the infusion. This may be related to continued redistribution of the drug from fat stores (23,26,36). Tachyphylaxis has been noted after infusions lasting more than 3 days. Benzodiazepines have been noted to cause dependence and withdrawal syndromes after prolonged use in some critically ill patients.

Metabolism: Midazolam is primarily metabolized in the liver by the oxidative pathway and also undergoes some hepatic glucuronidation. Midazolam has two

Table 7 Pharmacokinetics and Hepatic Enzyme Characteristics of Common Benzodiazepines in ICU Patients

Drug	Volume distribution (L/kg)	Half-life (hr)	Clearance (L/hr 70 kg)	Drug concentration to achieve sedation in ICU (μg/L)	Active metabolite(s)	Major hepatic enzyme system	Major enzyme inhibitors	Major enzyme enzymeinducers
Diazepam	2.9	72	1.2–1.8	> 100	Desmethyldiazepam; oxazepam	CYP2C19	Amiodarone; cimetidine; fluconazole; omeprazole; valproic acid	
Lorazepam	2.0	10–20	3–6	50–1500	None	Glucuronyl transferase	Chloramphenicol; valproic acid	Barbiturates; phenytoin; rifampin; carbamazepine; ritonavir
Midazolam	1.9	9.0	21–36	150–1000	α-Hydroxy midazolam	CYP3A4	Cimetidine; diltiazem; erythromycin; indinavir; ketoconazole; verapamil	Barbiturates; phenytoin; rifampin; carbamazepine

CYP, cytochrome P450 oxidative pathway.
Source: From Ref. 19.

active metabolites, alpha-hydroxymidazolam and alpha-hydroxymidazolam glucuronide. Small amounts (less than 1%) are excreted unchanged in the urine. A variety of drugs have been reported to prolong its duration of effect by interfering with its metabolism, including cimetidine, propofol, and diltiazem. Patients receiving cytochrome p450 inhibitors such as erythromycin and fluconazole will have reduced metabolism of midazolam (23). Hepatic disease will prolong its effect due to decreased metabolism. Renal failure may result in an increased effect as well due to an increase in the unbound portion of the drug. Healthy volunteers have a $t_{1/2}$ for midazolam of approximately 2 hr, whereas ICU patients have been found to have a $t_{1/2}$ of approximately $5\frac{1}{2}$ hr (19). Patients with multiple organ dysfunction are prone to prolonged effects.

Bolon et al. investigated midazolam disposition during continuous venovenous hemodialysis (CVVHD). Prolonged sedation has been observed in patients with severe renal failure who had been receiving long-term infusions of midazolam. The glucuronide metabolites of midazolam were previously assumed to be rapidly excreted and pharmacologically inactive; however, this has been found not to be the case. Prolonged sedation due to the accumulation of glucuronides has been described. The formation of glucuronide metabolites has also been found to be unaffected by hepatic failure.

The authors found that CVVHD was not effective for removing midazolam or 1-hydroxy midazolam from the plasma, likely due to the high protein binding of the drug. However, the water-soluble conjugated metabolite, 1-hydroxy-midazolam glucuronide, was effectively removed from plasma by CVVHD (51).

Dosing: Intermittent doses 0.02–0.08 mg/kg; infusion: 0.04–0.20 mg/kg/hr, after one or more bolus loading dose of 0.03 mg/kg (26,50).

Cardiovascular and respiratory: Benzodiazepines cause dose-related respiratory depression and may cause hypotension due to vasodilatation. These effects are more pronounced in patients whose cardiovascular status is more tenuous and after bolus administration. Large doses can cause vasodilatation and hypotension. Midazolam's relatively rapid onset is an advantage, enabling infusions to be more titratable compared to infusions of lorazepam. Its recent availability as a generic formulation has reduced its cost, making it a more appealing choice for prolonged infusions. Midazolam is an effective amnestic agent (6). Unlike lorazepam and diazepam, being water-soluble, midazolam is not in solution with the potentially toxic solvent propylene glycol. This may be viewed as an advantage for patients with renal insufficiency who require prolonged sedation.

A number of trials have been performed comparing infusions of midazolam to those of propofol. Many of these studies have involved sedation of postoperative cardiac surgical patients for less than 24 hr. Both agents have been found to provide adequate sedation. Propofol patients recover more quickly from sedation and were extubated earlier but tended to require more fluid resuscitation for hypotension than those receiving midazolam. There were no differences in postoperative ischemia or death (36). Midazolam is more effective than propofol in providing amnesia and may require fewer readjustments in infusion rates to achieve the desired level of sedation (6).

XXIII. LORAZEPAM

Lorazepam is a potent, intermediate-acting BZD that is approximately 90% protein-bound. It is less lipid-soluble than midazolam and diazepam, which decreases its capacity to accumulate in fat stores. This feature also causes lorazepam to traverse the blood–brain barrier more slowly, which delays onset (10–30 min vs. 3–5 min for midazolam) and also a longer duration of central effects, including longer amnestic activity (36,52). Lorazepam has a total body clearance rate of 1.05–1.1 mL/kg/min and a volume of distribution of 1.14–1.3 L/kg. It has a $t_{1/2}$ alpha of 3–20 min, a $t_{1/2}$ beta of 6–14 hr after bolus administration, and a duration of action of 12–32 hr after 72 hr of infusion (23,36). Compared to lorazepam, much larger doses of midazolam are required to produce equisedative effects. Lorazepam's relative potency is approximately 2–4 times that of midazolam (23). This cost-effective feature of lorazepam has been modified by the recent availability of midazolam in a generic formulation (52).

Metabolism: Lorazepam is metabolized by hepatic glucuronidation. This makes lorazepam unlikely to have drug interactions, which is an advantage over midazolam and diazepam. Lorazepam does not have active metabolites (19,36). Because of this, despite having a longer duration of action, recovery time compared with midazolam is faster after prolonged administration (26). The $t_{1/2}$ beta of lorazepam, normally 10–20 hr, is prolonged by hepatic and renal disease (19).

Available forms: Lorazepam may be administered orally, intravenously, or intramuscularly. Unlike diazepam, lorazepam is also absorbed dependably and rapidly after intramuscular injection. Intramuscular injections are relatively painless and provide dependable absorption, with a peak concentration within an hour after injection (19). Lorazepam may become unstable in solution and precipitate after 12 hr (23).

Neurological: Lorazepam increases the seizure threshold, as do midazolam and diazepam.

Cardiovascular: Modest reductions in arterial blood pressure occur, related to a decrease in systemic vascular resistance. Lorazepam tends to decrease blood pressure somewhat less than midazolam.

Respiratory: As with other BZDs, respiratory depression and apnea may occur in a dose-related manner. Elderly and debilitated patients are more likely to develop respiratory depression.

Dosing: Intermittent doses 0.02–0.06 mg/kg; infusion: 0.01–0.10 mg/kg/hr (50). Usual starting dose 0.044 mg/kg every 2–4 hr, prn, but this is highly variable. One or more loading doses are generally required with continuous infusion. Because lorazepam has a slightly delayed onset of action, a single dose of midazolam or diazepam may be utilized to initiate sedative therapy when rapid sedation is required. Drug requirements are significantly decreased in the elderly (26).

XXIV. LORAZEPAM AND PROPYLENE GLYCOL TOXICITY

Vehicle: Since lorazepam is insoluble in water, it is manufactured with propylene glycol as its vehicle in order to maintain a stable solution. Patients receiving high-dose lorazepam infusions have been reported to develop toxicity due to this solvent. Propylene glycol is metabolized by the liver to lactate and pyruvate by alcohol dehydrogenase. Approximately, 12–50% of propylene glycol administered is excreted by the kidneys. Thus, patients who have hepatic or renal dysfunction are predisposed to toxicity from this solvent, which has led some to recommend avoiding prolonged lorazepam infusions in patients with a creatinine clearances of less than 30 mL/min. Propylene glycol toxicity is manifested by the development of a lactic acidosis, hyperosmolarity and an elevated osmolal gap, and worsening renal insufficiency/acute tubular necrosis. Toxicity has been reported as early as 48 hr after initiation of a high-dose lorazepam infusion. Propylene glycol levels can be measured and can confirm the clinical diagnosis (53).

XXV. DIAZEPAM

Diazepam is a long-acting BZD that, being highly lipophilic, rapidly crosses the blood–brain barrier to produce an onset of effect within 2–3 min (26). Diazepam peaks in effect around 5 min after bolus administration. Its effect subsides afterwards as it undergoes peripheral redistribution. It is available in intravenous and oral forms. Due to its hydrophobic nature, it generally should not be mixed with other medications. Diazepam is now available in a sterile lipid emulsion rather than in a propylene glycol solvent.

Metabolism: Diazepam has a $t_{1/2}$ alpha of 30–66 min, and a $t_{1/2}$ beta of 24–57 hr. It has a volume of distribution of 0.7–1.7 L/kg, and a clearance of 0.24–0.53 mL/kg/min (23). Diazepam is metabolized by hepatic microsomal enzymes to desmethyldiazepam, which is an active metabolite with a very long $t_{1/2}$ of 100–200 hr. Desmethyldiazepam is ultimately eliminated by the kidneys. Diazepam is also metabolized to oxazepam, which has a $t_{1/2}$ of 10 hr. Advancing age increases the $t_{1/2}$ beta in a linear fashion. Infants and patients with liver disease will also have a prolonged half-life. Smoking, drugs, and nutritional status can also affect its metabolism (19).

Neurological: Diazepam produces antegrade amnestic effects and raises the seizure threshold, while reducing both $CMRO_2$ and cerebral blood flow as do the other BZDs (19).

Cardiovascular: Systemic vascular resistance is reduced slightly, producing a small decline in arterial blood pressure as do other members of this class (19).

Respiratory: Respiratory drive is minimally decreased by diazepam, however as with other BZDs, coadministration with opioids or other sedative-hypnotics will greatly potentiate its cardiovascular and respiratory depressant effects (19).

Dosing: Intermittent intravenous injection: 0.03–0.10 mg/kg. Infusions are not recommended, due to its prolonged half-life, and a requirement for dilution that results in large volumes of fluid being administered with the infusion. Diazepam is no longer recommended for routine use in the ICU. Even scheduled intermittent dosing may lead to excessive sedation.

XXVI. FLUMAZENIL

Flumazenil reverses the sedative and amnestic effects of BZDs by acting at the BZD binding site on the GABA receptor, due to its structural similarity to BZD agonists. It undergoes rapid clearance by hepatic metabolism, and its effects, which are seen immediately after administration, will dissipate with a $t_{1/2}$ beta of approximately 1 hr. The dosage is 0.2–1.0 mg intravenously. Caution is advised with use in patients receiving BZDs chronically, as it may precipitate withdrawal and seizure activity (19).

XXVII. PROPOFOL

Propofol (2,6-diisopropylphenol) is an intravenous anesthetic agent that has sedative, hypnotic, anxiolytic, and some anterograde amnestic properties at subanesthetic dosages. Its high lipid solubility results in rapid induction of anesthesia (26). The mechanism by which propofol produces hypnosis is not entirely clear, but it appears to enhance inhibitory synaptic transmission by activating the chloride channel of the beta-1 subunit of the GABA receptor. It also appears to inhibit excitatory synaptic transmission to a lesser extent, by inhibiting Ca^{2+}-dependent glutamate release that is evoked by secretogogues that involve voltage-gated Na^{+} channel activation. Indirect evidence exists that this appears to occur in multiple species by blockade of the presynaptic Na^{+} channels, making the nerve terminal unable to depolarize (54).

Propofol has three half-lives: the alpha half-life: 2–3 min (which represents distribution of the drug from the blood to the tissues after administration), a beta half-life: 30–60 min (elimination half-life), and a gamma half-life: 300–700 min (terminal half-life whereby the drug is mobilized and eliminated from adipose tissue) (30). When used as a sedative, administration by continuous infusion is recommended due to its rapid onset and offset. Time to awakening is rapid (15 min), (due to redistribution and rapid elimination), after short-term infusions but prolongs once infused for over 72 hr to 30–60 min (36). Propofol undergoes hepatic metabolism by conjugation to inactive glucuronide and sulfate forms, both of which are subsequently excreted by the kidney. Propofol has a volume of distribution of 5.4–7.8 L/kg, and a clearance of 26–29 mL/kg/min (23). Since propofol's clearance exceeds hepatic blood flow, extrahepatic metabolism has been suspected. Studies have indicated that the intestinal wall and the kidney may contribute to some of propofol's metabolism. Propofol's pharmacokinetics are generally unaffected by hepatic or renal disease (23,55). Long-term infusions result in accumulation within lipid stores, resulting in a prolonged elimination phase with a half-life of up to 300–700 min (26). However, subtherapeutic plasma concentrations are maintained after discontinuation of the drug by rapid clearance mechanisms (23,26). Propofol's rapid onset and offset make it particularly useful for short-term sedation.

Cardiovascular: Propofol decreases blood pressure by reducing vascular tone and by decreasing myocardial contractility. Bradycardia may be seen. Hypotension is less likely if intravascular volume is maintained (23,36,56).

Neurological: Propofol decreases CBF and decreases the cerebral metabolic requirement for oxygen, and thereby reduces intracranial pressure. Like alcohol, propofol effects both GABA-A and glutamate receptors, and has been used as an alternative to BZDs for the treatment of symptoms of alcohol withdrawal (23). Propofol has been used in the treatment of refractory status epilepticus (57). However, seizure-like phenomena have also been reported with the use of propofol, which usually occur upon induction or on emergence (58). Abnormal motor activity, including opisthotonos and dystonic reactions, have been seen and are presumed to be due to neuroexcitatory effects of the drug, possibly on subcortical structures (56,58).

Respiratory: Propofol has bronchodilatory properties in higher dose ranges (23). Respiratory depression is dose-related.

Hematological: Propofol may have some anti-inflammatory and antiplatelet effects (23). Propofol is manufactured as a lipid emulsion with 10% soybean oil, with a pH of approximately 7.5, an osmolarity of 250–350 mOsm, and contains 2.25% glycerol, and 1.2% purified egg phosphatide (50). This milieu makes propofol an attractive culture media for micro-organisms, and it is recommended that once a container of propofol has been opened, it should be used or discarded within 12 hr. If the solution is removed from its original container for administration via a syringe, it is recommended that it be discarded by 6 hr afterwards. Shortly, after the original formulation of propofol was introduced, a number of serious infections occurred in surgical patients, which were determined to have resulted from bacterial contamination of propofol. Formulations in the United States now contain 0.005% disodium edetate to impede the growth of bacteria or a generic formulation of propofol that contains sodium metabisulfite. The generic formulation may be less stable and somewhat more prone to bacterial contamination than the EDTA formulation, however the FDA considers them to be interchangeable (23). Anaphylaxis has been reported as well (36,56). Propofol use should be avoided in patients with allergies to eggs or soy, and the generic preparation should be avoided in patients with allergies to sulfites (59–61). Propofol commonly causes a transient burning sensation at the site of injection.

Hypertriglyceridemia may occur. Nutritional prescriptions need to account for the number of calories provided to the patient as lipid from the propofol infusion. There is potential for a fat embolism if the lipid emulsion becomes unstable, allowing fat droplets to coalesce (50). Propofol is manufactured as a 1% (10 mg propofol/mL) solution. A 2% propofol (20 mg/mL) solution has been developed, which would reduce by half the amount of lipid and volume administered to the patient. However, this solution is not currently available in the United States (50).

Prolonged administration may result in tolerance and the necessity for an increased dose and consequently larger volume of lipid vehicle administration (56). Propofol withdrawal syndrome and seizures have been reported after cessation of infusion. The incidence of this complication is unclear (56,62).

Propofol has been found to have antiplatelet effects in vitro and in vivo. This appears to be due to inhibition of platelet thromboxane A2, and an increase in synthesis of leukocyte nitric oxide, which has an antiplatelet effect (63). The clinical significance of this inhibition is unclear, but it may be a potential consideration when choosing a sedative regimen in cancer patients with severe thrombocytopenia.

Dosing: Initial infusion: 0.3–0.5 mg/kg/hr. The infusion rate may be rapidly titrated upwards in increments of 0.5 mg/kg/hr every 5–10 min, as required. Typical maintenance dosages range from 0.5–5.0 mg/kg/hr, depending upon the depth of sedation required and patient sensitivity. Pharmacokinetic and pharmacodynamic models have been devised for the ICU population to guide sedation with the use of target-controlled infusion devices (26,62).

Bolus dosing: Initial bolus doses of from 0.25 to 0.9 mg/kg may be administered prior to initiation of infusion, depending upon whether light or deep sedation is desired. The probability of developing hypotension is significantly greater in ICU patients after receiving a bolus of propofol. If a bolus is deemed necessary, administering it slowly over approximately 3 min may decrease the likelihood of developing hypotension (62).

Drug interactions: Propofol inhibits the cytochrome P450 system, and thus may potentially interact with drugs that are metabolized by these enzymes.

XXVIII. COMPARATIVE STUDIES

McCollam et al. (64) compared the sedation of 31 trauma patients in the ICU with midazolam vs. lorazepam vs. propofol. They found that adequate sedation occurred most frequently with midazolam, and oversedation most frequently with lorazepam, despite the fact that adequate sedation was achieved most quickly with propofol; undersedation was most frequently seen in those patients. Total drug costs were significantly higher for propofol. Other studies have shown that midazolam and propofol are equally effective as sedative agents in the critically ill (26).

Midazolam is considerably less expensive than propofol, however, and provides superior amnestic effects (6). Propofol has been favored for short-term infusions for patients who are anticipated to be ready for extubation within 24 hr of their ICU admission or sooner, such as fast-track cardiac surgical patients. The additional expense is felt to be offset by more rapid emergence and shorter times to extubation (19).

XXIX. PROPOFOL AND BRAIN INJURY

Propofol infusions have become favored for neurointensive care patients due to the rapid offset of propofol's sedative effects, enabling emergence for unobscured neurological examinations. Recovery times do lengthen on prolonged infusions, however (23).

Propofol may confer neuroprotection by decreasing concentrations of excitatory neurotransmitters such as glutamate, which can increase neuronal cell death provoked by brain ischemia, as well as other mechanisms (65).

XXX. PROPOFOL IN CHILDREN

Propofol infusions have been reported to cause mortality due to progressive myocardial failure and nonlactate metabolic acidosis in pediatric patients. Rhabdomyolysis, lipemia, ketonuria, bundle branch block, and arrhythmias have also been associated with this "propofol syndrome." Most commonly this has occurred when high doses (>4 mg/kg/hr) of propofol have been infused for more than 48 hr. Despite recognition of the causative process, symptoms have persisted and mortality has occurred despite discontinuation of the infusion and vigorous support (66–68).

In Britain, the Medicines Control Agency and Committee for Safety of Medicines has advised that propofol not be used for sedating children less than 16 years of age in ICUs. Others in the United States and Canada have also expressed concern regarding the use of propofol as a sedative in the pediatric ICU (66–69).

The mechanism of this syndrome, and reasons why it rarely occurs in adults, is unclear. Rat studies have shown that propofol acts to antagonize beta receptors in the rat myocardium in a dose-dependent, competitive manner, and that it also decrease myocardial contractility by a direct action on calcium channels (68). There has been some speculation that impaired fatty acid oxidation at the mitochondrial level may be a factor based on some clinical evidence from a case report (70). Propofol seems to be safe when used in relatively healthy children for procedural sedation or induction of general anesthesia; however, there have not been large randomized controlled trials to study this issue (71). Cornfield et al. (72) reported safe sedation of pediatric ICU patients maintaining the infusion rates less than 67 μg/kg/min.

XXXI. DEXMEDETOMIDINE

Dexmedetomidine (DEX) is a highly selective central alpha-2 agonist with a half-life of only 2.3 hr that has recently been approved for short-term (< 24 hr) use as a sedative in patients who are initially mechanically ventilated (46). Dexmedetomidine is 8–10 fold more potent than clonidine at the alpha-2 receptor, enabling it to be utilized at relatively high doses to cause sedation and analgesia, while avoiding adverse vascular effects resulting from activation of alpha-1 receptors (46,73).

Dexmedetomidine has some unique properties. It causes minimal respiratory depression, has both sedative and analgesic effects, and enables the patient to be easily aroused from sedation without the need to reduce or discontinue the infusion (36,74).

These features have encouraged its use in the ICU setting, often as an alternative to propofol in populations where frequent neurological examinations are indicated (44).

In the CNS, DEX acts at presynaptic nerve endings to inhibit the release of norepinephrine (NE), acetylcholine (ACh), serotonin, dopamine (DA), and Substance P. The reduction in central sympathetic activity results in hypotension and bradycardia. Dexmedetomidine reduces CBF, with no apparent change in cerebral oxygen consumption, thus potentially uncoupling CBF from metabolism. It does not appear to have an effect on intracranial pressure. Some experiments have shown potential neuroprotective effects with DEX administration (52). The sedative and anxiolytic effects of DEX are effected by binding to presynaptic alpha-2A adrenoceptors, resulting in inhibition of neuronal firing within the locus ceruleus, the chief noradrenergic nucleus in the brainstem. Analgesic effects of the drug arise from stimulation of alpha-2 adrenoceptors in the brain, spinal cord, and peripheral sites (46,52).

The bradycardic and hypotensive effects of alpha-2 agonists are thought to arise from their action at the medullary dorsal motor nucleus of the vagus, which has a high concentration of alpha-2 adrenoceptors. Drops in blood pressure in healthy volunteers reportedly are easily managed by increasing intravenous fluid administration. Dexmedetomidine does not have direct myocardial depressant effects; however, vasoconstriction may occur due to agonism at postsynaptic alpha-2 adrenoceptors located in arterial and venous smooth muscle. Vasoconstriction may then lead to transient hypertension and a decrease in cardiac index. Vasoconstriction becomes more pronounced with increasing doses of the drug (52,73). Infusions of DEX do not produce significant respiratory depression, although some respiratory depression may be seen with bolus doses. It produces some bronchodilation, and some attenuation of response to hypercapnia (52).

XXXII. PHARMACOKINETIC PROPERTIES

Dexmedetomidine clearance is essentially constant within therapeutic dose ranges. It has a rapid distribution phase half-life ($t_{1/2}$ alpha) of approximately 6 min and a terminal elimination half-life ($t_{1/2}$ beta) of approximately 2–2.5 hr. The pharmacokinetics of dexmedetomidine does not change with advancing age. Dexmedetomidine undergoes hepatic metabolism to a glucuronide, whereupon 95% is excreted in the urine. It is approximately 94% protein-bound. Dexmedetomidine clearance is decreased in the face of hepatic insufficiency, with clearance decreased by nearly 70% in advanced cirrhosis. The dose of DEX should be adjusted downwards in the presence of hepatic insufficiency (23,52).

Ebert et al. studied the effects of increasing plasma concentrations of DEX in healthy volunteers on hemodynamics, memory, and responses to cold pressor and baroreflex tests. Dexmedetomidine suppressed catecholamines by more than 40% at all doses, and eliminated the norepinephrine increase that is ordinarily seen during the cold pressor test. The authors noted a biphasic hemodynamic response to DEX infusions, with a lowering of MAP with no significant change in CVP, PA pressures, or PCWP at lower dose ranges, but found the onset of increasing MAP, CVP, PA pressures, and PCWP, and a decrease in cardiac output at higher doses, corresponding to a plasma DEX level of > 1.9 ng/mL. Dexmedetomidine potentiated baroreflex heart rate slowing to a phenylephrine challenge at both doses. Recall was preserved at lower doses of DEX, in the presence of sedation and analgesia, but began to decrease at higher dose ranges and was abolished at a plasma concentration of 1.9 ng/mL (73).

XXXIII. DEX IN THE ICU

Double-blind, placebo-controlled trials evaluating the efficacy of DEX as a sedative in the ICU have been performed, using midazolam and MSO4 or propofol and MSO4 as rescue agents. The patients receiving DEX were easily arousable and were able to continue DEX after extubation due to the lack of respiratory depression. Opioid requirements were reduced by half in the groups receiving DEX compared to those receiving placebo (52).

Venn et al. (75) compared the effects of postoperative infusions of propofol and dexmedetomidine on adrenocortical, endocrine, cardiovascular, and inflammatory responses. Endocrine effects were assessed since DEX is an imidazole compound, and thus has the potential to inhibit cortisol synthesis, as etomidate has been shown to do. Dexmedetomidine has been shown to inhibit cortisol synthesis in animal studies at plasma concentrations above 10^{-6} M, which is significantly higher than the therapeutic plasma range in humans of less than 10^{-9} M. There were no differences in serum cortisol or ACTH concentrations between patients receiving DEX and those on propofol.

Dexmedetomidine dosing and precautions: DEX has not been approved as yet for infusions lasting longer than 24 hr.

Infusion rates: 0.2–0.7 μg/kg/hr. Higher doses have been used; however, there is a ceiling effect such that higher infusion rates may not increase sedation any further.

Small bolus doses (0.25–1 μg/kg over 10 min) tend to drop blood pressure and cardiac output, while larger bolus doses (1–4 μg/kg) tend to transiently increase BP and cause a more significant bradycardia. Several bolus dose regimens have been employed by various groups (23). A bolus dose of 1 μg/kg over 30 min is utilized at the University of Wisconsin. Not all patients will require bolus doses, however. If speed of onset is not a major concern, maintenance infusions may be initiated without a bolus dose, and adjusted upward as necessary (23).

The most commonly observed adverse reactions include hypertension (during loading infusion due to its peripheral vascular effects), hypotension (due to its sympatholytic effects). Hypotension is more common in the presence of volume depletion. Bradycardia is common. Sinus arrest has been reported. Caution is advised in patients with advanced heart block. Nausea, fever, vomiting, hypoxia, and tachycardia have also been seen (36,52). Investigators studying the effects of DEX on patients undergoing coronary artery bypass grafting who were chronically on beta blockers did not note any significant further decrease in their heart rate, presumably since the mechanism for bradycardia with DEX administration is due to sympathetic blockade (76). Systemic and pulmonary hypertension may occur at higher dose ranges, which may compromise cardiac output, and should be kept in consideration with regards to patients who have severe hypertension, cardiomyopathy, pre-existing pulmonary hypertension, etc. Elderly patients, hypovolemic patients, and diabetics may be more likely to develop hypotension or bradycardia with administration.

A web site, www.dexmedetomidine.com, is available for drug information.

Dexmedetomidine is more costly than the other agents commonly used as sedatives in intensive care settings (44). Dexmedetomidine exhibits a ceiling on its sedative effect, which may limit its effectiveness as a single agent (36).

XXXIV. HALOPERIDOL

Haloperidol is a butyrophenone neuroleptic agent used to treat agitation and delirium. It is rapid in onset, with clinical effects being observed within 30–60 min of intravenous administration. Haloperidol easily crosses the blood–brain barrier and is believed to reduce agitation via central postsynaptic dopaminergic blockade (22). Haloperidol easily crosses the BBB and free drug concentrations in the CSF are 10 times greater than serum concentrations (22). Haloperidol is relatively devoid of cardiovascular or respiratory depressant effects and has essentially no active metabolites. It does not cause any musculoskeletal relaxation, or antegrade amnestic effects (22,77). Effects of bolus administration last approximately 4–8 hr, and the half-life of the drug is 18–54 hr (22,26).

Haloperidol is not yet approved by the FDA for intravenous administration; however, there is a long history of safety and efficacy with this route of administration, which maximizes its bioavailability. Although some have proposed that its effectiveness plateaus at 10 mg per dose, others have demonstrated that much higher doses have been well tolerated and efficacious (26).

Dopaminergic hyperfunction results in sensory and cognitive dissociation, resulting in a fearful and anxious state, characterized by dysfunctional reasoning, memory, and disorientation, and paranoia. This situation is exacerbated by stress and organ dysfunction. Haloperidol and other neuroleptic agents decrease CNS dopaminergic activity, and relieve anxiety and agitation if it is related to this type of aberrant neurochemistry. If a hyperdopaminergic state is not the cause of anxiety or agitation, haloperidol generally will not be efficacious. The converse is true as well, where BZDs will not be effective treatment for delirium or psychosis, as they have no ability to ameliorate the hyperdopaminergic state. In fact, the sedation from

BZDs may exacerbate the sensory disturbances associated with delirium (77).

As with other neuroleptics, haloperidol may result in extrapyramidal side effects, including dystonic reactions and akinesia. Laryngeal dystonia may occur and requires emergent treatment with diphenhydramine or benztropine mesylate. Benzodiazepines may also moderate the extrapyramidal effects of neuroleptics indirectly by an anticholinergic effect related to its GABA agonist activity. Extrapyramidal symptoms have been reported more frequently in patients infected with HIV (22). However, administration via the parenteral route reduces the incidence of extrapyramidal side effects. Thus this may be seen less frequently in the ICU than in other populations (22).

Neuroleptic malignant syndrome is seen more frequently with haloperidol than with other neuroleptics; however, it may have a lower mortality rate than with other drugs (22). Symptoms of neuroleptic malignant syndrome may persist for up to 10 days after discontinuing the drug (23). Haloperidol also reduces the seizure threshold (78). Haloperidol can cause QT interval prolongation on the electrocardiogram, which may predispose the patient to develop polymorphic ventricular tachycardia. It has been recommended that patients on continuous haloperidol infusions be in a monitored setting for this reason (22,26). Haloperidol must be used with caution with other drugs that may prolong the QT interval. Prolongation of the QT interval notoriously occurs with administration of Class I antiarrhythmics such as procainamide and quinidine. However, many drugs that are administered to patients in the ICU and critically ill cancer patients also prolong the QT interval, including antimicrobials (erythromycin, TMP/SMX, pentamidine, quinolones, amantadine), antifungals (ketoconazole, itraconazole), tricyclic antidepressants, Class II antiarrhythmics (sotalol, amiodarone), droperidol, and tacrolimus (79,80). Haloperidol should be discontinued if the QT interval prolongs by more than 25% of baseline, or to >450 msec (23).

Dose: The usual starting dose is 2–10 mg administered intravenously and the dosage is repeated every 2–4 hr (26).

Riker et al. (22) described a case series where patients, who had severe agitation refractory to intermittent injections of BZDs, opioids, and haloperidol, were treated with a continuous infusion of haloperidol, at a range of 3–25 mg/hr. No control group was used in this study. The infusions were continued for an average of 7 ± 3 days. They used the SAS to monitor the effectiveness of therapy. The SAS scores showed a consistent decreasing trend in their patients, who needed fewer bolus doses of sedatives. The authors felt that the protocol facilitated weaning the patients from the ventilator and controlled severe agitation. Less nursing time was spent procuring and administering bolus doses as well. One patient had an episode of monomorphic ventricular tachycardia that was hemodynamically significant and required cardioversion. However, the QT interval was not prolonged, and the patient had been receiving a dopamine infusion as well. The haloperidol infusion was resumed without incident. They found no correlation between severity of illness, survival, and length of stay with the sedative dose requirement.

XXXV. PROTOCOL FOR CONTINUOUS INFUSION OF HALOPERIDOL

Indications for Haloperidol

1. Critically ill patient for whom agitation or hemodynamic or respiratory depression may not be tolerated or may conflict with therapeutic goals.
2. Reversible causes of agitation have been excluded or treated.
3. Analgesia has been provided.
4. Other efforts at anxiolysis and control are ineffective.

Indications for Continuous Infusion of Haloperidol

1. More than eight 10 mg haloperidol boluses required in a 24 hr period or >10 mg/hr for >5 consecutive hours.

Guidelines for Preparing Haloperidol Infusion

Standard: 200 mg in 200 mL of 5% dextrose in water (1 mg/mL). Maximum concentration with normal saline to 0.75 mg/mL or 5% dextrose in water to 3 mg/mL.

Indications and Method to Start or Increase Infusion

1. Bolus dose of 10 mg, followed by 10 mg/hr initial infusion rate.
2. If agitation persists, can repeat bolus with 10 mg every 30 min accompanied by an increase in infusion rate by 5 mg/hr.
3. Consider addition of BZDs.

Indications and Method to Decrease Infusion

Once control attained with few or no boluses required for 24 hr, decrease infusion rate by half, or if Sedation–Agitation Scale is $\leq$–2, stop infusion and return to bolus infusions as required.

What to Monitor

1. Extrapyramidal symptoms and signs of neuroleptic malignant syndrome.
2. Vital signs and electrocardiogram (22).

XXXVI. OTHER AGENTS

Etomidate, ketamine, and barbiturates are not recommended for routine sedation of the critically ill (25).

XXXVII. ETOMIDATE

Etomidate would appear to be an ideal drug for sedation in the ICU due to its stable hemodynamic profile. However, European experience with etomidate infusions revealed an excessive mortality rate, which has been attributed to adrenocortical suppression caused by the drug. Even single doses of etomidate have been shown to result in reversible impairment of adrenocortical function due to inhibition of mitochondrial cytochrome P450 enzymes (25,75). In fact, infusions of etomidate have been used as a treatment for chronic severe hypercortisolism where patients have an occult, ectopic source of ACTH, and are unable to take oral medications (81). Although etomidate is not appropriate for continuous sedation, it remains very useful as an induction agent for intubation in the critically ill patient, due to its minimal cardiovascular depressant effects. The standard intubating dose used in the operating room for induction is 0.3 mg/kg; however debilitated, critically ill adults will often be induced with as little as 6–8 mg intravenously (82).

XXXVIII. BARBITURATES

Barbiturate use in the ICU has generally been limited to special circumstances, such as for treatment of patients with status epilepticus. Barbiturates are also used as a salvage protocol for patients with traumatic brain injury and a refractory increase in intracranial pressure, with the hopes of reducing secondary brain injury and minimizing "excitotoxicity" due to the excitatory neurotransmitter glutamate.

Barbiturates may have neuroprotective effects, via a decrease in cerebral metabolic requirement for oxygen, inhibition of lipid peroxidation due to free radical production, and preservation of cerebral energy stores of ATP and glycogen. Barbiturates modulate GABA receptor/chloride channel complexes resulting in prolonged presynaptic inhibition and potentiation of postsynaptic inhibition. Barbiturates also block glutamate receptors and decrease glutamate release (83).

Thiopental: Loading dose of 5–11 mg/kg followed by an infusion of 4–6 mg/kg/hr, to achieve a burst-suppression pattern on electroencephalography of 4–6 bursts/min. Thiopental has a $t_{1/2}$ of 11–120 hr (83).

Pentobarbital: Loading dose of 5 mg/kg over 30 min, maintenance infusion of 1–3 mg/kg/hr (84). Pentobarbital has the advantage of having a shorter half-life, approximately 8–48 hr, vs. that of thiopental, which will enable neurological examination sooner.

Barbiturate coma is fraught with a number of potentially serious side effects, including significant cardiovascular depression and immunosuppression. Mechanical ventilation is required, and hemodynamic support with vasopressors is often necessary. Many centers advise invasive hemodynamic monitoring with a pulmonary artery catheter if barbiturate coma is planned. Patients are also prone to developing septic complications, which may be more difficult to detect due to a hypothermic state often associated with the use of barbiturate coma. Neurological examinations are totally obscured under barbiturate coma, and may not be reliable for days after discontinuation of infusion, due to the prolonged elimination half-life of these drugs.

XXXIX. KETAMINE

Ketamine is a dissociative anesthetic that produces anesthetic and analgesic effects via blockade of CNS sodium channels and antagonism of the NMDA receptor. *N*-methyl-D-asparate antagonists suppress hyperalgesia in animal models. Animal studies also have suggested that ketamine provides antinociception via activation of the monoaminergic descending inhibitory system (85,86). Some of ketamine's analgesic effects may also be mediated by actions at opiate receptors.

Ketamine has not been commonly used in adult ICUs as a sedative agent; however, its analgesic effects, general lack of respiratory depression and depression of airway reflexes have made it attractive for use in burn units as a sedative and analgesic for dressing changes, and for pediatric sedation. Ketamine may be administered intramuscularly and has a rapid onset of approximately 3 min. This is an advantage of obtaining control of the situation with violent or uncontrollable patients where it becomes impossible to obtain intravenous access. Since ketamine can exacerbate hypertension and increase intracranial pressure, the risk–benefit ratio of the drug should be considered in such situations. Ketamine has also other qualities that are favorable in certain circumstances, such as its bronchodilatory effects, making it an option as an induction agent in patients with status asthmatics (87).

Ketamine doses for anesthetic induction: 1–2 mg/kg intravenously and 3–6 mg/kg intramuscularly. Duration of anesthetic effects after an intravenous bolus is approximately 15–30 min, and analgesic effects lasting longer. Ketamine infusions have been used with some chronic pain patients and also in patients with refractory bronchospasm. Doses of ketamine infusion: 20–60 μg/kg/min (87,88). Despite its apparent preservation of airway reflexes, the reflexes may not be protective. Adverse effects of ketamine include lacrimation and salivation. Excess salivation may predispose a patient, especially children, to laryngospasm. Thus, many patients receive an anticholinergic agent such as glycopyrollate to reduce secretions. Midazolam is also often coadministered with ketamine to decrease the likelihood of emergence reactions and vivid dreams associated with its use.

Ketamine has also been used as an infusion for refractory pain in cancer patients (86,89). Jackson et al. (89) did a multicenter open-label audit that revealed good responses for patients with both somatic and neuropathic types of pain to a "burst" infusion of 3–5 days of ketamine, with initial doses of 100 mg/24 hr, to a maximum of 500 mg/24 hr, achieving a 67% response rate.

XL. ANALGESIA

Analgesics are often used as adjuncts to sedative regimens in the ICU, since a significant number of patients will have some degree of pain or discomfort during their stay, either related to their presenting pathology or diagnostic and therapeutic maneuvers. It is important to account for noxious stimuli and pain as being a potential cause for agitation, and to avoid attempting to treat pain with sedative and hypnotic agents, which in fact have been shown to cause hyperalgesia in normal volunteers (52).

The physiological effects of pain can have detrimental effects, such as tachycardia and hypertension, resulting in an increase in myocardial oxygen consumption and potentially ischemic consequences, hypercoagulability, and immunosuppression (26).

The JCAHO, responding to concerns that pain is often underassessed and undertreated, has proclaimed that hospitals consider pain the "fifth vital sign," advising that it be assessed regularly and responded to appropriately, as one would to other physiological parameters (25).

The SCCM has published their recommendations for analgesia for critically ill patients.

1. Morphine is recommended for critically ill, hemodynamically stable patients due to its efficacy and low cost.
2. Fentanyl is recommended for patients who are hemodynamically unstable or have an allergy to MSO4 (26).
3. Meperidine is not recommended for use in the critically ill, since its active metabolite, normeperidine, may accumulate and produce CNS excitation or seizure activity.
4. Nonsteroidal anti-inflammatory drugs are generally best avoided due to their propensity to cause gastrointestinal bleeding, platelet inhibition, and renal insufficiency.

The use of opiate agonist–antagonists (such as nalbuphine and butorphanol) are not recommended for routine use in the critically ill (25,26).

The SCCM recommends the use of fentanyl, hydromorphone, or morphine if intravenous opioid analgesics are necessary in critically ill patients. Continuous infusions or scheduled doses of opioids are recommended over intermittent "PRN" regimens to maintain analgesic levels. Fentanyl is recommended for patients in acute distress due to its rapid onset. Fentanyl and hydromorphone are preferred agents in hemodynamically unstable patients, as they have minimal depressant effects on the cardiovascular system, and for those patients with renal insufficiency. Fentanyl is also recommended for patients with a history of morphine allergy. Morphine and hydromorphone are advised for use for intermittent therapy due to their longer duration of action compared to fentanyl (10,26,36,49,50).

XLI. OPIOIDS

The opiates produce analgesia and sedation via mu receptor agonism in the CNS. Mu-1 receptor agonism mediates supraspinal analgesia, whereas mu-2 receptor agonism is responsible for adverse effects such as ventilatory depression, bradycardia, and addiction. Opioids also can cause hypotension (especially in patients who are hemodynamically unstable or hypovolemic and those with elevated sympathetic tone), constipation, and urinary retention. Muscle rigidity and myoclonus may occur with higher doses. Opiates do not provide amnesia. They do not provide anxiolysis in low doses, however sedative effects occur at higher dose ranges (23,26,36).

XLII. REMIFENTANIL

Remifentanil is an opioid that is a piperidine derivative with a very rapid onset related to a short blood–brain equilibration time and rapid recovery due to hydrolysis of the drug by nonspecific esterases. This form of metabolism allows its pharmacokinetics to remain relatively unaffected by hepatic and renal insufficiency (52). Its main metabolite, which is relatively inactive, may accumulate after prolonged infusions in patients with renal failure.

Remifentanil has similar potency to fentanyl. It is 10 times less potent than sufentanil.

Due to its rapid offset, a continuous infusion is necessary in order to sustain its effect. Steady state is achieved in 10 min after initiation of an infusion at a constant rate. A plateau in its analgesic efficacy is reached at plasma concentrations of 5–8 ng/mL. It maintains a constant context-sensitive half-life of less than 15 min regardless of the duration of the infusion (52). Infusion doses range from 0.6 to 15 μg/kg/hr (49).

As with other opioids, its side effects include respiratory depression, hypotension, bradycardia, chest wall rigidity, pruritis, and nausea (52).

Remifentanil has been evaluated in the ICU in a number of different scenarios, although it has not been in extensive use in the ICU. When studied as a postoperative sedative regimen for neurosurgical patients, it showed no adverse effects on intracranial pressure or hemodynamic stability, and its rapid offset enabled neurological examinations to be performed within minutes of its discontinuation. In another study of its use in ventilated postoperative patients, the majority of patients required additional sedatives to reach the goal sedation score, but the majority were also extubatable within 15 min after discontinuing the infusion (52).

XLIII. FENTANYL

Fentanyl is a synthetic opioid that has a rapid onset and relatively short duration due to its rapid redistribution to peripheral compartments. Compared to morphine, it is more potent, more lipophilic, and less likely to cause hemodynamic instability. It has no significant metabolites (26,36). Dose: bolus administration, 1–2 μg/kg. Infusion: 1–2 μg/kg/hr, titrate to effect. Tachyphylaxis may occur, with a need for progressively larger doses over time. The $t_{1/2}$ increases significantly with prolonged infusions from 30–60 min to over 9 hr due to redistribution of stored drug from adipose tissue. Transdermal administration is not recommended for acute pain relief due to the 12–24 hr delay in onset of peak effect (26).

XLIV. HYDROMORPHONE

Hydromorphone is a high potency, semisynthetic opioid that has a half-life of approximately 2–3 hr. It is available in oral and parenteral forms and may be administered rectally as well. It has more sedative properties than morphine but causes less euphoria. Hydromorphone can accumulate in renal failure resulting in neuroexcitation. It does not cause histamine release and has no active metabolites (23,26,36).

Dose: Initial dose approximately 0.5 mg, titrate upward in 0.5 mg increments as necessary, typical intermittent dosing 1–2 mg q 1–2 hr (26).

XLV. MORPHINE SULFATE

Morphine is the most frequently used analgesic in the ICU due to its low cost and efficacy. It has a half-life of 1.5–3 hr in healthy adults, but the half-life increases in the presence of hepatic failure, burns, sepsis, and renal failure. Morphine-3 and morphine-6 glucuronides are significant active metabolites. Morphine-6 glucuronide, which has several times more opiate activity than its parent compound morphine sulfate, may accumulate in renal failure and prolong effects of narcosis (23,26,36).

Dose: Initial bolus dose of 0.05 mg/kg. Typical maintenance doses are 4–6 mg/hr. Intermittent dosing should be performed every 1–2 hr (26). Morphine sulfate may lead to hypotension due to vasodilatation or histamine release (36).

XLVI. NALOXONE

Opioid administration may produce excessive sedation and hypoventilation, which may result in apnea. Clinical criteria for opioid overdose have been described and include a GCS $\leq$12, respirations of $\leq$12 per minute, and miotic pupils (90). It must be remembered, however, that not all patients with respiratory depression due to opioids will have a slow respiratory rate.

Naloxone is a specific opioid antagonist that reverses sedation and respiratory depression induced by opioids. Naloxone's most potent effect is at opioid mu receptors. Initial doses of naloxone are 0.2–0.4 mg intravenously if overdose is suspected. Doses of up to 10 mg may be required to reverse the effects of agents such as propoxyphene and methadone. Lower doses (0.1–0.2 mg iv) may be used in opioid-dependent patients to avoid precipitating symptoms of opioid withdrawal. Most patients with respiratory depression related to opioids after anesthesia will require lower doses, 1–2 μg/kg intravenously. Onset of response is rapid, and the effect of naloxone will generally last 45–90 min after a bolus dose. Renarcotization may occur if the opioid that was reversed was long-acting. Naloxone infusions may be administered, with typical doses being 0.4–0.8 mg/hr (90). Low-dose naloxone infusions (5 μg/kg/hr) have also been used to help relieve pruritis associated with opioid analgesia without disrupting the analgesic efficacy of the opioid (91). Side effects may occur, including noncardiogenic pulmonary edema, which is more likely with higher doses of naloxone.

XLVII. DRUG INTERACTIONS IN CANCER PATIENTS

Many cancer patients will receive a variety of combinations of antibiotics, analgesics, antidepressants, antiseizure medications, sedatives, and anticoagulants. In addition to differences between ethnic groups, interindividual genetic variation exists such that some patients will be poor metabolizers and others may metabolize ultrarapidly. This makes it apparent that the same dose of drug for two patients of similar age and weight may undertreat one, and overtreat the other. The P450 enzyme system is responsible for metabolizing many of these drugs. Multiple forms of the cytochrome p450 system exist. Agents that are metabolized by hepatic glucuronidation, such as morphine sulfate, are less likely to interact with other drugs. Midazolam, methadone, imipramine, and fentanyl are cleared by CYP3A4. Phenytoin, which induces CYP3A4, may result in a reduction in efficacy of these agents or a need for dose escalation. Erythromycin and cimetidine can impede metabolism and prolong the effect of drugs cleared by CYP3A4. Of note, many chemotherapeutic agents, such as ifosphamide, tamoxifen, epipodophyllotoxins, taxol, and vinca alkaloids are also cleared by the CYP3A4 system (92,93).

Codeine achieves its effect by conversion to morphine by CYP2D6. The addition of haloperidol, which inhibits CYP2D6, to a patient on an analgesic regimen with codeine, will result in a loss of effect and a need for dose escalation. If haloperidol is subsequently removed from the regimen, this escalated dose will become excessive (92).

XLVIII. COST CONSIDERATIONS

Intensive care unit medications comprise a substantial proportion of hospital budgets, and sedatives and analgesics account for 10–15% of drug costs in medical and surgical ICUs (7,25,36).

Many of the commonly used sedatives in ICU practice have come off patent; however, cost remains a consideration in choosing an agent that will be appropriate for a patient's needs and circumstances. One must take into account both direct and indirect costs of these medications and individualize their use.

XLIX. POST-ICU DEPRESSION AND STRESS SYNDROMES

Nearly 30% of patients discharged from the ICU have been found to selfreport symptoms of post-traumatic stress disorder (PTSD), and 15% of patients meet diagnostic criteria for PTSD. This syndrome may last months or even years after discharge. In Schelling et al.'s (94) study of this phenomenon, higher PTSD scores correlated with longer ICU stays.

Capuzzo et al. (95) interviewed 152 adult patients who had been co-operative during their ICU stay 6 months after hospital discharge. Patients who were less critically ill and who had shorter ICU stays were less likely to remember their stay. The type of sedation (minimal, morphine alone, or morphine plus various combinations of propofol and/or BZDs) did not significantly affect the number of patients who reported that they had no recall. The most frequently reported memories included the endotracheal tube, being unable to speak and having difficulty breathing, discomfort, thirst, anxiety, nightmares, and hallucinations. Patients did not specifically recall pain unless prompted.

Rundshagen et al. (8) interviewed 289 patients who had been intubated and sedated in the ICU 48–72 hr after ICU discharge. Although sedation protocols were not followed in this ICU, the authors found that their younger patients were more likely to experience recall or dreams from their time in critical care. Patients who had short-term stays were more likely to report explicit recall. Those who required longer ventilation times and longer ICU stays were more likely to recall having had dreams. Patients who were critically ill in the ICU for a prolonged period of time were most likely to have experienced delusions, nightmares, and hallucinations.

Schelling et al. (94) reported that ARDS survivors who reported recalling multiple unpleasant experiences from their ICU stay were most likely to have psychomotor functional impairment, which affected the quality of their life. It is not known whether recent trends towards using lower levels of sedation will result in an increased incidence of recall of unpleasant events from the ICU stay (8). However, some contend that amnesia does not protect the patient from adverse psychological symptoms after critical illness, and that it may even impair the patient's ability to recuperate emotionally (95). Jones et al. (96) proposed that the development of PTSD in patients after critical illness may be related more to recall of delusions rather than to recall of real events. It is unclear whether alternating periods of wakefulness (during which the patient would be kept informed and given psychological support), with periods of sedation will reduce the likelihood of developing neurotic symptoms or PTSD after discharge.

L. WITHDRAWAL SYNDROMES

Cammarano et al. (97) retrospectively reviewed charts of 28 trauma/surgical patients at the San Francisco General Hospital requiring mechanical ventilation for more than a week. They found a 32% incidence of acute withdrawal syndrome after weaning of sedative, analgesic, and hypnotic drugs. They found significant correlations between the doses of fentanyl or lorazepam equivalents and the likelihood of developing a withdrawal syndrome. Patients who had ARDS were significantly more likely to suffer withdrawal syndromes. The use of neuromuscular blockade, propofol use for more than 1 day, and younger age were also significantly associated with the risk of withdrawal.

Withdrawal syndromes are more likely to occur when prolonged infusions, especially high dose infusions, are abruptly discontinued. Patients who had been receiving shorter-acting agents will generally manifest withdrawal symptoms sooner and more intensely than those who had received agents with longer half-lives. Patients withdrawing from BZDs may have seizure activity. Measures to decrease the likelihood of acute withdrawal syndrome include gradual tapering of the sedative and substitution with intermittent doses of longer-acting agents such as diazepam (19,25).

LI. REMOVAL OF LIFE SUPPORT

One of the most difficult processes that we undergo as physicians involves making the transition from aggressive care of a critically ill patient to palliative care of a terminally ill one. This realization of a need for a change of course is often a gradual one and is often not achieved simultaneously by different team members and family. Honest communication with family and with the patient, if possible, is imperative. It is best to maintain realistic expectations and frequently update family members so that they are not blindsided by news of a dismal prognosis. When the decision has been made that further aggressive or heroic measures are not to be undertaken, the plan for care transits from attempts to support vital functions and to achieve at least some short-term quality of life to that of removal of life support and palliation of pain and suffering. This is generally performed with the administration of analgesics and sedatives. There is often much concern and confusion about what constitutes palliative care and what represents euthanasia. Ethical and legal guidelines dictate that the intent of sedation and analgesia at the end of life should be to relieve pain and suffering, not to directly cause death. Patients who are on analgesic and sedative regimens prior to withdrawal of life support will generally receive higher doses of these agents upon removal of life support.

The Ethics Committee of the Society of Critical Care Medicine recently published recommendations for end-of-life care in the ICU. They distinguished between anticipatory and reactive dosing of sedative and analgesics. The Ethics Committee reasoned that as it can be anticipated that discomfort or distress may ensue upon extubation or withdrawal of support that it is more appropriate to anticipate that this will occur and dose the patient with analgesics and sedatives in an anticipatory fashion, as opposed to simply reacting to symptoms of distress after they occur. They suggested that as a general rule the hourly dose of sedative or analgesic that the patient had been receiving should be doubled or tripled and administered prior to extubation. The Ethics Committee distinguished between patients who are unconscious and unlikely to experience pain or suffering upon withdrawal of life support, and patients who are cognizant or conscious. They advised rapid withdrawal of life support in the unconscious patient and that the need for anticipatory, if any sedation should be individualized. The Ethics Committee recommended that conscious patients have more gradual withdrawal of support after sedatives and analgesics have been titrated to an optimally comfortable state. The committee advised that in almost all circumstances, neuromuscular blockade if present should be discontinued or reversed prior to removing life support. The presence of neuromuscular blockade masks symptoms of distress, which the physician and staff attempt to alleviate, and certainly provides no benefit to the patient in this situation. Control of symptoms of dyspnea or air hunger after extubation should be sought. Administration of oxygen may not be any more effective than administering air for the relief of dyspnea in cancer patients. Some patients may feel claustrophobic and more dyspneic with an oxygen mask on. Opioids help to palliate symptoms of dyspnea, due to their respiratory depressant and euphoric effects. Their vasodilatory properties may also help to relieve pulmonary vascular congestion. Nonpharmacological measures for a comforting environment should also be considered, including fans, positioning, music, reduced lighting, noise and monitors, in addition to religious support, and the presence and comfort of family members at the bedside (98).

LII. THE FUTURE OF INTENSIVE CARE SEDATION

The search for the ideal sedative continues. The true ideal sedative may also help improve outcome, first by decreasing length of stay (and thus decreasing the likelihood of developing secondary complications, and their associated morbidity and mortality) and second, by favorably modulating the body's neuroendocrine response to stress. We may achieve a less stressful ICU environment, gain more insight into nonpharmaceutical means for calming our patients, and find ways to minimize sleep disturbances that may trigger agitation and delirium. In the future, we will likely have a better understanding of genetic variations that will impact upon a patient's response to a particular drug regimen. We may also be able to implement more sophisticated means of delivering sedatives and analgesics, such as target-controlled delivery systems, and more objective means for monitoring their effects. With further advances in science and technology, sedation, a crucial component of humane intensive care, may truly become optimized.

REFERENCES

1. Udelsman R, Norton JA, Jelenich SE, Goldstein DS, Linehan WM, Loriaux DL, Chrousos GP. Responses of the hypothalamic–pituitary–adrenal and renin–angiotensin axes and the sympathetic system during controlled surgical and anesthetic stress. J Clin Endocrinol Metab 1987; 64(5):986–994.
2. Ng A, Tan SS, Lee HS, Chew SL. Effect of propofol infusion on the endocrine response to cardiac surgery. Anaesth Intensive Care 1995; 23(5):543–547.
3. Nilsson A, Persson MP, Hartvig P, Wide L. Effect of total intravenous anaesthesia with midazolam/alfentanil on the adrenocortical and hypoglycaemic response to abdominal surgery. Acta Anaesthesiol Scand 1988; 32(5):379–382.
4. Cohen D, Horiuchi K, Kemper M, Weissman C. Modulating effects of propofol on metabolic and cardiopulmonary responses to stressful ICU procedures. Crit Care Med 1996; 24(4):612–627.
5. Dorges V, Wenzel V, Dix S, Kuhl A, Schumann T, Huppe M, Iven H, Gerlach K. The effect of midazolam on stress levels during simulated emergency medical service transport: a placebo-controlled, dose–response study. Anesth Analg 2002; 95:417–422.
6. Weinbroum AA, Halpern P, Rudick V, Sorkine P, Freedman M, Geller E. Midazolam versus propofol for long-term sedation in the ICU: a randomized prospective comparison. Intensive Care Med 1997; 23(12):1258–1263.
7. Cohen L. Current issues in agitation management. Adv Stud Med 2002; 2(9):332–337.
8. Rundshagen I, Schnabel K, Wegner C, am Esch S. Incidence of recall, nightmares, and hallucinations during analgosedation in intensive care. Intensive Care Med 2002; 28(1):38–43.
9. Devlin J, Fraser G, Kanji S, Riker R. Sedation assessment in critically ill adults. Ann Pharmacother 2001; 35:1624–1632.
10. Berenholtz SM, Dorman T, Ngo K, Provonost PJ. Qualitative review of ICU quality indicators. J Crit Care 2002; 17(1):1–15.
11. Shaw A, Weavind L, Feeley T. Mechanical ventilation in critically ill cancer patients. Curr Opin Oncol 2001; 13:224–228.
12. Hallahan A, Shaw PJ, Rowell G, O'Connell A, Schell D, Gillis J. Improved outcomes of children with malignancy admitted to a pediatric ICU. Crit Care Med 2000; 28(11):3718–3721.
13. Sivan Y, Schwartz PH, Schonfield T, Cohen IJ, Newth CJ. Outcome of oncology patients in the pediatric ICU. Intensive Care Med 1991; 17:11–15.
14. Khassawneh BY, White P Jr, Anaissie EJ, Barlogie B, Hiller FC. Outcome from mechanical ventilation after autologous peripheral blood stem cell transplantation. Chest 2002; 121(1):185–188.
15. Dalrymple J, Levenback C, Wolf J, Bodurka D, Garcia M, Gershenson D. Trends among gynecologic oncology inpatient deaths: is end-of-life care improving? Gynecol Oncol 2002; 85:356–361.
16. Nelson JE, Meier DE, Oei EJ, Nierman DM, Senzel RS, Manfredi PL, Davis SM, Morrison RS. Self-reported symptom experience of critically ill cancer patients receiving intensive care. Crit Care Med 2001; 29(2):277–282.
17. Agrawal M, Emanuel E. Attending to psychologic symptoms and palliative care. J Clin Oncol 2002; 20(3): 624–626.
18. Morita T, Akechi T, Sugawara Y, Chihara S, Uchitomi Y. Practices and attitudes of Japanese oncologists and palliative care physicians concerning terminal sedation: a nationwide survey. J Clin Oncol 2002; 20(3):758–764.
19. Young C, Prielipp R. Benzodiazepines in the ICU. Crit Care Clin 2001; 17(4):843–862.
20. Kissin I. General anesthetic action: an obsolete notion? Anesth Analg 1993; 76(2):215–218
21. Martin MA, Barlow DH. Social and specific phobias. In: Tasman A, Kay J, Lieberman J A, eds. Psychiatry. 1st ed. Philadelphia: WB Saunders Company, 1997:1037.

22. Riker R, Fraser G, Cox P. Continuous infusion of haloperidol controls agitation in critically ill patients. Crit Care Med 1994; 22(3):433–440.
23. Agitation Roundtable Meeting Overview. CME Program. Management of the agitated ICU patient. Crit Care Med 2002; 30(1) (Suppl Management): S97–S123; quiz S:124–125.
24. Berkenbosch J, Fichter C, Tobias J. The correlation of the bispectral index monitor with clinical sedation scores during mechanical ventilation in the pediatric ICU. Anesth Analg 2002; 94(3):506–511.
25. Szokol JW, Vender JS. Anxiety, delirium, and pain in the ICU. Crit Care Clin 2001; 17(4):821–842.
26. Shapiro B, Warren J, Egol AB, Greenbaum DM, Jacobi J, Nasraway SA, Schein RM, Spevetz A, Stone JR. Practice parameters for intravenous analgesia and sedation for adult patients in the ICU: an executive summary. Crit Care Med 1995; 23(9):1596–1600.
27. Breitbart W, Strout D. Delirium in the terminally ill. Clin Geriatr Med 2000; 16(2):357–372.
28. Lawlor PG, Bruera ED. Delirium in patients with advanced cancer. Hematol Oncol Clin North Am 2002; 16(3):701–714.
29. Ely EW, Margolin R, Francis J, May L, Truman B, Dittus R, Speroff T, Gautam S, Bernard GR, Inouye SK. Evaluation of delirium in critically ill patients: validation of the Confusion Assessment Method for the ICU (CAM-ICU). Crit Care Med 2001; 29(7):1502–1512.
30. Hanania M, Kitain E. Melatonin for treatment and prevention of postoperative delirium. Anesth Analg 2002; 94(2):338–339.
31. Kober A, Scheck T, Schubert B, Strasser H, Gustorff B, Bertalanffy P, Wang SM, Kain ZN, Hoerauf K. Auricular acupressure as a treatment for anxiety in prehospital transport settings. Anesthesiology 2003; 98(6): 1328–1332.
32. Greif R, Laciny S, Mokhtarani M, Doufas AG, Bakhshandeh M, Dorfer L, Sessler DI. Transcutaneous electrical stimulation of an auricular acupuncture point decreases anesthetic requirement. Anesthesiology 2002; 96(2):306–312.
33. Epstein J, Breslow MJ. The stress response of critical illness. Crit Care Clin 1999; 15(1):17–33.
34. Crippen D. High-tech assessment of patient comfort in the ICU: time for a new look. Crit Care Med 2002; 30(8):1919–1920.
35. Myles PS, Hunt JO, Fletcher H, Watts J, Bain D, Silvers A, Buckland MR. Remifentanil, fentanyl, and cardiac surgery: a double-blinded, randomized controlled trial of costs and outcomes. Anesth Analg 2002; 95(4):805–812.
36. Brusco L. Choice of sedation for critically ill patients: a rational approach. Adv Stud Med 2002; 2(9):343–349.
37. Hansen-Flaschen J, Cowen J, Polomano RC. Beyond the Ramsay Scale: need for a validated measure of sedating drug efficacy in the ICU. Crit Care Med 1994; 22(5):732–733.
38. Marx C, Smith P, Lowrie L, Hamlett K, Ambuel B, Yamashita T, Blumer J. Optimal sedation of mechanically ventilated pediatric critical care patients. Crit Care Med 1994; 22(1):163–170.
39. Brattebo G, Hofoss D, Flaatten H, Muri AK, Gjerde S, Plsek PE. Effect of a scoring system and protocol for sedation on duration of patients' need for ventilator support in a surgical ICU. BMJ 2002; 324(7350): 1386–1389.
40. Domino KB, Posner KL, Caplan RA, Cheney FW. Awareness during anesthesia: a closed claims analysis. Anesthesiology 1999; 90(4):1053–1061.
41. Klessig HT, Geiger HJ, Murray MJ, Coursin DB. A national survey on the practice patterns of anesthesiologist intensivists in the use of muscle relaxants. Crit Care Med 1992; 20(9):1341–1345.
42. Murphy GS, Vender JS. Neuromuscular blocking drugs. Use and misuse in the ICU. Crit Care Clin 2001; 17(4):925–942.
43. Nasraway SA Jr, Wu EC, Kelleher RM, Yasuda CM, Donnelly AM. How reliable is the Bispectral Index in critically ill patients? A prospective, comparative, single-blinded observer study. Crit Care Med 2002; 30(7):1483–1487.
44. Triltsch A, Welte M , von Homeyer P, Grosse J, Genahr A, Moshirzadeh M, Sidiropoulos A, Konertz W, Kox WJ, Spies CD. Bispectral index-guided sedation with dexmedetomidine in intensive care: a prospective, randomized, double blind, placebo controlled phase II study. Crit Care Med 2002; 30(5):1007–1014.
45. Riker R, Fraser GL. Sedation in the ICU: refining the models and defining the questions. Crit Care Med 2002; 30(7):1661–1663.
46. Colombo JA. New agents, new monitors, same unanswered questions. Crit Care Med 2002; 30(5):1166–1167.
47. O'Connor MF, Daves SM, Tung A, Cook RI, Thisted R, Apfelbaum J. BIS monitoring to prevent awareness during general anesthesia. Anesthesiology 2001; 94(3): 520–522.
48. Gajraj RJ, Doi M, Mantzaridis H, Kenny GN. Analysis of the EEG bispectrum, auditory evoked potentials and the EEG power spectrum during repeated transitions from consciousness to unconsciousness. Br J Anaesth 1998; 80(1):46–52.
49. Jacobi J, Fraser GL, Coursin DB, Riker RR, Fontaine D, Wittbrodt ET, Chalfin DB, Masica MF, Bjerke HS, Coplin WM, Crippen DW, Fuchs BD, Kelleher RM, Marik PE, Nasraway SA Jr, Murray MJ, Peruzzi WT, Lumb PD. Task force of the American College of Critical Care Medicine (ACCM) of the Society of Critical Care Medicine. Clinical practice guidelines for the sustained use of sedatives and analgesics in the critically ill adult. Crit Care Med 2002; 30(1):119–141.
50. Driscoll D. Safety of parenteral infusions in the critical care setting. Adv Stud Med 2002; 2(9):338–342.
51. Bolon M, Bastien O, Flamens C, Paulus S, Boulieu R. Midazolam disposition in patients undergoing continuous

venovenous hemodialysis. J Clin Pharmacol 2001; 41: 95–96.
52. Maze M, Scarfini C, Cavaliere F. New agents for sedation in the ICU. Crit Care Clin 2001; 17(4):881–897.
53. Cawley MJ. Short-term lorazepam infusion and concern for propylene glycol toxicity: case report and review. Pharmacotherapy 2001; 21(9):1140–1144.
54. Lingamaneni R, Birch ML, Hemmings HC Jr. Widespread inhibition of sodium channel-dependent glutamate release from isolated nerve terminals by isoflurane and propofol. Anesthesiology 2001; 95(6):1460–1466.
55. Raoof AA, van Obbergh LJ, deVille deGoyet J, Verbeeck RK. Extrahepatic glucuronidation of propofol in man: possible contribution of gut wall and kidney. Eur J Clin Pharmacol 1996; 50(1–2):91–96.
56. Valente J, Anderson G, Branson RD, Johnson DJ, Davis K Jr, Porembka DT. Disadvantages of prolonged propofol sedation in the critical care unit. Crit Care Med 1994; 22(40):710–712.
57. Smith BJ. Treatment of status epilepticus. Neurol Clin 2001; 19(2):347–369.
58. Walder B, Tramer MR, Seeck M. Seizure-like phenomena and propofol. A systematic review. Neurology 2002; 58(9):1327–1332.
59. Nelson DB, Barkun AN, Block KP, Burdick JS, Ginsberg GG, Greenwald DA, Kelsey PB, Nakao NL, Slivka A, Smith P, Vakil N. American Society for Gastrointestinal Endoscopy. Technology Committee. Propofol use during gastrointestinal endoscopy. Gastrointest Endosc 2001; 53(7):876–879.
60. Hofer KN, McCarthy MW, Buck ML, Hendrick AE. Possible anaphylaxis after propofol in a child with food allergy. Ann Pharmacother 2003; 37(3):398–401.
61. Langevin PB. Propofol containing sulfite—potential for injury. Chest 1999; 116(4):1140–1141.
62. Barr J, Egan T, Sandoval N, Zomorodi K, Cohane C, Gambus P, Shafer S. Propofol dosing regimens for ICU sedation based upon an integrated pharmacokinetic–pharmacodynamic model. Anesthesiology 2001; 95(2):324–333.
63. Mendez D, De La Cruz JP, Arrebola MM, Guerrero A, Gonzalez-Correa JA, Garcia-Temboury E, Sanchez de la Cuesta F. The effect of propofol on the interaction of platelets with leukocytes and erythrocytes in surgical patients. Anesth Analg 2003; 96:713–719.
64. McCollam JS, O'Neil MG, Norcross ED, Byrne TK, Reeves ST. Continuous infusions of lorazepam, midazolam, and propofol for sedation of the critically ill surgery trauma patient: a prospective, randomized comparison. Crit Care Med 1999; 27(11):2454–2458.
65. Velly LJ, Guillet BA, Masmejean F, Nieoullon A, Bruder NJ, Gouin F, Pisano PM. Neuroprotective effects of propofol in a model of ischemic cortical cell cultures. Role of glutamate and its transporters. Anesthesiology 2003; 99(2):368–375.
66. Wooltorton E. Propofol: contraindicated for sedation of pediatric ICU patients. CMAJ 2002; 167(5):507.
67. Bray RJ. Propofol infusion for ICU sedation in children [letter to editor]. Anaesthesia 2002; 57(5):521.
68. Cannon M, Glazier S, Bauman L. Metabolic acidosis, rhabdomyolysis, and cardiovascular collapse after prolonged propofol infusion. J Neurosurg 2001; 96(6): 1053–1056.
69. Strickland RA, Murray M. Fatal metabolic acidosis in a pediatric patient receiving an infusion of propofol in the ICU: is there a relationship? Crit Care Med 1995; 23(2):405–409.
70. Wolf A, Weir P, Segar P, Stone J, Shield J. Impaired fatty acid oxidation in propofol infusion syndrome. Lancet 2001; 357:606–607.
71. Hatch DJ. Propofol-infusion syndrome in children. Lancet 1999; 353(9159):1117–1118.
72. Cornfield DN, Tegtmeyer K, Nelson MD, Milla CE, Sweeney M. Continuous propofol infusion in 142 critically ill children. Pediatrics 2002; 110(6):1177–1181.
73. Ebert T, Hall J, Barney J, Uhrich T, Colinco M. The effects of increasing plasma concentrations of dexmedetomidine in humans. Anesthesiology 2000; 93(2): 382–394.
74. Weinbroum A, Ben-Abraham R. Dextromethorphan and dexmedetomidine: new agents for the control of perioperative pain. Eur J Surg 2001; 167:563–569.
75. Venn RM, Bryant A, Hall GM, Grounds RM. Effects of dexmedetomidine on adrenocortical function, and the cardiovascular, endocrine, and inflammatory responses in postoperative patients needing sedation in the ICU. Br J Anaesth 2001; 86(5):650–656.
76. Jalonen J, Hynynen M, Kuitenen A, Heikkila H, Perttila J, Salmenpera M, Aantaa R, Kallio A. Dexmedetomidine as an anesthetic adjunct in coronary artery bypass grafting. Anesthesiology 1997; 86(2):331–345.
77. Crippen D, Ermakov S. Continuous infusions of haloperidol in critically ill patients [letter to the editor]. Crit Care Med 1995; 23(1):214–215.
78. Angelini G, Ketzler JT, Coursin DB. Use of propofol and other nonbenzodiazepine sedatives in the ICU. Crit Care Clin 2001; 17(4):863–880.
79. Khan IA. Clinical and therapeutic aspects of congenital and acquired long QT syndrome. Am J Med 2002; 112(1):58–66.
80. Dershwitz M. Droperidol: should the black box be light gray? J Clin Anesth 2002; 14(8):598–603.
81. Krakoff J, Koch C, et al. Use of a parenteral propylene-glycol containing etomidate preparation for the long-term management of ectopic Cushing's syndrome. J Clin Endocrinol Metab 2001; 86(9):4104–4108.
82. Aranda M, Hanson CW III. Anesthetics, sedatives, and paralytics. Understanding their use in the ICU. Surg Clin North Am 2000; 80(3):933–947.
83. Stover JF, Pleines UE, Morganti-Kossman MC, Stocker R, Kossman T. Thiopental attenuates energetic impairment but fails to normalize cerebrospinal fluid glutamate in brain-injured patients. Crit Care Med 1999; 27(7):1351–1357.

84. Biros MH, Heegaard W. Prehospital and resuscitative care of the head-injured patient. Curr Opin Crit Care 2001; 7(6):444–449.
85. Kawamata T, Omote K, Sonoda H, Kawamata M, Namiki A. Analgesic mechanisms of ketamine in the presence and absence of peripheral inflammation. Anesthesiology 2000; 93(2):520–528.
86. Vielhaber A, Portenoy RK. Advances in cancer pain management. Hematol Oncol Clin North Am 2002; 16(3):527–541.
87. Youssef-Ahmed MZ, Silver P, Nimkoff L, Sagy M. Continuous infusion of ketamine in mechanically ventilated children with refractory bronchospasm. Intensive Care Med 1996; 22(9):972–976.
88. Roberts JR, Geeting GK. Intramuscular ketamine for the rapid tranquilization of the uncontrollable, violent, and dangerous adult patient. J Trauma 2001; 51(5): 1008–1010.
89. Jackson K, Ashby M, Martin P, Pisasale M, Brumley D, Hayes B. "Burst" ketamine for refractory cancer pain: an open-label audit of 39 patients. J Pain Symptom Manage 2001; 23(4):834–842.
90. Mokhlesi B, Leikin JB, Murray P, Corbridge TC. Adult toxicology in critical care. Part II: specific poisonings. Chest 2003; 123(3):897–922.
91. Rawal N. Epidural and spinal agents for postoperative analgesia. Surg Clin North Am 1999; 79(2):313–344.
92. Bernard SA. The interaction of medications used in palliative care. Hematol Oncol Clin North Am 2002; 16(3):641–655.
93. Kivisto KT, Kroemer HK, Eichelbaum M. The role of human cytochrome P450 enzymes in the metabolism of anticancer agents: implications for drug interactions. Br J Clin Pharmacol 1995; 40:523–530.
94. Schelling G, Stoll C, Haller M, Briegel J, Manert W, Hummel T, Lenhart A, Heyduck M, Polasek J, Meier M, Preuss U, Bullinger M, Schuffel W, Peter K. Health-related quality of life and posttraumatic stress disorder in survivors of the acute respiratory distress syndrome. Crit Care Med 1998; 26(4):651–659.
95. Capuzzo M, Pinamonti A, Cingolani E, Grassi L, Bianconi M, Contu P, Gritti G, Alvisi R. Analgesia, sedation, and memory of intensive care. J Crit Care 2001; 16(3):83–89.
96. Jones C, Griffiths RD, MacMillan R, Palmer TEA. Psychological problems occurring after intensive care. Br J Intensive Care 1994; 2:46–53.
97. Cammarano W, Pittet JF, Weitz S, Schlobohm RM, Marks JD. Acute withdrawal syndrome related to the administration of analgesic and sedative medications in adult ICU patients. Crit Care Med 1998; 26(4): 676–684.
98. Truog R, Cist AF, Brackett SE, Burns JP, Curley MA, Danis M, DeVita MA, Rosenbaum SH, Rothenberg DM, Sprung CL, Webb SA, Wlody GS, Hurford WE. Recommendations for end-of-life care in the ICU: the Ethics Committee of the Society of Critical Care Medicine. Crit Care Med 2001; 29(12):2332–2348.

41

Cardiovascular Support

M. FANSHAWE

Departments of Anaesthesia and Perioperative Medicine and Anaesthesiology and Critical Care, Royal Brisbane Hospital, University of Queensland, Brisbane, Australia

S. G. TAN

Changi General Hospital, Singapore

JEFF LIPMAN

Departments of Intensive Care Medicine and Anaesthesiology and Critical Care, Royal Brisbane Hospital, University of Queensland, Brisbane, Australia

An abundance of monitoring equipment is used in modern operating rooms (ORs) and intensive care units to assist with cardiovascular support. Anesthetists and intensivists often go home after a busy but pleasing day at work, believing they have done well for their patients by using all the latest available monitoring facilities. It is a sobering thought, however, that there is little, if any, evidence to show that any of these monitors improves outcome (1). As clinicians, we use evidence based medicine to validate a new drug, requiring a large, positive randomized double-blind trial before we use it; yet we introduce technology at the merest hint of some proposed physiological benefit.

It is common practice to use invasive monitoring on very sick patients. Where is the evidence that it actually improves patient outcomes? There is none. This does not mean we should not apply invasive monitoring to obtain information for use with these patients. We should, however, always consider whether invasive monitoring is likely to benefit them.

In this chapter, we provide the reader with some guidance in the use of cardiovascular support in the critically ill oncology patient and to explain the rationale behind this advice.

I. INTRODUCTION

Circulatory function refers to the functioning of the entire circulatory system, including the heart, blood vessels, and blood volume. Circulatory failure is defined as the dysfunction of any or all of these systems. Circulatory support is therefore best conceptualized as treatment designed to minimize or reverse any dysfunction of the circulatory system (2).

There are both cardiac and vascular elements in circulatory failure. The endpoint of circulatory failure is shock, which can be defined as an imbalance between oxygen demand and oxygen supply such that cellular and organ dysfunction will occur (3,4). It is useful to identify the particular form of shock or circulatory failure that a patient is suffering in order to develop a logical and satisfactory treatment plan. Some patients will suffer from more than one form of shock. Ineffective tissue blood flow, rather than absolute measures of cardiac output (CO) or perfusion pressure, is the hallmark of shock (5). Treatment should therefore aim for adequate tissue or end-organ blood flow (5). Clinical endpoints, including urine output and peripheral perfusion, in response to an intervention such as a fluid challenge are of vital importance. There is no substitute for good clinical acumen (1).

Oncology patients constitute a challenging subgroup of critical care patients. Besides sepsis, there are innumerable other causes or complications which can contribute to circulatory failure (3). It is imperative to find and treat these causes if oncology patients are to have their best chance of a good outcome. (They are dealt with in detail later in the chapter.) The hemodynamic care of these patients perioperatively is also greatly influenced by these unique oncology issues. Adding to the conundrum is the higher risk associated with invasive hemodynamic monitoring in these patients, who frequently experience marrow failure resulting in low platelet counts and neutropenia (6). The use of noninvasive hemodynamic monitors should therefore be of benefit to them.

In this chapter, we consider the various monitoring modalities available for seriously ill patients; the causes of circulatory failure in oncology patients; perioperative optimization of care of oncology patients; and the treatment of oncology patients with circulatory failure.

II. HEMODYNAMIC MONITORING

Hemodynamic assessment is central to the effective, swift treatment of circulatory problems in the oncology patient. While the monitoring itself is not therapeutic (and provides no circulatory support), appropriate monitoring assists in the provision of effective circulatory support.

The form of hemodynamic monitoring to be chosen remains controversial, particularly since there is a lack of validation of most monitoring modalities (1).

Broadly, the types of monitoring available may be divided into invasive, minimally invasive, and noninvasive (Table 1). Interest in noninvasive or minimally invasive monitoring has recently increased (3,4,6–10).

Because oncology patients suffer from immunosuppression and thrombocytopenia, less invasive techniques are preferable to the use of lines such as pulmonary artery catheters, which have an even narrower therapeutic risk/benefit ratio than they do in nononcology patients.

In this chapter, we consider the following monitors: noninvasive blood pressure (NIBP), intra-arterial blood pressure (IAP), electrocardiography (ECG), central venous pressure (CVP), pulmonary artery catheter (PAC), transesophageal echocardiography (TEE), esophageal Doppler, pulse contour measurements, and other relatively noninvasive CO monitors. Since serum lactate levels are also useful to indicate inadequate cellular oxygenation, they will be considered.

Ideally, hemodynamic monitoring should provide data regarding contractility, preload, and afterload (6). In ASA III or IV patients, the degree of monitoring must be balanced between the extent of invasiveness and the ability to obtain rapidly and easily the information to manage hemodynamics (6).

A. Blood Pressure Monitoring

Studies have shown NIBP to be an unreliable monitor in patients suffering from circulatory failure. In addition, it does not provide beat-to-beat assessment of the blood pressure, making it less than ideal in patients receiving inotropes (4). We would therefore advocate the use of an IAP in oncology patients with circulatory failure. Intra-arterial blood pressure maintains accuracy during circulatory failure if used correctly, and allows beat-to-beat assessment of blood pressure. Intra-arterial blood pressure is a minimally invasive

Table 1 Monitoring Classification Based on Invasiveness

Invasive	Minimally invasive	Noninvasive
Pulmonary artery catheter	Transesophageal echocardiography	Clinical acumen, integration of all available data
Central venous pressure	Intra-arterial blood pressure	Continuous electrocardiography (ECG)
	Lactate, acid–base status, base excess	Urine output
	Pulse wave contour cardiac output (PiCCO®)	Peripheral perfusion
	Lithium dilution cardiac output	Transthoracic echocardiography
	Esophageal Doppler	Noninvasive blood pressure
		Noninvasive cardiac output

line, as it has a low rate of infection, thrombosis, and mechanical complication (11).

B. Electrocardiography

Continuous ECG monitoring is mandatory in all oncology patients suffering circulatory failure. It is a cheap, cost-effective monitor that is associated with almost no complications other than user (or interpretation) error. We would advocate a 5 lead ECG in preference to a 3 lead ECG, because even younger oncology patients are at increased risk of myocardial ischemia owing to their hypotension and chemotherapy treatment regimes. Electrocardiography also provides arrhythmia monitoring (12).

C. Central Venous Line

Central venous lines (CVL) can measure superior vena caval (SVC) pressures and provide a means of administering vasoactive drugs through a central vein. Femoral venous catheterization has been shown to trend SVC pressures adequately (13) and may therefore present an alternative route in the treatment of a thrombocytopenic patient where SVC cannulation is deemed to be significantly risky. There are few data demonstrating the superiority of one site of central venous access over another. Our unit tends to avoid femoral sites unless there is thrombocytopenia, for fear of higher infection risk. Subclavian central lines are associated with a lower infection rate than the internal jugular approach (14–19). One study, however, suggested that the right internal jugular approach had the highest success rate among residents (20). We feel that the difference between subclavian and internal jugular sites is largely a matter of personal experience and preference, particularly with the availability of antibiotic coated lines and increased awareness of aseptic techniques in the insertion and maintenance of these lines (21).

We would advocate the use of central lines (1) despite their complications in oncology patients with circulatory failure, because of the necessity to administer vasoactive drugs through a central vein. Because oncology patients frequently suffer significant cardiac disease, CVP is unlikely to be a reliable estimate of left ventricular preload. Certainly, absolute numbers obtained from a central line in guiding fluid management are, in our opinion, highly questionable (1,4). Central venous pressure trends are nevertheless often useful.

Preload responsiveness can be more useful than preload quantification. We would advocate judicious fluid challenges while assessing hemodynamic parameters and gas exchange changes. In many cases, there will be no decrement in gas exchange while there will be improvements in mean arterial pressure (MAP) and urine output with no significant changes in CVP. Such patients are preload responsive. Accurate quantification of preload with monitors such as CVP is not possible (1,4,7,22). The key for the clinician is to give serial fluid challenges while keeping a close eye on hemodynamic and respiratory parameters, including peripheral perfusion, to guide the assessment of adequate fluid loading (see in what follows).

Another benefit of a central line is that it enables measurement of central oxygen saturations (23). Studies have also shown that mixed venous saturations taken from the SVC are of comparable use to formal mixed venous saturations obtained from a PAC (23,24). Unfortunately, while low SvO_2 is associated with poor prognosis, it has not necessarily been demonstrated that the use of supranormal oxygen delivery and correction of the SvO2 improves prognosis (25,26).

D. Pulmonary Artery Catheter

Pulmonary artery catheter is often used in the monitoring, assessment, and treatment of critical care patients with circulatory failure. Nevertheless, some clinicians suggest that PACs may actually worsen patient outcome (27). This clinical equipoise was the motivation for a recently published randomized trial, which was unable to show benefit in terms of survival (28). There is no literature pertaining to their use in oncology patients with circulatory failure. We believe that, given the likelihood of immune compromised state, difficult access, thrombocytopenia and coagulopathy, the incidence of significant PAC related complications is likely to be even higher in the oncology subgroup (29,30). In our opinion, this would make the risk/benefit of their use even more marginal in this group than in other groups in which PACs are used. We therefore would not routinely use a PAC for oncology patients, preferring instead to use other, less invasive methods of assessment such as echocardiography or pulse contour wave technology.

E. Echocardiography

Echocardiography is useful as a less invasive means of assessing cardiovascular parameters in critical care. The choice rests between transthoracic echocardiography (TTE) and TEE. Transthoracic echocardiography is the less invasive of these methods and is therefore associated with the least number of iatrogenic mechanical complications. Transthoracic echocardiography is, however, less sensitive in detecting valvular vegetations, gives poorer assessment of the mitral valve apparatus, has a lower yield for embolic phenomenon, and is less sensitive in detecting aortic dissections than TEE (31,32).

The disadvantages of TEE include: a small but definite risk of esophageal perforation; laryngeal trauma; difficulty in swallowing; and accidental extubation (33). Given TEEs increased sensitivity to the detection of vegetations, each cancer patient admitted to critical care with circulatory failure should in our opinion have a TEE. Unless there are further major hemodynamic changes, further investigations could then reasonably be performed with TTE.

In comparison with PAC, a TEE will provide real time imaging and assessment of left ventricular end diastolic volume (LVEDV) and left atrial pressure (LAP); give a reasonably accurate measure of right ventricular systolic pressure (RVSP); allow the measurement of CO, which correlates well with PAC; and give a qualitative assessment of systemic vascular resistance (SVR) (34,35).

In addition to providing similar information to a PAC, echocardiography also provides diagnostic information. It allows an assessment of ischemia (via regional wall motion abnormalities), the exclusion of endocarditis, cardiac tamponade, pericardial effusion, ventricular septal defect (VSD), atrial septal defect (ASD), valvular pathology, and aortic pathology. It will also exclude massive pulmonary embolism. Therefore, a TEE is superior to a PAC in terms of its ability to provide diagnostic and monitoring information with less risk (36–39).

The disadvantages of echocardiography include significant set-up costs and a substantial investment in training for correct interpretation. The exact costs will vary from center to center depending on patient numbers (40,41). In our opinion, it is preferable to perform serial echocardiograms as clinical conditions dictate. Transesophageal echocardiography can also be used, in a sense, to "calibrate" the readings of the CVP and help assess whether they are likely to bear any correlation with LVEDV. In a study by Colreavy et al. (36), TEE revealed the cause of hypotension in 67% of cases. In 31% of cases, the hemodynamics improved after a TEE-mediated change in therapy, and in 32%, the TEE caused a change in management. These figures accord with our experience that TEE can have powerful dynamic influences on treatment and is a safer and more useful monitor in oncology patients than PAC.

Transesophageal echocardiography is of particular use in the accurate assessment of preload. In general, patients with a small left ventricular end diastolic area (LVEDA) have a low filling status. This indicator measure is unreliable in patients with left ventricular dilatation or a high preload state. Left ventricular end diastolic area has been shown to correlate well with blood loss, whereas pulmonary artery occlusion pressures have been shown to be a poor measure of preload. The left ventricle (LV) compliance curve means that when the LV is underfilled, LVEDA changes are large for a given change in pressure. In high preload states, Doppler methods provide a more accurate means of assessing preload and a Doppler transmitral E/A flow ratio of peaks >2 corresponds to a left ventricular end diastolic pressure (LVEDP) > 20 (37). Preload is considered decreased if LVEDA <9 $cm^2\ m^{-2}$ in transgastric short axis view or <15 $cm^2\ m^{-2}$ in transgastric long axis view.

In a study by Kolev et al. (38), the TEE was the catalyst for anti-ischemic management in 56% of OR cases, fluid administration in 28% of cases (4× greater fluid bolus interventions compared with pulmonary capillary wedge pressures), vasopressor/inotropic therapy in 16% or vasodilator therapy in 4% of cases. Transesophageal echocardiography also gives useful information about afterload and contractility.

The American Society of Anesthesiologists and the Society of Cardiovascular Anesthesiologists Task Force on TEE have divided the indications for TEE into three categories (39). Transesophageal echocardiography has been shown to have the most impact when used for Category 1 or 2 indications, which, broadly, mean that circulatory failure persists after the initial clinical assessment and treatment. It is therefore important to consider the indication for TEE in the critical care cancer patient before proceeding with TEE (6).

F. Other Measures of Cardiac Output

Other methods of measuring CO include bio-impedance cardiography, thoracic electrical bio-impedance, esophageal Doppler, and endotracheal techniques. These techniques potentially offer significant hemodynamic data in a less invasive manner than PAC and without requiring echocardiography expertise (8,10).

Bio-impedance cardiography is based on the "pulse contour CO" principle. This technology is currently marketed as the PiCCO® and LiDCO®. Unfortunately PiCCO® still requires a central arterial catheter such as a femoral artery or axillary artery, which means it is relatively invasive. It assumes a constant distensibility of the systemic arterial bed and is compromised in those patients with a high afterload. It also requires calibration via thermodilution and uses the area under the arterial line pressure trace in proportion to the stroke volume in order to calculate CO (6). It provides information on intrathoracic blood volume and extravascular lung water. These are used as surrogate markers of cardiac preload (10,22,42,43).

Pulse contour devices such as the PiCCO® need to be calibrated with a CO derived from another source. The use of lithium chloride dilution removes this problem. Lithium is injected into a vein and measured with a lithium sensitive electrode. Blood taken from the peripheral arterial system (an important advantage compared with the PiCCO®) may be used for this purpose (10). As this electrode is outside the artery, a sample of 3 mL of blood is required with each measurement. The CO is calculated using a dilution curve for lithium; the device can then be calibrated. Studies suggest CO measured with the lithium dilution CO monitor correlate well with PAC CO. Unlike with the thermodilution-derived pulse contour technique, there is no information about cardiac preload. To date, there are scant data validating this monitoring tool in critically ill patients.

Thoracic electrical bio-impedance measures the resistance of the thorax to a high frequency, low magnitude current. This measurement is indirectly proportional to the content of thoracic fluids. Changes in CO may be reflected in an overall change in bio-impedance. The determinants of overall thoracic bio-impedance are changes in pulmonary and venous blood induced by respiration and volumetric changes in aortic blood flow produced by myocardial contractility. There are many sources of measurement error in this technique. Recent studies have suggested that the technique is useful for trend analysis but not accurate enough for diagnostic determination (10).

The esophageal Doppler involves placing a probe in the esophagus and measuring flow velocity in the descending thoracic aorta (44). Because this vessel receives only 70% of CO, a correction factor is required, using a cross-sectional area as well as a velocity measurement. Because the area of a circle is πr^2, any error in measurement is squared (10).

The endotracheal method of CO measurement (NICO®) involves use of the indirect Fick method, which has been modified to use partial CO_2 rebreathing. Because the difference between mixed venous PCO_2 and $PaCO_2$ is small, any errors in measurement of these parameters can result in large changes in calculated CO. The method is valid only if $PaCO_2 > 30$ mmHg. It is best suited to monitor trends in critically ill patients with stable lung function (10).

Thoracic electrical bio-impedance, NICO®, esophageal Doppler, and lithium dilution techniques for measuring CO provide no information regarding preload, afterload, or contractility. While these techniques potentially have a place as noninvasive monitors of CO, their value is limited because they provide only CO data, with no reference to other central circulatory physiological parameters. In addition, clinical experience is required to validate their accuracy (6).

G. Lactate

Hyperlactatemia has been defined as a mild or moderate increase in blood lactate concentration (2–5 mmol/ L) without metabolic acidosis. Lactic acidosis has been defined as increased blood lactate levels, usually > 5 mmol/L, associated with metabolic acidosis. Hyperlactatemia that persists in stress states following adequate resuscitation suggests that mechanisms or abnormalities other than poor tissue perfusion or hypoxia may be involved (4,5,45–51).

The production and utilization of lactate is closely linked to the metabolic fate of pyruvate. Conditions resulting in increased production or decreased breakdown of pyruvate also cause hyperlactatemia (45,50). Pyruvate is derived intracellularly from three metabolic routes: (i) oxidation of lactate via dehydrogenase (LDH); (ii) proteolysis by various dehydrogenation and transamination reactions, contributing about 15%; and (iii) glycolysis. Glycolysis is quantitatively the most important means of production of pyruvate, and therefore lactate, and also results in the formation of adenosine triphosphate (ATP) and water. The major sources of lactate production are skin, red blood cells, skeletal muscle, and intestinal mucosa (45). The liver and kidney cortex are quantitatively the most important organs of lactate consumption. The normal blood lactate [mean (SD)] concentration in unstressed individuals is taken as 1.0 (0.5) mmol/L (45).

It therefore seems reasonable to assume that an increased lactate production is due to inadequate tissue perfusion or altered cellular metabolism. Despite this limitation, serum lactate can still be a useful clinical tool.

H. Recommendations

Our recommendations for hemodynamic monitoring would be: 5 lead ECG, CVP, intra-arterial line, and echocardiography (if there was an appropriate indication for it). We do not believe that the other noninvasive monitors of CO are yet sufficiently reliable. They also give no information regarding preload, afterload, or contractility (6). Appropriate assessment of preload responsiveness and adequate fluid loading is of prime importance in the management of oncology patients with circulatory failure. We would occasionally use the PiCCO® monitor, but are unable to recommend the use of PAC except in exceptional circumstances in these patients. We would also recommend the monitoring of serial serum lactate levels.

III. CAUSES OF CIRCULATORY FAILURE IN ONCOLOGY PATIENTS

Malignancy is a disease found across all age groups. The differential diagnosis of circulatory failure is broad, ranging from congenital heart disease in younger patients to coronary atherosclerosis in older patients. Oncology patients are at risk from all the usual causes of circulatory collapse as well as from those either related directly to their malignancy or resulting from a complication of oncology therapy (3).

Shock can be divided into four categories (4,7): hypovolemic, cardiogenic, obstructive, and distributive.

In oncology patients, hypovolemia is common, resulting from vomiting, bleeding into or from tumors, diarrhea, and poor oral intake (3). Clinicians must be alert for signs of hypovolemic shock, since many oncology patients are young and able to mask signs and symptoms until they are severely dehydrated.

Cardiogenic shock can occur in oncology patients for a number of reasons. Cancer and coronary artery disease or chronic untreated hypertension often coexist. Some chemotherapeutic agents produce cardiomyopathy (Table 2). The anthracyclines (daunorubicin, doxorubicin, epirubicin, and idarubicin) are associated with cardiomyopathy. Anthracycline cardiomyopathy is irreversible, can present at any time from a few days to 5 years after initiation of treatment, and leads to congestive cardiac failure with systolic dysfunction. Trastuzumab produces a potentially reversible cardiomyopathy. Cyclophosphamide can cause an acute hemorrhagic myo/pericarditis, and 5-fluorouracil can produce coronary vasospasm, myocarditis, and cardiomyopathy. A complete chemotherapeutic history of the oncology patient with circulatory failure is of vital importance (3).

Table 2 Chemotherapy Agents and Cardiac Complications

Agent class	Drug	Cardiac complications
Anthracyclines	Doxorubicin	Irreversible cardiomyopathy
	Daunorubicin	
	Epirubicin	
	Idarubicin	
	Trastuzumab	Partially reversible cardiomyopathy
	Cyclophosphamide	Acute hemorrhagic myo/pericarditis
	5-Fluorouracil	Coronary vasospasm, myocarditis, cardiomyopathy

Obstructive shock may also occur in oncology patients, some of whom present with hypercoagulable symptoms. Thromboembolic disorders such as pulmonary embolism must always be excluded. Other obstructive problems such as cardiac tamponade may cause circulatory failure. Intracardiac masses either from tumor metastases or thromboembolic phenomena may present in shock. Primary cardiac malignancies are rare, although even benign myxomas may also produce obstructive shock and death if left untreated. Myxomas are easily diagnosed with echocardiography and respond well to surgical treatment (52). Nonbacterial thrombotic endocarditis or marantic endocarditis, in which bland fibrin platelet thrombi occur on a cardiac valve, is known to occur in oncology (3,4,7).

The final category of shock is distributive shock. Septic shock is the most common cause of distributive shock and is common in oncology. These patients suffer immunosuppression, are burdened with necessary but often problematic long-term vascular access, and are subjected to cytotoxic therapy. They are also frequently admitted to hospitals carrying multiresistant organisms (53). In addition, busy health care professionals notoriously have poor hand hygiene (54). Oncology patients often suffer from malnutrition and leukocyte dysfunction along with cellular and humoral immune deficiencies.

For some patients, hematological or lymphoproliferative malignancies are the primary disorders. This combination makes them highly susceptible to episodes of sepsis, including infective endocarditis. It has been estimated that up to 70% of patients with chemotherapy-induced neutropenia will have at least one infective episode. In those with an absolute neutrophil count $<100/\text{mm}^3$, 20% will develop bacteremia with fever, with crude mortality figures of 47% compared with 14% mortality for those with a neutrophil count $>1000/\text{mm}^3$.

Besides sepsis, endocrine-mediated circulatory compromise may also cause distributive shock. The cause is usually a particular tumor such as pheochromocytoma, carcinoid syndrome, or it may be endocrine organ failure such as acute adrenal insufficiency (3,4,7).

Oncology patients may suffer circulatory collapse as a result of causes linked to all four categories of shock (Table 3). Many will have complex etiologies with causes relating to more than one category. They will suffer from acute and chronic medical conditions

Table 3 Classification of Shock Etiology in Cancer Patients

Category of shock	Common causes related to oncology
Hypovolemia	Bleeding into/from tumors Vomiting Diarrhea Poor oral intake
Cardiogenic	Coronary artery disease Hypertension Chemotherapy cardiomyopathy, myocarditis, vasospasm
Obstructive	Pulmonary embolism Cardiac tamponade Intracardiac masses—metastases, primary cardiac tumors, thrombus Nonbacterial thrombotic endocarditis
Distributive	Sepsis Acute adrenal insufficiency Endocrine tumors—pheochromocytoma, carcinoid

common to the general population (e.g., coronary artery disease) as well as conditions related directly to their cancer or cancer therapy. This combination is likely to make diagnosis and treatment very complex.

IV. PERIOPERATIVE OPTIMIZATION

The optimal preoperative preparation of the oncology patient with circulatory failure is a highly contentious issue. On the one hand, there are data to suggest that a regime of perioperative increase in oxygen delivery (DO_2) limits postoperative morbidity, but on the other hand, some researchers advocate the use of preoperative β blockade. Most would simply advocate appropriate preoperative investigations such as a chest roentogram (CXR), continuous ECG, echocardiography, and appropriate but not aggressive preoperative resuscitation.

Some clinicians endorse preoperative admission of a patient to a critical care environment for aggressive preparation. Still others support a "supranormal" oxygen delivery approach (26,55,56), particularly in septic patients (25). The literature on oncology patients does not specifically address this issue. To date, there is minimal evidence to suggest that preoperative optimization in a critical care unit is more effective than adequate ward management (25,26).

Systemic changes in sepsis include myocardial depression, increased oxygen demand, and altered oxygen extraction and distribution of flow. Initial studies by Shoemaker et al. (57) supported the hypothesis that supranormal cardiac indices with supranormal oxygen delivery improved survival. Hayes et al. (58) performed a randomized trial to test this hypothesis and produced increased mortality rates in the supranormal group. It may simply be that increases in cardiac indices and oxygen delivery reflect higher underlying physiological reserves in the patients who survive. Tuchschmidt et al. (59) tested only septic shock patients and obtained more positive results. Despite this finding, supranormal oxygen delivery cannot be routinely recommended because it is difficult to determine which patient group might benefit (4).

There is also the vexed question of perioperative β blockade in those elective patients at moderate or high risk of major cardiac events. Many oncology patients may fall into this group.

Perioperative cardiac events frequently complicate noncardiac surgery, resulting in significant morbidity and cost (60). Patients undergoing noncardiac surgery suffer the surgical stress response, which is characterized by increased levels of epinephrine, norepinephrine, cortisol, and free fatty acids, all of which are associated with increased heart rates and myocardial oxygen demands (61–63). A link between tachycardia and perioperative myocardial ischemia has been well established (64–66). β blockers reduce adrenergic activity and produce a reduction in free fatty acid levels. They also protect against tachycardia. There are now many trials showing a low rate of cardiac events as well as of mortality in absolute numbers (67–73). Mangano's randomized controlled trial of 200 patients suggested an apparent difference in mortality rates with β blocker therapy in the first year following surgery. However, if the events during the first 7 days (during which the β blocker group had a higher mortality) are included, no difference exists between the placebo and the β blocker group.

In summary, although some disagree (74), we do not believe that the trials to date provide definitive evidence for the use of routine perioperative β blockade of patients with cardiac histories who undergo noncardiac surgery. β Blocker therapy also has potential serious side effects, such as congestive heart failure, bradycardia, and hypotension. It is also worth noting that none of the information regarding β blockade relates specifically to patients with cancer or circulatory failure.

To complicate the issue even further, a recent meta-analysis suggests a perioperative benefit of α_2 agonists (75).

A. Recommendations

In summary, perioperative optimization remains a contentious area. Given the lack of clear trial based evidence and scarce critical care resources, we do not advocate preoperative admission to intensive care. The decision to use β blockers should be made on a case-by-case basis. We do not support supranormal oxygen delivery in oncology patients, because the evidence is equivocal. The risk of significant cardiac morbidity and mortality using this unproven strategy seems unjustifiable. Many cancer patients are likely to suffer from coexisting coronary artery disease or cardiomyopathies and would not sustain a supranormal CO for oxygen delivery.

Instead, we would advocate a more conservative approach, involving adequate ward assessment and resuscitation based on clinical indicators such as urine output, peripheral perfusion, mental state, acid–base status, and renal function. We believe the key is to avoid, or at least limit, critical organ dysfunction prior to surgery. Similarly, in the postoperative phase, we recommend assessment and resuscitation based on these clinical endpoints.

V. TREATMENT OF CIRCULATORY FAILURE

The central philosophy underlying treatment during circulatory failure must involve the support of organ perfusion and function while the cause of failure is found and treated. Patients in whom no treatable cause for the failure is found are unlikely to have a good outcome. Equally, if multiorgan failure has occurred by the time a treatable cause is found, a good outcome is also unlikely (4,5,7,25,26). In general, circulatory support should involve fluid resuscitation; inotropic agents; vasopressors; antibiotics; source control; ventilatory support (considered elsewhere in this book); and steroid therapy. Not all these treatments will be required in all patients.

A. Fluid Therapy

1. *Basic Principles*

The primary goal of fluid therapy is to provide optimal preload for maximal cardiac performance. Except for those suffering cardiogenic shock, most patients in circulatory failure have depleted intravascular fluid volume, which leads to suboptimal conditions for myocardial performance based on the Frank Starling principle (3,4,6,7,36–38). Cardiogenic shock often presents, however, with poor contractility and a subsequently elevated LVEDV (37,38). Difficulties arise when the picture is mixed: for example, sepsis with a low SVR requiring fluid administration and cardiogenic shock with poor contractility. Difficulties also arise when there is chronic cardiac failure with acute exacerbation, as these patients usually require an increased LVEDV for optimal cardiac performance. An assessment of optimal left ventricular filling can be difficult even with the aid of TEE (38,39). Our approach to fluid resuscitation is to use serial fluid challenges of 250–500 mL at a time and to assess the preload responsiveness with each fluid challenge. Some patients will be highly preload responsive and will immediately respond to fluid, showing a significant improvement in parameters such as heart rate and MAP. Others will be less responsive with either slight or no improvement. A third group will become worse. It therefore becomes necessary to find a suitable quantification of preload in order to guide appropriate fluid management. Changes in systolic arterial pressure and arterial pulse pressure often predict preload responsiveness (22,42,43).

We assess the following parameters with each fluid load: heart rate; pulse pressure; MAP; inspired oxygen requirements; chest auscultation; peripheral perfusion; urine output; and CVP (pressure and waveform) (1). The clinical endpoints are of prime importance and we would strongly counsel against using absolute CVP numbers as the sole guide to the adequacy of fluid resuscitation, for the reasons previously outlined (1,3,4,7,22).

In our opinion, early TEE is highly beneficial. As previously described, it gives a direct assessment of LVEDV and often diagnoses the cause of the hypotension. In a sense, we can calibrate the CVP to the TEE (especially, if the TEE indicates no reason why CVP would be an erroneous measure of LVEDP) (36–38). In those centers without access to TEE, we suggest using one of the noninvasive CO monitors discussed earlier (76). Some patients will not respond to fluid loading at all and will instead require an inotropic agent.

Because it is based on clinical endpoints, preload responsiveness is easier to assess than preload quantification. Preload quantification is the ultimate goal, but at present, there is no definitive method available. The best methods are constant clinical assessment and the use of echocardiography. Once a patient is optimally filled and demonstrated to be a preload nonresponder, inotropic agents or vasopressors are required for hemodynamic support (36–38).

2. *Crystalloids or Colloids*

The choice to be made during fluid resuscitation is between crystalloids and colloids. In a study by Rackow et al. (77), either crystalloids or colloids were titrated to the same filling pressure to restore tissue perfusion to the same degree. As expected, the crystalloid group required 2–4× more volume than the colloid group. Volume expansion is transient and fluid accumulates in the interstitial spaces, risking the development of pulmonary edema. However, to date, no difference in survival or outcomes has been demonstrated between crystalloid and colloid resuscitations (4). Our approach is to use crystalloids for fluid maintenance and to counteract ongoing fluid losses from, for example, abdominal wounds. We tend to use colloids for fluid challenges.

3. *Hemoglobin*

The optimal level of hemoglobin and hematocrit for patients in septic shock is unclear. A large study by Hebert et al. in ICU patients showed no benefit of transfusion to a hemoglobin of 10 vs. 7 g/dL. In fact, this trial showed improved survival in the Hb 7 g/dL group. Importantly, patients with coronary artery disease were excluded from this trial (78,79). In oncology, our approach would be to use a transfusion trigger of 7 g/dL Hb unless there were a history of coronary artery disease. Excessive tachycardia, very low mixed venous oxygen saturations (SvO_2), or ischemic ECG changes may also prompt us to consider a higher transfusion trigger of around 10 g/dL (4,80).

B. Inotropic/Vasopressor Agents

1. *Basic Principles*

Failure to respond to fluid loading is an indication for intensive care treatment with inotropic or vasopressor agents. The goal of hemodynamic support in these patients is to maintain vital organ function until the cause of the circulatory failure can be identified and treated (51). An inotropic agent is one that increases myocardial contractility via β_1 adrenergic receptors, whereas vasopressors are defined as agents that increase SVR via one of several mechanisms (81). In practice, many agents such as epinephrine or higher doses of dopamine have both inotropic and vasopressor actions. While there is no clear evidence supporting the use of one agent over another, it seems logical to identify the primary system that has failed and choose an agent that is likely to have the greatest effect on this system. For example, in primary cardiogenic shock, a pure β_1 agonist such as dobutamine would seem a logical choice, whereas in pure sepsis with a low SVR state norepinephrine (with its higher α agonist activity) would seem to be the drug of choice.

Central to the choice of inotropic support is, once again, constant reassessment of the patient's response to therapy. Parameters such as heart rate, MAP, pulse pressure, peripheral perfusion, urine output, inspired oxygen requirements, acid–base status, and lactate levels should be used to assess whether the chosen inotropic agent has been beneficial. It is not uncommon to find that a change from one agent to another can have beneficial therapeutic effects. If the situation involves both sepsis and cardiogenic complications, a combination of dobutamine and noradrenaline may also be beneficial. Again, in choosing a "logical" inotropic agent, it is important to determine the cause of circulatory failure. It is in these circumstances, we believe echocardiography to be most helpful (4,5,7,51).

The maintenance of renal function is a clear goal of critical care support of patients with circulatory failure, because renal failure has grim prognostic implications. No prospective randomized controlled studies have shown vasopressors to improve renal function significantly. However, if they are used with care, renal blood flow can be increased (82). Several open-label clinical series support an increase in renal perfusion pressure (83). Excessive doses of any vasopressor agent, however, are likely to shift the renal autoregulation curve to the right, necessitating a greater perfusion pressure for a specified renal blood flow. Target mean pressures should therefore be set at the minimal level required for adequate renal blood flow. Unfortunately, despite adequate filling and normalization of hemodynamic variables, some patients will remain oliguric. This state may be due to an absence of increased renal blood flow, a decrease in glomerular perfusion pressure, or irreversible ischemic renal lesions. Low dose dopamine has not been shown to have a beneficial effect on renal function in patients with sepsis (4,5,51,84).

2. *Vasopressin*

Part of the pathophysiology of vasodilatory shock is a vasopressin deficiency (85,86). Not unexpectedly, some clinicians have attempted to use the hormone in the management of this condition (87–92). Vasopressin will certainly produce vasoconstriction, particularly of arteriolar beds. Its effects on the splanchnic, muscular, and cutaneous vasculature are pronounced (89,92). It is probably best used in catecholamine-resistant vasodilatory conditions (89). Dosages should be kept relatively low, 0.02–0.04 IU/min, certainly not higher than 0.1 IU/min (89), since cutaneous and mucosal injury during its use has been documented (92).

Terlipressin, a long-acting synthetic analogue of vasopressin with a much longer half-life (6 hr), has also been similarly used (93).

3. *Inotropic Agents*

Many oncology patients have impaired cardiac function as a result of multiple mechanisms, as described previously. Even those with sepsis are likely to have impaired cardiac function because of changes in intracellular calcium homeostasis and in adrenergic signal transduction. Several inflammatory mediators such as cytokines, platelet activating factor, and nitric oxide have been shown to cause myocardial depression.

The available inotropic agents are dobutamine, epinephrine, dopexamine, phosphodiesterase inhibitors, calcium, and digoxin. Dobutamine increases cardiac index with concomitant increases in stroke volume and heart rate (94). Dopexamine does produce improved cardiac index and LV stroke work index (but is not available in the United States). Owing to the presence of hypotension and arrhythmias, amrinone and milrinone (phosphodiesterase inhibitors) have little place in the treatment of these patients. Calcium has shown no consistent beneficial hemodynamic effect and has been associated with increased mortality in animal models (95–97). Digoxin has been shown to significantly improve cardiac performance in hypodynamic septic patients but is associated with potential dosing problems and toxicity issues (5,51,95,96).

The potential for an inotropic agent to induce vasopressor-mediated splanchnic ischemia is a cause for concern (98). The effects on the gut of norepinephrine and epinephrine are unpredictable; and since gut mucosal ischemia may play a role in the development of multiorgan failure, it will affect clinical decision making. There is some evidence to suggest that a combination of norepinephrine and dobutamine may produce less splanchnic ischemia when used in cases of sepsis (5,51,94). It should only be used to restore normal MAP values, because higher values will produce an increase in afterload with potentially deleterious myocardial side effects. We prefer to use either dobutamine for cardiogenic problems or norepinephrine for low SVR problems and a combination of the two for mixed problems.

Epinephrine could also be used for mixed cardiogenic and low SVR problems (99). Disadvantages of epinephrine in this situation include unpredictable β_1 vs. α vs. β_2 effects, detrimental effects on splanchnic blood flow with potential mucosal ischemia (94,98), and an association with systemic and regional increases in lactate concentrations. The causes and significance of these increases are unclear but they reduce the usefulness of lactate as a marker of tissue perfusion (4,5,45,46,51).

Phenylephrine is also a vasopressor agent. Reinelt et al. (100) reported reduced splanchnic blood flow and oxygen delivery in six septic shock patients treated with phenylephrine compared to norepinephrine. On the basis of this finding, we would prefer to use norepinephrine rather than phenylephrine for continuous infusion.

4. *Recommendations*

We recommend the use of dobutamine and norepinephrine support as indicated by the cause of the circulatory failure (94). These agents may be used in combination if indicated by the patient's clinical condition. Constant assessment of fluid status and inotropic effect is mandatory. The goals and desired endpoints of inotropic therapy must be clearly defined and monitored, with therapy appropriately titrated. For patients with recalcitrant hypotension due to a low SVR state, we would also suggest the use of vasopressin [0.02–0.04 IU/min (85)] as the next line of management (4,85,88–90). If vasopressors were required for longer than 48 hr, we would consider adding steroids (see below) (101–104).

Because of a lack of data, no definitive recommendations can be made about the superiority of a particular vasopressor or inotropic agent (51).

C. Other Therapy

In addition to fluid resuscitation and management of inotropic and vasopressor agents, there are other important critical care therapies available for cancer patients with circulatory failure. These include antibiotics for sepsis, "source control," steroid therapy, and renal protection. Renal protection is dealt elsewhere in this book.

Bacterial infection is the most common cause of septic shock in patients with malignancy (3).

Antibiotic therapy must be coupled with source control. In all septic shock cases, the cause or source of infection must be identified and appropriate measures of elimination taken. They could be as simple as a line or catheter change or as complicated as major surgery, for example, for intra-abdominal sepsis. Without appropriate source control, antibiotic therapy during supportive resuscitation will be unsuccessful.

Renewed interest has recently been shown in the use of steroids in hemodynamic failure. Cancer patients are especially prone to adrenal insufficiency. Marik and Zaloga (101) demonstrated that serum cortisol levels <25 μ/dL are associated with steroid responsive hypotension. Recent literature suggests that patients with refractory hypotension, which persists despite the administration of fluids and vasopressors, often have a hemodynamic response to hydrocortisone 50 mg iv q6 hr, even if they do not suffer classical

Addison's disease (103,104). These doses lead to moderate supraphysiologic cortisol levels that may be important in overcoming tissue-specific corticosteroid resistance (101,102). One study in sepsis used fludrocortisone (105). Our approach in cancer patients would be to consider hydrocortisone therapy if the hemodynamics has not adequately responded to fluid and vasopressor therapy (see Appendix A).

VI. CONCLUSION

Cancer patients in circulatory failure pose significant challenges in critical care. The number of likely causes of failure is increased by virtue of the patients' primary cancer, their chemotherapy treatments, pro-coagulant tendencies, and possible surgical interventions. A thorough understanding of the possible causes and timely identification of the actual cause of circulatory failure is of paramount importance. For infections, source control treatment should be initiated and followed by supportive resuscitation with fluids and a vasopressor or inotropic agent. We would advocate the early use of echocardiography for both monitoring and diagnostic purposes. The choice of inotrope should be determined by considerations such as whether vasodilation, poor contractility or both constitute the cause of hypotension. The endpoints of supportive treatment should be based on clinical parameters such as urine output, peripheral perfusion, MAP, FiO2, and lactate levels.

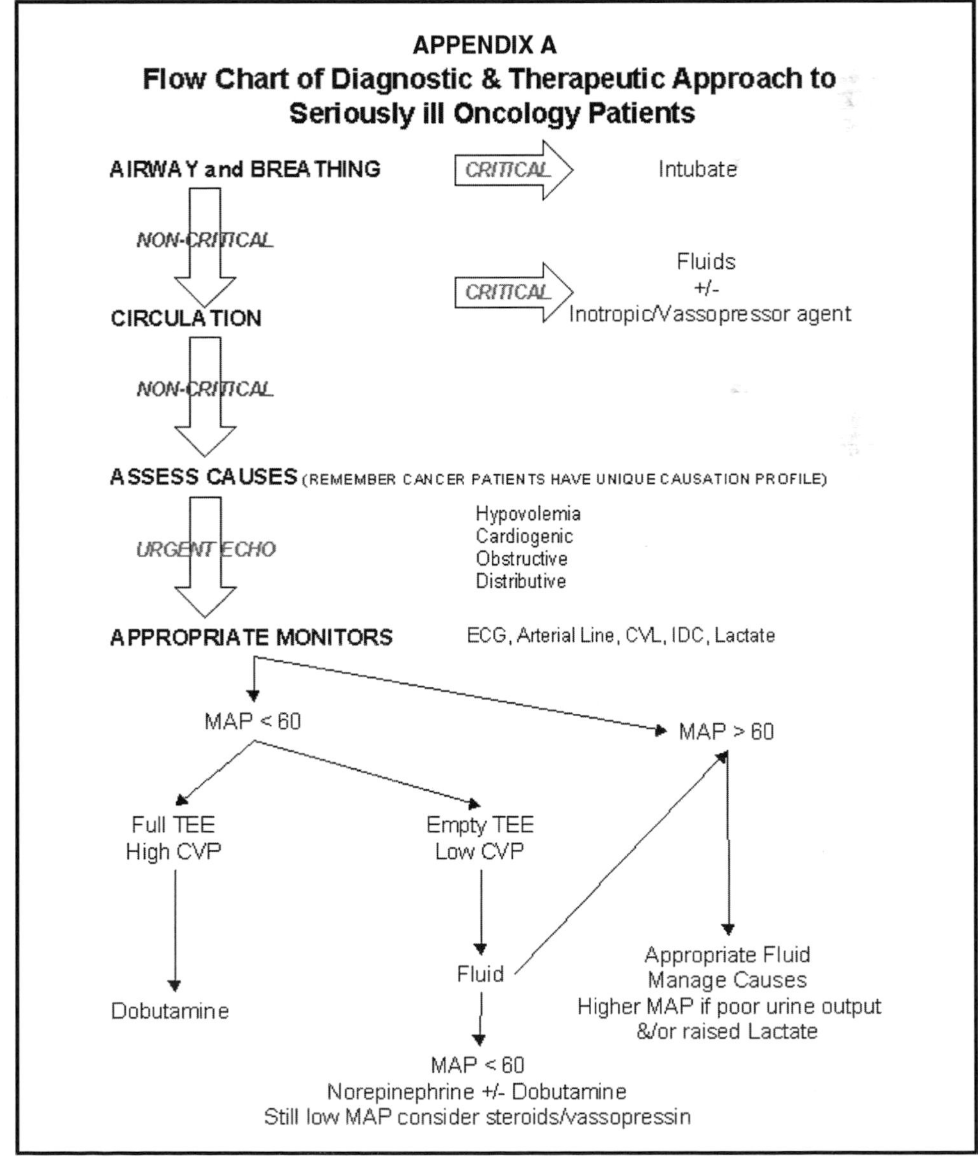

REFERENCES

1. Bellomo R, Uchino S. Cardiovascular monitoring tools: use and misuse. Curr Opin Crit Care 2003; 9(3): 225–229.
2. Thys DM, Dauchot P, Hillel Z. Advances in cardiovascular physiology. In: Kaplan JA, Reich DL, Konstadt SN, eds. Cardiac Anesthesia. 4th ed. Philadelphia: W.B. Saunders, 1999:217–240.
3. Bogolioubov A, Keefe DL, Groeger JS. Circulatory shock. Crit Care Clin 2001; 17(3):697–719.
4. Vincent JL. Hemodynamic support in septic shock. Intensive Care Med 2001; 27(suppl 1):S80–S92.
5. Kellum JA, Pinsky MR. Use of vasopressor agents in critically ill patients. Curr Opin Crit Care 2002; 8(3): 236–241.
6. Poelaert JIT. Haemodynamic monitoring. Curr Opin Anaesthesiol 2001; 14:27–32.
7. Hinds CJ, Watson D. ABC of intensive care: circulatory support. Br Med J 1999; 318(7200):1749–1752.
8. Caruso LJ, Layon AJ, Gabrielli A. What is the best way to measure cardiac output? Who cares, anyway? Chest 2002; 122(3):771–774.
9. Tibby SM, Murdoch IA. Measurement of cardiac output and tissue perfusion. Curr Opin Pediatr 2002; 14(3):303–309.
10. Chaney JC, Derdak S. Minimally invasive hemodynamic monitoring for the intensivist: current and emerging technology. Crit Care Med 2002; 30(10):2338–2345.
11. Shinozaki T, Deane RS, Mazuzan JE Jr, Hamel AJ, Hazelton D. Bacterial contamination of arterial lines. A prospective study. JAMA 1983; 249(2):223–225.
12. Griffin RM, Kaplan JA. Myocardial ischaemia during non-cardiac surgery. A comparison of different lead systems using computerised ST segment analysis. Anaesthesia 1987; 42(2):155–159.
13. Joynt GM, Gomersall CD, Buckley TA, Oh TE, Young RJ, Freebairn RC. Comparison of intrathoracic and intra-abdominal measurements of central venous pressure. Lancet 1996; 347(9009):1155–1157.
14. O'Grady NP, Alexander M, Dellinger EP, et al. Guidelines for the prevention of intravascular catheter-related infections. Infect Control Hosp Epidemiol 2002; 23(12):759–769.
15. Walder B, Pittet D, Tramer MR. Prevention of bloodstream infections with central venous catheters treated with anti-infective agents depends on catheter type and insertion time: evidence from a meta-analysis. Infect Control Hosp Epidemiol 2002; 23(12):748–756.
16. Polderman KH, Girbes AR. Central venous catheter use. Part 2: infectious complications. Intensive Care Med 2002; 28(1):18–28.
17. Polderman KH, Girbes AJ. Central venous catheter use. Part 1: mechanical complications. Intensive Care Med 2002; 28(1):1–17.
18. Mermel LA. Prevention of intravascular catheter-related infections. Ann Intern Med 2000; 132(5):391–402.
19. Merrer J, De Jonghe B, Golliot F, et al. Complications of femoral and subclavian venous catheterization in critically ill patients: a randomized controlled trial. JAMA 2001; 286(6):700–707.
20. Sessler CN, Glauser FL. Central venous cannulation done by house officers in the intensive care unit: a prospective study. South Med J 1987; 80(10):1239–1242, 1248.
21. Fraenkel DJ, Rickard C, Lipman J. Can we achieve consensus on central venous catheter-related infections? Anaesth Intensive Care 2000; 28(5):475–490.
22. Gunn SR, Pinsky MR. Implications of arterial pressure variation in patients in the intensive care unit. Curr Opin Crit Care 2001; 7(3):212–217.
23. Rivers EP, Ander DS, Powell D. Central venous oxygen saturation monitoring in the critically ill patient. Curr Opin Crit Care 2001; 7(3):204–211.
24. Lipman J, Roos CP, Eidelman J, Plit M. A comparison between right atrial and pulmonary arterial oxygen tensions. S Afr Med J 1986; 70(6):351–353.
25. Rivers E, Nguyen B, Havstad S, et al. Early goal-directed therapy in the treatment of severe sepsis and septic shock. N Engl J Med 2001; 345(19):1368–1377.
26. Kern JW, Shoemaker WC. Meta-analysis of hemodynamic optimization in high-risk patients. Crit Care Med 2002; 30(8):1686–1692.
27. Connors AF Jr, Speroff T, Dawson NV, et al. The effectiveness of right heart catheterization in the initial care of critically ill patients. SUPPORT Investigators. JAMA 1996; 276(11):889–897.
28. Sandham JD, Hull RD, Brant RF, et al. A randomized, controlled trial of the use of pulmonary-artery catheters in high-risk surgical patients. N Engl J Med 2003; 348(1):5–14.
29. Kelso LA. Complications associated with pulmonary artery catheterization. New Horiz 1997; 5(3):259–263.
30. Coulter TD, Wiedemann HP. Complications of hemodynamic monitoring. Clin Chest Med 1999; 20(2): 249–267, vii.
31. Ofili EO, Labovitz AJ. Transesophageal echocardiography: expanding indications for ICU use. How TEE can complement—or surpass—transthoracic techniques. J Crit Illn 1992; 7(1):85–96.
32. Pearson AC. Transthoracic echocardiography versus transesophageal echocardiography in detecting cardiac sources of embolism. Echocardiography 1993; 10(4): 397–403.
33. Seward JB, Khandheria BK, Oh JK, Freeman WK, Tajik AJ. Critical appraisal of transesophageal echocardiography: limitations, pitfalls, and complications. J Am Soc Echocardiogr 1992; 5(3):288–305.
34. Sutton DC, Cahalan MK. Intraoperative assessment of left ventricular function with transesophageal echocardiography. Cardiol Clin 1993; 11(3):389–398.
35. Darmon PL, Hillel Z, Mogtader A, Mindich B, Thys D. Cardiac output by transesophageal echocardiography using continuous-wave Doppler across the

aortic valve. Anesthesiology 1994; 80(4):796–805; discussion 25A.

36. Colreavy FB, Donovan K, Lee KY, Weekes J. Transesophageal echocardiography in critically ill patients. Crit Care Med 2002; 30(5):989–996.
37. Brown JM. Use of echocardiography for hemodynamic monitoring. Crit Care Med 2002; 30(6): 1361–1364.
38. Kolev N, Brase R, Swanevelder J, et al. The influence of transoesophageal echocardiography on intraoperative decision making. A European multicentre study. European Perioperative TOE Research Group. Anaesthesia 1998; 53(8):767–773.
39. Practice guidelines for perioperative transesophageal echocardiography. A report by the American Society of Anesthesiologists and the Society of Cardiovascular Anesthesiologists Task Force on Transesophageal Echocardiography. Anesthesiology 1996; 84(4):986–1006.
40. Benson MJ, Cahalan MK. Cost–benefit analysis of transesophageal echocardiography in cardiac surgery. Echocardiography 1995; 12(2):171–183.
41. Fanshawe M, Ellis C, Habib S, Konstadt SN, Reich DL. A retrospective analysis of the costs and benefits related to alterations in cardiac surgery from routine intraoperative transesophageal echocardiography. Anesth Analg 2002; 95(4):824–827; table of contents.
42. Tavernier B, Makhotine O, Lebuffe G, Dupont J, Scherpereel P. Systolic pressure variation as a guide to fluid therapy in patients with sepsis-induced hypotension. Anesthesiology 1998; 89(6):1313–1321.
43. Reuter DA, Felbinger TW, Schmidt C, et al. Stroke volume variations for assessment of cardiac responsiveness to volume loading in mechanically ventilated patients after cardiac surgery. Intensive Care Med 2002; 28(4):392–398.
44. Marik PE. Pulmonary artery catheterization and esophageal doppler monitoring in the ICU. Chest 1999; 116(4):1085–1091.
45. Pinder M, Lipman J. Interpretation of lactate levels in critical illness. S Afr J Surg 1998; 36(3):93–96.
46. Joynt GM, Lipman J, Gomersall CD, Tan I, Scribante J. Gastric intramucosal pH and blood lactate in severe sepsis. Anaesthesia 1997; 52(8):726–732.
47. Marecaux G, Pinsky MR, Dupont E, Kahn RJ, Vincent JL. Blood lactate levels are better prognostic indicators than TNF and IL-6 levels in patients with septic shock. Intensive Care Med 1996; 22(5):404–408.
48. Abramson D, Scalea TM, Hitchcock R, Trooskin SZ, Henry SM, Greenspan J. Lactate clearance and survival following injury. J Trauma 1993; 35(4):584–588; discussion 588–589.
49. Bakker J, Gris P, Coffernils M, Kahn RJ, Vincent JL. Serial blood lactate levels can predict the development of multiple organ failure following septic shock. Am J Surg 1996; 171(2):221–226.
50. Gore DC, Jahoor F, Hibbert JM, DeMaria EJ. Lactic acidosis during sepsis is related to increased pyruvate production, not deficits in tissue oxygen availability. Ann Surg 1996; 224(1):97–102.
51. Steele A, Bihari D. Choice of catecholamine: does it matter? Curr Opin Crit Care 2000; 6:347–353.
52. Pinede L, Duhaut P, Loire R. Clinical presentation of left atrial cardiac myxoma. A series of 112 consecutive cases. Medicine (Baltimore) 2001; 80(3):159–172.
53. Villegas MV, Hartstein AI. Acinetobacter outbreaks, 1977–2000. Infect Control Hosp Epidemiol 2003; 24(4):284–295.
54. Boyce JM, Pittet D. Guideline for hand hygiene in health-care settings. Am J Infect Control 2002; 30(8): 1–46.
55. Boyd O, Grounds RM, Bennett ED. A randomized clinical trial of the effect of deliberate perioperative increase of oxygen delivery on mortality in high-risk surgical patients. JAMA 1993; 270(22):2699–2707.
56. Wilson J, Woods I, Fawcett J, et al. Reducing the risk of major elective surgery: randomised controlled trial of preoperative optimisation of oxygen delivery. BMJ 1999; 318(7191):1099–1103.
57. Shoemaker WC, Appel PL, Kram HB, Waxman K, Lee TS. Prospective trial of supranormal values of survivors as therapeutic goals in high-risk surgical patients. Chest 1988; 94(6):1176–1186.
58. Hayes MA, Timmins AC, Yau EH, Palazzo M, Hinds CJ, Watson D. Elevation of systemic oxygen delivery in the treatment of critically ill patients. N Engl J Med 1994; 330(24):1717–1722.
59. Tuchschmidt J, Fried J, Astiz M, Rackow E. Elevation of cardiac output and oxygen delivery improves outcome in septic shock. Chest 1992; 102(1):216–220.
60. Mangano DT, Goldman L. Preoperative assessment of patients with known or suspected coronary disease. N Engl J Med 1995; 333(26):1750–1756.
61. Chernow B, Alexander HR, Smallridge RC, et al. Hormonal responses to graded surgical stress. Arch Intern Med 1987; 147(7):1273–1278.
62. Udelsman R, Norton JA, Jelenich SE, et al. Responses of the hypothalamic–pituitary–adrenal and renin–angiotensin axes and the sympathetic system during controlled surgical and anesthetic stress. J Clin Endocrinol Metab 1987; 64(5):986–994.
63. Clarke RS, Johnston H, Sheridan B. The influence of anaesthesia and surgery on plasma cortisol, insulin and free fatty acids. Br J Anaesth 1970; 42(4):295–299.
64. Mangano DT, Wong MG, London MJ, Tubau JF, Rapp JA. Perioperative myocardial ischemia in patients undergoing noncardiac surgery—II: incidence and severity during the 1st week after surgery. The Study of Perioperative Ischemia (SPI) Research Group. J Am Coll Cardiol 1991; 17(4):851–857.
65. Stone JG, Foex P, Sear JW, Johnson LL, Khambatta HJ, Triner L. Risk of myocardial ischaemia during anaesthesia in treated and untreated hypertensive patients. Br J Anaesth 1988; 61(6):675–679.
66. Stone JG, Foex P, Sear JW, Johnson LL, Khambatta HJ, Triner L. Myocardial ischemia in untreated hyper-

tensive patients: effect of a single small oral dose of a beta-adrenergic blocking agent. Anesthesiology 1988; 68(4):495–500.

67. Cucchiara RF, Benefiel DJ, Matteo RS, DeWood M, Albin MS. Evaluation of esmolol in controlling increases in heart rate and blood pressure during endotracheal intubation in patients undergoing carotid endarterectomy. Anesthesiology 1986; 65(5):528–531.
68. Magnusson J, Thulin T, Werner O, Jarhult J, Thomson D. Haemodynamic effects of pretreatment with metoprolol in hypertensive patients undergoing surgery. Br J Anaesth 1986; 58(3):251–260.
69. Poldermans D, Boersma E, Bax JJ, et al. The effect of bisoprolol on perioperative mortality and myocardial infarction in high-risk patients undergoing vascular surgery. Dutch Echocardiographic Cardiac Risk Evaluation Applying Stress Echocardiography Study Group. N Engl J Med 1999; 341(24):1789–1794.
70. Bayliff CD, Massel DR, Inculet RI, et al. Propranolol for the prevention of postoperative arrhythmias in general thoracic surgery. Ann Thorac Surg 1999; 67(1): 182–186.
71. Mangano DT, Layug EL, Wallace A, Tateo I. Effect of atenolol on mortality and cardiovascular morbidity after noncardiac surgery. Multicenter Study of Perioperative Ischemia Research Group. N Engl J Med 1996; 335(23):1713–1720.
72. Raby KE, Brull SJ, Timimi F, et al. The effect of heart rate control on myocardial ischemia among high-risk patients after vascular surgery. Anesth Analg 1999; 88(3):477–482.
73. Urban MK, Markowitz SM, Gordon MA, Urquhart BL, Kligfield P. Postoperative prophylactic administration of beta-adrenergic blockers in patients at risk for myocardial ischemia. Anesth Analg 2000; 90(6): 1257–1261.
74. Kertai MD, Klein J, Van Urk H, Bax JJ, Poldermans D. Cardiac complications after elective major vascular surgery. Acta Anaesthesiol Scand 2003; 47(6):643–654.
75. Wijeysundera DN, Naik JS, Scott Beattie W. Alpha-2 adrenergic agonists to prevent perioperative cardiovascular complications: a meta-analysis. Am J Med 2003; 114(9):742–752.
76. Imm A, Carlson RW. Fluid resuscitation in circulatory shock. Crit Care Clin 1993; 9(2):313–333.
77. Rackow EC, Falk JL, Fein IA, et al. Fluid resuscitation in circulatory shock: a comparison of the cardiorespiratory effects of albumin, hetastarch, and saline solutions in patients with hypovolemic and septic shock. Crit Care Med 1983; 11(11):839–850.
78. Hebert PC, Wells G, Blajchman MA, et al. A multicenter, randomized, controlled clinical trial of transfusion requirements in critical care. Transfusion Requirements in Critical Care Investigators, Canadian Critical Care Trials Group. N Engl J Med 1999; 340(6):409–417.
79. Hebert PC, Szick MHA. The anemic patient in the intensive care unit: how much does the heart tolerate? Curr Opin Crit Care 2000; 6:372–380.
80. Walsh TS, McClelland DBL. When should we transfuse critically ill and perioperative patients with known coronary artery disease? Br J Anaesth 2003; 90(6): 719–722.
81. Rudis MI, Basha MA, Zarowitz BJ. Is it time to reposition vasopressors and inotropes in sepsis? Crit Care Med 1996; 24(3):525–537.
82. Di Giantomasso D, May CN, Bellomo R. Norepinephrine and vital organ blood flow. Intensive Care Med 2002; 28(12):1804–1809.
83. Bellomo R, Giantomasso DD. Noradrenaline and the kidney: friends or foes? Crit Care 2001; 5(6):294–298.
84. Bellomo R, Chapman M, Finfer S, Hickling K, Myburgh J. Low-dose dopamine in patients with early renal dysfunction: a placebo-controlled randomised trial. Australian and New Zealand Intensive Care Society (ANZICS) Clinical Trials Group. Lancet 2000; 356(9248):2139–2143.
85. Holmes CL, Patel BM, Russell JA, Walley KR. Physiology of vasopressin relevant to management of septic shock. Chest 2001; 120(3):989–1002.
86. Landry DW, Oliver JA. The pathogenesis of vasodilatory shock. N Engl J Med 2001; 345(8):588–595.
87. Landry DW, Levin HR, Gallant EM, et al. Vasopressin pressor hypersensitivity in vasodilatory septic shock. Crit Care Med 1997; 25(8):1279–1282.
88. Dunser MW, Mayr AJ, Ulmer H, et al. Arginine vasopressin in advanced vasodilatory shock: a prospective, randomized, controlled study. Circulation 2003; 107(18):2313–2319.
89. Dunser MW, Wenzel V, Mayr AJ, Hasibeder WR. Management of vasodilatory shock: defining the role of arginine vasopressin. Drugs 2003; 63(3):237–256.
90. Holmes CL, Walley KR, Chittock DR, Lehman T, Russell JA. The effects of vasopressin on hemodynamics and renal function in severe septic shock: a case series. Intensive Care Med 2001; 27(8):1416–1421.
91. Patel BM, Chittock DR, Russell JA, Walley KR. Beneficial effects of short-term vasopressin infusion during severe septic shock. Anesthesiology 2002; 96(3): 576–582.
92. Dunser MW, Mayr AJ, Tur A, et al. Ischemic skin lesions as a complication of continuous vasopressin infusion in catecholamine-resistant vasodilatory shock: incidence and risk factors. Crit Care Med 2003; 31(5):1394–1398.
93. O'Brien A, Clapp L, Singer M. Terlipressin for norepinephrine-resistant septic shock. Lancet 2002; 359(9313):1209–1210.
94. Lisbon A. Dopexamine, dobutamine, and dopamine increase splanchnic blood flow: what is the evidence? Chest 2003; 123(90050):460S–463S.
95. Bongard FS. Shock and resuscitation. In: Bongard FS, Sue DY, eds. Current Critical Care Diagnosis & Treat-

ment. The McGraw-Hill Companies Inc.New York2003; 26(4):242–267.
96. Dellinger RP. Cardiovascular management of septic shock. Crit Care Med 2003; 31(3):946–955.
97. Malcolm DS, Zaloga GP, Holaday JW. Calcium administration increases the mortality of endotoxic shock in rats. Crit Care Med 1989; 17(9):900–903.
98. Reinhart K, Sakka SG, Meier-Hellmann A. Haemodynamic management of a patient with septic shock. Eur J Anaesthesiol 2000; 17(1):6–17.
99. Wilson W, Lipman J, Scribante J, et al. Septic shock: does adrenaline have a role as a first-line inotropic agent? Anaesth Intensive Care 1992; 20(4):470–474.
100. Reinelt H, Radermacher P, Kiefer P, et al. Impact of exogenous beta-adrenergic receptor stimulation on hepatosplanchnic oxygen kinetics and metabolic activity in septic shock. Crit Care Med 1999; 27(2): 325–331.
101. Marik PE, Zaloga GP. Adrenal insufficiency in the critically ill: a new look at an old problem. Chest 2002; 122(5):1784–1796.
102. Cooper MS, Stewart PM. Corticosteroid insufficiency in acutely ill patients. N Engl J Med 2003; 348(8): 727–734.
103. Briegel J, Forst H, Haller M, et al. Stress doses of hydrocortisone reverse hyperdynamic septic shock: a prospective, randomized, double-blind, single-center study. Crit Care Med 1999; 27(4):723–732.
104. Bollaert PE, Charpentier C, Levy B, Debouverie M, Audibert G, Larcan A. Reversal of late septic shock with supraphysiologic doses of hydrocortisone. Crit Care Med 1998; 26(4):645–650.
105. Annane D, Sebille V, Charpentier C, et al. Effect of treatment with low doses of hydrocortisone and fludrocortisone on mortality in patients with septic shock. JAMA 2002; 288(7):862–871.

42

Respiratory Failure and Mechanical Ventilation in Cancer Patients

TODD KELLY

Department of Critical Care, The University of Texas M.D. Anderson Cancer Center, Houston, Texas, U.S.A.

I. ETIOLOGIES OF RESPIRATORY FAILURE IN CANCER PATIENTS

The causes of respiratory failure are numerous and can result from primary pathological processes as well as from the treatments of these processes. It is imperative that a correct diagnosis of the cause of respiratory distress/failure be made so that the appropriate treatment can be initiated. In the cancer patient, respiratory failure can result from the cancer itself or from the surgical, radiation, or chemotherapeutic treatments of the cancer. In a study of 189 consecutive cancer patients referred to the intensive care unit (ICU) (103 with solid tumors and 86 with hematological malignancies), mechanical ventilation was required in 49.7%. The reasons for ICU referral were pneumonia (29.6%), sepsis (27.0%), fungal infection (11.1%), another infection (9.5%), gastrointestinal emergency (16.9%), treatment-related organ toxicity (6.9%), or other, noninfectious complications (43.9%) (1). In another study looking at 60 consecutive bone marrow transplantation (BMT) patients requiring mechanical ventilation at a major cancer center, the most frequent complication leading to respiratory failure was pneumonia (41%) followed by diffuse alveolar hemorrhage (33%) (Table 1) (2).

Inappropriate diagnosis and treatment will only delay recovery and possibly increase morbidity or mortality. In other words, all respiratory distress should not be managed with diuresis. Additionally, comorbid conditions such as cardiac or pulmonary dysfunction secondary to poorly controlled hypertension, vascular disease, and smoking can contribute to the development of respiratory failure. Their rapid identification and concurrent treatment is crucial to resolving the respiratory crisis.

It is important to identify cancer patients at risk for respiratory compromise early in the course of their evaluation and treatment. A thorough medical, family, surgical, and social history as well as a complete physical examination prior to any cancer treatments is crucial. Identifying a history of recent infections (including respiratory and urinary), neurologic impairments (stroke, swallowing or diaphragm dysfunction, alcoholism or other drug dependence, etc.), cardiac disease (coronary artery disease, valvular dysfunction, cardiomyopathy, congestive heart failure, and pulmonary hypertension), and pulmonary disease [asthma, chronic obstructive pulmonary disease (COPD), smoking, chronic bronchitis, or thoracic cage abnormalities] will stratify those patients who are at high risk for developing respiratory compromise.

Respiratory failure can result from the tumor burden itself or from the immune response to the tumor. Macroscopic tumor burden in the form of bulky space occupying lesions that compress surrounding tissues and impair respiratory function can result

Table 1 Outcome of Bone Marrow Transplantation Patients Requiring Mechanical Ventilation

Characteristics	Values (%)	ICU survival (%)	6-month survival (%)
Age (median ± SEM)	38.7±1.6	11 (18)	3 (5)
Gender			
Male	27 (45)	4 (15)	1 (4)
Female	33 (55)	7 (21)	2 (6)
Type of transplant			
Allogeneic	34 (57)	4 (12)	0 (0)
Autologous	26 (43)	7 (27)	3 (12)
Causes of respiratory failure (total = 80)			
Pneumonia	33 (41)	4 (12)	2 (6)
Diffuse alveolar hemorrhage	26 (32)	5 (19)	1 (4)
Pulmonary edema	7 (9)	6 (86)	2 (29)
ARDS	6 (8)	0 (0)	0 (0)
Other	8 (10)	1 (13)	1 (13)
Patients according to BMT mechanical ventilation interval (days)			
<30	31 (52)	10 (32)	2 (6)
30–100	17 (28)	0 (0)	0 (0)
>100	12 (20)	1 (8)	1 (8)
APACHE II score			
< 21	26 (44)	4 (15)	2 (8)
≥21	33 (56)	7 (21)	1 (3)

Abbreviations: ICU, intensive care unit; ARDS, acute respiratory distress syndrome; BMT, bone marrow transplantation; APACHE II, Acute Physiology and Chronic Health Evaluation II.
Source: From Ref. 2.

from numerous types of cancer. Microscopic tumor load can also impair respiratory function in the form of diffuse pulmonary tumor emboli from hepatic sinusoidal tumor burden that can present as sudden respiratory collapse (3). Eaton–Lambert syndrome (ELS), secondary to small cell lung cancer, is a neuromuscular disorder characterized by defective neurotransmitter release at presynaptic terminals caused by an IgG autoantibody reacting against voltage-gated calcium channels. It usually presents as progressive limb weakness over several months with rare ventilatory failure. Supportive care along with plasma exchange, chemotherapy, and possible surgical therapy can lead to dramatic improvement in symptoms (4).

Prior surgical history can also help identify those with increased risk of developing respiratory compromise. A history of lung, diaphragm, or chest wall resection can identify those with diminished pulmonary reserve. Past surgery for head and neck cancer might indicate difficult airway access or neurologic or functional deficit with an inability to protect the airway from secretions or aspiration. Prior brain tumor resection could have resulted in neurologic impairments in swallowing or airway protection and major spine resection could impair intercostal muscle function. Esophageal or gastric resections may increase the risk of reflux and aspiration.

Those patients with planned procedures known to impair respiratory reserve should undergo pulmonary function testing. Post-thoracic surgical cancer patients are at high risk of developing respiratory complications; therefore, it is important to identify those patients preoperatively who are likely to have complications. Patients undergoing lung resection surgery with a predicted postoperative FEV1 percentage less than 30% require special attention to postoperative management, as they are very high risk for pulmonary complications and death (5).

A review of current and past medications might assist with the diagnosis and treatment of respiratory failure or distress. Patients taking bronchodilators or steroids may be suffering from an exacerbation of asthma or COPD and may benefit from pulse steroid and bronchodilator therapy. Those chronically taking diuretics may need increased diuresis to remove excess lung water. Patients receiving thoracic radiation for tumors involving the breasts, chest wall, or intrathoracic structures can suffer from radiation pneumonitis (6–8), which often occurs within the first 4 weeks with large irradiated lung volumes and may not be detectable by chest x-ray (9). The CT findings of radiation-induced lung injury were variable including, homogeneous, patchy, or discrete pulmonary infiltrates (9). Some medications such as amiodarone (10–21), bleomycin

(22–24), or doxorubicin (25–27), as well as others (28), can cause pulmonary toxicity as well as initiate "recall pneumonitis" (medication induced reactivation of radiation pneumonitis) (29–32). Adriamycin can cause congestive heart failure (33–35). New cancer treating drugs are constantly being developed, many of them with significant cardiopulmonary side effects; thus, a discussion with the treating oncologist about the chemotherapeutic regimen and its side effects is very important.

A review of pertinent laboratory data, x-rays, as well as daily and cumulative fluid balance can also assist with the diagnosis and treatment of respiratory failure. An elevated white blood cell count and fevers could indicate an infectious process. Severe anemia can lead to respiratory distress secondary to low oxygen carrying capacity or cardiac ischemia. A review of the arterial blood gases may reveal isolated hypoxia resulting from pulmonary edema, pneumothorax, ARDS, pulmonary embolism, or pneumonitis. Isolated hypercarbia may be due to narcotic or benzodiazepine overdose, COPD exacerbation, overfeeding, or significant airway mucous plugging in patients with limited pulmonary reserve. Metabolic acidosis can result in compensatory respiratory alkalosis presenting as respiratory distress. The source of the metabolic acidosis must be sought out and treated appropriately. An infectious or necrotic source can present as a metabolic acidosis and result in systemic inflammatory response syndrome (SIRS), severe sepsis, or septic shock. Other causes of metabolic acidosis must be systematically excluded as well (i.e., uremia, lactic acidosis, drugs, methanol, paraldehyde, ethanol, renal tubular acidosis, and diarrhea). Anion and osmolar gap calculations can prove helpful in identifying the source of the metabolic acidosis. Hyponatremia may result from free water overload leading to pulmonary edema and subsequent respiratory difficulties. An elevated creatinine could indicate renal dysfunction predisposing to volume overload. Low serum protein concentration (i.e., albumin) result in poor plasma oncotic pressure and in the setting of increased hydrostatic pressures can lead to pulmonary edema or effusions. Low albumin can be secondary to hepatic dysfunction or malnutrition. Serum BNP levels can help differentiate cardiogenic from other causes of pulmonary edema (36–49). A chest x-ray can assist with the diagnosis of pneumothorax (if the patient is stable enough to wait for an x-ray), pneumonia, pulmonary edema, diaphragm dysfunction, cardiac tamponade, and pericardial effusion. A review of the daily and cumulative fluid balance can assist with the diagnosis of fluid overload.

A complete physical examination of the critically ill cancer patient is crucial to the diagnosis and treatment of respiratory failure. Depressed global neurologic function or specific neurologic deficits can lead to aspiration or poor respiratory muscle function with diminished functional residual capacity. Complaints consistent with coronary ischemia or new or loud murmurs, rubs, distant heart sounds with jugular venous distention, or the presence of a fourth heart sound may indicate pathologic cardiac dysfunction that warrants urgent additional work-up (i.e., echocardiogram, ECG, or cardiac enzymes), emergent treatment (pericardiocentesis or initiation of treatment for myocardial infarction), and specialist consultation. Pulmonary auscultation may reveal focal or diffuse rales, rhonchi, or wheezing, or diminished or absent breath sounds (pulmonary effusion, pneumothorax). Accessory respiratory muscle use may indicate impending respiratory failure and the need for urgent respiratory support. Asymmetric chest wall movement, a deviated trachea, and absent unilateral breath sounds are classic signs of tension pneumothorax and require immediate chest decompression. Abdomen examination may reveal peritoneal signs that may warrant surgical consultation and/or further radiographic evaluation.

II. PROGNOSIS OF MECHANICAL VENTILATION IN CANCER PATIENTS

The incidence of acute respiratory failure (ARF) in ICU patients has been estimated to be 77.6 cases per 100,000 in Sweden, Denmark, and Iceland, 110.8/100,00 residents aged >14 years old in Berlin (50,51), and 137.1/100.000 in the United States (51). In a retrospective review of the Nationwide Inpatient Sample, a database of all patients discharged from a representative sample of 904 nonfederal hospitals throughout the United States during 1994, 35.9 ± 0.3% of all patients with ARF did not survive to hospital discharge (Fig. 1). Median length of stay (LOS) (5th–95th percentile range) was 1.3 days (3–55 days) among survivors and 10 days (1–50 days) among nonsurvivors. Not surprisingly, however, it should be noted that in this survey, patients admitted to the hospital for BMT were excluded (51).

Critically ill cancer patients have an overall 30-day mortality of about 50% (52–56). Independent risk factors for ARF mortality in patients admitted to the ICU include older age (50,57–63), severe chronic comorbidities (HIV, active malignancy, and cirrhosis) (50,59,60,62,64,65), and certain precipitating events [trauma (59–61,66), drug overdose (60,67), bone marrow transplant (68), and multiple organ system dysfunction or failure (MODS) (58,66–69)]. In the

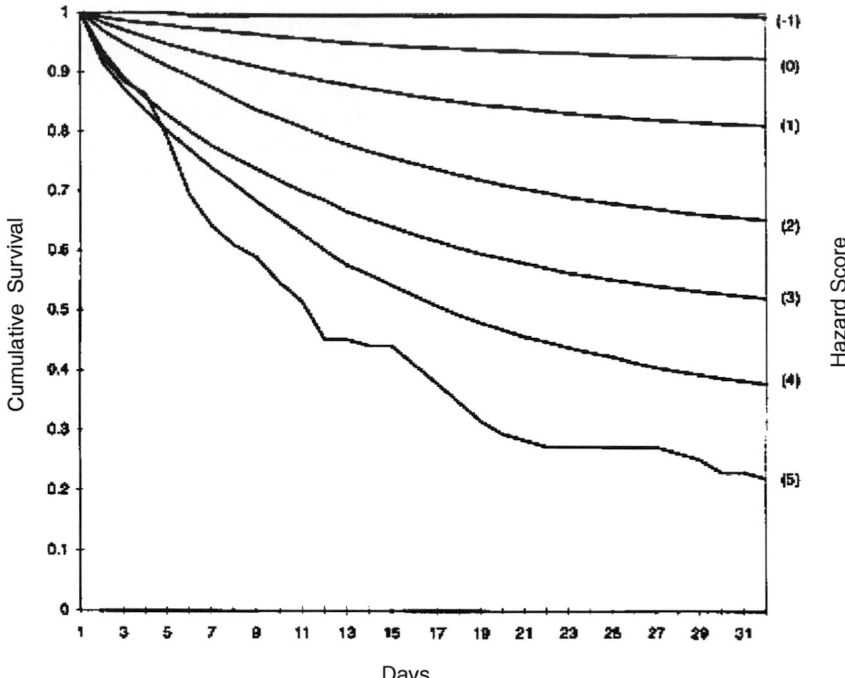

Figure 1 Survival of patients with ARF (1994 Nationwide Inpatient Sample). *Source*: From Ref. 51.

Nationwide Inpatient Sample, at the end of 3.1 days, hospital mortality among the cohort was 31.4 ± 0.2%. Hazards for 31-day mortality included age, MODS, HIV, chronic liver disease, and cancer. Cancer was a significant hazard until 80 years of age; thereafter, mortality among patients with and without cancer did not differ (51). Mortality rates among ARF patients with hematologic malignancy have been observed to be 63–83% (70,71) and 46% with solid tumors (70). An inception cohort study at four major cancer centers involving 1354 cancer patients surviving longer than 72 hr in the ICU found that mechanical ventilation resulted in an odds ratio of dying of 3.24 (coefficient = 1.1764, SE = 0.1739, 95% CI = 2.31–4.57). The authors concluded that the presence and degree of respiratory failure continues to be an important variable at 72 hr, as manifested by an increased risk of dying if the patient has a low PaO_2/FiO_2 and is intubated for any reason (70).

Often, respiratory failure is accompanied by other confounding clinical conditions resulting from the cancer or its treatments that may have a significant impact on prognosis. Chemotherapy and radiation therapy combined with cancer-related malnutrition can often lead to significant impairment of the immune system. Some of these patients will develop infections that can lead to pneumonia or other infections that can result in sepsis or septic shock leading to ARDS and severe respiratory failure. In a group of 88 cancer patients (80 with hematological malignancy and 8 with solid tumors) admitted to the ICU for septic shock, 30-day mortality was 65.5%. In this population of septic cancer patients, a univariable analysis of risk factors for 30-day mortality showed that mechanical ventilation resulted in an odds ratio of dying of 20.571 (95% CI = 5.247–80.648). Among the patients who needed vasopressors, mechanical ventilation, and dialysis on day 3, none survived, whereas one-third of the patients needing only mechanical ventilation on day 3 (i.e., who were weaned from vasopressors by day 3) were discharged alive from the hospital. Of the 68 patients who needed mechanical ventilation, the duration of mechanical ventilation was 3 (1–7) days in nonsurvivors and 11.5 (7–15) days in survivors (72). In another study by Maschmeyer, of 189 consecutive cancer patients referred to the intensive care unit (103 with solid tumors and 86 with hematological malignancies), mechanical ventilation was required in 49.7%. Sepsis, mechanical ventilation, vasopressor support, renal replacement therapy, and neutropenia were independent risk factors for fatal outcome (Table 2). The requirement of vasopressor support was the most significant single factor predicting ICU mortality and the ICU mortality rate showed a significant difference in favor of the nonventilated patients (ICU mortality rate, 75.3% vs. 35.7%, $P = 0.0044$). All patients with fungal infection who required vasopressor support and either had sepsis ($n = 13$) or needed mechanical

Table 2 Risk Factors for ARDS Outcome

Factor	*n*	Fatal outcome (%)	*P* value
Sepsis	51	62.8 versus 33.3	0.0003
Vasopressor support	95	69.5 versus 12.1	< 0.0001
Mechanical ventilation	94	68.1 versus 13.8	< 0.0001
Neutropenia	53	54.7 versus 35.8	0.0180
Treatment-related organ toxicity	13	15.4 versus 43.2	0.0495
Surgical treatment	51	27.4 versus 46.4	0.029
Haemodialysis/haemofiltration	50	60.0 versus 34.6	0.0018
Total	189	41.3	

Source: From Ref. 1.

ventilation ($n = 14$) died during ICU treatment, while all nonseptic patients who did not require mechanical ventilation survived. In neutropenic patients who required mechanical ventilation ($n = 36$), ICU mortality rate in these patients was significantly higher compared with the 17 neutropenic patients not being ventilated (ICU mortality rate, 72.2% vs. 17.6%, $P = 0.0001$). The subgroup of non-neutropenic patients with sepsis who did not require mechanical ventilation ($n = 6$) had a significantly lower ICU mortality compared with those who underwent mechanical ventilation ($n = 15$) (ICU mortality rates, 16.7% vs. 86.7%, $P = 0.002$) (Fig. 2). Patients without sepsis and who did not require mechanical ventilation ($n = 80$) had an ICU survival rate of 87.5%, compared with nonseptic, mechanically ventilated patients ($n = 57$) who had an ICU survival rate of 38.6% ($P < 0.0001$) (1).

A. Prognosis of Bone Marrow Transplant and Respiratory Failure

As previously mentioned, all cancers do not confer the same risk to mechanically ventilated patients. A retrospective chart review of 1301 patients who received autologous peripheral blood stem cell transplant found 78 patients (6%) received mechanical ventilation for ≥24 hr. In this group of patients, the median duration of mechanical ventilation was 7 days (range, 1–63 days) and hospital survival was 20 of 78 patients (26%) (73). Bone marrow transplantation patients with ARF requiring mechanical ventilation have a particularly poor prognosis. A review of the literature reveals that hospital or 30-day survival for BMT patients who required mechanical ventilation for respiratory failure is very low (4–13%) (63,74–86). In the largest study

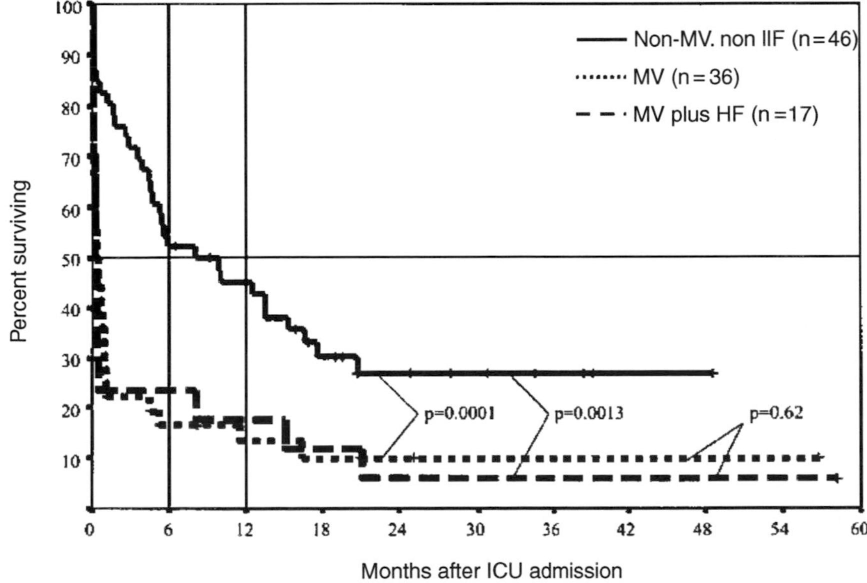

Figure 2 ICU mortality rates for patients with and without mechanical ventilation *Source*: From Ref. 71.

on the outcome of BMT patients receiving mechanical ventilation, the overall hospital survival was approximately 5%, and it was not dramatically affected by the type or number of organ failures (83).

A retrospective cohort study, involving 2776 patients in an ICU at a university cancer referral center, found that compared to patients with a solid tumor, leukemia, lymphoma, and patients with BMT had the highest APACHE III score at admission and had the highest frequency and duration of mechanical ventilation (71). The same author found that in this cohort of patients, overall ICU mortality was 44%, with significantly higher mortality in ventilated patients (74% vs. 12% in nonventilated patients ($P<0.001$) (Fig. 3). Multivariate analysis revealed mechanical ventilation and SAPS II as independent prognostic factors of both ICU mortality and long-term survival. Another study of BMT patients requiring mechanical ventilation found that only 18% of the patients were extubated and discharged from the ICU and only 5% were alive at 6 months (2). In the same study, a subgroup analysis revealed that none of the seven patients with acute lymphoblastic leukemia survived; 1 of 9 patients with acute myelogenous leukemia was weaned off the ventilator, as well as 2 of 16 patients with chronic myelocytic leukemia.

The most frequent complication leading to respiratory failure in BMT patients requiring mechanical ventilation at a major cancer center were pneumonia (41%) and diffuse alveolar hemorrhage (33%) (Table 1). Five of 26 patients with diffuse alveolar hemorrhage and 4 of 33 patients with pneumonia survived. In the infectious cause group, 3 of 12 patients with bacterial pneumonia survived as well as one of three patients with *Pneumocystis carinii pneumonia.* The mortality rate was 100% in the patients who had cytomegalovirus pneumonitis ($n=9$), aspergillosis ($n=5$), respiratory syncytial virus ($n=4$), and other viral infections ($n=1$). All four patients who experienced congestive heart failure/pulmonary edema survived, as did the only patient with documented drug-induced pneumonitis. None of the seven patients with idiopathic pneumonia syndrome (formerly called idiopathic interstitial pneumonitis), with bronchiolitis obliterans organizing pneumonia, multisystem organ failure, or recurrent malignancy survived. Graft vs. host disease was also predictor of a poor outcome with no survivors of 20 patients admitted to the ICU and mechanically ventilated (2).

The interval between BMT and the onset of mechanical ventilation might be an important prognostic indicator. Patients with respiratory failure within the first month after BMT had a 32% MICU survival rate compared with 3% when it occurred beyond the first month. The former were predominantly regimen-related toxicity or cardiogenic pulmonary edema. Those with late onset (>100 days after BMT) of pulmonary complications requiring

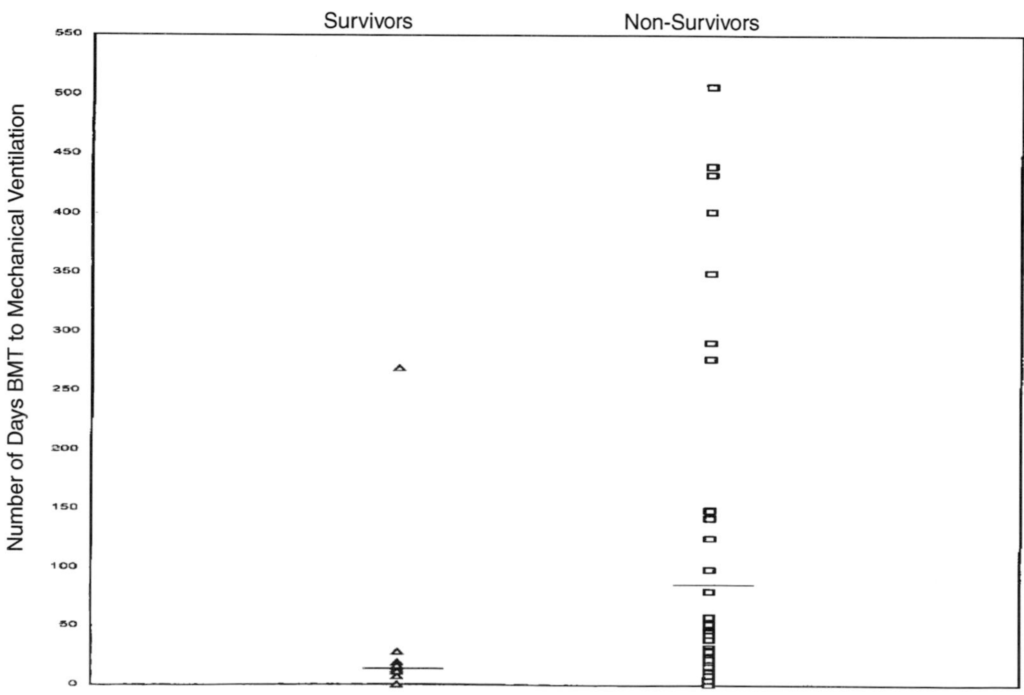

Figure 3 ICU mortality for BMT patients with and without mechanical ventilation. *Source*: From Ref. 2.

mechanical ventilation typically had infections or diffuse alveolar hemorrhage (Fig. 2) (2).

A major dilemma is how long to continue mechanical ventilation in this high mortality population of patients. Prolonged mechanical ventilation has been reported to be associated with a particularly poor outcome (87). However, other investigators have not confirmed this parameter as an independent, adverse prognostic factor (88,89). Several cut-off time periods have been reported to discriminate between survival and death, such as 4 days (77) or 7 days (90). Prolonged mechanical ventilation (>15 days) in a group of BMT patients resulted in an MICU survival rate of 5% (Fig. 4) (2).

III. MANAGEMENT OF RESPIRATORY FAILURE

A. Initial Management

Once the diagnosis of respiratory failure has been made as outlined above, the treatment centers around the concepts taught in Advanced Cardiac Life Support courses; the ABCs. If the patient is unable to breath without assistance, first open the airway with either the head tilt-chin lift or jaw thrust maneuver. Next, breathe for the patient using mouth-to-mouth or preferably bag-mask techniques and supplemental oxygen. Once airway and breathing have been established, check the circulation by feeling for a pulse and initiate chest compressions if necessary. Secondary procedures such as monitor placement and invasive intravenous access can now take place. These concepts may sound straightforward, but it is not unusual in the chaotic atmosphere of a code situation for even experienced care providers to forget the basics. Once the ABCs have been successfully completed, the next decision is whether or not to initiate mechanical ventilation.

There are four fundamental indications for mechanical ventilatory support in respiratory failure, regardless of the underlying cause: inability to oxygenate, inability to remove carbon dioxide (CO_2), inability to maintain a patent airway, and inability to effectively clear secretions (91). Any or all of these indications can be present in those cancer patients presenting to the ICU. Probably, the most common is a mixture of the first two classically referred to as Type II respiratory failure (failure to oxygenate with carbon dioxide retention). After the decision has been made to proceed with the implementation of mechanical ventilation, the next decision is whether to place an endotracheal tube (ETT) or attempt noninvasive positive-pressure ventilation (NPPV). The discussion to follow will present the merits and potential complications of each mode of ventilation.

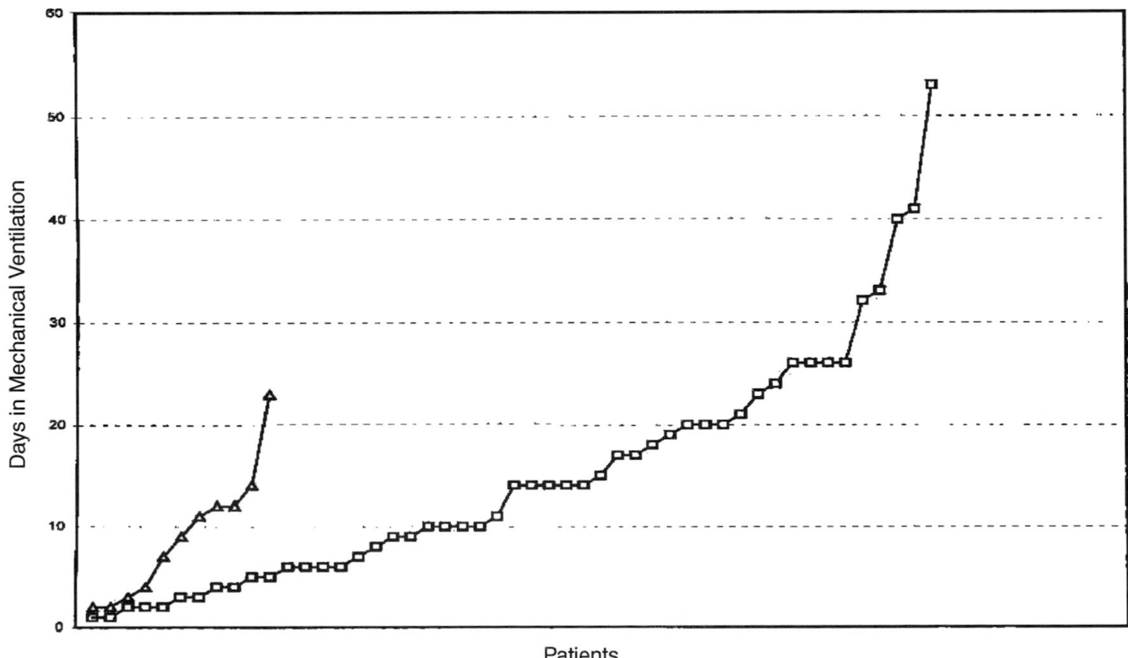

Figure 4 Duration of mechanical ventilation in survivors (*triangles*) and nonsurvivors (*squares*). There was no statistical difference between the two groups. *Source*: From Ref. 2.

B. Noninvasive Ventilation

Noninvasive positive-pressure ventilation is any form of ventilatory support applied without the use of an ETT. There are various modes of NPPV that include continuous positive airway pressure (CPAP), with or without inspiratory pressure support, as well as volume- and pressure-cycled systems, and proportional assist ventilation (PAV).

Patients suffering from both hypercarbia and hypoxemia stand to benefit from modes of ventilatory assistance that avoid the discomfort and risk associated with endotracheal intubation (ETI). A study out of the United Kingdom suggested up to 20% of hospitalized patients with COPD may be candidates for NPPV (92) while other studies indicate that 60–65% of patients with various forms of ARF can be successfully treated with NPPV (93,94). A survey of NPPV use in 42 medical ICUs in France, Switzerland, and Spain demonstrated that it was used prior to mechanical ventilation in 16% of cases (range, 0–67%) (93). The potential benefits of NPPV must be weighed against mask discomfort and risks specific to NPPV (i.e., inadequate ventilation or oxygenation, eye or nasal or skin trauma, or gastric distension/aspiration).

Noninvasive positive-pressure ventilation cannot be indiscriminately applied to all patients with ARF, and as stated above, the risks and potential benefits must be weighed. Experience has demonstrated that hypercarbic respiratory failure often responds more favorably to NPPV than hypoxic failure (94–96). Patients should be hemodynamically stable and able to protect their airway. Severe neurologic dysfunction or hemodynamic instability mandates airway control with intubation (Table 3).

For those in which NPPV is appropriate, reasonable therapeutic goals include avoidance of ETI, unloading respiratory muscles (which should decrease respiratory rate and the sensation of dyspnea, and increase patient comfort), improving alveolar gas exchange and thus oxygenation and acidosis, decreasing heart rate and improved hemodynamic status, decreasing ICU LOS and its associated complications (such as nosocomial infection), decreasing hospital stay, and reducing mortality. On the basis of these criteria, most patients with ARF should be considered for at least a trial of NPPV (97).

Table 3 Contraindications to NPPV

1. Cardiac or respiratory arrest
2. Nonrespiratory organ failure
   a. Severe encephalopathy (e.g., GCS < 10)
   b. Severe upper gastrointestinal bleeding
   c. Hemodynamic instability or unstable cardiac arrhythmia
3. Facial surgery, trauma, or deformity
4. Upper airway obstruction
5. Inability to cooperate/protect the airway
6. Inability to clear respiratory secretions
7. High risk for aspiration

Abbreviations: GCS, Glasgow Coma Scale.
Source: Ref. 97.

1. Application of NPPV and Complications

Noninvasive positive-pressure ventilation may be applied via a nasal or full-face mask secured via a head strap to the patient. The full-face mask allows higher ventilation pressures with fewer leaks, requires less patient co-operation, and permits mouth breathing. However, it is less comfortable, impedes communication, and limits oral intake. The nasal mask needs patent nasal passages and requires mouth closure to minimize air leaks. Gas leaks around the mask or from the mouth make monitoring the tidal volume difficult and are a frequent cause of failure of NPPV (98). Air leaks in patients with beards or with facial structural abnormalities after head and neck surgery can be particularly challenging and cause failure of NPPV. Persistent air leaks may also indicate low lung compliance or ventilation close to total lung capacity. Recent head and neck surgery, especially those cases involving flap reconstruction, is a contraindication to the application of NPPV due to possible flap injury secondary to the tight fitting straps used to hold the mask.

Although NPPV is relatively easy to use, patients must be carefully monitored to avoid potential complications. Both nasal and full-face masks can cause skin necrosis on the bridge of the nose or on the forehead (98). Caregivers must be very attentive to skin condition during NPPV and use cushioning materials (i.e., duoderm) and allow for "rest periods" off NPPV. The use of large face masks can increase dead space and the potential for rebreathing. To avoid this complication, dual tube (nonrebreathing) delivery circuits should be used. Gastric distension is a frequent complication and thus NPPV should be avoided in patients in whom this might be detrimental (i.e., recent esophagectomy, gastrectomy, or proximal small bowel surgery). Nasogastric decompression tubes may prevent this complication but may occasionally worsen air leak. Like all forms of positive-pressure ventilation (PPV), NPPV may be associated with adverse hemodynamic effects (99).

Some patients are unable to tolerate the mask due to discomfort, anxiety, or claustrophobia. The use of adjunctive anxiolysis can substantially enhance the success of NPPV. Medications that sedate without causing respiratory depression (i.e., dexmedetomidine) are particularly advantageous.

Failure to respond to NPPV may be demonstrated by persistently abnormal blood gases (100,101), abnormal or dysynchronous breathing patterns, tachypnea, accessory muscle use, respiratory muscle fatigue, hemodynamic instability, arrhythmias, altered mental status, or inability to tolerate the NPPV. Early recognition of failure to respond to NPPV is essential to prevent complications such as aspiration or excessive fatigue that can result in subsequent prolongation of intubation and mechanical ventilation with its inherent risks.

2. *Monitoring*

Although portable devices can provide NPPV, patients should be kept in an area where potential complications can be immediately recognized and appropriately managed. In spite of NPPV, subsequent ETI may be as high as 40% in hypoxemic ARF (102) and those with mask leaks may be associated with an even higher incidence of failure. Therefore, patients should be managed in an area where equipment and personnel qualified to manage the airway are immediately available.

The level of monitoring is determined by the patient's clinical condition and changes in respiratory, neurologic, and metabolic status must be frequently assessed. Continuous pulse oximetry should be employed to follow the oxygen saturation. Any deterioration of the patient's clinical condition including worsening neurologic status, hemodynamic instability, persistent, or worsening acidosis should be moved to a location where more aggressive monitoring and interventions can take place.

Noninvasive positive-pressure ventilation does not necessarily need to take place in the ICU and may be applied during the early stages of ARF or employed on an intermittent basis. Other locations in which NPPV can be employed include the emergency department, intermediate care unit, telemetry units, or the general wards provided adequate monitoring is available. In a randomized controlled trial (RCT) conducted in an intermediate care unit, NPPV led to a reduction in the need for intubation and duration of stay when compared with standard treatment of patients with COPD and community-acquired pneumonia (102). Observational and case-controlled studies indicate that NPPV administered in a general respiratory ward can reduce the need for ETI (103). Several RCTs of patients with acute exacerbations of COPD have been carried out in the general ward setting with mixed results (104,105). In a multicenter trial of patients with exacerbations of COPD (pH 7.25–7.35, $PaCO_2$ >45 mmHg, respiratory frequency >23), NPPV was initiated and maintained by the ward staff according to a strict protocol and after extensive training. Using prospectively defined criteria, NPPV reduced the need for ETI and hospital mortality (106). Additional benefits of NPPV outside the ICU include access to respiratory support for patients who would otherwise not be admitted to the ICU (100,107–109) and early intervention to prevent further respiratory deterioration (106).

3. *Ventilatory Modes*

Noninvasive positive-pressure ventilation can be either pressure or volume controlled. Continuous positive airway pressure alone can be used in spontaneously breathing patients with hypoxemic ARF. Pressure-support ventilation (PSV) can reduce the work of breathing (WOB) as the ventilator is triggered by the patient and assists inspiration until it senses expiration via a fall in inspiratory flow rate below a threshold value or at a preset time. When there are no spontaneous respirations or when inspiratory efforts are too small to trigger the ventilator pressure-controlled ventilation (PCV) can be utilized to set a respiratory rate and inspiratory-to-expiratory ratio. In pressure-controlled modes of ventilation, delivered tidal volumes (V_t) may vary from breath to breath as V_t is dependent on lung compliance. These modes of ventilation can be provided by most modern ventilators or by bilevel positive airway pressure generators that provide high-flow CPAP and cycle between a high inspiratory pressure and a lower expiratory pressure. Patients retain the ability to spontaneously breath at both pressure levels. Volume-limited ventilation may also be employed where the ventilator delivers a set tidal volume for each breath and inflation pressure may vary with each breath. The assist-control mode of ventilation (ACV) triggers the delivery of a full tidal volume with each detected respiratory effort. In volume support ventilation, the ventilator adjusts inspiratory pressures to deliver a preset tidal volume in response to inspiratory effort. A newer mode of NPPV is PAV, where the ventilator generates a pressure and volume in proportion to the patient's effort, thus resulting in a ventilatory pattern that matches the metabolic demand on a breath-by-breath basis (110). Proportional assist ventilation may result in a more efficient mode of ventilatory support, but to date, there are no conclusive data to recommend the use of PAV in NPPV.

Choosing the correct mode of NPPV for the patient depends on the clinical condition as each mode has advantages and disadvantages. Although volume-limited ventilation is generally well tolerated, peak mask pressure is not limited and thus mask leaks, gastric distension, pressure sores, and skin necrosis are more likely. Pressure-support ventilation improves patient comfort, minimizes side effects, and delivers reliable tidal volumes assuming constant lung compliance. However, patient–ventilator asynchrony may lead to prolonged inspiratory flow despite expiratory efforts resulting in leaks (111). Time-cycled, pressure-targeted modes can be used to improve patient–ventilator synchrony using sensitive triggering systems with short response times to decrease the WOB. Flow-triggered systems appear superior to pressure-triggered systems (112,113).

All modes of NPPV have been successfully implemented to improve respiratory failure. In ARF secondary to acute exacerbations of COPD, ACV, PSV, and PAV have all led to improvements in minute ventilation, respiratory rate, and arterial blood gases while unloading the respiratory muscles and relieving respiratory distress (114,115). Some investigators have found volume- and pressure-controlled modalities to reduce inspiratory workload better than PSV (116), while others have shown PSV to be equally efficient in reducing respiratory workload and improving physiological variables (99). Addition of positive end-expiratory pressure (PEEP) counteracts the effect of intrinsic PEEP, thereby reducing diaphragmatic effort and oxygen consumption.

Few studies have examined differences between the various NPPV modes in terms of physiological response. In acute hypercapnic exacerbations of COPD, two studies failed to find any differences in clinical outcome or arterial blood gas tensions between patients ventilated in ACV and PSV modes (117,118). Both modalities improved breathing pattern and provided respiratory muscle rest. Assist-control ventilation produced a lower respiratory workload, but with greater respiratory discomfort, more frequent loss of control of breathing, and diminished ability to compensate for mask leaks than PSV (116). In the absence of evidence favoring a specific ventilatory mode, choice should be based on local expertise and familiarity and tailored to the etiology, stage, and severity of the pathophysiologic process responsible for ARF. Although some advocate that controlled modes may be preferred for patients with severe respiratory distress, unstable ventilatory drive or respiratory mechanics, or apneas, it is probably prudent to electively perform ETI and initiate mechanical ventilation in these patients. Hypoventilation with a depressed mental status, resulting in an inability to protect the airway that not does quickly reverse with the application of NPPV, should lead to ETI and mechanical ventilation to prevent possible aspiration.

4. *NPPV in Certain Clinical Conditions*

ARF Due to Hypoventilation

In a randomized study, patients with acute exacerbations of COPD leading to hypoxemia and hypercapnia received either conventional treatment (CT) or CT plus volume-limited NPPV (105). Compared with CT, patients receiving NPPV displayed significant improvements in pH and $PaCO_2$ within the first hour of treatment. None of the patients randomized to NPPV required intubation and their 30-day mortality was significantly lower. Two other studies randomized patients with acute exacerbations of COPD to full-face mask PSV or standard therapy (119,120). Both reported significant improvements in vital signs and a reduced rate of intubation, length of hospital stay, in-hospital mortality, and other complications for those treated with NPPV. The majority of complications and deaths in the control group were attributable to intubation and subsequent mechanical ventilation (120). Another study compared PEEP plus PSV with standard therapy for patients stratified according to COPD or non-COPD-related disease (121). The rate of intubation was significantly lower with NPPV compared with standard therapy, although ICU mortality was similar for both treatment groups when considering patients with hypoxemic ARF.

ARF Due to Hypoxemia

Clinical studies in hypoxemic ARF of different etiologies indicate that NPPV can improve arterial blood gases, respiratory rate, dyspnea, and use of accessory muscles (122,123). There have been three randomized trials investigating whether NPPV prevents intubation in patients with hypoxemic ARF better than standard medical treatment. The first found no reduction in the overall rates of intubation or mortality in patients treated with NPPV. However, subset analysis revealed patients with $PaO_2 > 45\,mmHg$ had significantly decreased rates of intubation, ICU LOS, and mortality. Interestingly, all patients with pneumonia who received NPPV subsequently required intubation (124). Another study reported that NPPV was associated with a significant reduction in the rate of intubation and ICU LOS. However, NPPV did not change the duration of hospitalization or inpatient mortality in patients with ARF secondary to community-acquired pneumonia (102). In patients with hypoxemic ARF following solid organ transplantation, NPPV resulted in lower intubation rates, fewer fatal complications, reduced ICU LOS, and mortality. When compared with invasive ventilatory support in patients with hypoxemic ARF, NPPV was as effective in improving gas exchange and was associated with fewer serious complications and shorter ICU LOS. However, hospital mortality did not differ between NPPV and standard therapy groups (123). The investigators recommended that NPPV might substitute for invasive ventilatory support in such patients (123).

NPPV in Patients with CPE

Noninvasive positive-pressure ventilation is a very potent tool to treat patients admitted with acute respiratory insufficiency secondary to cardiogenic pulmonary edema. Two randomized controlled studies showed that CPAP alone (10–15 cm H_2O) administered via face mask rapidly decreases respiratory rate, corrects respiratory acidosis, and improves hemodynamics and oxygenation with a reduced need for intubation in patients with acute pulmonary edema (125,126). However, more recent investigators have found that CPAP with PSV might increase the rate of myocardial infarction in cardiogenic pulmonary edema (99).

NPPV to Assist with Weaning

Prolonged mechanical ventilation has been shown to increase the risk of nosocomial pneumonia, leads to prolonged ICU and hospital LOS, and is uncomfortable for patients (74,127,128). Some authors have advocated using NPPV as a bridge between intubation and mechanical ventilation to respiratory independence. Two randomized trials performed in Europe have investigated this potential for early extubation to NPPV in patients with acute exacerbations of chronic hypercapnic respiratory failure secondary to COPD (129,130). The patients had failed a T-piece trial after conventional mechanical ventilation via ETT for a period of 2–6 days and were randomized to receive standard weaning using PSV via an ETT or extubation to NPPV. Both studies showed a significant decrease in the period of mechanical ventilation when using the noninvasive approach with one demonstrating a significant increase in 3-month survival.

NPPV to Prevent Reintubation

Studies show that 2–25% (131,132) of patients fail extubation and approximately 3–14% of intubated patients undergo unplanned extubation (133–138) with 37–66% needing reintubation (134–140). These patients may potentially benefit from NPPV to avoid reintubation. Retrospective, controlled studies seem to confirm the utility of NPPV in the setting of failed extubation (141), although a randomized, controlled study did not find overall benefit (142).

Surgical Patients

After thoracic surgery for lung resection (143) or scoliosis (144), bilevel NPPV demonstrated short-term physiologic benefits on gas exchange without significant hemodynamic effects. Noninvasive positive-pressure ventilation was well tolerated, but no clinical end points were investigated. After upper abdominal surgery, NPPV (mask CPAP) increased lung volume more rapidly and decreased atelectasis 72 hr postoperatively compared with conventional therapy (145). In morbidly obese patients after gastroplasty, bilevel NPPV significantly improved arterial oxygenation on the first postoperative day, a physiological benefit associated with a more rapid recovery of pulmonary function (146).

Obesity Hypoventilation Syndrome

Pulmonologists have extensive experience using NPPV to manage obesity hypoventilation syndrome (OHS) and trials have shown it to be effective (147–149). If the patient presents with severe obstructive apnea, nasal CPAP and oxygen or bilevel PPV is indicated. If hypoventilation with central apnea or a hypopneic profile is present, NPPV with a volume-present respirator is safer as first line support (97).

Patients Deemed "Not to Be Intubated"

Many cancer patients in the terminal stages of their disease do not desire to be dependent on mechanical ventilation at the end of their life. For many patients, the ETT is identified as "being dependent on a machine to live." Noninvasive positive-pressure ventilation allows for mechanical respiratory support without patient perception of mechanical dependence. It may alleviate respiratory discomfort and allow patient–physician and patient–family interaction for these patients during the course of their respiratory insufficiency and possibly at the end of their life. The remaining family members are often grateful of the increased interaction they were able to have with their loved one, because they were on NPPV instead of being intubated. Studies suggest that NPPV in carefully selected patients with respiratory distress who do not desire intubation can reduce dyspnea and preserve patient autonomy (100,109).

C. Airway Management and Endotracheal Intubation

As discussed above, the initial step in assessment of the patient with respiratory distress is airway evaluation. If the patient needs assistance with respiration, the first step is to see that the airway is open before any other interventions are instituted. It is crucial that proper technique be utilized to open the airway. A gentle jaw thrust or head tilt-chin lift is usually all that is needed. Bag-mask ventilation with supplemental oxygen must be administered utilizing one of these two techniques to open the airway, otherwise ventilation will be ineffective and air will be shunted into the stomach thus increasing the risk of aspiration. This last point cannot be stressed enough that without effective pulmonary air exchange all other maneuvers are futile. Most patients can be adequately mask ventilated with cricoid pressure to prevent reflux until preparations for intubation can be completed. Other ACLS interventions can continue to take place during bag-mask ventilation.

Once the adequacy of air movement has been ensured, the next decision in respiratory management is whether the patient needs to have an oral or nasal ETT place or if NPPV can be initiated. If intubation is required because the patient does not meet the above-mentioned criteria for NPPV, careful preparation of both equipment and patient is essential to ensure successful intubation.

1. Intubation

Many patients will need to be intubated to provide PPV. It is inhumane (and dangerous) to endotracheally intubate patients without any sedation. As many of these patients are at high risk of aspiration due to full stomachs or air insufflation of the stomach from poor bag-mask technique, all patients should have cricoid pressure applied during induction and continued until confirmation of successful ETT placement. In order to adequately blunt the hemodynamic response to laryngoscopy and to prevent awareness, it is necessary to provide a short-term general anesthetic. Given the dangers of airway loss and the hemodynamic instability of many of these patients, it is wise to engage the help of a skilled anesthesiologist who has experience in airway management and anesthetizing sick patients. If possible, prior to the induction of anesthesia, the patient should be preoxygenated for 3–5 min to ensure adequate denitrogenation of the lungs and increase the margin of safety during ETI. Induction can be accomplished with a combination of etomidate (0.1–0.3 mg/kg) for anesthesia followed immediately with succinylcholine (1–1.5 mg/kg) for muscle relaxation and ETT placement. This combination provides the best compromise between hemodynamic instability (a consequence of general anesthesia in critically ill patients) and intubating conditions. Other drug combinations can be used and it is the manner (i.e., appropriate dosing) in which the drugs are given that is more important than the precise choice of agent. If the intubating person does not have expertise in airway management or with ETI, then muscle relaxants should be avoided as they leave the patient completely dependent on that provider for their airway and breathing. A regimen of high-dose benzodiazepine (i.e., 5–10 mg i.v.) may provide some relaxation and amnesia in these settings; however, there will be little blunting of the hemodynamic response to intubation.

Once the ETT has been observed to pass through the vocal cords, the tube position must be confirmed by bag ventilation while listening for equal breath sounds in either axilla, the presence of end-tidal CO_2 (as established by capnography or EasyCap), misting of the ETT with expiration, absence of breath sounds over the stomach, and adequate arterial oxygen saturation by pulse oximeter. Often, the latter may take a few minutes to recover to normal levels as there is often a lag in pulse oximetry SpO_2 determination and if the patient has incurred a significant oxygen debt. Once the ETT has been successfully placed and position confirmed the patient may be connected to the mechanical ventilator.

2. Concepts of Mechanical Ventilation

Although the initiation of PPV is often life saving, one must be aware of the deleterious effects that can follow. Given that our normal ventilatory pattern relies on negative pressure for inspiration, the implementation of PPV results in numerous nonphysiologic stresses on both the pulmonary and cardiovascular systems. Positive-pressure ventilation and ETI are injurious to the lungs and recent literature has focused on the detrimental effects of PPV and on the development of new ventilatory strategies that can help mitigate them.

Mechanisms of Lung Injury with Positive-Pressure Ventilation

Ventilator-induced lung injury (VILI) is a real risk of injudicious use of mechanical ventilation and has been demonstrated both experimentally in the lab (150) and clinically at the bedside (151–154). Numerous mechanisms have been attributed to VILI that include overpressurization or overdistension of alveoli as well as repeated alveolar collapse and reopening that results in stress-related injury to alveoli with the subsequent release of damaging inflammatory mediators.

INFLAMMATORY MEDIATORS AND LUNG INJURY: Inflammatory cells and mediators such as proinflammatory cytokines have been shown to contribute directly or indirectly to VILI (155–160). The lung damage may be a consequence of either systemic or pulmonary pathology. Systemic sources may lead to the SIRS with high levels of circulating cytokines, tumor necrosis factor alpha, and interleukins that can damage lung tissue. Local pulmonary pathology may lead to increased pulmonary concentrations of these same mediators that can cause an adverse feedback loop of worsening lung damage with a leak of these mediators into the systemic circulation that may lead to multiple organ dysfunction. Mechanotransduction describes intracellular signaling processes responding to external forces such as stretch and describes the mechanisms by which PPV activates the immune system. The evidence that PPV can trigger the inflammatory cascade is supported by a model of neutropenic surfactant depleted animals that demonstrated that inflammatory cells initiate or aggravate VILI (161). The concept of compartmentalization comprises the fact that the inflammatory response remains compartmentalized in the area of the body where it is produced. One consequence of the tissue destruction that occurs in lungs ventilated with high pressures and no PEEP is destruction of the barriers and decompartmentalization. As a result, local proinflammatory mediators, endotoxin, and bacteria are spread in the systemic circulation, and systemic factors enter the lung (162–164). Kolobow et al. (165) and Borelli et al. (166) found that sheep mechanically ventilated with lung overdistension for prolonged periods developed clinical features much like those seen in the syndrome of multiple organ failure. Thus, the inappropriate administration of PPV can cause or magnify the inflammatory release in the lungs (Table 4). These concepts have evolved into the "biotrauma" hypothesis, which states that lung injury caused by injurious ventilation strategies leads to excessive release of proinflammatory mediators and activation of the immune system (167,168). Lung protective ventilation strategies, however, appear to be associated with reduced markers of inflammation including proinflammatory cytokines (167–169).

Table 4 Principal Ways by which Ventilation Can Cause Release of Proinflammatory Mediators

1. Stress failure of plasma membrane (necrosis)
   a. Release of preformed mediators
   b. Proinflammatory effects of cytosol released from damaged cells
2. Stress failure of endothelial and epithelial barriers
   a. Loss of compartmentalization
   b. Hemorrhage and accumulation of leukocytes in the lungs
3. Overdistension without tissue destruction
4. Effects on the vasculature independent from stretch and rupture
   a. Increased intraluminal pressure
   b. Increased shear stress

Source: From Ref. 166a.

VOLUTRAUMA: Traditionally, V_t and/or end-inspiratory lung volume has been believed to be the main determinant of VILI (170,171). Numerous laboratory investigations have shown that alveolar overdistention or stretch results in the release of inflammatory cytokines. Vlahakis et al. (172) found that human alveolar epithelium cells subjected to mechanical stretch released significant amounts interleukin (IL-8), while Pugin et al. (173) made similar observations with alveolar macrophages. Experiments with isolated mouse lungs showed that cell stretching caused activation of the transcription factor nuclear factor (NF)-κB, an important step in mediator release (173,174). Tremblay et al. (169) examined cytokine levels in the bronchoalveolar lavage fluid of nonperfused isolated rat lungs ventilated with different end-expiratory pressures and V_t. High V_t ventilation (40 mL/kg body weight) with zero end-expiratory pressure resulted in the release of considerable amounts of TNF-α, IL-1β, and IL-6 and in macrophage inflammatory protein (MIP)-2, the rodent equivalent of human IL-8. The release of MIP-2 (or IL-8) by lung cells submitted to collapse and overstretch may explain the leukocyte recruitment in lungs during mechanical ventilation with large V_t (155,156,175–179). These findings have recently been challenged by several studies that found no increase in TNF-α in the BALF during experimental VILI (162,176,180).

Overinflating the lungs results in increased epithelial (181) and endothelial (171,182) permeability. Using an isolated perfused rat model, Parker et al. (183) showed that gadolinium, which blocks stretch-activated nonselective cation channels, annulled the increase in microvascular permeability induced by high airway pressure. This suggests that entry through stretch-activated channels and an increase in intracellular Ca^{2+} concentration may be the cause of this increase in permeability. This increase results in the activation of tyrosine kinases (184), activation of the Ca^{2+}/calmodulin pathway, and phosphorylation of myosin light chain kinase (185). Interestingly, they also found that the increase in microvascular permeability after short periods of overinflation, before the occurrence of cell lesions, is transient (186).

Recently, several clinical trials investigating ventilatory strategy to prevent VILI in ARDS patients showed that high tidal volumes (e.g., 12 mL/kg based on predicted or measured body weight) associated with high airway pressures (34 cm H_2O more) are harmful and should be avoided (151,154). Although a higher V_t strategy produces additional recruitment and a better PaO/FiO_2 ratio initially, it appears to result in worse outcomes (187) with the lower V_t group having a 22% reduction in mortality. It clearly appears that damage to lung cells and lung tissue structure by overdistension can initiate an inflammatory response in initially intact lungs.

Barotrauma: Barotrauma has long been considered to be injurious to the lung and can also promote an inflammatory state. Imanaka et al. (176) found significant upregulation of Mac-1 and ICAM-1 on alveolar macrophages in rats ventilated with 45 cm H_2O peak inspiratory pressure (PIP) compared with those from animals ventilated with 7 cm H_2O PIP. Mead et al. (188) calculated that the pressure in the tissue surrounding an atelectatic region might be very high as the whole lung expands, reaching approximately 140 cm H_2O for a transpulmonary pressure of 30 cm H_2O. Furthermore, high capillary transmural pressures may result in cell membrane rupture and endothelial and epithelial intracellular gaps that are sufficiently large to allow the passage of red blood cells in the air spaces (189,190). The plateau pressure is easily measured and arguably the best marker of the risk of overstretch with a tolerable threshold of 30–35 cm H_2O, the normal maximum transalveolar pressure at total lung capacity (191).

Stress failure of the plasma membrane: Both ventilation-induced volutrauma and barotrauma can lead to release of proinflammatory mediators resulting from stress failure of the plasma membrane or from stress failure of endothelial and epithelial barriers. Mechanical strain occurs when a force is applied to an elastic cell, causing a mechanical stretch or distortion. Shear stress is generated when fluids such as blood or air move across a cell surface. Recently, Vlahakis and Hubmayr (192) calculated that a typical plasma membrane can sustain strains between only 2% and 3% (in the plane of the membrane) before it breaks. Alveoli subjected to rapid transitions from being small and flooded at end exhalation to being large and air filled at end inspiration thus are at high risk of suffering injury from sheer stress.

Normal alveoli maintain a relatively constant volume during the respiratory cycle as demonstrated by Schiller et al. (193), who used in vivo video microscopy to directly observe and quantify the dynamic changes in alveolar size throughout the ventilatory cycle during tidal ventilation. In normal lungs, alveoli never collapsed in accordance with earlier results from Wilson and Bachofen (194). The loss of the surfactant monolayer resulting from various pathologic states contributes to a loss of alveolar patency and increases epithelial and endothelial strain resulting in further damage. Lungs depleted of surfactant by repeated bronchoalveolar lavage clinically appear similar to those with neonatal respiratory distress syndrome (195). Collapse and reopening as well as an increase in the alveolar size at end inspiration have been observed in surfactant-deactivated lungs (193). Surfactant-depleted lungs are thus prone to alveolar instability, atelectasis, and increased shear stress when ventilated at low lung volume. High shear stress generated during repeated closing and reopening of atelectatic areas, referred to as atelectotrauma (196), may result in deformation of the alveolar epithelium (197). Ventilation with high distending pressures in the absence of PEEP has been shown to cause tissue destruction (150,170,198,199) probably as a result of these sheer stresses and high levels of inflammatory mediator release (169). Sandhar et al. (200) showed that hyaline membrane formation was less important if rabbits subjected to saline lavage were ventilated with PEEP. Similarly, bronchiolar lesions have been observed in lavaged isolated lungs ventilated with low but not with high PEEP (201). These observations suggest that lung instability and the cyclic collapse and reopening of distal units may, in addition to overinflation, also promote VILI. Positive end-expiratory pressure can be used to maintain alveolar patency and surfactant monolayer integrity throughout the ventilatory cycle, thus improving the overall compliance of the alveolar unit resulting in a lower maximum distending pressure for a given V_t.

Strategies for Mechanical Ventilation

Traditional ventilator strategies revolved around large tidal volumes to reduce atelectasis and PEEP was applied to effectively reduce the fraction of inspired oxygen. More recent strategies for mechanical ventilation focus on techniques thought to cause the least amount of injury to the lung while providing adequate oxygenation until the patient is ready for extubation. These strategies attempt to use low V_t (5–7 cc/kg ideal body weight) to prevent volutrauma and limit peak airway pressures ($PIP < 40$ cm H_2O) to prevent barotrauma which, as discussed earlier, can lead to the release of inflammatory cytokines locally and into the systemic circulation resulting in distal organ dysfunction. The application of PEEP is crucial to these strategies as it prevents alveolar collapse and the resulting sheer stress. Positive end-expiratory pressure also helps optimize oxygenation by the preservation of adequate mean airway pressure during low-volume ventilation. Importantly, it has been recognized that physiologic improvement does not necessarily mean a better ultimate outcome. Ventilator settings should be frequently re-evaluated so that the lowest possible FiO_2 and ventilator pressures are used to minimize iatrogenic lung injury. Newer strategies revolve around the use of smaller tidal volumes and the appropriate application of PEEP.

Recent Clinical Trials

Clinical trials testing low tidal volumes (5–7 cc/kg) in acute lung injury (ALI) and adult respiratory distress syndrome (ARDS) have not shown uniform results (Table 5) (152,153,202). A recent meta-analysis (203) of ALI and ARDS trials testing low tidal volumes found three nonbeneficial trials and two beneficial trials. In the nonbeneficial trials, control tidal volumes were used that resulted in airway pressures of 28–32 cm H_2O, which some believe more accurately reflect contemporary ventilatory volume strategies with airway pressure of 29–31 cm H_2O (204). In these studies, low tidal volumes did not improve outcomes but instead showed a nonsignificant trend toward increased mortality (152,153,202).

The two beneficial trials compared low tidal volume ventilation with control arms with high airway pressures (34–37 cm H_2O) that many believe were potentially high enough to cause VILI. There was an increased odds ratio (1.56) of dying in the control groups that could have represented a significant increase in the number of ventilator-associated deaths in these patients due to inappropriately high control V_t (203). In this setting, it is possible that low tidal volumes appeared inaccurately beneficial.

The analysis of the beneficial trials clearly showed that high tidal volumes (e.g., 12 mL/kg based on predicted or measured body weight) associated with high airway pressures (34 cm H_2O or more) are harmful and should be avoided (151,154). In contrast, the three nonbeneficial trials (152,153,202) employed control arms that might more accurately reflect current practice of physicians treating patients with ALI and ARDS (151,154,204–207). These trials established that, as long as tidal volumes produce airway pressures between 28 and 32 cm H_2O, there may be no benefit from using low-volume ventilation. The ventilator management algorithm used by the ARDSnet trial is shown in Table 6 and has become the standard of care for management of patients with ARDS. However, further study in this area is required.

Open Lung Theory

With recent advancements in ventilator technology, it has become possible to easily and accurately determine the compliance of the lung and tailor the ventilatory strategy to suit the individual patient's needs. These technological advances, when combined with the increased understanding of VILI, have led to the development of the "open lung" concept (OLV) of mechanical ventilation. The "open lung" concept was first developed by Lachmann in 1992 (208). The idea behind OLV is to ventilate the lung along the open portion of its pressure–volume curve thus preventing stresses of repeated alveolar collapse and reopening and overdistension (Fig. 5). The idea is to protect those alveolar units at the top of the pressure–volume curve from overdistension (and VILl) while splinting open those units at the bottom of the curve thus recruiting more lung, preventing atelectasis, and reducing shunt fraction.

In this approach, the ventilator is set to ventilate the patient's lungs between the upper and lower inflection points of the pressure–volume curve (Fig. 6). These

Table 5 Tidal Volume Used in Clinical Trials of Lung Protective Ventilation Strategies in ALI or ARDS

	Reported tidal volumes		Mortality (%)	
Trial	Traditional	Lower	Traditional	Lower
Amato et al. (148)	$\leq 12^a$	$\geq 6^a$	71	38
NIH ARDS Network (151)	11.8^b	6.2^b	40	31
Brochard et al. (149)	10.3^c	7.1^c	38	47
Stewart et al. (150)	10.8	7.2^d	47	50
Brower et al. (199)	10.2^b	7.3^b	46	50

[a] Target tidal volumes expressed in mL/kg measured body weight as described in Methods.
[b] Tidal volumes expressed in mL/kg predicted body weight (PBW): male PBW (kg) = 50 + 2.3[(height in inches)–60]; female PBW (kg) = 45.5 + 2.3[(height in inches)–60].
[c] Tidal volumes expressed in mL/kg dry body weight (measured weight minus estimated weight gain from water and salt retention).
[d] Tidal volumes expressed in mL/kg ideal body weight (IBW): IBW = 25 × (Height in meters)^2.
ALI, acute lung injury; ARDS = acute respiratory distress syndrome.
Source: From Ref. 203a.

Table 6 Low Tidal Volume Ventilator Strategy NIH ARDS Network

Initial ventilator tidal volume and rate adjustments
A. Calculate predicted body weight (PBW)
  a. Male = 50 + 2.3 [height (inches)−60] or 50 + 0.91 [height (cm)−152.4]
  b. Female = 45.5 + 2.3 [height (inches)−60] or 45.5 + 0.91 [height (cm)−152.4]
B. Mode: volume assist-control
C. Set initial tidal volume to 8 mL/kg PBW
  a. Reduce tidal volume to 7 mL/kg after 1–2 hr and then to 6 mL/kg PBW after 1–2 hr
D. Set initial ventilator rate to maintain baseline minute ventilation (not >35 bpm)
Subsequent tidal volume adjustments
A. Plateau pressure goal: ≤30 cm H_2O
  a. Check inspiratory plateau pressure (P_{plat}) with 0.5 sec inspiratory pause at least every 4 hr and after each change in PEEP or tidal volume
  b. If P_{plat} >30 cm H_2O, decrease tidal volume by 1 mL/kg PBW steps to 5 or if necessary to 4 mL/kg PBW
  c. If P_{plat} <25 cm H_2O and tidal volume < 6 mL/kg, increase tidal volume by 1 mL/kg PBW until P_{plat} > 25 cm H_2O or tidal volume = 6 mL/kg
B. If breath stacking or severe dyspnea occurs, tidal volume may be increased (not required) to 7 or 8 mL/kg PBW if P_{plat} remains ≤30 cm H_2O
Arterial oxygenation
A. GOAL: PaO_2 55–80 mmHg or SpO_2 88–95%
  a. Use these FiO_2/PEEP combinations to achieve oxygenation goal

FiO_2	0.3	0.4	0.4	0.5	0.5	0.6	0.7	0.7	0.7	0.8	0.9	0.9	0.9	1.0
PEEP	5	5	8	8	10	10	10	12	14	14	14	16	18	20–24

Respiratory rate (RR) and arterial pH (GOAL: 7.30–7.45)
A. Acidosis management
  a. If pH 7.15–7.30
    i. Increase set RR until pH>7.30 or $PaCO_2$<25 (maximum set RR = 35)
    ii. If set RR = 35 and pH<7.30, $NaHCO_3$ may be given (not required)
  b. If pH<7.15
    i. Increase set RR to 35
    ii. If set RR = 35 and pH<7.15 and $NaHCO_3$ has been considered, tidal volume may be increased in 1 mL/kg PBW steps until pH>7.15 (P_{plat} target may be exceeded)
B. Alkalosis management: (pH>7.45)
  a. Decrease set RR until patient RR > set RR
  b. Minimum set RR = 6/min
C. *I:E* ratio
  a. GOAL: 1:1.0–1:3.0
  b. Adjust flow rate and inspiratory flow-wave form to achieve goal

These guidelines can be found at http://www.ardsnet.org/ along with a useful clinical synopsis.

points can be determined quickly and easily at the bedside. The lower inflection point is the pressure at which the compliance of the lung starts to increase as reflected by an increase in the slope of the pressure–volume curve. By setting the PEEP (or the PEEP low in bilevel ventilation) equal to the lower inflection point, atelectotrauma should be avoided (209,210). Positive end-expiratory pressure reduces the severity of VILI (211) and as mentioned above, may lessen the damage produced by the repeated collapse and re-expansion of lung units in surfactant-depleted lungs (201,212). However, using PEEP levels above the lower inflection point might increase lung injury and result in worse outcomes (213).

The pressure and the volume that are considered safe for some ARDS patients may cause lung overdistension in others (214–217) and the indiscriminate application of PEEP may favor overinflation if V_t is not reduced (150,218). The upper inflection point is the high inflation pressure at which the compliance of the lung starts to decrease as reflected by a decrease in the slope of the pressure–volume curve. The upper inflection point is often not seen in patients with compliant lungs as the usual volume used (15 cc/kg) to generate the pressure–volume curve is too small. The upper inflection point is usually seen in patients with less compliant lungs such as those with ARDS and has been ascribed to overinflation (216,217) or

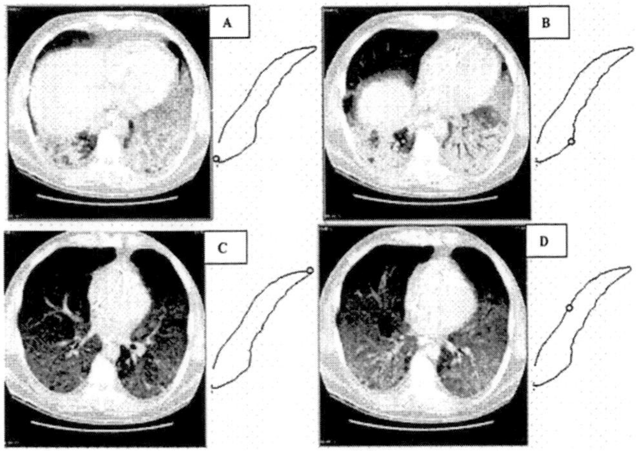

Figure 5 The thoracic tomography aspects of acute respiratory distress syndrome (ARDS) lungs at different levels of the inspiratory and expiratory pressure–volume curves. (A) Computed tomography scan at zero end-expiratory pressure showing gravitational-dependent lung opacities. (B) Computed tomography scan at the lower part of the point of inflection curve (L-Pflex) showing a more open lung but still with lung opacities in the gravitational-dependent regions. (C) A nearly fully recruited ARDS lung at the end of inspiration. (D) Computed tomography scan at the same airway pressure (L-Pflex) as in Panel (C) during expiration. The lungs are more aerated during expiration than during inspiration at the same pressure. Note the opening of the airways at the L-Pflex level. *Source*: From Ref. 151.

to the end of recruitment (219,220) during lung expansion. Therefore, by limiting the PIP (or PEEP high in the bilevel mode) in pressure control modes of ventilation or using smaller tidal volumes in volume control modes to keep pressures below the upper inflection point, volutrauma and barotrauma should be prevented (151,216,217).

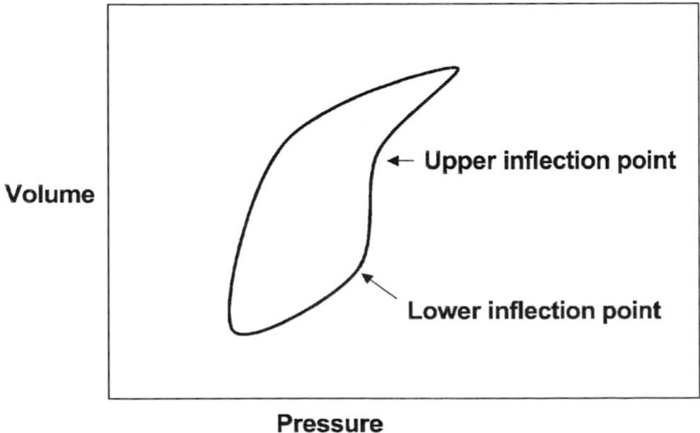

Figure 6 Pressure–volume curve demonstrating upper and lower inflection points. *Source*: From Ref. 91.

The open lung concept of alveolar recruitment can improve outcome in respiratory failure and ARDS. Even with the use of smaller tidal volumes (5–7 mL/kg for body weight), given the concepts discussed earlier in this chapter, we can see that these will generate biotrauma (cytokine release) in a nonopen lung. The goal of this technique is to minimize cyclic alveolar collapse and reopening (154,221), as the open lung is one in which there is little or no atelectasis and gas exchange is optimal. Experimental and clinical studies have demonstrated that techniques using the open lung approach can improve gas exchange, reduce time spent on mechanical ventilation, reduce mortality, and reduce ICU costs (222,223). A large trial comparing this approach with the current gold standard using low-volume ventilation is yet to be published.

ESTIMATING THE POTENTIAL FOR RECRUITMENT: The potential for recruitment mainly depends on the underlying lung pathology. If the pulmonary unit is filled with edema, fibrin, and cellular debris, reopening is likely to be impossible, regardless of the pressure applied (224). However, if the lung pathology is mainly interstitial edema resulting in increased lung weight, when combined with other compressive forces such as an increased abdominal pressure or heart weight, there is collapse of the small airways (loose atelectasis). With time, alveolar collapse follows due to gas reabsorption distal to small airway closure (sticky atelectasis). In this case, if sufficient pressure is applied to overcome the opening pressure, the pulmonaryunit may regain its aeration (225–227). However, intrue alveolar collapse, the pressure needed for alveolar recruitment may theoretically reach values of 60–70 cm H_2O (228) and attempts to rapidly rerecruit collapsed alveoli may cause significant lung injury.

Studies have shown that there is great potential for recruitment in laboratory models of ARDS such as lung lavage and oleic acid injury (226) as well as clinically in cases of secondary ARDS (ARDS from increased endothelial permeability driven by a distal source of inflammatory mediator release). However, in other conditions, such as experimental pneumonia, the potential for recruitment is much smaller (229). Some authors have unfortunately found as little as 5–10% of the lung parenchyma available for recruitment in ARDS when complicated by diffuse pneumonia (229). If all the pressure–volume points follow the same line in spite of increasing PEEP and plateau pressure while maintaining a constant V_t, this suggests low potential for recruitment (224,230).

Recruitment success should be checked with repeated graphic analysis of the pressure–volume curve

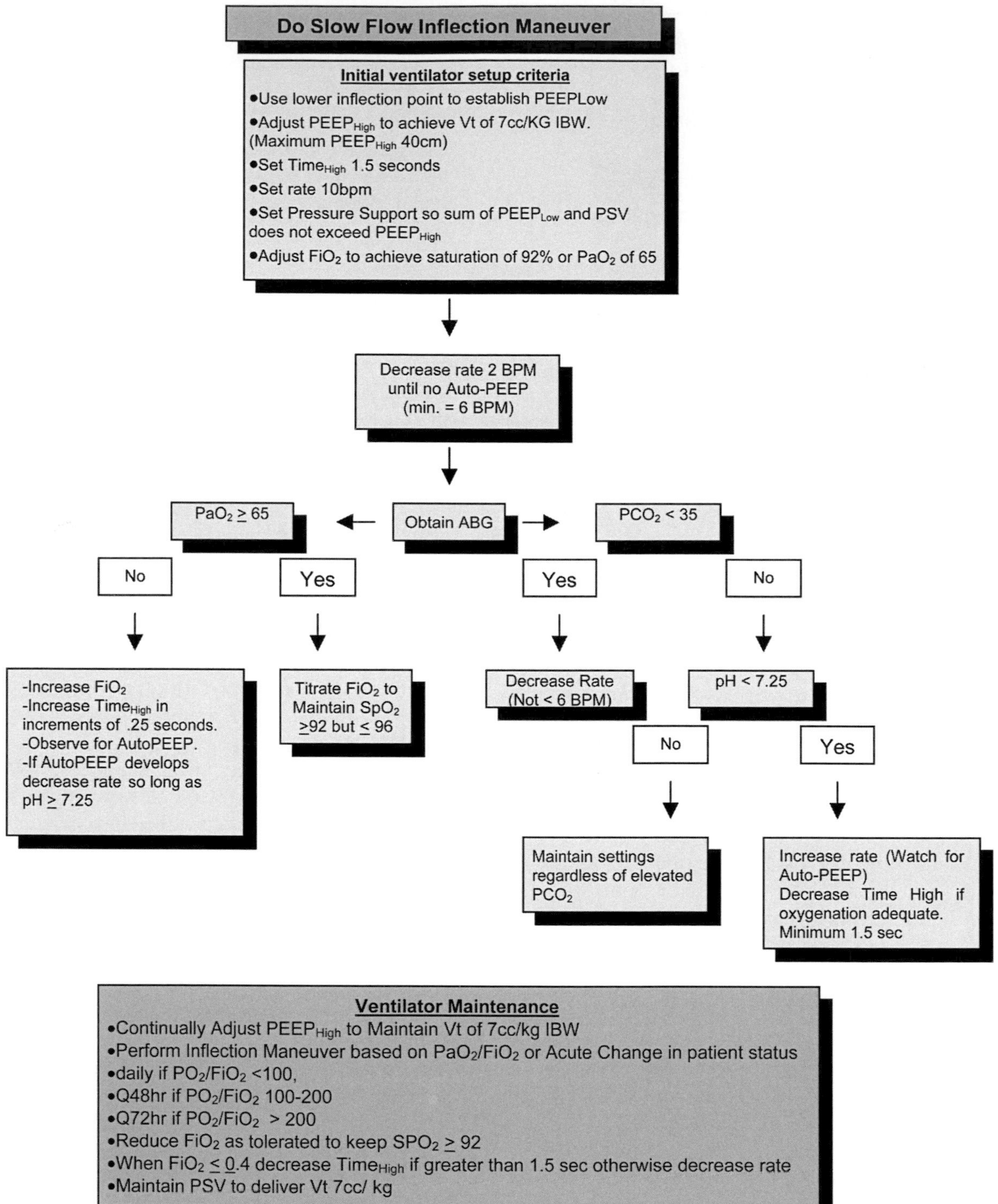

Figure 7 Bilevel ventilator management.

or with blood gas analysis and the ventilator adjusted appropriately to achieve the lowest possible ventilatory pressures and FiO_2. One such algorithm is illustrated in Fig. 7.

Modes of Ventilation

Traditional ventilatory techniques have relied on either volume- or pressure-controlled modes of ventilation. The initial choice of ventilatory mode for the critically ill patient depends less on the long-term effects of either mode and more on the initial delivery of adequate oxygen and hemodynamic stabilization. Often, it is desirable to minimize the patient's WOB while diagnostic evaluation and clinical stabilization are underway. This can be achieved by either volume-controlled modes such as continuous minute ventilation (CMV) or assist control (AC) as well as by synchronized intermittent mandatory ventilation (SIMV) with pressure support high enough to eliminate most of the WOB. Pressure control modes such as SIMV, bilevel, or airway pressure release ventilation (APRV) can be set at high enough respiratory rates to overcome the patients drive to spontaneously breathe or use high levels of pressure support such that the effective respiratory workload on the patient is minimal. The choice between modes and further discussions on the merits and details of each mode is beyond the scope of this chapter and can be found in numerous other textbooks on mechanical ventilation. The goal of therapy remains the same regardless of ventilatory mode and involves minimizing volutrauma, barotrauma, and sheer injury. Both Amato et al. (151) and Esteban et al. (231) used pressure control and found it effective, while the ARDS Network used volume control with improved outcomes (154).

With volume control ventilation (VCV), the delivered tidal volume is independent and the resultant ventilatory pressures are dependent. This means that the peak and mean airway pressures will vary as the compliance of the lung changes since a constant tidal volume will be delivered. Conversely, in pressure-controlled modes of ventilation, the pressure limits are preset and the tidal volume varies with lung compliance. Some believe that the rapid initial low pattern of the pressure-targeted breath may provide a better distribution of gas in the lung. If regional mechanics worsen, volume targeting will keep a constant V_t but plateau pressure will rise and the V_t will be preferentially distributed to healthier regions, increasing the risk of regional overdistention. V_e and carbon dioxide clearance, however, will be largely preserved. In contrast, with worsening of regional mechanics during pressure-targeted ventilation, the pressure limit is preserved, the overall V_t decreases (and thus carbon dioxide clearance is reduced), but the regional stretch in the healthier units is unchanged (187). In contrast to VCV, PCV generates no intrapulmonary redistribution of gas from other hyperdistended lung units, known as the "Pendeluft effect." Pressure-controlled modes thus generate an efficient system in which only fresh gas is entering the recruited alveoli (228,232,233).

There are several modes of pressure control ventilation. Airway pressure release ventilation, BIPAP, bilevel, and biphasic ventilatory support are all pressure-targeted, time-cycled modes with a pressure release mechanism that allows the patient to both exhale and inhale and still keep the ventilator's inflation pressure constant. Assist control and SIMV can also be manipulated to gain the advantages of pressure control by setting pressure limits that prevent high peak pressures. All provide good gas exchange and recruitment with less sedation than pressure-controlled inverse ratio ventilation (234). Although APRV puts a pressure limit on the ventilator stretch, spontaneous ventilation superimposed on the mechanical settings can add to V_t and thus the end-inspiratory stretch. This is especially important with machines that also provide pressure support above the set inflation pressure of APRV (187). With the bilevel mode of ventilation, 1.5 cm H_2O of pressure support is provided while at PEEP high, which limits the risk of overdistension.

Frequency and Tidal Volume

Alveolar (and thus arterial) PCO_2 and, to a degree, PO_2 are dependent on minute ventilation (V_e) and there needs to be a balancing of gas exchange goals against the risk of overstretching, especially of the healthier regions of the lung. In distributing the desired V_e between frequency and V_t, choose a V_t of around 6 mL/kg, as this is what the ARDSnet trial showed to be beneficial (154). The resultant V_t and inspiratory pressures should be below the threshold to cause injury to the lung as discussed previously. Although some institutions have chosen to ventilate all of their patients using the open lung concept and low tidal volumes, only patients with stiff, noncompliant lungs, such as those with ARDS, have been studied using these strategies. Patients with compliant lungs not expected to require long-term ventilation should do well even with more traditional higher volume ventilation strategies. However, as it is not always possible to predict those patients who will develop stiff lungs, it might prove wise to treat all intubated and mechanically ventilated patients as high risk and use lung protective strategies.

Choosing the frequency of mandatory breaths depends on the clinical situation. Initially, the mandatory breath rate should be set high enough to assume the entire WOB while diagnostic evaluation and hemodynamic stabilization is being undertaken. Given that low-volume ventilation is crucial to protect the lung from VILI, varying the rate of mandatory mechanical breaths becomes the only other respiratory means to control PCO_2 and thus pH. There are no good data to guide us as to the lowest tolerable pH. However, 7.2 is commonly quoted in the literature and 7.15 was the lower limit of acceptability in the ARDS Network trial (154). However, remember that as frequency (and V_e) goes up, the risk of air trapping and intrinsic PEEP increases as well.

Oxygen Concentration

During the initial period of evaluation and stabilization, set the fraction of inspired oxygen (FiO_2) at 1.0. Once the patient has been stabilized, attempt to wean the FiO_2 as near to room air concentration (0.21 at sea level) in order to minimize the risk of oxygen toxicity. It is typically safe to wean the FiO_2 to the minimum level required to keep the hemoglobin oxygen saturation $\geq$90–93%. A lower threshold can sometimes be used for patients with a history of COPD.

PEEP and Peak Inspiratory Pressure

As discussed previously, using PEEP to maintain alveolar patency and the surfactant monolayer throughout the ventilatory cycle improves the overall compliance of the alveolar unit such that a lower maximum distending pressure is required (233) which leads to improved survival (Fig. 8). Intrapulmonary shunt ideally should be less than 10% and this strategy minimizes shunt and permits a lower FiO_2 required to maintain hemoglobin oxygen saturation as mean airway pressure is preserved. Additionally, if sufficient PEEP is provided, repeated alveolar opening and collapse, an important contributor to VILI, is prevented.

The Law of Laplace links the pressure applied by the ventilator to the alveolar pressure (P) creating surface tension (T) and radius (R): $P = 2T/R$. Alveolar surfactant minimizes the surface forces at the air–liquid interface, thus improving alveolar stability at all alveolar sizes and minimizing surface tension. However, mechanical ventilation may cause varied levels of surfactant system dysfunction as a result of either direct ventilator effects or the indirect effect of the systemic inflammatory response. Given that appropriately applied PEEP can ameliorate atelectotrauma (200) and bronchiolar lesions (201) when surfactant function is abnormal, all patients should benefit from the application of PEEP.

In systemically induced ARDS (secondary ARDS), the lung injury is homogenous, and nonselective application of PEEP can produce homogeneous recruitment of collapsed alveolar units. ARDS from a primary lung injury such as pneumonia or trauma often creates focal, dense infiltrates. Under those conditions, PEEP will often distribute volume to the more compliant, healthier lung regions and may have little effect on recruiting injured regions.

The bilevel mode of ventilation (pressure control using the open lung strategy) uses the pressure–volume curve to determine the lower inflection point as described above. The low PEEP should be set equal to the lower inflection point. Earlier strategies that set the low PEEP several centimeters of H_2O above the lower inflection point might have resulted in worse

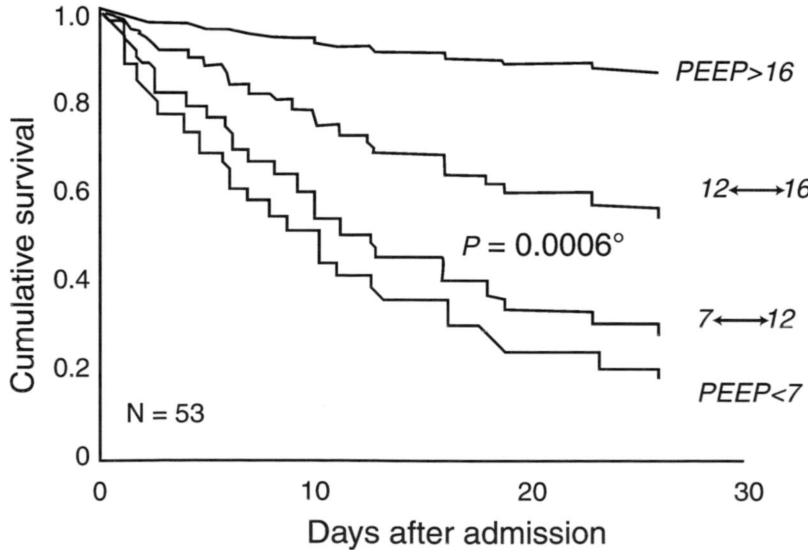

Figure 8 Survival according to PEEP levels during mechanical ventilation in acute respiratory distress syndrome patients (20).*Adjusted for acute physiology and chronic health evaluation II and plateau pressure. *Source*: From Ref. 234a.

outcomes in critically ill patients (213). Often, the upper inflection point is not seen on the pressure–volume curve generated with a 15-cc/kg breath, as most lungs are too compliant. Using the information learned from the ARDSnet trial (154), it is probably prudent to set the high PEEP (or PIP) so that the resultant tidal volume is around 6–7 cc/kg.

Although the proper utilization of PEEP can minimize positive-pressure-induced lung injury, injudicious application of PEEP can be detrimental. Exceedingly high levels of PEEP, particularly in noncompliant lungs, can result in reduced tidal volumes if the difference between the low PEEP and upper inflection point is too small to generate sufficient tidal volumes. This is the case because little volume may be added to the lung above the upper inflection point. In a model of mechanical ventilation of rats at high end-inspiratory pressure, the application of PEEP increased lung injury (amount of edema, Type I cell lysis, presence of hyaline membranes in alveolar spaces) and resulted in the reduction of V_t (211). In addition, higher PEEP may increase mean airway pressure enough to increase the size of the lung's West Zone 1, thus resulting in an increased dead space and worsening of ventilation and CO_2 removal.

Indiscriminate application of PEEP can have detrimental hemodynamic effects as cardiac preload may be diminished at high levels of PEEP due to a reduction in cardiac preload (235). In addition, high levels of PEEP should be avoided in cases of intracranial hypertension as PEEP can worsen intracranial pressure (236). In cases of bronchopleural fistulae, nonselective PEEP can worsen the air leak and attempts should be made to minimize airway pressures. Several investigators have demonstrated that plateau pressures should probably be limited to less than 35 cm H_2O to minimize barotrauma to the lung (151,154).

Inspiratory Flow and Pressure Support

Inspiratory flow can be administered in the form of constant (square wave), decelerating, or sinusoidal patterns. Many ventilators deliver a square wave pattern of flow with volume ventilation that might be beneficial in cases of cardiogenic pulmonary edema due to the higher mean airway pressures compared to other flow patterns. However, the decelerating pattern of flow has been shown to open alveoli better than a constant flow pattern and leads to better pulmonary gas exchange through better gas distribution (228,237,238).

Inspiratory flow must be set high enough to avoid increased WOB by the patient. Most patients at rest require around 60 L/min of inspiratory flow to breathe comfortably. Patients with an elevated ventilatory demand, such as those who are highly agitated or hypermetabolic will need significantly higher inspiratory flow rates to prevent excessive WOB. Conversely, patients with low respiratory drive, such as when sleeping, will need lower flow rates. Many modern ventilators have variable flow circuits that automatically adjust the inspiratory flow to match the patent's needs.

Pressure support is used to reduce the imposed WOB from the ventilatory circuit. The amount of pressure support should be enough to ensure that the patient receives an adequate tidal volume during spontaneous breaths, usually around 5 cc/kg. It is important to observe the patient for signs of discomfort or excessive WOB during spontaneous breaths as the amount of pressure support may need to be varied to ensure patient comfort. With very high levels of pressure support around 25–30 cm H_2O, it is possible to eliminate almost all of the WOB.

Spontaneous Breathing

The weaning process usually involves a rapid transition from controlled ventilation to spontaneous breathing. Diaphragm motion and gas distribution differ depending on whether the diaphragm is active or passive. Active ventilation is more evenly distributed and includes substantial dorsal aeration. With passive positive pressure ventilated, motion and ventilation are largely in the ventral regions. Because of this, an active diaphragm facilitates recruitment and reduces atelectasis; therefore, it may prove prudent to transition to spontaneous modes of ventilation as soon as the patient's clinical condition tolerates.

Recruitment Maneuvers

Intermittent mandatory sighs during PPV have been shown to reduce atelectasis and improve oxygenation (239). Forced recruitment maneuvers can involve inflations up to and above the upper inflection point on a pressure–volume curve for up to 1 or even 2 min. In true alveolar collapse, the pressure needed for alveolar recruitment may theoretically reach values of 60–70 cm H_2O (228), and there is the conceptual risk of overdistention injury as well as the potential for shear stress injury caused by markedly different regional volumes being delivered to adjacent lung units. Additionally, cardiovascular impairment can occur with the application of high intrathoracic pressures. For these reasons, the author does not recommend using high volume recruitment maneuvers unless needed for short-term salvage therapy during episodes of severe respiratory decompensation.

IV. WEANING

Thoughts of weaning the cancer patient off mechanical ventilation need to begin before the patient is intubated. Patients may be in the terminal stages of their cancer and may not want to spend their last days on a "breathing machine." In addition, many cancer patients may have significant comorbid illnesses that make the likelihood of successful extubation remote. Thus, thoughts of the potential for and the process of extubation need to begin before the insertion of the ETT.

Patients, and sometimes their surrogate decision makers, need to be presented with an honest assessment of the short- and long-term prognosis of recovery and survival from their cancer or its treatments and of the likelihood of being successfully weaned off mechanical ventilation. Some patients, when presented with this information, may choose to forego intubation and mechanical ventilation preferring instead the initiation of palliative comfort measures or risking death from respiratory failure as the terminal phase of their cancer.

For those patients who choose to be intubated and undergo mechanical ventilation, the weaning process should start as soon as the inciting factors have stabilized and the patient is hemodynamically stable. Factors to consider before starting the weaning process include adequacy of respiratory function (including both pulmonary gas exchange and respiratory muscle strength), neuropsychological factors, cardiovascular status, presence of bowel dysfunction, reversal of neuromuscular blockade, normothermia, low metabolic demands, the need for operative procedures, and the stability of the clinical condition.

A. Methods of Weaning from Mechanical Ventilation

There are numerous ways to wean a patient off mechanical ventilation as not all patients will wean in the same manner. The prognosis and clinical status will determine which method works best for each individual patient. Additionally, country and regional variations in clinical practice will influence the choice of the mode of weaning (205). Some of the modes of weaning include T-tube trials, synchronized intermittent minute ventilation (SIMV), PSV, and SIMV plus PSV. In one survey of a Spanish hospital, these methods were used in 24%, 18%, 15%, 9%, and some combination of two or more methods in succession in 33% of patients, respectively (240). During the last decade, 1990–2000, there was an increasing use of pressure-support ventilation and spontaneous breathing trials as compared to other methods of weaning (241). The ARDSnet group has published guidelines to assist the weaning process (Table 7).

Esteban et al. (240) showed that the time required for weaning ventilated ICU patients using a combination of SIMV and PSV was longer (17.8 days) than with other techniques (about 5 days). In another trial, the same author showed that a once-daily trial of spontaneous breathing led to extubation about three times more quickly than intermittent mandatory ventilation and about twice as quickly as pressure-support ventilation. Multiple daily trials of spontaneous breathing offered no benefit over once-daily trials (242). Conversely, Vitacca et al. (243) found that spontaneous breathing trials and decreasing levels of PSV were equally effective in difficult-to-wean patients with COPD.

Many adjunctive methods have been tried to shorten the duration of weaning from mechanical ventilation including biofeedback, ventilatory muscle strength training, and pharmacologic interventions. Holliday and Hyers (244) used daily frontalis electromyographic (EMG) relaxation feedback for anxiety reduction and improved respiratory muscle EMG efficiency as well as diaphragm EMG combined with tidal volume feedback (V_t) to reduce mean ventilator days to 20.6 vs. 32.6 days in the control group. Hypnosis has also been used in small trials to facilitate weaning in difficult-to-wean patients (245). In a small trial, Martin et al. (246) used inspiratory muscle strength training to successfully wean difficult-to-wean patients from mechanical ventilation. Pharmacologic manipulations include methylphenidate, a psychostimulant, and growth hormone. The former showed a possible benefit in two patients (247). One phase I trial with human growth hormone showed it to be safe and efficacious in promoting respiratory independence in difficult-to-wean surgical ICU patients (248).

B. Weaning Teams and Protocols

Patients receiving mechanical ventilation benefit from frequent evaluation of their continuing need for ventilatory support and should be removed from mechanical ventilation as soon as possible to minimize morbidity. Ely et al. (249) showed that daily screening of respiratory function by physicians, respiratory therapists, and nurses to identify those possibly capable of breathing spontaneously resulted in a reduction in ventilation from 6 to 4.5 days in a population of medical and coronary ICU patients. They also found a reduction in the rate of several mechanical ventilation complications including accidental ETT removal, reintubation, tracheostomy, and mechanical ventilation more than 21 days (20% vs. 41%). However, the

Table 7 ARDSnet Recommended Weaning Guidelines

A. Conduct A CPAP trial daily when:
1. $FiO_2 \leq 0.40$ and PEEP ≤ 8
2. PEEP and $FiO_2 \leq$ values of previous day
3. Patient has spontaneous breathing efforts (may decrease vent set rate by 50% for 5 min to detect effort)
4. Systolic BP ≥ 90 mmHg without vasopressor support
5. Conducting the CPAP trial:
   a. Set: CPAP = 5 cm H_2O, $FiO_2 = 0.50$
      i. If patient RR ≤ 35 for 5 min, advance to pressure support weaning (Section B)
      ii. If patient RR > 35, return to previous A/C settings and reassess for weaning next morning

B. Pressure support (PS) weaning procedure
1. Set PEEP = 5 and $FiO_2 = 0.50$
2. Set initial PS based on RR during CPAP trial:
   a. If CPAP RR < 25: set PS = 5 cm H_2O and go to Section C
   b. If CPAP RR = 25–35: set PS = 20 cm H_2O, then reduce by 5 cm H_2O at ≤ 5 min intervals until patient RR = 26–35, then go to Section C
   c. If initial PS not tolerated: return to previous A/C settings
3. Reducing PS: (no reductions made after 1,700 hr)
   a. Reduce PS by 5 cm H_2O at 1–3 hr
   b. If PS ≥ 10 cm H_2O not tolerated, return to previous A/C settings (If A. criteria O.K., resume last tolerated PS level next morning and go to Section C)
   c. If PS = 5 cm H_2O not tolerated, go to PS = 10 cm H_2O. If tolerated, PS of 5 or 10 cm H_2O may be used overnight with further attempts at weaning the next morning
   d. If PS = 5 cm H_2O tolerated for ≥ 2 hr, assess for ability to sustain unassisted breathing (Section C)

C. Unassisted breathing trial
1. Place on T-piece, trach collar, or CPAP < 5 cm H_2O
2. Assess for tolerance as below for 2 hr
3. If tolerated, consider extubation
4. If not tolerated, resume PS 5 cm H_2O

Source: http://www.ardsnet.org/

number of ICU and hospital days remained similar between the two groups.

Numerous groups have looked at the implementation of weaning protocols to reduce the duration of weaning. Weaning protocols, when developed in a multidisciplinary manner, are well tolerated by both the patients and care providers (250). Numerous authors have demonstrated a reduction in the duration of mechanical ventilation by implementing a systematic approach to weaning from mechanical ventilation. Henneman et al. (251,252) found that a collaborative weaning plan in the form of a weaning board and flowsheet resulted in a decrease in the length of ventilator time by 2.7 days and a decreased ICU LOS by 3.6 days and 1-year later had improved to 4.9 and 4.5 days, respectively. Kollef et al. (253) found that the median duration of mechanical ventilation was 35 vs. 44 hr for protocol directed vs. physician-directed. They also found that the rate of successful weaning was significantly greater in the protocol-directed group (risk ratio = 1.31), but hospital mortality rates were similar. Smyrnios et al.(254) also showed that ventilation weaning management protocol reduced mean days on mechanical ventilation from 23.9 to 17.5 days over a 2-year period in spite of a worsening of the average APACHE score in those same patients. They also demonstrated a decrease in the hospital LOS from 37.5 to 24.7 days and ICU LOS from 30.5 to 20.3 days in these same patients. However, not all studies have confirmed the apparent benefit of a weaning protocol. Duane et al. (255) found no differences in self-extubation rates, ventilatory days, ventilator charges, number of ICU days, or ICU charges with the implementation of a ventilator weaning protocol when patients requiring long-term mechanical ventilation were excluded.

Computerized protocols used to guide the weaning progress have also been developed and shown to speed up the weaning process. Linton et al. (256) used a closed-loop adaptive lung ventilation controller in 27 patients requiring prolonged mechanical ventilation who met standard weaning criteria to successfully wean patients to the point of extubation. Strickland and Hasson (257) also used a computer-directed weaning algorithm that resulted in shorter weaning times vs. physician directed weaning (18.7 ± 5.9 hr vs.

25.6 ± 5.6 hr), fewer arterial blood gases, and less time spent outside acceptable respiratory rate and tidal volume parameter. Iregui et al. (258) showed that by simply using a hand-held computer to guide respiratory therapist in the weaning process resulted in reduced time to spontaneous breathing trials, more patients were started on spontaneous breathing trials when meeting criteria, and ICU LOS was reduced when compared to the use of the same protocol without computer assistance.

Developing teams to supervise the weaning process has also been shown to benefit the weaning process. Cohen et al. (259) showed a 3.9-day reduction in the number of days on mechanical ventilation and a 3.3-day reduction in the number of ICU days by the use of a ventilatory management team consisting of an ICU attendant, nurse, and respiratory therapist who made daily ventilator management rounds. Several other investigators have demonstrated that nonphysician providers can effectively manage a well-designed protocol. Ely et al. (260) found that nonphysician respiratory care providers could appropriately perform and interpret a daily screen of mechanically ventilated patients 95% of the time. Marelich et al. (261) found that a ventilator management protocol driven by a respiratory care practitioner and a nurse resulted in decreased duration of mechanical ventilation, 124 vs. 68 hr, and a decrease in the incidence of ventilator-associated pneumonia in trauma patients. Scheinhorn et al. (262) reduced weaning time from 29 to 17 days with the implementation of a respiratory therapist-driven protocol. In a study of postcardiac surgery patients, Wood et al. (263) concluded that a respiratory initiated and directed intermittent mandatory ventilation weaning protocol could result in more rapid weaning (18.6 vs. 16.8 hr) without an increase in complications.

There are numerous barriers to successful weaning protocol implementation including physician unfamiliarity with the protocol, respiratory care provider inconsistency in seeking an order for advancing the patient when indicated by screening parameters, specific reasons cited by the physician for not weaning the patient, and inconsistent respiratory care provider coverage (260). Additionally, other patient factors may come into consideration when trying to successfully implement a weaning protocol. In neurosurgical patients, neurologic impairment may interfere with the successful implementation of a weaning protocol due to neurologic impairment (264).

Sedation protocols have shown a variable effect on weaning from mechanical ventilation in the literature. Duane et al. (255) found that a combined sedation and weaning protocol did not effect duration of weaning, number of ICU days, ICU charges, or self-extubation rates in 328 patients receiving mechanical ventilation. Similarly, Devlin et al. (265) found that although a sedation protocol promoting lorazepam over midazolam and propofol for breakthrough agitation did not alter the duration of weaning from mechanical ventilation but did significantly reduce total sedation drug cost by 75%. Since that study, however, propofol has come off patent and such cost saving may no longer be demonstrable. More recently, Kress et al. (266) demonstrated that in patients receiving mechanical ventilation, daily interruption of sedative–drug infusions decreased the duration of mechanical ventilation and the LOS in the ICU. Care must be taken when using any sedative regimen in mechanically ventilated patients as most tend to be respiratory depressants as illustrated by Khamiees et al. (267), who found that a propofol infusion resulted in significantly lower tidal volumes, higher rapid-shallow-breathing index (RSBI), and a higher respiratory rate when compared to the same patients without the infusion.

C. Cost–Benefit of Weaning Protocols

Weaning protocols have been shown to produce dramatic cost–savings in difficult-to-wean patients. Ely et al. (249) implemented once-daily screening of respiratory function to identify patients ready for a spontaneous breathing trial and reduced ICU costs. Cohen et al. (259) showed that a ventilatory management team supervising ventilatory management could save an estimated U.S.$ 1303.00 per episode of mechanical ventilation. Kollef et al. (253) found that protocol-guided weaning of mechanical ventilation, as performed by nurses and respiratory therapists, resulted in a U.S.$ 42,960.00 savings as compared to physician-directed weaning. Smyrnios et al. (254) started a multifaceted, multidisciplinary weaning management program and decreased total cost per case of from U.S.$ 92,933.00 to 63,687.00. However, some studies have failed to show any economic benefit to the implementation of weaning protocols or teams. Henneman et al. (251) found that although ICU LOS and ventilator time were reduced, there were no significant differences between groups related to cost or incidence of complications.

D. Evaluation for Extubation

When the patients' respiratory condition begins to improve and meets appropriate clinical criteria, they may be considered for extubation. Some commonly accepted criteria for consideration of discontinuation

Table 8 Criteria for Consideration for Discontinuation of Mechanical Ventilation and Extubation

1. Resolution of etiology of need for respiratory support
2. Adequate respiratory drive
3. Stable cardiovascular status with minimal or stable inotropes or pressors
4. $PaO_2/FiO_2 \geq 300$
5. PEEP ≤ 10 cm H_2O
6. Normothermia
7. No impending investigational studies that might require significant sedation
8. Ability to protect airway

Source: From Ref. 269a.

of mechanical ventilatory support can be seen in Table 8. Some authors have challenged these common sense guidelines and demonstrated that some patients might thrive off artificial ventilation in spite of poor respiratory function. In a study of 91 critically ill patients requiring prolonged mechanical ventilation, Khamiees et al. (268) found that patients with a PaO_2/FiO_2 (P:F) ratio of 120–200 were not less likely to be successfully extubated than those with P:F ratios of >200. Keep in mind that these are only general guidelines only and do not substitute for sound clinical judgment.

Numerous parameters have been measured and developed to assist the physician with predicting successful extubation and removal from mechanical ventilation. These extubation parameters can be divided into measures of neuromuscular function, measures of respiratory muscle load, and various integrative indices derived to predict successful liberation from mechanical ventilation, as well as weaning effects on other organs (269). In spite of the development of these parameters, clinical assessment of the patient's respiratory status and potential to thrive off mechanical ventilation remains essential in the evaluation for ETT removal (Table 9).

Table 9 Criteria to Predict Successful Removal of Endotracheal Tube

Mechanical factors
MV $<$ 15 L/min
NIF $<$ –25 cm H_2O
VC $>$ 10 cc/kg
Work $<$ 5 J/min (exclusive of endotracheal tube work)
Integrative factors
$f/V_t < 105$
CROP index $>$ 13
Weaning score based on compliance, resistance, VD/V_t, $PaCO_2$ and $f/V_t < 3$
Weaning index (PTI $\times$ MV for $PaCO_2$ of $40/V_t$) < 4
Neural network
PTI $<$ 0.15
Patient assessment
Absence of
Dyspnea
Accessory muscle use
Abdominal paradox
Agitation, anxiety, tachycardia

MV, minute ventilation; VC, vital capacity; PTI, pressure–time index; V_t, tidal volume; NIF, negative inspiratory force; f/V_t, frequency/tidal volume ratio (rapid shallow breathing index); CROP, compliance rate oxygenation pressure.
Source: Ref. 269a.

1. *Measures of Neuromuscular Function*

Many measures of the adequacy of neuromuscular function have been developed to predict sufficient respiratory muscle strength and endurance as well as cognitive function to protect the airway and participate in postextubation respiratory therapy to ensure successful extubation. The most commonly used parameters are the vital capacity (VC), minute ventilation (MV), airway occlusion pressure measured at 0.1 sec ($P_{0.1}$) after the start of inspiration, and the negative inspiratory force (NIF or $P_{0.1}$/maximal inspiratory pressure). Controversy exists in the literature as to which parameter is superior in predicting successful liberation from mechanical ventilation. The most commonly used measures are an MV $<$ 15 L/min, a VC $>$ 10 cc/kg, and an NIF $<$ –25 cm H_2O (270,271). Yang and Tobin (272) found the NIF to be one of the best predictors of failure and the most sensitive predictor (1.0) of successful weaning; it was, however, not very specific (0.11). Zeggwagh et al. (273) performed a multivariate analysis of 101 mechanically ventilated patients and found VC (threshold value = 635 mL) and NIF (threshold value = 28 cm H_2O) to offer accurate prediction of early extubation. Capdevila et al. (274) found that in 67 ready-to-wean long-term ventilated patients following a successful 20 min T-piece trial, the $P_{0.1}$ and the NIF predicted successful extubation in 88% and 98% of patients, respectively. They also found that the $P_{0.1}$ and the NIF were not influenced by tracheal tube resistance. Gandia and Blanco (275) found $P_{0.1}$ and NIF to predict weaning success with a diagnostic accuracy between 82% and 87%. Not all investigators have found these measures of neuromuscular function to be very sensitive or specific. Hilbert et al. (276) found that $P_{0.1}$ in COPD patients did not adequately predict postextubation respiratory failure.

One subjective measure of neuromuscular function has been investigated by Khamiees et al. (268), who found that an inability to clear secretions with a weak cough resulted in a fourfold increase in the risk of unsuccessful extubation.

2. Measures of Respiratory Muscle Load

The WOB imposed by the ETT and ventilator circuit can be measured by the use of an esophageal balloon (P_{es}, an estimate of pleural pressure) and can eventually lead to weaning failure (277). Muscle loads can be expressed as either work or pressure–time products (PTPs) per breath. The measured work can then be expressed as in relation to time (work/min) or ventilation (work/L), or to maximum muscle strength (PTP/NIF). As the former two values approach normal (5 J/min or 0.5 J/L), it becomes more likely that discontinuation of mechanical ventilation will be successful (277). The latter measure, PTP/NIF, can be multiplied by the inspiratory time fraction (T_I/tot), which gives the pressure–time index (PTI), which can predict fatigue above 0.15 (278). Kirton et al. (279) measured the WOB by integrating the change in intraesophageal pressure with tidal volume and concluded that the increased WOB during spontaneous ventilation may be misinterpreted as weaning failure (i.e., tachypnea) thus prolonging intubation. The ability to measure the contribution of imposed WOB by the ETT and ventilator circuit to the total WOB can identify those patients who may be safely extubated when the physiologic WOB (total WOB minus imposed WOB) is acceptable. Gluck et al. (280) evaluated clinical weaning vs. an esophageal balloon pressure manometry-guided protocol and found that the latter resulted in more aggressive weaning with a 1.68-day reduction in mechanical ventilation. However, Levy et al. (281) demonstrated that patient WOB was less accurate than conventional weaning parameters and clinical judgment for predicting successful extubation.

3. Integrative Indices

Successful liberation from mechanical ventilation remains challenging and it is often difficult to decide when and how to begin the process. Additionally, there are numerous published integrative indices with varying sensitivities and specificities and choosing among them can be confusing and difficult. The most common integrative indices are the rapid-shallow-breathing index (RSBI or f/V_t), the CROP index (compliance–rate–oxygenation–pressure), the weaning index (PTI $\times$ MV for $PaCO_2$ of $40/V_t$) < 4, and the weaning score. The RSBI and CROP were first described by Yang and Tobin (272), who found the former to be the most accurate predictor of failure, and its absence the most accurate predictor of success in weaning patients from mechanical ventilation. In their study, the RSBI had a sensitivity of 0.97 and a specificity of 0.64. Vassilakopoulos et al. (282) concluded that the TTI (the product of mean transdiaphragmatic pressure/maximum transdiaphragmatic pressure and the inspiratory duty cycle) and the RSBI are the major pathophysiologic determinants underlying the transition from weaning failure to weaning success. Capdevila et al. (274) found that following a successful 20 min T-piece trial, the RSBI predicted successful extubation in 73%. Numerous investigators have found the RSBI to have a positive predictive value of about 0.80 when ≤ 105 for weaning success (272,273,275,283,284), while some have found that a RSBI threshold value of ≤ 105 may not be specific enough to prevent extubation failure (285). However, most clinicians use still a RSBI threshold of < 105 as predicted successful liberation from mechanical ventilation. Keep in mind, when interpreting the RSBI, that gender differences may influence the choice of the threshold value. In 1996, Epstein and Ciubotaru (286) found that women, especially when breathing through small ETTs, have a higher RSBI (including likelihood of RSBI ≥ 100) than men, independent of extubation outcome. The weaning index was not found to be as sensitive as the RSBI in predicting successful from mechanical ventilation (287). The weaning score was an attempt by Gluck to improve upon the RSBI by combining static compliance, airway resistance, dead space to tidal volume ratio, $PaCO_2$, and frequency/tidal volume into a scoring system. These variables were chosen because they were the only ones found to have sufficiently low false-positive and false-negative prediction rates for successful weaning. A score greater than 3 was associated with failure to wean in all cases. A score less than 3 usually was associated with successful weaning but there were two false positives. The sensitivity, specificity, and positive predictive and negative predictive values for the scoring system were 1.0, 0.91, 0.83, and 1.0, respectively. None of the individual parameters included in the scoring system demonstrated equivalent statistical results (277).

Not all investigators have found these measures of neuromuscular function to be very sensitive or specific. Hilbert et al. (276) compared RSBI and $P_{0.1}$ in COPD patients and found that neither RSBI nor $P_{0.1}$ was able to adequately predict postextubation respiratory failure. Similarly, Khamiees et al. (268) demonstrated that the RSBI did not differ between successful and unsuccessful extubations.

4. Clinical Assessment

The final common pathway of all assessments of readiness for extubation is clinical evaluation of the patient's ability to support spontaneous ventilation prior to removal of the ETT. Comparisons have been made as to whether T-tube or pressure-support ventilation allows for better stratification of those being evaluated for extubation. Esteban et al. (288) found that T-piece evaluated patients failed the trial more than pressure-support patients but that the percentage of patients remaining extubated was the same. They concluded that spontaneous breathing trials with either pressure support or T-tube are suitable methods for successful discontinuation of ventilator support in patients without problems to resume spontaneous breathing.

The decision to measure weaning parameters as either as a spot check or after a period of spontaneous breathing has been investigated and the latter appears to be superior. Rivera and Weissman (289) noted that during an SIMV wean, the RSBI was higher in those patients who failed to wean thus allowing for an early determination of whether weaning would succeed. Vallverdu et al. (290) found that after a 2-hr T-piece trial, the RSBI, NIF, $P_{0.1}$, maximal expiratory pressure (MEP), and VC accurately classified 74.6% of weaning successes. Leitch et al. (291) found that after a successful 1-hr spontaneous breathing trial, only V_e (threshold > 10 L/min) and RSBI (threshold > 100) demonstrated a moderate sensitivity of 67% and 52% and specificity of 33% and 94%, respectively for predicting reintubation, whereas expired minute ventilation and NIF did not.

Chatila et al. (292) compared the RSBI, NIF, and spontaneous minute volume (V_e spont) before weaning and the RSBI 30 and 60 min after the onset of weaning. The patient's primary physician made weaning decisions. Initial RSBI sensitivity was 89%, specificity was 41%, positive predictive value was 72%, negative predictive value was 68%, and accuracy was 71%. The RSBI 30 and 60 min after the initiation of weaning sensitivity was 98%, specificity was 59%, positive predictive value was 83%, negative predictive value was 94%, and accuracy was 85%. Accuracies for the NIF and V_e spont were 66% and 62%, respectively. The area under the receiver–operator curve (RVR) for the RSBI at 30 min (0.92 ± 0.03) was higher than the RVR initial (0.74 ± 0.05), NIF (0.68 ± 0.06), and V_e (0.54 ± 0.06) ($P < 0.05$). They conclude that the RVR is more accurate than other commonly utilized clinical tools in predicting the outcome of weaning from mechanical ventilation and that the RVR measured at 30 min is superior to the RVR in the first minute of weaning.

Similar results were found by Krieger et al. (285), who showed in a retrospective analysis that the published threshold value for RSBI (≤105) had poor predictability for weaning success when measured at the beginning of the weaning trial. In the 9 of 10 patients who failed to wean in the retrospective review, the RSBI increased to > 130 as the trial progressed over 2–3 hr. These same authors also showed that delaying testing of the RSBI to later in the course of a spontaneously breathing trial can further increase the specificity of the RSBI to accurately predict extubation success. When the RSBI threshold value for prospectively predicting successful weaning was increased from ≤105 up to ≤130, the diagnostic accuracy, sensitivity, specificity, positive predictive value, and negative predictive value increased from 84%, 92%, 57%, 87%, and 67%, respectively, when measured at the beginning of the weaning trial to 92%, 93%, 89%, 97%, and 80%, respectively, when measured 3 hr later. The RVR for the RSBI also improved from 0.81 to 0.93 (285).

Thus, it is possible to increase the likelihood of predicting successful extubation if the weaning parameters are measured after a period of spontaneous breathing. However, it does not appear that prolonging the period of spontaneous breathing beyond 30 min significantly increases the predictive power of these measurements. Esteban et al. (293) also showed that successful 30- and 120-min spontaneous breathing trials equally predicted successful extubation and that there was no significant difference in the rate of success between once-daily trials and multiple trials of spontaneous breathing (242). Similarly, Perren et al.(294) found pressure-supported spontaneous breathing trials of 30 and 60 min to be equally effective in successfully predicting liberation from mechanical ventilation. Other investigators, however, did not find that spontaneous breathing trials offered any advantages in successfully predicting weaning outcome (295).

A careful clinical evaluation prior to extubation involves a thorough physical examination, with specific attention to neurologic and cardiopulmonary status, and a review of pertinent laboratory and radiologic examinations. Namen et al. (264) found that in 100 neurosurgical patients, the odds of successful extubation increased by 39% with each GCS score increment. A GCS score ≥ 8 at extubation was associated with success in 75% of cases, vs. 33% for a GCS score < 8. Implementation of a weaning protocol based on traditional respiratory physiologic parameters had practical limitations in neurosurgical patients, owing to concerns about neurologic impairment. Whereas, Khamiees et al. (268) discovered that patients with moderate-to-abundant secretions were more than eight times as likely to have unsuccessful extubations as those with no or mild secretions. Additionally, poor cough strength and significant endotracheal secretions were synergistic in predicting extubation failure. These same authors found that patients with hemoglobin levels ≤ 10 g/dL were more than five times as likely to have unsuccessful extubations as compared to those with hemoglobin levels > 10 g/dL. Although albumin concentration on ICU admission is not a predictor of the length of time spent receiving mechanical ventilation, its trend is important in determining the relative chance of being successfully weaned from the ventilator (296).

5. *Physiologic Response to Weaning and Weaning Failure*

Extubation failure rates range from 2% to 25% (131,132,291). Patients fail weaning and extubation for many reasons, including neurologic, cardiac, respiratory, neuromuscular, gastrointestinal, and anatomical. Weaning from mechanical ventilation can trigger alterations in the hemodynamic, respiratory, and metabolic systems that can impair weaning or lead to other adverse sequelae.

6. *Weaning Effects on Other Organs*

Neuromuscular

Having an awake and alert patient can certainly improve the likelihood of successful weaning and, conversely, a patient with a depressed mental status may prove difficult to wean. Namen et al. (264) found that in 100 neurosurgical patients, the odds of successful extubation increased by 39% with each GCS score increment. A GCS score ≥ 8 at extubation was associated with success in 75% of cases, vs. 33% for a GCS score < 8. It is common that the level of sedation is dramatically reduced prior to attempts at weaning. This may result in patient disorientation, agitation, and pain as their level of consciousness returns to normal. They are often in a new and unfamiliar environment and feelings of claustrophobia may begin as they do not yet recall why they are restrained with an ETT in place. Although agitation during the weaning process can be due to patient confusion or discomfort, it may also be a sign of early respiratory discomfort and impending weaning failure.

Severe muscle weakness from prolonged immobility or drugs [aminoglycosides (297), neuromuscular blockers (298,299), or steroids (300)] can lead to muscle atrophy or neuromuscular dysfunction referred to as critical illness polyneuropathy (CIP). In one study looking at patients with prolonged failure to wean from mechanical ventilation without identifiable pulmonary causes, all were found to have evidence of CIP regardless of the type of primary illness (301). Others have shown that CIP does not necessarily implicate difficult weaning from artificial ventilation (302). Although many weaning failure patients display diaphragmatic weakness, there is no evidence of low-frequency diaphragm fatigue (303).

Cardiovascular

The physiologic stress of weaning can increase the metabolic demands on the heart in cases with limited myocardial oxygen reserve and lead to myocardial ischemia and weaning failure. In postcardiovascular surgical patients, it has been observed that there is a rise in the cardiac index (CI) and a variable rise in the oxygen extraction ratio during weaning from mechanical ventilation (304). One study found that 6% of patients who fail to wean do so due to cardiac ischemia and this was more likely to occur in patients with coronary artery disease (305). Hurford and Favorito (306) similarly found that myocardial ischemia (as detected by a 24-hr, continuous Holter monitor) occurs frequently in ventilator-dependent patients and that the occurrence of ischemia was associated with failure to wean from mechanical ventilation. In a study of 83 patients with coronary artery disease being weaned from mechanical ventilation, Srivastava et al. (307) found that 9.6% of these patients experience ECG evidence of myocardial ischemia and the presence of ischemia significantly increased the risk of weaning failure (risk ratio = 2.1). Marcelino et al. (308) used echocardiography to measure heart function during weaning and found that isovolumetric relaxation time was a good predictor of successful weaning, thus illustrating the importance of diastolic changes with hemodynamic adaptation to negative pressure ventilation.

Respiratory

Obviously, failure to maintain adequate oxygenation due to significant intrapulmonary shunt (i.e., persistent pneumonia, ARDS, and pulmonary edema) or perfusion deficits (i.e., pulmonary embolism) will result in weaning failure. Hypoventilation can also lead to a failure of weaning with a rise in $PaCO_2$ and ultimately depressed mental status. Epstein et al. (309), in a study of elderly patients requiring more than 3 days of ventilation, found that although all patients had increases in oxygen consumption during weaning, those who were successfully weaned had decreases before extubation. Respiratory rate, NIF, the ratio of PaO_2 to fraction of inspired oxygen, and mean arterial pressure were higher in patients who could be weaned, while the oxygen cost of breathing and central venous pressure were lower. The mechanisms of postextubation failure in patients with COPD have been studied by Jubran and Tobin (310), who found that the development of acute respiratory distress during failed weaning attempts was due to worsening of pulmonary mechanics. This occurred in conjunction with rapid-shallow breathing that led to inefficient clearance of CO_2. An analysis of the inspiratory PTP revealed a 111% increase in the intrinsic PEEP (PEEPi), a 33% increase in the non-PEEPi elastic component, and a 42% increase in the resistive component. In spite of the rise in the PTP, most of the patients developed failure due to an increase in the $PaCO_2$. Another study looked at a broader spectrum of critically ill patients and found that patients unsuccessfully weaned exhibited more chaotic breathing patterns (i.e., increases in variation of tidal volumes, peak inspiratory flows, respiratory rate, and in entropy) when compared to those patients successfully weaned (311,312).

Gastrointestinal

Increased intraperitoneal volume secondary to ascities, bowel distension from ileus or bowel obstruction, organomegally, or tumor burden can lead to significant elevation of the diaphragms and a reduction in functional residual capacity and other lung volumes. Occasionally, a diaphragmatic hernia, most often on the left, can impair lung expansion and impede weaning (313).

Anatomical

Certain airway pathologies may not become apparent until they impair respiration after removal of the ETT. Prolonged ETI can lead to tracheal stenosis or tracheomalacia which may present as respiratory failure that does not become clinically evident until after removal of the ETT. In these patients, re-establishment of the airway with a longer tracheal tube or tracheal stent allowed most of the patients to be weaned (314). In a case report by St. John and Pacht (315), an unweanable COPD patient was found to have significant distal tracheal occlusion due to herpetic tracheitis and was successfully weaned once the tracheitis resolved with antiviral therapy. A noninterventional approach to overcome post-ETT removal airway obstruction has been investigated by some clinicians, who have advocated the use of a helium–oxygen mixture to improve patient comfort by decreasing the inspiratory effort (316). This mixture, however, did not improve gas exchange.

Inadequate Resources

The availability of adequate nursing and respiratory therapist resources is vitally important in optimally managing the critically ill mechanically ventilated patient. Thorens et al. (317) developed an "index of nursing" comparing the effective workforce of the nurses (number and qualifications) with the ideal workforce required by the number of patients and the severity of their diseases. A value of 1.0 represented a perfect match between the needed and the effectively present nurses, whereas a lesser value signified a diminished available workforce. This index was compared with the complications and duration of weaning from mechanical ventilation. During the first 5 years, the duration of mechanical ventilation increased progressively from 7.3 $\pm$ 8.0 to 38.2 $\pm$ 25.8 days ($P = 0.006$) and a significant inverse correlation between the duration of mechanical ventilation and the nursing index ($P = 0.025$) was found. In the sixth comparative year, the number of nurses increased (nursing index $= 1.05$) and the duration of mechanial ventilation decreased to 9.9 $\pm$ 13 days ($P = 0.001$), year 5 vs. year 6). They concluded that the quality of nursing appears to be a measurable and critical factor in the weaning from mechnical ventilation of patients with COPD. Below a thresold in the available workforce os ICU nurses, the weaning duration of patients with COPD increases dramatically and number of ICU nurses. Therefore, very close attention should be given to the education and number of ICU nurses.

V. ADVANCED VENTILATION

ARDS is a severe disease that carries a poor prognosis with an average mortality of 50% (318). Numerous therapeutic alternatives to conventional ventilation have been studied to improve outcome from ARDS, including high-frequency oscillatory ventilation (HF-OV), prone positioning, nitric oxide, and extracorporeal membrane oxygenation. The latter two will not be discussed as they remain in the experimental stages of development at this time. With severe unilateral lung disease, differential lung ventilation (DLV) has been advocated to improve ventilation/perfusion mismatching.

A. High-Frequency Ventilation

High-frequency ventilation (HFV) has been advocated for cases of severe respiratory insufficiency that fail conventional ventilation. Several modes of HFV have been developed. High-frequency positive-pressure ventilation (HFPPV) is achieved by increasing the respiratory rate to 60–100 breaths/min. High-frequency jet ventilation (HFJV) delivers frequencies of 100–600 breaths/min under high pressure via either a side channel of a special ETT or a small cannula passed through the ETT. High-frequency oscillatory ventilation involves passive gas flow (CPAP) with superimposed oscillation at a frequency of 1380–2400 breaths/min. Numerous case reports have been published describing survivors of ARDS who failed to respond to conventional ventilation measures and were subsequently treated with HFV (81,319). When compared to CMV and IMV conventional ventilation, HFV improves the PaO_2/FiO_2 ratio and reduces mean airway pressure (320), central venous pressure, and the need for sedatives and narcotics (321) but does not result in a reduction in mortality, ICU LOS, or barotrauma (320). In addition, HFOV has been shown to decrease inflammatory mediator release, which suggests reduced VILI (157,322–326). High-frequency ventilation has not definitively been shown to be superior to conventional ventilation, but many critical care practitioners managing patients dying of hypoxic respiratory failure have been impressed by its potential.

Several studies have demonstrated that HFV improves oxygenation in patients failing conventional ventilation (327). A group of 32 ARDS patients failing to improve on conventional ventilation were placed on HFV with a subsequent increase in PaO_2/FiO_2 ratio and mean airway pressure (328). In a group of six burn patients with ARDS, HFOV was initiated as "rescue therapy" and rapidly improved oxygenation and PaO_2/FiO_2 within 12 hr. Five of the six patients died, but none because of oxygenation failure (329). Sixteen ARDS patients were placed on HFOV with a subsequent improvement in PaO_2/FiO_2 and maintenance of hemodynamic stability (330). A group of five trauma patients who failed CMV were placed on HFOV and by 2 hr, the PaO_2/FiO_2 had improved significantly (52.2 ± 4.76 vs. 126.8 ± 21) and the mean and peak airway pressure were significantly reduced (34.6 ± 1.6 vs. 25.2 and 52.4 ± 3 vs. 35.8 ± 3.01, respectively) (331). Seventeen ARDS patients failing inverse ratio mechanical ventilation were placed on HFOV with incremental increases in mean airway pressure to achieve a $PaO_2 \geq 60$ Torr, with an $FiO_2 \leq 0.6$. Thirteen of the patients showed improved gas exchange and improvement in PaO_2/FiO_2 ratio in addition to reductions of the oxygenation index and FiO_2 (332). A patient who developed ARDS after a pneumonectomy for bronchogenic carcinoma failing to maintain oxygenation on conventional ventilation dramatically improved oxygenation after the initiation of HFOV with no negative side effects (333). In the largest randomized, controlled trial in acute respiratory distress syndrome patients ($n = 148$) to date comparing HFOV with a pressure-control ventilation strategy (PaO_2/FiO_2 ratio of $\leq$200 mmHg on PEEP of > 10 cm H_2O), there was an early (< 16 hr) improvement in PaO_2/FiO_2 ($P = 0.008$) in the HFOV group but no significant difference in oxygenation index between the two groups during the initial 72 hr of treatment. Thirty-day mortality was 37% in the HFOV group and 52% in the conventional ventilation group ($P = 0.102$). There was no significant difference between treatment groups in the prevalence of barotrauma, hemodynamic instability, or mucus plugging. This study suggests that HFOV is as effective and safe as the conventional strategy to which it was compared (334).

Early initiation of HFV in patients failing CMV may result in improved patient outcomes (332). In 24 adult patients with ARDS, HFOV survivors were mechanically ventilated for fewer days before institution of HFOV compared with nonsurvivors (1.6 ± 1.2 vs. 7.8 ± 5.8 days, $P = 0.001$) (327).

High-frequency ventilation is hemodynamically well tolerated as most studies have not demonstrated evidence of hemodynamic impairment with the implementation of HFOV (332). In a study of 10 ARDS patients failing conventional ventilation who were placed on high-frequency percussive ventilation (HFPV), there was an improvement in oxygenation and PaO_2/FiO_2 ratio without significant increases in PIP or changes in hemodynamic parameters (335). In another study, 32 ARDS patients failing to improve on conventional ventilation, initiation of HFPV resulted in a decrease in the PIP without changes to hemodynamic parameters (328). Other studies, however, have resulted in higher PAOP, CVP, and a reduction in CO without significant change in systemic or pulmonary pressure associated with HFOV (327). Ultrahigh-frequency ventilation has also been shown to improve PaO_2 and reduce PIP and PAW in ARDS patients failing conventional ventilation and did not result in any hemodynamic deterioration (336).

B. Combined High-Frequency Ventilation

Numerous methods of combining HFV with traditional low-frequency ventilation have been described and may be superior to HFV alone. Combined high-frequency ventilation (CHFV) involves a low respiratory rate (6–20 breaths/min), which allows for bulk flow of gas, with a superimposed high rate (250–1200 breaths/min), which adds diffusive flows characteristic of HFV. In several studies, low-frequency conventional mechanical ventilation has been superimposed on traditional HFV (337) and showed an improvement in oxygenation and a reduction of airway pressures in patients failing to improve with HFV alone (338). A 73-year-old man with ARDS due to multiple organ failure caused by *Chlamydia psittaci* failing to improve on conventional ventilation improved all ventilatory parameters after being placed on CHFV (339). This combination was well tolerated and in some cases, patients were able to continue to communicate with their families (337,340).

In patients with hemodynamic instability, combined HFV may be superior to either HFV or conventional ventilation alone. A study involving 35 patients with severe post-traumatic or septic-induced ARDS, who were refractory to conventional controlled mechanical ventilatory support were placed on CHFV which resulted in an increase in expired tidal volume, a reduction in mean airway pressure (PAW), respiratory index, and FiO_2. The reduction in PAW permitted a sustained or increased cardiac output with a rise in the DO_2/VO_2 ratio, thus allowing for a higher PaO_2 for any given level of pulmonary shunt (341). In a patient with severe myocardial and respiratory insufficiency unmanageable on conventional ventilation with high levels of PEEP and maximal inotropic support, implementation of CHFV lowered peak airway pressure and dramatically improved both cardiac and pulmonary function (342).

In an effort to further explore the possibility of additional benefits by combining HFV with ultra-high-frequency ventilation UHFV, El-Baz et al. (340) combined HFPPV at a rate of 250 breaths/min with HFOV at a rate of 2500 breaths/min and improved oxygenation over HFPPV alone and CO_2 retention in HFOV alone. This combined technique improves oxygenation by accelerated gas diffusion and facilitates CO_2 elimination by convection and is well tolerated hemodynamically. Unfortunately, 71% of the patients died of multisystem organ failure in spite of adequate oxygenation.

Currently, it has been recommended that some form of HFV be considered for clinical use in adults when FiO_2 requirements exceed 60% and mean airway pressure approaches 20 cm H(2)O or higher [or, alternatively, PEEP of >15 cm H(2)O] (343).

C. Prone Positioning

For many patients who are difficult to oxygenate, prone positioning may improve their V/Q mismatching leading to an improved PaO_2 (344–346). The posterior portions of the lung contain a proportionally larger percentage of the total lung volume than the anterior portions and thus receives the majority of cardiac output regardless of patient position. CT scanning has been used to show a progressive deflation of gas-containing alveoli along the gravity gradient (347), thus revealing that dependent portions of the lung collapse due to the weight of overlying structures. The improvement in oxygenation from prone positioning results from better gas flow to the nondependent posterior portions of the lung. Thus, the shunt fraction is reduced by placing the patient in the prone positioning by reducing posterior lung atelectasis and improving V/Q mismatching. In a study involving six patients with respiratory failure who were turned prone, there was a mean increase in the PaO_2 of 69 mmHg and a reduction of the FiO_2 in 4 of the 5 mechanically ventilated patients. Although the PaO_2 decreased in 12 of 14 instances after the patient was turned from prone to supine, no significant change in mean $PaCO_2$, respiratory rate, or effective compliance was observed (344). Mure et al. (345) found that 12 of 13 patients suffering from acute lung insufficiency demonstrated an increase in the oxygenation index and the alveolar–arterial oxygen gradient decreased dramatically with prone positioning.

Special care must be taken to position the patient properly when prone to prevent pressure ulceration and nerve stretch injury. All pressure points must be carefully padded. These pressure points include the face, shoulders, hips, elbows, knees, and feet. Additionally, special care must be taken to minimize abdominal pressure so as not to impair FRC. The shoulders should be adequately padded to prevent stretch of the brachial plexus. There are several commercially available devices to assist with proper prone positioning. However, with careful attention, the patient can be safely proned and padded using items commonly found in the ICU.

Prone positioning is reasonably well tolerated by most patients (346,348). There is a reduction in shunt fraction and chest wall compliance and, in some patients, an increase in FRC and lung compliance (346). Although obese patients may present some difficulty with patient positioning in the prone position, they also seem to benefit from this intervention (348). Brazzi et al.(346) demonstrated that obese patients could be safely proned and that although the chest wall compliance (C_{cw}) decreased, the FRC and lung compliance increased. They also demonstrated an improvement in the PaO_2 in this population. In the same study, they found that patients with ARF showed no difference in FRC, or respiratory system compliance (C_{rs}) despite a reduction in C_{cw} with proning. The position change improved PaO_2.

At our institution, we believe that patients benefit from earlier rather than later prone positioning. In order to maximize the benefits of better V/Q matching in the prone position, we typically prone patients for as long as possible during each 24-hr period. Typically, the patient is placed supine at 06:00 hr, so the patient can be examined before ICU rounds and reproned after ICU rounds are complete. The optimal duration of prone positioning lacks a consensus. Repeated prone positioning may confer some benefit (348). Kleinschmidt et al.

(349) showed that with repeated prone positioning in six patients, the oxygenation index improved significantly only during the first 2 days.

The transition from supine to prone, and vice versa, poses significant risk for the patient with severe respiratory insufficiency. Endotracheal tube displacement and hemodynamic impairment are significant risks associated with the transition from supine to prone positioning. Experience care providers, including those competent in airway management should be present when placing the patient in the prone position. Some patients will not hemodynamically tolerate the prone position and we avoid proning patients with impaired hemodynamics.

D. Differential Lung Ventilation

Unilateral lung disease that results in markedly different compliance between the affected and unaffected lung can be particularly difficult for the clinician to manage. Unilateral pulmonary contusion or pneumonia can lead to one lung that is very "stiff" compared to the unaffected lung. Gas preferentially flows to the most compliant regions of the lung possibly leading to their overdistension while less compliant areas are underfilled promoting alveolar collapse. This may result in volutrauma to the more compliant regions and alveolar collapse with increased shunt fraction and increased risk of infection in the less compliant regions. Nonselective application of PEEP may help open some areas of collapse but may also lead to further overdistension of already compliant regions. As discussed earlier, areas of pulmonary contusion may not be amenable to airway or alveolar opening due to fibrin deposition and occlusion of the airways (224). Differential lung ventilation allows for selective application of PEEP and PIPs or tidal volume to minimize lung trauma to both the compliant and noncompliant lung and reduce atelectasis (350,351) and improve V/Q mismatch (352,353). Each lung can be ventilated optimally on the compliant portion of its pressure–volume curve thus avoiding the trauma of overdistension to the more compliant lung, and alveolar shear stress to the less compliant lung. The use of appropriate distending pressures to each lung cannot only improve blood gases but also tidal volume, static compliance, and FRC of the diseased lung (354). Differential lung ventilation has proven to be hemodynamically well tolerated (355,356) and in some cases may actually improve hemodynamics compared to conventional ventilation (357).

The application of DLV and selective PEEP can result in an improvement of PaO_2 due to better V/Q matching (355,357). Talbot and Fu (358) found that in a case of traumatic unilateral lung contusion, the application of synchronized DLV revealed marked inequality in static compliance with the contused lung requiring 9 cm H_2O of PEEP while the noncontused lung required zero PEEP to equalize tidal volumes. Evident improvement in blood gases and chest radiograph was obtained within 30 min. They concluded that differential ventilation proved simple to use and highly effective in the management of severe unilateral pulmonary contusion. Alberti et al. (359) used nonsynchronized DLV in severe refractory unilateral atelectasis and demonstrated a progressive increase in compliance in the diseased lung, a fall in the required PEEP, and an improvement in the SvO_2, O_2AVI, PVRI, and Q_{va}/Q_t values. In addition, DLV has been used to successfully treat patients with unilateral bronchopleural fistula and massive unilateral pulmonary embolism (360) failing standard mechanical ventilation (351).

There is no advantage of synchronous over asynchronous DLV as demonstrated by East et al. (361) when they compared synchronous to asynchronous DLV in dogs with unilateral hydrochloric acid injury. There was no statistically significant difference in gas exchange [PaO_2, Q_{va}/Q_t, $PaCO_2$, P(A–a) O_2] or hemodynamics (mean arterial pressure, CVP, mean pulmonary arterial pressure, mean pulmonary arterial wedge pressure, cardiac output in triplicate, or heart rate) between the two groups.

Differential lung ventilation can be combined with other advanced ventilatory strategies to achieve the advantages of each. Miranda et al. (362) used DLV that combined HFPPV to the diseased lung and low-frequency conventional ventilation to the normal lung with success. Johannigman et al. (363) demonstrated that DLV combined with inhaled nitric oxide improved oxygenation in unilateral pulmonary contusion after trauma. Nishimura et al. (364) used DLV with the selective application of jet ventilation to the injured lung of a patient with massive atelectasis secondary to pulmonary hemorrhage and markedly improved arterial oxygenation.

VI. TERMINAL WEANING

The decision to withdraw all life sustaining interventions and initiate the terminal weaning process in the mechanically ventilated patient is one of the most difficult decisions patients, families, and physicians face. It is very important that patients and families be given very frank information regarding the current clinical condition and prognosis. Often, once confronted with the reality of their clinical condition, many patients and/or their families will come to the conclusion that it is time to allow the natural progression of their clinical condition to run its course. Once the decision to proceed with withdrawal of care has been made and appropriately documented in the medical record, it is crucial to assure the patient and/or the family that the entire focus of care from that point on will be to assure the comfort of both the patient and the family. Families need to be given time for the appropriate support structure to assemble, and visitation limits need to be liberalized. Often this involves awaiting the arrival of other family members, friends, or clergy. Once the patient's spiritual needs have been addressed and the patient and/or family are ready to begin withdrawing care, sedation and analgesia infusions are begun if not already present. An order should be placed in the chart to direct the nurse to titrate these medications to patient comfort. Nurses need to be comfortable titrating these medications and be able to promptly respond to signs of discomfort in order to assure a peaceful death.

Once the patient is comfortable, care may begin to be withdrawn. All the monitors and alarms in the room should be turned off if remote monitoring is available in ICU. If remote monitoring is not possible, then all monitors except the telemetry monitoring should be discontinued and all alarms suspended. This is important as the flashing numbers and recurrent alarms as the patient deteriorates will only serve as a source of stress for the family. All medications, except the analgesia and anxiolysis infusions, and laboratory studies are then discontinued.

If the patient is intubated, it is our practice to leave the ETT in place when withdrawing care. We have found that patients tend to exhibit less agonal or "fish-mouth" breathing which only distresses family mem-

Table 10 ICU End of Life Orders

- ☐ Verify DNR orders are consistent with a plan of care optimizing patient comfort.
- ☐ Titrate medications to alleviate the patient's signs & symptoms of discomfort.
- ☐ Contact Chaplain of family's choice for spiritual support

Transitional Care: (enact all orders unless otherwise specified)

- ☐ Discontinue neuromuscular blockade agents prior to weaning ventilator.
- ☐ Discontinue all tests and laboratory studies.
- ☐ Remove all monitoring equipment from the patient and patient's bedside except for the ECG.
- ☐ Suspend arrhythmia detection at bedside and central station.
- ☐ Suspend or decrease all auditory alarms at bedside and central station.
- ☐ Discontinue medications and fluids when appropriate:
  ☐ Hydration ☐ Vasoactive medication ☐ other________________
- ☐ Discontinue mechanical support devices:
  ☐ Dialysis ☐ IABP ☐ other________________
- ☐ Assess and monitor the patient for signs and symptoms of discomfort.
- ☐ Liberalize visitation.

Medications:

- ☐ Morphine drip at __________mg/hr **or** ☐ Fentanyl drip at __________mcg/hr.
- ☐ Lorazepam drip at __________mg/hr **or** ☐ Midazolam drip at __________mg/hr.
- ☐ Other medication drips (i.e. benzodiazepine, barbiturate, propofol):
  ☐ _______________mg/mcg/kg/hr ☐ ________________mg/mcg/kg/hr
- ☐ For signs of patient discomfort give IV bolus of medication equal to drip rate every 3-5 minutes until patient is comfortable.
- ☐ To **maintain** patient comfort, increase drip rate up to 50 % of prior rate.
- ☐ Contact physician and charge nurse regarding patient status.

Ventilator:

- ☐ Initiate ventilator wean once patient appears comfortable.
- ☐ Oscillatory Ventilation converted to conventional ventilator.
- ☐ Initial Ventilator setting: F_iO_2__________ Bilevel – High PEEP_____ Low PEEP_________
  PS_______IMV__________PEEP__________
- ☐ Reduce all ventilator alarms to minimum settings.
- ☐ Transition F_iO_2 to 0.21 and PEEP to zero.
- ☐ Assess for signs and symptoms of patient discomfort while decreasing the tidal volume and rate.
- ☐ When the patient is comfortable on minimal ventilator support, select one:
  ☐ extubate to room air ☐ T-piece ☐ remain on ventilator

bers at the bedside. However, some awake patients or families might request extubation prior to withdrawing care. Some authors have used bipap to successfully assist with respiratory discomfort during this process (100,109).

If the ETT is to remain in place, the next step is to remove all ventilatory supports. Although some authors will place the patient on a T-piece, we like to leave the patient attached to the ventilator. All ventilator alarms are suspended and apneic ventilation turned off. Finally, the patient is placed on CPAP with a pressure support and PEEP of zero and an FiO_2 of 0.21 (room air).

We have developed an order set, see Table 10, specially designed to assist with our terminal weaning process and assure that the dying experience is optimized for the patient and their family.

REFERENCES

1. Maschmeyer G, Bertschat FL, Moesta KT, et al. Outcome analysis of 189 consecutive cancer patients referred to the intensive care unit as emergencies during a 2-year period. Eur J Cancer 2003; 39(6): 783–792.
2. Huaringa AJ, Leyva FJ, Giralt SA, et al. Outcome of bone marrow transplantation patients requiring mechanical ventilation. Crit Care Med 2000; 28(4): 1014–1017.
3. Arisawa C, Fujii Y, Higashi Y, Owada F, Shimizu S, Kaneko K. Acute respiratory failure resulting from diffuse microscopic pulmonary tumor emboli by bladder cancer: a case diagnosed at autopsy. Hinyokika Kiyo 1993; 39:475–478.
4. Jiang JR, Shih JY, Wang HC, Wu RM, Yu CJ, Yang PC. Small-cell lung cancer presenting with Lambert–Eaton myasthenic syndrome and respiratory failure. J Formos Med Assoc 2002; 101:871–874.
5. Nakahara K, Ohno K, Hashimoto J, et al. Prediction of postoperative respiratory failure in patients undergoing lung resection for lung cancer. Ann Thorac Surg 1988; 46:549–552.
6. Nishioka A, Ogawa Y, Hamada N, Terashima M, Inomata T, Yoshida S. Analysis of radiation pneumonitis and radiation-induced lung fibrosis in breast cancer patients after breast conservation treatment. Oncol Rep 1999; 6:513–517.
7. Segawa Y, Takigawa N, Kataoka M, Takata I, Fujimoto N, Ueoka H. Risk factors for development of radiation pneumonitis following radiation therapy with or without chemotherapy for lung cancer. Int J Radiat Oncol Biol Phys 1997; 39:91–98.
8. Putterman C, Polliack A. Late cardiovascular and pulmonary complications of therapy in Hodgkin's disease: report of three unusual cases, with a review of relevant literature. Leuk Lymphoma 1992; 7:109–115.
9. Ikezoe J, Takashima S, Morimoto S, et al. CT appearance of acute radiation-induced injury in the lung. AJR Am J Roentgenol 1988; 150:765–770.
10. Sangha S, Uber PA, Mehra MR. Difficult cases in heart failure: amiodarone lung injury: another heart failure mimic? Congest Heart Fail 2002; 8:93–96.
11. Dimopoulou I, Marathias K, Daganou M, et al. Low-dose amiodarone-related complications after cardiac operations. J Thorac Cardiovasc Surg 1997; 114:31–37.
12. Copper JA Jr. Drug-induced lung disease. Adv Intern Med 1997; 42:231–268.
13. Pitcher WD. Amiodarone pulmonary toxicity. Am J Med Sci 1992; 303:206–212.
14. Pollak PT, Sharma AD, Carruthers SG. Relation of amiodarone hepatic and pulmonary toxicity to serum drug concentrations and superoxide dismutase activity. Am J Cardiol 1990; 65:1185–1191.
15. Martin WJ II. Mechanisms of amiodarone pulmonary toxicity. Clin Chest Med 1990; 11:131–138.
16. Smith GJ. The histopathology of pulmonary reactions to drugs. Clin Chest Med 1990; 11:95–117.
17. Kennedy TP, Gordon GB, Paky A, et al. Amiodarone causes acute oxidant lung injury in ventilated and perfused rabbit lungs. J Cardiovasc Pharmacol 1988; 12:23–36.
18. Martin WJ II, Rosenow EC III. Amiodarone pulmonary toxicity. Recognition and pathogenesis (part 2). Chest 1988; 93:1242–1248.
19. Cazzadori A, Braggio P, Barbieri E, Ganassini A. Amiodarone-induced pulmonary toxicity. Respiration 1986; 49:157–160.
20. Martin WJ, Howard DM. Amiodarone-induced lung toxicity. In vitro evidence for the direct toxicity of the drug. Am J Pathol 1985; 120:344–350.
21. Cantor JO, Osman M, Cerreta JM, Suarez R, Mandl I, Turino GM. Amiodarone-induced pulmonary fibrosis in hamsters. Exp Lung Res 1984; 6:1–10.
22. McCusker K, Dorman RA, Nicholson DP, Hough AJ. Reversible pulmonary injury after a small dose of bleomycin. South Med J 1983; 76:1447–1449.
23. Moseley PL, Shasby DM, Brady M, Hunninghake GW. Lung parenchymal injury induced by bleomycin. Am Rev Respir Dis 1984; 130:1082–1086.
24. Adamson IY, Bowden DH. Bleomycin-induced injury and metaplasia of alveolar type 2 cells. Relationship of cellular responses to drug presence in the lung. Am J Pathol 1979; 96:531–544.
25. Eisenbeis CF, Winn D, Poelman S, Polsky CV, Rubenstein JH, Olopade OI. A case of pulmonary toxicity associated with G-CSF and doxorubicin administration. Ann Hematol 2001; 80:121–123.
26. Baciewicz FA Jr, Arredondo M, Chaudhuri B, et al. Pharmacokinetics and toxicity of isolated perfusion of lung with doxorubicin. J Surg Res 1991; 50: 124–128.
27. Minchin RF, Johnston MR, Schuller HM, Aiken MA, Boyd MR. Pulmonary toxicity of doxorubicin

administered by in situ isolated lung perfusion in dogs. Cancer 1988; 61:1320–1325.

28. Cohen IJ, Loven D, Schoenfeld T, et al. Dactinomycin potentiation of radiation pneumonitis: a forgotten interaction. Pediatr Hematol Oncol 1991; 8:187–192.
29. Ma LD, Taylor GA, Wharam MD, Wiley JM. "Recall" pneumonitis: adriamycin potentiation of radiation pneumonitis in two children. Radiology 1993; 187:465–467.
30. Vegesna V, Withers HR, McBride WH, Holly FE. Adriamycin-induced recall of radiation pneumonitis and epilation in lung and hair follicles of mouse. Int J Radiat Oncol Biol Phys 1992; 23:977–981.
31. Son YH, Kapp DS. Esophago-pulmonary toxicity from concomitant use of adriamycin and irradiation. Conn Med 1981; 45:755–759.
32. Greco FA, Oldham RK. Adriamycin and radiation reactions. Ann Intern Med 1977; 86:655–656.
33. Singal PK, Li T, Kumar D, Danelisen I, Iliskovic N. Adriamycin-induced heart failure: mechanism and modulation. Mol Cell Biochem 2000; 207:77–86.
34. Monnet E, Orton EC. A canine model of heart failure by intracoronary adriamycin injection: hemodynamic and energetic results. J Card Fail 1999; 5:255–264.
35. Mettler FP, Young DM, Ward JM. Adriamycin-induced cardiotoxicity (cardiomyopathy and congestive heart failure) in rats. Cancer Res 1977; 37: 2705–2713.
36. Grantham JA, Borgeson DD, Burnett JC Jr. BNP: pathophysiological and potential therapeutic roles in acute congestive heart failure. Am J Physiol 1997; 272:R1077–R1083.
37. Clerico A, Iervasi G, Del Chicca MG, et al. Circulating levels of cardiac natriuretic peptides (ANP and BNP) measured by highly sensitive and specific immunoradiometric assays in normal subjects and in patients with different degrees of heart failure. J Endocrinol Invest 1998; 21:170–179.
38. Troughton RW, Frampton CM, Yandle TG, Espiner EA, Nicholls MG, Richards AM. Treatment of heart failure guided by plasma aminoterminal brain natriuretic peptide (N-BNP) concentrations. Lancet 2000; 355:1126–1130.
39. Yoshimura M, Yasue H, Ogawa H. Pathophysiological significance and clinical application of ANP and BNP in patients with heart failure. Can J Physiol Pharmacol 2001; 79:730–735.
40. Burger MR, Burger AJ. BNP in decompensated heart failure: diagnostic, prognostic and therapeutic potential. Curr Opin Investig Drugs 2001; 2:929–935.
41. Cowie MR, Mendez GF. BNP and congestive heart failure. Prog Cardiovasc Dis 2002; 44:293–321.
42. McCullough PA, Nowak RM, McCord J, et al. B-type natriuretic peptide and clinical judgment in emergency diagnosis of heart failure: analysis from Breathing Not Properly (BNP) Multinational Study. Circulation 2002; 106:416–422.
43. Lader E. BNP levels had high sensitivity but moderate specificity for detecting congestive heart failure in the emergency department. ACP J Club 2003; 138:23.
44. Shatzer M, Lauren S. Using a BNP test to identify heart failure. Nursing 2003; 33:68.
45. Pesola GR. The use of B-type natriuretic peptide (BNP) to distinguish heart failure from lung disease in patients presenting with dyspnea to the emergency department. Acad Emerg Med 2003; 10:275–277.
46. Hobbs RE. Using BNP to diagnose, manage, and treat heart failure. Cleve Clin J Med 2003; 70:333–336.
47. Maisel AS. The diagnosis of acute congestive heart failure: role of BNP measurements. Heart Fail Rev 2003; 8:327–334.
48. Maisel AS. Use of BNP levels in monitoring hospitalized heart failure patients with heart failure. Heart Fail Rev 2003; 8:339–344.
49. Cowie MR, Mendez GF. BNP and congestive heart failure. Curr Probl Cardiol 2003; 28:264–311.
50. Luhr OR, Antonsen K, Karlsson M, et al. Incidence and mortality after acute respiratory failure and acute respiratory distress syndrome in Sweden, Denmark, and Iceland. The ARF Study Group. Am J Respir Crit Care Med 1999; 159:1849–1861.
51. Behrendt CE. Acute respiratory failure in the United States: incidence and 31-day survival. Chest 2000; 118: 1100–1105.
52. Azoulay E, Recher C, Alberti C, et al. Changing use of intensive care for hematological patients: the example of multiple myeloma. Intensive Care Med 1999; 25: 1395–1401.
53. Azoulay E, Moreau D, Alberti C, et al. Predictors of short-term mortality in critically ill patients with solid malignancies. Intensive Care Med 2000; 26:1817–1823.
54. Blot F, Guiguet M, Nitenberg G, Leclercq B, Gachot B, Escudier B. Prognostic factors for neutropenic patients in an intensive care unit: respective roles of underlying malignancies and acute organ failures. Eur J Cancer 1997; 33:1031–1037.
55. Kress JP, Christenson J, Pohlman AS, Linkin DR, Hall JB. Outcomes of critically ill cancer patients in a university hospital setting. Am J Respir Crit Care Med 1999; 160:1957–1961.
56. Staudinger T, Stoiser B, Mullner M, et al. Outcome and prognostic factors in critically ill cancer patients admitted to the intensive care unit. Crit Care Med 2000; 28:1322–1328.
57. Lewandowski K, Metz J, Deutschmann C, et al. Incidence, severity, and mortality of acute respiratory failure in Berlin, Germany. Am J Respir Crit Care Med 1995; 151:1121–1125.
58. Stauffer JL, Fayter NA, Graves B, Cromb M, Lynch JC, Goebel P. Survival following mechanical ventilation for acute respiratory failure in adult men. Chest 1993; 104:1222–1229.
59. Knaus WA, Sun X, Hakim RB, Wagner DP. Evaluation of definitions for adult respiratory distress

syndrome. Am J Respir Crit Care Med 1994; 150: 311–317.
60. Cohen IL, Lambrinos J. Investigating the impact of age on outcome of mechanical ventilation using a population of 41,848 patients from a statewide database. Chest 1995; 107:1673–1680.
61. Gracey DR, Naessens JM, Krishan I, Marsh HM. Hospital and posthospital survival in patients mechanically ventilated for more than 29 days. Chest 1992; 101:211–214.
62. Pascual FE, Matthay MA, Bacchetti P, Wachter RM. Assessment of prognosis in patients with community-acquired pneumonia who require mechanical ventilation. Chest 2000; 117:503–512.
63. Epner DE, White P, Krasnoff M, Khanduja S, Kimball KT, Knaus WA. Outcome of mechanical ventilation for adults with hematologic malignancy. J Investig Med 1996; 44:254–260.
64. Swinburne AJ, Fedullo AJ, Bixby K, Lee DK, Wahl GW. Respiratory failure in the elderly. Analysis of outcome after treatment with mechanical ventilation. Arch Intern Med 1993; 153:1657–1662.
65. Knaus WA. Prognosis with mechanical ventilation: the influence of disease, severity of disease, age, and chronic health status on survival from an acute illness. Am Rev Respir Dis 1989; 140:S8–S13.
66. Vasilyev S, Schaap RN, Mortensen JD. Hospital survival rates of patients with acute respiratory failure in modern respiratory intensive care units. An international, multicenter, prospective survey. Chest 1995; 107: 1083–1088.
67. Epstein SK, Vuong V. Lack of influence of gender on outcomes of mechanically ventilated medical ICU patients. Chest 1999; 116:732–739.
68. Montaner JS, Hawley PH, Ronco JJ, et al. Multisystem organ failure predicts mortality of ICU patients with acute respiratory failure secondary to AIDS-related PCP. Chest 1992; 102:1823–1828.
69. Jimenez P, Torres A, Roca J, Cobos A, Rodriguez-Roisin R. Arterial oxygenation does not predict the outcome of patients with acute respiratory failure needing mechanical ventilation. Eur Respir J 1994; 7: 730–735.
70. Groeger JS, Glassman J, Nierman DM, et al. Probability of mortality of critically ill cancer patients at 72 h of intensive care unit (ICU) management. Support Care Cancer 2003.
71. Kroschinsky F, Weise M, Illmer T, et al. Outcome and prognostic features of intensive care unit treatment in patients with hematological malignancies. Intensive Care Med 2002; 28(9):1294–1300.
72. Larche J, Azoulay E, Fieux F, et al. Improved survival of critically ill cancer patients with septic shock. Intensive Care Med 2003.
73. Khassawneh BY, White P Jr, Anaissie EJ, Barlogie B, Hiller FC. Outcome from mechanical ventilation after autologous peripheral blood stem cell transplantation. Chest 2002; 121:185–188.
74. Gillespie DJ, Marsh HM, Divertie MB, Meadows JA III. Clinical outcome of respiratory failure in patients requiring prolonged (greater than 24 hours) mechanical ventilation. Chest 1986; 90:364–369.
75. Schuster DP. Everything that should be done—not everything that can be done. Am Rev Respir Dis 1992; 145:508–509.
76. Schuster DP, Marion JM. Precedents for meaningful recovery during treatment in a medical intensive care unit. Outcome in patients with hematologic malignancy. Am J Med 1983; 75:402–408.
77. Denardo SJ, Oye RK, Bellamy PE. Efficacy of intensive care for bone marrow transplant patients with respiratory failure. Crit Care Med 1989; 17:4–6.
78. Crawford SW, Schwartz DA, Petersen FB, Clark JG. Mechanical ventilation after marrow transplantation. Risk factors and clinical outcome. Am Rev Respir Dis 1988; 137:682–687.
79. Crawford SW, Petersen FB. Long-term survival from respiratory failure after marrow transplantation for malignancy. Am Rev Respir Dis 1992; 145:510–514.
80. Afessa B, Tefferi A, Hoagland HC, Letendre L, Peters SG. Outcome of recipients of bone marrow transplants who require intensive-care unit support. Mayo Clin Proc 1992; 67:117–122.
81. Faber-Langendoen K, Caplan AL, McGlave PB. Survival of adult bone marrow transplant patients receiving mechanical ventilation: a case for restricted use. Bone Marrow Transplant 1993; 12:501–507.
82. Paz HL, Crilley P, Weinar M, Brodsky I. Outcome of patients requiring medical ICU admission following bone marrow transplantation. Chest 1993; 104:527–531.
83. Rubenfeld GD, Crawford SW. Withdrawing life support from mechanically ventilated recipients of bone marrow transplants: a case for evidence-based guidelines. Ann Intern Med 1996; 125:625–633.
84. Jackson SR, Tweeddale MG, Barnett MJ, et al. Admission of bone marrow transplant recipients to the intensive care unit: outcome, survival and prognostic factors. Bone Marrow Transplant 1998; 21: 697–704.
85. Price KJ, Thall PF, Kish SK, Shannon VR, Andersson BS. Prognostic indicators for blood and marrow transplant patients admitted to an intensive care unit. Am J Respir Crit Care Med 1998; 158:876–884.
86. Groeger JS, White P Jr, Nierman DM, et al. Outcome for cancer patients requiring mechanical ventilation. J Clin Oncol 1999; 17:991–997.
87. Headley J, Theriault R, Smith TL. Independent validation of APACHE II severity of illness score for predicting mortality in patients with breast cancer admitted to the intensive care unit. Cancer 1992; 70:497–503.
88. Schapira DV, Studnicki J, Bradham DD, Wolff P, Jarrett A. Intensive care, survival, and expense of treating critically ill cancer patients. J Am Med Assoc 1993; 269:783–786.
89. Knaus WA, Wagner DP, Draper EA, et al. The APACHE III prognostic system. Risk prediction of

hospital mortality for critically ill hospitalized adults. Chest 1991; 100:1619–1636.

90. Torrecilla C, Cortes JL, Chamorro C, Rubio JJ, Galdos P, Dominguez de Villota E. Prognostic assessment of the acute complications of bone marrow transplantation requiring intensive therapy. Intensive Care Med 1988; 14:393–398.
91. Shaw A, Weavind L, Feeley T. Mechanical ventilation in critically ill cancer patients. Curr Opin Oncol 2001; 13(4):224–228.
92. Plant PK, Owen JL, Elliott MW. One year period prevalence study of respiratory acidosis in acute exacerbations of COPD: implications for the provision of non-invasive ventilation and oxygen administration. Thorax 2000; 55:550–554.
93. Carlucci A, Richard JC, Wysocki M, Lepage E, Brochard L. Noninvasive versus conventional mechanical ventilation. An epidemiologic survey. Am J Respir Crit Care Med 2001; 163:874–880.
94. Alsous F, Amoateng-Adjepong Y, Manthous CA. Noninvasive ventilation: experience at a community teaching hospital. Intensive Care Med 1999; 25:458–463.
95. Eremenko AA, Chaus NI, Levikov DI, Kolomiets V. Noninvasive mask ventilation of the lungs in the treatment of acute respiratory insufficiency in heart surgery patients in the postoperative period. Anesteziol Reanimatol 1997:36–38..
96. Heindl S, Karg O, Bullemer F, Kroworsch P, Pahnke J. Noninvasive ventilation in acute respiratory insufficiency. Med Klin (Munich) 1997; 92(suppl 1): 114–118.
97. International Consensus Conferences in Intensive Care Medicine: noninvasive positive pressure ventilation in acute respiratory failure. Am J Respir Crit Care Med 2001; 163(1):283–291.
98. Navalesi P, Fanfulla F, Frigerio P, Gregoretti C, Nava S. Physiologic evaluation of noninvasive mechanical ventilation delivered with three types of masks in patients with chronic hypercapnic respiratory failure. Crit Care Med 2000; 28:1785–1790.
99. Mehta S, Jay GD, Woolard RH, et al. Randomized, prospective trial of bilevel versus continuous positive airway pressure in acute pulmonary edema. Crit Care Med 1997; 25:620–628.
100. Meduri GU, Turner RE, Abou-Shala N, Wunderink R, Tolley E. Noninvasive positive pressure ventilation via face mask. First-line intervention in patients with acute hypercapnic and hypoxemic respiratory failure. Chest 1996; 109:179–193.
101. Antonelli M, Esquinas A, Conti G, et al. Risk factors for failure of non-invasive ventilation in acute hypoxemic respiratory failure: a multicenter study. Intensive Care Med 1999; 25.
102. Confalonieri M, Potena A, Carbone G, Porta RD, Tolley EA, Umberto Meduri G. Acute respiratory failure in patients with severe community-acquired pneumonia. A prospective randomized evaluation of noninvasive ventilation. Am J Respir Crit Care Med 1999; 160:1585–1591.
103. Vitacca M, Clini E, Rubini F, Nava S, Foglio K, Ambrosino N. Non-invasive mechanical ventilation in severe chronic obstructive lung disease and acute respiratory failure: short- and long-term prognosis. Intensive Care Med 1996; 22:94–100.
104. Barbe F, Togores B, Rubi M, Pons S, Maimo A, Agusti AG. Noninvasive ventilatory support does not facilitate recovery from acute respiratory failure in chronic obstructive pulmonary disease. Eur Respir J 1996; 9:1240–1245.
105. Bott J, Carroll MP, Conway JH, et al. Randomised controlled trial of nasal ventilation in acute ventilatory failure due to chronic obstructive airways disease. Lancet 1993; 341:1555–1557.
106. Plant PK, Owen JL, Elliott MW. Non-invasive ventilation in acute exacerbations of chronic obstructive pulmonary disease: long term survival and predictors of in-hospital outcome. Thorax 2001; 56:708–712.
107. Benhamou D, Muir JF, Melen B. Mechanical ventilation in elderly patients. Monaldi Arch Chest Dis 1998; 53:547–551.
108. Benhamou D, Girault C, Faure C, Portier F, Muir JF. Nasal mask ventilation in acute respiratory failure. Experience in elderly patients. Chest 1992; 102:912–917.
109. Meduri GU, Fox RC, Abou-Shala N, Leeper KV, Wunderink RG. Noninvasive mechanical ventilation via face mask in patients with acute respiratory failure who refused endotracheal intubation. Crit Care Med 1994; 22:1584–1590.
110. Younes M. Proportional assist ventilation, a new approach to ventilatory support. Theory. Am Rev Respir Dis 1992; 145:114–120.
111. Calderini E, Confalonieri M, Puccio PG, Francavilla N, Stella L, Gregoretti C. Patient–ventilator asynchrony during noninvasive ventilation: the role of expiratory trigger. Intensive Care Med 1999; 25:662–667.
112. Aslanian P, El Atrous S, Isabey D, et al. Effects of flow triggering on breathing effort during partial ventilatory support. Am J Respir Crit Care Med 1998; 157:135–143.
113. Giuliani R, Mascia L, Recchia F, Caracciolo A, Fiore T, Ranieri VM. Patient–ventilator interaction during synchronized intermittent mandatory ventilation. Effects of flow triggering. Am J Respir Crit Care Med 1995; 151:1–9.
114. Appendini L, Patessio A, Zanaboni S, et al. Physiologic effects of positive end-expiratory pressure and mask pressure support during exacerbations of chronic obstructive pulmonary disease. Am J Respir Crit Care Med 1994; 149:1069–1076.
115. Vitacca M, Clini E, Pagani M, Bianchi L, Rossi A, Ambrosino N. Physiologic effects of early administered mask proportional assist ventilation in patients with chronic obstructive pulmonary disease and acute respiratory failure. Crit Care Med 2000; 28:1791–1797.

116. Girault C, Richard JC, Chevron V, et al. Comparative physiologic effects of noninvasive assist-control and pressure support ventilation in acute hypercapnic respiratory failure. Chest 1997; 111:1639–1648.
117. Meecham Jones DJ, Paul EA, Grahame-Clarke C, Wedzicha JA. Nasal ventilation in acute exacerbations of chronic obstructive pulmonary disease: effect of ventilator mode on arterial blood gas tensions. Thorax 1994; 49:1222–1224.
118. Vitacca M, Rubini F, Foglio K, Scalvini S, Nava S, Ambrosino N. Non-invasive modalities of positive pressure ventilation improve the outcome of acute exacerbations in COLD patients. Intensive Care Med 1993; 19:450–455.
119. Kramer N, Meyer TJ, Meharg J, Cece RD, Hill NS. Randomized, prospective trial of noninvasive positive pressure ventilation in acute respiratory failure. Am J Respir Crit Care Med 1995; 151:1799–1806.
120. Brochard L, Mancebo J, Wysocki M, et al. Noninvasive ventilation for acute exacerbations of chronic obstructive pulmonary disease. N Engl J Med 1995; 333:817–822.
121. Martin TJ, Hovis JD, Costantino JP, et al. A randomized, prospective evaluation of noninvasive ventilation for acute respiratory failure. Am J Respir Crit Care Med 2000; 161:807–813.
122. Antonelli M, Conti G, Rocco M, et al. A comparison of noninvasive positive-pressure ventilation and conventional mechanical ventilation in patients with acute respiratory failure. N Engl J Med 1998; 339:429–435.
123. Antonelli M, Conti G, Bufi M, et al. Noninvasive ventilation for treatment of acute respiratory failure in patients undergoing solid organ transplantation: a randomized trial. J Am Med Assoc 2000; 283:235–241.
124. Wysocki M, Tric L, Wolff MA, Millet H, Herman B. Noninvasive pressure support ventilation in patients with acute respiratory failure. A randomized comparison with conventional therapy. Chest 1995; 107: 761–768.
125. Bersten AD, Holt AW, Vedig AE, Skowronski GA, Baggoley CJ. Treatment of severe cardiogenic pulmonary edema with continuous positive airway pressure delivered by face mask. N Engl J Med 1991; 325: 1825–1830.
126. Rasanen J, Heikkila J, Downs J, Nikki P, Vaisanen I, Viitanen A. Continuous positive airway pressure by face mask in acute cardiogenic pulmonary edema. Am J Cardiol 1985; 55:296–300.
127. Sladen A, Laver MB, Pontoppidan H. Pulmonary complications and water retention in prolonged mechanical ventilation. N Engl J Med 1968; 279: 448–453.
128. Meinders AJ, van der Hoeven JG, Meinders AE. The outcome of prolonged mechanical ventilation in elderly patients: are the efforts worthwhile? Age Ageing 1996; 25:353–356.
129. Nava S, Ambrosino N, Clini E, et al. Noninvasive mechanical ventilation in the weaning of patients with respiratory failure due to chronic obstructive pulmonary disease. A randomized, controlled trial. Ann Intern Med 1998; 128:721–728.
130. Girault C, Daudenthun I, Chevron V, Tamion F, Leroy J, Bonmarchand G. Noninvasive ventilation as a systematic extubation and weaning technique in acute-on-chronic respiratory failure: a prospective, randomized controlled study. Am J Respir Crit Care Med 1999; 160:86–92.
131. Rothaar RC, Epstein SK. Extubation failure: magnitude of the problem, impact on outcomes, and prevention. Curr Opin Crit Care 2003; 9:59–66.
132. Demling RH, Read T, Lind LJ, Flanagan HL. Incidence and morbidity of extubation failure in surgical intensive care patients. Crit Care Med 1988; 16: 573–577.
133. Hilbert G, Gruson D, Portel L, Gbikpi-Benissan G, Cardinaud JP. Noninvasive pressure support ventilation in COPD patients with postextubation hypercapnic respiratory insufficiency. Eur Respir J 1998; 11: 1349–1353.
134. Phoa LL, Pek WY, Syap W, Johan A. Unplanned extubation: a local experience. Singapore Med J 2002; 43:504–508.
135. Chen CZ, Chu YC, Lee CH, Chen CW, Chang HY, Hsiue TR. Factors predicting reintubation after unplanned extubation. J Formos Med Assoc 2002; 101:542–546.
136. de Lassence A, Alberti C, Azoulay E, et al. Impact of unplanned extubation and reintubation after weaning on nosocomial pneumonia risk in the intensive care unit: a prospective multicenter study. Anesthesiology 2002; 97:148–156.
137. Betbese AJ, Perez M, Bak E, Rialp G, Mancebo J. A prospective study of unplanned endotracheal extubation in intensive care unit patients. Crit Care Med 1998; 26:1180–1186.
138. Chevron V, Menard JF, Richard JC, Girault C, Leroy J, Bonmarchand G. Unplanned extubation: risk factors of development and predictive criteria for reintubation. Crit Care Med 1998; 26:1049–1053.
139. Epstein SK, Nevins ML, Chung J. Effect of unplanned extubation on outcome of mechanical ventilation. Am J Respir Crit Care Med 2000; 161:1912–1916.
140. Christie JM, Dethlefsen M, Cane RD. Unplanned endotracheal extubation in the intensive care unit. J Clin Anesth 1996; 8:289–293.
141. Kilger E, Briegel J, Haller M, et al. Effects of noninvasive positive pressure ventilatory support in non-COPD patients with acute respiratory insufficiency after early extubation. Intensive Care Med 1999; 25:1374–1380.
142. Jiang JS, Kao SJ, Wang SN. Effect of early application of biphasic positive airway pressure on the outcome of

extubation in ventilator weaning. Respirology 1999; 4:161–165.
143. Aguilo R, Togores B, Pons S, Rubi M, Barbe F, Agusti AG. Noninvasive ventilatory support after lung resectional surgery. Chest 1997; 112:117–121.
144. Norregaard O, Jensen TM, Vindelev P. Effects of inspiratory pressure support on oxygenation and central haemodynamics in the normal heart during the postoperative period. Respir Med 1996; 90:415–417.
145. Stock MC, Downs JB, Gauer PK, Alster JM, Imrey PB. Prevention of postoperative pulmonary complications with CPAP, incentive spirometry, and conservative therapy. Chest 1985; 87:151–157.
146. Joris JL, Sottiaux TM, Chiche JD, Desaive CJ, Lamy ML. Effect of bi-level positive airway pressure (BiPAP) nasal ventilation on the postoperative pulmonary restrictive syndrome in obese patients undergoing gastroplasty. Chest 1997; 111:665–670.
147. Shivaram U, Cash ME, Beal A. Nasal continuous positive airway pressure in decompensated hypercapnic respiratory failure as a complication of sleep apnea. Chest 1993; 104:770–774.
148. Sturani C, Galavotti V, Scarduelli C, et al. Acute respiratory failure, due to severe obstructive sleep apnoea syndrome, managed with nasal positive pressure ventilation. Monaldi Arch Chest Dis 1994; 49: 558–560.
149. Muir JF, Cuvelier A, Bota S, Portier F, Benhamou D, Onea G. Modalities of ventilation in obesity. Monaldi Arch Chest Dis 1998; 53:556–559.
150. Dreyfuss D, Saumon G. Ventilator-induced lung injury: lessons from experimental studies. Am J Respir Crit Care Med 1998; 157:294–323.
151. Amato MB, Barbas CS, Medeiros DM, et al. Effect of a protective-ventilation strategy on mortality in the acute respiratory distress syndrome. N Engl J Med 1998; 338:347–354.
152. Brochard L, Roudot-Thoraval F, Roupie E, et al. Tidal volume reduction for prevention of ventilator-induced lung injury in acute respiratory distress syndrome. The Multicenter Trail Group on Tidal Volume reduction in ARDS. Am J Respir Crit Care Med 1998; 158:1831–1838.
153. Stewart TE, Meade MO, Cook DJ, et al. Evaluation of a ventilation strategy to prevent barotrauma in patients at high risk for acute respiratory distress syndrome. Pressure- and Volume-Limited Ventilation Strategy Group. N Engl J Med 1998; 338:355–361.
154. The Acute Respiratory Distress Syndrome Network. Ventilation with lower tidal volumes as compared with traditional tidal volumes for acute lung injury and the acute respiratory distress syndrome. N Engl J Med 2000; 342:1301–1308.
155. Woo SW, Hedley-Whyte J. Macrophage accumulation and pulmonary edema due to thoracotomy and lung over inflation. J Appl Physiol 1972; 33:14–21.
156. Tsuno K, Miura K, Takeya M, Kolobow T, Morioka T. Histopathologic pulmonary changes from mechanical ventilation at high peak airway pressures. Am Rev Respir Dis 1991; 143:1115–1120.
157. Imai Y, Kawano T, Miyasaka K, Takata M, Imai T, Okuyama K. Inflammatory chemical mediators during conventional ventilation and during high frequency oscillatory ventilation. Am J Respir Crit Care Med 1994; 150:1550–1554.
158. Narimanbekov IO, Rozycki HJ. Effect of IL-1 blockade on inflammatory manifestations of acute ventilator-induced lung injury in a rabbit model. Exp Lung Res 1995; 21:239–254.
159. Takata M, Abe J, Tanaka H, et al. Intraalveolar expression of tumor necrosis factor-alpha gene during conventional and high-frequency ventilation. Am J Respir Crit Care Med 1997; 156:272–279.
160. Imai Y, Kawano T, Iwamoto S, Nakagawa S, Takata M, Miyasaka K. Intratracheal anti-tumor necrosis factor-alpha antibody attenuates ventilator-induced lung injury in rabbits. J Appl Physiol 1999; 87:510–515.
161. Kawano T, Mori S, Cybulsky M, et al. Effect of granulocyte depletion in a ventilated surfactant-depleted lung. J Appl Physiol 1987; 62:27–33.
162. Haitsma JJ, Uhlig S, Goggel R, Verbrugge SJ, Lachmann U, Lachmann B. Ventilator-induced lung injury leads to loss of alveolar and systemic compartmentalization of tumor necrosis factor-alpha. Intensive Care Med 2000; 26:1515–1522.
163. Murphy DB, Cregg N, Tremblay L, et al. Adverse ventilatory strategy causes pulmonary-to-systemic translocation of endotoxin. Am J Respir Crit Care Med 2000; 162:27–33.
164. Verbrugge SJ, Sorm V, van 't Veen A, Mouton JW, Gommers D, Lachmann B. Lung overinflation without positive end-expiratory pressure promotes bacteremia after experimental *Klebsiella pneumoniae* inoculation. Intensive Care Med 1998; 24:172–177.
165. Kolobow T, Moretti MP, Fumagalli R, et al. Severe impairment in lung function induced by high peak airway pressure during mechanical ventilation. An experimental study. Am Rev Respir Dis 1987; 135: 312–315.
166. Borelli M, Kolobow T, Spatola R, Prato P, Tsuno K. Severe acute respiratory failure managed with continuous positive airway pressure and partial extracorporeal carbon dioxide removal by an artificial membrane lung. A controlled, randomized animal study. Am Rev Respir Dis 1988; 138:1480–1487.
166a. Uhlig S. Mechanotransduction in the lung: ventilation-induced lung injury and mechanotransduction: stretching it too far? Am J Physiol Lung Cell Mol Physiol 2002; 282:L892–L896.
167. Tremblay LN, Slutsky AS. Ventilator-induced injury: from barotrauma to biotrauma. Proc Assoc Am Phys 1998; 110:482–488.
168. von Bethmann AN, Brasch F, Nusing R, et al. Hyperventilation induces release of cytokines from perfused mouse lung. Am J Respir Crit Care Med 1998; 157:263–272.

169. Tremblay L, Valenza F, Ribeiro SP, Li J, Slutsky AS. Injurious ventilatory strategies increase cytokines and c-fos m-RNA expression in an isolated rat lung model. J Clin Invest 1997; 99:944–952.
170. Webb HH, Tierney DF. Experimental pulmonary edema due to intermittent positive pressure ventilation with high inflation pressures. Protection by positive end-expiratory pressure. Am Rev Respir Dis 1974; 110:556–565.
171. Dreyfuss D, Basset G, Soler P, Saumon G. Intermittent positive-pressure hyperventilation with high inflation pressures produces pulmonary microvascular injury in rats. Am Rev Respir Dis 1985; 132: 880–884.
172. Vlahakis NE, Schroeder MA, Limper AH, Hubmayr RD. Stretch induces cytokine release by alveolar epithelial cells in vitro. Am J Physiol 1999; 277: L167–L173.
173. Pugin J, Dunn I, Jolliet P, et al. Activation of human macrophages by mechanical ventilation in vitro. Am J Physiol 1998; 275:L1040–L1050.
174. Held HD, Boettcher S, Hamann L, Uhlig S. Ventilation-induced chemokine and cytokine release is associated with activation of nuclear factor-κB and is blocked by steroids. Am J Respir Crit Care Med 2001; 163:711–716.
175. Sugiura M, McCulloch PR, Wren S, Dawson RH, Froese AB. Ventilator pattern influences neutrophil influx and activation in atelectasis-prone rabbit lung. J Appl Physiol 1994; 77:1355–1365.
176. Imanaka H, Shimaoka M, Matsuura N, Nishimura M, Ohta N, Kiyono H. Ventilator-induced lung injury is associated with neutrophil infiltration, macrophage activation, and TGF-beta 1 mRNA upregulation in rat lungs. Anesth Analg 2001; 92:428–436.
177. Markos J, Doerschuk CM, English D, Wiggs BR, Hogg JC. Effect of positive end-expiratory pressure on leukocyte transit in rabbit lungs. J Appl Physiol 1993; 74:2627–2633.
178. Matsuoka T, Kawano T, Miyasaka K. Role of high-frequency ventilation in surfactant-depleted lung injury as measured by granulocytes. J Appl Physiol 1994; 76:539–544.
179. Ohta N, Shimaoka M, Imanaka H, et al. Glucocorticoid suppresses neutrophil activation in ventilator-induced lung injury. Crit Care Med 2001; 29: 1012–1016.
180. Ricard JD, Dreyfuss D, Saumon G. Production of inflammatory cytokines in ventilator-induced lung injury: a reappraisal. Am J Respir Crit Care Med 2001; 163:1176–1180.
181. Egan EA. Lung inflation, lung solute permeability, and alveolar edema. J Appl Physiol 1982; 53:121–125.
182. Parker JC, Townsley MI, Rippe B, Taylor AE, Thigpen J. Increased microvascular permeability in dog lungs due to high peak airway pressures. J Appl Physiol 1984; 57:1809–1816.
183. Parker JC, Ivey CL, Tucker JA. Gadolinium prevents high airway pressure-induced permeability increases in isolated rat lungs. J Appl Physiol 1998; 84:1113–1118.
184. Parker JC, Ivey CL, Tucker A. Phosphotyrosine phosphatase and tyrosine kinase inhibition modulate airway pressure-induced lung injury. J Appl Physiol 1998; 85:1753–1761.
185. Parker JC. Inhibitors of myosin light chain kinase and phosphodiesterase reduce ventilator-induced lung injury. J Appl Physiol 2000; 89:2241–2248.
186. Dreyfuss D, Soler P, Saumon G. Spontaneous resolution of pulmonary edema caused by short periods of cyclic overinflation. J Appl Physiol 1992; 72:2081–2089.
187. MacIntyre NR. Invasive mechanical ventilation in adults: conference summary. Respir Care 2002; 47: 508–518.
188. Mead J, Takishima T, Leith D. Stress distribution in lungs: a model of pulmonary elasticity. J Appl Physiol 1970; 28:596–608.
189. Fu Z, Costello ML, Tsukimoto K, et al. High lung volume increases stress failure in pulmonary capillaries. J Appl Physiol 1992; 73:123–133.
190. Costello ML, Mathieu-Costello O, West JB. Stress failure of alveolar epithelial cells studied by scanning electron microscopy. Am Rev Respir Dis 1992; 145: 1446–1455.
191. Boussarsar M, Thierry G, Jaber S, Roudot-Thoraval F, Lemaire F, Brochard L. Relationship between ventilatory settings and barotrauma in the acute respiratory distress syndrome. Intensive Care Med 2002; 28: 406–413.
192. Vlahakis N, Hubmayr R. Cellular responses to capillary stress: plasma membrane stress failure in alveolar epithelial cells. J Appl Physiol 2000; 89: 2490–2496.
193. Schiller HJ, McCann UG II, Carney DE, Gatto LA, Steinberg JM, Nieman GF. Altered alveolar mechanics in the acutely injured lung. Crit Care Med 2001; 29:1049–1055.
194. Wilson TA, Bachofen H. A model for mechanical structure of the alveolar duct. J Appl Physiol 1982; 52: 1064–1070.
195. Ricard JD, Dreyfuss D, Saumon G. Ventilator-induced lung injury. Curr Opin Crit Care 2002; 8:12–20.
196. Slutsky AS. Lung injury caused by mechanical ventilation. Chest 1999; 116:9S–15S.
197. Tschumperlin DJ, Oswari J, Margulies AS. Deformation-induced injury of alveolar epithelial cells. Effect of frequency, duration, and amplitude. Am J Respir Crit Care Med 2000; 162:357–362.
198. Verbrugge SJ, Bohm SH, Gommers D, Zimmerman LJ, Lachmann B. Surfactant impairment after mechanical ventilation with large alveolar surface area changes and effects of positive end-expiratory pressure. Br J Anaesth 1998; 80:360–364.
199. Verbrugge SJ, de Jong JW, Keijzer E, Vazquez de Anda G, Lachmann B. Purine in bronchoalveolar

lavage fluid as a marker of ventilation-induced lung injury. Crit Care Med 1999; 27:779–783.
200. Sandhar B, Niblett D, Argiras E, et al. Effects of positive end-expiratory pressure on hyaline membrane formation in a rabbit model of the neonatal respiratory distress syndrome. Intensive Care Med 1988; 14: 538–546.
201. Muscedere JG, Mullen JB, Gan K, Slutsky AS. Tidal ventilation at low airway pressures can augment lung injury. Am J Respir Crit Care Med 1994; 149: 1327–1334.
202. Brower RG, Shanholtz CB, Fessler HE, et al. Prospective, randomized, controlled clinical trial comparing traditional versus reduced tidal volume ventilation in acute respiratory distress syndrome patients. Crit Care Med 1999; 27:1492–1498.
203. Eichacker PQ, Gerstenberger EP, Banks SM, Cui X, Natanson C. Meta-analysis of acute lung injury and acute respiratory distress syndrome trials testing low tidal volumes. Am J Respir Crit Care Med 2002; 166:1510–1514.
203a. Brower RG. Mechanical ventilation in acute lung injury and ARDS. Tidal volume reduction. Crit Care Clin 2002; 18(1):1–13.
204. Thompson BT, Hayden D, Matthay MA, Brower R, Parsons PE. Clinicians' approaches to mechanical ventilation in acute lung injury and ARDS. Chest 2001; 120:1622–1627.
205. Esteban A, Anzueto A, Alia I, et al. How is mechanical ventilation employed in the intensive care unit? An international utilization review. Am J Respir Crit Care Med 2000; 161:1450–1458.
206. Carmichael LC, Dorinsky PM, Higgins SB, et al. Diagnosis and therapy of acute respiratory distress syndrome in adults: an international survey. J Crit Care 1996; 11:9–18.
207. Esteban A, Anzueto A, Frutos F, et al. Characteristics and outcomes in adult patients receiving mechanical ventilation: a 28-day international study. J Am Med Assoc 2002; 287:345–355.
208. Lachmann B. Open up the lung and keep the lung open. Intensive Care Med 1992; 18:319–321.
209. Suter PM, Fairley B, Isenberg MD. Optimum end-expiratory airway pressure in patients with acute pulmonary failure. N Engl J Med 1975; 292:284–289.
210. Falke KJ, Pontoppidan H, Kumar A, Leith DE, Geffin B, Laver MB. Ventilation with end-expiratory pressure in acute lung disease. J Clin Invest 1972; 51: 2315–2323.
211. Dreyfuss D, Soler P, Basset G, Saumon G. High inflation pressure pulmonary edema. Respective effects of high airway pressure, high tidal volume, and positive end-expiratory pressure. Am Rev Respir Dis 1988; 137:1159–1164.
212. Argiras EP, Blakeley CR, Dunnill MS, Otremski S, Sykes MK. High PEEP decreases hyaline membrane formation in surfactant deficient lungs. Br J Anaesth 1987; 59:1278–1285.
213. Williams M, Wallace S, Akiwumi O, Munsell M, Shaw A. Pressure-determined mechanical ventilation may not be as protective as previously thought. Critic Care Med 2003; 31.
214. Gattinoni L, Pesenti A, Avalli L, Rossi F, Bombino M. Pressure–volume curve of total respiratory system in acute respiratory failure. Computed tomographic scan study. Am Rev Respir Dis 1987; 136:730–736.
215. Gattinoni L, Pelosi P, Crotti S, Valenza F. Effects of positive end-expiratory pressure on regional distribution of tidal volume and recruitment in adult respiratory distress syndrome. Am J Respir Crit Care Med 1995; 151:1807–1814.
216. Roupie E, Dambrosio M, Servillo G, et al. Titration of tidal volume and induced hypercapnia in acute respiratory distress syndrome. Am J Respir Crit Care Med 1995; 152:121–128.
217. Dambrosio M, Roupie E, Mollet JJ, et al. Effects of positive end-expiratory pressure and different tidal volumes on alveolar recruitment and hyperinflation. Anesthesiology 1997; 87:495–503.
218. Ranieri VM, Mascia L, Fiore T, Bruno F, Brienza A, Giuliani R. Cardiorespiratory effects of positive end-expiratory pressure during progressive tidal volume reduction (permissive hypercapnia) in patients with acute respiratory distress syndrome. Anesthesiology 1995; 83:710–720.
219. Hickling KG. The pressure–volume curve is greatly modified by recruitment. A mathematical model of ARDS lungs. Am J Respir Crit Care Med 1998; 158:194–202.
220. Jonson B, Richard JC, Straus C, Mancebo J, Lemaire F, Brochard L. Pressure–volume curves and compliance in acute lung injury: evidence of recruitment above the lower inflection point. Am J Respir Crit Care Med 1999; 159:1172–1178.
221. Dobb E. Second Asia Pacific Consensus Conference in Critical Care Medicine. Acute lung injury. Crit Care Shock 1999; 3:119–133.
222. Amato MB, Barbas CS, Medeiros DM, et al. Beneficial effects of the "open lung approach" with low ditending pressures in acute respiratory distress syndrome. A prospective randomized study on mechanical ventilation. Am J Respir Crit Care Med 1995; 152:1835–1846.
223. Anderson J, Papadakos P. Reducing mechanical ventilation time and cost in acute lung injury with pressure-regulated volume-controlled ventilation. Crit Care Shock 2000; 2:88–96.
224. Gattinoni L, Pelosi P, Suter PM, Pedoto A, Vercesi P, Lissoni A. Acute respiratory distress syndrome caused by pulmonary and extrapulmonary disease. Different syndromes? Am J Respir Crit Care Med 1998; 158: 3–11.
225. Crotti S, Mascheroni D, Caironi P, et al. Recruitment and derecruitment during acute respiratory failure: a clinical study. Am J Respir Crit Care Med 2001; 164:131–140.

226. Pelosi P, Goldner M, McKibben A, et al. Recruitment and derecruitment during acute respiratory failure: an experimental study. Am J Respir Crit Care Med 2001; 164:122–130.
227. Gattinoni L, Vagginelli F, Chiumello D, Taccone P, Carlesso E. Physiologic rationale for ventilator setting in acute lung injury/acute respiratory distress syndrome patients. Crit Care Med 2003; 31:S300–S304.
228. Bohm SH, Lachmann B. Pressure-control ventilation. Putting a mode into perspective. Int J Intensive Care 1996; 3:281–330.
229. Kloot TE, Blanch L, Melynne Youngblood A, et al. Recruitment maneuvers in three experimental models of acute lung injury. Effect on lung volume and gas exchange. Am J Respir Crit Care Med 2000; 161: 1485–1494.
230. Ranieri VM, Eissa NT, Corbeil C, et al. Effects of positive end-expiratory pressure on alveolar recruitment and gas exchange in patients with the adult respiratory distress syndrome. Am Rev Respir Dis 1991; 144:544–551.
231. Esteban A, Alia I, Gordo F, et al. Prospective randomized trial comparing pressure-controlled ventilation and volume-controlled ventilation in ARDS. For the Spanish Lung Failure Collaborative Group. Chest 2000; 117:1690–1696.
232. Jansson L, Jonson B. A theoretical study on flow patterns of ventilators. Scand J Respir Dis 1972; 53: 237–246.
233. Papadakos PJ, Lachmann B. The open lung concept of alveolar recruitment can improve outcome in respiratory failure and ARDS. Mt Sinai J Med 2002; 69: 73–77.
234. Kaplan LJ, Bailey H, Formosa V. Airway pressure release ventilation increases cardiac performance in patients with acute lung injury/adult respiratory distress syndrome. Crit Care 2001; 5:221–226.
234a. Barbas CSV, Medeiros DM, Magaldi RB, et al. High PEEP levels improved survival in ARDS patients. Am J Respir Crit Care Med 2002; 165:A218.
234b. Gattinoni L, Caironi P, Pelosi P, et al. What has computed tomography taught us about the acute respiratory distress syndrome? Am J Respir Crit Care Med 2001; 164:1701–1711.
235. Van Trigt P, Spray TL, Pasque MK, et al. The effect of PEEP on left ventricular diastolic dimensions and systolic performance following myocardial revascularization. Ann Thorac Surg 1982; 33:585–592.
236. Videtta W, Villarejo F, Cohen M, et al. Effects of positive end-expiratory pressure on intracranial pressure and cerebral perfusion pressure. Acta Neurochir Suppl 2002; 81:93–97.
237. Papadakos P, Lachmann B, Bohm SH. Pressure-control ventilation: review and new horizons. Clin Pulm Med 1998; 5:120–123.
238. Munoz J, Guerrero JE, Escalante JL, Palomino R, De La Calle B. Pressure-controlled ventilation versus controlled mechanical ventilation with decelerating inspiratory flow. Crit Care Med 1993; 21:1143–1148.
239. Pelosi P, Cadringher P, Bottino N, et al. Sigh in acute respiratory distress syndrome. Am J Respir Crit Care Med 1999; 159:872–880.
240. Esteban A, Alia I, Ibanez J, Benito S, Tobin MJ. Modes of mechanical ventilation and weaning. A national survey of Spanish hospitals. The Spanish Lung Failure Collaborative Group. Chest 1994; 106:1188–1193.
241. Frutos F, Alia I, Esteban A, Anzueto A. Evolution in the utilization of the mechanical ventilation in the critical care unit. Minerva Anestesiol 2001; 67:215–222.
242. Esteban A, Frutos F, Tobin MJ, et al. A comparison of four methods of weaning patients from mechanical ventilation. Spanish Lung Failure Collaborative Group. N Engl J Med 1995; 332:345–350.
243. Vitacca M, Vianello A, Colombo D, et al. Comparison of two methods for weaning patients with chronic obstructive pulmonary disease requiring mechanical ventilation for more than 15 days. Am J Respir Crit Care Med 2001; 164:225–230.
244. Holliday JE, Hyers TM. The reduction of weaning time from mechanical ventilation using tidal volume and relaxation biofeedback. Am Rev Respir Dis 1990; 141:1214–1220.
245. Treggiari-Venzi MM, Suter PM, de Tonnac N, Romand JA. Successful use of hypnosis as an adjunctive therapy for weaning from mechanical ventilation. Anesthesiology 2000; 92:890–892.
246. Martin AD, Davenport PD, Franceschi AC, Harman E. Use of inspiratory muscle strength training to facilitate ventilator weaning: a series of 10 consecutive patients. Chest 2002; 122:192–196.
247. Johnson CJ, Auger WR, Fedullo PF, Dimsdale JE. Methylphenidate in the 'hard to wean' patient. J Psychosom Res 1995; 39:63–68.
248. Knox JB, Wilmore DW, Demling RH, Sarraf P, Santos AA. Use of growth hormone for postoperative respiratory failure. Am J Surg 1996; 171:576–580.
249. Ely EW, Baker AM, Dunagan DP, et al. Effect on the duration of mechanical ventilation of identifying patients capable of breathing spontaneously. N Engl J Med 1996; 335:1864–1869.
250. Chan PK, Fischer S, Stewart TE, et al. Practicing evidence-based medicine: the design and implementation of a multidisciplinary team-driven extubation protocol. Crit Care 2001; 5:349–354.
251. Henneman E, Dracup K, Ganz T, Molayeme O, Cooper C. Effect of a collaborative weaning plan on patient outcome in the critical care setting. Crit Care Med 2001; 29:297–303.
252. Henneman E, Dracup K, Ganz T, Molayeme O, Cooper CB. Using a collaborative weaning plan to decrease duration of mechanical ventilation and length of stay in the intensive care unit for patients receiving long-term ventilation. Am J Crit Care 2002; 11: 132–140.

253. Kollef MH, Shapiro SD, Silver P, et al. A randomized, controlled trial of protocol-directed versus physician-directed weaning from mechanical ventilation. Crit Care Med 1997; 25:567–574.
254. Smyrnios NA, Connolly A, Wilson MM, et al. Effects of a multifaceted, multidisciplinary, hospital-wide quality improvement program on weaning from mechanical ventilation. Crit Care Med 2002; 30: 1224–1230.
255. Duane TM, Riblet JL, Golay D, Cole FJ Jr, Weireter LJ Jr, Britt LD. Protocol-driven ventilator management in a trauma intensive care unit population. Arch Surg 2002; 137:1223–1227.
256. Linton DM, Potgieter PD, Davis S, Fourie AT, Brunner JX, Laubscher TP. Automatic weaning from mechanical ventilation using an adaptive lung ventilation controller. Chest 1994; 106:1843–1850.
257. Strickland JH Jr, Hasson JH. A computer-controlled ventilator weaning system. Chest 1991; 100:1096–1099.
258. Iregui M, Ward S, Clinikscale D, Clayton D, Kollef MH. Use of a handheld computer by respiratory care practitioners to improve the efficiency of weaning patients from mechanical ventilation. Crit Care Med 2002; 30:2038–2043.
259. Cohen IL, Bari N, Strosberg MA, et al. Reduction of duration and cost of mechanical ventilation in an intensive care unit by use of a ventilatory management team. Crit Care Med 1991; 19:1278–1284.
260. Ely EW, Bennett PA, Bowton DL, Murphy SM, Florance AM, Haponik EF. Large scale implementation of a respiratory therapist-driven protocol for ventilator weaning. Am J Respir Crit Care Med 1999; 159: 439–446.
261. Marelich GP, Murin S, Battistella F, Inciardi J, Vierra T, Roby M. Protocol weaning of mechanical ventilation in medical and surgical patients by respiratory care practitioners and nurses: effect on weaning time and incidence of ventilator-associated pneumonia. Chest 2000; 118:459–467.
262. Scheinhorn DJ, Chao DC, Stearn-Hassenpflug M, Wallace WA. Outcomes in post-ICU mechanical ventilation: a therapist-implemented weaning protocol. Chest 2001; 119:236–242.
263. Wood G, MacLeod B, Moffatt S. Weaning from mechanical ventilation: physician-directed vs a respiratory-therapist-directed protocol. Respir Care 1995; 40:219–224.
264. Namen AM, Ely EW, Tatter SB, et al. Predictors of successful extubation in neurosurgical patients. Am J Respir Crit Care Med 2001; 163:658–664.
265. Devlin JW, Holbrook AM, Fuller HD. The effect of ICU sedation guidelines and pharmacist interventions on clinical outcomes and drug cost. Ann Pharmacother 1997; 31:689–695.
266. Kress JP, Pohlman AS, O'Connor MF, Hall JB. Daily interruption of sedative infusions in critically ill patients undergoing mechanical ventilation. N Engl J Med 2000; 342:1471–1477.
267. Khamiees M, Amoateng-Adjepong Y, Manthous CA. Propofol infusion is associated with a higher rapid shallow breathing index in patients preparing to wean from mechanical ventilation. Respir Care 2002; 47: 150–153.
268. Khamiees M, Raju P, DeGirolamo A, Amoateng-Adjepong Y, Manthous CA. Predictors of extubation outcome in patients who have successfully completed a spontaneous breathing trial. Chest 2001; 120: 1262–1270.
269. Manthous CA, Schmidt GA, Hall JB. Liberation from mechanical ventilation: a decade of progress. Chest 1998; 114:886–901.
269a. Shoemaker W. Textbook of Critical Care. W.B. Saunders, 2000.
270. Sahn SA, Lakshminarayan S. Bedside criteria for discontinuation of mechanical ventilation. Chest 1973; 63:1002–1005.
271. Morganroth ML, Morganroth JL, Nett LM, Petty TL. Criteria for weaning from prolonged mechanical ventilation. Arch Intern Med 1984; 144:1012–1016.
272. Yang KL, Tobin MJ. A prospective study of indexes predicting the outcome of trials of weaning from mechanical ventilation. N Engl J Med 1991; 324: 1445–1450.
273. Zeggwagh AA, Abouqal R, Madani N, Zekraoui A, Kerkeb O. Weaning from mechanical ventilation: a model for extubation. Intensive Care Med 1999; 25: 1077–1083.
274. Capdevila XJ, Perrigault PF, Perey PJ, Roustan JP, d'Athis F. Occlusion pressure and its ratio to maximum inspiratory pressure are useful predictors for successful extubation following T-piece weaning trial. Chest 1995; 108:482–489.
275. Gandia F, Blanco J. Evaluation of indexes predicting the outcome of ventilator weaning and value of adding supplemental inspiratory load. Intensive Care Med 1992; 18:327–333.
276. Hilbert G, Gruson D, Portel L, Vargas F, Gbikpi-Benissan G, Cardinaud JP. Airway occlusion pressure at 0.1 s (P0.1) after extubation: an early indicator of postextubation hypercapnic respiratory insufficiency. Intensive Care Med 1998; 24:1277–1282.
277. Gluck EH. Predicting eventual success or failure to wean in patients receiving long-term mechanical ventilation. Chest 1996; 110:1018–1024.
278. Bellemare F, Grassino A. Effect of pressure and timing of contraction on human diaphragm fatigue. J Appl Physiol 1982; 53:1190–1195.
279. Kirton OC, DeHaven CB, Morgan JP, Windsor J, Civetta JM. Elevated imposed work of breathing masquerading as ventilator weaning intolerance. Chest 1995; 108:1021–1025.
280. Gluck EH, Barkoviak MJ, Balk RA, Casey LC, Silver MR, Bone RC. Medical effectiveness of esophageal balloon pressure manometry in weaning patients from mechanical ventilation. Crit Care Med 1995; 23: 504–509.

281. Levy MM, Miyasaki A, Langston D. Work of breathing as a weaning parameter in mechanically ventilated patients. Chest 1995; 108:1018–1020.
282. Vassilakopoulos T, Zakynthinos S, Roussos C. The tension-time index and the frequency/tidal volume ratio are the major pathophysiologic determinants of weaning failure and success. Am J Respir Crit Care Med 1998; 158:378–385.
283. Epstein SK. Etiology of extubation failure and the predictive value of the rapid shallow breathing index. Am J Respir Crit Care Med 1995; 152:545–549.
284. Moody LE, Lowry L, Yarandi H, Voss A. Psychophysiologic predictors of weaning from mechanical ventilation in chronic bronchitis and emphysema. Clin Nurs Res 1997; 6:311–330; discussion 330–333.
285. Krieger BP, Isber J, Breitenbucher A, Throop G, Ershowsky P. Serial measurements of the rapid-shallow-breathing index as a predictor of weaning outcome in elderly medical patients. Chest 1997; 112: 1029–1034.
286. Epstein SK, Ciubotaru RL. Influence of gender and endotracheal tube size on preextubation breathing pattern. Am J Respir Crit Care Med 1996; 154: 1647–1652.
287. Jabour ER, Rabil DM, Truwit JD, Rochester DF. Evaluation of a new weaning index based on ventilatory endurance and the efficiency of gas exchange. Am Rev Respir Dis 1991; 144:531–537.
288. Esteban A, Alia I, Gordo F, et al. Extubation outcome after spontaneous breathing trials with T-tube or pressure support ventilation. The Spanish Lung Failure Collaborative Group. Am J Respir Crit Care Med 1997; 156:459–465.
289. Rivera L, Weissman C. Dynamic ventilatory characteristics during weaning in postoperative critically ill patients. Anesth Analg 1997; 84:1250–1255.
290. Vallverdu I, Calaf N, Subirana M, Net A, Benito S, Mancebo J. Clinical characteristics, respiratory functional parameters, and outcome of a two-hour T-piece trial in patients weaning from mechanical ventilation. Am J Respir Crit Care Med 1998; 158:1855–1862.
291. Leitch EA, Moran JL, Grealy B. Weaning and extubation in the intensive care unit. Clinical or index-driven approach? Intensive Care Med 1996; 22:752–759.
292. Chatila W, Jacob B, Guaglionone D, Manthous CA. The unassisted respiratory rate–tidal volume ratio accurately predicts weaning outcome. Am J Med 1996; 101:61–67.
293. Esteban A, Alia I, Tobin MJ, et al. Effect of spontaneous breathing trial duration on outcome of attempts to discontinue mechanical ventilation. Spanish Lung Failure Collaborative Group. Am J Respir Crit Care Med 1999; 159:512–518.
294. Perren A, Domenighetti G, Mauri S, Genini F, Vizzardi N. Protocol-directed weaning from mechanical ventilation: clinical outcome in patients randomized for a 30-min or 120-min trial with pressure support ventilation. Intensive Care Med 2002; 28: 1058–1063.
295. Koh Y, Hong SB, Lim CM, et al. Effect of an additional 1-hour T-piece trial on weaning outcome at minimal pressure support. J Crit Care 2000; 15:41–45.
296. Sapijaszko MJ, Brant R, Sandham D, Berthiaume Y. Nonrespiratory predictor of mechanical ventilation dependency in intensive care unit patients. Crit Care Med 1996; 24:601–607.
297. Hasfurther DL, Bailey PL. Failure of neuromuscular blockade reversal after rocuronium in a patient who received oral neomycin. Can J Anaesth 1996; 43: 617–620.
298. Booij LH. Neuromuscular transmission and its pharmacological blockade. Part 4: Use of relaxants in paediatric and elderly patients, in obstetrics, and in the intensive care unit. Pharm World Sci 1997; 19:45–52.
299. Geller TJ, Kaiboriboon K, Fenton GA, Hayat GR. Vecuronium-associated axonal motor neuropathy: a variant of critical illness polyneuropathy? Neuromuscul Disord 2001; 11:579–582.
300. Polsonetti BW, Joy SD, Laos LF. Steroid-induced myopathy in the ICU. Ann Pharmacother 2002; 36:1741–1744.
301. Hund EF, Fogel W, Krieger D, DeGeorgia M, Hacke W. Critical illness polyneuropathy: clinical findings and outcomes of a frequent cause of neuromuscular weaning failure. Crit Care Med 1996; 24:1328–1333.
302. Leijten FS, De Weerd AW, Poortvliet DC, De Ridder VA, Ulrich C, Harink-De Weerd JE. Critical illness polyneuropathy in multiple organ dysfunction syndrome and weaning from the ventilator. Intensive Care Med 1996; 22:856–861.
303. Laghi F, Cattapan SE, Jubran A, et al. Is weaning failure caused by low-frequency fatigue of the diaphragm? Am J Respir Crit Care Med 2003; 167:120–127.
304. De Backer D, El Haddad P, Preiser JC, Vincent JL. Hemodynamic responses to successful weaning from mechanical ventilation after cardiovascular surgery. Intensive Care Med 2000; 26:1201–1206.
305. Chatila W, Ani S, Guaglianone D, Jacob B, Amoateng-Adjepong Y, Manthous CA. Cardiac ischemia during weaning from mechanical ventilation. Chest 1996; 109:1577–1583.
306. Hurford WE, Favorito F. Association of myocardial ischemia with failure to wean from mechanical ventilation. Crit Care Med 1995; 23:1475–1480.
307. Srivastava S, Chatila W, Amoateng-Adjepong Y, et al. Myocardial ischemia and weaning failure in patients with coronary artery disease: an update. Crit Care Med 1999; 27:2109–2112.
308. Marcelino P, Fernandes AP, Marum S, Ribeiro JP. The influence of cardiac diastole on weaning from mechanical ventilation. Rev Port Cardiol 2002; 21:849–857.
309. Epstein CD, El-Mokadem N, Peerless JR. Weaning older patients from long-term mechanical ventilation: a pilot study. Am J Crit Care 2002; 11:369–377.

310. Jubran A, Tobin MJ. Pathophysiologic basis of acute respiratory distress in patients who fail a trial of weaning from mechanical ventilation. Am J Respir Crit Care Med 1997; 155:906–915.
311. Engoren M. Approximate entropy of respiratory rate and tidal volume during weaning from mechanical ventilation. Crit Care Med 1998; 26:1817–1823.
312. El-Khatib M, Jamaleddine G, Soubra R, Muallem M. Pattern of spontaneous breathing: potential marker for weaning outcome. Spontaneous breathing pattern and weaning from mechanical ventilation. Intensive Care Med 2001; 27:52–58.
313. Delgado Tapia J, Ramirez Sanchez A, Molina Moreno M, Palop Manjon-Cabeza E, Ferron Orihuela JA. Diaphragmatic hernia after transhiatal esophagectomy. Rev Esp Anestesiol Reanim 2000; 47:317–319.
314. Rumbak MJ, Walsh FW, Anderson WM, Rolfe MW, Solomon DA. Significant tracheal obstruction causing failure to wean in patients requiring prolonged mechanical ventilation: a forgotten complication of long-term mechanical ventilation. Chest 1999; 115:1092–1095.
315. St John RC, Pacht ER. Tracheal stenosis and failure to wean from mechanical ventilation due to herpetic tracheitis. Chest 1990; 98:1520–1522.
316. Jaber S, Carlucci A, Boussarsar M, et al. Helium–oxygen in the postextubation period decreases inspiratory effort. Am J Respir Crit Care Med 2001; 164: 633–637.
317. Thorens JB, Kaelin RM, Jolliet P, Chevrolet JC. Influence of the quality of nursing on the duration of weaning from mechanical ventilation in patients with chronic obstructive pulmonary disease. Crit Care Med 1995; 23:1807–1815.
318. Krafft P, Fridrich P, Pernerstorfer T, et al. The acute respiratory distress syndrome: definitions, severity and clinical outcome. An analysis of 101 clinical investigations. Intensive Care Med 1996; 22:519–529.
319. Flatau E, Barzilay E, Kaufmann N, Lev A, Ben-Ami M, Kohn D. Adult respiratory distress syndrome treated with high-frequency positive pressure ventilation. Isr J Med Sci 1981; 17:453–456.
320. Hurst JM, Branson RD, Davis K Jr, Barrette RR, Adams KS. Comparison of conventional mechanical ventilation and high-frequency ventilation. A prospective, randomized trial in patients with respiratory failure. Ann Surg 1990; 211:486–491.
321. Davey AJ, Leigh JM. High frequency venturi jet ventilation. Adult respiratory distress syndrome—a case report. Anaesthesia 1982; 37:670–674.
322. Hamilton PP, Onayemi A, Smyth JA et al. Comparison of conventional and high-frequency ventilation: oxygenation and lung pathology. J Appl Physiol 1983; 55:131–138.
323. McCulloch PR, Forkert PG, Froese AB. Lung volume maintenance prevents lung injury during high frequency oscillatory ventilation in surfactant-deficient rabbits. Am Rev Respir Dis 1988; 137:1185–1192.
324. Coalson JJ, deLemos RA. Pathologic features of various ventilatory strategies. Acta Anaesthesiol Scand Suppl 1989; 90:108–116.
325. Yoder BA, Siler-Khodr T, Winter VT, Coalson JJ. High-frequency oscillatory ventilation: effects on lung function, mechanics, and airway cytokines in the immature baboon model for neonatal chronic lung disease. Am J Respir Crit Care Med 2000; 162:1867–1876.
326. Imai Y, Nakagawa S, Ito Y, Kawano T, Slutsky AS, Miyasaka K. Comparison of lung protection strategies using conventional and high-frequency oscillatory ventilation. J Appl Physiol 2001; 91:1836–1844.
327. Mehta S, Lapinsky SE, Hallett DC, et al. Prospective trial of high-frequency oscillation in adults with acute respiratory distress syndrome. Crit Care Med 2001; 29:1360–1369.
328. Velmahos GC, Chan LS, Tatevossian R, et al. High-frequency percussive ventilation improves oxygenation in patients with ARDS. Chest 1999; 116:440–446.
329. Cartotto R, Cooper AB, Esmond JR, Gomez M, Fish JS, Smith T. Early clinical experience with high-frequency oscillatory ventilation for ARDS in adult burn patients. J Burn Care Rehabil 2001; 22:325–333.
330. Andersen FA, Guttormsen AB, Flaatten HK. High frequency oscillatory ventilation in adult patients with acute respiratory distress syndrome—a retrospective study. Acta Anaesthesiol Scand 2002; 46:1082–1088.
331. Claridge JA, Hostetter RG, Lowson SM, Young JS. High-frequency oscillatory ventilation can be effective as rescue therapy for refractory acute lung dysfunction. Am Surg 1999; 65:1092–1096.
332. Fort P, Farmer C, Westerman J, et al. High-frequency oscillatory ventilation for adult respiratory distress syndrome—a pilot study. Crit Care Med 1997; 25: 937–947.
333. Brambrink AM, Brachlow J, Weiler N, et al. Successful treatment of a patient with ARDS after pneumonectomy using high-frequency oscillatory ventilation. Intensive Care Med 1999; 25:1173–1176.
334. Derdak S, Mehta S, Stewart TE, et al. High-frequency oscillatory ventilation for acute respiratory distress syndrome in adults: a randomized, controlled trial. Am J Respir Crit Care Med 2002; 166:801–808.
335. Paulsen SM, Killyon GW, Barillo DJ. High-frequency percussive ventilation as a salvage modality in adult respiratory distress syndrome: a preliminary study. Am Surg 2002; 68:852–856; discussion 856.
336. Gluck E, Heard S, Patel C, et al. Use of ultrahigh frequency ventilation in patients with ARDS. A preliminary report. Chest 1993; 103:1413–1420.
337. Barzilay E, Lev A, Lesmes C, Fleck R, Khourieh A. Combined use of HFPPV with low-rate ventilation in traumatic respiratory insufficiency. Intensive Care Med 1984; 10:197–200.
338. Ip-Yam PC, Allsop E, Murphy J. Combined high-frequency ventilation (CHFV) in the treatment of acute lung injury—a case report. Ann Acad Med Singapore 1998; 27:437–441.

339. Barzilay E, Kessler D, Raz R. Superimposed high frequency ventilation with conventional mechanical ventilation. Chest 1989; 95:681–682.
340. El-Baz N, Faber LP, Doolas A. Combined high-frequency ventilation for management of terminal respiratory failure: a new technique. Anesth Analg 1983; 62:39–49.
341. Borg UR, Stoklosa JC, Siegel JH, et al. Prospective evaluation of combined high-frequency ventilation din post-traumatic patients with adult respiratory distress syndrome refractory to optimized conventional ventilatory management. Crit Care Med 1989; 17: 1129–1142.
342. Yeston NS, Grasberger RC, McCormick JR. Severe combined respiratory and myocardial failure treated with high-frequency ventilation. Crit Care Med 1985; 13:208–209.
343. Derdak S. High-frequency oscillatory ventilation for acute respiratory distress syndrome in adult patients. Crit Care Med 2003; 31:S317–S323.
344. Douglas WW, Rehder K, Beynen FM, Sessler AD, Marsh HM. Improved oxygenation in patients with acute respiratory failure: the prone position. Am Rev Respir Dis 1977; 115:559–566.
345. Mure M, Martling CR, Lindahl SG. Dramatic effect on oxygenation in patients with severe acute lung insufficiency treated in the prone position. Crit Care Med 1997; 25:1539–1544.
346. Brazzi L, Pelosi P, Gattinoni L. Prone position in mechanically-ventilated patients. Monaldi Arch Chest Dis 1998; 53:410–414.
347. Gattinoni L, Pelosi P, Vitale G, Pesenti A, D'Andrea L, Mascheroni D. Body position changes redistribute lung computed-tomographic density in patients with acute respiratory failure. Anesthesiology 1991; 74: 15–23.
348. Firodiya M, Mehta Y, Juneja R, Trehan N. Mechanical ventilation in the prone position: a strategy for acute respiratory failure after cardiac surgery. Indian Heart J 2001; 53:83–86.
349. Kleinschmidt S, Ziegenfuss T, Bauer M, Fuchs W. The effect of intermittent prone position on pulmonary gas exchange in acute lung failure. Anasthesiol Intensivmed Notfallmed Schmerzther 1993; 28:81–85.
350. Klingstedt C, Hedenstierna G, Lundquist H, Strandberg A, Tokics L, Brismar B. The influence of body position and differential ventilation on lung dimensions and atelectasis formation in anaesthetized man. Acta Anaesthesiol Scand 1990; 34:315–322.
351. Parish JM, Gracey DR, Southorn PA, Pairolero PA, Wheeler JT. Differential mechanical ventilation in respiratory failure due to severe unilateral lung disease. Mayo Clin Proc 1984; 59:822–828.
352. Zandstra DF, Stoutenbeek CP. Monitoring differential CO_2 excretion during differential lung ventilation in asymmetric pulmonary contusion. Clinical implications. Intensive Care Med 1988; 14:106–109.
353. Frostell C, Blomqvist H, Nilsson JA, Grenrot C, Baehrendtz S, Hedenstierna G. Differential ventilation with selective PEEP in bilateral lung disease. Intensive Care Med 1984; 10:265–267.
354. Rivara D, Bourgain JL, Rieuf P, Harf A, Lemaire F. Differential ventilation in unilateral lung disease: effects on respiratory mechanics and gas exchange. Intensive Care Med 1979; 5:189–191.
355. Baehrendtz S, Hedenstierna G. Differential ventilation and selective positive end-expiratory pressure: effects on patients with acute bilateral lung disease. Anesthesiology 1984; 61:511–517.
356. East TDt, Pace NL, Westenskow DR. Synchronous versus asynchronous differential lung ventilation with PEEP after unilateral acid aspiration in the dog. Crit Care Med 1983; 11:441–444.
357. Baehrendtz S, Santesson J, Bindslev L, Hedenstierna G, Matell G. Differential ventilation in acute bilateral lung disease. Influence on gas exchange and central haemodynamics. Acta Anaesthesiol Scand 1983; 27: 270–277.
358. Talbot AR, Fu CC. Clinical use of differential lung ventilation in the treatment of asymmetric lung injury: report of a case. Ma Zui Xue Za Zhi 1989; 27:67–73.
359. Alberti A, Valenti S, Gallo F, Vincenti E. Differential lung ventilation with a double-lumen tracheostomy tube in unilateral refractory atelectasis. Intensive Care Med 1992; 18:479–484.
360. Zandstra DF, Stoutenbeek CP. Treatment of massive unilateral pulmonary embolism by differential lung ventilation. Intensive Care Med 1987; 13:422–424.
361. East TDt, Pace NL, Westenskow DR, Lund K. Differential lung ventilation with unilateral PEEP following unilateral hydrochloric acid aspiration in the dog. Acta Anaesthesiol Scand 1983; 27:356–360.
362. Miranda DR, Stoutenbeek C, Kingma L. Differential lung ventilation with HFPPV. Intensive Care Med 1981; 7:139–141.
363. Johannigman JA, Campbell RS, Davis K Jr, Hurst JM. Combined differential lung ventilation and inhaled nitric oxide therapy in the management of unilateral pulmonary contusion. J Trauma 1997; 42: 108–111.
364. Nishimura M, Takezawa J, Nishijima MK, et al. High-frequency jet ventilation for differential lung ventilation. Crit Care Med 1984; 12:840 841.

43

Nutrition Support of the ICU Cancer Patient

TAMI JOHNSON, ANNE TUCKER, and TODD CANADA

Division of Pharmacy, The University of Texas M.D. Anderson Cancer Center, Houston, Texas, U.S.A.

I. INTRODUCTION

Protein–calorie malnutrition (PCM) is a common problem often observed in critically ill patients upon admission to the intensive care unit (ICU) (1). Cancer patients admitted to the ICU represent a unique challenge since malnutrition has been documented in up to 80% of this hospitalized population (2). The provision of nutrition support to critically ill cancer patients is considered controversial by some clinicians. It is unclear if nutrition support prevents starvation or decreases morbidity and mortality in this patient population. There is literature to corroborate that nutrition support may negate treatment (chemotherapy) and promote tumor growth in cancer (3,4). However, malnutrition has been associated with a higher incidence of poor wound healing, wound dehiscence, infection, impaired immune function, and respiratory dysfunction along with fluid and electrolyte disorders. Therefore, nutrition support appears to be a required supportive treatment in ICU and postoperative patients to prevent these complications. This chapter focuses on critically ill cancer patients and discusses important considerations when formulating nutrition support regimens.

II. ASSESSING AND MONITORING NUTRITIONAL STATUS

The cause of malnutrition in critically ill cancer patients is partially related to the length of time that nutrient provision does not meet the body's nutrient demands. Malnutrition in patients with cancer is often related to the type of malignancy (e.g., gastrointestinal) and treatments, such as chemotherapy or radiation. The degree and consequences of malnutrition can be obtained with a detailed clinical assessment. Subjective global assessment (SGA) has been used successfully to determine the severity of malnutrition and the risk of developing nutrition-related complications such as impaired wound healing, infections, or fluid and electrolyte disorders (5). The SGA is based solely upon patient history and physical examination. The goal is to diagnose PCM and to identify patients that would or would not likely benefit from nutrition support. Table 1 shows a detailed composite of multiple factors to help determine the risk of malnutrition. A weight history should always be obtained and used as part of the clinical assessment. Unfortunately, this may not be available in the ICU setting if the patient is

Table 1 Nutrition Assessment Components

Medical diagnoses	Evaluate any effect on nutrition status
History	Past medical, surgical, dietary, social, and medications focusing on chemotherapy and radiation therapies
Diet information	Allergies, nutrition intake and tolerance, dietary habits or restrictions, appetite history, intentional or unintentional weight loss, nutritional or herbal supplements, vitamins and trace elements
Physical examination	Cognitive function, functional status and activities of daily living, rashes, wounds, presence of hypotension or bradycardia, muscle wasting, cachexia, ascites, abdominal girth, edema, and tumor burden
Anthropometric data	Height, current weight and pretreatment weight, weight change and time period, tricep skinfold thickness, and midarm muscle circumference
Laboratory and biochemical data	Complete blood count including differential (screening for nutrition-related anemias), total lymphocyte count, serum electrolytes, glucose, total bilirubin, alkaline phosphatase, alanine aminotransferase, aspartate aminotransferase, serum creatinine, BUN, and visceral proteins (albumin, prealbumin)

obtunded or has no immediate contacts to provide additional information. The patient's usual body weight history can help determine changes in weight and the degree of malnutrition if weight loss has occurred (Table 2). Patients are at risk for malnutrition if any of the following is present: involuntary weight loss of greater than 5% in 1 month, 7.5% in 3 months, 10% in 6 months, body mass index (BMI) < 22 or >27 Kg/m^2, or a 20% weight change below ideal or usual body weight (6,7).

A number of serum markers for PCM are available to help determine nutritional status in the absence of the patient's history. Common measurable visceral serum proteins or markers include albumin, transferrin, prealbumin, retinol-binding protein, fibronectin, and C-reactive protein. Readily available visceral proteins used for nutrition assessment are albumin, prealbumin, and transferrin, due to their ease of analysis and rapid reporting. The serum levels of these three proteins reflect a balance between synthesis, distribution, and degradation. An acute increase in serum prealbumin or transferrin may reflect a positive nitrogen balance. However, a decrease may not indicate a negative nitrogen balance, as these are negative acute phase reactants. In critically ill cancer patients, liver export proteins (such as prealbumin) can be negatively altered

Table 2 Common Calculated Values to Determine Malnutrition

	Severity of malnutrition		
	Mild	Moderate	Severe
Percent (%) ideal body weight (IBW) Men 106 lb for 60 in. in height plus 6 lb for each additional inch	80–90%	70–79%	<70%
Women 100 lb for 60 in. in height plus 5 lb for each additional inch	80–90%	70–79%	<70%
BMI BMI = weight (kg)÷ [height (m)]^2	18.6–20 kg/m^2	16.5–18.5 kg/m^2	<16.5 kg/m^2
Percent (%) usual body weight (UBW) % UBW = [current weight ÷ usual weight] × 100	85–95%	75–84%	<74%
Percent (%) recent weight change (RWC) % RWC = [(usual weight – current weight) ÷ usual weight] × 100		1 week: 1–2%	1 week: >2%
		1 month: 5% 3 months: 7.5% 6 months: 10%	1 month: > 5% 3 months: >7.5% 6 months: >10%

lb = pounds; m = meter; 1 kg = 2.2 lbs; 1 inch = 2.54 cm; 1 meter =100 cm.

as a result of an acute phase response secondary to cytokines, inflammation, infection, surgery, or increased metabolic stress (Table 3).

Nitrogen balance studies may help determine the degree of stress or catabolism that the critically ill cancer patient is experiencing. Protein is 16% nitrogen; therefore each gram of nitrogen equals approximately 6.25 g of degraded protein. The nitrogen balance is determined by totaling the patient's dietary protein intake (in grams) by various routes (oral, enteral, and parenteral) and then dividing it by 6–6.25 g (depending on source) to calculate the patient's nitrogen intake. Concurrently, a 24-hr urine collection is performed to measure urinary urea nitrogen (UUN) with approximately 2–4 g added for insensible nitrogen losses from skin, hair, and feces for the patient's nitrogen output. Generally, most critically ill cancer patients will have UUN excretion rates of approximately 10–20 g/day; however, this is highly variable due to patient age and underlying lean body mass (LBM). The nitrogen balance is then calculated by subtracting the patient's nitrogen output from their nitrogen intake.

The main nutritional goal for every patient is to achieve a positive nitrogen balance (implying anabolism) in the range of 4–6 g/day to promote tissue and protein synthesis (1). A negative nitrogen balance (implying catabolism) indicates that there is ongoing tissue loss, primarily from skeletal muscle, due to inadequate nitrogen intake. Unfortunately, nitrogen balance studies are often difficult to calculate or interpret and sometimes impractical to collect for routine use in critically ill cancer patients. This is mainly due to the observation that only approximately 50% of delivered dietary protein is utilized in the critically ill and the rest is primarily excreted in the urine. Some additional limitations that may affect nitrogen balance studies are acute or chronic renal dysfunction, high-output fistulas (>500 mL/day) or ostomies (>1 L/day), moderate-to-severe diarrhea, and inadequate 24-hr urine collections. Another important detail that clinicians should understand when collecting a nitrogen balance for a critically ill cancer patient is that energy requirements and weight changes may not correlate with nitrogen losses, nitrogen retention, or nitrogen balance (8).

III. DETERMINATION OF ENERGY AND PROTEIN NEEDS

Determining energy and protein needs for cancer patients is challenging because energy expenditure in the presence of malignancy often manifests a different metabolic response than patients without malignancy. Normally during fasting, the body conserves energy and protein thereby decreasing energy expenditure and protein catabolism. However, in the presence of local or advanced cancer, energy expenditure and protein requirements may increase secondary to the malignancy itself above and beyond the basal energy and protein demands of the host. Thus, the cancer patient has an inability to physiologically adapt to fasting conditions.

A similar physiologic response occurs in critically ill patients experiencing starvation, as the body utilizes glycogen stores initially. Once glycogen stores are depleted (generally within 8–12 hr), muscle protein breakdown occurs secondary to gluconeogenesis thus preventing synthesis of tissue protein in various organs and muscle. Additionally, adipose tissue or fat stores are catabolized to fatty acids and eventually converted to ketone bodies by a lipid-mobilizing factor for energy (9). Often, the critically ill cancer patient is unable to adapt to severe metabolic stress due to lack of energy stores and pre-existing alterations in body composition, such as muscle wasting seen with cachexia. In cancer, protein catabolism and decreased protein synthesis may contribute to severe wasting of skeletal muscle as these patients have a 50% increase in protein turnover compared to noncancer patients (9,10). Furthermore, the metabolic changes occurring in cancer patients with cachexia are mediated by pro-inflammatory cytokines (primarily tumor necrosis factor, interleukin-1, and interleukin-6), neuroendocrine hormones, and tumor-derived factors such as proteolysis-inducing factor and lipid-mobilizing factor (11). The host response to cancer cachexia partially explains the wide variability in energy expenditure seen among cancer types and stages. An interesting study by Knox et al. (12) concluded that the presence of a tumor has considerable direct and indirect influences on resting energy expenditure. In the 200 patients with heterogeneous malignancies studied, 26% were found to be hypometabolic (<90% of predicted energy expenditure), 41% normometabolic, and 26% hypermetabolic (>110% of predicted energy expenditure). The duration of malignancy was found to have a role in the hypermetabolic patients.

Critically ill patients are often found to be hypermetabolic. Depending on the type of insult that occurs, energy expenditure may increase as high as 40–80% above baseline (13). When adding stress, infection or surgery to critically ill cancer patients, the metabolic response may be compounded. The response to stress manifests itself with increases in endogenous catecholamines, glucagon, glucocorticoids, cytokines, tissue ischemia, and acidosis, which further increase energy expenditure, catabolism, gluconeogenesis, and oxygen

Table 3 Visceral Serum Proteins Used in Nutrition Assessment

Serum protein	Normal value	Depletion			Half-life	Function	Clinical significance	Non-nutritional factors affecting value
		Mild	Moderate	Severe				
Albumin (g/dL)	3.5–5.0	2.9–3.5	2.1–2.8	<2.1	21 days	Maintain plasma oncotic pressure; carrier for amino acids, zinc, magnesium, calcium, free fatty acids, and certain drugs	Routinely available; useful in long-term nutritional assessment; limited value in ICU or acute care nutritional assessment (negative acute phase reactant)	Cytokines, surgery, infection, shock, acute hepatitis, cirrhosis, nephrotic syndrome, dialysis, heart failure, hydration status, chronic inflammation
Transferrin (mg/dL)	200–400	150–200	100–149	<100	7–9 days	Binds iron in plasma and transports to bone	Strongly influenced by iron status; limited value in ICU or acute care nutritional assessment (negative acute phase reactant)	Cytokines, surgery, infection, shock, iron deficiency anemia, acute hepatitis, cirrhosis, pregnancy, and chronic inflammation
Prealbumin (mg/dL)	16–40	10–15	5–10	<5	1–2 days	Binds thyroxine; carrier for retinol-binding protein	Associated with positive nitrogen balance if increasing; limited value in ICU or acute care nutritional assessment (negative acute phase reactant)	Cytokines, surgery, infection, shock, acute hepatitis, cirrhosis, renal failure, corticosteroids, and chronic inflammation

Table 4 Equations for Determining Energy Requirements

The Harris–Benedict energy equations	
Males: BEE = 66 + 13.8 (wt)+ 5 (ht)– 6.8 (age in years)	
Females: BEE = 655 + 9.6 (wt)+ 1.8 (ht)– 4.7 (age in years)	
Activity factor (AF): BEE × AF = REE	
Bedridden = 1.2 and ambulatory = 1.3	
Stress factors (SF): REE × SF	
Condition	Stress factor
Starvation	0.85–1.0
Maintenance	1.2–1.3
Severe stress, major surgery, infection	1.3–1.5
Bone marrow transplant	1.5–2.0
Clinically estimated energy expenditure	
Condition	Calories/kg/day
Mild or moderate illness	20–25
Sepsis, major surgery	25–30
Indirect calorimetry	
Abbreviated Weir formula for REE = [(3.9 × Vo_2) + (1.1 × VCO_2)] × 1.44	
Respiratory quotient (RQ) = VCO_2/VO_2	
Energy source	RQ
Starvation or ketosis	<0.6
Fat	0.7
Protein	0.8
Mixed fuel source	0.85
Carbohydrate	1.0
Net fat synthesis	>1.0

BEE, basal energy expenditure; REE, resting energy expenditure; wt, actual body weight (kg), use adjusted body weight (ABW) if >130% of ideal body weight (IBW), ABW, 0.25 (actual body weight – IBW)+ IBW; ht, height (cm); kg, actual body weight, use adjusted body weight (ABW) if >130% of ideal body weight (IBW); VCO_2, carbon dioxide production; VO_2, oxygen consumption.

consumption (13). This ultimately leads to a decrease in protein synthesis and an inability to reverse tissue catabolism. It has been determined that, in previously healthy postoperative ICU patients, depletion of lean tissue occurs at a rate of approximately 0.6 kg of lean tissue per day so nutrition may only be delayed for 5–7 days without significant host deterioration (14). The duration of tolerated starvation in critically ill cancer patients is unknown and depends on the available endogenous energy stores, muscle or lean tissue mass and the rate of endogenous protein and fat breakdown (4). Nutrition support in this patient population should ideally be initiated within 5–7 days of ICU admission to meet the metabolic demands of the body and prevent further nutrient losses.

The three most common methods to determine energy expenditure in the ICU are with the use of the Harris–Benedict basal energy expenditure equation with added stress factors, clinical estimation of energy expenditure (e.g., 20–30 cal/kg/day), and indirect calorimetry with a metabolic cart (Table 4). Accurately, feeding critically ill patients is difficult since both underfeeding and overfeeding may be detrimental. Underfeeding ICU patients may lead to impaired wound healing, prolonged mechanical ventilation, and host debilitation. Conversely, overfeeding may lead to respiratory compromise from excessive CO_2 production, hepatic dysfunction or steatosis, hyperglycemia, immunosuppression, electrolyte disorders, and azotemia (15). Providing excess calories to critically ill patients independent of nutrient source can lead to increased carbon dioxide production and a higher respiratory quotient. Indirect calorimetry offers the most accurate method for correctly assessing energy expenditure and may avoid complications from under- or overfeeding (16,17). The interpretation of indirect calorimetry should ideally incorporate a complete nutritional assessment and serial measurements may be more valuable than a single evaluation.

Normal protein requirements for critically ill patients are approximately 1.5 g/kg/day and often adjusted for severe renal and hepatic dysfunction (discussed later in this chapter under special ICU patient populations). Protein requirements may be as high as 2.5 g/kg/day for critically ill cancer patients with comorbidities such as enterocutaneous fistulas, chylothorax or postoperative chyle leaks > 500 mL/day, nonhealing wounds, or acute renal failure requiring continuous renal replacement therapy (CRRT) (18). Protein has a caloric density of 4 cal/g and ideally consumption should be in the range of 15–25% of total calories per day. Excessive protein intake above the body's requirements cannot be stored, so it is converted into energy and ammonia by the liver and ultimately excreted renally as urea. Since urea is a solute, its renal elimination draws water with it and may create a solute diuresis where dehydration is often an unfortunate complication. Adequate intravascular volume status must be maintained and urine output routinely monitored to prevent azotemia and subsequent dehydration or volume depletion in these patients.

The quantity of nonprotein calories supplied often helps determine how the body will utilize protein or nitrogen. Similarly, a nonprotein calorie to nitrogen ratio can be utilized to guide nutrition support in the ICU environment. Generally, hospitalized patients require approximately 100–150:1 and if severely metabolically stressed, protein (or nitrogen) requirements increase thereby reducing the ratio to approximately 50–80:1 (18).

Glucose is the most important carbohydrate in the body and preferential fuel for the brain, renal medulla, leukocytes, and erythrocytes. When exogenous carbohydrate is inadequate, the body quickly consumes liver and muscle glycogen stores while converting protein from muscle via gluconeogenesis to energy. The estimated consumption of glucose for these vital organs is approximately 150 g daily or approximately 2–3 g/kg/day (1). Therefore, it is crucial to administer adequate amounts of carbohydrate (and/or alternatively fat) to spare muscle protein from gluconeogenesis. Carbohydrates have a caloric density of 3.4–4 cal/g and consumption generally ranges from 30–50% of total calories per day depending on the patient's underlying medical condition (e.g., Type I or II diabetes mellitus) and comorbidities. Critically ill cancer patients are metabolically stressed with an accelerated rate of gluconeogenesis and a relative hyperglycemic state with peripheral insulin resistance (13).

When formulating a nutrition support plan, a hypocaloric, high protein composition may be required for patients with a history of diabetes mellitus, sepsis, hyperglycemia, pancreatitis, or obesity. A hypocaloric, high protein regimen consists of 20–25 cal/kg/day and 2 g protein/kg/day based upon the patient's ideal body weight provided their actual body weight is greater. Critically ill cancer patients manifest an inflammatory response with increased insulin resistance, glucose intolerance, and an impaired muscle glucose uptake. This further increases liver glucose production and despite the use of exogenous glucose infusions, gluconeogenesis is minimally inhibited in the critically ill (19). Intensive insulin therapy may be required to maintain appropriate blood glucose concentrations. In a 12-month study evaluating 1548 ICU patients, intensive insulin therapy to maintain blood glucose concentrations below 110 mg/dL reduced morbidity and mortality (20). However, the limitations of this study were that it was performed in a surgical ICU environment and only 31% of the patients had cancer. In critically ill cancer patients, a blood glucose goal of less than 110 mg/dL is often difficult to achieve due to hypermetabolism, insulin resistance, and corticosteroid use. A blood glucose goal of less than 150 mg/dL in this group of patients may be more realistic and more studies are needed in cancer patients.

Fat mobilization is often seen in host wasting with cancer cachexia. There are two dietary fatty acids considered essential for humans. If less than 4% of α-linolenic and linoleic acid are consumed in the diet of a healthy individual, an essential fatty acid deficiency (EFAD) may occur within approximately 4 weeks. An EFAD may present with a scaly dermatitis, alopecia, thrombocytopenia, anemia, and impaired wound healing; unfortunately, many of these critically ill patients may already manifest and confound the diagnosis of EFAD. Additionally, these EFAD signs and symptoms may present earlier in critically ill cancer patients with pre-existing malnutrition. Fat has a caloric density of 9 cal/g orally or enterally and the recommended daily fat intake is generally less than 30% of the total daily calories. Table 5 summarizes the total nutritional needs for critically ill cancer patients.

Table 5 Nutritional Needs for Critically Ill Cancer Patients

Substrate (caloric density)	Percentage (%) of total calories/day	Recommendations	Considerations	Monitoring parameters
Protein (1 g = 4 cal)	15–25	1.5 g/kg/day	↓With hepatic dysfunction with encephalopathy or severe azotemia ↑With high output fistulas, chyle leaks, CRRT, or nonhealing/large wounds	Prealbumin 24-hr UUN Urine output BUN Neurologic/ mental status
Carbohydrate Enteral/oral (1 g = 4 cal) Dextrose IV (1 g = 3.4 cal)	30–50	Dextrose infusion ≤4 mg/kg/min or ≤6 g/kg/day	Initiate slowly (2 g/kg/day) and gradually titrate to goal ↓ With hyperglycemia > 150 mg/dL	Electrolytes Serum glucose Urine output Pulmonary function Liver function tests
Fat Enteral/oral (1 g = 9 cal) Fat emulsion IV (10%-1 g = 11 cal; 20%-1 g = 10 cal)	10–25	IV infusion ≤1 g/kg/day (rate not to exceed 0.11 g/kg/hr)	IVPB hang time maximum of 12 hr if separate infusion Fat emulsion IV contains glycerin 10% solution = 1.1 kcal/mL 20% solution = 2 kcal/mL	Triglycerides Liver function tests

IV. ENTERAL VERSUS PARENTERAL NUTRITION

The ability to feed as early as possible to avoid prolonged starvation in critically ill patients has been a clinical challenge for several decades. A systematic review by Marik and Zaloga (21) on early enteral nutrition in acutely ill patients evaluated 15 randomized studies that compared early (<36 hr) vs. late (>36 hr) initiation of enteral feeding. Their findings showed a lower rate of infectious complications and reduced length of hospital stay with early enteral nutrition. Unfortunately, no significant difference in mortality or noninfectious complications was observed between the early vs. late initiation groups. A major limitation of this review was that it only included studies of patients with abdominal surgery, trauma, head injury, and burns. Additionally, no medical patients or the differentiation between cancer patients vs. noncancer patients were included in this systematic review.

Despite their ICU diagnosis, early enteral nutrition should be considered when a patient is hemodynamically stable and expected to be unable to eat by mouth for 5 days or more (22–25). Enteral nutrition offers the advantages of being more physiologic, minimizes atrophy of intestinal villi, stimulates gut-associated lymphoid tissue, and may prevent translocation of intestinal bacteria. When compared to parenteral nutrition (PN), enteral nutrition has fewer metabolic and mechanical complications (e.g., infection, thrombophlebitis, and pneumothorax), is less expensive, and may result in decreased hospital length of stay (23).

The ICU cancer patient requiring enteral nutrition for an anticipated time period of less than 2 weeks should have a small-bore (≤12 French) nasogastric or nasoduodenal feeding tube placed. For anticipated long-term feeding, a gastrostomy, gastrojejunostomy, or jejunostomy feeding tube should be considered and are often placed intraoperatively for surgical cancer patients. Pump-controlled continuous infusions are recommended in critically ill patients to prevent gastric distention, gastroesophageal reflex, dumping syndrome, and diarrhea.

Selecting an enteral nutrition formula is generally based on the patients' total nutrient requirements, need for fluid restriction, or the extent of normal digestion and absorption of the small intestine and colon present. There are several types of enteral formulas available commercially and each institution generally has developed their own formulary to meet their specific patient population requirements. Enteral nutrition is often classified by its protein content and these classifications include monomeric, oligomeric, and polymeric formulas. Monomeric (elemental) and oligomeric (semielemental) formulas contain high amounts of nitrogen as free amino acids or hydrolyzed proteins. These formulas also contain carbohydrates as glucose polymers and a lower content of fat from readily absorbable sources, such as medium-chain triglycerides. This combination requires minimal digestion, which leaves little residual for the colon and fortunately less diarrhea. Patients suffering from fat malabsorption, pancreatic exocrine insufficiency, and short bowel syndrome may benefit from these specific formulas.

Polymeric enteral formulas contain intact or partially hydrolyzed proteins and are generally considered isotonic (< 500 mOsm/kg). These polymeric formulas generally meet most patients' caloric needs and are lactose-free. Unfortunately, they often require additional protein supplementation to meet the nitrogen requirements of ICU patients. When compared to monomeric and oligomeric formulas, they are more palatable, do not require mixing or formulation, and are less expensive, making them a convenient choice. Additionally, administration of 1–2 L/day of most polymeric enteral formulas will meet the recommended adult dietary allowances for vitamins and minerals.

Specialized enteral formulas are commercially available for critically ill patients that target the cellular level to enhance immunity and minimize inflammation. Most contain one or more of the following immune-enhancing substrates: arginine, glutamine, nucleotides, and/or omega-3 fatty acids. Effects of theses agents are summarized in Table 6 (26). Arginine is a nonessential amino acid that is synthesized by the body in unstressed conditions to maintain growth and tissue repair. It is a potent anabolic hormone secretagogue, since growth hormone, glucagon, and insulin are increased with supplemental arginine. In metabolically stressed ICU patients, endogenous arginine synthesis is inadequate requiring dietary supplementation (23). Arginine supplementation may help maintain immune function and promote wound healing.

Nucleotides, which consist of purines and pyrimidines, are the structural components of deoxyribonucleic acid (DNA), ribonucleic acid (RNA), adenosine triphosphate, and multiple coenzymes. They are a small component [1–2 g/day] of a normal adult oral diet and are also available to the host via de novo synthesis or from degradation of DNA and RNA. The addition of nucleotides to enteral formulas may help maintain immunocompentence and GI mucosal function during periods of hypermetabolism and critical illness (26).

Glutamine is a nonessential amino acid that functions in many metabolic pathways (e.g., major substrate for gluconeogenesis, precursor of urinary ammonia, and nitrogen transport) and is considered conditionally essential in major catabolic states.

Table 6 Immune-Modulating Agents and Effects on the Host

Agent	Effects
Glutamine	Major fuel for enterocytes, colonocytes, lymphocytes, and macrophages Minimizes atrophy during PN and after chemotherapy and radiation Nitrogen shuttle Precursor of glutathione Role in hepatic visceral protein synthesis Substrate for renal ammonia production
Arginine	Suppression of T-cell-mediated immune function Positive effects on wound healing Increases insulin, IGF-1 Increases wound bed protein and hydroxyproline accumulation
Omega-3 polyunsaturated fatty acids	Modification of the inflammatory cascade (anti-inflammatory properties)
Docosahexaenoic acid	Alters eicosanoid and cytokine production
Eicosapentaenoic acid	Promotes T cell proliferation and cell-to-cell adhesion
Gamma linolenic acid	Modulates vascular dynamics, clotting, cell division, and growth

Glutamine is the primary fuel source in epithelial cells, lymphocytes, macrophages, and enterocytes of the intestinal mucosa. During injury or hypermetabolism, there is increased glutamine consumption primarily through the GI tract causing decreased plasma concentrations. Supplementation with glutamine may help maintain intestinal mucosal integrity and prevent bacterial translocation (26).

Fats, or commonly referred to as lipids, provide cell membrane structure and are precursors for the synthesis of eicosanoids. A typical Western oral diet is rich in polyunsaturated fatty acids, namely omega-6 fatty acids (e.g., linoleic acid). Interestingly, the source of fat has been shown to modulate the proinflammatory response to injury and hypermetabolism (26). Under normal metabolism, linoleic acid is finally desaturated to arachidonic acid that synthesizes eicosanoids via the cyclo-oxygenase and lipo-oxygenase pathways. This produces the proinflammatory and immune-suppressing 2-series prostaglandins and 4-series leukotrienes, which stimulate the production of tumor necrosis factor-alpha and interleukins-1, -2 and -6. Alternatively, linolenic acid, an omega-3 fatty acid, eventually desaturates into eicosapentaenoic acid, which produces the anti-inflammatory and immunomodulatory 3-series prostaglandins and 5-series leukotrienes (27,28). Additionally, the type of fats consumed can alter the composition of erythrocyte cell membranes in critically ill patients within 7 days (29).

Immune-enhancing formulas in critically ill cancer patients remain controversial. The immune-enhancing formulas commercially available often contain arginine that may be detrimental in patients that have ongoing systemic inflammatory response syndrome, sepsis, and organ failure. Arginine, as it is metabolized to citrulline, forms nitrous oxide that may lead to vasodilatation, transient hypotension, and an enhanced systemic inflammatory response (30). Arginine supplementation in postoperative patients has been shown to be beneficial given its association with reduced infectious risk, ventilator days, ICU, and hospital length of stay; however, it does not appear to be beneficial and may actually be harmful in critically ill patients with sepsis (30,31).

Only one randomized trial of immune-enhancing nutrition in the ICU has demonstrated a statistically significant difference in clinically important outcomes compared to a control group in an intention-to-treat analysis. Galban et al. evaluated 181 septic medical ICU patients fed enterally with Acute Physiology and Chronic Health Evaluation (APACHE) II baseline scores greater than 10 (32). Patients were randomized either to a standard or an immune-enhancing enteral formula containing omega-3 fatty acids, nucleotides, and arginine. The patients who received the immune-enhancing enteral formula experienced a reduction in mortality and number of bacteremic episodes. A reduction in mortality was only seen in patients with APACHE II scores less than 15, implying the least sick patients experience the most benefit (32). The patients in this study with an APACHE II baseline score greater than 15 observed no reduction in mortality compared to the control group leaving the effect of immune-enhancing nutrition in the most critically ill patients unanswered.

Unfortunately, most immune-enhancing ICU studies to date have excluded cancer patients; therefore, immune-enhancing formulas have no proven role in critically ill cancer patients (33). The cost for these specialized immune-enhancing formulas can be significantly higher than standard polymeric enteral formulas and the relative benefit must be considered before selection. Further research is clearly needed in this patient population before recommendations are developed.

Enteral nutrition is commonly associated with several patient complications, which can often be avoided if monitored appropriately. General monitoring parameters for patients receiving enteral nutrition include proper feeding tube placement, head of bed elevation to 30 degrees, daily weights and fluid balance, bowel function and consistency (constipation or diarrhea), glucose, electrolytes, gastric residuals (if gastrically placed feeding tube), nausea, vomiting, abdominal discomfort, cramping, and pain. Common mechanical complications include pulmonary aspiration of gastric contents, inadvertent tracheobronchial placement of the feeding tube, ulceration of the gastric mucosa, and feeding tube occlusion from medication administration. Feeding tube occlusion is often prevented by flushing pre- and postmedication administration with 10–30 mL of warm tap water and using elixir medication formulations when possible.

Aspiration of enteral nutrition is the most severe complication and precautions such as elevating the patients' head of bed to a minimum of 30 to preferably 45 degrees (if possible) are strongly recommended. Checking gastric residuals when gastric and duodenal feedings are used may also be helpful to prevent aspiration and feedings should be held when a high (>200 mL) residual is confirmed. Prokinetic medications, such as metoclopramide and erythromycin, may be beneficial for high gastric residuals along with positioning smaller (≤12 French) nasoenteric tubes beyond the pylorus. Unfortunately despite these precautions, pulmonary aspiration of gastric or oropharyngeal contents occurs frequently in critically ill patients requiring mechanical ventilation (34). Blue food dye has been regularly added in the past to enteral nutrition formulations to help detect aspiration in the mechanical ventilation circuit or tracheal secretions. This practice of adding the blue food dye has actually led to several cases of skin, plasma, and urine discoloration, as well as death in critically ill patients (34). Therefore, the practice of adding blue food dye in enteral nutrition formulations is strongly discouraged.

Diarrhea is a common problem in the ICU. Most patients in the ICU receiving enteral nutrition have multiple explanations for diarrhea since bacterial contamination of the enteral nutrition formulation itself may occur. Before discontinuing or holding enteral nutrition, other etiologies for diarrhea must be evaluated, such as multiple antibiotics altering the normal gastrointestinal bacterial flora, use of prokinetic medications or liquid medications containing sorbitol, and hypoalbuminemia (24). Critically ill cancer patients frequently suffer from diarrhea due to other causes, such as chemotherapy, radiation enteritis, typhilitis, multiple prior surgical resections of the small bowel and colon, graft-versus-host disease, and physiological changes that occur during critical illness.

PN is indicated for patients who cannot tolerate or meet their nutrient requirements through the gastrointestinal route. In general for ICU patients, PN should be reserved for patients who have diffuse peritonitis, intestinal obstruction, intractable vomiting, paralytic ileus, severe acute pancreatitis, high-output (>500 mL/day) enterocutaneous fistulas, severe diarrhea (>3 loose stools/day), and gastrointestinal ischemia. In 2001, the American Gastroenterological Association published their medical position statement on PN and its use in various patient populations including cancer and the critically ill (4). Overall, they cautioned that PN may be harmful if used inappropriately, such as in cancer patients undergoing chemotherapy since they found that 1 out of 14 patients treated would have no response to the chemotherapy and 1 out of every 6 patients would have an infectious complication. Unfortunately, the lack of randomized-controlled trials in critically ill cancer patients did not allow them a recommendation for its use in this population. However, patients with esophageal and gastric cancer who are severely malnourished benefit from preoperative PN since it reduces the rate of major postoperative complications.

The PN is usually given through a large, high flow central vein. The most common central access devices placed in the ICU are the percutaneous nontunneled jugular, femoral, or subclavian central venous catheters. The PN is often administered as a 3-in-1 admixture containing protein, dextrose, and fat emulsion or as a 2-in-1 admixture (protein, dextrose) with fat emulsion as a separate infusion. The advantage of administering fat emulsion as a separate infusion is the potential visual detection of small precipitates or particulates in the 2-in-1 admixture or other chemical incompatibilities if other medications are coinfused. Peripheral PN is not recommended in critically ill patients due to the increased fluid requirements needed and inability to provide adequate amounts of nutrition to prevent protein catabolism. Additionally, peripheral venous extravasation injury may result in tissue injury and necrosis.

The PN provides protein in the form of crystalline amino acids, carbohydrates as hypertonic dextrose, and fat emulsion as triacylglycerols. A variety of crystalline amino acids solutions are commercially available based upon their concentrations (3–20%) and balance between essential, nonessential, and semiessential amino acids. There are specialty amino acids for hepatic failure and critical illness that contain a higher percentage of branched-chain amino acids (BCAA). Unfortunately, there are currently no parenteral amino acids solutions in the United States that contain glutamine. Intravenous glutamine is heat sensitive, has limited stability, and a short shelf-life (35). In addition, glutamine is broken down into glutamic acid and ammonia, which could be detrimental in patients with liver failure.

Carbohydrate for intravenous use is available as dextrose in water in several concentrations ranging from 2.5–70%. Intravenous dextrose administration allows protein-sparing with minimal adverse effects when rates are $\leq$4 mg dextrose/kg/min or approximately 400 g/day for a 70 kg patient. Dextrose infusion rates in the ICU greater than 2–3 mg dextrose/kg/min may result in hyperglycemia and an increase in carbon dioxide production if underlying pulmonary dysfunction is present (36,37).

Fat for intravenous use is supplied as an oil-in-water emulsion of either soybean oil or a mixture of soybean and safflower oils. The soybean oil provides mainly omega-6 long-chain fatty acids (e.g., linoleic acid) and is commercially available in three concentrations of 10, 20 and 30%. However, the 30% is only for compounding and not direct intravenous infusion in its undiluted form. The caloric density of fat emulsion is slightly increased (11 cal/g for 10% and 10 cal/g for 20% and 30%) compared to enteral fat (9 cal/g) by the addition of glycerin and egg phospholipids as emulsifiers and to adjust the osmolarity of the oil-in-water emulsions. Intravenous fat emulsion must be used cautiously in patients who have serum triglyceride concentrations greater than 400 mg/dL, a history of type IV hyperlipidemia, and a severe egg allergy as fat emulsion contains egg phosphatides. The omega-6 long-chain fatty acids are precursors to eicosanoid synthesis and thus have the potential to be immunosuppressive and proinflammatory. Given these risks for the critically ill ICU patient, it is recommended that intravenous fat emulsion be administered in amounts less than 1 g/kg/day. When fat emulsion is administered intravenously, the maximal infusion rate should not exceed 0.11 g/kg/hr to prevent pulmonary gas diffusion abnormalities (38).

When initiating nutrition support in ICU patients who have not eaten for 7–10 days or in those with severe malnutrition, a complication known as "refeeding syndrome" may occur (39). Refeeding syndrome is defined as a total body depletion and compartmental shift of the primary intracellular electrolytes, phosphate, potassium, and magnesium. Chronic hypophosphatemia associated with the refeeding syndrome may be dangerous and potentially life threatening (Table 7). Other complications seen include alterations in glucose metabolism from thiamine deficiency with resulting lactic acidosis and volume overload. To avoid refeeding syndrome complications, initiate dextrose or carbohydrate infusion rates at less than 2 mg dextrose/kg/min or 200 g carbohydrate/day for a 70 kg patient and slowly increase to the patient's nutritional goals over 3–5 days as tolerated.

Table 7 Hypophosphatemia Adverse Effects

Cardiac dysfunction	Congestive heart failure
	Arrhthymias
	Sudden death
Neuromuscular dysfunction	Areflexic paralysis
	Confusion
	Lethargy
	Coma
Hematologic dysfunction	Altered red blood cells
	Altered white blood cells
	Hemolytic anemia
	Thrombocytopenia
Respiratory dysfunction	Decreased muscle contractility

V. NUTRITION SUPPORT IN SPECIAL PATIENT POPULATIONS

As mentioned earlier, the lack of available nutrition support information in critically ill cancer patients lends itself to the application of general nutrition principles in patients with underlying disease states such as hepatic, renal, and pulmonary failure. The following sections will be devoted to general principles on nutrient utilization and metabolism, effects on the host, assessment, and nutritional goals in special patient populations commonly encountered in the ICU.

VI. HEPATIC FAILURE

Chronic liver disease accounts for over 26,000 deaths annually and is the 7th leading disease-related cause of death in the United States (40). Acute decompensation or an abrupt decline in chronic liver disease was responsible for 356,000 hospital admissions and 1.56 million hospital days during the calendar year October 1996 to September 1997. It was estimated that of those admitted, 15% die within 30 days and have a 50% life expectancy within 4 years of their first admission to the hospital (41). In the ICU cancer patient, liver failure can be due to any of the following: primary malignancy, chemotherapy regimens, medications, vascular diseases, or hemodynamic collapse (Table 8) (42).

Many clinicians underestimate the value of the liver with respect to nutrition and metabolic homeostasis. The liver functions in the metabolism of carbohydrate,

Table 8 Causes of Liver Failure in Oncology

Malignancy	Hepatocellular carcinoma, metastatic infiltration of the liver
Chemotherapy	Cyclophosphamide, methotrexate, etoposide, cytarabine, asparaginase, nitrogen mustards, mercaptopurine, doxorubicin, taxanes, gemtuzumab, mitomycin C, and interleukin-2
Medications	Analgesics: acetaminophen, aspirin, and nonsteroidal anti-inflammatory drugs Steroids: estrogen, testosterone, and oral contraceptives Anticonvulsants: phenytoin, valproic acid, carbamazepine, and phenobarbital Antimicrobial agents: sulfonamides, erythromycin, penicillins, cephalosporins, rifampin, isoniazid, pentamidine, high dose tetracyclines, and fluoroquinolones Antifungal agents: ketoconazole, itraconazole, and fluconazole Cardiovascular agents: amiodarone, procainamide, diltiazem, quinidine, hydralazine, angiotensin-converting enzyme inhibitors, and methyldopa Oral hypoglycemic agents Antipsychotic agents: chlorpromazine, haloperidol, serotonin reuptake inhibitors, thioridazine, and fluphenazine Vitamin/Minerals: Vitamins A and E, iron salts, and niacin
Vascular disease	Veno-occlusive disorder
Hemodynamic	Sepsis, hypotension, hypovolemia, and congestive heart failure
Surgery	Hepatic resection
Other diseases	Antitrypsin deficiency, Wilson's disease, and hemachromatosis

amino acids, ammonia, cholesterol and lipids, the synthesis of numerous proteins and glycoproteins, and the detoxification of ingested compounds and hormones (43). The liver is very resilient, only in extreme cases of hepatic insufficiency (approximately $\leq$20% of functioning hepatocytes) will alterations in metabolic activity occur (44). These alterations are similar regardless of the type of insult, and commonly present as hyper- or hypoglycemia, mental status changes due to encephalopathy, muscle wasting, alterations in visceral protein concentrations, coagulation abnormalities, and unpredictable drug and hormonal effects.

Patients with liver failure are at a high risk of PCM and the degree of PCM noted corresponds to the severity of liver disease and outcome (45). It has been documented in the literature that 20% of patients with compensated liver failure and 80% of patients with decompensated liver failure have PCM (46). A VA Cooperative Study showed a 100% prevalence of PCM in severe alcoholic hepatitis patients (47). Liver transplantation remains the only treatment modality to halt protein catabolism and improve metabolic profiles in liver failure patients (48). Many factors lead to PCM in patients with liver failure including poor oral intake due to early satiety and unpalatable diets, malabsorption with resultant diarrhea, maldigestion, hormonal changes, and alterations in nutrient substrates (46).

This section will focus on the two major types of hepatic disease seen in critically ill cancer patients: acute liver failure (fulminant hepatitis and ischemic hepatitis) and chronic liver failure (compensated and decompensated cirrhosis). Acute liver failure is due to acute inflammation and necrosis of the liver with subsequent elevations in liver function tests. Fulminant hepatitis is a rare and devastating condition that occurs as a result of severe liver injury secondary to acute viral hepatitis, medications, toxins, and liver transplant failures. Excessive hepatic necrosis is the major characteristic of this type of acute liver failure and results in metabolic shutdown, coma, and death in as early as 1 week of injury (48). Other associated complications include cerebral edema, gastrointestinal hemorrhage, coagulopathy, and hypoglycemia. Ischemic hepatitis (also known as "shock liver") is characterized by centrilobular necrosis and an acute reversible elevation of serum aminotransferases. This is caused by a sustained period of hypotension and conditions associated with altered blood flow to the liver (49).

Chronic liver failure is caused by progressive degenerative changes within the liver resulting in an accumulation of nonfunctional scar tissue. Chronic viral hepatitis, chronic alcohol use, toxins, and certain metabolic and autoimmune diseases result in this condition (48). Patients with compensated cirrhosis usually show no signs of ascites, encephalopathy, alterations in serum albumin concentrations (albumin $\geq$3.5 g/dL), and have normal to slightly elevated serum total bilirubin levels (<1.5 mg/dL). Patients presenting with ascites, encephalopathy, hypoalbuminemia (serum albumin <3.5 g/dL), and elevated serum total bilirubin levels (>2.5 mg/dL) are classified as having decompensated cirrhosis (44).

Much of the data regarding the effects on substrate metabolism in liver failure have been gathered from the analysis of cirrhotic patients (Table 9) (46,48,50). Nutritional changes seen in liver failure patients include decreased glycogen stores, a lower respiratory quotient due to utilization of fat and protein for energy, attenuated protein synthesis, increased amino acid oxidation, and a normal to increased resting energy expenditure. Studies show that only 16–34% of cirrhotics have elevated energy expenditure (51) related to increased concentrations of catecholamines (52). Hunter et al. (53) compared results from indirect calorimetry to equations estimating energy expenditure in ICU patients, and noted that critically ill cirrhotic patients are not hypermetabolic on average.

Table 9 Effects on Substrate Metabolism in Liver Failure

Substrate affected	Effect in liver failure
Carbohydrate	Impairment in glucose and glycogen homeostasis
	Decreased glycogen stores in liver and muscle
	Normal to increased glucose consumption
	Hypoglycemia during periods of minimal fasting
	Insulin resistance
Protein	Increase in protein catabolism
	Low levels of BCAA
	High levels of AAA
	Imbalance in the production of urea and elimination of ammonia
	Depressed production of albumin
Fat	Increased lipolysis
	Enhanced turnover of nonesterified fatty acids
	Impairment of fatty acid storage as triglycerides
	Depletion of fat reserves
	Decreased maximal clearing ability of exogenous lipids
Other metabolic abnormalities	Increased insulin, glucagon, tumor necrosis factor, interleukins-1 and -6, catecholamines, growth hormone, and estradiol
	Decreased insulin-growth factor hormone-1 and cortisol

All patients with liver failure possess some defect in glucose homeostasis with the extent correlating to the amount of hepatic damage. Prolonged fasting is not recommended in critically ill liver failure patients due to their already depleted glycogen stores. Elevated growth hormone and depressed insulin-like growth factor-1 further contribute to diminished glycogen stores by decreasing glycogenesis and increasing protein catabolism (50). Generally, less than 12 hr of glycogen stores are present in liver failure patients and this obviously provides little substrate for maintaining baseline metabolic functions (48). Coincidentally, the rate of glucose consumption often remains unchanged and possibly increased due to cytokines (IL-1, IL-6, and TNF) and other counterregulatory hormones (insulin and glucagon). These patients require intravenous infusions of at least 10% dextrose early in their hospital admission or when signs and symptoms of hypoglycemia appear to prevent damage to vital organs, such as the brain. In contrast, cirrhotic patients receiving carbohydrates will exhibit hyperglycemia secondary to insulin resistance and defects in the metabolism and utilization of glucose (50).

With the increased rate of protein and fat metabolism used for energy, significant wasting of LBM and depletion of fat stores occurs. Changes in serum amino acids consistent with low concentrations of BCAA (leucine, valine, and isoleucine) and increased concentrations of aromatic amino acids (AAA) (phenylalanine, tyrosine, and tryptophan) are seen. There also is an imbalance in the production of urea and elimination of ammonia. These phenomena have commonly been associated with hepatic encephalopathy. Abnormalities in fat metabolism produce increased concentrations of fatty acids and ketone bodies with minimal elevations in serum triglyceride concentrations. This is primarily due to a decrease in lipoprotein lipase activity and increase in lipolysis (44,50).

Physical assessment and calculation of energy needs can be difficult in this subset of ICU patients. The SGA is a useful and accurate tool, and care must be taken not to overlook the presence of ascites, edema or anasarca, recent weight changes, and use of diuretics when determining a feeding weight (54). The use of traditional laboratory values for assessing malnutrition (serum albumin, prealbumin, and transferrin) is unreliable in liver failure secondary to reduced synthesis and volume imbalances. Indirect calorimetry and 24-hr nitrogen balance can also be used to guide therapy, the latter becoming more unreliable in patients with coexisting renal disease and decompensated liver failure.

The key to remember when providing nutrition support to critically ill patients with hepatic failure is to preserve LBM. Repletion or the attempt to support anabolism should not be the primary goal due to the inability of these patients to utilize large quantities of substrates administered to them over short periods of time (48). Use of the enteral route is preferred due to the beneficial effect on mucosal integrity and blunting of the stress response in critically ill patients. PN should be reserved for those unable to tolerate oral or enteral nutrition. Recommendations for nutrition support in patients with liver failure can be found in Tables 10–13 (44,48). Of note, patients undergoing elective hepatic resection are treated as typical post-operative patients unless hepatic encephalopathy or liver failure is present after surgery.

Prudent electrolyte management is important in this patient population since restrictions in sodium and fluid are mandated in patients with ascites and/or peripheral edema, as well as patients with fulminant hepatitis. Patients with fulminant hepatitis have coexisting cerebral edema, and the overzealous use of fluids may be fatal. The use of supplemental magnesium is often required in patients with a history of significant alcohol abuse, and documented magnesium deficiency is common in cirrhotics receiving diuretics. Hypophosphatemia is clinically significant in both acute liver failure and major hepatic resections since large quantities of oral and intravenous phosphate (>0.5 mmol/kg/day) may be necessary to provide homeostasis (48,55). Additionally, hypophosphatemia may be a risk factor for further hepatic injury and therefore supports aggressive supplementation for hepatic function and regeneration (56).

The administration of vitamins and trace elements to meet the recommended adult dietary allowances should be administered to all hepatic failure patients.

Table 10 Nutrition Support in Acute Liver Failure

Substrate	Fulminant and ischemic hepatitis
Energy	30–35 cal/kg/day
Protein	0.6 g/kg/day standard amino acids • If encephalopathy persists, change to enriched BCAA solution • Once mental status clears, increase protein to 1–1.5 g/kg/day and change to standard amino acids
Fluid restriction	Yes
Electrolytes	Sodium restriction and phosphate supplementation
Vitamins/minerals	Multivitamin and zinc

Table 11 Nutrition Support in Compensated Cirrhosis

Substrate	Compensated cirrhosis
Energy	30–35 cal/kg/day Frequent small meals and bedtime snack (utilizing complex carbohydrates) if taking oral diet
Protein	1–1.5 g/kg/day
Fluid restriction	Variable
Electrolytes	Sodium restriction if ascites or edema
Vitamins/minerals	Multivitamin and zinc

A history of alcohol abuse necessitates the initial administration of additional thiamine, folate, and potentially cyanocobalamin. Zinc deficiency is common in liver failure patients and should be supplemented at a dose up to 660 mg orally or enterally (30 mg IV) as the sulfate salt (50). Elevated serum total bilirubin concentrations warrant discontinuation of manganese and copper supplementation in PN to prevent the development of neurological adverse effects.

Hepatic encephalopathy presents as an alteration in mental status and is a sign of end stage liver failure that conveys a poor prognosis. The pathophysiology of hepatic encephalopathy is not completely understood, but is thought to involve imbalances in serum amino acid ratios (AAA to BCAA), the production of pathogenic neuroamines, and the liver's inability to eliminate nitrogenous compounds such as ammonia created by both the small intestine and colon (57–59). Arterial or venous ammonia concentrations can be used along with a thorough physical assessment to direct the diagnosis of hepatic encephalopathy. There are precipitating factors or "triggers" thought to instigate hepatic encephalopathy. These factors include gastrointestinal hemorrhage, infections, renal and electrolyte disorders, constipation, increased dietary protein, and acute liver decompensation. The goals of therapy in hepatic encephalopathy include correcting the underlying cause for decompensation, reducing the nitrogenous load in the intestinal system via bowel cleansing using nonabsorbing disaccharides (e.g., lactulose) with or without antimicrobials (e.g., neomycin), and preventing repeated episodes. Protein restriction is not appropriate (<0.6 g protein/kg/day) and leads to further iatrogenic protein malnutrition in cirrhotic patients with hepatic encephalopathy.

The use of intravenous solutions enriched with BCAA for patients with hepatic encephalopathy remains controversial. A meta-analysis conducted by

Table 12 Nutrition Support in Decompensated Cirrhosis

Substrate	Cirrhosis and acute encephalopathy	Cirrhosis and chronic encephalopathy
Energy	35 cal/kg/day	35 cal/kg/day
Protein	0.6–0.8 g/kg/day standard amino acids • If encephalopathy persists, change to branched-chain amino acid solution • Once mental status clears, may increase protein to 1–1.5 g/kg/day	0.6–0.8 g/kg/day standard amino acids Frequent small meals and bedtime snack if taking oral diet
Fluid restriction	Yes	
Electrolytes	Sodium restriction and add magnesium if alcohol history and phosphate as needed	
Vitamins	Multivitamin, thiamine, folic acid, vitamin K, and zinc	

Naylor et al. (60) comparing BCAA vs. standard amino acids solutions in PN showed faster rates of recovery from hepatic encephalopathy and a questionable mortality benefit. Eriksson and Conn (61) determined no clear benefit for both enteral and parenteral BCAA supplementation in a separate meta-analysis. The preferential use of these BCAA enriched solutions is clinically debatable and their increased costs may outweigh their benefits when patients have grade 2 or less hepatic encephalopathy. The recommendation from the American Society for Enteral and parenteral nutrition is that BCAA-enriched solutions should only be used in patients with refractory encephalopathy (62).

VII. RENAL FAILURE

Acute renal failure (ARF) is defined as an elevation of 50% over baseline in blood urea nitrogen (BUN) and serum creatinine occurring over a period of 1–2 days. This is commonly associated with a decrease or abrupt cessation of urine output. The ARF occurs in roughly 5% of hospitalized patients and is associated with a 50–90% mortality rate (63). The development of adverse consequences secondary to ARF occurs only after significant reductions in creatinine clearance ($\leq$20 mL/min). These adverse effects include fluid retention, electrolyte imbalances (hyperkalemia, hyperphosphatemia, and hypermagnesemia), metabolic acidosis, azotemia, and hyperglycemia.

Table 13 Nutrition Support in Liver Resection

Substrate	Post-liver resection
Energy	30–35 cal/kg/day
Protein	1.5 g/kg/day – If encephalopathy: 0.8 g/kg/day $\pm$ use of BCAA solution
Fluid	Variable
Electrolytes	Sodium restriction and phosphate supplementation
Vitamins	Multivitamin and zinc

Cancer patients are exposed to numerous agents that can lead to the development of ARF including aggressive chemotherapy protocols designed for cancer remission and cure. Other precipitating factors include nephrotoxic antimicrobial agents, intravenous contrast, hypovolemia, hemodynamic collapse, and associated oncology syndromes (thrombotic thrombocytopenia purpura, tumor lysis syndrome, hypercalcemia, and bone marrow transplantation). Table 14 provides an overview of medications that cause ARF (64,65).

Indications for acute hemodialysis include severe acidosis (pH < 7.20), electrolyte imbalances (serum potassium >6 mmol/L), volume overload, and severe uremia (BUN > 100 mg/dL). The decision for the use and type of hemodialysis is determined by the nephrologists and varies due to differing clinical experiences. Traditional hemodialysis, also referred to as intermittent hemodialysis (IHD), is the treatment modality of choice in patients who are hemodynamically stable. The IHD can be done in 3–6 hr sessions 3–7 days per week depending on patient specific characteristics such as blood pressure, volume to remove, and need for dialysis. Hemodynamically unstable patients with ARF often receive a form of CRRT known as sustained low-efficiency dialysis (SLED). CRRT has been shown to be safe for use in hemodynamically unstable patients due to the slower removal of fluid and improved solute control. The advantages of SLED over other continuous forms of hemodialysis (CAVHD, CVVHD) include decreased nursing time, use of a standard hemodialysis machine with modified software for

Table 14 Drug-Induced Acute Renal Failure in Oncology

Chemotherapy	Carmustine, cisplatin, carboplatin, ifosfamide, mitomycin, gemcitabine, methotrexate, pentostatin, aldesleukin, high dose cyclophosphamide, interferon alpha, and bleomycin/cisplatin
Medications	Cyclosporine, tacrolimus, NSAIDs, ACE inhibitors, aminoglycosides, amphotericin B, acyclovir, penicillins, cephalosporins, high dose tetracycline, intravenous immunoglobulin, diuretics, and mannitol

continuous dialysis, a bicarbonate-based dialysate solution, lower costs, and the ability of achieving higher urea clearances of 120–140 L/day (66).

It is generally implicit that critical illness, trauma, and multisystem organ dysfunction (MODS) are associated with increases in metabolism and catabolism (67,68). The incidence of ARF in these conditions is high and augments the metabolic and nutritional abnormalities observed. This is especially true when some form of hemodialysis is utilized (67). Table 15 provides an overview of the alterations in substrate homeostasis seen in critically ill patients with ARF (67–72). Upon discussion of substrate abnormalities in this patient population, clinicians should understand that the majority of effects are secondary to the underlying critical illness and presence of acute hemodialysis, not ARF (73). In the critically ill patient with ARF, elevations are seen in numerous hormones including insulin, glucagon, catecholamines, cortisol, and growth hormone (67,69). These endogenous hormones contribute to peripheral insulin resistance with resulting hyperglycemia that frequently necessitates the use of exogenous insulin during nutrition support. Increased hepatic production of acute phase proteins, utilization of skeletal muscle for gluconeogenesis, circulating proteolytic enzymes, and metabolic acidosis subsequently lead to further protein breakdown. The accumulation of nitrogenous waste products from these factors causes azotemia and uremia. The addition of IHD or CRRT accounts for additional protein losses. The IHD yields approximately 6–10 g of protein loss per session (73) and about 10–15% of infused amino acids per day are lost with CRRT (67,69). The clinical hypothesis that ARF patients should receive essential amino acid solutions as the sole protein source has not been shown to decrease renal recovery time, improve nitrogen balance or survival when compared to standard amino acids solutions containing both essential and nonessential amino acids (62,69).

Table 15 Effects of Renal Failure and Critical Illness on Substrate Homeostasis

Substrate affected	Effect in renal failure
Carbohydrate	Insulin resistance and hyperglycemia Decreased glycogen stores
Protein	Negative nitrogen balance Increased hepatic production of acute phase proteins Increased gluconeogenesis Increased circulating proteolytic enzymes and muscle protein catabolism Acidosis-related protein breakdown Impaired skeletal muscle protein synthesis due to impaired amino acid transport and uptake Azotemia/uremia
Fat	Impaired lipolysis Increased hepatic lipid production Decreased activity of lipoprotein lipase Hypertriglyceridemia
Other metabolic abnormalities	Increase in tumor necrosis factor, interleukin-1, glucagon, insulin, growth hormone, catecholamines and cortisol Decrease in tri-iodothyronine, testosterone, and ± insulin-growth factor hormone-1

The development of ARF during hospital admission has a high incidence of associated mortality (74,75). Malnutrition has not been identified as a risk factor despite an increased prevalence of malnutrition observed in hospitalized patients (76). A prospective cohort study by Fiaccadori et al. (77) assessed 309 ARF patients using SGA as well as traditional anthropometric assessment methods until death or hospital discharge. They found that 58% of patients were classified as malnourished and 42% were severely malnourished on admission. This subset of malnourished patients had a statistically significant increase in hospital mortality, hospital morbidity, and increased healthcare costs. This study suggests that severely malnourished ARF patients have a higher mortality and may warrant aggressive nutrition support; however, further research is needed to validate whether aggressive nutrition support reduces mortality in this patient population.

The nutrition assessment tool used frequently in ARF is the SGA. As with liver failure, physical assessments should include identification of volume overload

Table 16 Nutrition Support in Predialysis Renal Failure

Substrate	Predialysis
Energy	30–35 cal/kg/day
Protein	0.5–0.8 g/kg/day (adjust per BUN)
Fluid	Restrict
Electrolytes	As needed
Vitamins	Multivitamin

symptoms, recent weight changes, and signs and symptoms of nutrient deficiencies. The clinician should focus on the presence of comorbid disease states and any current treatment modalities used such as IHD, CRRT, and/or mechanical ventilation. The goals for nutrition support in ARF patients should not be confused with those for chronic renal failure (CRF). Protein restrictions of 0.6 g/kg/day as seen in CRF are not beneficial in ARF patients due to differences in protein homeostasis (63). Nutritional recommendations for patients with ARF can be found in Tables 16 and 17 (78).

Electrolyte management is guided by the use and type of hemodialysis. For predialysis patients, minimal to no electrolyte supplementation is employed due to decreased renal clearance. In fact, therapies may be employed to decrease the potential for adverse effects related to hyperkalemia, hypermagnesemia, and hyperphosphatemia. As needed, electrolyte supplementation with small gradual additions of scheduled daily electrolytes is a common practice in IHD patients. Our experience with 24-hr SLED has indicated that large amounts of magnesium (>0.5 mEq/kg/day) and phosphate (>0.5 mmol/kg/day) are usually needed within 24–48 hr of initiation of SLED due to the low concentrations of magnesium and lack of phosphate in the dialysate. Sodium and fluid restrictions are warranted to prevent volume overload and edema. Total serum calcium concentrations may be low in ARF patients due to hyperphosphatemia, reduced hydroxylation of vitamin D to 1,25-dihydroxyvitamin D (active form), low serum albumin concentrations, and hydration state (72). In these cases, measurement of serum ionized calcium concentrations is more clinically useful in managing symptomatic hypocalcemia.

Significant removal of water-soluble vitamins (B and C) occurs with hemodialysis, and renal diets with protein restrictions are also low in these vitamins. For these reasons, renal failure patients should receive daily multivitamins (79). However, in order to prevent oxalate deposition in the heart, kidney, and blood vessels, vitamin C supplementation should not exceed 200 mg/day in acute or CRF patients (72). If enteral feedings are being used, exogenous multivitamins will not be required as the majority of enteral nutrition products contain the recommended adult dietary allowances of vitamin and minerals when at least 1 L is used daily. Deficiencies or an excess of fat-soluble vitamins is rarely a concern in ARF due to the duration of this condition. There is literature suggesting deficiencies in vitamin E and selenium in ARF, but its clinical relevance is uncertain at this time (67). Iron studies should be assessed in anemic ARF or CRF patients on dialysis. Supplementation with 150 mg elemental oral iron daily or equivalent doses of parenteral iron should be administered if ferritin levels are <50 ng/dL (80).

VIII. PULMONARY FAILURE

Pulmonary failure is the primary reason for medical ICU admission and prolonged ICU stay. Pulmonary failure occurs due to the inability of the lungs to ventilate and subsequently oxygenate vital organs within the body. The use of mechanical ventilation is dependent upon the functional reserve of respiratory muscles in response to the patient's acute disease process. Acute respiratory failure in patients with chronic obstructive pulmonary disease (COPD), acute lung injury (ALI), and acute respiratory distress syndrome (ARDS) is frequently seen in the ICU and will be the topic of this section.

COPD is a group of pulmonary disorders characterized by airway obstruction caused by the destruction in the functional parenchyma of the lung

Table 17 Nutrition Support in Renal Failure with Dialysis

Substrate	IHD	SLED
Energy	30–35 cal/kg/day	25–30 cal/kg/day
Protein	1.2–1.5 g/kg/day	1.5–2.5 g/kg/day
Fluid	Restrict	No restriction
Electrolytes	Sodium restriction and supplement other electrolytes as needed	Increased requirements of potassium, magnesium, phosphate, and calcium
Vitamins	Multivitamin and carnitine (long term)	Multivitamin

Table 18 Causes of Acute Decompensated COPD and ALI/ARDS

	ALI/ARDS	
Acute decompensated COPD	Direct causes	Indirect causes
Respiratory infections	Gastric aspiration	Sepsis
Smoking	Toxic substance inhalation	Pancreatitis
Air pollution	High-inspired oxygen	Trauma
Toxic substance inhalation	Pneumonitis	Pulmonary embolus
Pulmonary embolus	Drugs	Shock
Left-sided heart failure	Pulmonary contusion	Disseminated intravascular coagulation
Pneumothorax	Radiation	Fat embolism
		Cardiac bypass

and/or excessive mucus secretion, plugging, and bronchial inflammation. Acute respiratory decompensation in patients with COPD accounts for over 660,000 hospital admissions annually and is the 4th leading cause of death in the United States (81). The most common cause of acute decompensation is the development of a respiratory infection that leads to further airway obstruction due to increases in volume and viscosity of purulent secretions. When pneumonia is ruled out, focus should be on left ventricular failure, pulmonary embolism, pneumothorax, and air pollution (Table 18) (25).

ALI and ARDS are two disorders resulting from acute severe lung injury and hypoxemia. The source of these disorders can be directly caused by aspiration, pneumonitis, toxic substance inhalation, high-inspired oxygen, pulmonary contusion, drugs, and radiation (Table 18). Indirect causes result from critical illnesses such as sepsis, severe acute pancreatitis, pulmonary embolism, disseminated intravascular coagulation, trauma, shock, fat embolism, and coronary artery bypass procedures (25). The diagnosis is centered on three criteria: a ratio of PaO_2/FiO_2 ($\leq$300 for ALI, $\leq$200 for ARDS) independent of the amount of positive end-expiratory pressure, bilateral lung infiltrates on chest x-ray, and pulmonary artery wedge pressure <18 mm Hg or no clinical evidence of elevated left atrial pressure per chest x-ray or clinical information (82). Characteristics of ALI and ARDS include increased pulmonary capillary permeability, pulmonary edema, destruction of alveoli, endothelial damage, and production of inflammatory mediators by macrophages (oxygen free radicals, cytokines, and eicosanoids) (83). Phospholipase A2 (PLA2) has been noted to play a vital role in the development of ALI and ARDS (84). When activated, PLA2 produces reduced amounts of functional surfactant and stimulates the cell membrane to release arachidonic acid (83). Supportive care and resolution of the underlying etiology remain the primary goals of therapy for both acute decompensation in COPD and ALI/ARDS.

Table 19 Nutrition-Related Effects on Pulmonary Function

Respiratory muscle wasting	Decreased respiratory contractility
Impaired ciliary function and pulmonary defense mechanisms	Decreased surfactant production and secretion
	Increases in inflammatory mediators (TNF, IL-1, and IL-6)
Hypoalbuminemia/pulmonary edema	
Decreased circulating antiproteinases	Immune system impairment
Altered respiratory drive	

Malnutrition is common in COPD patients and up to 50% have some degree of weight loss upon hospital admission primarily due to anorexia, decreased oral intake, corticosteroids, and an underlying hypermetabolic state (25). Inflammatory mediators and cytokines are elevated in COPD and often lead to higher energy requirements (85). Malnutrition and loss of LBM are prognostic variables for increased morbidity and mortality in this patient population. Malnutrition in ICU patients admitted with pulmonary failure yields a similar clinical scenario as up to 60% have been shown to be significantly malnourished upon ICU admission (25). This is important because nutrition-related adverse effects in patients with acute respiratory failure can be seen within days of ICU admissions (see Table 19) (25,83,86). Patients with ALI/ARDS are at a high risk of malnutrition due to their hypermetabolic underlying disease state, which warrants the use of early nutrition support to prevent malnutrition and loss of LBM.

Although there are minimal effects on substrate metabolism seen in patients with respiratory failure, certain guidelines are present to guide nutrition support and prevent untoward effects, which can be

Table 20 Nutrition Support in COPD and ALI/ARDS

Substrate	COPD	ALI/ARDS
Energy	25–30 cal/kg/day	25–30 cal/kg/day
Protein	1–1.5 g/kg/day	1.5–2 g/kg/day
Fluid	Restrict	Restrict as needed
Electrolytes	As needed	As needed
Vitamins	Multivitamins	Multivitamins, vitamins E, C, and beta carotene

found in Table 20 (86). The use of enteral nutrition is preferred to provide gut preservation in patients already at risk for malnutrition-induced immune dysfunction. Energy requirements are generally increased in critically ill patients with acute respiratory failure. The use of indirect calorimetry is the gold standard for this patient population and is useful in the prevention of over- and underfeeding. Carbohydrates should make up 50% of total daily calories and should be given intravenously at a rate not to exceed 4 mg dextrose/kg/min. Overfeeding should be avoided in order to prevent the development of hypercarbia that may lead to a negative impact when weaning from ventilatory support. If hyperglycemia or excessive carbon dioxide retention is noted, total calories may be reduced and higher doses of protein administered (1.5 g/kg/day). Administration of parenteral fat emulsion should be kept at ≤ 1 g/kg/day to prevent hypertriglyceridemia and potential immunosuppression.

The use of immune-enhancing agents, namely omega-3 polyunsaturated fatty acids, is of interest in ICU patient populations with ALI and ARDS where an increased activation of PLA2 causes the release of arachidonic acid from cell membranes leading to increased oxidative stress and inflammation. Studies ascertaining the effects of immune-enhancing enteral nutrition in patients with ARDS have been performed which showed a reduced number of ventilator days and length of stay (87,88). Gadek et al. (87) also showed a decrease in total number of neutrophils per milliliter of bronchoalveolar lavage fluid, an improvement in oxygenation, and a decrease in new organ dysfunction in ARDS patients. Unfortunately, no benefits in overall mortality were seen and patients with malignancy and those receiving chemotherapeutic agents were excluded from the study. Use of these specialized immune-enhancing enteral nutrition formulations is not clear in the critically ill cancer patient and necessitates well-designed randomized trials to evaluate both efficacy and safety.

Sodium and fluid restrictions may be necessary to prevent further pulmonary congestion or edema in an attempt to improve ventilation and oxygenation. The addition of diuretics in patients with acute respiratory failure is common and necessitates the close observation and repletion of sodium, potassium, magnesium, and calcium. Due to the increased incidence of malnutrition in patients with COPD and ALI/ARDS, refeeding syndrome with resultant hypophosphatemia can be common. Maintenance of phosphate homeostasis is important for the production of ATP to support diaphragmatic strength and other cellular functions. The recommended adult dietary allowances of vitamins and minerals should be administered to patients with respiratory failure. Additional supplementation of vitamins A, C, and E has been advocated to prevent immune dysfunction in ALI/ARDS (86).

IX. SUMMARY

Replenishing the malnourished critically ill cancer patient represents a difficult clinical dilemma. The presence of multiple organ failure may provide obstacles in formulating an adequate nutritional plan. It is generally accepted that nutrition has a supportive role in the ICU, however there is no universal agreement of when to start or stop, how to provide optimally, which route of administration is best, and how long to continue. There are unanswered questions regarding tumor growth rates with various forms of nutrition support in cancer patients, reductions in malnutrition-induced complications, and what impact nutrition support has on functional status or quality of life after ICU discharge. Many of the clinical trials in ICU patients have excluded patients with cancer leaving clinical guidelines for these patients unanswered. However, these should not be used as reasons for withholding nutrition and safely providing nutrition support should be the ultimate goal.

REFERENCES

1. Cerra FB, Benitez MR, Blackburn GL, Irwin RS, Jeejeebhoy K, Katz DP, et al. Applied nutrition in ICU patients. A consensus statement of the American College of Chest Physicians. Chest 1997; 111:769–778.

2. Kern KA, Norton JA. Cancer cachexia. JPEN J Parenter Enteral Nutr 1988; 2:286–298.
3. Canada T. Clinical dilemma in cancer: is tumor growth during nutrition support significant? Nutr Clin Pract 2002; 17:246–248.
4. Koretz RL, Lipman TO, Klein S. American gastroenterological association medical position statement: parenteral nutrition. Gastroenterology 2001; 121:970–1001.
5. Detsky AS, McLaughlin JR, Baker JP, Johnston N, Whittaker S, Mendelson RA, et al. What is subjective global assessment of nutrition status? JPEN J Parenter Enteral Nutr 1987; 11:8–13.
6. Ottery FD. Supportive nutrition to prevent cachexia and improve quality of life. Semin Oncol 1995; 22(suppl 3): 98–111.
7. Cresci GA. Nutrition assessment and monitoring. In: Shikora SA, Martindale RG, Schwaitzberg SD, eds. Nutritional Considerations in the Intensive Care Unit. Dubuque: Kendall/Hunt, 2002:21–30.
8. Brennan MF, Burt ME. Nitrogen metabolism in cancer patients. Cancer Treat Rep 1981; 65(suppl 5):67–78.
9. Tisdale MJ. Cancer anorexia and cachexia. Nutrition 2001; 17:438–442.
10. Souba WW, Copeland EM. Hyperalimentation in cancer. CA Cancer J Clin1989; 39:105–114.
11. Barber MD, Ross JA, Fearon KCH. Disordered metabolic response with cancer and its management. World J Surg 2000; 24:681–689.
12. Knox LS, Crosby LO, Feurer ID, Buzby GP, Miller CL, Mullen JL. Energy expenditure in malnourished cancer patients. Ann Surg 1983; 197:152–162.
13. Bauer P, Charpentier C, Bouchet C, Nace L, Raffy F, Gaconnet N. Parenteral with enteral nutrition in the critically ill. Intensive Care Med 2000; 26:893–900.
14. Shizgal HM, Milne CA, Spanier AH. The effect of nitrogen-sparing, intravenously administered fluids on postoperative body composition. Surgery 1979; 85: 496–503.
15. McClave SA, McClain CJ, Snider HL. Should indirect calorimetry be used as part of nutritional assessment? J Clin Gastroenterol 2001; 31:14–19.
16. Malone AM. Methods of assessing energy expenditure in the intensive are unit. Nutr Clin Pract 2002; 17: 21–28.
17. Petros S, Engelmann L. Validity of an abbreviated indirect calorimetry protocol for measurement of resting energy expenditure in mechanically ventilated and spontaneously breathing critically ill patients. Intensive Care Med 2001; 27:1164–1168.
18. Cerra FB. Hypermetabolism, organ failure, and metabolic support. Surgery 1987; 101:1–15.
19. Schwarz JM, Chiolero R, Revelly JP, Cayeux C, Schneiter P, Jequier E, et al. Effects of enteral carbohydrates on de novo lipogenesis in critically ill patients. Am J Clin Nutr 2000; 72:940–945.
20. Van den Berghe G, Wouters P, Weekers F, Verwaest C, Bruyninckx F, Schetz M, et al. Intensive insulin therapy in critically ill patients. N Engl J Med 2001; 345: 1359–1367.
21. Marik PE, Zaloga GP. Early enteral nutrition in acutely ill patients: a systematic review. Crit Care Med 2001; 29:2264–2270.
22. A.S.P.E.N. Board of Directors. Guidelines for the use of parenteral and enteral nutrition in adult and pediatric patients. JPEN J Parenter Enteral Nutr 1993; 17(suppl 4):1SA–26SA.
23. Heys SD, Walker LG, Smith I, Eremin O. Enteral nutritional supplementation with key nutrients in patients with critical illness and cancer. Ann Surg 1999; 229: 467–477.
24. American Gastroenterological Association Patient Care Committee. AGA technical review on tube feeding for enteral nutrition. Gastroenterology 1995; 108: 1280–1301.
25. McCarthy MS, Deal LE. Nutrition support in respiratory failure. In: Shikora SA, Martindale RG, Schwaitzberg SD, eds. Nutritional Considerations in the Intensive Care Unit. Dubuque: Kendall/Hunt, 2002: 187–197.
26. Schloerb PR. Immune-enhancing diets: products, components, and their rationales. JPEN J Parenter Enteral Nutr 2001; 25(suppl 2):S3–S7.
27. Bistrian BR. Clinical aspects of essential fatty acid metabolism. JPEN J Parenter Enteral Nutr 2003; 27: 168–175.
28. McCowen KC, Bistrian BR. Immunonutrition: problematic or problem solving? Am J Clin Nutr 2003; 77: 764–770.
29. Adams S, Yeh YY, Jensen GL. Changes in plasma and erythrocyte fatty acids in patients fed enteral formulas containing different fats. JPEN J Parenter Enteral Nutr 1993; 17:30–34.
30. Suchner U, Heyland DK, Peter K. Immune-modulatory action of arginine in the critically ill. Brit J Nutr 2002; 87(suppl 1):S121–S132.
31. Heyland DK, Samis A. Does immunonutrition in patients with sepsis do more harm than good? Intensive Care Med 2003; 29:669–671.
32. Galban C, Montejo JC, Mesejo A, Marco P, Celaya S, Sanchez-Segura J, et al. An immune-enhancing enteral diet reduces mortality rate and episodes of bacteremia in septic intensive care unit patients. Crit Care Med 2000; 28:643–648.
33. Barrera R. Nutrition support in cancer patients. JPEN J Parenter Enteral Nutr 2002; 26(suppl 5):S63–S71.
34. Maloney JP, Ryan TA, Brasel KJ, Binion DG, Johnson DR, Halbower AC, et al. Food dye use in enteral feeding: a review and a call for a moratorium. Nutr Clin Pract 2002; 17:169–181.
35. Kearns LR, Phillips MC, Ness-Abramof R, Apovian CM. Update on parenteral amino acids. Nutr Clin Pract 2001; 16:219–225.
36. Rosemarin DK, Wardlaw GM, Mirtallo J. Hyperglycemia associated with high, continuous infusion rates of

total parenteral nutrition dextrose. Nutr Clin Pract 1996; 11:151–156.

37. Burke JF, Wolfe RR, Mullany CJ, Mathews DE, Bier DM. Glucose requirements following burn injury. Ann Surg 1979; 190:274–283.
38. Klein S. A primer of nutrition support for gastroenterologists. Gastroenterology 2002; 122:1677–1687.
39. Solomon SM, Kirby DF. The refeeding syndrome: a review. JPEN J Parenter Enteral Nutr 1990; 14:90–97.
40. http://www.meridianhealth.com/index.cfm/Health Content/Adult/liver/stats.cfm accessed May 7, 2003.
41. http://www.cellectbio.com/html/liverdis.html accessed May 13, 2003.
42. Lee WM. Drug-induced hepatotoxicity. N Eng J Med 1995; 333:1118–1127.
43. Podolsky DK, Isselbacher KJ. Derangements of hepatic metabolism. In: Fauci AS, Martin JB, Braunwald E, Kasper DL, Isselbacher KJ, Hauser SL, Wilson JD, Longo DL, eds. Harrison's Principals of Internal Medicine. New York: The McGraw-Hill Companies Inc, 1998:1667–1672.
44. Teran JC, McCullough AF. Nutrition in liver diseases. In: Gottschlich MM, Fuhrman MP, Hammond KA, Holcombe BJ, Seidner DL, eds. The Science and Practice of Nutrition Support. Dubuque: Kendall/Hunt, 2000:537–551.
45. Mendenhall C, Anderson S, Weesner RE, Goldberg SJ, Crolic KA. Protein–calorie malnutrition associated with alcoholic hepatitis. A VA cooperative study group on alcoholic hepatitis. Am J Med 1984; 76:211–222.
46. Patton KAA, Aranda-Michel J. Nutritional aspects in liver disease and liver transplantation. Nutr Clin Pract 2002; 17:332–340.
47. Mendenhall CL, Moritz TE, Roselle GA, Morgan TR, Nemchausky BA, Tamburro CH, et al. A study of oral nutrition support with oxandrolone in malnourished patients with alcoholic hepatitis: results of a department of veterans affairs cooperative study. Hepatology 1993; 17:564–576.
48. Pomposelli JJ, Burns DL. Nutrition support in the liver transplant patient. Nutr Clin Pract 2002; 17:341–349.
49. Seeto RK, Fenn B, Rockey DC. Ischemic hepatitis: clinical presentation and pathogenesis. Am J Med 2000; 109:109–113.
50. Mizock BA. Nutritional support in hepatic encephalopathy. Nutrition 1999; 15:220–228.
51. McCullough AJ, Raguso C. Effect of cirrhosis on energy expenditure. Am J Clin Nutr 1999; 69: 1066–1068.
52. Muller MJ, Bottcher J, Selberg O, Weselmann S, Boker KHW, Schwarze M, et al. Hypermetabolism in clinically stable patients with liver cirrhosis. Am J Clin Nutr 1999; 69:1194–1201.
53. Hunter DC, Jaksic T, Lewis D, Benotti PN, Blackburn GL, Bistrian BR. Resting energy expenditure in the critically ill: estimations versus measurement. Br J Surg 1988; 75:875–878.
54. Hasse J, Strong S, Gorman MA. Subjective global assessment: alternative nutrition-assessment technique for liver-transplant candidates. Nutrition 1993; 24: 1422–1427.
55. George R, Shiu MH. Hypophosphatemia after major hepatic resection. Surgery 1992; 111:281–286.
56. Nanji AA, Anderson FH. Acute liver failure: a possible consequence of severe hypophosphatemia. J Clin Gastroenterol 1985; 7:338–340.
57. Blei AT, Cordoba J. Hepatic encephalopathy. Am J Gastroenterol 2001; 96:1968–1976.
58. Plauth M, Roske AE, Romaniuk P, Roth E, Ziebig R, Lochs H. Post-feeding hyperammonaemia in patients with transjugular intrahepatic portosystemic shunt and liver cirrhosis: role of small intestinal ammonia release and route of nutrient administration. Gut 2000; 46: 849–855.
59. James JH. Branched chain amino acids in hepatic encephalopathy. Am J Surg 2002; 183:424–429.
60. Naylor CD, O'Rourke K, Detsky AS, Baker JP. Parenteral nutrition with branched-chain amino acids in hepatic encephalopathy. a meta-analysis. Gastroenterology 1989; 97:1033–1042.
61. Eriksson LS, Conn HO. Branched chain amino acids in the management of hepatic encephalopathy: an analysis of variants. Hepatology 1989; 10:228–246.
62. Klein S, Kinney J, Jeejeebhoy K, Alpers D, Hellerstein M, Murray M, Twomey P. Nutrition support in clinical practice: review of published data and recommendations for future research directions. JPEN J Parenter Enteral Nutr 1997; 21:133–156.
63. Wolk R. Nutrition in renal failure. In: Gottschlich MM, Fuhrman MP, Hammond KA, Holcombe BJ, Seidner DL, eds. The Science and Practice of Nutrition Support. Dubuque: Kendall/Hunt, 2000:575–599.
64. Kapoor M, Chan GZ. Malignancy and renal disease. Crit Care Clin 2001; 17:571–598.
65. Kintzel PE. Anticancer drug-related kidney disorders. Incidence, prevention and management. Drug Safety 2001; 24:19–38.
66. Marshall MR, Golper TA, Shaver MJ, Alam MG, Chatoth DK. Sustained low-efficiency dialysis for critically ill patients requiring renal replacement therapy. Kidney Int 2001; 60:777–785.
67. Leverve X, Barnoud D. Stress metabolism and nutritional support in acute renal failure. Kidney Int 1998; 53:S62–S66.
68. Oldrizzi L, Rugiu C, Maschio G. Nutrition and the kidney: how to manage patients with renal failure. Nutr Clin Pract 1994; 9:3–10.
69. Kierdorf HP. The nutritional management of acute renal failure in the intensive care unit. New Horiz 1995; 3:699–707.
70. Charney P, Charney D. Nutrition support in acute renal failure. In: Shikora SA, Martindale RG, Schwaitzberg SD, eds. Nutritional Considerations in the Intensive Care Unit. Dubuque: Kendall/Hunt, 2002:209–217.

71. Sponsel H, Conger JD. Is parenteral nutrition therapy of value in acute renal failure patients? Am J Kidney Dis 1995; 25:96–102.
72. Druml W. Nutritional management of acute renal failure. Am J Kidney Dis 2001; 37(suppl 2):S89–S94.
73. Kopple JD. The nutrition management of the patient with acute renal failure. JPEN J Parenter Enteral Nutr 1996; 20:3–12.
74. Thadhani R, Pascual M, Bonventre JV. Acute renal failure. N Eng J Med 1996; 334:1448–1460.
75. Hou SH, Bushinsky DA, Wish JB, Cohen JJ, Harrington JT. Hospital-acquired renal insufficiency: a prospective study. Am J Med 1983; 74:243–248.
76. McWhirter JP, Pennington CR. Incidence and recognition of malnutrition in hospital. Br Med J 1994; 308: 945–948.
77. Fiaccadori E, Lombardi M, Leonardi S, Rotelli CF, Tortorella G, Borchetti A. Prevalence and clinical outcome associated with preexisting malnutrition in acute renal failure: a prospective cohort study. J Am Soc Nephrol 1999; 10:581–593.
78. Toigo G, Aparicio M, Attman PO. Expert working group report on nutrition in adult patients with renal insufficiency (Part 2 of 2). Clin Nutr 2000; 19:281–291.
79. Makoff R. Vitamin replacement therapy in renal failure patients. Miner Electrolyte Metab 1999; 25:349–351.
80. National Kidney Foundation. K/DOQI Clinical practice guidelines for anemia of chronic kidney disease, 2000. Am J Kidney Dis 2001; 37(suppl 1): S182–238.
81. http://www.copdinamerica.org/disease.html accessed May 27, 2003.
82. Bernard GR, Artigas A, Brigham KL, Carlet J, Falke K, Hudson L, et al. The American–European Consensus Conference on ARDS: definitions, mechanisms, relevant outcomes, and clinical trial coordination. Am J Respir Crit Care Med 1994; 149:818–824.
83. Mizock BA. Nutritional support in acute lung injury and acute respiratory distress syndrome. Nutr Clin Pract 2001; 16:319–328.
84. Anderson BO, Moore EE, Banerjee A. Phospholipase A2 regulates critical inflammatory mediators of multiple organ failure. J Surg Res 1994; 56:199–205.
85. Eid AA, Ionescu AA, Nixon LS, Lewis-Jenkins V, Matthews SB, Griffiths TL, et al. Inflammatory response and body composition in chronic obstructive pulmonary disease. Am J Respir Crit Care Med 2001; 164: 1414–1418.
86. Hogg J, Klapholz A, Reid-Hector J. Pulmonary Disease. In: Gottschlich MM, Fuhrman MP, Hammond KA, Holcombe BJ, Seidner DL, eds. The Science and Practice of Nutrition Support. Dubuque: Kendall/ Hunt, 2000:491–516.
87. Gadek JE, DeMichelle SJ, Karlstad MD, Pacht ER, Donahoe M, Albertson TE, et al. Effect of enteral feeding with eicosapentaenoic acid, gamma-linolenic acid, and antioxidants in patients with acute respiratory distress syndrome. Crit Care Med 1999; 27:1409–1420.
88. Atkinson S, Sieffert E, Bihari D. A prospective, randomized, double-blind, controlled clinical trial of enteral immunonutrition in the critically ill. Crit Care Med 1998; 26:1164–1172.

44

Nosocomial Infections and Antibiotic Therapy in Patients with Cancer

AMAR SAFDAR and ISSAM I. RAAD

Department of Infectious Diseases, Infection Control, and Employee Health, The University of Texas M.D. Anderson Cancer Center, Houston, Texas, U.S.A.

I. INTRODUCTION

Infection in hospitalized oncology patients pose a serious challenge and may lead to unfavorable impact on successful cancer treatment outcomes (1). In fact, nosocomial infections are among the important determinants of short-term survival in the critically ill patients with an underlying malignancy and recipients of hematopoietic stem cell transplantation (HSCT) (1–3). Bloodstream microbial invasion, systemic dissemination, and urinary and respiratory tract infections are frequent complications in hospitalized patients with an underlying malignancy; nosocomial infections are well-recognized predictors of prolonged hospital stay and increased the cost of healthcare (4–6).

In solid-organ cancer patients undergoing surgical procedures, postoperative infections are not uncommon. Most frequent infection in these patients is infected surgical wound site (7), which certainly may have a negative impact on short-term morbidity, resulting from delayed recovery and suboptimum postsurgical rehabilitation. Postoperative infections depend on surgical procedure, such as patients after abdominal surgery, are at the risk of intra-abdominal infected hematoma, body cavity abscesses, deep pelvic vein-infected phlebothrombosis, bowel anastomosis dehiscence leading to tertiary peritonitis, and secondary phenomenon such as aspiration pneumonia, infected decubitus ulcers, and/or intravenous access site infection, to name a few.

Opportunistic infections due to low-virulence, environmental saprophytic commensal micro-organisms may lead to serious systemic diseases in immunosuppressed patients with cancer (1,8). Specific defects in host's immune responses may predispose to life-threatening infections due to specific organisms that are rarely encountered in the absence of the specific defect in host's immune function (Table 1). Infections in this setting may be newly acquired organisms from hospital macro- and/or microflora, especially the emerging and re-emerging multidrug-resistant (MDR) nonfermentative, gram-negative bacilli such as *Pseudomonas aeruginosa*, *Acinetobacter*, *Stenotrophomonas maltophilia*, and *Alacligenes* spp., may pose serious treatment challenges in patients with chemotherapy-induced neutropenia [absolute neutrophil counts (ANC) < 500 cells/mm^3].

Patients during hospitalization may also present with recrudescence of previously acquired infection, such as inextricable human *Herpesviridae* infection due to human cytomegalovirus (HCMV), varicella-zoster virus (VZV), and herpes simplex virus (HSV), Epstein–Barr

Table 1 Infections Associated with Specific Immune Defects in Patients with an Underlying Malignancy

Immune defect	Bacteria	Fungi	Parasites	Viruses
Granulocytopenia	*Staphylococcus aureus*	*Candida albicans*, non-*albicans Candida* species		Herpes simplex virus I and II (HSV I and II)
	Streptococcus viridans	*Aspergillus fumigatus*, non-*fumigatus Aspergillus*		Varicella-zoster virus (VZV)
	Staphylococcus epidermidis	Non-*Aspergillus* hyalohyphomycosis such as*Pseudallescheria boydii, Fusarium solani*		
	Pseudomonas aeruginosa			
	Enterobacteriaceae	*Mucorales* (zygomycoses)		
	Escherichia coli	Dematiaceous (black) fungi such as *Alternaria*		
	Klebsiella species	*Bipolaris, Curvularia, Scedosporium apiospermum*		
	Stenotrophomonas maltophilia	*Scedosporium prolificans*		
	Acinetobacter species			
Cellular immune dysfunction	*Nocardia asteroides complex*	*Aspergillus* and non-*Aspergillus* filamentous molds	*Strongyloides stercoralis* (hyperinfection)	Human cytomegalovirsus
	Salmonella typhimurium	*Pneumocystis jiroveci* (*P. carini*)		Respiratory viruses
	Salmonella enteritidis	*Cryptococcus neoformans*	*Toxoplasma gondii*	Influenza A and Influenza B
	Rhodococcus equi	Endemic mycoses due to *Histoplasma capsulatum, Coccidioides immitis, Blastomyces dermatitidis*	Microsporidiosis	Parainfluenza
	Rhodococcus bronchialis		Leishmaniasis	Respiratory syncytial virus
	Listeria monocytogenes			Adenovirus
	Mycobacterium tuberculosis			VZV
	Nontuberculous mycobacteria			Human herpesvirus 6, human herpesvirus 8

Humoral immune dysfunction and splenectomy	*Streptococcus pneumoniae*	*Pneumocystis jiroveci* (*P. carini*) (rarely seen)	*Giardia lamblia*	VZV (systemic dissemination; rarely seen)
	Haemophilus influenzae *Neisseria meningitidis* *Capnocytophaga canimorsus* *Campylobacter*		*Babesia microti*	Echovirus Enterovirus
Mixed immune defects	*Streptococcus pneumoniae* *Staphylococcus aureus*	*Pneumocystis jiroveci* (*P. carini*) *Aspergillus* spp.	*Toxoplasma gondii* *Strongyloides stercoralis* (hyperinfection)	Herpes simplex virus I and II VZV (systemic dissemination)
	Haemophilus influenzae *Klebsiella pneumonia* *Pseudomonas aeruginosa* *Acinetobacter* spp.	*Candida* spp. *Cryptococcus neoformans* *Mucorales* (zygomycoses) Endemic mycoses (severe systemic dissemination)		Respiratory viruses Influenza Parainfluenza Respiratory syncytial virus
	Enterobacter spp. *Stenotrophomonas maltophilia* *Nocardia asteroides* complex *Mycobacterium tuberculosis* *Listeria monocytogenes* *Legionella* spp.			Adenovirus

Note: Patients with mixed immune defects includes recipients of allogeneic HSCT, acute or chronic GvHD, myelodysplastic syndrome, adult T-cell leukemia or lymphoma, antineoplastic agents like cyclophosphamide.

virus, human herpes virus-6 (HHV-6). Clinical features of *Toxoplasma gondii* reactivation involving the central nervous system (CNS), retinal, and/or lung are often indistinguishable from other opportunistic processes in patients with severe T-cell defects (9).

Patients with mucocutaneous excoriation following antineoplastic therapy are at risk of systemic invasion due to community- and/or hospital-acquired micro-organisms colonizing the orointestinal, respiratory tracts and/or part of normal cutaneous microflora; viridans streptococcus, *Streptococcus pneumoniae*, and coagulase-negative staphylococcus (CoNS) are prominent infections in this setting. *Candida* species bloodstream invasion is an important complication in patients, which remains neutropenic for a longer period; granulocytopenia for ≥ 5 days is considered as an independent risk for fungemia (1,8,10). In patients with rapid decline in peripheral blood neutrophil counts accompanied by ANC $<150\,\text{cells/mm}^3$, the risk of severe systemic infection (11) due to gram-positive (12) and gram-negative infections increases exponentially (13); a delay in appropriate empiric antimicrobial therapy in these patients with profound and severe drug-induced granulocytopenia results in unacceptably high mortality (14).

The near-exponential increase in the use of foreign, prosthetic devices during hospitalization has substantially contributed in the changing spectrum of infection seen in oncology centers worldwide. By far, the most prominent shifts in bloodstream infections (BSIs) observed in the last 25 years is the emergence of CoNS bacteremia, as a result of widespread use of indwelling central venous catheters (CVC) often seen in hospitalized patients receiving antineoplastic therapy (15).

Ineffective microbial bloodstream elimination in patients with splenic dysfunction or suboptimum opsonization due to B-cell defects seen in patients with multiple myeloma, Waldenstrom's macroglobulinemia, significantly increases the risk of fulminant infections due to encapsulated bacteria. Similarly, recrudescence of intracellular pathogens, as illustrated in Table 1, poses a serious challenge for patients with cancer-related and/or antineoplastic therapy-induced disruption in T-cell mediated cellular immune pathways. Cancer patients with cellular immune defects may present with distinct disease pattern compared to nononcology patients with adaptive cellular immune defects; for example, HCMV retinitis, often primary manifestation of HCMV disease in patients with advanced AIDS, is in fact rarely seen in patients with hematologic malignancies or recipients of allogeneic HSCT with cellular immune dysfunction.

It is imperative to note that in patients undergoing cancer therapy, especially in the era of accelerated near-cytoablative antineoplastic therapy, bioimmune therapy, stem cell transplantation, they may develop aberrances in more than one immune-response pathway. Similarly, presence of primary opportunistic infection such as HCMV may enhance risk of acquiring secondary infections due to organism-related (HCMV) and/or antimicrobial therapy-associated (ganciclovir) immune suppression (16–18). This is further complicated by the fact that in severely immunosuppressed patient, several opportunistic processes may coexists and present either simultaneously or sequentially during the same hospitalization (1,8).

In this chapter, we discuss common infections in hospitalized cancer with emphasis on recent changes in infection trends and shifts in treatment paradigm.

II. BLOODSTREAM INFECTIONS

Nosocomial bacteremia is a serious complication in the hospitalized patients and bloodstream infections in hospitalized patients are the 13th leading cause of death in the United States (19). In the past 20 years, >75% increase in age-adjusted mortality in patients with bloodstream infection has further increased awareness of this potentially fatal complication (19). Cancer patients constitute nearly 10% of all documented nosocomial bacteremia, and during last two decades, an overall decline in gram-negative bacteremia was associated with increased prevalence of hematogenous spread due to gram-positive cocci (GPC) (20). During the 1960s, in febrile neutropenic cancer patients, a rise in *Pseudomonas* species infection coincided with decline in infections due to *Staphylococcus aureus* (6,14,21–23). Despite recent shifts in the prevalence of GPC BSI, hematogenous *Pseudomonas* species infection remains important and formidable problem, especially in patients with severe granulocytopenia (ANC < 150 cells/mm^3) (11,13,24).

A. Gram-Positive Bacteremia

In the United States, nearly 60% of BSIs, community- and/or hospital-acquired infections, are due to GPC; most micro-organisms in this group consist of CoNS, α- and nonhemolytic streptococcus, *S. aureus*, and *Enterococcus* species (25,26). This overall trend in the United States has been consistently observed in febrile neutropenic patients with a positive blood culture (27). The near-exponential increase in the implantable or semi-implantable indwelling intravascular catheters has a prominent contribution in promoting this current trend (15). Similarly, decline in systemic gram-negative bacillaremia was in part attributed to widespread use of antipseudomonal fluoroquinolones often given as prophylaxis in individuals considered high-risk for GNB infections, such as patients with hematologic malignancy, and recipients of autologous or allogeneic HSCT (28).

1. *Gram-Positive Cocci*

Coagulase-negative staphylococcus has emerged as the most common blood culture isolate from hospitalized patients in the United States (26,29). Most infections are attributed in part due to an infected or colonized indwelling intravascular device. Other prosthetic implantable surgical materials such as heart valves, artificial joints, mechanical bridging, and spacer devices used in cancer patients undergoing tumor resection and/or reconstruction procedures may also lead to difficult-to-cure CoNS infections. Patients with bacteremia in this setting are febrile, albeit, unlike *S. aureus* or β-hemolytic streptococcal hematogenous spread, sepsis-like syndrome is seldom observed. Treatment includes systemic antibiotics given for 5–14 days for patients with uncomplicated bacteremia. Infected prosthetic devices are often removed in critically ill patients or in neutropenic patients in whom expected neutrophil recovery is slow. Catheter-related CoNS infection may be treated with catheter preservation techniques such as high concentration antibiotic catheter locks, although some reports suggest a higher infection relapse and possibly increased mortality (30).

Viridans group Streptococci, which are part of normal orointestinal microflora, may lead to severe systemic infection, and similar to experience in the pediatric population, adult cancer patients mostly with leukemia may present with rapidly evolving sepsis and/or septic shock early course of infection (12,31). Aggressive chemotherapy with antineoplastic agents such as cytosine-arabinoside that increases the likelihood of mucosal excoriation, causing widespread disruption of oral-gastrointestinal mechanical barriers, enhances patients' probability of developing hematogenous invasion due to commensal micro-organisms that are part of host's normal microflora (12,32). The increased incidence of *S. viridans* group bacteremia in patients with hematologic malignancies and HSCT may also be in part attributed to antimicrobial-related organism selection, such as patients receiving ciprofloxacin prophylaxis, a drug with suboptimum antistreptococcal activity, are at an increased risk to develop breakthrough streptococcal septicemia (33,34).

Similarly, bloodstream invasion due to *Stomatococcus* species is occasionally encountered in patients receiving quinolone prophylaxis; these infections commonly arise from hosts' intrinsic microflora, and primary bacteremia is the most common clinical presentation (35,36). Owing to neurotropism, patients with sustained or intermittent bacteremia may present with CNS involvement (37). Certainly, patients with sustained bacteremia due to any GPC, especially *S. aureus*, viridans streptococcus, *Stomatococcus*, and *Enterococcus* species, need a thorough diagnostic work-up to evaluate for underlying endovascular infection, such as native or prosthetic valve endocarditis. Patients with subacute endocarditis, especially infections resulting from a low virulence bacteria, often presents with nonspecific features such as fatigue, arthralgia, night sweats, headaches, and intermittent low-grade fever. Initial presentation as new onset back pain may herald septic embolic phenomenon resulting from diskitis and/or vertebral osteomyelitis; new often several hemorrhagic brain infarctions are few salient features that may prompt a diagnostic work-up for cryptic endovascular infection. A high-level of suspicion is critical in order to make correct diagnose and timely institution of appropriate, extended systemic antimicrobial therapy.

2. *Aerobic Gram-Positive Bacilli*

Corynebacterium jeikeium, *C. diphtheriae*, and non-*anthracis Bacillus* species are common constituents of normal skin flora; blood culture isolation may present a diagnostic dilemma, as it is not without suspicion to completely exclude true bacteremia from contamination during the culture process. In patients with indwelling CVC, a fivefold increase in bacterial isolation from CVC blood sample when compared with peripherally obtained blood specimens is regarded as diagnostic of true BSI and one indication that infected catheter is probably the source of infection (38). Features suggesting definite BSI include (a) higher bacterial count (>50–100 CFUs); (b) reproducibility, more than one blood culture obtained on separate occasions revealing identical organism; and (c) as mentioned earlier, in patients with indwelling intravascular catheter, fivefold higher bacterial counts in CVC blood when compared with peripheral blood culture sample (38–40). The infected catheters may be removed after a single episode of infection, especially in patients with high-grade, persistent (>72 hr) infection despite appropriate therapy (40). Alternatively in low-risk, non-neutropenic patients with unresolved bacteremia and CVC infection, instillation of high-concentration of antibiotics in the catheter lumen over a period of 8–12 hr may be attempted, although it must be emphasized that this antibiotic lock therapy is not proven standard of care and should be approached with cautions (41,42).

Listeria monocytogenes is an uncommon infection, and in cancer patients, advanced hematologic malignancy or certain solid-organ cancer, such as breast cancer, is considered at an increased risk for systemic *Listeria* infections (43). Among HSCT recipients, infection is seen in both autologous and allogeneic transplantation (16). The primary underlying immune defect is helper T-cell mediated cellular immune dysfunction; in patients with helper T-cell defects, 250–300% increased risk of systemic listeriosis has been reported compared with the general population (44). Fever is the most common clinical feature, and clinical findings suggest that *L. monocytogenes* meningitis or meningoencephalitis may be subclinical and not present on initial presentation. Therefore, it is currently recommended that all patients with evidence of systemic *Listerosis* should undergo diagnostic lumbar puncture (44). It is important to note that non-CNS end-organ involvement, such as listeric septic arthritis and deep cavity abscesses, is associated with extremely high mortality (>80%) when compared with nearly comparable *L. monocytogenes*-related deaths in patients with isolated bloodstream infection and those with CNS infections (43). Ampicillin plus gentamicin combination is regarded as treatment of choice; trimethoprim-sulfamethoxazole may be used in individuals with β-lactam intolerance. Clinical failures in patients treated with vancomycin and reports of breakthrough listerosis in patients receiving vancomycin therapy have cautioned against the use of vancomycin-based therapy in patients with serious allergies to β-lactam and sulfa (43). Carbapenems and newer fluorinated quinolones show excellent in vitro activity (45), although clinical validation is needed before routine use is advocated, albeit in patients with multiple-drug intolerance, these agents may be used in selective settings.

3. *Anaerobic Gram-Positive Bacteria*

Systemic *Clostridium* species infection is uncommon, although in patients with clostridial sepsis, presence of early-onset refractory hypotension, tachycardia, and disseminated intravascular coagulation may raise suspicion, especially in patients with known intestinal malignancies (1,46). In cancer patients with *C. perfringens* myonecrosis, preceding history of trauma, surgery, or other injuries may be conspicuously absent (47). Patients with intra-abdominal cancer, *Clostridium* species infections may initially present as rapidly progressive abdominal wall cellulitis and, if left unchecked or even slight delay in appropriate treatment, these infections can result in fatal necrotizing fascitis. Early and often, extensive surgical debridement plus high-dose penicillin (20–24 million units daily) are critical in patients with this grave infection. It is also important to realize that occasionally clostridial sepsis may be a part of polymicrobial processes and empiric treatment in appropriate individuals may include gram-negative coverage that may be re-evaluated for de-escalation therapy. *Clostridium septicum* bacteremia may be seen in otherwise asymptomatic patients; and in individuals with no known malignancy, a cancer diagnostic work-up is warranted, similar to patients with de novo *S. bovis* BSI (48).

B. Gram-Negative Bacteremia

The gram-negative bacteria (GNB) still pose a serious problem in hospitalized cancer patients, despite a decline in overall frequency. In hospitalized patients with profound granulocytopenia, *Pseudomonas* species remains as an important pathogen and often associated with febrile sepsis (21,24,49). A delay in initiation of appropriate combination of antipseudomonal therapy in febrile neutropenic patients with *Pseudomonas* bloodstream infections has been well recognized as an independent predictor of severely compromised outcome (14,23,50). Other GNB such as *Escherichia coli* and nonpseudomonas nonfermentators are common in non-neutropenic patients who remain hospitalized for extended duration; among these, patients who have undergone complicated surgical procedures and received extended care in critical care units are especially susceptible. Gram-negative bacteremia may accompany pneumonia, pyelonephritis, cholecystitis, diverticulitis, and body cavity abscesses such as intra-abdominal and deep pelvic abscesses, especially in patients with an underlying gastrointestinal and gynecologic malignancy.

For patients undergoing intra-abdominal surgical procedures such as bowel resection, urinary diversion operation including ileal conduit, cystostomy, neobladder surgery, or placement of chemotherapy delivery implantable devices to name a few, the risk of serious localized or systemic hematogenous infections due to nosocomially acquired GNB has been increased (1,10).

1. *Enterobacteriaceae*

Nearly 60–80% of all gram-negative bacteremia still belongs to this group; *E. coli* and *Klebsiella* species account for most systemic infections (1,10). They also predominate among gram-negative bacteremia isolated in febrile neutropenic patients; despite an overall decline in Enterobacteriaceae bloodstream infection, *E. coli* remains an important organism among hospitalized cancer patients (24). Most infections arise from patients' gastrointestinal tract; occasionally, bacteremia may accompany gram-negative pyelonephritis, perinephric abscesses, obstructive uropathies, and/or pneumonia. A secondary hematogenous seeding of an indwelling intravascular device may occur and these CVC gram-negative infections may be treated with appropriate systemic antimicrobials administered via all catheter lumens with favorable probability of salvage of the infected catheter. Most infections respond to appropriate therapy, although high mortality may occur in patients with pneumonia, enterocolitis, and deep pelvic or rectal abscesses, and polymicrobial infections (51).

2. *Nonfermentative Gram-Negative Bacteria*

Pseudomonas aeruginosa is the protagonist in this group and remains the leading cause of serious systemic infection in seriously ill hospitalized patients with cancer (13,14,24). Recently, there has been an overall decline in *P. aeruginosa* infections and currently accounts for nearly 20% of all nosocomial GNB infection. However, in patients with acute leukemia frequency of serious *Pseudomonas* species, infections have remained essentially unaltered in the last four decades (13). Some infections arise from host's intestinal tract, due to near-ubiquitous distribution of *Pseudomonas* in the micro- and macrohospital environment. Nonendogenous source of systemic bacterial invasion–infection includes catheter sites; surgical wounds; ventilator-duct and humidification systems; indwelling urinary catheters, nephrostomy tubes, biliary drainage catheters.

Another recent change in *Pseudomonas* infection was that patients had an increased frequency of community acquired *Pseudomonas* colonization. This fact cannot undermine the significance; however, that prolonged hospitalization increases intestinal colonization due to *Pseudomonas* among susceptible patients with cancer, such as 25% stool colonization in patients with leukemia increases to 50% after 4 weeks of hospitalization (10,21). Intestinal colonization and duration of colonization are both independent predictors of systemic invasion and disease (10,21). Profound (ANC <100 cells/mm^3) and prolonged (>5 days) neutropenia remains the most important predictor of systemic *Pseudomonas* infection; fever is present in nearly all patients with bacteremia and nearly one-third may either present with or develop septic shock during the course of hospitalization (52). Untreated *Pseudomonas* BSI in the setting of severe granulocytopenia is a near-universally fatal infection; prior to the availability of effective antipseudomonal antibiotics, mortality used to exceed 75% (14,53). Recently, 80% response in patients with *Pseudomonas* infection receiving appropriate therapy is encouraging (10,54). However, it is imperative that a combined antipseudomonal antimicrobial therapy is instituted promptly upon diagnoses and/or pre-emptively in the high-risk febrile neutropenic patients. In contrast to reports during the 1960s and the 1970s, presence of septic shock, pneumonia, and/or persistent granulocytopenia in patients with pseudomonal BSI does not gravely impact outcome if appropriate therapy is given in a timely manner (54).

In recent years, a decline in the classic cutaneous manifestation of ecthyma gangrenosum in patients with *Pseudomonas* sepsis may in part indicate widespread use of antipseudomonal antibiotics for prophylaxis and pre-emptive therapy in patients at risk of high-grade gram-negative bacteremia. These skin lesions are still occasionally encountered and may present either as a single or as a multiple erythematous, raised, and indurated lesion with a central area of necrosis. It is important to remember that disseminated infections due to *S. maltophilia*, noncholera *Vibrio* spp. patients with fungemia, especially *Fusarium* spp., and *Candida tropicalis* may present clinically indistinguishable lesions; diagnosis is confirmed by histological and microbiologic examination of full-thickness skin biopsy obtained at the edge of the evolving lesion.

C. Mycobacteriosis

Mycobacterial bloodstream infection in patients undergoing cancer treatment is often due to rapidly growing mycobacteria. Infections in this setting may present as uncomplicated hematogenous spread arising from infected indwelling intravascular catheter (55,56), although pneumonia (57), deep seated soft tissue abscesses, and infected prosthetic device infection are not uncommon (58). *Mycobacterium fortuitum-chelonae* and *M. abscessus* are most frequently associated with human infection; however, recent molecular-based diagnostic techniques have revealed an emerging array of new species of rapidly growing mycobacteria (59). Treatment includes a brief course of therapy (3 weeks), with a combination of two effective antimicrobial agents such as azalides and fluorinated quinolones for patients with uncomplicated bloodstream infection. In cases of CVC infection associated with rapidly growing mycobacterial pathogens, infected catheter needs to be removed and catheter salvage therapy is not recommended. Treatment is often extended for 3–6 months in patients with rapidly growing mycobacteria pulmonary infection and/or systemic dissemination. Again, antimicrobial combinations' approach is attempted to reduce the chances of acquired drug resistance. Antimicrobial options include fluorinated quinolones, tetracyclines, erythromycin group (azalides), amikacin, trimethoprim-sulfamethoxazole. In patients with severe and refractory disease, amikacin may be used in combination initially.

Mycobacterium avium–intracellulare complex (MAC) bacteremia is less frequent in cancer patients even with severe T-cell defects. This is in sharp contrast to HIV-I infected individuals with profound helper cell defects (60). Rarely, *M. avium* or *M. intracellulare* may lead to systemic infection in cancer patients with severe cellular immune defects, including individuals with refractory T-cell leukemia or lymphoma and recipients of high-risk allogeneic HSCT; infections in this setting remain mostly as uncomplicated bacteremia (61,62). Patients with hairy-cell leukemia are especially susceptible to systemic infection due to *M. avium–intracellulare*. These patients may present with clinical disease pattern not dissimilar compared to patients with advanced AIDS (63). Patient with solid-organ malignancy is also at risk for MAC disease; infections in this setting are often localized and bloodstream invasion is infrequent. Most infections involve the lung, and disease is chronic, insidious, and may remain undetected for an extended period (64); pulmonary nontuberculous mycobacteriosis is discussed later in this chapter.

In hospitalized allogeneic HSCT recipients, *M. avium* is not a common opportunistic infection, although when seen, infections are often widespread with evidence of bloodstream invasion, and tends to be refractory to multiple combinations of antimicrobial agents. In patients with specific cytokine defects, infection-related mortality remains high (65). Treatment includes antimicrobial combination consisting of two or more susceptible agents, such as combination of azithromycin or clarithromycin with ethambutol and rifamycins that may be used along with a fluorinated quinolone (ciprofloxacin, moxifloxacin, gatifloxacin) (66,67) or an aminoglycoside, such as amikacin. Infections due to MDR strains may pose serious treatment challenges, and all patients are given second- and third-line antimycobacterial therapy with or without immune augmentation with recombinant cytokines, such as interferon-γ, granulocyte macrophage-colony stimulating factors, interleukin (IL)-2, IL-12, etc. (68–70). Duration of treatment is often prolonged, and combination antimicrobials are often continued for 12–18 months.

D. Fungal Bloodstream Invasion

Candida species hematogenous invasion is the fourth leading cause of nosocomial bloodstream infection in the United States (71). Patients with candidemia have attributable-mortality of nearly 40%, which is twice as high as reported in patients with *P. aeruginosa* or *S. aureus* sepsis (72). *Candida albicans* remains the dominant *Candida* species associated with human disease (73). Although in certain patient population, such as patients with prior exposure to antifungal drugs, which includes HSCT recipients, hematologic malignancies, systemic yeast infections due to non-*albicans* *Candida* species have emerged in the last two decades (74,75). *Candida glabrata* that is frequently less susceptible to fluconazole and itraconazole has now evolved as the most common *Candida* species associated with infection in hospitalized cancer patients (76,77). In certain centers, a significant rise in *C. krusei* is alarming, as these *Candida* species exhibit intrinsic nonsusceptibility to commonly prescribed triazole-based antifungals (78).

The predominant source of nosocomial fungemia is host's endogenous gastrointestinal microflora or vascular catheter contamination by the hands of medical personnel. Prior colonization due to *C. glabrata* and *C. krusei*, especially involving multiple-body sites in high-risk patients with leukemia and/or HSCT, is associated with compromised short-term survival (79). As sensitivity of antemortem blood cultures is nearly 50%, most hospitalized cancer patients that have one or more risk factors, as outlined in Table 2, are commonly given empiric and/or pre-emptive antifungal therapy (74).

The important predictors of unfavorable outcome in patients with established *Candida* species bloodstream invasion includes (a) persistent severe granulocytopenia; (b) advanced underlying malignancy; (c) salvage, accelerated chemotherapy; (d) infections due to non-*albicans Candida*, especially *C. krusei* and *C. lusitaniae*; (e) severely ill patients with high APACHE-III score (77,80). Interestingly, admission to intensive care unit (ICU) or initial treatment with non-in vitro susceptible antifungal agents was not associated with a significant unfavorable impact on outcome (76). Treatment with amphotericin B-based preparation is considered as therapy of choice, especially in patients with severe neutropenia, although less critically ill patients with *C. albicans* and *C. parapsilosis* BSI may be candidates for high-dose fluconazole therapy. In patients with *C. lusitaniae*, a combination of amphotericin B plus fluconazole has been recommended (81). A recent prospective, comparative trial of caspofungin (Cancidas®) vs. amphotericin B for the treatment of systemic candidiasis showed that Cancidas® was at least as effective as amphotericin B and had significantly less toxicity profile when compared with adverse effects noted in patients treated with amphotericin B (82). It is important to appreciate that

Table 2 Predisposing Factors for Systemic Candidiasis

Intensive care unit (ICU)
Surgical, medical and neonatal: >5–7 days ICU stay
Indwelling intravascular devices (IVDs)
Implantable and semi-implantable IVDs, such as Hickman-Broviac, MediPort, HD catheters
Broad-spectrum antimicrobial therapy
> 2 Antibiotics
≥7 days
High-risk surgery
Complicated abdominopelvic surgery
Hollow viscus surgery
Cardiothoracic surgery
Hyperalimentation
Total parental nutrition
Prolonged hospitalization
≥3 weeks
Extensive trauma
Burns unit stay
Severe granulocytopenia
< 150 cells/mm^3
≥5–7 days
Candida spp. Colonization
High level of yeast burden in nonsterile sites (> 100,000 colony count)
Multiple body site colonization
Candida glabrata and *Candida krusei* colonization, especially in patients with leukemia, and HSCT
Corticosteroids
Cancer therapy (chemotherapy and radiation treatments) induced
Mucosal ulceration
Neutrophil dysfunction
Extremes of age
Diabetes mellitus (prolonged uncontrolled hyperglycemia)
Solid-organ transplant
Liver
Heart and lung
Hematopoietic stem cell transplant
Allogeneic HSCT with delayed engraftment and/or secondary graft failure
Graft rejection
Graft-vs.-host disease (GvHD)
Immunosuppressive GvHD therapy
Recurrent hematologic malignancy; refractory leukemia

Note: HD, hemodialysis.

during the same hospitalization, cancer patients may develop recurrent fungal bloodstream invasion due to different strains and/or yeast species with varying antimicrobial susceptibility profiles (83).

E. Polymicrobial Infections

Nearly one-fourth of nosocomial bacterial infections involve more than one micro-organism. Polymicrobial gram-negative infections are most frequently seen in hospitalized patients. Patients with advanced or refractory hematologic malignancies, especially individuals with leukemia, are at increased risk of polymicrobial septicemia (10). Gram-negative bacteria are common in this setting, whereas GPC, anaerobic bacteria, and fungi are uncommonly encountered (51). Interestingly, most catheter-related bloodstream infections (> 85%) are monomicrobial. Indeed, in patients with severe granulocytopenia and/or mixed immune defects, isolation of a single micro-organism does not exclude the possibility of an under-detected second or even third pathogen. An understanding of this phenomenon is important in determining and selecting empiric therapy for severely ill hospitalized patients that have failed initial empiric therapy. Patients at risk of polymicrobial bloodstream infection include prolonged granulocytopenia, severe orointestinal mucosal excoriation, necrotizing enterocolitis, ventilator-associated pneumonia (VAP), complicated peritonitis, complicated bowel surgery, perirectal abscesses. Polymicrobial bacteremia and/or fungemia in these patients are associated with higher mortality when compared with patients with similar end-organ disease and monomicrobial bloodstream invasion.

III. PNEUMONIA

Infections in severely immunocompromised patients with cancer or recipients of allogeneic transplants frequently involve the lungs (84–86). Neutropenia is an important underlying predisposing risk factor for cancer patients who may present with either community- or hospital-acquired lower respiratory tract infection (87,88). Nearly 10% of patients with febrile granulocytopenia may present with pulmonary infiltrate (89). Most infections are acquired by inhalation or aspiration of oropharyngeal contents. In certain situations, a small number of micro-organisms can lead to serious pneumonia, including (a) patients with disruption of respiratory tract lining resulting from antineoplastic and/or radiation therapy induced mucosal excoriation, which in turn compromises ciliary function leading to inadequate lower respiratory tract clearing and pulmonary stagnation of organisms and infection; (b) mechanical obstruction due to an endobranchial tumor or rapidly enlarging extraluminal mass may promote a favorable milieu for anaerobic bacteria to flourish leading to postobstructive pneumonia; (c) patients with reduced secretory and/or circulating immunoglobulins also increase risk of infections due to encapsulated bacterial such as *S. pneumoniae*, *Haemophilus influenzae*, and *Klebseilla* spp.; (d) defects in cellular immune functions involving disruption of lymphocyte–macrophage–lymphocyte cycle increase the risk of nontuberculous mycobacteriosis, invasive pulmonary mycosis, nocardiosis, and PCP (Table 1).

In addition, patients with febrile neutropenia have increased frequency of lung infection when compared with patients undergoing allogeneic HSCT, acute or refractory leukemia, and extended duration (>7 days) of severe (ANC < 150 cells/mm^3) neutropenia (1,90). Presence of an underlying pulmonary disease, chronic bronchiectasis, cystic fibrosis, and pulmonary fibrosis may further enhance the likelihood of infection. Infections may involve a single lung lobe, although diffuse consolidation is not uncommon; in patients with multicentric pulmonary infection, the risk of pneumonia-related death increases significantly (91). It is also important to appreciate that in most cases, due to multiple confounding factors, establishing correct etiology of ongoing lung infection is a daunting task. Currently, a number of hybrid diagnostic strategies are used to circumvent serious difficulty in early and correct diagnosis of pneumonia etiology in hospitalized patients receiving treatment for cancer (92–94).

A. Hospital-Acquired Pneumonia

Nosocomial pneumonia (NP) is defined as new pulmonary infection in patients ≥ 2 days after hospitalization. This does not include infections with long incubation period that may have been acquired prior to hospitalization (95). Patients receiving care in the ICU have a 20-fold higher risk of NP when compared with patients admitted to non-ICU setting (96). In the critically ill patients, two most important determinants of developing pneumonia are (a) duration of ICU stay and (b) presence of artificial airway (intubation) for mechanical ventilatory support (97,98). In fact, VAP is the most common cause of hospital-acquired pneumonia. In ICU, as many as 80% of lower respiratory tract infections are related to mechanical ventilation (99). Presence of VAP increases the duration of mechanical ventilation and duration of hospitalization by more than 10 days, which not inconceivably results in a substantial increase in healthcare coat. In 1999, VAP-incurred health care cost was estimated > $40,000 per patient (100). Interestingly, incidence of VAP has nearly doubled in surgical patients, especially following cardiothoracic surgery, when compared with patients receiving care in medical ICUs (101). Prior exposure to antimicrobials has also been identified as an important contributor in promoting the risk of NPs (102). Although short-term (<48 hr) exposure to systemic antibiotics prior to intubation in patients with VAP was recently shown to have modest protective role, albeit prolonged prior exposure paradoxically increases the risk of infection often to nosocomial resistant organisms, especially among patients requiring prolonged mechanical ventilation (103,104).

Presence of purulent respiratory secretions and early radiographic findings suggestive of pneumonia may be prominently absent in hospitalized oncology such as critically ill patients with hematologic malignancy with profound neutropenia (1,10). Early institution of appropriate antimicrobial therapy is critical in improving outcomes among patients with nosocomial pneumonia and VAP. It is paramount that microbiologic diagnosis must be pursued prior to the initiation of antibiotics when feasible, so as to improve diagnostic yield of lower respiratory samples. It is not always easy to correlate etiologic relevance of micro-organisms isolated from sputum, tracheal aspirate, and even bronchial wash, especially in individuals pretreated with antimicrobials, a common scenario in hospitalized cancer patients. However, identification of causative micro-organisms greatly improves ability to establish treatment strategies including escalation and de-escalation of antimicrobial therapy, when indicated (105,106).

In patients with no history of recent antimicrobial exposure, hospital-acquired pneumonia even in the setting of mechanical ventilation is frequently due to bacteria such as *H. influenzae* and *S. pneumoniae*, and methicillin-sensitive *S. aureus* are common (91). Patients with methicillin-resistant *S. aureus* were usually seen in those with prior antibiotic exposure (107), who were elderly, and receiving extended duration of ventilatory support. Although the recent rise in community-acquired MRSA has greatly influenced the pre-existing paradigm, MRSA infections in patients without stated risk are not an uncommon occurrence (108). Hospitalized patients are also at risk of gram-negative bacillary pulmonary infections. Organisms commonly isolated in this setting include *P. aeruginosa*, *Acinetobacter baumannii* complex, *Enterobacter* spp., and less commonly *S.* (*Xanthomonas*) *maltophilia*, *Burkholderia cepacia* complex, *Alcaligenes* (*Achromobacter*) spp. may be seen, especially in patients with prior extended multiple antibiotic exposure and/or those receiving prolonged mechanical ventilation (95). It is important to note that presence of severe neutropenia is an independent predisposing factor for NP due to nonfermentative gram-negative bacillary infection. These pathogens may gain access to the lower respiratory tract by aspiration of orointestinal contents, and/or hematogenous pulmonary seeding in patients with primary bacteremia arising from intestinal source is not uncommon. Hospital-acquired pneumonia due to MRSA and *P.*

aeruginosa, even though less common, are associated with disproportionably high mortality (109–112).

The treatment includes antimicrobial combination therapy, focusing on the probable pathogens involved. Vancomycin or linezolid may be used for MRSA, when applicable (113,114). For empiric therapy of nonfermentative gram-negative bacillary infections, individual hospital and community antibiograms may provide valuable information. Often, an antipseudomonal β-lactam is given with an aminoglycoside, although fluoroquinolones such as ciprofloxacin or gatifloxacin can be used as an alternative. For patients with MDR gram-negative bacillary infections, which tend to have in vitro resistance for a wide variety of antibiotics such as third and fourth generation cephalosporins (ceftazidime, cefepime), carbapenems (imipenem-cilastin, meropenem), quinolones, treatment options are greatly limited. High-dose trimethoprim-sulfamethoxazole, aminoglycosides (tobramycin, amikacin), antipseudomonal penicillins (ticarcillin-clavulanate, piperacillin-tazobactam), monobactam (aztreonam), and polymyxin B (colistin) may be used in various combinations depending upon the antimicrobial susceptibility profile. Duration of therapy is 2–3 weeks, although, recently, a shorter duration of treatment (8 days) was found to be comparable with 2-week antibiotic therapy (115). It is advisable that short treatment course must not be given to patients with profound neutropenia, severe pulmonary comorbidities, concurrent bacteremia, to high-risk patients such as those with leukemia, allogeneic HSCT recipients, and to patients with infection due to MDR micro-organism.

B. Pulmonary Mycobacteriosis

Mycobacterium tuberculosis is an uncommon infection in patients with cancer. Certain subpopulation of cancer patients, such as those with Hodgkin's disease and head, neck, or lung cancers, have been historically identified as having higher incidence of pulmonary tuberculosis (1,10,116). As most of the patients are with tuberculosis, infections are reactivation of remotely acquired latent *M. tuberculosis*. Although nosocomial spread of tuberculosis in hospitalized patients is rare (117), but occasional, outbreaks have been reported in health-care workers. It is important to note that hospitalized patients with cellular immune defect and those receiving systemic corticosteroids may present with *M. tuberculosis* reactivation that is clinically indistinguishable from other causes of NP. A high level of suspicion and prompt diagnostic work, including microbiologic and histological analysis of the involved area of lower respiratory tract, may provide accurate diagnosis for selected patients at risk. *Mycobacterium kansasii* leads to pulmonary disease, which is often clinically and radiographically indistinguishable from *M. tuberculosis*; patients with solid-organ and hematologic malignancy are susceptible (118). Owing to high rate of infection relapse and de novo drug resistance, patients with *M. kansasii* infection are often treated for >18 months with susceptible rifampin-based antimicrobial regimen (119).

C. Nontuberculous Mycobacteriosis

Infections due to MAC, *M. simiae*, and other slow-growing mycobacteria may lead to progressive, often multicentric lung disease that may be distinguish radiographically from other causes of pneumonia (64). Infections are insidious, although rapidly progressive fatal infections due to these low-virulence slow-growing mycobacteria are rarely seen in severely immunosuppressed recipients of allogeneic HSCT (62). Diagnosis is ascertained by clinical presentation of chronic cough, bronchiectasis, dyspnea on exertion, and characteristic radiographic findings and isolation of slow-growing mycobacteria from lower respiratory samples. Treatment includes a minimum of two effective antimycobacterial drugs that are given for 18–24 months. Recently, a selective cytokine defects has been described in patients with nontuberculous pulmonary mycobacteriosis (65,120), and in these patients, immune augmentation with recombinant cytokine may be cautiously attempted in the setting of refractory or relapsing disease.

D. Fungal Pneumonia

1. Pneumocystis jiroveci Pneumonia

Pneumocystis jiroveci (*P. carinii*) infections are seen in patients with severe underlying cellular immune defect; patients with leukemia, T-cell lymphoma, and recipients of allogeneic HSCT are especially at risk (1,10,121). Presentation is acute, rapidly progressive pneumonitis leading to respiratory failure and ARDS; more commonly, the disease pattern is slowly progressive interstitial pneumonitis that evolves over a period of weeks to months (1,10). During the early phase of infection, like viral pneumonia (1,10), PCP may be radiographically occult, and in order to make correct diagnosis, specialized imaging studies like noncontrast enhanced, high-resolution chest computed tomography are needed (122). Presence of exertional hypoxemia may further indicate presence of a cryptic *P. jiroveci* infection, although a host of other infections may have similar presentation including nonproductive cough, normal appearing chest radiograph, viral pneumonias due to respiratory viruses such as respiratory syncytial virus (RSV), influenza, parainfluenza, HCMV, and noninfectious lymphangitic lung metastasis, to name a few.

Bronchoalveolar lavage of the infected lung area has consistently been shown to have a high diagnostic yield (123), although in small number of patients with chronic PCP, diagnosis is made on histologic examination of infected lung tissue. Treatment includes high-dose (15–20 mg/kg daily) of TMP-SMX given for 3 weeks; for patients intolerant to sulfa, and have mild infection, oral atovaquone may be used (124). In seriously ill patients, intravenous pentamidine is considered alternative to TMP-SMX along with systemic corticosteroids.

2. *Invasive Pulmonary Mycosis*

Invasive fungal infection (IFI) involving lungs is a serious and well-recognized life-threatening infection (1,10). Invasive pulmonary aspergillosis (IPA) is the most common infection in this category (125,126) and mostly seen in patients with prolonged (>2 weeks) severe neutropenia, high-dose systemic corticosteroids given for extended periods (127); the non-neutropenic allogeneic HSCT recipients with graft-vs.-host disease (GvHD) are also at risk due to immunosuppressive therapy-induced defective T-cell mediated granulocyte recruitment at the site of infection (1,10,128). Radiographic features like "halo sign" and "crescent sign" may not be seen in most cases, although when present are highly suggestive of IFI (129–131). On CT scan, pulmonary fungal lesions often present as peripheral, pleural-based nodules, and in patients with advanced disease, localized or diffuse intra-alveolar hemorrhage may be present, which is difficult to distinguish from pulmonary congestion and/or ARDS, unless diagnosed and treatment promptly. Patients with diffuse intra-alveolar hemorrhage may rapidly progress to end-stage respiratory failure (1,10,125,126).

In the era of triazole-based antifungal prophylaxis and a recent decline in the use of amphotericin B-based therapy, IFI due to non-*Aspergillus* filamentous molds, including black molds, and pulmonary zygomycosis are being observed at an alarming rate in certain cancer and transplant centers. Infections due to these emerging and re-emerging molds tend to be less responsive to conventional antifungal agents (132–135). For definite diagnosis, demonstration of tissue fungal invasion is required. In most high-risk patients, the risk associated with lung biopsy procedure is considered unacceptable; therefore, at present, the majority of the antemortem invasive pulmonary mycoses are defined as probable infections on the basis of compatible clinical, radiographic, and microbiologic documentation of fungal infection. The evolving field of nonculture-based molecular diagnostic method (136,137) is presently undergoing intense scrutiny, and clinical relevance of the hybrid diagnostic protocols used in the detection of fungal (galactomannan) antigenemia (138,139) and/or DNA amplification remains uncertain (140,141).

Treatment for patients with invasive pulmonary mycosis includes any of the three lipid-based amphotericin B preparations available in the United States; both AmBisome® and Abelcet® have significant renal function preservation advantage when compared with Fungisome® (amphotericin B deoxycholate). Aminfusion-related adverse effect profile (142–144). Recently, a comparative study using voriconazole primary therapy for patients with IPA had a significant advantage over amphotericin B-based primary therapy (145). Infections due to non-*Aspergillus* spp. filamentous molds pose a serious treatment challenge, as most of dematiacious (black) molds such as *Alternaria*, *Curvularia*, *Bipolaris*, *Scedosporium prolificancs*, *Sc. apiospermum*, *Pseudallescheria boydii* are nonsusceptible to polyene-based antifungals (146), and treatment with either voriconazole or echinocandin-pneumocandin analogue (caspofungin; Cancidas®) may provide a much sort after treatment alternative (133,134). For patients with pulmonary zygomycosis, despite treatment with high-dose amphotericin B, outcome remains far from optimum. Preliminary analysis of treatment with posaconazole looks favorable, albeit prior to routine use is recommended and further clinical experience is needed (147). When possible, surgical excision may be attempted to remove infected necrotic tissue. However, most cancer patients with invasive systemic mycosis are poor surgical candidates, especially patients with either profound granulocytopenia or thrombocytopenia. Restitution of predisposing immune defect remains the pivotal determinant in successful recovery of patients with IFIs, and this observation has led to evaluations and experiments including adjuvant immunomodulatory therapy in the setting of systemic difficult-to-treat fungal infections; recombinant cytokines including IL-2, IL-12, IL-18, interferon-γ, G-CSF, GM-CSF, etc. (148–150). The role of adaptive immune augmentation is currently evolving and needs further clinical evaluation.

3. *Nocardiosis*

Nocardia asteroids complex is most commonly associated with systemic human disease. Pulmonary infection is the protean manifestation of disease and radiographically difficult to differentiate from other causes of opportunistic infection, especially invasive pulmonary mycosis, and noninfectious lymphomatous pulmonary infiltrates (151). Patients with cellular immune defects and those receiving prolonged high-dose systemic corticosteroids are at increased risk (152). Neutrotropism of Nocardia is entertained in working up patients with pulmonary infections, although similar to disseminated disease, *Nocardia* spp. brain abscesses are relatively uncommon even in patients with severe cellular immune defects (153). Trimethoprim-sulfamethoxazole (10–12 mg/Kg daily) is the treatment of choice and recommended for an extended period (>3 months). Patients with sulfa-based antimicrobial intolerance, a combination of carbapenems plus amikacin may be used as an alternative, although sulfa-desensitization may be considered in patients with serious infection; mortality in patients with systemic nocardiosis remains high despite institution of appropriate therapy (153).

E. *Viral Pneumonia*

Viral infections of the lower respiratory tract can often lead to serious morbidity and death, especially in patients with adaptive T-cell mediated immune dysfunctions, patients with acute myeloid leukemia, allogeneic HSCT; and patients receiving near-cytoablative therapy such as fludarabine-based antineoplastic regimen for chronic lymphocytic leukemia, T-cell lymphoma are at an increased risk (1,8,10). Human cytomegalovirus lung infection is the most frequent cause of opportunistic lung infection in this patient population, although rarely pneumonitis due to VZV, HHV-6 may be encountered (154,155). Another group of viruses that are associated with seasonal upper respiratory tract illness such as RSV, influenza A and B, and parainfluenza virus infection that may be acquired year round with a second peak during mid-summer months may also cause serious lung infection, which frequently progresses to respiratory failure and death if left untreated in the susceptible host (156,157).

Although chest radiography has low sensitivity and negative predictive value as a primary method of diagnosing viral pneumonia in the early stages of infection, noncontrast enhanced, high-resolution computed tomography has been shown to have near 90% sensitivity and >95% negative predictive value in diagnosing pneumonitis in the high-risk stem cell transplant recipients (129,130,151). Viral detection by either conventional culture methods, which may take >3 weeks, or the currently used rapid laboratory methods, including viral DNA amplification by polymerase chain reaction and antigenemia assay, commonly used to detect HCMV reactivation, may help in the early detection of viral presence in peripheral blood and/or lower respiratory tract samples such as bronchoalveolar lavage (158–160). It is imperative to recognize that the majority of patients with viremia even with a severe underlying immune dysfunction may not develop end-organ lung disease, although in high-risk patients with the evidence of viral presences, pre-emptive antiviral treatment is given to prevent the likelihood of life-threatening pneumonia (161,162).

Treatment for HCMV and VZV pneumonia involves a combination of antiviral agents, such as ganciclovir, foscarnet, cidofovir plus organism-specific (anti-HCMV, anti-VZV enriched), or nonspecific immunoglobulin (IVIG) (163–165). Antivirals are given at a higher (induction) dose for 14–21 days, and then dose is reduced to maintenance. Pneumonia due to RSV carries high mortality, and treatment requires inhaled ribavirin (6 g in 24 hr) plus RSV-specific immunoglobulins (palivizumab; Synagis®); for patients with influenza, the treatment for pneumonia includes early institution of oseltamivir or rimantadine or amantadine, as these drugs are effective drugs. The early phase of infected patients that are diagnosed with upper respiratory tract infection may be treated promptly to prevent lower respiratory tract progression of infection.

In conclusion, hospitalized critically ill oncology patients may present with a wide variety of infections. A keen understanding of the patterns of emerging and re-emerging pathogens, spectrum of antimicrobial drug resistance in hospital and community environment, and hosts' underlying immune dysfunction, which may interfere effective handling of infection on multiple levels, is critical in promoting optimum care for hospitalized patients with an underlying cancer.

REFERENCES

1. Safdar A, Armstrong D. Infectious morbidity in critically ill patients with cancer. Crit Care Clin 2001; 17(3):531–580.
2. Karchmer AW. Nosocomial bloodstream infections: organisms, risk factors, and implications. Clin Infect Dis 2000; 31(suppl 4):S139–S143.
3. Wenzel RP, Edmond MB. The impact of hospital-acquired bloodstream infections. Emerg Infect Dis 2001; 7:174–177.
4. Eggimann P, Pittet D. Infection control in the ICU. Chest 2001; 120:2059–2093.
5. Jarvis WR. Selected aspects of the socioeconomic impact of nosocomial infections: morbidity, mortality, cost, and prevention. Infect Control Hosp Epidemiol 1996; 17:552–557.
6. Hersh EM, Bodey GP, Nies BA, Freireich EJ. Causes of death in acute leukemia: a ten-year study of 414 patients from 1954–1963. JAMA 1965; 193:105–109.

7. Smith N. Sepsis: its causes and effects. J Wound Care 2003; 12:265–270.
8. Safdar A, Armstrong D. Infections in patients with neoplastic disease. In: Shoemaker WC, Grenvik M, Ayers SM, Holbrook PR, eds. Textbook of Critical Care. Philadelphia: WB Saunders, 2000:715–726.
9. Roemer E, Blau IW, Basara N, et al. Toxoplasmosis, a severe complication in allogeneic hematopoietic stem cell transplantation: successful treatment strategies during a 5-year single-center experience. Clin Infect Dis 2001; 32:E1–E8.
10. Rolston V, Bodey GP. Infections in patients with cancer. In: Holland JF, Frei E, eds. Cancer Medicine. 6th ed. Ontario: BC Decker, 2003:2633–2658.
11. Bodey GP. Infections in cancer patients. A continuing association. Am J Med 1986; 81(suppl 1A):11–26.
12. Eelting LS, Bodey GP, Keefe BH. Septicemia and shock syndrome due to viridans streptococci: a case–control study of predisposing factors. Clin Infect Dis 1992; 14:1201–1207.
13. Chatzinikolaou I, Abi-Said D, Bodey GP, Rolston KVI, Tarrand JJ, Samonis G. Recent experience with *Pseudomonas aeruginosa* bacteremia in patients with cancer. Arch Intern Med 2000; 160:501–509.
14. Schimpff S, Satterlee W, Young VM, et al. Empiric therapy with carbenicillin and gentamicin for febrile patients with cancer and granulocytopenia. N Engl J Med 1971; 284:1061–1065.
15. Raad II, Hanna HA. Intravascular catheter-related infections. Arch Intern Med 2002; 162:871–878.
16. Safdar A, Papadopoulous EB, Armstrong D. Listeriosis in recipients of allogeneic blood and marrow transplantation: thirteen year review of disease characteristics, treatment outcome and a new association with human cytomegalovirus infection. Bone Marrow Transplant 2002; 29:913–916.
17. Bilgrami S, Almeida GD, Quinn JJ, et al. Pancytopenia in allogeneic marrow transplant recipients: role of cytomegalovirus. Br J Haematol 1994; 87: 357–362.
18. Sparrelid E, Emanuel D, Fehniger T, et al. Interstitial pneumonitis in bone marrow transplant recipients is associated with local production of TH2-type cytokines and lack of T cell-mediated cytotoxicity. Transplantation 1997; 63:1782–1789.
19. National Nosocomial Infections Surveillance. NNIS system report, data summary from January 1992–April 2000. Issued June 2000. Am J Infect Control 2000; 28:429–448.
20. Wisplinghoff H, Seifert H, Wenzel RP, Edmond MB. Current trends in the epidemiology of nosocomial bloodstream infections in patients with hematological malignancies and solid neoplasms in Hospitals in the United States. Clin Infect Dis 2003; 36:1103–1110.
21. Bodey GP. Epidemiological studies of *Pseudomonas* species in patients with leukemia. Am J Sci 1970; 260:82–89.
22. Singer C, Kaplan MH, Armstrong D. Bacteremia and fungemia complicating neoplastic disease. A study of 364 cases. Am J Med 1977; 62:731–742.
23. Whimbey E, Kiehn TE, Brannon P, Blevins A, Armstrong D. Bacteremia and fungemia in patients with neoplastic diseases. Am J Med 1987; 82:723–730.
24. Rolston KV, Tarrand JJ . *Pseudomonas aeruginosa*—still a frequent pathogen in patients with cancer: 11-year experience at a comprehensive cancer center. Clin Infect Dis 1999; 29:463–464.
25. Pfaller MA, Jones RN, Doern GV, Kugler K, The SENTRY Participants Group. Bacterial pathogens isolated from patients with bloodstream infections: frequency of occurrence and antimicrobial susceptibility patterns from the SENTRY antimicrobial surveillance program (United States and Canada, 1997). Antimicrob Agents Chemother 1998; 42:1762–1770.
26. Pfaller MA, Jones RN, Doern GV, Sader HS, Kugler KC, Beach ML, The SENTRY Participants Group. Survey of bloodstream infections attributable to gram-positive cocci: frequency of occurrence and antimicrobial susceptibility of isolates collected in 1997 in the United States, Canada, and Latin America from the SENTRY Antimicrobial Surveillance Program. Diag Microbiol Infect Dis 1999; 33:283–297.
27. Hughes WT, Armstrong D, Bodey GP, et al. 2002 Guidelines for the use of antimicrobial agents in neutropenic patients with cancer. Clin Infect Dis 2002; 34:730–751.
28. Cruciani M, Rampazzo R, Malena M, et al. Prophylaxis with fluoroquinolones for bacterial infections in neutropenic patients. Clin Infect Dis 1996; 23:795–805.
29. Diekema DJ, Pfaller MA, Jones RN, et al. Age-related trends in pathogen frequency and antimicrobial susceptibility of bloodstream isolates in North America SENTRY Antimicrobial Surveillance Program, 1997–2000. Intern J Antimicrob Agents 2002; 20:412–418.
30. Raad I, Davis S, Khan A, Tarrand J, Elting L, Bodey GP. Impact of central venous catheter removal on the recurrence of catheter-related coagulase-negative0 staphylococcal bacteremia. Infect Control Hosp Epidemiol 1992; 13:215–221.
31. Okamoto Y, Ribeiro RC, Srivastava DK, Shenep JL, Pai CH, Razzouk BI. Viridans streptococcal sepsis: clinical features and complications in childhood acute myeloid leukemia. J Ped Hematol Oncol 2003; 25: 696–703.
32. Paganini H, Staffolani V, Zubizarreta P, Casimir L, Lopardo H, Luppino V. Viridans streptococci bacteremia in children with fever and neutropenia: a case–control study of predisposing factors. Euro J Cancer 2003; 39:1284–1289.
33. Rozenberg-Arska M, Dekker A, Verdonck L, Verhoef J. Prevention of bacteremia caused by alpha-hemolytic streptococci by roxithromycin (RU-28 965) in granulocytopenic patients receiving ciprofloxacin. Infection 1989; 17:240–244.

34. Rolston KV, Elting LS, Bodey GP. Bacteremia due to viridans streptococci in neutropenic patients [letter]. Am J Med 1995; 99:450.
35. Fanourgiakia P, Georgala A, Vekemans M, Daneau D, Heymans C, Aoun M. Bacteremia due to *Stomatococcus mucilaginosus* in neutropenic patients in the setting of a cancer institute. Clin Microbiol Infect Dis 2003; 9:1068–1072.
36. McWhinney P, Kibbler C, Gillespie S, et al. *Stomatococcus mucilaginosus*: an emerging pathogen in neutropenic patients. Clin Infect Dis 1992; 14:641–646.
37. Goldman M, Chaudharry UB, Greist A, Faucel CA. Central nervous system infections due to *Stomatococcus mucilaginosus* in immunocompromised hosts. Clin Infect Dis 1998; 27:1241–1246.
38. Maki DG, Weise CE, Sarafin HW. A semiquantitative culture method for identifying intravenous catheter infections. N Engl J Med 1977; 296:1305–1309.
39. Sheretz RJ, Raad II, Balani A, Koo L, Rand K. Three-year experience with sonicated vascular catheter cultures in a clinical microbiology laboratory. J Clin Microbiol 1990; 28:76–82.
40. Safdar A, Raad II. Management and treatment. In: O'Grady N, Pittet D, eds. Catheter-Related Infections in the Critically Ill. Kluwer series. In press, 2004; 99–112.
41. Gaillard JL, Merlino R, Pajot N, et al. Conventional and nonconventional modes of vancomycin administration to decontaminate the internal surface of catheters colonized with coagulase-negative staphylococci. JPEN J Parenter Enteral Nutr 1990; 14:593–597.
42. Douard MC, Arlet G, Leverger G, et al. Quantitative blood cultures for diagnosis and management of catheter-related sepsis in pediatric hematology and oncology patients. Intensive Care Med 1991; 17:30–35.
43. Safdar A, Armstrong D. Listeriosis in patients at a comprehensive cancer center, 1955–1997. Clin Infect Dis 2003; 37:359–364.
44. Lorber B. Listeriosis. Clin Infect Dis 1997; 24:1–11.
45. Safdar A, Armstrong D. Antimicrobial activity against 84 Listeria monocytogenes isolates from patients with systemic listeriosis at a comprehensive cancer center 955–1997). J Clin Microbiol 2003; 41:483–485.
46. Wynne JW, Armstrong D. Clostridial septicemia. Cancer 1972; 29:215–221.
47. Garcia-Suarez J, de Miguel D, Krsnik I, Barr-Ali M, Hernanz N, Burgaleta C. Spontaneous gas gangrene in malignant lymphoma: an underreported complication? Am J Hematol 2002; 70:145–148.
48. Momont SL, Overholt EL. Aortitis due to metastatic gas gangrene. Wis Med J 1989; 88:28–30.
49. Bodey Gp. *Pseudomonas aeruginosa* infections in cancer patients: have they gone away? Curr Opin Infect Dis 2001; 14:403–407.
50. Whitecar JP, Luna M, Bodey GP. *Pseudomonas bacteremia* in patients with malignant diseases. Am J Med Sci 1997; 260:216–222.
51. Elting LS, Bodey GP, Fainstien V. Polymicrobial septicemia in the cancer patient. Medicine 1986; 65:218–225.
52. Bodey GP, Jadeja L. *Pseudomonas bacteremia*: retrospective analysis of 410 episodes. Arch Intern Med 1985; 145:1621–1629.
53. Fishman LS, Armstrong D. *Pseudomonas aeruginosa* bacteremia in patients with neoplastic disease. Cancer 1972; 30:764–773.
54. Maschmeyer G, Braveny I. Review of the incidence and prognosis of *Pseudomonas aeruginosa* infections in cancer patients in the 1990s. Eur J Clin Microbiol Infect Dis 2000; 19:915–925.
55. Raad II, Vartivarian S, Khan A, Bodey GP. Catheter-related infections caused by the *Mycobacterium fortuitum* complex: 15 cases and review. Rev Infect Dis 1991; 13:1120–1125.
56. Levendoglu-Tugal O, Munoz J, Brudnicki A, Fevzi Ozkaynak M, Sandoval C, Jayabose S. Infections due to nontuberculous mycobacteria in children with leukemia. Clin Infect Dis 1998; 27:1227–1230.
57. Jacobson K, Garcia R, Libshitz H, et al. Clinical and radiological features of pulmonary disease caused by rapidly growing mycobacteria in cancer patients. Eur J Clin Microbiol Infect Dis 1998; 17:615–621.
58. Safdar A, Bains MS, Polsky B. Clinical microbiological case: refractory chest wall infection following reconstruction surgery in a patient with relapsed lung cancer. Clin Microbiol Infect 2001; 7:563–564, 577–579.
59. Safdar A, Han XY. *Mycobacterium lentiflavum*—A New Nontuberculous Mycobacterial Species in Patients with cancer. [Abstract #387]. The 41st Annual Meeting of Infectious Diseases Society of America. San Diego, CA October 9–12, 2003.
60. Tumbarello M, Tacconelli E, de Donati KG, et al. Changes in incidence and risk factors of *Mycobacterium avium* complex infections in patients with AIDS in the era of new antiretroviral therapies. Eur J Clin Microbiol Infect Dis 2001; 20:498–501.
61. Dube MP, Sattler FR. Catheter-related bacteremia due to *Mycobacterium avium* complex. Clin Infect Dis 1996; 23:405–406.
62. Roy V, Weisdorf D. *Mycobacterium* infections following bone marrow transplantation: a 20 year retrospective review. Bone Marrow Transplant 1997; 19:467–470.
63. Bennett C, Vardiman J, Golomb H. Disseminated atypical mycobacterial infection in patients with hairy cell leukemia. Am J Med 1986; 80:891–896.
64. Safdar A, White DA, Stover D, Armstrong D, Murray HW. Profound interferon-γdeficiency in patients with chronic pulmonary nontuberculous mycobacteriosis. Am J Med 2002; 113:756–759.
65. Horwitz ME, Uzel G, Linton GF, et al. Persistent *Mycobacterium avium* infection following nonmyeloablative allogeneic peripheral blood stem cell transplantation for interferon-γ receptor-1 deficiency. Blood 2003; 102:2692–2694.

66. Tomioka H, Sato K, Akaki T, Kajitani H, Kawahara S, Sakatani M. Comparative in vitro antimicrobial activities of the newly synthesized quinolone HSR-903, sitafloxacin (DU-6859a), gatifloxacin (AM-1155), and levofloxacin against *Mycobacterium tuberculosis* and *Mycobacterium avium* complex. Antimicrob Agents Chemother 1999; 43:3001–3004.
67. Tomioka H, Sano C, Sato K, Shimizu T. Antimicrobial activities of clarithromycin, gatifloxacin and sitafloxacin, in combination with various antimycobacterial drugs against extracellular and intramacrophage *Mycobacterium avium* complex. Int J Antimicrob Agents 2002; 19:139–145.
68. Holland SM. Immunotherapy of mycobacterial infection. Semin Respir Infect 2001; 16:47–59.
69. Greinert U, Ernst M, Schlaak M, Entzian P. Interleukin-12 as successful adjuvant in tuberculosis treatment. Eur Res J 2001; 17:1049–1051.
70. Raad I, Hachem R, Leeds N, Sawaya R, Salem Z, Atweh S. Use of adjuvant treatment with interferon-gamma in an immunocompromised patients who had refractory multidrug resistant tuberculosis of the brain. Clin Infect Dis 1996; 22:572–574.
71. Beck-Sague C, Jarvis WR. Secular trends in the epidemiology of nosocomial fungal infections in the United States, 1980–1990. National Nosocomical Infections Survellance System. J Infect Dis 1993; 167:1247–1251.
72. Pittet D, Wenzel RP. Nosocomial bloodstream infections. Secular trends in rates, mortality, and contribution to total hospital deaths. Arch Intern Med 1995; 155:1177–1184.
73. Safdar A, Chaturvedi V, Cross EW, et al. Prospective study of *Candida* species in patients at a comprehensive cancer center. Antimicrob Agents Chemother 2001; 45:2129–2133.
74. Safdar A, van Rhee F, Henslee-Downey JP, Singhal S, Mehta J. *Candida glabrata* and *Candida krusei* fungemia after high-risk allogeneic marrow transplantation: no adverse effects of low-dose fluconazole prophylaxis on incidence and outcome. Bone Marrow Transplant 2001; 28:873–878.
75. Bodey GP, Mardani M, Hanna HA, et al. The epidemiology of *Candida glabrata* and *Candida albicans* fungemia in immunocompromised patients with cancer. Am J Med 2002; 112:380–385.
76. Safdar A, Chaturvedi V, Koll BS, Larone DH, Perlin DS, Armstrong D. Prospective, multicenter surveillance study of *Candida glabrata*: fluconazole and itraconazole susceptibility profiles in bloodstream, invasive, and colonizing strains and differences between isolates from three urban teaching hospitals in New York City (*Candida* susceptibility trends study, 1998 to 1999). Antimicrob Agents Chemother 2002; 46:3268–3272.
77. Antoniadou A, Torres HA, Lewis RE, et al. Candidemia in a tertiary care cancer center. In vitro susceptibility and its association with outcome of initial antifungal therapy. Medicine 2003; 82:309–321.
78. Abbas J, Bodey GP, Hanna HA, et al. *Candida krusei* fungemia. An escalating serious infection in immunocompromised patients. Arch Intern Med 2000; 160:2659–2664.
79. Safdar A, Armstrong D. Prospective evaluation of *Candida* species colonization in hospitalized cancer patients: impact on short-term survival in recipients of marrow transplantation and patients with hematological malignancies. Bone Marrow Transplant 2002; 30:931–935.
80. Anaissie EJ, Rex JH, Uzun O, Vartivarian S. Predictors of adverse out-come in cancer patients with candidemia. Am J Med 1998; 104:238–245.
81. Minari A, Hachem R, Raad I. *Candida lusitaniae*: a cause of breakthrough fungemia in cancer patients. Clin Infect Dis 2001; 32:186–190.
82. Mora-Duarte J, Betts R, Rotstein C, et al. Comparison of caspofungin and amphotericin B for invasive candidasis. N Engl J Med 2002; 347:2020–2029.
83. Safdar A, Cross EW, Chaturvedi V, Perlin DS, Armstrong D. Prolonged candidemia in patients with cancer. Clin Infect Dis 2002; 35:778–779.
84. Neville K, Renbarger J, Dreyer Z. Pneumonia in the immunocompromised pediatric cancer patients. Semin Respir Infect 2002; 17:21–32.
85. Collin BA, Ramphal R. Pneumonia in the compromised host including cancer patients and transplant patients. Infect Dis Clin North Am 1998; 12:781–805.
86. Marschmeyer G, Link H, Hiddemann W, et al. Pulmonary infiltrations in febrile patients with neutropenia. Cancer 1994; 73:2296–2304.
87. Bodey GP, Buckley M, Sathe YS, et al. Quantitative relationships between circulating leukocytes and infection in patients with acute leukemia. Ann Intern Med 1966; 64:328–340.
88. Walsh TJ, Rubin M, Pizzo PA. Respiratory diseases in patients with malignant neoplasms. In: Shelhammer J, Pizzo PA, Parrillo JE, et al., eds. Respiratory disease in immunocompromised host. Philadelphia, PA: JB Lippincott, 1991:640–663.
89. Raad I, Whimbey E, Rolston K, et al. A comparison of aztreonam plus vancomycin and imipenem plus vancomycin as initial therapy for febrile neutropenic cancer patients. Cancer 1996; 77:1386–1394.
90. Ahmed S, Siddiqui AK, Rossoff L, Sison CP, Rai KR. Pulmonary complications in chronic lymphocytic leukemia. Cancer 2003; 98:1912–1917.
91. Rello J, Diaz E. Pneumonia in the intensive care unit. Crit Care Med 2003; 31:2544–2551.
92. Hauggaard A, Ellis M, Ekelund L. Early chest radiograph and CT in the diagnosis, management and outcome of invasive pulmonary aspergillosis. Acta Radiologica 2002; 43:292–298.
93. Kim K, Lee MH, Kim J, et al. Importance of open lung biopsy in the diagnosis of invasive pulmonary aspergillosis in patients with hematologic malignancies. Am J Hematol 2002; 71:75–79.

94. Wong PW, Stefanec T, Brown K, White DA. Role of fine-needle aspiration of focal lung lesions in patients with hematologic malignancies. Chest 2002; 121: 527–532.
95. American Thoracic Society. Hospital-acquired pneumonia in adults: diagnosis, assessment of severity, initial antimicrobial therapy, and preventive strategies; a consensus statement, American Thoracic Society, November 1995. Am J Respir Crit Care Med 1996; 153:1711–1725.
96. Leu HS, Kaiser DL, Mori M, et al. Hospital-acquired pneumonia: attributable morbidity and mortality. Am J Epidemiol 1989; 129:1258–1267.
97. Haley RW, Hooton TM, Culver DH, et al. Nosocomial infections in US hospitals, 1975–76: estimated frequency by selected characteristics of patients. Am J Med 1981; 70:947–959.
98. National Nosocomial Infections (NNIS) system: data summary from Jan 1992–June 2001. Am J Infect Control 2001; 29:408–421.
99. Vincent JL, Bihari DJ, Suter PM, et al. The prevalence of nosocomial infection in intensive care units in Europe: results of the European Prevalence of Infection in Intensive Care (EPIC) study. JAMA 1995; 274:639–644.
100. Rello J, Ollendorf DA, Oster G, et al. Epidemiology and outcomes of ventilator-associated pneumonia in a large US database. Chest 2002; 122:2115–2121.
101. Kollef MH. Ventilator-associated pneumonia: a multivariate analysis. JAMA 1993; 270:1965–1970.
102. Hubmayr RD. Statement of the 4th International Consensus Conference in Critical Care on ICU-acquired pneumonia—Chicago, Illinois, may 2002. Intensive Care Med 2002; 28:1521–1536.
103. Rello J, Diaz E, Roque M, et al. Risk factors for developing pneumonia within 48 hours of intubation. Am J Respir Crit Care Med 1999; 159:1742–1746.
104. Cook DJ, Walter SD, Cook RJ, et al. Incidence of and risk factors for ventilator-associated pneumonia in critically ill patients. Ann Intern Med 1988; 129:433–440.
105. Rolston KVI. The spectrum of pulmonary infections in cancer patients. Curr Opin Oncol 2001; 13:218–223.
106. Hoffken G, Niederman MS. Nosocomial pneumonia. The importance of a de-escalating strategy for antibiotic treatment of pneumonia in the ICU. Chest 2002; 122:2183–2196.
107. Pujol M, Corbella X, Pena C, et al. Clinical and epidemiologic findings in mechanically ventilated patients with methicillin-resistant *Staphylococcus aureus* pneumonia. Eur J Clin Microbiol Infect Dis 1998; 17: 622–628.
108. Dufour P, Gillet Y, Bes M, et al. Community-acquired methicillin-resistant *Staphylococcus aureus* infections in France: emergence of a single clone that produces panton-valentine leukocidin. Clin Infect Dis 2002; 35:819–824.
109. Rello J, Torres A, Ricart M, et al. Ventilator-associated pneumonia by *Staphylococcus aureus*: comparison of methicillin-resistant with methicillin sensitive episodes. Am J Respir Crit Care Med 1994; 150:1545–1549.
110. Rello J, Jubert P, Valles J, et al. Evaluation of outcome for intubated patients with pneumonia due to *Pseudomonas aeruginosa*. Clin Infect Dis 1996; 23: 973–978.
111. Kollef MH, Silver P, Murphy DM, et al. The effect of late onset ventilator-associated pneumonia in determining patient mortality. Chest 1995; 108:1655–1662.
112. Fagon JY, Chastre J, Hance AJ, et al. Nosocomial pneumonia in ventilated patients: a cohort study evaluating attributable mortality and hospital stay. Am J Med 1993; 94:281–288.
113. Stevens DL, Herr D, Lampiris H, Hunt JL, Batts DH, Hafkin B. Linezolid versus vancomycin for the treatment of methicillin-resistant *Staphylococcus aureus* infections. Clin Infect Dis 2002; 34:1481–1490.
114. Wunderink RG, Rello J, Cammarata SK, Croos-Dabrera RV, Kollef MH. Linezolid vs vancomycin – analysis of two double-blind studies of patients with methicillin-resistant *Staphylococcus aureus* nosocomial pneumonia. Chest 2003; 124:1789–1797.
115. Chastre J, Wolff M, Fagon J, et al. Comparison of 8 vs. 15 days of antibiotic therapy for ventilator-associated pneumonia in adults. JAMA 2003; 290: 2588–2598.
116. Kaplan MH, Armstrong D, Rosen P. Tuberculosis complicating neoplastic disease. A review of 201 cases. Cancer 1974; 33:850–858.
117. Larson JL, Lambert L, Stricof RL, Driscoll J, McGarry MA, Ridzon R. Potential nosocomial exposure to *Mycobacterium tuberculosis* from a bronchoscope. Infect Control Hosp Epidemiol 2003; 24: 825–830.
118. Jacobson KL, Teira R, Libshitz HI, et al. *Mycobacterium kansasii* infections in patients with cancer. Clin Infect Dis 2000; 31:628–631.
119. Griffith DE. Management of disease due to *Mycobacterium kansasii*. Clin Chest Med 2002; 23:613–621.
120. Safdar A, Armstrong D, Murray HW. A novel defect in interferon-gamma secretion in patients with refractory nontuberculous pulmonary mycobacteriosis. Ann Intern Med 2003; 138:521.
121. Roblot F, Le Moal G, Godet C, et al. *Pneumocystis carinii* pneumonia in patients with hematologic malignancies: a descriptive study. J Infect 2003; 47: 19–27.
122. Tanaka N, Matsumoto T, Miura G, Emoto T, Matsunaga N. HRCT findings of chest complications in patients with leukemia. Eur Radiol 2002; 12:1512–1522.
123. Huang L, Hecht FM, Stansell JD, Montanti R, Hadley WK, Hopewell PC. Suspected *Pneumocystis carinii* pneumonia with a negative induced sputum examination. Is early bronchoscopy useful? Am J Respir Crit Care Med 1995; 151:1866–1871
124. Varthalitia I, Meunier F. *Pneumocystis carinii* pneumonia in cancer patients. Cancer Treat Rev 1993; 19: 387–413.

125. Marr KA, Patterson T, Denning D. Aspergillosis. Pathogenesis, clinical manifestations, and therapy. Infect Dis Clin North Am 2002; 16:875–894.
126. Denning DW. Invasive aspergillosis. Clin Infect Dis 1998; 26:781–803.
127. Lionakis MS, Kontoyiannis DP. Glucocorticoids and invasive fungal infections. Lancet 2003; 362: 1828–1838.
128. Einsele H. Antigen-specific T cell for the treatment of infections after transplantation. Hematol J 2003; 4: 10–17.
129. Heussel CP, Kauczor HU, Heussel GE, et al. Pneumonia in febrile neutropenic patients and bone marrow and blood stem-cell transplant recipients: use of high-resolution computed tomography. J Clin Oncol 1999; 17:796–805.
130. Barloon JT, Galvin JR, Mori M, et al. High-resolution ultradast chest CT in the management of febrile bone marrow transplant patients with normal or nonspecific chest roentgenograms. Chest 1991; 99: 928–933.
131. Franquet T, Muller NL, Gimenez A, Guembe P, Torre J, Bague S. Spectrum of pulmonary aspergillosis: histologic, clinical, and radiologic findings. Radiographics 2001; 21:825–837.
132. Groll AH, Walsh TJ. Uncommon opportunistic fungi: new nosocomial threats. Clin Microbiol Infect 2001; 7(suppl 2):8–24.
133. Safdar A, Papadopoulos EB, Young JW. Breakthrough *Scedosporium apiospermum* (*Pseudallescheria boydii*) brain abscess during therapy for invasive pulmonary aspergillosis following high-risk allogeneic hematopoietic stem cell transplantation. Scedosporiasis and recent advances in antifungal therapy. Transplant Infect Dis 2002; 4:212–217.
134. Safdar A. Progressive cutaneous hyalohyphomycosis due to *Paecilomyces lilacinus*: rapid response to treatment with caspofungin and itraconazole. Clin Infect Dis 2002; 34:1415–1417.
135. Fleming RV, Walsh TJ, Anaissie EJ. Emerging and less common fungal pathogens. Infect Dis Clin North Am 2002; 16:915–933.
136. Reiss E, Obayashi T, Orle K, Yoshida M, Zancope-Oliveira RM. Non-culture based diagnostic tests for mycotic infections. Med Mycol 2000; 38(supp 11): 47–59.
137. Yeo SF, Wong B. Current status of nonculture methods for diagnosis of invasive fungal infections. Clin Microbiol Rev 2002; 15:465–484.
138. Maertens J, Verhaegen J, Lagrou K, Van Eldere J, Boogaert M. Screening for circulating galactomanna as a noninvasive diagnostic tool for invasive aspergillosis in prolonged neutropenic patients and stem cell transplantation recipients: a prospective validation. Blood 2001; 97:1604–1610.
139. Becker MJ, Lugtenburg EJ, Cornelissen JJ, van der Schee C, Hoogsteden HC, de Marie S. Galactomanna detection in computerized tomography-based croncho-alveolar lavage fluid and serum in haematological patients at risk for invasive pulmonary aspergillosis. Br J Haematol 2003; 121:448–457.
140. Pryce TM, Kay ID, Palladino S, Heath CH. Real-time automated polymerase chain reaction (PCR) to detect *Candida albicans* and *Aspergillus fumigatus* DNA in whole blood from high-risk patients. Diag Microbiol Infect Dis 2003; 47:487–496.
141. Hebart H, Loffler J, Reitze H, et al. Prospective screening by a panfungal polymerase chain reaction assay in patients at risk for fungal infections: implications for the management of febrile neutropenia. Br J Haematol 2000; 111:635–640.
142. Walsh TJ, Finberg RW, Arndt C, et al. Liposomal amphotericin B for empirical therapy in patients with persistent fever and neutropenia. N Engl J Med 1999; 340:764–771.
143. Bates DW, Su L, Yu DT, et al. Mortality and costs of acute renal failure associated with amphotericin B therapy. Clin Infect Dis 2001; 32:686–693.
144. Wingard JR, White MH, Anaissie E, et al. A randomized, double-blind comparative trial evaluating the safety of liposomal amphotericic B versus amphotericin B lipid complex in the empirical treatment of febrile neutropenia. Clin Infect Dis 2000; 31: 1155–1163.
145. Herbrecht R, Denning DW, Patterson TF, et al. Voriconazole versus amphotericin B for primary therapy of invasive aspergillosis. N Engl J Med 2002; 347: 408–415.
146. Safdar A. *Curvularia*—favorable response to oral itraconazole therapy in patients with locally invasive phaeohyphomycosis. Clin Infect Dis 2003; 9: 1219–1223.
147. Greenberg RN, Anstead G, Herbrecht R, et al. Posaconazole (POS) experience in the treatment of zygomycosis. Proceedings of the 43rd Interscience Conference on Antimicrobial Agents and Chemotherapy (abstract M-1757), Chicago, Illinois, Sept 14–17, 2003.
148. Safdar A, Dommers MP, Talwani R, Thompson CR. Intracranial perineural extension of invasive mycosis: a novel mechanism of disease propogation by *Aspergillus fumigatus*. Clin Infect Dis 2002; 35:e50–e53.
149. Roilides E, Lamaignere CG, Farmaki E. Cytokines in immunodeficient patients with invasive fungal infections: an emerging therapy. Int J Infect Dis 2002; 6: 154–163.
150. Farmaki E, Roilides E. Immunotherapy in patients with systemic mycoses: a promising adjunct. Biodrugs 2001; 15:207–214.
151. Wheeler JH, Fishman EK. Computed tomography in the management of chest infections: current status. Clin Infect Dis 1996; 23:232–240.
152. Young LS, Armstrong D, Blevins A, Lieberman P. Nocardia asteroids infection complicating neoplastic diseases. Am J Med 1971; 50:356–367.
153. Torres HA, Reddy BT, Raad II, et al. Nocardiosis in cancer patients. Medicine 2002; 81:388–397.

154. Taplitz RA, Jordan MC. Pneumonia caused by herpesviruses in recipients of hematopoietic cell transplants. Semin Respir Infect 2002; 17:121–129.
155. Konoplev S, Champlin RE, Giralt S, et al. Cytomegalovirus pneumonia in adult autologous blood and marrow transplant recipients. Bone Marrow Transplant 2001; 27:877–881.
156. Champlin R, Whimbey E. Community respiratory virus infections in bone marrow transplant recipients: The M.D. Anderson Cancer Center experience. Biol Blood Marrow Transplant 2001; 7:8S–10S.
157. Bowden RA. Respiratory virus infections after marrow transplant: the Fred Hutchinson Cancer Research Center experience. Am J Med 1997; 102:27–30.
158. Safdar A, Bruorton M, Henslee-Downey JP, van Rhee F. Role of quantitative human cytomegalovirus PCR in predicting antiviral treatment response among high-risk hematopoietic stem cell transplant recipients. Bone Marrow Transplant 2004; 33:463–464.
159. Nichols WG, Corey L, Gooley T, et al. Rising pp65 antigenemia during preemptive anticytomegalovirus therapy after allogeneic hematopoietic stem cell transplantation: risk factors, correlation with DNA load, and outcome. Blood 2001; 97:867–874.
160. Humar A, Lipton J, Welsh S, Moussa G, Messner H, Mazzulli T. A randomized trial comparing cytomegalovirus antigenemia assay vs screening bronchoscopy for the early detection and prevention of disease in allogeneic bone marrow and peripheral blood stem cell transplant recipients. Bone Marrow Transplant 2001; 28:485–490.
161. Gluckman E, Traineau R, Devergie A, Esperou-Bourdeau H, Hirsh I. Prevention and treatment of CMV infection after allogeneic bone marrow transplant. Ann Hematol 1992; 64(suppl 1):158–161.
162. Vij R, Khoury H, Brown R, et al. Low-dose short-course intravenous ganciclovir as pre-emptive therapy for CMV viremia post allo-PBSC transplantation. Bone Marrow Transplant 2003; 32:703–707.
163. Sokos DR, Berger M, Lazarus HM. Intravenous immunoglobulin: appropriate indications and uses in hematopoietic stem cell transplantation. Biol Blood Marrow Transplant 2002; 8:117–130.
164. Klaesson S, Ringden O, Markling L, Remberger M, Lundkvist I. Immune modulatory effects of immunoglobulins on cell-mediated immune responses in vitro. Scand J Immunol 1993; 38:477–484.
165. Ljungman P, Engelhard D, Link H, et al. Treatment of interstitial pneumonitis due to cytomegalovirus with ganciclovir and intravenous immunoglobulin: experience of European Bone Marrow Transplant Group. Clin Infect Dis 1992; 14:831–835.

45

Critical Care Imaging in Oncology Patients

CHAAN S. NG, SANJAY SINGH, and MYLENE T. TRUONG
Department of Radiology, The University of Texas M.D. Anderson Cancer Center, Houston, Texas, U.S.A.

Imaging plays a vital role in the management of oncologic patients in critical care ranging from the apparently routine, such as evaluation of percutaneous catheters, to the detection of unexpected and untoward abnormalities. The pathologic conditions and complications which affect this particular group of patients are wide, encompassing not only those which any critically ill patient may face, but also include conditions which are more specific to the oncologic population, in particular, dissemination of malignancy, complex surgery, and immuno- and myelosuppression. Although focus is directed toward oncologic-related conditions, by necessity some more common general conditions are also reviewed. Imaging often helps in the management of critically ill patients by assisting in the frequently difficult decisions of what, if anything, can be done, and when, and indeed whether to act at all (1). Because of constraints of space, this chapter limits discussion to the thorax, abdominopelvic cavity, and central nervous system (CNS), and restricts imaging to radiography, ultrasound, computed tomography (CT), and magnetic resonance imaging (MRI). However, we present a fuller review of the role of, and findings in, the chest radiograph (CXR) in view of its extensive use and role in the intensive care unit (ICU) setting.

I. COMPARISON OF IMAGING MODALITIES

Imaging of critically ill patients presents particular challenges, and inevitably there are compromises. As far as possible, it is sensible to undertake as much imaging "at the bedside" as is feasible. It has been reported that up to 70% of patients experience significant physiologic changes during transportation from ICU (2). However, it should be appreciated that bedside examinations impose constraints on image quality. Some practical considerations and comparative features between plain radiography, ultrasound, CT, and MRI are presented below and in Table 1.

A. Plain Radiographs

The great advantage of plain radiography is that it is portable to the patient and images can be obtained relatively rapidly. The advent of digital, as compared to conventional, radiography has improved the rapidity and consistency of image acquisition, and allows the potential for postprocessing image manipulation and incorporation into PACS systems (3). The disadvantages of digital radiography include poorer spatial resolution and more grainy images. Interpretation of plain radiographs can be extremely challenging; limiting factors include the two dimensional nature

Table 1 Table of Comparative Strengths and Weaknesses of Radiography, Ultrasound, CT, and MRI in the Critical Care Setting

	Radiography	Ultrasound	CT	MRI
Portability to patient	Good	Good	No	No
Anatomic extent of coverage	Limited	Good	Excellent	Limited
Real-time assessment	No	Yes	No	No
Duration of test	Short	Intermediate	Short/intermediate	Long
Operator/interpretational	Variable	High	Limited	Limited
Multiplanar information	No	Excellent	Limited	Yes
Tissue contrast information	Very limited	Some	Good	Excellent
Vascular information	No	Excellent	Good	Good
Scope for guiding	No	Excellent	Good	No
Contraindications—general	None	None	Unstable patients	Unstable patients ferromagnetic implants (Claustrophobia)
Contraindications—specific	No	No	Yes (IV contrast allergy)	Limited (IV contrast allergy)
Cost	Low	Moderate	Moderate/high	High

of images, inability to separate overlapping structures, and simply the practical constraints in obtaining the images (such as unconscious patients, patient rotation, poor lung expansion, and difficulty in obtaining orthogonal, erect and decubitus views).

B. Ultrasound

Ultrasound, unlike other cross-sectional imaging techniques, is portable to the patient. It allows real-time evaluation, and can be used to guide interventions. Doppler ultrasound allows excellent assessment of vascular structures. In addition, no ionizing radiation is involved. However, it requires an adequate "acoustic window" both in terms of access on the body surface (for example, bandages and wound sites) and absence of sound absorbing structures, for example, bone, bowel gas, and subcutaneous fat, and arguably suffers from "operator" variability.

C. Computed Tomography

CT is an extremely powerful cross-sectional imaging technique, which is able to evaluate the critical organs in a matter of seconds or minutes, and can also be used to guide interventions. However, to date, there are no portable CT machines (4,5), and the risks of transporting the patient have to be weighed against the potential benefits. For example, one study has reported that only 55% of examinations aided or altered the prestudy diagnosis, and more than 79% were of no benefit to the ICU patient (6). Unlike many trauma centers, CT scanners are frequently remote from ICU patients. Most indications for CT require iodinated intravenous contrast medium for a satisfactory evaluation, especially for lesion detection and assessment of vascular structures. Consideration needs to be given to the nephrotoxicity of these agents, particularly in patients who might already have renal impairment or be on nephrotoxic therapies. For studies below the diaphragm, gastrointestinal contrast (oral and/or rectal barium or Gastrografin) is generally required to aid in the delineation of bowel from other structures. Rectal contrast should be avoided in patients with a bleeding diathesis.

D. Magnetic Resonance Imaging

MRI is another extremely powerful cross-sectional imaging technique, which has relative strengths and weaknesses compared to CT. It has superior tissue characterization and multiplanar capability compared to CT, which are particularly valuable in CNS conditions. However, image acquisition is considerably longer, and there are often constraints on patient accessibility, which is a particular limitation in the case of unstable patients. Care is required in ensuring that there are no contraindications to imaging the patient e.g., cardiac pacemakers and other metallic devices (for example, aneurysm clips or orbital foreign bodies), and that all monitoring and ancillary equipment is MRI compatible (7). MRI is generally inferior to CT in evaluating acute hemorrhage. In comparison to CT, MRI intravenous contrast media (Gadolinium chelates) have no significant nephrotoxicity.

II. THORACIC IMAGING

The principal imaging modality in the diagnosis and monitoring of patients in the critical care setting is the portable CXR. In addition to evaluating the position of monitoring and therapeutic devices, CXRs are essential in assessing changes in cardiopulmonary status such as atelectasis, pneumonia, and pulmonary edema, as well as complication from ventilatory support such as barotrauma.

There is, however, some debate about the efficacy of CXRs in the ICU. Some investigators have reported that only 3.4% of patients in the surgical ICU had new chest film findings that resulted in a significant impact on management (8). In contrast, it has been reported that 65% of all CXRs (admission, routine, and for specific indications) in medical and surgical ICUs showed moderate-to-marked cardiopulmonary abnormalities or malposition of tubes or lines (9). It has also been reported that 43–45% of routine CXRs in respiratory care and medical ICUs reveal clinically unsuspected findings of either a change in cardiopulmonary status or malposition of a line or tube (10,11). The efficacy of the "routine daily" CXR is also debated, with some suggestions, that they should be reserved for initial admission, specific clinical indications, intubated patients, patients with pulmonary or cardiac diseases, and after placement of an invasive device.

Thoracic CT has a superior sensitivity and specificity compared to chest radiography, and may be of benefit in patients whose clinical course is not explained by the available clinical and radiographic information, or whose CXRs are difficult to interpret. For example, it has been shown that in leukemic patients with febrile neutropenia, CT is able to detect the pulmonary nodules of invasive aspergillosis, with their characteristic "halo" of edema, before chest radiographic abnormalities are identified (12). Other indications for CT include evaluation for pulmonary embolism, and complex pleuropulmonary problems, such as lung abscesses, empyemas, bronchopleural fistulas, and mediastinal abnormalities.

A. Monitoring and Therapeutic Devices

1. Endotracheal and Tracheostomy Tubes

One of the major indications for imaging in the ICU is the assessment of monitoring and therapeutic devices and complications arising from their placement. Treatment for respiratory failure entails establishing an airway and placing the patient on ventilatory support. The tip of the endotracheal tube (ETT) should be 5 ± 2 cm from the carina. With flexion and extension of the neck, the tube can move approximately 2 cm upward or downward. An ETT placed less than 2 cm from the carina may extend into the right main bronchus with neck flexion and prevent adequate ventilation of the left lung (Fig. 1). Physical examination has been shown to be inaccurate in detecting (13,14). Due to the high frequency of malpositioning of the ETT, daily CXRs are recommended in intubated

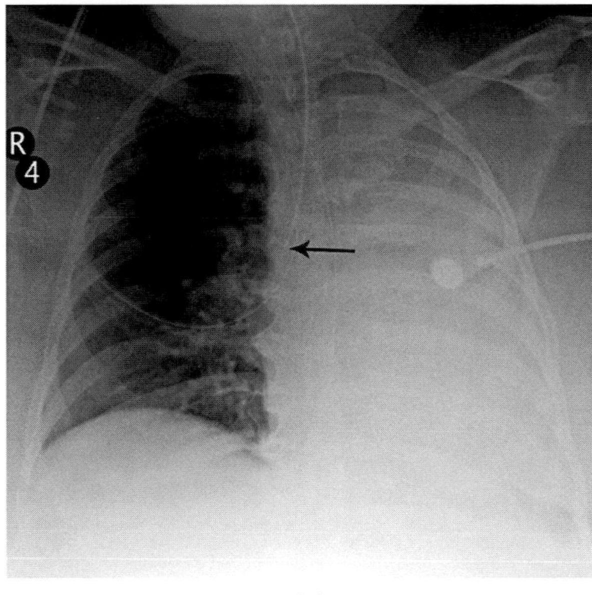

(a)

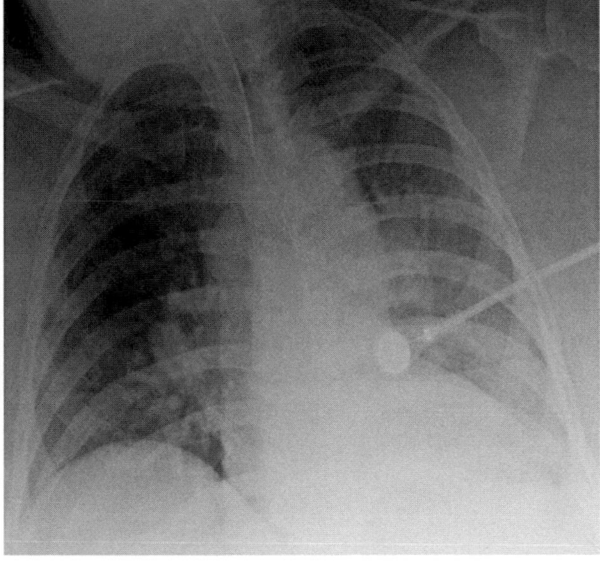
(b)

Figure 1 (a,b) An ETT in right main bronchus. 74-year-old woman with endometrial cancer. (a) CXR showing malposition of the ETT in the right main bronchus (*arrow*) preventing ventilation of the left lung. Atelectasis of the left lung is demonstrated by the opacity in the left hemithorax with shift of the heart and mediastinum to the left indicating volume loss. (b) Following repositioning the ETT, the left lung has re-expanded with the heart and mediastinum returning to normal position.

patients. To avoid long-term complications of the ETT, tracheostomy tubes are placed. The tip of the tracheostomy tube should be located one-half to two-thirds of the distance between the tracheal stoma and the carina at about the level of the T3 vertebra. The lumen of the tube should be about two-thirds of the tracheal diameter. Chest radiographs obtained after tracheostomy can assess for pneumomediastinum, subcutaneous emphysema, and pneumothorax.

2. Central Venous Pressure Monitors

In addition to ventilatory support, many ICU patients need monitoring of the circulatory blood volume. The catheters used for intravenous access may also be used for central venous pressure monitoring. In this case, the catheter tip should be located between the right atrium and the most proximal venous valves within the internal jugular and subclavian veins. These valves are approximately 2.5 cm from the point at which these veins join to form the brachiocephalic vein. The landmark for the last valve in the subclavian vein on a frontal CXR is the medial aspect of the anterior portion of the first rib. Complications of central line placement include pneumothorax, thrombus formation, venous perforation, mediastinal hematoma, and hemothorax (Figs. 2 and 3).

3. Chest Tubes

Chest tube tips should be placed cephalad and anterior within the pleural space, for treatment of pneumothoraces. For pleural fluid, chest tubes should be placed in the most dependent portion of the pleural space. Complications of chest tube insertion include inadvertent placement within the major fissure or lung, and placement of the catheter side-holes outside of the pleural space.

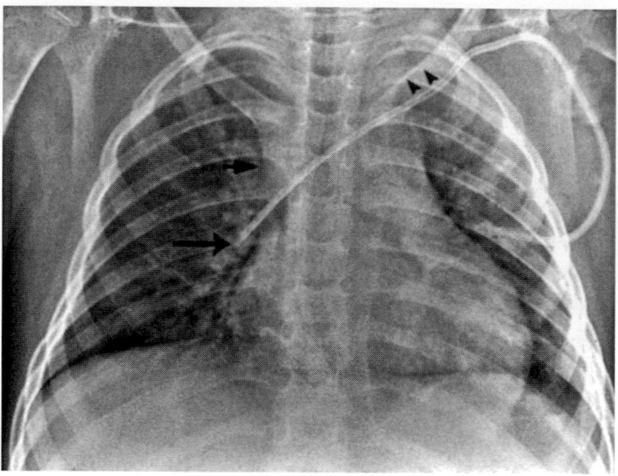

Figure 2 Superior vena cava (SVC) perforation. Five-year-old girl with aplastic anemia and graft-versus-host disease. The CXR showing the tip of a left subclavian catheter (*long arrow*) lying beyond the expected location of the SVC (*short arrow*). A left apical cap (*arrowheads*) suggests bleeding into the pleural space.

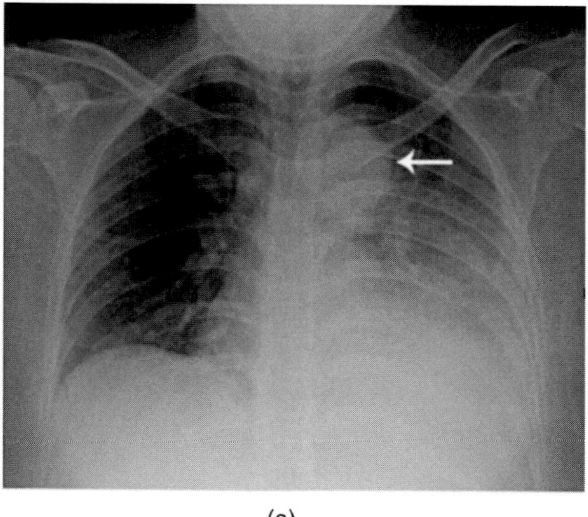

(a)

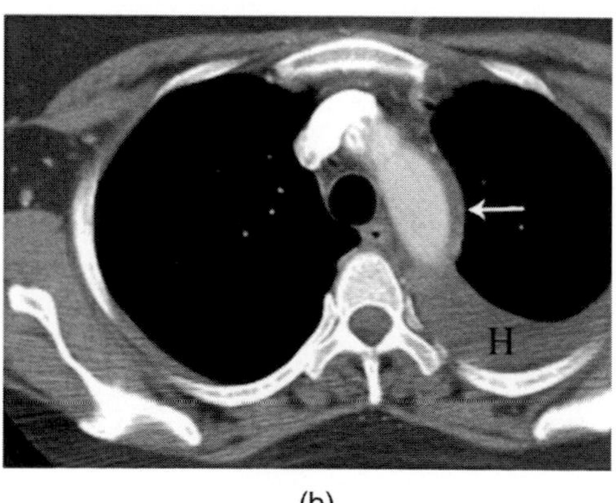

(b)

Figure 3 (a,b) Mediastinal hematoma following line placement. Forty-one-year-old woman with colon cancer and acute myelogenous leukemia. (a) The CXR following a failed central line attempt from a left subclavian approach. The aortic arch contour (*arrow*) is prominent and ill-defined suggesting a mediastinal hematoma. The hazy opacity in the left lower hemithorax is consistent with a left pleural effusion. (b) Chest CT confirms a mediastinal hematoma adjacent to the aortic arch (*arrow*) and left hemothorax (*H*) with an attenuation coefficient of 30 HU.

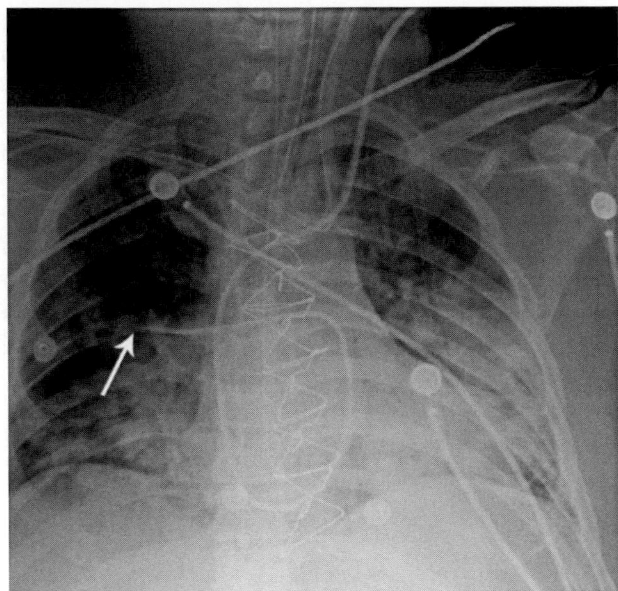

Figure 4 Swan-Ganz catheter malposition. Forty-three-year-old man with acute lymphocytic leukemia admitted to the ICU with respiratory distress and pneumonia. The CXR showing the Swan-Ganz catheter tip (*arrow*) located too far out distally and likely in a segmental branch of the right pulmonary artery.

4. *Pulmonary Capillary Wedge Pressure Monitors*

Pulmonary capillary wedge pressure (PCWP) is a more direct index of left atrial pressure than central venous pressure. These monitors aid in distinguishing cardiogenic and noncardiogenic pulmonary edema. The ideal location for the tip of the PCWP catheter is in the right, left or interlobar pulmonary arteries. The catheter can be floated into a "wedge" position with inflation of the associated balloon. A catheter tip in a more distal location increases the risk of pulmonary infarction and pulmonary arterial perforation (Fig. 4). Other complications include arrhythmia and knotting of the catheter.

5. *Intra-aortic Counterpulsation Balloon*

The intra-aortic counterpulsation balloon (IACB) was first used in the 1960s in the treatment of cardiogenic shock. The IACB inflates during diastole and deflates during systole. The rise in proximal aortic diastolic pressure increases blood flow and oxygen delivery via the coronary arteries to the myocardium, leading to improvement in cardiac function. The proximal tip of the catheter should be in the aorta just distal to the left subclavian artery origin but not so distal in the aorta as to have the inferior portion occlude the renal arteries.

6. *Transvenous Pacemakers*

The electrode lead of a transvenous pacemaker should be located with the distal tip in the apex of the right ventricle and should be directed inferiorly and toward the left. In the case of dual chamber pacemakers, the atrial lead should be deflected superiorly into the right atrial appendage. Complications include pneumothorax and malpositioning e.g., a lead within the coronary sinus. The latter can be recognized on a lateral radiograph by posterior, rather than anterior, orientation of the tip.

III. CARDIOPULMONARY DISORDERS

Common cardiopulmonary conditions seen in the ICU include atelectasis, aspiration, pneumonia, pulmonary edema, adult respiratory distress syndrome (ARDS), and barotrauma. Pulmonary embolism and drug toxicity are also important medical complications. Post operative complications include empyema, bronchopleural fistula and abscess formation in the mediastinum and lungs.

A. Atelectasis

Atelectasis is often associated with general anesthesia and is encountered most often after thoracic and abdominal surgery, particularly in patients with underlying lung disease, smokers, the obese, and the elderly. The incidence of atelectasis increases with prolonged anesthesia time (15–17). Atelectasis occurs most frequently in the left lower lobe (66%, Fig. 5), followed by the right lower lobe (22%), and the right upper lobe (11%) (18). Causes include mucus plugging, aspiration, splinting due to pain, ETT malposition, and pleural effusions. Radiographic signs include an opacity, which may be linear, platelike, patchy, or lobar in distribution. Signs of volume loss include displacement of a fissure or hilum, shift of the heart and mediastinum, elevation of the diaphragm, compensatory hyperinflation of an adjacent lobe or contralateral lung, and narrowing of the rib interspaces in the ipsilateral hemithorax (Fig. 6). The absence of air bronchograms in the area of consolidation suggests bronchial obstruction such as mucus plugging, which can be amenable to bronchoscopic clearing (19). With suctioning, atelectasis may clear in a matter of hours.

B. Aspiration

Aspiration can be associated with vomiting, nasotracheal intubation, tracheostomy, anesthesia, and CNS depression. Aspiration of gastric contents or oral

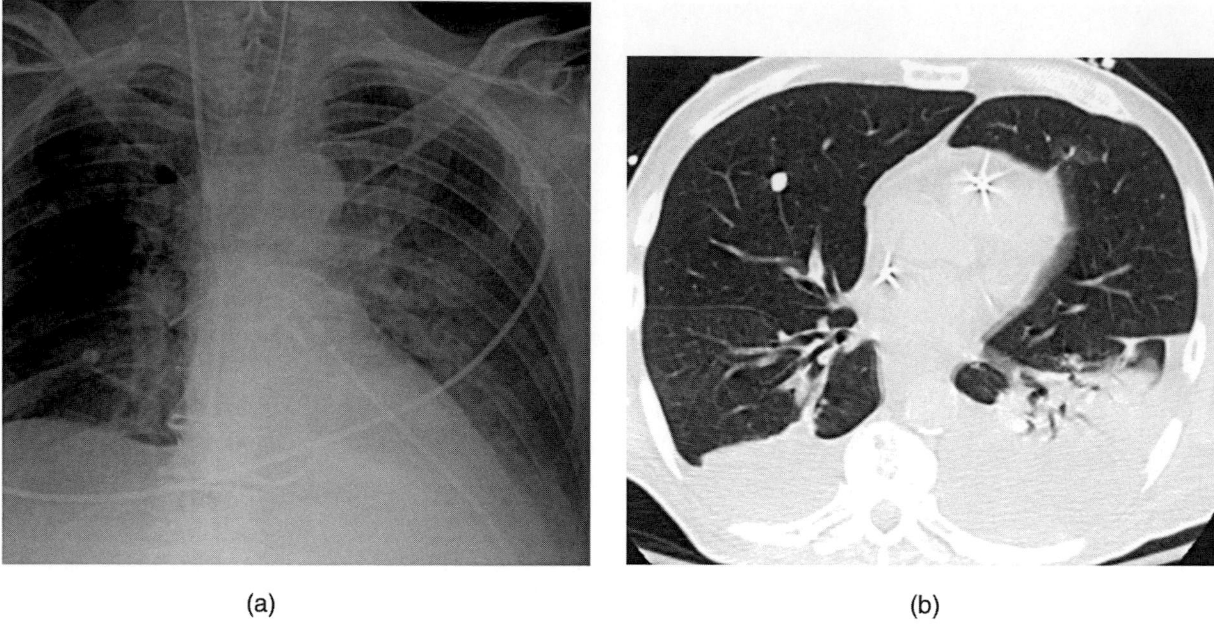

(a) (b)

Figure 5 (a,b) Left lower lobe collapse. Sixty-four-year-old man with esophageal cancer. (a) The CXR showing a dense left retrocardiac opacity consistent with atelectasis of the left lower lobe. (b) Chest CT confirms atelectasis due to compression from the pleural effusion.

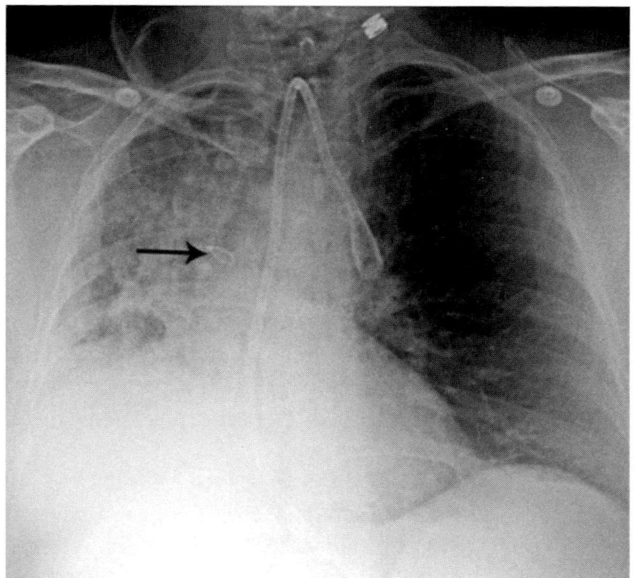

Figure 6 Aspiration of foreign body into right main bronchus. Fifty-nine-year-old woman with laryngeal cancer who aspirated her trachealesophageal prosthesis (*arrow*) into the right main bronchus causing airway obstruction. The CXR shows atelectasis of the right lung evidenced by opacity in the right hemithorax with signs of volume loss, demonstrated by elevation of the right hemidiaphragm and shift of the heart and mediastinum to the right. Emergent bronchoscopy was performed to remove the foreign body.

contrast material (particularly Gastrografin) may cause a chemical pneumonitis (Fig. 7). The distribution is usually in the superior or basilar segments of the lower lobes. Aspirated material usually clears within 1–3 days unless infection sets in.

C. Pneumonia

Findings of fever and leukocytosis together with new or progressive pulmonary opacities suggest pneumonia. However, these findings may not be reliable in immunocompromised patients or those on anti-inflammatory medications. The sensitivity for predicting pneumonia is only 60–64% and the specificity is 27–29% (20). Although typical patterns have been described, for example, lobar pneumonia and air bronchograms with pneumococcal pneumonia, consolidation associated with bulging pleural fissures with klebsiella pneumonia, and diffuse reticular pattern with bronchial wall thickening with viral pneumonia, radiographic patterns cannot reliably predict the causative organism. The time of onset of infection and the immune status of the patient may be useful: *Haemophilus influenzae* and *Streptococcus pneumoniae* pneumonias occur earlier in the ICU stay than methicillin resistant *Staphylococcus aureus* or Gram-negative pneumonias (21). In the oncologic setting, patients with acute myelogenous leukemia are susceptible to

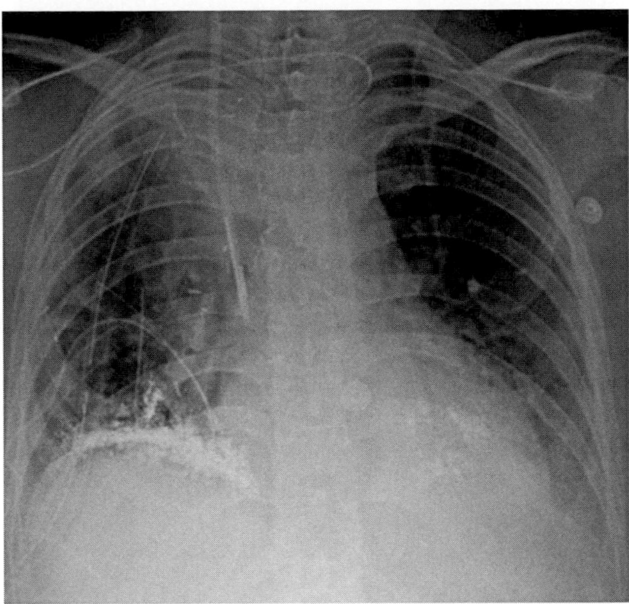

Figure 7 Aspiration of barium. Thiry-seven-year-old woman status post esophageal resection and repair of a tracheoesophageal fistula. The CXR showing aspirated barium in the bilateral lower lobes.

Aspergillus fumigatus infection particularly in the first month after bone marrow transplantation. The CT findings of angioinvasive aspergillosis include nodules surrounded by ground glass attenuation ("CT halo" sign), and during the phase of recovery of neutrophils, cavitation of the nodules ("air-crescent" sign) (Fig. 8) (22). Patients with indwelling catheters for chemotherapy are at risk for thrombosis, stenosis, and septic emboli. Radiographic findings of septic emboli include multiple peripheral nodules and patchy opacities, possibly with cavitation (Fig. 9).

D. Pulmonary Edema

Although pulmonary edema may be classified as cardiogenic or noncardiogenic, distinguishing the two entities may be difficult and a combination may exist in the same individual. Cardiogenic pulmonary edema is seen in patients with cardiac injury. Radiographic signs of this type of edema include cardiomegaly, redistribution, peribronchial cuffing, Kerley B lines, and pleural effusions. Noncardiogenic pulmonary edema is associated with many conditions, including in the ICU setting, uremia, aspiration, sepsis, fluid overload, neurogenic disorders, and allergic or drug reactions. Radiographically, noncardiogenic pulmonary edema is not associated with cardiomegaly, redistribution, or pleural effusions (Fig. 10).

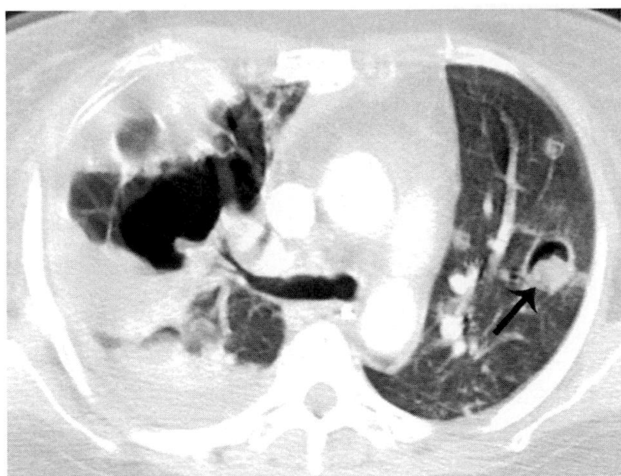

Figure 8 Invasive aspergillosis. Forty-nine-year-old woman with myelodysplastic syndrome and angioinvasive aspergillosis infection. Chest CT showing a left upper lobe cavitary nodule, with an "air-crescent" sign (*arrow*), and a large right lung abscess. In contrast to empyemas, lung abscesses are round, form acute angles with the interface of the chest wall, and have irregularly thickened walls.

E. Drug Toxicity

Drug-induced lung injury can be caused by numerous cytotoxic and noncytotoxic drugs. The time interval between the initiation of drug therapy and the onset of symptoms can be months to years. The diagnosis is frequently only suggested after infection, radiation injury, or recurrence of underlying disease have been

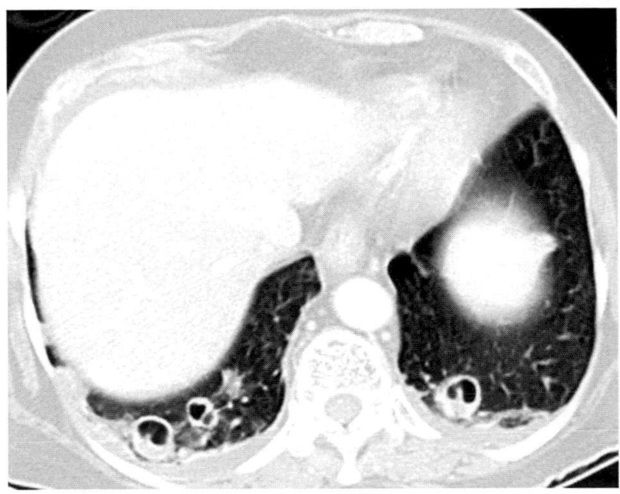

Figure 9 Septic emboli. Sixty-seven-year-old woman with CNS lymphoma. Chest CT showing multiple small peripheral cavitary lesions consistent with septic emboli from an infected indwelling central venous catheter.

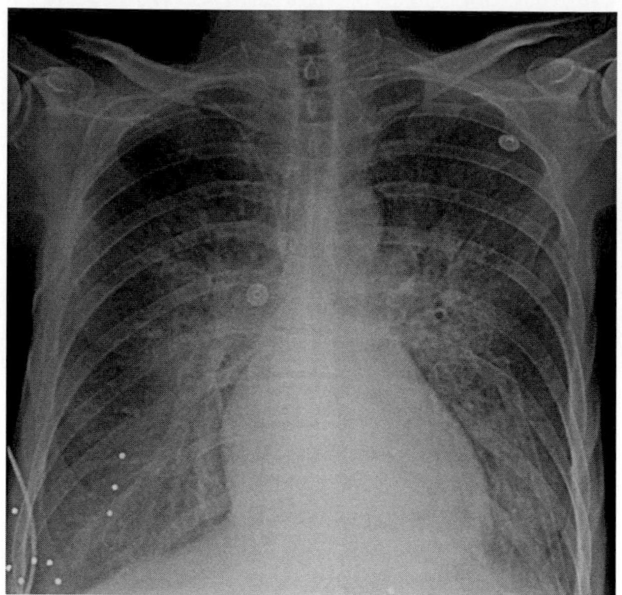

Figure 10 Noncardiogenic pulmonary edema. Fifty-nine-year-old man with mantle cell lymphoma treated with Ara-C. The CXR showing signs of noncardiogenic pulmonary edema. Note the normal heart size.

excluded. The most common patterns of drug-induced lung injury include noncardiogenic pulmonary edema, diffuse alveolar damage (DAD), nonspecific interstitial pneumonia (NSIP), bronchiolitis obliterans with organizing pneumonia (BOOP), eosinophilic pneumonia, and pulmonary hemorrhage (23). Chemotherapy-induced noncardiogenic pulmonary edema has been reported, not only most commonly with cytosine arabinoside (Ara-C) but also occurs with methotrexate, cyclophosphamide, vinblastine, and mitomycin (24). Noncardiogenic pulmonary edema and DAD can present as interstitial edema and can progress to an alveolar pattern in the exudative phase (Fig. 11). In the reparative phase, fibrosis and honeycombing may occur but can be reversible. The NSIP typically presents as basilar heterogeneous patchy opacities. The BOOP manifests as peripheral ground glass opacities and scattered areas of consolidation with bronchiectasis with an equal distribution to the upper and lower lobes. Eosinophilic pneumonia presents as peripheral areas of ground glass opacities and consolidation in an upper lobe distribution.

F. Adult Respiratory Distress Syndrome

Adult respiratory distress syndrome is a phrase used to describe a form of noncardiogenic pulmonary edema characterized by hypoxemia, diffuse pulmonary opacities, and reduced lung compliance. It may be associated with many conditions, including in the ICU setting, shock, sepsis, disseminated intravascular coagulation, and pancreatitis. Initially, the CXR is normal. Within the next 24–36 hr, interstitial

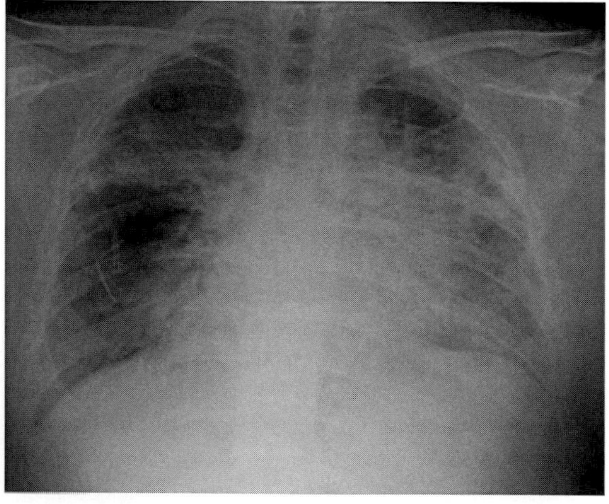

(a)

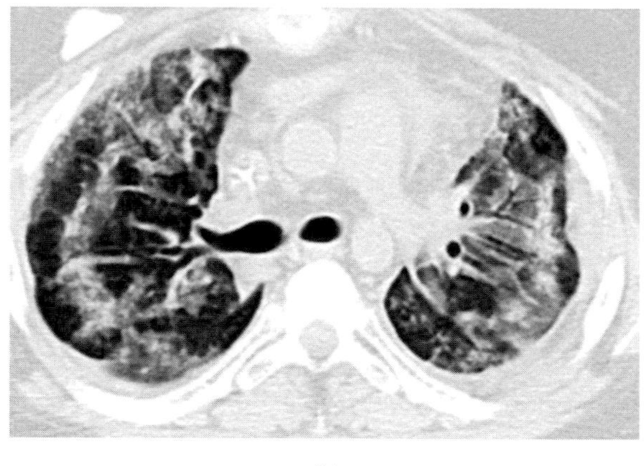

(b)

Figure 11 (a,b) Drug toxicity. Sixteen-year-old girl with Hodgkin's disease treated with chemotherapy and radiation. (a) The CXR showing radiation fibrosis in the paramediastinal portions of the lungs forming a characteristic geographic border. However, outside of the radiation port, patchy opacities are noted in both the upper and lower lobe distribution (b) Chest CT confirms the scattered foci of ground glass opacities and patchy consolidation. The differential diagnoses include infection, parenchymal lymphoma, and drug toxicity. Pathology at bronchoscopic biopsy revealed reactive bronchial epithelium consistent with therapy effect. No malignant cells or organisms were isolated.

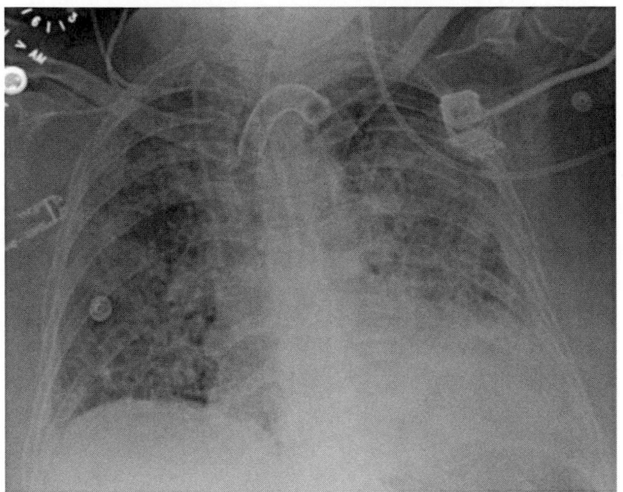

Figure 12 ARDS. Forty-five-year-old man with nonsmall cell lung cancer status post left upper lobectomy, and aspiration following tracheostomy. The CXR showing diffuse bilateral airspace disease consistent with ARDS.

pulmonary edema becomes evident. Over the next 24–48 hr, there is further worsening of oxygen saturation and more confluent diffuse bilateral air space opacities (Fig. 12). This pattern typically remains unchanged for days, unless complicated by barotrauma or infection.

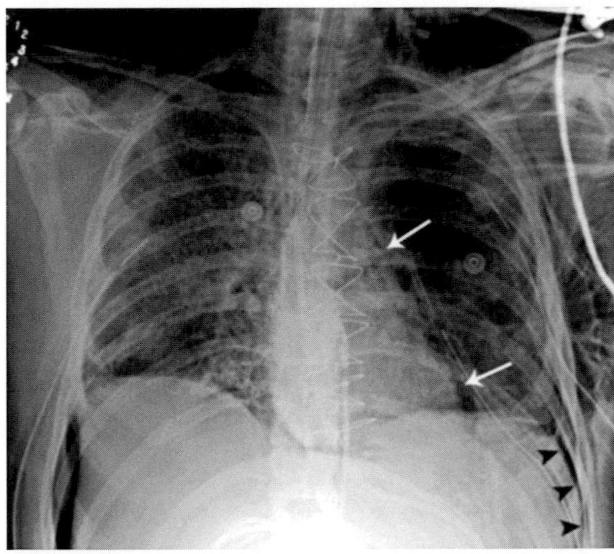

Figure 13 Barotrauma, with deep sulcus sign. Twenty-three-year-old man with nonseminomatous germ cell tumor with barotrauma. The CXR showing the "deep sulcus sign" (*black arrowheads*), indicating a left basal pneumothorax. Associated pneumomediastinum, indicated by streaks of air adjacent to the left heart border (*white arrows*). Extensive subcutaneous emphysema in the left side of the neck and chest is present. The patient is status post retroperitoneal lymph node dissection and partial resection of the inferior vena cava with air collection adjacent to the right lobe of the liver.

G. Abnormal Pleural Gas Collections

Barotrauma is a complication of mechanical ventilation, particularly in patients receiving positive end-expiratory pressure (PEEP). The spectrum of barotrauma includes interstitial pulmonary emphysema, pneumothorax, pneumomediastinum, and subcutaneous emphysema. Interstitial pulmonary emphysema presents as lucent streaks radiating from the hila to the periphery of the lungs. Subpleural blebs may rupture into the pleural space producing a pneumothorax. In recumbent patients, pleural air is located in an anteromedial or subpulmonic location; the thin white line of the visceral pleura may not be discernible. Increased lucency of the diaphragm, cardiac border, and lateral costophrenic sulcus ("deep sulcus" sign) may be the only clues (Fig. 13). Skin folds and bandages or sheets may mimic pneumothorax. When pneumothorax is suspected, evaluation with upright expiratory, decubitus (affected side in the nondependent position), or cross table lateral radiographs may be helpful.

The combination of a pneumothorax and mediastinal shift is radiographic evidence of a tension pneumothorax. Other radiographic signs of tension include depression of the hemidiaphragm, which is a reliable sign (Fig. 14), and flattening of the cardiac border and other vascular structures such as the SVC and IVC, reflecting impaired venous return, which is a specific sign (25). However, it is important to recognize that tension can be present in the absence of the above radiographic signs, for example, mediastinal shift may not occur in the context of ventilating noncompliant lungs, as in ARDS. In these circumstances, clinical suspicion is paramount.

Pneumomediastinum may be due to barotrauma, rupture of an airway or esophagus, dissection of air from the retroperitoneum following bowel perforation, or extension from the soft tissues of the neck due to pharyngeal or facial injuries. Air in the mediastinum may be seen in the postoperative period, following invasive procedures such as mediastinoscopy, endoscopic, or bronchoscopic biopsy. Radiographically, pneumomediastinum may be seen as lucent linear streaks outlining mediastinal structures. Air below the heart forms the "continuous diaphragm sign" of pneumomediastinum (Fig. 15). Subcutaneous emphysema may serve as an indicator of barotrauma, chest tube

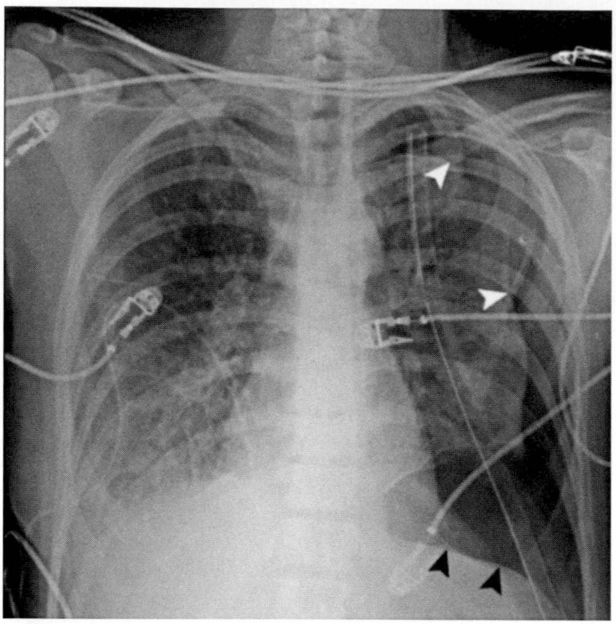

Figure 14 Pneumothorax left basal tension. Thirty-two-year-old woman with breast cancer status post pleurodesis. The CXR showing a moderate-to-large left pneumothorax under tension, evidenced by depression of the left hemidiaphragm (*black arrowheads*), and flattening of the left heart border. The visceral pleural line can be appreciated (*white arrowheads*).

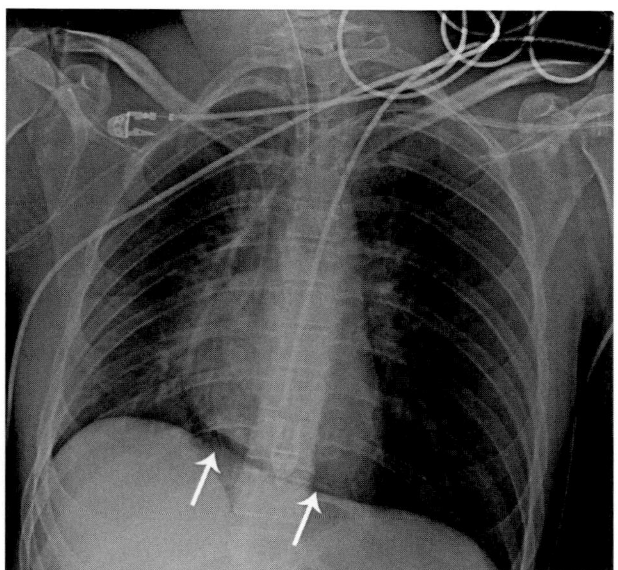

Figure 15 Pneumomediastinum, with continuous diaphragm sign. Eleven-year-old boy with Peutz–Jegers syndrome with evidence of barotrauma. The CXR showing pneumomediastinum evidenced by air outlining the base of the heart, forming the "continuous diaphragm sign" (*arrows*).

malfunction, airway, or esophageal injury during intubation. When severe, subcutaneous emphysema may obscure underlying disease in the lungs and pleural space.

H. Abnormal Pleural Fluid Collections

The most common pleural abnormality in the ICU is pleural effusion. Pleural effusions are seen in 60% of patients following upper abdominal operations (17). Pleural effusions can be associated with congestive heart failure, pneumonia, ARDS, pulmonary embolism, and pancreatitis. Radiographically, pleural fluid may present as a hazy homogeneous opacity in the lower thorax with loss of definition of the diaphragm, blunting of the costophrenic sulcus, an apical cap, or apparent elevation of the diaphragm (as in the case of subpulmonic fluid). The CT may help in determining the nature of the pleural fluid, attenuation coefficients of 0–20 Hounsfield Units (HU) suggest a transudate or exudate, whereas 25–60 HU may indicate hemorrhage. Other pleural abnormalities seen in the postoperative period, including empyema and bronchopleural fistula, are better assessed on CT.

I. Pulmonary Embolism

Chest radiographic findings of pulmonary embolic (PE) disease may include peripheral wedge-shaped pleural-based opacities indicating pulmonary infarction (Hampton's hump), atelectasis, pleural effusion, and focal oligemia (Westermark's sign). Since the sensitivity, specificity, and accuracy of CXRs for detection of PE are low, other modalities are routinely employed. Noninvasive ultrasound of the lower extremities has been used to diagnose deep venous thrombosis. Radionuclide ventilation/perfusion scanning has limitations in the presence of pulmonary and pleural disease, with a propensity for yielding indeterminate results, and is cumbersome in the ICU setting. Dynamic contrast-enhanced helical CT has emerged as the modality of choice in the detection of thrombi in the proximal pulmonary arteries out to the fourth order branches (26) (Fig. 16).

J. Empyema and Lung Abscess

CT can distinguish lung abscess from empyema. Lung abscesses are round, irregularly thick walled, form acute angles with the chest wall and do not compress the adjacent lung. Empyemas are lenticular in shape, have uniformly enhancing smooth thickened walls, form obtuse angles with the chest wall, compress

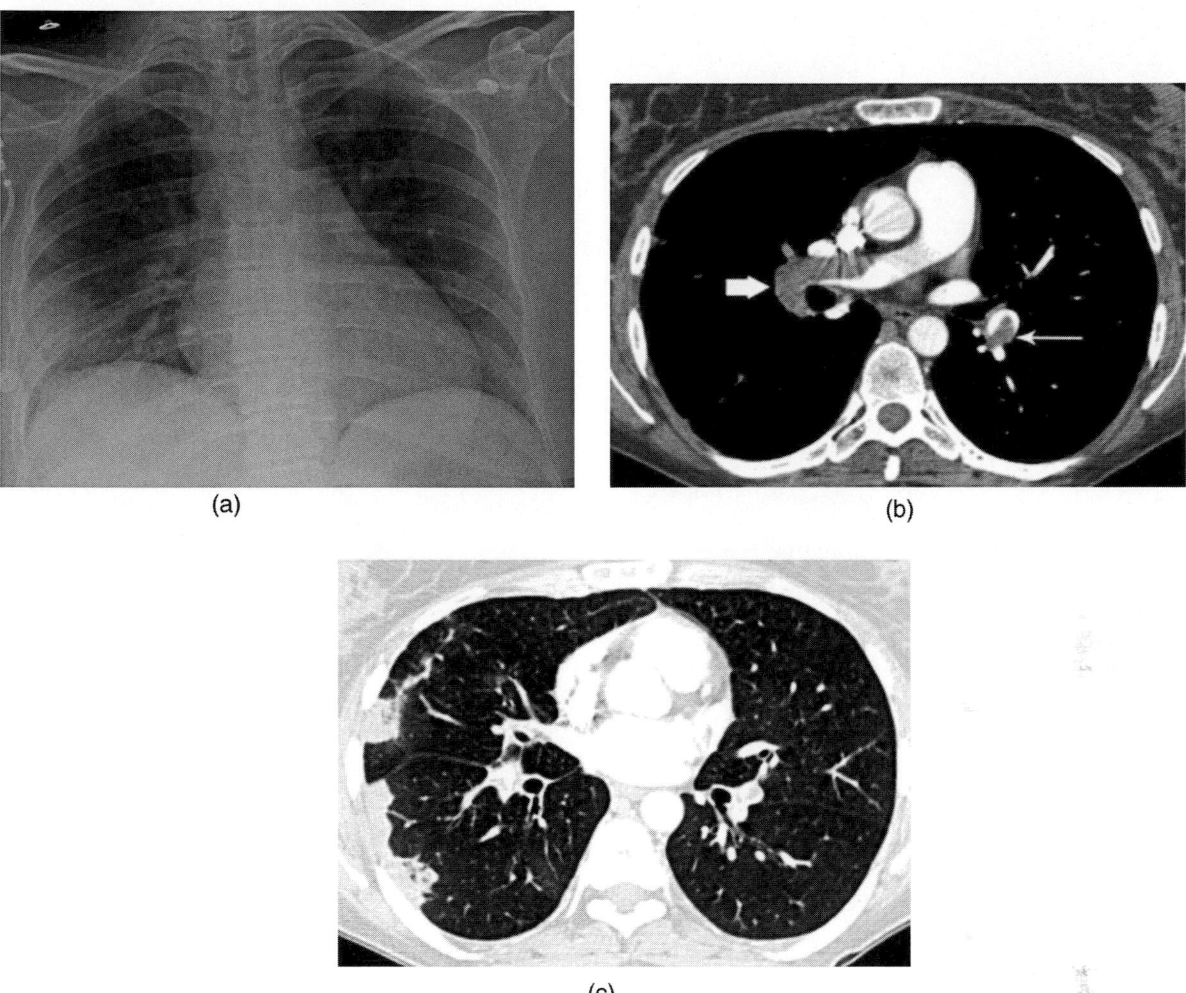

(a) (b) (c)

Figure 16 (a–c) Pulmonary embolism, with right lower lobe infarct. Thirty-four-year-old woman with acute lymphocytic leukemia. (a) The CXR showing a peripheral right lower lobe opacity abutting the pleura. (b) Dynamic contrast-enhanced helical chest CT demonstrates thrombus in the right pulmonary artery with extension into the right upper lobe and right interlobar pulmonary artery (*short arrow*). Nonocclusive thrombus is also seen in the left interlobar pulmonary artery (*long arrow*). (c) Chest CT with parenchymal lung windows showing areas of pulmonary infarction in the periphery of the right lower lobe.

the adjacent lung, and have separated visceral and parietal pleural surfaces (the "split pleura" sign) (27) (Fig. 17).

K. Bronchopleural Fistula

Although bronchopleural fistulae may occur as a complication of empyema draining spontaneously into the lung, a number of cases are seen after lung resection. Postsurgical fistulas occur with a frequency of 3%, and usually develop within 2 weeks of surgery (28). A bronchopleural fistula should be suspected with the postoperative development of fever, hemoptysis, cough, and a persistent large air leak in the presence of pleural drains. CT can be used to demonstrate anatomic detail of the communication between the bronchus and the pleural space (Figs. 18 and 19).

L. Mediastinal Abnormalities

CT can aid in the evaluation of mediastinal abnormalities such as mediastinal abscess and mediastinal hemorrhage (Fig. 20). Mediastinitis may present with infiltration and haziness of the mediastinal fat, fluid collection, small air bubbles, air–fluid levels, and pericardial thickening. It may be difficult to distinguish mediastinitis from the early, noninfected, and postoperative mediastinum. In the appropriate clinical setting, CT may guide the therapeutic drainage of abscesses.

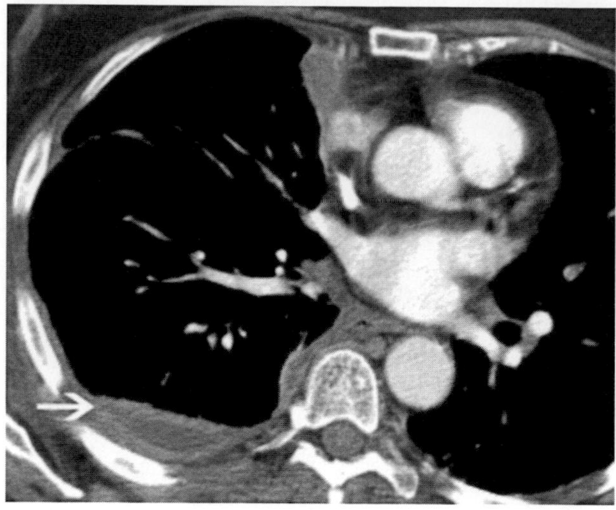

Figure 17 Empyema. Seventy-year-old woman status post-right upper lobectomy for nonsmall cell lung cancer who developed pneumonia and empyema from methicillin resistant *S. aureus* in the postoperative period. Chest CT showing enhancing, thickened visceral, and parietal layers of the pleura separated by a small amount of fluid, the "split pleura sign" (*arrow*).

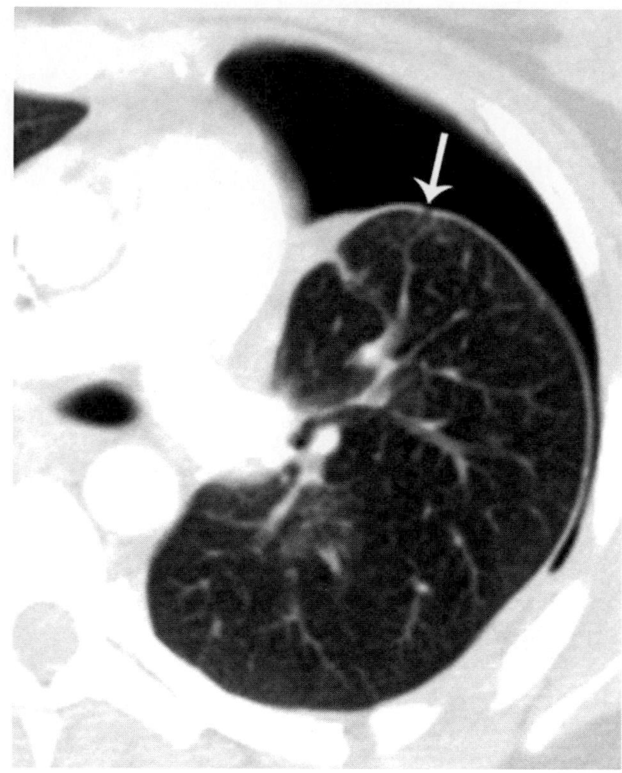

Figure 18 Bronchopleural fistula. Twenty-four-year-old woman with epithelioid sarcoma of the left anterior calf 3 weeks post wedge resection of the left lower lobe with persistent air leak due to bronchopleural fistula. Chest CT showing communication between a dilated bronchiole in the periphery of the left lower lobe and the left pleural space (*arrow*).

IV. ABDOMINOPELVIC DISORDERS

Common abdominal conditions that lead to admission to, or are seen in, ICU patients include bowel perforation and peritonitis, intestinal obstruction, collections, and solid organ disorders. The latter may be associated with sepsis or organ failure, for example, hepatic and renal dysfunction. Although relatively uncommon, oncologic patients are also prone to inflammatory conditions affecting the bowel.

A. Bowel Perforation and Peritonitis

Bowel perforation can be a challenging diagnosis in the critical care setting. A proportion may occur in a "silent" manner, particularly in patients on steroids. Perforations have also been described in docetaxel-based therapy (29).

The classical radiological investigations of an erect chest radiography, and abdominal series including decubitus films are frequently impractical in the critical care setting. The supine abdominal radiographic signs of free intraperitoneal gas are frequently subtle, and they include central abdominal lucency (the "football" sign) and unusual clarity of the bowel wall (Rigler's sign). CT has a much higher sensitivity for the detection of free intraperitonal air (Fig. 21). On a practical point, gastrointestinal contrast administered for the purposes of the CT may escape into the abdominal cavity, and therefore when a perforation is suspected, Gastrografin, and not barium, should be utilized.

In the context of patients in critical care, intraperitoneal free gas may not necessarily indicate a perforation; it may be related to recent surgery or intervention, and clinical details are essential for interpretation.

B. Intra-abdominal Collections

Intra-abdominal collections may be free (ascites) (Fig. 22) or loculated. They may consist of serous fluid (seroma), lymphatic fluid (lymphocele), blood (hemoperitoneum) or blood products (hematoma), pus (abscess), or malignant cells. Distinguishing between these, radiologically can be difficult, and may require diagnostic aspiration. Abscesses following surgery are not uncommon, particularly following the not infrequent major and complex surgery undertaken in oncologic patients that necessitates admission to the critical care unit (Fig. 23).

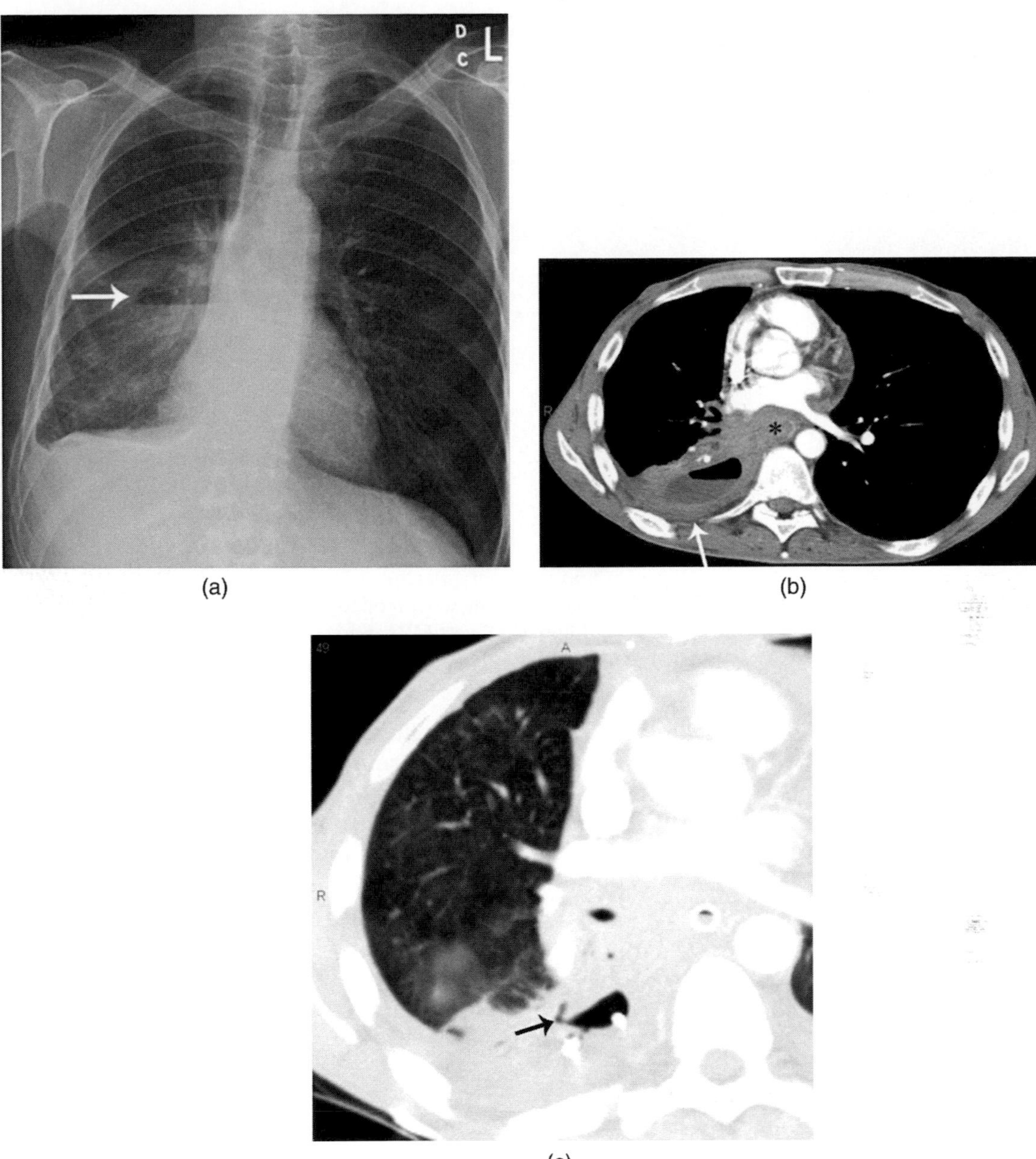

Figure 19 (a–c) Bronchopleural fistula. Forty-eight-year-old man with esophageal cancer within the stent invading the mediastinum and right lower lobe of the lung treated with radiation. (a) The CXR shows an air–fluid level in the right hemithorax located either in the lung or pleural space. (b) Chest CT localizes the air–fluid level in the right pleural space. The collection is lenticular in shape, with enhancing uniformly thickened pleura (*arrow*), and compression of the adjacent lung, consistent with empyema. Esophageal cancer (*asterisk*). (c) Chest CT with lung windows demonstrates anatomic detail of the bronchopleural fistula (*arrow*), namely direct communication between a bronchus in the peripheral aspect of the right lower lobe and the right pleural space.

Plain radiographs have little role in the detection of intra-abdominal abscesses. Ultrasound is reasonably sensitive at detecting ascites (Fig. 22) and may be able to identify large collections, but has a lower sensitivity than CT. Ultrasound is also able to identify pleural collections (Fig. 24). From a practical point of view, the accuracy of CT in detecting intra-abdominal collections is improved with intravenous contrast medium, and generous use of gastrointestinal contrast (Gastrografin or barium) administered orally and rectally.

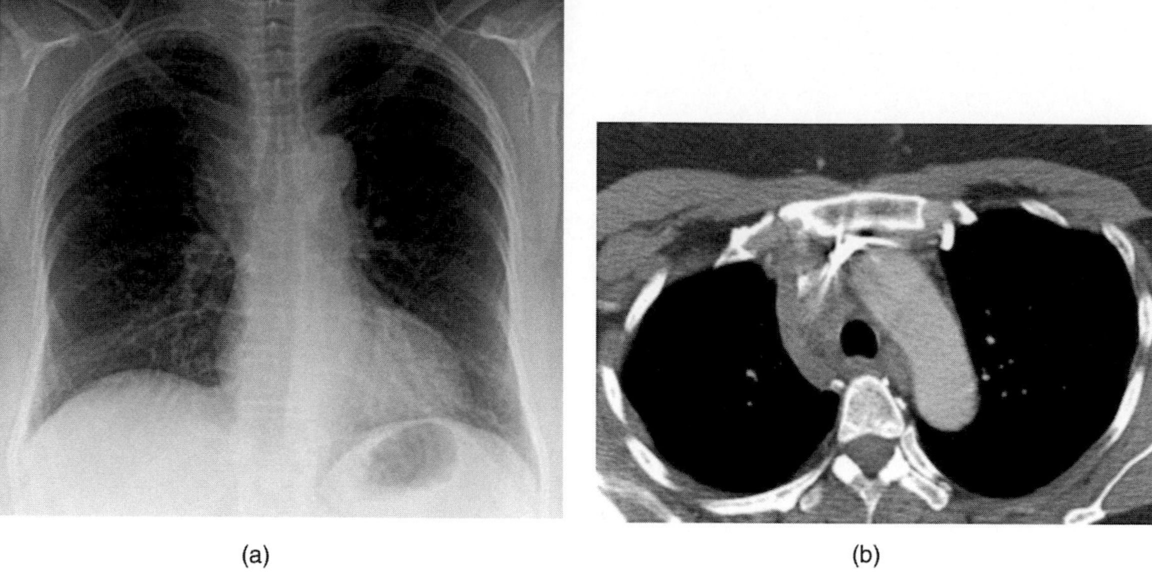

Figure 20 (a,b) Mediastinal hematoma. Fifty-seven-year-old woman with breast cancer following failed right subclavian catheter insertion. (a) The CXR showing a widened mediastinum. (b) Chest CT confirms a right paratracheal structure, with attenuation coefficient of 60 HU, consistent with a hematoma.

Evaluation for collections should include examination of both the abdomen and pelvis. The presence of gas within the collection(s) may be due to perforation, gas-forming organisms, or recent surgery, and careful clinical correlation is required.

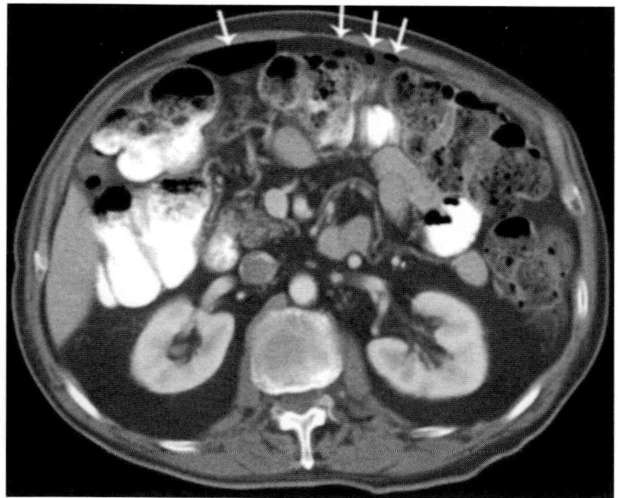

Figure 21 Intraperitoneal perforation. Sixty-eight-year-old male with spinal cord compression from metastatic prostate cancer, on high dose steroids. No acute abdominal symptoms or signs at the time of this staging abdominal CT, which shows free intraperitoneal gas (*arrows*). Surgery showed a perforated gastric ulcer.

C. Intestinal Obstruction, Intestinal Ileus, Pseudo-Obstruction

These conditions lead to abdominal distension, pain, nausea, vomiting, and constipation, and are not infrequently associated with a postsurgical status. The radiological feature common to these conditions is bowel distension, but distinguishing between them can be difficult. Generally, small bowel is considered to be dilated if the diameter is greater than 3.0 cm (Fig. 25); and large bowel, if greater than 5 cm. A transverse colonic diameter of greater than 6 cm, and a cecal diameter of greater than 9 cm, is generally considered to represent a risk for perforation (30). Classical plain radiographic signs on erect and decubitus firms include the "string of beads" sign, and multiple gas–fluid levels.

Of note, the absence of gas within the bowel lumen prevents plain film evaluation of bowel diameter. Although nonspecific, it is frequently a sign of bowel dysfunction (Fig. 26). CT has greater sensitivity and specificity than plain radiographs in the diagnosis of intestinal obstruction, in identifying the level of obstruction, and in identifying the cause, for example, adhesions, tumor, or intussusception (31–33).

Fecal impaction, which may be related to opiate administration, is one cause of large bowel obstruction in cancer patients. In comparison, pseudo-obstruction (Ogilvie's syndrome, or colonic ileus) is characterized by large bowel dilatation without a mechanical obstruction. The pathophysiologic cause is unknown, but

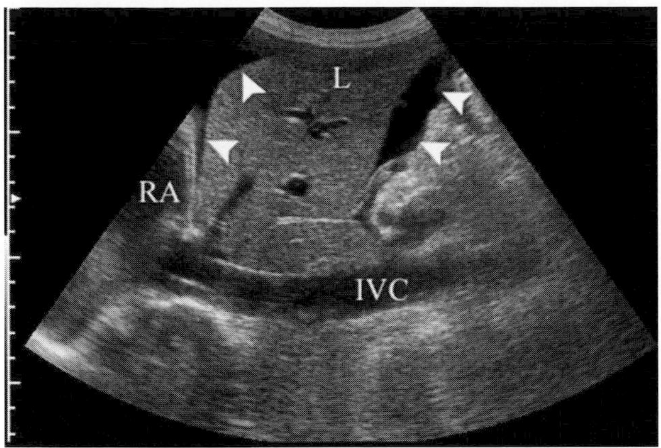

Figure 22 Ascites. Fifty-two-year-old man with primary amyloidosis, following bone marrow transplant. Midline sagittal abdominal ultrasound showing ascites around the liver (*arrows*). L, left lobe of liver; RA, right atrium; IVC, inferior vena cava.

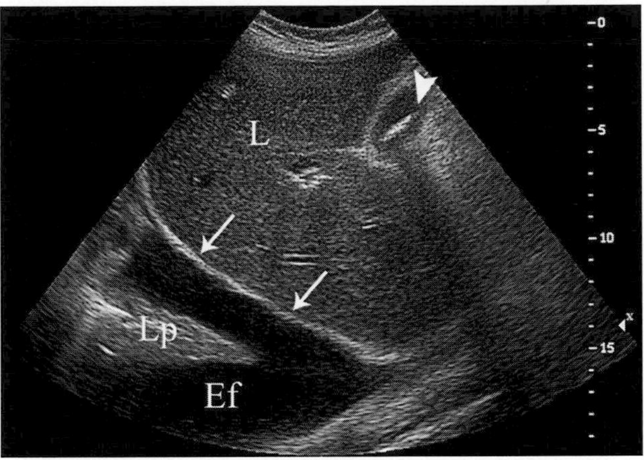

Figure 24 Pleural collection. Fifty-one-year-old woman with acute myeloid leukemia and abnormal liver function tests. Abdominal ultrasound of the right upper quadrant showing a right pleural collection (*Ef*). Diaphragm (*arrows*). Incidental calculus in the gallbladder (*arrowhead*). L, liver; Lp, atelectatic lung parenchyma.

is possibly related to an imbalance between sympathetic and parasympathetic colonic innervation (34). Ogilvie's syndrome is associated with postoperative patients. Colonoscopically placed tube decompression may be effective (35,36).

D. Neutropenic Enterocolitis (Typhlitis), Pseudomembranous Colitis, and Appendicitis

Neutropenic colitis (typhlitis) is typically associated, but not exclusively, with chemotherapy. The exact etiology is unclear, but is thought to be associated with mucosal breakdown due to inability to repair, and subsequent invasion by bacteria, and rapid progression to ischemia (37). The condition typically causes right-sided abdominal pain and diarrhea. It can be a difficult clinical diagnosis; CT is able to make a definite contribution by identifying colonic wall thickening, which is typically right-sided (Fig. 27). It is generally considered that the condition should be treated conservatively as far as possible (38).

Pseudomembranous colitis is caused by *Clostridium difficile* toxin, and is associated with antibiotic therapy.

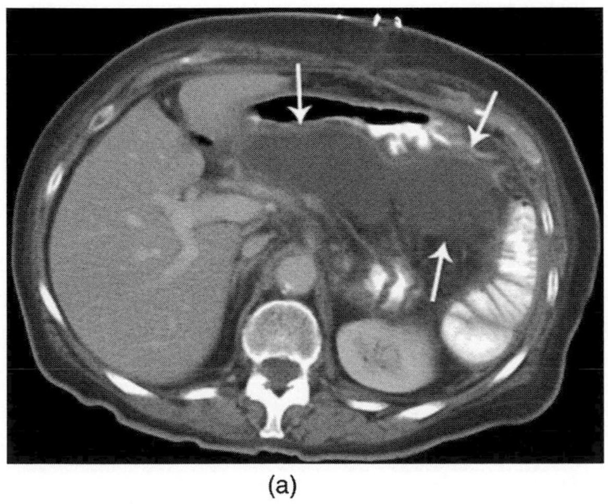
(a)

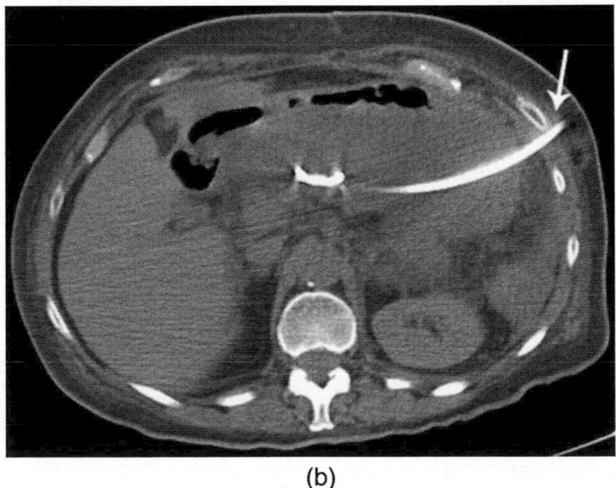
(b)

Figure 23 (a,b) Abscess collection, with percutaneous drainage. Sixty-six-year-old woman with left upper quadrant pain 2 weeks following a distal pancreatectomy and splenectomy for pancreatic carcinoma. (a) Abdominal CT showing an intra-abdominal collection (*arrows*). (b) CT following image guided percutaneous insertion of a catheter (*arrows*), which drained pus.

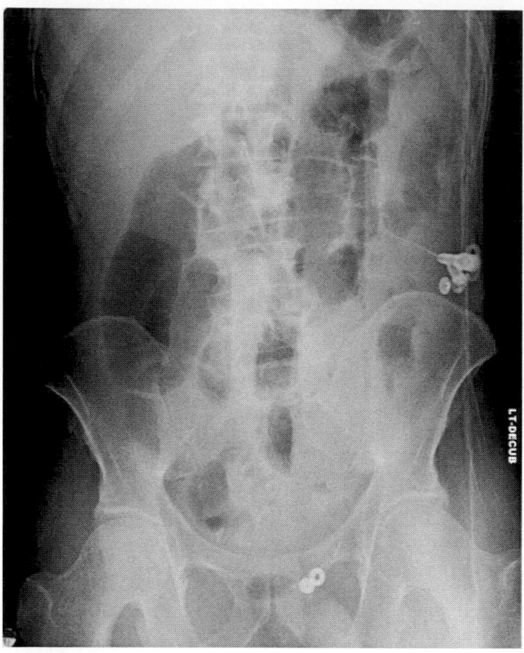

Figure 25 Small bowel obstruction. Sixty-three-year-old male with esophageal carcinoma, status post gastric pull up. Supine abdominal radiograph showing multiple dilated loops of small bowel.

Although the diagnosis is usually made by stool culture and/or the presence of pseudomembranes on endoscopy, the symptoms and signs can sometimes be entirely nonspecific (31); CT is able to suggest the diagnosis by identifying diffuse colonic wall thickening, frequently with a "target" and/or "accordion" sign (39) (Fig. 28).

Appendicitis can present with similar symptoms to typhlitis, both being predominantly right lower quadrant conditions (40). CT is highly accurate in detecting appendicitis (41).

E. Visceral Organ Disease

The liver, spleen, pancreas, and gallbladder can be evaluated at the bedside by ultrasound, which is an excellent screening modality for these organs.

The development of abnormal liver function tests in critically ill patients is not uncommon. Ultrasound is able to evaluate the biliary tree; in particular, biliary obstruction is effectively excluded in the absence of biliary dilatation (identifying the cause of obstruction, however can be more challenging) (Fig. 29). Ultrasound is also able to evaluate for focal liver lesions, such as metastases and abscesses. Parenchymal liver

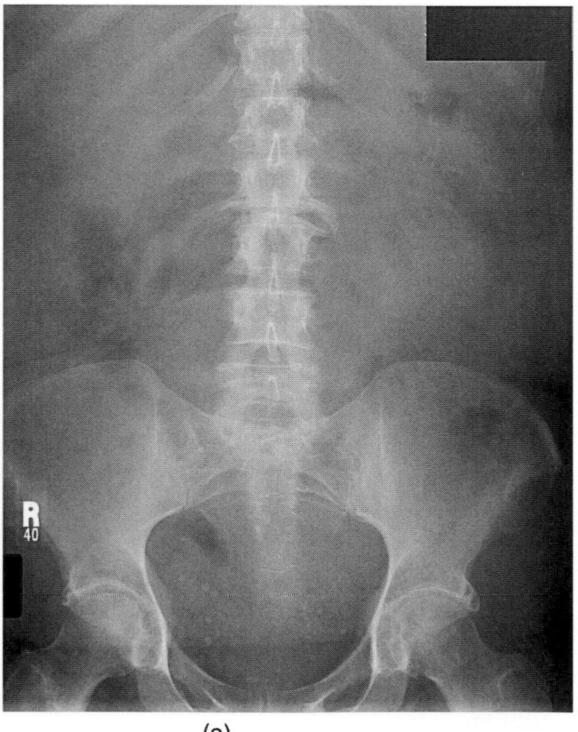

(a)

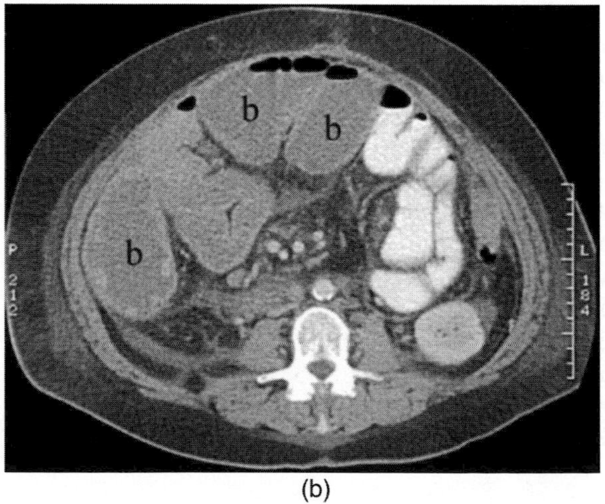

(b)

Figure 26 (a,b) Intestinal obstruction, inapparent on abdominal radiograph. Sixty-five-year-old female with ovarian cancer and abdominal pain. (a) Supine abdominal radiograph showing no evidence of dilated bowel, and is unremarkable. (b) Abdominal CT showing dilated fluid filled loops of large bowel (*b*).

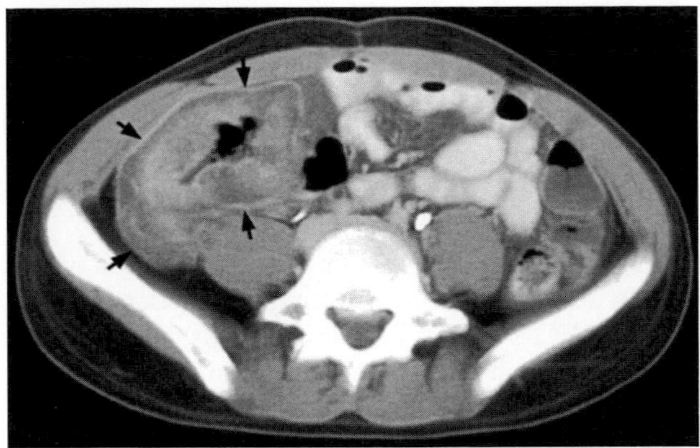

Figure 27 Typhlitis. Twenty-six-year-old male with leukemia and abdominal pain. Abdominal CT showing marked bowel thickening and edema in the ascending colon (*arrows*).

metastases are an unusual cause for abnormal liver function tests, unless associated with biliary duct obstruction. Microabscesses, typically of fungal or mycobacterial origin in immunosuppressed patients, can be difficult to detect by ultrasound, and CT may offer complementary information (6). Microabscesses, and other focal lesions, may also occur in the spleen and kidneys.

Cholecystitis may be calculus (Fig. 24) or acalculus in etiology, the latter being associated with debili tation, prolonged intubation, nasogastric suction, hyperalimentation, sepsis, and major surgery (6). Gallbladder wall thickening is the usual finding (Fig. 30).

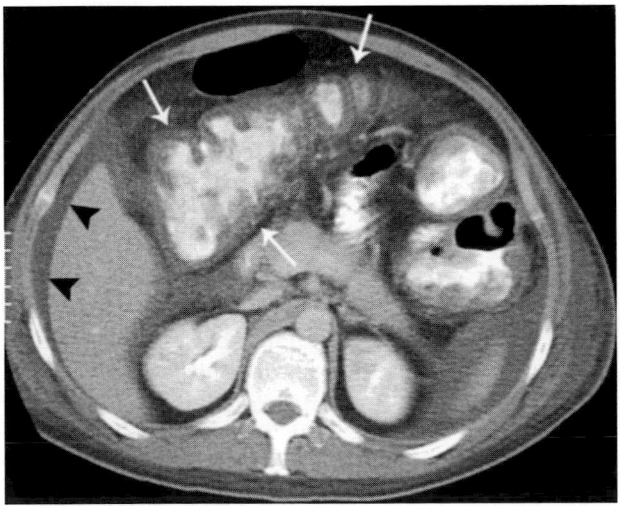

Figure 28 Pseudomembranous colitis. Fifty-six-year-old man with nonspecific abdominal pain. Abdominal CT showing bowel wall thickening and edema in the transverse colon (*arrows*), and also ascites (*arrowheads*). Note intraluminal gastrointestinal contrast.

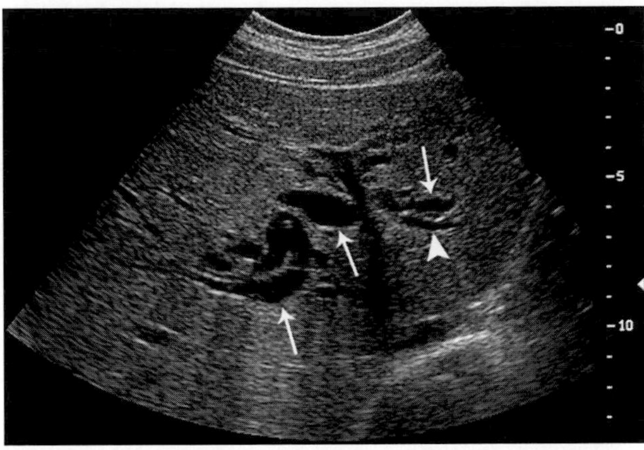

Figure 29 Biliary obstruction. Twenty-two-year-old man with lymphoma and elevated bilirubin despite a biliary stent. Ultrasound of the liver and porta hepatis region showing intrahepatic biliary duct dilatation (*arrows*). Portal vein (*arrowhead*).

Of note, gallbladder distension in isolation is a not uncommon finding in the intensive care patient, and is of limited significance. Ultrasound is superior to CT in the evaluation of gallbladder disease, and is able to identify pericholecystic collections, empyemas, emphysematous cholecystitis, and infarction. Cholecystostomy has been shown to be efficacious in selected patients (42–44).

Pancreatitis can sometimes be a difficult diagnosis, and it can vary widely in severity; steroid and L-asparaginase therapy, and raised intracranial pressure in brain tumors are established causes (45).

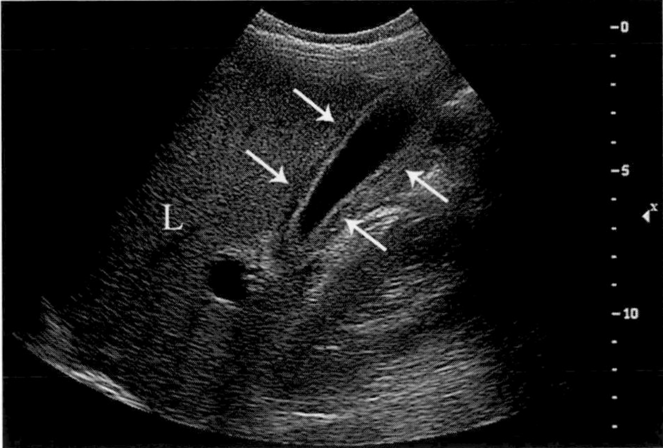

Figure 30 Cholecystitis. Twenty-one-year-old woman with leukemia, nausea and vomiting, abdominal pain, and right upper quadrant tenderness. Abdominal ultrasound of the right upper quadrant showing diffuse gallbladder wall thickening (*arrows*). L, liver parenchyma.

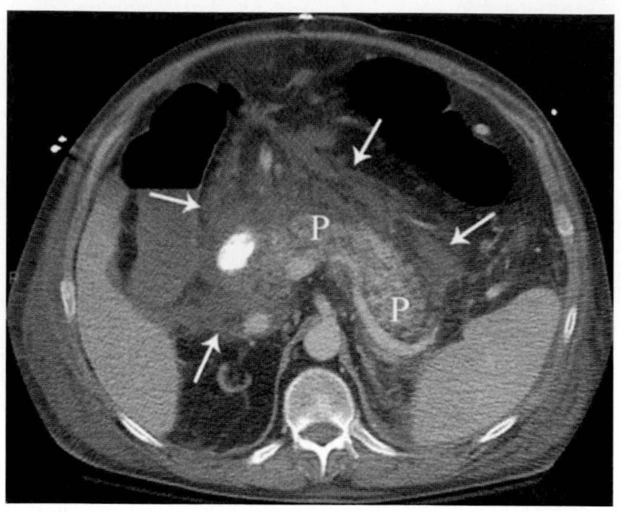

Figure 31 Acute pancreatitis. Fifty-five-year-old man with an elevated white count 7 days following a left nephrectomy. Abdominal CT showing extensive peripancreatic fluid (*arrows*) and an edematous pancreas (*p*). Note atrophic right kidney.

CT is superior to ultrasound in evaluation of the pancreas (Fig. 31). CT is able to delineate the extent of peripancreatic fluid collections and parenchymal necrosis (46–48).

Renal impairment may be due to urinary tract obstruction (e.g., from retroperitoneal or pelvic tumors, or blood clots, urolithiasis secondary to hyperuricemia and hyperphosphatemia, from tumor lysis) or parenchymal renal disease (e.g., from nephrotoxic drugs, or multisystem failure). Ultrasound is the initial investigation of choice to determine if there is hydronephrosis or hydroureter, which would be highly suggestive (but not necessarily diagnostic) of urinary tract obstruction (Fig. 32). The absence of hydronephrosis does not entirely exclude obstruction, but it would be most unlikely. In the event of urinary tract obstruction, CT is often better able to delineate the cause.

Doppler ultrasound is an excellent method of evaluating the larger intra-abdominal vessels, such as the aorta, IVC, portal veins, hepatic veins, and renal veins, some of which may be implicated in hepatic and renal dysfunction (Fig. 33).

V. CENTRAL NERVOUS SYSTEM DISORDERS

Patients in oncologic critical care are at risk from general neurologic problems, such as vascular disorders, but are frequently at added risk, for example, from metastases, infection (because of immuno-suppression and the sequelae of complex surgery), and specific conditions, such as posterior reversible edema syndrome (PRES).

A. Vascular Disorders

Vascular disease can be related to occlusion or narrowing of arterial or venous vessels. Acute cerebral ischemia is most often due to arterial disease with either thrombosis or embolus involving the artery in question. Cancer patients specifically can have embolization of noninfectious endocarditis vegetations

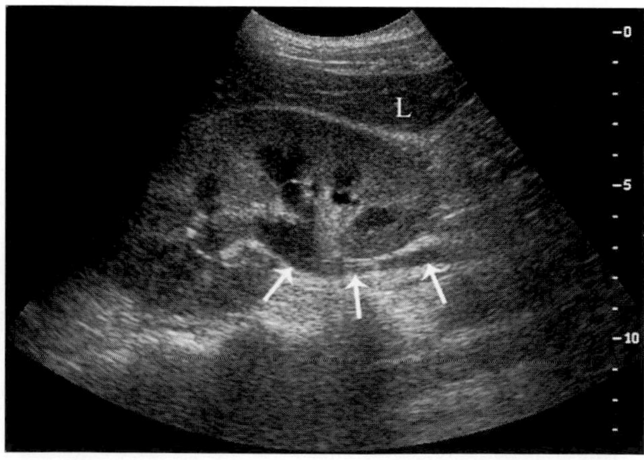

Figure 32 Hydronephrosis. Twenty-year-old woman with acute lymphoblastic leukemia and renal impairment. Renal ultrasound showing a dilated right pelvicaliceal system and proximal ureter (*arrows*). L, liver parenchyma. Found to have hemorrhagic cystitis on further evaluation.

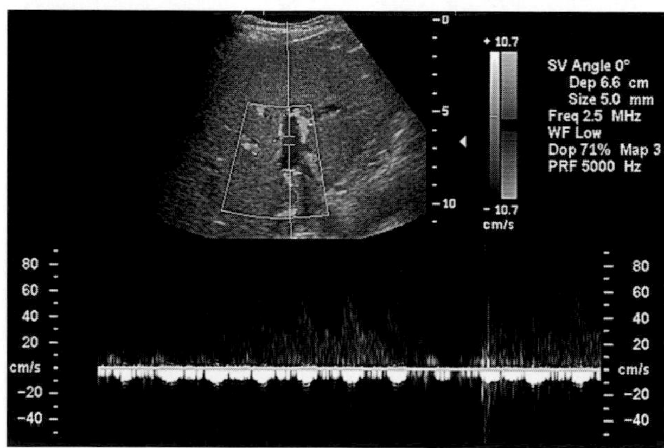

Figure 33 Reverse flow in the portal vein. Fifteen-year-old girl with acute lymphoblastic leukemia, nausea and vomiting, right upper quadrant tenderness, and abnormal liver function tests. Doppler ultrasound of the porta hepatis shows reverse flow in the portal vein (portal vein, and negative velocities in the Doppler trace). Findings suggestive of veno-occlusive disease.

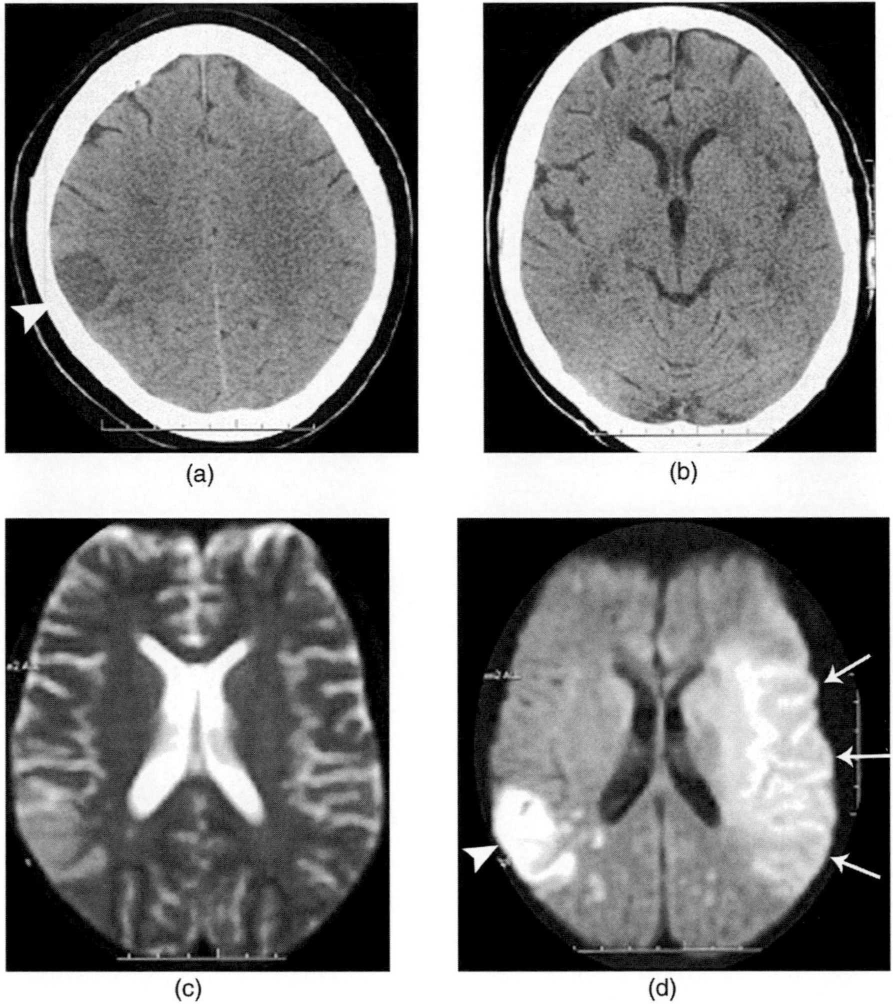

Figure 34 (a–d) Acute cerebral infarct. Fifty-year-old man with lung cancer and sudden right-sided weakness. (a,b) Noncontrast CT showing a subacute right parietal infarct (*arrowhead*), but no abnormality in the left cerebral hemisphere. (c) Axial T2-weighted MRI 1 hr later demonstrates the same findings. (d) However, axial diffusion-weighted MRI, undertaken at the same time, reveals large acute *left* middle cerebral artery infarct (*arrows*), in addition to the old right parietal infarct (*arrowhead*).

or vascular thrombosis because of an underlying coagulopathy (49). CT remains the study of choice because of its sensitivity for acute hemorrhage, noninvasiveness, and wide availability. Additionally, the extent of ischemia on the CT scan inversely correlates with the effectiveness of thrombolytic therapy (50). The early signs of ischemia on CT scanning include indistinctness of the insula and/or lentiform nucleus, gray–white matter hypodensity, and gyral swelling (51,52). MRI is able to detect ischemic changes earlier than CT (Fig. 34); in particular, diffusion-weighted MRI can detect ischemic changes in brain tissue within as little as 15 min of the acute event (53). MRI can confirm the diagnosis of ischemia and better define the full extent of injury. Also MR angiography and venography can noninvasively detect vascular occlusion and significant stenosis.

B. Infections

Infections of the CNS range from encephalitis to frank abscess formation. Infective processes outside of the brain parenchyma include leptomeningeal disease (meningitis) as well as epidural abscess. Epidural abscesses are often related to adjacent sinus or mastoid disease. Infections of the CNS can occur in the immuno-competent oncologic patient. However, infectious diseases are especially dangerous in immuno-compromised individuals such as leukemic patients. Opportunistic fungal infections such as aspergillus and candida can involve the brain in

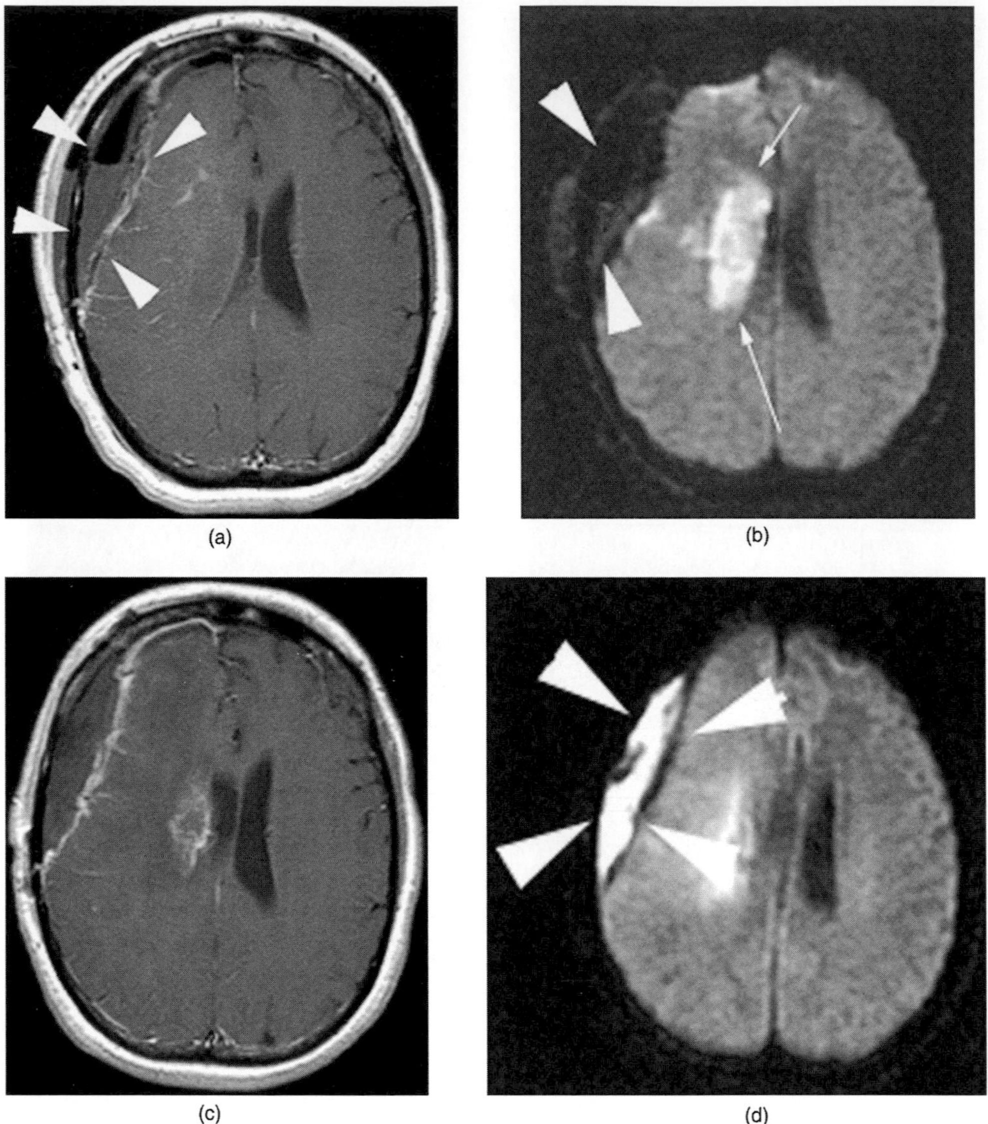

Figure 35 (a–d) Intracranial abscess. Fifty-five-year-old woman after a craniotomy for an anaplastic glioma. (a) Axial Tl-weighted MRI with intravenous Gadolinium and (b) axial diffusion-weighted MRI immediately after surgery showing right periventricular acute ischemic change (*arrows*) and rim-enhancing right frontoparietal extra-axial air/fluid collection on post-Gadolinium images, and with dark signal on diffusion-weighted image (*arrowheads*). (c,d) The MRI employing the same sequences 3 weeks later, showing bright signal (which was previously dark) on diffusion-weighted image within the extra-axial fluid collection (*arrowheads*), suggesting an abscess, which was confirmed at surgery.

immuno-compromised patients (54). CT allows prompt delineation of significant (potentially reversible) intracranial mass effect, but often MRI is required because of its increased sensitivity and specificity. The early stages of an encephalitis, such as herpes virus that affects the temporal lobes, are detected earlier with MRI than with CT, which is hampered by artifact from the bony walls of the middle cranial fossa. Furthermore, the addition of diffusion-weighted MRI is able to help in distinguishing abscesses from other necrotic appearing mass lesions, with the former appearing bright on diffusion-weighted images (55) (Fig. 35).

C. Seizures

Seizures often prompt imaging of the brain. CT scanning allows prompt evaluation for significant mass effect and hemorrhage, but MRI allows a more detailed evaluation. MRI should be tailored by the neurological findings including electroencephalo-

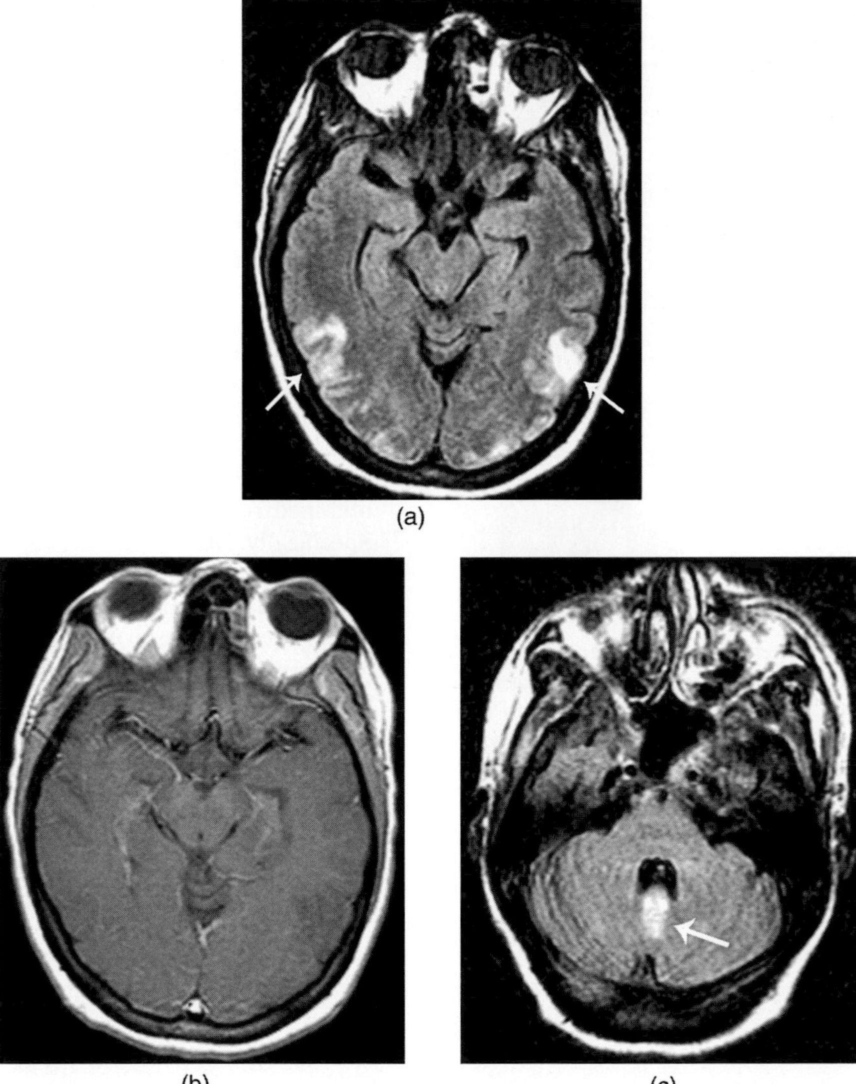

Figure 36 (a–c) PRES. Thirty-seven-year-old man who had undergone a bone marrow transplant and was on tacrolimus. (a) Axial fluid-attenuated inversion recovery (FLAIR) MRI showing abnormal signal in the posterior cerebrum that is both cortical and subcortical (*arrows*). (b) Axial Tl-weighted MRI with intravenous Gadolinium demonstrating absence of postcontrast enhancement. (c) Axial FLAIR MRI of the posterior fossa showing involvement of the cerebellar vermis as well (*arrow*).

graphy (EEG). If the clinical impression is consistent with temporal lobe origin, the MRI should include thin slice coronal images to delineate mesial temporal sclerosis (56). When neurologic deficits are persistent, a neoplastic cause of epilepsy should be considered. Both primary and metastatic tumors are well seen with MR imaging with intravenous contrast medium. The interpretation of MR images in the postictal period should be tempered by the realization that ephemeral areas of cortical and subcortical abnormality (possibly representing hyperemia) can be present (57).

D. Posterior Reversible Edema Syndrome

PRES can be confused with ischemia, encephalitis, or postictal hyperemia. PRES is an acute disorder of the posterior aspects of the brain (Fig. 36) thought to be secondary to fluid accumulation in the interstitium due to loss of autoregulation of cerebral perfusion (58). PRES is most often seen in the setting of hypertensive encephalopathy and eclampsia of pregnancy. In the oncologic setting, it has been related to chemotherapy in addition to immunosuppressive

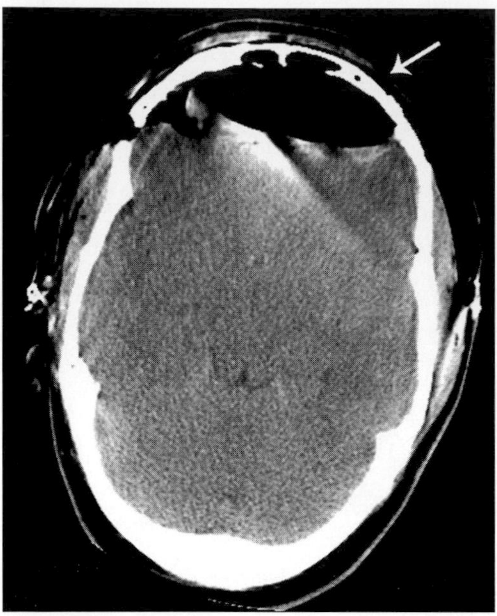

Figure 37 Postsurgical tension pneumocephalus. Forty-one-year-old woman after anterior skull base surgery for recurrent sinonasal undifferentiated carcinoma, with acute neurological deterioration. Axial noncontrast CT showing a large anterior air collection (*arrow*) that was relieved by direct aspiration.

therapy e.g., cyclosporine and tacrolimus (59). As the appearance of cortical and subcortical abnormalities can also be seen in venous thrombosis, careful scrutiny of the superior sagittal sinus must be undertaken.

E. Tumors

Brain neoplasms are either primary or metastatic. Brain tumors can present acutely due to a number of causes including hemorrhage and hydrocephalus. Hydrocephalus can be caused by a focal mass in the ventricular system or by diffuse leptomeningeal metastatic disease preventing resorption of cerebrospinal fluid (60). Again the initial imaging study should be a CT scan, which allows immediate evaluation for hemorrhage and mass effect. MRI can then be obtained based on the clinical and CT scan findings. Specifically, MRI with intravenous contrast is superior for detecting leptomeningeal metastatic disease (61). The evaluation of the brain immediately after craniotomy centers on identifying areas of ischemia, hemorrhage (both intraparenchymal and extra-axial), infection (Fig. 35), and, less emergently, residual or recurrent tumor (62). Rarely, pneumocephalus, especially after skull base surgery, can produce neurological deterioration (Fig. 37).

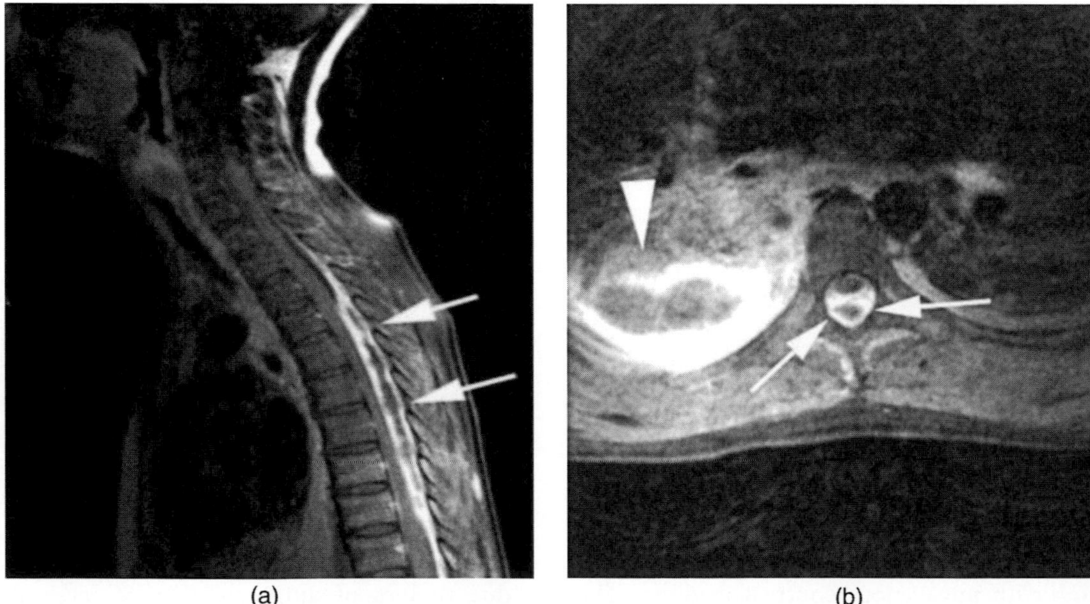

Figure 38 (a,b) Spinal abscess. Twenty-year-old man following recent thoracic surgery for a sarcoma, with an acute spinal cord syndrome. (a) Sagittal and (b) axial axial Tl-weighted MRI with intravenous Gadolinium showing an empyema in the right lung (*arrowhead*) and a dorsal enhancing epidural abscess in the cervical cervical and thoracic spine (*arrows*).

F. Spinal Disorders

The spine represents an additional area for emergent evaluation. In all cases, a careful neurological evaluation must precede any imaging. The reason is that a spinal cord level is an essential basis for guiding any imaging. A complete MRI evaluation of the entire spine is difficult particularly in a critically ill patient. The imaging must start at the clinically suspected level of the spine and continue superiorly to the foramen magnum. The most common location for lesions affecting the spinal column is the extradural space. Infections can be related to adjacent diskitis with secondary epidural abscess formation or primary epidural abscess (Fig. 38). Extradural neoplasms are most often osseous metastases with secondary extension into the epidural space. Spinal cord ischemia can occur in the setting of spinal/paraspinal surgery. In all these cases MR imaging is the study of choice (63).

REFERENCES

1. Blair SL, Schwarz RE. Critical care of patients with cancer. Surgical considerations. Crit Care Clin 2001; 17:721–742.
2. Indeck M, Peterson S, Smith J, Brotman S. Risk, cost, and benefit of transporting ICU patients for special studies. J Trauma 1988; 28:1020–1025.
3. Niklason LT, Chan HP, Cascade PN, Chang CL, Chee PW, Mathews JF. Portable chest imaging: comparison of storage phosphor digital, asymmetric screen-film, and conventional screen-film systems. Radiology 1993; 186:387–393.
4. Henry DA. Imaging in the new millennium. Crit Care Clin 2000; 16:579–599.
5. Lee SY, Frankel HL. Ultrasound and other imaging technologies in the intensive care unit. Surg Clin North Am 2000; 80:975–1003.
6. Zingas AP. Computed tomography of the abdomen in the critically ill. Crit Care Clin 1994; 10:321–339.
7. Shellock FG, Kanal E. Magnetic resonance: bioeffects, safety, and patient management. Philadelphia: Lippincott-Raven, 1996:xi, 342.
8. Silverstein DS, Livingston DH, Elcavage J, Kovar L, Kelly KM. The utility of routine daily chest radiography in the surgical intensive care unit. J Trauma 1993; 35:643–646.
9. Henschke CI, Pasternack GS, Schroeder S, Hart KK, Herman PG. Bedside chest radiography: diagnostic efficacy. Radiology 1983; 149:23–26.
10. Bekemeyer WB, Crapo RO, Calhoon S, Cannon CY, Clayton PD. Efficacy of chest radiography in a respiratory intensive care unit. A prospective study. Chest 1985; 88:691–696.
11. Greenbaum DM, Marschall KE. The value of routine daily chest x-rays in intubated patients in the medical intensive care unit. Crit Care Med 1982; 10:29–30.
12. Kuhlman JE, Fishman EK, Burch PA, Karp JE, Zerhouni EA, Siegelman SS. CT of invasive pulmonary aspergillosis. AJR Am J Roentgenol 1988; 150: 1015–1020.
13. Brunel W, Coleman DL, Schwartz DE, Peper E, Cohen NH. Assessment of routine chest roentgenograms and the physical examination to confirm endotracheal tube position. Chest 1989; 96:1043–1045.
14. Gray P, Sullivan G, Ostryzniuk P, McEwen TA, Rigby M, Roberts DE. Value of postprocedural chest radiographs in the adult intensive care unit. Crit Care Med 1992; 20:1513–1518.
15. Benjamin JJ, Cascade PN, Rubenfire M, Wajszczuk W, Kerin NZ. Left lower lobe atelectasis and consolidation following cardiac surgery: the effect of topical cooling on the phrenic nerve. Radiology 1982; 142: 11–14.
16. Goodman LR. Postoperative chest radiograph: I. Alterations after abdominal surgery. AJR Am J Roentgenol 1980; 134:533–541.
17. Goodman LR. Postoperative chest radiograph: II. Alterations after major intrathoracic surgery. AJR Am J Roentgenol 1980; 134:803–813.
18. Shevland JE, Hirleman MT, Hoang KA, Kealey GP. Lobar collapse in the surgical intensive care unit. Br J Radiol 1983; 56:531–534.
19. Pham DH, Huang D, Korwan A, Greyson ND. Acute unilateral pulmonary nonventilation due to mucous plugs. Radiology 1987; 165:135–137.
20. Winer-Muram HT, Rubin SA, Ellis JV, Jennings SG, Arheart KL, Wunderink RG, Leeper KV, Meduri GU. Pneumonia and ARDS in patients receiving mechanical ventilation: diagnostic accuracy of chest radiography. Radiology 1993; 188:479–485.
21. Singh N, Falestiny MN, Rogers P, Reed MJ, Pularski J, Norris R, Yu VL. Pulmonary infiltrates in the surgical ICU: prospective assessment of predictors of etiology and mortality. Chest 1998; 114:1129–1136.
22. Choi YH, Leung AN. Radiologic findings: pulmonary infections after bone marrow transplantation. J Thorac Imaging 1999; 14:201–206.
23. Erasmus JJ, McAdams HP, Rossi SE. Drug-induced lung injury. Semin Roentgenol 2002; 37:72–81.
24. Wesselius LJ. Pulmonary complications of cancer therapy. Compr Ther 1999; 25:272–277.
25. Tocino I. Chest imaging in the intensive care unit. Eur J Radiol 1996; 23:46–57.
26. Remy-Jardin M, Remy J, Wattinne L, Giraud F. Central pulmonary thromboembolism: diagnosis with spiral volumetric CT with the single-breath-hold technique—comparison with pulmonary angiography. Radiology 1992; 185:381–387.
27. Stark DD, Federle MP, Goodman PC, Podrasky AE, Webb WR. Differentiating lung abscess and empyema:

Radiography and computed tomography. AJR Am J Roentgenol 1983; 141:163–167.

28. Williams NS, Lewis CT. Bronchopleural fistula: a review of 86 cases. Br J Surg 1976; 63:520–522.

29. Ibrahim NK, Sahin AA, Dubrow RA, Lynch PM, Boehnke-Michaud L, Valero V, Buzdar AU, Hortobagyi GN. Colitis associated with docetaxel-based chemotherapy in patients with metastatic breast cancer. Lancet 2000; 355:281–283.

30. Brown K, Raman SS, Kallman C. Imaging procedures. In: Bongard FS, ed. Current Critical Care Diagnosis and Treatment. New York: McGraw-Hill Companies, Inc., 2003.

31. Cleary RK. *Clostridium difficile*-associated diarrhea and colitis: clinical manifestations, diagnosis, and treatment. Dis Colon Rectum 1998; 41:1435–1449.

32. Maglinte DD, Balthazar EJ, Kelvin FM, Megibow AJ. The role of radiology in the diagnosis of small-bowel obstruction. AJR Am J Roentgenol 1997; 168: 1171–1180.

33. Maglinte DD, Kelvin FM, Rowe MG, Bender GN, Rouch DM. Small-bowel obstruction: optimizing radiologic investigation and nonsurgical management. Radiology 2001; 218:39–46.

34. Rex DK. Acute colonic pseudo-obstruction (Ogilvie's syndrome). Gastroenterologist 1994; 2:233–238.

35. Stephenson KR, Rodriguez-Bigas MA. Decompression of the large intestine in Ogilvie's syndrome by a colonoscopically placed long intestinal tube. Surg Endosc 1994; 8:116–117.

36. Geller A, Petersen BT, Gostout CJ. Endoscopic decompression for acute colonic pseudo-obstruction. Gastrointest Endosc 1996; 44:144–150.

37. Katz JA, Wagner ML, Gresik MV, Mahoney DH Jr, Fernbach DJ. Typhlitis. An 18-year experience and postmortem review. Cancer 1990; 65:1041–1047.

38. Keidan RD, Fanning J, Gatenby RA, Weese JL. Recurrent typhlitis. A disease resulting from aggressive chemotherapy. Dis Colon Rectum 1989; 32:206–209.

39. Kawamoto S, Horton KM, Fishman EK. Pseudomembranous colitis: spectrum of imaging findings with clinical and pathologic correlation. Radiographics 1999; 19:887–897.

40. Skibber JM, Matter GJ, Pizzo PA, Lotze MT. Right lower quadrant pain in young patients with leukemia. A surgical perspective. Ann Surg 1987; 206:711–716.

41. Rao PM, Rhea JT, Novelline RA, McCabe CJ, Lawrason JN, Berger DL, Sacknoff R. Helical CT technique for the diagnosis of appendicitis: prospective evaluation of a focused appendix CT examination. Radiology 1997; 202:139–144.

42. Boland GW, Lee MJ, Leung J, Mueller PR. Percutaneous cholecystostomy in critically ill patients: early response and final outcome in 82 patients. AJR Am J Roentgenol 1994; 163:339–342.

43. Vauthey JN, Lerut J, Martini M, Becker C, Gertsch P, Blumgart LH. Indications and limitations of percutaneous cholecystostomy for acute cholecystitis. Surg Gynecol Obstet 1993; 176:49–54.

44. vanSonnenberg E, D'Agostino HB, Goodacre BW, Sanchez RB, Casola G. Percutaneous gallbladder puncture and cholecystostomy: results, complications, and caveats for safety. Radiology 1992; 183:167–170.

45. Kaste SC, Rodriguez-Galindo C, Furman WL. Imaging pediatric oncologic emergencies of the abdomen. AJR Am J Roentgenol 1999; 173:729–736.

46. Paulson EK, Vitellas KM, Keogan MT, Low VH, Nelson RC. Acute pancreatitis complicated by gland necrosis: spectrum of findings on contrast-enhanced CT. AJR Am J Roentgenol 1999; 172:609–613.

47. De Sanctis JT, Lee MJ, Gazelle GS, Boland GW, Halpern EF, Saini S, Mueller PR. Prognostic indicators in acute pancreatitis: CT vs Apache II. Clin Radiol 1997; 52:842–848.

48. Lee MJ, Wittich GR, Mueller PR. Percutaneous intervention in acute pancreatitis. Radiographics 1998; 18: 711–724; discussion 728.

49. Rogers LR. Cerebrovascular complications in cancer patients. Oncology (Huntingt) 1994; 8:23–30; discussion 31–22, 37.

50. von Kummer R, Allen KL, Holle R, Bozzao L, Bastianello S, Manelfe C, Bluhmki E, Ringleb P, Meier DH, Hacke W. Acute stroke: usefulness of early CT findings before thrombolytic therapy. Radiology 1997; 205:327–333.

51. Truwit CL, Barkovich AJ, Gean-Marton A, Hibri N, Norman D. Loss of the insular ribbon: another early CT sign of acute middle cerebral artery infarction. Radiology 1990; 176:801–806.

52. Tomura N, Uemura K, Inugami A, Fujita H, Higano S, Shishido F. Early CT finding in cerebral infarction: obscuration of the lentiform nucleus. Radiology 1988; 168:463–467.

53. Kucharczyk J, Mintorovitch J, Asgari HS, Moseley M. Diffusion/perfusion MR imaging of acute cerebral ischemia. Magn Reson Med 1991; 19:311–315.

54. Perfect JR, Durack DT. Fungal meningitis. In: Scheld WM, Whitley RJ, Durack DT, eds. Infections of the Central Nervous System. Philadelphia: Lippincott-Raven, 1997:721–739.

55. Lai PH, Ho JT, Chen WL, Hsu SS, Wang JS, Pan HB, Yang CF. Brain abscess and necrotic brain tumor: discrimination with proton MR spectroscopy and diffusion-weighted imaging. AJNR Am J Neuroradiol 2002; 23:1369–1377.

56. Margerison JH, Corsellis JA. Epilepsy and the temporal lobes. A clinical, electroencephalographic and neuropathological study of the brain in epilepsy, with particular reference to the temporal lobes. Brain 1966; 89:499–530.

57. Kramer RE, Luders H, Lesser RP, Weinstein MR, Dinner DS, Morris HH, Wyllie E. Transient focal

abnormalities of neuroimaging studies during focal status epilepticus. Epilepsia 1987; 28:528–532.

58. Covarrubias DJ, Luetmer PH, Campeau NG. Posterior reversible encephalopathy syndrome: prognostic utility of quantitative diffusion-weighted MR images. AJNR Am J Neuroradiol 2002; 23:1038–1048.
59. Ito Y, Arahata Y, Goto Y, Hirayama M, Nagamutsu M, Yasuda T, Yanagi T, Sobue G. Cisplatin neurotoxicity presenting as reversible posterior leukoencephalopathy syndrome. AJNR Am J Neuroradiol 1998; 19:415–417.
60. Ginsberg LE. Contrast enhancement in meningeal and extra-axial disease. Neuroimaging Clin N Am 1994; 4:133–152.
61. Singh SK, Agris JM, Leeds NE, Ginsberg LE. Intracranial leptomeningeal metastases: comparison of depiction at FLAIR and contrast-enhanced MR imaging. Radiology 2000; 217:50–53.
62. Sawaya R, Hammoud M, Schoppa D, Hess KR, Wu SZ, Shi WM, Wildrick DM. Neurosurgical outcomes in a modern series of 400 craniotomies for treatment of parenchymal tumors. Neurosurgery 1998; 42:1044–1055. Discussion 1055–1046.
63. Post MJ, Sze G, Quencer RM, Eismont FJ, Green BA, Gahbauer H. Gadolinium-enhanced MR in spinal infection. J Comput Assist Tomogr 1990; 14: 721–729.

46

Interventional Radiology in the Oncologic Critical Care Setting

MICHAEL J. WALLACE and DAVID C. MADOFF

Department of Interventional Radiology, The University of Texas M.D. Anderson Cancer Center, Houston, Texas, U.S.A.

I. INTRODUCTION

The interventional radiologist uses the standard imaging techniques that best define the target organ or lesion to guide minimally invasive vascular and nonvascular procedures. These procedures are adapted from standard surgical procedures to establish a diagnosis, initiate therapeutic management, or provide palliative care for patients with cancer. Minimally invasive approaches are often safer, less traumatic, and less painful but equally therapeutic and more cost effective than the surgical alternative for the patient and the health care provider. This is particularly important in the critically ill patient in the intensive care unit (ICU), in whom all procedures carry a higher than average risk. Procedures utilized in the care of patients with neoplasms include imaging-guided biopsy and drainage (gastrostomy, nephrostomy, biliary drain, and cholecystostomy); arterial interventions (infusion, embolization, chemoembolization, balloon angioplasty, and stent/stent-graft placement); and venous interventions (insertion and repositioning of long-term central venous access devices, stents, inferior vena caval filters; foreign body retrieval; thrombolysis; transjugular liver biopsy; and insertion of a transjugular intrahepatic portosystemic shunt [TIPS]), among others. State-of-the-art imaging modalities, including fluoroscopy, ultrasound, computed tomography (CT), and magnetic resonance imaging (MRI), are utilized to guide the placement of needles, catheters, and devices directly to the target site deep within the body through a small skin incision. These procedures often are performed under local anesthesia with intravenous sedation and typically do not require general anesthesia.

II. DRAINAGE PROCEDURES

Percutaneous catheter drainage is a major contribution of the interventional radiologist in the care of patients with malignancy, especially in the perioperative setting. Catheters are placed into obstructed genitourinary, biliary (including gallbladder and bilomas), and gastrointestinal tracts, as well as into collections of abnormal fluids such as abscesses, empyemas, urinomas, seromas, lymphocysts, and loculated ascites, under radiologic guidance by using the Seldinger technique, which makes use of a needle, guidewire, and catheter.

A. Percutaneous Abscess Drainage (PAD)

Care of a febrile patient is a common situation in the perioperative oncologic setting. Although febrile episodes have many causes, an intra-abdominal abscess may be life threatening and often results from perforation of a hollow viscus either by a neoplasm or as a postoperative complication. A septic episode is often accompanied by leukocytosis, cyclic or constant temperature elevation, and renal, pulmonary, or cardiovascular failure (1). When left untreated, intra-abdominal abscesses have a mortality rate of nearly 100% (2). Thirty-six percent of intra-abdominal abscesses are located within the peritoneal cavity, 38% within the retroperitoneum, and 26% within the viscera (3). Over the past 15–20 years, PAD has largely replaced surgical drainage as the treatment of choice for abscesses and other abnormal fluid collections such as biloma and urinoma (4–6). Percutaneous abscess drainage is less invasive than surgical drainage, better maintains the integrity of surrounding structures and overlying skin, and can be done at the time of initial diagnosis, thus saving time and expense. In addition, most PAD procedures are performed under intravenous conscious sedation (e.g., midazolam and fentanyl), obviating the need for general anesthesia care. Percutaneous abscess drainage also makes nursing care easier, as drainage systems are closed with no extensive surgical wound that requires frequent dressing changes.

Imaging, primarily ultrasound and CT, is essential for both diagnosis and intervention. The advantage of ultrasound is that it can be performed at the bedside for ICU patients who are not able to travel to the radiology department, especially when the abscess is superficial (5). While ultrasound can be used for real-time guidance of needle placement, limitations include degradation of images in the presence of intra-abdominal air-/gas resulting from postoperative intraperitoneal free air or intestinal air secondary to postoperative ileus. Ultrasound images are also of limited value in obese patients and for patients with overlying surgical dressings.

Computed tomography has emerged as the imaging modality of choice for the evaluation of patients with intra-abdominal sepsis (5). Availability of rapid acquisition multislice CT scanners now allows for adequate diagnostic examinations, even in critically ill patients who are unable to hold their breath. Computed tomography scans are better at determining the depth of the abscess, the cutaneous entry site, and the angle through which the collection is best approached so as to avoid adjacent vital structures such as bowel, organs, or major vessels. As in ultrasound, however, CT appearances of fluid collections are nonspecific, so that sterile collections cannot be differentiated from infected ones. Criteria used to identify an abscess include intracavitary gas (Fig. 1), thick or irregular walls, heterogenous internal debris, and contrast enhancement. Many studies report that CT is more accurate than ultrasound for identifying intra-abdominal fluid collections and abscesses with sensitivities reported between 90% and 100%, while the sensitivity of ultrasound has been reported at between 80% and 85% (5,7–11).

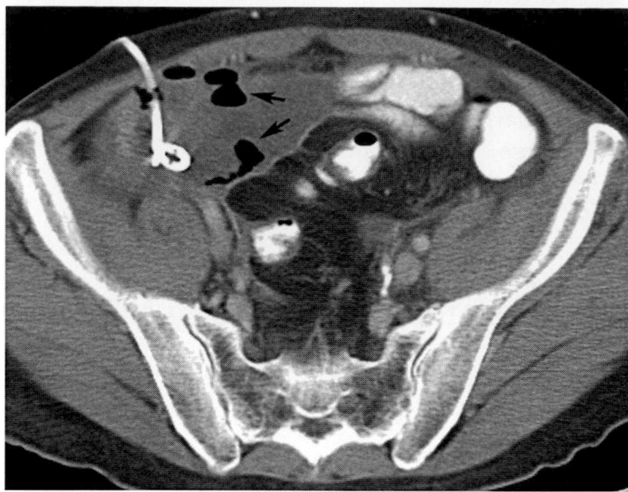

Figure 1 Computed tomographic (CT) image of the abdomen after CT guided drain insertion in a patient with a postoperative fluid collection in the right lower quadrant. Note the presence of air (*arrows*) within the collection suggesting the presence of an abscess.

The most important step in percutaneous drainage procedures is planning the access route (6). This is done after review of all pertinent imaging studies. In general, the shortest, straightest tract is the best approach. Care must be taken to avoid adjacent bowel, pleura, and major blood vessels. Diagnostic aspiration can be performed initially with an 18- to 22-gauge needle. The position of the needle is confirmed with ultrasound or CT, and the fluid is aspirated for culture, gram stain, and other pertinent laboratory studies. If frank pus is aspirated, the fluid can be drained immediately by inserting a catheter ranging from 10 to 20 F into the collection. Choice of the appropriate size of drainage catheter is based on the type and viscosity of fluid obtained on the initial aspiration.

Percutaneous abscess drainage is most successful when the fluid collection is well defined, unilocular, and free flowing, characteristics found in more than 90% of intra-abdominal collections (12). Postoperative abscesses have the best outcomes (13). When collections are more complex (e.g., abscess communication with bowel), the cure rate falls to between 80% and 90%. Pancreatic collections, abscesses infected with yeast, and tumors with abscess or phlegmon formation intermixed with necrosis are examples of situations in which percutaneous drainage is much less effective, with cure rates falling as low as 30–50% (6,14). Percutaneous drainage also may be helpful in less favorable situations (e.g., multilocular collection, necrotic debris), particularly when the patient is at a high surgical risk. In these less optimal circumstances, PAD may improve the patient's condition so that a more definitive surgical drainage can be performed at a later time (13).

The only absolute contraindication to PAD is the lack of a safe access route. This rarely is a problem when CT guidance is utilized. In very selected cases in which a fluid collection is deep within the pelvis, transrectal or transvaginal routes may be used, with endocavitary ultrasound probes providing guidance (15–17).

The overall complication rate for PAD in most series is 5% or less (6). Minor complications include transient bacteremia, skin infection, and minor bleeding. Major complications include frank hemorrhage requiring transfusion, peritonitis, sepsis, and bowel perforation. The recurrence rate following PAD is approximately 5%. Percutaneous abscess drainage compares favorably with surgical alternatives, whose mortality rates are 10–20% and recurrence rates 15–30%.

B. Chest Drainage

1. Pleural Drainage

Pleural fluid aspiration and drainage are the most common image-guided procedures performed on patients in the critical care setting (18). Pleural fluid accumulation occurs in as many as 75% of these bedridden and often mechanically ventilated patients. Most pleural effusions are small, gravity dependent, and not loculated; they usually are reactive or secondary to fluid overload or a pulmonary parenchymal process. As pleural fluid is often detected on routine imaging studies (i.e., chest radiograph), the clinician must have clear goals when a decision is made to aspirate or drain it. Thoracenteses are performed for diagnosis (e.g., empyema) and/or for therapeutic evacuation (e.g., shortness of breath) of noninfected serous fluid.

Drainage of large, nonloculated pleural effusions that fill nearly the entire hemithorax often require no image guidance, although transthoracic ultrasound or CT can direct needle or catheter placement if accessibility or precise localization is an issue. Complex pleural fluid collections can be evaluated with ultrasound or CT for identification of the best pocket or pockets for subsequent percutaneous catheter placement.

The imaging appearance of hemorrhagic fluid collections, loculated effusions, and empyemas consists of low-density pleural fluid, often surrounded by an enhancing thick or irregular rind of tissue, which may be located in nondependent locations. Frequently, these collections contain air bubbles, which may be dispersed throughout the fluid, suggesting thick or organized material. These collections can be treated with percutaneous catheter placement and water-sealed drainage at –20 cm of water suction. Loculated collections generally do not communicate with the remainder of the pleural space and can be managed by gravity drainage (18).

Chest tube patency is necessary to achieve adequate drainage, especially in ICU patients. Saline irrigation, performed two to three time daily, helps maintain catheter patency. Several reports have shown the benefit of infusing catheter-directed thrombolytics into the loculated collection to improve drainage (19,20). Although intracavitary thrombolytic administration increases fluid drainage and may hasten removal of the pleural catheter, there is no evidence that it reduces hospital stay, morbidity, or mortality (21). Percutaneous pleural drains are usually monitored clinically by chest radiograph and fluid output. If a patient does not respond clinically to chest tube drainage and the fluid output appears adequate, a CT scan of the chest should be performed to evaluate for additional collections or other signs of tube malfunction.

2. Lung Abscess

In the perioperative setting, processes that involve the lungs are generally diffuse including pulmonary edema, acute respiratory distress syndrome, pneumonitis, and occasionally, lung abscesses. Lung abscesses often occur after an episode of aspiration pneumonia with gram-negative organisms or with septic emboli associated with staphylococcal infections. While non-ICU patients can frequently clear the purulent material by coughing, the obtunded or ventilated patient cannot, leading to abscess formation. Such abscesses usually require surgical or percutaneous drainage. Although large, peripheral abscesses can be drained with fluoroscopic guidance, most require CT scan guidance to place the catheter into an optimal location. It is important that the affected lung be positioned in a dependent location, as purulent material may spread endobronchially during drainage when the involved lung is elevated, and abscess contents can spill into the contralateral lung during catheter manipulation. In addition, the lung should be accessed at a point where the abscess is juxtaposed to the pleura or where there is adjacent inflammation between the abscess and the pleura to minimize the risk of bronchopleural fistula formation. Following catheter placement, the abscess is evacuated as completely as possible and irrigated with normal saline. Catheters can typically be removed after 5–7 days (18).

C. Percutaneous Nephrostomy

In cancer patients, urinary tract obstruction usually develops as a result of compression or direct extension of primary or metastatic neoplasms in the pelvis or retroperitoneum. Less frequently, obstruction in these patients is caused by benign iatrogenic strictures from previous surgical intervention and/or radiation therapy or from urinary calculi. Percutaneous nephrostomy (PCN) tube placement is an established intervention for urinary diversion in patients with supravesical urinary tract obstruction, urinary fistulas or leaks, or hemorrhagic cystitis (22). Percutaneous renal access is also the initial maneuver for more complex urologic interventions such as percutaneous nephrolithotomy and other endourologic procedures.

Urinary obstruction may become evident because of azotemia or urinary sepsis, or it may be diagnosed incidentally after ultrasound or CT examination of the abdomen for other reasons. The diagnosis of an obstructed collecting system can be confirmed by any number of imaging modalities. Ultrasound is a good first-choice examination, especially when the patient's serum creatinine level is elevated and an obstructive uropathy is suspected.

Patients with pyonephrosis or infected hydronephrosis are at high risk for gram-negative sepsis (23–26). Under these circumstances, urinary diversion must be performed emergently. Patients often present with fever, flank pain, and evidence of urinary tract obstruction on cross-sectional imaging.

Percutaneous drainage has become the treatment of choice for initial decompression of an infected collecting system regardless of the underlying etiology. In the presence of obstruction without infection, urinary diversion can be used to preserve renal function. This is particularly important in patients whose therapy regimens include agents that depend on renal excretion and are potentially nephrotoxic (22). In patients with urinary leakage or fistulas, PCN tubes can be used to divert an adequate amount of urine to allow healing to occur. Similarly, percutaneous urinary diversion is one method of therapy for patients with hemorrhagic cystitis when more traditional local therapies have failed (27).

Overall success rates in excess of 98% have been reported for PCN tube placement (22). Success rates are often lower in patients with a nondilated collecting system and in patients with complex stone disease. The overall complication rate, including both major and minor complications, is approximately 10%. (22). Major hemorrhagic complications occur in approximately 2.5% of cases (28,29). Other potential complications include septic shock (23–25) and colon injury (30). Thoracic complications (pneumothorax, hydrothorax, hemothorax, and empyema) can occur when renal access is above the 12th rib (28).

D. Percutaneous Cholecystostomy

Elective cholecystectomy is a safe procedure for the treatment of acute cholecystitis in an otherwise healthy patient, with an operative mortality rate of 0–0.8% (31–33). However, the morbidity and mortality rates increase dramatically in ICU patients with multiorgan compromise (34–38). Percutaneous cholecystostomy has emerged as an alternative to standard surgical therapy. A very important advantage to this approach is that it can be done at the patient's bedside with no incision using only local anesthesia.

Indications for percutaneous cholecystostomy include acute calculous or acalculous cholecystitis in patients too ill to withstand surgical cholecystectomy and/or general anesthesia. In calculous disease, the gallbladder can be removed electively when the patient's condition stabilizes. Alternative approaches to operative cholecystectomy are percutaneous stone removal or dissolution therapy via the existing cholecystostomy tract. This is especially useful in patients who remain poor surgical candidates after transfer from the ICU (31,39).

Acute acalculous cholecystitis is increasingly being recognized in ICU patients. Unfortunately, its diagnosis is difficult to establish despite the use of advanced imaging techniques and laboratory analysis (40). Although ultrasound is extremely accurate in identifying cholelithiasis, it is considerably less reliable in diagnosing acute acalculous cholecystitis, with reported accuracy rates of 50–60%. The criteria used for nuclear medicine hepatobiliary scans are useful in evaluating cystic duct patency, but the false-positive rates are in the range of 25–30%. Generalized hepatocellular dysfunction, prolonged total parenteral nutrition (TPN), sepsis, and fasting all predispose to false-positive results on hepatobiliary scans (41).

In patients with acalculous cholecystitis, percutaneous cholecystostomy can confirm the diagnosis and serve as a definitive therapy. Prompt decompression can result in dramatic symptomatic relief. Typically, the cystic duct eventually opens, allowing tube removal without a formal cholecystectomy. Since results of bile gram stain and culture are helpful but not sensitive (30–50%), a cholecystostomy tube is inserted at the time of initial aspiration. Negative gram stain and culture results, however, do not exclude the diagnosis of acute cholecystitis, especially in patients who have received antibiotics (42). Catheters are left to drain by gravity. When the cystic duct is obstructed, the gallbladder normally produces 50–70 mL of clear mucus daily. Larger volumes of biliary drainage indicate cystic duct patency.

Percutaneous cholecystostomy placement is technically successful in over 95% of cases (43). Interestingly, as many as 20–30% of patients will not have acute cholecystitis, confirming the difficulty of diagnosing acute cholecystitis in critically ill patients. In a study by Boland et al. (38), approximately 60% of patients demonstrated clinical improvement following cholecystostomy in the setting of sepsis with suggestive ultrasonographic finding of a gallbladder source. England et al. (44) reported, however, that patients with localized signs and symptoms in the right upper quadrant were statistically more likely to respond to percutaneous cholecystostomy and patients in the ICU were less likely to respond. The response rates were 83% (34 of 41) in patients with signs and symptoms and 50% (9 of 18) in patients without pain and tenderness localized to the right upper quadrant. Interestingly, the response rate for patients in the ICU was 55% (17 of 31), whereas it was 93% (26 of 28) among patients outside the ICU. Despite these findings, percutaneous cholecystostomy still may be helpful in ICU patients because it excludes the diagnosis of acute cholecystitis and avoids unnecessary surgery. Response to percutaneous cholecystostomy depends not only on the presence of acute cholecystitis, but also on the patient's overall medical situation (34). When the gallbladder is the only focus of infection, the response is dramatic. A poor response is most likely due to severe concomitant systemic disease. Moreover, results of a recent study indicated that some patients with acalculous cholecystitis may respond to a 3-day trial of conservative management, obviating the need for percutaneous cholecystostomy (34).

With proper technique, complications from percutaneous cholecystostomy are few. When they do occur, they usually occur immediately or within days after the procedure and include hemorrhage, vagal reactions, sepsis, bile peritonitis, pneumothorax, intestinal loop perforation, secondary infection or colonization of the gallbladder, and catheter dislodgment (35,36,45). Late complications that have been reported include catheter dislodgment and recurrent cholecystitis (36). The overall major and minor complication rates were reported to range from 3% to 8% and 4% to 13%, respectively (35,36). Catheter dislodgment, reported as the most common complication, may be due to inadequate fixation of the catheter, patient movement, and/or failure to protect the catheter during patient transportation (46). Biliary peritonitis due to bile leakage occurs at a rate of 2.5% and may be prevented with catheter removal after formation of a mature tract. In recent publications, 30-day mortality rates varied from 0% to 25% (35,47,48). Fatal outcomes are often associated with a failure to clear sepsis and significant comorbid conditions forbidding definitive surgical therapy.

E. Percutaneous Biliary Drainage

Percutaneous drainage is an important adjunct to palliative treatment of patients with inoperable cancer, in whom it is performed to improve metabolic and nutritional status, provide relief of pruritus, and allow administration of chemotherapeutic agents that require unimpeded biliary excretion. In the ICU setting, percutaneous drainage is used to treat acute suppurative cholangitis, in failed biliary enteric bypass, and for diversion of bile flow in treating bile leaks (Fig. 2) and fistulas.

Endoscopic retrograde cholangiopancreatography (ERCP) has essentially replaced percutaneous transhepatic cholangiography (PTC) for diagnosis and has become the preferred method for therapy. The percutaneous alternative is usually reserved for situations in which the endoscopic approach has failed (49) or is

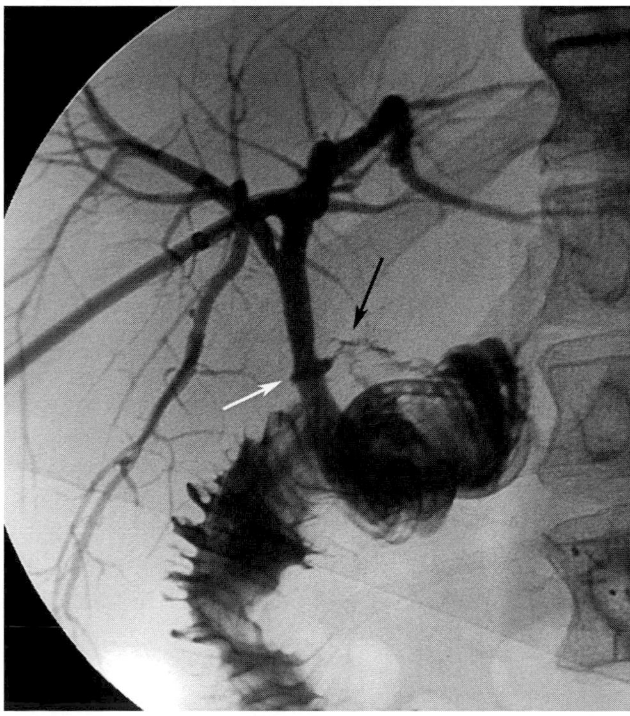

Figure 2 Cholangiogram following insertion of a transhepatic internal–external biliary drain demonstrates a bile leak (*black arrow*) arising from a biliary-enteric anastomosis (*white arrow*).

not feasible, as in patients with a history of partial gastrectomy or gastric outlet obstruction.

Three types of percutaneous biliary drainage are performed—external, combined external–internal, and internal drainage through indwelling plastic or metallic stents (50). With external drainage catheters, bile is completely diverted to an external reservoir. An internal–external biliary catheter extends from the skin through the hepatic parenchyma into the biliary system and across the obstruction, with the tip of the catheter situated within the small bowel. Multiple side-holes along the distal two-thirds of the catheter (the functional portion) allow either external drainage of bile or internal flow of bile into the small bowel. Internal biliary drainage can be accomplished with the use of plastic or metal stents that can be placed percutaneously or endoscopically. The stent extends above and below the obstruction, allowing bile to flow in the normal direction into the small bowel.

Major complication rates associated with PTC and percutaneous placement of external or internal–external biliary drainage catheters range from 5% to 25%, and the incidence of procedure-related deaths is 0–6% (51). The major complications include hemobilia necessitating blood transfusion and cholangitis associated with hypotension. Hemobilia is the most common serious cause of postprocedure morbidity, occurring in 3–10% of cases.

Complications of percutaneous transhepatic biliary stenting can be divided into short- and long-term. Short-term complications include cholangitis (5–7% of cases), hemobilia (2%), and bile leakage (2%) (52,53). The incidence of periprocedural cholangitis can be reduced with the use of prophylactic intravenous antibiotics. Delayed cholangitis occurs with stent occlusion, which occurs more frequently with plastic than with metalstents (54). Hemobilia is usually self-limiting and rarely necessitates blood transfusion. If bleeding persists and is severe, angiography and arterial embolization can be utilized (49). Bile leakage is rarely significant, but when it does occur, it may signify stent occlusion. Because bile takes the path of least resistance, if flows in retrograde fashion and tracks either out to the skin surface or into the perihepatic space, where it can give rise to a subhepatic or subphrenic abscess. Although not seen routinely in the ICU setting, long-term complications of percutaneous placement of biliary stents include stent occlusion and migration and duodenal ulceration.

F. Percutaneous Gastrostomy

Percutaneous gastrostomy catheters are placed for two distinct indications in the intensive care setting: nutritional support and gastric drainage. In providing nutrition, gastrostomy feeds are less expensive and require less nutritional support than TPN (55). Complications of TPN, including sepsis and venous thrombosis, are avoided. In addition, TPN may be unsuitable for some patients who have difficulty with the requirements for strict maintenance of their lines and infusions. Percutaneous gastrostomy is particularly useful in malignancy, offering a useful route for nutritional support in patients with unresectable esophageal cancer and in those who have undergone radiotherapy for head and neck neoplasms, which may compromise swallowing function and limit caloric intake. A number of reports have shown that patients who undergo percutaneous gastrostomy maintain their weights significantly better than similar patients who do not receive gastrostomy feeding (56–58). Although this may not always translate into prolonged survival, improved clinical outcomes would be a logical expectation if nutrition can be maintained.

Patients with gastric outlet obstruction or more distal intestinal obstruction (e.g., unresectable neoplasm or multiple enteric strictures secondary to irradiation) may receive substantial palliation from placement of a gastrostomy tube. Gastrostomy tubes are used for evacuation of gastric and other gastrointestinal secretions that otherwise accumulate and lead to repeated bouts of vomiting (59,60). Some patients may have gastroparesis secondary to neural invasion or diabetes, resulting in similar clinical scenarios. Patients with gastric outlet obstruction and ongoing nutritional concerns may benefit from a dual lumen gastrojejunostomy catheter. The gastric (proximal) port serves as a drainage route for retained oral and gastric secretions and the jejunal (distal) port serves as a conduit for nutrition.

Although previously considered surgical procedure, placement of gastrostomy tubes can be done by a percutaneous approach with fluoroscopic or endoscopic guidance in a vast majority of cases (61–63). Overall, the percutaneous fluoroscopic technique used to insert gastrostomy tubes is efficient and safe, with success rates of 98% or greater and minor and major complication rates ranging from 1% to 12% and 1% to 6%, respectively (61,64–66). In a review of 92 consecutive outpatient gastrostomy tube insertions at The University of Texas M.D. Anderson Cancer Center over a 6-month period, the success rate was 98%, with a major complication rate of 1% and a minor complication rate of 8% (61). Tube malfunctions were encountered in 13%.

III. ARTERIAL INTERVENTIONS

Over the past two decades, the role of the interventional radiologist has shifted from diagnosis to therapy in the care of patients with cancer. While direct percutaneous therapeutic options have attracted interest in the past several years, the transcatheter approach continues to play a significant role in the treatment of these challenging patients. These techniques have traditionally included intra-arterial infusion, embolization, and chemoembolization. The delivery of therapeutic agents via the arterial system requires selective vascular catheterization, which is accomplished by tailoring the catheter configuration to the vascular anatomy. With improvements in catheter technology, coaxial microcatheter systems that range from 2 to 3 F in outer diameter can be delivered through 4–5 F standard angiographic catheters to facilitate the technical challenges involved in small-vessel catheterization. An additional advantage of these microcatheter systems is their potential for reducing arterial injuries (e.g., dissection and perforation) that can occur with larger catheters. While these transarterial infusions and embolizations are employed most commonly in the treatment of hepatic malignancy, they are also helpful preoperative means of reducing tumor burden and intraoperative blood loss. Nonhepatic embolizations also have been utilized for pain palliation for patients who are not candidates for surgical resection. Neoplastic, iatrogenic, and treatment-related hemorrhage can be controlled effectively with embolization techniques. Intra-arterial treatment of patients with malignancy requires close collaboration among the interventional radiologist, surgeon, oncologist, and intensivist to ensure the maximum potential benefit from these minimally invasive therapeutic options.

A. Embolization

The control of hemorrhage in patients with neoplastic disease is often a life-saving procedure and may provide an opportunity for more specific antitumor therapy by surgery, irradiation, or chemotherapy. Transarterial embolization involves the deliberate occlusion of the arterial supply to a site of hemorrhage or neoplasm. In the presence of hemorrhage, embolization is an effective tool to treat the arterial injury and avoid surgical intervention. The goal of embolization for tumor therapy is to create ischemia and tumor necrosis and to arrest tumor growth. Large-vessel (proximal) occlusion is typically accomplished by the intra-arterial delivery of metallic coils and gel-foam pieces, and small-vessel (peripheral) occlusion is typically carried out by injecting particulate materials or liquid embolic agents. Agents that result in small-vessel (peripheral) embolization are preferred for tumor therapy over materials used to occlude the larger central vessels.

A central (proximal) occlusion of a vessel near its origin has an effect similar to a surgical ligation, with immediate formation of collateral circulation. The more proximal the occlusion, the more abundant is the development of collateral circulation. Proximal embolizations are not, however, the best approach for intra-arterial therapy to treat neoplasms directly, because this approach ultimately restricts the ability to re-treat the neoplasm from the same artery and requires pursuit of the technically challenging collaterals for further therapy. For the treatment of patients with bleeding (e.g., ulcer, diverticulum, or trauma), the central embolic approach is desirable to reduce the arterial pressure at the bleeding site sufficiently so that hemostasis can be achieved. Development of a collateral arterial supply subsequent to the embolization is an added benefit in this particular application. Use of peripheral embolic agents would increase the risk of undesired tissue necrosis.

The more peripheral the embolization is to the tumor, the less the opportunity for collateral circulation and the greater the likelihood of tumor necrosis. While tumor necrosis is a desired effect, necrosis of adjacent nontarget tissue is not. Microcatheter coaxial systems allow subselective embolizations to access tumor vessels and avoid embolization of nontarget tissues. Peripheral embolization produces small-vessel occlusion without sacrificing the main arteries, allowing future re-embolization when necessary.

The indications for transcatheter embolization of neoplasms are (1) to control hemorrhage, (2) to facilitate surgical resection by decreasing blood loss and operating time, (3) to inhibit tumor growth, and (4) to relieve pain by decreasing tumor bulk.

The complications that arise from embolization can be related to the catheterization (e.g., pseudoaneurysm, arteriovenous fistula, dissection, thrombosis, and perforation) or to occlusion effects on tumor or nontarget arterial supply (e.g., pain, ischemia/infarction, and abscess). In a series by Hemingway and Allison (67) representing a 10-year experience with 284 patients undergoing 410 embolizations, minor complications occurred in 16%, serious complications in 6.6%, and death in 2%. The postembolization syndrome (i.e., fever, elevated white blood cell count, and discomfort) occurred after 42.7% of the procedures. The underlying abnormality and its location usually determined the nature and risk of complications.

1. Gastrointestinal Hemorrhage

Gastrointestinal hemorrhage from neoplasms is uncommon but can occur secondary to (1) primary bowel neoplasms, (2) direct invasion (see Refs. 68–70), or (3) metastases (see Ref. 71), or (4) as a complication of therapy such as hepatic chemoembolization (see Ref. 72). Numerous case reports in the literature support the use of embolotherapy to aid in the management of these difficult problems. Embolization can result in cessation of bleeding or dramatically reduce transfusion requirements. Low-grade chronic bleeding from a neoplasm may be managed by the intra-arterial infusion of chemotherapy directly to the tumor. Otherwise, embolization may be necessary, but this too has its limitations and its effect may be only temporary.

The intravenous infusion of vasopressin (Pitressin), the preferred treatment for bleeding from esophageal varices, is at times effective in the management of diffuse gastrointestinal hemorrhage as seen in patients with leukemia or lymphoma. Vasopressin causes vasoconstriction and contraction of the bowel wall smooth muscle. It also has a weak antidiuretic effect. Once the site of bleeding has been identified, an infusion of vasopressin is started at a rate of 0.2 units per min; this can be increased in 0.1-unit increments up to 0.6 units per min, but this is seldom necessary. This dose can result in intestinal, myocardial, and/or peripheral vascular ischemic complications.

Vasopressin given intravenously or intra-arterially is usually ineffective in the control of gastrointestinal bleeding from malignant neoplasms because the blood vessels of cancerous tissue lack a vasoconstriction (73). It is still an option, however, in bleeding from benign lesions in patients who are also afflicted with cancer (e.g., ulcers or diverticular bleeding).

Selective transarterial embolization for malignancy-related gastrointestinal hemorrhage is the preferred alternative when surgical management is not considered a viable option. Even in patients with cancer, the vast majority of gastrointestinal embolization procedures are done for bleeding of benign etiology. In general, arterial embolization is safe in the upper gastrointestinal tract owing to the rich arterial collateral supply. Patients who have undergone visceral surgery or have severe atherosclerotic disease may be at a higher risk for ischemic complications following embolotherapy. Surgical resection remains the standard treatment for gastrointestinal bleeding distal to the ligament of Treitz. In the past decade, improvements in interventional techniques as well as in catheter manufacturing technology have allowed safer superselective embolization within the lower gastrointestinal tract. This must be done with great care because ischemia with infarction might be a catastrophic complication (69,74,75). In five studies whose results were reported over the past decade (73,76–81), no occurrence of bowel infarction was identified in 87 patients who underwent transarterial embolization of small and large bowel distal to the ligament of Treitz (Fig. 3). Bowel ischemia was evident, however, in as many as 24% in a series of 35 patients reported by Bandi et al. (78).

Gastrointestinal bleeding from neoplasms of the liver, stomach, duodenum, or rectosigmoid as well as from radiation injury is most readily controlled by embolization of the hepatic, left and right gastric, gastroduodenal, superior and inferior pancreaticoduodenal, superior and inferior mesenteric, and/or bilateral internal iliac arteries. Occasionally, extremely selective limited embolization of short segments of the superior and inferior mesenteric arteries with a few (1,2) small segments of gel-foam may be possible. Both internal iliac arteries (the middle hemorrhoidal arteries bilaterally) as well as the hemorrhoidal branches of the inferior mesenteric artery might be embolized to control bleeding from a rectal neoplasm.

2. *Genitourinary Hemorrhage*

Hemorrhage from genitourinary neoplasms has been treated successfully in patients with neoplasms of the bladder, uterine cervix, or corpus, as has bleeding caused by irradiation cystitis (75). Pelage et al. (82) reported the distribution of uterine pathology of 197 women who underwent embolization, which included leiomyoma (67.5%), primary and secondary postpartum hemorrhage (25%), postabortion hemorrhage (2.5%), postoperative hemorrhage (1%), adenomyosis (1.5%), uterine malformation (0.5%), and pelvic malignancy (2%).

Chronic low-grade bleeding from a neoplasm may be managed by intra-arterial infusion of chemotherapy directly to the tumor. Embolization can be beneficial in the treatment of patients with gynecologic neoplasms, but its effect may be only temporary. Kramer et al. (83) reported their experience with embolization for hemorrhage in a series of 13 patients with advanced cervical carcinoma. In nine of the 13 patients (69%), the bleeding was controlled immediately with a single bilateral embolization treatment. One patient (7.7%) died during therapy secondary to uncontrolled bleeding. The remaining three patients (23%) showed slight persistent or recurrent bleeding that was controlled on follow-up intervention.

Iatrogenic bleeding within the pelvis also can be managed by endovascular techniques. Severe hemorrhagic cystitis is estimated to occur in fewer than 5% of patients following radiotherapy to the pelvis. Bilateral internal iliac embolization has been employed to control hemorrhage (75), as have simple bladder irrigation; cystodiathermy; oral, parenteral, and intravesical agents; hyperbaric oxygen therapy; hydrodistension; urinary diversion; and cystectomy (84). Bleeding secondary to a ureteroarterial fistula can occur in the

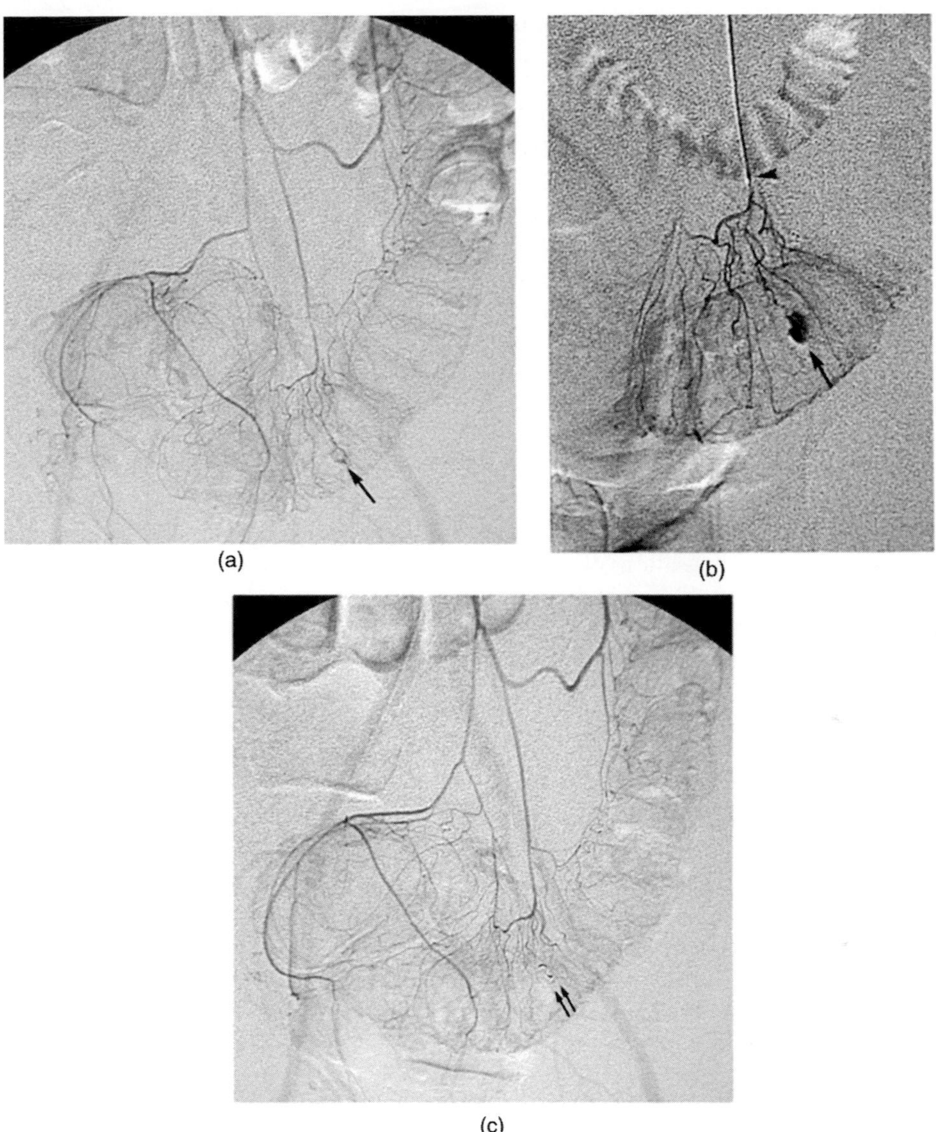

Figure 3 (a) Inferior mesenteric artery (IMA) arteriogram in a patient with a history of lower gastrointestinal bleeding demonstrates extralumenal pooling of contrast (*arrows*) in the rectosigmoid region of the large bowel representing the site of hemorrhage (a and b). (b) A superselective arteriogram with a 3 F microcatheter (arrowhead) in a sigmoid branch of the IMA. (c) IMA arteriography after microcoil (*double arrow*) embolization successful occlusion of the bleeding site.

presence of long-term ureterostomy diversion when the catheters erode into the adjacent iliac artery (85–87). Percutaneous management originally involved embolization of the affected iliac artery to control bleeding followed by extra-anatomic arterial bypass (85,87). More recently, covered stents have been used to exclude the fistula while maintaining patency of the involved iliac artery (86,88).

3. *Pulmonary Hemorrhage*

Pulmonary hemorrhage with blood loss of 600 mL/day is associated with a mortality rate of >50% (89), but even moderate hemoptysis with blood loss of 200 mL/day increases the risk of fatal hemorrhage. Bronchial artery embolization (BAE) has been utilized to control bleeding from malignancies, tuberculosis, bronchiectasis, arteriovenous malformations, mycetomas, and cystic fibrosis (90). Neoplasm as the cause of hemoptysis has ranged from 2% to 41% of cases in various studies (91–96). For patients with malignancy, the initial work-up should include CT in addition to bronchoscopy. Computed tomography can be utilized to assess the location and extent of malignancy to evaluate the pulmonary artery as an additional source of hemoptysis. Bronchoscopy is necessary to visualize and potentially treat the causative lesion or at least to localize the site of hemorrhage to the side or lobe of origin.

Technical success rates for BAE have ranged from 73% to 98% (91–96), and clinical success rate, defined as cessation of hemorrhage in the first 30 days after the procedure, from 51% to 85% (93–96). Rates of prolonged clinical success, defined as cessation of hemorrhage for longer than 30 days from embolization, have been reported as high as 82% (92), but the rate of recurrent hemorrhage requiring repeat embolization is approximately 16% (92,96).

Pulmonary hemorrhage secondary to irradiation even in the absence of residual or recurrent lung cancer can be controlled by selective embolization of the causative branches of the bronchial or pulmonary arteries. The site of bleeding can be established or confirmed by bronchoscopy. Frequently, extravasation of contrast material from a particular branch is not identified but there is local hypervascularity or abnormal vessels in the area of the bleeding. Embolization of these arteries may adequately control the hemorrhage.

IV. VENOUS INTERVENTIONS

Venous thromboembolic disease is a substantial health problem in the United States; the most lethal form, pulmonary embolus (PE), is diagnosed in 355,000 patients per year (97). Patients with malignancy are at greater risk for thromboembolic events than the general population. The clinical and imaging diagnosis of PE for ICU patients is often more problematic than its diagnosis among other less ill patients. The signs and symptoms along with ECG and chest x-ray findings are usually nonspecific. Furthermore, the sensitivity of clinical evaluation in the diagnosis of deep vein thrombosis (DVT) ranges from 60% to 96% and the specificity from 20% to 72% (98) stressing the need for supplemental diagnostic tools. Patients in the ICU are often ventilated and have more complex comorbid disease processes than the general patient, complicating the diagnosis of thromboembolic disease by noninvasive imaging techniques. Several options exist for documenting both DVT and PE, but controversies regarding diagnostic algorithms persist for all patients. The limitations of the available imaging modalities (ventilation perfusion [V/Q] scanning, spiral [helical] CT angiography [HCT], conventional pulmonary angiography, lower-extremity ultrasonography, and venography) necessitate correlation between the findings of these studies and the clinical pretest probability as part of a diagnostic algorithm.

A. Pulmonary Embolism and Thrombolysis

There is no clear consensus regarding the use of thrombolytic therapy in the management of patients with acute PE. Despite the effectiveness of heparin/warfarin, which has become the standard of care over the past three decades, the International Co-operative Pulmonary Embolism Registry in 1999 found a 17.4% 3-month mortality rate in its review of 2454 consecutive patients hospitalized for PE (99). This exemplifies the limitations of anticoagulation therapy and underscores the need for alternative therapeutic approaches. Traditional thrombolytic drugs include streptokinase (SK) and urokinase (UK), with more recent introduction of recombinant tissue plasminogen activators that include alteplase (t-PA), reteplase (r-PA), and tenecteplase (TNK). The potential advantages of these lytic agents include the rapid reduction in thrombus burden with restoration of pulmonary flow and subsequent improvement in gas exchange and hemodynamic compromise associated with PE.

Several studies have demonstrated rapid reductions in thrombus burden within the first several hours of lytic therapy but have failed to show any significant improvement after 24 hr with regards to clot resolution, PE recurrence, or morbidity when compared to conventional anticoagulation therapy (100–102). In a small series recently reported by Sharma et al. (103), 23 patients initially randomized to receive intravenous heparin or thrombolytic therapy were re-evaluated after a mean follow-up of 7.4 years. Their results demonstrated that resting pulmonary artery mean pressure and pulmonary vascular resistance were significantly higher in the heparin group. Both parameters increased significantly upon exercise in the heparin group but not in the thrombolytic group suggesting that thrombolytic therapy can preserve the normal hemodynamic response to exercise.

The most obvious benefit of thrombolytic therapy in the acute setting is in those patients with massive, life-threatening PE, and hemodynamic compromise. Jerjes-Sanchez et al. reported eight patients with hemodynamic instability who were randomized to receive either heparin ($n = 4$) or SK ($n = 4$). The four patients who received SK improved in the first hour after treatment, survived, and in 2 years of follow-up were without pulmonary arterial hypertension. All four patients treated with heparin alone died 1–3 hr after presentation ($P = 0.02$). Necropsy performed on three of the four patients demonstrated right ventricular infarction without evidence of coronary arterial obstruction.

The optimal thrombolytic agent, dosing regimen, and mode of delivery have yet to be determined.

Several series have demonstrated no significant differences in efficacy among SK, UK, and t-PA when equivalent doses were utilized (104–107). The mechanism of action of these agents revolves around the conversion, either directly or indirectly, of plasminogen to plasmin (108). Dosing regimens have included bolus administration, short infusion ($\leq$2 hr) and prolonged infusion for as long as 24–72 hr (109). The majority of reported series have utilized systemic administration of thrombolytic agents rather than intrapulmonary administration. The theoretical advantages of local delivery into the pulmonary circulation or into the thrombus itself is the potential for increasing the efficacy of lysis and lowering the total dose of the thrombolytic agents required, thus reducing hemorrhagic complications. The disadvantage of this technique is the procedural risk of inserting a catheter into the pulmonary artery and the risk of bleeding at the venous access site.

Only one randomized controlled study has compared intrapulmonary and systemic thrombolytic administration in patients with massive PE. Both groups received an initial dose of 50 mg over 2 hr with a repeat dose of 50 mg over 5 hr if insufficient improvement was identified on follow-up angiography. There were no significant differences in improvements in pulmonary artery pressure and pulmonary perfusion or in the risk of major hemorrhage between the two groups (110). In the past decade, transcatheter techniques have emerged in the management of DVT demonstrating their safety and efficacy (111,112). These catheter-based techniques were utilized in a small series of patients, where low-dose UK or t-PA was administered into the embolus in six patients with contraindications to systemic thrombolysis. Neither fibrinogenolysis nor bleeding occurred and all patients demonstrated at least 20% angiographic improvement by after 1 hr and 50–90% improvement after 24 hr (113). In a similar series of 13 patients reported by Molina et al. (114), UK administered at a dose of 2200 U/kg/hr into the thrombus for as long 24 hr resulted in complete lysis without hemorrhagic complications. While the currently available data do not support selective intrapulmonary or, more specifically, intrathrombus infusion of thrombolytic agents, further research is required to determine their places among the strategies for treating patients with PE.

In identifying patients who will benefit the most from thrombolytic therapy, right ventricular dysfunction is now being utilized as an indicator of PE severity and risk of death. Approximately 50% of patients with PE and normal systemic arterial pressure have signs of right ventricular hypokinesis at presentation. Patients with right ventricular hypokinesis are at a significantly higher risk for death from PE (99). The use of thrombolytic therapy in this subset of patients is supported by several studies (99,115), whose results show that mortality rates and recurrent PE rates were significantly better for patients receiving thrombolytic agents than for those receiving heparin alone. In one series of 719 patients (thrombolytics $n = 169$ and heparin $n = 550$), the 30-day mortality rate was significantly lower in the thrombolytic cohort (4.7% vs. 11.1%) (115).

The major limitation of thrombolytic therapy in the treatment of all patients with PE is the increased risk of major bleeding complications most notably intracranial hemorrhage. Pooled data suggest that the average incidence of hemorrhagic complications is 6.3% for thrombolysis and 1.8% for heparin-based therapy, with similar rates of bleeding demonstrated for SK, UK, and t-PA (109). Contraindications for thrombolytic therapy include recent cerebrovascular accident or intracranial surgery (<2 months), active intracranial abnormality (neoplasm, aneurysm, or vascular malformation), or recent major hemorrhage. Other relative contraindications include uncontrolled hypertension, recent major surgery or trauma, pregnancy pericarditis, and hemorrhagic retinopathy.

For patients with massive PE and a contraindication for thrombolysis and surgical embolectomy, other less invasive percutaneous approaches are available to debulk central emboli by fragmentation or aspiration. Fragmentation has been used to relieve central obstruction by redistributing emboli into peripheral pulmonary arteries to acutely improve cardiopulmonary hemodynamics and thus increase pulmonary blood flow and right ventricular function (116,117). Newer low-profile devices are now available to debulk emboli by various mechanisms. These devices, their mechanisms of action, and their clinical utility have been reported in the literature (118–120) and are beyond the scope of this discussion. The use of these devices and their "success" in the management of massive PE have been described only in case reports and small series (121–126).

B. Vena Cava Filters

Anticoagulation remains the therapy of choice for venous thromboembolic disease, with an expected risk of major hemorrhage of <5% in patients with no underlying sources of known active or potential bleeding (127). In this subset of patients, the inferior vena cava (IVC) filter is an effective method of reducing the risk of life-threatening PE in those with a contraindication to anticoagulation and those who experience PE despite adequate anticoagulation. The accepted indications for IVC filter placement include (1) contraindication to anticoagulation, (2) recurrent thromboembolic disease

Table 1 FDA Approved Inferior Vena Cava Filters

Filter	Manufacturer	FDA approved
Stainless steel Greenfield—original	Medi Tech	1973
Titanium Greenfield	Medi Tech	1989
Stainless steel Greenfield—low profile	Medi Tech	1995
Bird's Nest	Cook	1983
Simon Nitinol	Bard	1988
Vena Tech	B Braun	1989
Vena Tech—low profile	B Braun	2001
Trapease	Cordis	2000
Gunther Tulip	Cook	2001

despite anticoagulation therapy, and (3) significant complication from anticoagulation therapy. Relative indications include (1) large free-floating iliocaval thrombus, (2) chronic thromboembolic disease prior to pulmonary embolectomy, (3) thromboembolic disease with limited cardiopulmonary reserve (cor pulmonale), (4) poor compliance with medications,(5) prophylactic indications, that is, high risk for thromboembolic disease including massive trauma (head and spinal cord injury, pelvic and lower-extremity fractures), or history of thromboembolic disease with upcoming surgery, (6) recurrent PE despite IVC filter, and (7) DVT thrombolysis. Absolute contraindications to IVC filter placement include a chronically thrombosed IVC or lack of an adequate access route to place a filter.

The majority of IVC filters are placed by an interventional radiologist under fluoroscopic guidance. Since development of the Greenfield filter in 1972, nine

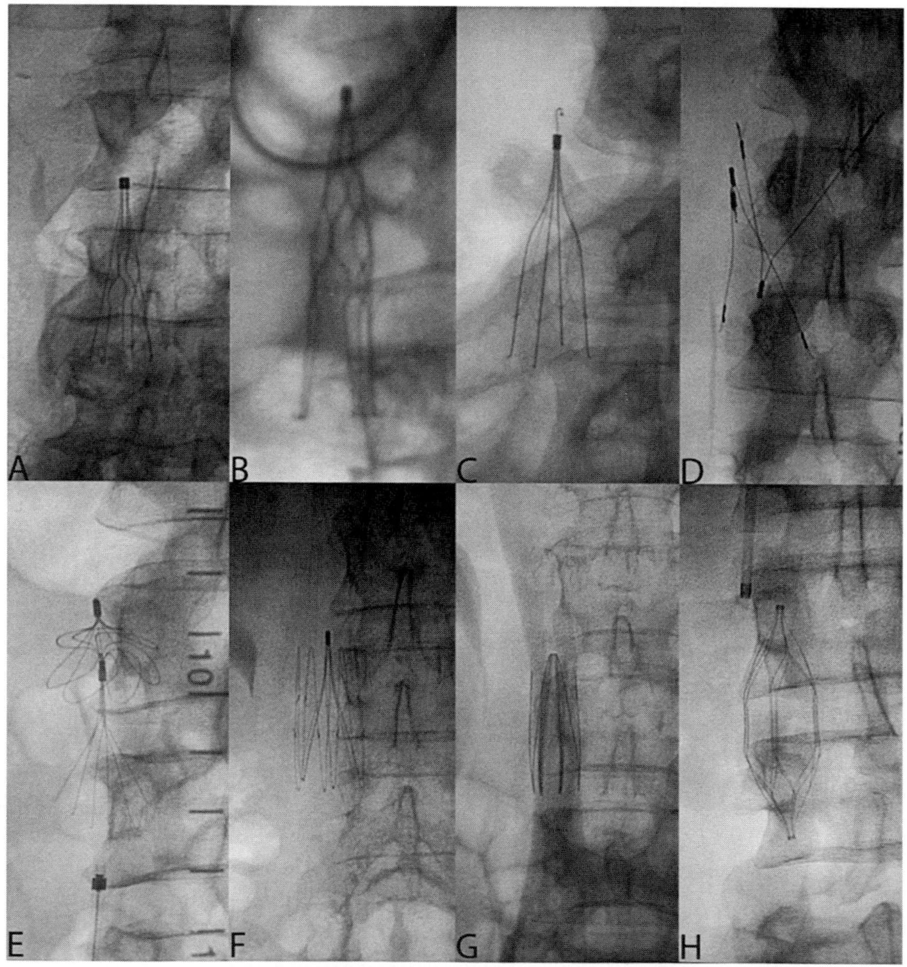

Figure 4 Frontal radiographic views of eight commercially available filters. (A) Stainless steel Greenfield filter, (B) Titanium Greenfield filter, (C) Gunther Tulip filter, (D) Bird's Nest filter, (E) Simon Nitinol filter, (F) Vena Tech-low profile filter, (G) Vena Tech filter, and (H) Trapease filter.

filters have been approved by the U.S. Food and Drug Administration and are available for use in the United States (Table 1 and Fig. 4). The delivery system of the initial version of the Greenfield filter was 29.5 F in outer diameter, while newer versions of the Greenfield filter are delivered through a 14 F system. Many of the delivery systems of the more recent filters range in outer diameter from 8 to 14 F and can be placed from the femoral, jugular, or antecubital vein approach. The majority of the available filters are constructed of non-ferromagnetic material and are considered safe for MRI imaging. Only the stainless steel Greenfield filter and the Bird's Nest filter are constructed of stainless steel and produce substantial MRI artifact. MRI can be performed safely in patients with these types of filters, but a delay as long as 6 weeks from implantation to imaging has been recommended by the manufacturer of the Bird's Nest filter.

In ex vivo tests, Katsamouris et al. (128) demonstrated that the Bird's Nest filter and the Simon Nitinol filter were the most efficient, while Hammer et al. (129) concluded that the Bird's Nest filter had the highest clot-trapping capacity. The reported rates of clinically relevant postfilter PE range from 3.3% to 5.6% (79,130,131), while just under 2.5% of these are fatal (130,131). No randomized clinical trial has stratified patients with associated risk factors and those on concomitant anticoagulation therapy to adequately compare the various filter designs with respect to recurrence of PE and other complications such as caval or access site thrombosis. IVC thrombosis can be caused by thrombus formation on the filter itself but is more likely due to entrapped thrombus that has embolized from the pelvis or lower extremities. The rate of caval thrombosis varies dramatically depending on the diligence of the follow-up and the definition. In several large series that used multiple filter designs, the thrombosis rate ranged from 2.7% to 19% (130,131).

REFERENCES

1. Sirinek KR. Diagnosis and treatment of intra-abdominal abscesses. Surg Infect (Larchmt) 2000; 1(1):31–38.
2. Branum GD, Tyson GS, Branum MA, Meyers WC. Hepatic abscess. Changes in etiology, diagnosis, and management. Ann Surg 1990; 212(6):655–662.
3. Altemeier WA, Culbertson WR, Fullen WD, Shook CD. Intra-abdominal abscesses. Am J Surg 1973; 125(1):70–79.
4. Men S, Akhan O, Koroglu M. Percutaneous drainage of abdominal abscess. Eur J Radiol 2002; 43(3): 204–218.
5. Lee MJ. Non-traumatic abdominal emergencies: imaging and intervention in sepsis. Eur Radiol 2002; 12(9):2172–2179.
6. vanSonnenberg E, Wittich GR, Goodacre BW, Casola G, D'Agostino HB. Percutaneous abscess drainage: update. World J Surg 2001; 25(3):362–369; discussion 370–372.
7. Knochel JQ, Koehler PR, Lee TG, Welch DM. Diagnosis of abdominal abscesses with computed tomography, ultrasound, and 111In leukocyte scans. Radiology 1980; 137(2):425–432.
8. Haaga JR, Alfidi RJ, Havrilla TR, Cooperman AM, Seidelmann FE, Reich NE, et al. CT detection and aspiration of abdominal abscesses. AJR Am J Roentgenol 1977; 128(3):465–474.
9. Dobrin PB, Gully PH, Greenlee HB, Freeark RJ, Moncada R, Churchill R, et al. Radiologic diagnosis of an intra-abdominal abscess. Do multiple tests help?Arch Surg 1986; 121(1):41–46.
10. Roche J. Effectiveness of computed tomography in the diagnosis of intra-abdominal abscess: a review of 111 patients. Med J Aust 1981; 2(2):85–86, 87–88.
11. Carroll B, Silverman PM, Goodwin DA, McDougall IR. Ultrasonography and indium 111 white blood cell scanning for the detection of intraabdominal abscesses. Radiology 1981; 140(1):155–160.
12. Bernini A, Spencer MP, Wong WD, Rothenberger DA, Madoff RD. Computed tomography-guided percutaneous abscess drainage in intestinal disease: factors associated with outcome. Dis Colon Rectum 1997; 40(9):1009–1013.
13. Cinat ME, Wilson SE, Din AM. Determinants for successful percutaneous image-guided drainage of intra-abdominal abscess. Arch Surg 2002; 137(7):845–849.
14. Freeny PC, Hauptmann E, Althaus SJ, Traverso LW, Sinanan M. Percutaneous CT-guided catheter drainage of infected acute necrotizing pancreatitis: techniques and results. AJR Am J Roentgenol 1998; 170(4): 969–975.
15. Alexander AA, Eschelman DJ, Nazarian LN, Bonn J. Transrectal sonographically guided drainage of deep pelvic abscesses. AJR Am J Roentgenol 1994; 162(5): 1227–1230; discussion 1231–1232.
16. Varghese JC, O'Neill MJ, Gervais DA, Boland GW, Mueller PR. Transvaginal catheter drainage of tuboovarian abscess using the trocar method: technique and literature review. AJR Am J Roentgenol 2001; 177(1): 139–144.
17. vanSonnenberg E, D'Agostino HB, Casola G, Goodacre BW, Sanchez RB, Taylor B. US-guided transvaginal drainage of pelvic abscesses and fluid collections. Radiology 1991; 181(1):53–56.
18. Walser E, Savage C, Zwischenberger JB. Thoracic imaging in the ICU. Interventional radiology. Chest Surg Clin N Am 2002; 12(2):209–226, v.
19. Moulton JS, Moore PT, Mencini RA. Treatment of loculated pleural effusions with transcatheter

intracavitary urokinase. AJR Am J Roentgenol 1989; 153(5):941–945.
20. Park CS, Chung WM, Lim MK, Cho CH, Suh CH, Chung WK. Transcatheter instillation of urokinase into loculated pleural effusion: analysis of treatment effect. AJR Am J Roentgenol 1996; 167(3):649–652.
21. Chin NK, Lim TK. Controlled trial of intrapleural streptokinase in the treatment of pleural empyema and complicated parapneumonic effusions. Chest 1997; 111(2):275–279.
22. Ramchandani P, Cardella JF, Grassi CJ, Roberts AC, Sacks D, Schwartzberg MS, et al. Quality improvement guidelines for percutaneous nephrostomy. J Vasc Interv Radiol 2001; 12(11):1247–1251.
23. Yoder IC, Pfister RC, Lindfors KK, Newhouse JH. Pyonephrosis: imaging and intervention. AJR Am J Roentgenol 1983; 141(4):735–740.
24. Yoder IC, Lindfors KK, Pfister RC. Diagnosis and treatment of pyonephrosis. Radiol Clin North Am 1984; 22(2):407–414.
25. Camunez F, Echenagusia A, Prieto ML, Salom P, Herranz F, Hernandez C. Percutaneous nephrostomy in pyonephrosis. Urol Radiol 1989; 11(2):77–81.
26. Pearle MS, Pierce HL, Miller GL, Summa JA, Mutz JM, Petty BA, et al. Optimal method of urgent decompression of the collecting system for obstruction and infection due to ureteral calculi. J Urol 1998; 160(4):1260–1264.
27. Zagoria RJ, Hodge RG, Dyer RB, Routh WD. Percutaneous nephrostomy for treatment of intractable hemorrhagic cystitis. J Urol 1993; 149(6):1449–1451.
28. Farrell TA, Hicks ME. A review of radiologically guided percutaneous nephrostomies in 303 patients. J Vasc Interv Radiol 1997; 8(5):769–774.
29. Lee WJ, Patel U, Patel S, Pillari GP. Emergency percutaneous nephrostomy: results and complications. J Vasc Interv Radiol 1994; 5(1):135–139.
30. Gerspach JM, Bellman GC, Stoller ML, Fugelso P. Conservative management of colon injury following percutaneous renal surgery. Urology 1997; 49(6): 831–836.
31. Akhan O, Akinci D, Ozmen MN. Percutaneous cholecystostomy. Eur J Radiol 2002; 43(3):229–236.
32. Gilliland TM, Traverso LW. Modern standards for comparison of cholecystectomy with alternative treatments for symptomatic cholelithiasis with emphasis on long-term relief of symptoms. Surg Gynecol Obstet 1990; 170(1):39–44.
33. Pickleman J, Gonzalez RP. The improving results of cholecystectomy. Arch Surg 1986; 121(8):930–934.
34. Hatzidakis AA, Prassopoulos P, Petinarakis I, Sanidas E, Chrysos E, Chalkiadakis G, et al. Acute cholecystitis in high-risk patients: percutaneous cholecystostomy vs conservative treatment. Eur Radiol 2002; 12(7): 1778–1784.
35. vanSonnenberg E, D'Agostino HB, Goodacre BW, Sanchez RB, Casola G. Percutaneous gallbladder puncture and cholecystostomy: results, complications, and caveats for safety. Radiology 1992; 183(1): 167–170.
36. van Overhagen H, Meyers H, Tilanus HW, Jeekel J, Lameris JS. Percutaneous cholecystectomy for patients with acute cholecystitis and an increased surgical risk. Cardiovasc Intervent Radiol 1996; 19(2): 72–76.
37. Mendez A, Mancera-Maldonado JL, Castaneda F. Complications of percutaneous cholecystostomy. Semin Intervent Radiol 1994; 11:283–286.
38. Boland GW, Lee MJ, Leung J, Mueller PR. Percutaneous cholecystostomy in critically ill patients: early response and final outcome in 82 patients. AJR Am J Roentgenol 1994; 163(2):339–342.
39. vanSonnenberg E, D'Agostino HB, Casola G, Varney RR, Ainge GD. Interventional radiology in the gallbladder: diagnosis, drainage, dissolution, and management of stones. Radiology 1990; 174(1):1–6.
40. Werbel GB, Nahrwold DL, Joehl RJ, Vogelzang RL, Rege RV. Percutaneous cholecystostomy in the diagnosis and treatment of acute cholecystitis in the high-risk patient. Arch Surg 1989; 124(7):782–785; discussion 785–786.
41. Menu Y, Vuillerme MP. Non-traumatic abdominal emergencies: imaging and intervention in acute biliary conditions. Eur Radiol 2002; 12(10):2397–2406.
42. McGahan JP, Lindfors KK. Acute cholecystitis: diagnostic accuracy of percutaneous aspiration of the gallbladder. Radiology 1988; 167(3):669–671.
43. McGahan JP, Lindfors KK. Percutaneous cholecystostomy: an alternative to surgical cholecystostomy for acute cholecystitis? Radiology 1989; 173(2):481–485.
44. England RE, McDermott VG, Smith TP, Suhocki PV, Payne CS, Newman GE. Percutaneous cholecystostomy: who responds? AJR Am J Roentgenol 1997; 168(5):1247–1251.
45. Gervais DA, Gazelle GS, Lu DS, Han PF, Mueller PR. Percutaneous transpulmonary CT-guided liver biopsy: a safe and technically easy approach for lesions located near the diaphragm. AJR Am J Roentgenol 1996; 167(2):482–483.
46. Patel M, Miedema BW, James MA, Marshall JB. Percutaneous cholecystostomy is an effective treatment for high-risk patients with acute cholecystitis. Am Surg 2000; 66(1):33–37.
47. Avrahami R, Badani E, Watemberg S, Nudelman I, Deutsch AA, Rabin E, et al. The role of percutaneous transhepatic cholecystostomy in the management of acute cholecystitis in high-risk patients. Int Surg 1995; 80(2):111–114.
48. Chang L, Moonka R, Stelzner M. Percutaneous cholecystostomy for acute cholecystitis in veteran patients. Am J Surg 2000; 180(3):198–202.
49. Cowling MG, Adam AN. Internal stenting in malignant biliary obstruction. World J Surg 2001; 25(3):355–359; discussion 359–361.
50. Madoff DC, Wallace MJ. Palliative treatment of unresectable bile duct cancer: which stent? Which

approach? Surg Oncol Clin N Am 2002; 11(4): 923–939.
51. Venbrux AC, Osterman FA, eds. Percutaneous Transhepatic Cholangiography and Percutaneous Biliary Drainage: Step by Step. Fairfax: The Society of Cardiovascular and Interventional Radiology, 1995.
52. Adam A, Chetty N, Roddie M, Yeung E, Benjamin IS. Self-expandable stainless steel endoprostheses for treatment of malignant bile duct obstruction. AJR Am J Roentgenol 1991; 156(2):321–325.
53. Nicholson AA, Royston CM. Palliation of inoperable biliary obstruction with self-expanding metal endoprostheses: a review of 77 patients. Clin Radiol 1993; 47(4):245–250.
54. Knyrim K, Wagner HJ, Pausch J, Vakil N. A prospective, randomized, controlled trial of metal stents for malignant obstruction of the common bile duct. Endoscopy 1993; 25(3):207–212.
55. Ho SG, Marchinkow LO, Legiehn GM, Munk PL, Lee MJ. Radiological percutaneous gastrostomy. Clin Radiol 2001; 56(11):902–910.
56. Lee JH, Machtay M, Unger LD, Weinstein GS, Weber RS, Chalian AA, et al. Prophylactic gastrostomy tubes in patients undergoing intensive irradiation for cancer of the head and neck. Arch Otolaryngol Head Neck Surg 1998; 124(8):871–875.
57. Lees J. Nasogastric and percutaneous endoscopic gastrostomy feeding in head and neck cancer patients receiving radiotherapy treatment at a regional oncology unit: a two year study. Eur J Cancer Care (Engl) 1997; 6(1):45–49.
58. Tyldesley S, Sheehan F, Munk P, Tsang V, Skarsgard D, Bowman CA, et al. The use of radiologically placed gastrostomy tubes in head and neck cancer patients receiving radiotherapy. Int J Radiat Oncol Biol Phys 1996; 36(5):1205–1209.
59. McFarland EG, Lee MJ, Boland GW, Mueller PR. Gastropexy breakdown and peritonitis after percutaneous gastrojejunostomy in a patient with ascites. AJR Am J Roentgenol 1995; 164(1):189–193.
60. Ho CS, Yeung EY. Percutaneous gastrostomy and transgastric jejunostomy. AJR Am J Roentgenol 1992; 158(2):251–257.
61. Beaver ME, Myers JN, Griffenberg L, Waugh K. Percutaneous fluoroscopic gastrostomy tube placement in patients with head and neck cancer. Arch Otolaryngol Head Neck Surg 1998; 124(10):1141–1144.
62. Ponsky JL, Gauderer MW, Stellato TA. Percutaneous endoscopic gastrostomy. Review of 150 cases. Arch Surg 1983; 118(8):913–914.
63. Preshaw RM. A percutaneous method for inserting a feeding gastrostomy tube. Surg Gynecol Obstet 1981; 152(5):658–660.
64. Hicks ME, Surratt RS, Picus D, Marx MV, Lang EV. Fluoroscopically guided percutaneous gastrostomy and gastroenterostomy: analysis of 158 consecutive cases. AJR Am J Roentgenol 1990; 154(4):725–728.
65. Ho CS, Gray RR, Goldfinger M, Rosen IE, McPherson R. Percutaneous gastrostomy for enteral feeding. Radiology 1985; 156(2):349–351.
66. Wills JS, Oglesby JT. Percutaneous gastrostomy. Radiology 1983; 149(2):449–453.
67. Hemingway AP, Allison DJ. Complications of embolization: analysis of 410 procedures. Radiology 1988; 166(3):669–672.
68. Hashimoto M, Watanabe G, Matsuda M, Yamamoto T, Tsutsumi K, Tsurumaru M. Case report: gastrointestinal bleeding from a hepatocellular carcinoma invading the transverse colon. J Gastroenterol Hepatol 1996; 11(8):765–767.
69. Yamada K, Tohyama H, Shizawa Y, Kohno M, Fukunishi Y, Tomoe M. Direct duodenal invasion of hepatocellular carcinoma. Intestinal hemorrhage treated by transcatheter arterial embolization. Clin Imaging 1998; 22(3):196–199.
70. Spinosa DJ, Angle JF, McGraw JK, Maurer EJ, Hagspiel KD, Matsumoto AH. Transcatheter treatment of life-threatening lower gastrointestinal bleeding due to advanced pelvic malignancy. Cardiovasc Intervent Radiol 1998; 21(6):503–505.
71. Gordon B, Lossef SV, Jelinger E, Barth KH. Embolotherapy for small bowel hemorrhage from metastatic renal cell carcinoma: case report. Cardiovasc Intervent Radiol 1991; 14(5):311–313.
72. Lin DY, Hung CF, Chen PC, Wu CS. Gastrointestinal bleeding after hepatic transcatheter arterial embolization in patients with hepatocellular carcinoma. Gastrointest Endosc 1996; 43(2 Pt 1):132–137.
73. Gordon RL, Ahl KL, Kerlan RK, Wilson MW, LaBerge JM, Sandhu JS, et al. Selective arterial embolization for the control of lower gastrointestinal bleeding. Am J Surg 1997; 174(1):24–28.
74. Srivastava DN, Gandhi D, Julka PK, Tandon RK. Gastrointestinal hemorrhage in hepatocellular carcinoma: management with transheptic arterioembolization. Abdom Imaging 2000; 25(4):380–384.
75. Schwartz PE, Goldstein HM, Wallace S, Rutledge FN. Control of arterial hemorrhage using percutaneous arterial catheter techniques in patients with gynecologic malignancies. Gynecol Oncol 1975; 3(4):276–288.
76. Peck DJ, McLoughlin RF, Hughson MN, Rankin RN. Percutaneous embolotherapy of lower gastrointestinal hemorrhage. J Vasc Interv Radiol 1998; 9(5):747–751.
77. Evangelista PT, Hallisey MJ. Transcatheter embolization for acute lower gastrointestinal hemorrhage. J Vasc Interv Radiol 2000; 11(5):601–606.
78. Bandi R, Shetty PC, Sharma RP, Burke TH, Burke MW, Kastan D. Superselective arterial embolization for the treatment of lower gastrointestinal hemorrhage. J Vasc Interv Radiol 2001; 12(12):1399–1405.
79. Greenfield LJ, Proctor MC. Twenty-year clinical experience with the Greenfield filter. Cardiovasc Surg 1995; 3(2):199–205.

80. Gupta S, Rajak CL, Sood BP, Gulati M, Rajwanshi A, Suri S. Sonographically guided fine needle aspiration biopsy of abdominal lymph nodes: experience in 102 patients. J Ultrasound Med 1999; 18(2):135–139.
81. Guy GE, Shetty PC, Sharma RP, Burke MW, Burke TH. Acute lower gastrointestinal hemorrhage: treatment by superselective embolization with polyvinyl alcohol particles. AJR Am J Roentgenol 1992; 159(3):521–526.
82. Pelage JP, Le Dref O, Soyer P, Jacob D, Kardache M, Dahan H, et al. Arterial anatomy of the female genital tract: variations and relevance to transcatheter embolization of the uterus. AJR Am J Roentgenol 1999; 172(4):989–994.
83. Kramer SC, Gorich J, Rilinger N, Heilmann V, Sokiranski R, Aschoff AJ, et al. [Interventional treatment of hemorrhages in advanced cervical carcinoma]. Radiologe 1999; 39(9):795–798.
84. Crew JP, Jephcott CR, Reynard JM. Radiation-induced haemorrhagic cystitis. Eur Urol 2001; 40(2):111–123.
85. Quillin SP, Darcy MD, Picus D. Angiographic evaluation and therapy of ureteroarterial fistulas. AJR Am J Roentgenol 1994; 162(4):873–878.
86. Feuer DS, Ciocca RG, Nackman GB, Siegel RL, Graham AM. Endovascular management of ureteroarterial fistula. J Vasc Surg 1999; 30(6):1146–1149.
87. Gheiler EL, Tefilli MV, Tiguert R, Friedland MS, Frontera RC, Pontes JE. Angiographic arterial occlusion and extra-anatomical vascular bypass for the management of a ureteral-iliac fistula: case report and review of the literature. Urol Int 1998; 61(1): 62–66.
88. Madoff DC, Toombs BD, Skolkin MD, Bodurka DC, Modesitt SC, Wood CG, et al. Endovascular management of ureteral-iliac artery fistulae with Wallgraft endoprostheses. Gynecol Oncol 2002; 85(1):212–217.
89. Jean-Baptiste E. Clinical assessment and management of massive hemoptysis. Crit Care Med 2000; 28(5): 1642–1647.
90. Remy J, Voisin C, Dupuis C, Beguery P, Tonnel AB, Denies JL, et al. [Treatment of hemoptysis by embolization of the systemic circulation]. Ann Radiol (Paris) 1974; 17(1):5–16.
91. Hayakawa K, Tanaka F, Torizuka T, Mitsumori M, Okuno Y, Matsui A, et al. Bronchial artery embolization for hemoptysis: immediate and long-term results. Cardiovasc Intervent Radiol 1992; 15(3):154–158; Discussion 158–159.
92. Cremaschi P, Nascimbene C, Vitulo P, Catanese C, Rota L, Barazzoni GC, et al. Therapeutic embolization of bronchial artery: a successful treatment in 209 cases of relapse hemoptysis. Angiology 1993; 44(4):295–299.
93. Ramakantan R, Bandekar VG, Gandhi MS, Aulakh BG, Deshmukh HL. Massive hemoptysis due to pulmonary tuberculosis: control with bronchial artery embolization. Radiology 1996; 200(3):691–694.
94. Mal H, Rullon I, Mellot F, Brugiere O, Sleiman C, Menu Y, et al. Immediate and long-term results of bronchial artery embolization for life-threatening hemoptysis. Chest 1999; 115(4):996–1001.
95. Swanson KL, Johnson CM, Prakash UB, McKusick MA, Andrews JC, Stanson AW. Bronchial artery embolization: experience with 54 patients. Chest 2002; 121(3):789–795.
96. Yu-Tang Goh P, Lin M, Teo N, En Shen Wong D. Embolization for hemoptysis: a six-year review. Cardiovasc Intervent Radiol 2002; 25(1):17–25.
97. Bick RL. Hereditary and acquired thrombophilia. Part I. Preface. Semin Thromb Hemost 1999; 25(3): 251–253.
98. Anand SS, Wells PS, Hunt D, Brill-Edwards P, Cook D, Ginsberg JS. Does this patient have deep vein thrombosis? JAMA 1998; 279(14):1094–1099.
99. Goldhaber SZ, Visani L, De Rosa M. Acute pulmonary embolism: clinical outcomes in the International Cooperative Pulmonary Embolism Registry (ICOPER). Lancet 1999; 353(9162):1386–1389.
100. Urokinase pulmonary embolism trial. Phase 1 results: a cooperative study. JAMA 1970; 214(12):2163–2172.
101. Levine M, Hirsh J, Weitz J, Cruickshank M, Neemeh J, Turpie AG, et al. A randomized trial of a single bolus dosage regimen of recombinant tissue plasminogen activator in patients with acute pulmonary embolism. Chest 1990; 98(6):1473–1479.
102. Dalla-Volta S, Palla A, Santolicandro A, Giuntini C, Pengo V, Visioli O, et al. PAIMS 2: alteplase combined with heparin versus heparin in the treatment of acute pulmonary embolism. Plasminogen activator Italian multicenter study 2. J Am Coll Cardiol 1992; 20(3):520–526.
103. Sharma GV, Folland ED, McIntyre KM, Sasahara AA. Long-term benefit of thrombolytic therapy in patients with pulmonary embolism. Vasc Med 2000; 5(2):91–95.
104. Urokinase-streptokinase embolism trial. Phase 2 results. A cooperative study. JAMA 1974; 229(12):1606–1613.
105. Goldhaber SZ, Kessler CM, Heit J, Markis J, Sharma GV, Dawley D, et al. Randomised controlled trial of recombinant tissue plasminogen activator versus urokinase in the treatment of acute pulmonary embolism. Lancet 1988; 2(8606):293–298.
106. Goldhabert SZ, Kessler CM, Heit JA, Elliott CG, Friedenberg WR, Heiselman DE, et al. Recombinant tissue-type plasminogen activator versus a novel dosing regimen of urokinase in acute pulmonary embolism: a randomized controlled multicenter trial. J Am Coll Cardiol 1992; 20(1):24–30.
107. Meneveau N, Schiele F, Metz D, Valette B, Attali P, Vuillemenot A, et al. Comparative efficacy of a two-hour regimen of streptokinase versus alteplase in acute massive pulmonary embolism: immediate clinical and hemodynamic outcome and one-year follow-up. J Am Coll Cardiol 1998; 31(5):1057–1063.

108. Hyers TM, Agnelli G, Hull RD, Morris TA, Samama M, Tapson V, et al. Antithrombotic therapy for venous thromboembolic disease. Chest 2001; 119 (1 suppl):176S–193S.
109. Arcasoy SM, Kreit JW. Thrombolytic therapy of pulmonary embolism: a comprehensive review of current evidence. Chest 1999; 115(6):1695–1707.
110. Verstraete M, Miller GA, Bounameaux H, Charbonnier B, Colle JP, Lecorf G, et al. Intravenous and intrapulmonary recombinant tissue-type plasminogen activator in the treatment of acute massive pulmonary embolism. Circulation 1988; 77(2):353–360.
111. Semba CP, Dake MD. Iliofemoral deep venous thrombosis: aggressive therapy with catheter-directed thrombolysis. Radiology 1994; 191(2):487–494.
112. Mewissen MW, Seabrook GR, Meissner MH, Cynamon J, Labropoulos N, Haughton SH. Catheter-directed thrombolysis for lower extremity deep venous thrombosis: report of a national multicenter registry. Radiology 1999; 211(1):39–49.
113. Tapson V, Davidson C, Bauman R, et al. Rapid thrombolysis of massive pulmonary emboli without systemic fibrinogenolysis: intra-embolic infusion of thrombolytic therapy (Abstract). Am Rev Respir Dis 1992; 145:A719.
114. Molina JE, Hunter DW, Yedlicka JW, Cerra FB. Thrombolytic therapy for postoperative pulmonary embolism. Am J Surg 1992; 163(4):375–380; discussion 380–381.
115. Konstantinides S, Geibel A, Olschewski M, Heinrich F, Grosser K, Rauber K, et al. Association between thrombolytic treatment and the prognosis of hemodynamically stable patients with major pulmonary embolism: results of a multicenter registry. Circulation 1997; 96(3):882–888.
116. Handa K, Sasaki Y, Kiyonaga A, Fujino M, Hiroki T, Arakawa K. Acute pulmonary thromboembolism treated successfully by balloon angioplasty–a case report. Angiology 1988; 39(8):775–778.
117. Fava M, Loyola S, Flores P, Huete I. Mechanical fragmentation and pharmacologic thrombolysis in massive pulmonary embolism. J Vasc Interv Radiol 1997; 8(2):261–266.
118. Sharafuddin MJ, Hicks ME. Current status of percutaneous mechanical thrombectomy. Part I. General principles. J Vasc Interv Radiol 1997; 8(6):911–921.
119. Sharafuddin MJ, Hicks ME. Current status of percutaneous mechanical thrombectomy. Part II. Devices and mechanisms of action. J Vasc Interv Radiol 1998; 9(1 Pt 1):15–31.
120. Sharafuddin MJ, Hicks ME. Current status of percutaneous mechanical thrombectomy. Part III. Present and future applications. J Vasc Interv Radiol 1998; 9(2):209–224.
121. Uflacker R, Strange C, Vujic I. Massive pulmonary embolism: preliminary results of treatment with the Amplatz thrombectomy device. J Vasc Interv Radiol 1996; 7(4):519–528.
122. Rocek M, Peregrin J, Velimsky T. Mechanical thrombectomy of massive pulmonary embolism using an Arrow- Trerotola percutaneous thrombolytic device. Eur Radiol 1998; 8(9):1683–1685.
123. Koning R, Cribier A, Gerber L, Eltchaninoff H, Tron C, Gupta V, et al. A new treatment for severe pulmonary embolism: percutaneous rheolytic thrombectomy. Circulation 1997; 96(8):2498–2500.
124. Voigtlander T, Rupprecht HJ, Nowak B, Post F, Mayer E, Stahr P, et al. Clinical application of a new rheolytic thrombectomy catheter system for massive pulmonary embolism. Catheter Cardiovasc Interv 1999; 47(1):91–96.
125. Brown DB, Cardella JF, Wilson RP, Singh H, Waybill PN. Evaluation of a modified arrow-trerotola percutaneous thrombolytic device for treatment of acute pulmonary embolus in a canine model. J Vasc Interv Radiol 1999; 10(6):733–740.
126. Peuster M, Bertram H, Windhagen-Mahnert B, Paul T, Hausdorf G. [Mechanical recanalization of venous thrombosis and pulmonary embolism with the Clotbuster thrombectomy system in a 12-year-old boy]. Z Kardiol 1998; 87(4):283–287.
127. Levine MN, Raskob G, Landefeld S, Kearon C. Hemorrhagic complications of anticoagulant treatment. Chest 1998; 114(5 suppl):511S–523S.
128. Katsamouris AA, Waltman AC, Delichatsios MA, Athanasoulis CA. Inferior vena cava filters: in vitro comparison of clot trapping and flow dynamics. Radiology 1988; 166(2):361–366.
129. Hammer FD, Rousseau HP, Joffre FG, Sentenac BP, Tran-Van T, Barthelemy RP. In vitro evaluation of vena cava filters. J Vasc Interv Radiol 1994; 5(6): 869–876.
130. Athanasoulis CA, Kaufman JA, Halpern EF, Waltman AC, Geller SC, Fan CM. Inferior vena caval filters: review of a 26-year single-center clinical experience. Radiology 2000; 216(1):54–66.
131. Ferris EJ, McCowan TC, Carver DK, McFarland DR. Percutaneous inferior vena caval filters: follow-up of seven designs in 320 patients. Radiology 1993; 188(3):851–856.

47

Care at the End of Life

C. LEE PARMLEY

The University of Texas M.D. Anderson Cancer Center, Houston, Texas, U.S.A.

I. INTRODUCTION/BACKGROUND

End-of-life (EOL) issues must be faced when dealing with cancer patients or others with terminal diseases. Despite improved surgical, medical, and preventive strategies, life comes to an end. For cancer patients, this may be life closing out after successful and curative treatment, or it may be somewhere during the course of the disease or its treatment. Society in general and cancer patients in particular should engage in planning how life will end. Patients expect their physicians to be confident and competent in providing care when they develop a life-threatening illness. Yet many physicians are uncomfortable communicating bad news and prognoses, and some fear addiction will result from control of symptoms (1).

The recent efforts of the American Medical Association to educate physicians on EOL care (EPEC) (2) demonstrate the recognized significance of this need. Patients need to deal with these issues, and physicians need to be prepared to provide EOL care as well as to guide patients and their family members into and through the process. Although a great deal of EOL care for cancer patients is provided in the hospice setting and with the assistance of palliative care programs, for purposes of this chapter, the focus will be on hospital-based care, in particular practices in the intensive care unit (ICU).

Within the ICU setting, it is common for the application of all known technological monitoring and mechanical support for organ function to fail in achieving the goal of cure or recovery. Patients are usually hospitalized at the time of death, and of deaths occurring in the hospital, many are in the ICU; up to 20% in the United States (3). About one-half of the patients who die in hospitals are cared for in ICU within three days of death, and about one-third spend 10 days or more in ICU prior to death (4). Of particular interest in this finding is that most of the time death follows soon after decisions are made by the physician and patient or surrogate decision maker.

Decisions are those associated with EOL care planning, and usually involve decisions to refocus care, limit or restrict therapies, refrain from escalation of treatment, withhold treatments, or withdraw treatments that sustain life. The underlying ethical principles and elements of the decision process will be reviewed in the context of what decisions need to be made, who should be involved in the process, and areas where conflict is likely to arise.

A. Ethical Principles

In order to deal with life and death issues, it is necessary to understand principles of biomedical ethics. Application of technology to sustain life involves interplay of moral, legal, and ethical values. Often a misunderstanding of legal aspects leads to treatment that might be challenged on ethical grounds. Fortunately, medical practice that is soundly based on ethical principles will readily be defendable from aspects of legal liability. The four basic ethical principles considered to be most compelling in EOL matters are beneficence, nonmaleficence, autonomy, and justice. These principles are reviewed here only briefly for purposes of subsequent discussion.

1. *Beneficence and Nonmaleficence*

Most basic of these principles are beneficence and nonmaleficence, founded within the statement "be of benefit and do no harm" attributed to Hippocrates. Beneficence can simply be thought of as the very purpose of the medical profession, to restore health and relieve suffering; to provide services that are of benefit. The fundamental role and responsibility of physicians are to cure disease when possible, to alleviate pain and suffering when cure is not possible.

Nonmaleficence is in essence the edict *primum non nocere*, "first, do no harm." There may be some degree of harm with nearly anything that is done for the benefit of a patient. For example, pain accompanies surgery. Current application of the beneficence–nonmaleficence principles weighs benefit against burden such that some burden is acceptable if the benefit outweighs it. If, on the other hand, the burden of a particular treatment is excessive in relationship to the potential benefit, it could be considered unethical to offer, provide, or continue the treatment.

2. *Autonomy*

Autonomy is the ethical principle directed at the respect of the identity of a human being as a person, and ones right to self-determination. A patient's right to self-determination is highly respected in American society. The United States (U.S.) Supreme Court wrote in 1891 "No right is held more sacred or is more carefully guarded by the common law than the right of every individual to the possession and control of his own person, free from all restraints or interference by others, unless by clear and unquestionable authority of law" (6).

The principle of autonomy is of particular interest in modern medical practice. Patients have the right of self-determination; to decide what they will accept or reject in terms of their medical treatment. A patient's autonomy includes the right to refuse treatment, even if the treatment will save the patient's life. This exercise of patient autonomy in modern medical practice is seen in contrast to the paternalistic practice of medicine, wherein healthcare decisions were made by the physician and imposed on the patient with little acknowledgement or respect for the patient's own identity. Physicians believed they knew what was best for their patients and set out to provide care along those lines. Patient autonomy is frequently cited as the reason for providing treatment deemed by physicians to be of no benefit to the patient, and as such can be seen as a basis for medical futility (5).

3. *Justice*

Justice is the fourth of the basic principles of medial ethics, and one that frequently remains unspoken. It deals with the fair allocation of resources for members of society, or distributive justice. Often justice is put into an economic perspective, that a treatment is very expensive, and has little chance of saving life. Unfortunately, this leads to the true but repugnant concept that the wealthy can have all of the expensive treatments, which might save life, while the poor will be left to die without the benefit of the same treatment. Another application of the principle of justice can be seen in the allocation of scarce resources such as intensive care beds, which might be occupied by patients who are unsalvageable. Therefore, the same beds are unavailable for patients who might be saved if the resource were available for them. The continued administration of blood components to a single patient, whose bleeding will not stop, may deplete resources that can sustain the lives of many others.

4. *Ethicists and Ethics Committees*

Clinical ethicists have entered the healthcare environment to assist practitioners with matters where analysis of ethical issues may help resolve conflicts or perhaps reach appropriate decisions. This has been particularly true where EOL decisions and conflicts surrounding them are involved. Ethicists may help identify or refine elements in conflict between healthcare providers and the patient, but more frequently between the surrogate decision maker and members of the healthcare team. At times, matters peripheral to the care of the patient detract from the issues needing attention. The ethicist may be able to help focus the parties involved on the benefit and burden of treatments under consideration, and to help sort out what the patient truly would want for him/herself, as opposed to what might be the desires of the surrogate as an individual.

Some ethicists lack sufficient clinical perspective to truly grasp the physician's dilemma and may engage in theoretical dialogue, which can fail to move the conflict toward resolution. One study on this perspective gathered and tabulated questionnaire responses from American physicians and nurses from both the

United States and United Kingdom which indicated significantly different beliefs from those of ethicists responding to the same questionnaire in regards to medical futility, withholding and withdrawing treatment and the distinction between heroic and ordinary interventions (7). Fortunately, this is not a uniform experience and should not detract from the potential value to be added by presence of the clinical ethicist.

The involvement of clinical ethicists on multidisciplinary ethics committees is a well-recognized value. Since the late 1970s, when conflicts arise between healthcare providers or their representatives, hospitals in the United States have relied more and more on the special committees, empanelled to assist in dealing with such complex issues. The significance of these ethics committees is well recognized and apparent in their requirement for accreditation for hospitals by Joint Commission of Accreditation Healthcare Organizations (JCAHO). Hospital policies under which ethics committees operate establish their function within a particular hospital, and specify how those seeking assistance may access the committee, whether they be patient, family member, or healthcare provider. Although it has been difficult to study the effect ethics committees have on EOL care processes, there is evidence that is measurable. One study of over 550 patients in 7 ICUs across the United States showed that, for patients who did not survive to hospital discharge, ethics committee consults were associated with significant reductions in treatments likely to lack benefit, without affecting the mortality (8).

5. *Autonomy, Informed Consent, and Surrogacy*

The process of informed consent is founded on the principle of autonomy. It involves the paternalistic physician setting forth what he/she deems to be the best treatment options for the patient, as well as discussion of the nontreatment options and alternative treatments. Based on the information provided, the patient reaches an understanding, then accepts and consents to a particular treatment. The informed consent will involve an understanding of the potential benefits and risks, the benefit/burden balance. Of course, the patient may well decide that the treatment is not wanted, and the physician cannot compel acceptance of the treatment. At the same time, if the patient wants a treatment that the physician deems inappropriate, the patient cannot compel the physician to provide treatment against medical judgment.

6. *Autonomy Via Surrogacy*

A patient's autonomy is not lost due to incompetence. When a patient is unable to speak on his own behalf, the law allows others to do so. On behalf of an incompetent patient, a surrogate decision maker can be identified by several means. Occasionally, a court of law may appoint a legal guardian. This is infrequent, and usually involves patients whose incompetence has been present for some time prior to the time of hospitalization. Short of a court-appointed guardian, a patient may authorize another individual to act as his/her agent by executing a legal document, often referred to as power of attorney for healthcare. The patient may have exercised his autonomy also by executing a directive to physicians, also known as a living will, which sets forth his/her desires for treatment in the event of incompetence, if diagnosed with a terminal or irreversible condition. Even if there is no guardian, directive, or power of attorney for healthcare, an incompetent patient's autonomy can still be protected through surrogate decision makers which the law identifies: the spouse, adult children, parents, and nearest living relative. One such individual would be expected to know the desires of the patient, if anyone would, and is authorized by law to consent on behalf of the incompetent patient.

In 1983, the Presidents' Commission for the Study of Ethical Problems in Medicine and Biomedical Research concluded that it was permissible for a competent patient to refuse treatment that would be life saving, and that this decision could also be made on behalf of an incompetent patient through substituted judgment. This is commonly through involvement of a surrogate decision maker (9).

II. PLANNING TERMINAL CARE

Dealing with EOL issues in the ICU presents numerous challenges. Most patients are admitted to the ICU due to critical not terminal illness. The advancements in technology and treatment provided for patients admitted to the ICU are intended to extend life for patients, whose very admission there indicates an increased risk of dying. Patients receiving aggressive life-sustaining treatments in the ICU who will ultimately not survive cannot always be identified. Often only in retrospect can we identify the terminal aspects of the critical illness for which they were admitted to the ICU, and thus it is extremely difficult to know when to shift from cure-oriented to comfort-oriented care. Unlike common ICU practice, traditional palliative care will develop a comfort-oriented care plan focusing on pain, discomfort, anxiety, sleep disturbances, depression, and dyspnea reported to be among common symptoms in dying patients. For patients in the ICU, pain is also known to accompany common interventions such as mechanical ventilation, the presence of urinary catheters, endotracheal, and nasogastric tubes, as well as turning and moving from ICU bed to chair (10).

It is important to carefully consider the dying process in an environment where ICU management is associated with symptoms which are not always well controlled, and where there are reports that often life-sustaining treatment is continued despite requests from patients or surrogates that it be stopped (11). To the primary goal of the ICU, which is to preserve meaningful life, we must add a goal directed at better care for the dying patient. In order to accomplish this, care givers truly must be able to move from what has become recognized as traditional heroic ICU efforts to meaningful EOL care.

A. Expectations and Resuscitative Rituals of Death

The closed-chest compressions and other maneuvers recognized as the hallmark of cardiopulmonary resuscitation (CPR) were developed to restore circulation for patients who suffered cardiac arrest as a result of anesthesia (12). This process of CPR has become widely incorporated into other settings, including its use on patients with terminal illnesses, and is recognizable as a ritual of death. Successful resuscitation has been colloquially defined as resuscitation, which returns a patient to taxpayer status. Efforts, which are technically successful at restarting the heart, despite the development of significant brain injury, instead represent a drain on the patient, the patient's family, and society (13).

CPR, as it is usually practiced, follows an algorithm that is intended to be basic, teachable, and memorable: the ABCs for airway, breathing, and circulation. Developers of advanced cardiac life support (ACLS) state that it is indicated to prevent the sudden, unexpected death (14). It is not indicated in cases of terminal illness and to provide it would only prolong the dying process, or temporarily interrupt it. Unfortunately, society has, in many areas of the world, developed an expectation that with continued application of technology, medication, and support, patients might, somehow, live on forever. This is reinforced by demonstrations and descriptions of resuscitative efforts in the media that unquestionably do not represent reality. Over time, there has developed a near-expectation that the declaration of death would only follow a full resuscitative effort.

Despite such an expectation, success with current resuscitation practices is clearly not what is seen in the entertainment world, where nearly 70% seem to survive CPR (15). Studies of success in real life practice report survival after cardiac arrest for hospitalized patients to be between 6.5% and 32% with significant decline in functional status in up to 44% of survivors (16). There is considerable variation in the patient populations studied; understandably, there are some where survival rates are extremely poor, and the quality of the survival is poor as well. Some patients have restoration of circulatory function, but have sustained anoxic neurological insult as a result of the prearrest conditions, resuscitative effort, or combination of factors. Recognition of this possibility has led to practices to restrict CPR in select cases.

B. Show, Slow, and No Codes

Early on, do not resuscitate (DNR) decisions and practices were neither the topic of open conversation nor decision-making shared with the patient/surrogate. Systems of passing on the DNR decision to healthcare practitioners evolved in a near-underground manner, and special terminology regarding the quality of the resuscitative effort surfaced. Terms such as "slow code," "show code," "chemical code," and other expressions were used to indicate that when a cardiopulmonary arrest occurred there would be something less than a genuine effort toward resuscitation. The idea was to fool the family or others into believing that death could be declared because the resuscitative ritual, although unsuccessful, was completed. The concept of allowing patients to die without full resuscitative effort has been the foundation for further EOL decision-making and advance care planning. Not surprising, in ICU practice, a very high proportion of deaths occurs after decisions are made to limit treatment and refocus care (17).

C. Values and Quality Factors

Developing an appropriate plan for EOL care should involve discussions with a procedure-based approach, which identifies patient's goals and focuses on what interventions will be performed. This may include time-limited trials of dialysis or mechanical ventilation, while underlying conditions are being treated. Redirection of care at the EOL must emphasize measures to promote comfort, not prolong life. "There is nothing more we can do" is an example of language to be avoided, and exchanged for expressions of what can be done to protect dignity and provide comfort such as "Your loved one will be comfortable and free from pain" (18).

Family members who respond to questionnaires pertaining to the experience of the process of dying in the ICU as experienced by their loved one focus on comfort, compassion, communication, and shared decision-making as significant to them (19).

These values are in line with ones identified in efforts seeking to improve the delivery of EOL care in the ICU setting or the seven domains for ICU EOL care: (1) patient- and family-centered decision-making, (2) communication, (3) continuity of care, (4) emotional and practical support, (5) symptom management and comfort care, (6) spiritual support, and (7) emotional and organizational support for ICU clinicians (20). These domains represent areas where the energy focused will tend to optimize quality of the EOL experience for terminal patients in the ICU.

Patients suffering from life-threatening illnesses expect to experience multiple symptoms in addition to dealing with psychological, social, spiritual, and practical issues (1). Family members' expectations of a patient suffering are also the same. Patients with cancer who are hospitalized experience more symptoms than outpatients, 12.5% as compared to 9.7%, respectively (21). Pain, nausea and vomiting, constipation, and breathlessness are among these prevalent symptoms. Psychological distresses including anxiety, worry, fear, sadness, hopelessness, and depressions are commonly reported as well. With weight loss, patients become weak and easily fatigued, losing function and independence that may be a source of suffering (1).

Functional decline tends to differ between certain patient populations, and has been compared in four types of illness: sudden death, cancer death, death from organ failure, and frailty. For purposes of comparison, decline in physical function is defined in terms of a patient's ability to perform activities of daily living (ADLs) within one year prior to death. Such ADLs include walking across a small room, bathing, grooming, dressing, eating, transferring from bed to chair, and using the toilet. Among the four patient groups compared, cancer patients were highly functional early in their final year but were markedly more disabled three months prior to death. This suggests that progressive ADL dependency is among circumstances heralding death for the older cancer patient (22).

The fear of loss of function, progressive dependency, and being a burden on others is associated with requests for assisted death (23). Understandably, patients at the EOL are troubled by the idea of being financial, social, or care burden on family and friends. Many times one or more family members will have to quit work or make other major life changes in order to provide care for dying loved ones (24). One study of families of cancer patients found that 40% became impoverished providing care (25).

Despite the concern about impact and burden on family, patients would prefer to die at home. And for cancer patients it is deemed highly important for death to occur at the preferred place (26). Despite the preference for death at home, the preponderance of death in the United States occurs in hospitals and a large number of those deaths are in the ICU setting. The majority of deaths in ICUs involve the decision to withhold or withdraw life-sustaining treatment (4). This pattern is true in American as well as European communities, although there is variation in terminology as well as overall ICU utilization and other medical practices (27).

D. Palliative Care

Palliative care in the critical care setting requires special consideration. Unfortunately, measures intended to preserve organ function for the benefit of survival are often highly leveraged against the burdens of pain and violations of human dignity. With cure, or even short-term survival as the treatment goal, the balance of benefit against burden will allow healthcare providers to continue efforts despite the burden to the patient. The understanding is that the patient accepts this burden when consideration is in conjunction with the potential benefit. Once it becomes clear, or even when it starts becoming apparent, that survival is not to be expected, or that the hope of even short-term survival is unlikely, and the cost is tremendous in terms of burden to the patient, the treatment can be refocused.

The conversion from goals of cure and recovery to that of providing comfort and protecting dignity demonstrates the overlap and coexistence of intensive care and palliative care. These areas of medical practice must be recognized as supplemental rather than mutually exclusive. Many believe that all ICU patients, being at increased risk of death, can benefit from aspects of palliative care in their management. The transition from curative to palliative care has been shown schematically (Fig. 1) by Ferris (28) in a manner that demonstrates the interplay of patient, family, and health care providers. Within this scheme, the role of intensive care practice should be only a small portion of the overall system providing care for the terminal patient.

Some have suggested two phases for the delivery of care at the EOL. The first phase is one of shared decision-makings that involve the shift of care from cure and recovery to one of comfort, dignity, and freedom from pain. The second phase concerns the actions taken once the decision to refocus care has been made. The time spent in each phase is highly variable, and can range from hours to weeks (28). While patient comfort and dignity should constitute the foundation of medical care, the accepted encroachments on this foundation are recognized as necessary in order to sustain a patient, especially in the ICU. Redirecting

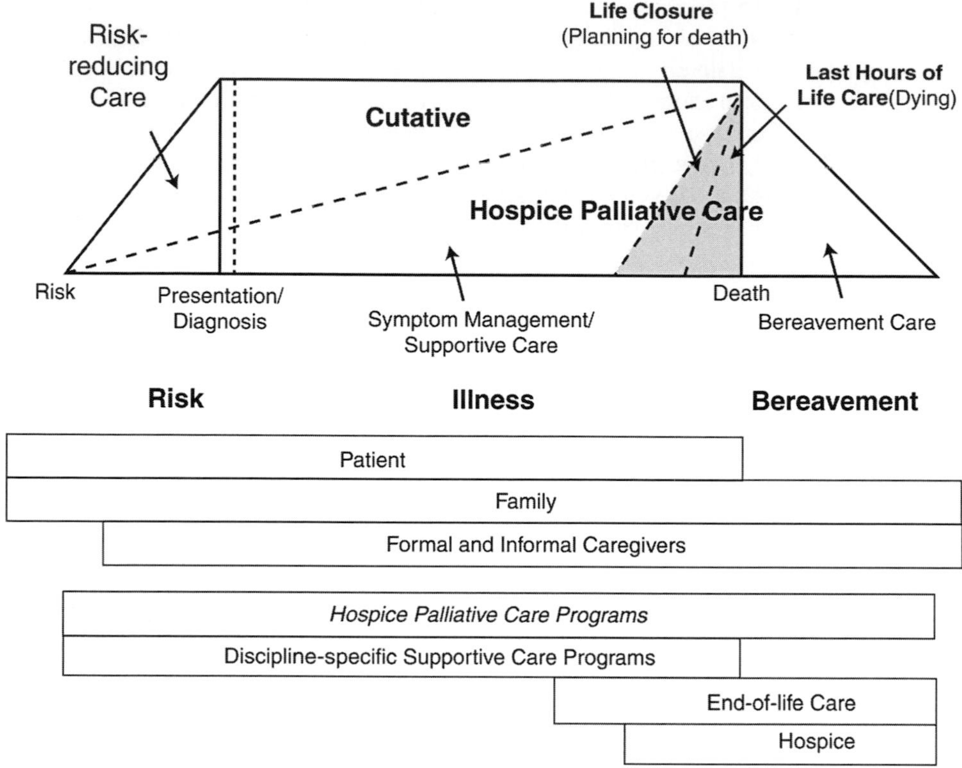

Figure 1 Palliative care within the experience of illness, bereavement, and risk. *Source*: From Ref. 28.

care to provide comfort and dignity requires decisions that are often difficult to make. For the protection of patient autonomy, the patient's participation in the decision-making process is necessary.

E. Directives and Decisions

Until the last half-century, most people died before reaching old age and were not particularly sick until shortly before death. Currently, however, most Americans die while old, sick, and after a substantial period of disability. Since our care system does not yet match our new demographics, in order to avoid unnecessary costs, suffering, and loss of dignity, advance care planning is needed to improve management of patients suffering from fatal chronic illnesses (29). A quality indicator for judging care for vulnerable patients should be appropriate advance care plans implemented across sites and times (30).

Prognostic factors for cancer patients are of extreme importance in making plans to deal with EOL issues, and prognostication is known to be complex, but this should not prevent discussions to develop appropriate plans for EOL care (31). When admitted to the ICU, it will likely be too late to afford a patient optimal involvement in the process. Ultimately, there should be planning well in advance, with decisions and plans implemented in writing.

Advance directives allow patients to set forth their decisions for management of their care at EOL. Living wills and healthcare proxy designation are two forms of advance directives. Advance care planning will allow a person to discuss with loved ones and healthcare providers how EOL care is to be provided before the emotional upheaval associated with the dying process occurs (18).

Traditional language of a living will or directive to physicians and family sets forth the situation in which it is to take effect and the decisions the patient has made regarding certain treatments, usually those considered life sustaining. Nearly, all living wills are designed to take effect when the patient is incompetent and unable to speak on his/her own behalf. The specific conditions to be present in order for decisions to be effectuated are usually that the patient's condition is terminal, or in the alternative, the condition is irreversible and without certain life-sustaining treatment, the patient would die.

Patients, who have taken the time and invested the effort needed to execute a living will or directive to physicians and family, usually instruct that life-sustaining treatment is to be with held or withdrawn in the event of their incompetence with a diagnosis of terminal or irreversible condition. The patient's right to make decisions and for healthcare provider to execute such decisions are recognized ethically under the principle of autonomy, and legally within a privacy right cited even prior to the Karen Quinlan case in 1976. Living will statutes and Natural Death Acts establish appropriate practices within the United States, where some variation is seen, although all acknowledge the patient's right to refuse life-sustaining treatment. Despite some variation with its application, the general principle is that decisions should be consistent with the patient's wishes, if known, and if not, those who know the patient can give the best idea of the patient's values.

III. DECISIONS IN EOL CARE

Using technology and expertise, critical care practitioners support patients through illnesses threatening survival. Often the question arises as to whether or not it is appropriate to continue life-sustaining therapy. Patients themselves rarely participate in the decision-making process, because they are heavily sedated or just too ill. As a result, the decision-making falls to the family members or the patient's surrogate, in consultation with the medical team. Effective communication includes sharing the burden of decision-making between physicians and family members, and seeking a patient-focused consensus (32).

Some ICU patients linger neither improving nor acutely dying, and showing dwindling capacity to recover. Decision-making is usually done without the direct participation of the patient through surrogates in conjunction with the healthcare team. The stressful nature of these matters may compromise patient care and engender guilt among family members involved in the decision-making. Focusing on consistent and effective communication can help alleviate this to some degree and give a sense of shared burden for decision-making. A shift from individual responsibility to patient-focused consensus may help family members gain understanding and move into a situation of letting go of life-sustaining interventions (32).

A. Resuscitation and Intubation

The resuscitative ritual at the EOL can be eliminated with an order to withhold CPR. This DNR order should only preclude resuscitative efforts in the event of cardiopulmonary arrest and should not influence other therapeutic interventions that may be appropriate for the patient (33). The evolution of DNR practices has grown through phases where decisions were made but not written, rather passed along by word of mouth. This was followed by the development of order sets, which combine additional treatment options with the DNR, apparently to clarify that the DNR decision was not a demonstration that all hope for the patient was lost.

The decision regarding CPR is pivotal and likely represents a threshold to be crossed as EOL care planning takes place. Unlike most decisions in medicine, the one regarding CPR must be made in advance, in fact, CPR is the only medical therapy that requires an order to be with held (18). While there may be some controversy regarding how the DNR decision is reached, the general rule is that effort should be made to resuscitate patients who suffer cardiac or respiratory arrest except when circumstances indicate that CPR would be inappropriate or not in accord with the desires or best interest of the patient (33). Patients do not have rights to useless treatment and CPR should not be used if there is no reasonable prospect of success (34).

Similar to a decision not to resuscitate is a decision not to intubate. For patients whose pulmonary disease is end-stage, the use of endotracheal intubation and mechanical ventilation must be carefully considered. The natural progression of the pulmonary disease would lead to hypoxemia and resultant organ failure, including the central nervous system and heart. If untreated or at least unsupported, the hypoxemia would predictably lead to loss of mental function followed at some point by hypoxic cardiac arrest. If supported with supplemental oxygen and thereafter with intubation and eventual mechanical ventilation, the natural course of the disease is interrupted, and death is delayed but now will occur on a ventilator, probably in an ICU. In situations such as this, a routine DNR order will not prevent the intubation in response to worsening respiratory distress. In some cases, it is important to recognize the progression of disease and make appropriate EOL decisions that take effect prior to a full cardiac or respiratory arrest.

A "Do Not Intubate" order should be accompanied by a DNR order. One of the first actions in CPR is the establishment of an airway; the A of the ABCs for basic life support. Patients on life support that includes mechanical ventilation already have the A and B of the ABCs taken care of, so a DNR essentially means waiting for the C or cardiac component of the arrest.

B. Withholding and Withdrawing Life-Sustaining Treatments

1. Patient's Choice

The American Medical Association's statement regarding the withholding or withdrawing of life-sustaining treatment reviews the duties of physicians to sustain life and relieve suffering. In that context, however, where the performance of one's duty conflicts with the other, patient preferences should prevail. Physicians must respect a competent patient's decision to forego life-sustaining treatment (35).

In the process of making decisions regarding interventions to extend life, the potential benefit of the interventions should be based on scientific evidence, the consensus of society, and standards of the medical profession rather than on individual bias regarding the quality of life or other subjective matters (36). Treatment judged to have no realistic likelihood of benefit should not be offered, and physicians are under no ethical obligation to provide such treatments (36). Likewise, decisions to withhold treatments should be made with careful consideration of potential risks, patient preferences, and family wishes in conjunction with scientific evidence of the likelihood of medical or other benefits. When interventions are withheld, special efforts directed at comfort, support and counseling for the patient, family, and friends must be continued as well as ongoing efforts to maintain effective communication (36).

2. *Withholding*

More often than not, death in the ICU is subsequent to decisions to refocus treatment goals, and to limit, withhold, or withdraw certain interventions. Clearly, a simple DNR order for patients on full mechanical life support falls short of the overall decision to refocus treatment on EOL care. Unfortunately, the concept of DNR has been taken in this context. This confusion of the true meaning of DNR orders has made the initial threshold DNR decision more troublesome than it would otherwise be. While a DNR order is a tiny piece of an EOL care plan, not all patients with DNR orders are appropriate for other decisions needed for such planning. Truly, ICU patients with DNR orders may well be expected to survive their ICU stay; the order merely means that, in the event of cardiac arrest, resuscitation will not be initiated.

A decision to withhold or withdraw life-sustaining treatment for a patient with a terminal or irreversible condition lies at the heart of the living will or directive to physicians and family. State statutes pertaining to living wills often called advance directive or Natural Death Acts establish the legality of such practices. Law acknowledges a patient's right to refuse treatment, and to die naturally. Unfortunately, death that occurs in an ICU is far from what occurs in the natural dying process. Natural death resulting from respiratory failure or sepsis-induced circulatory failure will involve a process during which oxygenation and perfusion inadequacies result in progressive organ failure. Mental functions deteriorate in the process that renders a patient less acutely aware of and perplexed by the impending death. Intensive care management will seek to maintain oxygenation and restore perfusion to preserve organ function. This process may be unsuccessful at restoring health, but it is usually somewhat successful at delaying organ failure and death, which when it does occur, is far from natural.

Withholding and withdrawing the interventions initiated to preserve and maintain organ function are appropriate when we determine that the criteria for conditions of terminal or irreversible are met. Criteria for these conditions vary to some extent from state to state, but in general a terminal condition is one where death is expected from the condition within 6 months, even with treatment in accordance with standard medical practice. An irreversible condition is one that can be treated but never cured, and for purposes of living will and directives, the irreversible condition is such that because of it the patient would die without the application of life-sustaining treatment. If a patient knows she/he has such conditions, he can refuse life-sustaining treatments, and if they are already being provided, she/he can demand that they be stopped. If the individual is incompetent, and has executed a directive so stating, life-sustaining treatment can and in fact must be withheld and/or withdrawn in accordance with the directive. Even without a directive, the same decision can be made on behalf of the incompetent patient who has a terminal or irreversible condition. Such decision-making is supported by legal statutes and ethical principles.

3. *Withdrawing*

"There is no ethical distinction between withdrawing and withholding life-sustaining treatment" (35). Regrettably, there has been a reluctance to withdraw life-sustaining treatments that are already being provided, while it has been easier to make the similar decision to withhold the same treatment, which had not yet been initiated. Some have concerns that the act of withdrawal of the treatment is an intentional act, which will cause death, and as such could be considered some form of homicide. Such is not the case. The act of withdrawal of life-sustaining treatment rather than causing death merely stops the delay of death. Death is allowed to occur through the natural process that was underway, but interrupted, by the medical care interposed. There is a long-standing recognition that there is no legal, moral, or ethical distinction between withholding or withdrawing treatment that is of no benefit to a patient.

Additional controversy has revolved around the distinction between artificial nutrition and hydration as life-sustaining treatment when contrasted with mechanical modalities such as ventilation and dialysis. Some argue against what they consider the inhumanity of starvation of patients who are terminally ill. Loss of appetite, however, seems to accompany terminal illness, and force-feeding of a patient whose organs are shutting down can be the source of discomfort. Attention to the patient's comfort and dignity can be the best guide for EOL decisions; thirsty patients should drink, hungry patients should eat. If nutrition and hydration are provided for comfort, they cannot be discontinued. However, if they are provided as life-sustaining treatment, they must be stopped.

Comfort measures are appropriate and should be included in EOL care plans. Measures to provide comfort and protect dignity include good hygiene, nursing care, and access to family members and others that would be a source of comfort and provide a sense of well-being. The ICU environment is not conducive to open access to family and friends, but accommodations are often possible to improve the quality of the EOL experience.

4. *Terminal Care*

With or without a written directive, decision to withhold or withdraw life-sustaining treatment in the ICU will culminate in an EOL care plan. The plan must have considerations for the patient, family members, and the healthcare team. Management of pain and distress of the patient must have highest priority. The patient and family members may be reassured by the knowledge that treatment will be provided with respect and dignity through out the dying process and afterward. Acknowledging and respecting religious and cultural expectations are also of value. The presence of clergy and the opportunity to perform religious rites and services may afford meaning for the EOL experience.

Family members often want to be present at the bedside and be of help to dying loved ones. They seek information about what is being done and for what reason. In addition to requiring assurance that the patient is comfortable, family members needed to be comforted as well. They need to express their emotions and deal with the reality of the dying process and decisions required at the EOL. The decisions will be ones about the discontinuation or administration of medications, about tubes and monitors, and about the handling of mechanical support. These decisions and how they are carried out will have an impact on the healthcare providers as well as the patient and family members.

Family members at the bedside as well as the healthcare providers must continue to assess the patient's appearance of comfort. Dying in one's sleep, viewed as a natural way to depart this life, stands in contrast to dying in the ICU following a decision to refocus care. The interventions instituted to promote cure and recovery and to preserve organ function must be considered in a different light when cure and recovery are no longer realistic goals. Measures implemented to support circulatory and respiratory function for purposes of survival require specific attention. The hypoxemia and hypercarbia from respiratory depression as well as the hypoperfusion from circulatory compromise accompanying critical illness are associated with decreased cerebral function and unconsciousness as part of the dying process. While these natural physiologic processes may contribute to the comfort of dying patients, the effects are not uniform, and some patients may be more uncomfortable as mental function lapses. Control of pain and distress will guide administration of medications at EOL.

5. *Medications*

Despite the evidence that appropriate administration of medications can ameliorate pain without intolerable side effects in 70–95% of terminally ill patients (37), many terminally ill patients are inadequately treated for their pain (38,39). Many physicians, remarkably, fear that such patients will develop narcotic abuse while under their treatment. Lack of awareness of the current ethical and legal consensus regarding palliative care at the EOL may make physicians reluctant to freely administer pain-relieving medications; even if such will hasten death, its administration is appropriate if the underlying intention is to provide comfort (40).

The term "double effect" for medications administered for symptom control refers to the additional effect that may be to depress respiratory or other vital functions. Liberal administration of medications for control of symptoms, despite the double effect, is widely recognized as acceptable practice (41–43).

Opioid analgesics are the mainstay for managing pain and suffering of the dying patient. Morphine remains popular for this purpose in ICU practice, but alternative agents such as fentanyl and hydromorphone are also useful (Table 1). The effect of opioids to invoke analgesia is well known, as are the effects of euphoria and sedation, which may be favorable in the EOL setting. Respiratory depression, constipation, urinary retention, and nausea are side effects that may present, but should not preclude administration to an end point of pain control and comfort.

In addition to opioid analgesics, sedative agents may be useful in assuring comfort. Such agents

Table 1 Opiod Analgestics

Medication	Equianalgesic dosing (IV)	Typical starting dose adult (IV)	Typical starting dose, pediatric (IV)	Duration (hr)	Typical starting infusion rate	Comments
Morphine	1	2–10 mg	0.1 mg/kg	3–4	0.05–0.1 mg/kg^{-1} hr^{-1}	Histamine release (caution in asthma, vasodilation, and hypotension)
Hydromorphone	0.15	0.3–1.5 mg	—	3–4	—	Less pruritus, nausea, sedation, and euphoria than morphine
Pentanyl	0.01	50–100 μg	1–5 μg/kg	0.5–2.0	1–10 μg/kg^{-1} hr^{-1}	Minimal hemodynamic effects, duration of action short when given by intermittent bolus, half-life prolonged when administered chronically
Meperidine	10	25–100 mg	1 mg/kg	2–4	—	Not recommended for chronic use; catastrophic interaction with MAO inhibitors; tachycardia; seizures

Table 2 Adjunctive Sedative Agents

Medication	Typical starting dose, adult (IV)	Typical starting dose, pediatric (IV)	Duration (hr)	Typical starting infusion rate, adult	Typical starting infusion rate, pediatric	Comments
Lorazepam	1–3 mg	0.05 mg/kg	2–4	0.025–0.05 mg/kg^{-1} hr^{-1}	0.05–0.1 mg/kg^{-1} hr^{-1}	Longer acting, ideal for long-term administration
Midazolam	1 mg	0.1 mg/kg	1.5–2	1–5 mg/hr	0.05–0.1 mg/kg^{-1} hr^{-1}	Well tolerated but fairly expensive
Haloperidol	0.5–20 mg	—	2–4	3–5 mg/hr IV	—	Not often used in pediatrics because extrapyramidal effects more frequent
Propofol	1 mg/kg	1 mg/kg	10–15 min	0.5–3.0 mg/kg^{-1} hr^{-1}	0.5–3.0 mg/kg^{-1} hr^{-1}	Hypotension, lipid base lead to hyperlipidemia, painful on injection
Pentobar bital	150 mg	2–6 mg/kg	2–4	3–5 mg/kg^{-1} hr^{-1}	3–5 mg/kg^{-1} hr^{-1}	Propofol should replace pentobarbital in most EOL situation

(Table 2) can cause amnesia, limit anxiety, and help control suffering which is not responsive to opioids alone. Dosing of one or multiple agents must be based on the intention to provide sedation and analgesia, and titrated to effect rather than to maximal dosage limit. Recognized side effects such as respiratory depression should not limit dosage titration in EOL care. The 'double effect' of a medication is an effect that may hasten death, when comfort is the primary effect sought in its administration. Documenting the purpose or intent in the medical record and specifying the indication for administration of the medication in the orders will decrease the likelihood of misinterpretation or abuse.

Occasionally, the traditional methods of controlling pain and suffering fail, so other options must be considered. "Terminal sedation" is the term applied to the practice of sedating patients to the point of unconsciousness, and may be necessary as a last resort to assure comfort and the EOL. In the ICU setting such patients are usually supported with mechanical ventilation, and the terminal aspect of the sedation is associated with the discontinuation of other support.

6. *Mechanical Ventilation*

Decisions to refocus ICU care at the EOL often involve withdrawal of mechanical ventilation. The two commonly used approaches are referred to as "terminal extubation" and "terminal wean" both of which achieve the same end point of discontinuation of mechanical support. Terminal extubation usually follows bolus administration of sedative and analgesic medications. While this method may not mask the effects of stridor, airway obstruction, and air hunger, it does allow the patient to be free from the unnatural intervention of an endotracheal tube, and does not prolong the dying process. By contrast, the process of a terminal wean does allow the patient to remain intubated and thus avoids the appearance of distress which may be unsettling to family members and others at the bedside.

Terminal weaning occurs with considerable variability and may take place over several minutes or several days. In general, the process involves the gradual reduction in oxygen concentration and minute ventilation as medications are titrated to maintain comfort. Obvious advantages are that the appearance of discomfort from air hunger, airway obstruction, and agonal respirations are avoided. Choice of this option should not be viewed as something other than a decision to withdraw support in the process of refocusing care at the EOL. The choice of terminal wean over terminal extubation should not operate to prolong the dying process and extend suffering and loss of dignity of the patient.

IV. CONFLICTS OVER TERMINAL CARE

Management of terminal ICU patients has been the source of conflict and controversy in regard to medical futility and physician-assisted death (PAD). Cancer patients dying on life support in multiple organ failure present a clear representation of medical futility. The circumstances attending the decision to initiate life-sustaining treatment may be remote to the moment at hand, where a surrogate decision maker on behalf of the patient insists that full aggressive treatment be continued. Equally troubling is the request for assistance in dying coming from a patient who survives in misery, yet deterioration of organ function and overall decline suggest that death is not at hand. In both settings, the request for assistance in dying and the demand for unwarranted treatment, the physician must face the conflict over what is being asked and what should be done.

A. Evolution of Medical Futility

The American Medical Association has addressed medical futility as follows:

> Physicians are not ethically obligated to deliver care that, in their best professional judgment, will not have a reasonable chance of benefiting their patients. Patients should not be given treatments simply because they demand them. Denial of treatment should be justified by reliance on openly stated ethical principles and acceptable standards of care ... not on the concept of "futility," which cannot be meaningfully defined. (44)

The very term "medical futility" is difficult to define (44), and as such makes uniform or even consistent approaches to the concept difficult. The recognized phenomenon, however, touches all aspects of care delivery within the ICU, involving physicians, nursing staff, and other health care providers in allocation of scarce resources and cost-containment (45). Despite the current difficulty with a consistent definition, the concept of medical futility can be seen even in ancient Hippocratic writings which suggest three major goals for medicine, which include not only cure and relief of suffering, but also to treat those who are overmastered by their diseases (46). Those would be ones who are dying despite efforts at cure and relief of suffering.

In American practice, the 1970s and 1980s were seen as times when controversies centered on patients' right to refuse treatment that was keeping them alive contrary to their wishes, usually as expressed by surrogates. By contrast, the 1990s have shown a trend moving into the era of limitation on patients' rights to demand treatment that physicians deem inappropriate (18). The promotion of patient autonomy in an era of rapidly developing technology has led to this area of conflict.

A patient exercising his/her autonomous right chooses options that include the most advanced treatment modalities available, hoping to live on indefinitely. While this exercise of autonomy is commonly seen in situations of medical futility, it is clearly quite different from cases that brought patient autonomy to the forefront. In American practice, decisions about life-sustaining treatment are often tracked back to a New Jersey case involving a neurologically injured young lady, Karen Quinlan. The court acknowledged her right to refuse treatment even though it was keeping her alive, and validated the expression of her desire in this regard as expressed by her father. The concept of patient autonomy and self-determination is well founded in American medical practice, and supported by the Quinlan case and a line of cases that followed.

The treatments in question in cases such as Quinlan, most of which involved neurologic injury, are treatments that sustain life, but do not restore lost function. Another way to consider the situation is that function will not be restored because the condition is irreversible, but by sustaining life the treatments merely delay the moment death, or even prolong the dying process. In the context of irreversible conditions, be they neurologic or organ failure from cancer or its treatments, life-sustaining treatments must be considered in relationship to the overall treatment goal. When recovery is not to be expected, and without the application of life-sustaining treatments the death would occur naturally, the treatments merely delay the moment of death. Clearly, the patient should be able to choose not to have death delayed needlessly, and refusing the continuation of life-sustaining treatments is understandable. The patient has a right to refuse this treatment that may well be considered futile.

By contrast, the patient does not have the right to demand treatment that is futile or of no benefit, and certainly physicians should not offer treatment that is medically inappropriate. The determination of futility can be seen as a judgment call, not of the patient, but of the physician (47). The common setting is one where an ICU patient has been on life support for some period of time, and it has become apparent that underlying conditions cannot be reversed, and recovery and survival are no longer expected; the illness is terminal. Despite this prognosis, there is an insistence on continuation of life support usually coming from family or surrogate rather than the patient him/herself.

At this point, new treatment goals must be established with the prognosis and use of life support in proper perspective. Life support that was initiated and appropriate early on now acts only to delay the moment of death or prolong the dying process. With good communication throughout the period of critical illness, this progression is often recognized by the patient or surrogate, and a smooth transition into EOL care occurs with the development of new treatment goals. Demands for treatments where goals are controversial are often resolved through open communication and negotiations, but at times will require conflict-resolution techniques (48).

B. Futility Policies and Practices

The cost of futile care for the dying is great, measured not only in monetary costs of such care, but also in its negative effects on staff members, and the burden it creates in allocating limited resources. This is among the reasons that institutions have worked to develop a better understanding of futility and strategies for decreasing nonbeneficial care (47). In addition, the idea of discontinuing medical treatment contrary to a patient's wishes or contrary to the wishes expressed by a surrogate led to fear of legal consequences. Concerns about legal consequences were counterbalanced by ethical requirement to provide treatment that is of benefit and that causes no harm. Frequently, hospital ethics committees have been called upon to help deal with such situations, and can readily rely on provisions in the Code of Ethics of the American Medical Association.

In the early 1990s, some hospitals developed policies that set forth procedures whereby treatments, which physicians deemed medically appropriate, would be reviewed. Two paths were the focus, the persistent vegetative state (PVS) patients, and those presumed to be terminal, wherein therapy directed at a specific goal is being demanded despite its unlikely ability to achieve that goal (18). The review processes provided for an outcome that allowed discontinuation of treatment found to be medically inappropriate. Reasonable physicians practicing with an institution would be expected to follow appropriate hospital policies, and the policies dealing within futility set forth what a reasonably prudent physician would be expected to do. As such, it was expected that futility policies would provide a means to defend against legal action that might follow

When further intervention to prolong the life of a patient becomes futile, physicians have an obligation to shift the intent of care toward comfort and closure. However, there are necessary value judgments involved in coming to the assessment of futility. These judgments must give consideration to patient or proxy assessments of worthwhile outcome. They should also take into account the physician or other provider's perception of intent to treatment, which should not be to prolong the dying process without benefit to the patient or to others with legitimate interests. They may also take into account community and institutional standards, which in turn may have used physiological or functional outcome measures.

Nevertheless, conflicts between the parties may persist in determining what is futility in the particular instance. This may interrupt satisfactory decision-making and adversely affect patient care, family satisfaction, and physician–clinical team functioning. To assist in fair and satisfactory decision-making about what constituted futile interventions:

1. All health care institutions, whether large or small, should adopt a policy on medical futility; and
2. Policies on medical futility should follow a due process approach. The following seven steps should be included in such a due process approach to declaring futility in specific cases.
   a. Earnest attempts should be made in advance to deliberate over and negotiate prior understandings between patient, proxy, and physician or what constitutes futile care for the patient, and what falls within acceptable limits for the physician, family, and possible also the institution.
   b. Joint decision-making should occur between patient or proxy and physician to the maximum extent possible.
   c. Attempts should be made to negotiate disagreements if they arise, and to reach resolution within all parties' acceptable limits, with the assistance of consultants as appropriate.
   d. Involvement of an institutional committee such as the ethics committee should be requested if disagreements are irresolvable.
   e. If the institutional review supports the patient's position and the physician remains unpersuaded, transfer of care to another physician with the institution may be arranged.
   f. If the process supports the physician's position and the patient/proxy remains unpersuaded, transfer to another institution may be sought and, if done, should be supported by the transferring and receiving institution.
   g. If transfer is not possible, the intervention need not be offered.

Figure 2 Medical futility in EOL care. *Source*: From Ref. 49.

discontinuation of futile treatment contrary to the wishes or demands of the patient or family.

Futility policies that evolved varied to some degree, but in general they involved a mechanism to review the treatments being demanded yet deemed by the physician to be futile. If unsuccessful at resolving the dispute to the agreement of all, the review process would support discontinuation of treatments if they were found to be futile, as deemed by the physician. Institutional ethics committees represent the forum for dispute resolution in most institutions, which is in compliance with recommendations of the "AMA's Code of Medical Ethics 2.037. Medical Futility in End-of-Life Care" (Fig. 2).

Texas rewrote its Natural Death Act in 1999 and incorporated in it new provisions that provide protection from civil and criminal liability in cases where life-sustaining treatment is with held or withdrawn contrary to patient or family demands. The new law, the Advance Directives Act of 1999, establishes and sanctions an extrajudicial process for resolving disputes over EOL care (50). A review of treatments by a medical or ethics committee may find them to be medically inappropriate, and if so they can be discontinued after a specified amount of time. The provisions in the Texas law are consistent with those set forth in the AMA's Code of Ethics.

V. PHYSICIAN-ASSISTED DEATH (PAD) IN THE UNITED STATES AND ELSEWHERE

Another area of conflict between patients and physicians is in the area of euthanasia or assisted death. PAD is similar to futility by virtue of the fact that the patient is asking for treatment only to meet resistance from the healthcare provider. In addition to the similarity with futility PAD has underlying principles that are associated with other actions that take place in routine EOL care. Ultimately, the distinction lies in the underlying purpose or intent of a particular act.

Clearly, there are distinctions that must be made. Involuntary passive euthanasia is a practice where, without the knowledge or involvement in the decision to do so, a patient's life is ended through the action of another individual. Theoretically, this could take place in EOL care, if the intent of medication administration is to cause or hasten death, rather than to provide comfort. Voluntary passive euthanasia is similar to this only the patient's wish is known, and essentially being carried out through another individual whose actions end the patient's life. This is similar to assisted suicide, although distinguishable in that the life-ending act is performed by another individual rather than the patient himself. The patient's actions are responsible for ending life in assisted suicide, but as the term suggests, assistance is required. When a physician provides the assistance such as prescribing medications and/or giving instructions, the suicide is physician-assisted. A physician or other individual can provide the assistance, just as they can be the one participating in euthanasia.

The AMA states that euthanasia is fundamentally incompatible with the physician's role as healer, and would pose serious societal risks. Physician-assisted suicide is seen in the same light. Regulations governing nursing practice also prohibit euthanasia (51). Despite the position of these professional bodies and societal condemnation, there is fairly wide belief that such practices do take place, and that they are appropriate in select settings. Anonymous reports prior to any form of legalized PAS in the United States revealed incidents of assisted suicide being practiced with a relatively high prevalence among oncologists (52,53). The United States physicians report receiving and honoring requests for assistance in hastening patient death. When asked to describe the characteristics of their most recent patient making such a request, 1902 physicians responded. A total of 379 described 415 instances of refusal and 80 instances where the request was granted. Those requesting assistance with death were seriously ill, near death, with physical discomfort and the burden of pain being significant. Nearly half were described as depressed, and most of them made the request themselves along with their family. Physicians were more inclined to honor a request for assistance with death if the patient was in severe pain or discomfort, had less than one month to live, and if the patient was not believed to be depressed at the time the request was made (54).

One study of 1210 oncology nurses in the United States found 47% indicating they would vote to legalize PAD, and 16% indicating willingness to follow a physicians order for administration of a lethal injection to a competent, terminally ill patient who requested such assistance (55). Anonymous reporting from 1139 nurses, 71% of whom worked exclusively in ICUs in the United States disclosed interesting experiences involving assisting with death. Patient and family requests for euthanasia or assisted suicide were reported by 17% of these ICU nurse, and 16% reported they had engaged in such practices. A smaller number (4%) reported that they had hastened a patient's death by pretending to provide life-sustaining treatments that were ordered by physicians (56).

Anonymous questionnaires returned from internal medicine residents found one-third believing that some form of PAD should be legalized, and that it is ethically appropriate in some situations. Two-thirds agreed with terminal sedation for refractory pain in terminal illness, and 85% agreed with aggressive analgesia for terminally ill patients, even if such might hasten death (57).

In the Code of Medical Ethics pertaining to both euthanasia and physician-assisted suicide, the AMA states that physicians must aggressively respond to the needs of patients at the EOL, including adequate pain control. In fact, the AMA states that "physicians have an obligation to relieve pain and suffering and to promote the dignity and autonomy of dying patients in their care. This includes providing effective palliative treatment even though it may foreseeable hasten death" (35). Clearly, it is acceptable, and even necessary to liberally administer medications for comfort of the terminally ill patient. Reducing the burden of suffering is not only acceptable but also it is an obligation. Even opponents of PAS (58) as well as the U.S. Supreme Court have recognized the administration of sedatives and analgesics in escalating doses in order to control discomfort as ethically and professionally sound; even when seeking to achieve terminal sedation, where the patient's death is likely to occur because of the dosage of medication (41).

Assisted death by the medical profession is legal in some countries, and legislatures within others are in discussions on the topic. In order to guide legislative actions, it is helpful to understand why patients might choose to end their lives, and whether better EOL care planning might change their view (59). Euthanasia in Europe has been accepted in the Netherlands for several years. Patient who request termination of their life have certain characteristics in common. Not all patients who make a request have it granted, and overall there seems to be little criticism of the practice as being inappropriately utilized.

The Dutch, a population which has a high incidence of terminal cancer, has openly practiced PAD for three decades with the Dutch parliament granting physician immunity from prosecution, if the patient has repeatedly requested euthanasia freely, has suffering that cannot be relieved, and the physician reports the true cause of death to the coroner. One study of the Dutch practice published in 1990 found that 2,700 of 130,000 deaths were from euthanasia, and of these, 99% were expected to die within one month. Physicians were also found to have rejected more than two-thirds of patient requests for PAD (60). Reasons given by patients requesting PAD were loss of dignity, pain, discomfort, fear of pain and discomfort, dependency, and "tired of life." When more than one reason was given for making the request, more than half of the time loss of dignity was given, followed by pain. A 1995 publication reviewing the Dutch practice found an increase in the request for PAD while the percentage of requests granted had decreased slightly (61).

In addition to the Netherlands, Belgium has legalized PAD. Other countries are not there yet. Two cases from the British courts in 2002 found it acceptable to withdraw ventilator support from a quadraplegic patient in order for death to occur; but for another patient, not on life support, the court denied authority to administer a lethal dose of medication (62).

The state of Oregon put into effect the first American law that supported the practice of physician-assisted suicide. Evidence from the early phases of Oregon's Death With Dignity Act indicates that during 1998–2000 there was no bias on the basis of race or gender although requesters tended to be better educated than most patients (63). The debates over PAS bring patient self-determination to the forefront in EOL care planning. Preliminary evidence suggests that under controlled circumstances PAS is relatively free from abuse and bias (64). A second physician's opinion is required by both Oregon and the Netherlands. Some believe there should be involvement of a psychiatrist to address the impact of depression (65). Of 165 patients in Oregon who had requested PAS, 20% showed evidence of depressions, and none of those were granted lethal prescriptions. In addition, only one in sixty requests for PAS actually resulted in suicide (63).

VI. CONCLUSION

The management of dying patients in the practice of modern medicine has become increasingly complex. This is due in part to the advancement in technology that has improved our capability to sustain life through support of organ function. Intensive care admission is usually due to life-threatening illness; an illness, which may develop into conditions which are terminal. In such a setting, the potential benefits of life-sustaining technology must always be balanced against the burdens of pain, suffering, and indignity associated with them. The ethical principles of beneficence and nonmaleficence must be respected. Likewise, respect for patient autonomy is crucial. Shared decision-making is the ideal mode for planning EOL care; the patient's involvement is best, and respect for his/her values is necessary in any regard.

Autonomy does not require providing treatment that is of no value, and CPR is not indicated for terminal patients where death is expected. Continuation of life-sustaining treatments when there is no hope of recovery is also inappropriate and consideration must be directed at how to reach an agreement on converting to EOL care. Policies providing review of futile treatment, and involvement of institutional ethics committees will be helpful when a patient or surrogate is unrealistic and continues to demand unwarranted treatment. Ultimate decision-making may involve refocusing goals from cure and recovery to comfort and dignity.

Discontinuation of life-sustaining treatment must be accomplished with care to provide comfort and protect dignity. Appropriate and generous administration of medications to assure patient comfort is appropriate, and must not be confused with causing death or euthanasia. The acceptable double effect of sedative and analgesic medications that may even hasten death should not limit administration when the intent is to provide comfort. A patient focused model with ultimate respect for a patient's comfort and dignity should be the foundation for providing EOL care for the patient with cancer.

REFERENCES

1. Emanuel LL, vonGunten CF, Ferris FD. Gaps in end-of-life care. Arch Fam Med 2000; 9(10):1176–1180.
2. Education for Physicians on End-of-Life Care (EPEC): An Initiative of the American Medical Association's Institute for Ethics. Supported by a grant from the Robert Wood Johnson Foundation EOEC Project, 1999.
3. Linde-Zwirble W, Angus DC, Griffin M, Watson RS, Clermont G. ICU care at the end-of-life in America: an epidemiologic study. Crit Care Med 2000; 28:A34.
4. Rocker GM, Curtis JR. Caring for the dying in the intensive care unit: in search of clarity. JAMA 2003; 290:820–822.
5. Gazelle G. The slow code—should anyone rush to its defense? NEJM 1998; 338:467–469
6. Union Pacific Railway Co v. Botsford, 141 US 250, 1891.

7. Dickenson DL. Are medical ethicists out of touch? Practitioner attitude in the US and UK towards decisions at the end of life. J Med Ethics 2000; 26: 254–260.
8. Schneiderman LJ, Gilmer T, Teetzel HD, Dugan DO, Blustein J, Cranford R, Briggs KB, Komatsu GI, Goodman-Crews P, Cohn F, Young EWD. Effect of ethics consultations on nonbeneficial life-sustaining treatments in the intensive care setting: a randomized controlled trial. JAMA 2003; 290:1166–1172.
9. President's Commission for the Study of Ethical Problems in Medicine and Biomedical and Behavioral Research: Deciding to Forego Life-Sustaining Treatment: A Report on the Ethical, Medical, and Legal Issues in Treatment Decisions. Washington, DC: US Government Printing Office, 1983:73–77, 141–145.
10. Nelson JE, Danis M. End-of-life care in the intensive care unit: where are we now? Crit Care Med 2001; 29(suppl 2):N2–N9.
11. Asch DA, Hansen-Flashen J, Lanken P. Decisions to limit or continue life-sustaining treatment by critical care physicians in the United States: conflicts between physicians' practices and patients' wishes. Am J Respir Crit Care Med 1995; 151:288–292.
12. Burns JP, Edwards J, Johnson J, Cassem NH, Truog R. Do-not-resuscitate order after 25 years. Crit Care Med 2003; 31:1543–1550.
13. Bircher NG. Resuscitation research and consent: ethical and practical issues. Crit Care Med 2003; 31(suppl5): S379–S384.
14. Standards for cardiopulmonary resuscitation and emergency cardiac care. JAMA 1974; 227(suppl):833–868.
15. Diem SJ, Lantos JD, Tulsky JA. Cardiopulmonary resuscitation on television: miracles and misinformation. N Engl J Med 1996; 334:1578–1582.
16. Zoch TW, Desbiens NA, DeStefano F, Stueland DT, Layde PM. Short- and long-term survival after cardiopulmonary resuscitation. Arch Intern Med 2000; 160:1969–1973.
17. Pendergast TJ, Luce JM. Increasing incidence of withholding and withdrawal of life support from the critically ill. Am J Respir Crit Care Med 1997; 155:15–20.
18. Waisel DB, Truog RD. The end-of-life sequence. Anesthesiology 1997; 87(3):676–686.
19. Heyland DK, Rocker GM, O'Callaghan CJ, Dodek PM, Cook DJ. Dying in the ICU: perspectives of family members. Chest 2003; 124:392–397.
20. Clarke EB, Curtis JR, Luce JM, Levy M, Danis M, Nelson J, Solomon MZ. Quality indicators for end-of-life care in the intensive care unit. Crit Care Med 2003; 31:2255–2262.
21. Portenoy RK, Thaler HT, Kornblith AB, et al. Symptom prevalence, characteristics and distress in a cancer population. Qual Life Res 1994; 3:183–189.
22. Lunney JR, Lynn J, Foley DJ, Lipson S, Guralnik JM. Patterns of functional decline at the end of life. JAMA 2003; 289:2387–2392.
23. Lorenz K, Lynn J. Moral and practical challenges of physician-assisted suicide. JAMA 2003; 289:2282.
24. Institute of Medicine. Approaching Death: Improving Care at the End of Life. Washington, DC: National Academy Press, 1997:14–49.
25. Covinsky KE, Goldman L, Cook EF, et al. The impact of serious illness on patients' families. JAMA 1994; 272:1839–1844.
26. Tang ST. When Death Is Imminent: Where Terminally Ill Patients With Cancer Prefer to Die and Why? Cancer Nurs 2003; 26(3):245–251.
27. Sprung CL, Cohen SL, Sjokvist P, Baras M, Bulow H, Hovilehto S, Ledoux D, Lippert A, Maria P, Phelan D, Schobersberger W, Wennberg E, Woodcock T. End-of-life practices in European intensive care units: the ethicus study. JAMA 2003; 290:790–797.
28. Truog RD, Cist AFM Bracket SE, et al. Recommendations for end-of-life care in the intensive care unit: the Ethics Committee of the Society of Critical Care Medicine. Crit Care Med 2001; 29(12):2332–2348.
29. Lynn, Joanne MD, Goldstein NE. Advance care planning for fatal chronic illness: avoiding commonplace errors and unwarranted suffering. Ann Intern Med 2003; 138(10):812–818.
30. Wenger NS, Rosenfeld K. Quality indicators for end-of-life care in vulnerable elders. Ann Intern Med 2001; 134:677–685.
31. Lamont EB, Christakis NA. Complexities in prognostication in advanced cancer: "to help them live their lives the way they want to." JAMA 2003; 290:98–104.
32. Pendergast TJ, Puntillo KA. Withdrawal of life support: intensive caring at the end of life. JAMA 2002; 288:2732–2740.
33. AMA Code of Medical Ethics 2.22. "Do-Not-Resuscitate Orders."
34. Saunders J. Perspectives on CPR: resuscitation or resurrection. Clin Med 2001; 1:457–460.
35. AMA Code of Medical Ethics 2.20. "Withholding or Withdrawing Life-Sustaining Treatment."
36. Marco CA, Larkin GL, Moskop JC, Derse AR. Determination of "futility" in emergency medicine. Ann Emerg Med. 2000; 35:604–612.
37. Jadad AR, Brownman GP. The WHO analgesic ladder for cancer pain management: stepping up the quality of its evaluation. JAMA 1994; 274:1870–1873.
38. Buchan ML, Tolle SW. Pain relief for dying persons: dealing with physicians' fears and concerns. J Clin Ethics 1995; 6:53–61.
39. Foley KM. Competent care for the dying instead of physician-assisted suicide. N Engl J Med 1997; 337: 54–59.
40. Solomon MZ, et al. Decisions near the end of life: professional views on life-sustaining treatments. Am J Public Health 1993; 83:14–23.
41. Compassion in Dying v State of Washington, 79 F3d 790 (9th cir), 1996.
42. Vacco v Quill, 521 US 793, 1997.

43. New York State Task Force on Life and the Law. When Death Is Sought: Assisted Suicide and Euthanasia in the Medical Context. New York, NY: New York State Task Force on Life and Law, 1994.
44. AMA Code of Medical Ethics 2.035. "Futile Care".
45. Cogliano JF. The medical futility controversy: bioethical implications for the critical care nurse. CC Nurs Quar 1999; 22:81–88.
46. Jecker NS. Knowing when to stop: the limits of medicine. Hastings Cent Rep 1991; 21:5–8.
47. Coppa S. Futile care: confronting the high costs of dying. J Nurs Adm 1996; 26:18–23.
48. Weijer C, Singer PA, Dickens BM, Workman S. Bioethics for clinicians: dealing with demands for inappropriate treatment. CMAJ 1998; 159:817–821.
49. AMA Code of Medical Ethics 2.037. "Medical Futility in End-of-Life Care."
50. Fine RL, Mayo TW. Resolution of futility by due process: early experience with the Texas Advance Directives Act. Ann Intern Med 2003; 138:743–746.
51. AMA Code of Medical Ethics 2.21 "Euthanasia". AMA Code of Medical Ethics 2.211 "Physician-Assisted Suicide".
52. Meier DE, Emmons CA, Wallenstein S, Quill T, Morrison RS, Cassel CK. A national survey of physician-assisted suicide and euthanasia in the United States. N Engl J Med 1998; 338:1193–1201.
53. Emanuel EJ, Fairclough DL, Slutsman J, Alpert H, Baldwin D, Emmanuel LL. Assistance from family members, friends, paid cargivers, and volunteers in the care of terminally ill patients. N Engl J Med 1998; 341:956–963.
54. Meier DE, Emmons CA, Litke NM, Wallenstein S, Morrison RS. Characteristics of patients requesting and receiving physician-assisted death archives of internal medicine. 2003; 163:1537–1542.
55. Young A, Volker D, Rieger PT, Thrope DM. Oncology nurses' attitudes regarding voluntary, physician-assited dying for competent, terminally ill patients. Oncol Nurs Forum. 1993 Apr; 20(3):445–451.
56. Asch DA. The role of critical care nurses in euthanasia and assisted suicide. N Eng J Med 1996; 335(13):971–974.
57. Kaldiian LC, We B, Kirkpatrick JN, Thomas-Geevarghese A, Vaughan-Sarrazin M. Medical House Officers' attitudes toward aggressive analgesia, terminal sedation, and assisted suicide in end-of-life care: are there associations with training, demographic, and religious factors?. J Gen Intern Med 2003; 18:245.
58. Hamerly JP. Views on assisted suicide: perspectives of the AMA and the NHO. Am J Health Syst Pharm. 1998; 55:543–547.
59. Mak YYW, Elwyn G, Finlay IG. Patients' voices are needed in debates on euthanasia. BMJ 2003; 327: 213–215.
60. van der Maas PJ, et al. Euthanasia and other medical decisions concerning the end of life. Lancet 1991; 338:669–674.
61. van der Maas PJ, et al. Euthanasia, physician-assisted suicide, and other medical practices involving the end of life in the Netherlands, 1990–1995. N Engl J Med 1996; 335(22):1699–1705.
62. Batlle JC. Legal status of physician-assisted suicide. JAMA 2003; 289:2279–2281.
63. Ganzini L, Nelson HD, Schmidt TA, Kraemer DF, Delorit MA, Lee MA. Physicians' experiences with the Oregon Death With Dignity Act. NEJM 2000; 342:557–563.
64. Sullivan AD, Hedberg K, Hopkins D. Legalized hysician-assisted suicide in Oregon, 1998–2000. NEJM 2001; 344:605–607.
65. Baile WF, Dimaggio JR, Schapira CV, et al. The request for assistance in dying: the need for psychiatric consultation. Cancer 1993; 72:2786–2791.

48

Legal Considerations: Liability, Consent, Risk Management, Withdrawing Life Support

I. McLELLAN and J. TRING

University Hospitals of Leicester NHS Trust, University of Leicester, Leicester, U.K.

I. INTRODUCTION

This chapter is aimed to bring together some of the differing practicalities and views in legal areas. In this, we will be comparing some of the similarities and differences between systems, outlook, and the law between the United Kingdom and the United States of America. There are of course differences in the legal system between individual states in the United States (1). In the United Kingdom also, these do occur between the four main constituent countries, but these are at present mainly similarities and only four variations. However, the U.K. is liable for some control under the European Law.

Because of space limitations, there will be restriction of the subject matter that can be covered and we will be using "snapshots." We hope this chapter encourages clinicians to be analytical about the legal issues arising in this area of patient care.

II. LIABILITY

There are two main areas that there is liability involved in the care of the patient in these circumstances.

Firstly, there is a liability in a health care system for providing availability of care. Different systems will have different targets depending on factors involved with resource allocation. In the perfect world, all treatments in reality would be freely available for all patients. This is of course not so as resources are restricted no matter how the system is organized. The basic issue of resources is of money to pay for the treatment. Health care systems are broadly funded by allocations that are taxation or insurance based.

There is also a group of patients found in these systems who are not covered by either and these must be considered to be a third group "self-pay patients." There is also a fourth group, those patients who cannot afford to pay and so do not get treatment. Is there a difference between the two main resource systems of the United States and the U.K.? It is widely believed in the United Kingdom that the National Health Service provides an all-encompassing care for patients in the cancer and oncology category. This is seen as providing a deeper level of care particularly for the older patient with cancer than insurance-based systems, which may limit care. However, even in Britain limitations are put on care and potential treatments limited by resources. This was shown in the Courts in the U.K., where in this case a health authority—the provider—declined to pay for a child to undergo further therapy because of the cost and the authority had other priorities (2).

This group of patients who may have a limited prognosis is vulnerable to resource pressures. This has become apparent in both the United States and the U.K. It becomes most obvious when there are two reasons for a limited life span such as cancer and the patient being elderly. In the U.K., this had been evidenced by the needs of the elderly being championed by the health service tsar—a National Director of Older People Services with a National Service Framework for Older People (3) and the setting up of the NHS Cancer Plan (4).

Resources in the United States affect the care planning of patients. Some will pay full independent costs, others will be covered by health maintenance organizations, preferred provider organizations, or independent practice associations. As these are driven by cost as well as quality, there are vulnerable groups and some providers may not provide a service to these at all. This provides opportunity for others in a business sense for providing the needs of specialist groups. Other citizens may not be covered by any of the above systems and may have limited financial resources. This had lead to some U.S. citizens seeking part of their care from Canada as evidenced by the issue of online prescription drug ordering (5).

At the heart of liability to provide services is cost/benefit ratio. In Oregon (6), this has been developed into a priority setting using the above but also taking into account the public's views. Of course, this will change with different circumstances and as such requires regular updating. Financial resources become significant and the treatments would have been limited (7). Cancer of the esophagus was one condition, which would have been so low in the priority list that it would not be on the treatment schedule.

In the U.K., there has been a need to take legal action on the part of patients to ensure that health services required for an area population are provided. This was, however, unsuccessful (8) and was repeated in 1988, when the Court of Appeal rejected an application as the courts could not rule on resource distribution to and use within the National Health Service (9). The variation in medical opinion also allows patients to fall into a gap in provision of service. This was shown in the U.K. by R v Cambridge Health Authority, exp B, where a 10-year old lymphoma sufferer was denied the financial resources for treatment by the health authority, as there was a much more limited prognosis given by their experts than by others sought out by the father. The Courts upheld the health authorities right to decide priorities. The child was, in fact, treated due to an anonymous financial gift and survived for over a year (2).

It may well be that future decisions may be affected by Article 2 of the Human Rights Act—the right to life (10).

A. Individual Liability

There is liability for health care professionals to treat patients in their best interests. In general, the requirements on doctors to treat the oncology patient are the same all over the world. Doctors may be restricted in what they can offer by the resources that are available on a particular site, but should have the requirement to refer care on if treatments are only available in limited centers.

There does need to have fully informed consent particularly where the cost/benefit ratio is high, treatment being high cost with low benefit. The patient needs to take into account the information given and have the ability to comprehend it.

Does patients' demand influence care? The patient who wishes to be treated by a doctor, even when that doctor considers that outcome is limited, does not have a right to treatment but again should be referred on for a second opinion. Pressure from the educated patient may, however, cause the doctor to treat. On first impressions, there are more patients in the United States who may be in this category than in the U.K.

III. CONSENT

The term "consent" in medical practice has profound legal and ethical connotations. In a legal sense, consent is a common law defense to a civil or criminal action, which may arise as a result of physical contact between two people. The consent provides a justification for the contact, providing it is given freely without "force, fear, or fraud" (11).

In the practice of medicine, contact between patient and doctor is likely to be unavoidable and indeed forms an essential element of the intimate nature of the doctor–patient relationship. But this necessity for contact does not exempt the medical profession from the general legal principles relating to assault and consent (12). In these times of increasing litigation, obtaining consent is sometimes viewed by health workers as part of a legal bureaucracy that has been thrust upon them in recent years. This is to misunderstand fundamentally the function of the consent process, which is first and foremost to protect the patient's right to self-determination.

In the United Kingdom, the law has repeatedly emphasized the importance of this principle. However, there have been relatively few cases where a patient has successfully sued their doctor for battery on the grounds that consent to being touched was not given. The law in both the United States and U.K. has interpreted failure to obtain consent as a basis for negligence rather than assault or battery and indeed state-funded indemnity schemes restrict funding to claims for negligence only (13). Much emphasis has been placed on the extent and nature of the process by which *information* has been given to the patient during the process of obtaining consent and this appears to be of more concern to legal systems worldwide than the potential for tortious claims for battery.

A legally valid consent consists of the following elements:

- It is given by a competent person
- It is given voluntarily
- It is an adequately informed consent

A. What Is Competence?

A three-stage test has evolved in English law for establishing a patient's capacity to decide (14,15). The stages are:

- Can the patient comprehend and retain the necessary information?
- Does the patient believe the information they have been given?
- Is the patient able to weigh the information, balancing risks and needs, so as to arrive at a decision?

The establishment of a patient's competence to make decisions can be difficult, particularly in situations where a patient's level of consciousness is clouded as a result of drugs or illness. In such instances of fluctuating competence where retention of information is a problem, U.K. medical defense organizations recommend that any decisions the patient makes while competent should be recorded, together with any discussion that may have taken place. Over a period of time, when sustained competence may return, those decisions should be reviewed to establish whether they are consistently held (16).

Although the idea of self-determination is fundamental to legal systems worldwide, the decision as to whether a patient has the capacity to make decisions still lies with the physician. Patient autonomy is, paradoxically, granted by the doctor who may be seeking consent.

In North America, a proxy may be appointed to make decisions on behalf of the incompetent patient. No such provision exists in England, Wales, or Northern Ireland.

B. Is Consent Given Voluntarily?

Consent cannot be valid if it is obtained under duress or coercion. This may seem obvious but coercion, where consent is obtained but not freely, can be an unintentional result of a physician's enthusiasm for a particular course of action or the way in which information is given to the patient. The balance of power and knowledge almost always lies with the physician and this may adversely affect the patient's autonomy, albeit unintentionally (17).

C. Informed Consent

In the United States, the communication process by which informed consent is obtained is both an ethical and legal obligation set out in statute and case law in all 50 states. In the U.K., a statutory obligation is imposed in very few instances, but the abundance of case law pertaining to the failure to obtain informed consent imposes a common law duty on doctors to follow the process.

The concept of informed consent stems from the basic ethical principles, which were set out in the Nuremburg Code after human experimentation during World War Two. This code was further supplemented by the Declaration of Helsinki of the World Medical Association in 1964. Specifically, it states with respect to research that "In any research on human beings, each potential subject must be adequately informed of the aims, methods, anticipated benefits and potential hazards of the study and the discomfort it may entail." This has become extended to apply to the practice of medicine in general. The American Medical Association has set down strict guidelines to be followed during the consent process (18). The emphasis is very much on creating an exchange of ideas and information between doctor and patient. In 1998, the U.K. General Medical Council issued guidelines on good practice, which broadly reflect those of the AMA.

Informed consent can only be effectively obtained if the patient has received sufficient information on which to base a decision. This should include information about the diagnosis, the nature and purpose of a proposed treatment, the risks and benefits of a proposed treatment or procedure, alternatives, the risks and benefits of the alternatives, and the effects of having no treatment.

Consent should be obtained by the physician providing or performing the treatment or procedure, although in the U.K. this person can delegate to a suitably qualified person (19). How frequently a complication has to occur before the patient needs to be informed is a difficult question. An incidence of between 1% and 2% is often quoted, but it seems a simplistic approach to apply this in all situations. The medical profession has long exercised its own judgment in this matter and courts appear more concerned with usual practice rather than absolute frequency of risk. In everyday situations, most doctors will be influenced by a combination of factors such as the patient's age, general prognosis, and the nature of the risk. Providing the basic information required by the statutory regulating bodies is provided to the patient, assessment of the need to know is frequently made by the attending physician. Obtaining consent involves a continuing dialogue between doctor and patient, which keeps them both aware of any changing circumstances. Patients often require more information than is currently provided and the way in which information is given to patients has been the cause of much discussion, particularly with regard to the explanation of risk (20). Leaflets, Internet websites, and liaison nurses have all been used to provide an information service to patients with great effect.

The onus on how much information should be provided to the patient lies with the doctor, but, providing information is given sympathetically, facts which may dissuade the patient from opting for treatment or which may frighten them if disclosed should not be witheld if it is deemed important for the patient to know.

It is interesting to note that some ethicists believe that we should be using the term "informed request" for treatment. This would appear to be more in keeping with clinical reality. Patients ask doctors for treatment, doctors do not ask patients to submit to treatment. Although it may be an interesting ethical question, the process of information provision is likely to be indistinguishable.

D. Clinical Trials

Autonomy is the central theme of valid consent—the ability of an individual to determine what happens to his or her own body. Clinical trials when applied to critically ill patients open up a vast array of ethical and legal dilemmas. The critically ill are a population who may benefit most from the fruits of medical research, yet they are often unable to give consent.

Modern legislation applying to human research depends on the principles outlined in the Declaration of Helsinki and the Belmont Report, a federal commission document produced in 1974, which is used to educate Institutional Review Boards (IRBs) in the United States. (The IRB is an independent body that supervises clinical research, similar to an Ethics Committee in the U.K.) The Belmont Report defined the difference between clinical practice and research and recommended that human research fulfill three basic ethical principles:

1. Respect for the patient
2. A risk/benefit analysis where the benefits sought clearly outweigh the attendant risks
3. Justice—so there is a fair distribution of both burden and benefit of human investigation

Thus, easily accessible populations are not preferentially targeted.

These broad principles are adhered to in almost every country, but significant differences arise in the application of the law of consent in the critical care population between the United States and Europe.

Research in critical care falls into two main categories: *clinical trials* of new treatments and *observational studies* that require the gathering of patient data and samples, the so-called "nontherapeutic" research. In situations where the patient is unable to give consent, inclusion in clinical research is becoming ethically permissible. The Council of Europe recommendation (90) 3 (21) states that research is possible without consent, provided there is at least the potential of direct benefit for the individual. The Council also recommended that consent for studies in incompetent patients could be given by a legally authorized representative. In the U.K., however, the principle that an individual has rights that the law protects and which nobody can infringe for the public good still holds true. There is no provision in English law for surrogate decision making in such circumstances. The Medical Research Council statement in 1962–1963, which required that any person taking part in observational studies must volunteer fully, has, however, been amended in recognition of the unique problems facing critical care researchers. The MRC now recommends that "the person must not object or appear to object" to the study. This may be difficult in a sedated and ventilated patient. As an added safeguard, the Local Ethics Committee must agree that the patient's welfare and safety are being upheld and, in an attempt to preserve the patient's autonomy, retrospective consent is needed whereby research subjects are given full information on their recovery and are given the opportunity to withdraw.

In the United States, the idea of a patient-designated surrogate does not appear to have substantially reduced the problems of obtaining consent because proxies do not accurately express the unknown wishes of the patient (22). Few people discuss in advance their feelings about participating in clinical research and most surrogates do not know with certainty the position of the patient on these issues. Retrospective consent was formerly used in the United States in the 1980s, but the U.S. Office of Protection from Research Risks judged that it was impossible to consent to something that had already happened.

The current U.S. position on this issue has replaced the need for retrospective consent with a permission to waive the need for consent, provided certain criteria are met: the research must pose no more than minimal risk, the waiver does not adversely affect the participant's rights, informed consent or proxy consent is not feasible, and the participant must be provided with additional information after participation (23). This has at least addressed some important issues such as the realization that obtaining informed consent is sometimes an impossible prerequisite. In Europe, a proxy may be appointed but in the U.K. the law does not even provide for that. The Medical Research Council has attempted to make its approach more flexible, yet has to work within the confines of the fundamental legal principle of patient autonomy. This approach will undoubtedly restrict critical care research in the U.K., but it does preserve the fundamental basis of the doctor–patient relationship, namely, the right to self-determination.

In summary, possible solutions to these problems include the waiver of consent under the auspices of the IRB/ Local Ethics Committees, prospective consent, or retrospective consent. Waiving the need for consent may be the easiest way of resolving the question for nontherapeutic research, where data collection does not interfere with the care of the patient but it undermines patient autonomy, which is one of the most important concepts in medical law.

Prospective consent, or a living will, may give a false impression of a patient's wishes. How can a decision made in good health accurately reflect a patient's wishes when something as fundamental as mental state or level of consciousness becomes affected? Retrospective consent would appear to be a contradiction in terms and would be unobtainable if the patient dies (24,25).

Critical care patients thus present a huge dilemma. Inherent in civilized medical practice since the 1940s is the principle of patient autonomy and yet the availability of new and innovative treatments to this group may become restricted if the law fails to provide the critical care community with a suitable legal and ethical framework.

IV. RISK MANAGEMENT

A. Introduction

Risk Management is a process that seeks to identify, control, and prevent any event that may result in adverse consequences. It forms an essential part of the ethos of clinical governance, which has been introduced in an attempt to improve standards of medical care. Many see it as a device for protecting patients and preventing litigation. It owes its origins to commercial organizations, which were affected by a series of high-profile financial and operational disasters during the 1970s and 1980s. Out of these events, the concept of *governance* and the principles of *corporate governance* were established in the Cadbury and Greenbury reports, which specified structures for the organization of company boards (26). These, or similar, structures have been implemented in hospitals throughout the U.K. and United States. Risk Management has been imported from the private sector into health systems worldwide because of the spiraling costs of healthcare and increasing alarm at the apparently high incidence of errors in medical care. The National Center for Patient Safety estimates that as many as 180,000 deaths occur in the United States each year due to preventable medical errors. It has been estimated that a hospital patient has a one in 200 chance of being the victim of serious error, compared with one in 2,000,000 on an aeroplane (27).

In the U.K. during the late 1990s, political exposure of high-profile failures in medical care gave cause for concern amongst the public about standards generally (28).

In a response to this situation in the United States, over 90 public and private bodies, which purchase health care on behalf of their workers across the country, formed a group called the Leapfrog Initiative, which works with medical experts to identify and propose solutions that will improve the delivery of health care. Patients, or consumers, can view the results of various hospitals and those failing to implement proposed solutions may lose funding from the third party payers.

In the U.K., where the government funds the bulk of healthcare through taxation, statutory bodies such as the Commission for Health Improvement have been set up to assess and oversee the performance of hospitals and to ensure that current standards of medical care are met. A National Institute of Clinical Excellence (NICE) was established as a Special Authority for England and Wales in 1999 to "provide patients, health professionals and the public with authoritative, robust and reliable guidance on current best practice" and also to develop and disseminate clinical audit methodologies (29). The United States and U.K. have therefore addressed the problem in different ways: third party payers in the United States use a financial tool with which to control improvements in the health care system, whilst in the U.K. a political approach has been used via government agencies.

B. Risk Management Structures

A physician setting up a basic risk management structure should consider the following elements:

- Risk identification
- Risk analysis
- Risk control
- Economic aspects of risk management

1. Risk Identification

This involves considering sources of potential error or mishap and then assessing under what circumstances the mishap may occur. An appraisal of the effects of the event should be made. This will allow an appropriate degree of importance to be apportioned.

2. Risk Analysis

The National Center for Patient Safety recommends the process of root cause analysis to determine what happened, why did it happen, what do you do to prevent it from happening again? It is a tool for identifying prevention strategies and forms part of an overall effort to create a culture of safety. It should be an interdisciplinary approach involving those who are most familiar with the situation, where changes that need to be made to the system are identified impartially. It is essential to consider human and system factors as well as analyzing underlying causes through continual enquiry as to why an action was performed.

3. Risk Control

This involves an assessment of how risks can be eliminated and if they cannot, then how may their effects be reduced? A consideration should also be given to how a system may be able to absorb the consequences of the remaining risks.

4. Economic Aspects of Risk Management

The cost of identifying, analyzing, and controlling a risk should be set against the likely impact of the risk occurring and a cost/benefit analysis performed. However, although this may be appropriate in nonclinical situations, actual risk to patients should be reduced wherever possible.

But the systems for risk management are only part of the climate of safety, which should be promoted in a hospital. A philosophy of quality improvement, a culture of cooperation and information sharing, and the recruitment of personnel who are able to lead teams as part of the overall governance strategy is essential. An effective risk management team will allow clinicians the opportunity to submit evidence of potential or actual risk in a "no blame" environment. This information should be collected at regular intervals and reviewed by a trained risk physician. A system by which these reports are analyzed and graded according to severity should be used. In the U.K., the National Patient Safety Agency has devised a categorization scheme for incidents based on the potential for harm occurring to the patient. These graded forms should be reviewed by a trained Risk Manager and clinicians and managers together should formulate a response. In the U.K., hospitals submit all adverse health incident reports to a National Patient Safety Agency. According to the grading of the incident, the agency has discretion to investigate any event. It is hoped that the central collection of information will aid audit and communication throughout the health network and promote an environment of openness.

Potential solutions may be financial or organizational. Clinical staff should link in with managerial staff to ensure an effective action. The type of response will depend upon the problem, but evidence-based medicine has now largely superseded opinion and a good risk management structure should ensure best practice guidelines are instituted where necessary (30).

C. Strategies for Improving Standards

In the U.K., hospitals are expected to demonstrate a range of activities designed to ensure quality of care such as clinical audit programs, the routine application of evidence-based medicine, and high-quality record keeping. This mirrors the approach taken in the United States, which uses comprehensive clinical quality improvement programs (31). Other mechanisms that have been introduced as part of risk management responses include examination of the appropriateness of clinical interventions (32), efforts to improve physicians' behavior (33), and the implementation of practice guidelines (34).

D. Practice Guidelines

The response of a risk management team to a perceived problem may be to formulate practice guidelines. A practice guideline may be defined as a standardized specification for medical care developed by a formal process that incorporates the best scientific evidence of effectiveness with expert opinion (35). Some risk managers may perceive guidelines as an ideal way in which to achieve uniformity of care, but there are certain problems associated with them. It must first be established whether the guideline has been introduced to offer physicians choice, advice, and suggestions or whether it is an attempt to direct their practice. In this circumstance, especially where a third party payer is seeking to introduce the guideline, the lessons from Wickline vs. State of California should be remembered. In this case, it was established that the physician is ultimately responsible for all medical decisions in a patient's care. If there is deviation from the guideline the doctor risks financial loss, whereas compliance may lead to a clinical negligence claim. This represents a potential disadvantage of the insurer-led U.S. health reform.

The legal authority of guidelines is unclear. It is undesirable that they automatically establish the standard of care, but their authority will depend upon the context to which they are to be applied and the degree to which the wording expresses the intention that the guideline should be followed (35).

V. WITHDRAWING LIFE SUPPORT

This subject is full of emotional, ethical and legal issues. It involves the treatment team, not only the medical staff but also the nurses, the therapists, in fact all who are treating the patient. Obviously, it must involve the patient, their relatives, a patient's advocate, and take into account any advance directives or living wills.

There are two areas that have to be considered: treatment which when withdrawn allows to the disease process to advance slowly and the patients dies in weeks or months which is seen as a normal way of dying and the second area where withdrawal mean the disease and its secondary manifestations will lead to the patient dying within days. Why is there a difference? Surely this is because the first allows the patient to come to terms and organize their affairs, whereas the second may not allow that and also death will be part of immediate episode for the clinical treatment team.

When making the decision to withdraw treatment timing must be right and there has to be good strategy and tactics. Full information about the situation and the options must be made clear to the patient. They must have time to reflect on these and if necessary ask the treatment team any questions.

Withdrawal of treatment is carried out when treatment is futile and the benefit/burden ratio falls. Burden should be considered as primarily the effect of treatment on the patient, but may both in the public and insured/private sector include the financial cost of treatment.

Futility is an overused word. In this chapter, it is considered to be the treatment that is not having an effective action on the disease process and is reinforced if the treatment has significant side effects.

It is a decision taken by the doctors in conjunction with the other clinical staff. It should be shared with the patients and with their consent, to avoid breaking confidentiality, their relatives also. That, of course, is in the case of the competent patient. With the incompetent patient, not only should treatment be in their "best interests" but so also should breaking confidentiality and discussion with the patients or patients' advocate.

In both situations above, it may be necessary to arrange a case conference and with any dissention a second opinion should be sought. The patient's wishes should be respected, but a doctor does not have to treat a patient if the treatment is felt by that doctor not to be in the patient's best interests. However, in that situation, the patient's care should be handed over to another practitioner.

When withdrawing treatment, the clinician has to be aware of the possible consequences. As discussed above, treatment is withdrawn because of futility and increasing burdens on the patient. The clinician must see withdrawal as being in the patient's best interest. In general, the clinician would be aware that withdrawal could lead to the earlier death of the patient. In withdrawal, like the prescription of some drugs this issue of earlier death should be considered under "double effect." This is the concept that an action with good intent in the best interests of the patient may lead to hastening their death. This is lawful as long as that was not the primary intention, or the method by which the good intent was affected.

In the United States, withdrawal of treatment is considered more to be part of the family's responsibility in the competent patient. It is possible to take example from the Quinlan judgment, which involved the father, the attending physicians, and the hospital ethics committee (36). Further judgements in Cruzan (37) and Fiori (38) supported the intention of the family with the attending physicians in decision making. In fact, in the latter so long as there was agreement between the family and the physicians there was no need for court involvement.

The above issues in the incompetent patient bring up again the consent issues. There is, in the U.S. cases above, acceptance of the concept of the family being able to consent on behalf of the patient as reasoned in the President's Commission report in 1983 (16). In the U.K., other than Scotland, there is no authority for relatives to make decisions on patient's behalf. Consent also should be considered in discussing treatment and the patient's condition. At the start of treatment and at regular intervals, particularly at significant clinical events, the patient's wishes about disclosing the facts to their relatives or other nominated persons should be rechecked. It would be necessary to record such wishes in the patient's notes. The patient should also be asked what they want disclosed or discussed if they become incompetent. As again, information given to relatives and other persons is breaking confidentiality, one of the bases of medical practice.

In considering when a clinician withdraws treatment, there are other aspects to this decision. Above the question of criminal law and withdrawal has been briefly touched on. There is a widely perceived difference in the quantity of litigation in the Civil Courts between the United States and the U.K. This is reflected in differences in the indemnity insurance premiums between these countries. They are being used as examples, with other countries also showing differences. The effect of a higher level of litigation in the United States has lead to a belief in the U.K. that clinicians in the United States are far less likely to withdraw treatment than those in the U.K. This leads to more heroic treatment being carried out in the United States than in the U.K., as not only does the clinician want to serve the patient but also the fear is that withdrawal will lead to malpractice litigation not only by the patient but also by the family. The clinician must decide what is best for the patient.

The decision of withdrawal has to be made balancing what is possible in terms of organ and body support and what is useful to the patient. Of course, this also brings in the question of available resources and puts more pressure on the clinician to decide what are "best interests" (39). The clinician not only has to decide what in that patient's interests but also will have to consider their other patients from whom resources are being withheld. This is not an easy ethical debate. Of course, external influences such as the state, insurance companies, and even the patients own resources may not only influence but also direct what is available. Although clinicians should act in the "best interests" of individual patients, there must be effective limits in how much of the health care resources is used.

Where then can the clinician go? The pathway must be in consensus with patient and family. The withdrawal of treatment if court directed can only bring about a break up of trust between patient and the clinicians and must be a last resort. So far the competent patient who does not wish withdrawal against the advice of the clinicians has not been considered. All efforts must be made to agree this with the patient and relatives. There should be a protocol for this path, using repeated case conferences, outside assessors, and only, finally, the courts.

What has not yet been tested is Article 2 of the Human Rights Act—the right to life (10). Patients in the U.K. may use this to gain treatment by putting on pressure and the law into the doctor's decision. Of course, too active treatment could be considered to be against Article 3—the prohibition of torture and inhumane treatment. This is especially true if consent is questionable. This has been tested in a critical care decision over ventilation (40).

VI. CONCLUSION

This chapter has touched on several aspects of the legal considerations that involve patients undergoing treatment for cancer. The subject is large and full of potential pitfalls for the clinician. We hope this chapter will clarify some points, show ways forward, and support the clinical staff in their vision of the patient and their treatment.

REFERENCES

1. Kroll DA. Medico-legal aspects: an American perspective. In: Healey TEJ, Cohen PJ , eds.Wyhe and Churchill. Davidson's a Practice of Anaesthesia. 6th ed. London: Edward Arnold, 1449:1454.
2. R v Cambridge Health Authority, exp B (1995) 25. BMLR 5. (1995) 23. BMLR.1.CA.
3. National Service Framework for Older People. www.doh.gov.uk/nsf/olderpeople.htm.
4. NHS Cancer Plan. London.
5. BMJ. Drug importation to USA. BMJ 2003; 326:618. Department of Health, 2000.
6. Dixon J, Gilbert Welch H. Priority setting. Lessons from Oregon. Lancet 1991; 337:891–894.
7. Ham C. Retracing the Oregon trail: the experience of rationing and the Oregon Health Plan. BMJ 1998; 316:1965–1969.
8. Brahms D. Enforcing a duty of care for patients in the NHS. Lancet 1984; 2:1224–1225.
9. Brahms D. Seeking increased NHS resources. Through the courts. Lancet 1988; 1:133–134.
10. Human Rights Act, 1998.
11. Smith JS, Hogan B. Criminal Law Cases and Materials 6th ed. London: Butterworths.
12. Malette v Shulman (1990) 67 DLR (4th) 321 (Ont CA).
13. Kennedy I, Grubb A. Medical Law. 3rd ed. London: Butterworths.
14. Re C (a minor) (detention for medical treatment) [1997] 2 FLR 180 (Fam Div).
15. Gillick v West Norfolk and Wisbech AHA (1985) 3 All ER 402.
16. Medical Protection Society, U.K., 2003.
17. President's Commission, Making Health Care Decisions, 1983.

18. America Medical Association, Informed Consent, 2003.
19. Department of Health. Good practice in Consent Implementation Guide: Consent to Examination or Treatment. London: The Stationery Office, 2001.
20. Edwards A, Elwyn G, Mulley A. Explaining risks: turning numerical data into meaningful pictures. BMJ 2002; 34:827.
21. Council of Europe. Recommendation R(90)3 of the committee of ministers to the member states concerning medical research on human beings. 1990.
22. Coppolino M, Ackerson L. Do surrogate decision makers provide accurate consent for intensive care research? Chest 2001; 119:603–612.
23. Protection of Human Subjects United States Department of Health and Human Services, 1981: Title45, Code of Federal Regulations, Part, 46.116(d).
24. Reade MC, Young JD. Consent for observational studies in critical care: time to open Pandora's box [editorial]. Anaesthesia 2003; 58.
25. Bigatello LM, George E, Hurford W. Ethical considerations for research in critically ill patients. Crit Care Med 2003; 31(3).
26. Committee on Corporate Governance. Final Report. London: Gee Publishing, 1997.
27. Hopkins Tanne J. AMA moves to tackle medical errors. BMJ 1997; 315:970.
28. Horton R. Doctors, the General Medical Council, and Bristol [editorial]. Lancet 1998; 351:1525–1526.
29. National Institute for Clinical Excellence, 2000.
30. Evidence-based Medicine Working Group. Evidence-based medicine: a new approach to teaching the practice of medicine. JAMA 1992; 268:2420–2425.
31. Kassirer J. The quality of care and the quality of measuring it. N Engl J Med 1993; 329:1263–1265.
32. Phelps C. The methodologic foundations of studies of the appropriateness of medical care. N Engl J Med 1993; 329:1241–1245.
33. Greco P, Eisenberg J. Changing physicians' practices. N Engl J Med 1993; 329:1271–1274.
34. Lomas J, Anderson G, Domnick-Pierre K, Vayda E, Enkin M, Hannah W. Do practice guidelines guide practice? The effect of a consensus statement on the practice of physicians. N Engl J Med 1989; 321: 1306–1311.
35. West JC. Risk management and medical practice guidelines: what is risk management's proper role? J Healthcare Risk Manage 1994; 14:3
36. Re Quinlan. 355. A2d. 647. (NJ 1976).
37. Cruzan v Director, Missouri. Department of Health. 110. S Ct. 2841 (1990).
38. Re Fiori. 652. A 2d. 1350. (Pa 1995).
39. McLellan I. Withdrawal of Treatment in the Competent Patient. M. Phil. Dissertation, University of Glasgow, U.K., 2001.
40. B v An NHS Hospital Trust (2002) EWHC 429. Fam.

49

Perioperative Care of Children with Cancer: An Overview

ALAN I. FIELDS and RODRIGO MEJIA

Division of Pediatrics, The Children's Cancer Hospital at the University of Texas M.D. Anderson Cancer Center and Division of Anesthesiology and Critical Care, The University of Texas M.D. Anderson Cancer Center, Houston, Texas, U.S.A.

JAMES D. WILKINSON

Department of Epidemiology and Public Health, University of Miami School of Medicine, Miami, Florida, U.S.A.

The prognosis and outcome for pediatric oncology patients have improved considerably over recent decades (1–12). Earlier published reports indicated pessimistic outcomes for oncology patients admitted to the pediatric intensive care unit (PICU) and some even concluded that the application of intensive care therapies was futile (1). As a result, pediatric oncology units, especially those that offered stem cell transplants, developed a very broad therapeutic repertoire. Patients with a severity-of-illness, which would have ordinarily dictated a PICU admission, remained in these units for treatment, including attempts at hemodynamic support for early septic and/or hypovolemic shock and renal replacement therapies (9). Admission to the PICU was reserved for those children requiring mechanical ventilation, usually for acute respiratory failure. This philosophy often resulted in delayed PICU admission and use of appropriately aggressive interventions until "late in the spiral of multisystem organ failure" (7), if a PICU admission was offered at all.

More recently, a more aggressive therapeutic approach with earlier application of invasive therapies has resulted in improved outcomes for pediatric oncology patients admitted to the PICU. Outcomes for patients with liquid and solid tumors (excepting stem cell transplants), who receive mechanical ventilation for respiratory disease or shock, are now comparable to those of the general PICU population (Fig. 1). Indeed, Kutko et al. (13) noted that oncologic illness, in the absence of bone marrow transplantation, does not appear to be associated with an increased mortality for children with septic shock.

Perioperative mortality, especially for those patients receiving postoperative mechanical ventilation, has remained fairly low over the last two decades (1,7). In the case of solid tumors, both improved survival and functional outcomes have been ascribed to improved chemotherapy and secondarily to improved radiation therapy, more conservative (less mutilating) surgical treatment, and more judicious use of analgesia and sedation (14). Thus, we may expect to find that future advances in treatment for the perioperative pediatric oncology patient will be focused on decreasing morbidity, rather than

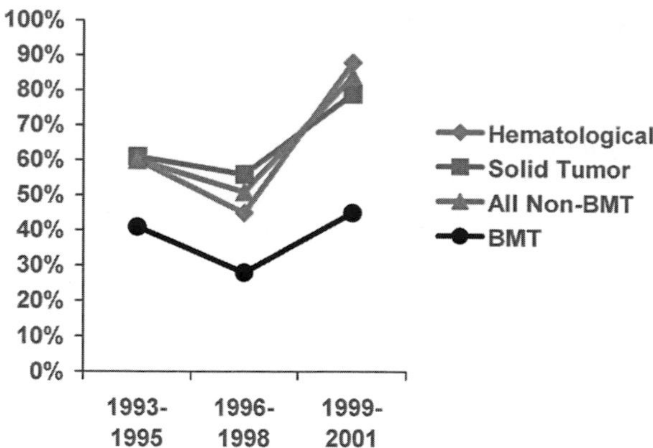

Non-BMT [a] patients outcome 64% vs. BMT patients 36% ($p < 0.0001$)
Odds Ratio of ICU survival 99-01 vs. 93-98: 1.45% (95% C.I. 1.09, 1.98)
[a] Bone marrow transplantation
* Adapted with permission RF Tamburro

Figure 1 ICU survival of respiratory failure in pediatric oncology patients at St. Judes Children's Research Hospital (Sillos, 2002). (Adapted from Tamburro RF.)

significantly decreasing already low perioperative mortality.

Although perioperative mortality may remain low, extrapolating from experimental data we may speculate that long-term mortality may still be affected by our surgical and anesthetic approaches. It has been shown both experimentally and clinically that surgery causes transient immunosupression (15–17), which may be associated with the implantation of surgically disseminated tumor cells and the growth of micrometastases. Experimentally, both management of perioperative pain (18) and various regional anesthetic techniques, such as spinal blockade (17) and epidural anesthesia (19), may protect against surgery-induced decreases in host resistance against metastasis. The clinical significance of attenuating postoperative immunosupression by the use of regional anesthesia and effective perioperative pain management is unclear. However, with pain now considered being the "fifth vital sign," the more judicious use of conscious and deep sedation for diagnostic and therapeutic procedures remains important, nonetheless. Formerly, lumbar punctures and bone marrow aspirations were frequently performed with physical restraint and, at best, local anesthesia and little or no sedation. This approach was associated with a risk of significant anxiety, pain, and even injury. With the availability of better intravenous anesthetics/analgesics and monitoring practices, application of appropriate levels of conscious or deeper sedation for invasive procedures should be the standard of care for pediatric oncology patients.

Among oncology patients admitted to the PICU, the stem cell transplantation patient continues to present the greatest challenges. A review of recent literature on this population indicates improved PICU and short-term hospital outcomes (6,11) (Table 1). Comparison of these studies and the resulting treatment recommendations are made difficult due to differences in patient populations (e.g., some include transplants for genetic and metabolic disorders in addition to oncology patients), PICU admission criteria, severity of illness, and clinical thresholds for implementing

Table 1 Outcomes Of Bone Marrow Transplant Patients (BMT) Admitted to the Pediatric Intensive Care Unit (ICU) for Acute Respiratory Failure (ARF)

Ref.	Years of study	No. of BMT pts.	No. of pts. (ICU admits)	No. of pts. intubated for ARF	No. of pts. with pneumonia (ICU survivors %)	PRISM score[a] (20)	Ventilated survival to ICU discharge (%)	Hospital survival at 6 months (%)
Bojko et al. (3)	1986–1993		43	43	9	19.4	5 (12)	1 (2)
Keenan et al. (8)	1983–1996	1080	121	74	55 (6)		19 (16)	8 (7)
Todd et al. (2)	1973–1990	285	111	54	35 (6)		6 (11)	4 (7)
Rossi et al. (6)	1986–1995	355	39 (41)	39		11.4	17 (44)	14 (36)
Hallahan et al. (7)	1987–1996		28 (34)	20		10	(54)	(32)
Diaz de Heredia et al. (5)	1991–1995	176	31	26	12 (25)		12 (46)	6 (23)
Diaz et al. (10)	1993–2001	240	42	37			13 (21.4)	14.2
Jacobe et al. (12)	1994–1998	210	40 (57)	31		12–24		11 (12.9)
Schneider et al. (9)	1989–1998	180	28	28		11–16	(36)	(14)

[a] Pediatric risk of mortality.
Abbreviation: pts., patients.

intensive therapies. The studies are usually retrospective, from a single institution, and with inadequate power to identify significant risk factors for mortality. Therefore, the results of these studies, using evidenced-based methodology, are inconclusive regarding clear identification of treatment strategies associated with decreased mortality. However, some suggestive themes do emerge from examination of these study results. Studies by Hallahan et al. (7) and Rossi et al. (6) suggest that early intervention for patients with lower PRISM (20) illness severity scores upon PICU admission are associated with better outcomes. Although inclusion of less severely ill patients could not be ruled out, these studies are consistent in finding that mortality increases as more organ systems fail. Thus, based on current knowledge, we believe that intervention before end organ failure has occurred is a prudent therapeutic goal, as once three or more organ systems fail, survival markedly decreases (12,21).

An example of the potential for improved outcomes for stem cell transplantation patients with earlier intervention is acute respiratory failure. Traditionally, stem cell transplantation patients who received endotracheal intubation for acute respiratory failure, especially in the presence of pneumonia, had poor outcomes (2,8,12). More recently, improved outcomes for these patients are postulated to be related to the use of "lung protective" conventional ventilation strategies. Subsequent application of therapies such as high frequency oscillatory ventilation (HFOV) after failure of "lung protective" conventional ventilation appear associated with probable mortality (11,12). However, in the study by Hagen et al. (11), use of HFOV within the first 6 hr of respiratory failure was associated with improved survival, once again suggesting that earlier intervention in the acute lung injury process may improve survival.

Many studies have identified various clinical variables, which predict poor patient outcomes, but presently there are no such variables, which reliably predict mortality with certainty, especially at the time of PICU admission. In spite of individual studies that found no survivors in their populations based on criteria such as specific oxygen index values (at 96 hr of ventilation) (11) or duration of mechanical ventilation (8), other investigators have identified patients who have survived even when they exceeded these clinical parameters. This lack of agreement among mortality studies does not support recent suggestions by some to deny PICU admission and/or limit supportive therapies for a subgroup of patients based solely on mortality predictors from specific retrospective patient studies (10). Rather, we recommend that decisions regarding limitation of care be made based on an ongoing assessment of the individual patient's clinical course in terms of the goals of therapy, or if there is progression of multisystem organ failure in spite of treatment.

Care for the pediatric oncology patient in the perioperative period requires ongoing multidisciplinary communication and planning by all members of the patient care team. Except for stem cell transplantation patients, mortality and morbidity for pediatric oncology patients in the PICU should be comparable to that of the general PICU population. Based on current knowledge, consideration of admission to the PICU, and application of aggressive supportive therapies should occur as earlier as possible in the context of a child's declining clinical course and impending multisystem organ dysfunction. Decisions on therapy should be continuously re-evaluated based on the patient's clinical course to assure a more informed discussion among caregivers, patients, and families concerning the continuation, limitations, or even withdrawal of PICU care. Robust, prospective outcomes research for specific oncology subpopulations, such as stem cell transplant patients, is needed to better inform both therapeutic recommendations and prognoses.

REFERENCES

1. Butt W, Barker G, Walker C, Gillis J, Kilham H, Stevens M. Outcome of children with hematologic malignancy who are admitted to an intensive care unit. Crit Care Med 1988; 16:761–764.
2. Todd K, Wiley F, Landaw E, et al. Survival outcome among 54 intubated pediatric bone marrow transplant patients. Crit Care Med 1994; 22:171–176.
3. Bojko T, Notterman DA, Greenwald BM, De Bruin WJ, Magid MS, Godwin T. Acute hypoxemic respiratory failure in children following bone marrow transplantation: an outcome and pathologic study. Crit Care Med 1995; 23:755–759.
4. van Veen A, Karstens A, van der Hoek AC, Tibboel D, Hahlen K, van der Voort E. The prognosis of oncologic patients in the pediatric intensive care unit. Intensive Care Med 1996; 22:237–241.
5. Diaz de Heredia C, Moreno A, Olive T, Iglesias J, Ortega JJ. Role of the intensive care unit in children undergoing bone marrow transplantation with life-threatening complications. Bone Marrow Transplant 1999; 24:163–168.
6. Rossi R, Shemie SD, Calderwood S. Prognosis of pediatric bone marrow transplant recipients requiring mechanical ventilation. Crit Care Med 1999; 27: 1181–1186.
7. Hallahan AR, Shaw PJ, Rowell G, O'Connell A, Schell D, Gillis J. Improved outcomes of children with malignancy admitted to a pediatric intensive care unit. Crit Care Med 2000; 28:3718–3721.

8. Keenan HT, Bratton SL, Martin LD, Crawford SW, Weiss NS. Outcome of children who require mechanical ventilatory support after bone marrow transplantation. Crit Care Med 2000; 28:830–835.
9. Schneider DT, Lemburg P, Sprock I, Heying R, Gobel U, Nurnberger W. Introduction of the oncological pediatric risk of mortality score (O-PRISM) for ICU support following stem cell transplantation in children. Bone Marrow Transplant 2000; 25: 1079–1086.
10. Diaz MA, Vicent MG, Prudencio M, et al. Predicting factors for admission to an intensive care unit and clinical outcome in pediatric patients receiving hematopoietic stem cell transplantation. Haematologica 2002; 87:292–298.
11. Hagen SA, Craig DM, Martin PL, et al. Mechanically ventilated pediatric stem cell transplant recipients: effect of cord blood transplant and organ dysfunction on outcome. Pediatr Crit Care Med 2003; 4:206–213.
12. Jacobe SJ, Hassan A, Veys P, Mok Q. Outcome of children requiring admission to an intensive care unit after bone marrow transplantation. Crit Care Med 2003; 31:1299–1305.
13. Kutko MC, Calarco MP, Flaherty MB, et al. Mortality rates in pediatric septic shock with and without multiple organ system failure. Pediatr Crit Care Med 2003; 4:333–337.
14. Andrassy RJ. Advances in the surgical management of sarcomas in children. Am J Surg 2002; 184:484–491.
15. Salo M. Effects of anaesthesia and surgery on the immune response. Acta Anaesthesiol Scand 1992; 36: 201–220.
16. Colacchio TA, Yeager MP, Hildebrandt LW. Perioperative immunomodulation in cancer surgery. Am J Surg 1994; 167:174–179.
17. Bar-Yosef S, Melamed R, Page GG, Shakhar G, Shakhar K, Ben-Eliyahu S. Attenuation of the tumor-promoting effect of surgery by spinal blockade in rats. Anesthesiology 2001; 94:1066–1073.
18. Page GG, Ben-Eliyahu S. Natural killer cell activity and resistance to tumor metastasis in prepubescent rats: deficient baselines, but invulnerability to stress and beta-adrenergic stimulation. Neuroimmunomodulation 2000; 7:160–168.
19. Koltun WA, Bloomer MM, Tilberg AF, et al. Awake epidural anesthesia is associated with improved natural killer cell cytotoxicity and a reduced stress response. Am J Surg 1996; 171:68–72; discussion 72–73.
20. Pollack MM, Ruttimann UE, Getson PR. Pediatric risk of mortality (PRISM) score. Crit Care Med 1988; 16:1110–1116.
21. Wilkinson JD, Pollack MM, Ruttimann UE, Glass NL, Yeh TS. Outcome of pediatric patients with multiple organ system failure. Crit Care Med 1986; 14:271–274.

50

Perioperative Care of Children with Cancer

KERRI J. GEORGE and NANCY L. GLASS

Baylor College of Medicine and Texas Children's Hospital, Houston, Texas, U.S.A.

I. INTRODUCTION

Pediatric cancer occurs relatively infrequently, being diagnosed in only 1 in 7000 children 0–14 years old, each year (1). The incidence of cancer in adolescence, aged 15–19 years, is even more uncommon (2). Although cancer in pediatric patients is uncommon, it still represents a major cause of death in childhood. Cancer is only secondary to accidents as the most common cause of death in patients 0–14 years old, and is the fourth most common cause of death in 15–19 year olds ranking behind accidents, homicide, and suicide (1,2). There is a marked difference found in the age-distribution of various cancers within the first 19 years of life. Figure 1 illustrates the different patterns of cancer occurring in young children and adolescents (1,2). The most common types of cancer occurring in children 0–14 years old include acute lymphoblastic leukemia (ALL), accounting for 23.5% of childhood cancers, central nervous system (CNS) tumors, accounting for 22.1% of childhood cancers, and non-CNS solid tumors (1,3). Non-CNS solid tumors, including neuroblastoma, Wilm's tumor, and non-Hodgkin's lymphoma (NHL), account for 20% of childhood cancers (1). Adolescents exhibit a different spectrum of cancers. Hodgkin's disease (HD) is the most common cancer, representing almost 20% of adolescent cancer, followed by germ cell tumors, CNS tumors, NHL, acute leukemias, bone and soft tissue sarcomas, malignant melanoma, and thyroid carcinoma. Altogether, these cancers account for nearly 90% of the cancers diagnosed in adolescence (2,4).

Many risk factors for various cancers have been identified, both environmental and genetic. Down's syndrome (DS) has been associated with an increased risk of both ALL and acute megakaryoblastic leukemia, along with an increased risk of germ cell tumors of the testis and brain (2,3,5,6). There seems to be a genetic component to some cancers, including Hodgkin's disease, which occurs more commonly in children with an affected sibling (2,7,8). Prior history of radiation treatment may also increase the risk of some cancers including thyroid cancer (2,9), whereas excessive exposure to ultraviolet light has been associated with malignant melanoma (2,10).

Over the past several decades, the survival rates for childhood cancer have improved dramatically. Prior to the 1970s, the survival rates were dismal with an overall 5-year survival rate below 30% (1). With improvements in cancer treatments, including aggressive medical and surgical management, along with advances in chemotherapy and supportive care, the 5-year survival rates now range from 40% to 99%, depending on the type of cancer (Table 1) (1–4,11). The overall 5-year survival rate for all pediatric cancer is 75% (1–3).

With an increase in survival rates for childhood cancer, the cancer patient may present to the operating

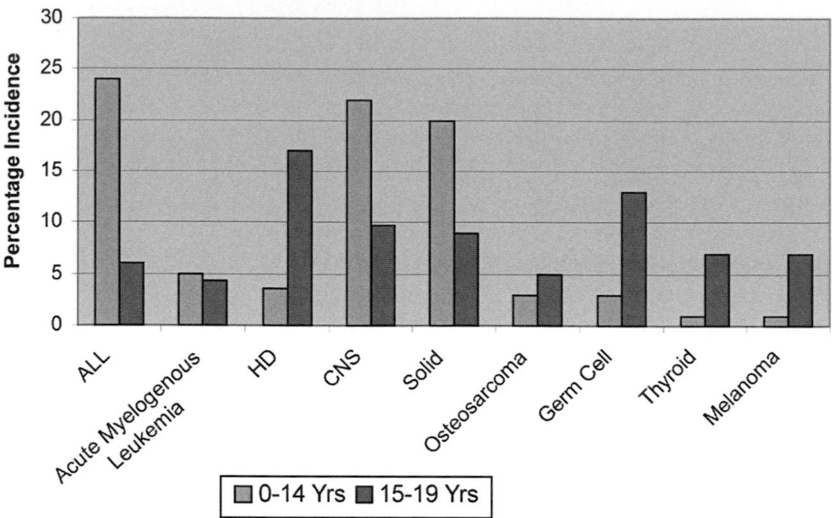

Figure 1 Distribution of pediatric and adolescent cancers. *Source*: Adapted from Refs. 1–3.

room (OR) during the course of cancer therapy, as well as for other routine procedures in the years following the cancer diagnosis and treatment. The challenges that these patients present to perioperative physicians include ongoing or residual effects from the cancer, treatment complexity, coexisting conditions, and treatment-related side effects.

Table 1 Five-Year Survival Rates for Pediatric and Adolescent Cancers

Type of tumor	0–14 years (%)	15–19 years (%)
Total	75	75
Acute lymphocytic leukemia	69–82	51
Acute nonlymphocytic leukemia	44	42
Hodgkin's disease	87–94	90
Non-Hodgkin's lymphoma	78	69
Central nervous system	65–71	75
Osteosarcoma	68	60
Ewing's sarcoma	63	56
Rhabdomyosarcoma	71	35
Germ cell tumors	86–92	90
Thyroid tumors	99–100	99
Melanoma	93–96	92
Wilm's tumor	83	NA

Source: Adapted from Refs. 1, 3, 11.

II. ANESTHETIC PERSPECTIVES

The advances in chemotherapy and radiation have increased the frequency with which pediatric-cancer patients come through the OR during the course of therapy. Cancer patients present to the OR for placement of central lines necessary for the administration of chemotherapy or nutrition, for gastrostomy-tube placement to facilitate enteral nutrition, for primary or secondary tumor resection, and for palliative procedures (12,13). The frequency with which these patients require surgical intervention demands a complete understanding by both the surgeons and the anesthesiologists about the physiologic effects of cancer and metastatic disease, the side effects of chemotherapy and radiation, as well as the interactions between anesthetic and chemotherapeutic agents.

A. Chemotherapy and Radiation

Advances in chemotherapeutic drugs and radiation are largely responsible for increasing the survival rates from childhood cancers (14). Chemotherapeutic drugs not only act in rapidly dividing cancer cells, but also affect normal tissue (12). These agents virtually affect every organ system, but the gastrointestinal tract, lymphoreticular system, and the bone marrow are most regularly affected (12). Normal cells recover more quickly than the cancer cells allowing for the administration of repeated courses of chemotherapy. Combinations of chemotherapeutic agents are usually used, allowing for a lower dose of each individual drug, thus decreasing the drug resistance, increasing the effectiveness, and decreasing the side effects. Common side effects of chemotherapy include nausea, vomiting, mucosal irritation, and bone marrow toxicity (12). The OR team, including the anesthesiologist, the surgeon, and the perioperative physician, must know the chemotherapeutic agents and doses administered, schedule of administration, expected toxicities, risk of side effects, and dates of all scheduled therapy before caring for these patients (15).

Radiation therapy is also used to treat pediatric malignancies, including stage I Hodgkin's disease, brain tumors, and other tumors that have failed to respond to conventional treatment. The effectiveness of the radiation depends on the patient's age, tumor site and size, and tumor sensitivity (12). Guidelines for radiation administration include using the lowest effective dose, treating the smallest possible volume of tissue, and employing appropriate time determinants for treatment schedules (12). Radiation also affects normal tissue and can cause the acute side effects of diarrhea and skin reactions. Common skin reactions include inflammation, necrosis, and fibrosis. These local skin reactions may cause postoperative complications by compromising wound healing. Along with the acute side effects from radiation, chronic effects may also occur.

B. Effects of Chemotherapy

A detailed list of types of cancer, chemotherapeutic agents, and their side effects is shown in Table 2.

1. Cardiovascular System

Cancer patients may develop cardiac toxicity from chemotherapeutic agents including cyclophosphamide, cisplatin, and especially the anthracyclines, doxorubicin and daunorubicin (13,14,16,17). Pediatric cancer patients appear to demonstrate an increased sensitivity to the cardiotoxic effects of these drugs, including the anthracyclines (17). The anthracyclines are effective antileukemic agents that have been used in pediatric cancer treatment for the last 30 years. Patients may present with clinical signs of cardiac toxicity, including congestive heart failure (CHF), or may demonstrate evidence of cardiac toxicity on a screening electrocardiogram (ECG), including supraventricular tachycardia, atrial or ventricular extrasystoles, decreased QRS voltages, and ST-T wave changes (13). An echocardiogram (ECHO) may also demonstrate decreased myocardial contractility (13).

Because of the severity and potential irreversibility of the effects of the anthracyclines, these agents have been vigorously studied. Toxicity is related to the total dose delivered, concomitant radiation to the heart, and the coadministration of cyclophosphamide (13–16,18). Patients usually present with an irreversible cardiomyopathy months to years after the last dose of anthracycline was given. Lipshultz et al. (19) studied 115 children with ALL, who were in remission and had been treated with doxorubicin 1–15 years earlier. None of the patients received radiation or had received cardiotoxic doses of other chemotherapeutic agents. A total of 57% of the patients had evidence of an increase in left ventricular afterload or a decreased contractility on ECHO. A total of 10% (11/115) of the patients developed CHF within 1 year of treatment. All 11 patients initially responded to medical therapy; but five of the 11 patients suffered a recurrence of CHF and two patients eventually required heart transplantation. Treatment factors associated with the development of an increased left ventricular afterload included total cumulative dose, a longer interval between completion of doxorubicin therapy and follow up, and younger age at the time of treatment. Among these factors, the cumulative dose was the most important.

Ali et al. (17) studied the relationship between doxorubicin-associated cardiotoxicity in children and viral infections. They concluded that viral infections might depress myocardial function, triggering (or exacerbating) the doxorubicin-related myocardial dysfunction. They postulated that other stressors, including physical exercise, drugs, anemia, alcohol, poor nutrition, and fever, also contribute to cardiac dysfunction when combined with doxorubicin treatment. Once again, the strongest indicator of cardiac dysfunction was a higher cumulative dose, postulating that a threshold must be reached before myocardial dysfunction occurs.

Finally, Dearth et al. (16) reported a series of 112 children given either doxorubicin or daunorubicin evaluated by an ECG and an ECHO. Six of the 112 patients developed cardiomyopathy and symptoms of CHF. Five of the six patients were also receiving cyclophosphamide, whereas two of the six patients had received previous radiation therapy. Five of the six patients died within 1–6 months of diagnosis, despite medical treatment. The authors concluded that patients who received >400 mg/m^2 of the anthracycline had a 28% risk of developing CHF, whereas those who received <400 mg/m^2 were at a lower risk for developing this complication.

Radiotherapy treatments can also damage the pericardium, myocardium, or vasculature (12,14,20). Patients may present with pericarditis, myocarditis, advanced coronary artery disease, or a pericardial effusion. The degree of risk correlates with younger

Table 2 Cancer, Chemotherapeutic Agents, and Side Effects

Tumor	Agent	Side effects
Wilm's tumor	Vincristine	Peripheral neuropathy
		Constipation
		Local cellulitis
		Seizures
		Syndrome of inappropriate antidiuretic hormone secretion (SIADH)
	Actinomycin-D	Hepatic fibrosis
		Esophagitis
		Stomatitis
		Soft tissue necrosis
	Doxorubicin	Cardiomyopathy
		Arrhythmias
		Esophagitis
		Skin necrosis
		Radiation dermatitis
		Nausea, vomiting, diarrhea
	Cyclophosphamide	Cardiac toxicity
		Pulmonary toxicity
		Hemorrhagic cystitis
		Sterility
		Water retention
		Myelosuppression
Neuroblastoma	Vincristine	See above
	Cisplatinum	Nephrotoxicity
		Neurotoxicity
		Myelosuppression
		Ototoxicity
		Nausea, vomiting
	Etoposide	Neurotoxicity
		Nausea, vomiting
		Mucositis
		Secondary leukemia
	Cyclophosphamide	See above
Rhabdomyosarcoma	Vincristine	See above
	Actinomycin-D	See above
	Cyclophosphamide	See above
Hodgkin's disease (MOPP)	Mechlorethamine	Myelosuppression
		Nausea, vomiting
		Mucositis
		Infertility
	Vincristine	See above
	Procarbazine	Hepatic fibrosis
		Nausea, vomiting
		Mucositis
	Prednisone	Leukemia
		Lymphoma
Hodgkin's disease (ABVD)	Adriamycin (doxorubicin)	See above
	Bleomycin	Pulmonary fibrosis
		Hypersensitivity skin reaction
		Pneumonitis
		Fever
		Raynaud's phenomenon
		Nausea, vomiting

(*Continued*)

Table 2 Cancer, Chemotherapeutic Agents, and Side Effects (*Continued*)

Tumor	Agent	Side effects
	Vinblastine	Neuropathy
		Myositis
		Leukopenia
	Dacarbazine	Nausea, vomiting, flu-like syndrome
		Hepatic toxicity
		Myelosuppression
	Prednisolone	Lymphoma
		Leukemia
		Cushing's syndrome
		Diabetes
		Hypertension
		Avascular necrosis
	Radiation	See above
Leukemia (acute	Prednisolone	See above
lymphocytic leukemia)	Vincristine	See above
	L-Asparaginase	Allergic reaction
		Pancreatitis
		Hyperglycemia
		Hepatic fibrosis
		CNS toxicity
		Platelet dysfunction
		Coagulopathy
	Daunorubicin	Nausea, vomiting, diarrhea
		Cardiomyopathy
		Bone marrow toxicity
	CNS irradiation	Neurocognitive dysfunction
		Impaired intellectual and psychomotor function
		Hypothalamic–pituitary dysfunction
	Intrathecal methotrexate	Pulmonary toxicity
		Arachnoiditis
		Encephalopathy
		Myelopathy
		Paraplegia
		Hepatotoxicity
	Cyclophosphamide	See above
Acute myelogenous leukemia	Cytarabine (Ara C)	Nausea, vomiting, flu-like illness
		Bone marrow suppression
		Conjunctivitis
		Mucositis
		CNS dysfunction
	Daunomycin	Cardiomyopathy
	Etoposide	See above
	Bone marrow transplant	Graft versus host disease, immunosuppression, growth problems, sterility, secondary malignancies

Source: Adapted from Refs. 12, 13, 15, 22, 34, 120.

age, total radiation dose, schedule of radiation doses, and site of irradiation (12,14,20,21). Both children and the elderly share an increased risk of cardiac damage. Children and adolescents treated for Hodgkin's disease are at a very high risk of developing cardiovascular complications because of their young age at the time of treatment (12,20). Those who received doxorubicin and cyclophosphamide in addition to radiation were reported to have a higher risk for toxicity than those who received radiation alone (13). Dearth et al. (16) showed that the patients who received radiation to the mediastinum, along with doxorubicin or daunorubicin, were at an increased risk for developing CHF.

2. Respiratory System

Pulmonary involvement may occur from the primary cancer, metastases to the lungs, or pulmonary disturbances caused by either chemotherapy or radiation (12–14,22). Pulmonary tissues are vulnerable to damage caused by chemotherapy and radiation. Radiation may cause acute radiation pneumonitis within 6 weeks of treatment or chronic involvement manifested by a decrease in vital capacity, total lung capacity, and diffusing capacity (12,14). Radiation side effects occur more frequently in patients receiving higher radiation doses and in patients whose chemotherapy regimen includes bleomycin (14,15,23).

Pulmonary fibrosis may be seen, following the administration of agents including bleomycin, cyclophosphamide, methotrexate, procarbazine, and carmustine (BCNU) (13,14,22–24). Common characteristics of pulmonary involvement include dyspnea, a nonproductive cough, fever, evidence of rales on physical exam, evidence of hypoxemia on arterial blood gas, and a pattern of restrictive lung disease on pulmonary function tests (PFTs) (15,18,22,24). Steroid therapy may reverse some of these changes, but the toxic drug should be stopped immediately. Bleomycin, which is used in the treatment of germ cell tumors, NHL, Hodgkin's disease, hepatocellular carcinoma, and osteogenic sarcoma, has been the most extensively studied chemotherapy agent with respect to pulmonary toxicity (23). Bleomycin causes severe damage to the lungs by binding to DNA and causing conversion of a ferrous ion to the ferric state, liberating electrons. Both superoxide and oxygen free radicals are formed when oxygen accepts the electrons (23). The lungs are particularly susceptible to bleomycin toxicity because of the high oxygen concentration in the lung and the low concentration of the enzyme that inactivates bleomycin (23,25). A delayed toxicity pattern consisting of headache, malaise, dyspnea, fever, and a nonproductive cough may be seen following the bleomycin treatment (15).

Chung (13) found that 5–10% of patients treated with bleomycin had some measure of pulmonary dysfunction, ranging from minimal alterations in PFTs to severe pulmonary fibrosis. These complications were dose related, and doses >500 mg caused the most severe reactions. The onset of toxic effects generally occurred 4–10 weeks after the initiation of therapy; prominent signs and symptoms included dyspnea, tachypnea, and rales. Co-treatment with cyclophosphamide and high-inspired oxygen concentrations were shown to have synergistic effects with bleomycin (13,14,23). Severe respiratory distress after anesthesia has also been discovered in some of the patients treated with bleomycin (23). Goldiner and Schweizer (26) reported an increased mortality rate and respiratory complications in patients who received $>40\%$ inspired oxygen concentration during surgery. As postoperative respiratory distress did not occur in patients who received $<25\%$ inspired oxygen (26), several authors have recommended that anesthesiologists limit the inspired oxygen concentration to the lowest level compatible with adequate oxygen delivery, maintaining oxygen saturations between 95% and 97% (14,22,23,26,27). The addition of positive end-expiratory pressure to increase oxygenation, along with the addition of aggressive chest physiotherapy postoperatively, may allow for the administration of a lower oxygen concentration (22).

Eigen (23) reported the case of a 3 year old with a history of embryonal cell carcinoma metastatic to the lungs, and treated with bleomycin. In the OR, the patient developed laryngospasm requiring treatment with 100% oxygen; the patient immediately developed pulmonary edema, required admission to the intensive care unit (ICU), and died 3 months later secondary to cardiopulmonary arrest. Eigen concluded that the cause of pulmonary toxicity was due to the high dose of bleomycin, and that the risk of toxicity was further increased by cotreatment with cyclophosphamide, radiation to the chest, and treatment with inspired concentrations of oxygen exceeding 40%.

The risk of pulmonary fibrosis after treatment with bleomycin persists for up to 12 months after administration. To decrease the risk of pulmonary fibrosis, it is recommended that the total bleomycin dose be the lowest amount effective in tumor lysis, cyclophosphamide or radiation treatment only be used with caution, and the lowest possible concentration of oxygen be used if oxygen therapy is needed (23).

3. Endocrine System

Endocrinopathy is a significant consequence of childhood cancers. The abnormalities in endocrine function may be due to the tumor causing direct damage to the hypothalamic–pituitary gland or from the treatment of the primary tumor with radiation or chemotherapy (28–30). Endocrine effects of chemotherapy and radiation have been noted in 20–50% of survivors of childhood cancer, with an increased incidence in patients treated for CNS tumors (28,31).

The CNS radiation effects to the endocrine system are common and are related to the total dose administered, dosing regimen, and duration of treatment (28,29). Younger children are especially vulnerable to the toxic effects of radiation treatment, with hypothalamic–pituitary dysfunction occurring in many children treated with radiation therapy for CNS tumors or total body radiation (28,29). The most frequent anterior pituitary abnormality is a deficiency in growth hormone (GH) release causing growth retardation, which becomes evident $\geq$2 years following CNS radiation (28,29,32). Growth abnormalities are even more prominent following irradiation of the epiphyseal plate (29). Other abnormalities include early pubertal development after low doses of CNS radiation, gonadotropin insufficiency with high doses of CNS radiation, thyroid deficiency, obesity, osteopenia/osteoporosis, and hyperprolactinemia (28,29). Thyroid disease is particularly common, following head and neck irradiation for Hodgkin's disease, CNS irradiation, or total body irradiation because of the radiosensitivity of the thyroid gland (28,29,33). Hypothyroidism is the most frequent abnormality following thyroid gland irradiation, but hyperthyroidism, thyroid nodules, and thyroid cancer may also occur. Elective surgery should be cancelled until the patient is euthyroid, but emergency surgery should proceed with extra caution.

Signs and symptoms of hypothyroidism include lethargy, intolerance to cold, bradycardia, decreased cardiac output, and peripheral vasoconstriction. Hypothyroid patients may demonstrate exaggerated responses to myocardial depressant drugs and hypovolemia, and may also exhibit evidence of prolonged gastric emptying. One good choice for anesthetic induction in the hypothyroid patient might be ketamine, as the resultant sympathetic stimulation may be helpful in maintaining cardiac output. Opioids and muscle relaxants would also be appropriate in this setting, although they should be administered judiciously, since hypothyroidism increases the sensitivity of the myocardium to drug-induced depression. Muscle relaxants should also be titrated carefully, as these patients may have coexisting skeletal muscle weakness that might mimic the effects caused by muscle relaxants (34). Normothermia should be maintained throughout.

Hyperthyroidism may present as anxiety, fatigue, skeletal muscle weakness, tachycardia, and cardiac arrhythmias. These patients may benefit from the administration of a short-acting beta-adrenergic antagonist to decrease heart rate and blood pressure prior to surgery. Choices for the induction of general anesthesia include thiopental, which has intrinsic antithyroid activity, volatile anesthetic agents, and opioids; muscle relaxants without cardiovascular effects would be preferable in this setting. Isoflurane is commonly selected because it inhibits sympathetic stimulation without sensitizing the heart to the effects of endogenous catecholamine release. Temperature monitoring is necessary, as these patients may be prone to the development of hyperthermia (34).

Endocrine abnormalities are also apparent after cancer treatment with chemotherapy alone. Approximately a quarter of childhood cancer survivors who were treated with only chemotherapy developed GH deficiency and central hypothyroidism, whereas another 44% of this group had evidence of some type of hypothalamic–pituitary dysfunction (29). As adrenal insufficiency following cancer treatment is common and the patient is frequently asymptomatic, it is important to monitor and treat each patient for these abnormalities. A number of patients will come to the OR while receiving hormone replacement therapy, and the anesthetic technique should be altered as necessary.

4. *Renal System*

Nephrotoxicity has been reported as a side effect of numerous chemotherapeutic agents including BCNU, *cis*-diamminedichloroplatinum (II), ifosfamide, cisplatin, and methotrexate, and may be a dose-limiting toxicity of some drugs (12–15). Cell breakdown following chemotherapy leads to the formation of uric acid crystals and produces a diffuse tubular block (12,35). Maintaining an adequate intravascular volume and brisk urine output, along with administration of allopurinol and urinary alkalinization, will promote dissolution and excretion of uric acid crystals and may prevent renal damage. Cisplatinum may cause acute tubular necrosis, whereas cyclophosphamide causes hemorrhagic cystitis (12).

Radiation to the kidney area, often used in the treatment of Wilm's tumor and Hodgkin's disease, and the combination of chemotherapy and radiation are particularly damaging. Creatinine clearance was impaired in 27.4% of patients with Wilm's tumor after nephrectomy and abdominal irradiation. The severity and degree of impairment correlated with the total radiation dose (14).

5. *Gastrointestinal System*

The gastrointestinal tract is one of the most sensitive organ systems in the body to the hazardous effects of chemotherapy and radiation. The mucosal lining of the gastrointestinal tract has a very rapid cell turnover, making it particularly vulnerable to the effects of chemotherapy (12). Gastrointestinal toxicity presents as mucositis, nausea, vomiting, and diarrhea, resulting in fluid and electrolyte abnormalities (13,15). Most chemotherapeutic agents have the potential to cause nausea, vomiting, and diarrhea, but many other drugs also have the capacity to damage the oral or gastrointestinal mucosa (12,13,15). Doxorubicin and actinomycin

D commonly cause oral or esophageal mucositis, whereas methotrexate may cause hemorrhagic colitis or mucositis (15). Other agents causing mucositis include adriamycin, bleomycin, and vinblastine, whereas an autonomic neuropathy resulting in constipation may follow treatment with vincristine and vinblastine.

Cancer, or its treatment, may also cause cachexia, poor nutrition, and a decreased albumin level (13). Albumin binds acidic drugs, like barbiturates, and renders them inactive. If the albumin level is decreased, there is more unbound drug available for tissue uptake, and the amount of circulating active drug is greater. In these cases, the amount of drug given must be decreased to prevent the effects of overdose (36,37). It is very important for the anesthesiologist to check the preoperative fluid and electrolyte status of any operative patient and to correct any significant abnormalities before entering the OR.

Radiation treatment to the abdomen may also cause both acute and chronic side effects. Symptoms of nausea, vomiting, and diarrhea are common initial complaints from the mucosal irritation caused by radiation treatment. Malabsorption, bowel obstruction, or stricture, resulting from radiation-induced compromise of the blood supply to the bowel, may also develop after a period of time (12).

6. *Central Nervous System*

Chemotherapy and CNS radiation are frequently administered together to treat or prevent CNS disease. Vincristine, vinblastine, and cisplatin have all been reported to cause a peripheral neuropathy, presenting with pain or paresthesias, decreased deep tendon reflexes, or muscle weakness (13,15). Intrathecal methotrexate, used to treat patients with brain tumors or as CNS prophylaxis in patients with leukemia, may result in chronic leuko-encephalopathy (12,15). Radiation is also a concern, as young patients who receive head and neck radiation may have early demyelination, leading to radiation necrosis, brain atrophy, and developmental delay (12,38). For this reason, radiation as the first line treatment in very young children is used less than in previous years. Likewise, CNS radiation for the prevention of CNS complications or for the treatment of tumor relapse is considered routine only for high-risk patients.

7. *Hepatic System*

Liver dysfunction in children with cancer results from the cancer itself, damage caused by the chemotherapy drugs, and damage caused by infections (39). Liver dysfunction and damage may produce undesirable effects of the chemotherapy drugs, including a decrease in their effectiveness and an increase in toxicity. Hepatic fibrosis has been seen following administration of methotrexate, procarbazine, cyclophosphamide, adriamycin, and l-asparaginase. However, hepatic failure rarely develops, and liver function tests usually normalize after the drug is discontinued (12,13,15). Hepatic cirrhosis has also been found in pediatric leukemia patients treated with methotrexate (13). Risk factors for cirrhosis include total duration of therapy, the use of small frequent doses, and the total dose of the drug administered (13). Many studies have been done attempting to determine a dose regimen that will decrease the side effects of the chemotherapy agents without decreasing the efficacy of the drug. Wiela-Hojenska et al. (39) studied 21 patients with ALL, examining the effects of various chemotherapy regimens on liver function. They found that all of the anticancer drugs they used decreased metabolic liver activity, specifically the hepatic mixed function oxidase system; the most dramatic decline in function followed treatment with high dose methotrexate.

The decrease in liver activity is important, because there will be some inhibition of drug metabolism when the metabolic activity of the liver is decreased (39). This change will lead to an increase in the amount of circulating drug left in the active form and an increase in toxicity of drugs metabolized by the hepatic mixed function oxidase system (39). The drugs' duration of action may also be increased with a decrease in liver metabolic activity. Therefore, the degree of liver dysfunction must be evaluated, and the dose of drugs must be adjusted in patients receiving chemotherapeutic drugs that affect hepatic function (15,39).

8. *Hematological System*

Bone marrow suppression manifested by anemia, thrombocytopenia, and neutropenia is the most common toxicity seen with chemotherapy agents, commonly occurring between 7 and 14 days post-treatment (15). The resultant anemia is a normocytic, normochromic anemia, similar to that of chronic disease (40). The primary cause of the anemia in children is bone marrow replacement by tumor cells, with chemotherapy-induced causes following (40). Lack of adequate erythropoietin production in response to decreased hemoglobin may also be a factor in the development of anemia (41–43). Nearly half of the children with acute lymphocytic leukemia present with anemia at the time of diagnosis, as infiltration of the bone marrow by leukemic cells decreases hematopoietic cells, resulting in a lower hemoglobin level(40).

Although transfusion is still the standard treatment for cancer-associated anemia, there are no set guidelines to determine when a transfusion should be administered. Children tolerate a lower hemoglobin level better than adults do, especially if the anemia has developed over time. Most patients with hemoglobin levels less than 7 g/dL will require a transfusion, but individual assessment of each patient is required (40). The patient with additional risk factors, such as a low platelet count, a history of bleeding, or a surgical candidate, may need a transfusion at a hemoglobin level well above 7 g/dL.

Although transfusions are frequently required in cancer patients, they are not without risks, including transfusion reactions, viral transmission, and alloimmunization (42). Alternatives to transfusions have been studied, including recombinant human erythropoietin (rHuEPO), to decrease the need for erythrocyte transfusions (41–43). Porter et al. (42) studied 24 pediatric patients with solid tumors, randomly assigned to receive either placebo or rHuEPO. The group receiving EPO required fewer packed red blood cell transfusions and was exposed to fewer donors than the placebo group. One disadvantage of rHuEPO treatment is the length of time required for a clinical response. There is no significant increase in hemoglobin levels prior to 4 weeks of therapy, so transfusions may still be required in the peri-operative period (41–43).

9. *Immunologic System*

The incidence of infections is increased in patients with cancer because of the immunosuppression produced by the chemotherapeutic agents (12). Strict hand washing and attention to aseptic technique for invasive procedures are important in this population. These patients not only have an increased incidence of common infections, but also have an increased risk of developing opportunistic or hospital-acquired infections. Common pathways for these infections include indwelling foley catheters, venous access catheters, and nasogastric tubes. Other infections frequently seen in cancer patients include lung infections (bacterial, viral, or fungal), CNS infections (including meningitis), liver infections, and bowel infections (typhlitis) (12).

10. *Graft-vs.-Host Disease*

The incidence of graft-vs.-host disease (GVHD) is increasing because an increasing number of bone marrow transplantations are being performed in children with leukemia following relapse after their initial remission. Two distinct clinical syndromes have been described: acute GVHD and chronic GVHD (44). Acute GVHD occurs within the first 2 weeks to 2 months after bone marrow transplantation. Risk factors include gender mismatch between the donor and the recipient, HLA mismatch, the use of unrelated donor marrow, and older age of the recipient (25,44,45). Acute GVHD generally involves the skin, liver, and gastrointestinal systems (12,44). Skin involvement manifests as a rash that begins with a maculopapular pattern on the palms and soles. Jaundice signals hepatic involvement, with an increase in plasma alkaline phosphatase and transaminase levels. Diarrhea, abdominal pain, and nausea may be the manifestations of gastrointestinal involvement, but these symptoms are less specific.

Chronic GVHD occurs more frequently in patients who have experienced acute GVHD and presents (by definition) more than 100 days after bone marrow transplantation (44). The most important risk factor is HLA mismatch; but a history of acute GVHD and older age at transplant also increase the risk of chronic GVHD. Again, the most common organ systems involved are the skin, mouth, eyes, and liver (12,44). Occasionally, one may see the involvement of the respiratory tract, manifested by cough, recurrent pulmonary infections, and bronchiolitis obliterans. The musculoskeletal system, neurologic system, and gastrointestinal tract are less commonly involved. All patients with GVHD must be considered immunocompromised either from the cancer itself or from the chemotherapy treatment. Because these patients are immunocompromised, there is an increased risk for all types of infections including bacterial, viral, and fungal (12,44). Careful surveillance for infections, along with attention to aseptic technique, is required for this population.

C. Associated Anomalies

There has been some evidence of both hereditary and environmental causes being responsible for cancer occurrences. Patients with DS have an atypical distribution of cancer types, while some families may reveal an excess number of cancers or carry a predisposing genetic trait (46). Environmental factors may also contribute to more than 70% of all cancers (46)

1. *Down Syndrome (DS)*

Patients with DS have a unique distribution of cancers, with an increased risk of leukemia, including a greatly increased risk of myelodysplastic syndrome, acute myelocytic leukemia (AML) and acute megakaryocytic leukemia, but a decreased incidence of solid tumors (2). Leukemia in patients with DS accounts for about 60% of all cancers and usually presents during the first

4 years of life (5,6). Down syndrome was found to be the most frequent condition associated with childhood AML, with about 50% of the cases being diagnosed at 1 year of age (6). There are also different clinical and laboratory manifestations of AML and myelodysplastic syndrome in children with DS when compared with normal children, including clinical presentation at a younger age with thrombocytopenia and neutropenia (6). Hasle et al. (5) surveyed nearly 3000 individuals with DS and found that although the overall risk of cancer in these individuals was not higher than the population at large, the distribution of cancer types was remarkably different. The incidence of solid tumors was much lower in this population, but there was an 18-fold increased risk of leukemia, especially in children less than 5 years of age. Acute megakaryocytic leukemia occurred much more frequently in the patient with DS when compared with the general population. Although the exact cause for these findings is not known, some investigators think that there are tumor suppressor genes on chromosome 21, leading to the decreased incidence of solid tumors, along with leukemogenic genes on chromosome 21 leading to a similar increase in the incidence of leukemias (5).

Interestingly, children with DS have a higher survival rate for AML when compared with normal children, with survival rates well over 80% for this diagnosis (5,6). It appears that the myeloblasts in DS patients are more sensitive to the chemotherapeutic agents used in the treatment of AML than those in non-DS patients (5,47). For this reason, some investigators recommend that less time-intensive therapy be given to decrease the risk of side effects from the treatment drugs (5).

2. *Genetics*

A small percentage of pediatric cancer cases may be due to heritable causes. The child's family may have a large number of cancers noted on review of the family tree or they may have a gene that is recognized to predispose family members to particular cancers. There may also be nongenetic explanations for the occurrence of cancer in a familial pattern, including environmental exposures, or history of previous antineoplastic treatment (48). Narod et al. (46) did a 13-year study, attempting to relate the incidence of childhood cancer with genetic predisposition, reporting that between 3.07% and 4.2% of all reported cancers had some underlying genetic component. The most common cancers with a heritable fraction were bilateral retinoblastoma, DS, neurofibromatosis, Wilm's tumor, and tuberous sclerosis. Early age of onset and bilateral tumors were the features of familial cancers that differentiated them from sporadic cancers.

III. PREOPERATIVE ASSESSMENT

Overall survival rates from childhood cancer have improved dramatically in the past several years. More than 90% of these children come to the OR for therapeutic or palliative treatment. Children with cancer often have other medical problems related to their malignancy or to their current or previous treatment (Table 3). As increasing numbers of these patients present to the OR, it is imperative for the operative team to understand the potential problems arising from pediatric cancer and its treatment. A thorough preoperative assessment is the foundation for high quality perioperative care.

A. Preoperative History

The anesthesiologist should obtain a detailed medical history for the cancer patient, with an emphasis on assessing the patient's functional status (49,50). Some patients are ambulatory and able to participate in daily activities, whereas other patients are severely debilitated. The patient's functional status reflects the type of cancer, treatment side effects, stage of disease, presence of metastases, underlying medical conditions, or a combination of the above (18). The patient may be malnourished because of decreased intake related to pain, nausea and vomiting, chemotherapy-associated stomatitis or mucositis, tumor location, or clinical depression. An active, well-nourished patient generally recovers uneventfully following the surgery, and requires little in the way of preoperative workup. On the other hand, the child with a recent change in activity, energy level, oral intake, or weight loss may be exhibiting functional deterioration such that the perioperative physician should consider a more detailed workup prior to surgery.

A thorough history should also include an inquiry into the type and location of the cancer, prior medical treatment, including therapeutic drugs, total doses received, date of the last treatment, and history of glucocorticoid administration (15,49). It is important to know the precise location of tumors and lymph nodes in the oropharynx, neck, and thorax, as lesions in the upper airway and anterior mediastinum may result in precipitous airway obstruction during the induction of anesthesia (18,51).

The presence of a large abdominal mass requires a special scrutiny, as the tumor's bulk may prevent normal gastric emptying, obstruct venous return to the heart (49,50), or compromise pulmonary gas exchange. Patients with abdominal distension from tumors may be at an increased risk for regurgitation and aspiration

Table 3 Medical Problems in Cancer Patients

Organ system	Potential medical issues	Recommended preoperative screening tests
Cardiovascular	Drug-induced cardiomyopathy or congestive failure Drug-induced arrhythmias Pericardial effusion	Electrocardiogram/Echocardiogram/ Chest radiograph
Respiratory	Drug-induced pulmonary fibrosis Restrictive lung disease Pneumonitis Pleural effusion	Chest radiograph/Pulmonary function tests/ Arterial blood gas
Endocrine and metabolic	Pituitary dysfunction Growth hormone deficiency Hypothyroidism Electrolyte abnormalities	Serum electrolytes/Calcium/Glucose/ Serum magnesium level
Renal	Renal dysfunction Electrolyte abnormalities Hemorrhagic cystitis	Serum electrolytes/BUN/creatinine
Gastrointestinal	Mucositis Malnutrition Cachexia Hemorrhagic colitis	Serum albumin level/Serum electrolytes
Central and peripheral nervous system	Peripheral neuropathy Encephalopathy Brain metastases Mass lesion with an increased ICP Developmental delay Altered level of consciousness	Computed tomography/Magnetic resonance imaging
Hepatic	Hepatic damage Fibrosis Cirrhosis	Liver function tests (AST, ALT, PT, Alk Phos)/ Liver ultrasound or CT scan
Hematologic	Bone marrow suppression Anemia Granulocytopenia Thrombocytopenia Hypercoagulable state	Complete blood count/Platelet count/Bone marrow aspiration and/or biopsy/PT/PTT

Source: Adapted from Refs. 13, 15, 121.

of gastric contents (52). The tumor may invade the inferior vena cava directly or may compress the cava, decreasing venous return and leading to hypotension. Such patients may not tolerate the supine position, requiring lateral displacement of the mass to facilitate patient comfort, to ease respiratory effort, and to improve cardiac output.

Many cancer patients receive myelosuppressive chemotherapy in anticipation of surgical therapy. The surgeon and the anesthesiologist must know when maximal myelosuppression is most likely to occur and should plan elective surgery when sufficient time has elapsed for the bone marrow to recover. Reviewing the details of previous surgical procedures, including surgical or anesthetic complications, perioperative problems, and effective analgesics regimens is helpful in planning for subsequent surgical interventions. A history of radiation therapy, including total radiation dose, timing of last dose, location of irradiated area, and side effects of radiation, should be obtained.

Current laboratory data should be reviewed, and a physical exam should be performed. A focused exam may reveal organ dysfunction or abnormalities that may make securing the airway, vascular access, or ventilation more difficult (50). Radiation complications including inflammation, necrosis, and fibrosis at the site of irradiation may cause alterations in wound healing or anatomic distortion of the airway (36,51). Even though a thorough review of medical records may inform the anesthesiologist about whether or not the patient's airway was difficult to manage during the previous procedure, it is also wise to remember that the child's anatomy may change significantly from one anesthetic to the next.

As other medical conditions may also occur in pediatric cancer patients, a history of heart, lung, liver, renal, or endocrine diseases should be obtained. The presence of coexisting conditions may suggest the need for additional preoperative testing. Finally, the patient's pain level and basal analgesic regimen should be reviewed preoperatively, because pre-existing opioid tolerance may affect intraoperative and postoperative opiate requirements.

B. Preoperative Testing

Preoperative laboratory testing (Table 3) is rarely indicated for routine pediatric surgery, but the pediatric cancer patient presents with a more complex set of problems. Even so, the preoperative history and physical exam should guide the decision to perform lab studies. Specific tests should be ordered to look for complications of chemotherapy, to identify correctable problems, or to facilitate anesthetic planning. Laboratory tests may help physicians make the decision to postpone surgery until hematologic or metabolic abnormalities can be corrected.

If the patient has recently received chemotherapy, radiation, or bone marrow transplantation, a complete blood count should be performed (49,50). Thrombocytopenia is common due to immunosuppressive drugs or bone marrow infiltration from the cancer. For surgical procedures, a platelet count $>50{,}000/\text{mm}^3$ is recommended to prevent excessive surgical bleeding (18,49,50). Ideally, hemoglobin levels should be >10 g/dL, but compensatory physiologic changes take place in the face of chronic anemia, allowing the threshold for transfusion to be lower in chronically anemic patients. Each patient's adaptation should be considered individually; judgment about preoperative transfusion should be made on the basis of expectations for surgical bleeding, the degree of compensation for the anemia, and the patient's cardiorespiratory function. If the patient has a history of easy bruisability or nontraumatic bleeding, a coagulation profile should be obtained.

Electrolyte abnormalities are common in pediatric cancer patients. Patients receiving nephrotoxic drugs including methotrexate and cyclophosphamide, and those receiving parenteral nutrition should have a serum electrolyte panel drawn, along with a calcium and magnesium level (36,49,50). Hypercalcemia occurs in 5% of all cancer patients (18) and may be due to bony metastases or secretion of humoral mediators, such as parathyroid hormone-like substances, cytokines, or prostaglandins (18,51). The serum creatinine level is a good indicator of renal function and hydration status; a baseline value helps guide fluid management in the OR (36). Liver function tests should be checked in patients who have received hepatotoxic agents, those who are poorly nourished, and those who have been receiving parenteral nutrition. Liver function abnormalities may alter the metabolism of local, systemic, and inhalational anesthetics, reducing the tolerated doses of drugs that the anesthesiologist might administer (15,49).

Since the anthracycline derivatives, doxorubicin and daunorubicin have the potential to cause cardiac toxicity, patients who have received these agents should have a preoperative ECG to look for evidence of toxicity (13,15,50). Acute toxicity may cause nonspecific ST-T wave changes, a decreased QRS voltage, or arrhythmias, whereas chronic toxicity may demonstrate evidence of CHF on the ECG. If the history and/or physical exam suggest cardiac toxicity or if the patient has received high doses of the anthracycline derivatives, a preoperative ECHO should be performed in order to determine the patient's ventricular function (15,49). Results of the ECHO may guide the selection of invasive hemodynamic monitors for intraoperative care and may influence decisions regarding the use of specific anesthetic agents.

A chest radiograph should be obtained for patients presenting with a productive cough, dyspnea, or bibasilar rales on physical exam, particularly in those children who have received bleomycin, nitrosoureas, cyclophosphamide, or methotrexate (13,15,49,50). Similarly, patients with significant lymphadenopathy or mediastinal masses should have a chest radiograph and possibly a chest CT before surgery, as tracheal deviation or compression may impact airway management and ventilation (see discussion later) (18,53). Pulmonary function tests and baseline arterial blood gases may also be indicated in the patient with evidence of significant pulmonary toxicity.

Although anesthesiologists rarely order head CT scans or MRI scans in patients with suspected CNS disease, it is helpful to review these scans and their interpretation. Nonspecific symptoms such as headache, nausea, vomiting, lethargy, and confusion may be caused by the primary tumor or its metastasis, or by the tumor treatment (15,18). If the patient presents with evidence of increased intracranial pressure (ICP) reflecting tumor growth or metastatic disease, then the patient's condition may be considered terminal, and the treatment plan may not include surgery (15).

C. Consultations

Additional preoperative consultations may be indicated if the consulted service can provide recommendations for improving the patient's condition prior to surgery. Anticipating the patient's expected physiologic response to the hemodynamic and metabolic changes that may occur during surgery, the consultant may provide valuable advice for minimizing the adverse effects of surgery (36). Further consultations are not necessary if the patient is already in optimal condition.

D. NPO Guidelines

The NPO guidelines for pediatric cancer patients are the same as NPO guidelines for healthy pediatric patients (Table 4), although certain clinical circumstances may require extra precautions to prevent regurgitation and aspiration during the induction of anesthesia. Large abdominal masses including Wilm's tumor, lymphoma, and neuroblastomas may cause abdominal distention and obstruction that may delay the normal emptying process (50,54). Patients who are in pain, those receiving opiate therapy, and those presenting for urgent or emergent procedures all have delayed gastric emptying and may still be at risk for regurgitation and aspiration, even if they have been NPO for an appropriate length of time.

E. Psychological Preparation

In addition to the normal childhood fears of surgery including separation anxiety, the pediatric cancer patient must also deal with peer reaction/treatment, physical impairment, pain, functional impairment, learning disabilities, depression, withdrawal, and a sense of mortality (49,54). It is important that the anesthesiologist explain the anticipated plan with the patient and family, considering the patient's developmental stage. Age-appropriate toys, books, and videos are often helpful, along with OR tours. The most important task is to make the surgical experience as stress-free and surprise-free as possible, as these children are likely to return to the OR for additional procedures.

Table 4 NPO Guidelines

Clear liquids	May offer until 2 hr before procedure
Breast milk	May offer until 4 hr before procedure
Formula, milk, solid foods	Must discontinue at least 6 hr before procedure

Source: Adapted from Refs. 49, 122.

F. Premedication

Recognizing that children may demonstrate behavioral changes related to the stress of surgery and anesthesia, anesthesiologists should consider sedative premedication prior to the induction of anesthesia (55,56). Administration of sedative premedication should be individualized, as the child's age, personality, previous experiences, and parental expectations all play a role in determining which children need or might benefit from premedication (50). Available routes for administration of sedatives include the oral, intramuscular, intravascular, rectal, and intranasal routes. Rectal administration is inadvisable in neutropenic patients, as rectal trauma could lead to infection (34). Intramuscular injections are relatively contraindicated in coagulopathic or thrombocytopenic patients, and they are not popular with young children. Consequently, intramuscular sedation, using pentobarbital, midazolam, or ketamine, is generally reserved only for the most recalcitrant patient who cannot be managed by any other technique. Although techniques for instilling intranasal midazolam, ketamine, and sufentanil have been described, these agents cause a burning sensation in the nasopharynx, limiting their popularity; intranasal sufentanil has been associated with respiratory depression (57–62).

Oral sedation is the most accepted route of administration for young children who are accustomed to taking oral medications for cancer treatment. Oral transmucosal fentanyl has been used in cancer patients for painful procedures and may be appropriate for some patients presenting to the OR (63). The use of the fentanyl Oralet® does necessitate respiratory monitoring, as some patients may demonstrate oxygen desaturation. However, in our experience, the frequency with which nausea and vomiting occur in the preoperative period limits the clinical usefulness of this technique. Another choice for sedative premedication is oral ketamine, more popular in Europe than in the United States. Oral ketamine has a bitter taste like midazolam, which must be masked by dilution with some kind of sweet syrup. By far, the most commonly administered preoperative sedation is oral midazolam (64). For children with intravenous (IV) access, IV midazolam, titrated to effect, is even more convenient. Patients who present in the preoperative period with pain should be treated with opiates before the induction of anesthesia.

Parental presence during the induction of anesthesia is an alternative or an adjunct to sedative premedication at some institutions; parents are either invited into an induction room adjacent to the OR or into the OR itself (50,54). There is a wealth of literature on the effects of parental presence on child and parental anxiety. Kain (65) found that in children who are randomly assigned to receive either the oral midazolam, parental presence during induction, or no intervention at all, the treatment with oral midazolam was more effective than either parental presence or no intervention in diminishing the anxiety of both children and parents. However, when those same children returned to the OR for subsequent surgeries, the parents were offered a choice of interventions. More than 80% chose to be present in the OR, whereas only 23% chose for their child to receive midazolam alone (66).

Decisions regarding parental presence in the OR reflect institutional cultures, facilities, and comfort level of anesthesiologists and other caregivers. Clearly, the goals for both preoperative sedation and parental presence in the OR are the same: facilitating separation from the parents, minimizing the stress of induction, and preventing subsequent behavioral changes. A variety of techniques should be available for managing the child's anxiety, and care should be individualized.

Other patients who may need additional medications before surgery include patients receiving glucocorticoid therapy and patients with a full stomach or delayed gastric emptying. Patients who have received >2 weeks of glucocorticoid therapy in the preceding year should receive a stress dose of steroids before surgery to prevent an adrenal crisis caused by pituitary–adrenal axis suppression (18,51). Practically speaking, this is generally administered in the OR after IV access is secured. For patients with a full stomach or delayed gastric emptying, the clinician should consider administering a nonparticulate antacid like sodium bicarbonate (Bicitra®). Alternatively, metoclopramide or an H-2 blocking agent like ranitidine may be administered (67).

IV. INTRAOPERATIVE MANAGEMENT

Planning the intraoperative management of the pediatric cancer patient requires an understanding of the underlying cancer, previous therapy, and ongoing treatment. Vigilance and precision are critical, as pediatric patients may experience rapid changes in clinical condition during surgery.

A. Monitors

Monitoring the pediatric cancer patient is similar to monitoring any other pediatric surgical patient. Standard ASA monitoring guidelines should be observed. An ECG not only monitors heart rate and rhythm, but also validates the readings of the pulse oximeter. Temperature monitoring and pulse oximetry are also considered routine. Pulse oximetry is useful for confirming adequate oxygenation and ventilation; it also functions as an indirect monitor of cardiovascular status. For short procedures, most clinicians monitor axillary or skin temperature; for more invasive procedures, temperature probes monitor core temperature at the tympanic membrane, the rectum, or in the distal esophagus. Rectal probes are not recommended for neutropenic patients for reasons mentioned earlier. End-tidal carbon dioxide (CO_2) tension should also be monitored during all anesthetics to confirm adequacy of ventilation. The presence of end-tidal CO_2 confirms placement of the endotracheal tube in the trachea, adequacy of mask ventilation, or proper placement of a laryngeal mask airway. In addition, a sudden rise in end-tidal CO_2 is the most sensitive indicator for the onset of malignant hyperthermia.

Noninvasive blood pressure monitoring is appropriate for most physiologically stable patients and for procedures in which intravascular volume is expected to remain stable. Examples of procedures for which invasive blood pressure monitoring is indicated might include those procedures with the potential for significant blood loss, in which sudden hemodynamic changes are expected, or the patient with significant underlying cardiorespiratory disease (50). The placement of an arterial line also facilitates frequent laboratory testing during surgery or in the postoperative period.

The placement of a central venous catheter is indicated for some procedures. The advantages of placing a central line in a pediatric patient include (a) the ability to monitor central venous pressure to guide IV fluid and blood product administration, (b) a ready source for blood sampling, and (c) a secure access to the central circulation for the administration of vasoactive drugs or parenteral nutrition (49). The central line may not replace a large-bore peripheral line as a route for the rapid infusion of drugs or fluid, as the narrow radius and long length of the catheter increase resistance to flow. Access to the central circulation may be attained via the internal or external jugular veins, the subclavian veins, or the femoral veins. In most cases, the choice between subclavian and jugular catheters is an institutional and/or operator preference. For procedures below the level of the diaphragm, most clinicians prefer the jugular or subclavian approach, since tumor mass, invasion of the inferior vena cava, or massive blood loss may compromise the reliability of femoral access.

Although rarely used in pediatric cancer surgery, patients with an increased ICP may require a subarachnoid drain or an ICP monitor prior to surgery. All of the monitors mentioned are important during the operative course, but none is a substitute for the vigilant anesthesiologist.

B. Fluid Management and Intravascular Access

The requirement for secure intravascular access cannot be overstated. Placement of suitable lines may be among the most difficult parts of the anesthetic care, as many of these patients have already had multiple intravascular lines for chemotherapy. Fortunately, many patients come to the OR with a central line for chemotherapy or parenteral nutrition already in place. Using sterile technique, the central line may be accessed for the induction of anesthesia, following which additional peripheral lines may be placed if needed. At least one large bore peripheral IV is needed in cases where there is anticipated blood loss or fluid shifts.

Because the patient may present to the OR with significant fluid deficits secondary to nutritional depletion, nausea and vomiting, or a prolonged NPO period, it is important to assess the preoperative fluid status and replace the calculated deficit along with the maintenance fluids. Estimated fluid requirements can be calculated using the 4:2:1 guidelines (Table 5). Surgical losses, including blood, evaporative losses, and third space redistribution should also be measured or estimated, and replaced throughout the case. For the stable patient with a hemoglobin level >10 g/dL, blood loss is replaced initially with a balanced salt solution. When anemia becomes significant enough to cause hemodynamic changes, colloid solutions or packed red blood cells may be needed. Blood loss may be rapid or unexpected during some procedures, resulting in large fluid shifts (50).

C. Temperature Management

Maintaining normothermia for pediatric patients in the OR is more challenging than for adult patients.

Table 5 Maintenance Fluid Requirements

Weight (kg)	Maintenance requirements
0–10	4 mL/kg/hr
10–20	4 mL/kg/hr for the first 10 kg plus 2 mL/kg/hr for each kilogram between 10 and 20 kg
>20	4 mL/kg/hr for the first 10 kg plus 2 mL/kg/hr for each kilogram between 10 and 20 kg plus 1 mL/kg/hr for each kilogram over 20 kg

Source: Adapted from Ref. 123.

Significant reductions in temperature occur secondary to redistribution, conduction, convection, radiation, and evaporation (68). Clinical factors contributing to hypothermia include cold ORs, large exposed skin areas, open body cavities, and the use of cold irrigant solutions and skin cleansers. Anesthesia itself inhibits normal thermoregulatory function and decreases metabolic heat production (50,68,69). The initial drop in temperature following induction of anesthesia results primarily from redistribution of heat from the core tissues to the periphery, but the other mechanisms of heat transfer are also important. Children have an increased surface area-to-volume ratio compared with adult patients, explaining the rapidity with which heat is lost to the environment. In the awake patient, the hypothalamus responds to temperature changes and maintains core body temperature within a narrow range, but general anesthesia blunts this response and increases the threshold temperature. The anesthesiologist should aggressively prevent heat loss by minimizing skin exposure, warming fluid and blood products, incorporating active or passive warming devices into the breathing circuit, and using forced-air warming devices (50,68,69).

D. Anesthetic Technique

Pediatric cancer patients should be evaluated in the same manner as any other patient with respect to the selection of the anesthetic technique (Table 6). A complete understanding of the drug interactions between anesthetic agents and chemotherapy drugs, along with evaluation of the patient's cardiovascular, respiratory, renal, and hepatic function, will help determine which agents are indicated and which should be avoided. Although a complete review of the effects of anesthetic agents on organ function is beyond the scope of this chapter, some specific examples will be cited.

1. *Induction of Anesthesia*

The most common routes for induction of anesthesia include inhalation or IV. Factors influencing the induction technique include the presence of an IV line, hemodynamic stability, and concerns about a potentially difficult airway. An inhalation induction is frequently selected when the child does not have an IV, as most young children do not want to be stuck with needles. Flavoring the mask with candy oil facilitates the child's tolerance of the mask, as does beginning the induction with nitrous oxide and oxygen before gradually introducing the volatile anesthetic. The selection of the volatile anesthetic is individually tailored to the characteristics of the agent (49) and to some extent, by the experience and preference of the practitioner.

Table 6 Influence of Chemotherapeutic Agents on Anesthetic Technique

Chemotherapeutic agent	Anesthetic agent or technique	Anesthetic implication
Bleomycin	High inspired oxygen concentration	Pulmonary edema Acute respiratory distress syndrome Oxygen toxicity
Doxorubicin/daunorubicin	Thiopental Propofol	Myocardial depression
	Halothane	Myocardial depression
Cyclophosphamide	Succinylcholine	Prolonged apnea
	Drugs metabolized by cytochrome P-450 system: volatile anesthetic agents, fentanyl, alfentanil, sufentanil, benzodiazepines, lidocaine, and ropivacaine	Increased sensitivity, may require dose adjustment
Procarbazine	Barbiturates	Enhanced CNS depressant effects
Mithramycin	Succinylcholine	Prolonged apnea
Antimetabolites Methotrexate Mercaptopurine Cytarabine Fluorouracil	Nondepolarizing muscle relaxants	Decreased effect, requiring higher dose

Source: Adapted from Refs. 13, 49.

All inhalational anesthetics may produce some degree of myocardial depression, although this effect is most pronounced with halothane. Isoflurane or sevoflurane causes little direct myocardial depression; but in a patient who has received cardiotoxic agents such as the anthracyclines, or a patient with a history of thoracic radiation to the heart area, it may be wise to avoid inhalational anesthetics or, alternatively, to pick the agent with the least possible myocardial depression (49).

Induction of anesthesia with a volatile agent is ideal for the child whose larynx may be difficult to visualize or to intubate, as spontaneous ventilation during attempts at laryngoscopy prevents hypoxia and loss of the airway. Oral fiberoptic intubation or intubation through a laryngeal mask airway is easier to accomplish in the spontaneously breathing patient.

When the child presents to the OR with IV access already in place, the simplest technique is an IV induction using sodium thiopental, propofol, etomidate, or ketamine. Selection of an agent depends, in part, on the patient's hemodynamic status, as the administration of thiopental and propofol may be accompanied by a significant reduction in blood pressure unless the induction dose is titrated slowly to the clinical effect. Propofol is an ideal agent for short procedures, as arousal from anesthesia is rapid, and nausea and vomiting are uncommon. The discomfort of propofol injection can be minimized by the coadministration of a small dose of lidocaine or ketamine. Etomidate and ketamine are suitable alternatives for patients who are hypovolemic or who have significant myocardial dysfunction. Fentanyl is frequently also administered at the time of induction to blunt the hemodynamic response to induction, and the administration of midazolam with ketamine may prevent adverse emergence events.

Application of local anesthetic cream [EMLA: (eutectic mixture of local anesthetic)] on the dorsal surface of the hands facilitates the insertion of an IV when the child needs a rapid sequence induction of anesthesia. Preoxygenation, injection of the hypnotic agent and a rapid-acting muscle relaxant, and the application of cricoid pressure during laryngoscopy all serve to protect the airway of the patient who is at risk for regurgitation and aspiration of gastric contents.

2. *Maintenance of Anesthesia*

Techniques for the maintenance of anesthesia include inhalational anesthetics, IV anesthetics, or regional anesthetics (alone or combined with general anesthesia); the most commonly used technique, termed "balanced anesthesia," combines IV opiates and adjuncts with volatile anesthetics and muscle relaxants. This technique decreases the total amount of each drug needed, thus minimizing the side effects. Inhalational agents should be used with caution in several situations. In patients with renal dysfunction, sevoflurane should be avoided because its metabolism releases a free fluoride ion (50). Patients with cardiac toxicity may need to avoid inhalational agents, as all of these agents produce some degree of myocardial depression. Halothane has the most negative inotropic effect, so that an alternative agent should be selected (49,50). Nitrous oxide is commonly administered along with volatile agents because it contributes analgesic and amnestic properties, without cardiac or respiratory depression (49). Using nitrous oxide is also an effective strategy for minimizing the inspired concentration of oxygen for patients who have received pulmonary toxic drugs like bleomycin.

Opioids are an important component of a balanced anesthetic technique. Opioids blunt the stress response to surgery and provide analgesia. Although any opioids can be administered in the OR, fentanyl is the most commonly administered agent; morphine is sometimes given at the end of procedures for postoperative analgesia. Because pediatric cancer patients may have been receiving chronic opioids before surgery, they may demonstrate tolerance to these agents, increasing their dose requirements.

The pharmacology of commonly used neuromuscular blocking (NMB) agents (muscle relaxants) can be altered by cancer and cancer therapy (13,49). For example, the duration of action of succinylcholine may be prolonged in patients who have received cyclophosphamide, so that such a patient might demonstrate prolonged or unexpected apnea (13,35,49). There are two explanations for this observation: (i) chemotherapy-related hepatic dysfunction may result in decreased synthesis of pseudocholinesterase necessary for the inactivation of succinylcholine and (ii) depression of the hepatic system can occur from the cancer itself, whether or not chemotherapy has been given (49). The dose of nondepolarizing muscle relaxants may also need to be altered in these patients. Neuromuscular blocking drugs that rely on renal clearance, such as pancuronium, may need to be decreased in patients with altered renal function (50), or an alternative NMB agent should be selected. Immunosuppressive therapy may decrease the potency of NMB, requiring two to four times the normal dose to achieve muscle relaxation (13).

Electrolyte abnormalities occur commonly in cancer patients and may affect the administration and metabolism of muscle relaxants. The administration of an intubating dose of the depolarizing muscle relaxant, succinylcholine, will increase serum potassium levels by 0.5–1.0 mEq/L, an effect that is well tolerated in healthy patients. However, in pediatric cancer patients in whom tissue breakdown has already resulted in an increased potassium level, the administration of succinylcholine may cause a dramatic increase in potassium, leading to symptomatic cardiac arrhythmias or cardiac arrest. Prolongation of the P-R interval, prolongation of the QRS complex, S-T segment elevation, and peaked T waves may herald cardiac collapse, but these arrhythmias may respond to aggressive treatment with glucose, insulin, sodium bicarbonate, calcium chloride, and furosemide. Hypokalemia in pediatric cancer patients results from poor oral intake, vomiting, and diarrhea related to chemotherapy (13). Moderate hypokalemia is usually asymptomatic, but a severe deficit may present with skeletal muscle weakness, fatigue, and cramps, and with ECG changes including S-T segment depression, the appearance of U waves, and PR and QRS prolongation (70). Hypokalemia must be corrected slowly and carefully in order to avoid overcorrection. Treatment includes oral or IV replacement and avoidance of glucose-containing solutions, as glucose will stimulate insulin secretion and drive potassium into the cells (70,71).

Hypercalcemia may result from bony metastases or bone lysis, whereas hypocalcemia may occur after treatment with chemotherapeutic agents including cisplatinum (15,50). Hypercalcemia, occurring in roughly 5% of cancer patients, presents as fatigue, nausea, abdominal pain, anxiety, and depression (18,70). Shortening of the Q-T interval and other arrhythmias may appear on the ECG. Treatment with IV fluids and diuresis with furosemide in the perioperative period should be continued, pending normalization of the intravascular fluid volume and the serum calcium level (70,71).

Hypocalcemia may also occur, most commonly during tumor lysis syndrome (TLS) secondary to hyperphosphatemia. The TLS occurs when large numbers of dying tumor cells are released into the circulation (72). Electrolyte abnormalities include hyperuricemia, hyperkalemia, and hyperphosphatemia, leading to hypocalcemia. The TLS usually begins within 12–72 hr after the onset of treatment. Acute renal failure may ensue, limiting electrolyte excretion. Treatments consisting of aggressive hydration, allopurinol, and alkalinization of the urine help prevent the development of hyperkalemia. Dialysis may be required if supportive care fails (72). Although calcium facilitates acetylcholine release and muscular contractions, the effect of calcium abnormalities on the response to muscle relaxants in the clinical setting is unpredictable (71).

It may also be appropriate in a patient with cardiovascular or pulmonary compromise to use a regional technique as the primary anesthetic, in combination with general anesthesia, or as a means for providing postoperative analgesia (49). Regional anesthesia has minimal effects on the cardiovascular function of children and will decrease the amount of supplemental inhalational or IV medication required when using a combined technique with general anesthesia (49).

3. *Emergence from Anesthesia*

Planning for emergence from anesthesia begins in the OR with discontinuation of the volatile agent or IV infusion, reversal of muscle relaxation, and evaluation of the patient's suitability for extubation. For most procedures, extubation of the trachea is expected. In other cases, particularly prolonged or major intra-abdominal, intrathoracic, or intracranial procedures, the anesthesiologist and surgeon may agree that a period of postoperative mechanical ventilation is warranted. Generally speaking, such a decision is based on the patient's preoperative condition, the location and extent of the surgical dissection, the amount of blood loss and fluid replacement, as well as unexpected intraoperative complications. The patient's body temperature at the end of surgery may influence the extubation decision, as hypothermia delays the elimination of volatile agents and slows the metabolism of fixed agents.

V. POSTOPERATIVE CARE

Postoperative care may be initiated in the Post-Anesthesia Care Unit (PACU) or Pediatric Intensive Care Unit (PICU). For patients undergoing routine procedures, the PACU is the logical site for recovery from anesthesia. Following longer or more complex procedures, recovery and ongoing care may require intensive care. By institutional protocol or custom, critically ill or unstable patients may be stabilized in the PACU initially or may be transferred directly from the OR to the PICU.

A. The Post-Anesthesia Care Unit

Once the patient has been safely extubated, transport to the PACU initiates the recovery process. During the early recovery period, the major issues include airway obstruction and hypoventilation, cardiovascular stability, temperature maintenance, the assessment of ongoing fluid losses and replacement, and postoperative pain management. Assessing the adequacy of post-operative analgesia can be challenging in the early recovery period, as expressions of confusion and disorientation may mimic pain in the young or preverbal child. Agitation can also be caused by a distended bladder, hypoxia and/or hypercarbia, hypothermia, and hypoglycemia; in addition, the anxiety of separation may become more apparent, as the child becomes more aware of his/her surroundings.

Intermittent IV administration of opioids remains the gold standard for early postoperative pain management. Titration of opioid therapy to patient comfort should be done before initiation of patient-controlled analgesia, as smaller interval doses may not be sufficient for managing acute postoperative pain. Opioid analgesia may be supplemented with a variety of adjuncts including oral nonsteroidal anti-inflammatory agents (NSAIDs) or acetaminophen, if the patient is tolerating oral fluids. Intravenous ketorolac may be an alternative choice for patients who are not at an increased risk for perioperative bleeding.

For patients whose anesthetic included placement of an epidural or peripheral nerve sheath catheter, the effectiveness of the block must be assessed in the PACU. An inadequate dermatomal level, a unilateral sensory or motor block, an excessive motor block, or an early onset of side effects like pruritus and nausea may require additional dosing of the epidural or changing the continuous infusion. Those adjustments are best made while the patient is still in the PACU.

Discharge from PACU, either to home or to an inpatient unit, requires that the patient meet institutional guidelines, which include the ability to maintain the airway independently, the ability to maintain adequate oxygen saturation (with or without supplemental oxygen), stable vital signs, and effective management of pain, nausea and/or vomiting. Arousal from anesthesia is required, although inpatients may remain somewhat somnolent from analgesics administered in the PACU. Use of scoring systems like the Aldrete score assures consistency and uniformity of discharge criteria within an institution (73).

B. Acute Pain Management

1. Opioids

The principles of postoperative pain management in cancer patients are the same as in children without malignancy. Children who have previously been receiving opioid medications should receive their daily opioid dose plus additional opioids as needed in the immediate post-operative period for pain control (74,75). Many patients are under-medicated because they are only treated for their postoperative pain, without regard for the opioid tolerance that they may have developed in the preoperative period. For this reason, the authors recommend continuing long-acting oral opioids in the perioperative period, transitioning to parenteral medication if the patient cannot tolerate the oral preparation. This strategy minimizes sudden decreases in plasma levels. Titrating intermittent opioids to effect in the early postoperative period should result in a calm, easily arousable, and comfortable child. Once the patient is comfortable, patient-controlled analgesia may be instituted (or resumed) in the PACU.

2. Regional Analgesia

Epidural anesthesia offers analgesia that may be superior in quality to that of IV opioids with fewer side effects, in addition to other physiologic benefits in the postoperative patient (76,77). Although only a few studies have evaluated the effectiveness of epidural anesthesia for postoperative pain relief in pediatric oncology patients, evidence in the adult literature points to positive effects on postoperative cardiovascular, respiratory, and metabolic function (76). Effective postoperative pain relief prevents or minimizes the postoperative surge in circulating catecholamines that causes an increased blood pressure, heart rate, and oxygen consumption. Epidural analgesia blunts these responses just as it blocks pain sensations (76). Postoperative respiratory function is also improved in patients with epidural catheters, because minimizing pain promotes preservation of functional residual capacity (FRC) and prevents the development of atelectasis (78).

Potential problems associated with the placement of epidural catheters include difficult placement, infection, bleeding, accidental dural puncture, inadvertent overdose of local anesthetic, and excessive motor or sympathetic blockade. Fortunately, development of an epidural hematoma leading to paralysis represents a rare complication (76). Local anesthetics such as lidocaine, bupivacaine, or ropivacaine are injected into the epidural space to block transmission of pain impulses at the spinal cord level. These agents produce dose-dependent, titratable sensory and motor blockade. Older children may exhibit hypotension caused by sympathetic blockade, although this finding is less common in younger children. Adding an opiate to the local anesthetic infusion allows for the administration of a lower dose of local anesthetic, minimizing local anesthetic toxicity, motor block, and sympathetic blockade.

Epidural opiates, like systemic opiates, may cause urinary retention, pruritus, nausea, and vomiting. Less commonly, the administration of epidural opiates may be accompanied by respiratory depression. The relative risk for this complication, as well as the expected timing of depression, depends on the opiate administered. The lipophilic agent fentanyl is least likely to cause respiratory depression, hydromorphone is intermediate in its effects, and epidural morphine is the agent most likely to result in late respiratory depression (76,79). The respiratory depression may be biphasic: the initial (early) respiratory depression represents systemic absorption of the opioid, whereas the delayed response results from absorption of the agent into the CSF with cephalad spread up to the brainstem. Systemic effects will occur within 2 hr of injection, whereas CSF spread may cause respiratory depression 6–12 hours later (80). Although monitoring guidelines will vary by institution, we believe that patients receiving epidural morphine or hydromorphone should be monitored for at least the first 24 hr due to the potential for respiratory depression. We monitor all infants <1 year of age with indwelling epidural catheters, irrespective of the infusion. Monitoring should include periodic assessment of the respiratory rate and level of consciousness; some advocate routine ECG and pulse oximetry as well (81).

Although few studies have examined outcomes from epidural analgesia in pediatric oncology patients, Tobias et al. (76) retrospectively reviewed the course of 60 such patients, aged 4 months to 19 years, whose postoperative pain was managed using an epidural catheter placed in the OR, following the induction of general anesthesia. Catheter placement was successful in 97% of the patients. There were no catheter complications, and analgesia was maintained for the first several postoperative days. They concluded that epidural anesthesia was an effective way to provide postoperative analgesia in the pediatric oncology patient. There have not been any direct comparisons of the efficacy of epidural analgesia compared with traditional opioids in pediatric cancer patients.

VI. SPECIFIC CLINICAL CASES

A. Abdominal Masses

The most common solid tumor in infancy is neuroblastoma, although Wilm's tumor is the most frequent primary malignant renal tumor of childhood (50,82). The majority of neuroblastomas and Wilm's tumors present as abdominal masses. As concomitant thoracic involvement or extension of the tumor is not unusual, it is important to determine the full extent of tumor involvement. Tumor extension into the chest may negatively impact ventilation, and superior vena cava (SVC) or right atrial involvement may adversely affect cardiac function. If the tumor involves the thoracic cavity or if there is a large amount of ascites displacing the diaphragm superiorly, FRC may be decreased, and the patient may behave like a patient with restrictive lung disease. Such patients are prone to rapid oxygen desaturation during laryngoscopy and tracheal intubation.

A tumor involving the vena cava or right atrium is particularly concerning for the anesthesiologist, as surgical manipulation of the tumor may dramatically alter venous return to the heart, resulting in wide swings in blood pressure and heart rate. Rapid and massive blood loss during tumor resection, tumor embolism into the heart, or occlusion of the inferior vena cava may occur. Establishing vascular access in the upper extremity assures access to the circulation even if the inferior vena cava must be cross-clamped for control of surgical bleeding. An arterial catheter and central venous access are important in these cases for monitoring beat-to-beat changes in the arterial pressure and intravascular volume.

Compression and displacement of the stomach by the abdominal mass warrants special attention by the anesthesiologist because compression may delay gastric emptying, even if the patient has observed standard NPO guidelines. These patients should have a rapid sequence induction of anesthesia to minimize the risk of regurgitation and aspiration of gastric contents. Nitrous oxide is avoided in abdominal surgery, as its diffusion into closed air spaces will promote intestinal distention, which may compromise respiratory function, increase intra-abdominal pressure, and increase the difficulty of closing the abdominal incision.

B. Thoracic Tumors

Most cancerous lung masses in children are metastatic lesions requiring pulmonary wedge resection. The major anesthetic consideration in these patients is the selection of a technique for providing single-lung ventilation, in order to facilitate surgical exposure. Although one-lung ventilation is possible in children, it is more difficult than in adults because of the smaller size of most pediatric endotracheal tubes and the more limited selection of devices available for isolating the lungs. Some older, larger adolescents may be appropriate candidates for a standard adult double-lumen endotracheal tube (DLT). The smallest commercially available DLT is a 28 French tube with an outside diameter of 9.8 mm, which correlates to a sized 7.0 standard endotracheal tube. An endotracheal tube of this size can only be placed in children >8 years (83). A traditional double-lumen tube allows for the separate application of continuous airway pressure to the deflated lung, which may help maintain adequate oxygenation during lung compression.

Another option for lung isolation is the use of a bronchial blocker. The patient's trachea is intubated by direct laryngoscopy, and then the bronchial blocker is passed through the endotracheal tube. A fiberoptic bronchoscope placed within the endotracheal tube at the same time is used to confirm correct placement of the bronchial blocker. The smallest bronchial blocker will pass through a sized 4.5 endotracheal tube, appropriate for most 2-year-old children. However, the bronchial blocker does not allow for the application of continuous positive airway pressure to the deflated lung. The third option for lung isolation is the use of a Univent® tube, which differs from a bronchial blocker such that the bronchial blocker is built directly into the wall of the tube. Again, the endotracheal tube is passed through the vocal cords by direct laryngoscopy, and the blocker is guided to the correct position using a fiberoptic bronchoscope. The smallest Univent® tube has an inside diameter of 3.5 mm with an outside diameter of 7.5 mm, corresponding to a 5.5 standard endotracheal tube.

For the smallest infants and toddlers, a deliberate mainstem intubation is often the simplest technique. Placement of the endotracheal tube into the right mainstem bronchus is easy when the tumor involves the left lung, but intubation of the left bronchus is more difficult. One strategy is to turn the infant's head to the right while advancing the tube and another is to use the neonatal fiberscope to direct the placement of the tube under direct vision.

C. Anterior Mediastinal Masses

Anterior mediastinal masses present special challenges for the anesthetist, as sudden tracheal or bronchial obstruction may develop in the supine patient; pulmonary edema and SVC obstruction have also been reported (49,51). Condition permitting, the preoperative evaluation includes both a chest X-ray and a chest CT scan, although particularly symptomatic children may not tolerate being supine long enough for the CT scan. The CT scan may help localize and measure the mass effect, but it is not a particularly good predictor of dynamic airway or pulmonary changes that may occur when the patient assumes the supine position, receives a muscle relaxant, or is ventilated with positive pressure (50). An ECHO may be performed to look for any evidence of cardiac invasion or compression by the mass. Although PFTs may be helpful in stable patients for evaluating changes in respiratory function in different body positions, many patients with rapidly progressive disease and respiratory distress, particularly in younger children, will not be able to cooperate for pulmonary function studies. Specific symptoms of concern include dyspnea, nonproductive cough, orthopnea, or symptoms of SVC obstruction including venous engorgement and edema of the head, neck, and arms (51). Evidence of rales on chest auscultation may be present in severe cases.

Ferrari and Bedford (53) did a study of anterior mediastinal masses in patients with both Hodgkin's lymphoma and NHL. They reviewed the cases of 163 patients over a 4-year period that presented with anterior mediastinal masses, evaluating 44 patients who received general anesthesia for a diagnostic biopsy before radiation treatment. After reviewing the patient's history for symptoms of airway compromise, an IV was placed in a lower extremity to avoid concerns about the SVC, and then an induction technique was selected based on the presence or absence of airway distress. Anesthesia was induced in the sitting position in symptomatic patients using inhalational agents, whereas asymptomatic patients had an IV induction. If it was possible to manually ventilate the patient with positive pressure, then a muscle relaxant was administered to facilitate tracheal intubation. If positive pressure ventilation was difficult or impossible, tracheal intubation was performed without relaxant.

Two of the nine patients with preoperative respiratory symptoms developed airway obstruction after the administration of a muscle relaxant, while two of the asymptomatic patients developed airway obstruction during the maintenance phase of anesthesia. Three other asymptomatic patients could not be extubated in the OR, requiring radiation and chemotherapy prior to extubation in the ICU. After reviewing their experience, the authors recommended inhalational induction of anesthesia in the sitting position for patients with anterior mediastinal masses. They also advised IV placement in a lower extremity prior to induction, maintenance of spontaneous ventilation until the anesthesiologist demonstrated the ability to successfully assist ventilation with positive pressure, and immediate availability of a rigid bronchoscope in the event of tracheal compression.

Although most anterior mediastinal masses are exquisitely sensitive to radiation, it is important to get a precise tissue diagnosis before beginning the radiation therapy. In some cases, it may be possible to get a biopsy of a lymph node in the supraclavicular area using local anesthesia alone, thereby avoiding the airway issues just described. If not, a general anesthetic will be necessary. Despite the use of the aforementioned caveats, airway compromise may still occur when muscle tone decreases during induction, or during the maintenance phase. Airway obstruction may also result from compression of the airways distal to the endotracheal tube caused by the tumor itself. Finally, airway obstruction may occur during emergence from anesthesia, as the bulk of the tumor has usually not been removed (18,49,51). Strategies for dealing with the airway obstruction during anesthesia may include changing the patient's position, altering the ventilation technique, or advancement of the endotracheal tube beyond the obstruction. In emergent situations, it may be necessary to place the patient on femoral–femoral bypass to maintain arterial pressure, oxygenation, and ventilation until the airway obstruction can be relieved by surgical resection (51).

D. Airway Tumors

Although primary airway tumors in pediatric patients are rare, their presentation may pose considerable difficulties for the anesthesiologist. Head and neck cancer may cause distortion of the normal airway anatomy, creating a challenge for the anesthesiologist when securing the airway. Hodgkin's disease may present with cervical adenopathy, causing tracheal deviation or obstruction, as well as symptoms of SVC syndrome including tracheal obstruction secondary to venous engorgement. Airway management may be extremely difficult. Alternate approaches and equipment for intubation should be available and prepared, including a variety of endotracheal tube sizes and laryngoscope blades, a pediatric fiberoptic bronchoscope, and an intubating laryngeal mask airway; a surgeon skilled in performing pediatric tracheostomies should be available as well (50,51).

Among the most challenging patients the anesthesiologist will manage is the cancer patient who has received head and neck irradiation (Fig. 2). Radiation causes acute swelling and anatomical distortion, leading to restricted mobility of the jaw and/or neck.

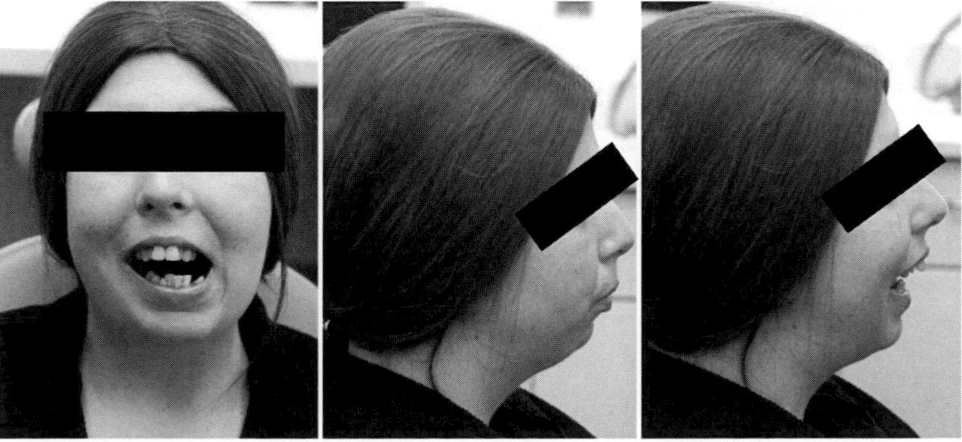

Figure 2 Adolescent patient who received radiation to the head and neck for nasopharyngeal carcinoma. Notice the malocclusion and decreased range of motion of the TMJ. The patient also had retrognathia and limited neck extension.

Mouth opening may be so limited that visualization of the larynx and intubation of the trachea by direct laryngoscopy may be impossible. Having anticipated and identified the site of difficulty, the anesthesiologist must develop an alternative plan for securing the airway. Alternatives to standard tracheal intubation may include intubation through a laryngeal mask, use of specialized laryngoscope blades or handles, awake fiberoptic intubation, or even the establishment of a tracheostomy before surgery. The reader is referred to the ASA difficult airway algorithm (84). An awake fiberoptic intubation or even a presurgical tracheostomy may represent the safest technique for a given patient, although both of these techniques are difficult in the very young child. Postoperative problems may also occur secondary to laryngeal edema and swelling at the surgical site (50,51), such that prolonged intubation and steroid treatment may be required.

E. Bone Tumors

Pain is the presenting symptom for most children with bone cancer and may predate the diagnosis by >2 months (85). Osteosarcoma and Ewing's sarcoma are the most common primary bone tumors in children, and both present with bone pain as a frequent symptom at the time of diagnosis. Other pediatric cancers that may present with bone pain include leukemias and neuroblastomas (86). The preoperative pain should be managed the same way as other cancer pain, with attention to the World Health Organization (WHO) ladder for pain management. There is some suggestion that preoperative pain predicts the presence and severity of phantom limb pain after amputation (87).

Other issues in the perioperative management of bone tumors include the possibility of considerable bleeding during resection, especially from long bone tumors. Adequate venous access, availability of a sufficient number of units of blood for transfusion, and the use of a tourniquet may minimize the physiologic impact of the blood loss. Bleeding from raw bone surfaces is difficult to control; the anesthesiologist may consider using a hypotensive technique to minimize blood loss (88).

Epidural anesthesia is particularly helpful in the perioperative management of patients undergoing limb salvage procedures and major amputations. We place epidural catheters in the OR following the induction of general anesthesia and use both local anesthetic and opiate to provide surgical anesthesia. A supplemental "light" general anesthetic provides hypnosis and amnesia for the procedure. Selection of agents for continuous epidural infusion following surgery depends on the patient's condition and the plan for postoperative physical therapy. If the surgeon plans to use a continuous passive motion device postoperatively, we select an agent (bupivacaine) and a concentration (0.125%) likely to provide a dense motor block and muscle relaxation. If, on the other hand, the plan is for early postoperative mobilization and ambulation, we use ropivacaine instead, in order to minimize motor block. In most cases of lower extremity surgery, fentanyl is the most appropriate opioid for the infusion, as the catheter tip is located close to the nerve roots requiring anesthesia.

F. Intracranial Tumors

Tumors of the CNS represent a large number of pediatric cancer cases. Specific concerns for CNS tumors include elevated ICP, blood loss, patient monitoring, and patient positioning. Symptoms of elevated ICP include nausea, vomiting, headaches, lethargy, changes in mental status, and coma (49,89). Prior to anesthesia, the patient may have an external ventricular drain placed to allow cerebral spinal fluid drainage and decrease ICP. Anesthetic management includes hyperventilation, diuresis, mild hypothermia, and maintaining high-normal mean arterial pressures. All IV induction agents, with the exception of ketamine, decrease cerebral metabolic rate, cerebral blood flow, and intracranial pressure; a nondepolarizing muscle relaxant that is not associated with histamine release should be selected, such as vecuronium, rocuronium, or *cis*-atracurium. Although all volatile agents produce some degree of vasodilation, this effect may be abolished by hyperventilation. Isoflurane may be the volatile agent of choice because it causes minimal cerebral vasodilation.

Bleeding may be a concern in some neurosurgical cases so an adequate IV access and an arterial line are indicated. An arterial line will allow beat-to-beat monitoring of blood pressure changes, along with frequent arterial blood gas measurements as needed. Positioning is most commonly in the prone or supine position depending on the tumor location. Careful padding of bony prominences is important to prevent nerve injuries, along with careful eye protection, including lubricant and eye covering (90). The most common eye complication is a corneal abrasion from dircct trauma, but ischemic optic neuropathy may occur. This can cause permanent visual loss due to infarction of the optic nerve. Risk factors include hypotension and anemia plus an additional factor such as venous obstruction. It is important to monitor blood loss and keep these patients normotensive.

Infrequently, the patient may be placed in a sitting position with the head above the heart. This helps minimize blood loss and facilitates surgical exposure (90). The sitting position may impair venous return to the heart, decreasing blood pressure, and has a higher incidence of venous air embolism. A central line should be placed in these patients to allow air aspiration from the right atrium in the event of a venous air embolism, and either a Doppler ultrasound or transesophageal ECHO should be used to detect venous air embolism. Management of venous air embolism includes notifying the surgeon, so that they can flood the surgical field with normal saline, ventilation with 100% oxygen, discontinuation of nitrous oxide, aspiration of air from the central venous line, jugular venous compression, lowering the head of the bed, and providing hemodynamic support as needed (90).

VII. ANESTHESIA OUTSIDE THE OPERATING ROOM

The pediatric cancer patient may require general anesthesia for diagnostic or therapeutic procedures outside of the OR including the radiology suite, cancer clinic procedure rooms, echocardiology laboratory, and the bone marrow transplant unit. Anxiety and fear accompany the pain of the procedure and may be associated with long-term behavioral changes. Consequently, the goal for the conduct of the procedure is to make the child physically and psychologically comfortable (91). Management should begin with measures to alleviate the fear and anxiety, including behavioral interventions, psychological interventions, and a complete discussion with the family and child (91).

Applicable anesthetic techniques in these locations are dependent on the specific sedation quality and requirements for the procedure. For long, painless procedures like magnetic resonance imaging, reliable sedation, immobility, and amnesia are necessary. For short but painful procedures, the goals for therapy may include rapid onset, rapid arousal, and effective analgesia.

Regardless of the specific techniques employed, regulatory requirements mandate that patients receiving general anesthesia in a nonsurgical area receive the same level of care with respect to physiologic and safety monitoring that they would receive in the OR. Safety guidelines must be followed at these outside locations including the availability of resuscitation equipment, ASA monitors, and pediatric equipment (50,92). Anesthesia protocols must address preoperative assessment, NPO guidelines, postoperative recovery, and quality assurance such that the care delivered outside the OR environment meets the same standards as that in the OR.

A number of studies have compared general anesthesia to conscious sedation techniques for bone marrow aspirations and lumbar punctures in pediatric cancer patients. Propofol has been used because of its rapid onset, easy titration, rapid emergence, and antiemetic properties. Although propofol is an appropriate drug for some patients, it must be used with caution in patients with myocardial dysfunction or hypovolemia because of its myocardial depressant properties. For such children, an alternative drug such as ketamine or etomidate may be a better choice.

Ljungman et al. (92) studied 25 children with leukemia and NHL who required 15–20 lumbar punctures for aggressive intrathecal chemotherapy. One group received a general anesthetic with fentanyl and propofol. The other group received a conscious sedation technique that included the local application of EMLA cream and injection of local anesthesia at the lumbar puncture site, along with a combination of meperidine and midazolam. At the time of the next procedure, the groups were switched, so that each child served as his/her own control. The patient and family each completed a questionnaire after the second procedure. There were no differences in side effects, the level of patient distress, or discomfort. Patients and their families preferred the conscious sedation technique, but there were more sedation failures in this group attributed to a lack of cooperation, particularly in the younger patients.

Fortney et al. (93) studied patients requiring external beam radiation therapy with and without general anesthesia. General anesthesia was needed in the majority of patients under the age of 3 years, but older patients did well with sedation only. Using educational interventions, behavior modification techniques, and visual aids, the investigators were able to reduce the number of patients requiring general anesthesia.

Finally, Jayabose et al. (94) studied sedation for 355 procedures with propofol or propofol plus combinations of fentanyl and midazolam for imaging studies, radiation therapy, bone marrow aspiration and biopsies, and lumbar punctures. After propofol administration, oxygen was provided by facemask or nasal cannula, and vital signs were recorded every 5–10 min. Mild hypoxia (SaO_2: 85–94%) was seen in six of the 355 procedures; one patient had a brief period of laryngospasm, requiring supplemental oxygen, oral suctioning, and hydrocortisone. No patient required tracheal intubation. He concluded that propofol administered by an anesthesiologist is a safe and effective way to achieve anesthesia for these painful procedures.

In our practice, anesthesiologists administer propofol as the sole agent to children undergoing lumbar punctures and bone marrow aspiration, with or without biopsy. We provide this service in the PACU for cancer patients who cannot be managed in the clinic setting using an institutional protocol of midazolam and fentanyl. Total propofol doses much higher than traditional induction doses are required, even when local anesthesia is injected at the bone marrow site. During these brief procedures, we provide oxygen from the wall outlet using a facemask connected to a Jackson-Rees circuit; suction and intubation equipment are immediately available. As it is not uncommon for us to see apnea even while the child is still moving vigorously, we believe that the use of propofol should be limited to those skilled in airway management.

VIII. DO NOT RESUSCITATE ORDERS AND THE TERMINALLY ILL CHILD

Patients and their families have a right to refuse medical treatment. Twelve thousand new cases of pediatric cancer are diagnosed yearly in the United States, and 25% of these children die from their disease (95). Surgery may be performed on a terminally ill child for palliative reasons, including the reduction of pain, placement of lines or devices to help with feeding, or relief of an obstruction caused by the cancer (95,96). The arrival of a child with a "do not resuscitate" (DNR) order on the chart to the operating suite may provoke questions and anxiety among the OR staff. Previously, DNR orders were "automatically" suspended when patients came to the OR, but that is not necessarily the case now. The surgeon and anesthesiologist should discuss possible outcomes and scenarios with the family, involving them in decisions about appropriate limits to care (95–97). As anesthesia affects not only consciousness but also cardiorespiratory function, it is important to explain to the family that common anesthetic effects might exacerbate cardiopulmonary dysfunction or hasten death in the terminally ill patient. Similarly, the anesthesiologist must try to identify for the family which effects might be anesthesia-related, and might require an attempt to reverse, and which might be attributed to the patient's underlying condition (95–97). A careful and frank discussion with the patient and the family may help them decide if they want to suspend the DNR orders or maintain the orders during surgery.

IX. CHRONIC PAIN IN THE PEDIATRIC CANCER PATIENT

Pain is one of the most frequent and feared complications in the pediatric cancer patient. Pain may result from metastasis or direct extension of the primary tumor, from treatment, or from diagnostic or therapeutic procedures (75,98,99) (Table 7). Treatment-related pain is much more common in children than adults and includes postoperative pain, procedural pain, mucositis, infection, chemotherapy-related pain, and phantom limb pain (75,100). Children with cancer may undergo numerous procedures requiring brief periods of sedation and analgesia, or general anesthesia.

There are a number of reasons why childhood cancer victims are often under medicated and under treated, creating additional stress and suffering for the patients and their families. Admittedly, the assessment of pain in the very young or nonverbal child can be quite difficult, especially in young infants, preverbal, or cognitively impaired children. Self-reporting pain tools used in older children are not applicable in these patients; physicians must rely on physiologic and behavioral measures including hemodynamic responses, facial expressions, body movement and position, and vocalizations. Many physicians are fearful of respiratory depression and other side effects from potent pain medications, so, they prescribe inadequate therapy that is less aggressive than the analgesic treatment of adult patients (98). Others are afraid of creating addicted patients, but true addiction is extremely rare when opioids are used correctly (79).

Chronic pain in pediatric cancer patients should be addressed in a stepwise fashion. The first approach may include nonpharmacologic management, including physical therapy, acupuncture, massage, and heat and cold treatments, as well as behavioral and cognitive interventions (75,79). These modalities may help

Table 7 The Etiology and Causes of Pediatric Cancer Pain

Tumor-related pain: 15–25%	Metastases into bone, nerve, or soft tissue
	Compression of bone, nerve, or solid organ
	Obstruction of blood vessels
Treatment-related pain: 40–50%	Postoperative pain
	Mucositis
	Phantom limb pain
	Postchemotherapy pain
	Postradiation pain
	Infection
	Postdural puncture headache
	Avascular necrosis
Procedure-related pain: 35%	Bone marrow aspiration and biopsy
	Lumbar puncture
	Central line placement and removal
	PICC line insertion

Source: Adapted from Refs. 75, 79, 98, 100.

alleviate the patient's anxiety and improve the ability to deal with the stress of diagnosis and treatment. The decision to use nonpharmacologic treatment before medications depends on numerous factors, including the patient's age, level of understanding, coping ability, expectations, past history, and cause of pain. The main goal in treating the patient with cancer pain is to identify the source of the pain and prepare a treatment to help decrease the painful experience (79,101).

A. Opioids and Other Analgesic Drugs

The WHO has described a graduated "ladder" strategy for the treatment of pain in cancer patients (79,100). It recommends a stepwise advancement in strength of pain medication from acetaminophen and nonsteroidal anti-inflammatory drugs, first adding mild opioids, then stronger opioids and finally, adjunctive agents are added if necessary (75,79). The mainstay in treatment for cancer pain is analgesic drugs, including nonsteroidal anti-inflammatory drugs, weak opioids, and strong opioids.

Nonsteroidal anti-inflammatory drugs include aspirin, acetaminophen, and ibuprofen. These drugs inhibit prostaglandin synthesis and prevent inflammation. All of these drugs, except acetaminophen, cause gastric irritation and the possibility of gastric bleeding by inhibiting platelet function (75,79,100). For this reason, acetaminophen is the first drug of choice in the cancer patient. Because it has a high therapeutic index, there is a low risk of toxic side effects for most patients (102). The agents in this class all have antipyretic activity and must be used with caution in the patient who is immunocompromised or neutropenic, as their use may obscure the recognition of infection (75,100). Nonsteroidal anti-inflammatory drugs exhibit a ceiling effect such that increasing the dose does not increase effectiveness, but may increase toxicity. Although acetaminophen and NSAIDs may offer basal analgesia, more than half of pediatric patients with progressive cancer will require pain relief beyond that which can be achieved with these agents.

If pain is unrelieved by acetaminophen and nonsteroidal agents, then weak opioids, such as codeine, may be added. Administered orally, these drugs may be administered alone to manage mild to moderate pain or may be combined with NSAIDs. They are more commonly used with a nonopioid analgesic because they potentiate the effect of the nonopioid, by acting centrally, whereas the NSAIDs primarily act on the periphery (79). As commercial preparations frequently combine the weak opioid with acetaminophen, it is important to check the total dose of acetaminophen to avoid overdosing on that component. If the patient is still in pain following the addition of a weak opioid, a stronger opioid should be substituted.

Morphine remains the gold standard for the management of severe cancer pain, and its use has been well studied in children (98,102). Starting doses vary depending on the clinical situation and the age of the patient. Clearance of morphine during the first 3 months of life is delayed compared with older children, so, the starting dose in the newborn period should be reduced to ~25% of the dose that would be administered to an older child (75,98). Doses should be scheduled at intervals frequent enough that the next available dose might be administered before the effect of the previous dose has worn off. Controlled-release morphine offers the convenience of 12-hr dosing, but oral absorption can be unpredictable, and dosing adjustments may be necessary. The administration of an immediate-release morphine preparation may be used to supplement analgesia or to manage breakthrough pain. For some patients, side effects from morphine, including nausea, vomiting, constipation, pruritus, somnolence, and respiratory depression, are distressing enough that alternatives should be considered.

Practical alternatives to parenteral morphine include hydromorphone, fentanyl, meperidine, and methadone. Hydromorphone is five to eight times more potent than morphine, whereas fentanyl is 50–100 times more potent than morphine; both may be used in the setting of dose-limiting side effects from morphine. The high lipid solubility of fentanyl, accounting for its rapid onset and short duration of action, makes it a good agent to use for patient- or parent-controlled analgesia (PCA) therapy, particularly for patients who develop pruritus with morphine. The administration of meperidine has fallen out of favor in the last few years, as practitioners have become more familiar with the CNS excitation (tremors, hallucinations, dysphoria, and seizures) that accompanies accumulation of its primary metabolite, normeperidine (103). In our institution, we have discontinued the availability of meperidine PCA, and recommend that meperidine administration be limited to <48 hr. The CNS effects of meperidine are exaggerated in patients with renal impairment, as reduced excretion facilitates accumulation of normeperidine (75). Finally, IV or oral methadone may be helpful when opiate requirements are stable or when patients prefer the convenience of less frequent dosing intervals. However, effective titration of methadone offers additional challenges, since increasing the dose may result in delayed sedation (103).

The WHO guidelines are effective in almost 90% of patients with chronic cancer pain, but in the remaining 10%, an alternative strategy for pain management must be attempted (104). These may include periodic rotation of pain medications, parenteral administration, transdermal opioids, and regional techniques, including peripheral nerve blocks, epidural analgesia, or intrathecal opiates (75,98,100,104–107). Alternative routes may need to be considered when oral administration is not possible because of patient refusal, ileus, bowel obstruction, nausea, vomiting, painful swallowing, or young age. Intravenous administration of opioids offers the most rapid onset of analgesia and may be the most efficient route while the caregivers are trying to identify an effective oral regimen. Intermittent scheduled doses, continuous infusions, or PCA may all be appropriate for given clinical situations. Enting et al. (104) studied 100 patients with advanced cancer and pain that was intolerable in spite of the treatment with oral or transdermal opioids. They found that nearly three quarters of those who had severe pain while receiving oral or transdermal opioids achieved effective analgesia with parenteral opioids.

Although parenteral administration of narcotics is most frequently used when oral medications provide inadequate analgesia, another less intensive approach to the treatment of cancer pain is the application of transdermal fentanyl. Providing a constant release of fentanyl through the skin, the transdermal patch minimizes pain and anxiety with minimal side effects (108–110). Noyes and Irving (109) studied 13 patients, aged 3–18 years, who transitioned from oral opioids to transdermal fentanyl because of bothersome side effects from oral medications. Effective pain relief was achieved in 11 of the 13 children, with minimal side effects. The main difficulties encountered included skin irritation, difficulties with patch adhesion, irritability when changing the patch, and withdrawal when stopping the fentanyl (109). Collins et al. (111) studied 11 patients, 7–18 years old, with cancer and cancer pain requiring opioid treatment. They started all patients on transdermal fentanyl and determined that this approach was well tolerated and effective in most patients.

If pain relief is still not adequate despite aggressive opiate administration, adjuvant therapy may be added (75,79) (Table 8). Adjuvants may enhance the effects of other analgesics, decrease pain symptoms, or decrease pain in specific syndromes (75,79). These agents may also decrease the depression and anxiety that are common in cancer patients (79). Commonly administered adjuvants include tricycle antidepressants, psychostimulants, corticosteroids, anticonvulsants, and neuroleptics. Although these adjuvants are not generally considered analgesics when given alone, they have been found to be helpful analgesics in specific situations. Tricyclic antidepressants improve sleep quality, and augment opiate analgesia. Psychostimulants, such as methylphenidate, counter the sedative effects of opiates (103). We tend to add methylphenidate in the setting of escalating opioid requirements in terminal patients, in order to facilitate communication and interaction between the patient and family. Corticosteroids may play a role in managing the pain related to bone, brain, or spinal cord tumors (75). It is important to administer these adjuvants at scheduled intervals, recognizing that additional doses of opiates must still be available for the management of breakthrough pain.

B. Neuropathic Pain

Neuropathic pain in pediatric cancer patients is not uncommon. Characteristics that distinguish neuropathic pain from somatic pain include a burning or electrical quality to the pain, allodynia, and paroxysms of severe, shooting pain. These features are seen in the setting of tumors with neural components, or tumors invading or compressing nerves, including neuroblastomas. One of the newest therapies for advanced stage neuroblastoma, anti-GD_2, is a monoclonal antibody that targets gangliosides on the tumor cells; it also attacks other neural tissue (112). The pain associated with the infusion of the antibody is very intense and requires high dose opiate therapy. Wallace et al. reported the continuous infusion of lidocaine in a small group of patients receiving anti-GD_2therapy. Patients received either a morphine bolus followed by a morphine infusion or a lidocaine bolus followed by a lidocaine infusion; both groups received additional morphine for breakthrough pain. The patients who received lidocaine required significantly less morphine, not only on the day of the infusion, but also on the following 3 days. In another report, Massey et al. (113) reported the use of a continuous infusion of lidocaine in a 5-year-old child with terminal retinoblastoma and pain refractory to aggressively escalating doses of morphine (113). The authors combined lidocaine with background methadone, resulting in marked symptom relief with improved alertness.

Finally, the administration of vincristine may result in a severe peripheral neuropathy, requiring high dose opiates. Adjunctive therapies, including tricyclic antidepressants or gabapentin, have been reported to be effective, although large-scale studies have not been performed in pediatric patients (75). Some of these same patients may develop a more chronic neuropathic pain syndrome. Interestingly, some of the patients who have developed neuropathic pain during vincristine therapy have been found to have other previously undiagnosed neuropathies, including Charcot–Marie-Tooth disease and hereditary neuropathy with liability to pressure palsies (114,115).

Table 8 Adjuvant Therapy for Chronic Cancer Pain

Adjuvant	Condition	Miscellaneous
Antidepressants Amitriptyline Imipramine	Neuropathic pain Depression	Consider ECG if hx of cardiac dysfunction or if patient has been treated with cardiotoxic agents
Psychostimulants Dextroamphetamine Methylphenidate	Advanced cancer	Potentiates opioid effects, no useful alone for analgesia Improves sleep quality Minimize sedative effects of potent opioids
Corticosteroids Dexamethasone	Bone pain Cerebral edema with an increased ICP Spinal cord compression	Adds analgesia related to anti-inflammatory effects Decreases tumor edema Use with caution in patients receiving NSAIDs, as combination may increase risk of GI bleeding
Anticonvulsants Carbamazepine Phenytoin Valproic acid Gabapentin	Neuropathic pain, including phantom limb pain	May affect clotting studies and liver functions Neutropenia
Radionuclides	Bone metastases	May cause thrombocytopenia and cystitis
Neuroleptics	Cancer pain associated with anxiety, nausea, vomiting, and/or restlessness	May increase level of sedation
Methotrimeprazine		

Source: Adapted from Refs. 75, 79, 100, 103.

Another form of neuropathic pain in children is phantom pain following amputation. Krane and Heller (87), as well as Wilkins et al. (116), have investigated the prevalence of both phantom sensations and phantom pain in pediatric cancer patients. Phantom sensations are nearly universal in the early postoperative period, although severe burning pain indication is less common in children. Unlike the pattern in adult amputees, there is generally resolution of the phantom pain over time. A number of treatment modalities have been described for the management of phantom pain in children, including gabapentin (117), amitriptyline (118), carbamazepine, baclofen, and ketamine (119). Regional analgesic techniques may be appropriate for severe pain refractory to other agents. Whether preoperative epidural analgesia decreases the subsequent presentation of phantom pain is not clear. Aggressive chemotherapy, early mobilization and use of a prosthetic limb, and meticulous stump care may also influence the development and severity of phantom limb pain.

C. Regional Analgesic Techniques

Some children with advanced malignancies may benefit from regional analgesic techniques like epidural or subarachnoid infusions to improve pain relief. Indications for epidural or subarachnoid infusions include excessive side effects from systemic pain medications, opioid resistance, and severe pain no longer responsive to IV opioids (105,106). Other considerations include the patient/parent's desires, effects of the tumor or treatment including coagulation status, tumor spread (especially spinal involvement), and severity of the pain and suffering. Collins et al. (105) evaluated 11 cancer patients, aged 5 months to 16 years, who received either epidural or subarachnoid infusions to manage their pain. Complications included motor and bladder dysfunction, postdural puncture headache (PDPH), respiratory depression, and infection; some patients required doses of local anesthetic that were at the upper limit of the recommended range for safety. The authors found that the regional techniques provided effective analgesia while preserving alertness and activity levels better than with opioids alone. They emphasized a role for supplemental medications for managing breakthrough pain.

Other regional analgesic techniques, including peripheral nerve injections and continuous catheter techniques, have been used for controlling cancer pain. Selection criteria for these techniques vary by institution. Factors that inform the decision to recommend a regional technique in a given patient include the location and severity of the pain, response to standard analgesics, other treatment options, risks of the proposed nerve block, life expectancy, and the skill and experience of the person performing the block (79). Regional blocks are not performed as often in pediatric cancer pain management, because the children and their parents are reluctant to accept additional potentially uncomfortable procedures and because the placement and securing of indwelling catheters in small children is more difficult than in adults. In addition, the presence of a coagulopathy is a contraindication to the placement of most peripheral nerve blocks. Heavy sedation or general anesthesia is recommended when performing regional techniques on pediatric patients (102). Regional nerve blocks that may be useful in children include celiac plexus block, peripheral nerve blocks of the extremities, intrathecal blocks, and intercostal nerve blocks.

D. Postdural Puncture Headache (PDPH)

Although the most common side effects of cancer pain treatment have already been discussed, one deserves special mention. Postdural puncture headache may occur in pediatric cancer patients following a lumbar puncture or placement of an epidural catheter. Even though the incidence of PDPH is inversely related to age in the adult literature, that finding cannot be extended into the pediatric age group. Until recently, there were very few reports of PDPH in children (99). Bolder (99) studied 26 children with the diagnosis of cancer aged 3–17 years old, requiring a lumbar puncture. Postdural puncture headaches occurred more commonly in children over 13 years old and were normally mild, lasting <48 hr. The author (N.L.G.) treated one preschool boy who developed a severe PDPH following lumbar puncture with a 22-G spinal needle with a Quincke tip. He required an epidural blood patch for management of his headache after failing conservative therapy, but the boy has had no subsequent headaches since his lumbar punctures have been performed using a 22-G pencil-point Whitacre needle. Similarly, we managed a young adult who had several debilitating postdural headaches after lumbar puncture performed with a 20-G spinal needle. The young adult responded to an epidural blood patch and has had no recurrences with use of the Whitacre needle. Needle size, tip shape, and bevel orientation are recognized factors contributing to the incidence of PDPH, but relatively large spinal needles are necessary in cancer patients in order to obtain sufficient CSF sample volume, and to facilitate the injection of chemotherapeutic agents. Number of attempts, operator skill, and level of sedation may also affect the incidence PDPH in young children.

X. CONCLUSION

Survival rates from childhood cancer have improved over the last two decades with advances in aggressive and targeted therapy; improvements in supportive care have also contributed to this success. Throughout the perioperative period, conscientious care requires a thorough understanding of the presentation, physiologic effects, and complications of the various cancers and their treatments. Similarly, a sophisticated approach to the prevention and management of pain incorporates multiple modalities to minimize the stress and suffering of young patients and their families.

REFERENCES

1. Smith MA, Ries LAG. Childhood cancer: incidence, survival, and mortality. In: Pizzo PA, Poplack DG, eds. Principles and Practice of Pediatric Oncology. Philadelphia: Lippincott Williams and Wilkins, 2002:1–12.
2. Stiller C. Epidemiology of cancer in adolescents. Med Pediatr Oncol 2002; 39:149–155.
3. Miller RW, Young JL Jr, Novakovic B. Childhood cancer. Cancer 1995; 75:395–405.
4. Smith MA, Gurney JG, Ries LAG. Cancer among adolescents 15–19 years old. In: Ries LAG, Smith MA, Gurney JG, et al., eds. Cancer Incidence and Survival among Children and Adolescents: United States SEER Program 1975–1995. Bethesda: National Cancer Institute, 1999:157–164.
5. Hasle H, Clemmensen IH, Mikkelsen M. Risks of leukaemia and solid tumours in individuals with Down's syndrome. Lancet 2000; 355:165–169.
6. Hasle H. Pattern of malignant disorders in individuals with Down's syndrome. Lancet Oncol 2001; 2: 429–436.
7. Grufferman S, Barton JW III, Eby NL. Increased sex concordance of sibling pairs with Behcet's disease, Hodgkin's disease, multiple sclerosis, and sarcoidosis. Am J Epidemiol 1987; 126:365–369.
8. Mack TM, Cozen W, Shibata DK, et al. Concordance for Hodgkin's disease in identical twins suggesting genetic susceptibility to the young–adult form of the disease. N Engl J Med 1995; 332:413–418.
9. Ron E, Lubin JH, Shore RE, et al. Thyroid cancer after exposure to external radiation: a pooled analysis of seven studies. Radiat Res 1995; 141:259–277.
10. Armstrong BK, Kricker A. How much melanoma is caused by sun exposure? Melanoma Res 1993; 3: 395–401.
11. Stiller C. Epidemiology of childhood cancer. Arch Dis Child 1999; 81:283E.
12. MacKenzie JR. Complications of treatment of paediatric malignancies. Eur J Radiol 2001; 37:109–119.
13. Chung F. Cancer, chemotherapy and anaesthesia. Can Anaesth Soc J 1982; 29:364–371.
14. Green DM. Effects of treatment for childhood cancer on vital organ systems. Cancer 1993; 71:3299–3305.
15. McClay EF, Bellet RE. Preoperative evaluation of the oncology patient. Med Clin North Am 1987; 71: 529–540.

16. Dearth J, Osborn R, Wilson E, et al. Anthracycline-induced cardiomyopathy in children: a report of six cases. Med Pediatr Oncol 1984; 12:54–58.
17. Ali MK, Ewer MS, Gibbs HR, et al. Late doxorubicin-associated cardiotoxicity in children. The possible role of intercurrent viral infection. Cancer 1994; 74: 182–188.
18. Manzullo EF, Weed HG. Perioperative issues in patients with cancer. Med Clin North Am 2003; 87:243–256.
19. Lipshultz SE, Colan SD, Gelber RD, et al. Late cardiac effects of doxorubicin therapy for acute lymphoblastic leukemia in childhood. N Engl J Med 1991; 324:808–815.
20. Adams MJ, Hardenbergh PH, Constine LS, Lipshultz SE. Radiation-associated cardiovascular disease. Crit Rev Oncol Hematol 2003; 45:55–75.
21. Carmel RJ, Kaplan HS. Mantle irradiation in Hodgkin's disease. An analysis of technique, tumor eradication, and complications. Cancer 1976; 37:2813–2825.
22. Klein DS, Wilds PR. Pulmonary toxicity of antineoplastic agents: anaesthetic and postoperative implications. Can Anaesth Soc J 1983; 30:399–405.
23. Eigen H, Wyszomierski D. Bleomycin lung injury in children. Pathophysiology and guidelines for management. Am J Pediatr Hematol Oncol 1985; 7:71–78.
24. Kaplan E, Sklar C, Wilmott R, et al. Pulmonary function in children treated for rhabdomyosarcoma. Med Pediatr Oncol 1996; 27:79–84.
25. Nash RA, Pepe MS, Storb R, et al. Acute graft-versus-host disease: analysis of risk factors after allogeneic marrow transplantation and prophylaxis with cyclosporine and methotrexate. Blood 1992; 80:1838–1845.
26. Goldiner PL, Schweizer O. The hazards of anesthesia and surgery in bleomycin-treated patients. Semin Oncol 1979; 6:121–124.
27. Goldiner PL, Carlon GC, Cvitkovic E, et al. Factors influencing postoperative morbidity and mortality in patients treated with bleomycin. Br Med J 1978; 1:1664–1667.
28. Cohen LE. Endocrine late effects of cancer treatment. Curr Opin Pediatr 2003; 15:3–9.
29. Diamond FB Jr, Bercu BB. Endocrine sequelae of cancer therapy in childhood. J Endocrinol Invest 2001; 24:648–658.
30. Sklar CA. Childhood brain tumors. J Pediatr Endocrinol Metab 2002; 15(suppl 2):669–673.
31. Sklar CA. Endocrine complications of the successful treatment of neoplastic disease in childhood. Growth Genet Horm 2001; 17:37–42.
32. Shalet SM. Radiation and pituitary dysfunction. N Engl J Med 1993; 328:131–133.
33. Gleeson HK, Shalet SM. Endocrine complications of neoplastic diseases in children and adolescents. Curr Opin Ped 2001; 13:346–351.
34. Maxwell LG, Zuckerberg AL, Motoyama EK, et al. Systemic disorders in pediatric anesthesia. In: Motoyama EK, Davis PJ, eds. Smith's Anesthesia for Infants and Children. St. Louis: Mosby, 2003: 827–874.
35. Dillman JB. Safe use of succinylcholine during repeated anesthetics in a patient treated with cyclophosphamide. Anesth Analg 1987; 66:351–353.
36. Mihalo RM, Cagle CK, Cronau LH Jr, Sassoon PM. Preanesthetic evaluation of the cancer patient. Int Anesthesiol Clin 1998; 36:1–8.
37. Sullivan KM, Agura E, Anasetti C, et al. Chronic graft-versus-host disease and other late complications of bone marrow transplantation. Semin Hematol 1991; 28:250–259.
38. Moskowitz MD, Parker RB. Complications of cancer therapy. Miller JH, White L, eds. Imaging in Paediatric Oncology. Baltimore: Williams and Wilkins, 1985:472–499.
39. Wiela-Hojenska A, Gorczynska E, Orzechowska-Juzwenko K, et al. Metabolic functions of the liver during chemotherapy in children with acute lymphoblastic leukemia. Int J Clin Pharmacol Ther 2001; 39:246–250.
40. Ruggiero A, Riccardi R. Interventions for anemia in pediatric cancer patients. Med Pediatr Oncol 2002; 39:451–454.
41. Miller CB. The use of erythropoietin in cancer patients. Hem/Onc Annals 1994; 2:288–296.
42. Porter JC, Leahey A, Polise K, et al. Recombinant human erythropoietin reduces the need for erythrocyte and platelet transfusions in pediatric patients with sarcoma: a randomized, double-blind, placebo-controlled trial. J Pediatr 1996; 129:656–660.
43. MacMillan ML, Freedman MH. Recombinant human erythropoietin in children with cancer. J Pediatr Hematol Oncol 1998; 20:187–189.
44. Arai S, Vogelsang GB. Management of graft-versus-host disease. Blood Rev 2000; 14:190–204.
45. Weisdorf D, Hakke R, Blazar B, et al. Risk factors for acute graft-versus-host disease in histocompatible donor bone marrow transplantation. Transplantation 1991; 51:1197–1203.
46. Narod SA, Stiller C, Lenoir GM. An estimate of the heritable fraction of childhood cancer. Br J Cancer 1991; 63:993–999.
47. Ravindranath Y, Abella E, Krischer JP, et al. Acute myeloid leukemia (AML) in Down's syndrome is highly responsive to chemotherapy: experience on Pediatric Oncology Group AML Study 8498. Blood 1992; 80:2210–2214.
48. Doll R, Peto R. The causes of cancer: quantitative estimates of avoidable risks of cancer in the United States today. J Natl Cancer Inst 1981; 66:1191–1308.
49. Hall SC, Stevenson GW. Anesthetic considerations in the pediatric cancer patient. Semin Surg Oncol 1990; 6:148–155.
50. McDowall RH. Anesthesia considerations for pediatric cancer. Semin Surg Oncol 1993; 9:478–488.

51. Lefor AT. Perioperative management of the patient with cancer. Chest 1999; 115:165S–171S.
52. Davis PJ, Hall S, Deshpande JK, Spear RM. Anesthesia for general, urologic, and plastic surgery. In: Motoyama EK, Davis PJ, eds. Smith's Anesthesia for Infants and Children. St. Louis: Mosby, 1996:571–604.
53. Ferrari LR, Bedford RF. General anesthesia prior to treatment of anterior mediastinal masses in pediatric cancer patients. Anesthesiology 1990; 72:991–995.
54. Mulhern RK, Wasserman AL, Friedman AG, Fairclough D. Social competence and behavioral adjustment of children who are long-term survivors of cancer. Pediatrics 1989; 83:18–25.
55. Kain ZN, Mayes LC, Wang SM, Hofstadter MB. Postoperative behavioral outcomes in children: effects of sedative premedication. Anesthesiology 1999; 90: 758–765.
56. Kain ZN, Wang SM, Mayes LC, et al. Distress during the induction of anesthesia and postoperative behavioral outcomes. Anesth Analg 1999; 88:1042–1047.
57. Karl HW, Rosenberger JL, Larach MG, Ruffle JM. Transmucosal administration of midazolam for premedication of pediatric patients. Comparison of the nasal and sublingual routes. Anesthesiology 1993; 78:885–891.
58. Kogan A, Katz J, Efrat R, Eidelman LA. Premedication with midazolam in young children: a comparison of four routes of administration. Paediatr Anaesth 2002; 12:685–689.
59. Diaz JH. Intranasal ketamine preinduction of paediatric outpatients. Paediatr Anaesth 1997; 7:273–278.
60. Geldner G, Hubmann M, Knoll R, Jacobi K. Comparison between three transmucosal routes of administration of midazolam in children. Paediatr Anaesth 1997; 7:103–109.
61. Zedie N, Amory DW, Wagner BK, O'Hara DA. Comparison of intranasal midazolam and sufentanil premedication in pediatric outpatients. Clin Pharmacol Ther 1996; 59:341–348.
62. Weksler N, Ovadia L, Muati G, Stav A. Nasal ketamine for paediatric premedication. Can J Anaesth 1993; 40:119–121.
63. Streisand JB, Stanley TH, Hague B, et al. Oral transmucosal fentanyl citrate premedication in children. Anesth Analg 1989; 69:28–34.
64. Feld LH, Negus JB, White PF. Oral midazolam preanesthetic medication in pediatric outpatients. Anesthesiology 1990; 73:831–834.
65. Kain ZN, Mayes LC, Wang SM, et al. Parental presence during induction of anesthesia versus sedative premedication: which intervention is more effective? Anesthesiology 1998; 89:1147–1156.
66. Kain ZN, Caldwell-Andrews AA, Wang SM, et al. Parental intervention choices for children undergoing repeated surgeries. Anesth Analg 2003; 96:970–975.
67. Krane EJ, Davis PJ, Smith RM. Preoperative preparation. In: Motoyama EK, Davis PJ, eds. Smith's Anesthesia for Infants and Children. St. Louis: Mosby, 1996:213–228.
68. Bissonnette B, Davis PJ. Thermal regulation—physiology and perioperative management in infants and children. In: Motoyama EK, Davis PJ, eds. Smith's Anesthesia for Infants and Children. St. Louis: Mosby, 1996:139–158.
69. Sessler DI. Temperature regulation. In: Gregory GA, ed. Pediatric Anesthesia. New York: Churchill Livingstone, 1994:47–82.
70. Dabbagh S, Ellis D, Gruskin AB. Regulation of fluids and electrolytes in infants and children. In: Motoyama EK, Davis PJ, eds. Smith's Anesthesia for Infants and Children. St. Louis: Mosby, 1996:105–138.
71. Torres NE. Calcium. In: Faust RJ, Cucchiara RF, Rose SH, Spackman TN, Wedel DJ, Wass CT, eds. Anesthesiology Review. Philadelphia: Churchill Livingstone, 2002:34–36.
72. Rheingold SR, Lange BJ. Oncologic emergencies. In: Pizzo PA, Poplack DG, eds. Principles and Practice of Pediatric Oncology. Philadelphia: Lippincott Williams & Wilkins, 2002:1177–1204.
73. Aldrete JA. Modifications to the postanesthesia score for use in ambulatory surgery. J Perianesth Nurs 1998; 13:148–155.
74. Berde CB, Billett AL, Collins JJ. Symptom management in supportive care. In: Pizzo PA, Poplack DG, eds. Principles and Practice of Pediatric Oncology. Philadelphia: Lippincott Williams & Wilkins, 1997:1301–1332.
75. Collins JJ, Weisman SJ. Management of pain in childhood cancer. In: Schechter NL, Berde CB, Yaster M, eds. Pain in Infants, Children, and Adolescents. Philadelphia: Lippincott Williams & Wilkins, 2003:517–533.
76. Tobias JD, Oakes L, Rao B. Continuous epidural anesthesia for postoperative analgesia in the pediatric oncology patient. Am J Pediatr Hematol Oncol 1992; 14:216–221.
77. Dalens B, Tanguy A, Haberer JP. Lumbar epidural anesthesia for operative and postoperative pain relief in infants and young children. Anesth Analg 1986; 65:1069–1073.
78. Tyler DC. Respiratory effects of pain in a child after thoracotomy. Anesthesiology 1989; 70:873–874.
79. Ashburn MA, Lipman AG. Management of pain in the cancer patient. Anesth Analg 1993; 76:402–416.
80. Carns PE. Neuraxial opioids. In: Faust RJ, Cucchiara RF, Rose SH, Spackman TN, Wedel DJ, Wass CT, eds. Anesthesiology Review. Philadelphia: Churchill Livingstone, 2002:267–268.
81. Rice LJ. Regional anestheia and analgesia. In: Motoyama EK, Davis PJ, eds. Smith's Anesthesia for Infants and Children. St. Louis: Mosby, 1996: 403–444.
82. Vietti TJ, Steuber CP. Clinical assessment and differential diagnosis of the child with suspected cancer. In: Pizzo PA, Poplack DG, eds. Principles and Practice

of Pediatric Oncology. Philadelphia: Lippincott Williams & Wilkins, 2002:149–159.
83. Steven JM, Cohen DE, Sclabassi RJ. Anesthesia equipment and monitoring. In: Motoyama EK, Davis PJ, eds. Smith's Anesthesia for Infants and Children. St. Louis: Mosby, 1996:229–280.
84. Stone DJ, Gal TJ. Airway management. In: Miller RD, ed. Anesthesia. Philadelphia: Churchill Livingstone, 2000:1414–1451.
85. Collins JJ, Berde BB. Management of cancer pain in children. In: Pizzo PA, Poplack DG, eds. Principles and Practice of Pediatric Oncology. Philadelphia: Lippincott-Raven, 1997:1183–1199.
86. Trueworthy RC, Templeton KJ. Malignant bone tumors presenting as musculoskeletal pain. Pediatr Ann 2002; 31:355–359.
87. Krane EJ, Heller LB. The prevalence of phantom sensation and pain in pediatric amputees. J Pain Symptom Manage 1995; 10:21–29.
88. Zuckerberg AL, Yaster M. Anesthesia for orthopedic surgery. In: Motoyama EK, Davis PJ, eds. Smith's Anesthesia for Infants and Children. St. Louis: Mosby, 1996:605–632.
89. Strother DR, Pollack IF, Fisher PG, et al. Tumors of the central nervous system. In: Pizzo PA, Poplack DG, eds. Principles and Practice of Pediatric Oncology. Philadelphia: Lippincott Williams & Wilkins, 2002: 751–824.
90. Krane EJ, Domino KB. Anesthesia for neurosurgery. In: Motoyama EK, Davis PJ, eds. Smith's Anesthesia for Infants and Children. St. Louis: Mosby, 1996:541–570.
91. Zeltzer LK, Altman A, Cohen D, et al. American Academy of Pediatrics Report of the Subcommittee on the Management of Pain Associated with Procedures in Children with Cancer. Pediatrics 1990; 86:826–831.
92. Ljungman G, Gordh T, Sorensen S, Kreuger A. Lumbar puncture in pediatric oncology: conscious sedation vs. general anesthesia. Med Pediatr Oncol 2001; 36:372–379.
93. Fortney JT, Halperin EC, Hertz CM, Schulman SR. Anesthesia for pediatric external beam radiation therapy. Int J Radiat Oncol Biol Phys 1999; 44:587–591.
94. Jayabose S, Levendoglu-Tugal O, Giamelli J, et al. Intravenous anesthesia with propofol for painful procedures in children with cancer. J Pediatr Hematol Oncol 2001; 23:290–293.
95. Santos KG, Fallat ME. Surgical and anesthetic decisions for children with terminal illness. Semin Pediatr Surg 2001; 10:237–242.
96. McGraw KS. Should do-not-resuscitate orders be suspended during surgical procedures? AORN J 1998; 67:794–796, 799.
97. Goldberg S. Do-not-resuscitate orders in the OR—suspend or enforce? AORN J 2002; 76:296–299.
98. Babul N, Darke AC. Evaluation and use of opioid analgesics in pediatric cancer pain. J Palliat Care 1993; 9:19–25.
99. Bolder PM. Postlumbar puncture headache in pediatric oncology patients. Anesthesiology 1986; 65: 696–698.
100. Miser AW, Miser JS. The treatment of cancer pain in children. Pediatr Clin North Am 1989; 36:979–999.
101. Miser AW, Dothage JA, Wesley RA, Miser JS. The prevalence of pain in a pediatric and young adult cancer population. Pain 1987; 29:73–83.
102. Berde C, Ablin A, Glazer J, et al. American Academy of Pediatrics Report of the Subcommittee on Disease-Related Pain in Childhood Cancer. Pediatrics 1990; 86:818–825.
103. Berde CB, Sethna NF. Analgesics for the treatment of pain in children. N Engl J Med 2002; 347:1094–1103.
104. Enting RH, Oldenmenger WH, van der Rijt CC, et al. A prospective study evaluating the response of patients with unrelieved cancer pain to parenteral opioids. Cancer 2002; 94:3049–3056.
105. Collins JJ, Grier HE, Sethna NF, et al. Regional anesthesia for pain associated with terminal pediatric malignancy. Pain 1996; 65:63–69.
106. Smitt PS, Tsafka A, Teng-van de Zande F, et al. Outcome and complications of epidural analgesia in patients with chronic cancer pain. Cancer 1998; 83: 2015–2022.
107. Schug SA, Zech D, Dorr U. Cancer pain management according to WHO analgesic guidelines. J Pain Symptom Manage 1990; 5:27–32.
108. Hunt A, Goldman A, Devine T, Phillips M. Transdermal fentanyl for pain relief in a paediatric palliative care population. Palliat Med 2001; 15:405–412.
109. Noyes M, Irving H. The use of transdermal fentanyl in pediatric oncology palliative care. Am J Hosp Palliat Care 2001; 18:411–416.
110. Miser AW, Narang PK, Dothage JA, et al. Transdermal fentanyl for pain control in patients with cancer. Pain 1989; 37:15–21.
111. Collins JJ, Dunkel IJ, Gupta SK, et al. Transdermal fentanyl in children with cancer pain: feasibility, tolerability, and pharmacokinetic correlates. J Pediatr 1999; 134:319–323.
112. Wallace MS, Lee J, Sorkin L, et al. Intravenous lidocaine: effects on controlling pain after anti-GD2 antibody therapy in children with neuroblastoma—a report of a series. Anesth Analg 1997; 85:794–796.
113. Massey GV, Pedigo S, Dunn NL, et al. Continuous lidocaine infusion for the relief of refractory malignant pain in a terminally ill pediatric cancer patient. J Pediatr Hematol Oncol 2002; 24:566–568.
114. Chauvenet AR, Shashi V, Selsky C, et al. Vincristine-induced neuropathy as the initial presentation of charcot-marie-tooth disease in acute lymphoblastic leukemia: a Pediatric Oncology Group study. J Pediatr Hematol Oncol 2003; 25:316–320.
115. Kalfakis N, Panas M, Karadima G, et al. Hereditary neuropathy with liability to pressure palsies emerging during vincristine treatment. Neurology 2002; 59:1470–1471.

116. Wilkins KL, McGrath PJ, Finley GA, Katz J. Phantom limb sensations and phantom limb pain in child and adolescent amputees. Pain 1998; 78:7–12.
117. Rusy LM, Troshynski TJ, Weisman SJ. Gabapentin in phantom limb pain management in children and young adults: report of seven cases. J Pain Symptom Manage 2001; 21:78–82.
118. Rogers AG. Use of amitriptyline (Elavil) for phantom limb pain in younger children. J Pain Symptom Manage 1989; 4:96.
119. Dangel T. Chronic pain management in children. Part I: cancer and phantom pain. Paediatr Anaesth 1998; 8:5–10.
120. Balis FM, Holcenberg JS, Blaney SM. General principles of chemotherapy. In: Pizzo PA, Poplack DG, eds. Principles and Practice of Pediatric Oncology. Philadelphia: Lippincott Williams & Wilkins, 2002: 237–308.
121. Stoelting RK, Dierdorf SF. Cancer. In: Stoelting RK, Dierdorf SF, eds. Anesthesia and Co-existing Disease. Philadelphia: Churchill Livingstone, 1993:485–500.
122. van Vlymen JM, White PF. Outpatient anesthesia. In: Miller CB, ed. Anesthesia. Philadelphia: Churchill Livingstone, 2000:2213–2240.
123. Siker D. Pediatric fluids, electrolytes, and nutrition. In: Gregory GA, ed. Pediatric Anesthesia. New York: Churchill Livingstone, 1994:83–118.

51

Perioperative Care of Children with Cancer: Intensive Care Perspectives

H. MICHAEL USHAY

Division of Pediatric Critical Care Medicine, Weill Medical College of Cornell University and Laura Rosenberg Pediatric Observation Unit, Memorial Sloan-Kettering Cancer Center, New York, New York, U.S.A.

BRUCE M. GREENWALD

Division of Pediatric Critical Care Medicine, Weill Medical College of Cornell University, New York, New York, U.S.A.

I. INTRODUCTION

Advances in pediatric surgical oncology have increased the complexity of perioperative management. Modern intensive care has helped facilitate many of these advances. Intensive care may be delivered in the post-anesthesia care unit (PACU), the pediatric intensive care unit (PICU) or the transitional care unit (TCU), extending the ability to perform careful monitoring and quick intervention from the operating room (OR) into the patient's recovery phase. Research has consistently shown that pediatric oncology patients, including recipients of hematopoietic cell transplants (HCT), benefit from intensive care for medical and surgical reasons (1–4).

The perioperative PICU population with oncologic illness is diverse. Patients range from a child recovering from an extensive thoracoabdominal neuroblastoma resection to an adolescent with severe mucositis recovering from HCT with airway obstruction after a relatively minor operative procedure. Children are admitted to the PICU at the time of diagnosis of central nervous system (CNS) tumors and return for care after surgical resection.

The intensive care needs of the perioperative pediatric oncology patient encompass all of pediatric critical care medicine. In this chapter, the effort has been made to correlate the practical knowledge obtained from an extensive practice of postoperative intensive care of pediatric oncology patients with research-based guidelines. Evidence-based clinical practice guidelines are starting to appear in the pediatric critical care medicine literature, but do not exist for most clinical scenarios involving perioperative care of the child with cancer.

II. GENERAL PRINCIPLES OF PERIOPERATIVE CARE

A. Who Comes to the ICU? What Level of Care Is Required?

One of the first decisions to be made in the care of the perioperative patient is an assignment of the location for delivery of care (5,6). The surgeon, anesthesiologist, and intensivist should decide collaboratively, sometimes within the framework of written guidelines, the level of care required and the site where it should be delivered. The choices of location may include the PACU, a transitional care (step up/step down) unit (TCU) or the PICU. Efforts have been made to create statistical models that might predict the need for postoperative intensive care in pediatric surgery patients (7,8). An example of guidelines used in our institution for deciding whether to care for postoperative patients in a transitional care unit or transfer them to the PICU is found in Table 1. The Society of Critical Care Medicine (SCCM) continues to refine guidelines for the level of care to be provided and the patient population to be served in PICUs and intermediate care units (9).

B. PACU vs. PICU

The PACU of a children's hospital may be appropriately child centered, but the PACUs of most general hospitals are not oriented to the care of a child. When reasonable, a pediatric patient should not be kept in a PACU longer than is necessary. This recommendation is based upon the premise that optimal care of children is best provided in a unit that is dedicated specifically to the care of children. If postoperative PICU care is anticipated, it may be best to move the patient directly from the operating room to the PICU. In that way, the PICU provides both postoperative stabilization and longitudinal care. Alternatively, a surgeon may want to observe a particular patient closely for an event that might require emergent return to the OR; and that patient may benefit from remaining in the PACU prior to transfer to the PICU.

C. Preoperative Assessment

Postoperative intensive care begins with a careful review of the patient's preoperative history. Much of the extensive resective oncologic surgery that leads to postoperative PICU admission is performed during the course, or following the completion, of multiple rounds of combination chemotherapy. Previous chemotherapy, radiation, and surgical therapies, responses to therapy, as well as the cumulative toxicities of therapy need to be considered as the patient's postoperative course progresses. Therapy-related injuries to the heart, lungs,

Table 1 Criteria Used in One Institution for Deciding which Postoperative Patients Are Cared for in the TCU vs. the PICU

Admission criteria for TCU	Criteria for immediate or subsequent transfer to the PICU	Criteria for transfer to inpatient unit
All surgery: Children >1 year of age who are recovering from major abdominal or thoracic surgery deemed at risk for:	1. Patients with a requirement for extended mechanical support or ventilation	1. Stable airway
(a) Airway compromise, pneumothorax or acute respiratory deterioration	2. Patients whose cardiovascular condition is not improving as anticipated	2. Stable status after a minimum of 12 hr observation with epidural catheters
(b) Major shifts in fluids from intravascular to extravascular compartments or vice versa	3. Patients requiring a pulmonary artery catheter	3. Pain and fluid management within normal guidelines
(c) Acute blood loss		
Neurosurgery: Children >1 year of age who are recovering from neurosurgical procedures to debulk or remove supra- and infratentorial tumors.	1. 1, 2, 3 above as per guidelines for other postoperative cases	4. Stable neurologic exam in neurosurgical patients
Children recovering from spinal surgery designed for tumor removal or insertion of catheters for pain control exhibiting potential for hemodynamic instability	2. Patients exhibiting deterioration in neurological status, which is not an anticipated part of normal postoperative course	5. No externalized CSF drains

kidneys, liver, GI tract, and hematopoietic systems may have an impact on the postoperative course. Preoperative assessments of cardiac, pulmonary, renal, and hematopoietic function will permit the team caring for the patient postoperatively to anticipate challenges that may be present in the postoperative period (10,11).

D. Perioperative Monitoring in Children

Critically ill children benefit from a range of invasive and noninvasive monitoring techniques (12,13). Careful interpretation of data obtained from physiologic monitoring permits caregivers to anticipate clinical deterioration and intercede proactively. All pediatric intensive care unit patients require, at a minimum, continuous cardiorespiratory monitoring and pulse oximetry. In the perioperative population, people-intensive monitoring such as frequent assessment of neurologic status in a postoperative neurosurgery patient or noting changes in distal perfusion in a patient who has undergone limb salvage surgery are as important to the respective patients as technology-intensive modalities like invasive hemodynamic monitoring.

E. Noninvasive Monitoring Modalities

1. Pulse Oximetry

Continuous pulse oximetry is a standard of care in PICUs and oxygen saturation is included in the vital signs. New-generation pulse oximeters permit uninterrupted and accurate monitoring of oxygen saturation in the face of patient movement and compromised perfusion. In the perioperative patient, pulse oximetry facilitates weaning of supplemental oxygen and indicates the efficacy of pulmonary toilet in preventing and treating postoperative atelectasis. The accuracy of pulse oximetry as a measurement of the hemoglobin oxygen saturation is limited in certain clinical situations; e.g., by jaundice, which is common in oncology patients.

2. Capnography

End tidal CO_2 ($ETCO_2$) monitoring (capnography) is a useful adjunct in caring for the pediatric patient (14). Low dead space in-line monitors as well as side stream monitors that require small volumes of aspirated gas have increased the utility of capnography in the PICU. The implementation of nasal cannulae with side stream $ETCO_2$ technology has added to the intensivist's ability to monitor the extubated patient (15,16). Capnography is recommended for confirming tube placement in emergency and elective endotracheal intubations.

Increases in pulmonary dead space and the presence of ventilation perfusion mismatch limit the accuracy of $ETCO_2$ monitoring in patients with parenchymal lung disease. However, capnography can be very useful in the typical perioperative patient who does not have severe parenchymal lung disease. Comparing the capnographic CO_2 level with a measured arterial $PaCO_2$ determines the accuracy of the $ETCO_2$. Following trends in $ETCO_2$ permits intermediate steps in weaning mechanical ventilation without the need for an arterial blood gas with every ventilator change (17,18). Side stream capnography is also useful in monitoring patients undergoing procedural sedation (19).

3. Echocardiography

M-mode and 2D echocardiography are employed in the PICU for assessment of children with myocardial dysfunction. Echocardiography is particularly useful in the evaluation of chamber size and contractility in critically ill children who have received cardiotoxic therapy (20). Transesophageal Doppler cardiography has demonstrated some utility in following cardiac output and response to volume resuscitation in critically ill children (21,22).

F. Invasive Monitoring Modalities

Invasive monitoring of the cardiovascular, respiratory, and neurologic systems is a key component of pediatric critical care medicine (23,24).

1. Arterial Catheterization

Insertion of an arterial catheter is indicated in patients who require continuous blood pressure monitoring or repeated arterial blood gas analyses. Arterial catheters may be placed in the radial, dorsalis pedis, posterior tibial, femoral, and axillary arteries. The use of the axillary artery for indwelling catheterization is safe and efficacious in infants and children in whom other sites are not available (25). In infants and small children (weight less than 20 kg), 22 gauge catheters are appropriate for all sites. In larger children, 20 gauge catheters may be employed. The radial and pedal arteries can usually be catheterized using a catheter-over-needle method. The Seldinger technique is generally employed for femoral and axillary arterial insertions. Table 2 provides information regarding appropriate catheter, needle, and wire sizes for children.

2. Central Venous Catheterization

Central venous access in the form of tunneled silastic catheters and port-type devices is very common in pediatric oncology. These devices may be used for obtaining central venous pressure measurements as well

Table 2 Equipment for Arterial and Central Venous Catheterization in Infants and Children[a]

Site	Weight (kg)	Entry needle (gauge)	Guide wire diameter (in.)	Catheter size
Arterial				
Radial, pedal	3–20	21 or 22	0.018	22 gauge
	20–30	21 or 22	0.018	22 gauge
	> 30	20	0.025	20 gauge
Femoral, axillary	3–20	21 or 22	0.018	22 gauge
	20–30	20	0.025	20 gauge
	> 30	20	0.025	20 gauge
Central venous				
Double lumen: Internal jugular, Subclavian, Axillary	3–30	21 or 22	0.018	4 or 5 Fr 5–15 cm
Femoral	3–30	21 or 22	0.018	4 or 5 Fr 15–30 cm
Triple lumen: Internal jugular, Subclavian	3–30	20	0.025	5 Fr, 5–15 cm
Axillary	> 30	18	0.035	7 Fr, 15 cm
Femoral	3–30	20	0.025	5 Fr, 15–30 cm
	> 30	18	0.035	7 Fr, 30–45 cm

0.018 in = 0.46 mm; 0.025 in = 0.64 mm; 0.035 in = 0.89 mm.
[a] These values are representative. Needle, wire, and catheter sizes may vary with the manufacturer.

as their primary purpose of secure venous access for blood drawing and infusion of vesicant medications (26).

Percutaneous central venous catheterization and monitoring is indicated for the management of patients with shock states associated with abnormalities of central venous pressure. Central access is also indicated for infusion of hypertonic solutions, pressor amines, or calcium salts. Sites of insertion include the femoral, internal jugular, subclavian, and axillary veins. Central venous access as well as monitoring capability can also be obtained through the use of peripherally inserted central catheters (PICC) (27). The risk of vascular injury is minimized by the use of the Seldinger technique. When performed by experienced physicians, both the internal jugular and subclavian veins can be safely cannulated, even in infants (28). Subclavian catheterization should be approached cautiously in patients with thrombocytopenia or a coagulation disorder. Despite the possibility of significant complications, subclavian catheters have the advantage of being more comfortable than internal jugular and femoral catheters in patients who are able to move around. Appropriate sizes and lengths for catheters, needles, and guide wires are provided in Table 2. Evidence-based guidelines on the insertion and management of central venous catheters in children and adults have been published by the Centers for Disease Control (CDC) (29–32).

3. *Pulmonary Artery Catheterization*

Pulmonary artery (PA) thermodilution catheters are used much less frequently in the present era of critical care medicine as compared to the past. The effectiveness of PA catheter use in adults has been questioned and a lack of consistent interpretation of pulmonary artery catheter derived data has been demonstrated among adult ICU physicians (33,34). However, in a pediatric oncology patient with severely compromised cardiac function complicating hypoxemic respiratory failure, a pulmonary artery catheter can provide valuable information and aid in management. A meta-analysis of published articles in which pulmonary artery catheters were used in pediatric patients suggested that substantial valuable information was derived from the use of PA catheters (35). Education programs detailing indications, techniques for safe placement, and data interpretation are available (36). General indications for placement of a flow-directed pulmonary artery catheter include shock states that are refractory to intravascular volume expansion and infusion of moderate dosages of dopamine, epinephrine, or norepinephrine (37). Application of high levels of end expiratory pressure (more than 15 cm H_2O) creates difficulty evaluating the adequacy of left ventricular filling clinically or by measurement of CVP. Under such conditions, measurement of pulmonary artery wedge pressure (PAWP) and cardiac output with a PA catheter may be of value. Perioperative states that are likely to meet the indications for PA catheter placement include septic shock complicated by chemotherapy or sepsis-induced myocardial failure, acute respiratory distress syndrome requiring high levels of positive end-expiratory pressure (PEEP), and other causes of distributive and cardiogenic shock. Use of norepinephrine to treat distributive shock, and epinephrine to treat cardiogenic shock can be guided by measurement of cardiac output and systemic vascular resistance. Data support the use of the pulmonary artery catheter to guide goal-directed therapy in fluid refractory septic shock (38).

A 5-French, 75 cm catheter (15 cm proximal port) is used for children weighing less than 30 kg; 7 or 7.5 French, 110 cm (30 cm proximal port) is used in larger children. Children as small as 5–7 kg have been catheterized at the bedside; visual guidance with 2-D echocardiography or fluoroscopy may shorten procedure time, but is not absolutely necessary.

Complications of pulmonary artery catheterization in children include vascular injury at the site of insertion, pneumothorax, dysrhythmia, pulmonary infarction, pulmonary artery rupture, catheter knotting within the heart, and infection (39,40). In addition, inflation of the balloon may compromise pulmonary blood flow when PA catheters are employed in small infants.

III. SYSTEM-SPECIFIC ISSUES IN THE CARE OF THE PERIOPERATIVE PEDIATRIC ONCOLOGY PATIENT IN THE PICU

Although each tumor and specific operation results in a particular set of perioperative issues, extensive replication would occur if each were discussed separately. For this reason, general principles of perioperative intensive care are discussed in the following sections. In our institution, the thoracoabdominal resection (TAR) of neuroblastoma is the operation and tumor that presents the greatest perioperative challenge and serves as the basis for many of the recommendations found in this chapter.

A. Airway and Respiratory Support

1. Introduction

Airway and respiratory issues are among the most frequent indications for admission of the perioperative patient to the PICU. Airway and respiratory crises can be sudden, life threatening and the appropriate intervention lifesaving. Continual practice, education, and reinforcement of airway management skills are necessary to maintain a successful perioperative environment.

2. Upper Airway Obstruction

The pediatric oncology patient is subject to many of the same congenital and infectious causes of upper airway obstruction as the nononcology patient. To these are added etiologies of upper airway obstruction germane to the oncology patient such as severe mucositis of the oropharynx, pharyngeal masses adjacent to or involving the airway, edema following extensive head and neck tumor resections, superior vena cava syndrome, scarring of airway tissues from radiation therapy, and postextubation stridor.

Airways partially obstructed by masses, severe mucositis, or edema can be supported, to an extent, by positioning, racemic epinephrine, steroids, and helium: oxygen (heliox) mixtures. The vasoconstricting action of racemic epinephrine temporarily shrinks swollen soft tissues in the upper airway. Although evidence-based data are lacking, dexamethasone is considered part of the pharmacologic management of airway edema and has a prophylactic role in the prevention of postextubation stridor (41). In severe mucositis, diligent attention is paid to keeping the mouth and pharynx clear of debris as well as administering appropriate analgesia.

In cases of airway obstruction, heliox gas mixtures ease airflow by increasing the laminar flow characteristics of the gas (42). In a randomized comparison in children with steroid-treated viral croup, heliox and racemic epinephrine effected similar decreases in croup score (43). Currently, 80:20, 70:30, and 60:40 mixtures of helium:oxygen are available. Nasal and facial positive pressure administered as continuous positive airway pressure (CPAP) or bilevel positive airway pressure (BiPAP) can reduce the work of breathing and increase comfort in patients with airway obstruction (44,45). The combination of noninvasive positive pressure and heliox has been used successfully (46).

3. Airway Management

The patient with a compromised airway must be carefully monitored. Patients frequently maintain adequate oxygenation and ventilation despite a compromised airway until the moment respiratory failure occurs, either due to worsening anatomic obstruction or exhaustion. In the patient with partial upper airway obstruction and a difficult airway, management should occur in a multidisciplinary manner. The most experienced person performs the intubation and a general surgeon or otolaryngologist should be immediately available in the event a surgical airway is needed. Physicians caring for patients with difficult airways should be prepared to perform needle cricothyroidotomy, if necessary.

The oncology patient presents special problems in securing and maintaining the airway. Thrombocytopenia puts the patient at risk for bleeding with instrumentation of the pharyngeal and tracheal mucosa. Severe mucositis may render the airway partially obstructed and make recognition of airway anatomy difficult. Therefore, careful planning and skilled execution are required for intubating. A rapid sequence technique with an inducing agent such as thiopental or propofol and a rapid acting paralytic agent such as rocuronium allows the operator to preoxygenate the patient with bag-valve-mask (BVM) ventilation, position the patient appropriately, laryngoscope the airway, and suction under direct vision prior to insertion of the endotracheal tube. Use of a PEEP valve on the BVM resuscitator improves the operator's ability to oxygenate a hypoxemic patient both prior to and immediately after intubation. Etomidate and ketamine have been associated with less myocardial depression than thiopental and propofol and may be considered as alternative induction agents (47,48).

If severe perioperative airway issues are anticipated (for example, after extensive head and neck surgery), the surgeon may perform an elective tracheostomy in order to provide a stable airway in the perioperative period. The care of a new tracheostomy aside, the presence of a stable surgical airway removes airway-related issues from the patient's problem list (49).

4. *Mediastinal Masses*

The presence of an anterior mediastinal mass (as seen in Hodgkin's or non-Hodgkin's lymphoma) presents a particular challenge in airway management (11). In one series of 45 children admitted to a PICU with mediastinal masses, 21 were admitted emergently with 19/21 having respiratory distress (50). Once a patient's respiratory effort is blocked by sedation and/or pharmacologic paralysis, the respiratory physiology changes from inspiration generated negative intrathoracic pressure to positive pressure-driven air entry. The mechanics of a mass anterior to the airway is such that obstruction of the airway may occur during this transition from negative inspiratory force to positive inspiratory pressure. Once this obstruction occurs, it can be difficult to break and may result in hypoxemia-induced cardiac arrest. In managing the patient with an anterior mediastinal mass, all members of the team should be prepared with a plan should the mass compromise the airway (51,52). Management strategies include intubation in the upright position, use of PEEP via BVM or ETT to maintain the airway, and use of a rigid bronchoscope to stent open the trachea (53,54). Heliox may be useful in the anesthetic management of the child with an anterior mediastinal mass (55).

5. *Perioperative Ventilatory Support*

The surgical oncology patient may require postoperative assisted ventilation for several reasons. Duration and depth of anesthesia, extent of fluid shifts and blood transfusion, surgery of the head, neck, chest ,or abdomen, or a need to transport the patient to a unit remote from the OR are all reasons a pediatric patient may need to remain intubated postoperatively. The surgeon, anesthesiologist, and intensivist should have a common understanding as to why the patient requires postoperative ventilatory support.

6. *Intrahospital Transport*

Transport of the intubated postoperative patient from the OR or PACU to the PICU requires appropriate personnel, equipment, and monitors in order to avoid adverse events (56). Significant alterations in ventilation can occur when a patient is ventilated by hand as compared with a mechanical ventilator during transport to the PICU (57). These alterations can be prevented by close monitoring of oxygen saturation and $ETCO_2$ during transport (58). The transport of intubated pediatric patients from the PICU to diagnostic tests such as CT and MR demands the same attention to detail in order to avoid adverse events.

7. *Cuffed Endotracheal Tubes*

Cuffed endotracheal tubes are very useful in surgical patients who may require a significant course of perioperative mechanical ventilation. When cuffed endotracheal tubes were used in a PICU population, there was no increase in postextubation stridor compared with children in whom uncuffed tubes were used (59). The concerns of potential subglottic stenosis or other tracheal injury from the use of cuffed tracheal tubes are usually outweighed by the real risk of refractory atelectasis and inadequate ventilation that a significant air leak around the tracheal tube can precipitate. Lungs that are compliant and easy to ventilate in the OR may become much less compliant during the postoperative period. Moreover, an elective change to a cuffed endotracheal tube in an edematous postoperative patient presents risks that could be avoided by using a cuffed tube from the start. The risk of subglottic injury is decreased by using a tube with a low pressure cuff, inflating the cuff only when necessary, monitoring the pressure of the cuff, and insuring that cuff deflation produces a leak around the endotracheal tube.

B. Surgical Issues Affecting Postoperative Respiratory Function

1. *Abdominal Surgery*

From a respiratory standpoint, children do not tolerate extensive abdominal surgery as well as adults. Postoperative abdominal distension and abdominal wall edema may necessitate mechanical support of respiration. Developmentally, the child is dependent on the diaphragm as the primary muscle of respiration. Adults have a less compliant rib cage and greater development of intercostal musculature and therefore can tolerate diaphragmatic dysfunction better. In the postoperative child, diaphragmatic dysfunction may lead to atelectasis, exhaustion, and hypoxemia. In some situations, noninvasive supportive techniques such as nasal or facemask CPAP or BiPAP may provide the necessary support to prevent or treat atelectasis (60,61).

2. *Pleural Effusions*

Pleural effusions have a deleterious effect on postoperative respiratory function. If effusions are evident radiographically while the patient is intubated, they will worsen upon extubation when negative intrathoracic pressures are generated by spontaneous respiration. A moderate-sized right-sided pleural effusion that is present in a ventilated patient after extensive liver surgery or thoracoabdominal resection (TAR) of neuroblastoma, will become larger upon the removal of positive pressure. Addressing a pleural effusion by diuresis (spontaneous or pharmacologic-assisted) or by drainage will result in a smoother postextubation course. The Seldinger technique can be used to insert 16 gauge single lumen side hole or 7–8.5 French pigtail catheters, which are then attached to a drainage system, thus avoiding the need for classical tube thoracostomy in many cases (62). The smaller, softer tubes are less painful both to insert and to maintain in place. Alteplase has been used to facilitate the drainage of a complicated pleural effusion through a 16-gauge side hole catheter (63).

3. *Thoracotomy*

Although thoracic surgery is increasingly being performed by minimally invasive video-assisted thoracoscopic techniques (VATS), the open thoracotomy remains a frequent operation in pediatric oncologic surgery. Many patients can be extubated immediately after thoracotomy, but pain management and pulmonary toilet are of paramount importance. Pain related to the presence of a thoracostomy tube often causes significant splinting with resultant atelectasis. See below for a discussion of pain management in the thoracotomy patient.

C. Duration of Mechanical Ventilation

The length of time that a postoperative patient requires mechanical ventilation depends on the time to resolution of the issues that require postoperative respiratory support. In patients remaining intubated pending clearance of anesthetic agents or transport to the site of definitive care, the time can be short. If patients require support due to abdominal or chest edema or pleural effusions, the duration of ventilatory support can be much longer. In cases of neuroblastoma, desmoplastic small round cell tumor, hepatoblastoma, osteosarcoma, Ewing's sarcoma, and Wilm's tumor, patients are exposed to multiple rounds of intensive chemotherapy prior to definitive surgery, and they generally recover more slowly than patients who had not been exposed to chemotherapy. The precise timing of extubation is multifactorial and complex and it is best not to make promises in advance about when it will occur.

D. Principles of Mechanical Ventilation

Comprehensive discussions of pediatric mechanical ventilation can be found in several excellent reviews (64–68). The type of ventilator used for the pediatric perioperative patient is a matter of institutional preference. Several ventilators are marketed that provide sophisticated technology that can be applied across the age spectrum from infancy to adulthood. The mode of ventilation is also a matter of choice. Synchronized intermittent mandatory ventilation (SIMV) with or without pressure support (PS), assist control (AC), and pressure-regulated volume control (PRVC) are available modalities. Evidence-based guidelines do not yet exist for selecting the best mode of mechanical ventilation for children.

In our center, volume-assured ventilation in the SIMV mode with PS is the standard modality for routine postoperative patients. Tidal volumes in the range of 10–12 mL/kg and age-appropriate respiratory rates are chosen. A minimum PEEP of 5 cm of water is set and FiO_2 is weaned rapidly to ≤ 0.60. When necessary, the PEEP is increased to sustain this FiO_2. If significant atelectasis or pulmonary edema is present, the PEEP is increased incrementally to recruit and maintain lung volume. If the ABG (and/or pulse oximetric hemoglobin oxygen saturation and $ETCO_2$) shows acceptable ventilation and oxygenation, the settings can be decreased. Typically, the ventilator rate is decreased first in order to allow the patient to assume more of the respiratory work. In general, patients are permitted to breathe spontaneously when the PEEP is $\leq$10 cm H_2O, and are deeply sedated and receive neuromuscular blocking agents when the PEEP is $>$10 cm H_2O.

The use of pressure-supported (PS) breaths helps decrease work of breathing, takes advantage of a patient's respiratory drive, and increases comfort on the ventilator. The optimal level of pressure support is not known and individual practices vary. One strategy is to set the PS at 10 cm H_2O for patients on SIMV and decrease it to 5 cm H_2O for spontaneous breathing trials in preparation for extubation. Another is to adjust the pressure support to provide a spontaneous tidal volume that is 50% of the set tidal volume in SIMV. Removal of PS prior to extubation is controversial. Pressure support may overcome additional work imposed by the presence of the endotracheal tube. Conversely, removal of the endotracheal tube may reverse a stenting effect provided by the tube. When coupled with postextubation edema, the extubated airway may in fact be narrower than the intubated one. Thus, removal of PS prior to extubation may provide a better reflection of the work that will be required of the patient when the tube is removed (68).

In 2000, the ARDSNet low tidal volume trial was published. This study demonstrated a significant mortality reduction in adults with acute respiratory distress syndrome (ARDS) who were ventilated at tidal volumes approaching 6 ml/kg compared with a tidal volume of 12 ml/kg (69). Although the reduction of cyclic high volume inflation and deflation of the lung makes sense physiologically as a means of reducing ventilator-associated lung injury, it is unclear how well this translates to the pediatric population. Children have more compliant rib cages than adults and, as a result, are more prone to develop atelectasis when the closing volume of lung units is greater than functional residual capacity. As compensation for greater rib cage compliance, infants and small children use end expiratory muscle tone and partial closure of the vocal cords to maintain end expiratory lung volume above closing volume (70). Anesthesia, sedation, and pain often remove these compensatory mechanisms. Thus, the infant and young child is more prone to atelectasis than the adult (71). In many postoperative patients, atelectasis is a difficult problem that requires both PEEP and high volume expansion of the lungs to reverse. Particularly in the postoperative child, low tidal volume high respiratory rate ventilatory methods may not be effective.

E. Weaning and Liberation from Mechanical Ventilation

In most cases, patients tolerate a gradual decrease in ventilatory support and can be successfully extubated when the following criteria are met: (1) resolution of the process that led to the mechanical ventilatory support (anesthesia/atelectasis/fluid overload/ pneumonia, etc.); (2) adequate spontaneous respiratory drive; (3) adequate airway protective reflexes; and (4) ability to oxygenate adequately—$PaO_2 > 100$ mmHg on $FiO_2 < 50\%$ ($PaO_2/FiO_2 > 200$) is a standard criterion.

F. Protocol-Based Weaning of Mechanical Ventilation

Studies in adult patients have shown that protocol-based weaning of ventilatory support results in improved outcomes compared with the use of individual practices. Evidence-based guidelines for weaning and discontinuing ventilatory support in adult patients have been published (68,72,73). Although no evidence-based guidelines for weaning of mechanical ventilation in children exist, clinical trials have been performed. In one randomized, controlled trial comparing pressure support ventilation, volume support ventilation and no protocol at all, there was no difference in time to extubation (74). However, another prospective randomized trial in children comparing protocol- vs. physician-directed weaning showed a reduction in weaning time in the protocol-driven group (75).

Objective criteria to direct extubation and predict outcome in children are not widely used but could be helpful in complex situations. The rapid shallow breathing index (RSBI) and the compliance, resistance, oxygenation, and pressure index (CROP index) have been shown to be useful predictors of extubation success (76). The RSBI (breaths/mL/kg) is the spontaneous respiratory rate divided by the spontaneously measured tidal volume indexed for weight while intubated on CPAP of 4 cm H_2O (RR/sVt). An RSBI of $\leq$8 breaths/mL/kg was a sensitive and specific indicator for predicting extubation success. The CROP index (mL/kg/breaths/min), calculated from parameters measured while the patient is receiving ventilator breaths and breathing spontaneously on a CPAP of 4 cm H_2O, is the product of the dynamic compliance (Cdyn), the negative inspiratory force (NIF), and PaO_2/PAO_2 divided by the RR. [(Cdyn)(NIF)(PaO_2/PAO_2)/RR]. Cdyn is calculated by dividing the exhaled tidal volume from a ventilator breath by the difference of the peak inspiratory pressure (PIP) and the PEEP [Cdyn = Vt(vent breath)/(PIP−PEEP)]. The

NIF is a standard measured parameter in intubated patients. The PAO_2 is calculated from the alveolar gas equation and the PaO_2 is from an ABG. A CROP index value ≥ 0.15 mL/kg/breaths/min had sensitivity similar to the RSBI and somewhat lower specificity for predicting extubation success.

The ratio of physiologic dead space, $V(D)$, to tidal volume, $V(T)$, is another method that can be used to predict extubation success in pediatric patients. A $V(D)/V(T)$ ratio of ≤ 0.50 reliably predicted successful extubation. A dead space to tidal volume ratio > 0.65 identified patients at risk for respiratory failure following extubation (18).

G. The Recently Extubated Patient

Airway and ventilation issues in the recently extubated patient are sometimes more complex than the preceding course of mechanical ventilation. Interventions mentioned earlier for the partially obstructed airway are relevant in the management of postextubation stridor. In addition to aggressive chest percussion and postural drainage, postextubation atelectasis can be treated with intermittent positive pressure breathing (IPPB), facial or nasal BiPAP, and high-frequency chest wall oscillation (HFCWO) administered by a chest vest device (77). Although the above modalities are applied aggressively in postoperative patients to treat atelectasis and prevent reintubation, studies have not conclusively proved their effectiveness (78).

H. Nonconventional Mechanical Ventilation

1. *High-Frequency Oscillatory Ventilation*

In the event of a complicated perioperative ventilator course, nonconventional techniques may be considered (79). It is recognized that high tidal volumes, high peak airway pressures, high PEEP, and high-inspired oxygen concentrations are deleterious to the lung and may contribute to multiorgan system dysfunction. High-frequency oscillatory ventilation (HFOV) is a modality that is well established in the neonatal and pediatric age groups (80–83). In HFOV, oxygenation is manipulated by adjusting the mean airway pressure (MAP), which is maintained by a constant flow of gas that is regulated by a flow-restricting valve. The oscillator allows the maintenance of a high MAP and an acceptable level of oxygenation without the concomitant peaks in airway pressure seen with conventional volume ventilation. Eliminating cyclic inflation and deflation of the lungs has been theorized to reduce the amount of ventilator-associated lung injury (84). The Viasys/Sensormedics 3100A high-frequency oscillatory ventilator has been used most often in the neonatal and pediatric patients and the newer 3100B has been approved for use in patients > 40 kg (85–87).

2. *Inhaled Nitric Oxide*

Inhaled nitric oxide (iNO) is employed in the treatment of pulmonary hypertension and improves oxygenation by means of amplifying cGMP-induced smooth muscle relaxation in the pulmonary capillaries. Its role in the management of pediatric surgical oncology patients has not been well studied. Studies in adults and children with hypoxemic respiratory failure have shown significant temporary increases in oxygenation but no demonstrable change in outcome or mortality (88). The addition of iNO in patients who are on HFOV has been shown to result in an amplified increase in oxygenation (89,90). Pediatric oncology patients with acute hypoxemic respiratory failure (AHRF) respond with a similar frequency and degree of improved oxygenation to nononcology patients. Inhaled nitric oxide has been used with reported success in the treatment of postpneumonectomy pulmonary edema in an adult with lung cancer (91).

3. *Prone Positioning*

Prone positioning has been used successfully for improving oxygenation and facilitating pulmonary toilet in perioperative patients including pediatric oncology patients. Patients can be moved from supine to prone safely. The mechanism of action for improving oxygenation includes redistribution of perfusion to well-ventilated lung units. In the supine position, the anterior lung regions are better ventilated but less well perfused than the posterior segments. The posterior lung units are more prone to atelectasis. Upon rotating the patient from supine to prone, the previously anterior, better ventilated, lung units become dependent and receive increased, gravity-dependent, blood flow resulting in improved matching of ventilation and perfusion. There are insufficient data to prove a benefit in outcome following prone positioning in patients with hypoxemic respiratory failure (79).

I. Complicated Perioperative Mechanical Ventilation

The pediatric oncology patient who develops intrinsic lung disease prior to surgery or postoperatively necessitating a prolonged course of mechanical ventilatory support presents a diagnostic and therapeutic challenge (92). Causes of parenchymal lung disease include viral or bacterial pneumonia, pulmonary contusion, or hemorrhage, exacerbation of reactive airways disease, atelectasis, pulmonary edema, exacerbation of treatment-related lung diseases such as bronchiolitis obliterans organizing pneumonia (BOOP) (93) or acute hypoxemic respiratory failure (AHRF).

Initiation of mechanical ventilation in the patient with worsening respiratory distress who is in need of an invasive diagnostic procedure such as a bronchoscopic bronchoalveolar lavage (BAL) or open lung biopsy is often delayed due to the concern that intubation, anesthesia and the procedure itself will put the patient "over the edge." In most cases, these procedures are tolerated well and the patient can be extubated quickly. Flexible fiberoptic bronchoscopy with BAL and open lung biopsy can be performed safely once a patient is on a ventilator, even at high settings (94,95). The yield of BAL in children may not be as great as in adult patients and in a significant percentage of cases, open lung biopsy reveals an infectious etiology for respiratory failure that was not present on BAL (96).

J. Mechanical Ventilation after Hematopoietic Cell Transplantation

Pediatric patients who develop AHRF following hematopoietic cell transplantation (HCT) have an extremely high mortality rate whether bone marrow, umbilical cord blood, or peripheral blood was transplanted. Our center reported a mortality rate of 0.88 between 1988 and 1993 in 43 pediatric patients who underwent bone marrow transplantation and developed AHRF (97). More recently, a study in children requiring ICU admission after bone marrow transplant (BMT) showed that 41.6% of patients who were intubated could be extubated, but there were no survivors among patients who had pulmonary infections and required mechanical ventilation for >48 hr (98). A mortality rate of 96% in 74 pediatric BMT patients who received mechanical ventilation for respiratory failure was reported in 2000 (99). Survival of only one of 20 pediatric patients who fulfilled specified criteria for lung injury after BMT was also reported (100). A recent study comparing the outcome of mechanical ventilation in pediatric patients with umbilical cord blood transplant with bone marrow transplant showed that the umbilical cord transplant recipients had a poorer outcome than the BMT recipients, with survival 37% and 47%, respectively. In this report, prognosticators of survival included mechanical ventilation for seizures or airway obstruction and lack of significant hepatic disease (101).

K. Extracorporeal Membrane Oxygenation

Extracorporeal membrane oxygenation (ECMO) is a therapeutic option for treating overwhelming lung failure in pediatric patients (102–104). The role of ECMO in the pediatric oncology patient and particularly the perioperative patient has yet to be clarified although its use has been described in case reports (105–107).

L. Analgesia

Many pediatric oncology patients have received opiate analgesic medications and sedative hypnotics prior to admission to the PICU for perioperative care. The potential requirement for prodigious amounts of opiates and sedatives must be anticipated as one plans an analgesic and sedative regimen for postoperative care. The intubated postoperative patient benefits from continuous infusions of an opiate such as fentanyl with supplemental anxiolysis and sedation provided by a benzodiazepine such as lorazepam or midazolam administered either continuously by infusion or intermittently. The use of epidural analgesia by continuous infusion while sedated, with transition to patient-controlled analgesia (PCA) when awake is effective and minimizes the side effects seen with systemic opiate administration (108).

Following painful procedures in the abdomen and chest, excellent analgesia is obtained with the addition of the parenteral nonsteroidal anti-inflammatory agent ketorolac to an epidural or systemic opiate PCA regimen. Published studies have confirmed the efficacy and safety of ketorolac when it is used within recommended dosing and duration of therapy guidelines (109–111). Little to no increase in bleeding has been observed (112). Some surgeons feel strongly that nonsteroidal analgesic agents should not be used in patients whose surgeries put them at an elevated risk of bleeding and especially bleeding into a closed space. Therefore, it is prudent to solicit the surgeon's opinion prior to starting nonsteroidal analgesia and to avoid parenteral NSAIDS altogether in postoperative neurosurgery patients.

Although the pediatric intensivist is usually well versed in pain management and sedation techniques, the assistance of a pain service with pediatric expertise can be extremely valuable in the management of postoperative oncology patients (113).

M. Analgesia and Sedation for Mechanical Ventilation

In the absence of an epidural catheter, intubated patients receive intravenous fentanyl starting a 1–2 μg/kg/hr and intravenous lorazepam at 0.05–0.1 mg/kg every 2–4 hr. Continuous midazolam starting at 0.04 mg/kg/hr can be used in place of intermittent lorazepam. In patients receiving epidural analgesia, IV fentanyl is not administered but a benzodiazepine is continued to provide anxiolysis, sedation, and amnesia.

The use of propofol for prolonged sedation in the PICU is proscribed by a manufacturer's warning due to reports of unexplained metabolic acidosis and death. However, this rapid acting sedative can be useful for short periods of time when patients are carefully monitored (114). Propofol is a useful adjunct in preparing patients for extubation due to its short half-life and easy titratability. A longer acting agent such as a benzodiazepine should be used if the duration of mechanical ventilation is to be more than several hours.

N. Abstinence Syndromes

Abstinence syndromes resulting from abrupt cessation of opiates and benzodiazepines can occur if the postoperative opiate and/or benzodiazepine requirement is prolonged. An additional consideration in the development of abstinence syndromes in the pediatric oncology population is duration of opiate analgesia received prior to surgery. Strategies for prevention and management of abstinence syndromes in the ICU include the use of oral methadone and lorazepam (115,116).

IV. APPROACH TO PERIOPERATIVE CARDIOVASCULAR AND ORGAN SYSTEM SUPPORT

A. Impact of Operative Course

Intraoperative fluid management is a subject of continuing discussion. Efforts are sometimes made, particularly in thoracic cases, to restrict the volume of fluid administered intraoperatively in order to minimize edema and facilitate early extubation. Although the patient may be less edematous at the end of the surgery, excessive fluid limitation can lead to a hemodynamically precarious patient, as tissue edema and third space fluid loss leads to intravascular volume depletion. Invasive monitoring plays an important role in guiding the operative and postoperative fluid management of such patients.

B. Repletion and Maintenance of Intravascular Volume

Intravascular volume repletion is an important part of general postoperative care as well as a key component of cardiovascular support in the perioperative pediatric patient. Reasons for inadequate intravascular volume include failure to keep up with sensible and insensible intraoperative fluid losses, bleeding in the postoperative period due to inadequate operative hemostasis or uncorrected coagulopathy, and ongoing third space fluid losses exacerbated by capillary leak syndromes. Careful repletion of intravascular volume should be the first component of the correction of cardiovascular insufficiency in the postoperative patient.

Signs of inadequate intravascular volume include diminishing urine output, cool extremities with delayed capillary refill, tachycardia, and, ultimately, decreasing blood pressure. An elevated blood urea nitrogen, metabolic acidosis and, in surgeries involving the liver, rising transaminases are laboratory findings that suggest hypovolemia. The approach to correction of intravascular volume depletion in pediatrics is based on provision of maintenance fluid supplemented by repletion of estimated deficits and replacement of ongoing losses.

Our standard management is to provide maintenance fluid calculated by standard methods supplemented with boluses of isotonic crystalloid (normal saline or lactated ringers) as indicated to maintain a minimum urine output of 0.5–1.0 mL/kg/hr. Measurement of CVP is a key component in monitoring the intravascular volume and is very helpful in postoperative situations where extensive third spacing is seen or anticipated. A low CVP (<5 mmHg) suggests decreased intravascular volume and in the presence of clinical and laboratory signs of intravascular hypovolemia, indicates that fluid administration is required. While in the cases of thoracic surgery and neurosurgery there may be an effort made to restrict fluids and "keep the patient dry," there are other situations where maintenance of a generous intravascular volume may be beneficial. Hepatic lobe resection or division and reanastamosis of the renal vasculature in resection of perinephric neuroblastoma are examples of extensive abdominal vascular surgery following which maintenance of adequate or even generous intravascular volume may be important in the prevention of thrombosis. In the face of end organ dysfunction after the vascular supply to that organ system has been manipulated, color Doppler ultrasound may reveal the presence of thrombosis that could be addressed with thrombolysis (117). There is no literature that indicates an ideal central venous pressure in postoperative children.

C. Third Space Fluid Losses

Intravascular dehydration and electrolyte disorders related to third spacing occur frequently in the surgical patient. Third spacing occurs when tissue bed capillary leak results in the movement of fluid from the vascular to the extravascular space. This extravasation of fluid is an insensible water loss that is often underappreciated and can result in significant intravascular volume depletion. It is often assumed that intraoperative radiation therapy (IORT) increases tissue bed inflammation and results in increased third space losses, but this has not been well described (118,119). Hyponatremia results from intravenous replacement of third spaced fluid with a solution with a lower sodium concentration than that of the plasma fluid exuded into tissue beds. The signs of third spacing are those of intravascular volume depletion with the addition of weight gain and edema. This process responds to volume replacement with isotonic crystalloid solutions.

D. Perioperative Use of Dopamine in the Pediatric Oncology Patient

There are frequent occasions in postoperative management of pediatric oncology patients in which signs of inadequate tissue perfusion and/or unacceptable hemodynamics such as tachycardia or hypotension persist despite aggressive repletion of intravascular volume. In these situations, patients may benefit from the use of dopamine as an inotropic and vasopressor agent. Dosages ranging from 0.5 to 10 μg/kg/min are used. This perioperative state is analogous to compensated shock and may be related to the surgical intervention, preexisting therapy-related injury to the cardiovascular system, or the onset of sepsis or septic shock, which must be considered in the immunocompromised patient.

The use of dopamine in "renal doses" in order to increase renal and splanchnic circulation has been practiced widely in pediatric surgery patients without evidence supporting its actual benefit to the kidneys. It remains unproven whether the improvement in urine production seen upon administration of dopamine to the postoperative patient is due to activation of the D1 and D2 receptors as has been hypothesized or due to an improvement in inotropic state and vascular tone that occurs through stimulation of $\beta 1$ and $\alpha 1$ receptors (120). The specific D1 receptor agonist fenoldopam is a vasodilator that has been used as an antihypertensive agent in children (121) and has been shown to preserve renal function in situations of potential renal ischemia in adults (122). Its role in supporting postoperative renal function and splanchnic blood vessel perfusion in children after oncologic surgery has not yet been demonstrated.

E. The Hemodynamic Effects of Surgery on Catecholamine Secreting Tumors

Tumors including pheochromocytoma, neuroblastoma, and adrenal cortical carcinoma are associated with the secretion of catecholamines (123). Pheochromocytoma, a relatively uncommon tumor in children, is frequently associated with flushing, tachycardia, arrhythmias, and hypertension. Those patients with hypertension require alpha blockade with phentolamine and/or phenoxybenzamine preoperatively to prevent complications related to catecholamine excess and to provide for a stable operative course. Postoperatively, removal of the catecholamine-secreting tumor, relative intravascular volume depletion due to long-term vasoconstriction, and persistence of therapeutic alpha blockade often produce a requirement for aggressive volume administration and vasopressor support with norepinephrine (124,125).

Neuroblastoma, the most common nonintracranial solid tumor of childhood, is associated with secretion of norepinephrine in approximately 70% of cases. Patients with neuroblastoma may be hypertensive at diagnosis, but this and other signs of catecholamine excess usually resolve with chemotherapy and are only rarely present by the time patients undergo definitive tumor resection surgery (126,127). An exception occurs when infants with presumed neuroblastoma require surgery urgently (e.g., for spinal cord compression). In a series of young children diagnosed with neuroblastoma by mass urine screening, elevations in blood pressure as well as plasma levels of catecholamines were noted with tumor manipulation (128). Approximately 45% of patients in one series, though not hypertensive during surgery, had clinically important episodes of hypotension following neuroblastoma resection (129). In most of these cases, hypotension resolved with volume resuscitation. However, some neuroblastoma patients remain hypotensive despite postoperative fluid resuscitation and require dopamine or norepinephrine to stabilize their hemodynamics. The presence of a catecholamine requirement postoperatively may represent hemodynamic changes related to removal of catecholamine-secreting tumor tissue.

Another potential cause of hemodynamic instability after resection of abdominal neuroblastoma is acute adrenal insufficiency. Resection of a mass involving one or both adrenal glands or compromise of the adrenal blood supply secondary to tumor involvement may lead to hypotension that is resistant to fluid administration and vasopressor agents. Administration of stress doses of corticosteroids (most often hydrocortisone) followed by physiologic replacement may reverse the hemodynamic changes.

Some postoperative neuroblastoma patients manifest misleadingly robust perfusion related to disruption of the sympathetic chain and a resultant partial surgical sympathectomy to one or more extremities.

F. Hematologic Issues in the Perioperative Patient

Anemia and thrombocytopenia are common in pediatric oncology patients and may be present perioperatively. Coagulopathy may develop in patients who have undergone massive transfusion, have an underlying coagulation factor deficiency, or who have undergone extensive liver surgery. Platelets and fresh frozen plasma are transfused in response to excessive bleeding associated with thrombocytopenia and abnormal coagulation studies, respectively. Cryoprecipitate is added in patients with persistent bleeding associated with hypofibrinogenemia. The colloid osmotic pressure provided by these products may also help to minimize postoperative fluid leak and edema. Vitamin K may be used for isolated prothrombin time prolongation.

Evidence-based guidelines do not exist for transfusion of packed red blood cells (RBC) in children. Minimizing the use of blood products is desirable due to declining supply, infectious risk, and data in both critically ill adults (130) and children (131,132) indicating that RBC transfusion may not be associated with improved outcome. Due to repetitive cycles of chemotherapy as well as chronic illness, oncology patients may not possess the compensatory reserve provided by a healthy bone marrow and liver. Local experience supports aggressive use of blood products in the replacement of deficits and ongoing losses in postoperative oncology patients as well as those with sepsis and septic shock.

G. Splanchnic and Visceral Issues

Acute hepatic necrosis is a known side effect of extensive hepatic resection and cross clamping of the hepatic blood vessels in the Pringle maneuver. Routine monitoring of transaminiases, bilirubin, and prothrombin time are important in liver surgery patients. A serum ammonia level should be obtained if questions arise about the adequacy of hepatic function. Hepatic blood vessel Doppler ultrasonography can be used to follow changes in blood flow in the liver vasculature after surgery.

The presence of ascites may slow ventilator weaning or impact negatively on the postoperative respiratory status of the spontaneously breathing patient. Pressure exerted on the renal veins by ascitic fluid can decrease glomerular filtration rate (GFR) resulting in azotemia and declining urine output. Small catheter paracentesis of abdominal ascites performed by Seldinger technique is useful diagnostically and therapeutically. In the event of persistent chylous ascites, octreotide has been reported to have a beneficial effect in decreasing fluid production (133).

Preoperative chemotherapy and antibiotics increase the likelihood of renal insufficiency in the postoperative oncology patient. Decreases in preoperative GFR can be amplified by perioperative hypovolemia secondary to inadequate resuscitation or replacement of third space losses. Special attention needs to be paid to the patient whose abdominal resection involved division and reanastomosis of the renal artery and vein. In renal replacement therapy is required, continuous veno venous hemodiafiltration (CVVHDF) may provide sufficient fluid balance and metabolic control in a patient who is not a good candidate for dialysis.

H. Metabolic and Fluid Balance Issues

Fluid balance and electrolyte disorders occur frequently in pediatric oncology patients, both pre- and postoperatively. General reviews of fluid and electrolyte physiology in the postoperative child are available (134). During the perioperative period, hypokalemia, hypocalcemia, and hypomagnesemia are common problems attributable to chemotherapy-induced renal tubular injury, particularly following *cis*-platinum. These electrolyte deficiencies usually respond to the addition of appropriate supplemental salts to intravenous fluids.

One difference between oncologic and nononcologic surgical patients is the potential role of diuretics in the mobilization of retained fluids postoperatively. Traditional surgical dogma is to permit the body to mobilize fluids spontaneously at the point in the recovery process when it is physiologically appropriate. This approach prevents iatrogenic dehydration from occurring in the patient with inadequate urine output due to intravascular volume depletion. Diuretics are thought to place the tissue beds at risk by compromising perfusion. The oncology patient, on the other hand, often has compromised glomerular filtration secondary to chemotherapy and may not appropriately mobilize fluids and diurese. In these patients, pharmacologic diuresis may be beneficial in stimulating removal of retained fluid once adequate intravascular volume and adequate tissue bed perfusion are assured.

I. Hyponatremia

Hyponatremia occurs frequently in critically ill children. In the nonoperative patient, hyponatremia is most often due to water excess. In the operative patient, however, third space fluid losses must be considered. Hyponatremia secondary to inappropriate antidiuretic hormone secretion (SIADH) should be distinguished from hyponatremia secondary to third space losses. The syndrome of inappropriate antidiuretic hormone secretion is manifested by hypertonic urine with an elevated urine sodium and absence of dehydration (low BUN and serum uric acid). The treatment of SIADH is fluid restriction and in extreme circumstances, sodium supplementation to address critically symptomatic hyponatremia. When hyponatremia is related to third space fluid and electrolyte losses, the urine sodium is low, and the patient has relative intravascular volume depletion (elevated BUN and serum uric acid) that exists in the face of tissue edema. The treatment is fluid and electrolyte replenishment with a goal of minimizing administration of free water. Urinary electrolytes must be interpreted cautiously in patients who may have chemotherapy-related renal tubular injuries and associated renal concentrating defects.

J. Nutrition

Many pediatric oncology patients go into surgery intolerant of enteral feeds, on total parenteral nutrition (TPN). In these patients, it is reasonable to restart TPN early in the postoperative course after stabilization of fluid balance and electrolyte issues. Early initiation of parenteral nutrition has been shown to have positive effects on the anabolic response of pediatric patients recovering from extensive abdominal surgery (135). Duodenal placement of a silastic feeding tube is accomplished easily in the PICU when the patient is intubated, and may permit utilization of enteral nutrition in the patient who had previously been TPN dependent. Transpyloric feeding is well tolerated in sedated and pharmacologically paralyzed pediatric patients (136). Duodenal placement insures a decreased risk of aspiration. Enteral nutrition through a transpyloric feeding tube may be continued through the process of weaning from ventilatory support and even extubation without risk of aspiration (137). Multiple techniques are used to pass the feeding tube through the pylorus into the small intestine (138,139). Although a duodenal or jejunal feeding tube can be blindly placed, a pH-guided technique increases the chance of first attempt transpyloric placement (140,141).

V. CARDIOVASCULAR SUPPORT AND SHOCK

A. Introduction

Cardiovascular dysfunction is present in varying degrees in many pediatric oncology patients after major surgery. The impact of this cardiovascular dysfunction on the postoperative course depends on several factors including the preoperative status, the extent of tissue injury inflicted by the operation and the adequacy of intraoperative resuscitation. The management of cardiovascular dysfunction in the perioperative oncology patient is analogous to the management of shock. Any degree of baseline cardiovascular dysfunction can be exacerbated by sepsis and septic shock, perioperative complications that are frequently encountered in immunocompromised patients.

B. Developmental Considerations

Infants and children exhibit fundamental differences from adults in the manner with which their cardiovascular systems respond to stress (120,142,143). These differences have several important implications for the critical care management of the child less than 1 year of age: (1) intravascular volume loading may increase atrial and ventricular pressures without significantly increasing end diastolic volume (preload); thus stroke volume may not increase as expected. (2) The functional inotropic state of the infant's heart is near maximal even at rest. Therefore, it is difficult to augment the inotropic state of the infant's myocardium and improvement in cardiac output often depends upon increasing heart rate. (3) Infants respond initially to volume depletion with tachycardia and increases in systemic vascular resistance. Once the limit of this response has been reached, blood pressure falls suddenly and precipitously.

C. Impact of Previous Treatment on Cardiovascular Condition

Cardiomyopathy due to chemotherapy in the pediatric oncology patient has been well studied. Doxorubicin and daunorubicin are anthracycline agents that produce acute and chronic dose-related reductions in cardiac function (20,144). Cardiomyopathy occurs in as many as 30% of patients receiving cumulative dosages greater than 600 mg/m^2(145). Cyclophosphamide and mediastinal radiation are associated with an increased risk of cardiomyopathy in patients receiving anthracyclines (146), and high-dose cyclophosphamide (120–240 mg/kg) alone is associated with cardiotoxicity. Knowledge of preoperative echocardiographic studies may be helpful in dissecting out a treatment-related component of cardiovascular dysfunction. The possible presence of therapy-related myocardial dysfunction might lead the intensive care physician to be more aggressive in perioperative hemodyamic monitoring and management.

In the present era, few patients exceed the recommended limits for anthracyline dosages (147,148) and the iron chelating agent dexrazoxane has been shown to be useful in ameliorating the cardiotoxic effects of anthracyclines (149). However, it is not known what effect subcardiotoxic burdens of anthracyclines may have when the heart is exposed to the metabolic stress of surgery (150).

Children who develop chemotherapy-associated cardiac dysfunction present with signs of congestive heart failure. Echocardiographically, anthracycline cardiomyopathy is as likely to be restrictive as dilated in children. In the extreme, this presentation blends into one of cardiogenic shock, and the patient displays acrocyanosis, poor peripheral perfusion, cardiomegaly, and evidence of pulmonary congestion.

D. Sepsis and Septic Shock

Postoperative sepsis and septic shock are potential concerns in the immunocompromised patient. Chemotherapy and cytoreductive regimens often expose patients to extended periods of neutropenia. Permanent central venous access devices (Broviac, Hickman, infusaport) and prosthetic materials (biologic and nonbiologic) used in reconstructive surgery amplify the already high risk of infection (151,152). Fortunately, septic shock in children is associated with improved outcome compared with a previous era (153).

There are differences in the way the cardiovascular systems of infants and children respond to the stress of sepsis. While adults who are septic manifest severe dysregulation of vascular tone that is amenable to vasopressor therapy, younger pediatric patients often manifest a mixed picture of inotropic and vascular dysfunction. Compensated or early septic shock in children is characterized by low systemic vascular resistance and high cardiac output (154). Late or uncompensated shock is characterized by worsening tissue perfusion, critical reductions in cardiac output, progressive acidosis, and multiple organ failure (155,156). Contrary to the adult experience, low cardiac output, not low systemic vascular resistance is associated with mortality in pediatric septic shock (157–165).

E. Principles of Septic Shock Management

Recently published clinical practice guidelines for the management of septic shock in pediatric patients are evidence and consensus based (37,166). Septic shock is a life-threatening condition and management should proceed with precision and alacrity. Hemodynamic and respiratory supportive therapies are supplemented by antimicrobials, removal of potentially infected catheters or materials, appropriate surgical intervention, and hemodynamic and respiratory support. In the neutropenic child who presents to the PICU with an acute hemodynamic disturbance, therapy is usually initiated with vancomycin, an aminoglycoside and a third- or fourth-generation cephalosporin; local practice and sensitivity testing should govern the specific choices (167). Sepsis due to fungal or viral organisms is considered in patients with negative blood cultures who do not show signs of improvement on antibacterial therapy. In such patients, treatment with an amphotericin-containing product should be started (168,169).

The decision to remove a Broviac catheter, infusaport, or surgical prosthesis is often difficult. In hemodynamically stable patients with blood stream infections and permanent indwelling vascular access devices, many authorities recommend a trial of medical management prior to removing the device (170,171). However, in the patient with poor perfusion or other evidence of shock such as hypotension, it is wise to remove the catheter if shock cannot be reversed promptly.

Adjunctive treatment of septic shock with corticosteroids continues to be a subject of discussion (172,173). Patients at high risk of adrenal insufficiency include those with *Purpura fulminans* and the Waterhouse–Friedrichsen syndrome, children with hypopituitarism or adrenal tumors and those who have received chronic steroid therapy. Adult data suggest that all patients with septic shock are at risk for adrenal insufficiency (174–177). A committee of pediatric experts adopted as a definition of adrenal insufficiency a total cortisol level between 0 and 18 mg/dL and recommended that the administration of hydrocortisone be considered in patients with fluid and catecholamine refractory septic shock and a serum cortisol level in this range (37). To date, there have been no adequate pediatric trials of steroids in the treatment of septic shock. The practice guideline consensus group recommended (level III) hydrocortisone dosages that range from 1–2 mg/kg/day for replacement therapy to 50 mg/kg/day for shock. The consensus group also stressed the importance of correcting serum calcium, glucose, and thyroid function abnormalities in patients with septic shock.

F. Hemodynamic Support of Children with Shock

The goal of hemodynamic support of the failing circulation is improvement in organ perfusion and correction of associated metabolic abnormalities. Data in adult patients have indicated that it may be advantageous to treat shock by elevating cardiac output and oxygen delivery to supranormal values (178,179). Pollack reported a series of pediatric patients with septic shock in whom there was a lower mortality rate among those patients in whom oxygen utilization (VO_2), arteriovenous O_2 content difference, and O_2 extraction ratio became greater than normal during therapy. In a study involving a group of 90 pediatric patients, including those with septic and cardiogenic shock, Carcillo et al. (180) showed that oxygen utilization increases in response to increases in oxygen delivery, and recommended that therapy be aimed at increasing oxygen delivery. Subsequently, Ceneviva et al. (38) showed that attaining a cardiac index (CI) of 3.3–6.0 L/min/m^2 as a therapeutic goal might result in improved survival.

Initial management of the hemodynamic abnormalities associated with shock is aimed at restoration of intravascular volume and ventricular preload. In the hypotensive patient with poor peripheral perfusion, 20 mL/kg of isotonic crystalloid or 10 mL/kg of colloid is infused over 5–10 min and repeated immediately if the patient does not improve. Volumes up to and over 60 mL/kg may be necessary. Hypoglycemia and hypocalcemia must be corrected. If administration of 60 mL/kg of isotonic crystalloid or 30 mL/kg of colloid does not result in improved perfusion, then placement of a central venous catheter is indicated for the measurement of CVP and the administration of catecholamine agents. An arterial catheter should also be inserted for accurate, continuous monitoring of blood pressure. Fluid administration can continue as long as signs of congestive heart failure do not supervene. The major goal is attainment of normal perfusion and blood pressure. For the child with cardiogenic shock, or distributive shock complicated by chemotherapy-associated myocardial dysfunction, insertion of a pulmonary artery catheter should be considered.

The controversy regarding infusion of crystalloid and colloid in treatment of shock has been reviewed without resolution (181–183). A Cochrane Group metaanalysis implied harmful effects of colloid use in critical illness, but evaluated no studies examining fluid resuscitation in children with septic shock (184). Clinical practice guidelines for hemodynamic support of pediatric patients with septic shock recommend either crystalloid or colloid for initial fluid resuscitation in cases of septic shock (37).

G. Inotropic and Vasopressor Agents for the Failing Circulation

Inotropic and vasopressor agents are employed to treat children who do not improve adequately with restoration of intravascular volume. A detailed discussion of the pharmacology of these agents in children is available (120).

Dopamine is generally employed as a first-line agent to treat cardiogenic or distributive shock associated with mild to moderate degrees of hypotension. Its versatility is due to the fact that it stimulates both α_1 and β_1 adrenergic receptors (as well as β_2 and dopaminergic receptors) and therefore depending upon dosage possesses vasodilator, inotropic, and vasopressor activity. The usual starting dosage for patients with cardiac dysfunction is 5 μg/kg/min, and 10 μg/kg/min for patients with distributive shock. If the desired therapeutic effect is not achieved with a dosage of 20 μg/kg/min, it is unlikely that further increases in infusion rate will be beneficial and epinephrine or norepinephrine should be added depending upon evaluation of hemodynamic abnormalities.

In patients with distributive shock associated with significant hypotension, low systemic vascular resistance, and elevated or normal cardiac output (warm shock), *norepinephrine* is an appropriate vasopressor to choose (185,186). Norepinephrine acts upon the α_1 and β_1 receptors. It increases systemic vascular resistance, blood pressure, and tissue perfusion without a major increase in heart rate. The improvement in blood pressure and renal perfusion often leads to an increase in urine output. The starting dosage of norepinephrine in the treatment of distributive shock is 0.1 μg/kg/min and the infusion is titrated to desired effect.

Arginine vasopressin has found a role as a vasopressor agent in recent years because its effect does not depend on the α receptor, and efficacy is not limited by downregulation of the α receptor (187,188). Likewise, vasopressin does not stimulate the β1 receptor and therefore does not increase myocardial oxygen consumption, as does norepinephrine. An initial dose of 0.5 milliunit/kg/min of arginine vasopressin has been effective and may be titrated up or down to effect.

Myocardial dysfunction without hypotension may be treated with dopamine, dobutamine, or milrinone. When myocardial dysfunction is complicated by hypotension or is unresponsive to dopamine, dobutamine, or milrinone, then epinephrine should be employed. Nitroprusside may be used in combination with dobutamine or epinephrine, as adjunctive afterload reducing therapy for patients with hypertension or elevated systemic vascular resistance.

Dobutamine is thought to act as a β_1-adrenergic agonist, increasing stroke volume, stroke work, and cardiac index (189). Dobutamine should be started at 5–10 μg/kg/min and increased as necessary to 20–30 μg/kg/min. For patients who require afterload-reducing therapy, nitroprusside may be added at a dosage of 0.5 μg/kg/min and titrated to effect.

Milrinone produces improvement in cardiac performance by increasing the inotropic state of the heart and by reducing afterload. Treatment may be initiated with a loading dose of 50–75 μg/kg over 5 min, followed by a continuous infusion of 0.5–0.75 μg/kg/min (some practitioners have employed dosages up to 1.0 μg/kg/min). In patients with unstable blood pressure, the loading dose may be omitted (190).

Epinephrine is used in the treatment of cardiogenic shock that is refractory to therapy with dopamine, dobutamine, or milrinone. It is also indicated in the treatment of septic shock with myocardial dysfunction (formerly called cold shock). The starting dosage is 0.05–0.1 μg/kg/min. Activation of β_1 receptors produces an increase in stroke volume, heart rate, and cardiac index. At low dosage (generally less than 0.2 μg/kg/min), epinephrine activates β_2 receptors, relaxing vascular smooth muscle and lowering systemic vascular resistance. As the dosage of epinephrine is increased, cardiac performance continues to improve, and α_1 receptors are stimulated, leading to a net increase in vascular tone. At high dosages (0.5–1.0 μ/kg/min or more) epinephrine produces severe vasoconstriction, increased systemic vascular resistance and compromised blood flow to renal and peripheral vascular beds.

VI. THE NEUROSURGICAL ONCOLOGY PATIENT

A. Introduction

Tumors of the CNS are the most common solid tumors in the pediatric population. Children with CNS masses are admitted to the PICU before and after surgery. Other frequent neurologic and neurosurgical emergencies in pediatric oncology patients include acute alterations in mental status, signs and symptoms of increased intracranial pressure or herniation, ventriculoperiotoneal (VP) shunt infection or malfunction, seizures and status epilepticus, and spinal cord compression syndromes. It is common for central nervous system neoplasms to present with subacute onset of neurologic abnormalities, leading to PICU admission. Acute changes in mental status in the oncology patient can be secondary to CNS infection, mass effect or chemotherapy-related toxicities. Respiratory and autonomic insufficiency related to progression of brain stem tumors is another, more unfortunate reason for admission to the PICU.

B. Monitoring in Neurointensive Care

1. *Continuous Electroencephalography*

Neurointensive care monitoring includes the use of electroencephalography (EEG) and intracranial pressure monitoring (191,192). With the recognition that decreased levels of consciousness can be related to nonconvulsive status epilepticus, the use of one-time and continuous EEG has assumed greater importance (193–195). Continuous EEG monitoring aids in the titration of anticonvulsant medications in refractory status epilepticus.

2. *Intracranial Pressure Monitoring*

Measurement of intracranial pressure (ICP) is indicated when elevation in ICP is suspected based upon the presence of clinical signs of intracranial hypertension (dilating pupil, hypertension with bradycardia). In addition, customary indications for placing an ICP monitor in oncology patients include meningitis or meningoencephalitis with evidence of progressive neurologic injury and elevated ICP, acute obstructive hydrocephalus, and intracranial hemorrhage with elevated ICP (196). Although several indirect indicators of ICP are used (CT scan, palpation of anterior fontanelle), there is no procedure or test that substitutes for actual measurement of pressure. Intracranial pressure monitoring is not, at present, indicated in the management of global cerebral hypoxic ischemic injury. Although elevations of ICP are often present in this context, treatment directed at controlling ICP has not been demonstrated to improve long-term neurologic outcome.

Pediatric brain tumors, especially those of the posterior fossa, may present with hydrocephalus that requires emergent ventriculostomy and placement of an externalized ventricular drain (EVD). The management of increased intracranial pressure with external ventricular drainage often relieves many of the presenting symptoms, permits a systematic approach to the patient's disease, and avoids an emergent surgical procedure. Following surgical resection, patients may return from the OR to the PICU with a ventriculostomy in place for monitoring pressure and to provide early recognition of postoperative hydrocephalus. An EVD may also be left in place to assess the effectiveness of an endoscopic third ventriculostomy. The presence of a drain serves to decompress the operative bed and permit wound healing without the development of a CSF leak.

Several techniques are available for monitoring intracranial pressure (197). Historically, the two most frequently employed devices have been the intraventricular catheter and the subarachnoid (Philadelphia bolt, Richmond screw) bolt. In current practice, parenchymal fiber optic devices (Camino) are available that do not require ventricular placement. There are also devices available with both fiber optic pressure monitoring and ventricular drainage capabilities. In most circumstances, we favor use of an intraventricular device. Placement of a catheter not only provides continuous information regarding intraventricular pressure, but also permits drainage of cerebrospinal fluid as the foundation of management of increased intracranial pressure. Relative contraindications are thrombocytopenia and coagulopathy. With the use of a guide developed by Ghajar (198), these catheters can be placed at the bedside even when compressed "slit-like" ventricles are present. Complication rates of ICP monitoring, including hemorrhage are low (199). The general goal of therapy of elevated ICP in children is to prevent the pressure from exceeding 20–25 mmHg, and to maintain the cerebral perfusion pressure greater than 50 mmHg.

The watchword in postoperative neurosurgical care is diligent longitudinal assessment of the neurologic exam in close coordination with the neurosurgical team (196,200). Pediatric patients with newly discovered CNS neoplasms may be admitted to the PICU for close observation, initiation of corticosteroid therapy, and, in some cases, placement of an EVD to relieve acute hydrocephalus. Dexamethasone at a dose of 0.1–0.5 mg/kg IV every 6 hr is generally initiated for tumor-associated edema (201,202). For acute worsening of neurologic condition, dexamethasone may be administered in increasing amounts up to a 2 mg/kg bolus followed by 2 mg/kg/day in divided doses. Further neurointensive care interventions including tracheal intubation to gain airway and ventilatory control, placement of EVD to relieve hydrocephalus, and mannitol can help to stabilize the failing brain tumor patient preoperatively (203). In many cases, these interventions will prevent the need to perform emergency surgery. Although the use of steroids may provide significant relief of symptoms related to tumor-related edema, the potential side effects including gastrointestinal bleeding, steroid-induced myopathy, and altered immunologic function must be kept in mind and the lowest possible effective dose should be used. It is routine to begin gastrointenstinal bleeding prophylaxis with an H2-receptor antagonist or a proton pump inhibitor at the time steroid therapy is initiated.

After some neurosurgical procedures, the patient may remain in the PACU for monitoring in close proximity to the operating room. This is done so that the patient can be returned to the OR rapidly to treat acute neurologic deterioration, drain malfunctions or unexpected significant increases in intracranial pressure. In some cases, the surgical team will take the patient for immediate postoperative imaging and return the patient to the PACU for emergence from anesthesia.

A smooth emergence from anesthesia without coughing, gagging, or vomiting is desirable in neurosurgical patients. Coughing and agitation both cause increase in intracranial pressure that can result in leakage of CSF and blood through areas where the dura was incised, manipulated, and reopposed (204). The effort to obtain a smooth extubation by performing the extubating in a partially anesthetized patient must be counterbalanced by the imperative to avoid hypoventilation and resultant hypercarbia. Hypercarbia causes cerebral vasodilatation, which results in an increase in cerebral blood flow and may result in elevated intracranial pressure.

C. Perioperative Hypertension in the Neurosurgical Patient

Intraoperative and perioperative hypertension are common in neurosurgical patients. Although hypertension may be related to pain or agitation, other etiologies must be considered. Normally, cerebral blood flow remains relatively constant within the mean blood pressure range of 50–150 mmHg due to cerebral blood flow autoregulation (197). However, autoregulation may be temporarily disrupted after craniotomy and increases in mean arterial pressure may be associated with significant increases in cerebral blood flow and intracranial pressure. Elevated ICP and increased cerebral blood flow produce a risk of bleeding into the operative bed (a closed space), and a risk of CSF leak through the incision site as well. CSF leaks do not generally close spontaneously, and if persistent and untreated, increase the risk of postoperative meningitis. It is of paramount importance to know if postoperative hypertension is due to the loss of cerebral autoregulation or is an appropriate compensatory response to increased or rising ICP secondary to cerebral edema or bleeding. In the latter situation, antihypertensive treatment without first addressing the elevated ICP would compromise cerebral perfusion and could be disastrous for the patient. Most neurosurgical oncology patients do not return to the PICU with ICP monitors so the caregiver must rely on the neurologic examination and imaging.

Hypertension due to loss of cerebral autoregulation in the pediatric neurosurgical patient can be managed with one of several pharmacologic modalities (205–207). Intravenous agents that can be used judiciously to control blood pressure include labetalol and nitroprusside. Although the use of these agents in pediatric hypertension is well described, there is limited published information analyzing efficacy and safety in postneurosurgical hypertension in children. Nitroprusside is a balanced arterial and venodilator with a short duration of action, which when administered by continuous infusion provides for facile titration of the blood pressure. Although a very potent agent, the short elimination half-life provides a significant safety advantage over longer acting agents. Accurate and continuous blood pressure measurements are best obtained with arterial catheter monitoring in neurosurgical patients in whom nitroprusside and other potent antihypertensive agents are employed. Nitroprusside is administered by continuous IV infusion starting at a dose of 0.3–0.5 μg/kg/min and increased as necessary to as high as 8–10 μg/kg/min. The use of nitroprusside for prolonged periods of time or in patients with impaired renal function may result in a significant accumulation of cyanide, thiocyanate, and methemoglobin.

Labetalol, an alpha- and beta-blocking agent, has a longer half-life than nitroprusside and can be administered either intermittently or by continuous infusion. Labetalol is the agent used most frequently in our center intraoperatively for the management of neurosurgical hypertension and it is continued, when necessary, in the PICU. Labetalol lowers blood pressure within 5–10 min after intravenous administration. The beta- and alpha-receptor blocking effects of labetalol are in the ratio of approximately 3:1. Labetalol is not as potent a vasodilator as nitroprusside, and the reflex tachycardia induced by the vasodilation is tempered by its beta-adrenergic blocking activity. It can be used safely and effectively within a wide range of renal function(208). Labetalol has been demonstrated to have favorable effects on ICP and cerebral perfusion pressure in adults (209). A disadvantage of labetalol is the possible exacerbation of bronchospasm in patients with asthma. The use of a beta-blocker in patients who have received significant doses of cardiotoxic chemotherapy is also a concern. Labetalol is administered in dosages of 0.2–1.0 mg/kg every 10 min until the blood pressure is controlled or by continuous IV infusion of 0.25–3.0 mg/kg/hr. If necessary, labetalol can be transitioned from IV to an oral formulation.

In the event of severe postoperative hypertension or when there are contraindications to the use of nitroprusside and labetalol, nicardipine is an appropriate alternative agent. Nicardipine is a dihydropyridine calcium channel blocker that is administered by continuous IV infusion. Nicardipine has been used safely and effectively in the management of hypertension in adult patients recovering from craniotomy for tumor surgery (210). It has been shown to lower blood pressure safely and effectively in pediatric patients with a wide range of diagnoses and degrees of renal function (211–214). Although concerns exist regarding the potential for elevated ICP related to its use, no increases were seen in pediatric patients with ICP monitors in place when nicardipine was used (215–217). Recommended starting dosages are 0.5–1.0 μg/kg/min with upward titration to a maximum dose of 3.0 μg/kg/min. Significant side effects include flushing, tachycardia, thrombophlebitis, and hypotension.

D. Fluid Balance and Electrolyte Abnormalities in Neurosurgical Patients

Abnormalities in water and electrolyte balance that follow neurosurgery and specifically brain tumor resection can present a significant challenge to clinicians charged with caring for the patient in the perioperative setting. In a retrospective analysis of 122 children operated on for various brain tumors, abnormalities of water homeostasis were seen in 15 patients (12%). Of these 15 cases, 10 manifested diabetes insipidus (DI) with or without the syndrome of inappropriate antidiuretic hormone secretion (SIADH) and SIADH alone was seen in five patients (218).

In order to avoid hyponatremia and possible exacerbation of neuronal and cerebral edema, efforts are made to minimize free water intake during and after neurosurgical procedures. Normal saline or normal saline with 5% dextrose is administered perioperatively at a rate equal to two-thirds of the calculated maintenance requirement (219). At the same time that free water is minimized, efforts are made to insure that the intravascular volume is adequate to provide appropriate tissue perfusion and nutrient delivery. Inappropriate dehydration can be as deleterious as free water overload. In the course of postoperative care it is important to follow and address alterations in serum sodium.

E. Diabetes Insipidus

Central DI is a known complication of resection of intracranial tumors. The resection of tumors involving the hypothalamic–pituitary region of the brain (craniopharyngioma and germinoma) is the most common cause of DI in the pediatric neurosurgical population. In a retrospective review of 39 children who underwent resection of craniopharyngioma, 94% of patients without preoperative evidence of DI developed DI either intra- or immediately postoperatively (220). Diabetes insipidus, caused by the inability of the hypothalamus to secrete adequate amounts of arginine vasopressin (antidiuretic hormone, ADH), is manifested by the production of large quantities of dilute urine ($SG < 1.005$) with a concomitant rise in serum sodium. In a patient with an intact thirst mechanism and availability of sufficient liquids, serum chemistries often remain relatively normal. In patients who are intubated and obtunded or are otherwise unable to drink, DI will, if unchecked, result in severe intravascular volume depletion and complications associated with a hyperosmolar state. Attempts at management using equal volume replacement of urine output with 5% dextrose in water (D5W) as a source of free water may result in acceptable serum electrolytes. However, the amount of dextrose administered often causes hyperglycemia, producing an additional source of free water loss through osmotic diuresis. The treatment of choice for central DI is replacement of ADH, which can be done by the IV, SQ, enteral, or intranasal routes. In the perioperative period, safe and effective control of DI can be obtained by a continuous infusion of aqueous vasopressin starting at 0.5 milliunits/kg/min with titration upward or downward based on serum sodium, serum osmolality, and the urine output (221,222). The major advantage of a continuous infusion is that it provides for a carefully titratable response. Associated with treatment is the risk of transitioning the patient from DI to hyponatremia and water intoxication if the response to vasopressin is too vigorous or if the DI resolves (223). Coexistence of adrenal corticotropic hormone (ACTH) deficiency and partial ADH deficiency may clinically mask polyuria as cortisol is required for free water excretion. Following corticosteroid treatment with dexamethasone for postsurgical edema, partial DI can become manifest (224). Once the extent and permanence of the DI is known, the patient can be transitioned to intranasal or oral vasopressin.

F. Hyponatremia

Hyponatremia in the postoperative neurosurgical patient can be a result of excessive free water administration, SIADH, excessive administration of vasopressin or the controversial entity of cerebral salt wasting (CSW). Although any postoperative patient is at risk for hyponatremia from third space losses this is more likely to occur following major abdominal surgery as compared with neurosurgery. The feared consequence of hyponatremia in the neurosurgical patient is influx of water into the intracellular space, resulting in cellular swelling, diffuse cerebral edema, and encephalopathy. As mentioned above, administration of free water is to be avoided in the perioperative neurosurgical patient. Management includes the use of isotonic IV fluids and avoidance of IV fluids or medications in hypoosmolar solution. Administration of exogenous vasopressin can result in accumulation of free water and result in hyponatremia. Postoperative DI may resolve spontaneously after 3–5 days, be persistent, be followed by SIADH, which then resolves (biphasic pattern), or be followed by SIADH and then return of DI (triphasic pattern) (218). The resolution of DI or transitioning into SIADH from DI puts the patient at risk for hyponatremia, especially when vasopressin administration is continued.

Syndrome of inappropriate antidiuretic hormone secretion can occur in many clinical scenarios in children, especially when the central nervous system is affected (225). Syndrome of inappropriate antidiuretic hormone secretion is caused by elevated ADH secretion in the absence of a hyperosmotic state or hypovolemia. The biochemical characteristics of SIADH are low plasma osmolality (urine to plasma osmolality ratio > 1), hyponatremia with urine sodium concentration > 20 mmol/L, and low to normal values for plasma renin activity, hematocrit, urea, and uric acid concentrations. The overall volume status of the patient is normal to slightly increased. Fluid restriction is the hallmark of management of SIADH and is successful by itself in most mild to moderate cases. If the serum sodium continues to drop in the face of fluid restriction or if the patient becomes symptomatic due to hyponatremia, more aggressive interventions including elimination of all free water, loop diuretics, and administration of hypertonic saline are useful. Hyponatremic seizures can be treated safely with an IV bolus of 4–6 mL/kg of 3% saline, which will increase the serum sodium 4–6 mmol/L and effectively stop the seizures (226). An alternative to bolus therapy is to infuse 3% saline (500 mmol/L) at 1–2 mL/kg/hr (0.5–1 mmol/kg/hr) for 2–3 hr, followed by conservative measures to limit the rate of correction to less than 12 mmol/L/day (224). Assuming that total body water comprises 50% of total body weight, 1 mL/kg of 3% sodium chloride in water will raise the plasma sodium by about 1 mmol/L. Excessively rapid correction of hyponatremia is associated with central pontine myelinolysis.

G. Cerebral Salt Wasting

Cerebral salt wasting (CWS) is described in patients in whom there is extracellular fluid depletion and hyponatremia caused by progressive natriuresis with concomitant diuresis. Cerebral salt wasting is frequently described in the literature, but remains controversial with respect to its actual incidence (227,228). The main biochemical findings in CSW are low serum osmolality with high urine osmolality (urine to serum osmolality ratio > 1), hyponatremia with urine sodium concentration greater than 20 mmol/L, a normal to high hematocrit, and elevated blood urea concentration. Cerebral salt wasting is also associated with a normal serum uric acid level and a plasma renin activity that can be normal, elevated, or low. It has been hypothesized that secretion of atrial natriuretic peptide may be responsible for CWS. In practice, the difference between CWS and SIADH is that intravascular volume is normal or expanded in SIADH and contracted in CSW. Clinical signs of dehydration and a low or dropping central venous pressure in the presence of diuresis and high urine sodium concentration support the diagnosis of CSW. The importance of distinguishing CSW from SIADH lies in the management. In patients with SIADH, water intake must be restricted, while in those with CSW extracellular volume must be restored. Management of CSW includes replacement of the extracellular volume deficit along with urinary sodium losses (229). As in other cases of hyponatremia, a slow increase in plasma sodium is desirable for the nonsymptomatic patient.

VII. CONCLUSION

In this chapter, an effort has been made to summarize some of the many issues confronting the team caring for a pediatric oncology patient in the perioperative setting.

REFERENCES

1. Hallahan AR, Shaw PJ, Rowell G, O'Connell A, Schell D, Gillis J. Improved outcomes of children with malignancy admitted to a pediatric intensive care unit. Crit Care Med 2000; 28(11):3718–3721.
2. Heying R, Schneider DT, Korholz D, Stannigel H, Lemburg P, Gobel U. Efficacy and outcome of intensive care in pediatric oncologic patients. Crit Care Med 2001; 29(12):2276–2280.
3. van Veen A, Karstens A, van der Hoek AC, Tibboel D, Hahlen K, van der Voort E. The prognosis of oncologic patients in the pediatric intensive care unit. Intensive Care Med 1996; 22(3):237–241.
4. Ben Abraham R, Toren A, Ono N, Weinbroum AA, Vardi A, Barzilay Z, Paret G. Predictors of outcome in the pediatric intensive care units of children with malignancies. J Pediatr Hematol Oncol 2002; 24(1): 23–26.
5. Maxwell LG, Yaster M. Perioperative management issues in pediatric patients. Anesthesiol Clin North Am 2000; 18:601–632.
6. Meyer-Pahoulis E, Williams SL, Davidson SI, McVey JR, Mazurek A. The pediatric patient in the post anesthesia care unit. Nurs Clin North Am 1993; 28:519–530.
7. American Academy of Pediatrics Committee on Hospital Care. Guidelines and levels of care for pediatric intensive care units. Crit Care Med 1993; 21:1077–1086.
8. Anand KJS, Hopkins SE, Wright JA, et al. Statistical models to predict the need for postoperative intensive care and hospitalization in pediatric surgery patients. Intensive Care Med 2001; 27:873–883.
9. Jaimovich DG, Hauser GJ, Witte MK, et al. Guidelines for developing admission and discharge policies for the pediatric intensive care unit. Crit Care Med 1999; 27:843–845.
10. Balis FM, Holcenberg JS, Blaney SM. General principles of chemotherapy. Pizzo PA, Poplack DG, eds. Principles and Practice of Pediatric Oncology. Philadelphia: Lippincott, 2002:237–308.
11. McDowall RH. Anesthesia for the pediatric patient. Chest Surg Clin North Am 1997; 7:831–868.
12. Lowrie L, Difiore JM, Martin RJ. Monitoring in pediatric and neonatal intensive care units. Tobin MJ, ed. Principles and Practice of Intensive Care Monitoring. New York: McGraw-Hill, 1998:1223–1235.
13. DeNicola LK, Kissoon N, Abram HS Jr, Sullivan KJ, Delgado-Corcoran C, Taylor C. Noninvasive monitoring in the pediatric intensive care unit. Pediatr Clin North Am 2001; 48:573–588.
14. Hess DR. Capnometry. In: Tobin MJ, ed. Principles and Practice of Intensive Care Monitoring. New York: McGraw-Hill, 1998:377–400.
15. Bhende MS. End-tidal carbon dioxide monitoring in pediatrics—clinical applications. J Postgrad Med 2001; 47:215–218.
16. Mason KP, Burrows PE, Dorsey MM, Zurakowski D, Krauss B. Accuracy of capnography with a 30 foot nasal cannula for monitoring respiratory rate and end-tidal CO2 in children. J Clin Monit Comput 2000; 16:259–262.
17. Morley TF, Giaimo J, Maroszan E, Bermingham J, Gordon R, Griesback R, Zappasodi SJ, Giudice JC. Use of capnography for assessment of the adequacy of alveolar ventilation during weaning from mechanical ventilation. Am Rev Respir Dis 1993; 148:339–344.
18. Hubble CL, Gentile MA, Tripp DS, Craig DM, Meliones JN, Cheifetz IM. Deadspace to tidal volume ratio predicts successful extubation in infants and children. Crit Care Med 2000; 28:2034–2040.
19. McQuillen KK, Steele DW. Capnography during sedation/analgesia in the pediatric emergency department. Pediatr Emerg Care 2000; 16:401–404.
20. Giantris A, Abdurrahman L, Hinkle A, Asselin B, Lipshultz SE. Anthracycline-induced cardiotoxicity in children and young adults. Crit Rev Oncol Hematol 1998; 27:53–68.
21. Tibby SM, Hatherill M, Durward A, et al. Are transesophageal Doppler parameters a reliable guide to pediatric hemodynamic status and fluid management? Intensive Care Med 2001; 27:201–205.
22. Mohan UR, Britto J, Habibi P, de MC, Nadel S. Noninvasive measurement of cardiac output in critically ill children. Pediatr Cardiol 2002; 23:58–61.
23. Wetzel RC, Tabata BK, Rogers MC. Hemodynamic monitoring considerations in pediatric critical care. In: Rogers MC, ed. Textbook of Pediatric Intensive Care. 2nd ed. Baltimore: Williams and Wilkins, 1992:614–635.

24. Greenwald BM, Ghajar J, Notterman DA. Critical care of children with acute brain injury. Adv Pediatr 1995; 42:47–89.
25. Greenwald BM, Notterman DA, DeBruin WJ, McCready M. Percutaneous axillary artery catheterization in critically ill infants and children. J Pediatr 1990; 117:442–444.
26. Blot F, Laplanche A, Raynard B, Germann N, Antoun S, Nitenberg G. Accuracy of totally implanted ports, tunnelled, single- and multiple-lumen central venous catheters for measurement of central venous pressure. Intensive Care Med 2000; 26:1837–1842.
27. Black IH, Blosser SA, Murray WB. Central venous pressure measurements: peripherally inserted catheters versus centrally inserted catheters. Crit Care Med 2000; 28:3833–3836.
28. Venkataraman ST, Orr RA, Thompson AE. Percutaneous infraclavicular subcalvian vein catheterization in critically ill infants and children. J Pediatr 1988; 113: 480–485.
29. O'Grady NP, Alexander M, Dellinger EP, Gerberding JL, Heard SO, Maki DG, Masur H, McCormick RD, Mermel LA, Pearson ML, Raad II, Randolph A, Weinstein RA. Guidelines for the prevention of intravascular catheter-related infections. Centers for Disease Control and Prevention. MMWR Recomm Rep 2002; 51(RR-10):1–29.
30. Garland JS, Henrickson K, Maki DG. 2002 Hospital Infection Control Practices Advisory Committee Centers for Disease Control and Prevention. The 2002 Hospital Infection Control Practices Advisory Committee Centers for Disease Control and Prevention guideline for prevention of intravascular device-related infection. Pediatrics 2002; 110: 1009–1013.
31. O'Grady NP, Alexander M, Dellinger EP, Gerberding JL, Heard SO, Maki DG, Masur H, McCormick RD, Mermel LA, Pearson ML, Raad II, Randolph A, Weinstein RA. Guidelines for the Prevention of Intravascular Catheter-Related Infections. Vol. 110. The Hospital Infection Control Practices Advisory Committee, Center for Disease Control and Prevention, U.S. Pediatrics, 2002:e51.
32. McGee DC, Gould MK. Current concepts: preventing complications of central venous catheterization. N Engl J Med 2003; 348:1123–1133.
33. Connors AF Jr, Speroff T, Dawson NV, Thomas C, Harrell FE Jr, Wagner D, Desbiens N, Goldman L, Wu AW, Califf RM, Fulkerson WJ Jr, Vidaillet H, Broste S, Bellamy P, Lynn J, Knaus WA. The effectiveness of right heart catheterization in the initial care of critically ill patients. SUPPORT Investigators. JAMA 1996; 276:889–897.
34. Connors AF Jr. Right heart catheterization: is it effective? New Horiz 1997; 5:195–200.
35. Thompson AE. Pulmonary artery catheterization in children. New Horiz 1997; 5:244–250.
36. Society of Critical Care Medicine, American College of Chest Physicians. Pulmonary artery catheter education project (PACEP). http://www.pacep.org.
37. Carcillo JA, Fields AI. Task Force Committee Members. Clinical practice parameters for hemodynamic support of pediatric and neonatal patients in septic shock. Crit Care Med 2002; 30:1365–1378.
38. Ceneviva G, Paschall JA, Maffei F, Carcillo JA. Hemodynamic support in fluid-refractory pediatric septic shock. Pediatrics 1998; 102:e19.
39. Elliott CG, Zimmerman GA, et al. Complications of pulmonary artery catheterization in the care of critically ill patients: a prospective study. Chest 1979; 76:647.
40. Smith-Wright DL, Green TP, Lock JE, et al. Complications of vascular catheterization in critically ill children. Crit Care Med 1984; 12:1015.
41. Markovitz BP, Randolph AG. Corticosteroids for the prevention and treatment of post-extubation stridor in neonates, children and adults. Cochrane Database Syst Rev 2000; 2:CD001000.
42. Gluck HE, Onorato DJ, Castriotta R. Helium–oxygen mixtures in intubated patients with status asthmaticus and respiratory acidosis. Chest 1990; 98:693–698.
43. Weber JE, Chudnofsky CR, Younger JG, Larkin GL, Boczar M, Wilkerson MD, Zuriekat GY, Nolan B, Eicke DM. A randomized comparison of helium–oxygen mixture (Heliox) and racemic epinephrine for the treatment of moderate to severe croup. Pediatrics 2001; 107(6):E96.
44. Bruppacher H, Reber A, Keller JP, Geidushek J, Erb TO, Frei FJ. The effects of common airway maneuvers on airway pressure and flow in children undergoing adenoidectomies. Anesth Analg 2003; 97:29–34.
45. Reber A, Paganoni R, Frei FJ. Effect of common airway manoeuvers on upper airway dimensions and clinical signs in anaesthetized, spontaneously breathing children. Br J Anaesth 2001; 86:217–222.
46. Chatmongkolchart S, Kacmarek RM, Hess DR. Heliox delivery with noninvasive positive pressure ventilation: a laboratory study. Respir Care 2001; 46(3):248–254.
47. McDowall RH, Scher CS, Barst SM. Total intravenous anesthesia for children undergoing brief diagnostic or therapeutic procedures. J Clin Anesth 1995; 7: 273–280.
48. Guldner G, Schultz J, Sexton P, Fortner C, Richmond M. Etomidate for rapid-sequence intubation in young children: hemodynamic effects and adverse events. Acad Emerg Med 2003; 10:134–139.
49. Gluth MB, Maska S, Nelson J, Otto RA. Postoperative management of pediatric tracheostomy: results of a nationwide survey. Otolaryngol Head Neck Surg 2000; 122:701–705.
50. Freud E, Ben-Ari J, Schonfeld T, Blumenfeld A, Steinberg R, Dlugy E, Yaniv I, Katz J, Schwartz M, Zer M. Mediastinal tumors in children: a single institution experience. Clin Pediatr 2002; 41:219–223.

51. Shamberger RC, Holzman RS, Griscom NT, Tarbell NJ, Weinstein HJ. CT quantitation of tracheal cross-sectional area as a guide to the surgical and anesthetic management of children with anterior mediastinal masses. J Pediatr Surg 1991; 26:138–142.
52. Shamberger RC, Holzman RS, Griscom NT, Tarbell NJ, Weinstein HJ, Wohl ME. Prospective evaluation by computed tomography and pulmonary function tests of children with mediastinal masses. Surgery 1995; 118:468–471.
53. Azizkhan RG, Dudgeon DL, Buck JR, Colombani PM, Yaster M, Nichols D, Civin C, Kramer SS, Haller JA Jr. Life-threatening airway obstruction as a complication to the management of mediastinal masses in children. J Pediatr Surg 1985; 20:816–822.
54. Benumof JL, Alfery DD. Anesthesia for thoracic surgery. In: Miller RD, ed. Anesthesia. Vol 2. 5th ed. Philadelphia: Churchill Livingstone, 2000:1736–1738.
55. Polaner DM. The use of heliox and the laryngeal mask airway in a child with an terior mediastinal mass. Anesth Analg 1996; 82:208–210.
56. Wallen E, Venkataraman ST, Grosso MJ, Kiene K, Orr RA. Intrahospital transport of critically ill pediatric patients. Crit Care Med 1995; 23:1588–1595.
57. Dockery WK, Futterman C, Keller SR, Sheridan MJ, Aki BF. A comparison of manual and mechanical ventilation during pediatric transport. Crit Care Med 1999; 27:802–806.
58. Venkataraman ST. Intrahospital transport of critically ill children—should we pay attention? Crit Care Med 1999; 27:694–695.
59. Deakers TW, Reynolds G, Stretton M, Newth CJ. Cuffed endotracheal tubes in pediatric intensive care. J Pediatr 1994; 125:57–62.
60. Tobias JD. Noninvasive ventilation using bilevel positive airway pressure to treat impending respiratory failure in the postanesthesia care unit. J Clin Anesth 2000; 12:409–412.
61. Fortenberry JD, Del Toro J, Jefferson LS, Evey L, Haase D. Management of pediatric acute hypoxemic respiratory insufficiency with bilevel positive pressure (BiPAP) nasal mask ventilation. Chest 1995; 108:1059–1064.
62. Roberts JS, Bratton SL, Brogan TV. Efficacy and complications of percutaneous pigtail catheters for thoracostomy in pediatric patients. Chest 1998; 114:1116–1121.
63. Bishop NB, Pon S, Ushay HM, Greenwald BM. Alteplase in the treatment of complicated parapneumonic effusion: a case report. Pediatrics 2003; 111:e188–e190.
64. Venkataraman ST, Orr RA. Mechanical ventilation and respiratory care. In: Fuhrman BP, Zimmerman JJ, eds. Pediatric Critical Care. 2nd ed. St. Louis: Mosby, 1998:538–561.
65. Martin LD, Rafferty JF, Walker LK, Gioia FR. Principles of respiratory support and mechanical ventilation. In: Rogers MC, ed. Textbook of Pediatric Intensive Care. 2nd ed. Baltimore: Williams and Wilkins, 1992:134–203.
66. Hemmila MR, Jirschl RB. Advnances in ventilatory support of the pediatric surgical patient. Curr Opin Pediatr 1999; 11:241–248.
67. Hirschl RB. Mechanical ventilation in pediatric surgical disease. In: Ashcraft KW, ed. Pediatric Surgey. 2nd ed. Philadelphia: W.B. Saunders, 2000:72–94.
68. Tobin MJ. Advances in mechanical ventilation. N Engl J Med 2001; 344:1986–1996.
69. The Acute Respiratory Distress Syndrome Network. Ventilation with lower tidal volumes as compared with traditional tidal volumes for acute lung injury and the acute respiratory distress syndrome. N Engl J Med 2000; 342:1301–1308.
70. Mortola JP, Milic-Emili J, Noworaj A, et al. Muscle pressure and flow during expiration in infants. Am Rev Respir Dis 1984; 129:49–53.
71. Winnie GB. Preoperative and postoperative care. In: Loughlin GM, Eigen H, eds. Respiratory Disease in Children. Baltimore: Williams and Wilkins, 1994:805–812.
72. MacIntyre NR, Cook DJ, Ely EW Jr, Epstein SK, Fink JB, Heffner JE, Hess D, Hubmayer RD, Scheinhorn DJ, American College of Chest Physicians, American Association for Respiratory Care, American College of Critical Care Medicine. Evidence-based guidelines for weaning and discontinuing ventilatory support: a collective task force facilitated by the American College of Chest Physicians; the American Association for Respiratory Care; and the American College of Critical Care Medicine. Chest 2001; 120(6 suppl): 375S–395S.
73. Tobin MJ, Alex CG. Discontinuation of mechanical ventilation. In: Tobin MJ, ed. Principles and Practice of Mechanical Ventilation. New York: McGraw-Hill, 1994:1177–1206.
74. Randolph AG, Wypij D, Venkataraman ST, Hanson JH, Gedeit RG, Meert KL, Luckett PM, Forbes P, Lilley M, Thompson J, Cheifetz IM, Hibberd P, Wetzel R, Cox PN, Arnold JH, Pediatric Acute Lung Injury and Sepsis Investigators (PALISI) Network. Effect of mechanical ventilator weaning protocols on respiratory outcomes in infants and children: a randomized controlled trial. JAMA 2002; 288(20):2561–2568.
75. Schultz TR, Lin RJ, Watzman HM, Durning SM, Hales R, Woodson A, Francis B, Tyler L, Napoli L, Godinez RI. Weaning children from mechanical ventilation: a prospective randomized trial of protocol-directed versus physician-directed weaning. Respir Care 2001; 46:772–782.
76. Thiagarajan RR, Bratton SL, Martin LD, Brogan TV, Taylor D. Predictors of successful extubation in children. Am J Respir Crit Care Med 1999; 160:1562–1566.
77. Fink JB, Mahlmeister MJ. High-frequency oscillation of the airway and chest wall. Respir Care 2002; 47:797–807.
78. Flenady VJ, Gray PH. Chest physiotherapy for preventing morbidity in babies being extubated from mechanical ventilation. The Cochrane Database of Sysytematic Reviews 2002, Issue 2. Art. No: CD000283. DOI: 10. 1002/14651858. CD000283.

79. Marraro GA. Innovative practices of ventilatory support with pediatric patients. Pediatr Crit Care Med 2003; 4(1):8–20.
80. Arnold JH, Truog RD, Thompson JE, Fackler JC. High-frequency oscillatory ventilation in pediatric respiratory failure. Crit Care Med 1993; 21(2):272–278.
81. Priebe GP, Arnold JH. High-frequency oscillatory ventilation in pediatric patients. Respir Care Clin North Am 2001; 7(4):633–645.
82. Arnold JH, Anas NG, Luckett P, Cheifetz IM, Reyes G, Newth CJ, Kocis KC, Heidemann SM, Hanson JH, Brogan TV, Bohn DJ. High-frequency oscillatory ventilation in pediatric respiratory failure: a multicenter experience. Crit Care Med 2000; 28:3913–3919.
83. Arnold JH, Hanson JH, Toro-Figuero LO, Gutierrez J, Berens RJ, Anglin DL. Prospective, randomized comparison of high-frequency oscillatory ventilation and conventional mechanical ventilation in pediatric respiratory failure. Crit Care Med 1994; 22:1530–1539.
84. Slutsky AS, Drazen JM. Ventilation with small tidal volumes. N Engl J Med 2002; 347:630–631.
85. Derdak S. High-frequency oscillatory ventilation for acute respiratory distress syndrome in adult patients. Crit Care Med 2003; 31:S317–S323.
86. Singh JM, Stewart TE. High-frequency oscillatory ventilation in adults with acute respiratory distress syndrome. Curr Opin Crit Care 2003; 9(1):28–32.
87. Derdak S, Mehta S, Stewart TE, Smith T, Rogers M, Buchman TG, Carlin B, Lowson S, Granton J, Multicenter Oscillatory Ventilation For Acute Respiratory Distress Syndrome Trial (MOAT) Study Investigators. High-frequency oscillatory ventilation for acute respiratory distress syndrome in adults: a randomized, controlled trial. Am J Respir Crit Care Med 2002; 166:801–808.
88. Bohn D. Permissive hypoxemia and inhaled nitric oxide in ARDS. In: Randolph AG, ed. Current Concepts in Pediatric Critical Care—2003. Chicago: The Society of Critical Care Medicine, 2003:105–110.
89. Dobyns EL, Anas NG, Fortenberry JD, Deshpande J, Cornfield DN, Tasker RC, Liu P, Eells PL, Griebel J, Kinsella JP, Abman SH. Interactive effects of high-frequency oscillatory ventilation and inhaled nitric oxide in acute hypoxemic respiratory failure in pediatrics. Crit Care Med 2002; 30:2425–2429.
90. Mehta S, MacDonald R, Hallett DC, Lapinsky SE, Aubin M, Stewart TE. Acute oxygenation response to inhaled nitric oxide when combined with high-frequency oscillatory ventilation in adults with acute respiratory distress syndrome. Crit Care Med 2003; 31:383–389.
91. Rabkin DG, Sladen RN, DeMango A, Steinglass KM, Goldstein DJ. Nitric oxide for the treatment of post-pneumonectomy pulmonary edema. Ann Thorac Surg 2001; 72:272–274.
92. Reichenberger F, Habicht J, Kaim A, Dalquen P, Bernet F, Schlapfer R, Stulz P, Perruchoud AP, Tichelli A, Gratwohl A, Tamm M. Lung resection for invasive pulmonary aspergillosis in neutropenic patients with hematologic diseases. Am J Respir Crit Care Med 1998; 158:885–890.
93. Mathew P, Bozeman P, Krance RA, Brenner MK, Heslop HE. Brochiolitis obliterans organizing pneumonia (BOOP) in children after allogeneic bone marrow transplantation. Bone Marrow Transplant 1994; 13:221–223.
94. Ben-Ari J, Yaniv I, Nahun E, Stein J, Samra Z, Schonfeld T. Yield of bronchoalveolar lavage in ventilated and non-ventilated children after bone marrow transplantation. Bone Marrow Transplant 2001; 27:191–194.
95. Huaringa AJ, Leyva FJ, Signes-Costa J, Morice RC, Raad I, Darwish AA, Champlin RE. Bronchoalveolar lavage in the diagnosis of pulmonary complications of bone marrow transplant patients. Bone Marrow Transplant 2000; 25:975–979.
96. Kornecki A, Shemie SD. Open lung biopsy in children with respiratory failure. Crit Care Med 2001; 29: 1247–1250.
97. Bojko T, Notterman DA, Greenwald BM, DeBruin WJ, Magid MS, Godwin T. Acute hypoxemic respiratory failure in children following bone marrow transplantation: an outcome and pathologic study. Crit Care Med 1995; 23:755–759.
98. Jacobe SJ, Hassan A, Veys P, Mok Q. Outcome of children requiring admission to an intensive care unit after bone marrow transplantation. Crit Care Med 2003; 31(5):1299–1305.
99. Keenan HT, Bratton SL, Martin LD, Crawford SW, Weiss NS. Outcome of children who require mechanical ventilatory support after bone marrow transplantation. Crit Care Med 2000; 28:830–835.
100. Hayes C, Lush RJ, Cornish JM, et al. The outcome of children requiring admission to an intensive care unit following bone marrow transplantation. Br J Haematol 1998; 102:666–670.
101. Hagen SA, Craig DM, Martin PL, Plumer DD, Gentile MA, Schulman SR, Cheifetz IM. Mechanically ventilated pediatric stem cell transplant recipients: effect of cord blood transplant and organ dysfunction on outcome. Pediatr Crit Care Med 2003; 4:206–213.
102. O'Rourke PP, Stolar CJ, Zwischenberger JB, Snedecor SM, Bartlett RH. Extracorporeal membrane oxygenation: support for overwhelming pulmonary failure in the pediatric population. Collective experience from the extracorporeal life support organization. J Pediatr Surg 1993; 28:523–528.
103. Morton A, Dalton H, Kochanek P, Janosky J, Thompson A. Extracorporeal membrane oxygenation for pediatric respiratory failure: five-year experience at the University of Pittsburgh. Crit Care Med 1994; 22:1659–1667.
104. Green TP, Timmons OD, Fackler JC, Moler FW, Thompson AE, Sweeney MF. The impact of extracorporeal membrane oxygenation on survival in pediatric patients with acute respiratory failure. Pediatric Critical

Care Study Group. Crit Care Med 1996; 24:323–329.
105. Farmer DI, Cullen ML, Philippart AI, Rector FE, Klein MD. Extracorporeal membrane oxygenation as salvage in pediatric surgical emergencies. J Pediatr Surg 1995; 30:347–348.
106. Leahey AM, Bunin NJ, Schears GJ, Smith CA, Flake AW, Sullivan KE. Successful use of extracorporeal membrane oxygenation (ECMO) during BMT for SCID. Bone Marrow Transplant 1998; 21:839–840.
107. Linden V, Karlen J, Olsson M, Palmer K, Ehren H, Henter JI, Kalin M. Successful extracorporeal membrane oxygenation in four children with malignant disease and severe pneumocystis carinii pneumonia. Med Pediatr Oncol 1999; 32:35–31.
108. Tobias JD, Oakes L, Rao B. Continuous epidural anesthesia for postoperative analgesia in the pediatric oncology patient. Am J Pediatr Hematol Oncol 1992; 14:216–221.
109. Lieh-Lai MW, Kauffman RE, Uy HG, Danjin M, Simpson PM. A randomized comparison of ketorolac tromethamine and morphine for postoperative analgesia in critically ill children. Crit Care Med 1999; 27:2786–2791.
110. Houck CS, Wilder RT, McDermott JS, Sethna NF, Berde CB. Safety of intravenous ketorolac in children and cost savings with a unit dosing system. J Pediatr 1996; 129:292–296.
111. Burd RS, Tobias JD. Ketorolac for pain management after abdominal surgical procedures in infants. South Med J 2002; 95:331–333.
112. Forrest JB, Heitlinger EL, Revell S. Ketorolac for postoperative pain management in children. Drug Saf 1997; 16:309–329.
113. Tobias JD, Rasmussen GE. Pain management and sedation in the pediatric intensive care unit. Pediatr Clin North Am 1994; 41:1269–1292.
114. Cornfield DN, Tegtmeyer K, Nelson MD, Milla CE, Sweeney M. Continuous propofol infusion in 142 critically ill children. Pediatrics 2002; 110:1177–1181.
115. Anand KJ, Arnold JH. Opioid tolerance and dependence in infants and children. Crit Care Med 1994; 22:334–342.
116. Tobias JD. Tolerance, withdrawal, and physical dependency after long-term sedation and analgesia of children in the pediatric intensive care unit. Crit Care Med 2000; 28:2122–2132.
117. Fusaro F, Cecchetto G, Boglino C, Inserra A, Zanon GF, Giusti F, Dall'Igna P. Measures to prevent renal impairment after resection of retroperitoneal neuroblastoma. Pediatr Surg Int 2002; 18:388–391.
118. Merchant TE, Zelefsky MJ, Sheldon JM, LaQuaglia MP, Harrison LB. High-dose rate intraoperative radiation therapy for pediatric solid tumors. Med Pediatr Oncol 1998; 30:34–39.
119. Haas-Kogan DA, Fisch BM, Wara WM, Swift PS, Farmer DL, Harrison MR, Albanese C, Weinberg V, Matthay KK. Intraoperative radiation therapy for high-risk pediatric neuroblastoma. Int J Radiat Oncol Biol Phys 2000; 47:985–992.
120. Notterman DA. Pharmacology of the cardiovascular system. In: Fuhrman BP, Zimmerman JJ, eds. Pediatric Critical Care. 2nd, ed. St. Louis : Mosby, 1998: 329–346.
121. Stauser LM, Pruitt RD, Tobias JD. Initial experience with fenoldopam in children. Am J Ther 1999; 6: 283–288.
122. Mathur VS. The role of the DA1 receptor agonist fenoldopam in the management of critically ill, transplant, and hypertensive patients. Rev Cardiovasc Med 2003; 4:S35–S40.
123. Koch CA, Pacak K, Chrousos GP. Endocrine tumors. In: Pizzo PA, Poplack DG , ed. Principles and Practice of Pediatric Oncology. 4th ed. Philadelphia: Lippincott Williams & Wilkins, 2002:1115–1148.
124. Turner MC, Lieberman E, DeQuattro V. The perioperative management of pheochromocytoma in children. Clin Pediatr 1992; 31:583–589.
125. Hack HA. The perioperative management of children with phaeochromocytoma. Pediatr Anesth 2000; 10: 463–476.
126. Sendo D, Katsuura M, Akiba K, Yokoyama S, Tanabe S, Wakabayashi T, Sato S, Otaki S, Obata K, Yamagiwa I, Hayasaka K. Severe hypertension and cardiac failure associated with neuroblastoma: a case report. J Pediatr Surg 1996; 31:1688–1690.
127. Kain ZN, Shamberger RS, Holzman RS. Anesthetic management of children with neuroblastoma. J Clin Anesth 1993; 5:486–491.
128. Fujimura H, Kitamura S, Kawahara R, Takada Y, Ohnishi Y, Maeda L. Serum catecholamine concentrations and hemodynamics during operations on 23 children with neuoblastoma. Masui 1992; 41:919–924.
129. Haberkern CM, Coles PG, Morray JP, Kennard SC, Sawin RS. Intraoperative hypertension during surgical excision of neuroblastoma—case report and review of 20 years' experience. Anesth Analg 1992; 75:854–858.
130. Hébert PC, Wells G, Blajchman MA, Marshall J, Martin C, Pagliarello G, Tweeddale M, Schweitzer I, Yetisir E, The Transfusion Requirements in Critical Care Investigators for the Canadian Critical Care Trials Group. A multicenter, randomized, controlled clinical trial of transfusion requirements in critical care. N Engl J Med 1999; 340:409–417.
131. Goodman AM, Pollack MM, Patel KM, Luban NLC. Pediatric red blood cell transfusions increase resource use. J Pediatr 2003; 142:123–127.
132. Bratton SL, Annich GM. Packed red blood cell transfusions for critically ill pediatric patients: when and for what conditions? J Pediatr 2003; 142:95–97.
133. Bhatia C, Pratap U, Slavik Z. Octreotide therapy: a new horizon in treatment of iatrogenic chyloperitoneum. Arch Dis Child 2001; 85:234–235.
134. Rice HE, Caty MG, Glick PL. Fluid therapy in the pediatric surgical patient. Pediatr Clin North Am

1998; 45:719–727.
135. Rebollo MVB, Castillo-Duran CD, Lopez MT, Sanabria MS, Moraga FM, Castro F, Barrera FQ. Controlled study of early postoperative parenteral nutrition in children. J Pediatr Surg 1999; 34: 1330–1335.
136. Panadero E, Lopez-Herce J, Caro L, Sanchez A, Cueto E, Bustinza A, Moral R, Carrillo A, Sancho L. Transpyloric enteral feeding in critically ill children. J Pediatr Gastroenterol Nutr 1998; 26:43–48.
137. Lyons KA, Brilli RJ, Wieman RA, Jacobs BR. Continuation of transpyloric feeding during weaning of mechanical ventilation and tracheal extubation in children: a randomized controlled trial. J Parenter Enteral Nutr 2002; 26:209–213.
138. Joffe AR, Grant M, Wong B, Gresiuk C. Validation of a blind transpyloric feeding tube placement techique in pediatric intensive care: rapid, simple, and highly successful. Pediatr Crit Care Med 2000; 1:151–155.
139. DaSilva PS, Paulo CS, de Oloveira Iglesias SB, de Carvalho WB, Santana e Meneses F. Bedside transpyloric placement in the pediatric intensive care unit: a modified insufflation air technique. Intensive Care Med 2002; 28:943–946.
140. Krafte-Jacobs B, Persinger M, Carver J, Moore L, Brilli R. Rapid placement of transpyloric feeding tubes: a comparison of pH-assisted and standard insertion techniques in children. Pediatrics 1996; 98:242–248.
141. Dimand RJ, Veereman-Wauters G, Braner DA. Bedside placement of pH-guided transpyloric small bowel feeding tubes in critically ill infants and small children. J Parenter Enteral Nutr 1997; 21:112–114.
142. Notterman DA. Cardiovascular support—pharmacologic. In: Holbrook PR, ed. Textbook of Pediatric Critical Care. Philadelphia: W.B. Saunders, 1993:288–315.
143. Greenwald BM, Notterman DA. Care of the critically ill child. In: Groeger JS, ed. Critical Care of the Cancer Patient. 2nd. ed. St. Louis: Mosby Year Book, 1991:299–319.
144. Singal PK, Iliskovic N. Doxorubicin-induced cardiomyopathy. N Engl J Med 1998; 339:900–905.
145. Lefrak EA, Pitha J, Rosenheim S, et al. A clinicopathologic analysis of adriamycin cardiotoxicity. Cancer 1973; 32:302.
146. Minow RA, Benjamin RS, Lee ET, et al. Adriamycin cardiomyopathy—risk factors. Cancer 1977; 39:1397.
147. Zucchi R, Danesi R. Cardiac toxicity of antineoplastic anthracyclines. Curr Med Chem Anti-Cancer Agents 2003; 3:151–171.
148. Sorensen K, Levitt GA, Bull C, Dorup I, Sullivan ID. Late anthracycline cardiotoxicity after childhood cancer: a prospective longitudinal study. Cancer 2003; 97:1991–1998.
149. Wexler LH. Ameliorating anthracycline cardiotoxicity in children with cancer: clinical trials with dexrazoxane. Semin Oncol 1998; 25(4 suppl 10):86–92.
150. Kremer LC, van der Pal HJ, Offringa M, van Dalen EC, Voute PA. Frequency and risk factors of subclinical cardiotoxicity after anthracycline therapy in children: a systematic review. Ann Oncol 2002; 13:819–829.
151. Wurzel CL, Halom K, Feldman JG, Rubin LG. Infection rates of Broviac–Hickman catheters and implantable venous devices. Am J Dis Child 1988; 142: 536–540.
152. Fratino G, Molinari AC, Mazzola C, Giacchino M, Saracco P, Bertocchi E, Castagnola E. Prospective study of indwelling central venous catheter-related complications in children with Broviac or clampless valved catheters. J Pediatr Hematol Oncol 2002; 24:657–661.
153. Kutko MC, Calarco MP, Flaherty MB, Helmrich RF, Ushay HM, Pon S, Greenwald BM. Mortality rates in pediatric septic shock with and without multiple organ system failure. Pediatr Crit Care Med 2003; 4:333–337.
154. MacLean LD, Mulligan WG, McLean APH, et al. Patterns of septic shock in man—a detailed study of 56 patients. Ann Surg 1961; 166:544.
155. Parker MM, Parrillo JE. Septic shock: hemodynamics and pathogenesis. JAMA 1983; 250:3324.
156. Pollack MM, Fields AI, Ruttimann UE. Distributions of cardiopulmonary variables in pediatric survivors and nonsurvivors of septic shock. Crit Care Med 1985; 13:454.
157. Pollack MM, Fields AI, Ruttimann UE, et al. Sequential cardiopulmonary variables of infants and children in septic shock. Crit Care Med 1984; 12:554–559.
158. Pollack MM, Fields AI, Ruttimann UE. Distributions of cardiopulmonary variables in pediatric survivors and nonsurvivors of septic shock. Crit Care Med 1985; 13:454–459.
159. Monsalve F, Rucabado L, Salvador A, et al. Myocardial depression in septic shock caused by meningococcal infection. Crit Care Med 1984; 12:1021–1023.
160. Mercier JC, Beaufils F, Hartmann JF, et al. Hemodynamic patterns of meningococcal shock in children. Crit Care Med 1988; 16:27–33.
161. Simma B, Fritz MG, Trawoger R, et al. Changes in left ventricular function in shocked newborns. Intensive Care Med 1997; 23:982–986.
162. Walther FJ, Siassi B, Ramadan NA. Cardiac output in newborn infants with transient myocardial dysfunction. J Pediatr 1985; 107:781–785.
163. Ferdman B, Jureidini SB, Mink RB. Severe left ventricular dysfunction and arrhythmias as complication of gram positive sepsis: rapid recovery in children. Pediatr Cardiol 1998; 19:482–486.
164. Feltes TF, Pignatelli R, Kleinert S, et al. Quantitated left ventricular systolic mechanics in children with septic shock utilizing noninvasive wall stress analysis. Crit Care Med 1994; 22: 1647–1659.
165. Ceneviva G, Paschall JA, Maffei F, et al. Hemodynamic support in fluid refractory pediatric septic shock. Pediatrics 1998; 102:e19.
166. Carcillo JA. Pediatric septic shock and multiple organ failure. Crit Care Clin 2003; 19:413–440.

167. Alexander SW, Walsh TJ, Freifeld AG, Pizzo PA. Infectious complications in pediatric cancer patients. In: Pizzo PA, Poplack DG, eds. Principles and Practice of Pediatric Oncology. 4th ed. Philadelphia: Lippincott Williams & Wilkins, 2002:1239–1283.
168. Pizzo PA, Robichaud KJ, Gill FA, et al. Empiric antibiotic and antifungal therapy for cancer patients with prolonged fever and granulocytopenia. Am J Med 1982; 72:101.
169. Walsh TJ, Pappas P, Winston DJ, Lazarus HM, Petersen F, Raffalli J, Yanovich S, Stiff P, Greenberg R, Donowitz G, Schuster M, Reboli A, Wingard J, Arndt C, Reinhardt J, Hadley S, Finberg R, Laverdiere M, Perfect J, Garber G, Fioritoni G, Anaissie E, Lee J, National Institute of Allergy and Infectious Diseases Mycoses Study Group. Voriconazole compared with liposomal amphotericin B for empirical antifungal therapy in patients with neutropenia and persistent fever. N Engl J Med 2002; 346:225–234.
170. Hiemenz J, Skelton J, Pizzo A. Perspective on the management of catheter-related infections in cancer patients. Pediatr Infect Dis 1986; 5:6.
171. Press OW, Ramsey PG, Larsen EB, et al. Hickman catheter infections in patients with malignancies. Medicine 1984; 63:189.
172. Brilli RJ. The role of steroids, vasopressin, and activated protein C in the treatment of patients with sepsis. In: Randolph AG, ed. Current Concepts in Pediatric Critical Care—2003. Chicago: The Society of Critical Care Medicine, 2003:111–121.
173. Cooper MS, Stewart PM. Corticosteroid insufficiency in acutely ill patients. N Engl J Med 2003; 348: 727–734.
174. Marik PE, Zaloga GP. Adrenal insufficiency in the critically ill, a new look at an old problem. Chest 2002; 122:1784–1796.
175. Marik PE, Zaloga GP. Adrenal insufficiency during septic shock. Crit Care Med 2003; 31:141–145.
176. Kenyon N. Defining adrenal insufficiency in septic shock. Crit Care Med 2003; 31:321–323.
177. Annane D, Sebille V, Charpentier C, Bollaert P-E, Francois B, Korach J-M, Capellier G, Cohen Y, Azoulay E, Troche G, Chaumert-Riffaut P, Bellissant E. Effect of treatment with low doses of hydrocortisone and fludorcortisone on mortality in patients with septic shock. JAMA 2002; 288:862–871.
178. Shoemaker WC, Appel PL, Waxman K, et al. Clinical trial of survivors' cardiopulmonary patterns as therapeutic goals in critically ill postoperative patients. Crit Care Med 1982; 10:390.
179. Abraham E, Bland RD, Cobo JC, et al. Sequential cardiorespiratory patterns associated with outcome in septic shock. Chest 1984; 85:75.
180. Carcillo JA, Pollack MM, Ruttimann UE, et al. Sequential physiologic interactions in pediatric cardiogenic and septic shock. Crit Care Med 1989; 17:12.
181. Falk JL, Rackow EC, Weil MH. Colloid and crystalloid fluid resuscitation. In: Shoemaker WC, Ayres S, Grenvik A, et al., eds. Textbook of Critical Care. Philadelphia: W.B. Saunders Company, 1989:1055.
182. Rainey TG, English JF. Pharmacology of colloids and crystalloids. In: Chernow B, ed. The Pharmacologic Approach to the Critically Ill Patient. Baltimore: William and Wilkins, 1988:219.
183. Shoemaker WC. Diagnosis and treatment of shock and circulatory dysfunction. In: Shoemaker WC, Grenvik A, Ayres SM, Holbrook PR, eds.Textbook of Critical Care. 4th ed. Philadelphia: W.B. Saunders, 2000:92–114.
184. Cochrane Injuries Group Albumin Reviewers. Human albumin administration in critically ill patients: systematic review of randomized clinical trials. BMJ 1998; 317:235–240.
185. Desjars P, Pinaud M, Potel G, et al. A reappraisal of norepinephrine therapy in human septic shock. Crit Care Med 1987; 15:2.
186. Meadows D, Edwards D, Wilkins R, et al. Reversal of intractable septic shock with norepinephrine therapy. Crit Care Med 1988; 16:663.
187. Yunge M, Petros A. Angiotensin for septic shock unresponsive to noradrenaline. Arch Dis Child 2000; 82:388–389.
188. Rosenzweig EB, Starc TJ, Chen JM, Cullinane S, Timchak DM, Gersony WM, Landry DW, Galantowicz ME. Intravenous arginine–vasopressin in children with vasodilatory shock after cardiac surgery. Circulation 1999; 100(19 suppl):11182–11186.
189. Leier CV, Unverferth DV. Dobutamine. Ann Intern Med 1983; 99:4.
190. Barton P, Garcia J, Kouatli A, Kitchen L, Zorka A, Lindsay C, Lawless S, Giroir B. Hemodynamic effects of i.v. milrinone lactate in pediatric patients with septic shock. A prospective, double-blinded, randomized, placebo-controlled, interventional study. Chest 1996; 109:1302–1312.
191. Scheuer ML. Continuous EEG monitoring in the intensive care unit. Epilepsia 2002; 43(suppl 3): 114–127.
192. Claassen J, Mayer SA. Continuous electroencephalographic monitoring in neurocritical care. Curr Neurol Neurosci Rep 2002; 2(6):534–540.
193. Ruegg SJ, Dichter MA. Diagnosis and treatment of nonconvulsive status epilepticus in an intensive care unit setting. Curr Treat Options Neurol 2003; 5(2):93–110.
194. Filloux F, Dean JM, Kirsch JR. Monitoring the central nervous system. In: Rogers MC, eds. Textbook of Pediatric Intensive Care. 2nd ed. Baltimore: Williams and Wilkins, 1992:667–697.
195. Claassen J, Hirsch LJ, Emerson RG, Bates JE, Thompson TB, Mayer SA. Continuous EEG monitoring and midazolam infusion for refractory nonconvulsive status epilepticus. Neurology 2001; 57(6):1036–1042.
196. Greenwald BM, Ghajar J, Notterman DA. Critical care of children with acute brain injury. Adv Pediatr 1995; 42:47–87.

197. Dean JM, Rogers MC, Traystman RJ. Pathophysiology and clinical management of the intracranial vault. In: Rogers MC, ed. Textbook of Pediatric Intensive Care. Baltimore: Williams and Wilkins, 1992:639–666.
198. Ghajar JB. A guide for ventricular catheter placement. J Neurosurg 1985; 63:985.
199. Blaha M, Lazar D, Winn RH, Ghatan S. Hemorrhagic complications of intracranial pressure monitors in children. Pediatr Neurosurg 2003; 39(1):27–31.
200. Hammer GB, Krane EJ. Perioperative care of the neurosurgical pediatric patient. Int Anesthesiol Clin 1996; 34:55–71.
201. Strother DR, Pollack IF, Fisher PG, Hunter JV, Woo SV, Pomeroy SL, Rorke LB. Tumors of the central nervous system. In: Pizzo PA, Poplack DG, eds. Principles and Practice of Pediatric Oncology. 4th ed. Philadelphia: Lippincott, 2002:750–824.
202. Wen PY, Marks PW. Medical management of patients with brain tumors. Curr Opin Oncol 2002; 14:299–307.
203. Bilsky M, Posner JB. Inensive and postoperative care of intracranial tumors. In: Ropper AH, eds. Neurological and Neurosurgical Intensive Care. 3rd ed. New York: Raven Press, 1993:309–329.
204. Drummond JC, Patel PM. Neurosurgical anesthesia. In: Miller RD, eds. Anesthesia. 5th ed. Philadelphia: Churchill Livingstone, 2000:1895–1933.
205. Sinaiko A. Hypertension in children. N Engl J Med 1996; 335:1968–1973.
206. Fivush B, Neu A, Furth S. Acute hypertensive crises in children: emergencies and urgencies. Curr Opin Pediatr 1997; 9:233–236.
207. Temple ME, Nahata MC. Treatment of pediatric hypertension. Pharmacotherapy 2000; 20:140–150.
208. Bunchman TE, Lynch RE, Wood EG. Intravenously administered labetalol for treatment of hypertension in children. J Pediatr 1992; 120:140–144.
209. Orlowski JP, Shiesley D, Vidt DG, Barnett GH, Little JR. Labetalol to control blood pressure after cerebrovascular surgery. Crit Care Med 1988; 16:765–768.
210. Kross RA, Ferri E, Leung D, Pratila M, Broad C, Veronesi M, Melendez JA. A comparative study between a calcium channel blocker (nicardipine) and a combined α–β-blocker (labetalol) for the control of emergence hypertension during craniotomy for tumor surgery. Anesth Analg 2000; 91:904–909.
211. Flynn JT, Mottes TA, Brophy PD, Kershaw DB, Smoyer WE, Bunchman TE. Intravenous nicardipine for treatment of severe hypertension in children. J Pediatr 2001; 139:38–43.
212. Michael J, Groshong T, Tobias JD. Nicardipine for hypertensive emergencies in children with renal disease. Pediatr Nephrol 1998; 12:40–42.
213. Tenney F, Sakarcan A. Nicardipine is a safe and effective agent in pediatric hypertensive emergencies. Am J Kidney Dis 2000; 35:E20.
214. Tobias JD, Lowe S, Deshpande JK. Nicardipine: perioperative applications in children. Paediatr Anaesth 1995; 5:171–176.
215. Nishikawa T, Omote K, Namiki A, Takhashi T. The effects of nicardipine on cerebrospinal fluid pressure in humans. Anesth Analg 1986; 65:507–510.
216. Groshong T. Hypertensive crises in children. Pediatr Ann 1996; 25:368–376.
217. Tobias JD. Nicardipine to control mean arterial pressure in a pediatric intensive care unit population. Am J Anesthesiol 1996; 23:109–112.
218. Blumberg DL, Sklar CA, Wisoff J, David R. Abnormalities of water metabolism in children an adolescents following craniotomy for a brain tumor. Child Nerv Syst 1994; 10:505–508.
219. Moritz ML, Ayus JC. Prevention of hospital-acquired hyponatremia: a case for using isotonic saline. Pediatrics 2003; 111:227–230.
220. Lehrnbecher T, Muller-Scholden J, Danhauser-Leistner I, Sorensen N, von Stockhausen H-B. Perioperative fluid and electrolyte management in children undergoing surgery for craniopharyngioma. Child Nerv Syst 1998; 14:276–279.
221. Sklar CA. Diabetes insipidus. In: Zimmerman SS, Gildes JH, eds. Critical Care Pediatrics. Philadelphia: Saunders, 1985:249–256.
222. McDonald JA, Martha PM, Kerrigan J, Clarke WL, Rogol AD, Blizzard RM. Treatment of the young child with central diabetes insipidus. Am J Dis Child 1989; 143:201–204.
223. Rizzo V, Albanese A, Stanhope R. Morbidity and mortality associated with vasopressin replacement therapy in children. J Pediatr Endocrinol Metab 2001; 14:861–867.
224. Albanese A, Hindmarsh P, Stanhope R. Management of hyponatremia in patients with acute cerebral insults. Arch Dis Child 2001; 85:246–251.
225. Moritz ML, Ayus JC. Disorders of water metabolism in children: hyponatremia and hypernatremia. Pediatr Rev 2002; 23:371–379.
226. Sarnaik AP, Meert K, Hackbarth R, Fleischman L. Management of hyponatremic seizures in children with hypertonic saline: a safe and effective strategy. Crit Care Med 1991; 19:758–762.
227. Bussmann C, Bast T, Rating D. Hyponatremia in children with acute CNS disease: SIADH or cerebral salt wasting?. Child Nerv Syst 2001; 17:58–63.
228. Singh S, Bohn D, Carlotti APC, Cusimano M, Rutka JT, Halperin ML. Cerebral salt wasting: truths, fallacies, and challenges. Crit Care Med 2002; 30: 2575–2579.
229. Berkenbosch JW, Lentz CW, Jimenez DF, Tobias JD. Cerebral salt wasting syndrome following brain injury in three pediatric patients: suggestions for rapid diagnosis and therapy. Pediatr Neurosurg 2002; 36:75–79.

52

Pediatric Surgical Oncology

MARTIN L. BLAKELY
Division of Pediatric Surgery, The University of Tennessee Health Science Center, Memphis, Tennessee, U.S.A.

RICHARD J. ANDRASSY
The University of Texas, M.D. Anderson Cancer Center, Houston, Texas, U.S.A.

I. INTRODUCTION

Modern care of the pediatric oncology patient requires a multidisciplinary team approach. Depending on the specific diagnosis, the pediatric surgeon may have a primary role or a supportive role. In either case, surgical input is needed in almost all patients in order to provide optimal care.

Survival rates for children with many solid tumors have steadily increased over the past 3 decades, largely as a result of the multimodal approach to therapy (1). Improvements in the effectiveness of chemotherapy regimens and radiation therapy have allowed for more conservative, less mutilating surgical procedures to be utilized. There have also been direct improvements in surgical technique, e.g., improved methods of liver resection, chest wall reconstruction, use of newly available prosthetic devices, and utilization of minimally invasive surgical techniques for biopsy and resection of tumor masses. Improvements in all these areas have contributed to the improved outcome for pediatric oncology patients.

The purpose of this chapter is to review the various roles of the pediatric surgeon, depending on the specific diagnosis of the patient. In general, for nonsolid tumors, such as leukemia and lymphoma, duties of the pediatric surgeon include establishing vascular access for chemotherapy, obtaining tissue for biopsy with many lymphomas, and at times providing surgical care for complications of aggressive medical therapy, e.g., neutropenic colitis (typhlitis). Outside the scope of this chapter is pediatric surgeon involvement in benign hematologic conditions. An example is splenectomy for hereditary spherocytosis or other hematologic condition.

For solid tumors, primarily Wilms' tumor, neuroblastoma, sarcoma, germ cell tumors, and hepatoblastoma, the pediatric surgeon is critical in patient management throughout the patient's course, as will be reviewed in detail below.

II. SUPPORTIVE CARE FOR NON-SOLID TUMORS

The most common type of cancer in children and adolescents is leukemia, with acute lymphoblastic leukemia (ALL) accounting for 24% of all cancer in children aged 0–14 years (2). The pediatric surgeon's role in central nervous system (CNS) solid tumors is also supportive in nature. This is relevant because, CNS tumors combined with leukemias comprise 50% of all childhood cancer diagnosis, indicating the large number of patients in whom the pediatric surgical oncologist primarily provides supportive care.

For non-solid tumors, as well as many solid tumors, aggressive chemotherapy is the initial, and often, sole treatment modality. For children to receive long-term, uninterrupted chemotherapy, surgical vascular access is the preferred approach. Vascular access devices also provide a reliable means for frequent blood samples, administration of blood or blood products, routes for parenteral nutrition, as well as for antibiotics or intravenous fluids when needed. There are multiple central venous catheters available and proper selection depends on the therapeutic plan, duration of chemotherapy administration, age and size of the patient, and preferences of the patient and the parents. In general, central venous catheters used for oncology patients are external, tunneled catheters, or internal (subcutaneous) catheters known generally as "portacaths." Both catheter types typically require general anesthesia and have similar risk profiles as reviewed below. Another alternative is the peripherally inserted central catheter ("picc") that is typically performed by a dedicated nursing team at the bedside with local anesthesia, usually with conscious sedation. This catheter type has not been proved to be reliable in children due to difficulty in obtaining access, increased phlebitic changes due to small caliber peripheral veins, and other causes of dysfunction (3).

A large prospective study ($n = 1019$) from the Children's Cancer Study Group reported that 72% of central venous catheters were external and 28% were portacaths (4). Over time, however, portacaths have become increasingly utilized even for infants. Currently, at M.D. Anderson Cancer Center, totally implantable portacaths are utilized for the majority of patients. In infants, 4–5 French (Fr), low-profile ports are utilized. In older children and adolescents, 7 Fr ports are the most commonly used size. Advantages of totally implantable portacath include less restriction of physical activity (e.g., swimming), decreased catheter maintenance, improved cosmesis and body image, and potentially less risk for infection (5).

Despite their widespread use, complications related to any of these vascular access devices are not infrequent. The most common complications are infection and catheter-related sepsis, catheter thrombosis or occlusion, catheter dislodgment, and complications during insertion.

Infectious complications include both site-related infections (20–50% of all infectious complications) and catheter-related blood stream infections or bacteremia (6). Bacteremia is usually due to coagulase-negative staphylococci, but may also include other gram-positive organisms as well as gram-negative or fungal organisms. Factors that increase the infectious risk in children include neutropenia (<1000 absolute neutrophil count) and the failure to use prophylactic systemic antibiotics (6).

In addition to establishing vascular access for non-solid tumor pediatric oncology patients, pediatric surgeons at times play other important supporting roles. These activities include establishment of external feeding access (gastrostomy or jejunostomy) for patients unable to tolerate oral feeding; evaluation of abdominal pain, for example, secondary to chemotherapy-induced pancreatitis; and management of neutropenic entercolitis (typhlitis).

III. DIAGNOSIS OF SOLID TUMORS

The pediatric surgeon plays a critical role in establishing (or excluding) a definitive diagnosis for patients with solid tumors. The distribution of specific cancer diagnoses (Fig. 1) indicates that the most common solid tumor diagnosis is partly age-dependent. For younger children (<15 years of age), the most common non-CNS solid tumors are neuroblastoma, Wilms' tumor, non-Hodgkin's lymphoma, followed by soft tissue sarcomas [rhabdomyosarcoma (RMS) and nonrhabdosarcoma soft-tissue sarcoma] and more rare types (2). Among adolescents, germ-cell tumors, non-RMS soft-tissue sarcomas, non-Hodgkin's lymphoma, malignant melanoma, and thyroid cancers become more common.

Various biopsy techniques are available, each having advantages and disadvantages. These include fine-needle aspiration (FNA), core-needle biopsy, and minimally invasive (e.g., laparoscopic or thoracoscopic) directed biopsy. Consultation with other members of the multimodal team is very important in determining the optimal biopsy technique based on suspected histology and tumor site.

Advantages of FNA and core-needle biopsy include rapidity, the ability to do these in the outpatient clinic, radiology suite, or operating room, and their minimally invasive nature (1). Because several pediatric tumors have the histologic appearance of "small, round, blue-cell tumors," immunohistochemical staining may be required to make a definitive diagnosis. In 156 patients undergoing FNA biopsy at M.D. Anderson Cancer Center, a diagnosis was obtained in 90% of patients with solid tumors, but in only 47% of those with lymphoma (7). A negative biopsy result or insufficient tissue should be considered nondiagnostic and should be followed by open biopsy when clinical suspicion for malignancy is high. Core-needle

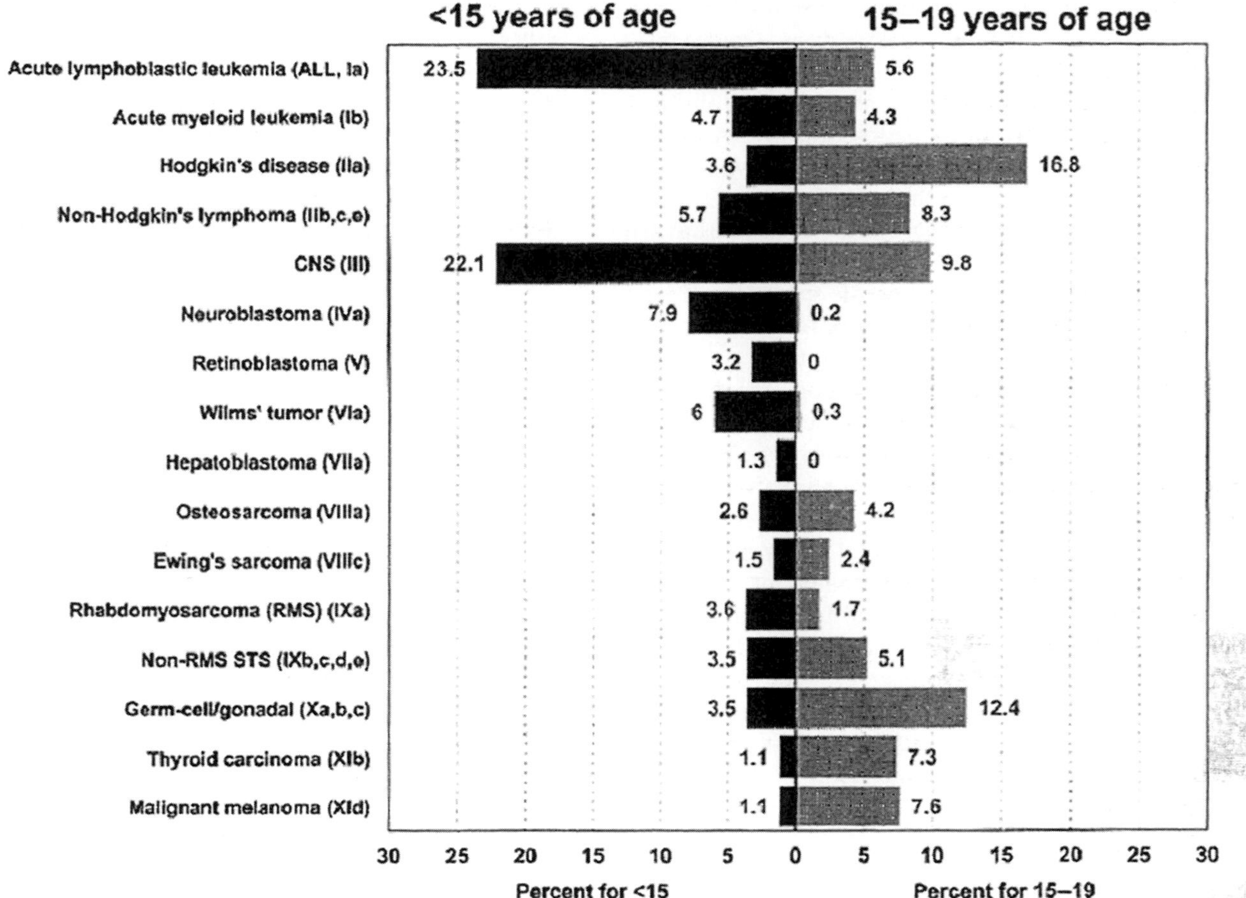

Figure 1 Distribution of specific cancer diagnosis for children (0–14 years) and adolescents (15–19 years), 1990–1997. Percent distribution by international classification of childhood cancer diagnostic groups and subgroups for, 15 years and 15–19 years of age (all cases and both sexes). CNS, central nervous system; RMS, rhabdomyosarcoma; STS, soft tissue sarcoma. (Incidence data are from the Surveillance, Epidemiology, and End Results Program, National Cancer Institute.)

biopsy may be performed in many of the same situations as FNA and can provide tissue with intact architecture that is helpful for pathologic evaluation.

Biopsy of any lesion may involve the need for reoperation and wide tumor excisions. Longitudinal incisions are preferred over transverse incisions, especially in extremities. This allows subsequent wide excision to include the initial biopsy site more easily, with a less invasive surgical approach.

More traditional solid tumor biopsy techniques include excisional biopsy, in which the entire tumor is included in the specimen, and incisional biopsies, in which only a portion of the tumor is included. With excisional biopsy, margins should be carefully marked to allow reresection should the biopsy reveal positive histologic margins. For large or invasive solid tumors, incisional biopsy is more appropriate.

Wilms' tumors (nephroblastoma) have traditionally been resected without biopsy, because it was believed that any breach of the tumor capsule would promote intraperitoneal spread. Effective chemotherapy makes this possibility lower, but this policy (no biopsy) continues because the likelihood of performing an unnecessary nephrectomy in this setting is very low. FNA, core-needle, or incisional biopsy is useful to confirm the diagnosis in patients with bilateral Wilms' tumors who will receive preoperative chemotherapy to allow for minimal resection, leaving enough residual kidney tissue to provide adequate renal function. The approach may also be utilized with massive unilateral Wilms' tumors thought to be unresectable with neoadjuvant chemotherapy.

The diagnosis of neuroblastoma is frequently established by urine or serum studies prior to any manipulation of the primary tumor. However, in other patients, biopsy is required to differentiate neuroblastoma from other abdominal or thoracic tumors.

The diagnosis of RMS is usually made by open, incisional biopsy, because no helpful serum markers or specific imaging studies are available. The pathologist is expected to identify the histologic subgroups of RMS to allow adequate staging, which, in turn, dictates therapeutic alternatives. Several grams of tissue are required for this, typically. Biopsies of genitourinary RMS are frequently done endoscopically. Although these are most commonly embryonal subtypes, large biopsies are still helpful to the pathologist.

The needle biopsies that are performed to establish the diagnosis of prostatic RMS are difficult to interpret and must include several core needle specimens. Trunk and extremity RMS should be approached through excisional or incisional biopsy techniques.

In patients with ovarian solid tumors, the diagnosis is frequently suggested by serum biochemical marker analyses. A biopsy or an oophorectomy for biopsy purposes may be indicated if the tumor involves most of the ovary. If a malignant or teratoid tumor is identified by this procedure, the contralateral ovary is inspected and biopsied or incised longitudinally for inspection of its interior. Potential abdominal tumor implants or omental nodules should also be biopsied in these patients. Teratomas and other germ-cell tumors are high-risk for sampling error, which may lead to failure to identify malignant elements adequately. If feasible, excisional biopsies are recommended.

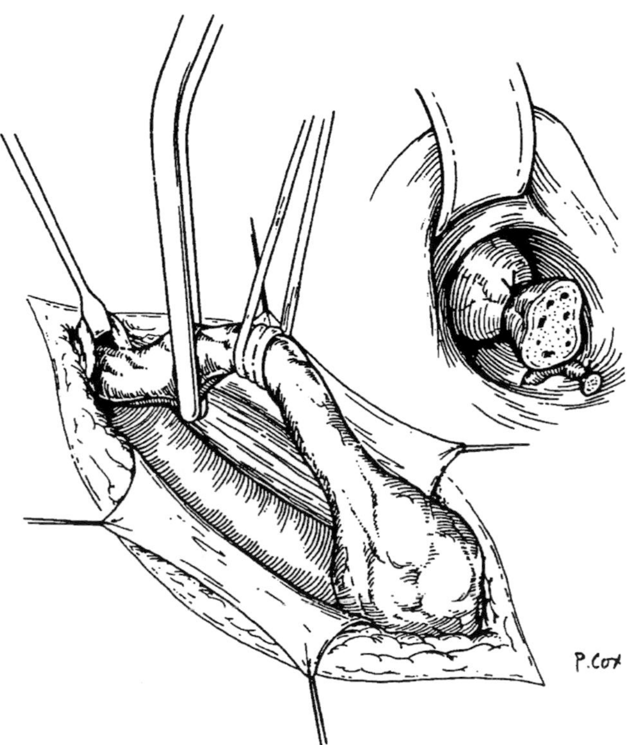

Figure 2 Inguinal orchiectomy for paratesticular tumor with complete resection of the spermatic cord strictures at the level of the internal inguinal ring.

For testicular masses, typically scrotal ultrasound will allow differentiation of solid from cystic masses. For solid testicular or paratesticular masses, an inguinal approach is recommended rather than a scrotal approach. In this procedure, after the inguinal incision the spermatic vessels are temporarily occluded near the internal inguinal ring. The testicle is then mobilized from the scrotum and if a solid tumor is confirmed an inguinal orchiectomy is performed (Fig. 2).

IV. RESECTION OF SOLID TUMORS

A. Wilms' Tumor

The management of Wilms' tumor has been the model by which the multimodal approach to cancer therapy for all tumors has been judged. Surgical resection of the tumor remains the cornerstone of Wilms' tumor management; however, a dramatic improvement in overall survival rate has resulted from the coordinated use of surgery, multiagent chemotherapy, and radiation therapy. Nephroblastoma usually presents as a painless abdominal mass in an otherwise well child. Radical nephrectomy is the primary treatment of unilateral Wilms' tumor. The presence of extensive caval extension of tumor (proximal to the hepatic veins), bilateral disease, tumor in a solitary kidney, or massive tumor is indication for biopsy, chemotherapy, and delayed partial or total nephrectomy.

For Wilms' tumor resection, a transverse upper abdominal incision is utilized to facilitate complete exposure of both kidneys. Abdominal contents are examined for liver or peritoneal spread. The contralateral kidney is fully mobilized and examined on both anterior and posterior surfaces to potentially detect previously unsuspected bilateral disease. If the disease is found to be unilateral, the colon and mesentery are dissected from the anterior surface of the kidney and reflected medially. Complete resection of the kidney and ureter down to the pelvic brim is then done, being careful not to allow tumor spillage. Perihilar and aortocaval lymph nodes are then sampled as an important part of the surgical staging system.

B. Neuroblastoma

Neuroblastoma is the most common extracranial solid tumor in children. Surgical therapy may be diagnostic, therapeutic, and/or palliative. Preoperative surgical evaluation is critically important to aid in operative decisions, such as the approach and extent of resection.

When suspected neuroblastoma patients present with extensive or metastatic disease, the most accessible tissues are chosen for biopsy. Fine-needle aspiration or core-needle biopsies, or percutaneous bone marrow biopsy are being done with increasing frequency. Also, adequate tissue (1–5 g) for biologic or cytogenetic studies is becoming more important in the selection of appropriate therapy for neuroblastoma. Staging for neuroblastoma can be clinical (preoperative), operative (surgical), or postoperative. Several staging systems, including the Evans, the previous Pediatric Oncology Group (POG), and the International Neuroblastoma Staging System (INSS), have been described.

For stages 1–3 with resectable disease, initial complete resection is performed. For patients with stages 2–4 (Evans) with unfavorable histology and N-myc amplification (>3 copies), neoadjuvant chemotherapy and delayed excision is the usual therapy. For stage 4 disease patients, initial tumor resection does not appear to increase survival duration. However, after complete clinical response has been achieved by chemotherapy, delayed excision of the primary tumor is performed if feasible.

Abdominal tumors are usually approached through a generous transverse incision, depending on the exact location of the tumor. Adrenal tumors are generally more easily resected than central retroperitoneal tumors. Tumors in the central retroperitoneum typically surround or are intimately attached to the celiac axis or mesenteric vessels. Extreme caution must be used to avoid injury to the kidney, liver, vena cava, aorta, or other adjacent structure.

Thoracic neuroblastomas are generally approached through a standard posterolateral thoracotomy. These posterior thoracic tumors can occasionally require posterior laminectomy for tumor near the spinal foramina and cooperation with neurosurgeons on these cases is beneficial. In other cases, chest wall resection and reconstruction may be indicated.

Unfortunately, for high-risk neuroblastoma with poor prognosis biologic factors, survival is rare (<5%).

C. Sarcoma

Childhood soft-tissue sarcoma is categorized as either RMS or the heterogeneous group of non-RMS soft tissue sarcomas (NRSTS). Rhabdomyosarcoma is more common in younger children and can occur at essentially any anatomic location. Surgical treatment of RMS is site-specific and precise details are available in other publications (8). There are, however, several important surgical principles in the management of RMS. Complete wide excision of the primary tumor should be performed while preserving cosmesis and function if possible. Incomplete excision, or debulking, is not thought to be beneficial (possible exception—pelvis) and mutilating or debilitating resections should not be done initially. Although many RMS tumors are massive at presentation and preclude initial complete resection, many will respond dramatically to initial multiagent chemotherapy and/or radiation. This allows subsequent resection to be more easily performed and to more likely result in negative resection margins.

For RMS in particular, initial evaluation of regional draining lymph nodes is an important part of surgical staging. Positive regional lymph nodes upstage patients and dictate that more aggressive chemotherapy and radiation be given. This is especially a concern for RMS of the extremity, perineum, and paratesticular region, sites known to have a high rate of lymph node spread.

An important principle in RMS (especially extremity tumors) is that of primary reexcision (PRE). This specifically refers to a second attempt at resection of a tumor that has either positive or indeterminate margins after an initial limited excision. This strategy frequently downstages patients, allows negative margins to be obtained, and improves survival (9). In general, the surgical approach to RMS, at many sites, has become more conservative over the past 20–30 years with improved patient outcomes rather than extremely aggressive initial operations that frequently resected organs (e.g., hysterectomy, cystectomy, vaginectomy). Initial biopsy of large tumors followed by chemotherapy, possible radiation, and second-look operation is recommended.

For older children and adolescents, NRSTS become more common. The most common sites of involvement are the extremities and trunk (pelvic and retroperitoneum). These tumors are not as chemosensitive as RMS and initial surgical resection allows the best outcome, if feasible. The usual approach for STS is wide local resection, generally with local radiation therapy. Surgical therapy for these tumors is site-specific and the general principles described for RMS are also valid for STS.

D. Hepatoblastoma

Hepatoblastomas are the most frequent malignant liver tumors in children. Hepatocellular carcinoma tends to occur in older children. The most common symptoms of primary liver malignancies are an upper abdominal mass or generalized abdominal enlargement. Preoperative evaluation includes determining the extent of intrahepatic disease, potential for hepatic resectability, and the presence or absence of extrahepatic disease.

The usual evaluation should include history and physical examination and routine laboratory tests, including liver function studies, coagulation profile, CT scan of the abdomen and chest, alpha-fetoprotein (AFP) measurement, and chest x-ray. Occasionally, MRI with 3-D reconstruction will allow more precise determination of the location of the tumor in relation to the portal venous branches.

Surgical resection continues to be the mainstay of therapy, although most commonly preoperative chemotherapy is utilized initially. Preoperative chemotherapy usually reduces tumor size, allowing hepatic resection to be performed more easily and safely (10). Reresection is indicated for locally recurrent hepatic tumors or for inadequate margins after an initial resection. Hepatoblastoma metastasizes most frequently to the lungs and aggressive resection of these metastases is indicated (11).

Alpha-fetoprotein is a valuable marker for monitoring the residual, recurrent, or metastatic disease after resection of the primary tumor or for monitoring the response of an unresectable primary tumor to therapy. Overall, newer intraoperative techniques and preoperative chemotherapy combined with extensive resection have improved local control, increased survival, and decreased postoperative complications.

E. Germ-Cell Tumors

Malignant germ-cell tumors account for approximately 3% of all childhood malignancies. They occur in gonadal and extragonadal sites. Extragonadal and testicular tumors predominate in children younger than 3 years of age; gonadal location is more common in prepubescent or postpubescent patients (12). Teratomas represent the most common histologic type of pediatric germ-cell tumor. The anatomic and age distribution of these tumors are as follows: sacrococcygeal, 42% (newborns); ovary, 35% (median-age = 13 years); head and neck, 6% (newborns); retroperitoneum, 5% (median age = 5 months); mediastinum, 4% (infants); brain and spinal cord, 4% (median age = 2.5 years); and testes, 3% (median age = 3.5 years) (13). In general, the treatment of mature teratomas consists of excision alone.

Human chorionic gonadotropin (HCG) and AFP are useful tumor markers with germ-cell tumors. Alpha-fetoprotein is a sensitive marker when endodermal sinus tumor forms a portion of a malignant germ-cell tumor. Beta-hCG serves as a tumor marker when syncytiotrophoblasts are present, especially with choriocarcinoma. Lactate dehydrogenase (LDH) is a nonspecific tumor marker that is elevated in many germ-cell tumors.

Detailed descriptions of optimal surgical management of the various germ-cell tumors have been previously described (14) and are beyond the scope of this chapter.

V. SURGICAL THERAPY FOR SOLID TUMOR METASTASES

An important aspect of pediatric surgical oncology is the diagnosis and therapeutic resection of metastatic disease. The impact of metastatic disease on patient outcome varies with tumor type and is summarized in Table 1 (15). In general, surgical resection of metastatic disease is restricted to pulmonary or hepatic metastases in selected tumor types. Consideration for aggressive resection of metastatic disease should be given when the primary tumor has been resected (local control achieved), there is no evidence of either locally recurrent or other distant disease, and the metastatic disease in question is completely resectable. The most

Table 1 Impact of Metastases on Outcome in Patients with Pediatric Solid Tumors

Tumor type	Percent of patients with metastases at diagnosis	Common metastatic sites	Survival rate for stage 4 patients (sec)
Neuroblastoma	60	Bone, liver, marrow	25[a]
Wilms' tumor	15	Lung, liver	63–69[b]
Rhabdomyosarcoma	10–20	Lung, bone, liver	43–62[c]
Osteogenic sarcoma	10–20	Lung, bone	30–40[a]
Ewing's sarcoma	14–50	Lung, bone	33[a]
Primary hepatic tumors	20	Lung, bone	0

[a] Three-year survival.
[b] Two-year survival.
[c] Of those responding to therapy.

common clinical scenario in which pediatric surgeons resect pulmonary metastases is in osteosarcoma. The majority of patients who have distant relapse with osteosarcoma have pulmonary metastases. Many of these have lung-only metastases, and an aggressive strategy of complete surgical resection of all imaging-detected and occult metastatic nodules will allow a long-term survival rate of 30%. Many of these patients will undergo multiple thoracotomies, as recurrence after initial thoracotomy is not uncommon. Prognostic variables that have been shown to predict outcome after pulmonary metastasectomy include number of nodules, time of occurrence (synchronous or metachronous), and most importantly completeness of resection. When incompletely resected, chances of long-term are essentially nil. Because of the importance of complete resection, even of nodules that are not seen on preoperative CT imaging, but that are detectable with palpation at thoracotomy, thoracoscopic approaches are strongly discouraged for most osteosarcoma patients with lung metastases. Possible indications for thoracoscopic resection of osteosarcoma lung metastases include patients with a long disease-free interval (2 years after original diagnosis) who have 1–2 peripheral nodules on CT scan, when osteosarcoma metastasizes to other anatomic locations (brain, other bone). In adult series, a similar aggressive approach of surgical resection of isolated pulmonary metastases is recommended for soft-tissue sarcomas. More limited information is available from children and adolescents due to the rarity of the disease. In general, surgical resection should be considered (as with osteosarcoma) for soft-tissue sarcoma patients who have isolated, resectable pulmonary metastases that do not disappear with aggressive multiagent chemotherapy.

For Wilms' tumor, pulmonary metastases are more commonly treated with whole-lung radiation and systemic chemotherapy. It is generally thought that surgical resection of lung metastases in this condition is not beneficial and does not confer a survival advantage over that seen with chemotherapy and radiation alone. If isolated pulmonary lesions can be surgically removed and whole-lung irradiation avoided, however, then surgical resection may be beneficial. This emphasizes the importance of keeping surgical considerations within the broader context of the multidisciplinary team approach. Broad recommendations often do not apply to individual patients and treatment should be carefully considered with each individual patient.

Hepatoblastoma is another condition in which isolated pulmonary metastases should have aggressive surgical resection. Although there is no high-quality study comparing resection vs. no resection for hepatoblastoma lung metastases, a strategy of resection is recommended if the local tumor has been completely resected and there is no evidence of other metastatic disease.

VI. INVOLVEMENT IN CLINICAL AND BASIC RESEARCH

The pediatric surgeon is in a unique position to facilitate the conduct of research protocols. As the person most responsible for procurement and handling of tumor specimens, it is imperative upon pediatric surgeons to cooperate fully with ongoing biology protocols and to facilitate enrollment of all patients into clinical trials. Many advances have been realized over the past 20 years through the widespread cooperation in the Children's Oncology Group (and its predecessors), as well as the International Society of Pediatric Oncology (SIOP). Only with the continued efforts of such groups, and other clinical trials, will further progress be made. There are also many specific surgical questions that have never been adequately studied and that would serve as important research questions to be considered in prospective clinical studies.

REFERENCES

1. Andrassy RJ. General principles. In: Andrassy RJ, ed. Pediatric Surgical Oncology. Chapter 2. Philadelphia: W. B. Saunders Company, 1998:13–34.
2. Smith MA, Ries LAG. Childhood cancer: incidence, survival, and mortality. In: Pizzo PA, Poplack DG, eds. Principles and Practice of Pediatric Oncology. 4th ed. Chapter 1. Philadelphia: Lippincott Williams & Wilkins, 2002:1–12.
3. Duerkson DR, Papineau N, Siemens J, et al. Peripherally inserted central catheters for parenteral nutrition: a comparison with centrally inserted catheters. J Parent Ent Nutr 1999; 23:85–89.
4. Wiener ES, McGuire P, Stolar CJ, et al. The CCSG prospective study of venous access devices: an analysis of insertions and causes for removal. J Pediatr Surg 1992; 27(2):155–163.
5. Horwitz JR, Lally KP. Vascular access. In: Andrassy RJ, ed. Pediatric Surgical Oncology. Chapter 8. Philadelphia: W. B. Saunders Company, 1998:137–153.
6. Shaul DB, Scheer B, Rohhsar S, et al. Risk factors for early infection of central venous catheters in pediatric patients. J Am Coll Surg 1998; 186:654–658.
7. Smith MB, Katz R, Black CT, et al. A rational approach to the use of fine-needle aspiration biopsy in the evaluation of primary and recurrent neoplasms in children. J Pediatr Surg 1993; 28:1245–1247.
8. Blakely MS, Harting MT, Andrassy RJ. Rhabdomyosarcoma. In: Asbcraft KW, Holcomb GWIII, Murphy JP, eds. Pediatric Surgery 4th ed. Chapter 70. Philadelphia: Elsevier Inc, 2005:1019–1027.

9. Hays DM, Lawrence WJ, Wharam M, et al. Primary re-excision for patients with "microscopic residual" tumor following initial excision of sarcomas of trunk and extremity sites. J Pediatr Surg 1989; 24:5–10.
10. Black CT, Cangir A, Choroszy M, et al. Marked response to preoperative high-dose cisplatinum in children with unresectable hepatoblastoma. J Pediatr Surg 1991; 26:1070–1073.
11. Black CT, Luck SR, Musemeche CA, et al. Aggressive excision of pulmonary metastases is warranted in the management of childhood hepatic tumors. J Pediatr Surg 1991; 26:1082–1086.
12. Dehner LP. Gonadal and extragonadal germ-cell neoplasia of childhood. Hum Pathol 1983; 14:493.
13. Lack EE, Young RH, Scully RE. Pathology of ovarian neoplasms in childhood and adolescence. Pathol Annu 1992; 27:281.
14. Rescorla FJ. Pediatric germ-cell tumors. In: Andrassy RJ, ed. Pediatric Surgical Oncology. Chapter 13. Philadelphia: W. B. Saunders Company, 1998:239–266.
15. Saenz NC, LaQuaglia MP. Metastases from solid tumors. In: Andrassy RJ, ed. Pediatric Surgical Oncology. Chapter 22. Philadelphia: W. B. Saunders Company, 1998:405–417.

53

Symptom Assessment

ANTHONY H. RISSER, KAREN O. ANDERSON, TITO R. MENDOZA, and CHARLES S. CLEELAND

Department of Symptom Research, The University of Texas M.D. Anderson Cancer Center, Houston, Texas, U.S.A.

I. INTRODUCTION

Patients undergoing surgical treatment for cancer experience a number of acute as well as persisting symptoms that can include pain, fatigue, altered mood, disturbed sleep, and cognitive problems (1). These symptoms occur alongside the specific local symptoms that are related to the type and location of the cancer that is the object of surgical intervention and the acute symptoms that will depend upon both the surgical procedure per se and the adequacy of symptom management in the postoperative recovery period. Perioperative symptoms are of concern to surgeons and anesthesiologists in contemporary medicine; specific procedures and surgical sites can be anticipated to be associated with acute perioperative symptoms (2), especially pain (3,4). Traditionally for many, these concerns were usually considered to be the transient consequences of having undergone surgery. We now know that concern extends beyond the acute postoperative recovery period to include the risk of developing chronic postsurgical pain syndromes that may last for months or years (5). Post-breast-surgery syndromes, such as postmastectomy pain syndrome and phantom-breast pain syndrome (6), post-thoracotomy syndrome (7), and postamputation phantom-limb pain syndrome (8) are the most common examples of these conditions.

Actually, most cancer patients will fall between these extremes of patients whose symptom experience is only a transitory one and those who are diagnosed with a specific chronic syndrome. Hence, the formal assessment of symptoms is desirable for all cancer patients undergoing treatment; this remains a best practice, rather than established practice. The task is a sizeable one. While many local and procedure-based symptoms can be anticipated by cancer specialists, the longitudinal measurement of postsurgical symptoms, as well as guidelines for the management of persisting symptoms, are still developing (9). Not recognizing or underestimating these symptoms can become a barrier to patient care, but one that a reasonable assessment approach can help overcome (e.g., Ref. 10), even, for example, in the simple implementation of notations of pain-intensity ratings placed in patient charts (11). Attempts to develop this knowledge base through systematic clinical research efforts have made substantial progress over the past 20 years, not only in surgical therapy but also for radiation therapy (e.g., Ref. 12) and chemotherapy (e.g., Refs. 13, 14).

Progress has resulted in clinical guidelines, such as the World Health Organization guidelines for cancer pain relief (15) and the National Comprehensive Cancer Network guidelines for cancer-related pain (16), fatigue (17), and psychosocial distress (18). Application of these treatment guidelines depends upon recognition (i.e., assessment) of the presence and severity of symptoms. Considerable progress has been made over the past 20 years in the rapid assessment and interpretation of symptoms. Assessment of symptoms is also important for additional reasons: better understanding of the medical condition per se and a more complete understanding of cancer's impact upon individual daily functioning. Perioperatively, the prediction of who might develop chronic postoperative syndromes also can be of benefit, given concern for examining whether preoperative and perioperative factors alter the risk for postsurgical persistent symptoms (5,7,19).

Tools of symptom assessment rely on the self-report of patients, given the subjective nature of symptoms. These tools are useful to the degree that they are standardized in their administration and scoring, have demonstrated reliability and validity, and are consistent with actual clinical need (20,21). Reliability and validity are traditional psychometric properties that instruments need to meet and are goals of good test construction, standardization, and revision. Statistical standards such as Cronbach's alpha and test–retest reliability provide ways to determine if a tool is reliable in its measurement. Several measures of validity, such as construct, criterion, and known-groups validity, can be performed to assess whether the tool is measuring what it is purported to measure. Details about these procedures can be found in psychometric sources, such as Ref. 22.

We explore cancer-related symptom assessment and its role in management in this chapter, placing emphasis on pain, which has been the area of symptom expression to be explored most fully to date, but also covering the assessment of fatigue and mood. Given the perioperative context of this book, we place our emphasis on one aspect of assessment: basic screening to ascertain the presence and severity of symptoms. The surgical environment, for obvious reasons, is not the one most conducive to a detailed assessment of these types of symptoms, yet the need to appreciate symptoms related to cancer and its treatment is prerequisite to their adequate management.

The clinician seeking to incorporate symptom information into patient care is faced with a basic benefit-cost decision: the perceived benefit of the information needs to be balanced against the predicted expenditure of time and effort to obtain that information. At one end of the assessment spectrum, one can obtain basic information in a very short period of time measured in minutes while, at the other, one can obtain comprehensive information gained through an assessment process that may take considerably longer. In this chapter, we examine the basic-information/short-time end of the spectrum. Understanding and treating cancer-related symptoms benefits from comprehensive examination, but the perioperative period is not the most practical time to consider performing that type of assessment. Coverage of a more in-depth approach to symptom assessment can be examined in Ref. 23 for pain and Ref. 24 or 21 for fatigue.

II. MULTIDIMENSIONAL SYMPTOM ASSESSMENT

A multidimensional, broad-based approach to symptom assessment begins with the recognition that the particular set of symptoms experienced by an individual varies from person to person and, for any one individual, from time period to time period, but that the symptoms of those with a given cancer receiving the same treatment may be similar. A multidimensional approach also recognizes the need to capture the influence or impact of symptoms on the individualized daily-life functioning of patients with cancer.

A brief screening for symptoms benefits from using an instrument with content that anticipates the likely spectrum of potential symptoms. One practical benefit of having patients complete these types of instruments is that it may give the patient some guidance to report symptoms that the physician may not formally ask about, an important concern given that research on clinician–patient communication in cancer care often finds that its structure and direction remain predominantly under the clinician's control (e.g., Ref. 25). Another practical benefit of multidimensional symptom assessment is that it minimizes any clinical bias toward considering one symptom (usually, pain) as the primary one and all others as being associated and secondary ones, which may be inconsistent with both the patient's experience and the underlying etiology. The simultaneous assessment of different symptoms using instruments that are structured to allow direct comparisons between symptoms is a relatively new advance and only a few standardized tests are available to do so (1).

We conceptualize this rapid assessment as a process having four sequential steps (26). This approach is outlined in Table 1. An integrated, multiple-symptom screening comprises the first step. Where clinical need exists and when time permits, the results of this initial screening leads one directly to a second assessment step: the fuller evaluation of the severity (intensity) of the specific symptoms that were identified during the first step—an evaluation still characterized by its brevity, but using instruments designed specifically for that symptom. Third and fourth steps can follow from

Table 1 Symptom Assessment

Assessment step	Nature	Goal	Test examples
Step One	Integrated initial screening	Identification of specific symptoms. Proceed to Step Two, as needed	MDASI, MSAS-SF
Step Two	Specific symptom severity	Mild, moderate, or severe. Interference in daily life	BPI, BFI, BDI-II
Step Three	Specific symptom characteristics	Location, quality, temporal pattern, history, physical and mental facets, etc.	MFI-20, interview
Step Four	Functional and quality-of-life impact	Intrapersonal, interpersonal (social), and vocational impact of symptoms	QLQ-C30, FACT-G
Iteration step	Reentry at any prior step, as needed	Assess improvement or decrement over time and/or to assess impact of treatment and management.	—

there: in-depth characterization of the symptom and, finally, its functional impact and influence over an individual's quality of life. Steps Two, Three, and Four are derived from the decision-analysis model presented for pain assessment by Cleeland and Syrjala (26) and, more recently, by Anderson and colleagues (10). Within this model, the assessment procedure is broken into steps, with selective branching into more specific questioning based upon initial responses, leading to differential treatment and patient-education options. This assessment process is an iterative one, with any step repeated as required by changes in patient status. Simple assessment, if it becomes routine and frequent during clinic visits, allows for rapid identification of emerging symptoms or symptoms that are responding to appropriate treatment.

III. STEP ONE: INITIAL IDENTIFICATION OF SYMPTOMS

Several single and multiple symptom scales have been developed that permit rapid assessment of symptom presence and severity, placing minimal burden on clinical practice. The development of standards of application of symptom scales is likely to ensure their increasing use in practice, such as the Joint Commission on Accreditation of Healthcare Organizations requirement that pain be frequently assessed during clinical encounters (27). Here, we will review some of these scales and their application.

The M.D. Anderson symptom inventory (MDASI) (28), developed for use with cancer patients, is an example of a broad-based, brief screening tool. There are a small number of similar instruments, such as the Memorial symptom assessment scale (MSAS) (29) and its short-form variant (MSAS-SF) (30), the Edmonton symptom assessment scale (ESAS) (31), and the symptom distress scale (SDS) (32). The goals leading to the development and standardization of these instruments include targeting symptoms that occur most frequently and are the most distressing, brief administration time, easy to understand and complete (even in the presence of severe levels of pain and fatigue), applicable to both clinical and research settings, repeatable, simple paper-and-pencil format but convertible into new technologies, and easy to translate into different languages.

In a surgical setting, a screening measure like this may be administered preoperatively to document symptom features leading up to the time of surgical intervention and potentially have a role in surgical and anesthesiological planning. With repeat assessment during early postoperative recovery, acute and fluctuating changes in symptoms can be identified and managed. Symptom data may prove useful for predischarge planning and for follow-up appointments, as well as documenting the persistence or resolution of symptoms as part of evaluating long-term outcome.

The MDASI is a measure of the severity and impact of a core group of cancer-related symptoms and, when required, additional supplementary items to allow for coverage of symptoms that are specific to certain cancers, stages of illness, or type of treatment (28). Details of the MDASI's psychometric development are available in Ref. 28. The MDASI core consists of 13 symptom items: pain, fatigue, nausea, disturbed sleep, emotional distress, shortness of breath, lack of appetite, drowsiness, dry mouth, sadness, vomiting, difficulty remembering, and numbness/tingling. Each symptom is rated on an 11-point scale, with 0 being "not present" and 10 being "as bad as you can imagine." The MDASI also contains six items for patients to report how much the symptoms have interfered with different aspects of their lives during the past 24 hr: general activity, mood, walking ability, normal work (including both work outside the home and housework), relations with other people, and enjoyment of life. Each interference item is rated on an 11-point scale, with 0 being "does not interfere" and 10 being "completely interferes."

The MDASI requires patients to rate each symptom at its worst in the last 24 hr, deferring additional ratings of symptom distress and duration that may be included in longer symptom scales for the sake of brevity, simplicity, and acceptability to very ill patients and to their service providers under tight schedule constraints.

The MSAS-SF (30) requires patients to rate 32 physical and psychological symptoms on a five-point scale from 0 ("no symptom") to 4 ("very much"). Physical symptoms include pain, lack of energy, lack of appetite, feeling drowsy, vomiting, nausea, dry mouth, change in taste, and constipation. Psychological symptoms include sadness, worrying, irritability, and feeling nervous.

If the administration of the MDASI, MSAS-SF, or a similar instrument yields a set of symptoms that the patient is experiencing, these symptoms can then be explored in more detail to determine their severity, performed in Step Two.

IV. STEP TWO: ASSESSING SYMPTOM SEVERITY/INTENSITY

Symptom severity often has the highest priority in a screening assessment—even more so when time is limited. Severity (intensity) is initially determined during Step One on a measure like the MDASI. Getting a fuller sense as to a specific symptom's severity is the goal of Step Two. Standardized instruments have been created to examine the severity of cancer-related symptoms in a more detailed manner than those used in Step One, albeit with the expectation that they will remain brief in time expenditure. Symptom scales specific to pain, fatigue, and mood make it possible to assess the experience of these symptoms on a routine basis and repeatedly, even with the surgical inpatient. We present some of these scales below.

A. Pain

A recent review reports the presence of over 100 possible instruments to examine cancer-related pain (1). The brief pain inventory (BPI) (33) in original and short forms and the McGill pain questionnaire in its original 78-item (MPQ) (34) and short 15-item (SF-MPQ) (35,36) forms are two instruments commonly used to assess pain. The BPI was designed specifically for cancer-related pain and the MPQ is used predominantly for chronic noncancer pain, but has seen use in assessing cancer-related pain (20,37,38). Standard assessment of the multidimensional aspects of cancer pain makes it clear that pain severity is the primary factor determining the impact of pain on the patient and the urgency of the treatment process (10).

Though the most frequent reason among people actually seeking medical attention, pain is common in everyday life and, typically, is benign and does not lead to medical encounters (39). Patients with cancer function effectively even when a background level of some pain is present. As pain severity increases, however, it passes a threshold to become disruptive to many aspects of the patient's life. At very high levels, pain becomes a primary focus of attention and prohibits most functional activity (40). In a surgical setting, obtaining baseline and/or acute recovery levels of pain may prove useful in anticipation of the postoperative recovery period and may possess predictive value for the later occurrence of postsurgical pain syndromes (5). As one example, Katz and colleagues (7) found that pain intensity measured on a verbal rating scale and MPQ scores obtained 24 and 48 hr after thoracotomy were actually predictive of chronic pain 1.5 years later.

The BPI (33) assesses self-reported pain across 15 items, allowing patients to rate the intensity and functional interference of pain over the previous 24 hr. A longer version of the test also is available. The BPI rates intensity of pain at its worst, least, average, and "right now" at the time of test completion. Research on the BPI has been performed in a diverse set of cancer diagnoses and cancer-treatment settings (e.g., Refs. 33, 41, 42). Several studies have explored the BPI in postoperative patients: Zalon (43), Tittle et al. (44), and Mendoza et al. (45). Mendoza and colleagues have shown that the short version of the BPI is a psychometrically valid and reliable tool to use in longitudinally assessing postoperative pain in patients who have had coronary artery bypass graft (CABG) surgery. A practical finding by Tittle and colleagues was their report that BPI average scores possessed less utility than other BPI intensity ratings, given acute fluctuations in postoperative pain levels.

One of the primary goals of using the BPI is to determine whether the patient's reported pain is "mild," "moderate," or "severe," as ranges of responses on the numeric rating of pain at its worst or at its usual (average) level. These categories of pain severity are based on the degree of interference with function associated with each category and possess management implications (10,40). The use of mild, moderate, and severe classifications is a simple means of describing pain and could be a particularly meaningful outcome measure in designing clinical trials. For example, if the majority of patients experience only minor pain in the early postoperative period (as in the case of CABG patients), design of long-term clinical trials of postoperative pain control may be more efficient and cost-effective if the focus is placed upon the subset of patients with persistent moderate or severe pain. These severity categories have been replicated in patients with phantom-limb pain (46) and in postoperative CABG patients (47). The studies by Mendoza and colleagues also showed that the longer BPI version may not be appropriate for the first 24–48 hr after surgery, but that the short version demonstrated good reliability and validity for up to 14 days after the first 48-hr period.

Mild pain (1–4 "worst" pain; 1–3 "average" pain, on the BPI) in a patient with cancer may call for a "mild" analgesic (acetaminophen or a nonsteroidal antiinflammatory), or "moderate" analgesic such as hydrocodone or oxycodone. The patient with mild pain can benefit from education about the need to report pain when it occurs, when it gets worse, or if it is not relieved by current treatment. A mild pain level requires the least assessment at subsequent steps, since it causes the least interference with function. In clinical practice, it is valuable to also assess the impact of pain when the level is 3 or 4, because a small proportion of patients will underrepresent their pain levels. Also, if the pain etiology is understood, the clinician can determine whether the self-reported pain is likely to be transient, progressive, or subject to frequent exacerbations.

Moderate pain (5–6 "worst" pain, 4–6 "average" pain) calls for a more aggressive analgesic program and indicates the need to complete Steps Three and Four of the assessment process.

When pain is severe (7–10 "worst" or "average" pain) the steps are similar to moderate pain, except that the analgesic selection and titration need to be aggressive, and reassessment needs to occur, typically within 24 hr after the initial assessment is made. In cases like this, frequent reassessment of intensity can be a part of acute medical management and aid in decision making.

B. Fatigue

Though less routinely examined than pain, cancer-related fatigue is actually a more prevalent symptom (48). As with pain, it is important to evaluate cancer- and treatment-related fatigue symptoms over time in order to monitor changes in severity and response to treatment. Cancer-related fatigue appears across the various disease diagnoses and all its major therapies. A severe level of fatigue is significantly more common in cancer patients than in the normal population and has qualitative differences that further distinguish it from fatigue in otherwise healthy individuals. For example, while everyone experiences tiredness and exhaustion, obtaining sleep lacks the same restorative value for cancer-related fatigue (49). In a study of multiple symptoms, fatigue and related problems were the most severe symptoms reported by a large sample of outpatients with a variety of cancers and treatments in a comprehensive cancer center (28).

In the perioperative context, fatigue needs to be examined in terms of its presence and intensity in the time leading up to surgery, in the postoperative recovery period, the postdischarge recovery period, and in the longer term. Postoperative fatigue is the most frequently reported symptom after major surgery, such as thoracic surgery, and can be prolonged for months. Salmon and Hall (50–53) have examined the relative contributions of physiological and psychological influences on postoperative fatigue, including the role of preoperative levels of fatigue.

Fatigue can occur at any phase of cancer and result from any kind of cancer therapy. However, the clinical research literature about fatigue is far more detailed in the context of chemotherapy or radiotherapy than for cancer surgery. In a recent review of treatment-related fatigue, only one of 26 studies that explored fatigue during treatment was a surgical one (14). This single study (54) explored a specific facet of fatigue (i.e., the so-called "attentional fatigue") in patients hospitalized for breast-cancer surgery. Subsequent studies by Cimprich and Ronis (55,56) have explored this facet in further detail. More recently, Cooley et al. (57) studied symptom prevalence in lung cancer and included a subset of patients who were examined subsequent to surgical treatment.

Gradually increased fatigue severity levels can be observed during chemotherapy (58) or preoperative chemoradiotherapy (59) or—if not increasing—higher during treatment than before it began (e.g., Ref. 60). Nadir-associated fatigue can occur if significant myelosuppression develops during bone marrow transplantation (61). Decreasing percentages of patients reporting "high distress" about fatigue and insomnia during the same period as first decreasing and then increasing percentages of "high distress" about the frequency and severity of pain have been reported in postsurgical lung-cancer patients (57). Finally, persisting fatigue may be present among cancer survivors (14,62,63).

Three instruments specific to cancer-related fatigue with the rating of severity (intensity) being their primary goal are the brief fatigue inventory (BFI) (64), the cancer-related fatigue distress scale (CRFDS) (65), and the fatigue symptom inventory (FSI) (60,66–68).

The BFI (64) assesses self-reported fatigue across nine items over the 24-hr period leading up to the test's administration: the severity of fatigue at its worst, at the current time (of test administration), and at its usual level and the interference caused by fatigue on general activity, mood, walking ability, work (both vocational and daily chores), relationships with others, and enjoyment of life.

A mean fatigue score is calculated from the nine ratings; a mean interference score also is calculated. The "fatigue worst" item can be used as a general index of symptom severity. As with the BPI, categorizing BFI "fatigue worst" scores as reflecting one of three severity levels (i.e., mild, moderate, and severe) has been explored; the result being somewhat clearer for establishing a boundary between moderate and severe fatigue (i.e., severe indexed by a score of 7 or above) than for one between mild and moderate fatigue. Thirty-five percent of the sample of cancer patients in the Mendoza et al. (64) study reported fatigue corresponding to the severe level.

The BFI has been validated in a variety of cancer types and treatments. Studies include a sample of patients attending a specialty cancer fatigue clinic (69), patients undergoing preoperative chemoradiation for resectable rectal cancer (59), and patients being treated for leukemia or for non-Hodgkin's lymphoma (70). Community-dwelling healthy adults and noncancer patients with clinical depression have also been examined (71). The measure is able to distinguish cancer patients from normal controls and discriminates between patient groups expected to have differing levels of fatigue. The simple wording of the instrument makes it easy to understand for patients with limited educational backgrounds as well making it easy to translate.

C. Mood

Although most patients with cancer do not develop mood disorders, it is important to screen for possible depression, anxiety, and level of adjustment. When an individual's affect appears to be outside the parameters of normal limits (as might be found, e.g., during Step One with a rating for the item "sad" on the MDASI of 5 or greater), a differential diagnosis of mental disorders might be suggested. This diagnostic workup would be beyond the standard practice of the surgical or anesthesiologist cancer specialist and support team. However, short of that, there are facets of mood changes that can be discerned by the clinician with the aid of screening instruments, bedside interview, and history review. Two such scales (among many) are the Beck depression inventory-II (BDI-II) (72) and the profile of mood states (POMS) in its original format (73) and in two short forms: 11-item (74) and 37-item [(75); validated for cancer patients by Baker et al. (76)] versions. The BDI-II assesses symptoms of depressed mood using 21 items on four-point rating scales, covering the 2 weeks prior to self-report. Examples of items queried include sadness, suicidal thinking, loss of pleasure, tiredness/fatigue, and irritability. The POMS includes, but is not limited to, depressed mood in its coverage, with items such as feelings of being sad, blue, worthless, helpless, angry, grouchy, on edge, and fatigued.

As with pain, understanding mood and distress in the time leading up to surgery in general is becoming an active area of interest among anesthesiologists and surgical teams. This is perhaps best seen in efforts to understand the effectiveness (or lack of effectiveness) of the modality of patient-controlled analgesia (PCA) during the early postoperative period. For example, Özalp and colleagues (77) reported that higher preoperative Beck depression inventory ratings were associated with more intense postoperative pain and more opioid consumption, but with less satisfaction with PCA, than those reporting lower preoperative levels of depressed mood in a sample of breast-cancer patients undergoing modified radical mastectomies.

Recently, Uchitomi and colleagues (78) examined the clinical diagnosis of depression, as well as symptoms of depression and distress as measured on the POMS, in a sample of over 200 patients over the first postoperative year after curative resection for non-small-cell lung cancer. Though far less prevalent than self-reported depression in a sample of noncurative lung-cancer patients undergoing palliative care (e.g., Ref. 79), clinical depression was present in the sample at a rate of roughly 5–8%.

The majority of individuals adjust to the stresses of cancer and its symptoms without clinically diagnosable syndromes related to depression, anxiety, or other mental disorders (80,81). However, patients with pain report significantly more depression and anxiety than those without pain (82–84). Pretreatment general performance status and presence of fatigue possess predictive value for depressive symptoms after treatment has been completed (e.g., Ref. 79). Any relation between mood disorder and fatigue is a problematic one, as fatigue may itself be a feature of depressed mood per se and is one of the criteria for the diagnosis of clinical depression. For this (and other reasons), mood disorders can be among the most difficult to identify among the many symptoms possible during the course of cancer. Difficulty in recognizing mood disruptions results from the similarity of presentation of some mood symptoms and common disease-related somatic complaints, such as fatigue and weight loss. Assessment of mood in cancer patients with other symptoms such as pain and fatigue requires a focus on the affective components of mood disturbance, with somewhat more cautious evaluation of cognitive and behavioral components and with awareness, but not emphasis, on somatic components.

Though the first two assessment steps may prove useful in documenting cancer-related pain and fatigue without necessarily looking at each in more detail, mood is less easily gauged in this manner. The severity of the mood disturbance per se is not one and the same as the clinical diagnosis of, for example, a depressive disorder. Screening mood during these assessment stages, therefore, needs to be done with caution and, even with the use of specific mood questionnaires, the actual diagnosis of a mood disorder requires additional diagnostic work-up or—at least—a careful clinical interview. Palmer and Coyne (85) outline the pitfalls of relying only on screening data about mood disorders for individuals examined in medical settings. If performed, should mood screening indicate a possible disorder, then a referral to a psychiatrist, psychologist, or other mental health professional with experience in medical populations is indicated.

V. STEP THREE: ASSESSING SYMPTOM CHARACTERISTICS

Whether to proceed beyond Step Two in a given clinical setting with a specific patient is an important decision-making node in a formal symptom-assessment approach. Clinical need balanced against time and staff resource allocation—and the physical capacity of the patient—may result in a decision to proceed or a decision to defer further assessment at the time. If the decision is to defer the two steps that follow, however, rudimentary information about symptom characteristics (Step Three) and functional impact (Step Four) often can be gleaned from the results of the first two steps.

In practice, with the completion of the first two steps, Step Three is limited to the subset of symptoms found to be present and usually only those present at a moderate-to-severe level of intensity. Information about aspects of cancer symptoms other than severity makes the relation between different types of symptoms more understandable and helps refine management plans. Much of this information can be gathered through the use of additional standardized questionnaires and short follow-up interviewing for clarification or elaboration to guide the patient's subjective reports. We examine these characteristics for pain, fatigue, and mood below.

A. Pain

Beyond severity, characteristics of pain to be considered are its location, temporal pattern, quality, and history. These features are described in detail by Anderson et al. (10). Though a body diagram is usefully employed to document location, most of these features can be elicited through questioning the patient. Localization is most easily accomplished by asking the patient to mark on the body diagram the location(s) of pain. In the surgical context, this includes consideration as to anticipated regions of pain as a result of the operation. This can provide a wealth of information about possible physical mechanisms contributing to the pain. It may also help to determine why pain is more of a problem with particular movements or positions. Temporal pattern may help determine the regularity of changes in severity over the course of the typical day and, as a result, may help identify atypical or "breakthrough" symptoms. Pain quality is often the more difficult characteristic to explore, as people often find it difficult to spontaneously describe their pain. Word lists of potential descriptors help the patient portray pain quality. For example, pain caused by destruction of nerve pathways may be described as "numb," "pins and needles," "burning," or "shooting." Pain from tumor destruction of soft tissue or bone is often described as "aching." Establishing the qualities of a pain is an essential part of establishing the physical basis of the pain, which will, in turn, determine the types of therapies to be considered. Finally, pain history may be useful to consider or rule out any premorbid somatization tendencies and to help define the patient's response to prior pain treatment, impact on quality of life, and prognosis. When assessing response to prior analgesic treatments, the patients' adherence to their prescribed analgesic medications also must be determined, along with beliefs that might dictate future adherence (10).

B. Fatigue

Parameters of fatigue include its duration, its own pattern and its relation to sleep patterns, distinguishing its physical and mental facets, and understanding the individual's general activity level. Most of these features can be obtained through the use of any one of a collection of instruments often grouped together under the label of "multidimensional fatigue" tools. They include the multidimensional fatigue inventory (MFI-20) (86), revised Piper fatigue scale (R-PFS) (87), fatigue assessment instrument (FAI) (88), multidimensional fatigue symptom inventory (MFSI) (89), and the Schwartz cancer fatigue scale (SCFS) (90). Multidimensional fatigue measures typically distinguish physical from mental fatigue and commonly also include affective/mood and activity-level dimensions—distinctions that are important to consider at a more comprehensive level of outpatient assessment than warranted in a surgical setting. However, one of these scales is short enough to merit mention in this chapter: the multidimensional fatigue inventory.

The MFI-20 (86) is comprised of 20 items that are each rated on a five-point scale anchored "yes, that is true" to "no, that is not true." The timeframe for responding relates to how much fatigue one is experiencing "lately." These items populate five specific dimensions: general fatigue, physical fatigue, mental fatigue, reduced motivation, and reduced activity. The instrument was initially used in a tracking study of 250 patients as they progressed through radiotherapy, with a follow-up 9 months later (91,92). The MFI-20 showed a gradual increase in fatigue over the course of therapy and a decrease upon its ending, with fatigue scores after the course of treatment "slightly, though significantly" higher than at pretreatment levels. As a group, disease-free patients at 9 months were not significantly different than the general population, albeit with the presence of individual differences and potential "response shift" attributional issues.

Although proper interpretation of the MFI-20's five factors has been debated (93,94), the instrument is one of the more commonly used measures of cancer-related fatigue. Its format is a simple one and the language and attentional demands of the test appear to be minor. Use of such a measure can provide information as to whether a given level of fatigue severity is shared equally by physical demands as by mental ones in the patient's daily life.

The level of detail about cancer-related fatigue that can be obtained at this level of assessment may prove quite useful for intervention-based clinical research, which includes pharmacological and exercise-based treatment modalities (e.g., Ref. 95). Whether proposed interventions are found to have a general impact on fatigue or an impact specific to certain of its facets (e.g., physical fatigue) will be an important consideration in exploring management options with patients.

C. Mood

Parameters of mood disorder beyond screening for the severity of depressed mood include understanding the premorbid psychosocial history of the patient prior to cancer diagnosis, current psychopharmacological medications, the effectiveness of any prior medical and/or psychotherapeutic treatments, the temporal pattern of the mood disorder (i.e., whether chronic, episodic, or in response to specific events or circumstances), coping strategies, and available psychosocial support and resources. A psychologist or psychiatrist, who will perform both a thorough clinical interview with the patient and additional testing, can explore these features through specialty consultation. These parameters are useful in that they allow a differential diagnosis to unfold to, if symptoms warrant, identify the type of mood disorder that is present and direct treatment efforts. Examples of specific mood disorders include major depressive disorder, mood disorder due to a general medical condition, dysthymic disorder, and adjustment disorder with depressed mood. The Diagnostic and Statistical Manual of Mental Disorders, IVth edition (DSM-IV) (96), provides guidance for this diagnostic process.

Palmer and Coyne (85) concluded that screening for current mood in medical settings at a level that appears generally consistent with that noted for Steps One and Two would be most suitable for those patients who have already been diagnosed with one of the mood disorder clinical syndromes. In that circumstance, the additional medical condition generates the need to monitor symptoms of that known mental disorder during the course of adjustment to the medical condition and its treatments. A study by Kudoh et al. (97) provides an example of the possible complications that medically treated mood disorders may present. In examining patients with preexisting major depressive disorders treated with antidepressant medication and those without a psychiatric diagnosis over the initial hours of recovery from undergoing abdominal surgery with general anesthesia, Kudoh et al. reported that patients with depression reported significantly higher pain scores 8 and 16 hr post termination of anesthesia and that these pain scores were correlated with presurgical scores on the Hamilton Depression Scale. Group differences dissipated by postoperative days 2–4.

VI. STEP FOUR: ASSESSING SYMPTOM FUNCTIONAL IMPACT

Step four of symptom assessment measures the degree to which symptoms interfere with the patient's life and the degree to which symptoms or problems interact to disrupt the patient's treatment or functioning. The suggested assessment here is again tailored to elicit information that will lead to specific treatment recommendations. At a practical level, the basic information about interference in daily functions available from the use, for example, of the MDASI at Step One or the BDI or the BFI at Step Two may suffice for tracking symptom-related interference during the perioperative period, with a fuller evaluation planned for after the patient recovers from the acute impact of any cancer-related surgery.

The need for this type of clinical data in the overall management of the cancer patient is straightforward, although deciding what test to employ and what the results of that test indicate is difficult for many clinicians (e.g., Ref. 98). Impact assessment recognizes that additional factors other than cancer burden and symptom burden will figure into the subjective experience of every patient as an individual: premorbid lifestyle, level of psychosocial engagement with others, roles within families and peer groups, vocational and avocational successes, etc. These usually ill-defined factors are often among the most important for the patient as he or she grapples with cancer, treatment regimens, and short- and long-term outcomes.

Additionally, although occurring late in the symptom-assessment process described here, there are occasions when quality-of-life (QOL) assessment is the sole purpose of an assessment, for needs that go beyond examining the impact of specific symptoms (98,99).

There are a number of specific QOL test instruments that can be considered for use during this step. Two of the ones commonly administered to patients with cancer are the EORTC quality of life questionnaire QLQ-C30 (100) and the functional assessment of cancer therapy, in its general version (FACT-G) (101) and in other versions, such as its breast cancer format (102).

Quality-of-life assessment may seem removed from the care provided during the perioperative period. However, studies are beginning to explore acute changes to self-perception of QOL during the early postoperative period. Wu et al. (103), for example, tracked the impact of pain and the side effects of analgesics in patients undergoing elective hip or knee replacement surgery over the first 14 days post surgery. Severity of pain correlated with decreased physical and mental QOL during this time period. Importantly, the QOL literature suggests that certain scenarios exist, which place QOL considerations squarely in the surgical realm; for example, when surgical options exist and both physician and patient have to weigh these options before reaching a decision. Research about different surgical procedures for breast cancer, for example, addresses QOL concerns directly (102).

VII. IMPLEMENTATION OF SYMPTOM ASSESSMENT

The availability of symptom-based consultation services, staff training programs (e.g., Ref. 11), and developments in communications and computer technology can provide ways to support implementation of symptom assessment in contemporary cancer care and in the specific support of surgical services. Experience in the use of these services in chemotherapy, radiation therapy, and general cancer (e.g., Ref. 69) settings can offer some precedent for similar uses in surgical settings. Successes in providing anesthesiology-directed perioperative pain management services (e.g., Ref. 104) and with patient-controlled analgesic pumps and their preoperative patient training (e.g., Ref. 2) also can reinforce the introduction of broader symptom assessment services. Staff in-services, access to specialists in symptom assessment/research, case conferences, and promotion of available clinical-practice guidelines can help raise staff awareness of the need to identify symptoms. As reported for analyses of favorable acute-pain-management program implementation in hospital settings, firm institutional resources, administrative planning to integrate practice guidelines into formal patient outcomes/satisfaction programs, and perceived economic and legal incentives for the institution can play significant roles (105).

Recent developments in communications and computer technology offer new opportunities for the assessment of symptoms. Although the so-called "digital divide" exists in terms of more-limited access to the Internet for the disadvantaged and while the validity/quality of online information can be uncertain or minimal, the percentage of individuals who access Internet websites for information about medical conditions continues to increase (106,107). As a result, the use of computer technologies is viewed by some as now being a facet of contemporary cancer care expected by patients and their families (108,109).

Tablet computers, laptops, touch-screens, personal digital assistants (PDAs), and other electronic recording devices have been used for the assessment of symptoms in hospital and during outpatient appointments (e.g., Refs. 110, 111) and in home and work environments (e.g., Ref. 112). Both Allenby et al. (110) and Ruland et al. (111) offer basic program evaluations of the automated collection of symptom data in cancer settings in its impact on subsequent clinician–patient interactions. Allenby and colleagues document that such technologies in the clinic are generally met with interest by patients, even those who are not computer literate, and that task-to-completion times are consistent with the demands of busy practice settings. Ruland and colleagues found that if touch-screen symptom information is obtained prior to an appointment and then automatically printed for the physician to have at hand and review prior to the face-to-face appointment with the patient, a closer consonance exists between patient and physician understanding of current symptoms than if the information were collected via the technology but not printed for the physician prior to the appointment time.

Computer-administered versions of symptom ratings scales have been used successfully to screen for psychological symptoms (e.g., Ref. 113) and to collect QOL information (e.g., Ref. 114). The computer versions of symptom scales appear to be reliable, valid, cost-effective instruments that provide data equivalent to interview or self-administered scales (115,116). Given that memory for pain and other symptoms is often poor and subject to shifting attribution, the "real time" assessment of symptoms can provide accurate data regarding symptom patterns and changes over time as they take place. Identity-protected Internet-based portals to collect data from individuals in their daily-life environment provide a means to collect that type of ongoing information outside the hospital setting.

The development of telephone-based interactive voice response systems (IVRs) presents an attractive alternative to personal computer or PDA assessment systems. Such systems are based on a centralized computer software system that calls patients at home at appropriate intervals. Patients use the keypad of their touch-tone telephone to rate severity for symptoms highly prevalent for persons with a particular condition or treatment. Symptom interference, such as that represented in the MDASI (28), can also be rated. Patients can pick a time of the day that they prefer to receive the call. The computer system can be programmed to repeat the call at specified intervals, and document calls that are unanswered for manual follow-up by staff. Patients can also call the system to preclude the programmed call. The server can be set at predetermined thresholds to give immediate feedback when symptoms become moderate to severe. Threshold-crossing symptom feedback can be sent automatically to service providers by pager or e-mail, together with contact information for the patient. Such a system may have special advantages for tracking postsurgical patients in the first days after discharge. In a pilot study at M. D. Anderson Cancer Center, patients were administered the BPI and a provider was paged when pain severity exceeded a preset threshold (117). Patients reported a high level of satisfaction with the system, and there was at least preliminary evidence that readmissions and emergency visits for pain were reduced for those patients using the system.

REFERENCES

1. National Institutes of Health State-of-the-Science Panel. National Institutes of Health state-of-the-science conference statement: Symptom management in cancer: Pain, depression, and fatigue. J Natl Cancer Inst 2003; 95:1110–1117.
2. Ready LB. Acute perioperative pain. In: Miller RD, ed. Anesthesia. 5th ed. Philadelphia: Churchill Livingstone, 2000.
3. Carr DB, Jacox AK, Chapman RC, et al. Acute Pain Management: Operative or Medical Procedures and Trauma—Clinical Practice Guideline. Rockville, MD: Agency for Health Care Policy and Research, 1992.
4. Rosenquist RW, Rosenberg J. Postoperative pain guidelines. Regional Anesth Pain Med 2003; 28: 279–288.
5. Perkins FM, Kehlet H. Chronic pain as an outcome of surgery: a review of predictive factors. Anesthesiology 2000; 93:1123–1133.
6. Jung BF, Ahrendt GM, Oaklander AL, Dworkin RH. Neuropathic pain following breast cancer surgery: proposed classification and research update. Pain 2003; 104:1–13.
7. Katz J, Jackson M, Kavanaugh BP, Sandler AN. Acute pain after thoracic surgery predicts long-term post-thoracotomy pain. Clin J Pain 1996; 12:50–55.
8. Smith J, Thompson JM. Phantom limb pain and chemotherapy in pediatric amputees. Mayo Clin Proc 1995; 70:357–364.
9. Green CR, Wheeler JRC. Physician variability in the management of acute postoperative and cancer pain: a quantitative analysis of the Michigan experience. Pain Med 2003; 4:8–20.
10. Anderson KO, Syrjala KL, Cleeland CS. How to assess cancer pain. In: Turk DC, Melzack R, eds. Handbook of Pain Assessment. 2nd ed. New York: Guilford Press, 2001:579–600.
11. Rhodes DJ, Koshy RC, Waterfield WC, Wu AW, Grossman SA. Feasibility of quantitative pain assessment in outpatient oncology practice. J Clin Oncol 2001; 19:501–508.
12. Jacobsen PB, Thors CL. Fatigue in the radiation therapy patient: current management and investigations. Semin Radiat Oncol 2003; 13:372–380.
13. Richardson A, Ream E. The experience of fatigue and other symptoms in patients receiving chemotherapy. Eur J Cancer Care 1996; 5:24–30.
14. Servaes P, Verhagen C, Bleijenberg G. Fatigue in cancer during and after treatment: prevalence, correlates and interventions. Eur J Cancer 2002; 38:27–43.
15. World Health Organization. WHO Guidelines for Cancer Pain Relief. Geneva: World Health Organization, 1996.
16. Benedetti C, Brock C, Cleeland C, Coyle N, Dube JE, Ferrell B, et al. NCCN practice guidelines for cancer pain. Oncology 2000; 14(11A):135–150.
17. Mock V, Atkinson A, Barsevick A, Cella D, Cimprich B, Cleeland C, Donnelly J, Eisenberger MA, et al. National Comprehensive Cancer Network practice guidelines for cancer-related fatigue. Oncology 2000; 14:151–161.

18. Holland JC, Jacobsen PB, Riba MB, et al. NCCN practice guidelines for the management of psychosocial distress. Oncology 1999; 13:113–147.
19. Wallace MS, Wallace AM, Lee J, Dobke MK. Pain after breast surgery: a survey of 282 women. Pain 1996; 66:195–205.
20. Jensen MP. The validity and reliability of pain measures in adults with cancer. J Pain 2003; 4:2–21.
21. Wang XS, Risser AH. Measurement of cancer-related fatigue. In: Simmonds M, ed. Measuring and Managing Patients, Practitioners and Therapies in Rehabilitation. Elsevier Press. In press.
22. Nunnally JC, Bernstein IH. Psychometric Theory. New York: McGraw-Hill, 1994.
23. Turk DC, Melzack R, eds. Handbook of Pain Assessment. 2nd ed. New York: Guilford Press, 2001.
24. Richardson A. Measuring fatigue in patients with cancer. Supportive Care Cancer 1998; 6:94–100.
25. Berry DL, Wilkie DJ, Thomas CR, Fortner P. Clinicians communicating with patients experiencing cancer pain. Cancer Invest 2003; 21:374–381.
26. Cleeland CS, Syrjala KL. How to assess cancer pain. In: Turk DC, Melzack R, eds. Handbook of Pain Assessment. New York: Guilford Press, 1992.
27. Cohen MZ, Easley MK, Ellis C, Hughes B, Ownby K, Rashad BG, Rude M, Taft E, Westbrooks JB. Cancer pain management and the JCAHO's pain standards: an institutional challenge. J Pain Symptom Manage 2003; 25:519–527.
28. Cleeland CS, Mendoza TR, Wang XS, Chou C, Harle MT, Morrissey M, Engstrom MC. Assessing symptom distress in cancer patients: the M.D. Anderson Symptom Inventory. Cancer 2000; 89:1634–1646.
29. Portenoy RK, Thaler HT, Kornblith AB, Lepore JM, Friedlander-Klar H, Kiyasu E, Sobel K, Coyle N, Kemeny N, Norton L, et al. The memorial symptom assessment scale: an instrument for the evaluation of symptom prevalence, characteristics and distress. Eur J Cancer 1994; 30A:1326–1336.
30. Chang VT, Hwang SS, Feuerman M, Kasimis BS, Thaler HT. The memorial symptom assessment scale short form (MSAS-SF): validity and reliability. Cancer 2000; 89:1162–1171.
31. Bruera E, Kuehn M, Miller MJ, Selmser P, Macmillan K. The Edmonton symptom assessment system (ESAS): a simple method for the assessment of palliative care patients. J Palliat Care 1991; 7:6–9.
32. McCorkle R. The measurement of symptom distress. Semin Oncol Nurs 1987; 3:248–256.
33. Cleeland CS, Nakamura Y, Mendoza TR, Edwards KR, Douglas J, Serlin RC. Dimensions of the impact of cancer pain in a four country sample: new information from multidimensional scaling. Pain 1996; 67: 267–273.
34. Melzack R, Katz J. The McGill pain questionnaire: appraisal and current status. In: Turk DC, Melzack R, eds. Handbook of Pain Assessment. New York: Guilford Press, 1992:152–168.
35. Melzack R. The short-form McGill pain questionnaire. Pain 1987; 30:191–197.
36. Caffo O, Amichetti M, Ferro A, Lucenti A, Valduga F, Galligioni E. Pain and quality of life after surgery for breast cancer. Breast Cancer Res Treat 2003; 80:39–48.
37. Caraceni A. Evaluation and assessment of cancer pain and cancer pain treatment. Acta Anaesthesiol Scand 2001; 45:1067–1075.
38. Caraceni A, Cherny N, Fainsinger R, Kaasa S, Poulain P, Radbruch L, DeConno F. The Steering Committee for the EAPC Research Network. Pain measurement tools and methods in clinical research in palliative care: recommendations of an expert working group of the European Association of Palliative Care. J Pain Symptom Manage 2002; 23:239–255.
39. Petrie KJ, Weinman J. More focus needed on symptom appraisal (editorial). J Psychosomatic Res 2003; 54:401–403.
40. Serlin RC, Mendoza TR, Nakamura Y, Edwards KR, Cleeland CS. When is cancer pain mild, moderate or severe? Grading pain severity by its interference with function. Pain 1995; 61:277–284.
41. Cleeland CS. Measurement of pain by subjective report. In: Chapman CR, Loeser JD, eds. Advances in Pain Research and Therapy. Vol. 12. Issues in Pain Measurement. New York Raven Press, 1989:391–403.
42. Cleeland CS, Gonin R, Hatfield AK, Edmonson JH, Blum RH, Stewart JA, Pandya KJ. Pain and its treatment in outpatients with metastatic cancer. N Engl J Med 1994; 330:592–596.
43. Zalon ML. Comparison of pain measures in surgical patients. J Nurs Meas 1999; 7:135–152.
44. Tittle MB, McMillan SC, Hagan S. Validating the brief pain inventory for use with surgical patients with cancer. Oncol Nurs Forum 2003; 30:325–330.
45. Mendoza TR, Chen C, Brugger A, Hubbard R, Snabes M, Palmer SN, Zhang Q, Cleeland CS. The utility and validity of the modified brief pain inventory in a multiple-dose postoperative analgesic trial. Clin J Pain. In press.
46. Jensen MP, Smith DG, Ehde DM, Robinson LR. Pain site and the effects of amputation pain: further clarification of the meaning of mild, moderate, and severe pain. Pain 2001; 91:317–322.
47. Mendoza TR, Chen C, Brugger A, Hubbard R, Snabes M, Palmer SN, Zhang Q, Cleeland CS. Lessons learned from a multiple-dose postoperative analgesic trial. Pain. In press.
48. Glaus A, Crow R, Hammond S. A qualitative study to explore the concept of fatigue/tiredness in cancer patients and in healthy individuals. Supportive Care Cancer 1996; 4:82–96.
49. Richardson A. Fatigue in cancer patients: a review of the literature. Eur J Cancer Care 1995; 4:20–32.
50. Hall GM, Salmon P. Physiological and psychological influences on postoperative fatigue. Anesth Analg 2002; 95:1446–1450.

51. Salmon P, Hall GM. A theory of postoperative fatigue: an interaction of biological, psychological, and social processes. Pharmacol Biochem Behav 1997; 56: 623–628.
52. Salmon P, Hall GM. Postoperative fatigue is a component of the emotional response to surgery: results of multivariate analysis. J Psychosomatic Res 2001; 50: 325–335.
53. Salmon P, Hall GM, Peerbhoy D, Shenkin A, Parker C. Recovery from hip and knee arthroplasty: patients' perspective on pain, function, quality of life, and well-being up to 6 months postoperatively. Arch Phys Med Rehab 2001; 82:360–366.
54. Cimprich B. Attentional fatigue following breast cancer surgery. Res Nurs Health 1992; 15:199–207.
55. Cimprich B, Ronis DL. Attention and symptom distress in women with and without breast cancer. Nurs Res 2001; 50:86–94.
56. Cimprich B, Ronis DL. An environmental intervention to restore attention in women newly diagnosed with breast cancer. Cancer Nurs 2003; 26:284–294.
57. Cooley ME, Short TH, Moriarty HJ. Symptom prevalence, distress, and change over time in adults receiving treatment for lung cancer. Psycho-Oncology 2003; 12: 694–708.
58. Knobel H, Loge JH, Nordoy T, Kolstad AL, Espevik T, Kvaloy S, Kaasa S. High level of fatigue in lymphoma patients treated with high dose therapy. J Pain Symptom Manage 2000; 19:446–456.
59. Wang XS, Janjan NA, Guo H, Johnson BA, Engstrom MC, Crane CH, Mendoza TR, Cleeland CS. Fatigue during preoperative chemoradiation for resectable rectal cancer. Cancer 2001; 92(6 suppl):1725–1732.
60. Jacobsen PB, Hann DM, Azzarello LM, Horton J, Balducci L, Lyman GH. Fatigue in women receiving adjuvant chemotherapy for breast cancer: characteristics, course, and correlates. J Pain Symptom Manage 1999; 18:233–242.
61. Lawrence CC, Gilbert CJ, Peters WP. Evaluation of symptom distress in a bone marrow transplant outpatient environment. Ann Pharmacother 1996; 30: 941–944.
62. Andrykowski MA, Curran SL, Lightner R. Off-treatment fatigue in breast cancer survivors: a ontrolled comparison. J Behav Med 1998; 21:1–18.
63. Bower JE, Ganz PA, Desmond KA, Rowland JH, Meyerowitz BE, Belin TR. Fatigue in breast cancer survivors: occurrence, correlates, and impact on quality of life. J Clin Oncol 2000; 18:743–753.
64. Mendoza TR, Wang XS, Cleeland CS, Morrissey M, Johnson BA, Wendt JK, Huber SL. The rapid assessment of fatigue severity in cancer patients: use of the brief fatigue inventory. Cancer 1999; 85:1186–1196.
65. Holley SK. Evaluating patient distress from cancer-related fatigue: an instrument development study. Oncol Nurs Forum 2000; 27:1425–1431.
66. Hann DM, Jacobsen PB, Martin SC, Kronish LE, Azzarello LM, Fields KK. Fatigue in women treated with bone marrow transplantation for breast cancer: a comparison with women with no history of cancer. Supportive Care Cancer 1997; 5:44–52.
67. Hann DM, Garovoy N, Finkelstein B, Jacobsen PB, Azzarello LM, Fields KK. Fatigue and quality of life in breast cancer patients undergoing autologous stem cell transplantation: a longitudinal comparative study. J Pain Symptom Manage 1999; 17:311–319.
68. Hann DM, Denniston MM, Baker F. Measurement of fatigue in cancer patients: further validation of the fatigue symptom inventory. Qual Life Res 2000; 9: 847–854.
69. Escalante CP, Grover T, Johnson BA, Harle M, Guo H, Mendoza TR, Rivera E, Ho V, Lee EU, Cleeland CS. A fatigue clinic in a comprehensive cancer center. Cancer 2001; 92(suppl 6):1706–1713.
70. Wang XS, Giralt SA, Mendoza TR, Engstrom MC, Johnson BA, Peterson N, Broemeling LD, Cleeland CS. Clinical factors associated with cancer-related fatigue in patients being treated for leukemia and non-Hodgkin's lymphoma. J Clin Oncol 2002; 20: 1319–1328.
71. Anderson KO, Getto CJ, Mendoza TR, Palmer SN, Wang XS, Reyes-Gibby CC, Cleeland CS. Fatigue and sleep disturbance in patients with cancer, patients with clinical depression, and community-dwelling adults. J Pain Symptom Manage 2003; 25:307–318.
72. Beck AT, Steer RA, Brown GK. Beck Depression Inventory-II (BDI-II). San Antonio, TX: Psychological Corporation, 1996.
73. McNair DM, Lorr M, Droppleman LF. Manual for the Profile of Mood States. San Diego: Educational and Industrial Testing Service, 1992.
74. Cella DF, Jacobsen PB, Orav EJ, Holland JC, Silberfarb PM, Rafla S. A brief POMS measure of distress for cancer patients. J Chronic Dis 1987; 40: 939–942.
75. Shacham S. A shortened version of the profile of mood states. J Personality Assess 1983; 47:305–306.
76. Baker F, Denniston M, Zabora J, Polland A, Dudley WN. A POMS short form for cancer patients: psychometric and structural evaluation. Psycho-Oncology 2002; 11:273–281.
77. Özalp G, Sarioglu R, Tuncel G, Aslan K, Kadiogullari N. Preoperative emotional states in patients with breast cancer and postoperative pain. Acta Anaesthesiol Scand 2003; 47:26–29.
78. Uchitomi Y, Mikami I, Nagai K, Nishiwaki Y, Akechi T, Okamura H. Depression and psychological distress in patients during the year after curative resection of non-small-cell lung cancer. J Clin Oncol 2003; 21:69–77.
79. Hopwood P, Stephens RJ. Depression in patients with lung cancer: prevalence and risk factors derived from quality-of-life data. J Clin Oncol 2000; 18:893–903.
80. McDaniel JS, Musselman DL, Porter MR, Reed DA, Nemeroff CB. Depression in patients with cancer: diagnosis, biology, and treatment. Arch Gen Psychiatry 1995; 52:89–99.

81. Raison CL, Miller AH. Depression in cancer: new developments regarding diagnosis and treatment. Biol Psychiatry 2003; 54:283–294.
82. Ahles TA, Blanchard EB, Ruckdeschel JC. The multidimensional nature of cancer-related pain. Pain 1983; 17:277–288.
83. Glover J, Dibble SL, Dodd MS, Miaskowski C. Mood states on oncology outpatients: does pain make a difference? J Pain Symptom Manage 1995; 10: 120–128.
84. Heim HM, Oei TP. Comparison of prostate cancer patients with and without pain. Pain 1993; 53:159–162.
85. Palmer SC, Coyne JC. Screening for depression in medical care: pitfalls, alternatives, and revised priorities. J Psychosomatic Res 2003; 54:279–287.
86. Smets EMA, Garssen B, Bonke B, de Haes JCJM. The multidimensional fatigue inventory (MFI) psychometric qualities of an instrument to assess fatigue. J Psychosomatic Res 1995; 39:315–325.
87. Piper BF, Dibble SL, Dodd MJ, Weiss MC, Slaughter RE, Paul SM. The revised piper fatigue scale: psychometric evaluation in women with breast cancer. Oncol Nurs Forum 1998; 25:677–684.
88. Schwartz JE, Jandorf L, Krupp LB. The measurement of fatigue: a new instrument. J Psychosomatic Res 1993; 37:753–762.
89. Stein KD, Martin SC, Hann DM, Jacobsen PB. A multidimensional measure of fatigue for use with cancer patients. Cancer Practice 1998; 6:143–152.
90. Schwartz AL. The Schwartz cancer fatigue scale: testing reliability and validity. Oncol Nurs Forum 1998; 25:711–717.
91. Smets EM, Visser MRM, Willems-Groot AFMN, Garssen B, Oldenburger F, van Tienhoven G, de Haes JCJM. Fatigue and radiotherapy: (A) experience in patients undergoing treatment. Br J Cancer 1998; 78: 899–906.
92. Smets EM, Visser MRM, Willems-Groot AFMN, Garssen B, Schuster-Uitterhoeve ALJ, de Haes JCJM. Fatigue and radiotherapy: (B) experience in patients 9 months following treatment. Br J Cancer 1998; 78: 907–912.
93. Meek PM, Nail LM, Barsevick A, Schwartz AL, Stephen S, Whitmer K, Beck SL, Jones LS, Walker BL. Psychometric testing of fatigue instruments for use with cancer patients. Nurs Res 2000; 49:181–190.
94. Schneider RA. Reliability and validity of the multidimensional fatigue inventory (MFI-20) and the Rhoten fatigue scale among rural cancer outpatients. Cancer Nurs 1998; 21:370–373.
95. Lucia A, Earnest C, Pérez, M. Cancer-related fatigue: can exercise physiology assist oncologists? Lancet Oncol 2003; 4:616–625.
96. American Psychiatric Association. DSM-IV: Diagnostic and Statistical Manual of Mental Disorders. 4th ed. Washington, DC: APA Press, 1995.
97. Kudoh A, Katagai H, Takazawa T. Increased postoperative pain scores in chronic depression patients who take antidepressants. J Clin Anesth 2002; 14: 421–425.
98. Fallowfield L. Quality of life: a new perspective for cancer patients. Nat Rev Cancer 2002; 2:873–879.
99. Movsas B. Quality of life in oncology trials: a clinical guide. Semin Radiat Oncol 2003; 13:235–247.
100. Aaronson NK, Ahmedzai S, Bergman B, et al. The European Organization for Research and Treatment of Cancer QLQ-C30: a quality of life instrument for use in international clinical trials in oncology. J Natl Cancer Inst 1993; 85:365–376.
101. Cella DF, Tulsky DS, Gray G, Sarafian B, Linn E, Bonomi A, Silberman M, et al. The functional assessment of cancer therapy scale: development and validation of the general measure. J Clin Oncol 1993; 11: 570–579.
102. Nissen MJ, Swenson KK, Ritz LJ, Farrell JB, Sladek ML, Lally RM. Quality of life after breast carcinoma surgery: a comparison of three surgical procedures. Cancer 2001; 91:1238–1246.
103. Wu CL, Naqibuddin M, Rowlingson AJ, Lietman SA, Jermyn RM, Fleisher LA. The effect of pain on health-related quality of life in the immediate postoperative period. Anesth Analg 2003; 97:1078–1085.
104. Ready LB, Ashburn M, Caplan RA, Carr DB, Connis RT, Dixon CL, Hubbard L, Rics LJ. Practice guidelines for acute pain management in the perioperative setting: a report by the American Society of Anesthesiologists task force on pain management, acute pain section. Anesthesiology 1995; 82:1071–1081.
105. Jiang HJ, Lagasse RS, Ciccone K, Jakubowski MS, Kitain EM. Factors influencing hospital implementation of acute pain management practice guidelines. J Clin Anesth 2001; 13:268–276.
106. Fox S, Rainie L. Vital Decisions: How Internet Users Decide What Information to Trust When They or Their Loved Ones Are Sick. Washington, DC: Pew Foundation, 2002.
107. Murray E, Lo B, Pollack L, Donelan K, Catania J, White M, Zapert K, Turner R. The impact of health information on the Internet on the physician-patient relationship: patient perceptions. Arch Internal Med 2003; 163:1727–1734.
108. Metz JM, Devine P, DeNittis A, Jones H, Hampshire M, Goldwein J, Whittington R. A multi-institutional study of Internet utilization by radiation oncology patients. Int J Radiat Oncol Biol Phys 2003; 56:1201–1205.
109. Norum J, Grev A, Moen M-A, Balteskard L, Holte K. Information and communication technology (ICT) in oncology: Patients' and relatives' experiences and suggestions. Supportive Care Cancer 2003; 11:286–293.
110. Allenby A, Matthews J, Beresford J, McLachlan SA. The application of touch-screen technology in screening for psychosocial distress in an ambulatory oncology setting. Eur J Cancer Care 2002; 11:245–253.
111. Ruland CM, White T, Stevens M, Fanciullo G, Khilani SM. Effects of computerized system to support shared decision making in symptom management of cancer

patients: preliminary results. J Am Med Inform Assoc. In press.

112. Lewis B, Lewis D, Cumming G. Frequent measurement of chronic pain: an electronic diary and empirical findings. Pain 1995; 60:341–347.
113. Boyes A, Newell S, Girgis A. Rapid assessment of psychosocial well-being: are computers the way forward in a clinical setting? Qual Life Res 2002; 11:27–35.
114. Taenzer P, Bultz BD, Carlson LE, Speca M, DeGagne T, Olson K, Doll R, Rosberger Z. Impact of computerized quality of life screening on physician behavior and patient satisfaction in lung cancer outpatients. Psycho-Oncology 2000; 9:203–213.
115. Lofland JH, Schaffer M, Goldfarb N. Evaluating health-related quality of life: cost comparison of computerized touch-screen technology and traditional paper systems. Pharmacotherapy 2000; 20: 1390–1395.
116. Velikova G, Wright EP, Smith AB, Cull A, Gould A, Forman D, Perren T, Stead M, Brown J, Selby PJ. Automated collection of quality-of-life data: a comparison of paper and computer touch-screen questionnaires. J Clin Oncol 1999; 17:998–1007.
117. Chandler SW, Payne R. Computerized tools to assess and manage cancer pain. Highlights Oncol Pract 1997; 14:114–117.

54

Pathophysiology of Cancer Pain

P. M. DOUGHERTY

Department of Anesthesiology and Pain Medicine, The University of Texas M.D. Anderson Cancer Center, Houston, Texas, U.S.A.

I. INTRODUCTION

The sensation of pain is normally a response associated with the application of noxious or injurious stimuli. In the setting of the cancer patient, pain stimuli occur as a result of trauma secondary to surgical/medical procedures, due to invasion and compression of tumor cells into peripheral nerves and spinal cord, and finally due to cancer chemo- and radiation therapy. Thus, pain in cancer patients involves multiple components and mechanisms including those mediating acute somatic pain, mediating primary and secondary hyperalgesia, and those mediating neuropathic pain (1,2). In this chapter, the basic physiology of the neural apparatus that responds to noxious stimuli is reviewed. This is followed by a synopsis of the neural mechanisms and neurochemical mediators of acute primary and secondary hyperalgesia and finally by a review of the mechanisms of neuropathic pain. The context is to provide an informed basis for intervention strategies for each of these sources of pain.

II. PAIN FROM UNINJURED TISSUE

A. Peripheral Neural Mechanisms

The initial neural encoding of pain is dependent upon the properties of nociceptors, a distinct class of primary afferent fibers that respond selectively to noxious stimuli. The responses of these fibers to natural stimuli correlate with the pain reported by subjects to the same stimuli. Primary afferent nociceptors are generally subdivided according to whether the parent nerve fiber is unmyelinated (C-fiber) or myelinated (A-fiber).

1. C-Fiber Nociceptors

In monkey, cutaneous C-fiber nociceptors typically are responsive to stimuli over a receptive field area of about 20 mm^2. Most C-fiber nociceptors respond to a number of different stimulus modalities including heat, chemical, and mechanical stimuli and so are often termed *polymodal* (3–6). Several lines of evidence indicate that C-fiber nociceptors are essential for the normal perception of pain. C-fiber nociceptors recorded from monkey (7) and from humans (8) exhibit a monotonically increasing discharge frequency with heat applied to skin that correlate to changes in human judgments of pain. The latency for heat pain sensations following step temperature changes applied to skin matches the calculated conduction time of C-fiber nociceptors (9). Intraneural electrical stimulation of presumed single identified C-fiber nociceptors in humans elicits pain (10) and selective C-fiber block prevents thermal pain perception at the normal heat pain threshold (11,12). Pain stimulus interaction effects observed in psychophysical studies are accounted by C-fiber nociceptors. For example, when two identical heat stimuli are applied to the skin 30 sec apart, the second stimulus is perceived to be about half as painful, and the response of the C-fiber nociceptors is about half as much (5). Finally, in patients with congenital insensitivity to pain, microscopic examination of the peripheral nerves indicates an absence of C fibers (10).

2. *A-Fiber Nociceptors*

A-fiber nociceptors also respond to mechanical, heat, and chemical stimuli and therefore are polymodal in nature like C-fibers. Two types of A-fiber nociceptors have been identified based on their profile of response to heat stimuli. Type I A-fiber nociceptors have very high thresholds under normal circumstances, and, because of this, are referred to as high-threshold mechanoreceptors by many investigators (13–15). However, many of these nociceptors also respond well to intense heat stimuli (16), and therefore are likely involved in signaling the pain associated with intense heat. Type I A-fiber nociceptors are particularly prevalent on the glabrous skin of the hand in monkey (17) and have also been described in cat, rabbit, and man (18,19). The mean conduction velocity for Type I A-fiber nociceptors in monkey is 30 m/sec and extends as high as 55 m/sec. Thus, by conduction velocity criteria, these nociceptors fall into a category between that of Aδ and Aβ fibers.

Type II A-fiber nociceptors are found exclusively on hairy skin. The major distinguishing feature of Type II A-fiber nociceptors is that their threshold to heat is substantially lower than that of Type I A-fiber nociceptors. In addition, their mean conduction velocity, 15 m/sec, is also lower than that of the Type I A-fibers. In hairy skin, stepped heat stimuli evoke a fast onset sharp pricking sensation, followed by a slower onset burning sensation (9). Type II A-fiber nociceptors have several characteristics that make them ideally suited to signal this first pain sensation. The thermal threshold of Type II fibers is near the threshold temperature for first pain (20). The receptor utilization time (time between stimulus onset and receptor activation) of these fibers is short (21) and the conduction velocity of myelinated afferent fibers corresponds to the latency of response to first pain (9). Type II A-fiber nociceptors yield a burst of activity at the onset of a heat stimulus that is consistent with the percept of a momentary pricking sensation (21). Finally, the absence of a first pain sensation to heat stimuli applied to the palm of the human hand (9) correlates with the failure to find Type II A-fiber nociceptors in glabrous skin.

3. *Mechanically Insensitive Afferents*

Not all cutaneous nociceptors respond to mechanical stimuli. Recent evidence suggests that about half of A-fiber nociceptors and 30% of C-fiber nociceptors either have very high mechanical thresholds or are unresponsive to mechanical stimuli (3,22–24). These nociceptors are referred to as mechanically insensitive afferents. Similar afferent fibers have been reported in knee joint (25), viscera (26), and cornea (27). Some cutaneous mechanically insensitive afferents may be chemospecific receptors (3,24,28,29). Others respond to intense cold or heat stimuli (3,24,30).

B. Central Mechanisms

Following transduction by peripheral afferents, nociceptive information flows to the central nervous system (CNS) where it is processed, registered, and a reaction formulated. Figure 1 shows a schematic diagram of the flow of somatosensory information through the neuraxis. The spinal dorsal horn and to a much lesser extent the dorsal column nuclei provide the first link in the central nociceptive pathways. From here, nociceptive information is distributed to sites in the brainstem, midbrain, hypothalamus, thalamus, and finally sensory and the so-called limbic cortices (31–33).

1. *The Spinal Dorsal Horn*

The cells of the dorsal horn are arranged in layers that are defined by anatomic and physiologic methods first described by Rolando, and later schematized by Rexed (34). Figure 2 shows a sketch of a representative dorsal horn with Rexeds layers included. Under this scheme, the dorsal horn consists of layers I–VI. Primary afferent fibers make stereotyped connections with dorsal horn neurons (35–39). Fine myelinated (Aδ) and unmyelinated (C) afferents primarily terminate in the most superficial dorsal horn (layers I and II outer). The targets include cells intrinsic to the dorsal horn (interneurons) as well as cells whose axons leave the spinal cord and ascend (project) to more rostral targets in the brainstem and diencephalon. The larger myelinated afferents end upon cells deeper in the dorsal horn, especially layers III–V and perhaps the inner aspect of II.

The functional properties of cells in the dorsal horn reflect the innervation pattern of the primary afferent fibers. Many of the neurons in the superficial laminae respond exclusively to noxious inputs (40). These cells are often called nociceptive specific (NS) or high-threshold neurons (41,42). Nociceptive specific neurons, like most neurons in CNS sensory pathways studied in an anesthetized preparation, tend to have

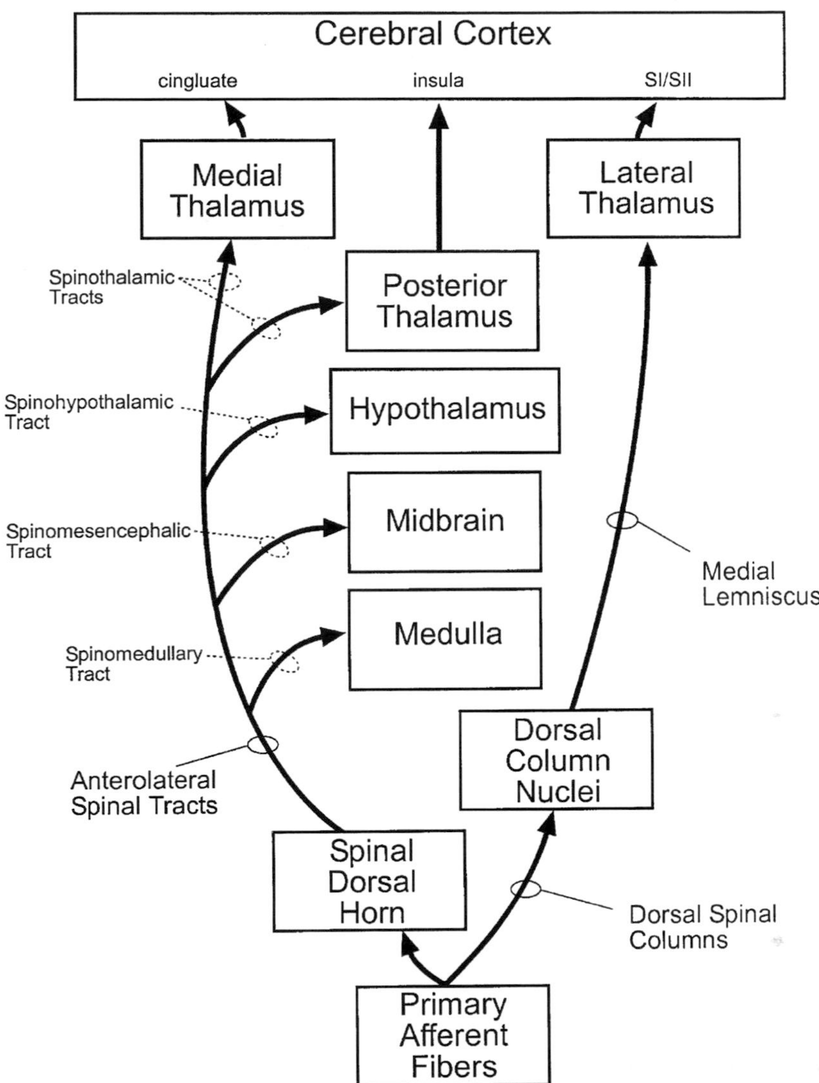

Figure 1 Schematic diagram of the central nociceptive pathways. Each box represents the discrete anatomical locations at which noxious stimuli are processed and/or registered. The lines indicate the neural pathways that interconnect each of the anatomical locations.

ongoing background activity (this is not the case in awake preparations, see Ref. 43). However, NS cells have a lower level of spontaneous activity than most other cells, averaging around 2 Hz as a group (44). Nociceptive specific cells also tend to have relatively small excitatory receptive field sizes, often confined to a single digit or small patch of skin. Many NS cells show polymodal responses to both cutaneous mechanical, heat chemical, and in some cases cooling stimuli (41,42,44,45).

Two other classes of cells are also found in the dorsal horn. Low-threshold (LT) cells respond only to nonnoxious stimuli (33), whereas wide dynamic range (WDR) or multireceptive cells respond to both noxious as well as nonnoxious stimuli (44,45).

Wide dynamic range and LT cells have a higher mean level of spontaneous activity (in the anesthetized preparation) than NS neurons, averaging around 10 Hz (44,45). The excitatory receptive fields are usually larger than for HT cells, often covering two or more digits, and often covering both glabrous and hairy skin. Low-threshold cells are especially prevalent in laminae II, and many of these may be inhibitory interneurons. Low-threshold tract neurons project from the spinal cord primarily to the dorsal column nuclei, with relatively few of these cells projecting to the brainstem, midbrain, or diencephalon.

The WDR cells in laminae I–VI are both intrinsic and projection neurons. The inputs from nociceptors to these cells may be passed via contacts from more

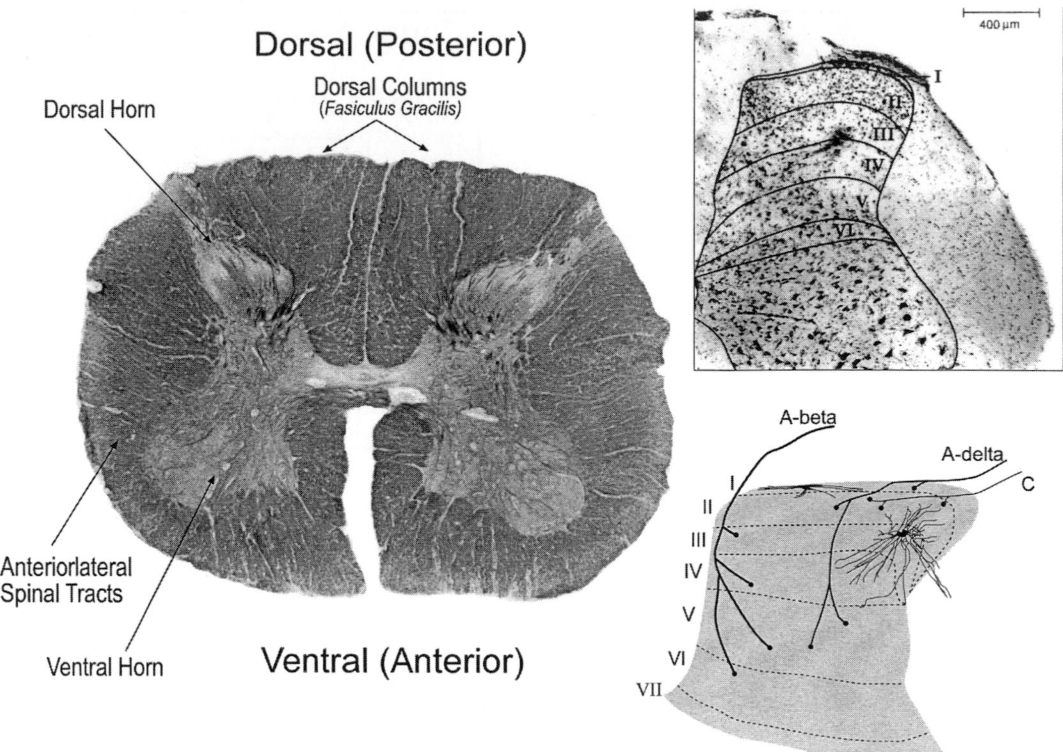

Figure 2 Histological sections and schematic diagrams of the spinal dorsal horn. The histological section at left from human lumbar spinal cord is labeled to show the relationship between the major spinal somatosensory structures. The histological section at right is from rat spinal cord. The outer heavy lines show the boundary of the spinal gray matter, while the inner heavy lines show the boundaries of Rexeds laminae. These boundaries are established by the histological characteristics of each zone, and the layers are identified by the numerals at the right of the dorsal horn boundary. Finally, the schematic at the bottom illustrates the pattern of primary afferent innervation to the nonhuman primate spinal dorsal horn. The large myelinated (A-beta) fibers segregate to the dorsal aspect of an entering rootlet and then course medially in the dorsal horn and terminate in layers III–V. The small myelinated (A-delta) fibers and C-fibers that carry nociceptive information segregate ventrally in the entering roots, course laterally in the dorsal horn, and then largely terminate in the more superficial layers (I and II) of the dorsal horn. The cell profiles inserted in laminae I and II–IV are representative of superficial and deep classes of spinothalamic neurons.

superficial intrinsic cells or may be passed via contacts of afferents on dorsal dendrites that penetrate into the superficial laminae. WDR neurons found in lamina I may be the key neural substrates for the transmission of cooling and warm (nonnoxious thermal) stimuli (23,41,46). Wide dynamic range cells in laminae III–V show responses to both cutaneous mechanical and heat stimuli, but rarely show responses from deep tissues. Wide dynamic range projection neurons in these laminae are found to innervate all rostral targets of the spinal cord. Cells in laminae VI and VII tend to especially show responses from deep tissue and visceral receptors.

The responses of typical NS, WDR, and LT neurons to different intensities of mechanical stimuli are shown in Fig. 3. As mentioned above, WDR neurons show responses to both noxious as well as nonnoxious stimuli. Indeed, many of these cells show responses that are graded with the intensity of the cutaneous stimuli. Many NS neurons, on the other hand, respond only to stimuli well above the intensity needed to provoke the sensation of pain, to stimuli that are sufficient to cause tissue damage. Based on these observations, it was suggested that WDR neurons provide the neural substrate for the detection and discrimination of noxious from nonnoxious stimuli. This property allows the organism to detect cutaneous stimuli as they approach an intensity that would be tissue damaging and so allow a reaction to be formed to avoid actual damage (47,48). Nociceptive specific cells under this scheme only inform the organism that actual tissue damage has occurred (49). Another possibility is that WDR cells provide a "nonspecific alerting or conditioning input," which primes more rostral neurons for the more specific inputs of the NS neurons (50).

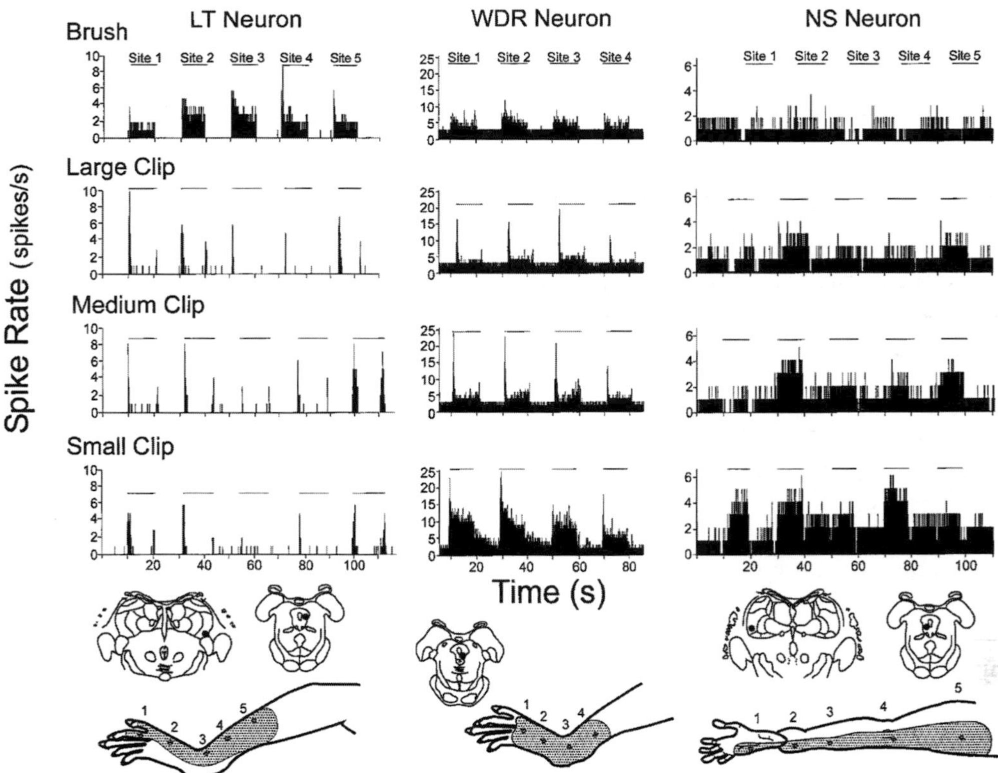

Figure 3 The rate histograms show responses of primate spinothalamic tract neurons representative of LT, WDR, and NS classes. The responses of these cells were evoked by application of a series of mechanical stimuli of graded intensity to multiple sites across the receptive field for each cell. The times and sites of each stimulus application are indicated by the lines and labels at the top of each histogram. The brush stimulus was provided by a soft camel hair brush, while the large, medium, and small clip stimuli were provided by applications of increasingly intense compressive arterial clips to the skin. The WDR cell in the center of the figure shows responses that are graded with the intensity of the stimuli. The NS neuron shows no significant responses to any stimuli but the most intense, while the LT neuron responds to innocuous brushing of the skin alone (the transient responses with the application and removal or the arterial clips are due to the touch stimuli provided at contact). The diagrams of the brain cross sections shown at the bottom indicate the locations from which each cell was antidromically activated (two had double projections to thalamus and the midbrain). Finally, the diagrams of the hindlimbs show the receptive field locations of each neuron (shaded region) and the sites on skin where each of the mechanical stimuli were applied (spots and numerals).

2. *The Dorsal Column Nuclei*

Some neurons resident in the spinal dorsal horn project to a number of more rostral brain targets. In addition to the primary afferent input to the dorsal column nuclei, there is also input to this site from at least two groups of dorsal horn projection neurons, the postsynaptic dorsal column pathway and the spinocervical tract (31,33). The cells of the dorsal column nuclei largely respond to innocuous stimuli alone. The lemniscal system in primates does not appear to encode painful stimuli. The information carried in this path is primarily from hair follicle receptors, pacinian corpuscles, and Types I and II slowly adapting receptors (32,33). In addition, the nucleus cuneatus (but not gracilis) shows responses to muscle afferents (spindles and golgi tendon organs). However, there are several lines of evidence, which suggest a role of the dorsal column nuclei in nociceptive transmission. For example, the recurrence of pain after lesion of the anterolateral spinal quadrant (51) and the reference of pain to other regions of the body immediately after anterolateral chordotomy is often cited (52). Although most afferent input to the dorsal column nuclei is from large myelinated afferents, neuropathic pains are in fact largely conveyed by myelinated fiber inputs (53). In addition, an input from nonmyelinated afferents to the dorsal column nuclei has also been shown (54–58) and a small number of nociceptive dorsal column neurons have been reported (59,60). Although not yet demonstrated in man, the two spinal tracts that ascend to the dorsal column nuclei mentioned above are often nociceptive (61,62). Finally, research suggests the presence of a novel pain pathway running in the dorsal columns that mediates the perception of visceral pain (63,64).

3. *Rostral CNS Areas Involved in Pain Perception*

Other dorsal horn neurons project to the medullary reticular formation (spinoreticular tract), the mesencephalic periaqueductal gray and neighboring area (spinomesencephalic), the hypothalamus (spinohypothalamic tract), and finally, the sensory regions of thalamus (spinothalamic tract) including the ventral posterior-lateral (VPL) nucleus, the posterior-inferior thalamic region, and to a more limited extent the central-lateral nucleus (32).

Among the higher nociceptive centers, the thalamus and the spinothalamic tract are the most studied (32). One reason for this intense study is the observation that neurons of the spinothalamic tract encode stimuli in a way that matches well with the perceptions of humans to noxious stimuli. This characteristic is well illustrated by comparison of the psychophysical ratings of humans and the physiological responses of spinothalamic neurons in primates to graded intensities of cutaneous stimuli. Figure 4 shows that the responses of spinothalamic neurons to graded heat stimuli applied to the skin correlate well with the rating of pain intensity given by

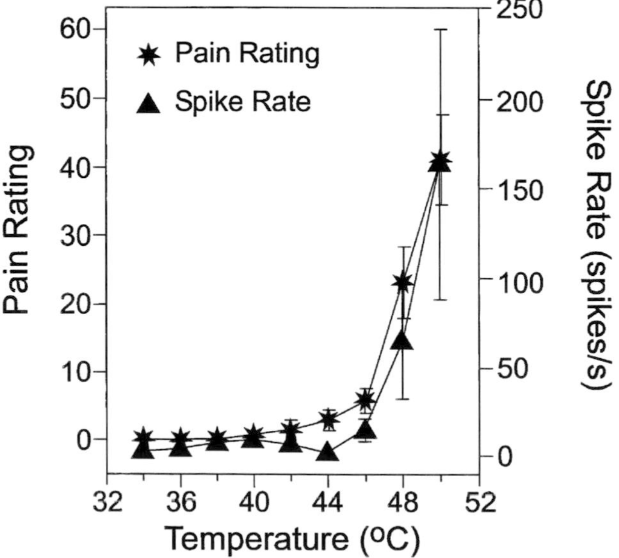

Figure 4 Comparison of pain ratings of human subjects (stars) to graded heat stimuli with the discharges of monkey spinothalamic neurons (triangles) to the identical stimuli. The *y*-axis is labeled in units for the pain ratings on the left and for the neuron discharge rates on the right. *Source*: From Ref. 65.

human subjects to the same stimuli (65). The other spinal pathways (e.g., the spinoreticular, spinomesencephalic, and spinohypothalamic tracts) each has some neurons that show responses profiles, which resemble those for the spinothalamic cells. But these additional pathways also include subsets of cells that do not show this close correlation with human ratings of pain intensity. For example, many of the cells in these pathways have receptive fields that are spread over very large body areas and that show complex responses to cutaneous stimuli that do not resemble human ratings of stimulus intensity (32). The specific functions of these pathways remain poorly defined, but are suggested to include the affective/motivational and vegetative (autonomic and neuroendocrine) aspects of nociception.

Each of the primary targets of spinal projection neurons in turn projects to more rostral targets. The dorsal column nuclei project via the medial lemniscus to an area of the ventralposterior thalamus just anterior to the termination of the spinothalamic tract (66,67). This region is often termed the "core" of the ventralposterior nucleus. Neurons in thalamus in turn project to the SI, SII, and retroinsular cortexes, with those thalamic cells receiving lemniscal inputs especially projecting to the more rostral SI and SII areas and the cells receiving spinothalamic input especially projecting to the posterior-inferior retroinsular area (66,67). The rostral targets of the brainstem reticular formation, the mesencephalic gray, and the hypothalamus are very diffuse, and outputs of these structures may also include pathways that descend back to the spinal cord.

The same types of neurons present in the spinal dorsal horn have also been described for each of these higher sites in the central nociceptive pathways. For example, Fig. 5 shows the responses of a WDR neuron in the chief sensory nucleus of nonhuman primate thalamus to graded thermal, mechanical, and cooling stimuli (68). Also present in the thalamus, but not illustrated, are low- and high-threshold neurons as described previously for the dorsal horn. The low-threshold neurons are especially prevalent in the "core" or "rod zone" of the ventral posterior nucleus, which largely receives inputs from the medial lemniscus via the dorsal column nuclei. The NS types of neurons in thalamus are especially concentrated in the posterior-inferior area of the thalamus, which some term the matrix area of the thalamus.

C. Neurochemistry of Somatosensory Transmission

As illustrated in Fig. 6, there are multiple neurotransmitters and neuropeptides involved in somatosensory neurotransmission. The main excitatory neurotransmitters in the somatosensory system are the amino

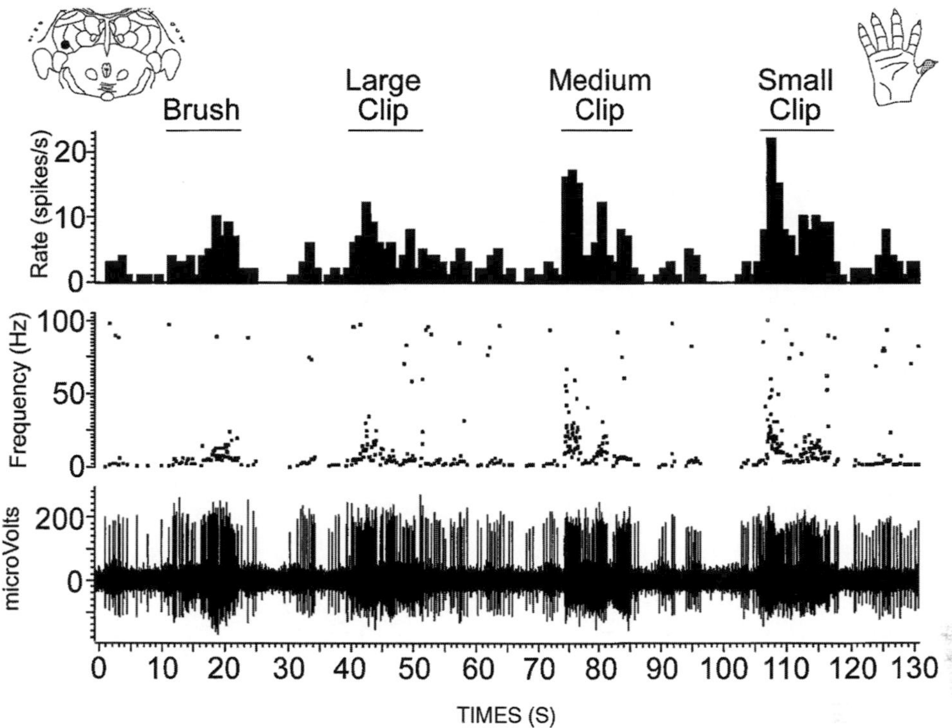

Figure 5 Responses of a WDR neuron in the nonhuman somatosensory thalamus (VPL) to noxious and nonnoxious mechanical stimuli. The bottom line shows an oscilloscope sweep of analog recordings of the cell to the mechanical stimuli, while compiled rate histograms and instantaneous frequency plots for each of the stimuli are shown in the top and middle lines. The outline at top left shows the estimated recording site in thalamus and the drawing of the forepaw at top right shows the location of the neuron's receptive field.

acids glutamate and aspartate (69–71). These excitatory amino acids appear to mediate the transmission at each of the afferent connection in the somatosensory system, including the synaptic connection between primary afferent fibers and spinal neurons, from spinal neurons to thalamic neurons, etc. There are four receptor types for glutamate and aspartate in the somatosensory system (72–76). These receptors are named for the synthetic agonists by whom they are best activated. Thus, one class of receptors best activated by *N*-methyl-D-aspartate (NMDA) is termed the NMDA glutamate receptor. A second class of receptors not activated by NMDA (non-NMDA receptors) include three subtypes, a kainate receptor, an AMPA [(*R,S*)-α-amino-3-hydroxy-5-methylisoxazole-4-proprionic acid] receptor and an ACPD (*trans*-(±) -1-amino-cyclopentane-1,3-dicarboxylate) receptor. The AMPA and kainate receptors are linked to sodium channels and are considered to mediate the majority of the fast synaptic afferent signaling in this system for all modalities and intensities of stimuli. The NMDA receptor is usually considered as recruited only by intense and/or prolonged somatosensory stimuli. This characteristic is due to the NMDA receptor's well-known magnesium block that is only relieved by prolonged depolarization of the cell membrane. The NMDA receptor is linked to a calcium ionophore that when activated results in many long-term changes in excitability of sensory neurons (sensitization). The AMPA/kainate and NMDA receptors are also frequently considered to mediate mono- and polysynaptic contacts of primary afferent fibers to dorsal horn neurons. Finally, the ACPD site, often termed the metabotropic glutamate receptor, is a G-protein-linked site that when activated results in liberation of ionositol phosphate resulting in liberation of cytosolic calcium. It is unclear what role the ACPD receptor plays in somatosensory signaling.

A second type of excitatory substance that may have a transmitter role in the somatosensory system is adenosine triphosphate (ATP) (77,78). Adenosine triphosphate excited some dorsal horn neurons in an in vitro preparation. Excitation of ATP in vivo was found to be rather specific for cells receiving only low-threshold mechanoreceptive inputs in spinal laminae II and III.

The primary inhibitory neurotransmitters of the somatosensory system include the amino acids glycine and gamma-amino-butyric acid (GABA). Glycine is

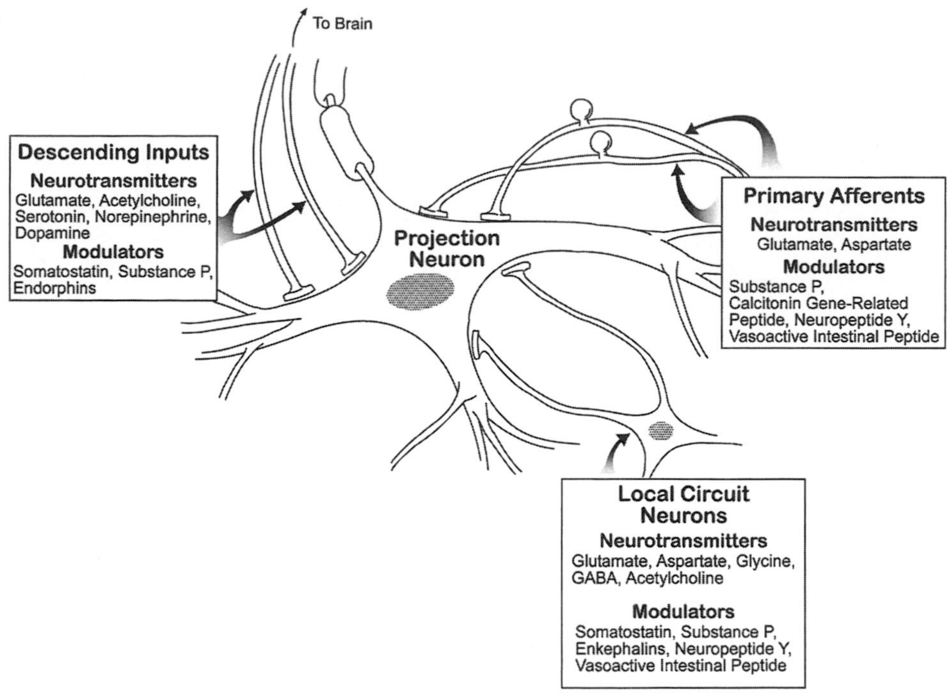

Figure 6 The schematic summarizes the neurochemical pathways involved in somatosensory neurotransmission in the dorsal horn. Intrinsic sources of each transmitter are indicated by each of the labeled boxes.

particularly important at spinal levels, while GABA is the predominate inhibitory transmitter at higher levels (79–82). Glycine has two receptor sites: a chloride-linked strychnine-sensitive inhibitory receptor as well as a strychnine-insensitive modulatory site on the NMDA glutamate receptor complex. Gamma-amino-butyric acid also has two receptor sites. The GABA-A receptor is a chloride-linked ionophore that is also the site of action for barbiturates and benzodiazepines. The GABA-B receptors are linked to either potassium channels or to activation of G-proteins.

Alterations in the functions of the inhibitory neurotransmitters may be particularly important with the induction of hyperalgesia and following the development of neuropathic pain. For example, a GABA-A-mediated link between large myelinated fibers and C-fiber nociceptors has been proposed as a mechanism for the development of allodynia following intradermal injection of the irritant capsaicin. Additionally, a selective loss of inhibitory interneurons at both spinal and thalamic levels has been suggested as contributing to some neuropathic pain conditions.

Norepinephrine is an important inhibitory neurotransmitter in descending brainstem projections to the dorsal horn (83,84). The adrenergic receptors include two broad classes termed the alpha- and beta-receptors, each of which in turn has several subtypes. The alpha 2 adrenergic receptor is the primary form found in the spinal dorsal horn that provides an inhibitory function of neurotransmission of sensory information. However, it should be noted that the function of norepinephrine following injury to the nervous systems might become reversed from an inhibitory, analgesic role into one of promoting and or sustaining an ongoing chronic pain state.

Another important secondary inhibitory neurotransmitter at spinal levels is the purine adenosine (85). There are at least two types of adenosine receptors termed the A1 and A2 sites. Occupation of these sites by adenosine results in G-protein-mediated alterations of cyclic AMP levels in target cells. However, both elevations as well as decreases in cAMP formation have been reported in various conditions. Adenosine may mediate a portion of the analgesia produced by brainstem norepinephrine projections to the spinal cord and appears to have especially robust analgesic properties in neuropathic pain conditions.

Acetylcholine is yet another neurotransmitter that appears to mediate antinociception at the level of the spinal dorsal horn. The antinociceptive effects appear to be mediated by the muscarinic and not by the nicotinic acetylcholine receptor subtypes (86).

Finally, serotonin has been proposed as an inhibitory transmitter in pathways descending to the spinal dorsal horn from the midbrain raphe nuclei (87–89). There are multiple serotonin receptor subtypes including 5HT-1, -2 and -3 receptors. Each of these major types also has several subtypes. Controversy remains concerning which of these subtypes mediate the analgesic properties of serotonin. In part, this controversy may be due to the fact that some serotonin receptor subtypes, in fact, promote nociception while others are inhibitory.

There are multiple neuropeptides that contribute to signaling of somatosensory information. The excitatory neuropeptides in the somatosensory system include substance P and neurokinin A (90–93). These peptides are especially concentrated in primary afferent fibers, but also may be present in intrinsic neurons of the spinal dorsal horn and thalamus. The receptors for these peptides include the neurokinin 1 and 2 sites, each of which has been associated with elevation of intracellular calcium levels, perhaps through liberation of ionositol phosphate. At the spinal level, these peptides are only released following application of noxious stimuli, which are sufficient to produce sustained discharges in C-nociceptors, although some small myelinated (Aδ) fibers may also contain substance P. These peptides do not appear to signal as synaptic transmitters but rather as transsynaptic transmitters. Thus, once released, the peptides are not confined to a site of action on the immediate postsynaptic membrane, but instead tend to spread throughout the dorsal horn potentially acting on multiple synapses at some distance from their point of release. It has been suggested that stimuli of particular modalities (e.g., mechanical vs. thermal) are associated with selective release of one peptide vs. another; however, this suggestion has not been corroborated. Activation of neurokinin 1 and/or 2 receptors by substance P and/or neurokinin A is agreed as key step needed for the induction of sensitization and hence the expression of hyperalgesia following cutaneous injury. It has been further proposed that the mechanism of neurokinin receptor involvement in the expression of sensitization is through facilitation of the synaptic actions of the excitatory amino acid neurotransmitters.

The inhibitory neuropeptides at spinal levels include somatostatin, the enkephalins, and possibly dynorphin (94–97). These peptides are contained in both intrinsic neurons of the dorsal horn and in the fibers descending to the dorsal horn from various brainstem nuclei. At thalamic levels, the inhibitory neuropeptides also include the endorphins, which are contained in ascending antinociceptive pathways. The receptor types for the opioid peptides include the mu, delta, and kappa receptor subtypes at all levels of the somatosensory system. These receptors are associated with modulation of both intracellular cAMP and potassium levels. There is also an important cooperative functional link between mu opioid and alpha 2 adrenergic receptors that have yet to be fully exploited for clinical applications.

Finally, there are a number of neuropeptides that are present in the somatosensory system that yet to have clear functions identified and so, for now, need to be considered as a third category. These peptides include calcitonin gene-related peptide (CGRP), vasoactive intestinal peptide (VIP), neuropeptide Y (NPY), and cholecystokinin (CCK), among others. Future volumes such as this will no doubt have more to say about the role of these peptides in the neurochemistry of synaptic transmission in the somatosensory system.

III. HYPERALGESIA FOLLOWING TISSUE INJURY AND INFLAMMATION

Hyperalgesia develops after injury or inflammation of cutaneous and deep tissue such as that occurring with surgery in the cancer patient. Hyperalgesia is characterized by a decrease in pain threshold, an increased pain to suprathreshold stimuli, and ongoing pain. Hyperalgesia occurs not only at the site of injury but also in the surrounding uninjured area. Hyperalgesia at the site of injury is termed *primary hyperalgesia*, while hyperalgesia in the uninjured skin surrounding the injury is termed *secondary hyperalgesia* (98).

The characteristics of primary and secondary hyperalgesia differ. A burn to the glabrous skin of the hand leads to a marked hyperalgesia to heat and to mechanical stimuli applied at the injury site (16). The pain threshold for both modalities is dramatically reduced, and pain to suprathreshold stimuli is greatly increased in this primary zone of hyperalgesia. In contrast, when stimuli are applied away from the site of injury, hypersensitivity to mechanical stimuli but not to thermal stimuli is found present in the zone of secondary hyperalgesia (99). Indeed, at least two forms of mechanical hyperalgesia have been reported in the secondary zone (100,101). Hyperalgesia to light touch or stroking stimuli is often referred to as allodynia (102–104) and hyperalgesia to sharp stimuli such as VonFrey probes referred to as punctate hyperalgesia are both present and appear to have different neural mechanisms (100,101).

A. Primary Afferent Sensitization and Primary Hyperalgesia

Primary hyperalgesia is mediated by sensitization of nociceptors (16,105). *Sensitization* is defined as a leftward shift of the stimulus-response function that relates magnitude of the neural response to stimulus intensity. Sensitization is characterized by a decrease in threshold, an augmented response to suprathreshold stimuli, and ongoing spontaneous activity (106–108). The changes in responses of primary afferent fibers recorded in anesthetized monkeys after injury correlates to the changes in subjective ratings of pain in humans following the same injury (16). Test heat stimuli were applied to the glabrous skin of the hand before and after a burn that led to prominent hyperalgesia in human subjects. C-fiber nociceptors showed a decreased response following the burn, whereas the Type I A-fiber nociceptors were markedly sensitized. Thus, A-fiber nociceptors play an important role in primary hyperalgesia in glabrous skin. In contrast, C-fiber nociceptors in hairy skin are sensitized following injury and so C- and A-fiber nociceptors mediate primary hyperalgesia that occurs in hairy skin (109). In the knee joint, mechanically insensitive afferents become responsive to mechanical stimuli after inflammation (110). Similar sensitization to mechanical stimuli after administration of inflammatory agents or after cutaneous injury has also been observed in cutaneous mechanically insensitive afferents (22,24,28). Thus, mechanically insensitive afferents also have an important role in the mechanical hyperalgesia following both cutaneous and deep tissue injury.

B. Spinal Neuron Sensitization and Secondary Hyperalgesia

The idea that sensitization of spinal neurons accounts for secondary hyperalgesia remained controversial for a prolonged period. Lewis (98) first proposed that spreading sensitization of primary afferents, wherein activation and sensitization of an initial nociceptor leads to sensitization of neighboring nociceptors due to the effects of a sensitizing substance released from the initial nociceptor, accounted for secondary hyperalgesia. However, injury adjacent to a nociceptors receptive field or indeed even to one-half of a receptive field does not produce sensitization of the nociceptor fibers outside the area of injury (111–113). Similarly, antidromic stimulation of nociceptive fibers does not cause sensitization of primary afferent endings (112,114).

Psychophysical studies provided the earliest evidence that spinal neurons mediate secondary hyperalgesia. Intradermal injection of capsaicin, the active ingredient in hot peppers, produces intense pain at the injection site and a large zone of secondary hyperalgesia surrounding the injection site. When capsaicin is administered under conditions of a proximal anesthetic nerve block to spare the spinal cord from the nociceptive barrage generated at the time of injection but leaving the peripheral nervous system effects of the capsaicin unaffected, no secondary hyperalgesia is present even after the block has worn off (101). An alteration in central processing therefore plays a major role in secondary hyperalgesia. When the capsaicin injection site is cooled or anesthetized after the injection, signs of secondary hyperalgesia to light touch are eliminated or substantially reduced, while hyperalgesia to punctate stimuli remains largely unaffected (101). Thus, ongoing input from primary afferent neurons at the site of injury is required to maintain some types of secondary hyperalgesia, while other types become independent of nociceptor input after the provoking nociceptor barrage. These two forms of secondary mechanical hyperalgesia are transmitted by different primary afferent types. Selectively blocking large myelinated fibers using pressure causes pain to light touch to disappear when touch sensation is lost but heat and cold sensations are still present (100,101). Similarly, intraneural microstimulation of large diameter (Aβ) fibers in awake human subjects evoked tactile paresthesias in normal skin, but pain in skin made hyperalgesic with capsaicin (115). Meanwhile, other lines of psychophysical evidence indicate that punctate secondary mechanical hyperalgesia is mediated by small diameter (Aδ) fibers (116).

Neurophysiological investigations have shown that the characteristics of secondary hyperalgesia are well explained by properties of dorsal horn neurons after injury (44,65,117,118). As mentioned above, the responses of spinothalamic cells to noxious stimuli correlate well with the pain ratings of humans to the same stimuli (65). Similarly, spinothalamic cell responses after injury also correlate with the development of secondary hyperalgesia. As shown in Fig. 7, the responses of dorsal horn neurons to mechanical stimuli are increased in magnitude to a given stimulus following an injury. In addition, the receptive field areas of single neurons become expanded. This expansion of receptive field area results in a greater number of cells responding to a stimulus delivered to any given area of skin. Thus, both more pain signaling cells are responding to a given mechanical stimulus and these responses are increased in magnitude. Meanwhile, the response to heat of dorsal horn neurons is enhanced only for stimuli applied in the area of primary hyperalgesia at the site of injury, but either unchanged or even reduced for heat stimuli applied in the adjacent secondary hyperalgesia areas of undamaged skin (119).

Controversy still remains regarding the specific roles that functional subsets of dorsal horn neurons play in generating secondary hyperalgesia. Most WDR dorsal horn neurons are sensitized by a variety of peripheral injuries, suggesting that this subtype of neurons are important for the detection and discrimination of tissue damaging stimuli and in the generation of secondary hyperalgesia. Nociceptive specific cells sensitize less frequently after peripheral injury than do WDR neurons and so NS cells have often been assigned a less prominent role in the generation of secondary

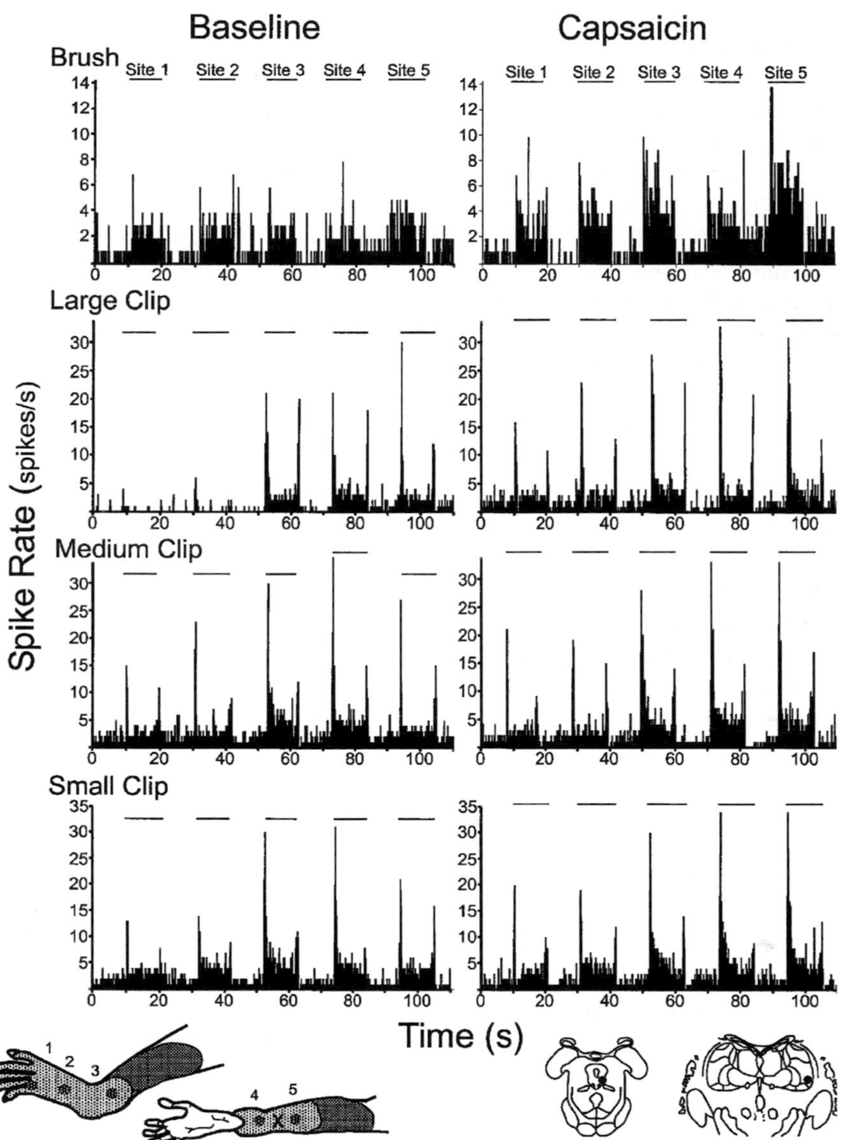

Figure 7 The rate histograms show the background activity and responses of a representative wide dynamic range spinothalamic tract neuron to mechanical stimulation of the hindlimb before and following an intradermal injection of capsaicin. The baseline responses to the mechanical stimuli are shown in the left-hand column, while the matching records after capsaicin are shown in the right-hand column. The mechanical stimuli were applied to the sites shown on the drawing of the leg at the bottom of the figure. The "X" shows the site at which capsaicin was delivered. The lightly stippled area shows the receptive field during the baseline recordings, while the heavily stippled area shows the expansion in receptive field induced by capsaicin.

hyperalgesia (48). However, since even the signaling of nonsensitized NS cells would be superimposed on that of sensitized WDR cells, a role for NS cells in secondary hyperalgesia should not be minimized (50). Low-threshold cells have not been reported to acquire nociceptive inputs following injury, but rather often show a loss of all excitatory responses (120). At first blush, this data suggests that this group of neurons appears to have little or no role in the generation of secondary hyperalgesia. Yet, some characteristics of secondary hyperalgesia, such as the uniform intensity of pain throughout the zone and the sharp borders to the zone of hyperalgesia, could involve a subtraction-type of signal like that shown by LT neurons.

C. Hyperalgesia and Plasticity in Rostral CNS Structures

Finally, neurons in higher CNS areas also show enhanced responses after injury. For example, the responses of neurons in the thalamus and cortex of rats to cutaneous mechanical stimuli have been shown to increase with the induction of both experimental arthritis and experimental neuropathy (121,122). Similarly, the neuronal activity in the thalamus of humans with chronic pain also shows alterations (68,123–125). Although these changes in responses of thalamic and cortical neurons may just reflect changes that have taken place in the primary afferents and spinal cord neurons under each of these conditions, it should be noted that anatomical and neurochemical changes also take place in the thalamus and cortex under each of these conditions (126,127). Thus, neuronal substrates exist to support a third or even fourth component to hyperalgesia.

D. Neurochemistry of Primary Afferent and Central Sensitization

Mechanistically, primary afferent fibers are sensitized by the release of the inflammatory soup arising from damaged tissues and from activated immune and inflammatory cells (128). These mediators, many of which directly cause pain (129), include bradykinin, serotonin, histamine, prostaglandins, leukotrienes, excitatory amino acids, adenosine triphosphate, substance P, cytokines, nerve growth factor, nitric oxide, and various physiochemical stimuli (128,130). Specific primary afferent fibers are often sensitive to only one or a few of these substances and specific substances often produce hyperalgesia to only a specific modality of sensation. For example, bradykinin only produces thermal hyperalgesia when injected to human skin (128). Other components of the soup, most notably the prostaglandins, do not directly cause pain or hyperalgesia, but sensitize the fibers to other mediators of the soup (130). Nevertheless, a final common biochemical pathway shared by most all these mediators in their effects on primary afferent fibers through is activation of adenyl cyclase (131).

The wide variety of chemical mediators involved in regular sensory neurotransmission as reviewed above can all influence the sensitization process in the spinal dorsal horn. However, as illustrated in Fig. 8, the key event in spinal sensitization is facilitation of excitatory amino acid neurotransmission between primary afferent fibers and dorsal horn neurons by coreleased neuropeptides (44,117). Tachykinin neuropeptides, substance P, and neurokinin A released from C-fibers with noxious stimulation produce an immediate increase in the postsynaptic effects of the excitatory amino acids, glutamate, and aspartate, that are released from either nociceptive or nonnociceptive primary afferents. Facilitation of responses by tachykinins at AMPA-type glutamate receptors requires continuous activation at tachykinin receptors, and thus provides a neurochemical mechanism for the signs of secondary hyperalgesia that are readily reversible with anesthesia of the site of injury. In contrast, facilitation of responses by tachykinins at NMDA-type glutamate receptors is often very long lasting after a single coordinated coactivation of these receptors by both types of ligands. Thus, neurokinin-induced facilitation of glutamate NMDA receptors provides a neurochemical mechanism for the characteristics of secondary hyperalgesia such as punctuate hyperalgesia that outlast anesthesia of the injury site.

IV. HYPERALGESIA FOLLOWING NERVE INJURY

A. Symptomology and Psychophysics of Neuropathic Pain

Traumatic injury to soft-tissue, bone, and/or nerve leads, in certain cases, to a chronic pain state that is characterized by ongoing pain and hyperalgesia (132–134). Intriguingly, in some patients the pain and hyperalgesia are dependent on sympathetic innervation of the affected area (sympathetically maintained pain, SMP (135)), while in others the pain is independent of the sympathetics [SIP (53,111)]. Clinically, both SMP and SIP patients often present with similar signs and symptoms (136).

Several lines of evidence indicate that activity in low-threshold mechanoreceptors can evoke pain in neuropathic pain patients. For example, touch-evoked pain disappears during a selective A-fiber block (53). Further, the latency for touch-evoked pain is short and requires that the primary afferent signal be conducted in Aβ fibers (53,133). Finally, in patients with SMP, weak electrical stimulation of the involved peripheral nerve such that only Aß fibers were activated evoked pain before, but only tingling after, a sympathetic block (137).

Although primary afferent nociceptor sensitization accounts for certain aspects of hyperalgesia in tissue injury (see above), the touch-evoked pain commonly seen in neuropathic pain states appears to be due to a central sensitization. Central neurons, activity in which leads to the sensation of pain, develop an enhanced response to input from nonnociceptive afferents such as low-threshold mechanoreceptors. Such a central sensitization of dorsal horn neurons following cutaneous injury has been demonstrated by several investigators (see above). This central sensitization may be selective in that mechanical hyperalgesia can be present in the absence of hyperalgesia to heat (99,138). Thus, the mechanical hyperalgesia observed in neuropathic pain is similar to the secondary hyperalgesia observed after cutaneous injury.

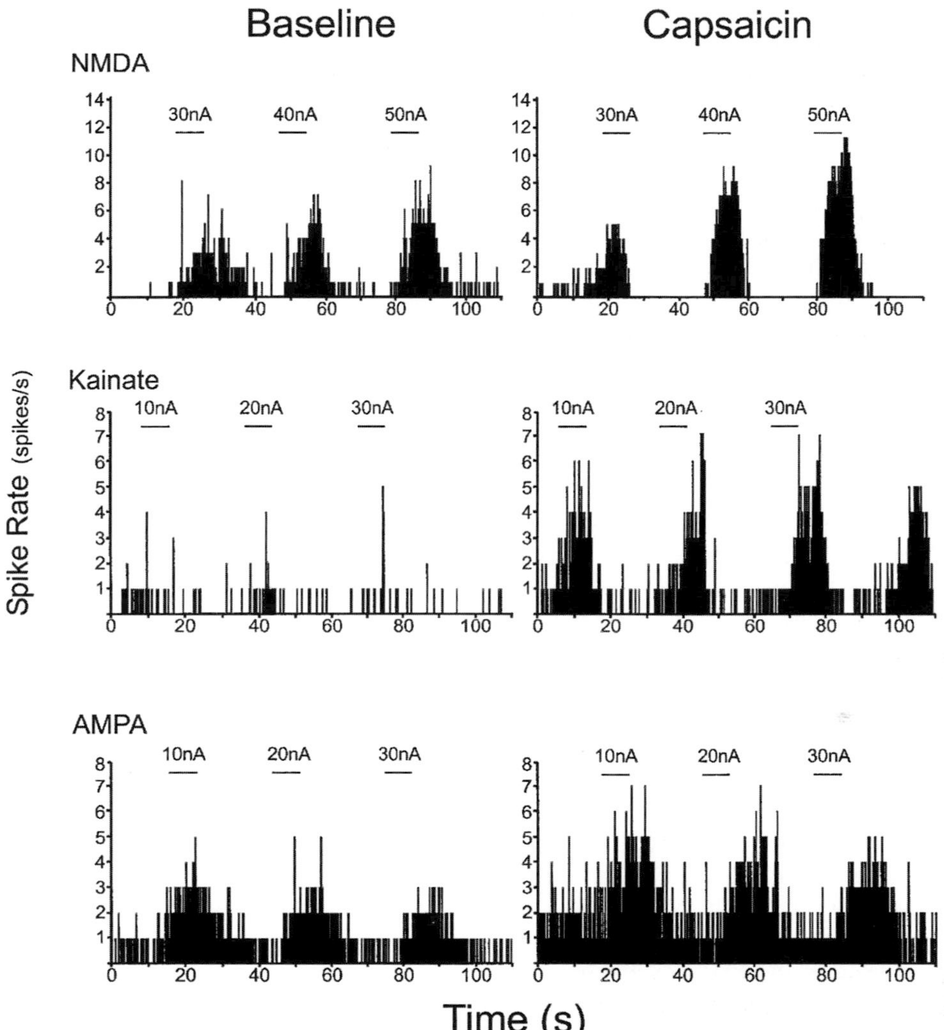

Figure 8 The rate histograms show the responses to excitatory amino acids applied by microiontophoresis onto the same cell shown in Fig. 7 before (left column) and then following sensitization by capsaicin (right column). The times of each drug application are shown by the lines over each set of histograms. NMDA = *N*-methyl-D-aspartate, AMPA = α-amino-3-hydroxy-5-methyl-isoxazolepropionic acid.

B. Animal Models for the Study of Neuropathic Pain

Plasticity in the nervous system after nerve injury has been studied following axotomy (139,140), rhizotomy (141–144), and more recently following various types of partial injuries to nerves innervating the hindlimbs (145–147).

Justification of these injuries as models for the study of human neuropathic pain is based on the behaviors shown by animals with these injuries. For example, a few days to a week after rhizotomy or axotomy, animals show an increased sensitivity to mechanical stimuli (148) and may self-mutilate the deafferented limb (autotomy) (143,149), cf. Refs. 150–152. In contrast, animals with partial nerve injury rarely autotomize yet do exhibit other behavioral changes consistent with a neuropathic pain state. These symptoms are observed within hours (146,147) or several days after the partial nerve injury (153). The posture of the rats is altered so that the hindlimb appears to be maintained in a "guarded" position (145–147). In addition, the rats exhibit enhanced behavioral responses to noxious thermal, mechanical, and sometimes cooling stimuli (145–147).

C. Physiologic Changes in Peripheral Nerves After Nerve Injury

Peripheral nerves show an initial afferent barrage when injured that may be briefly quite intense, but which usually resolves within no more than several minutes (140,154). This injury barrage appears to be a very important event in provoking many of the sequelae of nerve injury. Although an injury barrage following partial nerve injury models has not been directly measured, indirect evidence suggests that such an injury barrage does, in fact, take place with these models. For example, anesthesia of the sciatic nerve prior to injury reduces both the severity and duration of the thermal hyperalgesia that develops later (155). Similarly, administration of MK-801, an antagonist for the NMDA-type glutamate receptor activated by intense afferent barrages, reduces the severity of partial nerve injury induced hyperalgesia (156,157) as do antagonists for the nitric oxide cascade (158).

Once the injury discharges subside, the injured axons enter a period of quiescence. The transected axons are clearly no longer connected to the peripheral transducers. Similarly, many axons in partially injured nerves fail to conduct through the nerve injury site (159), and the dorsal root potentials and afferent volleys are reduced (160).

Three to five days following axotomy, rhizotomy, or partial nerve injury, spontaneous discharges develop in the severed nerves (139,154,159,161–166). This activity following overt nerve section reaches a peak frequency at about day 14 after injury and then slowly tapers to a low level, which is sustained for many weeks. Most of the spontaneously active fibers have conduction velocity of small myelinated fibers, although some unmyelinated fibers also show spontaneous discharges. Ectopic discharges arise from sites both at the cut ends of fibers in the neuroma as well as near the cell bodies in the dorsal root ganglia. Many fibers in a neuroma are sensitive to mechanical or chemical stimuli, some alter their discharge rates upon heating or cooling, and some may form direct electrical (ephaptic) connections with neighboring fibers within the neuroma (167). However, it is not clear whether the ectopic activity in neuroma or injured axons parallels the behaviors shown by animals with nerve injuries (154,168).

D. Physiological Changes in Central Neurons After Nerve Injury

Central nervous system neurons, like primary afferents, also show a large discharge at the time of nerve transaction (169). The time course of the injury discharges observed in the CNS parallels that found in primary afferents. Once the injury discharges subside, spinal neurons also enter a period of quiescence, which is characterized by a decrease in excitatory inputs. Indeed, for many spinal neurons, the decrease in excitatory input is global so that receptive fields become more difficult to identify in the dorsal horn, especially for cells immediately contiguous to the entry zone of the severed nerve.

A few days following nerve injury, many CNS neurons develop changes in spontaneous activity (e.g., Refs. 141,142,144,149,163,169,170). These changes lag behind the development of spontaneous discharges in afferent fibers by 1–3 days. Cells either show a continuous, regular discharge of high frequency, or are relatively silent except for sudden high-frequency bursts. Most of the cells showing these changes after nerve section are in the center of a deafferented zone and have no defined peripheral receptive field. However, some cells at the margins of the deafferented zones exhibit responses to cutaneous stimuli as well as changes in spontaneous activity. Higher percentages than normal of these cells respond only to noxious stimuli. Similar changes in the spontaneous activity of dorsal horn cells were also shown after partial nerve injury, although most dorsal horn cells retained receptive fields (171–173). Altered spontaneous discharges develop in the dorsal horn and dorsal column nuclei as soon as a week following peripheral nerve injury, while similar changes in the thalamus and cortex are not reported until later time points (174–176). Moreover, alterations in spontaneous activity are not limited to experimental animals, but have also been shown in the human spinal cord and thalamus after nerve injury (123–125,177).

Reappearance of receptive fields for dorsal horn neurons that were originally deafferented occurs about 1–2 weeks after injury (142,162,178,179). Many of these new receptive fields are somatotopically inappropriate, usually located in body areas corresponding to dermatomes neighboring the deafferented areas (cf. Refs. 180,181). The receptive fields often have unusual sizes varying from very large to very small, and are often split. Many of these neurons respond only to low-intensity mechanical stimuli. The development of inappropriate somatotopy has also been reported to take place in the human thalamus following nerve injury (182) and in the cortex of experimental animals (183–185).

Dorsal horn neurons studied in animals with partial nerve injuries do not usually show altered receptive fields. Instead, these neurons have elevated baseline firing rates and a propensity for very prolonged after discharges (171,172) (Fig. 9). Cells in monkeys with partial nerve injuries show elevated responses to all cutaneous stimuli at the margins of the nerve-injured zone (172).

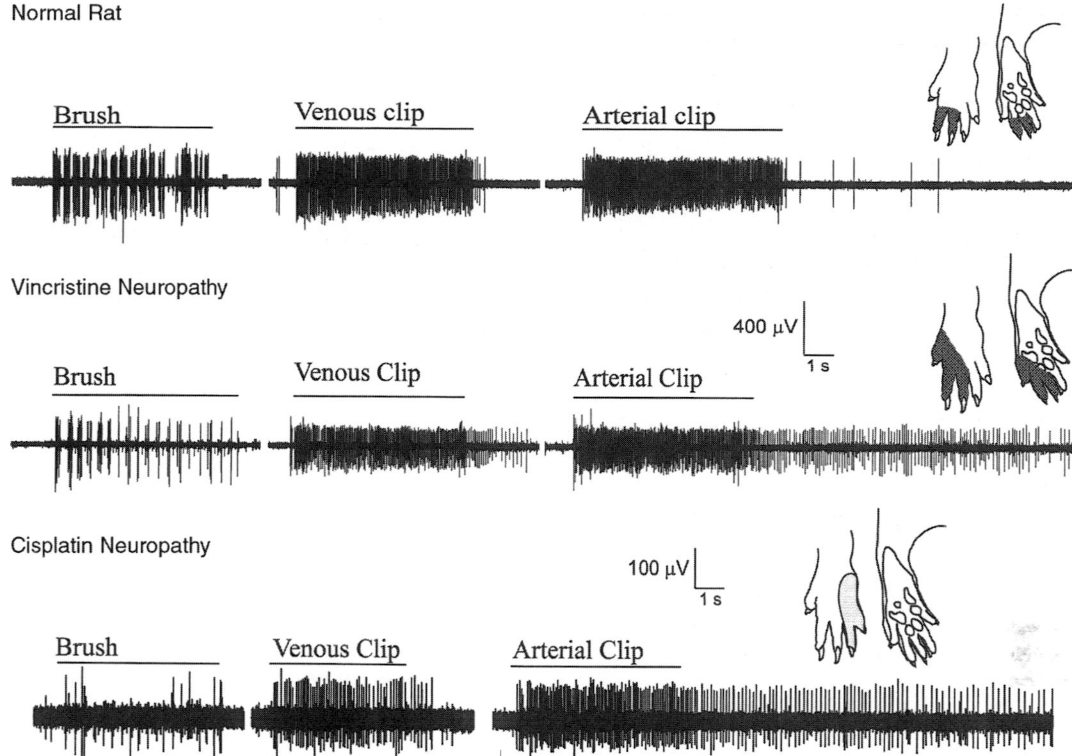

Figure 9 The analog recordings of neuron activity from spinal cord show excess afterdischarges to cutaneous stimuli in rats with hyperalgesia after being treated for 3–5 days with vincristine or cisplatin. The times of each stimulus application are indicted by the lines over each trace and the receptive field location are shown in the drawings at the right.

E. Neurochemistry of Neuropathic Pain

The neurochemistry underlying neuropathic pain shares much in common with that underlying acute primary and secondary hyperalgesia reviewed above. Thus, inflammatory mediators near primary afferent nerve endings produce sensitization of these fibers and excitatory amino acids and neurokinin peptides contribute to sensitization of spinal neurons. However, given that neuropathic pain by definition involves damage to the nervous system, it should not be surprising that this neurochemistry is further complicated due to both degenerative (186) as well as regenerative processes in both primary afferent and central neurons (187). Not only does cell loss and attempted regrowth complicate the neurochemical milieu in the somatosensory system but the morphological responses to injury and attempted tissue repair are also likely culprits that underlie the refractory and long-term nature of neuropathic pain.

The most obvious of the degenerative changes occurring with peripheral nerve damage is the loss of primary afferent drive to the spinal dorsal horn. The gate theory of pain control posits that inputs in large-diameter fibers inhibit spinal processing of signals from small-diameter nociceptors (188). A disinhibition of pain signaling in cells that normally have convergent input could easily be envisaged as a consequence of nerve damage that preferentially affects large fiber inputs to this cell or group of cells. A less obvious degenerative change thought to contribute to neuropathic pain after peripheral nerve injury is the transsynaptic loss of inhibitory neurons in the spinal cord following peripheral nerve injury (189,190). A similar loss of inhibitory neurons in the thalamus may contribute to central pain following spinal cord injury (191). Wallerian degeneration of peripheral axons and digestion of lost central neurons provokes the activation of both central and peripheral glial elements as well as inflammatory cells. Activation of these cells results in increases in the levels of perineural inflammatory cytokines that can further activate nociceptive neurons and generate pain (192–195).

Following the phase of axonal/neuronal degeneration due to injury is the stimulation of regrowth of surviving injured axons and proliferation of neurons that adjoin deafferented neural and peripheral targets. Neurons that are injured will attempt to restore connectivity that is lost to an original innervation target and uninjured neurons will attempt to establish innervation to targets that have become deprived of neural input. Competition between these two sets of growing neurons almost ensures that inappropriate connectivity both within the central nervous system and in the periphery will result. In addition, as neurons grow they discharge spontaneously, thus increasing signal traffic throughout the somatosensory axis. Gene expression is also changed in neurons (196–198) that results in changes in cell phenotype that may include alteration of cell surface ion channels (199,200) neurotransmitter and neuropeptide receptors (189) surface growth-associated proteins (187) and changes in neurotransmitter and neuropeptide content and synaptic release. Invasion of dorsal root ganglia by sympathetic nerves and the de novo expression of adrenergic receptors on peripheral nerves is one example of a phenotypic change resulting in pain (186,201). Finally, the expression of nerve growth factors is upregulated with neuronal proliferation, which directly produces pain when administered to experimental animals (202–204).

V. SUMMARY

The physiological basis of pain sensation from skin can be summarized as a series of neuronal linkages that run from the skin to the spinal cord and then on to a number of more rostral centers located in the brainstem, midbrain, diencephalons, and finally the cortex. Cancer pain occurs as a result of alterations in the usual manners in which both noxious and nonnoxious stimuli are processed by these networks of neurons and involves the routine processing of acute nociceptive stimuli, processes of short-term sensitization of peripheral and central neurons, and long-term processes associated with neuropathic pain. Each of these pain processes shares signaling pathways and has shared as well unique neurochemical and physiological components. Thus, treatment of pain in cancer patients requires identification of the specific pain mechanisms that have been activated and subsequently a tailoring of treatment to best remedy for each specific pain component.

REFERENCES

1. Schwei MJ, Honore P, Rogers SD, Salak-Johnson JL, Finke MP, Ramnaraine ML, et al. Neurochemical and cellular reorganization of the spinal cord in a murine model of bone cancer pain. J Neurosci 1999; 19(24): 10,886–10,897.
2. Wilkie D, Huang H-Y, Reilly N, Cain K. Nociceptive and neuropathic pain in patients with lung cancer: a comparison of pain quality descriptors. J Pain Symptom Manage 2002; 22(5):899–910.
3. Kress M, Koltzenburg M, Reeh PW, Handwerker HO. Responsiveness and functional attributes of electrically localized terminals of cutaneous C-fibers in vivo and in vitro. J Neurophysiol 1992; 68:581–595.
4. Lynn B, Baranowski R. A comparison of the relative numbers and properties of cutaneous nociceptive afferents in different mammalian species. In: Schmidt RF, Schaible HG, Vahle-Heinz C, eds. Fine Afferent Nerve Fibers and Pain. Weinheim: VCH, 1987:86–94.
5. LaMotte RH, Campbell JN. Comparison of responses of warm and nociceptive C-fiber afferents in monkey with human judgments of thermal pain. J Neurophysiol 1978; 41:509–528.
6. Ochoa J, Torebjork E. Sensations evoked by intraneural microstimulation of single mechanoreceptor units innervating the human hand. J Physiol 1983; 342:633–654.
7. Meyer RA, Campbell JN. Peripheral neural coding of pain sensation. J H A P L Tech Digest 1981; 2:164–171.
8. Torebjork HE, LaMotte RH, Robinson CJ. Peripheral neural correlates of magnitude of cutaneous pain and hyperalgesia: simultaneous recordings in humans of sensory judgements of pain and evoked responses in nociceptors with C-fibers. J Neurophysiol 1984; 51: 325–339.
9. Campbell JN, LaMotte RH. Latency to detection of first pain. Brain Res 1983; 266:203–208.
10. Bischoff A. Congenital insensitivity to pain with anhidrosis. A morphometric study of sural nerve and cutaneous receptors in the human prepuce. In: Bonica JJ, Liebeskind JC, Albe-Fessard DG, eds. Advances in Pain Research and Therapy. New York: Raven Press, 1979:53–65.
11. Sinclair DC, Hinshaw JR. A comparison of the sensory dissociation produced by procaine and by limb compression. Brain 1950; 73:480–498.
12. Torebjork HE, Hallin RG. Perceptual changes accompanying controlled preferential blocking of A and C fibre responses in intact human skin nerves. Exp Brain Res 1973; 16:321–332.
13. Burgess PR, Petit D, Warren RM. Receptor types in cat hairy skin supplied by myelinated fibers. J Neurophysiol 1968; 31:833–848.
14. Burgess PR, Perl ER. Myelinated afferent fibres responding specifically to noxious stimulation of the skin. J Physiol 1967; 190:541–562.
15. Perl ER. Myelinated afferent fibers innervating the primate skin and their response to noxious stimuli. J Physiol 1968; 97:593–615.
16. Meyer RA, Campbell JN. Myelinated nociceptive afferents account for the hyperalgesia that follows a burn to the hand. Science 1981; 213:1527–1529.
17. Campbell JN, Meyer RA. Sensitization of unmyelinated nociceptive afferents in monkey varies with skin type. J Neurophysiol 1983; 49:98–110.
18. Fitzgerald M, Lynn B. The sensitization of high threshold mechanoreceptors with myelinated axons by repeated heating. J Physiol 1977; 265:549–563.

19. Roberts WJ, Elardo SM. Sympathetic activation of unmyelinated mechanoreceptors in cat skin. Brain Res 1985; 339:123–125.
20. Dubner R, Price DD, Beitel RE, Hu JW. Peripheral neural correlates of behavior in monkey and human related to sensory-discriminative aspects of pain. In: Anderson, Matthews, eds. Pain in the Trigeminal Region. Amsterdam: Elsevier, 1977:57–66.
21. Meyer RA, Campbell JN, Raja SN. Peripheral neural mechanisms of cutaneous hyperalgesia. In: Fields HL, Dubner R, Cervero F, eds. Advances in Pain Research and Therapy. New York: Raven Press, 1985; 9:53–71.
22. Schmelz M, Schmidt R, Ringkamp M, Handwerker HO, Torebjork HE. Sensitization of insensitive branches of C nociceptors in human skin. J Physiol 1994; 480(Pt 2): 389–394.
23. Handwerker HO, Kobal G. Psychophysiology of experimentally induced pain. Physiol Rev 1993; 73:639–671.
24. Meyer RA, Davis KD, Cohen RH, Treede RD, Campbell JN. Mechanically insensitive afferents (MIAs) in cutaneous nerves of monkey. Brain Res 1991; 561:252–261.
25. Schaible HG, Schmidt RF. Effects of an experimental arthritis on the sensory properties of fine articular afferent units. J Neurophysiol 1985; 54:1109–1122.
26. Habler HJ, Jänig W, Koltzenburg M. A novel type of unmyelinated chemosensitive nociceptor in the acutely inflamed urinary bladder. Agents Actions 1988; 25: 219–221.
27. Tanelian DL. Cholinergic activation of a population of corneal afferent nerves. Exp Brain Res 1991; 86: 414–420.
28. Davis KD, Meyer RA, Campbell JN. Chemosensitivity and sensitization of nociceptive afferents that innervate the hairy skin of monkey. J Neurophysiol 1993; 69(4):1071–1081.
29. LaMotte RH, Simone DA, Baumann TK, Shain CN, Alreja M. Hypothesis for novel classes of chemoreceptors mediating chemogenic pain and itch. In: Dubner R, Gebhart GF, Bond MR, eds. Proceedings of the Vth World Congress on Pain. Amsterdam: Elsevier Science Publishers, 1988:529–540.
30. LaMotte RH, Thalhammer JG. Response properties of high-threshold cutaneous cold receptors in the primate. Brain Res 1982; 244:279–287.
31. Wall PD, Melzack R. Textbook of Pain. 3rd ed. New York: Churchill Livingstone, 1994.
32. Willis WD. The Pain System. The Neural Basis of Nociceptive Transmission in the Mammalian Nervous System. Basel: Karger, 1985.
33. Willis WD, Coggeshall RE. Sensory Mechanisms of the Spinal Cord. New York: Plenum Press, 1991.
34. Rexed B. The cytoarchitectonic organization of the spinal cord in the cat. J Comp Neurol 1952; 96: 415–466.
35. Ralston HJI, Ralston DD. The distribution of dorsal root axons in laminae I, II and III of the macaque spinal cord: a quantitative electron microscope study. J Comp Neurol 1979; 184:643–684.
36. Ralston HJ III, Ralston DD. The distribution of dorsal root axons to laminae IV, V, and VI of the macaque spinal cord: a quantitative electron microscopic study. J Comp Neurol 1982; 212:435–448.
37. Woolf CJ. Central terminations of cutaneous mechanoreceptive afferents in the rat lumbar spinal cord. J Comp Neurol 1987; 261:105–119.
38. Woolf CJ, Fitzgerald M. Somatotopic organization of cutaneous afferent terminals and dorsal horn neuronal receptive fields in the superficial and deep lamine of the rat lumbar spinal cord. J Comp Neurol 1986; 251: 517–531.
39. Light AR, Trevino DL, Perl ER. Morphological features of functionally defined neurons in the marginal zone and substantia gelatinosa of the spinal dorsal horn. J Comp Neurol 1979; 186:151–172.
40. Cervero F, Bennett GJ, Headley PM. Processing of sensory information in the superficial dorsal horn of the spinal cord. New York: Plenum Press, 1989.
41. Craig AD, Kniffki KD. Spinothalamic lumbosacral lamina I cells responsive to skin and muscle stimulation in the cat. J Physiol 1985; 365:197–221.
42. Han ZS, Zhang ET, Craig AD. Nociceptive and thermoreceptive lamina I neurons are anatomically distinct. Nat Neurosci 1998; 1:218–225.
43. Collins JG. A descriptive study of spinal dorsal horn neurons in the physiologically intact, awake, drug-free cat. Brain Res 1987; 416:34–42.
44. Dougherty PM, Willis WD. Enhanced responses of spinothalamic tract neurons to excitatory amino acids accompany the generation of capsaicin-induced hyperalgesia in the monkey. J Neurosci 1992; 12:883–894.
45. Dougherty PM, Palecek J, Paleckova V, Sorkin LS, Willis WD. The role of NMDA and non-NMDA excitatory amino acid receptors in the excitation of primate spinothalamic tract neurons by mechanical, thermal, chemical, and electrical stimuli. J Neurosci 1992; 12:3025–3041.
46. Craig AD, Hunsley SJ. Morphine enhances the activity of thermoreceptive cold-specific lamina I spinothalamic neurons in the cat. Brain Res 1991; 558:93–97.
47. Dubner R, Kenshalo DR Jr, Maixner W, Bushnell MC, Oliveras JL. The correlation of monkey medullary dorsal horn neuronal activity and the perceived intensity of noxious heat stimuli. J Neurophysiol 1989; 62:450–457.
48. Willis WD. Mechanical allodynia: a role for sensitized nociceptive tract cells with convergent input from mechanoreceptors and nociceptors? Am Pain Soc J 1993; 2:23–33.
49. Surmeier DJ, Honda CN, Willis WD. Responses of primate spinothalamic neurons to noxious thermal stimulation of glabrous and hairy skin. J Neurophysiol 1986; 56:351–369.
50. Perl ER. Multireceptive neurons and mechanical allodynia. Am Pain Soc J 1993; 2:37–41.

51. Vierck CJ. Can mechanisms of central pain syndrome be investigated in animals models? Casey KL, ed. Pain and Central Nervous System Disease: The Central Pain Syndromes. New York: Raven Press, 1991: 129–141.
52. Nagaro T, Amakawa K, Kimura S, Arai T. Reference of pain following percutaneous cervical cordotomy. Pain 1993; 53:205–211.
53. Campbell JN, Raja SN, Meyer RA, Mackinnon SE. Myelinated afferents signal the hyperalgesia associated with nerve injury. Pain 1988; 32:89–94.
54. Conti F, De Biasi S, Giuffrida R, Rustioni A. Substance P-containing projections in the dorsal columns of rats and cats. Neuroscience 1990; 34:607–621.
55. Fabri M, Conti F. Calcitonin gene-related peptide-positive neurons and fibers in the cat dorsal column nuclei. Neuroscience 1990; 35:167–174.
56. Garret L, Coggeshall RE, Patterson JT, Chung K. Numbers and proportions of unmyelinated axons at cervical levels in the fasciculus gracilis of monkey and cat. Anat Rec 1992; 232:301–304.
57. Patterson JT, Coggeshall RE, Lee WT, Chung K. Long ascending unmyelinated primary afferent axons in the rat dorsal column: immunohistochemical localizations. Neurosci Lett 1990; 108:6–10.
58. Patterson JT, Chung K, Coggeshall RE. Further evidence for the existence of long ascending unmyelinated primary afferent fibers with the dorsal funiculus: effects of caosaicin. Pain 1992; 49:117–120.
59. Cliffer KD, Hasegawa T, Willis WD. Responses of neurons in the gracile nucleus of cats to innocuous and noxious stimuli: basic characterization and antidromic activation from the thalamus. J Neurophysiol 1992; 68:818–832.
60. Ferrington DG, Downie JM, Willis WD Jr. Primate nucleus gracilis neurons: responses to innocuous and noxious stimuli. J Neurophysiol 1988; 59:886–907.
61. Brown AG, Brown PB, Fyffe REW, Pubols LM. Receptive field organization and response properties of spinal neurones with axons ascending the dorsal columns in the cat. J Physiol 1983; 337:575–588.
62. Brown AG, Franz DN. Responses of spinocervical tract neurones to natural stimulation of identified cutaneous receptors. Exp Brain Res 1969; 7:231–249.
63. Al-Chaer ED, Westlund KN, Willis WD. Nucleus gracilis: an integrator for visceral and somatic information. J Neurophysiol 1997; 78:521–527.
64. Al-Chaer ED, Feng Y, Willis WD. A role for the dorsal column in nociceptive visceral input to thalamus of primates. J Neurophysiol 1998; 79:3143–3150.
65. Simone DA, Sorkin LS, Oh U, Chung JM, Owens C, LaMotte RH, et al. Neurogenic hyperalgesia: central neural correlates in responses of spinothalamic tract neurons. J Neurophysiol 1991; 66:228–246.
66. Jones EG. The Thalamus. New York, London: Plenum Press, 1985.
67. Jones EG, Burton H. Cytoarchitecture and somatic sensory connectivity of thalamic nuclei other than the ventrobasal complex in the cat. J Comp Neurol 1974; 154:395–432.
68. Lenz FA, Seike M, Lin YC, Baker FH, Rowland LH, Gracely RH, et al. Neurons in the area of human nucleus ventralis caudalis (Vc) respond to painful heat stimuli. Brain Res 1993; 623:235–240.
69. Ottersen OP, Storm-Mathisen J. Glutamate- and GABA-containing neurons in the mouse and rat brain, as demonstrated with a new immunocy tochemical technique. J Comp Neurol 1984; 229: 374–392.
70. Fagg GE, Foster AC. Amino acid neurotransmitters and their pathways in the mammalian central nervous system. Neuroscience 1983; 9:701–719.
71. Greenamyre JT, Young AB, Penney JB. Quantitative autoradiographic distribution of l-[3h] glutamate-binding sites in rat central nervous system. J Neurosci 1984; 4(8):2133–2144.
72. Cotman CW, Iversen LL. Excitatory amino acids in the brain—focus on NMDA receptors. Trends Neurosci 1987; 10:263–302.
73. Aanonsen LM, Lei S, Wilcox GL. Excitatory amino acid receptors and nociceptive neurotransmission in rat spinal cord. Pain 1990; 41:309–321.
74. Cotman CW, Monaghan DT, Ottersen OP, Storm-Mathisen J. Anatomical organization of excitatory amino acid receptors and their pathways. Trends Neurosci 1987; 10:273–280.
75. Davies J, Quinlan JE, Sheardown MJ. Mediation of excitatory transmission in specific brain pathways by amino acids acting at NMDA and non-NMDA receptors. In: Hicks TP, Lodge D, McLennan H, eds. Excitatory Amino Acid Transmission. New York: Alan R. Liss, Inc., 1987:277–284.
76. Mayer ML, Westbrook GL. The physiology of excitatory amino acids in the vertebrate central nervous system. Prog Neurobiol 1987; 28:197–276.
77. Fyffe REW, Perl ER. Is ATP a central synaptic mediator for certain primary afferent fibers from mammalian skin? Proc Natl Acad Sci USA 1984; 81: 6890–6893.
78. Li J, Perl ER. ATP modulation of synaptic transmission in the spinal substantia gelatinosa. J Neurosci 1995; 15(5):3357–3365.
79. Berger SJ, Carter JG, Lowry OH. The distribution of glycine, GABA, glutamate and aspartate in rabbit spinal cord, cerebellum and hippocampus. J Neurochem 1977; 28:149–158.
80. Bowery NG, Hudson AL, Price GW. GABA-A and GABA-B receptor site distribution in the rat central nervous system. Neurosci Lett 1987; 20:365–383.
81. Malcangio M, Bowery NG. GABA and its receptors in the spinal cord. TIPS 1996; 17:457–462.
82. Ryall RW. Amino acid receptors in CNS. I. GABA and glycine in spinal cord. In: Iverson, Snyder, eds. Handbook of Psychopharmacology. New York: Plenum Press, 1975:83–128.

83. Hylden JL, Wilcox GL, Antinociceptive effect of morphine and norepinephrine on rat spinothalamic tract and other dorsal horn neurons. Neuroscience 1986; 19:393–401.
84. Archer T, Jonsson G, Minor BG, Post C. Noradrenergic–serotonergic interactions and nociception in the rat. Eur J Pharmacol 1986; 120:295–307.
85. Aran S, Proudfit HK. Antinociception produced by interactions between intrathecally administered adenosine agonists and norepinephrine. Brain Res 1990; 513: 255–263.
86. Yaksh TL, Dirksen R, Harty GJ. Antinociceptive effects of intrathecally injected cholinomimetic drugs in the rat and cat. Eur J Pharmacol 1985; 117(1): 81–88.
87. Carstens E, MacKinnon JD, Guinan MJ. Serotonin involvement in descending inhibition of spinal nociceptive transmission produced by stimulation of medial diencephalon and basal forebrain. J Neurosci 1983; 3:2112–2120.
88. Messing RB, Lytle LD. Serotonin-containing neurons: their possible role in pain and analgesia. Pain 1977; 4:1–21.
89. Sorkin LS, McAdoo DJ, Willis WD. Raphe magnus stimulation-induced antinociception in the cat is associated with the release of amino acids as well as serotonin in the lumbar dorsal hom. Brain Res 1993; 618:95–108.
90. Barber RP, Vaughn JE, Slemmon R, Salvaterra PM, Roberts E, Leeman SE. The origin distribution and synaptic relationships of substance P axons in rat spinal cord. J Comp Neurol 1979; 184:331–352.
91. Henry JL, Krnjevic K, Morris ME. Substance P and spinal neurones. Can J Physiol Pharmacol 1975; 53: 423–432.
92. Krnjevic K. Effects of substance P on central neurons in cats. In: VonEuler US, Pernow B, eds. Substance P. New York: Raven Press, 1977:217–230.
93. Pederson-Bjergaard U, Nielsen LB, Jensen K, Edvinsson L, Jansen I, Olesen J. Algesia and local responses induced by neurokinin A and substance P in human skin and temporal muscle. Peptides 1989; 10:1147–1152.
94. Betoin F, Ardid D, Herbet A, Aumaitre O, Kemeny JL, Duchene-MArullaz P, et al. Evidence for a cental long-lasting antinociceptive effect of vapreotide, an analog of somatostatin, involving an opioidergic mechanism. J Pharm Exp Ther 1994; 269(1):7–14.
95. Kuraishi Y, Hirota N, Sato Y, Hino Y, Satoh M, Takagi H. Evidence that substance P and somatostatin transmit separate information related to pain in the spinal dorsal horn. Brain Res 1985; 325:294–298.
96. Akil H, Richardson DE, Barchas JD. Pain control by focal brain stimulation in man: relationship to enkephalins and endorphins. In: Beers RF, Bassett EG, eds. Mechanisms of Pain and Analgesic Compounds. New York: Raven Press, 1979:239–247.
97. Iadarola MJ, Douglass J, Civelli O, Naranjo JR. Differential activation of spinal cord dynorphin and enkephalin neurons during hyperalgesia: evidence using cDNA hybridization. Brain Res 1988; 455:205–212.
98. Lewis T. Pain. New York: Macmillan, 1942.
99. Raja SN, Campbell JN, Meyer RA. Evidence for different mechanisms of primary and secondary hyper-algesia following heat injury to the glabrous skin. Brain 1984; 107:1179–1188.
100. Koltzenburg M, Lundberg LER, Torebjork HE. Dynamic and static components of mechanical hyperalgesia in human hairy skin. Pain 1992; 51:207–219.
101. LaMotte RH, Shain CN, Simone DA, Tsai E-FP. Neurogenic hyperalgesia: psychophysical studies of underlying mechanisms. J Neurophysiol 1991; 66: 190–211.
102. LaMotte RH. Subpopulations of "nociceptor neurons" contributing to pain and allodynia, itch and allokinesis. APS J 1992; 1:115–126.
103. Merskey H. Pain terms: A supplementary note. Pain 1982; 14:205–206.
104. Meyer RA, Treede RD, Raja SN, Campbell JN. Peripheral versus central mechanisms for secondary hyperalgesia: is the controversy resolved? APS J 1992; 1:127–131.
105. LaMotte RH, Thalhammer JG, Torebjork HE, Robinson CJ. Peripheral neural mechanisms of cutaneous hyperalgesia following mild injury by heat. J Neurosci 1982; 2:765–781.
106. Beck PW, Handwerker HO, Zimmermann M. Nervous outflow from the cat's foot during noxious radiant heat stimulation. Brain Res 1974; 67:373–386.
107. Beitel RE, Dubner R. Response of unmyelinated (C) polymodal nociceptors to thermal stimuli applied to monkey's face. J Neurophysiol 1976; 39:1160–1175.
108. Bessou P, Perl ER. Response of cutaneous sensory units with unmyelinated fibers to noxious stimuli. J Neurophysiol 1969; 32:1025–1043.
109. LaMotte RH, Thalhammer JG, Robinson CJ. Peripheral neural correlates of magnitude of cutaneous pain and hyperalgesia: a comparison of neural events in monkey with sensory judgments in human. J Neurophysiol 1983; 50:1–26.
110. Grigg P, Schaible HG, Schmidt RF. Mechanical sensitivity of group III and IV afferents from posterior articular nerve in normal and inflamed cat knee. J Neurophysiol 1986; 55:635–643.
111. Campbell JN, Khan AA, Meyer RA, Raja SN. Responses to heat of C-fiber nociceptors in monkey are altered by injury in the receptive field but not by adjacent injury. Pain 1988; 32:327–332.
112. Reeh PW, Kocher L, Jung S. Does neurogenic inflammation alter the sensitivity of unmyelinated nociceptors in the rat? Brain Res 1986; 384:42–50.
113. Thalhammer JG, LaMotte RH. Heat sensitization of one-half of a cutaneous nociceptor's receptive field does not alter the sensitivity of the other half. In: Bonica JJ, Lindblom U, eds. Advances in Pain,

Research and Theraphy. Vol. 5. New York: Raven Press, 1983:71–75.

114. Meyer RA, Campbell JN, Raja SN. Antidromic nerve stimulation in monkey does not sensitize unmyleinated nociceptors to heat. Brain Res 1988; 441:168–172.
115. Torebjork HE, Lundberg LER, LaMotte RH. Central changes in processing of mechanoreceptive input in capsaicin-induced secondary hyperalgesia in humans. J Physiol 1992; 448:765–780.
116. Cervero F, Meyer RA, Campbell JN. A psychophysical study of secondary hyperalgesia: evidence for increased pain to input from nociceptors. Pain 1994; 58:21–28.
117. Dougherty PM, Palecek J, Willis WD Jr. Does sensitization of responses to excitatory amino acids underlie the psychophysical reports of two modalities of increased sensitivity in zones of secondary hyperalgesia? APS J 1993; 2(4):276–279.
118. Woolf CJ. Evidence for a central component of post-injury pain hypersensitivity. Nature 1983; 306: 686–688.
119. Dougherty PM, Willis WD, Lenz FA. Transient inhibition of responses to thermal stimuli of spinal sensory tract neurons in monkeys during sensitization by intradermal capsaicin. Pain 1998; 77:129–136.
120. Dougherty PM, Schwartz A, Lenz FA. Responses of primate spinomesencephalic tract cells to intradermal capsaicin. Neuroscience 1999; 90: 1377–1392.
121. Guilbaud G, Benoist JM, Jazat F, Gautron M. Neuronal responsiveness in the ventrobasal thalamic complex of rats with an experimental peripheral mononeuropathy. J Neurophysiol 1990; 64:1537–1554.
122. Guilbaud G, Kayser V, Attal N, Benoist J-M. Evidence for a central contribution to secondary hyperalgesia. In: Willis WD, ed. Hyperalgesia and Allodynia. New York: Raven Press, 1992:187–201.
123. Lenz FA, Kwan HC, Dostrovsky JO, Tasker RR. Characteristics of the bursting pattern of action potentials that occurs in the thalamus of patients with central pain. Brain Res 1989; 496:357–360.
124. Lenz FA, Tasker RP, Dostrovsky JO, Kwan HC, Gorecki J, Hirayama T, et al. Abnormal single-unit activity recorded in the somatosensory thalamus of a quadriplegic patient with central pain. Pain 1987; 31: 225–236.
125. Lenz FA, Tasker RR, Dostrovsky JO, Kwan HC, Gorecki J, Hirayama K, et al. Abnormal single-unit activity and responses to stimulation in the presumed ventrocaudal nucleus of patients with central pain. Pain Res Clin Manage 1988; 3:157–164.
126. Casey KL. Pain and central nervous system disease: a summary and overview. In: Casey KL, ed. Pain and Central Nervous System Disease: the Central Pain Syndromes. New York: Raven Press, Ltd., 1991:1–11.
127. Rausell E, Cusick CG, Taub A, Jones EG. Chronic deafferentation in monkeys differentially affects nociceptive and non-nociceptive pathway distinguished by specific calcium-binding proteins and down-regulates gamma-aminobutyric acid type A receptors at thalamic levels. Proc Natl Acad Sci USA 1992; 89: 2571–2575.
128. Meyer RA, Raja SN, Campbell JN. Neural mechanisms of primary hyperalgesia. In: Belmonte C, Cervero F, eds. Neurobiology of Nociceptors. Oxford, New York, Tokyo: Oxford University Press, 1996:370–389.
129. Keele CA, Armstrong D. Substances Producing Pain and Itch. London: Edward Arnold, 1964.
130. Kress M, Reeh PW. Chemical excitation and sensitization in nociceptors. In: Belmonte C, Cervero F, eds. Neurobiology of Nociceptors. Oxford, New York, Tokyo: Oxford University Press, 1996:258–297.
131. Kress M, Rodl J, Reeh PW. Stable analogues of cyclic AMP but not cyclic GMP sensitize unmyelinated primary afferents in rat skin to heat stimulation but not to inflammatory mediators, in vitro. Neuroscience 1996; 74(2):609–617.
132. Bonica JJ. Causalgia and other reflex sympathetic dystrophies. Bonica JJ, ed. Advances in Pain Research and Therapy. New York: Raven Press, 1979:141–166.
133. Lindblom U, Verrillo RT. Sensory functions in chronic neuralgia. J Neurol Neurosurg Psychiat 1979; 42:422–435.
134. Sunderland S. Pain mechanisms in causalgia. J Neurol Neurosurg Psychiat 1976; 39:471–480.
135. Roberts WJ. A hypothesis on the physiological basis for causalgia and related pains. Pain 1986; 24:297–311.
136. Frost SA, Raja SN, Campbell JN, Meyer RA, Khan AA. Does hyperalgesia to cooling stimuli characterize patients with sympathetically maintained pain (reflex sympathetic dystrophy)? In: Dubner R, Gebhart GF, Bond MR, eds. Proceedings of the Vth World Congress on Pain. Amsterdam: Elsevier Science Publishers , 1988:151–156.
137. Price DD, Bennett GJ, Rafii A. Psychophysical observations on painful peripheral neuropathies that are relieved by a sympathetic block. Pain 1989; 36: 273–288.
138. Price DD. Characterizing central mechanisms of pathological pain states by sensory testing and neurophysiological analysis. In: Casey KL, ed. Pain and Central Nervous System Disease: the Central Pain Syndromes. New York: Raven Press, 1991:103–115.
139. Kirk EJ, Denny-Brown D. Functional variation in dermatomes in the macaque monkey following dorsal root lesions. J Comp Neurol 1970; 139(307):320.
140. Wall PD, Waxman S, Basbaum AI. Ongoing activity in peripheral nerve: injury discharge. Exp Neurol 1974; 45:576–589.
141. Basbaum AI. Effects of central lesions on disorders produced by multiple dorsal rhizotomy in rats. Exp Neurol 1974; 42:490–501.
142. Basbaum AI, Wall PD. Chronic changes in the response of cells in adult cat dorsal horn following partial deafferentation: the appearance of responding cells in a previously non-responsive region. Brain Res 1976; 116:181–204.

143. Denny-Brown D, Kirk E. Hyperalgesia from spinal and root lesions. Trans Am Neurol Assoc 1968; 93:116–120.
144. Merrill EG, Wall PD. Factors forming the edge of a receptive field: the presence of relatively ineffective afferent terminals. J Physiol 1972; 226:825–846.
145. Bennett GJ, Xie YK. A peripheral mononeuropathy in rat that produces disorder of pain sensation like those seen in man. Pain 1988; 33:87–107.
146. Kim SH, Chung JM. An experimental model for peripheral neuropathy produced by segmental spinal nerve ligation in the rat. Pain 1992; 50:355–364.
147. Seltzer Z, Dubner R, Shir Y. A novel behavioral model of neuropathic pain disorders produced by partial sciatic nerve injury. Pain 1990; 43:205–218.
148. Kingery WS, Vallin JA. The development of chronic mechanical hyperalgesia, autotomy and collateral sprouting following sciatic nerve section in rat. Pain 1989; 38:321–332.
149. Coderre TJ, Grimes RW, Melzak R. Deafferentation and chronic pain in animals: an evaluation of evidence suggesting autotomy is related to pain. Pain 1986; 26:61–84.
150. Levitt M. Dysesthesias and self-mutilation in humans and subhumans: a review of clinical and experimental studies. Brain Res Rev 1985; 10:247–290.
151. Rodin BE, Kruger L. Deafferentation in animals as a model for the study of pain: an alternative hypothesis. Brain Res Rev 1984; 7:213–228.
152. Sweet WH. Animal models of chronic pain: their possible validation from human experience with posterior rhizotomy and congenital analgesia. Pain 1981; 10: 275–295.
153. Bennett GJ, Xie YK. An experimental peripheral neuropathy in rat that produces abnormal pain sensation. In: Dubner R, Gebhart GF, Bond MR, eds. Proceedings of the Vth World Congress on Pain. Amsterdam: Elsevier Science Publishers BV (Biomedical Division), 1988:129–134.
154. Govrin-Lippmann R, Devor M. Ongoing activity in severed nerves: source and variation with time. Brain Res 1978; 159:406–410.
155. Dougherty PM, Garrison CJ, Carlton SM. Differential influence of local anesthetic upon two models of experimentally-induced peripheral mononeuropathy in the rat. Brain Res 1992; 570:109–115.
156. Davar G, Hama A, Deykin A, Vos B, Maciewicz R. MK-801 blocks the development of thermal hyperalgesia in a rat model of experimental painful neuropathy. Brain Res 1991; 553:327–330.
157. Mao J, Price DD, Mayer DJ, Lu J, Hayes RL. Intrathecal MK-801 and local nerve anesthesia synergistically reduce nociceptive behavior in rats with experimental peripheral mononeuropathy. Brain Res 1992; 576:254–262.
158. Meller ST, Pechman PS, Gebhart GF, Maves TJ. Nitric oxide mediates the thermal hyperalgesia produced in a model of neuorpathic pain in the rat. Neuroscience 1992; 50:7–10.
159. Kajander KC, Bennett GJ. Onset of a painful neuropathy in rat: a partial and differential deafferentation and spontaneous discharge in AB and Aδ primary afferent neurons. J Neurophysiol 1992; 68: 734–744.
160. Laird JMA, Bennett GJ. Dorsal root potentials and afferent input to the spinal cord in rats with an experimental peripheral neuropathy. Brain Res 1992; 584:181–190.
161. Burichel KJ. Effects of electrical and mechanical stimulation on two foci of spontaneous activity which develop in primary afferent neurons after peripheral axotomy. Pain 1984; 18:249–265.
162. Devor M, Bernstein JJ. Abnormal impulse generation in neuromas, electrophysiology and ultrastructure. In: Culp WJ, Ochoa J, eds. Abnormal Nerves and Muscles as Impulse Generators. London: Oxford University Press, 1982:363–380.
163. Matzner O, Devor M. Contrasting thermal sensitivity of spontaneously active a- and c- fibers in experimental nerve-end neuromas. Pain 1987; 30:373–384.
164. Papir-Kricheli D, Devor M. Abnormal impulse discharge in primary afferent axons injured in the peripheral versus the central nervous system. Somatosens Motor Res 1988; 6(1):63–77.
165. Wall PD, Devor M. Sensory afferent impulses originate from dorsal root ganglia as well as from the periphery in normal and nerve injured rats. Pain 1983; 17:321–339.
166. Wall PD, Gutnick M. Ongoing activity in peripheral nerves: the physiology and pharmacology of impulses originating from a neuroma. Exp Neurol 1974; 43: 580–593.
167. Seltzer Z, Devor M. Ephaptic transmission in chronically damaged peripheral nerves. Neurology 1979; 29:1061–1064.
168. Scadding JW. Ectopic impulse generation in experimental neuromas: behavioral, physiological and anatomical correlates. In: Culp WJ, Ochoa J, eds. Abnormal Nerves and Muscles as Impulse Generators. New York: Oxford University Press, 1982:533–552.
169. Devor M. Central changes mediating neuropathic pain. In: Dubner R, Gebhart GF, Bond MR, eds. Proceedings of the Vth World Congress on Pain. New York: Elsevier Science Publishers, 1988:114–128.
170. Mendell LM, Sassoon EM, Wall PD. Properties of synaptic linkage from long ranging afferents onto dorsal horn neurones in normal and deafferented cats. J Physiol 1978; 285:299–310.
171. Laird JM, Bennett GJ. An electrophysiological study of dorsal horn neurons in the spinal cord of rats with an experimental peripheral neuropathy. J Neurophysiol 1993; 69:2072–2085.
172. Palecek J, Paleckova V, Dougherty PM, Carlton SM, Willis WD. Responses of spinothalamic tract cells to mechanical and thermal stimulation of the skin in rats with an experimental peripheral neuropathy. J Neurophysiol 1992; 67:1562–1573.

173. Palecek J, Dougherty PM, Kim SH, Lekan HA, Carlton SM, Chung JM. et al. Responses of spinothalamic tract neurons to mechanical and thermal stimuli in an experimental model of peripheral neuropathy in primates. J Neurophysiol 1993; 68:1951–1966.
174. Albe-Fessard D, Rampin O. Neurophysiological studies in rats deafferented by dorsal root section. In: Nashold BS Jr, Ovelmen-Levitt J, eds. Deafferentation Pain Syndromes: Pathophysiology and Treatment. New York: Raven Press, 1991:125–139.
175. Dostrovsky JO, Millar J, Wall PD. The immediate shift of afferent drive of dorsal column nucleus cells following deafferentation: a comparison of acute and chronic deafferentation in gracile nucleus and spinal cord. Exp Neurol 1976; 52:480–495.
176. Millar J, Basbaum AI, Wall PD. Restructuring of the somatotopic map and appearance of abnormal neuronal activity in the gracile nucleus after partial deafferentation. Exp Neurol 1976; 50:658–672.
177. Loeser JD, Ward AA Jr, White LE Jr. Chronic deafferentation of human spinal cord neurons. J Neurosurg 1968; 29:48–50.
178. Devor M, Wall PD. Plasticity in the spinal cord sensory map following peripheral nerve injury in rats. J Neurosci 1981; 1:679–684.
179. Devor M, Wall PD. Reorganisation of spinal cord sensory map after peripheral nerve injury. Nature 1978; 276:75–76.
180. Pubols LM, Brenowitz GL. Maintenance of dorsal horn somatotopic organization and increased high-threshold response after single-root or spared-root deafferentation in cats. J Neurophysiol 1982; 47: 103–112.
181. Pubols LM, Goldberger ME. Recovery of function in dorsal horn following partial deafferentation. J Neurophysiol 1980; 43:102–117.
182. Lenz FA, Gracely RH, Baker FH, Richardson RT, Dougherty PM. Reorganization of sensory modalities evoked by microstimulation in region of the thalamic principal sensory nucleus in patients with pain due to nervous system injury. J Comp Neurol 1998; 399:125–138.
183. Kaas JH, Merzenich MM, Killackey HP. The reorganization of somatosensory cortex following peripheral nerve damage in adult and developing mammals. Ann Rev Neurosci 1983; 6:325–356.
184. Pons TP, Garraghty PE, Ommaya AK, Kaas JH, Taub E, Mishkin M. Massive cortical reorganization after sensory deafferentation in adult macaques. Science 1991; 252:1857–1860.
185. Wall JT, Cusick CG. Cutaneous responsiveness in primary somatosensory (S-1) hindpaw cortex before and after partial hindpaw deafferentation in adult rats. J Neurosci 1984; 4:1499–1515.
186. Ramer MS, French GD, Bisby MA. Wallerian degeneration is required for both neuropathic pain and sympathetic sprouting into the DRG. Pain 1997; 72: 71–78.
187. Cameron AA, Cliffer KD, Dougherty PM, Garrison CJ, Willis WD, Carlton SM. Time course of degenerative and regenerative changes in the dorsal horn in a rat model of peripheral neuropathy. J Comp Neurol 1997; 379:428–442.
188. Melzack R, Wall PD. Pain mechanisms: a new theory. Science 1965; 150:971–979.
189. Bennett GJ, Kajander KC, Sahara Y, Iadarola MJ, Sugimoto T. Neurochemical and anatomical changes in the dorsal horn of rats with an experimental painful peripheral neuropathy. In: Cervero F, Bennett GJ, Headley PM, eds. Processing of Sensory Information in the Superficial Dorsal Horn of the Spinal Cord. 1988:1–23.
190. Sugimoto T, Bennett GJ, Kajander KC. Transsynaptic degeneration in the superficial dorsal horn after sciatic nerve injury: effects of a chronic constriction injury, transection, and strychnine. Pain 1990; 42(2):205–213.
191. Ralston DD, Dougherty PM, Lenz FA, Weng HR, Vierck CJ, Ralston HJ. Plasticity of the inhibitory circuits of the primate ventrobasal thalamus following lesions of the somatosensory pathways. In: Devor M, Rowbotham MC, Wiesenfeld-Hallin Z, eds. Proceedings of the 9th World Congress on Pain. Seattle: IASP Press, 2000:427–434.
192. Milligan ED, Twining C, Chacur M, Biedenkapp J, O'Connor K, Poole S, et al. Spinal glia and proinflammatory cytokines mediate mirror-image neuropathic pain in rats. J Neurosci 2003; 23(3):1026–1040. Ref Type: Generic.
193. DeLeo JA, Colburn RW, Rickman AJ. Cytokine and growth factor immunohistochemical spinal profiles in two animal models of mononeuropathy. Brain Res 1997; 759:50–57.
194. Sorkin LS, Doom CM. Epineurial application of TNF elicits an acute mechanical hyperalgesia in the awake rat. J Peripher Nerv Syst 2000; 5(2):96–100.
195. Sakaue G, Shimaoka M, Fukuoka T, Hiroi T, Inoue T, Hashimoto N, et al. NF-kB decoy suppresses cytokine expression and thermal hyperalgesia in a rat neuropathic pain model. Neuroreport 2001; 12(10): 2079–2084.
196. Marchand JE, Wurm WH, Kato T, Kream RM. Altered tachykinin expression by dorsal root ganglion neurons in a rat model of neuropathic pain. Pain 1994; 58:219–231.
197. Nahin R, Ren Ke, De Leon M, Ruda M. Primary sensory neurons exhibit altered gene in a rat model of neuropathic pain. Pain 1994; 58:95–108.
198. Okamoto K, Martin DP, Schmelzer JD, Mitsui Y, Low PA. Pro- and anti-inflammatory cytokine gene expression in rat sciatic nerve chronic constriction injury model of neuropathic pain. Exp Neurol 2001; 169:386–391.
199. Dib-Hajj SD, Fjell J, Cummins TR, Zheng Z, Fried K, LaMotte R, et al. Plasticity of sodium channel expression in DRG neurons in the chronic constriction injury model of neuropathic pain. Pain 1999; 83:591–600.

200. Okuse K, Chaplan SR, McMahon SB, Luo ZD, Calcutt NA, Scott BP, et al. Regulation of expression of the sensory neuron-specific sodium channel SNS in inflammatory and neuropathic pain. Mol Cell Neurosci 1997; 10(3–4):196–207.
201. Petersen M, Zhang J, Zhang J-M, LaMotte RH. Abnormal spontaneous activity and responses to norepinephrine in dissociated dorsal root ganglion cells after chronic nerve constriction. Pain 1996; 67:391–397.
202. Kanaan SA, Saade NE, Karam M, Khansa H, Jabbur SJ, Jurjus AR. Hyperalgesia and upregulation of cytokines and nerve growth factor by cutaneous leishmaniasis. Pain 2000; 85:477–482.
203. Lewin GL, Ritter AM, Mendell LM. Nerve growth factor-induced hyperalgesia in the neonatal and adult rat. J Neurosci 1993; 13(5):2136–2148.
204. Woolf CJ, Allchorne A, Safieh-Garabedian B, Poole S. Cytokines, nerve growth factor and inflammatory hyperalgesia: the contribution of tumor necrosis factor α. Br J Pharmacol 1997; 121:417–424.

55

Epidemiology of Pain and Cancer-Related Symptoms

CIELITO C. REYES-GIBBY and CHARLES S. CLEELAND

Department of Symptom Research, The University of Texas M.D. Anderson Cancer Center, Houston, Texas, U.S.A.

I. INTRODUCTION

Patients with cancer typically experience multiple symptoms related to cancer and cancer treatment. These symptoms can include physical (e.g., pain, shortness of breath), cognitive (e.g., delirium, memory problems, impaired concentration), and affective (e.g., depression, anxiety) experiences associated with the disease and its treatments (1). *Symptoms* are the side effects and "toxicities" of treatment, as well as the direct product of the disease process itself. Symptoms are what patients report to clinicians as the subjective negative feelings of physical and mental changes produced by both disease and treatment. Symptom severity is related to the extent of disease and the aggressiveness of therapy. Common symptoms of cancer and cancer treatment significantly impair the daily function and quality of life of patients. Symptoms that are unrecognized by treatment teams may also become so severe that emergency room visits or hospitalization are required for management, adding substantially to the cost of treatment and to the disruption of the patients' routines and those of their families. Untreated symptoms may also negatively influence treatment effectiveness by interrupting treatment (2). Multiple and severe symptoms present a significant challenge to the resources of those who care for and manage cancer patients. For example, intensive cancer therapies produce severe and sometimes life-threatening side effects, resulting in patients' inability to care for themselves and in total dependence on caregivers (3). Undertreatment of symptoms has become a major health problem in its own right.

In this chapter, we review epidemiologic studies of pain and other cancer-related symptoms; present the few studies that examined methods of improving the practice of cancer pain management; discuss how new therapies might impact the epidemiology of symptoms and discuss potential research challenges; and offer recommendations on the conduct of pain and symptom research.

II. EPIDEMIOLOGY AND DESCRIPTIVE RESEARCH: PREVALENCE OF CANCER PAIN AND OTHER CANCER-RELATED SYMPTOMS

Pain is prevalent for large numbers of patients with cancer (4–8). Approximately 55% of outpatients with metastatic cancer have disease-related pain, and 36% have pain of sufficient severity to impair their function and quality of life (5). Despite national and international guidelines for its management, many patients with pain are not prescribed an analgesic appropriate to the severity of their pain. Multicenter studies indicate that approximately 40% of patients with cancer pain are not prescribed analgesics potent enough to manage their pain, with additional patients not receiving sufficient dosing of the analgesic prescribed (7).

Clinically, severe symptoms are almost never expressed in isolation. In one symptom study of cancer patients, the most common symptom cluster (pain, dyspnea, and anxiety) comprised the majority of the symptom burden: hierarchical multiple regression model of symptoms explained 48% of the variance in functional status (9). Portenoy et al. (6) found that the most frequently reported symptoms in a random sample of inpatients and outpatients with cancer were lack of energy, worry, sadness, and pain. Another prospective study (10) ($N = 1635$) of cancer patients found that in addition to pain, patients reported an average of more than three other symptoms. The most common were insomnia, anorexia, and constipation. One in five patients also reported sweating, nausea and vomiting, dyspnea, dysphagia, and neuropsychiatric symptoms. Gaston-Johansson et al. (11) in a study of 127 women with stages II, III, or IV breast cancer found a high prevalence of fatigue (91%), pain (47%), and depression (54%) that were significantly correlated to each other and to total health status.

Studies document cancer-related symptoms associated with aggressive treatments such as chemotherapy and radiotherapy. For example, Schwartz and colleagues (12) described the patterns of cancer-related fatigue (CRF) and vigor in a sample of patients receiving chemotherapy and radiotherapy. They found that patterns of CRF and vigor differed for patients receiving chemotherapy vs. radiotherapy. Chemotherapy-related fatigue peaks in the days after chemotherapy, whereas radiotherapy-related fatigue gradually accumulates over the course of treatment. Other studies also found that the majority of patients undergoing chemotherapy or radiotherapy report significant fatigue and other symptoms during the course of treatment (13–15). In a recent study of over 500 patients in active treatment, more than 20% of patients reported a variety of severe symptoms, including fatigue, worry, distress, poor sleep, lack of appetite, and dry mouth (15).

Symptoms following surgical therapy have not been well studied. Despite the thousands of cancer patients who undergo curative surgery, very little is known about the prevalence, duration and functional impact of treatment-related symptoms in this patient population. Most studies of symptom prevalence, severity and impact have been done with cancer patients who have more advanced disease. Patients not only suffer from the side effects of the chemotherapy or radiotherapy before surgery for their cancer but may also develop serious postsurgical symptoms.

For example, the majority of lung cancer patients (80%) present with nonsmall cell lung cancer (NCSLC). Earlier staged patients (UICC stages I, II, and some IIIA) (16) are believed to eventually achieve some survival benefit from local and systemic interventions, such as surgery alone or surgery following chemotherapy or radiotherapy. It is less well known, however, that clinically significant depression occurs in approximately 15% of NSCLC patients even after successful surgical treatment (17).

Salmon and Hall (18) document that postoperative fatigue is the most frequently reported symptom after major surgery, such as thoracic surgery, and can be prolonged for several months. Perttunen et al. (19) followed patients for up to 1 year after thoracotomy, using standard pain measures every 3 months. Thirty-four percent of this sample had moderate to severe postsurgical pain at 3 months, 30% at 6 months and 16% at 1 year. More than 50% of patients reported that postoperative pain interfered with normal daily life at 3 and 6 months. These studies suggest that although postthoracic surgery pain, fatigue, and depression are common, these symptoms are infrequently assessed and are usually dismissed as very transient postoperative sequelae (20).

Among breast cancer patients, studies document that the incidence of chronic pain following breast cancer surgery may even exceed 50% (21). Amichetti and Caffo (22) surveyed patients ($n = 348$) who had conservative breast surgery (quadrantectomy) with radiotherapy. Results showed that 141 patients reported pain as a consequence of treatment. Pain generally started within 3 months after the completion of therapy, was localized in the axillary region and was intermittent. The pain was mainly described as aching (59%), tender (51%), and cramping (43%). Jung and colleagues (21), in their review of symptoms associated with breast cancer surgery, suggest that postoperative sensations reported by patients can be transient or long-lasting, and can include pain, phantom sensations, and sensory loss or changes.

Other studies have also examined the multiple symptoms of cancer patients in advanced stage. In a prospective study among 1000 cancer patients, Donnelly and Walsh (23) found pain, fatigue, and anorexia to be among the 10 most prevalent symptoms at all 17 primary sites studied. When pain, anorexia, weakness, anxiety, lack of energy, severe fatigue, early satiety, constipation, and dyspnea were present, a majority of patients rated them as moderate or severe.

Other studies (24) found that fatigue, weakness, pain, sleepiness, and cognitive impairment were frequent symptoms of terminal patients enrolled in a supportive care program, with fatigue (58%) and pain (54%) as the most prevalent symptoms. Similarly, a prospective study of cancer patients in palliative care centers in Europe, Australia, and the United States found that over half the patients reported pain and weakness (25). Weight loss, anorexia, constipation, nausea, and dyspnea were also common.

As part of the SUPPORT studies, McCarthy et al. (26) evaluated over 1000 cancer patients during the 3 days before death and also at 1–3 months before death, and 3–6 months before death. As expected, as they progressed toward death, their estimated 6-month prognosis decreased significantly and the severity of their disease worsened. Patients' functional status also declined significantly as they approached death, such that most patients had four or more symptoms within the 3 days before death. Patients with cancer experienced significantly more pain and confusion as death approached. Severe pain was common; more than one-quarter of patients with cancer experienced significant pain 3–6 months before death and more than 40% were in significant pain during their last 3 days of life.

It is less well recognized that many cancer survivors continue to experience physical, affective, or cognitive symptoms even when their disease is in remission or treatment has ended. These symptoms may be due to physiological changes associated with prior treatments, delayed side effects of treatment, or long-term consequences of the disease. For example, survivors of bone marrow transplantation may report cognitive impairment, physical symptoms, or emotional distress many years after the transplant (27–29). Bush et al. (30) found in a descriptive study of 125 bone marrow transplant (BMT) survivors that 10 years or more post-transplantation, long-term survivors continued to experience a moderate incidence of lingering complications and demands, including emotional and sexual dysfunction, fatigue, eye problems, sleep disturbance, general pain, and cognitive dysfunction. Molassiotis and colleagues (31) found that long-term autologous bone marrow transplant (ABMT) survivors report symptoms of anxiety (20%), had signs of clinical depression (10%), and had not returned to full-time employment (20%). Similarly, McQuellon et al. (28) found in study of 52 breast cancer patients undergoing high-dose chemotherapy, with ABMT that 30% of patients following ABMT had problems with sexuality, fatigue, and depressive symptoms.

While it is recognized that undertreatment of symptoms is prevalent, evidence suggests that the elderly, women, and patients from minority groups may have an even greater risk for undertreatment of symptoms (7,32). Minority patients seen at clinics serving minority clients were found to be three times more likely to be undermedicated with analgesics than patients treated in nonminority community treatment settings (5). Patients treated at centers seeing primarily African Americans, Hispanics, or both, as well as patients treated at university centers were more likely to receive inadequate analgesia than patients treated in nonminority community treatment settings (77% vs. 52%). Minority patients had the severity of their pain underestimated by their physicians, reported that they needed stronger pain medication and felt that they needed to take more analgesics than their doctors had prescribed. Assessing differences within the minority groups, more Hispanic patients reported lower levels of pain relief compared to African Americans.

A more recent study (32) also examined the pain treatment needs of socioeconomically disadvantaged African-American and Hispanic patients with recurrent or metastatic cancer. One hundred and eight African-American and Hispanic patients with metastatic or recurrent cancer and pain completed a pain assessment form (Brief Pain Inventory, BPI) and a survey about their attitudes toward analgesic medications. Physicians rated the patient's pain and the adequacy of the patient's current analgesic prescriptions was assessed. Results showed that approximately 28% of the Hispanic and 31% of the African-American patients received analgesics of insufficient strength to manage their pain.

Although few disagree that painful conditions should be treated regardless of age, studies document undertreatment of cancer pain in older populations. In a study of 4003 elderly cancer patients (24%, 29%, 38% of those aged ≥85, 75–84, and 65–74 years, respectively), Bernabei and colleagues (33) found that more than a quarter (26%) of patients in daily pain did not receive any analgesic agent. Patients aged 85 years and older were found less likely to receive morphine or other strong opiates than those aged 65–74 years (13% vs. 38%, respectively) and were also more likely to receive no analgesia. African-American elderly patients were also at a higher risk for undertreatment, suggesting that the disparity in pain treatment is compounded for elderly minority patients. Our study (5), which looked at undertreatment of pain for ambulatory patients with metastatic cancer, also showed that older age (70 years or older) was a significant predictor of inadequate analgesia according to the World Health Organization guidelines (34) for treatment of patients with cancer pain.

III. FACTORS ASSOCIATED WITH INADEQUATE TREATMENT AND CONTROL OF PAIN AND OTHER SYMPTOMS

A number of factors predict inadequate symptom control. These factors have been studied in the area of cancer pain management. Poor pain assessment remains the most salient barrier. Although quantitative pain assessment has demonstrated its feasibility and validated pain assessment tools are available, recent data from a community-based oncology setting (35) still show a virtual absence of documentation of quantitative pain assessment (only in 0–5% of medical and radiation oncology physicians' notes). Twenty-eight percent of patients with significant pain had no mention of pain in the physicians' notes and 48% had no documented analgesic treatment. This points to the critical role of adequate assessment and monitoring for the control of pain, and for other symptoms.

Many cancer specialists recognize that symptom control is often suboptimal. Medical oncologists were surveyed about their treatment of cancer pain in a study conducted by the Eastern Cooperative Oncology Group (ECOG) (4). Only half of the physicians surveyed indicated that cancer pain control was good or very good in their practice setting. Seventy-five percent of the physicians indicated that the most important barrier to cancer pain management was inadequate pain assessment. Over 60% reported that physicians' reluctance to prescribe analgesics and patients' unwillingness to report pain or take opioids were barriers to adequate pain treatment. Inadequate knowledge about cancer pain management was reported by over 50% of the ECOG physicians surveyed. The survey acknowledged that a substandard level of education about cancer pain management and a reluctance to address it in practice existed at all levels of professional health care. Cleeland and colleagues (36) repeated the ECOG study format with physician members of the Radiation Therapy Oncology Group. Although there has been some improvement in the use of stronger analgesics, many barriers to good pain control remain, and poor pain assessment is still seen as the major barrier to good pain management.

Due to the influence of managed care, cancer therapy has shifted to the ambulatory setting in recent years, while at the same time therapy has become much more aggressive with a greater burden of treatment-related symptoms. As a result, more responsibility for symptom management has moved from the healthcare professional to patients and their families. The patient and family are increasingly responsible for initial symptom assessment, initial home-based symptom management, and active contacts with care providers. Families have varying resources, abilities, and assertiveness in contacting health care professionals. However, patient and family reluctance to report symptoms, even when they are severe, is probably the norm. In fact, patient reluctance to report pain is identified by both oncologists (4,7) and oncology nurses (37) as one of the major barriers to the adequate control of cancer pain. A major barrier to the recognition of depression is that cancer patients are reluctant to report depression for many of the same reasons that they are unwilling to report pain (38). Patients may be reluctant to report symptoms to their physicians or nurses because of fear of the meaning of the symptoms, fear of complicating their treatment by taking additional drugs, or fear of the psychoactive component of symptom management drugs. Patients may also think that complaining of symptoms will distract their health care providers from focusing their efforts to cure the disease (39,40). We have found that patients' reluctance to report symptoms is often compounded by the difficulty of finding time for adequate symptom assessment in a busy clinic (32). Patients may also be reluctant to bother their health care providers with symptoms that they consider an expected part of their disease (41).

IV. IMPROVING CONTROL OF CANCER PAIN AND OTHER CANCER-RELATED SYMPTOMS

In spite of the recent concerns over symptom management, there is substantial evidence that symptoms that could, in principle, be well managed are undertreated, especially for patients who are still in active treatment. Many symptoms could be more adequately controlled if we systematically applied the knowledge that we now have about symptom management.

There is at least preliminary evidence that improving assessment can improve pain management, and may improve the management of other symptoms as well. Trowbridge et al. (42) conducted a randomized controlled trial of 320 patients and 13 oncologists. Patients were asked to complete assessments of their pain, their pain regimens, and the degrees of relief received and were later surveyed by mail 4 weeks after their clinic visits. The intervention group's clinical charts contained a summary of the completed pain scales and the oncologists who treated these patients were instructed to review the summary sheet prior to an evaluation. This summary was not available for the oncologists treating the patients in the control group. Results showed a significant difference ($p = 0.0162$) in the physicians' prescription patterns.

In the control group, prescriptions for 86% of the patients did not change, with no decrease in analgesic prescriptions. In the intervention group, analgesic prescriptions changed for 25% of the patients, decreasing for 5% and increasing for 20%. A decrease in the incidence of pain described as more than life's usual aches and pains was found for the intervention group ($p = 0.05$). The findings from this study suggest that standardized pain assessment leads to improved cancer pain management.

Beginning with the publication of the World Health Organization's Cancer Pain Management guidelines in 1986 (34), there have been several guidelines issued for the practice of cancer pain management, including the Agency for Healthcare Research and Quality (AHRQ) Guideline for Cancer Pain Management (43), guidelines from the American Society of Anesthesiologists (44), and, more recently, guidelines from the National Cancer Center Network. There is, however, only one published study that evaluates the effectiveness of adherence to a pain management guideline for cancer pain (45). In this study, 81 cancer patients were enrolled in a prospective, longitudinal, randomized controlled study from outpatient clinics of 26 medical oncologists in western Washington. A multilevel treatment algorithm based on the AHRQ Guidelines for Cancer Pain Management was compared with standard-practice (control) therapies for pain and symptom management used by community oncologists. The primary outcome of interest was pain. Patients randomized to the pain algorithm group achieved a statistically significant reduction in usual pain intensity when compared with standard community practice.

In a recently completed study done in the Eastern Cooperative Oncology Group (unpublished data), we also found that the institutional use of a protocol for pain management improved pain control in lung and prostate cancer patients, but failed to improve the pain management of other patients (breast cancer and patients with myeloma) in the same institutions who were *not* specifically treated by the pain protocol. Forty-eight percent of patients with lung and prostate cancer in the institutions that used a protocol for pain management reported statistically significant reduction in moderate and severe pain ($p < 0.02$).

Finally, a recent randomized trial (46) also showed that a computerized reminder system for physicians significantly increased the rate of delivery of preventive care in inpatient settings. The results of these studies, taken together, suggest that improved assessment of symptoms alone, or symptom assessment coupled with symptom management guidelines and protocols, should improve symptom management for cancer patients.

Other studies have also examined the effectiveness of improving the practice of cancer pain management through training and education programs. A training program that includes the active participation of health care professionals and includes "role models" has demonstrated lasting changes in the cancer pain management knowledge of physicians and nurses (47,48). Although these studies did not examine patient report of pain as an outcome variable, they did suggest that durable change in knowledge was possible.

A second study evaluating the effects of a cancer pain education program (49) also used pain as an outcome variable. The effectiveness of a pain education program in cancer patients with chronic pain was investigated in a randomized clinical trial. A multimethod approach was used in which verbal instruction, written material, an audio cassette tape, and the use of a pain diary were combined to inform and instruct patients about pain and pain management. The pain education program consisted of three elements: (1) educating patients about the basic principles regarding pain and pain management; (2) instructing patients how to report their pain in a pain diary; and (3) instructing patients how to communicate about pain and how to contact health care providers. Patients in the intervention group participated in the pain education program in the hospital, and 3 and 7 days postdischarge by telephone. Results showed a significant increase in pain knowledge and a significant decrease in pain intensity in patients who received the pain education program.

More recently, a systems improvement approach was used to improve pain management in a national healthcare system (50), with some reported success. A joint collaborative effort of the Veterans Health Administration and the Institute for Healthcare Improvement (VHA-IHI), the focus of the project was to achieve rapid improvements in pain management in the clinical and operational areas in the national VHA system. An underlying premise was the spread of existing knowledge to multiple sites. A total of 70 teams were formed and were asked to identify their goals and to implement changes in their practice setting. Changes that were implemented included the development of new assessment forms to increase the number of patients with documented assessment and follow up for treatment plan; development of guidelines and/or protocols; formation of one-on-one, group provider, or computer-based educational methods to improve both assessment and follow-up, and/or ways to effectively link provider education with other system changes such as drug ordering or assessment processes; and development of innovative ways to link primary care physicians with pain specialists.

In terms of outcomes, the following were reported: moderate or severe pain on study units dropped from 24% to 17%; pain assessment increased from 75% to 85%; pain care plans for patients with at least mild pain increased from 58% to 78%; and number of patients provided with pain educational materials increased from 35% to 62%. Importantly, faculty involved in the initiative developed the attributes of an ideal pain management system (Table 1).

V. LIMITATIONS OF LITERATURE ON CANCER-RELATED SYMPTOMS

Overall, studies of cancer-related symptoms have a number of limitations. Symptoms, as described and "labeled," are often assessed and treated as separate and mutually exclusive entities (for instance, pain, fatigue, and depression). When symptoms are grouped, the grouping often is done intuitively rather than empirically (51,52). Physical symptoms (pain, nausea, diarrhea, fatigue, wasting/cachexia) commonly are

Table 1 Attributes of an Ideal Pain Management System

1. Assessment routine and timely
   - A pain assessment that includes a pain intensity rating is performed on all patients on admission and is included in the patient's medical record
   - Pain intensity ratings, like other vital signs, are recorded in the patient's medical record during every clinical encounter including telephone follow-ups and after drug administration
   - Protocols for assessment are developed at the local level and consistent with good clinical practice
2. Access to an appropriate level of treatment
   - Pain management is provided by a multidisciplinary team with the primary care provider as the central link in the system
   - Responsibility for action is determined from the pain assessment
   - Specialty consults are available to the primary care provider
   - Referrals to specialized pain clinics are made when needed
3. Treatment Protocols in place and understood
   - Protocols, specific to the setting and usable by different providers, are available for the most common conditions and are used to establish care plans. Protocols include recommended analgesics and, when possible, methods for the prevention of pain
   - When a diagnosis specific protocol is unavailable, a general protocol is used that requires the inclusion of pain management in the plan of care
   - Reminders for adherence to the care plan are built into the system
   - PRN medication form includes pain drugs
   - Standards for time between assessment of pain and action and response time for medication requests are established
4. Health care providers knowledgeable regarding state of the art principles of pain management as consistent with their scope of practice
   - An educational plan is in place at the institutional level
   - Different strategies including one-on-one consultations, unit-based programs, and grand rounds are considered
   - Providers have competencies to manage 80% of the conditions they see
5. Patients and families knowledgeable regarding pain management
   - A plan for educational interventions is in place
   - Educational information about pain is supplied to all patients
   - Education includes the caregiver
   - Educational information is provided prior to admission or surgery
   - The impact of the education is monitored and the need for additional interventions determined
   - Pain management is part of discharge planning
6. Pain management standards in place
   - A facility-wide policy for pain is established that meets JCAHO standards
   - A standard nursing policy is established for pain that includes standard definitions and beliefs about pain management
   - Limits are set for acceptable variation for key parameters within the system. Standards should be considered even though resources (e.g., PCAs, epidurals) may not be currently available
7. Outcomes monitored, reviewed and a plan for specific improvements in place
   - System goals for key outcomes are agreed upon
   - A schedule for review of progress is established
   - Necessary improvements to the system are identified and implemented

Source: From Ref. 50.

dissociated from cognitive symptoms (poor problem solving, memory, attention) and affective symptoms (anxiety and depression). Often, symptoms are evaluated and reported without stratifying for heterogeneity with respect to disease type, disease treatment, and response to disease treatment (53). Durations of symptoms may be days, months, or years, but assessments often are performed cross-sectionally rather than longitudinally, thus failing to assess patterns and symptom trajectories.

Furthermore, studies of predictors of cancer-related symptoms have traditionally focused on disease-related variables (stage of disease), clinical health status (performance status, comorbid conditions) and sociodemographic characteristics (age, gender, race, marital status), failing to perform mechanism-based assessments.

The State of Science Report by the National Institute of Health (53) "Symptom Management in Cancer: Pain, Depression and Fatigue," calls for the application of epidemiologic principles in the study of symptoms of cancer. Limitations of current literature on symptoms include the following:

- Conceptualization and measurement of pain, depression, and fatigue:
  - Heterogeneity of conditions or phenomena defined as pain, depression, and fatigue
  - Lack of consensus on the criteria to define these symptoms individually or in combination
  - Lack of consensus on the "best" measure(s) in terms of validity and reliability for each of the symptoms separately and in combination
- Weaknesses in research methodology include:
  - Lack of clarity regarding the difference between incidence (rate of new symptom development over a defined period) and prevalence (number of symptoms at a moment in time) and failure to consider the effects of the strengths and weaknesses of different study designs (e.g., case series, cross-sectional, case-control, and cohort) on estimates of incidence and prevalence
  - The lack of well-defined study populations
  - Failure to adequately describe study settings, study designs, and lack of standardization of study procedures
  - Lack of appropriate comparison group(s) to assess whether the incidence or prevalence of pain, fatigue, and depression is in fact higher among cancer patients compared with other ill populations and with general population samples
  - Potential impact of study design bias, confounding, and chance on estimates of the occurrence of these symptoms
  - Lack of information on the role that coexisting conditions and patient characteristics play in the development of pain, depression, and fatigue in cancer patients

VI. FUTURE DIRECTIONS: RESEARCH AND TREATMENT

Studies of the prevalence, severity, and treatment of pain present a model of the epidemiologic research that needs to be done in other areas of symptom management. First, we need to determine the prevalence and severity of various symptoms in patients throughout the course of their disease: at diagnosis, during treatment, when cancer is in remission, and near the end of life. We need to explore whether symptoms experienced by cancer patients differ quantitatively and qualitatively with that of noncancer populations. Incidence studies that will provide clinicians with information regarding the likelihood of occurrence, severity, and duration of these symptoms after a diagnosis of cancer will also be useful in determining the epidemiology of cancer symptoms. Since symptoms do not occur in isolation, mechanism-based classifications of cancer symptoms that will identify common biological mechanisms by using imaging, molecular, and innovative techniques will help improve our understanding of cancer-related symptoms. Second, we need to include longitudinal designs so that we can determine changes in these symptom patterns over time. Third, we need to identify the current adequacy of care for these symptoms, including identifying what factors (e.g., patient-related, clinician-related, system-related) are predictive of poor symptom management.

Over the last 20 years, changes in the treatment of cancer-related pain have been significant. However, the approach to the treatment of other symptoms in cancer, such as fatigue, depression, and sleep disturbance, is less systematically developed than the treatment of pain. For further development in this area, researchers must first establish that a single symptom or combined set of symptoms is prevalent and of a severity to cause distress as well as loss of function to significant numbers of patients. Evidence that supports the effectiveness of treatment for these symptoms must be demonstrated. Effective symptomatic treatments, since they can be viewed as elective, need to minimize negative side effects. For example, a treatment for fatigue that causes significant sleep disturbance would be unacceptable. Guidelines for both the assessment of these symptoms (when to treat) and treatment (how to treat) need to be in place, and established as standards. Finally, data describing the cost and benefit of symptom reduction need to be available for public debate and the consideration of approval and funding agencies.

REFERENCES

1. Cleeland CS. Cancer-related symptoms. Semin Radiat Oncol 2000; 10(3):175–190.
2. Borden EC, Parkinson D. A perspective on the clinical effectiveness and tolerance of interferon-alpha. Semin Oncol 1998; 25:3–8.
3. Sarna L, McCorkle R. Burden of care and lung cancer. Cancer Pract 1996; 4(5):245–251.
4. Von Roenn JH, Cleeland CS, Gonin R, Hatfield AK, Pandya KJ. Physician attitudes and practice in cancer pain management. A survey from the Eastern Cooperative Oncology Group. Ann Intern Med 1993; 119(2): 121–126.
5. Cleeland CS, Gonin R, Hatfield AK, Edmonson JH, Blum RH, Stewart JA, Pandya KJ. Pain and its treatment in outpatients with metastatic cancer. N Engl J Med 1994; 330(9):592–596.
6. Portenoy RK, Thaler HT, Kornblith AB, Lepore JM, Friedlander-Klar H, Coyle N, Smart-Curley T, Kemeny N, Norton L, Hoskins W, et al. Symptom prevalence, characteristics and distress in a cancer population. Qual Life Res 1994; 3(3):183–189.
7. Cleeland CS, Gonin R, Baez L, Loehrer P, Pandya KJ. Pain and treatment of pain in minority patients with cancer. The Eastern Cooperative Oncology Group Minority Outpatient Pain Study. Ann Intern Med 1997; 127(9):813–816.
8. Cleeland CS. Undertreatment of cancer pain in elderly patients. JAMA 1998; 17, 279(23):1914–1915.
9. Dodd MJ, Miaskowski C, Paul SM. Symptom clusters and their effect on the functional status of patients with cancer. Oncol Nurs Forum 2001; 28(3):465–470.
10. Grond S, Zech D, Diefenbach C, Bischoff A. Prevalence and pattern of symptoms in patients with cancer pain: a prospective evaluation of 1635 cancer patients referred to a pain clinic. J Pain Symptom Manage 1994; 9(6):372–382.
11. Gaston-Johansson F, Fall-Dickson JM, Bakos AB, Kennedy MJ. Fatigue, pain, and depression in pre-autotransplant breast cancer patients. Cancer Pract. 1999; 7(5):240–247.
12. Schwartz AL, Nail LM, Chen S, Meek P, Barsevick AM, King ME, Jones LS. Fatigue patterns observed in patients receiving chemotherapy and radiotherapy. Cancer Invest 2000; 18:11–19.
13. Irvine D, Vincent L, Graydon JE, Bubela N, Thompson L. The prevalence and correlates of fatigue in patients receiving treatment with chemotherapy and radiotherapy. A comparison with the fatigue experienced by healthy individuals. Cancer Nurs 1994; 17(5):367–378.
14. Smets EM, Garssen B, Cull A, de Haes JC. Application of the multidimensional fatigue inventory (MFI-20) in cancer patients receiving radiotherapy. Br J Cancer 1996; 73(2):241–245.
15. Cleeland CS, Mendoza TR, Wang XS, Chou C, Harle MT, Morrissey M, Engstrom MC. Assessing symptom distress in cancer: the M. D. Anderson Symptom Inventory. Cancer 2000; 89(7):1634–1646.
16. Pollock RE, ed. Manual of Clinical Oncology. International Union Against Cancer. 7th ed. A. John Wiley & Sons, Inc. Publication, 1999.
17. Uchitomi Y, Mikami I, Kugaya A, Akizuki N, Nagai K, Nishiwaki Y, Akechi T, Okamura H. Depression after successful treatment for non small cell lung carcinoma. Cancer 2000; 89(5):1172–1179.
18. Salmon P, Hall GM. A theory of postoperative fatigue: an interaction of biological, psychological, and social processes. Pharmacol Biochem Behav 1997; 56(6): 623–628.
19. Perttunen K, Tasmuth T, Kalso E. Chronic pain after thoracic surgery: a follow-up study. Acta Anaesthesiol Scand 1999; 43(5):563–567.
20. Dajczman E, Gordon A, Kreisman H, Wolkove N. Long-term post-thoracotomy pain. Chest 1991; 99:270–274.
21. Jung BF, Ahrendt GM, Oaklander AL, Dworkin RH. Neuropathic pain following breast cancer surgery: proposed classification and research update. Pain. 2003; 104(1–2):1–13.
22. Amichetti M, Caffo O. Pain after quadrantectomy and radiotherapy for early-stage breast cancer: incidence, characteristics and influence on quality of life. Results from a retrospective study. Oncology 2003; 65(1):23–28.
23. Donnelly S, Walsh D. The symptoms of advanced cancer. Semin Oncol 1995; 22:67–72.
24. Coyle N, Adelhardt J, Foley KM, Portenoy RK. Character of terminal illness in the advanced cancer patient: pain and other symptoms during the last four weeks of life. J Pain Symptom Manage 1990; 5(2):83–93.
25. Vainio A, Auvinen A. Prevalence of symptoms among patients with advanced cancer: an international collaborative study. Symptom Prevalence Group. J Pain Symptom Manage 1996; 12(1):3–10.
26. McCarthy EP, Phillips RS, Zhong Z, Drews RE, Lynn J. Dying with cancer: patients' function, symptoms, and care preferences as death approaches. J Am Geriatr Soc 2000; 48(5 suppl):S110–S121.
27. Andrykowski MA, Bruehl S, Brady MJ, Henslee-Downey PJ. Physical and psychosocial status of adults one-year after bone marrow transplantation: a prospective study. Bone Marrow Transplant 1995; 5(6): 837–844.
28. McQuellon RP, Craven B, Russell GB, Hoffman S, Cruz JM, Perry JJ, Hurd DD. Quality of life in breast cancer patients before and after autologous bone marrow transplantation. Bone Marrow Transplant 1996; 18(3):579–584.

29. Prieto JM, Saez R, Carreras E, Atala J, Sierra J, Rovira M, Batlle M, Blanch J, Escobar R, Vieta E, Gomez E, Rozman C, Cirera E. Physical and psychosocial functioning of 117 survivors of bone marrow transplantation. Bone Marrow Transplant 1996; 17(6):1133–1142.
30. Bush NE, Haberman M, Donaldson G, Sullivan KM. Quality of life of 125 adults surviving 6–18 years after bone marrow transplantation. Soc Sci Med 1995; 40(4):479–490.
31. Molassiotis A, van den Akker OB, Milligan DW, Goldman JM, Boughton BJ, Holmes JA, Thomas S. Quality of life in long-term survivors of marrow transplantation: comparison with a matched group receiving maintenance chemotherapy. Bone Marrow Transplant 1996; 17(2):249–258.
32. Anderson KO, Mendoza TR, Valero V, Richman SP, Russell C, Hurley J, DeLeon C, Washington P, Palos G, Payne R, Cleeland CS. Minority cancer patients and their providers: pain management attitudes and practice. Cancer 2000; 88(8):1929–1938.
33. Bernabei R, Gambassi G, Lapane K, Landi F, Gatsonis C, Dunlop R, Lipsitz L, Steel K, Mor V. Management of pain in older adults patients with cancer. SAGE Study Group. Systematic Assessment of Geriatric Drug Use via Epidemiology. JAMA 1998; 279(23):1877–1882.
34. World Health Organization. Cancer Pain Relief. Geneva: World Health Organization, 1986.
35. Rhodes DJ, Koshy RC, Waterfield WC, Wu AW, Grossman SA. Feasibility of quantitative pain assessment in outpatient oncology practice. J Clin Oncol 2001; 19(2):501–508.
36. Cleeland CS, Janjan NA, Scott CB, Seiferheld WF, Curran WJ. Cancer pain management by radiotherapists: a survey of radiation therapy oncology group physicians. Int J Radiat Oncol Biol Phys 2000; 47(1): 203–208.
37. Larson PJ, Viele CS, Coleman S, Dibble SL, Cebulski C. Comparison of perceived symptoms of patients undergoing bone marrow transplant and the nurses caring for them. Oncol Nurs Forum 1993; 20(1):81–87.
38. Valente SM, Saunders JM, Cohen MZ. Evaluating depression among patients with cancer. Cancer Pract 1994; 2(1):65–71.
39. Anderson KO, Bradley LA, Turner RA, Agudelo CA, Pisko EJ, Salley AN Jr, Fletcher KE. Observation of pain behavior in rheumatoid arthritis patients during physical examination. Relationship to disease activity and psychological variables. Arthritis Care Res 1992; 5(1):49–56.
40. Ward SE, Goldberg N, Miller-McCauley V, Mueller C, Nolan A, Pawlik-Plank D, Robbins A, Stormoen D, Weissman DE. Patient-related barriers to management of cancer pain. Pain 1993; 52(3):319–324.
41. Anderson KO, McDaniel LK, Young LD, Turner RA, Agudelo CA, Keefe FJ, Pisko EJ, Snyder RM, Semble EL. The assessment of pain in rheumatoid arthritis: validity of a behavioral observation method. Arthritis Rheumatism 1987; 30:36–43.
42. Trowbridge R, Dugan W, Jay SJ, Littrell D, Casebeer LL, Edgerton S, Anderson J, O'Toole JB. Determining the effectiveness of a clinical-practice intervention in improving the control of pain in outpatients with cancer. Acad Med 1997; 72(9):798–800.
43. Jacox A, Carr DB, Payne R, et al. Management of Cancer Pain. Clinical Practice Guideline No. 9. AHCPR Publication No. 94–0592. Rockville, MD: Agency for Health Care Policy and Research, U.S. Department of Health and Human Services, Public Health Service, 1994.
44. Practice guidelines for acute pain management in the perioperative setting. ©1995 American Society of Anesthesiologists, Inc. J.B. Lippincott Company, Philadelphia. Anesthesiology 1995; 82:1071–1081.
45. Du Pen SL, Du Pen AR, Polissar N, Hansberry J, Kraybill BM, Stillman M, Panke J, Everly R, Syrjala K. Implementing guidelines for cancer pain management: results of a randomized controlled clinical trial. J Clin Oncol 1999; 17(1):361–370.
46. Dexter PR, Perkins S, Overhage, JM, Maharry K, Kohler RB, McDonald CJ. A computerized reminder system to increase the use of preventive care for hospitalized patients. N Engl J Med 2001; 453(13):965–970.
47. Weissman DE, Dahl JL, Beasley JW. The cancer pain role model program of the Wisconsin cancer pain initiative. J Pain Symptom Manage 1993; 8(1):29–35.
48. Janjan NA, Martin CG, Payne R, Dahl JL, Weissman DE, Hill CS. Teaching cancer pain management: durability of educational effects of a role model program. Cancer 1996; 77(5):996–1001.
49. de Wit R, van Dam F, Zandbelt L, van Buuren A, van der Heijden K, Leenhouts G, Loonstra S. A pain education program for chronic cancer pain patients: follow-up results from a randomized controlled trial. Pain 1997; 73(1):55–69.
50. Cleeland CS, Reyes-Gibby CC, Schall M, Nolan K, Paice J, Rosenberg JM, Tollett JH, Kerns RD. Rapid improvement in pain management: the Veterans Health Administration and the Institute for Healthcare Improvement collaborative. Clin J Pain 2003; 19(5): 298–305.
51. Cleeland CS, Reyes-Gibby CC. When is it justified to treat symptoms? Measuring symptom burden. Oncology 2002; 16(9 suppl 10):64–70.
52. Cleeland CS, Bennett GJ, Dantzer R, Dougherty PM, Dunn AJ, Meyers CA, Miller AH, Payne R, Reuben JM, Wang XS, Lee BN. Are the symptoms of cancer and cancer treatment due to a shared biologic mechanism? A cytokine-immunologic model of cancer symptoms. Cancer 2003; 97(11):2919–2925.
53. National Institute of Health (2002). http://consensus.nih.gov/ta/022/022_ statement.htm.

56

Perioperative Pain in Cancer Patients

ALICIA KOWALSKI, DENISE DALEY, THAO P. BUI, and PETER NORMAN

Department of Anesthesiology and Pain Management, The University of Texas M.D. Anderson Cancer Center, Houston, Texas, U.S.A.

I. BACKGROUND

In the cancer setting, surgical intervention is frequently a component of treatment. Depending on the tumor pathology, it may occur before or after chemotherapy, and/or radiotherapy. Pain is an expected consequence of all surgery and is influenced by many variables. Unfortunately, these compounding factors are frequently exacerbated when a patient has a diagnosis of cancer (1). With appropriate understanding of the patient's history, patient education, and institutional collaboration, reasonable expectations regarding pain management can be met. This, in turn, results in better surgical outcome, improved patient satisfaction, and, sometimes, faster discharge from the hospital, ultimately impacting overall cost.

A. Etiology of Pain: A Review

According to the International Association for the Study of Pain, the definition of pain is an unpleasant sensory and an emotional experience, associated with actual or potential tissue damage.

1. Sensory Component

For review, the sensory component of pain is transmitted via three different nocioceptors: mechanoreceptors, thermoreceptors, and polymodal nocioreceptors. Surgical trauma results primarily in stimulation of the polymodal nocioceptors. Initially, the cells damaged from incision release substance P (SP) and a number of autocoids (histamine, bradykinin, and 5-hydroxytryptamine), which results in inflammation and stimulation of the small, myelinated, "fast pain" fibers, A-delta. This often prompts a reflexive withdrawal of the injured body part.

Nerve endings in the surgical region continue to be sensitized by prostaglandins and stimulated by the autocoids. Separate nerve fibers, unmyelinated C fibers, carry this "slow pain" message. The C fibers are also responsible for transmitting visceral pain stimulation. Importantly, the neurotransmitter mediating synaptic activity in C fibers is SP, the presynaptic release of which can be inhibited by endogenous enkephalins.

These two types of nerve fibers, A-delta and C, travel to the spinal cord, where they synapse to second-order neurons in the dorsal horn laminae II–IV and V. These second-order neurons cross the midline and pass up the contralateral spinothalamic tract to the thalamus.

In order to modulate the incoming signals of excitability, there are a number of mechanisms at various levels throughout the central nervous system. The first is a *central descending control system*, originating in the brain. This antinociceptive tract begins in the periventricular and periaqueductal gray areas of the

Table 1 Physiologic Mechanisms for Modulation of Incoming Excitation Signals

Descending control system	Periventricular and periaqueductal gray	Enkephalins inhibit SP
Spinal control mechanism	Spinal cord	Exogenous opioids inhibit SP Baclofen and benzodiazepines work via GABA and serotonin systems
Peripheral nerve fibers	Spinal cord	Directly inhibit spinal cord cells

Source: From Ref. 1.

hypothalamus and midbrain, where the incoming stimulus terminates. It extends to the dorsal horn laminae where the incoming signals initially synapse. Within this descending tract, the release of enkephalins occurs, resulting in the presynaptic inhibition of SP release at the level of the periaqueductal gray and the substantia gelatinosa, thus attenuating the pain signal input to the brain.

The second modulator is at the level of the spinal cord, and is known as a *spinal control mechanism*. This control method works by impacting a number of neurotransmitter systems. Exogenous opioids applied to the spinal cord by intrathecal or epidural injection result in the inhibition of SP release (6). Further, serotonin and GABA (affected by baclofen and benzodiazepines) systems are also involved at this spinal cord level (7).

Finally, there are *peripheral nerve fibers*, which inhibit the spinal cord cells excited by injury (8). These subsidiary pathways involve catecholamines, and hence the analgesia benefit obtained from antidepressants (6) (Table 1).

Beyond impacting neurotransmitter activity as a way of modulating pain, there are external mechanisms that can influence signal input along the sensory path. Stimulation of large A-beta fibers, via mechanoreceptors, can attenuate pain transmission through the dorsal horn. This "distraction" mechanism is addressed with the use of transcutaneous electrical nerve stimulation (TENS) (7). Acupuncture is thought to share a similar mechanism. Finally, the transmission of a signal along nerve fibers such as A-delta and C can be abolished by the local anesthetic agents.

2. *Emotional Component*

The emotional component of pain perception can be impacted by a number of variables including anxiety, mood, sleep, and environment (9–12). Fixed contributors to the emotional component include the patient's age and personality. A combination of all these variables exists for any individual patient, with a potential for change in quality or degree of any given component (Fig. 1).

These emotional components of postsurgical pain have particular relevance in the cancer setting. Alone the diagnosis of "cancer" carries a tremendous impact of fear, anxiety, and uncertainty (13). There is likewise a potential for depression, which has a tremendous correlation with postoperative pain (14). Furthermore, sleep patterns are greatly disturbed in people with pain and/or life-threatening illness (15). Over time, living with a chronic disease can intensify these emotional states.

Each patient carries concerns and fears about the surgical procedure itself. There may be upsetting memories of previous perioperative experiences, which would bias the patient, making one more sensitive to perceiving an uncomfortable stimulus as pain. For cancer patients, surgery may be especially stressful, as the findings at surgery often have a major impact on further management, and the ultimate prognosis. Expectations of pain control may also be unreasonable. Finally, for those patients admitted to the hospital, being in an unfamiliar environment with new and continuous visual and auditory stimulation can dramatically impact a patient's orientation and emo-

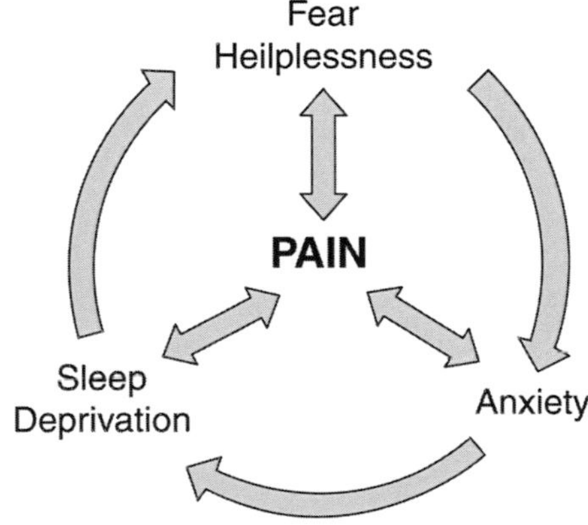

Figure 1 Vicious cycle of pain, anxiety, sleep deprivation. If pain persists unrelieved for several days, anger and depression also begin to contribute to the vicious circle, as patients become demoralized and lose confidence in the ability (and motivation) of their medical attendants to relieve their pain. Sleeplessness compounds the problem. *Source*: From Cousins MJ, Phillips GD. Acute Pain Management, p. 46.

tional state. With insight and education, the patient develops coping skills and reasonable goals for pain management, controlling anxiety, and obtaining sleep, all of which facilitate a faster and more favorable recovery.

II. ANESTHETIC PERSPECTIVES

A. Pain: Specific Pain Management Indications, Techniques, and Considerations

Postoperative pain varies considerably with each type of surgical case: somatic pain, visceral pain, or a combination of the two. Somatic pain is due to input from nocioreceptors involving striated muscle, joints, periosteum, bones, and nerve trunks (16). Visceral pain is due to hollow viscus smooth muscle spasms; distortion of a solid organ's capsule; inflammation; chemical irritation resulting in trauma to mesentery (i.e., intraperitoneal hyperthermic perfusion); and ischemia, necrosis, or encroachment of tumors (16). Compounding this variability is the fact that many cancer-related surgical procedures involve more than one surgical site, such as the mediastinoscopy prior to the thoracotomy, or the lower extremity sarcoma resection with rectus abdominous flap repair.

Although it is beyond the scope of this chapter to discuss specifically each cancer-related procedure, general comments can be made regarding resections in various anatomical locations and their relative degrees of stimulation. As well, physiological considerations are highlighted, where relevant.

1. Oral

In general, straightforward, intraoral procedures have satisfactory pain management with minimal opioid requirements. Dental procedures have the advantage of lending themselves to intraoperative injection of local anesthetic. Further pain can be well controlled with enteral opioids (oral or via feeding tube), rarely requiring intravenous (IV) medication for breakthrough pain.

2. Central Nervous System

Intracranial procedures are considered to cause relatively minimal pain. With the exception of the frontal area, craniotomies result in less postoperative pain than that of other surgical procedures (17). This phenomenon can be explained by a number of reasons. Typical craniotomy incisions are in areas with a low density in pain fibers. In addition, the dura is not richly innervated, and the brain is considered insensible to pain (17).

Typical pain management techniques include IV opioids for a short, immediate postoperative period, followed by transition to oral medications. It is important to remember that a basal infusion of opioids can confuse a clinical picture of altered mental status resulting from an intracranial process, or surgical complication.

In an opioid-dependent patient, the patient's preoperative opioid requirements should be carefully assessed and provided as a baseline postoperative requirement, plus additional dosing to cover the acute surgical pain (see Chapter 10 for more details on this topic). Further, more vigilant monitoring of the patient should be used in this unique population, with increased awareness of the pain management requirements on the part of the bedside nurse.

Major neurosurgical spine procedures such as vertebrectomy cause significant postoperative pain. Further, this patient population frequently has experienced chronic pain, with the associated emotional components and opioid tolerance. Postoperative analgesic requirements are commonly heightened, with a frequent need for adjuvants. Neuraxial analgesia is not usable in these patients due to the extensive spinal ablative surgery.

3. Chest Wall

Mastectomies without immediate reconstruction are often performed on an outpatient basis. The most common procedure is a segmental mastectomy, with or without intraoperative lymph node mapping. Pain resulting from this procedure is well managed with oral opioids; nonsteroidal anti-inflammatory drugs (NSAIDs) are a useful adjuvant.

There is evidence for a potential major cost savings when pain is managed with a unilateral paravertebral block. The benefit manifests as good pain control, minimizing pharmacy costs, and reduced risk of nausea from opioid administration (18). Although the use of this technique may be valid, it is not currently widely practiced.

For more extensive breast resections, or those with axillary node dissections, postoperative pain may be heightened. A 23-hr overnight observation may be prudent, also allowing for IV opioid supplementation.

Occasionally, there are indications for extensive tumor resection involving the external chest wall, with a reconstructive flap. These procedures are very painful for reasons similar to those discussed in the Intrathoracic section. In these instances, a regional analgesic catheter is an appropriate option. Supplementation with IV opioids may be necessary if the graft donor site is not controlled within the distribution of the neuraxial regimen.

4. *Intrathoracic*

Intrathoracic cancer procedures are most frequently performed without cardiopulmonary bypass. These include thoracotomies, esophagectomies, and pneumonectomies (intrapleural and extrapleural). Patients undergoing these procedures have frequently undergone treatment of their cancer preoperatively, involving chemotherapy and/or radiation, and they are likely to have decreased lung reserve from comorbid conditions. Preserving respiratory function in this population is critical.

Postoperatively, a chest tube can cause intense pain, as it passes through the ribs where it abuts the intercostal nerve during respiration and movement. In addition, the tip of the chest tube can irritate the pleura within the chest cavity. This is particularly painful. Incisional pain, as well as pain, due to the chest tube(s) and/or drains are best managed with a regional analgesic catheter.

Following thoracotomy, 75–85% of patients have ipsilateral shoulder pain. The differential diagnosis of this includes ligament or joint distraction from patient positioning, stretching of the brachial plexus, referred pain due to chest tube placement, transection of a major bronchus, and referred pain via the phrenic nerve (19,20).

Although there are several accepted techniques for providing post-thoracotomy analgesia, most institutions (including ours) currently favor thoracic epidural analgesia (Table 2). An infusion of a combination of dilute local anesthetic coupled with an opioid works best (21,22). The synergism between the two drugs is beneficial, along with less likelihood hypotension from a sympathetic blockade. Adjuvants, such as NSAIDs, work well in the postoperative setting, in conjunction with the epidural infusion.

The duration of epidural analgesia varies between institutions, but generally ranges between 48 and 96 hr. Once the chest tube is removed, a major painful stimulus is gone with incisional healing progressing also. At this point, the epidural can be removed, and the patient can easily transit to enteral or oral opioids. There are a few exceptions. Patients who have their chest tube(s) removed within the first 48–72 hr after surgery may show continued benefit from a full 72 hr of epidural infusion. Pneumonectomy patients typically do not have chest tubes beyond 24 hr, but they show continued benefit to their pulmonary effort with a longer infusion via a regional anesthesia technique.

An intercostal nerve block performed by the surgeon intraoperatively is an alternative to epidural analgesia. However, there are a number of disadvantages of this technique: the duration is short, lasting only 3–6 hr; unless a catheter is placed, it does not impact any stimulus caused by the tip of the chest tube within the chest cavity; and the actual incision may not be fully anesthetized. A good setting for the intercostal block is in the patient for whom systemic heparinization was anticipated but not required. The surgeon can place an intercostal block to keep the patient comfortable in the immediate recovery phase, until an epidural can be placed.

Finally, it is important to recognize that there are a number of intrathoracic procedures, which have more than one incision and/or an incision that covers a large number of dermatomes (esophagectomies, thoracotomies preceded by a mediastinoscopy, and clamshell thoracotomies). In these instances, IV opioid supplementation may prove warranted and beneficial.

Table 2 Summary of Regional Analgesia Techniques for Post-Thoracotomy Pain

Technique	Ease of insertion	Analgesic efficacy	Preservation of pulmonary function	Modification of stress response	Hypotension	Motor blockade	Urinary retention	Respiratory depression
Intercostal nerve blocks	+++	+	+	−	−	−	−	−
Interpleural analgesia	++++	±	±	−	−	−	−	−
Thoracic paravertebral block	++	+	++	+	−	−	−	−
Epidural analgesia[a]	++	+	+	−	−	±	++	±

[a] With opioid/low-dose local anesthetic infusions.
Source: From Ref. 19.

In those intrathoracic procedures, in which cardiopulmonary bypass is indicated, traditional practice dictates avoidance of neuraxial anesthetic techniques with systemic heparinization. For more discussion regarding coagulation, please refer to the section on epidurals.

5. Intra-abdominal

Upper Abdominal Cavity

Many cancer resections involve the upper abdominal cavity: hepatic resections, bowel procedures, splenectomies, retroperitoneal tumor resections, intraperitoneal hyperthermic perfusions, and others. Because of the intimate proximity to the diaphragm, postoperative respiratory compromise is a concern. Another concern is referred pain to the shoulder, which is very common following hepatic resections particularly, and occurs via the phrenic nerve.

In addition to the earlier-mentioned variables, there are physiologic changes within the body that occur as a direct result of the surgical procedure. Hepatic resections result in a deficiency of coagulation factor production, which presents as an elevation in PT (or INR). Occasionally, patients also exhibit a decrease in platelet count following hepatic resections. Typically, the peak in abnormal coagulation value is 48–72 hr postoperatively (just around the time for the neuraxial catheter to come out), and the intensity and duration correlate directly with the amount of liver resected (23).

Pain management options in upper abdominal surgical procedures include IV patient-controlled analgesia (PCA) and/or epidural infusion [also administered in a patient-controlled method, known as patient-controlled epidural analgesia (PCEA)]. For the unique hepatic resection population and all their associated postoperative physiologic implications, IV PCA is a reasonable option, although in some centers epidural analgesia is utilized in spite of the added risks.

From the information supported by the limited literature available to date, the relative benefits from an epidural, in a patient undergoing hepatic resection, may outweigh the potential associated risks (24).

Furthermore, because of the removed hepatic tissue, metabolic pathways are impacted. This can be presented as an increase in side effects from any opioids the patient is receiving. In patients with an epidural catheter infusing local anesthetics and opioids, hypersomnolence often manifests around 24 hr postoperatively.

The impact of hepatic resection on local anesthetics is not as dramatic. Although there is a potential for decreased metabolism, resulting in an increased plasma concentration of these drugs, clinically, this author has not experienced a higher incidence of toxicity following hepatic resections (and this includes those with $>50\%$ of tissue removed). This may be attributed to the very small overall dose of local anesthetic (i.e., 0.07–0.125% bupivacaine at 4–8 cm^3/hr infusion), or the plasma esterase levels are not impacted by the loss of liver tissue during the time of ester local anesthetic infusion (4).

Lower Abdominal Cavity

Malignancies of the lower abdominal cavity can be particularly painful. Approximately 60% of cancer patients with disease originating in the lower abdomen (the cervix, uterus, vagina, colon, rectum, and other tissues in women, and from penile, prostate, and colorectal carcinoma and sarcoma in men) have associated neuropathic pain due to sacral plexus involvement (16). This baseline neuropathic pain can compound the pain management requirements for a postoperative regimen.

Cancer resections of the lower abdominal cavity encompass a wide range of surgical procedures: simple hysterectomies, varying degrees of colon resections, cystectomies, pelvic exenteration, and others. The primary concerns postoperatively for pain management include facilitating ambulation, respiratory function, and return of bowel motility.

In order to accomplish these goals, IV PCA is effective, as are neuraxial techniques. Again, the anesthesiologist needs to evaluate the patient as a whole entity and determine which method has advantages that outweigh any risks for a given patient. In general, studies show that epidurals have benefits over other pain management options.

Ileus resolution, as defined by stool output or bowel sounds, was found to occur earlier with epidural vs. IV analgesia (25). Further, placement of an epidural at the thoracic level (above T12), as opposed to the lumbar level, allowed the infusion of local anesthetic coupled with opioid without significantly impacting gut motility. Thus, a more profound analgesia is obtained while avoiding hindrance of the return of bowel function (25–27). Further comparison of epidural use in abdominal cases shows stress responses to be more attenuated following lower abdominal procedures than upper abdominal procedures (28). One justification for this profound difference is accessory pathways (which occur with upper abdominal procedures), such as phrenic or thoracic somatosensory afferents, are less easily blocked by epidural analgesia (29).

Cancer resections of the lower abdomen frequently have additional associated concerns. Particularly stimulating are the procedures involving the anus. It is beneficial to incorporate stool softeners, dietary manipulation, and local anesthetic suppositories into the pain management regimen (29). Particularly, in anorectal procedures, muscle tension can compound pain. Relaxation techniques may be especially helpful in this population, with a concomitant improvement in sleep and decrease in anxiety (12).

B. Modalities of Pain Management

1. World Health Organization Ladder

Although the World Health Organization's ladder for analgesia is intended for disease-related cancer pain, a similar stepwise approach to analgesia may be useful in postoperative pain management. For opioid naïve patients having minimally painful procedures, hydrocodone with acetaminophen is a reasonable option. The clinician needs to maintain a willingness to supplement with, or convert to, stronger opioids including oxycodone or morphine if needed (Fig. 2)

For opioid-tolerant patients in the postoperative setting, often supplementing their baseline regimen with additional doses of their oral opioid is effective. Our formula is to provide the patient with their baseline opioid regimen plus a 10–30% increase in breakthrough medications, either oral or parenterally (see Chapter 10).

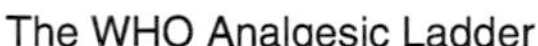

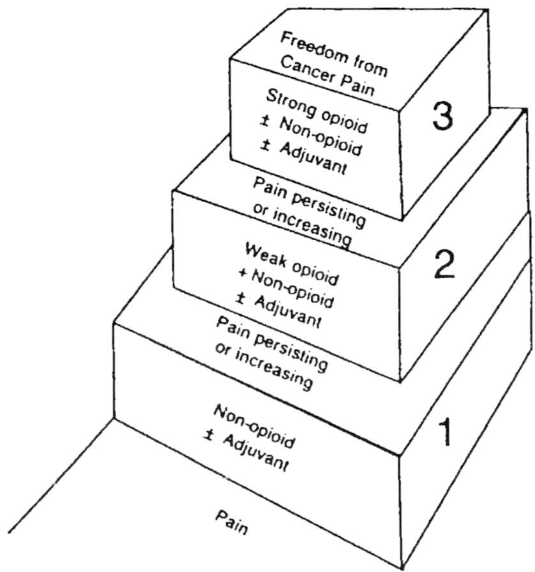

Figure 2 World Health Organization—advocated ladder approach toward cancer pain relief that relies primarily on pain intensity and, to a lesser extent, pain mechanism as determinants of therapy. *Source*: From World Health Organization. Cancer Pain Relief. Geneva: WHO, 1986 and From Abram SE, Haddox JD. The Pain Clinic Manual. 2nd ed, p. 307.

2. Routes of Administration

Oral

The oral route of medication administration is still the mainstay in pain management regimens. Along with the traditional oral medications, a newer form of fentanyl, oral transmucosal fentanyl citrate, may be a good choice in breakthrough pain situations when the IV route is unavailable (as an alternative to IM).

Transdermal

This form of fentanyl is not recommended for postoperative pain management because of difficulty with titration. Adverse events may be easily reversed with naloxone, but systemic effects may continue for up to 12 hr after removal of the patch. For those chronic pain patients on this preoperatively, continuance of the "baseline" regimen offers a beneficial contribution to the pain management regimen.

Intravenous

Introduced in 1970, now the most widely utilized form of medication administration is the IV PCA. The theory is that smaller doses are required to control pain, if they are available at frequent intervals. This frequent administration of the opioid allows maintenance of a steady blood level within the therapeutic range (Fig. 3).

The PCA therapy is based on a negative feedback loop: as pain is reduced, there is no further demand. The program provides a designated dose at a given time interval, obtained by a patient's trigger. A continuous basal infusion of medication may or may not be coadministered. If utilized, current recommendations are for the basal infusion to be no more than 20–30% of the total analgesic dose (30).

Many advantages of PCA include ease of titration and adjustment for the caregivers, high quality of analgesia, autonomy without delay in drug delivery due to nursing or pharmacy issues, crucial safety mechanism in the patient seeking one's own balance of analgesia vs. sedation, and a lower incidence of side effects. Disadvantages of the technique include the requirement for patient insight, the need for appropriate multistep programming, and the potential for equipment malfunction or disconnect (31–34).

Regional Anesthesia

In certain cases, regional techniques offer effective pain control. The use of local anesthesia minimizes requirements for opioids and, consequently, their

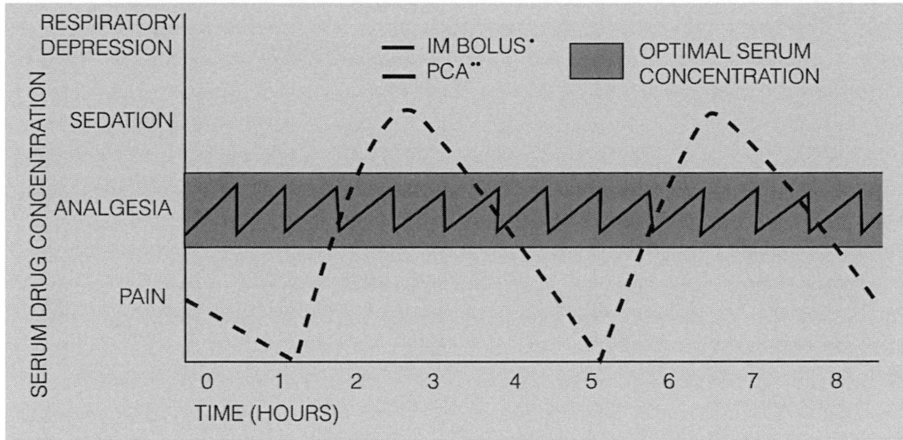

Figure 3 Harmful effects of unrelieved acute pain. *Source*: From Sevarino FB, Preble LM, Weeks JG, Sinatra RS. A Manual for Acute Postoperative Pain Management. New York: Raven Press, 1992.

related side effects. Although there are many forms of regional anesthesia, the mainstay of postoperative pain management in this author's institution is epidural.

Because of the potential for more than one surgical site within any one given cancer resection, there is a possibility that techniques may have to be integrated. For example, a patient with a mediastinoscopy prior to the thoracotomy may not have sufficient pain control at the neck incision with an epidural regimen alone. Infusion of pure local anesthetic via the epidural, coupled with an IV PCA opioid, works very well to maintain comfort levels. An exceptional overview of all routes of administration is seen in the table taken from Alexander and Hill, Postoperative Pain Control (Fig. 4).

3. *Regional Anesthesia*

Blocks

Interpleural analgesia is a reasonable option for patients in whom thoracic epidurals are contraindicated.

Continuous spinal catheters are uncommonly used in the perioperative setting, but may be useful for certain cancer pain syndromes (see Chapter 10). Peripheral nerve catheters (brachial plexus, femoral, sciatic) are excellent analgesic techniques, but often are not viable with an axillary node resection, or groin dissection, which are frequently components in cancer excisions.

Epidural catheters are widely used in thoracic, upper abdominal, and extensive pelvic cancer surgeries. Epidural analgesia has been shown to be superior to IV PCA for thoracic and upper abdominal analgesia by several parameters (26,35–37). The epidural infusion may be administered by caregiver boluses at given intervals, or more commonly on an infusion via a PCEA technique. The same PCA theory works in the epidural setting when accompanied by a basal rate programmed with the prn dose.

Drugs

Although a thorough review of all local anesthetics is beyond the scope of this section, a cursory review is warranted. Of the many local anesthetics available, the most common choice over the last couple of decades has been the amide, bupivacaine. Bupivacaine is a racemic solution that provides a good sensory and motor block. Accepted infusion doses typically have a concentration of 0.125%. More dilute concentrations, as low as 0.075%, have been used successfully when coupled with opioids.

In 1996, ropivacaine became available. It is a solution of the isolated *s*-enantiomer of bupivacaine's racemic mixture. It offers equipotent sensory block with less profound motor block and exhibits less potential for cardiac toxicity than bupivacaine.

Epinephrine in low concentrations may be added to regional anesthesia solutions. This decreases the systemic absorption of the other drugs (19,38,39), and potentially enhances the effectiveness of the block. The alpha-2 stimulation by the epinephrine itself may further contribute to pain relief (19). Potential disadvantages include hypertension, tachycardia, and exacerbation of opioid-related side effects, when used in conjunction with opioids (19,41,42).

Clonidine produces analgesic effects via its alpha-2 agonist activity, decreasing sympathetic outflow. In comparison with IV administration, analgesia is twice as potent when added to epidural solutions. It also extends the duration of regional anesthetic blockade. The most common side effects include hypotension and sedation.

CHOICES IN MANAGEMENT OF POSTOPERATIVE PAIN

Route of Administration	Proportion of Drug Absorbed Into Systemic Circulation	Rate of Absorbtion	Effect of Stress, Anxiety, Shock or Hypotension	Is Sterility Required?	Advantages
Intravenous	All - directly	Immediate	Higher proportion of drug delivered to heart and brain - reduced rate of metabolism and excretion	Yes	Most rapid and reliable form of administration. Does can be titrated against pain. It is the preferred route in shock, as absorption does not depend on regional blood flow. Rapid effect makes it suitable for patient-controlled analgesia (PCA)
Intramuscular	All - directly	Moderate	Absorption delayed	Yes	Absorption slower, peak effect less, and duration of effect longer.
Subcutaneous	All - directly	Slow - can be varied	Absorption greatly delayed	Yes	Effect even more constant and prolonged than above.
Transdermal	Variable unless occlusive dressing used - directly	Slow	Absorption greatly delayed	No	Non-invasive, painless administration
Oral	Very variable - via portal circulation and liver	Moderate to slow - rate can be reduced by slow-release preparations.	Absorption delayed to a variable extent[2]	No	Non-invasive, painless, easy to administer[3]. Relatively inexpensive, no additional equipment required.
Sublingual	Variable depending on how much of the dose is swallowed - directly	Moderate	Absorption slightly delayed	No	Relatively inexpensive tablet form which enters the systemic circulation directly.
Nasal	Slightly variable, some may be exhaled - directly	Moderate to rapid	Little effect	No	Convenient administration, which enters the systemic circulation directly.
Pulmonary	Variable, most of the gas is expired, - directly	Rapid	Slight - because of altered ventilation - perfusion ratio	No	Rapid onset of peak effect. Self-administration device inherently safe because of the need to make an airtight seal to inhale gas at subatmospheric pressure
Rectal	Variable, some may be evacuated before absorption. - directly	Moderate	Delayed, but less than with oral route	No	Suitable for concious or unconcious patient

Route of Administration	Disadvantages	Appropriate Person to Administer Drug	Analgesic Techniques Feasible by This Route	Drugs Available by This Route
Intravenous	Onset of peak rate of biotransformation and excretion also rapid, therefore duration of effect relatively short. Requires trained staff to administer drug. Therefore drug may not be immediately available.	Doctor or patient (for PCA)	Bolus injection on demand. Regular bolus injections. Continuous on computer-controlled infusions. Patient-controlled analgesia (PCA)	Opioids, Some NSAIDs *(e.g. lysine acid salicylate, ketorolac)*, Nefopam, ketamine
Intramuscular	Rate of absorption dependent on regional blood flow to muscle; some drugs painful on injection, e.g. diclofenac. Pain more likely when muscles wasted. Risk of inadvertent vascular or neural puncture. Concurrent anticoagulation may lead to extensive bruising.	Doctor or nurse	Bolus injection on demand. Regular bolus injections.	Opioids, Some NSAIDs *(e.g. lysine acid salicylate, ketorolac, diclofenac)*, Nefopam, ketamine
Subcutaneous	Rate of absorption dependent on skin blood flow and even more dependent than above on shock, anxiety, sedation, or hypoventilation. Some irritant drugs cause ulcers or abscesses.	Doctor or nurse	Bolus injection on demand[4]. Regular bolus injections. Continuous infusions.	Opioids, ketamine
Transdermal	Absorption too slow to allow titration of drug against pain. Few drugs available for this use.	Doctor, nurse or patient	Regular application	Hyoscine *(for muscle spasm)*. Flyceryl trinitrate *(for angina)*, fentanyl
Oral	In the postoperative period, the patient may be stuporous or the laryngeal reflexes may be sluggish. Oral administration may then lead to inhalation of the drug. Oral ingestion may cause nausea and vomiting. Gastric emptying may be delayed following stress, pain, opioids, or anaesthesia absorption from the small intestine would be delayed. Gastric irritants, e. g. aspirin, more irritant to the empty stomach.	Doctor, nurse or patient	On demand or regular administration.	Paracetamol, NSAIDs, Opioids, Ketamine
Sublingual	Excessive salivation leads to swallowing, like the oral route, this route is not safe unless the larynx is competent. Few drugs are available for this route of absorption.	Doctor, nurse or patient	On demand or regular administration.	buprenorphine, phenazocine, glyceryl, trinitrate.
Nasal	Drugs must be in fine powder or mist form. Conscious effort required. Inappropriate during bouts of the common cold or if mucosa altered by cocaine.	Patient	On demand or regular administration.	Diamorphine, morphine and cocaine 'snorted' by addict population
Pulmonary	Bulky equipment required. Effect short-lasting. Dry gases lead to retrosternal soreness. Hyperventilation leads to dizziness. Exhaled gases cause environmental contamination. Continuous administration needs continuous supervision.	Patient/nurse: physiotherapist for PCA: anaesthetist for continuous	On demand administration. Continuous administration. Patient-controlled analgesia	Nitrous oxide/oxygen, Trichloroethylene[5], morphine, diamorphine.[6]
Rectal	Proportion of dose unknown, especially when intestinal hurry present. Application may initiate evacuation. May cause proctitis. Aesthetically unpleasing to the majority of British patients.	Doctor, nurse or patient.	On demand or regular administration.	Some NSAIDs *(e.g. indomethacin, piroxicam)*, Some opioids *(e.g. morphine, dextromoramide)*

Notes:

1 This depends not only on the route of administration but also on the solubility and dissociation constant of the drugb, the acidity of the environment, and the surface area and the regional blood flow of the absorptive area.

2 Systemic absorption from the gastrointestinal tract depends on:
- a) The site of absorption - stomach or small intestine
- b) The rate of passage and dissolution of the drug in a patient who may be dehydrated and recumbent.
- c) The rate of gastric emptying.
- d) The amount of drug which traverses the hapatic circulation without biotransformation.

3 Unless the patient is uncooperative, in which case great skill is required.

4 The insertion of a plastic, low-volume cannula subcutaneously in children during the operative procedure and general anaesthetic allows painless post-operative injection of many drugs

5 Tricholoroethylene, although more long-lasting than nitrous oxide, is rarely used because of the induced nausea, tachycardia and tacypnoea.

6 In the 19th century, the distillation and inhalation of opium was used by postoperative patients (and their attendants), but now morphine and diamorphine are smoked only by the addict population (chasing the dragon).

Figure 4 Postoperative pain control. *Source*: From Alexander JI, Hill RG. Postoperative Pain Control. Blackwell, 1987:119–121.

The opioids, fentanyl and morphine, are often combined with local anesthetics for epidural infusions. These two agents differ in their lipophilicity, with fentanyl being highly lipophilic, whereas morphine is hydrophilic. Thus, fentanyl is rapidly absorbed into the blood stream, but morphine stays within the CNS, with some delayed rostral spread and associated delayed sedation. Any opioid-related side effects (nausea, pruritus, sedation) usually respond to low-dose naloxone; a dilute infusion or small IV dose frequently minimizes, if not abolishes, the side effects without interfering with analgesia.

Side Effects/Risks

With any technique or medication, there are side effects and possible complications. Intravenous access must be established prior to all catheter or neural blockade procedures. Furthermore, resuscitative equipment must be available at the time of placement including drugs and equipment for intubation (43).

Cancer patients are frequently immunocompromised from chemotherapy and/or steroids. This identifies a high-risk population for epidural abscess. Other compounding risk factors include catheter duration for >7 days and diabetes (44–46). In all of these scenarios, it is critical to give heightened attention to sterile technique during placement of the catheter, as well as postoperative care of the insertion site for the duration of the catheter.

There are a few case reports in the literature of spinal cord infarct from epidural-associated hypotension. With a sympathectomy from a well-functioning epidural, a drop in blood pressure can be compounded by a change in the patient's position (sitting up in a chair) and/or hypovolemia (especially common in the thoracic surgical population). Vigilant monitoring and early intervention are critical on the part of the caregiver when motor block occurs in the face of sensory preservation, the classic physical signs of spinal cord infarction.

Perioperative anticoagulation is a concern in those patients receiving epidural catheters because of the potential for epidural hematoma. The incidence of preoperative therapy with drugs affecting coagulation is increasing, and the clinician needs to have a heightened level of awareness in deciding whether to place a neuraxial catheter. Postoperatively, anticoagulation therapy (when indicated) in surgical patients is a standard of practice for certain types of surgery. Again, concern rises in the face of concurrent therapy with epidural catheters. A summary of recommendations with various medications (Tables 3 and 4) is given in what follows.

Contraindications

Absolute contraindications to regional anesthetic techniques include patient refusal, infection at the site of insertion, allergy to the medication for infusion, and a lack of resuscitative equipment. Relative contraindications include cardiac conduction disorders and vertebral metastasis, and concern about a comorbid state interfering with the efficacy of the technique to be utilized, anticoagulation, and multiple sclerosis.

4. *Opioid-Tolerant Patients*

Patients requiring opioid therapy preoperatively should have their regimen continued perioperatively, as much as possible. Those patients using fentanyl patch should have their regimen maintained, with vigilant monitoring and adjustment of the postopera-

Table 3 Epidural Management in Patients Receiving Agents Affecting Coagulation Preoperatively

Agent	Insertion recommendations	Laboratory tests before insertion
Subcutaneous unfractionated heparin (1000 U q 8–12 hr)	Insert EP ≥4 hr after last dose	aPTT if cachetic or liver dysfunction Platelets if heparin for >4 days
LMWH heparin	Insert EP ≥12 hr (ideally 24 hr) after last dose	None recommended
Intravenous heparin	Insert EP ≥2–4 hr after last dose	aPTT Platelets if heparin for more than 4 days
Coumadin	Insert EP ≥4–7 days after last dose	PT, INR
Thrombolytics and Fibrinolytics (e.g., streptokinase, t-PA)	Insert EP ≥1–2 days after last dose	Fibrinogen
Ticlopidine	Insert ≥7 days	None recommended

Source: Information compiled from Heit JA. Low-molecular-weight heparin: biochemistry, pharmacology, and concurrent drug precations. Reg Anesth Pain Med 1998; 23(6) (suppl 2:) 135–139.

Table 4 Epidural Management in Patients to Receive Agents Affecting Coagulation Perioperatively

Agent	Initiation of agent	Removing epidural catheter	Laboratory tests before removing epidural catheter
Subcutaneous unfractionated heparin (1000 U q 8–12 hr)	Start ≥1 hr after EP insertion	Remove ≥4 hr after last dose	aPTT if cachetic or liver dysfunction Platelets if heparin for >4 days
LMWH heparin	Start ≥4 hr after EP insertion	Remove ≥12 hr (ideally 24 hr) after last dose Wait ≥2 hr after removal before injecting next dose	None recommended
Intravenous heparin	Start ≥1 hr after EP insertion	Remove ≥2–4 hr after last dose	aPTT Platelets if heparin for >4 days
Coumadin	Insert >7 days	No specific recommendations	PT, INR

Note: The use of EP catheters in patients who will receive thrombolytics and fibrinolytics is strongly discouraged.
Source: Information compiled from Heit JA. Low-molecular-weight heparin: biochemistry, pharmacology, and concurrent drug precautions. Reg Anesth Pain Med 1998; 23(6)(suppl 2):135–139.

tive regimen to accommodate "new" pain from surgery. Consideration of the cancer pain control regimen as a "baseline" for functioning justifies continuance through the recovery phase. Furthermore, any decrease in opioid administration, and associated withdrawal, can be avoided. Our usual strategy is to continue to providc the patients basal dose of opioids analgesics plus between a 10% and 30% increase in total daily opioids generally in the form of an IV PCA.

5. Adjuvant Medications

Knowing that eicosanoids mediate inflammation, interfering with their production can be beneficial. The pathway for production involves the cyclo-oxygenase enzyme, which regulates the conversion of arachidonic acid to prostaglandins. Nonsteroidal anti-inflammatory drugs inhibit cyclo-oxygenase. There are two identifiable isoenzymes: cox-1 and cox-2. Cox-1 modulates platelet activity, gastrointestinal cytoprotection, and renal function (especially in hypovolemic states), and cox-2, inducible by inflammatory stimuli, is involved in inflammation and pain. A nonselective cox-inhibitor, ketorolac, can be associated with side effects, such as postop bleeding, gastric ulceration, and renal dysfunction. Currently, the advantage of this drug is its availability in the IV form. A selective cox-2 inhibitor, such as rofecoxib, celecoxib, or valdecoxib, allows for protection against the earlier-mentioned side effects, with maintenance of benefits. The drawback is that its availability is limited to the enteral route; currently, the IV form is undergoing FDA trials. Overall, NSAIDs show a therapeutic benefit and opioid sparing effect (19,47).

6. Nonpharmacological Techniques

There are many nonpharmacological interventions patients use to help cope with pain. Some are intuitive (immobilizing, guarding, massage) and others require effort for application (TENS, heat, or ice). Use of any of these techniques has been shown to facilitate pain control (13,48–51) (Table 5).

Transcutaneous electrical nerve stimulation exerts its benefit via sensory input at the dorsal horn, which modulates painful sensation favorably. A greater effect is seen with reduction in somatic over visceral pain (51,52). Current literature reports shorter durations of IV PCA use when coupled with TENS and a decrease in opioid consumption by 15–30% (7,51,53).

C. Emotional Considerations

1. Anxiety

The perception of pain is highly influenced by non-nocioceptive factors. It is imperative that these factors

Table 5 Nonpharmacological Pain Control Techniques

Relaxation techniques—breathing, imagery, music, meditation, spiritual practices
Positioning/immobilizing/guarding
Distraction/moaning
Cold/heat
Eating/drinking
Acupressure/massage
Herbs/vitamins
TENS

Source: From Refs. 13, 48–51.

be taken into account in the assessment of any given patient. Patients with a large anxiety or depression contribution to their report of "severe pain" will often report "10/10" pain in spite of repeated attempts at adjusting their analgesics. Until their overall emotional situation is addressed, it may be close to impossible to control their pain with analgesics alone. Anxiety may be present as a result of "fear of the unknown," feelings of loss of control, or a combination of the two. A patient may not even realize or admit that he/she is anxious. As a clinician, it is important to recognize clues that anxiety might be present including knowing the patient's diagnosis, whether the surgery was successful, hearing the patient ask the same question(s) repeatedly without integrating the answer, recognizing the patients' focus on worries outside of their control (i.e., the spouse's lost glasses, whether the yard man came), irritability, fidgeting, and facial expression (54).

For an optimal recovery, anxiety must be addressed. Education for the patient about their disease, what was accomplished during surgery, expectations about outcome, and identification of short-term recovery goals all lend to cognitive coping skills. The emotional component of anxiety can be addressed with reassurance for the patient, friendly visitors, giving the patient back the control to handle routine daily living tasks as quickly as tolerated, and encouragement. Finally, benzodiazepines (newly prescribed or continuance of preoperative therapy) are reasonable pharmacological adjuvants to recovery in patients needing this degree of intervention.

2. Mood

Mood can play a major role in a patient's recovery. For those who had a favorable diagnosis and outcome from the surgical intervention, there is relief and often elation. Obviously, this tone can dramatically facilitate a patient's tolerance of pain and discomfort; it can motivate recovery exercises and alleviate other psychological and emotional burdens. For those unfortunate patients with more advanced disease, who receive disappointing news, there may be a sense of hopelessness and helplessness. Such devastation can interfere with a patient's coping skills for participation in and even desire for a recovery.

Clinicians need to be sensitive to the patient's shock, sadness, and grief for a "loss"—whether it is a lost limb or a lost hope. Tearfulness, irritability, insomnia, anger, and unwillingness to participate in recovery exercises all should raise the clinician's level of concern that the patient is experiencing depression. Psychological and pharmacological intervention may be implemented to widen the patient's repertoire of coping mechanisms, realizing that antidepressants take up to 4 weeks to begin working.

3. Sleep

Historically, the importance of adequate sleep in the postoperative period has been neglected (55). Some researches have shown that quality sleep is a critical factor in the recovery phase following surgery (12).

There are a multitude of factors that potentially interfere with a patient maintaining a normal sleep pattern. Pain, fever, drains, nursing duties, physiotherapy, drugs, emotions, concerns, and visitors often keep patients awake. Aside from the obvious benefits of feeling rested on awakening, there are measurable physiological detriments to sleep deprivation. For patients deprived of rapid eye movement (REM) sleep over a period of about 48 hr, there is a compensatory increase in REM sleep during subsequent sleep periods. These compensations are associated with ventilatory disturbances, central apnea attacks, and episodic hypoxia. It has been postulated that the increase in myocardial infarction on the third postoperative day may be attributed to this phenomenon (55).

Unfortunately, opioids themselves may interfere with normal sleep patterns. High-dose opioid regimens have been shown to alter sleep patterns for some days in the postoperative period (33). Optimizing the therapeutic dose, along with potential adjuvants, can help minimize this side effect. Co-ordinating nursing interventions during the night can also promote longer sleep intervals. Modifying environmental variables for optimal impact may be challenging, but invaluable, as described in what follows. Finally, this is another area where pharmacological intervention, in the form of short acting sleep medications, may be necessary in some patients. Notably, the sedative hypnotic agents must be used very cautiously in the immediate postoperative period due to their sedative synergy with the opioids.

4. Environment

Intertwined with sleep is the impact the hospital environment has on the recovering patient. Noise levels, particularly in the ICU, are elevated, and continue 24 hr a day. Visual stimulation is often similarly heightened around the clock with factors such as light, movement of staff, and monitors. The effort on the part of the hospital staff to minimize stimulation to a patient during the night helps promote good sleep periods and maintain orientation (Fig. 5).

Lack of ultraviolet light stimulation can deprive patients of day–night cycles. Thus, it is important for patients to have exposure to a window, if at all possi-

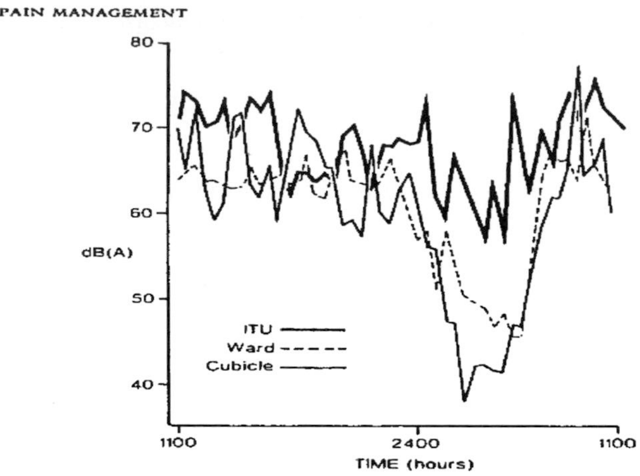

Figure 5 Noise levels in various clinical areas, with excessive noise persisting at night in ICU. *Source*: From Bentley S, Murphy F, Dudley H. Perceived noise in surgical wards and an intensive care area: an objective analysis. Fr Med J 1977; 2:1503 and from Cousins MJ, Phillips GD. Acute Pain Management, p. 46.

ble. Studies show that a lack of windows in an ICU environment contributes to a two to three times higher incidence of postoperative delirium (56,57). During the day, the patient should be encouraged to turn on the lights in their room, watch TV, read, exercise, and ambulate in the halls. At night, stimulation should be minimized with the lights and TV turned off, the door closed, and hospital staff minimizing variables within their control. Families can help maintain their loved one's orientation by bringing in family pictures, familiar music, a clock, and making sure the patient has own glasses and/or hearing aid(s) from home. The overall benefit of an alert and oriented patient is the facilitation of a faster, less complicated recovery course.

D. Clinical Practice

The American Society of Anesthesiologists' Task Force on Pain Management developed practice guidelines for acute pain management. They defined "acute pain in the perioperative setting as pain that is present in a surgical patient because of the pre-existing disease, the procedure, or a combination of both" of these sources (29). A broad overview of the guidelines includes proactive planning, education, and an interdisciplinary approach toward pain management. This last component includes frequent assessment, 24-hr availability of anesthesiologists, standardized institutional policies and procedures, and a multimodality approach of pain management as outlined elsewhere in this chapter.

1. Proactive Planning

In planning for perioperative pain management in a cancer patient, there are a number of unique considerations. First, and foremost, is the type of procedure the patient will have. Various surgical interventions are associated with varying degrees of postoperative pain. Further consideration includes prior chemotherapy and/or radiotherapy. These treatments, particularly radiotherapy, can cause tissues to be damaged and wound healing to be compromised. In such instances, the duration of postoperative pain signals can be prolonged and intensified.

The incidence of chronic opioid use is higher in the cancer patient population than in the general public undergoing surgery. Pain due to cancer can be attributed to those causes listed in what follows (Table 6).

Opioid-tolerant cancer patients will likely have unique and challenging postoperative pain management issues. Our strategy is to continue, when possible, the patients' preoperative opioids and adjuvant regimen. Then, an IV PCA or epidural catheter is added to this baseline regimen to cover the increased perioperative pain.

A final consideration in this planning stage is who is going to manage the patient's pain. Although most capable and conscientious surgeons can manage pain for their patients, optimal care combines these efforts with interdisciplinary programs. Such collaboration has been advocated by pain societies worldwide, along with the U.S. Federal Government. According to the American Society of Anesthesiology Task Force on Acute Pain Management, and authorities through-

Table 6 Pathophysiology of Pain in the Cancer Patient

Cancer pain caused by direct infiltration and tissue damage
Necrosis and inflammation, infection, and ulceration
Invasion of bone and/or periosteum or nerves by tumor
Obstruction of body organs or ducts
Occlusion of blood or lymphatic vessels
Stretching of the peritoneum
Pain caused by (cancer treatment) surgery, radiotherapy, and/or chemotherapy
Postoperative pain
Neuropathic pain
Stump/phantom pain
Causalgia/reflex sympathetic dystrophy
Chemotherapy
Other conditions that may exacerbate pain:
Constipation from pain medications, insomnia, and nausea and vomiting

Source: From Hamill RJ, Rowlingson JC. Handbook of Critical Care Pain Management. New York: McGraw-Hill, Inc., 1994:483.

out the literature, the anesthesiologist is the most uniquely qualified professional to provide leadership for comprehensive programs within institutions (5,29,58,59).

If there is a regional anesthetic catheter, the anesthesiology department typically will manage the therapy. However, there is often a gray zone in cancer patients who are not receiving an anesthetic catheter. Some patients do well with routine IV PCA management, but for others this does not suffice. Many opioid-tolerant patients are managed on an outpatient basis by a pain management group. Because of their high opioid requirements, the surgeons may not be comfortable with the high-dose IV PCA regimens required, and it is feasible that a pain management team should follow these patients postoperatively.

2. *Education*

Patient and family education is a critical part of the postoperative pain management process. Many patients assume that pain is something to be tolerated as part of recovery, not knowing that there are physiologic detriments to unmanaged pain. It is important to emphasize the expectation of exercises during recovery (incentive spirometry, ambulation, physical therapy, etc.), and the beneficial role pain management can have to facilitate these activities. Discussion and education about the nature of activity-related postoperative pain and healing will encourage the patient to use adequate "break-through" medications. If a patient has a fear of addiction, this should be addressed with education as to the rarity of this condition in postoperative pain management.

The various techniques for pain management, and the risks and benefits of each, can be discussed with the patient prior to surgery. Many patients do not realize that there are options for pain management techniques. The potential side effects and their management should also be addressed with the patient. Frequently, educational tools including a handout or video can act as a reference for the patient and the patient's family.

If a surgeon has a bias toward a particular method of pain management, it is helpful for this to be disclosed in the surgeon's preoperative visit with the patient. Most patients have a more extensive relationship with their surgeon and thus their recommended approach to postoperative pain management will lend credibility to the suggested regimen, thereby laying a foundation for a "team approach" between the surgeon and anesthesiologist. Conversely, if a surgeon has a strong bias against epidural catheters (for example), it may be unwise to strongly recommend this approach to the patient.

Finally, it is important to recognize that patients, who require opioids to control their cancer-related pain preoperatively, may expect to be "pain free" once their tumor is removed. Candor with these patients that this is not likely, coupled with reassurance that their medications will be tapered as quickly as tolerated, is a successful approach. Consequently, patients develop more realistic expectations regarding comfort levels during their recovery and duration of opioid dependence.

Education is not limited to the patients. The hospital staff must be educated in the various expectations, pain assessments, and management methods as well. This awareness contributes to a consistency of patient care. Ongoing educational in-services are important addressing skills for pain assessment, various pain management techniques, and appropriate interventions to modify and individualize the patients' regimens (29).

3. *Interdisciplinary Approach*

Assessment

All members of the patient care team (nurses, house officers, pharmacists, physician extenders, and physicians) should all be familiar with a standard method of evaluating a patient's pain and the effects of the pain therapy. Consistent use of a single method avoids undue confusion to the patient, improves reliability of the patient's report(s), and provides the caregivers with a report history for relative comparison. Frequent assessment of the patient is critical. JCAHO has recently classified a pain score as the "fifth vital sign," along with blood pressure, pulse, respiratory rate, and oxygen saturation. The pain score provides the health care team with information necessary to facilitate adequate pain treatment. If pain is not adequately controlled, or significant side effects are impacting the patient, an intervention can be made.

There are subjective and objective ways to evaluate pain control. Subjectively, the patient is responsible for factually reporting their pain at rest and during activity (i.e., coughing, getting from chair to bed). Many standard methods for assessing subjective pain exist, such as verbal scales, visual scales, numerical scales, and drawings. The most commonly used pain measurement tool for an adult patient is the visual analog scale (VAS) (60,61), represented by a 10-cm line with opposite ends designated "no pain" (given a corresponding 0) and "worst imaginable" (given a corresponding 10) (Fig. 6).

The validity of the VAS is supported by a large body of the literature. Many of its advantages include a high number of response options, simple and quick to use, reproducible results, applicable in a wide variety of settings, and scores that can be statistically analyzed. Disadvantages include its requirement of a

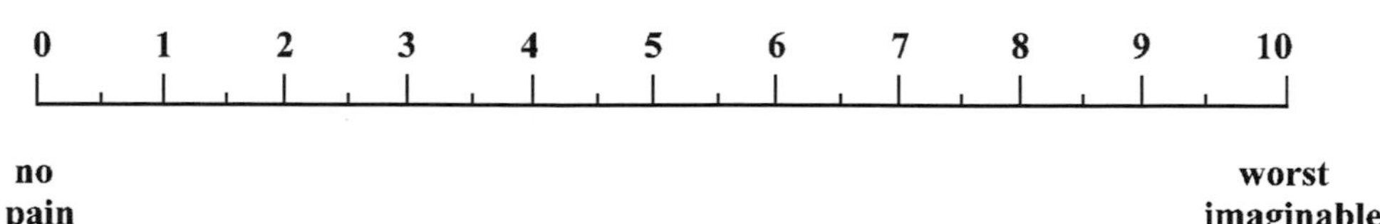

Figure 6 Visual analog pain scale. *Source*: From Hamill RJ, Rowlingson JC. Handbook of Critical Care Pain Management. New York: McGraw-Hill, Inc., 1994:20.

certain level of cognitive functioning and limited use in children (58).

From an objective standpoint, the goals of pain management are to facilitate postoperative pulmonary exercises, ambulation, activities of daily living, and physical therapy. A bedside incentive spirometer gives numeric, quantitative feedback on a patient's capability for diaphragmatic excursion. In addition, evaluation of the patients' cough effort is valuable feedback regarding their ability to clear pulmonary secretions. Observation of a patient ambulating or participating in physical therapy is another useful method of evaluating the adequacy of pain management. Behaviors such as splinting, guarding, distorted posture, limited mobility, and insomnia should alert the clinician to consider poorly controlled pain. However, unexpected, acute onset of intense pain accompanied by hemodynamic or respiratory changes should warrant evaluation of more critical conditions (i.e., dehiscence, tension pneumothorax).

Physician Availability

For those patients who have a regional anesthetic catheter, along with the assessments of the bedside nursing staff, the pain management service should evaluate the patient on a regular basis (minimum once per day, more often if unstable) and be available for interventions. At this author's institution, a handbook was published for the nursing staff on the postoperative pain service, where practice guidelines are delineated in algorithmic fashion for interventions as they arise (Fig. 7). This postoperative pain team should consist of an anesthesiologist available 24 hr/day with support as needed from house staff, physician extenders, and nurses. The primary responsibility of this service is to manage patients with interventional pain management techniques and offer support for those patients requiring additional attention for pain not relieved by conventional treatment.

The postoperative pain service should continue with patient education at the bedside. Expectations should be reinforced, as well as what interventions are available for additional breakthrough pain and/or side effects. Finally, as a consult service that is ultimately responsible for the patient's analgesic therapy, it is essential that the pain management team be the ultimate authority to approve additional medications such as sedative hypnotic agents. Hence, should patient compromise occur, the anesthesiologist's team is aware of the patient's therapeutic regimen.

Standardized Institutional Policies, Procedures, and Orders

A standardized clinical practice within a given institution promotes safety and yet lays a foundation for individualization of care (62). Such consistent practice allows the patient to transfer seamlessly from the PACU or ICU to the ward, allows nursing staff to float from unit to unit, and throughout the hospital, clear and identified consistent practices are in place. Any institution utilizing various pain management techniques should develop standardized policies, procedures, and orders for administering, discontinuing, and (when appropriate) transferring responsibility for the pain management. Such consistency facilitates integration of interdisciplinary contributions to care.

All standardized orders for pain management techniques should include drug(s), concentration(s), route of administration, pump settings, any loading dose, instructions for breakthrough pain, the treatment of side effects, monitoring parameters with triggers to call the pain management team, contact name and number for issues if they arise, and a statement for the pain service to authorize those CNS depressant drugs ordered by other services (63) (Fig. 8).

VARIOUS ALGORITHMS FOR PAIN MANAGEMENT DECISION

- Decision Tree for Pain *(see example below)*
- Epidural Management New Post-OP Patients
- Decision Tree for Pruritus
- Decision Tree for Numbness or Motor Block
- Decision Tree for Respiratory Depression
- Decision Tree for Hypotension
- Decision Tree for Epidural Catheter Disconnect
- Decision Tree for Down Stream Occlusion
- Blood Patch Guidelines

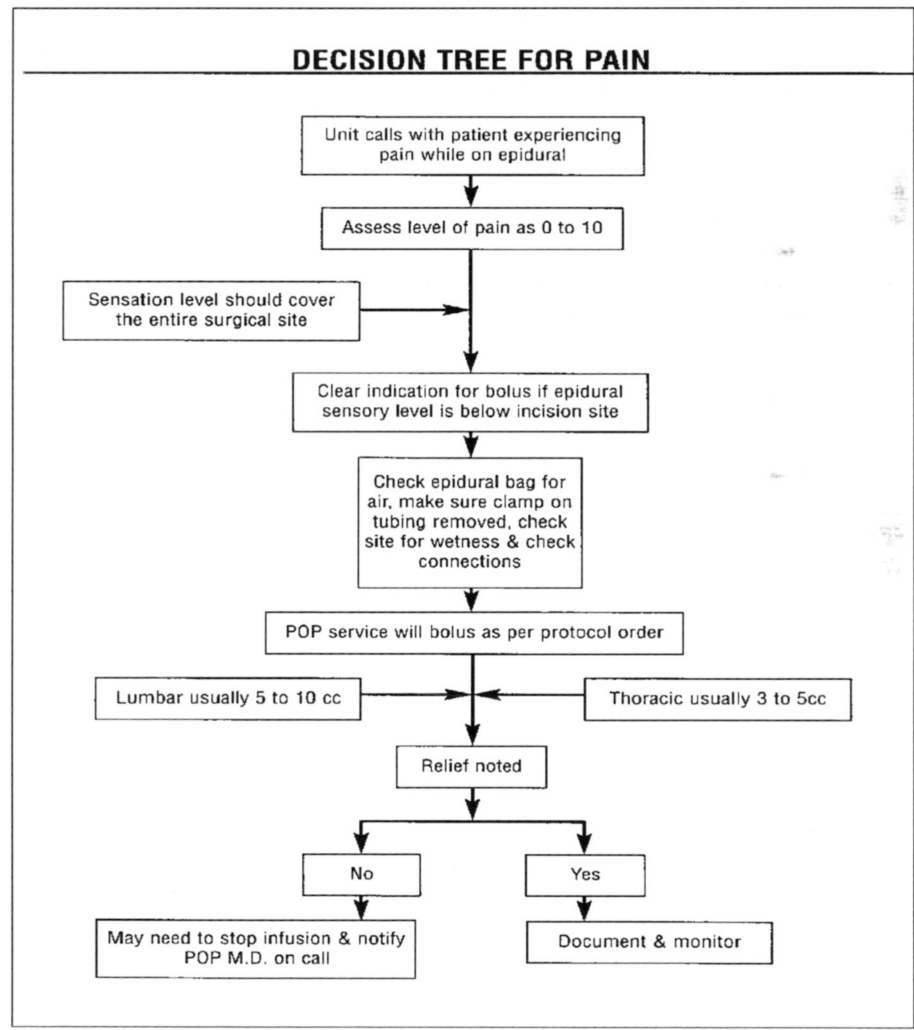

Figure 7 Pain management decision trees for patients with epidurals.

Multimodality Approach

Although the anesthesiologist is the pain management leader in the hospital, successful pain-related care (i.e., optimizing comfort and safety) involves the collaboration of surgeons, nurses, pharmacists, physical therapists, and other health care providers. For example, knowing he/she

THE UNIVERSITY OF TEXAS
MD ANDERSON
CANCER CENTER

Inpatient Physician Orders

Epidural Orders

Postoperative Pain Service (PPS) Pager 713-404-2264

Allergies: ____

MD's signature indicates all orders are activated. To delete an order, draw one line through the item, write delete and initial your entry.

DO NOT ADMINISTER THE FOLLOWING MEDICATIONS until Post Operative Pain Service (PPS) is notified: no IV or PO narcotics, CNS depressants, antiplatelets, anticoagulants, including IV or SC heparin and low molecular weight heparin.

Treatment *Notify PPS when patient arrives in SICU or PACU.*

1. Record drug use on Daily Epidural Record.
2. Record respiration rate, O_2 saturation %, pain, sedation, numbness, lower extremity weakness on Daily Epidural Record every 4 hours for the duration of therapy.
3. Continuous pulse oximeter for first 24 hours of therapy, then q4h until epidural discontinued.
4. Notify PPS if:
   a. Sedation scale = 4, RR < 10, and/or O_2 saturation < 90% for 2 minutes. Place on O_2 per N/C at 4L/minute if O_2 saturation < 90%.
   b. Catheter connector comes off – STOP infusion.
   c. Epidural dressing becomes loose/wet – cover cath with sterile 4x4 and tape.
   d. Patient has urinary retention (only if patient has no Foley catheter in).
   e. Patient has leg weakness or numbness.
   f. Pain control is inadequate.
5. DO NOT change epidural dressing.

IV Fluids If IV fluids discontinued, maintain IV access with heparin lock until epidural infusion discontinued.

Activity Ambulate with assistance according to surgeon's post-op orders.

Medications

1. Heparin Lock IV with 100 units q shift when IV fluids are discontinued.
2. Naloxone 0.4 mg with 10 ml syringe and 10 ml sterile NS available at all times during epidural therapy. In an emergency, select "override" to access Naloxone from Pyxis.
3.

Standard Formulations:*	Non-Standard Formulations:*	PPS RNs only:
☐ Fentanyl **5 mcg/ml** with Bupivacaine 0.075%	☐ Fentanyl ________ mcg/ml	☐ Follow Thoracic Epidural Protocol
☐ Fentanyl **10 mcg/ml** with Bupivacaine 0.075%	☐ Bupivacaine 0.075 %	☐ Follow Lumbar Epidural Protocol
☐ Fentanyl **20 mcg/ml** with Bupivacaine 0.075%	☐ Bupivacaine 0.125 %	
	☐ Ropivacaine 0.2 %	

***Selected items above to be prepared in preservative free (PF) NS 100ml and administered via epidural pump.**

Basal Rate _____ ml/hr	**PCA Dose** ____ml	**Delay Interval** ______min (5-15 min)	**Hourly Limit (optional)**______ml/hr

Medications as needed (prn)

- ☐ Ondansetron 4-8 mg ☐ IV Push or ☐ in 50 ml NS IVPB q6h prn for nausea/vomiting. Note: if 4 mg given, repeat 4 mg to a maximum dose of 8 mg within 6 hours. Notify pain MD if patient has no relief.
- ☐ Diphenhydramine 12.5 mg in 50 ml NS IVPB q4h prn severe itching. Notify pain MD if patient has no relief.
- ☐ In PACU, RN may bolus 5ml Epidural x 2, 15 min. apart and notify PPS of bolus.
- ☐ RN may give 5ml Epidural bolus 15 min. prior to OOB or activity if BP stable. Recheck BP after 15min.

Physician's Signature/Number: ______________________ **Date:** __________ **Time:** __________

Pager: ______________

Orders transcribed by:________**Date/time:**_______ **Orders verified by:**__________**Date/time:**_______

FAX and COPY COMPLETED ORDERS TO PHARMACY

File under: Physician Orders Page 1 of 1 POS Inst 00015 V6 4/9/03

Figure 8 Example of standardized orders for pain management.

Table 7 Organizational Aspects of an Anesthesiology-Based Postoperative Pain Program

Education (initial, updates)
Anesthesiologists
Surgeons
Nurses
Pharmacists
Patients and families
Hospital Administrators
Health insurance carriers
Areas of regular administrative activity
Maintenance of clear lines of communication
Human resources: 24-hr/day availability of pain service personnel
Evaluation of equipment
Secretarial support
Economic issues
Quality Improvement
Resident teaching (if applicable)
Related research (if applicable)
Collaboration with nursing services
Job description of pain service nurses
Nursing policies and procedures
Nurses' in-service and continuing education
Definition of roles in patient care
Institutional administrative activities
Quality improvement
Related research (if applicable)
Elements of documentation
Preprinted orders
Policies
Procedures
Bedside pain management flow sheet
Daily consult notes
Educational packages

Source: From Ref. 29.

is going to treat an orthopedic patient in recovery exercises, a physical therapist can call the bedside nurse and request the patient receive an "as needed" bolus to prepare for the therapy. Another example is the pharmacist who anticipates the epidural bag volume and prepares a replacement without delay (Table 7).

III. SURGICAL PERSPECTIVES

From a surgical perspective, the goal of postoperative pain management is to facilitate recovery and, ultimately, a judicious discharge. To contribute to the healing process, adequate pain management should help to minimize global sympathetic tone and potential postoperative complications. Beyond the ethical obligation of the practitioner to address pain, good postoperative pain management results in an increase in patient satisfaction and quality of care. Finally, any benefit of medical care, which leads to an earlier return to normal activity, decreases costs to the patient, the healthcare system, and ultimately society.

Table 8 Summary of the Actual Trends in Various Hormones and Chemical Messengers

Hormones that are increased in the surgical stress response
Prolactin
Growth hormone
LH/FSH
Renin/angiotensin II/ADH
Aldosterone
Cortisol
ACTH
Glucagon
Prostaglandins E2 and I2
Beta-endorphin
Thromboxane-A2
Dopamine
Noradrenaline
Adrenaline
Hormones that are decreased in the surgical stress response
Testosterone
Estradiol
Insulin

Source: From Refs. 9, 29, and Smith G, Covino BG. Acute Pain. Boston: Butterworths & Co. Ltd., 1985.

A. Humoral Stress Response

The surgically induced stress response results in a number of neuroendocrine and immunologic changes. Ultimately, the increase in adrenergic activity and energy expenditure results in an increase in metabolic rate, a tendency toward body tissue breakdown, impaired immune function, delayed return of normal gastric and bowel function, sodium and water retention, blood clotting, and negative emotions triggered by the "fight or flight" response (64). A summary of the actual trends in various hormones and chemical messengers (Table 8) is given in what follows.

Such undesirable tissue breakdown and immunosuppression, as mentioned earlier, can be attenuated. Studies show overwhelming evidence that the stress response can be blunted by neuraxial local anesthetics. Plasma levels of these hormones are reduced postoperatively in patients with epidurals infusing local anesthetic. Granted, this is not to convey total abolishment of the sympathoadrenergic response. However, the decrease in levels is significant enough to favor the healing process (29,65).

Additionally, early enteral feeding has shown surprisingly important contributions to recovery. Besides blunting the surgical stress response, there is improvement in wound healing and a reduction in postoperative complications (66). Finally, the surgical literature prioritizes ileus resolution postoperatively, based on the theory that there is a beneficial reduction in any surgically induced immunosuppressive state (67).

Evidence shows that an epidural with local anesthetic not only blunts the surgical stress response, but also facilitates relatively earlier return of bowel function. This promotes healing and further suppression of the adrenergic response. In patients for whom the gastrointestinal tract is not an option for nutrition, epidural therapy still has favorable effects. When compared with IV PCA, patients with epidural analgesia, who require administration of nutrient substrates, show a greater level of protein synthesis (65).

Finally, although the benefits of adequate postoperative pain management far outweighs the potential drawbacks, IV opioids have been shown to exert immunosuppressive effects, particularly in the cancer population (64). Further, a delay in gut motility can lead to the earlier-mentioned consequences, and it is a well-known fact that opioids delay bowel function.

B. Postoperative Complications

Other than complications related to dehiscence, or a technical aspect of surgery, the most concerning postoperative complications are ileus, insufficient pulmonary function, nausea and vomiting, and immobility with associated potential sequelae. Pain can have physiologic, as well as psychological, impacts, responsible for increasing the risks of complications during the postoperative course (12).

1. *Ileus*

As a result of surgical stress and the physical manipulation of the bowel, organized propulsive motility is inhibited. Moreover, pain initiates a spinal reflexive arc that further inhibits gut motility, compounding the ileus (26,27,68).

Epidural infusion of local anesthetics may improve bowel motility via inhibition of nocioceptive input on the afferent limb, plus blockade of the spinal sympathetic efferent limb. Another advantage of the sympathetic blockade obtained with neuraxial local anesthetics is a potential increase in colonic blood flow, which aids in the reduction of ileus (27,66). In one study following patients after various large bowel resections, blood flow was found to be increased in patients who received epidural bupivacaine (69).

Many studies in postoperative abdominal surgical populations illustrate the physiologic benefit of epidurals. Ahn et al. (70) measured transit time through the intestinal tract, following resection of the left colon or rectum. Patients who were receiving epidural analgesia had a mean transit time through the tract of 35 hr vs. 150 hr in the IV PCA control group. Carli et al. (26) also compared bowel motility between epidural and IV PCA groups. Earlier, bowel return as identified by flatus or bowel movement occurred in the epidural group. In a population of women following hysterectomy, postoperative ileus has been shown to resolve faster in patients receiving epidural analgesia with bupivacaine for pain relief than those treated with IV PCA opioids (71). Earlier resolution of ileus results in fewer days of nasogastric tube therapy, an ability to tolerate solid foods earlier, and a shorter hospital stay (66).

2. *Pulmonary Dysfunction*

Beyond the impact on the complication of an ileus, epidural analgesia has benefits on pulmonary function. Meta-analysis of controlled trials has demonstrated improved pulmonary outcome in those patients who received postoperative pain management with epidural analgesia (72,73).

3. *Nausea and Vomiting*

Minimizing the perioperative use of opioids, patients can have a postoperative course characterized by a lower incidence of nausea and vomiting. Less nausea is a more comfortable state, which promotes faster return to activity, and a more favorable recovery.

4. *Immobility*

Any immobility can predispose to venous stasis, platelet aggregation, and ultimately deep venous thrombosis with pulmonary embolus. Adequate pain management facilitates mobilization. Current literature supports a lower incidence of deep venous thrombosis in the orthopedic population that recovers with epidurals. Such benefit is directly attributed to a "hyperkinetic effect" on lower limb blood flow (74,75). Further studies show that bupivacaine inhibits coagulation in vitro, perhaps contributing to the favorable decrease in thrombosis (76).

C. Quality of Care, Patient Satisfaction, and Cost to Patient

Not only are short-term objective benefits obtained from adequate postoperative pain control, but also long-term results may also be favorably impacted.

Although long-term follow-up studies are limited, there is literature supporting a correlation between decreased death rate overtime and effective postoperative pain management (35). In addition, the subjective measure of patients' satisfaction is higher with minimized fatigue and functional impairment (77). Moreover, a positive effect predominates when patients are comfortable, and this is even more favorably impacted in those patients utilizing pharmacological, as well as nonpharmacological, treatment modalities. Such a positive disposition toward surgery and recovery is critical, especially in cancer patients who frequently require multiple resections for disease management. Today's medical practice is challenged to keep the cost of care in the consideration of treatment. Adequate postoperative pain control (particularly with epidural analgesia) has been shown to promote earlier discharge from the hospital and substantial cost savings (29,66,78).

IV. ICU PERSPECTIVES

Despite the compromised medical condition of the ICU patient, it is important to safely optimize pain control, thus improving outcome and preventing occurrence of long-term pain syndromes. Assessment and treatment of pain may take a lower priority in the ICU settings shown in several studies, which show that the ICU nursing assessment of pain is often inadequate (79,80). Assessment of pain in critically ill ICU patients is very difficult involving a complex interplay of nociception, anxiety, and multiple painful stimuli in patients with sedation or other neurologic compromise. Many ICU patients have some form of hemodynamic or respiratory compromise. Thus, the ICU team is presented with a difficult challenge: balancing patient comfort and patient safety. Often patients in the ICU require sedation; thus, the care providers must juggle the side effects of both the sedatives and the analgesics.

Despite sedation, there is a potential for recall; thus, it is paramount to adequately control pain (81). The technique of pain management can be impacted by whether or not the patient is receiving sedation. For example, IV PCA and PCEA require patient awareness for the prn utilization. Conversely, a basal infusion of analgesic agent without additional supplementation, or a nursing administered prn dose of medication, may be preferable in sedated patients (82). Regardless of the technique, adequate pain management must not be overlooked. In one study of over 400 cancer patients requiring ICU care, epidural pain management promoted earlier weaning from mechanical ventilation, earlier transfer out of the unit, and lower costs (78).

In addition to pain, ICU patients also have a great deal of anxiety. The patient and the patient's family

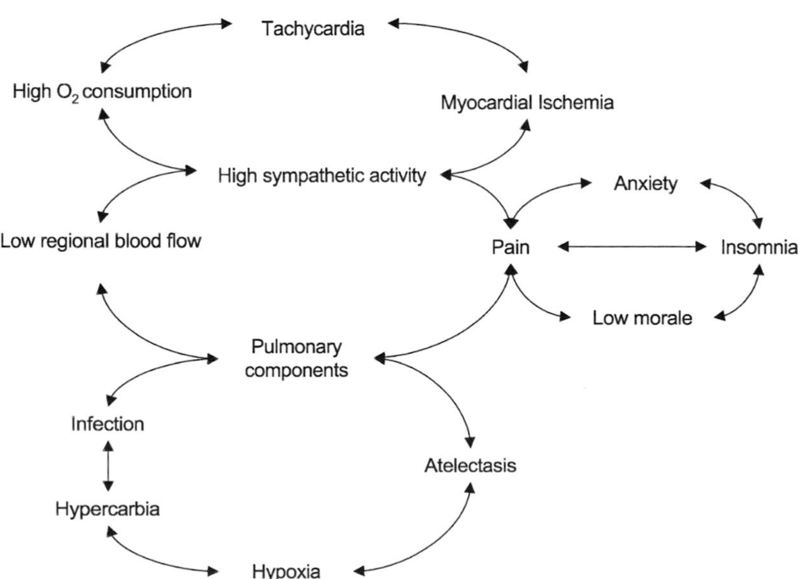

Figure 9 Harmful effects of unrelieved acute pain. *Source*: From Sevarino FB, Preble LM, Weeks JG, Sinatra RS. A Manual for Acute Postoperative Pain Management. New York: Raven Press, 1992.

may perceive the patient's situation to be life threatening and associate the ICU stay with end of life issues. The ICU environment is very disruptive to sleep and frequently leads to disorientation. Often, for those patients requiring ventilatory support, communication is hindered. Finally, there is an increased dependence on the caregiver, which can lead to an emotionally regressed state, more distress to the patient, and diminished coping capabilities (9). All of this leads to additional stress (83). Along with adequate pain management, it is important to also manage the anxiety. Staying in the ICU for a few days could push older patients into "ICU Psychosis" (84,85) (see Chapter 10). The use of haloperidol and decreasing the use of opioids by using adjuvants (like ketorolac) (86) may help with this challenge.

A new drug for pain control in ICU is dexmedetomidine, which provides analgesia and sedation without respiratory depression (88). A selective alpha-2 agonist results in sedation without the associated hemodynamic effects of alpha-1 activity. Because of its short half-life, dexmedetomidine is an ideal sedative for the ICU setting, where safety and efficacy are critical with an option for quick reversal (88).

V. CONCLUSIONS

Uncontrolled postoperative pain is highly detrimental. Undertreated pain leads to physiologic and psychological consequences, which worsen surgical outcome (89,90). A standardized postoperative pain service that provides individualized care for each patient will help optimize perioperative pain control. As physicians and medical caregivers, adequate pain control is an ethical obligation as part of the overall treatment process (Fig. 9).

A summary of favorable benefits from good postoperative pain management in the postoperative setting (Table 9) (91) is given in what follows.

To provide pain management in the hospital setting, a designated pain service is essential, with the integrated multimodality support of institutional resources. Such collaboration of care must be a priority in the cancer setting, where pain is a major symptom: approximately two-thirds of patients with advanced cancer have pain associated with their disease (1,92,93).

Table 9 Benefits from Adequate Postoperative Pain Control

Benefits
Improvement in postoperative pulmonary function
Decreased length of postoperative ventilation and ICU stay
Attenuation of the stress response to surgery
Associated improvement in the metabolic response to injury
Maintenance of immunocompetence
Earlier mobilization, which may lead to a decreased incidence of thrombotic sequelae
Heightened patient satisfaction, independence, coping mechanisms, sense of control
Greater ease in participation with recovery exercises
Less anxiety, disorientation, dependence, stress
Better sleep quality
Costs savings
Prevention of long term pain syndromes

Source: From Sevarino FB, Preble LM, Weeks JG, Sinatra RS. A Manual for Acute Postoperative Pain Management, 1992.

REFERENCES

1. Ponte J, Green David W. Handbook of Anaesthetics and Perioperative Care. Philadelphia: W.B. Saunders Co. Ltd., 1994:263.
2. Ponte J, Green David W. Handbook of Anaesthetics and Perioperative Care. Philadelphia: W.B. Saunders Co. Ltd., 1994:235.
3. Cousins MF, Phillips GD. Acute Pain Management. New York: Churchill Livingstone, 1986:47.
4. Dodson ME. The Management of Postoperative Pain. Baltimore: Edward Arnold, 1985:234–235.
5. Sevarino FB, Preble LM, Weeks JG, Sinatra RS. A Manual for Acute Postoperative Pain Management. New York: Raven Press, 1992:3.
6. Ponte J, Green David W. Handbook of Anaesthetics and Perioperative Care. Philadelphia: W.B. Saunders Co. Ltd., 1994:238.
7. Cousins MF, Phillips GD. Acute Pain Management. New York: Churchill Livingstone, 1986:37.
8. Cousins MF, Phillips GD. Acute Pain Management. New York: Churchill Livingstone, 1986:25.
9. Hamill RJ, Rowlingson JC. Handbook of Critical Care Pain Management. New York: McGraw-Hill, Inc., 1994:4–5.
10. Cousins MF, Phillips GD. Acute Pain Management. New York: Churchill Livingstone, 1986:32.
11. Alexander JI, Hill RG. Postoperative Pain Control. Boston: Blackwell Scientific Publications, 1987:32.
12. Renzi C, Peticca L, Pescatori M. The use of relaxation techniques in the perioperative management of proctological patients: preliminary results. Int J Colorectal Dis 2000; 15(5–6):313–316.
13. Kwekkeboom KL. Pain management strategies used by patients with breast and gynecologic cancer with postoperative pain. Cancer Nurs 2001; 24(5):378–386.
14. Egan KJ, Ready LB, Nessly M, Greer BE. Self-administration of midazolam for postoperative anxiety: a double blinded study. Pain 1992; 49(1):3–8.
15. Cousins MF, Phillips GD. Acute Pain Management. New York: Churchill Livingstone, 1986:40.

16. Rigor BM Sr. Pelvic cancer pain. J Surg Oncol 2000; 75(4):280–300.
17. Dunbar PJ, Visco E, Lam AM. Craniotomy procedures are associated with less analgesic requirements than other surgical procedures. Anesth Analg 1999; 88: 335–340.
18. Coveney E, Weltz CR, Greengrass R, Iglehart JD, Leight GS, Steele SM, Lyerly HK. Use of paravertebral block anesthesia in the surgical management of breast cancer: experience in 156 cases. Ann Surg 1998; 227(4): 496–501.
19. Franco P. Post-thoracotomy pain management. New Advances in Thoracic Surgery. Submitted for publication.
20. Cousins MF, Phillips GD. Acute Pain Management. New York: Churchill Livingstone, 1986:35.
21. Rogers MC, Tinker JH, Covino BG, Longnecker DE. Principles and Practice of Anesthesiology. Chicago: Mosby Year Book, 1993:1467.
22. Ashburn M, Fine P, Stanley T. Pain management in anesthesiology. Papers presented at the 43rd Annual Postgraduate Course in Anesthesiology. Boston: Kluwer Academic Publishers, Feb 1998:85.
23. Daley MD, Norman PH, Hogervost, S, Kowalski AM, Srejic U, Popat KU, Arens JF, Kennamer D, Curley S, Vauthey J. Epidural analgesia for non-transplant liver surgery. Can J Anesth 2003; 50:A48.
24. Matot I, Scheinin O, Ahmed E, Jurim O. Epidural anesthesia and analgesia in liver resection. Anesth Analg 2002; 95:1179–1181.
25. Scott AM, Starling JR, Ruscher AE, DeLessio ST, Harms BA. Thoracic versus lumbar epidural anesthesia's effect on pain control and ileus resolution after restorative proctocolectomy. Surgery 1996; 120(4): 668–695; discussion 695–697.
26. Carli F, Trudel JL, Belliveau P. The effect of intraoperative thoracic epidural anesthesia and postoperative analgesia on bowel function after colorectal surgery: a prospective, randomized trial. Dis Colon Rectum 2001; 44(8):1083–1089.
27. Liu SS, Carpenter RL, Mackey DC, Thirlby RC, Rupp SM, Shine TSJ, Feinglass NG, Metzger PP, Fulmer JT, Smith SL. Effects of perioperative analgesic technique on rate of recovery after colon surgery. Anesthesiology 1995; 83(4):757–765.
28. Kehlet H. The stress response to surgery: release mechanisms and the modifying effect of pain relief. Acta Chir Scand Suppl 1989; 550:22–28.
29. Ready LB, Ashburn M, Caplan RA, Carr DB, Connis RT, Dixon CL, Hubbard L, Rice LJ. Practice guidelines for acute pain management in the perioperative setting: a report by the American Society of Anesthesiologists Task Force on Pain Management, Acute Pain Section. Anesthesiology 1995; 82(4): 1071–1081.
30. Welchew E, Hahn CEW, Adams AP. Principles and Practice Series: Patient Controlled Analgesia. BMJ Publishing, 1995:14.
31. Welchew E, Hahn CEW, Adams AP. Principles and Practice Series: Patient Controlled Analgesia. BMJ Publishing, 1995:20.
32. Ponte J, Green David W. Handbook of Anaesthetics and Perioperative Care. Philadelphia: W.B. Saunders Co. Ltd., 1994:247–248.
33. Heath ML, Thomas VJ. Patient-Controlled Analgesia: Confidence in Postoperative Pain Control. New York: Oxford University Press, 1993:102, 112.
34. Ashburn M, Fine P, Stanley T. Pain management in anesthesiology. Papers presented at the 43rd Annual Postgraduate Course in Anesthesiology. Boston: Kluwer Academic Publishers, Feb 1998:106–107.
35. Whooley BP, Law S, Murthy SC, Alexandrou A, Wong J. Analysis of reduced death and complication rates after esophageal resection. Ann Surg 2001; 233(3): 338–344.
36. Hubbell MR. Pain management and spirometry following thoracotomy: a prospective, randomized study of four techniques. J Cardiothoracic Vascular Anesth 1993; 7(5):529–534.
37. Basse L, Hjort Jakobsen D, Billesbolle P, Werner M, Kehlet H. A clinical pathway to accelerate recovery after colonic resection. Ann Surg 2000; 232(1):51–57.
38. Baron CM, Kowalski SE, Greengrass R, Horan TA, Unruh HW, Baron CL. Epinephrine decreases postoperative requirements for continuous thoracic epidural fentanyl infusions. Anesth Analg 1996; 82:760–765.
39. Niemi G, Breivik H. Adrenaline markedly improves thoracic epidural analgesia produced by a low-dose infusion of bupivacaine, fentanyl and adrenaline after major surgery. A randomized, double-blind, cross-over study with and without adrenaline. Acta Anaesthesiol Scand 1998; 42:897–909.
40. Robertson K, Douglas MJ, McMorland GH. Epidural fentanyl, with and without epinephrine for post-caesarean section analgesia. Can Anaesth Soc J 1985; 32(5):502–505.
41. Welchew EA. The optimum concentration of epidural fentanyl: a randomized, double-blind comparison with and without 1:200,000 adrenaline. Anaesthesia 1983; 38:1037–1041.
42. Bromage PR, Camporesi EM, Durant PA, Nielsen CH. Influence of epinephrine as an adjunct to epidural morphine. Anesthesiology 1983; 58:257–262.
43. Alexander JI, Hill RG. Postoperative Pain Control. Boston: Blackwell Scientific Publications, 1987: 158–159.
44. Reihaus E, Waldbaur H, Seeling W. Spinal epidural abscess: a meta-analysis of 915 patients. Neurosurg Rev 2000; 23(4):175–204.
45. Wang LP, Schmidt JF. Severe infections after epidural catheterization. Ugeskr Laeger 1998; 160(22):3202–3206.
46. Linnemann MU, Bulow HH. Infections after insertion of epidural catheters. Ugeskr Laeger 1993; 155(30): 2350–2352.
47. Dodson ME. The Management of Postoperative Pain. Baltimore: Edward Arnold, 1985:84–86.

48. Wilkie et al. Cancer pain control behaviors: description and correlation with pain intensity. Oncol Nurse Forum 1988; 15:723–773.
49. Eisenberg et al. Unconventional medicine in the United States. N Engl J Med 1993; 328:246–252.
50. Sparber et al. Use of complimentary medicine by adult patients participating in cancer clinical trials. Oncol Nurse Forum 2000; 27:623–630.
51. Hmaza et al. Effect of frequency of transcutaneous electrical nerve stimulation on the postoperative opioid analgesic requirement and recovery profile. Anesthesiology 1999; 91(5):1232–1238.
52. Smith CM, Guralnick MS, Gelfand MM, Jeans ME. The effect of transcutaneous electrical nerve stimulation on post-caesarian pain. Pain 1986; 27(2):181–193.
53. Ashburn M, Fine P, Stanley T. Pain management in anesthesiology. Papers presented at the 43rd Annual Postgraduate Course in Anesthesiology. Boston: Kluwer Academic Publishers, Feb 1998:145.
54. Alexander JI, Hill RG. Postoperative Pain Control. Boston: Blackwell Scientific Publications, 1987:41.
55. Heath ML, Thomas VJ. Patient-Controlled Analgesia: Confidence in Postoperative Pain Control. New York: Oxford University Press, 1993:165.
56. Cousins MF, Phillips GD. Acute Pain Management. New York: Churchill Livingstone, 1986:43.
57. Keep PJ. Stimulus deprivation in windowless rooms. Anaesthesia 1977; 32:598.
58. Hamill RJ, Rowlingson JC. Handbook of Critical Care Pain Management. New York: McGraw-Hill, Inc., 1994:19–21.
59. Ponte J, Green David W. Handbook of Anaesthetics and Perioperative Care. Philadelphia: W.B. Saunders Co. Ltd., 1994:255–256, 259.
60. Ponte J, Green David W. Handbook of Anaesthetics and Perioperative Care. Philadelphia: W.B. Saunders Co. Ltd., 1994:257.
61. Hamill RJ, Rowlingson JC. Handbook of Critical Care Pain Management. New York: McGraw-Hill, Inc., 1994:21.
62. Holritz K, Lucas A. Implementation of an anesthesia pain management service program. Cancer Practice 1993; 1(2):129–136.
63. Ready LB, Ashburn M, Caplan RA, Carr DB, Connis RT, Dixon CL, Hubbard L, Rice LJ. Practice guidelines for acute pain management in the perioperative setting: a report by the American Society of Anesthesiologists Task Force on Pain Management, Acute Pain Section. Anesthesiology 1995; 82(4). Tables 2, 3.
64. Sacerdote P, Bianchi M, Gaspani L, Manfredi B, Maucione A, Terno G, Ammatuna M, Panerai AE. The effects of tramadol and morphine on immune responses and pain after surgery in cancer patients. Anesth Analg 2000; 90(6):1411–1414.
65. Schricker T, Wykes L, Eberhart L, Lattermann R, Mazza L, Carli F. The anabolic effect of epidural blockade requires energy and substrate supply. Anesthesiology 2002; 97(4):943–951.
66. de Leon-Casasola OA, Karabella D, Lema MJ. Bowel function recovery after radical hysterectomies: thoracic epidural bupivacaine-morphine versus intravenous patient-controlled analgesia with morphine: a pilot study. J Clin Anesth 1996; 8(2):87–92.
67. Basse L, Hjort Jakobsen D, Billesbolle P, Werner M, Kehlet H. A clinical pathway to accelerate recovery after colon resection. Ann Surg 2000; 231(1):51–57.
68. Livingston EH, Passaro EP Jr. Postoperative ileus. Digest Dis Sci 1990; 35(1):121–132.
69. Johansson K, Ahn H, Lindhagen J, Tryselius U. Effect of epidural anaesthesia on intestinal blood flow. Br J Surg 1988; 75(1):73–76.
70. Ahn H, Bronge A, Johansson K, Ygge H, Lindhagen J. Effect of continuous postoperative epidural analgesia on intestinal motility. Br J Surg 1988; 75(12):1176–1178.
71. Wattwil M, Thoren T, Hennerdal S, Garvill JE. Epidural Analgesia with bupivacaine reduces postoperative paralytic ileus after hysterectomy. Anesth Analg 1989; 68(3):353–358.
72. Rawal N. Epidural and spinal agents for postoperative analgesia. Surg Clin North Am 1999; 79(2):313–344.
73. Ashburn M, Fine P, Stanley T. Pain management in anesthesiology. Papers presented at the 43rd Annual Postgraduate Course in Anesthesiology. Boston: Kluwer Academic Publishers, Feb 1998:71.
74. Dalldorf PG, Perkins FM, Totterman S, Pellegrini VD Jr. Deep venous thrombosis following total hip arthroplasty. Effects of prolonged postoperative epidural anesthesia. J Arthroplasty 1994; 9(6):611–616.
75. Ragucci MV, Leali A, Moroz A, Fetto J. Comprehensive deep venous thrombosis prevention strategy after total-knee arthroplasty. Am J Phys Med Rehabil 2003; 82(3):164–168.
76. Kohrs R, Hoenemann CW, Feirer N, Durieux ME. Bupivacaine inhibits whole blood coagulation in vitro. Reg Anesth Pain Med 1999; 24(4):326–330.
77. Bardram L, Funch-Jensen P, Jensen P, Crawford ME, Kehlet H. Recovery after laparoscopic colonic surgery with epidural analgesia, and early oral nutrition and mobilization. Lancet 1995; 345(8952):763–764.
78. deLeon-Casasola OA, Parker BM, Lema MJ, Groth R, Orsini-Fuentes, J. Epidural analgesia versus intravenous patient controlled analgesia. Differences in postoperative course of cancer patients. Regional Anesth 1995; 20(6):549.
79. Puntillo KA. Pain experiences of intensive care unit patients. Heart Lung 1990; 19(5 Pt 1):526–533.
80. Tittle M, McMillan SC. Pain and pain-related side effects in an ICU and on a surgical unit: nurses' management. Am J Crit Care 1994; 3(1):25–30.
81. Cheng EY. Recall in the sedated ICU patient. J Clin Anesth 1996; 8:675–678.
82. Rundshagen I, Kochs E, Standl T, Schnabel K, Schulte am Esch J. Subarachnoid and intravenous PCA versus bolus administration for postoperative pain relief in orthopaedic patients. Acta Anaesthesiol Scand 1998; 42(4):1215–1221.

83. Guirardello EB, Romero-Gabriel CA, Pereira IC, Miranda AF. The patients' perception during their stay in the intensive care unit. Revista Escola de Enfermagem da USP 1999; 33(2):123–129.
84. Weber RJ, Oszko MA, Bolender BJ, Grysiak DL. The intensive care unit syndrome: causes, treatment, and prevention. Drug Intell Clin Pharm 1985; 19(1):13–20.
85. Nadelson T. The psychiatrist in the surgical intensive care unit. I. Postoperative delirium. Arch Surg 1976; 111(2):113–117.
86. Carney DE, Nicolette LA, Ratner MH, Minerd A, Baesl TJ. Ketorolac reduces postoperative narcotic requirements. J Pediatr Surg 2001; 36(1):76–79.
87. Venn RM, Hell J, Grounds RM. Respiratory effects of dexmedetomidine in the surgical patient requiring intensive care. Critical Care 2000; 4(5):302–308.
88. Hall JE, Uhrich TD, Barney JA, Arain SR, Ebert TJ. Sedative amnestic and analgesic properties of small-dose dexmedetomidine infusions. Anesth Analg 2000; 90:699–705.
89. Sevarino FB, Preble LM, Weeks JG, Sinatra RS. A Manual for Acute Postoperative Pain Management. New York: Raven Press, 1992:5.
90. Cousins MF, Phillips GD. Acute Pain Management. New York: Churchill Livingstone, 1986:21.
91. Hamill RJ, Rowlingson JC. Handbook of Critical Care Pain Management. New York: McGraw-Hill. Inc., 1994:6.
92. Ventafridda V, Saita L, Ripamonti C, De Conno F. WHO guidelines for the use of analgesics in cancer pain. Int J Tissue React 1985; 7:93–96.
93. Portenoy RK, Kornblith AB, Wong G, Vlamis V, Lepore JM, Loseth DB, Hakes T, Foley KM, Hoskins WJ. Pain in ovarian cancer patients. Prevalence, characteristics, and associated symptoms. Cancer 1994; 74(3):907–915.

SUGGESTED READINGS

Dodson ME. The Management of Postoperative Pain. Baltimore: Edward Arnold, 1985.

Welchew E, Hahn CEW, Adams AP. Principles and Practice Series. Patient Controlled Analgesia. BMJ Publishing, 1995.

57

Cancer Pain

HEMANT N. SHAH and ALLEN W. BURTON

Section of Cancer Pain Management, Department of Anesthesiology and Pain Medicine, The University of Texas M.D. Anderson Cancer Center, Houston, Texas, U.S.A.

OSCAR DE LEON-CASASOLA

Department of Anesthesiology, University at Buffalo and Department of Anesthesiology and Pain Medicine, Roswell Park Cancer Institute, Buffalo, NewYork, U.S.A.

I. INTRODUCTION

Cancer pain is defined as pain that is attributable to cancer or its therapies (1). A more general and accepted definition of pain is "an unpleasant sensory and emotional experience associated with actual or potential tissue damage, or described in terms of such damage (2)." Cancer pain is a problem that has attained a rising level of recognition among the health care community. Optimal management involves careful assessment, optimal analgesia, intensive follow-up, and a proactive approach to treatment. Adequate control of pain can be achieved in the majority of patients with a rigorous and aggressive application of a treatment algorithm that is ultimately quite straightforward (3,4). Control of pain and related symptoms promotes an enhanced quality of life, improved functioning, better compliance, and a means for patients to focus on those things that give meaning to life (5). In addition to their salutary effects on quality of life, mounting evidence suggests that good pain control influences survival (6,7).

II. EPIDEMIOLOGY

Approximately 6.35 million new cases of cancer are diagnosed worldwide annually, half of which originate in developing nations (8). The WHO estimates that by the year 2021, there will be 15 million new cases of cancer worldwide annually. This will lead to an increased number of patients with cancer related pain.

1.3 million new diagnosis of cancer are made annually in the United States (9). 556,000 people, or one of every four deaths in the United States is a result of cancer, which is approximately 1500 cancer related death daily (10). The incidence of cancer increases with age and is particularly problematic, given our rapidly aging population.

It is estimated that up to 50% of patients undergoing treatment for cancer and up to 90% of patients with advanced cancer have pain (11). Most (70%) cancer pain is due to tumor involvement of organic structures, notably bone, neural tissue, viscera, or others. Up to 25% of cancer pain is due to therapy, including chemotherapy, radiotherapy, or surgery. Up to 10% of "cancer pain" is accounted for by common chronic pain syndromes, including back pain and headaches, which might have been exacerbated by the ongoing growth or treatment of cancer (12).

Overall, cancer cure rates have not changed markedly over the past four decades: the overall 5-year survival rate for patients diagnosed with cancer in the United States is still only about 40–50% and as a result of inadequate early detection, is less then one-third worldwide (8). The annual mortality rate is about 4.3 million worldwide and about 510,000 in the United States (9). Palliative treatment, which may extend survival, is often more successful than therapies with curative intent, and as a result there is an increasing trend for patients to have lingering advanced disease with associated chronic pain.

III. CANCER PAIN DATA

Together with anorexia and fatigue, pain is among the most common symptoms associated with cancer (13,14). Significant pain is present in up to 25% of patients in active treatment and in up to 90% of patients with advanced cancer (11,15–19). According to several studies including a survey of oncologists in the Eastern Cooperative Oncology Group (ECOG) and a survey of 1103 consecutive admission to a U.S. tertiary care cancer hospital, 73% of patients in active treatment admitted to pain with 38% reporting severe pain (11,20). Despite the availability of simple, cost-effective treatment (21,22), inadequately controlled pain remains a significant problem.

Studies following the WHO cancer pain ladder (e.g., oral analgesics and careful follow-up) have achieved favorable outcomes in the 70–90% range (23) suggesting that the key to achieving more effective global cancer pain relief involves applying known technology more effectively rather than development of new medical technologies or drugs. While a variety of such factors have been identified, authorities agree that the so-called "opiophobia," a reluctance to use opioids, largely because of exaggerated concerns of addiction and regulatory reprisal, exerts a potent influence at all levels and probably is the single most important impediment to better symptom control globally. In general, in Western developed sectors, barriers are largely educational and attitudinal in nature, while in developed nations a multitude of resource and access problems are operant.

Indirect effects on survival may stem from the negative influence of pain on performance status. Performance status, as measured by the ECOG and Karnofsky scales (see Table 1), is a global rating of patients overall functional status. When performance status is low, as is often the case when pain is severe, patients may find it difficult to tolerate recommended

Table 1 Methods of Assessing Performance Status

ECOG		Karnofsky	
0	Fully active, able to carry on all predisease performance without restriction	100	Normal; no complaints, no evidence of disease
1	Restricted in physically strenuous activity but ambulatory and able to carry out light or sedentary work (e.g., light housework, office work)	90	Able to carry on normal activity; minor signs or symptoms of disease
2	Ambulatory and capable of all self-care but unable to work; up and about more then 50% of waking hours	80	Normal activity with effort; some signs or symptoms of disease
3	Capable of only limited self-care, confined to bed or chair more than 50% of waking hours	70	Cares for self; unable to carry on normal activity or to do active work
4	Completely disabled, cannot carry on any self-care, totally confined to bed or chair	60	Requires occasional assistance but is able to care for most needs
5	Dead	50	Requires considerable assistance and frequent medical care
		40	Disabled, requires special care and assistance
		30	Severely disabled, hospitalization indicated; death not imminent
		20	Very sick; hospitalization necessary; active supportive treatment necessary
		10	Moribund; fatal processes; progressing rapidly
		0	Dead

chemotherapy, indeed they may not be considered candidates for chemotherapy. Further benefits of good pain management often include improvements in nutrition, rest, and mood, all of which contribute to quality of life and have the potential to influence the outcome of antineoplastic therapy.

IV. ASSESSMENT

Pain is always subjective and is experienced only by the patient. Over the past 20 years, the assessment of pain has been the subject of much research and refinement of techniques and instruments. A cursory review is presented in this section, the reader is directed to Chapter X for more details on the assessment of cancer pain.

V. SCREENING INSTRUMENTS

Many pain clinics utilize a questionnaire to aid in and standardize assessment. The Wisconsin brief pain inventory (BPI) (24,25) and memorial pain assessment card (26) are well-accepted and standard tools for assessing cancer pain. At the University of Texas M. D. Anderson Cancer Center, an institutionally approved M. D. Anderson questionnaire (modified BPI) is used for initial and follow-up assessment of patients.

Numerous tools are available for assessing cancer-related pain including:

1. Wisconsin brief pain inventory:
   a. Fifteen-minute questionnaire, which can be self-administered.
   b. Includes several questions about the characteristics of the pain, including its origin and their effects of prior treatments.
   c. It incorporates two valuable features of the McGill Pain Questionnaire, a graphic representation of the location of pain and groups of qualitative descriptors. Severity of pain is assessed by a series of visual analog scale (VAS) that score pain at its best, worst, and on average. The perceived level of interference with normal function is quantified with VAS also.
   d. Preliminary evidence suggests that the BPI is cross-culturally valid (24,25) and is useful, particularly when patients are not fit to complete a more thorough or comprehensive questionnaire.
2. Memorial pain assessment card:
   a. It is a simple efficient, and valid instrument that provides rapid clinical evaluation of the major aspects of pain experienced by cancer patients (26).
   b. It is easy to understand and use and can be completed by experienced patients in 20 sec.
   c. It consists of two-sided $8.5 \times 11\,\text{inch}^2$ card that is folded so that four separate measures are created.
   d. It features scales intended for the measurements of pain intensity, pain relief, mood, and a set of descriptive adjectives.
3. Edmonton staging system:
   a. It is performed by health care providers.
   b. It was developed to predict the likelihood of achieving effective relief of pain in cancer patients (27,28).
   c. The system's originators have provided validation that treatment outcome can be accurately predicted according to five clinical features (neuropathic pain, movement-related pain, recent history of tolerance to opioids, psychological distress, and a history of alcoholism or drug abuse).
   d. Staging requires only 5–10 min and requires no special skills.
   e. Its value lies in prospective identification of potentially problematic patients, further legitimizing clinical research on symptom control by introducing better standardization and improving our ability to assess critically the results of various therapeutic interventions in large population of patients.
4. Pediatric cancer pain assessment: This includes Beyer's the Oucher, Eland's color scale-body outline, Hester's poker chip tool, McGrath's faces scale (see Fig. 1), and others (29–32).
5. Numerical pain rating scale (NRS) or visual analog scale (VAS): Often pain is assessed on an 11-point numerical rating scale from 0 (no pain) to 10 (worst pain imaginable) (see Fig. 1). The VAS is a 10 cm line without markings from no pain to worst pain; the patient marks their pain score and a measurement in cm defines their level of pain. Objective observations of grimacing, limping, and vital signs (tachycardia) may be useful in assessing the patient, but these signs are often absent in patients with chronic cancer pain. Pain evaluation should be integrated with a detailed oncological, medical, and psychological assessment. The initial evaluation should include evaluation of person, his or her feelings and attitudes

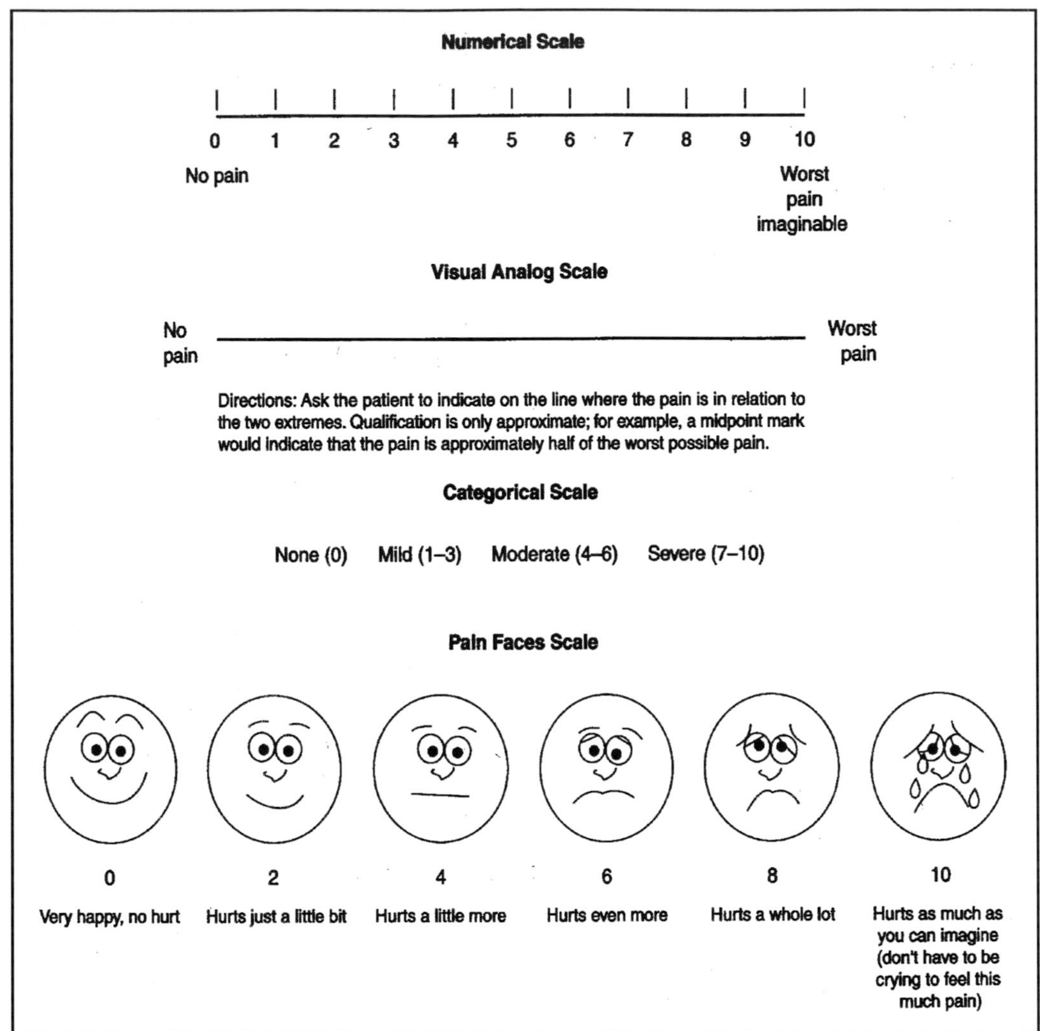

Figure 1 Conventional pain assessment scales.

about the pain and disease, family concerns, and the patient's premorbid psychological history. A comprehensive but objective approach to assessment instills confidence in the patients and family that will be valuable throughout treatment.

A comprehensive evaluation of the patients with cancer pain includes the following:

- The chief complaint is obtained to ensure appropriate triage (i.e., severe pain with a bowel obstruction may need to be sent to the emergency center for urgent treatment).
- Next, the oncologic history is obtained to gain the context of the pain problem. The oncologic history includes diagnosis and stage of disease, therapy and outcome—including side effects, and the patient's understanding of the disease process and prognosis.
- The pain history should include any premorbid chronic pain and for each new pain site: onset and evolution, site and radiation, pattern (constant, intermittent, or unpredictable), intensity (best, worst, average, current) 0–10 scales, quality, exacerbating and relieving factors, pain interference with usual activities, neurological and motor abnormalities (including bowel and bladder continence), vasomotor changes, current and past analgesics (use, efficacy, side effects). Prior analgesic use, efficacy, and side effects should be cataloged. Prior treatments for pain should be noted (radiotherapy, nerve blocks, physiotherapy, etc.).
- Review of medical record and radiological studies: Many of the treatments for cancer can

cause pain themselves (eg. chemotherapy and radiotherapy-induced neuropathies or post-operative pain syndromes; postthoracotomy pain syndromes and postmastectomy pain syndrome) (see Table 2), and many specific cancers can cause well-established pain patterns due to known likely sites of metastasis: (a) breast to long bones, spine, chest wall, brachial plexus, and spine; (b) colon to pelvis, hips, lumbar plexus, sacral plexus, and spine; and (c) prostate to long bones, pelvis, hips, lung, and spinal cord.

- Psychological history: This should include marital and residential status, employment history and status, educational background, functional status, activities of daily living, recreational activities, support systems, health and capabilities of spouse or significant others, past history of (or current) drug or alcohol abuse.
- Medical history (independent of oncological history) including coexisting systemic disease, exercise intolerance, allergies to medications and medication use, prior illness and surgery, and a thorough review of systems, including the following systems:
  - General (including anorexia, weight loss, cachexia, fatigue, weakness, insomnia)
  - Neurologic (including sedation, confusion, hallucination, headache, motor weakness, altered sensation, incontinence)
  - Respiratory (including dyspnea, cough, pneumonia)
  - Gastrointestinal (including dysphagia, nausea, vomiting, dehydration, constipation, diarrhea)
  - Psychological (including irritability, anxiety, depression, dementia, and suicidal ideation)
  - Genitourinary (including urgency, hesitancy, or hematuria)

Physical examination: The physical examination must be thorough although at times it is appropriate to perform a focused examination. In patients with spinal pain and known or suspected metastatic disease, a complete neurologic examination is mandatory. Gonzales and colleagues (33) found new evidence of metastatic disease in 64% of patients and this resulted in antitumor therapy for 18% of patients evaluated by their pain service.

- Determination of need for further studies.
- Formulate clinical impression (diagnosis). Multiple diagnosis usually applies and it is optimal to use the most specific known diagnosis. For example: 1. T-11 compression fracture (pathologic vs. osteoporotic) with severe pain; 2. metastatic breast carcinoma (with known bony metastasis); 3. nausea with inanition; 4. constipation.
- Formulate recommendations (plan) and alternatives for each problem. For example (related to the above problem list): 1. MRI of the T-Spine

Table 2 Common Cancer Pain Syndrome

Pain syndrome	Associated signs and symptoms	Affected nerves
Tumor infiltration of a peripheral nerve	Constant burning pain with dysesthesia in an area of sensory loss. Pain is radicular and often unilateral	Peripheral
Postradical neck dissection	Tight, burning sensation in the area of sensory loss. Dysesthesias may occur. Second type of pain is not unusual	Cervical plexus
Postmastectomy pain	Tight, constricting, burning pain in the arm, axial, and anterior chest wall. Pain exacerbated by arm movement	Intercostobrachial
Postthoracotomy pain	Aching sensation in the distribution of the incision with or without autonomic changes. Trigger point. CRPS I may develop	Intercostal
Postnephrectomy pain	Numbness, fullness, or heaviness in the flank, anterior abdomen, and groin. Dysesthesias are common	Superficial flank
Postlimb amputation	Phantom limb pain. Stump pain several months/years postsurgery. Burning dysesthesia that is exacerbated by movement	Peripheral endings and central projections
Cranial neuropathies	Severe head pain with cranial nerve dysfunction. Leptomeningeal disease. Base skull metastasis	Cranial V, VII, IX, X, XI, and XII most common
Acute and PHN	Painful paresthesia and dysesthesia. Constant burning and aching pain. Shocklike paroxysmal pain. Immunosuppression is a risk factor. Incidence increases with age	Thoracic and cranial (VI) are most common

with consideration of vertebroplasty if appropriate; 2. oxycodone slow release 10 mg twice daily, with oral transmucosal fentanyl citrate for breakthrough pain; 3. management including further chemotherapy, radiotherapy, or bisphosphonates in coordination with the patient's oncologist; 4. metoclopramide 10 mg po 30 min prior to meals and as needed for nausea; 5. addition of senekot-S twice daily for constipation.

- A call to the referring oncologist and/or primary care provider helps ensure good communication between all of a patient's physicians.
- Exit interview:
  - Explain the probable cause of symptoms in terms the patient can understand.
  - Discuss prognosis for symptom relief, management options and specific recommendations. In addition to writing prescriptions, oral and written instructions must be provided. Educational material regarding medications, pain management strategies, procedures, or others should be provided. Potential side effects should be discussed.
  - Arrange for follow-up with clinic contact information.
  - A dictated summary should be sent to referring and consulting physicians to keep them appraised of the patient's present status and treatment offered.

VI. CLASSIFICATION OF CANCER PAIN

A. Chronicity:

a. Acute pain: It is frequently associated with sympathetic hyperactivity and heightened distress. It is often temporally associated with the onset or recrudescence of primary or metastatic disease, and its presence should motivate the clinician to seek its cause aggressively and need for more potent analgesics.

b. Subacute pain: The pain that some patients experience for 4–6 weeks after a major surgical procedure. This type of pain is largely undertreated and deserves special attention as it may affect patient's ability to perform activities of daily living after being discharged from the hospital.

c. Chronic pain: Treating pain of a chronic nature mandates a combination of palliation, adjustment, and acceptance. With time, a biological and behavioral adjustment to symptoms occurs, and hopefully associated symptoms are blunted. Chronic pain with superimposed episodes of acute pain (breakthrough pain) is probably the most common pattern observed in patients with ongoing cancer pain.

B. Intensity: The consistent use of measurements of pain intensity aids in following a patient's progress and may serve as a basis for interpatient comparisons. High pain scores may alert the clinician to the need for more aggressive treatment (see Fig. 2, MD Anderson Cancer Center (MDACC) treatment algorithm).

C. Pathophysiology: This approach is useful when formulating the initial approach to treatment.

a. Somatic nociceptive pain is described as a constant, well-localized pain often characterized as aching, throbbing, sharp, or gnawing. It tends to be opioid responsive and amenable to relief by interruption of proximal pathways by neural blockade when indicated.

b. Visceral nociceptive pain originates from injury to organs. This pain is transmitted via fibers in the sympathetic nervous system. Visceral pain is characteristically vague in distribution and quality and is often described as deep, dull, aching, dragging, squeezing, or pressure-like sensation. When acute, it may be paroxysmal and colicky and can be associated with nausea, vomiting, diaphoresis, and alterations in blood pressure and heart rate. Mechanisms of visceral pain include abnormal distension or contraction of the smooth muscle walls (hollow viscera), rapid capsular stretch (solid viscera), ischemia of visceral muscle, serosal or mucosal irritation by algesic substances and other chemical stimuli, distension and traction or torsion on mesenteric attachments and vasculature, and necrosis (34). The viscera are, however, insensitive to simple manipulation, cutting and burning. Visceral involvement often produces referred pain (35) (e.g., phrenic nerve-mediated shoulder pain of hepatic origin).

c. Neuropathic pain is defined as pain emanating from the nervous system due to injury or irritation to some element of the nervous system. Examples of neuropathic pain syndromes associated with cancer are depicted in Table 2.

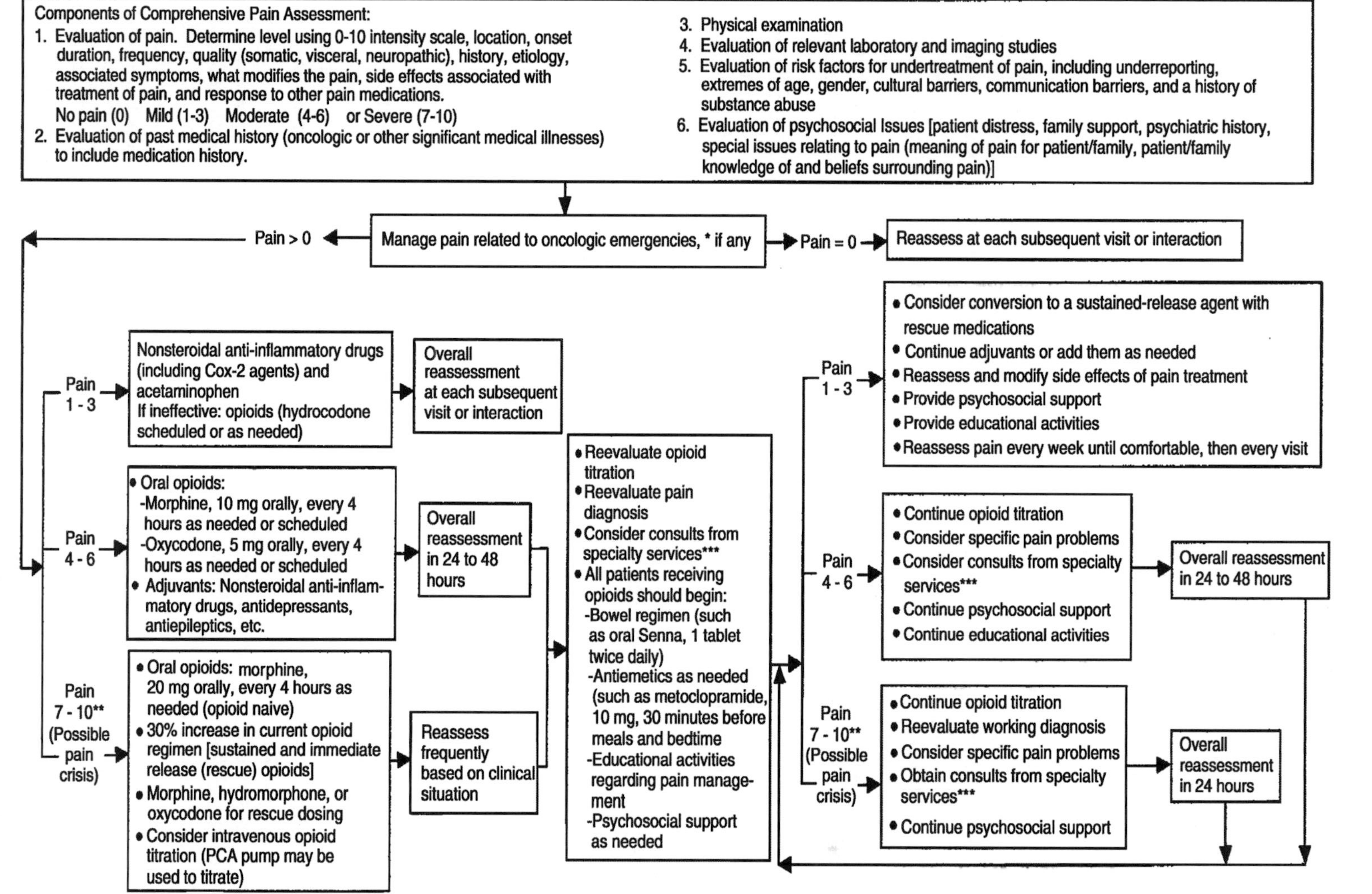

*Pain related to an oncologic emergency requires assessment and treatment (e.g. surgery, steroids, radiotherapy, antibiotics) along with an emergent consultation. Oncologic emergencies include:

- Bowel obstruction/perforation
- Brain metastasis
- Epidural metastasis/spinal cord compression
- Fracture or impending fracture of weight-bearing bone
- Leptomeningeal metastasis
- Pain related to infection

**Some patients with chronic pain syndromes will report high pain scores on an ongoing basis. Generally, this situation is not a crisis.

***Consult the Postoperative Pain Service, Cancer Pain Section, Department of Symptom Control and Palliative Care, or other specialties needed (i.e. Radiotherapy).

(V3 10/25/01)

Figure 2 MD Anderson Cancer Center (MDACC) treatment algorithm.

Neuropathic pain is often resistant to standard analgesic therapies and often requires an approach utilizing opioids, anticonvulsants, oral or topical local anesthetics, corticosteroids, NMDA blockers, and others.

D. Temporal aspects of pain:

a. Constant pain: This pain is most amenable to drug therapy administered around the clock, contingent on time rather then symptoms. It is best managed by long-acting analgesics or in selected cases, infusion of analgesics.
b. Breakthrough pain and incident pain: Breakthrough pain that is related to a specific activity, such as eating, defecation, socializing, or walking is referred to as incident pain. Breakthrough pain is best managed by supplementing the preventative around-the-clock regimen with analgesics with a rapid onset of action and a short duration. Once a pattern of incident pain is established, escape or rescue, doses of analgesics can be administered in anticipation of the pain-provoking activity. Breakthrough pain that occurs consistently prior to the next scheduled dose of around-the-clock opioids is called "end of dose failure" and is related to the decrease in plasma concentrations of the analgesics below minimum effective analgesic concentrations (MEAC). "End of dose failure" is ideally managed by increasing the dose of the basal analgesic or reducing the intervals between doses. Refractory incident pain often is responsive to stabilization, such as fixation of a pathologic fracture or vertebroplasty for a vertebral compression fracture (VCF).
c. Intermittent pain: This is very unpredictable and can be best managed by administration of immediate release potent analgesics of rapid onset and short duration.

E. Specific cancer pain syndromes:

a. Osseous invasion or tumor infiltration of the bone is cited as the most common cause of cancer pain and is most often seen in metastatic carcinoma of the prostate, breast, thyroid, lung, or kidney (36–38). The presentation of one metastasis pain is variable, usually a constant deep dull ache, often greatest at night and with movement or weight bearing, complicated by paroxysms of stabbing pain. Approximately 25% of patients with bone metastasis experience severe pain. Somatic and sympathetic fibers carry pain. A bone scan (isotope scanning, scintigraphy) is preferred for detecting most bone metastasis.

   Prostaglandin E2 (PGE2) and other cytokines are elaborated by osseous metastasis. These cytokines are felt to contribute to pain by sensitization of peripheral periosteal nociceptors in addition to causing central sensitization (39–41). Nonsteroidal anti-inflammatory drugs (NSAIDs) and steroids are postulated to reduce pain from bony metastasis via inhibition of the cyclooxygenase (COX) pathway of arachidonic acid breakdown, thus decreasing the formation of PGE2. The cox-2-selective anti-inflammatories have been shown in a murine sarcoma bone metastasis model to effectively inhibit spontaneous and movement-related bone pain, reduce biochemical markers of peripheral and central sensitization, reduce tumor-induced osteoclastic proliferation, and finally to reduce overall tumor burden (40). As deposits enlarge, stretching of the periosteum, pathological fracture, and perineural invasion contribute to pain and requirements for analgesics increase. Palliative radiation is commonly successfully employed to relieve pain emanating from bony metastasis. Hormonal therapy (chemotherapy such as tamoxifen or leuprolide, orchiectomy, or rarely hypophysectomy) often reduces bony pain in patients with hormonal-dependent disease (breast, prostate). In general, the hormone refractory breast and prostatic carcinomas are less responsive to treatment (42,43).
b. Vertebral body metastasis is most commonly associated with metastatic carcinoma of the lung, breast, and prostate. Localized paraspinal, radicular, or referred pain is usually the first sign of metastasis to the bony vertebral column. The pain is often described as severe local, dull, steady, aching, often exacerbated by recumbence, sitting, movement, and local pressure; may be relieved by standing; local midline tenderness may be present; associated nerve compression may

produce radiating dermatomal pain and corresponding neurological changes; may be associated with epidural-spinal cord compression (44).

c. Base of skull metastasis: Usually present with headache and a spectrum of neurological findings, especially involving cranial nerves. Symptomatic metastasis to the skull is usually but not always a late finding (45). Plain x-ray, scintigraphy, and CT scan are helpful for diagnosis of bony disease, while MRI and lumbar puncture are useful to evaluate the soft tissue and to detect leptomeningeal disease, respectively (46).

d. Visceral pain is usually seen in gastrointestinal malignancies due to direct tumor and invasion of visceral structures. This pain is transmitted via fibers in the sympathetic nervous system (35). Visceral pain is characteristically vague in distribution and quality, and is often described as deep, dull, aching, dragging, squeezing, or pressure-like sensation. When acute, it may be paroxysmal and colicky and can be associated with nausea, vomiting, diaphoresis, and alterations in blood pressure and heart rate. Mechanisms of visceral pain include abnormal distension or contraction of the smooth muscle walls (hollow viscera), rapid capsular stretch (solid viscera), ischemia of visceral muscle, serosal or mucosal irritation by algesic substances and other chemical stimuli, distension and traction or torsion on mesenteric attachments and vasculature, and necrosis. The classic cancer visceral pain syndrome is pancreatic cancer-related pain. This pain is described as relentless, mid-epigastric aching, which radiates through to the mid-back, often relieved by the fetal position and worsened by recumbence.

e. Musculoskeletal pain is probably underdiagnosed in cancer patients (46). Underrecognition is probably due in part to the inability of standard radiographic technique to document muscle injury, as well as the varied, sometimes vague, and usually nonneurological constellation of characteristic symptoms.

f. Nerve invasion: Typically constant, burning dysesthetic pain, often with an intermittent lancinating, electrical component; may be associated with neurologic deficit or diffuse hyperesthesia or hypesthesia and localized parasthesia; muscle weakness and atrophy may be present in mixed or motor nerve syndromes (47,48).

g. Leptomeningeal metastasis, meningeal carcinomatosis: Most common with primary malignancies of breast and lung; lymphoma and leukemia; it is secondary to diffuse infiltration of meninges. About 40% of patients have headache or back pain, presumably due to traction on the pain-sensitive meninges, cranial, and spinal nerves and/or raised intracranial pressure (49,50). Headache is most common presenting complaint; characteristically unrelenting; may be associated with nausea, vomiting, nuchial rigidity, and mental status changes associated neurological abnormalities may include seizures, cranial nerve deficits, papilledema, hemiparesis, ataxia and cauda syndrome; diagnosis confirmed with lumbar puncture and CSF analysis, which revealed the presence of malignant cells, and may also be remarkable for an increased opening pressure, raised protein, and decreased glucose (51). CT or MRI are also recommended and may reveal plaque like tumor. The natural history of patients with leptomeningeal metastasis is gradual decline and death over 4–6 weeks, although survival is often extended to 6 months or more when treatment with radiation therapy and/or intrathecal chemotherapy is instituted (52). Steroids may be useful in the management of headache (46).

h. Spinal cord compression is usually heralded by pain in the presence of neurological changes. An urgent radiological workup is mandatory in the face of neurological deficits, particularly motor weakness, bandlike encircling pain or incontinence. Prompt treatment in form of radiotherapy or spinal stabilization may limit neurologic morbidity (44).

i. Plexopathies are syndromes of tumor invasion into the nerve plexus in the upper or lower extremity. Cervical plexopathy is most commonly caused by local invasion of head and neck cancers or from enlarged lymph nodes. Symptoms are primarily sensory in the distribution of plexus, experiencing as aching preauricular, postauricular, or neck pain. Brachial plexopathy is most common due to upper lobe lung cancer (called the Pancoast syndrome or superior sulcus syndrome), breast cancer, or lymphoma; pain is an early symptom, usually preceding neurological findings by up to 9 months (47). The lower cord of the plexus (C8-T1) is affected most frequently, and pain is usually diffuse aching in shoulder girdle, radiating down arm, often to the elbow and medial (ulnar) aspect of the hand (48). When the upper trunk is involved (C5-6), pain is usually in the shoulder girdle and upper arm, radiating to the thumb and index finger. Horner's syndrome, dysesthesias, progressive atrophy, and neurological impairment (weakness and numbness) may occur. In some situations, the clinical presentation may be difficult to differentiate from radiation fibrosis, which characteristically is less severe, less often associated with motor changes, tends to involve the upper trunks, and may be associated with lymphedema without a Horner's sign. Brachial plexus invasion may be associated with contiguous spread to the epidural space (53–55). Lumbosacral plexopathy may be due to local soft tissue invasion or compression occurring most commonly with tumors of the rectum, cervix, breast, sarcoma, and lymphoma; pain is usually the presenting symptom in 70% of patients (56). The pain is usually described as aching or pressure-like and only rarely dysesthetic (56). Depending on the level involved, pain is referred to the low back, abdomen, buttock, or lower extremity (56,57). Reflex asymmetry and mild sensory and motor changes, when present, were relatively early findings, whereas impotence and incontinence are relatively rare. This syndrome must be differentiated from spinal cord invasion or cauda equina syndrome in which urgent diagnosis and treatment is mandatory.

j. Chemotherapy related:

   i. Oral mucositis usually occurs in 1–2 weeks of the initiation of chemotherapy. This condition is most common with the use of methotrexate, doxorubicin, daunorubicin, bleomycin, etoposide, 5-fluorouricil, and dactinomycin (58). Mucositis is often most severe when chemotherapy is combined with radiation treatments to the head and neck region.
   ii. Painful polyneuropathy occurs most commonly with vincristine (motor and sensory involvement), vinblastine, taxol taxotere, the platinum derivative (predominantly sensory involvement), and navelbine (59). Symptoms commonly include burning, dysesthetic pain in the hands and feet.

k. Postsurgical chronic pain syndromes are most common after mastectomy, thoracotomy, radical neck dissection, nephrectomy, and amputation (60). The clinical characteristics usually include aching, shooting, or tingling pain in distribution of peripheral nerves (e.g., intercostals-brachial, intercostals, cervical plexus) with or without skin hypersensitivity. In one of the study (61), the incidence of postmastectomy pain was higher after conservative surgery than modified radical mastectomy (33% vs. 17%). In this same study, 25% of patients experienced postoperative phantom breast pain. The exact incidence of postsurgical pain syndromes is unclear, but appears to be in the 25–50% range by some estimates (60).
l. Headache is present in 60% of patients with a primary or metastatic brain tumor, half of whom classified as their primary complaint (62). It is typically steady, deep, dull, and aching with moderate intensity and that is rarely rhythmic or throbbing. It is usually intermittent and may be worse in the morning and with coughing-straining. Symptoms often improve with radiation therapy, nonsteroidal anti-inflammatories, or corticosteroids (63–65).
m. Cervicofacial pain syndromes are most common in patients with head and neck cancers. The head and neck are richly innervated by contributions from cranial nerves V, VII, IX, X, and upper cervical nerves, so pain varies in character. When cranial nerves are involved, symptoms represent those of trigeminal, glossopharyngeal, and/or intermittent neuralgia, with sudden, severe lancinating pain radiating to the face, throat, or ear, respectively.
n. Radiation therapy may be associated with both acute and chronic pain syndromes.

Acutely, mucositis, cutaneous burns may be seen. Chronically, postradiation syndromes include osteoradionecrosis, myelopathy, plexopathy, soft-tissue fibrosis, and the emergence of new secondary neurogenic tumors (67–69).

VII. TREATMENT

The goal of treatment of cancer pain is to relieve pain by modifying its source, interrupting its transmission, or modulating its influence at brain or spinal cord sites. This can be achieved with various means and combination of following available modalities.

Treatment modalities available for cancer pain patients:

A. Antineoplastic treatment
B. Pharmacological management
    a. NSAIDs
    b. Opioids
    c. Adjuvant analgesics
        i. Sequential drug trials
        ii. Antidepressant
        iii. Anticonvulsants
        iv. Baclofen
        v. Oral local anesthetics
        vi. Amphetamine
        vii. Corticosteroid
        viii. *N*-Methyl-D-aspartate antagonists
        ix. Alpha-2 adrenergic antagonists
        x. Others
    d. Interventional pain management:
        i. Continuous parenteral infusion of opioids
        ii. Neuraxial analgesia—epidural or intrathecal infusions
        iii. Vertebroplasty
        iv. Nerve blocks
            - Local anesthetic nerve block
            - Neurolytic nerve block
        v. Neuromodulation
    e. Behavioral Pain Management
    f. Other intervention
    g. Home-based and hospice care

A. Antineoplastic Treatment

The most effective form of treatment of any cancer-related pain is treatment of the cancer itself, which in the majority of cases will reduce or eliminate the pain. Once diagnosed, the pathological process responsible for pain can often be altered with surgical extirpation, external beam radiation therapy (targeted fractioned or single-dosed therapy, hemibody or total body irradiation) radionuclides (e.g., strontium-89, samarium) chemotherapy, hormonal treatment, and even whole-body hyperthermia. The majority of patients require some form of primary analgesic therapy even when pursuing antitumor therapy.

B. Pharmacological Management

The control of pain involves three basic principles: modifying the source of the pain, altering the central perception of pain, and blocking the transmission of the pain to the central nervous system. In addition, any new pain in a patient with cancer is assumed disease progression or recurrence until proven otherwise.

Oral analgesics are the mainstay of therapy for patients with cancer pain. An estimated 70–90% of patients can be rendered relatively free of pain when straightforward guidelines-based participles applied in a thorough, careful manner (1,4,59).

The World Health Organization (WHO) has developed a three-step ladder approach (see Fig. 3) to cancer pain management that relies exclusively on the administration of oral agents and that is usually effective (69,70). When more conservative therapies produce inadequate results, escalating doses or alternative therapy should be sought. The role of more invasive forms of analgesia, ranging from parenteral analgesics to neural blockade or neuraxial analgesia, should be considered judiciously.

Before initiation of therapy, assessment of problems and setting realistic goals that are acceptable to the patient should be established along with a treatment plan and contingencies.

The noninvasive route should be maintained as long as possible for reasons that include simplicity, maintenance of independence and mobility, convenience, and cost. Treatment should be directed towards relief of pain and suffering, which includes consideration of all aspects of function (e.g., disturbance of sleep, appetite, mood, activity, posture, and sexuality), and attention should be paid not only to physical but also to emotional, psychological, and spiritual aspects of suffering.

The University of Texas M. D. Anderson Cancer Center published a modified and condensed version of the NCCN guidelines (see Figs. 2,4,5), the general theme is of stronger opioids and adjuvants with more frequent reassessment for higher pain levels. Some basic principles to manage large population of patients

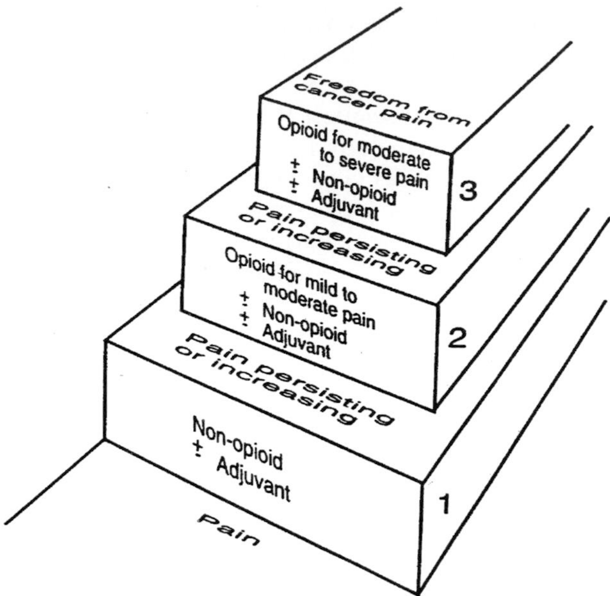

Figure 3 World Health Organization step ladder model for pain intensity and treatment modality.

are described here as pearls for cancer pain therapeutics (see Table 3).

1. Nonsteroidal Anti-Inflammatory Drugs

Nonsteroidal anti-inflammatory drugs are most effective for pain of inflammatory (e.g., bone metastasis) origin by virtue of interference with prostaglandin (PG) synthesis (41). Consider the regular (around-the-clock) administration of an NSAID as the sole treatment for mild pain or in combination with opioid analgesic for moderate or severe pain (1,4,37). Potential for benefit should be balanced against potential for toxicity (which includes upper GI irritation, renal insufficiency, platelet dysfunction, and masking of fever), which is pertinent in the context of recent antitumor therapy and advanced age (71). Consider avoiding NSAIDs all together or instituting prophylaxis (e.g., misoprostol) in patients predisposed to gastropathy.

The nonacetylated salicylate (sodium salicylate, choline magnesium trisalicylate) are associated with a favorable toxicity profile, since they fail to interfere with platelet aggregation, are rarely associated with GI bleeding, and are well tolerated by asthmatic patients (72,73). A parenteral formulation of ketorolac is equianalgesic to low doses of morphine in some settings, but is associated with the same range of side effects as oral NSAIDs (74).

Nonsteroidal anti-inflammatory drugs are associated with ceiling effects, above which dose escalations produce toxicity but no greater analgesia. However, the ceiling dose for a given drug differs from patient to patient, allowing some potential for dose titration. When efficacy is poor, the clinician may consider rotating to another NSAID, usually from a different biochemical class because it is clear that for a given patient, clinical response differs among various agents (interindividual variability), and there is recent evidence that various classes of NSAIDs may exert their anti-PG effects on different subtypes of COX (75), the enzyme primarily responsible for PG degradation. There may be a better safety profile of the newer COX-2 inhibitors in cancer patients vs. the traditional NSAIDs, which are nonspecific inhibitors of COX-1 and COX-2.

The use of COX-2 inhibitors will be particularly important in patients with the following problems:

- History of perforation, ulcer, or bleeding.
- Concomitant anticoagulant therapy.
- Use of oral corticosteroids.
- Longer duration of NSAID therapy.
- Advanced age.
- Poor general health status.

If a patient has two or more of these problems, the risk of intestinal bleeding will be greater than expected in the general population.

2. Opioids

"Weak Opioids"

When NSAIDs provide insufficient relief, are contraindicated, are poorly tolerated, or when pain is severe at presentation, the addition or substitution of a so-called "weak" opioid (e.g., codeine, propoxyphene, hydrocodone, or dihydrocodone preparations) is recommended as an analgesic of intermediate potency (3). These medications are almost exclusively formulated as combination products; these agents are weak only insofar as the inclusion of aspirin, acetaminophen, or ibuprofen results in a ceiling dose above, which the incidence of toxicity increases.

While the weak opioids are appropriate for mild or intermittent pain, physician often rely excessively on these agents, frequently continuing their use after they are no longer effective in an ill-advised attempt to avoid prescribing more potent opioids that are also more highly regulated. The potency of hydrocodone and dihydrocodone preparations is greater than that of codeine and propoxyphene (76). These agents have perceived advantage of not requiring triplicate prescriptions (DEA Class C-III vs. C-II), although the clinician must be cautious not to exceed the usual recommended dose of acetaminophen (4 g/day) as opioid requirements increase.

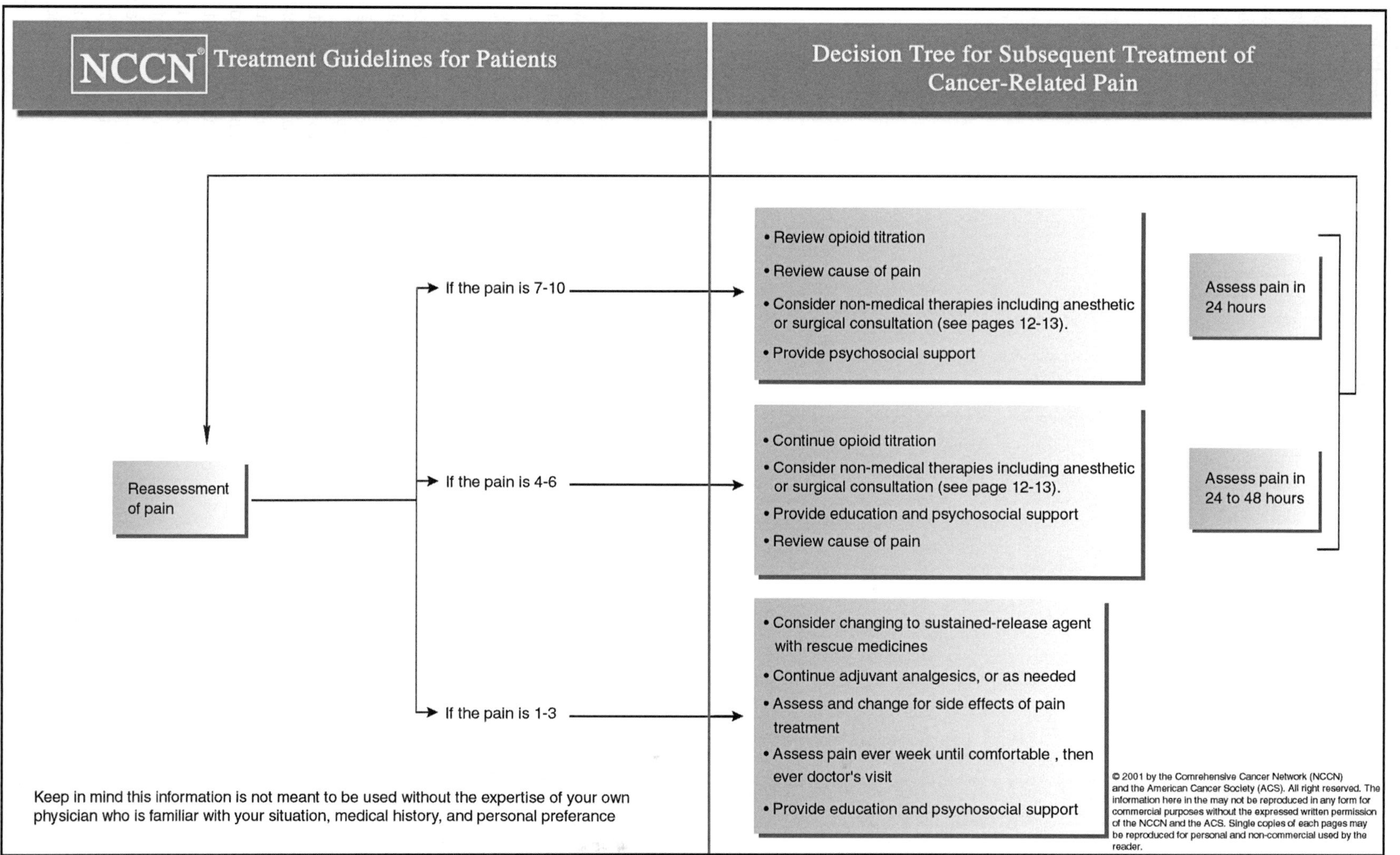

Figure 4 NCCN treatment algorithm.

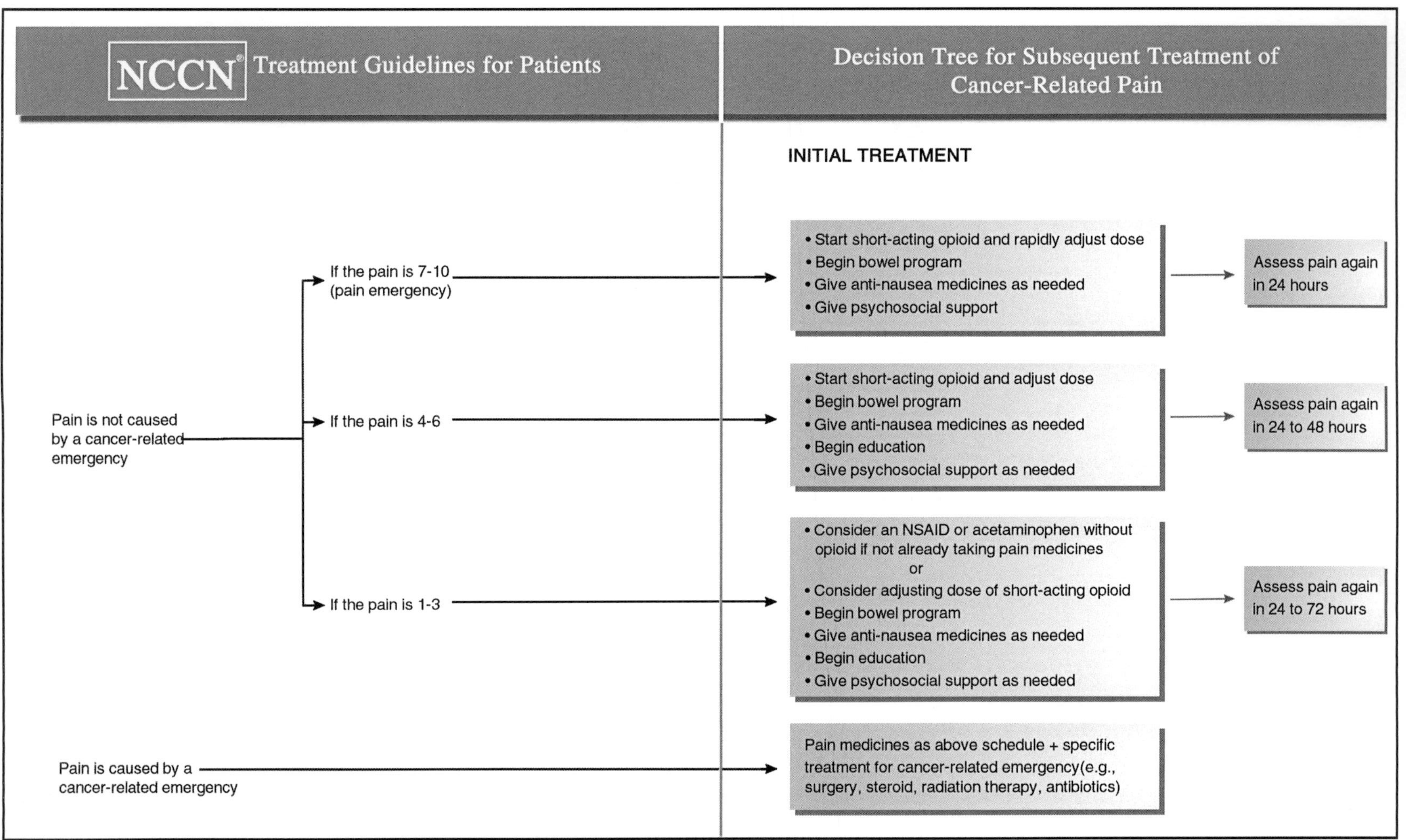

Figure 5 NCCN treatment algorithm.

Table 3 Pearls for Cancer Pain Therapeutics

1. Individualize the route, dosage, and schedule
2. Administer analgesics regularly (not only prn) if pain is present most of the day.
3. Become familiar with the dose and time course of several strong opioids
4. Give infant and children adequate opioid doses
5. Follow patient closely, particularly when beginning or changing analgesic regimens
6. When changing to a new opioid or a different route, first use the equianalgesic doses to estimate the new dose. Then, modify the estimate based on the clinical situation and the specific drugs
7. Recognize and treat side effects
8. Do not use placebo to assess the nature of pain
9. Watch for development to tolerance and treat appropriately
10. Be aware of the development of physical dependence and prevent withdrawal
11. Do not label a patient addicted (i.e., psychologically dependant), if you merely mean physically dependant on or tolerantto opioids
12. Be alert to the psychological state of the patient

"Potent Opioids"

When combinations of weak opioids and adjuvants provide insufficient analgesia or when pain is severe at presentation, more potent opioids should be considered (69). Morphine, hydromorphone, transdermal fentanyl, and oxycodone are appropriate first-line opioids for the treatment of moderate to severe pain. Methadone, although inexpensive, and to a lesser extent levorphanol are usually reserved for special circumstances because their half-lives are long and unpredictable, introducing the potential for accumulation, especially in the presence of advanced age and altered renal function (77).

Dosing Guidelines

Pharmacological therapy should be individualized in light of the specific characteristics and needs of each patient (87). The correct dose of an opioid is the one that effectively relieves pain without inducing unacceptable side effects. Opioids should initially be introduced in low doses, since the early development of side effects will impair compliance, but they should be rapidly titrated to effect. If side effects ensue before adequate pain relief is established, they are treated aggressively in an algorithmic fashion or other strategies should be applied, which are described later in this chapter.

1. *Calculation of morphine equivalent daily dose (MEDD)*: If the patient is already on opioid medication, it is recommended to calculate the MEDD in order to administer an equianalgesic dose of an alternate opioid if desired. Opioid dose conversion tables may helpful for calculation, but should be followed cautiously allowing for interpatient variability in opioid side effect sensitivity (see Tables 4 and 5).

2. *Basal and rescue dosing guidelines*: If analgesics are withheld until pain becomes more severe, sympathetic arousal occurs and then even potent analgesics may be ineffective. Thus, a time-contingent schedule for the administration of analgesics is generally preferred to symptom-contingent administration. With prolonged administration on demand, patterns of anticipation and memory of pain become established and may contribute to suffering, even during periods of adequate analgesia. Around-the-clock administration of appropriate analgesics maintains more even therapeutics blood levels and decreases the likelihood of intolerable pain. Compliance and overall quality of analgesia are enhanced by the regular administration of long-acting opioid analgesics for basal pain control, supplemented by a short-acting opioid analgesic administered as needed for breakthrough and incident pain. In practice, controlled-release morphine, controlled-release oxycodone, or transdermal fentanyl are available which cannot be broken, crushed, or chewed. When these agents are poorly tolerated, methadone or levorphanol may be prescribed, but careful monitoring is required, particularly in elderly patients.

A drug of relatively high potency, short onset, and brief duration, such as immediate-release morphine, hydromorphone, oxycodone, or oral transmucosal fentanyl citrate is selected for as-needed administration to manage exacerbation of pain (78). These agents should be prescribed every 2–4 hr as needed. When breakthrough medications are used more then 2–3 times over 12 hr consistently, the dose of basal, long-acting analgesic may be increased. If incident pain is a significant problem, the patient should be instructed to take the breakthrough dose in anticipation of pain-provoking activity. A new formulation of oral transmucosal fentanyl citrate has been shown to produce meaningful relief of breakthrough pain within 5 min of initiating consumption, an onset that mimics

Table 4 Calculation of MEDD

Conversion from another opioids to morphine: To determine the total amount of opioids that effectively controls pain in 24 hr; use the conversion factor in table below. Give 50% less of the new opioid to avoid partial cross-tolerance. Divide by the number of doses/day (14).

Opioid	From IV opioids to IV morphine	From same IV opioid to oral opioid	From oral opioid to oral morphine	From oral morphine to oral opioid
Morphine	1.0	3.0	1.0	1.0
Hydromorphone	5.0	3.0	5.0	0.2
Meperidine	0.13	3.0	0.1	10.0
Oxycodone	–	–	1.5	0.7
Hydrocodone	–	–	0.15	7.0
Methadone	–	1.0	10.0[a]	0.1
Codeine	–	–	0.15	7.0

[a] Methadone conversion is probably not linear, and may be closer to 1:1 with morphine at low doses, and as high as 10:1 at higher doses.

intravenous administration, despite the noninvasive character of this therapy (79,80).

3. Agonist–antagonists: Agonist–antagonist and partial agonist opioid should generally be avoided for a variety of reasons, the most important of which is the presence of a ceiling effect, or dose above which toxicity but not analgesia increases.

Route of Administration

1. Oral: When possible, analgesics should be administered orally or by a similarly noninvasive route (transdermal, rectal, transmucosal) to promote independence and mobility and for ease of titration. In the presence of a functional, intact GI system, once the dose is adjusted to account for the hepatic first-pass effect, oral administration provides analgesia that is as effective as parenteral administration. The sublingual route of administration was favored in the hospice setting, but erratic absorption of morphine is problematic. Buccal administration of fentanyl in the form of oral transmucosal fentanyl citrate has become a valuable option for rapid analgesia in patients with severe breakthrough pain (80).

2. Transdermal: When pain control is inadequate with oral analgesics or the oral route is contraindicated, alternative means of drug delivery route should be explored. Transdermal fentanyl provides steady plasma level of analgesic for 72 hr per applied patch. The system's rate-controlling membrane regulates drug release at a slower rate than average skin flux, ensuring that the delivery system rather than the skin is the main determinant of absorption. Temperature is the most important factor in the determinant of absorption, so patients should be cautioned not to place a heating pad directly over the patch. Although low level of fentanyl can be detected in the bloodstream just an hour after administration, a consistent, near-peak level is not obtained for 12–18 hr after treatment is initiated. In addition, as a result of the formation of a skin depot (I am not sure that this is true, the depot is the fatty tissues) of drug, effects persist for 12–18 hr following removal of the patch. Because of the lag between dose and response, transdermal fentanyl analgesia is best suited for patients with relatively stable dose requirements and is particularly useful when the oral route is contraindicated.

3. Rectal: Rectal route is reliable for short-term use except in the presence of diarrhea, fistula, or other anatomical abnormalities. Morphine and hydromorphone are available in rectal preparations, and oxymorphone rectal suppositories provide 4–6 hr of potent analgesia

Table 5 Conversion Table for Fentanyl Patch

Conversion from/to transdermal fentanyl: To determine the 24-hr morphine equivalent dose requirement, select the μg/hr dose according to the ranges listed below. For dosage requirement >100 μg/hr, multiple patches can be used (patch duration = 72 hr). To titrate the dose effectively, prescribe a dose of morphine or other opioids as needed, especially during the first 12 hr. The patch will take 18 hr to achieve the peak dose. Increase the dose based on the additional amount of opioids required during the 72-hr period.

IV morphine (mg/24 hr)	Fentanyl equivalent (μg/hr)
8–22	25
23–37	50
38–52	75
53–67	100
68–82	125
83–97	150

(81). Rectal methadone is also available in compounded form but should be used judiciously.

4. Others: Continuous subcutaneous or intravenous infusions of opioids by means of a pump, IV, or subcutaneous patient-controlled analgesia (PCA), and intrathecal or epidural opioids administered via an externalized catheter or internalized pump (see Interventional pain section below).

Side Effects

Constipation and miosis are the only two opioid-mediated effects to which significant tolerance appears never to develop. Usually, a combined mild laxative and softener (Senokot-S) is prescribed when opioid therapy started. Patients should be instructed about sliding-scale regimen until a regular bowel habit develops. An osmotic agent (e.g., Lactulose) is the usual second-line agent of choice for refractory constipation. Severe constipation may leads to fecal impaction requiring manual disimpaction or nausea/vomiting requiring rehydration.

Opioid-induced nausea and vomiting usually resolve spontaneously with continued opioid use, and thus patients should be reassured and encouraged to adhere to their prescribed regimen of analgesics. The properistaltic agent metocloprapramide is our first choice for opioids-related emesis, after ensuring constipation is not the cause. Metoclopramide is particularly effective when gastric stasis is suggested by nausea, bloating, and early satiety. Haloperidol, prochlorperazine, and chlorpromazine are other reasonable choices, especially when cost is consideration (82). Ondansetron, a 5-HT3 anatagonist, is commonly used as an adjunct to emetic chemotherapies, is sometimes useful, but is very expensive. Dronabinol and corticosteroids are other treatments for refractory nausea.

Opioid-induced sedation that fails to improve with time can often be managed effectively with a psychostimulant such as methylphenidate or dextroamphetamine (83).

When side effects are refractory to above-mentioned medications trials, opioid rotation should be considered, since side effects are often idiosyncratic and may not be triggered by agents that are in other respects quite similar. If patients have persistent refractory side effects, more invasive modalities should be considered.

Opioid addiction is always a fear in patients receiving opioid medication, which is defined as a psychobehavioral phenomenon with possible genetic influence characterized by overwhelming drug use, nonmedical drug use, and continued use despite the presence or threat of physiological or psychological harm. Physicians should be able to differentiate addiction from tolerance, which is defined as the need for increasing dosages over time to maintain a desired effect, and physical dependence, a state characterized by the onset of characterized withdrawal symptoms when a drug is precipitously stopped or a specific antagonist is administered. Tolerance and physical dependence are biophysical phenomenon that are inevitable and should be regarded as pharmacological effects. Patient and family education should clarify these issues to aid in patient compliance with the prescribed regimen. This education is an essential element of a successful pain relief program.

Chronic administration of meperidine leads to accumulation of normeperidine, a metabolite, which may lead to frank seizure activities, especially when renal function is impaired (84). Thus, meperidine has fallen from favor as a useful analgesic agent in the treatment of cancer-related pain.

3. Adjuvant Analgesics

The aim of adjuvant therapy is to elicit an additive or synergistic effect or to diminish the toxicity of the primary therapy. In context of cancer pain, either it enhances opioid-mediated analgesia, diminishes opioid-mediated side effects or improves other symptoms associated with cancer. This analgesics are heterogeneous group of medications originally developed for purposes other then relief of pain that have observed to promote analgesia in specific clinical settings.

Important facts to remember are that (a) not every agent belonging to each component drug class appears to posses analgesic properties, (b) even agents with confirmed analgesic properties relieve only specific types of pain derived from specific selected conditions, and (c) even then, pain relief does not accrue in all affected patients.

Sequential Drug Trials

The recognition that neuropathic pain often fails to respond adequately to the routine administration of opioid and often responds in a binary fashion (no response or partial response) to many adjuvants titrated over time underlies the contemporary concept of sequential trials. Candidates are best initiated singly in low doses and titrated upward over time (4–6 weeks) until analgesia is achieved, side effects supervene, or the agent under trial can be excluded and a new trial can be commenced.

Antidepressants

The efficacy of selected antidepressant as analgesics per se, independent of their effects on mood and nighttime sleep, has been demonstrated mostly in noncancer models, although utility has been demonstrated for some agents in cancer patients as well (85–91). The antidepressant characteristically induces analgesia in responders with doses generally considered insufficient to relieve depression argues for a direct, independent underlying mechanism of effect. In addition, although onset is not immediate, analgesia is generally established more rapidly than are antidepressant effects (typically 3–7 days vs. 14–21 days). The operant mechanism for antidepressant-mediated analgesia presumably relates to increased circulating pools of norepinephrine and serotonin induced by reductions in the postsynaptic uptake of these neurotransmitters. It is also observed that coadministration of at least amitriptyline and clomipramine increases plasma morphine levels (90).

Tricyclic antidepressants are used for patients with neuropathic pain (e.g., postherpetic neuralgia, central pain, diabetic neuropathy), headache, arthritis, chronic low-back pain, and psychogenic pain. The main indication is neuropathic pain that is relatively constant and unrelenting and that is not predominantly intermittent, lancinating, jabbing, or shocklike. Paroxysmal neuropathic pain may also be treated effectively with tricyclic antidepressants, but is often first treated with an anticonvulsant.

Amitriptyline and to a lesser extent imipramine remain the most extensively studied of these agents, and as a result they are the usual first choices. Although relatively innocuous, side effects are especially prominent with these agents. Their metabolites include nortriptyline and desipramine, both of which have a better side effects profile. Some physicians may prefer to start with nortriptyline or desipramine as a first-line therapy. Since the newer class of antidepressants, the SSRIs (fluoxetine, paroxitine, sertraline, and others) are less effective for treating pain then above-mentioned agents, they may have efficacy in treating depression associated with pain.

Usually, amitriptyline, nortriptyline, or desipramine is started at 10–25 mg nightly and gradually titrated upward, usually to a range of 50–125 mg and occasionally higher, until toxicity occurs or analgesia is established. Dry mouth, constipation, drowsiness, and dysphoria are the most prominent of a wide range of side effects, which include urinary retention and cardiac dysrhythmia. Unlike the opioids, the development of tolerance is less robust, and side effects are less readily reversible. So if side effects are more prominent than analgesia, the offending agent is usually discontinued and a pharmacological analog or a drug from another class is started. The newer SSRIs may be preferred over the heterocyclic agents for fragile elderly patient, or in patients predisposed to developing anticholinergic side effects, patients whose multiple trials of tricyclics have failed because of side effects, and when depression is a prominent comorbidity.

Anticonvulsants

Carbamazepine, phenytoin, valproate, clonazepam, and most recently gabapentin, alone or in combination with the tricyclic antidepressants, have been shown to successfully treat neuropathic pain (91). Most authorities consider them as first choice for neuropathic pain and second-line therapy for relatively steady, constant neuropathic pain when tricyclic antidepressants are poorly tolerated, ineffective, or only partially effective. Anticonvulsants dampen ectopic foci of electrical activity and spontaneous discharge from injured nerves, in a manner analogous to their salutary effects in seizure disorders.

Although carbamazepine therapy has been the most thoroughly studied anticonvulsant for the treatment of neuropathic pain, it has largely been replaced by the newer and safer anticonvulsants including gabapentin. Gabapentin is a newer anticonvulsant and considered efficacious and well tolerated for neuropathic pain (92). It should be started in low dose at 100 mg/day and subsequently slowly increased up to 900 mg three or four times a day until analgesia obtained or side effects developed. Occasionally, patients respond to much higher doses of gabapentin without side effects. Felbamate is also known to interact with NMDA receptors, but its use is limited secondary to aplastic anemia. Other well-tolerated newer anticonvulsants include topiramate, levitiracetam, tiagabine, oxcarbazepine, lamotrigine, and zonisamide.

Baclofen

Baclofen is a γ-amino butyric acid (GABA) agonist, which although generally used for spasticity, has been reported to be effective for lancinating, ticlike neuropathic pain. It is usually started at 5 mg twice or three times day or and may be titrated up to 30–90 mg/day, as tolerated. It is also useful for spasticity; especially due to spinal cord injury and multiple sclerosis in the intrathecal route (93).

Oral Local Anesthetics

Oral mexiletine is usually regarded as a second- or third-line agent for continuous or intermittent neuropathic pain disorders. Several studies have shown disappointing efficacy and a high rate of side effects.

Amphetamines

The most widely accepted use for amphetamines in the treatment of cancer pain is as a means to reverse opioids-induced sedation (94). Research suggests that dextroamphetamine and methylphenidate possess some analgesic properties and are excellent antidepressants (95). The amphetamines are well tolerated by cancer patients and instead of inducing anorexia these agents typically have a paradoxical effect of increasing appetite by enhancing alertness. Nervousness and agitation are the most common side effects.

Corticosteroids

Corticosteroids are known for its efficacy for treatment of acute pain resulting from raised intracranial pressure and spinal cord compression secondary to its effect in reducing peritumoral edema and inflammation with consequent relief of pressure and traction on nerves and other pain-sensitive structures. Improvements in symptoms are often rapid and dramatic but usually depend on continued administration. These effects are short-lived and usually level off in few weeks.

Dexamethasone is the usual drug of choice because it has less potent mineralocorticoid effects. Side effects ranged from dysphoria and diabetes mellitus to florid psychosis. For oncologic emergencies, 100 mg of dexamethasone should be administered as bolus dose, followed by intravenous maintenance dose. The large bolus dose produces severe but transient perineal burning via unknown mechanism. For nonemergencies, dose is 2–6 mg three or four times a day.

N-Methyl-D-Aspartate Antagonists

The NMDA receptor has been well described and implicated in the transmission of pain. Ketamine and dextromethorphan, partial NMDA antagonists, appear to mediate pain by this mechanism. Subanesthetic doses of ketamine have been administered for prolonged periods with fair success in a small number of patients with refractory neuropathic cancer pain (96,97). Because of side effects, ketamine infusion should be regarded as a late treatment for highly refractory pain.

Alpha-2 Adrenergic Agonists

The centrally acting antihypertensive clonidine has been observed to promote analgesia for neuropathic pain when administered near the neuraxis. Epidural administration has received U.S. Food and Drug Administration (FDA) approval. In a prospective randomized study of 38 patients with severe cancer pain (98) that persisted despite large doses of spinal opioids, the addition of epidural clonidine was associated with significant improvement in 45% of patients overall and 56% of patients with neuropathic pain. Hypotension during the initiation and rebound hypertension during withdrawal are the main potential risk of treatment.

Others

Strontium is an analogue of calcium and is taken up by the skeleton into active sites of bone remodeling and metastasis. A large clinical trial demonstrated that a 10 μCi IV dose was an effective adjuvant to local radiotherapy, and that it reduced disease progression, decreased new sites of pain, and decreased systemic analgesics use (99). It is also a useful adjuvant for diffuse metastatic bone pain. The latency of response can be as long as 2–3 weeks, in which case patients must be instructed to continue analgesic therapy.

The bisphosphonate pamidronate disodium inhibits osteoclastic bone resorption and has been shown to reduce pain and skeletal complications, such as pathological fracture in breast cancer patients and multiple myeloma (100,101). The drug is administered in a 90 mg intravenous infusion in 2 hr approximately every 4 weeks.

4. *Interventional Pain Management*

When a comprehensive trial of pharmacological therapy fails to provide adequate analgesia or leads to unacceptable side effects, consideration should be given to alternative modalities.

Continuous Subcutaneous Infusion (CSCI) of Opioids

It is an excellent option for patients whose medical condition precludes the use of the oral route or whose pain is poorly controlled despite large doses of oral opioids (102,103).

Starting doses are calculated based on the 24-hr dose requirement of intravenous morphine with a conversion table (see Table 4) and divide it by 24, which gives the hourly rate. Tissue irritation is minimized when volumes under 1–2 mL/hr are prescribed (by concentrating the mixture). A 27-gauge butterfly needle is inserted subcutaneously anywhere with the most preferred sites including the infraclavicular fossa or chest wall for the ease of ambulation.

Absorption of subcutaneously administered opioids is rapid, and steady-state plasma levels are generally approached within an hour (103). Most parenteral opioids are suitable for CSCI, although morphine and hydromorphone are used most commonly and meperidine, methadone, and pentazocine should be avoided because of the potential for tissue irritation.

Rescue doses should be given as subcutaneous injection equal to the hourly dose to be administered every 1–2 hr as needed.

Continuous Intravenous Infusion (CII) of Opioids

This modality is indicated in a group of patients including intolerance of the oral route because of GI obstruction, malabsorption, opioid-induced vomiting, dysphagia, or the requirement of large number of pills. It is also indicated in a patient getting prominent bolus effect with intermittent injection, the necessity for rapid titration and requirement of bolus injections that exceed nursing capabilities. It is very similar to CSCI, although CSCI is preferred in the home care setting unless a permanent vascular access device is already in place (103).

Patient-controlled analgesia is a similar version and excellent option, but is reserved for patients with the capacity to understand and use this modification correctly. Dose should be adjusted upward until pain relief is adequate or side effects become intolerable.

Intraspinal Analgesia

Neuraxial analgesia is achieved by the epidural or intrathecal administration of an opioid alone or in combination with other agents. With the use of neuraxial analgesia, pain relief is obtained in a highly selective fashion with an absence of motor, sensory, and sympathetic effects, making these modalities highly adaptable to the home care environment (104–108). The principle of neuraxial opioid therapy is that introducing minute quantities of opioids in close proximity to their receptors (substantia gelatinosa of the spinal cord) achieves high local concentrations (105,109). With this therapy, analgesia may be superior to that achieved when opioids are administered by other routes, and since the absolute amount of drug administered is reduced, side effects are minimized. Our algorithm for choosing intrathecal or epidural with or without an implanted pump are described in figure form (see Fig. 2).

The neuraxis can be accessed via an intrathecal, epidural, or intraventricular approach, although the intraventricular route is used infrequently, primarily for intractable head and neck pain, and then usually when an access device (Ommaya reservoir) is already in place (110). The most important aspect of this therapy is its reversibility and the reliability and simplicity of advance screening measures to confirm efficacy. Screening can generally be accomplished on an outpatient basis by observing the patient's response either to a morphine infusion via a temporary percutaneous epidural catheter or a single-shot intrathecal injection. If improved pain control and reduced side effects are sufficiently profound to warrant more prolonged therapy either with temporary catheter for period of days to weeks or replacement with a permanent implanted catheter along with implanted medication deliverable pump.

Chronic administration of epidural opioids can be accomplished by intermittent bolus administered by the patient, family members, nursing personnel, or more commonly by continuous infusion via a standard PCA portable infusion pump connected to the epidural port. Continuous infusion is a preferred means of administration because intervals of pain between injections are avoided. More commonly, a combination of epidural opioids and dilute local anesthetic agents has been determined to be safe and are often beneficial for pain that is refractory to opioids alone (111).

Subarachnoid catheter placement is an alternative to epidural administration. Opioid requirements are less than with epidural administration because of more direct access to the spinal cord. Many factors are considered in the decision for an external pump system vs. an implantable pump. These include factors that lead us to an external system: a short life expectancy (<3 months), the need for frequent patient-controlled doses (such as with severe incident pain), the need for an epidural infusion (which generally requires infusion volumes too great for the implanted pump), the lack of reprogramming/refilling capabilities near the patient's home, or payor constraints. We use a variety of catheters for our external systems including a tunneled Arrow Flex-Tip® catheter, the Du Pen's® epidural catheter, and the Sims® epidural portacath. Our decision tree for neuraxial analgesia is presented in Fig. 6.

Factors that lead us to consider an implantable intrathecal pump include a longer life expectancy (>3 months), access to pump refill/reprogramming capabilities, diffuse pain (e.g., widespread metastasis), and favorable response to an intrathecal trial. We use a programmable (Synchromed®, Medtronic, Inc., Minneapolis, MN) pump for permanent implantation (Fig. 7).

A recently published multicenter prospective randomized clinical trial by Smith et al. (112) compared intrathecal therapy to continued medical management revealing a slight trend toward better analgesia in the intrathecal group (not statistically significant), but improved side effect profile and increased survival in the intrathecal group. Our group reported our outcome utilizing the algorithm in Fig. 6 in 79 patients for refractory cancer pain. We found a significant improvement in pain scores, a lowering of oral opioid

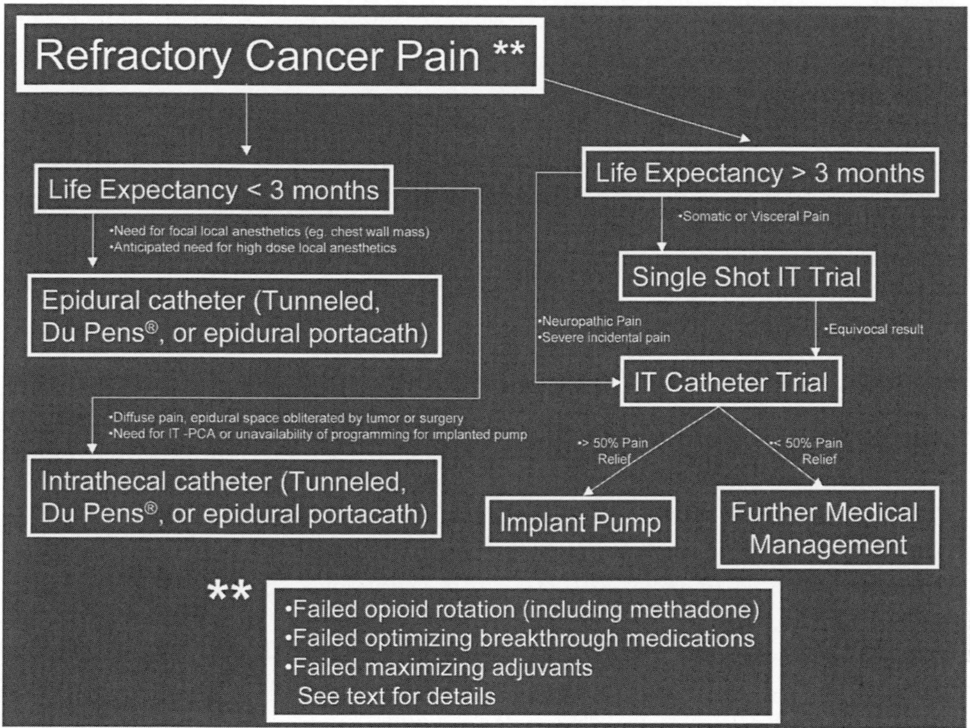

Figure 6 MDACC algorithm for the use of neuraxial analgesia in treating refractory cancer related pain.

intake, and an improvement in mental clouding and drowsiness (113).

Neuraxial medication is expensive, particularly as to whether an implanted pump is a justifiable expense in a patient with a limited life expectancy. Two studies evaluated the external vs. internal pump, with the ongoing costs of external pump lease and tubing vs. the high initial cost of the implanted pump. These analyses show a "break even" point at approximately 3 months (114,115).

Recently, Hassenbusch and colleagues published current practice data on intrathecal medication management. A survey of 413 physicians managing 13,342 patients was performed. It showed a variety of medications being used in the intrathecal pump including: morphine (48%), morphine/bupivacaine (12%), hydromorphone (8%), morphine/clonidine (8%), hydromorphone/clonidine (8%), morphine/clonidine/bupivacaine (5%), morphine/baclofen (3%), and others (<3%). Other drugs mentioned included: fentanyl, sufentanil, ziconotide, meperidine, methadone, ropivacaine, tetracaine, ketamine, midazolam, neostigmine, droperidol, and naloxone (116).

Side effects in forms of nausea, respiratory depression, pruritus, urinary retention, dysphoria are common for opioid-naïve patients, but are extremely rare in opioid-tolerant individuals (104).

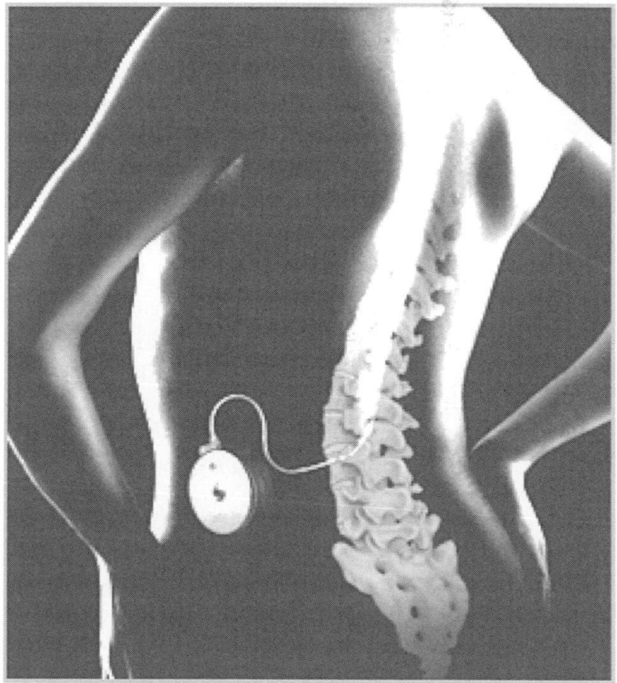

Figure 7 Schematic view of implanted intrathecal pump. (Courtesy of Medtronic, Inc.)

Nerve Blocks

1. *Local anesthetic nerve block*: Local anesthetic injections can be broadly classified as being applicable for diagnostic, and/or therapeutic purposes (117–120).

a. *Diagnostic blocks*: Diagnostic blocks help to characterize the underlying mechanism of pain (nociceptive, neuropathic, sympathetically mediated) and to discern the anatomical pathways involved in pain transmission. Its main indication is as a preliminary intervention conducted prior to a therapeutic nerve block or other definitive therapy. This helps the clinician to determine the potential for subsequent neurolysis if indicated. While results often have good predictive value, they are not entirely reliable.
b. *Therapeutic blocks*: The role of this block in cancer patients is limited typically because of transient nature of attendant pain relief. Therapeutic injections of local anesthetics, with or without corticosteroid, into trigger points, subcutaneous foci of localized muscle spasm, may provide lasting relief of myofascial pain. This bedside procedure is particularly useful when muscle spasm arise as a result of prolonged bed rest and for pain that follows thoracotomy, mastectomy, or radical neck dissection. Diffuse subcutaneous injection of corticosteroids and local anesthetics may be useful in acute herpes zoster or postherpetic neuralgia. Epidural steroid–local anesthetics injection are unlikely to provide lasting relief for back pain due to progressive neoplastic lesions. Local anesthetic injections administered in a series may contribute to lasting pain relief in the setting of post-traumatic sympathetically maintained pain (e.g., reflex sympathetic dystrophy or complex regional pain syndrome) (118,119). Although infrequent, such symptoms may arise as a result of tumor invasion of nervous system structure (e.g., brachial or lumbosacral plexopathy), in which case either local anesthetic blockade of the stellate ganglion or lumbar sympathetic chain has been used with some success to relieve pain.

2. *Neurolytic nerve block*: Neurolytic blocks have played an important role in the management of intractable cancer pain. This modality should be offered when pain persists despite thorough trials of aggressive pharmacological management or when drug therapy produces unwanted and uncontrollable side effects. Patient selection is important, including: (a) severe pain, (b) pain is expected to persist, (c) pain cannot be modified by less invasive means, (d) pain is well localized, (e) pain is well characterized, (f) pain is not multifocal, (g) pain is of somatic or visceral origin, (h) patient with limited life expectancy.

Alcohol and phenol are the only agents commonly used to produce chemical neurolysis. Ethyl alcohol is a pungent, colorless solution that can be readily injected through small-bore needles and that is hypobaric with respect to CSF. For peripheral and subarachnoid blocks, alcohol is generally used undiluted (referred to as 100% alcohol, dehydrated alcohol, or absolute alcohol), while a 50% solution is used for celiac plexus block. It should not be exposed to atmosphere, because absorbed moisture dilutes it. Alcohol injection is typically followed by intense burning pain and occasionally erythema along the targeted nerve distribution. Denervation and pain relief sometimes accrue over a few days following injection.

Phenol is fairly unstable at room temperature. It lasts at least 1 year when refrigerated and kept away from light. Phenol can be used in 3–15% concentration and with saline, water, and glycerol or radiological dye. It is relatively insoluble in water, and as a result concentration in excess of 6.7% cannot be obtained at room temperature without adding glycerine to increase its solubility in water. Phenol with glycerine is hyperbaric (vs. alcohol being hypobaric) in CSF, but is so viscid that even when warmed, it is difficult to inject through needles smaller than 20 gauge. Phenol has a biphasic action—its initial local anesthetic action produces subjective warmth and numbness that usually give way to chronic denervation over a day's time. Hypoalgesia after phenol is typically not as dense as after alcohol, and quality and extent of analgesia may fade slightly within the first 24 hr of administration.

Subarachnoid (intrathecal) injections of alcohol or phenol continue to play an important role in the management of intractable cancer pain in carefully selected patients. Neurolytic neuraxial block produces pain relief by chemical rhizotomy. Since alcohol and phenol destroy nervous tissue indiscriminately, careful attention to the selection of the injection site, volume and concentration of injectate, and selection and positioning of the patient are essential to avoid neurological complications (121,122). Most authorities agree that neither alcohol nor phenol offers a clear advantage except insofar as variations in baric properties facilitate positioning of the patient (123,124). Except for perineal pain, alcohol is usually preferred, since most patients are unable to lie on their painful side, as is required for intrathecal phenol neurolysis. In one of the analysis of 13 published series documenting treatment with intrathecal rhizolysis of more than 2500 patients, Swerdlow reported that 58% of patients obtained "good" relief; "fair" relief was observed in an additional 21%, and in 20% of patients "little or no relief" was noted (123). Average duration of relief is estimated at 3–6 months, with a wide range of distribution. Reports of analgesia persisting 1–2 years are fairly common (125). In representative series using alcohol ($n = 252$) and phenol ($n = 151$), a total of 407 and 313 blocks were performed, respectively (126,127). In these two series, neither motor weakness nor fecal incontinence occurred, and of eight patients with transient urinary dysfunction, incontinence persisted in just one.

Subarachnoid neurolysis can be performed at any level up to the mid-cervical region, above which the risk of drug spread to medullary centers and the potential for cardiorespiratory collapse increases (128). Blocks in the region of the brachial outflow are best reserved for patients with preexisting compromise of upper limb function. Similarly, lumbar injections are avoided in ambulatory patients, as are sacral injections in patients with normal bowel and bladder function. Hyperbaric phenol saddle block is relatively simple and is particularly suitable for many patients with colostomy and urinary diversion. Until recently, epidural neurolysis was performed infrequently. Results were inferior to those obtained with sub arachnoid blockade, presumably because the dura acts as a barrier to diffusion, resulting in limited contact between the drug and targeted nerves (125,129).

Sympathetic blockade also produces prolonged relief of pain in cases where the pain is sympathetically mediated (118). When local anesthetic sympathetic blocks provide only temporary relief or when clinical findings suggest visceral or sympathetically mediated pain, consideration of chemical sympathectomy is warranted.

Celiac plexus block continues to be one of the most efficacious and common nerve blocks employed in patients with cancer pain (130). It has great potential for relieving upper abdominal and referred back pain secondary to malignant neoplasm involving structures derived from the foregut (distal esophagus to mid-transverse colon, liver, biliary tree, and adrenal glands). The most common indication for celiac axis block is pancreatic cancer. Celiac axis block is most commonly performed by positioning needles bilaterally either antero- or retrocrurally via a posterior percutaneous approach (Figs. 8 and 9, respectively). The retrocrural technique is more accurately called a splachnic nerve block. Despite the proximity of major organs (aorta, vena cava, kidneys, pleura) and the requirements for a large volume of neurolytic (30–50 mL of 50% alcohol in the anterocrural technique, much less volume in the retrocrural) complication rates are uniformly low, although some complications are serious (130–133). In contemporary practice, most authorities consider radiological guidance mandatory to verify needle placement (149). Traditionally, fluoroscopy has been used, but CT guidance is increasing in popularity because vascular structures, viscera, and masses can be visualized (132). Although studies have been criticized for methodological deficiencies, 85–94% incidence of good to excellent relief of pain has been obtained in large series of patients undergoing one or more neurolytic celiac plexus blocks for pain from pancreatic cancer, or a vari-

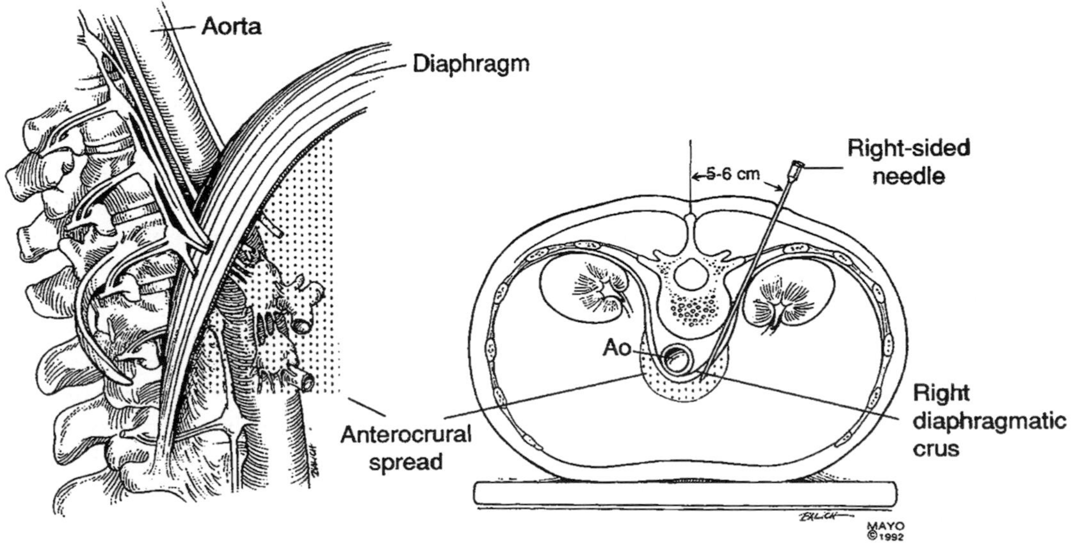

Figure 8 Anterocrural celiac plexus block.

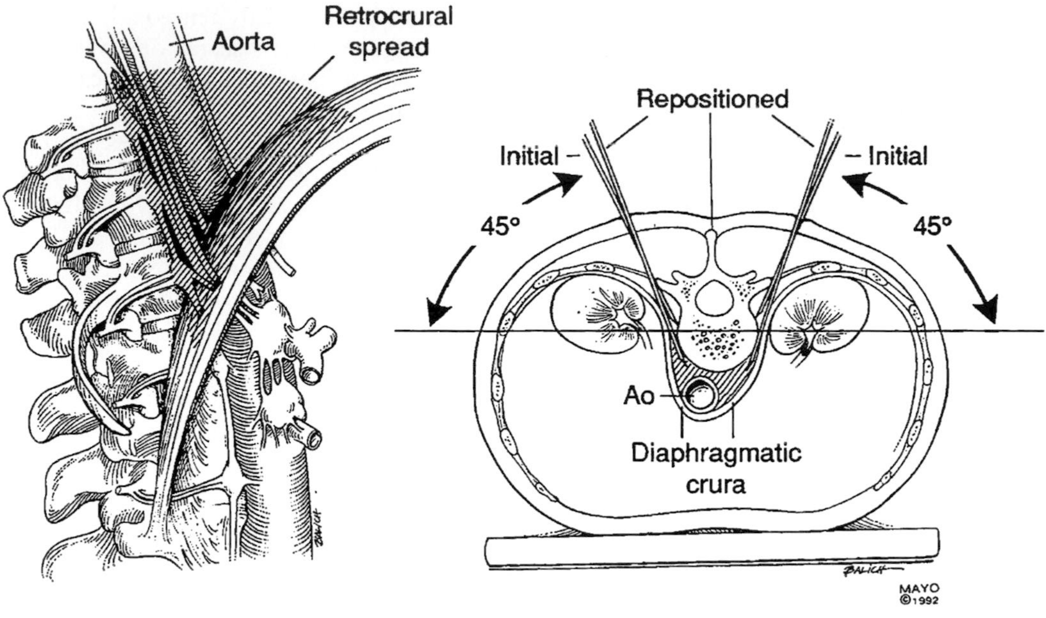

Figure 9 Retrocrural celiac plexus block or splachnic nerve block.

ety of intraabdominal neoplasms (131). In one of the randomized double-blind, placebo-controlled study of intraoperative celiac neurolysis demonstrated that treated patients had not only improved pain control, reduction in opioid use and improved function but also statistically significant improvement in survival (7). Wong and colleagues reported significantly improved pain control with the celiac plexus block versus medical management in an elegant double-blind, randomized study comparing the two techniques in patients with abdominal pain due to pancreatic cancer (133).

Stellate ganglion block, with repeated local anesthetic of the sympathetic outflow to the head, neck, and arm, often provide persistent relief of sympathetically maintained pain affecting these regions. Stellate ganglion neurolysis is hazardous because of the close proximity of other important structures (brachial plexus, laryngeal nerves, epidural and subarachnoid space, vertebral artery) and the potential for injury because of inaccurate needle placement. If local anesthetic injections have been documented to provide temporary relief of pain, surgical extirpation of the ganglia may be considered, or neurolysis may be performed cautiously using radiological guidance and small volumes of injectate (134).

Neurolytic lumbar sympathetic block is most applicable for pain in the lower extremities due to lymphedema or reflex sympathetic imbalance, although it has also been applied for rectal and pelvic pain in anecdotal fashion (117).

Superior hypogastric plexus block (135) is generally preferred for intractable chronic pelvic or rectal pain of neoplastic origin. In contrast to subarachnoid injection, risks of bowel, bladder, and motor dysfunction with either lumbar sympathetic or hypogastric block, even when performed bilaterally, are extremely low, particularly with radiological guidance.

In the first published study of superior hypogastric block (135), 28 patients with intrapelvic neoplasms or radiation enteritis were studied, and all had significant or complete relief of pain with no complications. In all but two patients with pain due to neoplasm, relief persisted until death (3–12 months). In another study of 26 cancer patients with severe (10 out of 10 intensity) intractable pelvic pain, 70% had satisfactory relief (less than four out of 10 intensity) and the remaining patients, moderate relief (4–7 of 10) (136). Complications were not observed, and no patients with satisfactory relief required repetition out to a 6-month follow-up.

The ganglion impar is a solitary retroperitoneal structure at the level of the sacrococcygeal junction that marks the termination of the paired paravertebral sympathetic chains. Although the anatomical interconnections of the ganglion impar are rarely described in any detail, even in the anatomy literature, the sympathetic component of perineal pain syndromes appears to derive at least in part from this structure. The first report of interruption of the ganglion impar for the relief of anal, genital, or perineal cancer-related pain appeared in 1990 (137). Of 16 patients, eight had complete, durable relief of pain, and the remainder had significant reductions in pain. Blocks were repeated in two patients with further improvement. No complications occurred, and follow-up, which depended on survival, was carried out for 14–120 days. The technique entails the use of a 20- or 22-gauge spinal needle that is manually bent near its hub at about 30°. The needle is introduced through the anococcygeal ligament with its concavity oriented toward the concavity of the sacrum and coccyx. Under fluoroscopic guidance, the needle is advanced until its tip lies near the anterior surface of the junction of the sacrum and coccyx, posterior to the rectum where injection takes place.

More recently, radiofrequency-generated thermal lesions are another effective means of inducing therapeutic nerve injury and when directed to the tumor itself, it can have a tumoricidal effect often with salutary effects on symptoms (138). An optimal result requires the judicious use of fluoroscopy for placement of needle and application of simple but essential adjuncts including the use of a nerve stimulator to avoid the motor root if applicable.

3. Peripheral/cranial nerve blocks: Peripheral nerve blockade has a limited role in the management of cancer pain (120). Neoplastic head and neck pain is many times difficult to control because of rich sensory innervations of the structures. In selected patients, blockade of involved cranial and/or upper cervical nerves is very helpful. Blockade of trigeminal nerve within the foramen ovale at the base of skull or its branches may be beneficial for facial pain (139) (see Fig. 10). If neural blockade is not effective, intraspinal opioid therapy by means of an implanted cervical epidural catheter or intraventricular opioid therapy may be considered (140,141).

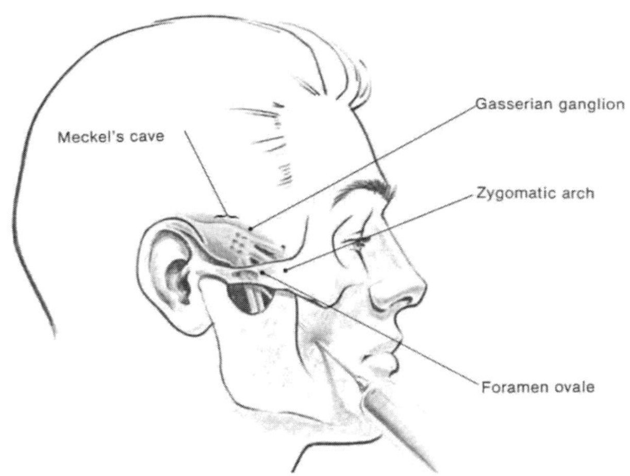

Figure 10 Gasserian ganglion injection.

Vertebroplasty

Many cancer patients with metastatic VCFs or osteoporotic VCFs present with movement-related back pain. Percutaneous vertebroplasty (PV) is a minimally invasive procedure involving injecting an opacified bone cement (usually polymethymethacrylate or PMMA) into the fractured vertebral body to alleviate the pain and perhaps enhance structural stability (see Fig. 11a and b). This procedure is performed by placing needles under fluoroscopic guidance with a uni- or bipedicular approach. PMMA is injected in a carefully controlled manner to avoid unintended cement spread into the spinal canal. Injection is stopped as soon as cement starts approaching in posterior on third of vertebral body. Percutaneous vertebroplasty has been shown efficacious in treating VCF-related pain in cancer patients (142).

Neuromodulation

Spinal cord stimulation is widely popularized for refractory neuropathic chronic pain states. It has limited applicability in cancer pain states, except in ongoing chronic neuropathic pain states. Selection of this patient population is very important in cancer group, as MRI is contraindicated after this devise is placed.

a. Neurosurgical palliative techniques have fallen into less favor as more medications and reversible, titratable, lower risk techniques have largely replaced these procedures. Pituitary ablation entails destruction of the gland by means of the injection of a small quantity of alcohol through a needle positioned transnasally under light general anesthesia. This technique is effective in relieving pain originating from disseminated bony metastases, particularly secondary to hormone-dependent tumors (breast and prostate) (143). Commissural myelotomy has been reported to be efficacious in cancer pain refractory to more conservative therapy (144). Percutaneous cordotomy produces a thermal lesion within the substance of the spinal cord and reliably relieves unilateral truncal and lower limb pain (145). As with pituitary ablation, it necessitates a high degree of skill and expertise, but pain relief is often profound and the rigors of a major neurosurgical procedure are avoided.

Behavioral Pain Management

Different behavioral pain management techniques have been used in patients with cancer includes hypnosis, relaxation, biofeedback, sensory alteration, guided imagery, and cognitive strategies (146). Relaxation and

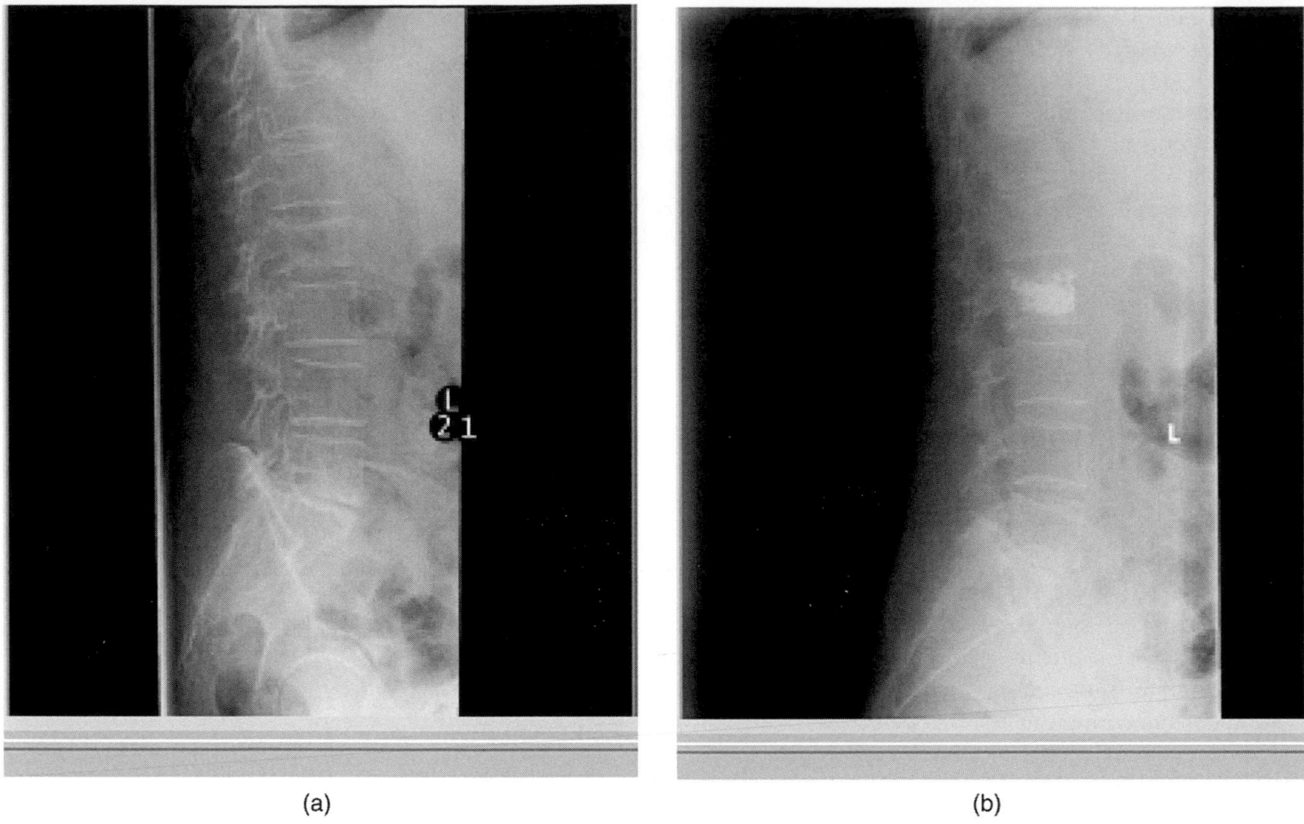

(a) (b)

Figure 11 (a) L2 vertebral compression fracture, lateral image. (b) Postvertebroplasty lateral radiograph of L2.

imagery training significantly reduce visual analog scale scores in patients who have mucositis during bone marrow transplant (147). This training is probably most effective for patients who have no significant psychological or psychiatric problems (148) and in insightful psychology-minded patients.

Home-based and hospice care:

For years together, hospice is often incorrectly regarded as a place people go to die, but correctly it is a philosophy of care that is "a blend of clinical pharmacology and applied compassionate psychology" (149,150). In the United States, hospice care has developed primarily as a home-based service, with a minority of institutions offering short inpatient stays to stabilize refractory symptoms and to provide respite for overwhelmed families.

The principles of home-based pain management are in most respects similar to those that apply to ambulatory and inpatient pain management. Differences generally relate to a recognition that further curative therapy is futile rather than that care is being provided at home. No compromise in quality of care based on where it is delivered is justified.

Hospice care is comfort oriented, focusing specifically on alleviating symptoms rather than necessarily treating their underlying cause or causes. Factors that influence the selection of home treatment are advanced, incurable disease, realization and acceptance of the appropriateness of palliative care (care directed at preserving comfort and the quality of life rather than at curing the tumor and extending life), and a desire to die in familiar surroundings. Many difficulties associated with providing intensive palliative care at home can be reconciled by education and orientation of the family and that can be performed with coordination with health care institutions, home care nursing, laboratory, and pharmacy services. See Chapter 58 for more details regarding palliative care.

VIII. SUMMARY

Acute and chronic pain occurs in a high frequency of cancer patients. Inadequate assessment and treatment of pain and other distressing symptoms may interfere with primary antitumor therapy and markedly detract from the quality of life. While a strong focus on pain control is important independent of disease stage, it is a special priority in patients with advanced disease who are no longer candidates for potentially curative therapy.

While rarely eliminated altogether, pain can be controlled in the vast majority of patients, usually with the careful application of straightforward pharmacological measures combined with diagnostic acumen and conscientious follow-up. In the small but significant proportion of patients whose pain is not readily controlled with noninvasive analgesics, a variety of alternative measures, when selected carefully, are also associated with a high degree of success. An increasingly large cadre of anesthesiologists have come to recognize that far from an exercise in futility, caring for patients with advanced irreversible illness can be a highly satisfying endeavor that is usually met with considerable success. Thus, no patient should ever wish for death as a result of inadequate control of pain or other symptoms, and clinicians need never communicate overtly or indirectly that nothing more can be done. Comprehensive cancer care is best regarded as a continuum that commences with prevention and early detection, focuses intensely on curative therapy, and ideally is rendered complete by a seamless transition to palliation and attention of quality of life.

The future of cancer pain relief is bright, as much mechanistic research is looking into different groups of specifically targeted medications including tumor necrosis alpha receptor antagonists, inhibitors of glutamate release, substance P inhibitors, nitric oxide synthetase inhibitors, and other novel compounds.

REFERENCES

1. American Society of Anesthesiologists. Practice guidelines for cancer pain management—a report by the American Society of Anesthesiologists task force on pain management, Cancer Pain Section. Anesthesiology 1996; 84:1243–1257.
2. Merskey H, ed. Classification of chronic pain: description of chronic pain syndromes and definitions of pain terms. Pain 1986; (suppl 3):S127.
3. American Pain Society. Principles of Analgesic Use in the Treatment of Acute Pain and Chronic Cancer Pain. 3rd ed. Skokie, IL: APS, 1992.
4. Jacox A, Carr DB, Payne R, et al. Management of Cancer Pain: Clinical Practice Guideline 9. Agency for Health Care Policy and Research Pub. 94-0592. Rockville, MD: ACHPR, 1994.
5. Ferrell BR, Wisdon C, Wenzl C. Quality of life as an outcome variable in management of cancer pain. Cancer 1989; 63:2321.
6. Smith TJ, Staats PS, Deer T, et al. Randomized clinical trial of an implantable durg delivery system with comprehensive medical management for refractory cancer pain: Impact on pain, durg-related toxicity, and survival. J Clin Oncology 2002; 20(19):4040–4049.
7. Lillemoe KD, Cameron JL, Kaufman HS, et al. Chemical splanchnicectomy in patients with unresectable pancreatic cancer. Ann Surg 1993; 217:447–457.
8. Ferlay J, Bray F, Pisani P, Parkin DM. Globocan 2000: Cancer incidence, mortality, and prevalence worldwide. IARC CancerBase No 5. Lyon: IARC Press, 2001.
9. Silverberg E, Boring CC, Squires TS. Cancer statistics, 1990. CA Cancer J Clin 1990; 40:9.
10. American Cancer Society. Cancer Facts and Figures: 1994. Atlanta: ACS, 1994.
11. Cleeland CS, Gonin R, Hatfield AK, et al. Pain and its treatment in outpatients with metastatic cancer. N Engl J Med 1994; 330:592–596.
12. Higginson IJ. Innovation in assessment: epidemiology and assessment of pain in advanced cancer. In: Janson TS, Turner JA, Wiesenfeld-hallin Z, eds. Proceedings of the 8th World Congress on Pain; Progress in Pain Research and Therapy. Seattle: IASP Press, WA Patel, 1997:707–716.
13. Walsh TD. Oral morphine in chronic cancer pain. Pain 1984; 18:1.
14. Bruera E. Malnutrition and asthenia in advanced cancer. Cancer Bull 1991; 43:387.
15. Bonica JJ. Management of cancer pain. Rec Res Cancer Res 1984; 89:13.
16. Daut RL, Cleeland CS. The prevalence and severity of pain in cancer. Cancer 1982; 50:1913.
17. Mumford JW, Mumford SP. The care of cancer patients in a rural South Indian hospital. Palliat Med 1988; 2:157.
18. World Health Organization. Cancer Pain Relief. Geneva: WHO, 1986.
19. Portenoy RK. Cancer pain: epidemiology and syndromes. Cancer 1989; 63:2307.
20. Brescia FJ, Adler D, Gray G, Ryan MA. A profile of hospitalized advanced cancer patients. J Pain Symptom Manage 1990; 5:221.
21. Swerdlow M, Stjernsward J. Cancer pain relief: an urgent problem. World Health Forum 1982; 3:325–330.
22. Burton AW, Cleeland CS. Cancer pain: Progress since the WHO Guidelines. Pain Practice 2001; 1(3): 236–242.
23. Zech DFG, Grong S, Lynch J, et al. Validation of the World Health Organization guidelines for cancer pain relief: a 10-year prospective study. Pain 1996; 63: 65–76.
24. Daut RL, Cleeland CS, Flannery RC. Development of the Wisconsin brief pain questionnaire to access pain in cancer and other diseases. Pain 1983; 17:197.
25. Cleeland CS. Assessment of pain in cancer. Adv Pain Res Ther 1990; 16:47.
26. Fishman B, Pasternak S, Wallenstein S, et al. The memorial pain assessment card: a valid instrument for the evaluation of cancer pain. Cancer 1987; 60:1151.

27. Bruera E, MacMillan K, Hanson J, et al. The Edmonton staging system for cancer pain: preliminary report. Pain 1989; 37:203.
28. Bruera E, Schoeller T, wenk R, et al. A prospective multicenter assessment of the Edmonton staging system for cancer pain. J Pain Symptom Manage 1995; 10:348–355.
29. Beyer J, Aradine C. Content validity of an instrument to measure young children's perceptions of the intensity of their pain. J Pediatr Nurs 1986; 1:386.
30. Eland J. Eland color scale. In: McCaffery M, Beebe A, eds. Pain: Clinical Manual for Nursing Practice. St. Louis: Mosby, 1989.
31. Hester N, Foster R, Kristensen K. Measurement of pain in children: generalizability and validity of the pain ladder and the poker chip tool. In: Tyler D, Krane E, eds. Advances in Pain Research and Therapy: Pediatric Pain. Vol. 1. New York: Raven Press, 1990:79.
32. McGrath PA. Pain in Children: Nature, Assessment and Treatment. New York: Guilford, 1990.
33. Gonzales GR, Elliot KJ, Portenoy RK, Foley KM. The impact of a comprehensive evaluation in the management of cancer pain. Pain 1991; 47:141–144.
34. Procacci P, Maresca M. Pathophysiology of visceral pain. Adv Pain Res Ther 1990; 13:123.
35. Cervero F. Visceral pain. In: Dubner R, Gebhart GF, Bond MR, eds. Proceedings of the VI World Congress on Pain. Amsterdam: Elsevier, 1988:216.
36. Enneking WF, Conrad EU III. Common bone tumors. Clin Symptom 1989; 41:1.
37. Foley KM. Pain syndromes in patients with cancer. Adv Pain Res Ther 1979; 2:59.
38. Schneck D, Frankel SO, et al. Bone metastasis and bone pain in breast cancer. JAMA 1979; 2242:1747–1748.
39. Bennett A. The role of biochemical mediators in peripheral nociception and bone pain. Cancer Surv 1998; 7:55–67.
40. Sabino MAC, Ghilardi JR, Jongen JLM, Keyser CP, Luger NM, Mach DB, Peters CM, Rogers SD, Scwei MJ, Felipe C, Mantyh PW. Simultaneous reduction in cancer pain, bone destruction, and tumor growth by selective inhibition of cyclo-oxygenase-2. Cancer Res 2002; 62:7343–7349.
41. Clohisy DR, Mantyh PW. Bone cancer pain. Cancer 2003; 97:866–73S.
42. Kuru B, Camlibel M, Ali Gulcelik M, Alagol H. Prognostic factors affecting survival and disease free survival in lymph node negative breast carcinomas. J Surg Oncol 2003; 83(3):167–172.
43. David A, Khwaja R, Hudes G. Treatments for improving survival of patients with prostate carcinoma. Drugs Aging 2003; 20(9):683–699.
44. Gokaslan ZL. Spine surgery for cancer. Curr Opin Oncol 1996; 8:178–181.
45. Greenberg HS, Deck MDF, Vikram B, et al. Metastases to the base of the skull: clinical findings in 43 patients. Neurology 1981; 31:530.
46. Elliot K, Foley KM. Neurologic pain syndromes in patients with cancer. Crit Care Clin 1990; 6:393.
47. Foley KM. Brachial plexopathy in patients with breast cancer. In: Harris JR, Hellman S, Henderson IC, et al, eds. Breast Diseases. Philadelphia: Lippincott, 1987.
48. Kori SH, Foley KM, Posner JB. Brachial plexus lesions in patients with cancer: 100 cases. Neurology 1981; 31:45.
49. Olson ME, Chernik NL, Posner JB. Infiltration of the leptomeninges by systemic cancer: a clinical and pathologic study. Arch Neurol 1930: 122.
50. Wasserstrom WR, Glass JP, Posner JB. Diagnosis and treatment of leptomeningeal metastases from solid tumor: experience with 90 patients. Cancer 1982; 49:759.
51. Schild SC, Wasserstrom WR, Fleischer M, et al. Cerebrospinal fluid biochemical markers of central nervous metastases. Ann Neurol 1980; 8:597.
52. Glass JP, Foley KM. Carcinomatous meningitis. In: Harris JR, Hellman S, Henderson IC, et al., eds. Breast Diseases. Philadelphia: Lippincott, 1987:497.
53. Cascino TL, Kori S, Krol G, et al. CT scan of the brachial plexus in patients with cancer. Neurology 1983; 33:1553.
54. Kanner RM, Martini N, Foley KM. Epidural spinal cord compression in Pancoast syndrome (superior pulmonary sulcus tumor): clinical presentation and outcome. Ann Neurol 1981; 10:77.
55. Foley KM. Overview of cancer pain and brachial and lumbosacral plexopathy. In: Foley KM, ed. Management of Cancer Pain. New York: Memorial Sloan Kettering Cancer Center, 1985:25.
56. Jaekle KA, Young DF, In: Foley KM. The natural history of lumbosacral plexopathy in cancer. Neurology 1985; 35:8–15.
57. Pettigrew LC, Glass JP, Maor M, et al. Diagnosis and treatment of lumbosacral plexopathy in patients with cancer. Arch Neurol 1984; 41:1282.
58. Shubert MM, Sullivan KM, Morten TH, et al. Oral manifestations of chronic graft-versus-host disease. Arch Intern Med 1984; 144:1591.
59. Dougherty PM, Cata JP, Cordella JV, Burton AW, Weng HR. Taxol-induced sensory disturbance is characterized by preferential impairment of myelinated fiber function in cancer patients. Pain 2004; 109(1–2): 132–142.
60. Perkins, Kehlet H. Chronic pain syndromes after surgery: a review of predicitive factors. Anesthesiology 2000.
61. Tasmuth T, von Smitten K, Kalso E, et al. Pain and other symptoms during the first year after radical and conservative surgery for breast surgery. Br J Cancer 1996; 74:2024–2031.
62. Rushton JG, Rooke ED. Brain tumor headache. Headache 1962; 2:147.
63. Zimm S, Wampler GL, Stablein D, et al. Intracerebral metastases in solid tumor patients: natural history and results of treatment. Cancer 1981; 48:384.

64. Black P. Brain metastasis: current status and recommended guidelines for management. Neurosurgery 1979; 5:617.
65. Guitin PH. Corticosteroid therapy in patients with brain tumor. Natl Cancer Inst Monogr 1977; 46:151.
66. Reuther T, Schuster T, Mende U, Kubler A. Osteoradionecrosis of the jaws as a side effect of radiotheraphy of head and neck tumour patients-a report of a thirty year retrospective review. Int Oral Maxillofac Surg 2003; 32:289–295.
67. Fathers E, Thrush D, Huson SM, Norman A. Radiation-induced brachial plexopathy in women treated for carcinoma of the breast. Clin Rehabil 2002; 16:160–165.
68. Nagler RM. Effects of head and neck radiotheraphy on major salivary glands-animal studies and human implications. In Vivo 2003; 17:369–375.
69. Foley KM. Treatment of cancer pain. N Engl J Med 1985; 313:84.
70. Grond S, Zech D, Diefenbach C, et al. Assessment of cancer pain: a prospective evaluation in 2266 patients referred to a pain service. Pain 1996; 64:107–114.
71. Schlegel SI, Paulus HE. Nonsteroidal and analgesic use in the elderly. Clin Rheum Disease 1986; 12:245.
72. Rothwell KG. Efficacy and safety of a non-acetylated salicylate, choline magnesium trisalicylate in the treatment of rheumatoid arthritis. J Int Med Res 1983; 11:343.
73. Leonards JR, Levy G. Gastrointestinal blood loss from aspirin and sodium salicylate tablets in man. Clin Pharmacol Ther 1973; 14:61.
74. Buckley MMT, Brogden RN. Ketorolac: a review of its pharmacodynamic and pharmacokinetic properties and therapeutic potential. Drugs 1990; 39:86–109.
75. Needleman P, Isakson PC. The discovery and function of COX-2. J Rheumatol 1997; 24(suppl 49):6–8.
76. Hopkinson JH III. Vicodin: a new analgesic: clinical evaluation of efficacy and safety of repeated doses. Curr Ther Res 1978; 24:633– 645.
77. Ettinger DS, Vitale PJ, Trump DL. Important clinical pharmacologic considerations in the use of methadone in cancer patients. Cancer Treat Rep 1979; 63:457.
78. Portenoy RK. Breakthrough pain: definition and management. Oncology 1983; 3:25–29.
79. Fine PG, Marcus M, De Boer AJ, Van der Oord B. An open label study of oral transmucosal fentanyl citrate(OTFC) for the treatment of breakthrough cancer pain. Pain 1991; 45:149–153.
80. Burton AW, Driver LC, Mendoza TR, Syed G. Oral Transmucosal in the outpatient management of severe cancer pain crises: a retrospective case series. Clin J Pain 2004; 20(3):195–197.
81. Baines M. Nausea and vomiting in the patient with advanced cancer. J Pain Symptom Manage 1988; 3:81–85.
82. Bruera E, Chadwick S, Brenneis C, et al. Methylphenidate associated with narcotics for the treatment of cancer pain. Cancer Treat Rep 1987; 71:67–70.
83. Kaiko RF, Foley KM, Grabinski PY, et al. Central nervous system excitatory effects of meperidine in cancer patients. Ann Neurol 1983; 13:180–185.
84. Portenoy RK, Kanner RM. Nonopioid and adjuvant analgesics. In: Portenoy RK, Kanner RM, eds. Pain Management: Theory and Practice. Philadelphia: Davis, 1996:219–247.
85. Watson C, Evans R, Reed K, et al. Amitriptyline versus placebo in post-herpetic neuralgia. Neurology 1982; 32:671–673.
86. Kishore-Kumar R, Max MB, Schafer SC, et al. Desipramine relieves post-herpetic neuralgia. Clin Pharmacol Ther 1990; 47:305–372.
87. Sindrup SH, Ejlertsen B, froland A, et al. Imipramine treatment in diabetic neuropathy: relief of subjective symptoms without changes in peripheral and autonomic nerve function. Eur J Clin Pharmacol 1989; 37:151–153.
88. Sindrup SH, Gram LF, Skjold T, et al. Clomipramine vs desipramine vs placebo in the treatment of diabetic neuropathy symptoms: a double blind crossover study. Br J Clin Pharmacol 1990; 30:683–691.
89. Walsh TD. Controlled study of imipramine and morphine in chronic pain due to cancer. Proc Am Soc Clin Oncol 1986; 5:237.
90. Vantafridda V, Bianchi M, Ripamonti C, et al. Studies on the effects of antidepressant drugs on the antinociceptive action of morphine on plasma morphine in rat and man. Pain 1990; 43:155–162.
91. Hatangdi VS, Boas RA, Richard EG. Postherpetic neuralgia: management with antiepileptic and tricyclic drugs. Adv Pain Res Ther 1976; 1(1):583–587.
92. Mellegers MA, et al. Gabapentin: a meta-analysis. Clin J Pain 2001.
93. Ordia JI, Fischer E, Adamski E, Spatz EL. Chronic intrathecal delivery of baclofen by a programmable pump for the treatment of severe spasticity. J Neurosurg 1996; 85:452–457.
94. Bruera E, Chadwick S, Brenneis C. Methylphenidate associated with narcotics for the treatment of cancer pain. Cancer Treat Rep 1987; 71:120.
95. Forrest WH Jr, Brown BM Jr, Brown CR. Dextroamphetamine with morphine for the treatment of prospective pain. N Engl J Med 1977; 13:712–715.
96. Mercadante S, Lodi F, Sapio M, et al. Long-term ketamine subcutaneous continuous infusion in neuropathic cancer pain. J Pain Symptom Mgmt 1995; 10:564–567.
97. Yang CY, Wong CS, Chang JY, Ho ST. Intrathecal ketamine reduces morphine requirements in patients with terminal cancer pain. Can J Anaesth 1996; 43:379–383.
98. Eisenach JC, DuPen S, Dubois M, et al. Epidural clonidine analgesia for intractable cancer pain. Pain 1995; 61:391–399.
99. Porter AT, McEwan AJB, Powe JE, et al. Results of a randomized phase-III trial to evaluate the efficacy of strontium adjuvant to local field external beam irra-

diation in the management of endocrine resistant metastatic prostate cancer. Int J Radiat Oncol Biol Phys 1993; 25:805–813.
100. Hortobagyi GN, Theriault RL, Porter L, et al. Efficacy of pamidronate in reducing skeletal complications in patients with breast cancer and lytic bone metastases. New Engl J Med 1996; 335:1785–1791.
101. Berenson JR, Lichtenstein A, Porter L, et al. Efficacy of pamidronate in reducing skeletal events in patients with advanced multiple myeloma. New Engl J Med 1996; 334:488–493.
102. Bruera E. Subcutaneous administration of opioids in the management of cancer pain. In: Foley K, Ventafridda V, eds. Recent Advances in Pain Research. Vol. 16. New York: Raven Press, 1990:203–218.
103. Bruera E, Ripamonti C. Alternate routes of administration of narcotics. In: Patt RB, ed. Cancer Pain. Philadelphia: Lippincott, 1993:161.
104. Cousins MJ, Mather LE. Intrathecal and epidural administration of opioids. Anesthesiology 1984; 61:276–310.
105. Yaksh TL. Spinal opiates: a review of their effect on spinal function with an emphasis on pain processing. Acta Anaesthesiol Scand 1987; 31(suppl 85):25.
106. Smith DE. Spinal opioids in the home and hospice setting. J Pain Symptom Mgmt 1990; 5:175.
107. Boersma FP, Buist AB, Thie J. Epidural pain treatment in the northern Netherlands: organizational and treatment aspects. Acta Anaesthesiol Belg 1987; 38:213.
108. Crawford ME, Andersen HB, Augustenborg G, et al. Pain treatment on outpatient basis using extradural opiates: Danish multicenter study comprising 105 patients. Pain 1983; 16:41.
109. Snyder SH. Opiate receptors in the brain. N Engl J Med 1977; 296:266–271.
110. Roquefeuil B, Benezech J, Blanchet P, et al. Intraventricular administration of morphine in patients with neoplastic intractable pain. Surg Neurol 1984; 21:155–158.
111. Du Pen S, Kharasch ED, Williams A, et al. Chronic epidural bupivacaine–opioid infusion in intractable cancer pain. Pain 1992; 49:293–300.
112. Smith TJ, et al. Randomized comparison of intrathecal drug delivery system (IDDS) + comprehensive medical management (CMM) vs. CMM alone for unrelieved cancer pain. J Clin Oncol.
113. Burton AW, Rajagopal A, Shah HN, Mendoza T, Cleeland CS, Hassenbusch SJ, Arens JF. Epidural and intrathecal analgesia is effective in treating refractory cancer pain. Pain Medicine 2004; 5(3):239–247.
114. Bedder MD, Burchiel KJ, Larson A. Cost analysis of two implantable narcotic delivery systems. J Pain Symptom Mgmt 1991; 6:368.
115. Hassenbusch SJ, Bedder M, Patt RB, Bell GK. Current status of intrathecal therapy for nonmalignant pain management: clinical realities and economic unknowns. J Pain Symptom Mgmt 1997; 14:S36–S48.
116. Hassenbusch, et al. Current practice in IT therapy. JPSM 2000.
117. Cousins MJ. Anesthetic approaches in cancer pain. Adv Pain Res Ther 16; 1990:249–273.
118. Payne R. Neuropathic pain syndromes, with special reference to causalgia and reflex sympathetic dystrophy. Clin J Pain 1986; 2:59–73.
119. Warfield CA, Crews DA. Use of stellate ganglion blocks in the treatment of intractable limb pain in lung cancer. Clin J Pain 1987; 3:13.
120. Doyle D. Nerve blocks in advanced cancer. Practitioner 1982; 226:539–544.
121. Peyton Wt, Semansky EJ, Baker AB. Subarachnoid injection of alcohol for relief of intractable pain with discussion of cord changes found at autopsy. Am J Cancer 1937; 30:709.
122. Smith MC. Histological findings following intrathecal injections of phenol solutions for relief of pain. Br J Anaesth 1963; 36:387–406.
123. Swerdlow M. Intrathecal neurolysis. Anaesthesia 1978; 33:733–740.
124. Katz J. The current role of neurolytic agents. Adv Neurol 1974; 4:471–476.
125. Swerdlow M. Subarachnoid and extradural blocks. Adv Pain Res Ther 1979; 2:325–337.
126. Hay RC. Subarachnoid alcohol block in the control of intractable pain. Anesth Analg 1962; 41:12–16.
127. Stovner J, Endresen R. Intrathecal phenol for cancer pain. Acta Anaesthesiol Scand 1972; 16:17–21.
128. Holland AJC, Youssef M. A complication of subarachnoid phenol blockade. Anaesthesia 1979; 34:260–262.
129. Racz GB, Heavner J, Haynsworth R. Repeat epidural phenol injections in chronic pain and spasticity. In: Lipton S, Miles J, eds. Persistent Pain. Vol. 5. Orlando: Grune & Stratton, 1985:157–179.
130. Brown BL, Bulley CK, Quiel EC. Neurolytic celiac plexus block for pancreatic cancer pain. Anesth Analg 1987; 66:869–873.
131. Eisenberg, Carr DB. Celiac plexus block for abdominal pain associated with malignancy: a meta-analysis. Anesth Analg 1995; 80:290–295.
132. Matamala AM, Lopez FV, Martinez LI. Percutaneous approach to the celiac plexus using CT guidance. Pain 1988; 34:285–288.
133. Wong GY, Schroeder DR, Carns PE, et al. Effect of neurolytic celiac plexus block on pain relief, quality of life, and survival in patients with unresectable pancreatic cancer: a randomized controlled trail. JAMA 2004; 291:1092–1099.
134. Racz GB, Holubec JT. Stellate ganglion phenol neurolysis. In: Racz GB, ed. Techniques of Neurolysis. Boston: Kluwer, 1989:133–143.
135. Plancarte R, Amescua C, Patt R, et al. Superior hypogastric plexus block for pelvic cancer pain. Anesthesiology 1990; 73:236.
136. De Leon-Casasola OA, Kent E, Lema MJ. Neurolytic superior hypogastric plexus block for chronic pelvic pain associated with cancer. Pain 1993; 54:145–151.

137. Plancarte R, Amescua C, Patt RB. Presacral blockade of the ganglion impar (ganglion of Walther). Anesthesiology 1990; 73:A751.
138. Patti JW, Neerman Z, Wood BJ. Radiofrequency ablation for cancer-associated pain. J Pain 2002; 3(6): 471–473.
139. Madrid JL, Bonica JJ. Cranial nerve blocks. In: Bonica JJ, Ventafridda V, eds. Adv Pain Res Ther. Vol. 2. New York: Raven Press, 1979:463–468.
140. Waldman SD, Feldstein GS, Allen ML, et al. Cervical epidural implantable narcotic delivery systems in the management of upper body pain. Anesth Analg 1987; 66:780–782.
141. Lobato RD, Madrid JL, Fatela LV, et al. Intraventricular morphine for intractable cancer pain: rationale, methods, clinical results. Acta Anaesthesiol Scand 1987; 31:68–74.
142. Fourney DR, Schomer DF, Nader R, Chlan-Fourney J, Suki D, Ahrar K, Rhines LD, Gokaslan ZL. Percutaneous vertebroplasty and kyphoplasty for painful vertebral body fractures in cancer patients. J Neurosurg (Spine 1) 2003; 98:21–30.
143. Lahuerta J, Lipton S, Miles J, et al. Update on percutaneous cervical cordotomy and pituitary alcohol neuroadenolysis: an audit of our recent results and complications. In: Lipton S, Miles J, eds. Persistent Pain. Vol. 5. New York: Grune & Stratton, 1985: 197–223.
144. Watling CJ, Payne R, Allen RR, Hassenbusch S. Commissural myelotomy for intractable cancer pain: report of two cases. Clin J Pain 1996; 12:151–156.
145. Lipton S. Percutaneous cordotomy. In: Wall PD, Melzack R, eds. Textbook of Pain. New York: Churchill Livingstone, 1984:632–638.
146. Mount BM. Psychological and social aspects of cancer pain. In: Wall PD, Melzack R, eds. Textbook of Pain. Edinburgh: Churchill Livingstone, 1984:460–471.
147. Syrjala KL, Donaldson GW, Davis MW, et al. Relaxation and imagery and cognitive-behavioral training reduce pain during cancer treatment: a controlled clinical trial. Pain 1995; 63:189–198.
148. Angarola RT, Wray SD. Legal impediments to cancer pain treatment. Adv Pain Res Ther 1089; 11:213.
149. Smith JL. Care of people who are dying: the hospice approach. In: Patt R, ed. Cancer Pain Management: a Multidisciplinary Approach. Philadelphia: Lippincott, 1993:543–552.
150. Doyle D. Education and training in palliative care. J Palliat Care 1987; 2:5.

58

Palliative Care

SURESH K. REDDY, AHMED ELSAYEM, and
RUDRANATH TALUKDAR

Department of Palliative Care and Rehabilitation for Medicine, The University of Texas M.D. Anderson Cancer Center, Houston, Texas, U.S.A.

The term palliative care may be defined as the interdisciplinary care of patients and families focused on the relief of suffering and improving quality of life. This can occur in cancer as well as in other advanced diseases, where symptoms predominate both during treatment as well as toward the end of life.

Palliative care differs from other specialties in terms of approach, which is predominantly interdisciplinary in nature, and geared both toward patients and families. The main disciplines are medicine, nursing, social work, and chaplaincy. Pharmacists, physical and occupational therapists, nutritionist, speech therapist, volunteers, bereavement counselors, psychologists, and those from other disciplines are also frequently included. Disciplines are sometimes tailored to the needs of the patients.

The World Health Organization has put forth a definition of palliative medicine (1): "Palliative care is an approach that improves the quality of life of patients and their families facing the problem associated with life-threatening illness, through the prevention and relief of suffering by means of early identification and impeccable assessment and treatment of pain and other problems, physical, psychosocial and spiritual."

I. PRINCIPLES OF SYMPTOM CONTROL: ASSESSMENT AND TREATMENT

A. Assessment

A multidisciplinary assessment is the key to the successful management of symptoms in advanced cancer. The domains that need to be assessed include:

1. *Intensity of symptoms* on a 0–10 scale with a simple tool of Edmonton Symptom Assessment Scale (2). This scale provides graphical display of all symptoms in real time and helps decision-making on a day-to-day basis.
2. *Psychosocial assessment* includes questions pertaining to loss of autonomy, family conflicts, financial issues, social standing, fear of death, depression, and anxiety. Cognitive function is assessed by the mini mental state examination (3).
3. *Spiritual assessment* includes questions pertaining to meaning of life, God, hope, "Why me?" and "God will heal everything."

Table 1 List of Symptoms in Cancer

Fatigue
Pain
Dyspnea
Delirium
Anorexia/cachexia
Nausea/vomiting
Depression
Anxiety
Constipation
Insomnia

B. Principles of Treatment

1. Pharmacotherapy
2. Interventional management
3. Counseling
4. Behavioral management
5. Spiritual management
6. Bereavement care

Symptoms in patients with advanced incapacitating illness include fatigue, pain, anorexia, nausea, dyspnea, constipation, anxiety, depression, and cachexia (see Table 1.)

1. Fatigue

Fatigue is one of the most common symptoms in cancer patients (4), experienced by 70–100% in patients receiving cancer treatment (5). Fatigue refers to a subjective sense of decreased vitality in physical and/or mental functioning that usually occurs in the setting of medical disease. The physical dimension is usually described as a perception of muscle weakness or a tendency to fatigue rapidly. Physical activity is difficult to sustain and in some cases dyspnea accompanies minimal exertion. Rest or sleep does not return perceived strength or stamina to normal. The mental component is described as lack of interest or motivation in objects or activities. Other symptoms include difficulty in concentrating or maintaining attention. Mood may be flat or depressed. Lethargy or tendency to somnolence may be noted, but there is not a need for excessive sleep. Rest or sleep may improve symptoms, but do not eliminate them. Fatigue is experienced both during treatment as well as during terminal stages. For patients with advanced cancer, however, fatigue may be a severe symptom that either decreases their capacity for physical and mental work or renders them completely unable to function normally. Fatigue gets worse as the disease progresses toward the end stage. The presence of fatigue may also magnify other symptoms affecting the patient. The causes of fatigue are multifactorial and interrelated. These include problems related to the cancer itself, treatment side effects or toxicities, underlying systemic pathophysiologic disorders, and other causes (Fig. 1).

Assessment of Fatigue

The severity of fatigue can be measured on a scale of 0–10 (where 0 equals no fatigue and 10 equals the worst fatigue imaginable), as in ESAS, or by other numeric or verbal rating scales. Like other symptoms in cancer, the assessment of fatigue should focus on the multidimensional aspect. The impact of fatigue on activities, function, and the quality of life should be assessed. Laboratory investigations and imaging studies should be based upon indications derived from the patient history and physical examination.

Management of Fatigue

As with other problematic symptoms in advanced cancer patients, management of fatigue should address possible underlying etiologies as well as the patient's expression of symptoms (3,6).

Treat underlying problems: pain, depression, anxiety, stress, or sleep disturbances. Dehydration should be corrected and an attempt should be made to treat cachexia in appropriate cases. Simplify the medication regimes, and treat infections as well as anemia with transfusions where appropriate. Administer epoetin alpha 10,000 U subcutaneously three times weekly as indicated (7). Low-dose steroids may alleviate some of the symptoms of fatigue in advanced cancer patients (8,9). Psychostimulants, like methylphenidate 5–10 mg in the morning and same dose at noon, may be useful if the patient is experiencing concomitant problems such as depression, hypoactive delirium, or drowsiness due to opioids (10,11). Some antidepressants, like serotonin-specific reuptake inhibitors, may improve energy levels in some fatigued patients, though their benefit is unproven. Recently, there is increasing evidence that hypogonadism in cancer patients on chronic opioid therapy may suffer from fatigue (12). Replacement therapy with testosterone may improve fatigue in these patients, but needs to be studied in future. Bruera et al. (13) showed that patient-controlled methylphenidate administration rapidly improved fatigue and other symptoms.

2. Dyspnea

Dyspnea is defined as the "uncomfortable awareness of breathing" (14). It is described in terms of air hunger, suffocation, choking, or heavy breathing. It

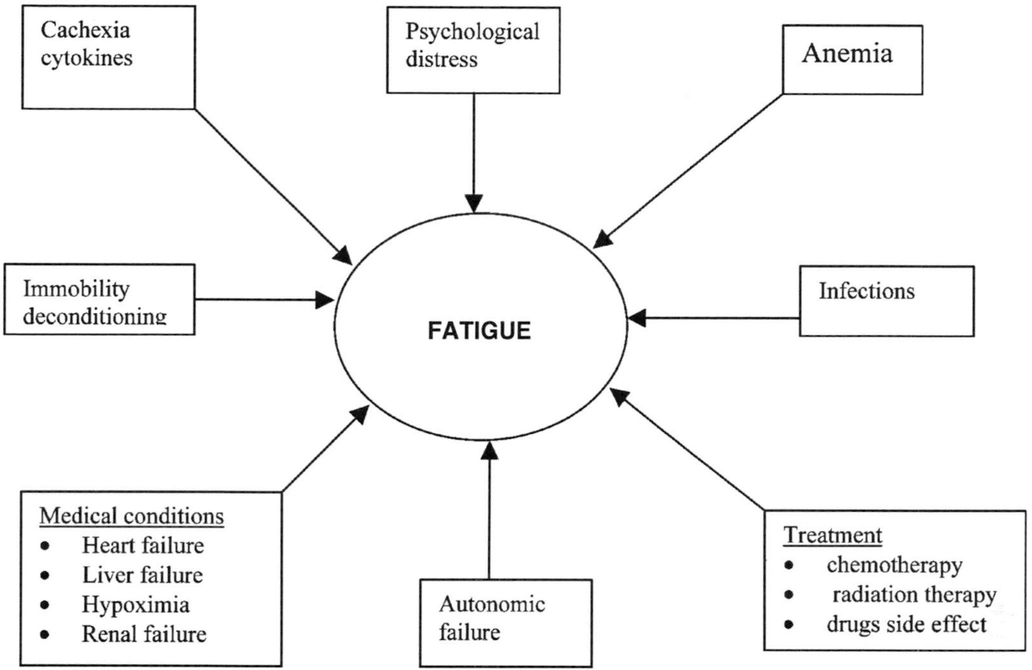

Figure 1 Causes of fatigue.

is a subjective sensation, associated with and impacted by factors such as location and progression of the tumor, psychosocial phenomenon (15), and preexisting chronic lung pathology like chronic obstructive airway disease, asthma, and congestive heart failure. The frequency and severity of dyspnea depend on the stage of the disease, and it increases in frequency when death is imminent.

Dyspnea as a lonely symptom or in association with other parameters is a bad prognostic indicator of survival (16,17). Dyspnea is a multidimensional symptom influenced by factors such as anxiety, tumor location, fatigue, and other factors. Dyspnea can be caused by a number of clinical conditions, but the cause mainly falls into two categories:

1. Dyspnea with abnormal mechanics of ventilation, e.g., cachexia, asthenia, myasthenia syndrome, Eaton Lambert syndrome, etc., and
2. Dyspnea with the normal mechanics of ventilation. This category may be subdivided into a respiratory and no respiratory causes of dyspnea (see Table 2).

Assessment of Dyspnea

Dyspnea is a complex symptom, caused by various factors, some not well understood. But a thorough history, with physical examination, with appropriate laboratory and imaging studies should be undertaken to assess dyspnea. Some of the factors that contribute to dyspnea include anxiety, phobia, pain, and fatigue.

Treatment of Dyspnea

The aim of the dyspnea treatment is a subjective improvement in the patient's perception. Treatment involves treating the cause and the symptoms as well as managing psychosocial issues contributing to dyspnea.

Treatment of the Cause

Treating of the underlying cause is attempted as an initial step. Various treatments may include thoracentesis for pleural effusion, blood transfusion for anemia, corticosteroids for carcinomatosis lymphangitis, anticoagulants for pulmonary embolism, and antibiotics for pneumonia.

Symptomatic Treatment

OXYGEN THERAPY: Long-term oxygen therapy has been shown to have beneficial effects on the outcome of patients with chronic obstructive pulmonary disease (18,19). Studies in cancer dyspnea suggest beneficial effects of oxygen in cancer patients in cross-over trials (20,21). Oxygen may be given by nasal cannula and may be humidified whenever feasible. Oxygen treatment towards the end of life may lead to anxiety

Table 2 Causes of Dyspnea in Cancer Patients[a]

Dyspnea with abnormal mechanisms of ventilation	Dyspnea with normal mechanisms of ventilation
Asthenia	*Direct effect of the tumor*
Cachexia	Primary or metastatic tumor
Myasthenia gravis	Pleural effusion/pericardial infusion
Eaten Lambert syndrome	Superior vena cava syndrome
Rib fracture	Carcinomatous lymphangitis
Chest wall deformity	Atelectasis
Neuromuscular disease (motor neuron disease)	Phrenic nerve palsy
	Trachael obstruction
	Trachael-esophageal fistula
	Carcinomatous infiltration of the chest wall (carcinoma en cuirasse)
	Effect of therapy
	Postactinic fibrosis
	Postpneumectomy
	Mitomycin-vinca alkaloid (acute dyspnea syndrome)
	Bleomycin-induced fibrosis
	Adriamycin- and cyclophosphamide-induced cardiomyopathy
	Not directly related to the tumor or therapy
	Anemia
	Ascites
	Metabolic acidosis
	Fever
	COPD
	Asthma
	Pulmonary embolism
	Pneumonia
	Pneumothorax
	Heart failure
	Obesity
	Thyrotoxicosis
	Psychosocial distress (i.e., anxiety, somatization)
	Unknown

[a] Physician to check off causes of dyspnea. More than one may be checked.

among family members, who sometimes interpret this as a way of prolonging life and suffering. Counseling of family members about this issue is of paramount importance.

Drug therapy: A number of pharmacological agents have been tried effectively to relieve the perception of dyspnea in terminal cancer patients. The major drugs are opioids, corticosteroids, and benzodiazepines. Many studies found that opioids of different types, doses, and routes of administration are capable of relieving dyspnea (22,23). Nebulized opioids have also been shown to be effective in some studies (24–28). There are some conflicting studies about the use of nebulized opioids to treat dyspnea (29). Opioids act possibly by reducing the subjective sensation of dyspnea without reducing respiratory rate or oxygen saturation. They also possibly cause venodilation of pulmonary vessels, thereby reducing preload to the heart and improve breathing. Corticosteroids are only useful if dyspnea is caused by carcinomatosis lymphangitis, or in superior vena cava syndrome. They also may play a role if associated COPD or asthma coexist in a patient (30). Benzodiazepines have a limited role in dyspnea, except when anxiety and apprehension is the cause of dyspnea. Subsequently, they are commonly used medications for terminal dyspnea in hospice settings. Bronchodilators play a role if dyspnea is caused by bronchospasm. Both nebulized and oral agents are used. In a study by Congleton and Muers (31), bronchodilators provided significant relief of dyspnea in patients with lung carcinoma and airflow obstruction. Sometimes phenothiazines such as chlorpromazine may help in drying secretions and help in reducing anxiety (32).

General supportive measures: A number of measures can be implemented for the support of both the patient and the family. Relaxation techniques or a guided imagery provide relief in patients with anticipatory or anxiety-driven dyspnea. Assist devices can be used to minimize muscle effort. Maneuvers such as postural drainage and incentive spirometry can help in special situations.

3. *Delirium*

Delirium is defined as a transient organic brain syndrome characterized by the acute onset of disordered attention (arousal) and cognition, accompanied by disturbances of psychomotor behavior and perception (33). Delirium is common with progressive disease and is common in patients with pancreatic cancer near death. It may signal a new and serious medical complication, markedly impair the function and comfort of the patient, and increase the family's distress (34). The prevalence of delirium in hospitalized medical and surgical patients is approximately 10% and the prevalence in hospitalized cancer patients ranges from 8% to 40% (35–37). Causes of delirium are listed in Table 3.

Clinical Features

The symptoms and signs of delirium fluctuate; therefore, careful attention should be paid to the mental status examination. The diagnosis is established by a new onset of cognitive dysfunction, accompanied by a disturbance of arousal or clouding of consciousness. Three clinical variants have been described based on the type of arousal disturbance: hypoalert-hypoactive, hyperalert-hyperactive, and mixed type (38,39). The presenting features include memory impairment or confusion, dysphoria, hypomania, illusions, hallucinations, and altered arousal state. The DSM-IV American Psychiatric Association (40) criteria for delirium have been considered gold standard for diagnosis of delirium. These include impairment in responsiveness and alertness as manifested by fluctuating inability to maintain or shift attention to external stimuli, cognitive dysfunction of recent onset, development of the disturbance over a short period of time, evidence from history, physical examination, or laboratory findings etiologically related to the disturbance.

Table 3 Causes of Delirium

Tumor related
Primary brain tumor or metastatic brain metastasis
Leptomeningeal disease
Paraneoplastic syndromes
Seizure
Metabolic
Electrolyte imbalance
Metabolic encephalopathy secondary organ failure
Hypercalcemia
Medications
Chemotherapeutic agents, e.g., ifosfamide
Opioid medications
Benzodiazepines
Antiemetics
Steroids
Anticholinergics
Infection
Sepsis
Pneumonia
Vascular:
Thromboembolic phenomenon
Intracranial hemorrhage

Assessment

Delirium is a frequently missed diagnosis and more frequently it is misdiagnosed as insomnia, anxiety, or depression because the presenting symptoms may mimic any of these conditions. Understanding the patient baseline, listening to the family members' and nurses' observations will help pick up the diagnosis of delirium before the condition is florid and out of control. The cause of the delirium should be investigated if possible since the treatment will depend on correction of the cause. The history is of utmost importance, especially the acute onset of the condition. Medications particularly opioids, benzodiazepines, some antiemetics, and corticosteroids are frequent causes of delirium. Physical examination may reveal signs of dehydration or increased intracranial pressure. Laboratory examinations may show hypercalcemia, hyponatremia, renal or hepatic failure.

Treatment of Delirium

If the diagnosis of delirium is suspected, the clinician should act immediately to establish the diagnosis and remove inciting medication if this is the likely cause. Safety is of paramount importance, especially in the agitated (hyperactive) type, since patients may endanger themselves by removing intravenous lines, fall, or walkout. Educating family members and nurses is important. The appropriate management includes identifying and treating the underlying causes. Other reversible causes should be identified and corrected. If opioids is the cause, dosage reduction or rotation to a different opioid should be attempted. Treating infection, hydrating a dehydrated patient, or correcting hypercalcemia may be all what is needed to treat the delirious patient. Symptomatic treatment to control agitation is achieved by the use of neuroleptics. Haloperidol remains the drug of choice for the treatment of delirium. It is a dopamine blocker with less sedative effects and low incidence of cardiovascular and anticholinergic side effects. Mostly, haloperidol in the dosage of 1–3 mg/day is effective in treating agitation paranoia and fear. A higher dose may be needed in special circumstances. Sometimes, acute dystonias and extrapyramidal side effects are seen with haloperidol, in which case beztropine can be administered. Methotrimeprazine is sometimes used effectively to control agitation. It has also been shown to be an analgesic. Newer novel antipsychotics such as olanzapine (41) are as effective and may be useful in patient with anxiety and depressive symptoms. Sometimes, a combination of haloperidol with benzodiazepine is useful. In a study by Brietbart et al. (42), lorazepam alone was ineffective in the treatment of delirium and, in fact, contributed to the worsening of delirium and increased cognitive impairment. In severe cases, a palliative care consultation is important and if the condition proves to be refractory to antipsychotic in terminal cases, sedation will be considered.

4. *Depression*

Depression is a common and devastating problem for patients with cancer and other terminal diseases. Major depression can affect from 25% to 35% of cancer patients (43). This prevalence touches 77% in those with advanced disease (44). Pancreatic cancer is more likely to be associated with depression. The depression in pancreatic cancer will have even greater loss of appetite, weight loss, low energy, etc. Thus, it can be critically important to diagnose and treat depression early, thereby ameliorating some of the physiological changes that are inevitable with advanced cancer. The cause of depression in pancreatic cancer is unclear, may be caused by indirect effect of cancer on serotonergic function of brain, or may result from psychological reaction to cancer (45). Pain has a close correspondence to psychiatric illness. It is twice as likely that patients reporting pain will have a psychiatric diagnosis (46).

The cardinal features of depression include loss of interest or pleasure, impaired decision-making ability, changes in appetite, sleep, psychomotor activity, decreased energy, feeling of guilt and/or worthlessness. Mild episodes may be masked by increased effort on the part of the individual.

Assessment of Depression

Diagnosis is confounded by the presence of normal sadness and grief and also by delirium. Anhedonia can be mistaken for the fatigue that occurs in cancer patients. Assessing depression quickly and accurately is important. There are no clear-cut guidelines on assessing depression in terminal cancer patients. A recent report by Fisch et al. (47) suggested the usefulness of a brief two-question assessment of depression in advanced cancer patients with the primary objective being to measure the quality of life after intervention with fluoxetine and the secondary objective being to assess the reduction in depression. Other validated measures of assessing depression in the primary care setting include the WHO-5 Well Being Index (48), HAM-D (Hamilton rating scale for depression), and MADRS (Montgomery Asberg depression rating scale). The patient should be evaluated for depressive episodes and substance abuse, family history of depression and suicide, concurrent life stressors, losses secondary to cancer, and availability of social support.

Delirium, particularly in the early stages, is often misidentified as depression and is treated as such with poor effects (49). The key is to accurately diagnose the clinical problem. In doubtful situations, a consultation with a palliative care physician or a psychiatrist should be obtained.

Treatment

A combination or a balanced approach of supportive psychotherapy and pharmacotherapy is key to the optimal treatment of depression. Individual or group counseling has been shown to be useful (50). Other methods include relaxation techniques, guided imagery (50), and music therapy (51). Counseling both patients and their family is crucial to treat depression successfully. This helps to reduce anxiety, allows patients to express their fears and disappointments in a "safe" way and enhances well being.

Pharmacotherapy

The mainstay of treatment of depression is pharmacotherapy.

The agents commonly employed include newer selective serotonin reuptake inhibitors (SSRIs), tricyclic antidepressants (TCAs), and psychostimulants. The SSRIs fluoxitene hydrochloride, sertraline hydrochloride, paroxitene hydrochloride, citalopram, and recently escitalopram have gained popularity due to fewer side-effect profile compared to TCAs. For mild depression, SSRIs are very useful. They however take weeks to effect a change. Some, such as escitalopram have a lower profile of side effects and work a little faster than the first generation SSRIs such as fluoxetine. The side effects are generally mild and include problematic ones such as reduced appetite, nausea, and anxiety. These tend to be limited in duration and have not been a limiting factor in their application in cancer patients. Other problems arise from their mechanism of action and include diarrhea, fatigue, sexual dysfunction. If a switch from an SSRI to another medication, especially MAO-I (monoamine oxidase inhibitors) is considered, the wash-out period of various SSRIs will need to be taken into account. As such, it may be useful to have a patient take SSRIs such as sertraline or escitalopram, which have a shorter wash-out, compared with older one's such as fluoxetine. Our experience has shown methylphenidate to be particularly useful especially in patients with a limited life expectancy, where a few weeks may be too much to ask (51). Methylphenidate also helps to reduce the symptoms of fatigue, a common problem in cancer patients, and that makes it a potentially useful medication for a number of reasons (52).

Tricyclic antidepressants have been used and work faster than SSRIs; however, they have more side effects, some of which (like the anticholinergic effects) can be a major problem for older cancer patients. They do offer additional benefits for patients suffering from neuropathic pain. For that reason, these medications should be started at a low dose and slowly escalated as tolerated. Desipramine and nortryptiline are generally better tolerated in the older population as compared to amitryptiline and imipramine.

In a recent study, mirtazapine was found to be effective in ameliorating symptoms of depression in cancer patients (53). Some additional benefits of mirtazapine may accrue from its beneficial effects on chemotherapy-induced nausea/vomiting (CINV) and insomnia (54).

5. *Constipation*

Constipation is the infrequent and difficult passage of hard stool. It is a very common cause of morbidity in the palliative care setting and is thought to affect the overwhelming majority (>95%) of patients consuming opioids for cancer-related pain syndromes (55,56). Constipation can be a difficult condition to assess and treat because of the wide variety of presenting symptoms. Patients may report a feeling of incomplete evacuation, bloating, decreased appetite, or generalized abdominal discomfort or pain. Due to the wide variability in normal bowel movement patterns in individual patients, the diagnosis of constipation can only be made in comparison with an individual's normal pattern (57).

Causes

The most common causes of constipation include opioid medication, and progressive disease. Other causes include anorexia/ cachexia, bowel obstruction, immobility, hypercalcemia and dehydration. In the palliative care setting, careful attention must be given to the multifactorial nature of constipation. The common causes of constipation are outlined in Table 4.

Complications

Although constipation is often overlooked in the setting of other comorbid conditions, it is not necessarily a benign condition and some of the complications of unrelieved constipation can indeed be life-threatening (58). Severe constipation can lead to bowel obstruction with attendant issues of severe morbidity. In patients who are neutropenic, severe constipation can lead to bacterial transfer across the colon with bacteremia and sepsis.

Table 4 Causes of Constipation in Advanced Cancer Patients

Structural abnormalities
Obstruction
Pelvic tumor mass
Radiation fibrosis
Painful anorectal conditions
Anal fissure, hemorrhoids, perianal abscess
Drugs
Opioids
Agents with antichlinergic actions
Anticholinergics
Antispasmodics
Antidepressants
Antipsychotics (e.g., phenothiazines, haloperidol)
Antiacids (aluminum-containing)
Antiemetics (e.g., ondansetron)
Diuretics
Anticonvulsants
Iron
Antihypertensive agents
Anticancer drugs (e.g., vinca alkaloids)
Metabolic disturbances
Dehydration (vomiting, fever, polyuria, poor fluid intake, diuretic use)
Hypercalcemia
Hypokalemia
Uremia
Diabetes
Hypothyroidism
Neurological disorders
Cerebral tumors
Spinal cord compression
Sacral nerve infiltration
Autonomic failure

Diagnosis

The diagnosis of constipation begins with a careful history of the patient's recent bowel movements. Specific topics to be queried include the date of the last bowel movement, the characteristics of the stool (hard vs. soft, loose vs. formed, "ribbon-like" vs. "pellet-like"), the degree of straining and pain involved, and whether or not the movement felt complete. Related questions include whether or not there was blood in the stool (possibly identifying tumor mass or a hemorrhoid) or an urge to defecate at all (suggesting colonic inertia).

After the history, a careful physical examination should include the abdominal examination (distension, firmness, tenderness, the presence or absence of bowel sounds) and a rectal examination. The rectal examination should assess the presence of hard stool in the vault and may reveal the presence of masses, hemorrhoids, fissures, or fistulae. Caution should be exercised in performing a rectal examination on anyone with neutropenia or thrombocytopenia.

In addition to the history and physical examination, a simple "constipation score" (59) may also be obtained. A flat abdominal radiograph of the abdomen is obtained and the colon is divided into four quadrants (ascending, transverse, descending, and sigmoid) by drawing a large X with the umbilicus in the middle. Each quadrant is assigned a score from 0 to 3 based on the degree of stool in the lumen. A score of 0 indicates no stool, a score of 1 indicates "less than 50%" occupancy, a score of 2 indicates "greater than 50% occupancy" and a score of 3 indicates complete occupancy of the lumen with stool. Scores may range from 0 to 12 and score of 7 (or greater) indicates severe constipation.

Prevention and Treatment

Prevention of constipation includes patient education on the various reasons for constipation, encouragement of adequate fluid intake, and prescribing stool softeners and laxatives. In addition, a high degree of vigilance should be maintained regarding the patient's other medications that may cause constipation.

Initial treatment of constipation includes starting the patient on a stool-softening agent (e.g., docusate 100–240 mg/os twice daily) with a laxative agent (e.g., senna 1–2 tablets twice daily). Refractory constipation may be managed with lactulose 30 mL/os every 6 hr until a large bowel movement occurs. Intractable cases may require a bisacodyl suppository, milk-and-molasses enema, or Fleets enema. Proximal impaction may require magnesium citrate. In rare cases, where hard stools are present in the vault, manual disimpaction may be necessary. In refractory cases opioid antagonist, naloxone, given orally may result in laxation (60–62). Mild opioid withdrawal may be seen with naloxone. Recently, methylnaltrexone, given parenterally, is showing promising effects on opioid-induced constipation (63,64).

6. *Chronic Nausea*

Nausea and vomiting are highly unpleasant symptoms that affect between 40% and 70% of patients in the palliative care setting (65–67). In the cancer setting, nausea is prevalent in patients under the age of 65, females and patients with breast, stomach, or gynecologic cancers. The etiology of chronic nausea is often multifactorial and can be due to the underlying disease, its treatment, or as a side effect of medications that treat cancer-related pain (e.g., opioids) (Fig. 2). The underlying cause of nausea should be ascertained, if possible, and the selection of the antiemetic agent should be tailored to maximize therapeutic value (65). Table 5 lists the common causes of nausea in the cancer setting. Medication side effects and chronic constipation are the most common causes. As shown Figure 3, the experience of nausea and vomiting is generated as a result of the complex interrelationship between the chemoreceptor trigger zone (CTZ) and the vomiting center (VC). Chemoreceptor trigger zone can be affected directly by drugs, toxins, or metabolites or receives afferent impulses from chemoreceptors and mechanoreceptors originating in the gastrointestinal tract, chest, or pelvis and subsequently influence the vomiting center. The VC also receives direct input from the cerebral cortex.

Assessment

The etiology of nausea should be determined, if at all possible, since proper management will depend on identifying and treating the underlying cause. The assessment of the patient with nausea should be part of the multidimensional approach to assess multiple symptoms simultaneously. It begins by taking detailed history including the onset of the nausea, duration, frequency of episodes, and severity of the episode, on a 0–10 scale of ESAS. In addition, since chronic constipation is one of the main causes of nausea, bowel function should also be assessed. The list of medications should be reviewed for possible medication side effects.

The examination of the patient should focus on life-threatening complications related to dehydration such as hypotension and tachycardia and if present should be corrected promptly. The abdominal exam, looking for signs of obstruction or constipation, the CNS exam to rule out raised intracranial pressure, and possibly

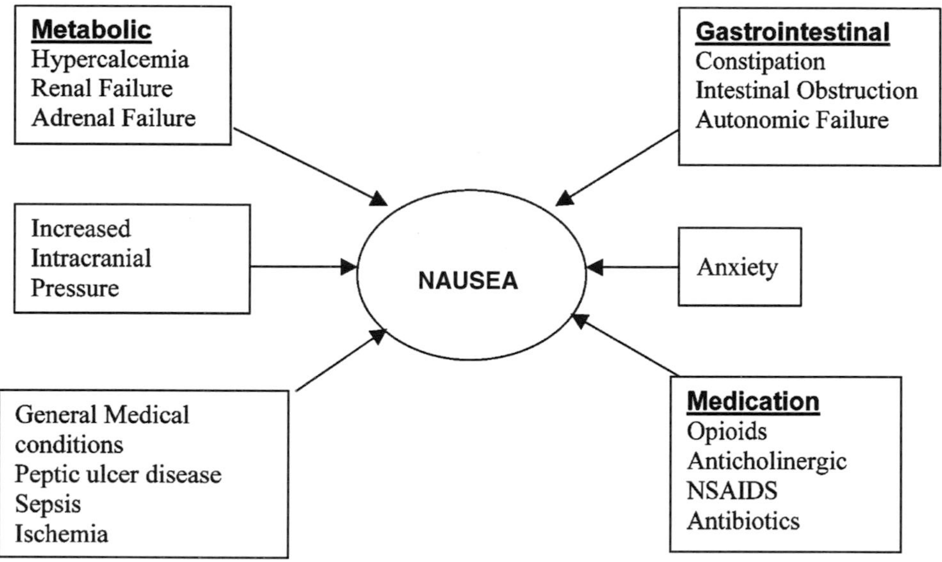

Figure 2 Causes of nausea.

even the cardiac exam to rule out initial symptoms for a major cardiac event should be performed.

Diagnostic tests include serum evaluation of electrolytes, serum calcium, liver and renal function tests. Abdominal x-rays may be obtained to gauge the degree of constipation (see the Constipation section). Brain imaging may be considered if clinically appropriate.

Treatment

Correction of the underlying problem should be attempted if a cause could be found. Treating constipation or removing the inciting medication may relieve the nausea if it is caused by any of them. Steroids or radiation may help nausea caused by increased intracranial pressure. If opioids is the cause adding antiemetic may help, but rarely opioid rotation may be required.

Table 5 Causes of Nausea in Cancer Patients

Metabolic
Hypercalcemia
Renal Failure
Adrenal Failure
Increased intracranial pressure
General Medical conditions
Peptic ulcer disease
Sepsis
Gastrointestinal
Constipation
Intestinal obstruction
Autonomic failure
Anxiety
Medication
Opioids
Anticholinergic
NSAIDS

Pharmacological Therapy

Pharmacological therapy should be directed towards the underlying problem. Table 6 lists the most commonly used antiemetics. For most chronic, opioid-related nausea, a prokinetic agent such as metoclopramide (10 mg/os/intravenous/subcutaneous every 4–6 hr) is helpful. The antidopaminergic properties of haloperidol (1–2 mg/os/intravenous/subcutaneous every 4–8 hr) may help certain forms of refractory nausea. The 5HT3 antagonists (e.g., ondansetron 4–8 mg/os/intravenous/subcutaneous) may help chemotherapy-related nausea (65,66), but is less helpful in chronic nausea. Moreover, these agents are expensive and constipating. Octreotide, a somatostatin analogue that reduces gastric motility and secretions is helpful in nausea caused by intestinal obstruction. Benzodiazepines and other H1 antagonists may help anxiety-provoked nausea. Finally, steroids have been shown to be helpful for nausea both with a direct effect (e.g., in certain chemotherapy or opioid-related problems with nausea) and by an indirect effect (e.g., reducing intracranial pressure in patients with intracranial neoplasms) (67,68).

7. *Cachexia*

The cachexia syndrome, characterized by a marked weight loss, anorexia, asthenia, and anemia, is invari-

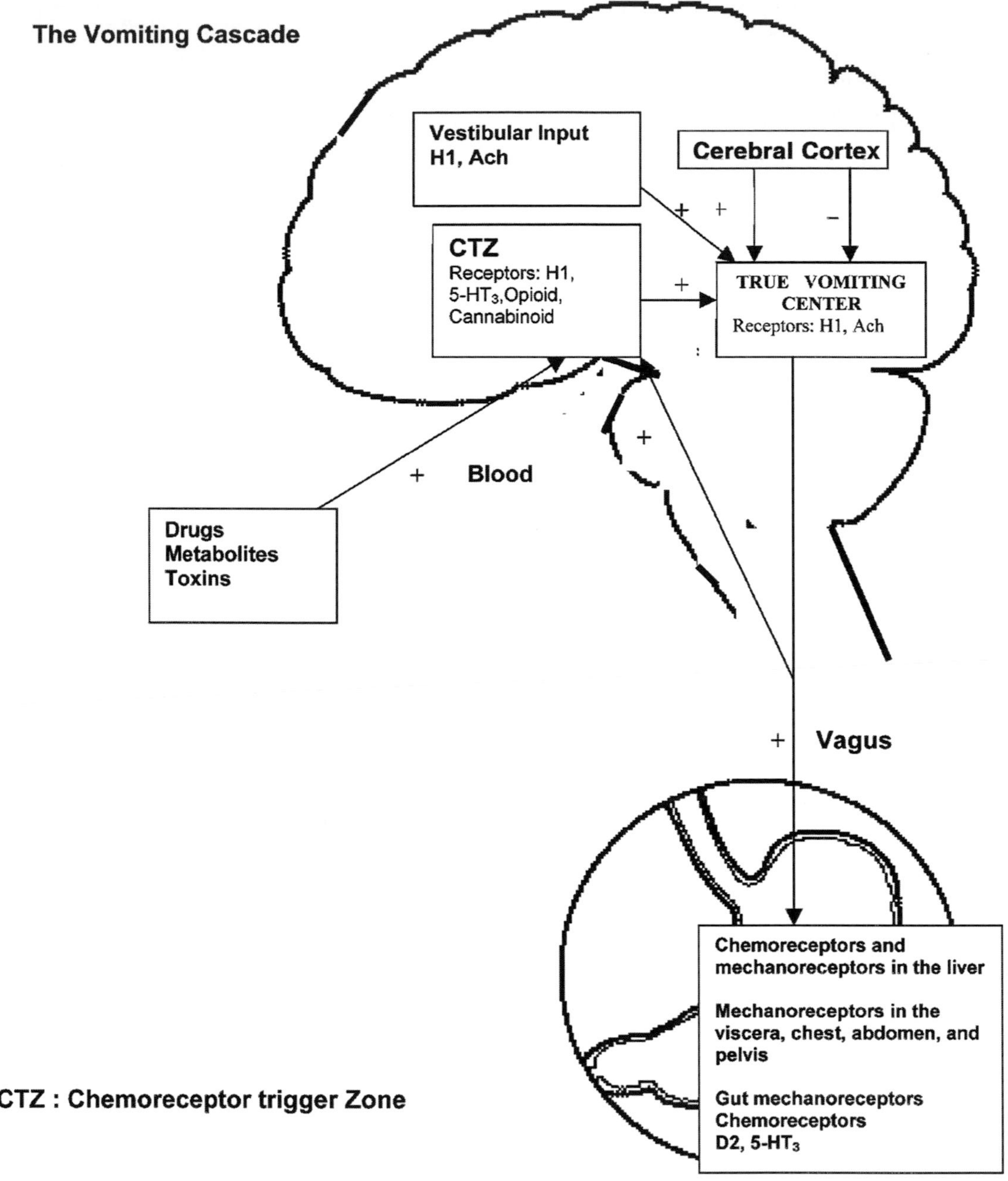

Figure 3 The vomiting cascade.

ably associated with the growth of a tumor and leads to a malnutrition status caused by the induction of anorexia or decreased food intake. In addition, the competition for nutrients between the tumor and the host results in an accelerated catabolism state, which promotes severe metabolic disturbances in the patient. Cachexia is a complex metabolic syndrome characterized clinically by progressive involuntary weight loss, which can lead to the death of the host. The mechanism is not precisely known, but represents abnormalities of carbohydrate, fat, protein, and energy metabolism. Cachexia is found in majority of patients with advanced cancer, and is a major contributing factor of death in about 50% of these patients (69). Cachexia leads to diminished appetite, weight loss, severe lethargy, fatigue, and generalized weakness known as asthenia. Patients with this syndrome are prone to have side effects and respond poorly to treatment. Cachexia commonly tends to occur in patients with solid tumors, in children, and in elderly

Table 6 Antiemetic Drugs: Drugs Useful for the Treatment of Chronic Nausea

Drug[a]	Main receptor	Main indication	Starting po dose/route	Equivalent price[b]	Side effects
Metoclopramide	D2	Opioid induced; gastric stasis	10 mg every 4 hr; po, sc, iv	1	EPS (akathisia, dystonia, dyskinesia)
Prochlorperazine	D2	Opioid induced	10 mg every 6 hr; po, iv	3	Sedation hypotension
Cyclizine	H1	Vestibular causes intestinal obstruction	25–50 mg every 8 hr; po, sc, pr	—	Sedation, dry mouth, blurred vision
Promethazine	H1	Vestibular, motion sickness, obstruction	12.5 mg every 4 hr; po, pr, iv	2	Sedation
Haloperidol	D2	Opioid, chemical, metabolic	1-2 mg bid; po, iv, sc	1	Rarely EPS
Ondansetron	5 HT_3	Chemotherapy	4–8 mg every 8 hr; po, iv	84	Headache constipation
Diphenhydramine	H1, Ach	Intestinal obstruction, vestibular, ICP	25 mg every 6 hr; po, iv, sc	0.2	Sedation, dry mouth, blurred vision
Hyoscine	Ach	Intestinal obstruction, colic, secretions	0.2–0.4 mg every 4 hr; sl, sc, td	0.4	Dry mouth, blurred vision, urine retention, agitation

[a] Corticosteroids not included because of varied doses and limited indications (see text).
[b] Prices are compared to metoclopramide 10 mg tablets orally for 10 days based on the formulary prices at M.D. Anderson Cancer Center November 2001.
pr, per rectum; td, transdermal; sl, sublingual; D2, dopamine; H1, histamine; Ach, acetylcholine; ICP, intracranial pressure; EPS, extrapyramidal symptoms.
Source: From Elsayem A, Driver L, Bruera E, eds. M.D. Anderson Palliative Care Handbook. 2nd ed. Houston, Texas: M.D. Anderson, 2002.

patients. The etiology is multifactorial. The main cause tends to be due to tumor by-products and host cytokines, such as tumor necrosis factor, proteolysis inducing factor, lipid mobilizing factor, and interleukins (70,71).

In patients with this syndrome, the basal metabolic rate is increased. The liver produces acute-phase proteins that play a role in the inflammatory and antitumor process but draw their energy from muscle break down. Glucose turnover is increased and at the same time there is a relative glucose intolerance in the muscle with insulin resistance. There is suppression of de novo lipogenesis and peripheral activation of lipolysis, whereas central (hepatic) lipogenesis is increased. Whole body protein turnover is increased and liver protein synthesis is directed towards increase in the production of acute-phase proteins and lower production of albumin. Thus, cachexia is characterized by an *increase* in energy expenditure, protein synthesis (largely acute-phase proteins at the expense of muscle proteins), proteolysis, lipolysis, glucose turnover, and a decrease in muscle proteins, lipogenesis, and increased ketone bodies (71).

Feeding of the patient with cancer cachexia was found to increase acute-phase protein production without influencing the rate of albumin synthesis (72). Other contributory factors include nausea, dysphagia, bowel obstruction, or constipation. Sometimes food aversion, depression, and apathy play a role.

Assessment

The clinical assessment includes a careful history that is focused on nutritional issues and a physical exam. A 5 lb weight loss in the previous 2 months and/or an estimated daily calorie intake of less than 70 cal/kg is a simple diagnostic indicator. Simple and inexpensive tests are available to assess the body composition, such as: anthropometric measurements, skinfold thickness, arm muscle circumference and area, and weight and body mass index (BMI). Biochemical measurements are also available, such as serum albumin, transferring, and prealbumin. Careful clinical assessment and laboratory tests, especially serum sodium, are the keystones for diagnosis and effective management. Bioelectrical impedance (BEI) is an easy way to assess both nutrition status and fluid deficits in advanced cancer and should be used more often (73).

Management

The approach to management consists of identifying the etiology and treating the underlying cause.

The nutritionist should advise on the dietary options to maximize nutritional intake. Small frequent meals are less intimidating than usual large three meals a day.

The pharmacological treatment consists of symptom control of the contributory factors and appetite stimulation. Chronic nausea or early satiety is treated within metoclopramide 10 mg every 4-6 hr. Appetite stimulants include progestational agents, corticosteroids, cannabinoids, or adjuvant agents. Progestational agents include megestrol acetate; 40–120 mg po QID will improve appetite in up to 80% of patients and induce weight gain in many patients (74,75). Symptomatic improvement in appetite occurs in less than 1 week; however, weight gain may take several weeks. Appetite stimulation with these agents lasts longer than with corticosteroids. Caution is exercised in patients with venous thrombosis, pulmonary embolism, or severe cardiac disease. Corticosteroids may stimulate appetite and decrease nausea (76,77). The effect does not last long. A cannabinoid, dronabinol, is approved for appetite stimulation and is dosed at 2.5 mg po bid, and may produce concurrent antiemetic effects, but may also produce central nervous system side effects (78). Antidepressants, tricyclic antidepressants, and serotonin-specific reuptake inhibitors may help with appetite in patients with depression. Thalidomide has been studied and has been shown to improve appetite, nausea, and well being (79). Synthetic and semisynthetic testosterone derivatives have been studied especially in terminal AIDS patients and have been shown to benefit appetite and weight loss (80).

Enteral and parenteral nutrition are inappropriate for most patients with advanced cancer (81) other than in patients who have a starvation component to cachexia such as severe dysphagia or bowel obstruction. They do not enhance response to antineoplastic therapy or significantly abate its toxicity, and do not improve survival or quality of life. They can be burdensome to patients and families and may offer an obstruction for transition to a hospice setting.

Nonpharmacological Therapy

Counseling of the patient and their family and loved ones is very important in assuring them that their fears and needs have a outlet to be expressed and acted upon. In addition, it provides a venue to reframe the condition from that of "starving to death" to the more complex one of irreversible (usually) metabolic abnormalities and the futility of pushing nutrition. This reframing can decrease the distress in both patients and families and can maintain the social benefit of mealtimes. Exercise has benefit both for maintaining muscle and reducing depression; leaving the confines of the hospital room and being in sunlight have benefits for mood, depression, and over all sense of well being.

8. Hypercalcemia

Hypercalcemia is a common life-threatening complication of cancer affecting 10–20% of patients and is more common in certain cancers such as squamous cell of lung or head and neck, renal cell, breast, and multiple myeloma (82–84). The usual cause of hypercalcemia is humoral secretion of the parathyroid hormone-related protein (PTHrP), and the clinical syndrome mimics hyperparathyroidism biochemically, except that the serum PTH is suppressed. Less frequent causes include ectopic production of parathyroid hormone itself. Clinically, the disorder contrasts with primary hyperparathyroidism. Hypercalcemia is abrupt in onset and is often severe, and the associated neoplasm is usually obvious. It is usually unnecessary to measure the serum PTHrP levels to confirm the diagnosis; a determination of PTH will rule out intercurrent primary hyperparathyroidism. In multiple myeloma, it is caused by direct activation of bone resorption by cytokines secreted from myeloma cells in the bone marrow. Lymphomas can cause hypercalcemia by a similar local osteolytic mechanism or by conversion of vitamin D to 1,25-dihydroxyvitamin D.

Clinical Presentation

Early symptoms are mild and include anorexia, nausea and vomiting, constipation, fatigue, weakness, polydipsia, and polyuria (nephrogenic diabetes insipidus). Late symptoms are usually severe and include dehydration, altered mental status, generalized weakness, progressive gastrointestinal symptoms, and cardiac arrhythmias, especially when serum calcium levels rise rapidly. A high index of suspicion is required and the diagnosis is established by measurement of the ionized calcium or the corrected serum calcium since it is highly protein bound.

Treatment of Hypercalcemia

Treatment of hypercalcemia should be aimed both at lowering the serum calcium concentration and, if possible, correcting or decreasing the underlying disease (85,86). Hypercalcemia impairs both the glomerular filtration rate and urinary concentration, and with the resultant azotemia and dehydration, the renal route for clearance of calcium is compromised. The mainstay of acute therapy of hypercalcemia is correction of dehydration, institution of saline diuresis to increase the renal excretion of calcium, and the use of agents to decrease bone resorption (87). Intravenous infusion of 100–200 mL/hr can effectively replenish fluid volume and decrease serum calcium in 15–30% of the patients.

Treatment with bisphosphonate is usually required if the patient is symptomatic or the corrected serum calcium is above 12 mg/dL (88). Pamidronate is given in a dose of 90 mg in 500 mL normal saline over 2–4 hr. Pamidronate decreases bone resorption by the inhibition of the osteoclast activity (89). Renal function should be monitored both before and after pamidronate therapy, since this agent is relatively contraindicated in renal failure patients. Zoledronic acid has emerged as another bisphosphonate with superior results to pamidronate in some clinical trials (90). Zoledronic acid is given at a dose of 4 mg over 15 min. The peak effect of bisphosphonates is reached after 5–7 days and the dose is repeated at 4 weeks intervals.

In severe hypercalcemia, rapid lowering of calcium levels may be achieved by subcutaneous administration of calcitonin 100–200 U tid for 3–6 doses (91). Serum calcium should be evaluated 1 day after calcitonin treatment. The other available agents for treatment of acute hypercalcemia are less useful (etidronate disodium, gallium nitrate) or toxic (plicamycin).

II. CONCLUSION

While the medical profession continues to make major discoveries of the causes and treatment of a number of diseases, there remains a challenge to provide medical care of comfort to patients who suffer from incurable diseases like cancer. There is an urgent need for the health care providers to develop a better appreciation of patient's distress beyond physical nature of symptoms. An interdisciplinary, Palliative-care team that is able to understand the complex symptomatology, and provide a compassionate and competent care to the patient and families, both during active treatment as well as in advanced stages of the disease, is an ideal model to care for these patients.

REFERENCES

1. World Health Organization. Cancer Pain Relief and Palliative Care: Report of a WHO Expert Committee. Geneva, Switzerland: WHO. Technical Bull 1990; 804:11–12.
2. Bruera E, Kuehn N, Miller MJ, Selmser P, MacMillan K. The Edmonton symptom assessment system: a simple method for the assessment of palliative care patients. J Palliative Care 1991; 7:6–9.
3. Portenoy RK, Itri LM. Cancer-related fatigue: guidelines for evaluation and management. Oncologist 1999; 4:1–10.
4. Stone P, Richards M, Hardy J. Fatigue in patients with cancer. Eur J Cancer 1998; 34:1670–1676.
5. Jacobsen PB, Hann DM, Azzarello LM, et al. Fatigue in women receiving adjuvant chemotherapy for breast cancer: characteristics, course, and correlates. J Pain Symptom Manage 1999; 18:233–242.
6. Cella D, Peterman A, Passik S, et al. Progress toward guidelines for the management of fatigue. Oncology 1998; 12:369–377.
7. Demetri GD, Kris M, Wade J, et al. Quality of life benefit in chemotherapy patients treated with epoetin alfa is independent of disease response or tumor type: results from a prospective community oncology study. Oncology 1998; 16:3412–3425.
8. Bruera E, Roca E, Cedaro L, et al. Action of oral methyl prednisolone in terminal cancer patients: a prospective randomized double-blind study. Cancer Treat Rep 1985; 69:751–754.
9. Tannock I, Gospodarowicz M, Meakin W, et al. Treatment of metastatic prostate cancer with low dose prednisone: evaluation of pain and quality of life as pragmatic indices of response. J Clin Oncol 1989; 7:590–597.
10. Bruera E, Brenneis C, Paterson AH, Mac Donald RN. Use of methylphenidate as an adjuvant to narcotic analgesics in patients with advanced cancer. J Pain Symptom Manage 1989; 4:3–6.
11. Katon W, Raskind M. Treatment of depression in the medically ill elderly with methylphenidate. Am J Psychiatry 1980; 137:963–965.
12. Rajagopal A, Vassilopoulou-Sellin R, Palmer JL, Kaur G, Bruera E. Symptomatic hypogonadism in male survivors of cancer with chronic exposure to opioids. Cancer 2004; 100(4):851–858.
13. Bruera E, Driver L, Barnes EA, et al. Patient-controlled methylphenidate for the management of fatigue in patients with advanced cancer: a preliminary report. J Clin Oncol 2003; 23:4439–4443.
14. Wasserman K, Casaburi R. Dyspnea and physiological and athophysiological mechanisms. Annu Rev Med 1988; 39:503–515.
15. Farncombe M. Dypsnea: assessment and treatment. Support Care Cancer 1997; 5:94–99.
16. Hardy JR, Turner R, Saunders M, A'Hern R. Prediction of survival in a hospital-based continuing care unit. Eur J Cancer 1994; 30:284–288.
17. Escalante CP, Martin CG, Elting LS, et al. Dyspnea in cancer patients: etiology, resource utilization, and survival. Cancer 1996; 78:1314–1319.
18. Anthonisen NR. Long-term oxygen therapy. Ann Intern Med 1983; 99:519–527.
19. Nocturnal Oxygen Therapy Trial Group. Continuous or nocturnal oxygen therapy in hypoxemic chronic

obstructive lung disease. Ann Intern Med 1980; 93: 391–398.
20. Bruera E, De Stoutz N, Velasco-Leiva, et al. The effects of oxygen on the intensity of dyspnea in hypoxemic terminal cancer patients. Lancet 1993; 342:13–14.
21. Bruera E, Scholler T, MacEachern T. Symptomatic benefit of supplemental oxygen in hypoxemic patients with terminal cancer: the use of the N of 1 rando mized control trial. J Pain Symptom Manage 1992; 7:365–368.
22. Bruera E, MacEachern T, Ripamonti C, et al. Subcutaneous morphine for dyspnea in cancer patients. Ann Intern Med 1993; 119:906–907.
23. Bruera E, MacMillan K, Pither J, et al. The effects of morphine on the dyspnea of terminal cancer patients. J Pain Symptom Manage 1990; 5:341–344.
24. Cohen MH, Johnston Anderson A, Krasnow SH, et al. Continuous intravenous infusion of morphine for severe dyspnea. South Med J 1991; 84:229–234.
25. Davis CL, Hodder C, Love S, et al. Effect of nebulised morphine and morphine-6-glucuronide on exercise endurance in patients with chronic obstructive pulmonary disease. Thorax 1994; 49:393.
26. Farncombe M, Chater S, Gillin A. The use of nebulized opioids for breathlessness: a chart review. Palliative Med 1994; 8:306–312.
27. Farncombe M, Chater S. Clinical application of nebulized opioids for treatment of dyspnoea in patients with malignant disease. Support Care Cancer 1994; 2(3):184–187.
28. Zeppetella G. Nebulized morphine in the palliation of dyspnoea. Palliat Med 1997; 11(4):267–275.
29. Coyne PJ, Viswanathan R, Smith TJ. Nebulized fentanyl citrate improves patients' perception of breathing, respiratory rate, and oxygen saturation in dyspnea. J Pain Symptom Manage 2002; 23(2):157–160.
30. Weir DC, Gove RI, Robertson AS, et al. Corticosteroids trials in nonasthmatic chronic airflow obstruction: a comparison of oral prednisolone and inhaled bechomethasone diproprionate. Thorax 1991; 45:112–117.
31. Congleton J, Meurs MF. The incidence of airflow obstruction in bronchial carcinoma, its relation to breathlessness, and response to bronchodilator therapy. Respir Med 1995; 89:291–296.
32. Neil PA, Morton PB, Stark RD. Chlorpromazine—a special effect on breathlessness? Br J Clin Pharmacol 1985; 19:793–797.
33. Lipowski ZJ. Delirium (acute confusional states). JAMA 1987; 258(13):1789–1792.
34. Rabins PV. Psychosocial and management aspects of delirium. Int Psychogetriatr 1991; 3:39–324.
35. Derogatis LR, Morrow GR, Fetting J, et al. The prevalence of psychiatric disorders among cancer patients. JAMA 1983; 249:751–757.
36. Levine PM, Silberfarb PM, Lipowski ZJ. Mental disorders in cancer patients: a study of 100 psychiatric referrals. Cancer 1978; 42:1385–1391.
37. Stiefel F, Finsinger R, Bruera E. Acute confusional states in patients with advanced cancer. J Pain Symptom Manage 1992; 7:94–98.
38. Lipowski ZJ. Delirium in the elderly patient. N Engl J Med 1989; 320:578–582.
39. Liptzin B, Levkoff SE. An empirical study of delirium subtypes. Br J Psychiatry 1992; 161:843–845.
40. American Psychiatric Association. Diagnostic and Statistical Manual of Mental Disorders. 4th ed. Washington, DC: American Psychiatric Association, 1994.
41. Voruganti L, Cortese L, Owyeumi L, Kotteda V, Cernovsky Z, Zirul S, Awad A. Switching from conventional to novel antipsychotic drugs: results of a prospective naturalistic study. Schizophr Res 2002; 57(2–3): 201–208.
42. Briebart W, Marotta R, Platt MM, et al. A double-blinded trial of haloperidol, chlorazepam, and lorazepam in the treatment of delirium in the hospitalized AIDS patients. Am J Psychiatry 1996; 153:231–237.
43. Derogatis LR, Marrow GR, Fettig J, et al. The prevalence of psychiatric disorders among cancer patients. JAMA 1983; 249:751–757.
44. Wilson KG, Chochinov HM, de Faye B, et al. Diagnosis and management of depression in palliative care. In: Chochinov HM, Breitbart W, eds. Handbook of Psychiatry in Palliative Care. Oxford, United Kingdom: Oxford University Press, 2000:25–49, 106.
45. Green AI, Austin PV. Psychopathology of pancreatic cancer: a psychobiologic probe. Psychosomatics 1993; 34:208.
46. Massie MJ, Holland J. The cancer patient with pain; psychiatric complications and their management. Med Clin North Am 1987; 71:243.
47. Fisch MJ, Loehrer PJ, Kristeller J, Passik S, Jung SH, Shen J, Arquette MA, Brames MJ, Einhorn LH. Hoosier Oncology Group. Fluoxetine versus placebo in advanced cancer outpatients: a double-blinded trial of the Hoosier Oncology Group. J Clin Oncol 2003; 21(10):1937–1943.
48. Bonsignore M, Barkow K, Jessen F, Heun R. Validity of the five item WHO Well Being Index (WHO-5) in an elderly population. Eur Arch Psychiatry Clin Neurosci 2001; 251(suppl 2):II27–II31.
49. Massie MJ, Popkin MK. Depressive disorders. In: Holland JC, ed. Psycho-Oncology. New York, NY: Oxford University Press, 1998:518–540.
50. Holland JC, Morrow G, Schmale A, et al. Reduction of anxiety and depression in cancer patients by alprazolam or by a behavioural technique [abstr]. Proc Am Soc Clin Oncol 1988; 6:258.
51. Vickers AJ, Cassileth BR. Unconventional therapies for cancer and cancer-related symptoms. Lancet Oncol 2001; 2(4):226–232. Review. Lancet Oncol 2001; 2(4): 226–232.
52. Pereira J, Bruera E. Depression with psychomotor retardation: diagnostic challenges and the use of psychostimulants. J Palliat Med 2001; 4(1):15–21.
53. Theobald DE, Kirsh KL, Holtsclaw E, Donaghy K, Passik SD. An open-label, crossover trial of mirtazapine (15 and 30 mg) in cancer patients with pain and

other distressing symptoms. J Pain Symptom Manage 2002; 23(5):442–447.
54. Kast R. Mirtazapine may be useful in treating nausea and insomnia of cancer chemotherapy. Support Care Cancer 2001; 9(6):469–470.
55. Sykes NP. Constipation and diarrhoea. In: Doyle D, Hanks GWC, MacDonald N, eds. Oxford Textbook of Palliative Medicine. 2nd ed. Oxford, England: Oxford University Press, 2001:513–526.
56. Mancini I, Bruera E. Constipation in advanced cancer patients. Support Care Cancer 1998; 6:356–364.
57. Mercadante S. Diarhea, malabsorption, and constipation. In: Berger AM, Portenoy RK, Weismann DE, eds. Principles and Practice of Supportive Oncology. Philadelphia: Lippincott-Raven Publishers, 1998: 191–206.
58. Mercadante S, Casuccio A, et al. The course of symptom frequency and intensity in advanced cancer patients followed at home. J Pain Symptom Manage 2000; 20:104–112.
59. Bruera E, Suarez-Almazor M, et al. The assessment of constipation in terminal cancer patients admitted to a palliative care unit: a retrospective review. J Pain Symptom Manage 1994; 9:515–519.
60. Sykes NP. An investigation of the ability of oral naloxone to correct opioids-related constipation in patients with advanced cancer. Palliat Med 1996; 10:135–144.
61. Latasch L, Zimmerman M, Eberhart B, et al. Oral naloxone antagonizes morphine-induced constipation. Anesthetist 1997; 46:191–194.
62. Meissner W, Schimdt U, Hartman M, et al. Oral naloxone reverses opioids-associated constipation. Pain 2000; 84:105–109.
63. Yuan CS, Foss JF, O'Connor M, Osinski J, Karrison T, Moss J, Roizen MF. Methylnaltrexone for reversal of constipation due to chronic methadone use: a randomized controlled trial. JAMA 2000; 283(3):367–372.
64. Stephenson J. Methylnaltrexone reverses opioid-induced constipation. Lancet Oncol 2002; 3(4):202.
65. Mannix KA. Palliation of nausea and vomiting. In: Doyle D, Hanks GWC, MacDonald N, eds. Oxford Textbook of Palliative Medicine. 2nd ed. Oxford, England: Oxford University Press, 2001:489–499.
66. Driver LC, Bruera E. The M. D. Anderson Palliative Care Handbook. Houston, Texas: The University of Texas Health Science Center at Houston Printing Services, 2000:55.
67. Bruera ED, Roca E, Cedaro L, et al. Improved control of chemotherapy-induced emesis by the addition of dexamethasone to metoclopramide in patients resistant to metoclopramide. Cancer Treat Rep 1983; 67: 381–383.
68. Mercadante S, Fulfaro F, Casuccio A. The use of corticosteroids in home palliative care. Support Care Cancer 2001; 9:386–389.
69. DeWys WD, Begg D, Lavin PT. Prognostic effect of weight loss prior to chemotherapy in cancer patients. Am J Med 1980; 69:491–499.
70. Tisdale MJ. Loss of skeletal muscle in cancer: biochemical mechanisms. Front Biosci 2001; 6:D164–D174.
71. Belizario JE, Katz M, Chenker E, Raw I. Bioactivity of skeletal muscle proteolysis-inducing factors in the plasma proteins from cancer patients with weight loss. Br J Cancer 1991; 63(5):705–710.
72. Barber MD, Fearon KC, McMillan DC, et al. Liver export protein synthetic rates are increased by oral meal feeding in weight losing cancer patients (115). Am J Physiol Enocrinol Metabol 2000; 279: E707–E714.
73. Sarhill N, Mahmoud FA, Christie R, Tahir A. Assessment of nutritional status and fluid deficits in advanced cancer. Am J Hosp Palliat Care 2003; 20(6): 465–473.
74. Loprinzi CL, Ellison NM, Schaid DJ, et al. Phase III evaluation of four doses of megestrol acetate as therapy for patients with cancer anorexia and/or cachexia. J Clin Oncol 1993; 11:762–767.
75. Feliu J, Gonzales-Baron M, Berrocal A, et al. Usefulness of megestrol acetate in cancer cachexia and anorexia. Am J Clin Oncol 1992; 15:436–440.
76. Popiela T, Lucchi R, Giongo F. Methylprednisolone as an appetite stimulant in patients with cancer. Eur J Cancer Clin Oncol 1989; 25:1823–1829.
77. Wilcox J, Corr J, Shaw J, et al. Prednisolone as an appetite stimulant in patients with cancer. Br Med J 1984; 27:288–290.
78. Sacks N, Hutcheson JR, Watts JM, Webb RE. Case report: the effect of tetrahydrocannabinol on food intake during chemotherapy. J Am Coll Nutr 1990; 9:630–632.
79. Bruera E, Neumann CM, Pituskin E, et al. Thalidomide in patients with cachexia due to terminal cancer: preliminary report. Ann Oncol 1999; 10:857–859.
80. Mulligan K, Schambelan M. Anabolic treatment with GH, IGF-I, or anabolic steroids in patients with HIV-associated wasting. Int J Cardiol 2002; 85(1): 151–159.
81. Bozzetti F, Gavazzi C, Ferrari P, et al. Effect of total parenteral nutrition on the protein kinetics of patients with cancer cachexia. Tumori 2000; 86:408–411.
82. Mundy GR, Guise, TA. Hypercalcemia of malignancy. Am J Med 1997; 103:134–145.
83. Heys SD, Smith, IC, et al. Hypercalcaemia in patients with cancer: aetiology and treatment. Eur J Surg Oncol 1998; 24:139–142.
84. Bower M, Brazil L, Coombes R. Endocrine and metabolic complications in advanced cancer. In: Doyle D, Hanks G, MacDonald N, eds. Oxford Textbook of Palliative Medicine. 2nd ed. Oxford, England: Oxford University Press, 1998:709–712.
85. Bilezikian, JP. Management of acute hypercalcemia. N Engl J Med 1992; 326:1196–1203.
86. Bilezikian, JP. Hypercalcemia. Curr Ther Endocrinol Metab 1994; 5:511–514.
87. Kovacs CS, MacDonald SM, et al. Hypercalcemia of malignancy in the palliative care patient: a treatment strategy. J Pain Symptom Manage 1995; 10:224–232.

88. Riccardi A, Grasso D, Danova M. Bisphosphonates in oncology: physiopathologic bases and clinical activity. Tumori 2003; 89(3):223–236.
89. Gucalp R, Theriault R, et al. Treatment of cancer-associated hypercalcemia. Double-blind comparison of rapid and slow intravenous infusion regimens of pamidronate disodium and saline alone. Arch Intern Med 1994; 154:1935–1944.
90. Neville-Webbe H, Coleman RE. The use of zoledronic acid in the management of metastatic bone disease and hypercalcaemia. Palliat Med 2003; 17(6):539–553.
91. Ljunghall S. Use of clodronate and calcitonin in hypercalcemia due to malignancy. Recent Results Cancer Res 1989; 116:40–45.

Index

ABOUT THE EDITORS

ANDREW D. SHAW is Assistant Professor, Department of Critical Care Medicine, The University of Texas M.D. Anderson Cancer Center, Houston. He received his medical degree from St. Bartholomew's Hospital Medical College, University of London, England.

BERNHARD J. RIEDEL is Associate Professor of Anesthesiology and Critical Care, The University of Texas M.D. Anderson Cancer Center, Houston. He received his medical degree from the University of the Free State, South Africa.

ALLEN W. BURTON is Associate Professor and Section Chief of Cancer Pain Management, Department of Anesthesiology and Pain Medicine, The University of Texas M.D. Anderson Cancer Center, Houston. He received the M.D. degree from Baylor College of Medicine, Houston, Texas.

ALAN I. FIELDS is Professor of Pediatrics, and Anesthesiology and Critical Care Medicine, and Director of Pediatric Critical Care Services, The University of Texas M.D. Anderson Cancer Center, Houston. He received the M.D. degree from the State University of New York Downstate Medical Center, New York.

THOMAS W. FEELEY is Helen Shafer Fly Distinguished Professor of Anesthesiology and Vice President, Medical Operations and, Head of the Division of Anesthesiology and Critical Care, The University of Texas M.D. Anderson Cancer Center, Houston. He received the M.D. degree from Boston University, Massachusetts.